AF674767

Cardiodiabetes Update

A Textbook of Cardiology

DISCLAIMER

The views and opinions expressed in this book are solely those of the original contributor(s)/author(s) and do not necessarily represent those of editor(s) of the book.

All brand names and product names used in this book are trade names, service marks, trademarks or registered trademarks of their respective owners. The publisher is not associated with any product or vendor mentioned in this book.

Medical knowledge and practice change constantly. This book is designed to provide accurate, authoritative information about the subject matter in question. However, readers are advised to check the most current information available on procedures included and check information from the manufacturer of each product to be administered, to verify the recommended dose, formula, method and duration of administration, adverse effects and contraindications. It is the responsibility of the practitioner to take all appropriate safety precautions. Neither the publisher nor the author(s)/editor(s) assume any liability for any injury and/or damage to persons or property arising from or related to use of material in this book.

This book is sold on the understanding that the publisher is not engaged in providing professional medical services. If such advice or services are required, the services of a competent medical professional should be sought.

Every effort has been made, where necessary, to contact holders of copyright to obtain permission to reproduce copyright material. If any has been inadvertently overlooked, the publisher will be pleased to make the necessary arrangements at the first opportunity.

Cardiodiabetes Update

A Textbook of Cardiology

Editors

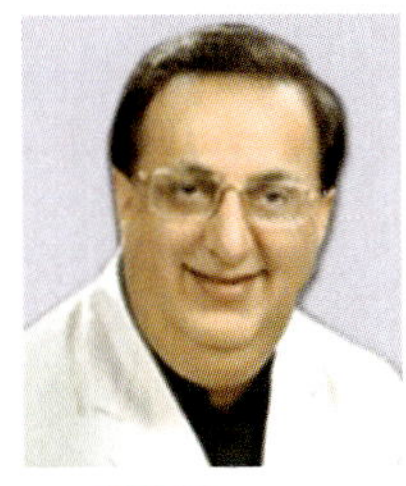

HK Chopra
Chairman, National CSI Affairs Advisory Committee
National President, IAE- 2017, CSI -2015
Chairman, World Wellness Foundation
Country Head, American Heart Association
Sr Consultant Cardiologist
Moolchand Medcity
New Delhi, India

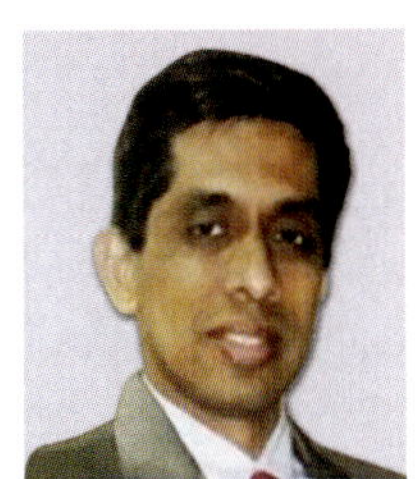

Shashank R Joshi
'Padma Shri' Awardee
Sr Endocrinologist, Joshi Clinic
Lilavati Hospital
Apollo Sugar Clinic and Bhatia Hospital
Mumbai, Maharashtra, India
National President, API–2015
Vice President, PCOS Society
Secretary, Indian Thyroid Society
Editor Emeritus, JAPI
President, IAD & HSI

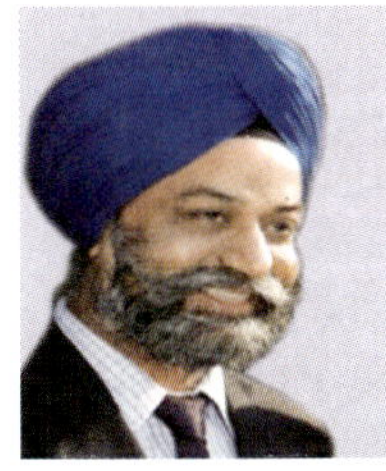

GS Wander
'Dr BC Roy' Awardee
President, API–2017
Chief Coordinator and Head
Department of Cardiology
Hero DMC Heart Institute
Unit of DMC and Hospital
Ludhiana, Punjab, India

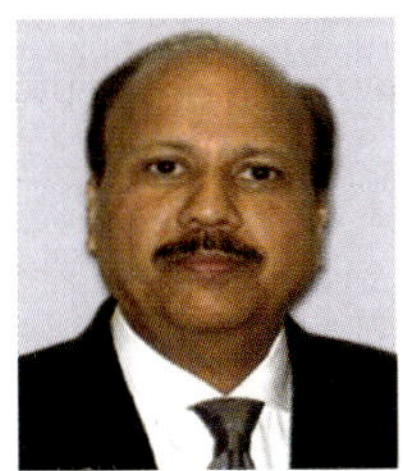

Ravi R Kasliwal
Chairman, Clinical and Preventive Cardiology
Medanta Heart Institute
Medanta–The Medicity
Gurugram, Haryana, India

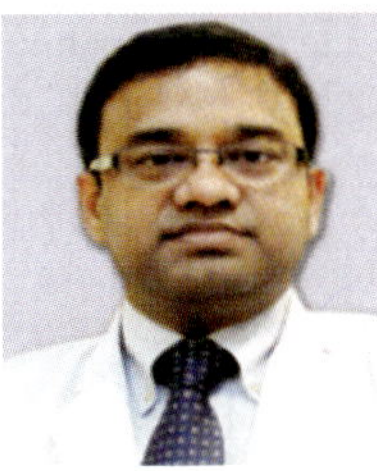

Viveka Kumar
Director, Cath Lab
Senior Consultant Interventional Cardiologist and Electrophysiologist
Max Super Speciality Hospital
New Delhi, India

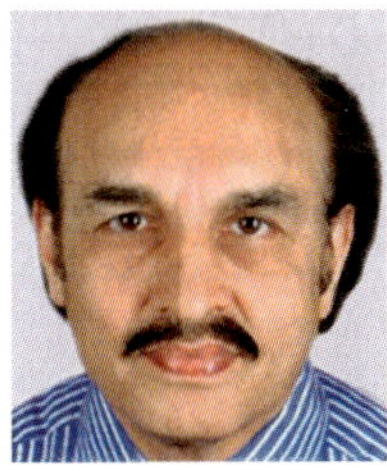

AK Pancholia
Head, Department of Clinical and Preventive Cardiology
Arihant Hospital and Gokuldas Heart Center
Indore, Madhya Pradesh, India

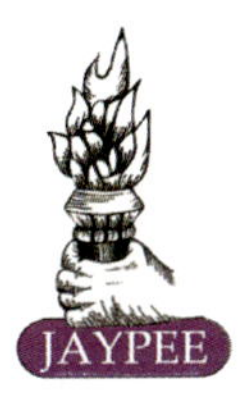

The Health Sciences Publisher
New Delhi | London | Panama

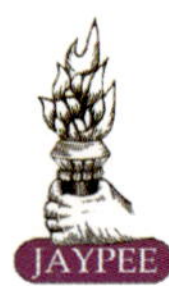

Jaypee Brothers Medical Publishers (P) Ltd

Headquarters
Jaypee Brothers Medical Publishers (P) Ltd
4838/24, Ansari Road, Daryaganj
New Delhi 110 002, India
Phone: +91-11-43574357
Fax: +91-11-43574314
Email: jaypee@jaypeebrothers.com

Overseas Offices

J.P. Medical Ltd
83 Victoria Street, London
SW1H 0HW (UK)
Phone: +44 20 3170 8910
Fax: +44 (0)20 3008 6180
Email: info@jpmedpub.com

Jaypee-Highlights Medical Publishers Inc
City of Knowledge, Bld. 235, 2nd Floor, Clayton
Panama City, Panama
Phone: +1 507-301-0496
Fax: +1 507-301-0499
Email: cservice@jphmedical.com

Jaypee Brothers Medical Publishers (P) Ltd
17/1-B Babar Road, Block-B, Shaymali
Mohammadpur, Dhaka-1207
Bangladesh
Mobile: +08801912003485
Email: jaypeedhaka@gmail.com

Jaypee Brothers Medical Publishers (P) Ltd
Bhotahity, Kathmandu, Nepal
Phone: +977-9741283608
Email: kathmandu@jaypeebrothers.com

Website: www.jaypeebrothers.com
Website: www.jaypeedigital.com

Inquiries for bulk sales may be solicited at: jaypee@jaypeebrothers.com

Cardiodiabetes Update: A Textbook of Cardiology

First Edition: **2018**

ISBN: 978-93-5270-304-3

Printed at Sanat Printers

Co-Editors

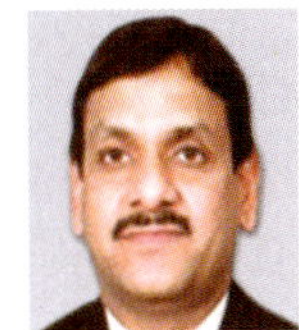

Satyendra Tewari
Professor
Department of Cardiology
SGPGIMS
Lucknow, Uttar Pradesh, India

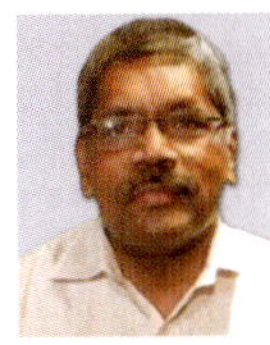

PP Mohanan
Director and Head
Department of Cardiology
Westfort Hitech Hospital
Thrissur, Kerala, India

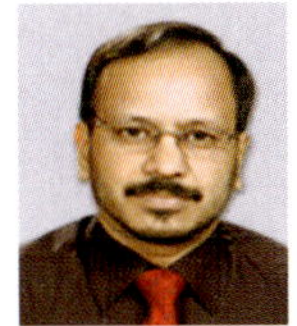

Rakesh Gupta
Director and Chief Cardiologist
JROP Healthcare
New Delhi, India

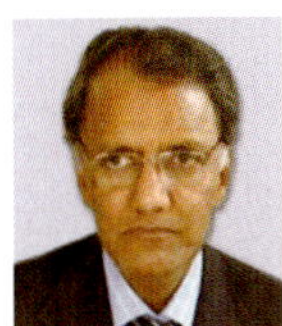

Rajeev Gupta
Sr Consultant Cardiologist
Department of Internal Medicine and Preventive Cardiology
Eternal Heart Care Center and Research Institute
Mount Sinai, New York, Affiliate
Jaipur, Rajasthan, India

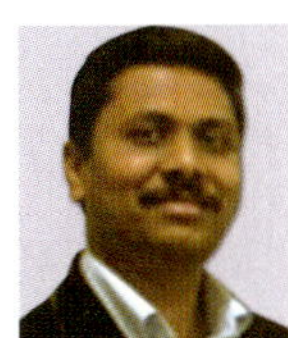

Manish Bansal
Associate Director
Department of Cardiology
Medanta–The Medicity
Gurugram, Haryana, India

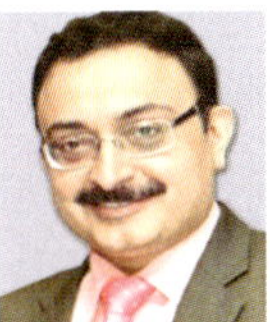

NN Khanna
Sr Consultant, Interventional Cardiology and Vascular Interventions
Indraprastha Apollo Hospital
New Delhi, India

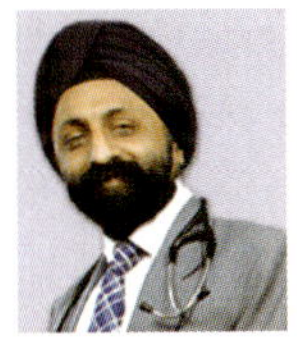

JPS Sawhney
Chairman, Department of Cardiology
Sir Ganga Ram Hospital
New Delhi, India

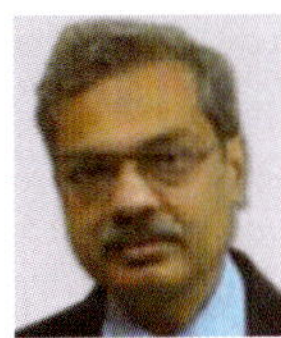

Sameer Shrivastava
Director, Noninvasive Cardiology
Fortis Escorts Heart Institute
New Delhi, India

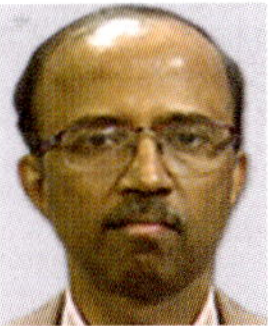

CK Ponde
Sr Consultant Cardiologist
PD Hinduja National Hospital and MRC
Mumbai, Maharashtra, India

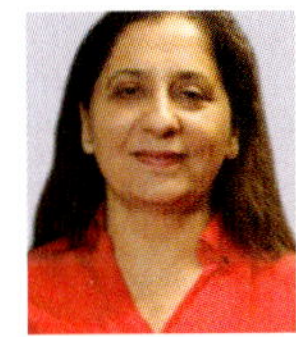

Poonam Malhotra Kapoor
Professor, Department of Cardiac Anesthesia
Cardio-Neuro Center (CNC)
All India Institute of Medical Sciences (AIIMS)
New Delhi, India

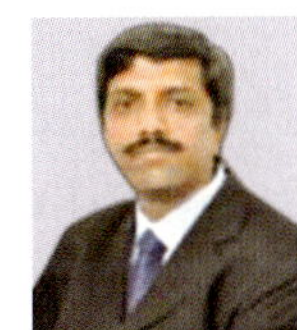

S Ramakrishnan
Professor, Department of Cardiology
All India Institute of Medical Sciences (AIIMS)
New Delhi, India

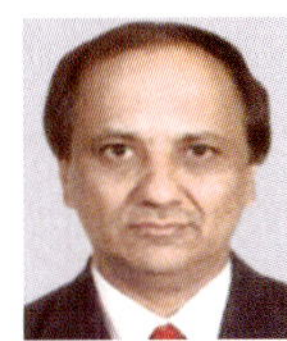

Vidyut Jain
Sr Consultant Cardiologist
Choithram Hospital
Indore, Madhya Pradesh, India

Dedicated to

Cardiological Society of India, our parents, our teachers, all the members of CSI, our colleagues, patients, students and our families.

Contributors

Aashish Contractor
Head, Rehabilitation and Sports Medicine
Sir HN Reliance Foundation Hospital
Mumbai, Maharashtra, India

Abhimanyu Bhatia
Clinical Associate
Critical Care
Moolchand Medcity
New Delhi, India

Abhirup Chatterjee
Vivekananda Institute of Medical Sciences
Kolkata, West Bengal, India

Adel A Farhoud
Division of Cardiovascular Disease
University of Alabama at Birmingham
Birmingham, Alabama, USA

Aditya Kapoor
Professor
Department of Cardiology
Sanjay Gandhi Postgraduate Institute of
Medical Sciences (SGPGIMS)
Lucknow, Uttar Pradesh, India

A Gupta
Department of Cardiology
Govind Ballabh Pant Institute of Postgraduate
Medicine and Research
New Delhi, India

Ahmed Abdelhaleem
Division of Cardiovascular Disease
University of Alabama at Birmingham
Birmingham, Alabama, USA

Ajay Kumar Sinha
Head, Department of Cardiology
Paras HMRI Hospital
Patna, Bihar, India

Akash Nair
Government TD Medical College
Alappuzha, Kerala, India

AK Bali
Sr Consultant Physician
Moolchand Medcity
New Delhi, India

AK Pancholia
Head
Department of Clinical and Preventive
Cardiology
Arihant Hospital and Gokuldas Heart Center
Indore, Madhya Pradesh, India

Anand Gopal
Cardiac Care
Paras HMRI Hospital
Patna, Bihar, India

Aneesa Kapadia
Jaslok Hospital and Research Centre
Mumbai, Maharashtra, India

Anil Bhan
Deputy Chairman
Department of CTVS
Medanta-The Medicity
Gurugram, Haryana, India

Anil Kumar
Honorary Professor
Department of Cardiology
Grant Government Medical College and
Sir JJ Group of Hospitals
Mumbai, Maharashtra, India

Aniruddha Pawar
Seth GS Medical College and
KEM Hospital
Mumbai, Maharashtra, India

Anita Dhar
Professor
Department of Surgical Disciplines
All India Institute of Medical Sciences
New Delhi, India

Ankit Bansal
Department of Cardiology
GB Pant Hospital
New Delhi, India

Ankit Kumar Sahu
Department of Cardiology
Sanjay Gandhi Postgraduate Institute of
Medical Sciences (SGPGIMS)
Lucknow, Uttar Pradesh, India

Apoorv Mittal
Sr Consultant Interventional Cardiologist
Moolchand Medcity
New Delhi, India

Arindam Pande
Consultant Interventional Cardiologist
Medica Superspecialty Hospital
Kolkata, West Bengal, India

Arjun Sreekumar
Dharma Vira Heart Center
Sir Ganga Ram Hospital
New Delhi, India

Arpit Agarwal
King George's Medical University
Lucknow, Uttar Pradesh, India

Arun Sharma
Cardiac Radiology
All India Institute of Medical Sciences
New Delhi, India

Arvind Lal
Chairman and Managing Director
Dr Lal Path Labs Limited
Gurugram, Haryana, India

Arvind Sethi
Consultant
Department of Interventional Cardiology
Fortis Hospital
New Delhi, India

Asha Moorthy
Sr Cardiologist, GG Multispeciality Hospital
Chennai, Tamil Nadu, India

Ashokan Nambiar
Sr Consultant and Head
Department of Cardiology
Baby Memorial Hospital
Kozhikode, Kerala, India

Ashok Jaiswal
Head, Medical Affairs
Zydus Recovery
Ahmedabad, Gujarat, India

Asim Perwez
Cardiac Care
Paras HMRI Hospital
Patna, Bihar, India

Auriom Kar
Department of Cardiology
NRS Medical College
Kolkata, West Bengal, India

Avani Jain
Choithram Hospital and Research Centre
Indore, Madhya Pradesh, India

Avi Kumar
Sr Consultant Pulmonologist
Moolchand Medcity
New Delhi, India

Aviraj Chaudhary
Department of Cardiology
Institute of Medical Sciences, BHU
Varanasi, Uttar Pradesh, India

Ayman Battisha
Division of Cardiovascular Disease
University of Alabama at Birmingham
Birmingham, Alabama, USA

Bahekar Anurag D
Department of Cardiology
Pushpagiri Medical College
Thiruvalla, Kerala, India

Balaji Lohiya
Department of Cardiology
Institute of Medical Sciences, BHU
Varanasi, Uttar Pradesh, India

Balbir Singh
Chairman
Department of Cardiology
Medanta-The Medicity
Gurugram, Haryana, India

Binoy John
Director and Head
Department of Interventional Cardiology
Advanced Heart Diseases, Heart Failure and Cardiac Transplant Medicine
MIOT International
Chennai, Tamil Nadu, India

Biswadev Basu
Department of Cardiology
NRS Medical College
Kolkata, West Bengal, India

Biswajit Paul
Associate Director and Head
Department of Noninvasive Cardiology
Jaypee Hospital
Noida, Uttar Pradesh, India

Biswaranjan Mishra
Chief Consultant Cardiologist
Max Diagnostic Centre
Cuttack, Odisha, India

BP Singh
Professor and Head
Department of Cardiology, IGIMS
Patna, Bihar, India

Brian Pinto
Chief Cardiologist
Holy Family Hospital
Mumbai, Maharashtra, India

Brij Mohan Makkar
Diabetologist and Obesity Specialist
Diabetes and Obesity Centre
Honorary Secretary, RSSDI
New Delhi, India

C Elamaran
Assistant Professor
Department of Cardiology
Madras Medical College
Chennai, Tamil Nadu, India

Chandril Chugh
Senior Consultant and Head
Interventional Neurology
Max Super Speciality Hospital
New Delhi, India

Charu Paruthi
Consultant, Department of Radiology
Moolchand Medcity
New Delhi, India

Chetan P Shah
Director, Department of Cardiology
Zynova Heart Hospital and Kohinoor Hospital
Mumbai, Maharashtra, India

Chockalingam A
Associate Professor, Clinical Medicine
Division of Cardiovascular Medicine
University of Missouri
Columbia, USA

Chockalingam P
Clinical Director, Cardiac Wellness Institute
Chennai, Tamil Nadu, India

Chockalingam V
Professor Emeritus
Department of Cardiology
Dr MGR Medical University
Chennai, Tamil Nadu, India

CK Ponde
Sr Consultant Cardiologist
PD Hinduja National Hospital and MRC
Mumbai, Maharashtra, India

CN Manjunath
Professor and Head
Department of Cardiology
Director
Sri Jayadeva Institute of Cardiovascular Sciences and Research
Bengaluru, Karnataka, India

C Venkata S Ram
World Hypertension League/South Asia Office
Apollo Hospitals, Hyderabad, Telangana, India
University of Texas Southwestern Medical School
Dallas, Texas, USA

Debabrata Roy
Sr Consultant Cardiologist and Academic Coordinator, NH-RTIICS
Kolkata, West Bengal, India

Deepak K Jumani
Assistant Professor
Department of Medicine
Sir JJ Group of Hospitals and Grant Medical College
Consultant Sexual Health Physician, Mumbai Police Hospital
Consultant Sexual Health Physician, Apollo Sugar Clinic
Mumbai, Maharashtra, India

Deep Chandh Raja
Associate Consultant
Department of Cardiology
Madras Medical Mission
Chennai, Tamil Nadu, India

Deepti Siddharthan
All India Institute of Medical Sciences
New Delhi, India

Dev Pahlajani
Head, Department of Interventional Cardiology
Breach Candy Hospital
Mumbai, Maharashtra, India

Dharmendra Jain
Assistant Professor, Department of Cardiology
IMS, BHU
Varanasi, Uttar Pradesh, India

Dinanath Kumar
Cardiac Care
Paras HMRI Hospital
Patna, Bihar, India

Dinesh Parikh
Holy Family Hospital
Mumbai, Maharashtra, India

Dipak Ranjan Das
Assistant Professor, Department of Cardiology
SCB Medical College
Cuttack, Odisha, India

DS Rana
'Padma Shri' Awardee
'Dr BC Roy' National Awardee
Chairman, Board of Management
Chairman, Department of Nephrology
Trustee, Sir Ganga Ram Trust Society
Sir Ganga Ram Hospital
New Delhi, India

Gaurav M Ganeshwala
Ruby Hall Clinic
Pune, Maharashtra, India

Gaurav Mohan
Assistant Professor, Department of Medicine
Sri Guru Ram Das Institute of Medical Sciences and Research
Amritsar, Punjab, India

Gauri Gupta
Department of Radiology
Moolchand Medcity
New Delhi, India

Geetha Subramanian
Head, Department of Cardiology
Institute of Medical Sciences, BHU, Varanasi
Professor Emeritus of Cardiology
Tamil Nadu Dr MGR Medical University
Former Head, Department of Cardiology
Madras Medical College
Chennai, Tamil Nadu, India

George Koshy
Professor, Department of Cardiology
Pushpagiri Medical College
Thiruvalla, Kerala, India

GN Mahapatra
Senior Consultant and Head
Department of Nuclear Medicine
PET-CT and SPECT-CT
Seven Hills Hospital
Mumbai, Maharashtra, India

GS Sainani
Director Emeritus
Department of Medicine
Jaslok Hospital and Research Centre
Mumbai, Maharashtra, India

Gulshant Panesar
Sr Consultant Dermatologist
Moolchand Medcity
New Delhi, India

GS Wander
'Dr BC Roy' Awardee
President, API–2017
Chief Coordinator and Head
Department of Cardiology
Hero DMC Heart Institute
Unit of DMC and Hospital
Ludhiana, Punjab, India

G Vijayaraghavan
Dean, Postgraduate Medical Studies
Kerala Institute of Medical Studies
Trivandrum, Kerala, India

Hakim Irfan Showkat
Department of Cardiology
National Heart Institute
New Delhi, India

Harinder K Bali
Director, Department of Cardiology
Fortis Hospital
Mohali, Punjab, India

Harmeet Singh
Head
Department of Emergency and Urgent Care
Moolchand Medcity
New Delhi, India

Harsh Wardhan
Head, Department of Cardiology
Primus Super Speciality Hospital
Formerly, Professor, Consultant and Head
Department of Cardiology
RML Hospital and PGIMER
New Delhi, India

Harvinder Kaur
Department Continuing Nursing Education
Dr Ram Manohar Lohia Hospital
New Delhi, India

Hassan Kamel
Division of Cardiovascular Disease
University of Alabama at Birmingham
Birmingham, Alabama, USA

Hiteshi KC Chauhan
Department of Cardiology
Fortis Hospital, Mohali, Punjab, India

HK Chopra
Chairman, National CSI Affairs Advisory Committee
National President, IAE- 2017, CSI -2015
Chairman, World Wellness Foundation
Country Head, American Heart Association
Sr Consultant Cardiologist
Moolchand Medcity
New Delhi, India

IB Vijayalakshmi
Professor, Department of Pediatric Cardiology
Bengaluru Medical College and Research Institute, Bengaluru, Karnataka, India

I Sathyamurthy
Sr Interventional Cardiologist
Director, Department of Cardiology
Apollo Hospitals
Chennai, Tamil Nadu, India

Jabir A
Sr Consultant Cardiologist
Lisie Hospital
Kochi, Kerala, India

Jaideep C Menon
Amrita Institute of Medical Sciences
Kochi, Kerala, India

Jamshed J Dalal
Centre for Cardiac Sciences
Kokilaben Hospital
Mumbai, Maharashtra, India

Jasjeet S Wasir
Senior Consultant
Division on Endocrinology and Diabetes
Medanta–The Medicity
Gurugram, Haryana, India

Jatin Yadav
Fortis Escorts Heart Institute and Research Centre
New Delhi, India

Jayesh Suresh
Department of Surgical Disciplines
All India Institute of Medical Sciences
New Delhi, India

Jimit Vadgama
Clinical Associate
Department of Diabetes, Endocrine and Metabolism
Lilavati Hospital and Research Centre
Mumbai, Maharashtra, India

JPS Sawhney
Chairman, Department of Cardiology
Sir Ganga Ram Hospital
New Delhi, India

Jugal Bihari Gupta
Department of Internal Medicine
Eternal Heart Care Centre
and Research Institute
Jaipur, Rajasthan, India

Jugal Kishore Sharma
Medical Director and
Senior Consultant
Central Delhi Diabetes Centre
New Delhi, India

Kajal Ganguly
Professor and Head
Department of Cardiology
NRS Medical College
Kolkata, West Bengal, India

Kapil Sharma
Bench to Bedside Engineering Co-President
Department of Bioengineering
University of Utah Center of Medical Innovation
Salt Lake City, Utah, USA

Kartik Ganga
Cardiac Radiology
All India Institute of Medical Sciences
New Delhi, India

Kewal C Goswami
Senior Professor
Department of Cardiology
All India Institute of Medical Sciences
New Delhi, India
President-Elect, National CSI

KK Kapur
Chief and Sr Consultant
Noninvasive Cardiology
Apollo Hospital
New Delhi, India

KN Srinivasan
Sr Interventional Cardiologist
Apollo Hospitals
Chennai, Tamil Nadu, India

Krishna CK
Department of Cardiology
National Heart Institute
New Delhi, India

Krishnam Raju P
Sr Consultant Cardiologist
CARE Hospital
Hyderabad, Telangana, India

Kunal Sinkar
Holy Family Hospital
Mumbai, Maharashtra, India

Kushal Madan
Cardiac Rehabilitation Consultant
Dharma Vira Heart Center
Sir Ganga Ram Hospital
New Delhi, India

K Venugopal
Professor, Department of Cardiology
Pushpagiri Medical College
Thiruvalla, Kerala, India

Lal C Daga
Consultant, Department of Cardiology
Fortis Hospital
Noida, Uttar Pradesh, India

Madhumanti Panja
Rabindranath Tagore
International Institute of Cardiac Sciences
Kolkata, West Bengal, India

Mahim Saran
Department of Cardiology
King George Medical University
Lucknow, Uttar Pradesh, India

Manisha Sawhney
Jaslok Hospital and Research Centre
Mumbai, Maharashtra, India

Manish Bansal
Associate Director
Department of Cardiology
Medanta–The Medicity
Gurugram, Haryana, India

Manotosh Panja
Director
Department of Cardiology
Bellevue Hospital
Course Director, DNB (Cardiology)
BM Birla Heart Research Institute
Kolkata, West Bengal, India

Mary Anne Joseph
Consultant
Department of Nuclear Medicine,
PET-CT and SPECT-CT
Seven Hills Hospital
Mumbai, Maharashtra, India

Maulik Parekh
Department of Cardiology
PD Hinduja National Hospital
Mumbai, Maharashtra, India

Md Saiyed Rana
Sr Post-Doctoral Fellow
NH-RTIICS
Kolkata, West Bengal, India

Meeta Maheshwari
Max Super Speciality Hospital
New Delhi, India

Meghna Gupta
Kishori Ram Hospital and Diabetes Care Centre
Bathinda, Punjab, India

Mohamed S Mahmoud
Division of Cardiovascular Disease
University of Alabama at Birmingham
Birmingham, Alabama, USA

Mohammad Jibran
Lifeline Superspeciality Hospital and Heart Centre
Jhansi, Uttar Pradesh, India

Mohammed J Arisha
Division of Cardiovascular Disease
University of Alabama at Birmingham
Birmingham, Alabama, USA

Mohit D Gupta
Professor
Department of Cardiology
Govind Ballabh Pant Institute of Postgraduate Medicine and Research
New Delhi, India

Mohsin Wali
Senior Physician and Consultant
Ram Manohar Lohia Hospital
New Delhi, India
Physician to the President of India

Mona Bhatia
Head
Department of Radiology and Imaging
Fortis Escorts Heart Institute
New Delhi, India

MP Girish
Professor
Department of Cardiology
Govind Ballabh Pant Institute of Postgraduate Medicine and Research
New Delhi, India

Mrinal Kanti Das
Sr Consultant Cardiologist
BM Birla Heart Research Centre
Kothari Medical Centre
Kolkata, West Bengal, India

M Somasundaram
Department of Cardiology
Apollo Hospitals
Chennai, Tamil Nadu, India

Nagesh S Waghmare
Associate Professor
Department of Cardiology
Grant Government Medical College and Sir JJ Group of Hospitals
Mumbai, Maharashtra, India

Naresh Trehan
Chairman and Managing Director
Department of Cardiothoracic and Vascular Surgery
Medanta–The Medicity
Gurugram, Haryana, India

Naveen Garg
Clinical Cardiologist, BK Hospital
Faridabad, Haryana, India

Naveen Mittal
Professor, Department of Endocrinology
Dayanand Medical College and Hospital
Ludhiana, Punjab, India

Navin C Nanda
Professor
Division of Cardiovascular Disease
University of Alabama at Birmingham
Birmingham, Alabama, USA
President, ISCU
Chairman, Board of Directors, AACIO
Editor-in-Chief, Echocardiography Journal

Neelam Bisht
Senior Consultant
National Heart Institute
New Delhi, India

Neeraj Desai
Holy Family Hospital
Mumbai, Maharashtra, India

Neeraj Tyagi
Sr Consultant, Department of Neurosciences
Moolchand Medcity
New Delhi, India

Neha Gupta
Sr Consultant, Fetal Medicine
Jaypee Hospital
Noida, Uttar Pradesh, India

Nikhil Bhat
Associate Consultant Critical Care
Moolchand Medcity
New Delhi, India

Nimmi Kansal
Head, Department of Biochemistry
Dr Lal Path Labs Limited
Gurugram, Haryana, India

Nirav Kumar
Associate Professor
Department of Cardiology
IGIMS
Patna, Bihar, India

Nishant Tripathy
Associate Professor, Department of Cardiology
IGIMS
Patna, Bihar, India

Nitin Aggarwal
Consultant Cardiologist
Action Balaji Hospital
Visiting Cardiologist
Rajiv Gandhi Cancer Institute and Research Centre
New Delhi, India

Nitin Burkule
Sr Consultant Cardiologist
Jupiter Hospital
Mumbai, Maharashtra, India

Nitin Joshi
Jaslok Hospital and Research Centre
Mumbai, Maharashtra, India

NN Khanna
Sr Consultant, Interventional Cardiology and Vascular Interventions
Indraprastha Apollo Hospital
New Delhi, India

Omar Tageldin
Division of Cardiovascular Disease
University of Alabama at Birmingham
Birmingham, Alabama, USA

Om J Lakhani
Department of Endocrinology and Metabolism
Sir Ganga Ram Hospital
New Delhi, India

OP Yadava
CEO and Chief Cardiac Surgeon
National Heart Institute
New Delhi, India

Pankaj Kumar
Sr Consultant, Department of Critical Care
Fortis Hospital
New Delhi, India

Pankaj Manoria
Chief Interventional Cardiologist
Manoria Heart and Critical Care Hospital
Bhopal, Madhya Pradesh, India

Paras Aggarwal
Consultant
Division of Endocrinology and Diabetes
Medanta-The Medicity
Gurugram, Haryana, India

Paul N Hopkins
Professor
Division of Cardiovascular Medicine
University of Utah School of Medicine
Salt Lake City, Utah, USA

Pawan K Sharma
Assistant Professor
Division of Cardiovascular Medicine
University of Utah School of Medicine
Salt Lake City, Utah, USA

PB Jayagopal
Director and Senior Interventional Cardiologist
Lakshmi Hospital
Palakkad, Kerala, India

PC Manoria
Director and Chief Cardiologist
Manoria Heart and Critical Care Hospital
Bhopal, Madhya Pradesh, India

PC Mondal
Consultant Interventional Cardiologist
Apollo Gleneagles Hospitals
Kolkata, West Bengal, India

Poonam Malhotra Kapoor
Professor
Department of Cardiac Anesthesia
Cardio-Neuro Center (CNC)
All India Institute of Medical Sciences (AIIMS)
New Delhi, India

PP Mohanan
Director and Head
Department of Cardiology
Westfort Hitech Hospital
Thrissur, Kerala, India

Prabhavathi
Sri Jayadeva Institute of Cardiovascular Sciences and Research
Bengaluru, Karnataka, India

Prafulla Kerkar
Consultant Cardiologist
Department of Cardiology
Seth GS Medical College and KEM Hospital
Mumbai, Maharashtra, India

Prasad SG
Department of Telemedicine
CARE Foundation
Hyderabad, Telangana, India

Praveen Jain
Professor Emeritus
Department of Cardiology
Maharani Laxmibai Medical College
Jhansi, Uttar Pradesh, India

Preeti Gupta
Assistant Professor
Department of Cardiology
VMMC and Safdarjung Hospital
New Delhi, India

Priya Jagia
Professor
Department of Cardiovascular Radiology and Endovascular Interventions
All India Institute of Medical Sciences
New Delhi, India

Priyank Mody
Somaiya and Gurunanak Hospital
Mumbai, Maharashtra, India

Rabin Chakraborty
Sr Consultant
Interventional Cardiologist and Electrophysiologist
Senior Vice Chairman
Medica Superspecialty Hospital
Kolkata, West Bengal, India

Rahul Gupta
RMM Global Hospital Trauma Center
Rajasthan, Jaipur, India

Rahul Mehrotra
Principal Consultant and Head
Noninvasive Cardiology
Max Super Speciality Hospital
New Delhi, India

Rajan Joseph Manjuran
Professor Emeritus
Department of Cardiology
Pushpagiri Medical College
Thiruvalla, Kerala, India
Past President, CSI & IAE

Rajat Jain
Vardhman Mahavir Medical College
Safdarjung Hospital
New Delhi, India

Rajeeve Kumar Rajput
Sr Consultant Cardiologist and Interventionist
Coordinator, Heart Failure Program
Indraprastha Apollo Hospital
New Delhi, India

Rajeev Gupta
Sr Consultant Cardiologist
Department of Internal Medicine and Preventive Cardiology
Eternal Heart Care Center and Research Institute
Mount Sinai, New York, Affiliate
Jaipur, Rajasthan, India

Rajendra Kumar Agarwal
Consultant
Department of Interventional Cardiology and Electrophysiology
Max Heart and Vascular Institute
New Delhi, India

Rajesh Sainani
Jaslok Hospital and Research Centre
Mumbai, Maharashtra, India

Raj Kumar Dahiya
Consultant, Noninvasive Cardiology
Max Super Speciality Hospital
New Delhi, India

Rakesh Varma
Professor and Chief Cardiologist
Additional Medical Superintendent
Vardhman Mahavir Medical College
Safdarjung Hospital
New Delhi, India

Ramesh Hotchandani
Director and Head
Department of Nephrology
Dialysis and Kidney Transplant
Moolchand Medcity
New Delhi, India

Ravina Sharma
Dayanand Medical College and Hospital
Ludhiana, Punjab, India

Ravi R Kasliwal
Chairman, Clinical and Preventive Cardiology
Medanta Heart Institute
Medanta-The Medicity
Gurugram, Haryana, India

Ravi Vishnu Prasad
Associate Professor, Department of Cardiology
IGIMS
Patna, Bihar, India

Reeta Kanaujiya
Department of Radiology
Moolchand Medcity
New Delhi, India

Rekha Mishra
Consultant Noninvasive Cardiologist
National Heart Institute
New Delhi, India

Rekha Sharma
Former Chief Dietician
All India Institute of Medical Sciences
New Delhi, India
President and Director, Nutrition and Dietetics
Diabetes Foundation (India)
President, Indian Dietetic Association (2011-2014)
Country Representative and Director
International Confederation of Dietetic Associations (2012-2016)

RK Saran
Former Head, Department of Cardiology
King George Medical University
Lucknow, Uttar Pradesh, India

Rohin Vinayak
Dayanand Medical College and Hospital
Ludhiana, Punjab, India

Rohit Walia
Head of the Department
Super Specialty Pediatric Hospital and Post Graduate Teaching Institute
Noida, Uttar Pradesh, India

Ruchi Tandon
Consultant
Department of Obstetrics and Gynecology
Infertility Specialist
Moolchand Medcity
New Delhi, India

Ruvan Al Ekanayaka
Consultant Cardiologist, Norris Clinic
Nawaloka Hospital
Sri Lanka

RVA Ananth
Consultant Cardiologist
Jeyalakshmi Heart Centre
Madurai, Tamil Nadu, India

Sagri Negi
Programme Coordinator
Research Division
Public Health Foundation of India
New Delhi, India

Sajan Ahmad
Assistant Professor
Department of Cardiology
Pushpagiri Medical College
Thiruvalla, Kerala, India

Sameer Shrivastava
Director, Noninvasive Cardiology
Fortis Escorts Heart Institute
New Delhi, India

Sandeep Bansal
Professor and Head
Department of Cardiology
VMMC and Safdarjung Hospital
New Delhi, India

Sanjay Kalra
Department of Endocrinology
Bharti Hospital
Karnal, Haryana, India

Sanjay Mittal
Director, Clinical Cardiology and Research
Medanta-The Medicity
Gurugram, Haryana, India

SanJeev Asotra
Senior Consultant Cardiologist
National Heart Institute
New Delhi, India

Sanjeev Kumar
Senior Consultant Neurosurgeon
Batra Hospital and Medical Research Center and Moolchand Medcity
New Delhi, India

Sanjiv Sharma
Department of Cardiology
Batra Hospital and Medical Research Centre
New Delhi, India

Santanu De
Department of Cardiology
NRS Medical College
Kolkata, West Bengal, India

Santanu Guha
Professor and Head, Department of Cardiology
Medical College
Kolkata, West Bengal, India
Past President, CSI

Satish Kr Gupta
RMM Global Hospital Trauma Center
Rajasthan, Jaipur, India

Satya Nand Pathak
Sr Consultant, Interventional Cardiology
Moolchand Medcity
New Delhi, India

Satyanarayan Routray
Professor and Head, Department of Cardiology
SCB Medical College
Cuttack, Odisha, India

Satyendra Tewari
Professor
Department of Cardiology, SGPGIMS
Lucknow, Uttar Pradesh, India

Saumitra Ray
Professor
Vivekananda Institute of Medical Sciences
Sr Consultant Interventional Cardiologist
AMRI and Woodland Hospitals
Kolkata, West Bengal, India

Saurabh Bagga
Department of Cardiology
GB Pant Hospital
New Delhi, India

SC Manchanda
Senior Consultant
Department of Cardiology
Dharma Vira Heart Center
Sir Ganga Ram Hospital
New Delhi, India

Shaheen Ahmad
Cardiac Care
Paras HMRI Hospital
Patna, Bihar, India

Shashank R Joshi
'Padma Shri' Awardee
Sr Endocrinologist, Joshi Clinic
Lilavati Hospital
Apollo Sugar Clinic and Bhatia Hospital
Mumbai, Maharashtra, India
National President, API-2015
Vice President, PCOS Society
Secretary, Indian Thyroid Society
Editor Emeritus, JAPI
President, IAD & HSI

Shirish (MS) Hiremath
President, CSI
Director, Cath Lab, Ruby Hall
Pune, Maharashtra, India

Shishu Shankar Mishra
Professor and Director
Department of Cardiology
Hi-Tech Medical College
Bhubaneswar
Director and Sr Consultant Cardiologist
Med 'N' Heart Clinic
Cuttack, Odisha, India

Shivani Aggarwal
Cardiac Anesthesia
Cardiothoracic Centre
All India Institute of Medical Sciences
New Delhi, India

Shivya Tucker
Consultant
Department of Radiology
Moolchand Medcity
New Delhi, India

Shraddha Ranjan
Medanta–The Medicity
Gurugram, Haryana, India

Simran Sawhney
Department of Medicine
St Stephen's Hospital
New Delhi, India

Smita Mishra
Associate Director
Department of Pediatric Cardiology
Jaypee Hospital
Noida, Uttar Pradesh, India

Soumitra Kumar
Professor and Head
Department of Cardiology
Vivekananda Institute of Medical Sciences
Kolkata, West Bengal, India

S Ramasamy
EECP Consultant
Heart Failure Clinic
Frontier Lifeline Hospital
Dr KM Cherian Heart Foundation
Chennai, Tamil Nadu, India

Srikanth Sola
Senior Consultant
Sri Sathya Sai Institute of Higher Medical Sciences
Bengaluru, Karnataka, India

Srikant Sharma
Sr Consultant Physician
Moolchand Medcity
New Delhi, India

S Shanmugasundaram
Professor Emeritus
Department of Cardiology
Tamil Nadu Dr MGR Medical University
Convenor
Council for Preventive Cardiology
CSI
Sr Consultant, Billroth Hospitals
Chennai, Tamil Nadu, India

SS Iyengar
Sr Consultant Cardiologist
Manipal Hospital
Bengaluru, Karnataka, India

Sulthan Raslin Salih
Department of Cardiology
Pushpagiri Medical College
Thiruvalla, Kerala, India

Suman Bhandari
Director and Head
Department of Cardiology
Fortis Hospital
Noida, Uttar Pradesh, India

Sumanta Chatterjee
Consultant Cardiologist
AMRI Hospital
Kolkata, West Bengal, India

Suparna Rao
Clinical Associate
Department of Cardiology
Indraprastha Apollo Hospitals
New Delhi, India

Surabhi Awasthi
Head
Department of Critical Care
Moolchand Medcity
New Delhi, India

Surabhi Chhabra
Department of Emergency and Urgent Care
Moolchand Medcity
New Delhi, India

Surender Kumar
Honorary Endocrinologist to the President of India
President, SAARC Diabetes Association
Chairman, Department of Endocrinology
Sir Ganga Ram Hospital
New Delhi, India

Swetha Srialluri
Division of Cardiovascular Disease
University of Alabama at Birmingham
Birmingham, Alabama, USA

Tanu Satija
Noida Medicare Centre Ltd
Noida, Uttar Pradesh, India

Tapan Sinha
Consultant Cardiologist
Kothari Medical Centre
Kolkata, West Bengal, India

Tarannum Bano
Division of Endocrinology and Diabetes
Medanta–The Medicity
Gurugram, Haryana, India

Tejas Kamat
Clinical Associate
Department of Diabetes, Endocrine and Metabolism
Lilavati Hospital and Research Centre
Mumbai, Maharashtra, India

Thachathodiyl Rajesh
Department of Cardiology
School of Medicine
Kochi, Kerala, India

Tiny Nair
Head, Department of Cardiology
PRS Hospital
Trivandrum, Kerala, India

T Kallarakkal Jain
Interventional Cardiologist
St Mary's Hospital
Thodupuzha, Kerala, India

Ulhas M Pandurangi
Chief, Department of Electrophysiology
Madras Medical Mission
Chennai, Tamil Nadu, India

Umesh C Samal
Ex Professor of Cardiology and Head
Medicine, PMCH
Patna, Bihar, India
Past Member, Senate, Patna University and MCI
Past Member, ACC-Indian Board of Advisors
Permanent Invitee, ICC HFFI
Permanent Honorary General Secretary
ICC Heart Failure Foundation of India

Upendra Kaul
Dean and Executive Director
Clinical Research, Fortis Healthcare
New Delhi, India

V Amuthan
Professor Emeritus
Department of Cardiology
Tamil Nadu Dr MGR Medical University
Former Professor and Head
Department of Cardiology
Madurai Medical College
Director of 3D Echocardiography
Jeyalakshmi Heart Centre
Senior Interventional Cardiologist
Vadamalayan Hospital
Madurai, Tamil Nadu, India

Varsha Koul
Department of Cardiology
Batra Hospital and Medical Research Centre
New Delhi, India

Varun Gupta
Department of Cardiology
Batra Hospital and Medical Research Centre
New Delhi, India

Vasudha Jain
Assistant Professor, Department of Medicine
Era's Lucknow Medical College and Hospital
Lucknow, Uttar Pradesh, India

Vatchsala Sree Varadharajan
Senior Research Fellow
Sri Sathya Sai Institute of Higher Medical Sciences, Bengaluru
Cardiologist, Muhil Heart Centre
Vellore, Tamil Nadu, India

Vidyut Jain
Sr Consultant Cardiologist
Choithram Hospital
Indore, Madhya Pradesh, India

Vijay Panikar
Department of Diabetes, Endocrine and Metabolism
Lilavati Hospital and Research Centre
Mumbai, Maharashtra, India

Vikas Agrawal
Associate Professor, Department of Cardiology
Institute of Medical Sciences, BHU
Varanasi, Uttar Pradesh, India

Vikas Singh
Heart Hospital, Patna, Bihar, India

Vinod Sharma
Senior Consultant Cardiologist
National Heart Institute
New Delhi, India

Vitull K Gupta
Sr Consultant Physician
Kishori Ram Hospital and Diabetes Care Centre
Professor and Unit Head
Department of Medicine, AIMSR
Bathinda, Punjab, India

Viveka Kumar
Director, Cath Lab
Senior Consultant
Department of Interventional Cardiology and Electrophysiology
Max Super Speciality Hospital
New Delhi, India

Vivek Chaturvedi
Professor, Department of Cardiology
GB Pant Hospital
New Delhi, India

Vivek Kumar
Consultant
Department of Interventional Cardiology
Max Super Speciality Hospital
New Delhi, India

Yugal Mishra
Director
Department of Cardiovascular Surgery
Fortis Escorts Heart Institute and Research Centre
New Delhi, India

Foreword

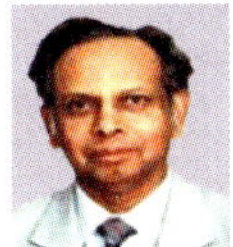 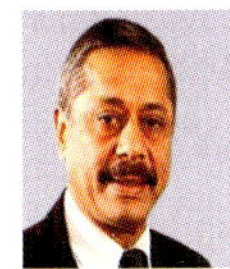 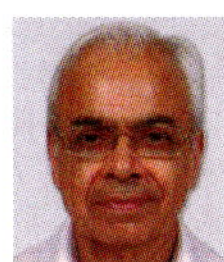 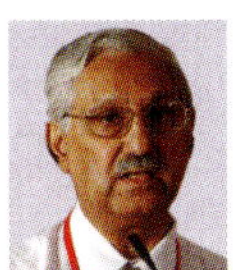 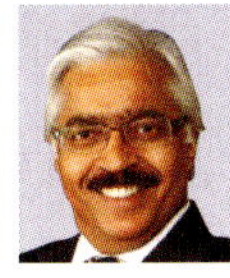 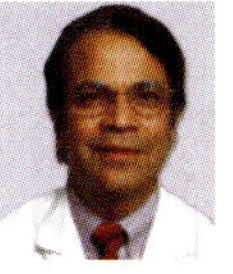 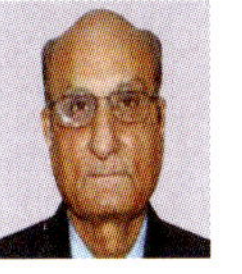 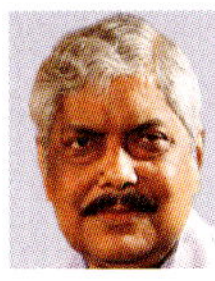 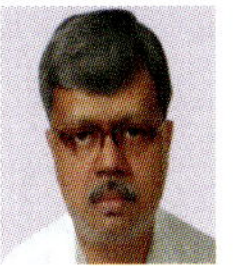 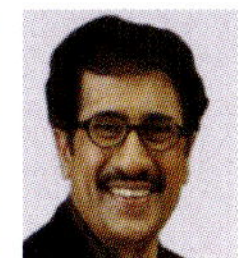

We are honored and have a great pleasure to write the Foreword for the state-of-the-art *Cardiodiabetes Update: A Textbook of Cardiology,* being released on the occasion of inaugural function of 69th Annual Conference of Cardiological Society of India (CSI) at Kolkata, West Bengal, India. This textbook was long due considering the wealth of the data and new strategies to treat the most common metabolic disease encountered in clinical practice. It is one of the most needed, comprehensive, illustrative, and well-structured books, published for the 'first-time ever' from India and presented to cardiology, endocrinology, nephrology, neurology, imaging community, all over the world.

The management of cardiodiabetes has evolved rapidly over the last few years. The enormous benefits are shown by non-pharmacological, pharmacological, oral antidiabetic, insulin therapy and various cardiovascular therapies, including drugs such as beta blockers, calcium channel blockers, aspirin, statins, ACEIs, ARBs, especially azilsartan with thiazide-like diuretics such as chlorthalidone and recently introduced cardiometabolic drugs such as SGL2 inhibitors and meticulous control of diabetes has a definite impact by reducing cardiovascular-inflicted morbidity and mortality in cardiodiabetes besides various interventional modalities. The emerging new scientific discipline: cardio-diabetology, has a team which includes cardiologist, endocrinologist, nephrologist, neurologist, lipidologist, peripheral vascular expert, ophthalmologist, pediatrician, pediatric surgeon, cardiovascular surgeon, dermatologist, gynecologist, imaging expert and nutritionist to enhance cardiodiabetes care and reduce cardiovascular-inflicted morbidity and mortality.

This book is an excellent and outstanding educational initiative by the joint efforts of 6 editors, 12 co-editors and over 250 contributing authors. It comprises nine sections, including *Clinical Spectrum, Diagnosis, Management Strategies, Nutraceutical and Obesity Care, Arrhythmia Management, Intervention, Cardiac Surgery, Rehabilitation, and Future Directions,* including a total of 132 chapters. Each chapter addresses a separate and distinct issue of clinical relevance. The chapters are well-outlined, organized, well-written and referenced. The writing style of every chapter is vivid, concise and practical. There are excellent graphics, tables and figures and flow charts that present the relevant information. The printing and binding is of excellent quality. This book will represent a milestone for cardiodiabetes management strategies in the world.

We congratulate the editors HK Chopra, Shashank R Joshi, GS Wander, Ravi R Kasliwal, Viveka Kumar, and AK Pancholia, all the co-editors, and the contributors, for accomplishing this prodigious achievement of great clinical relevance in cardiology practice today.

M Khalilullah
Director and Senior Consultant Cardiologist
The Heart Centre
New Delhi, India
Past President, National CSI

Naresh Trehan
Chairman and Managing Director
Medanta–The Medicity
Gurugram, Haryana
India

SC Manchanda
Senior Consultant
Department of Cardiology
Dharma Vira Heart Centre
Sir Ganga Ram Hospital
New Delhi, India

Amal Kumar Banerjee
Past President, National CSI, API and SAARC CS
Kolkata, West Bengal
India

Ashok Seth
'Padma Bhushan' and 'Padma Shri' Awardee
Chairman, Fortis Escorts Heart Institute
New Delhi, India
Past President, National CSI

C Venkata S Ram
Director, Apollo Institute for Blood Pressure Management
World Hypertension League South Asia Office
Apollo Hospitals, Hyderabad
Telangana, India

SK Parashar
Director, ECHO Lab
Metro Hospitals and Heart Institute
New Delhi, India
Past President
National CSI and IAE

PK Deb
Formerly, Chief Cardiologist
ESI PG Institute of Medical Sciences
Kolkata, West Bengal, India
Past President, National CSI

Santanu Guha
Professor and Head
Department of Cardiology
Medical College
Kolkata, West Bengal
India
President, National CSI

Shirish (MS) Hiremath
President, CSI
Director, Cath Lab
Ruby Hall
Pune, Maharashtra, India

Preface

Cardiodiabetes: An Enigma of Global Concern

In the world, the scenario of prevalence of cardiometabolic syndrome varies from 60% to 90%. The prevalence of cardiometabolic syndrome in India varies from 40% to 65% and is prevalent, to a large extent, in Punjab and Kerala, in India. The prevalence rate of central obesity in the cardiometabolic syndrome varies from 80% to 90%; and, hypertension 70% to 80%. The rising menace of this hidden medical terrorist has reached pandemic proportions worldwide. It is a predictor of premature abnormal 'cardiovascular thrombo-inflammatory chain'. Hypertension, diabetes mellitus, dyslipidemia, inflammation, thrombosis, and micro and macro vasculopathy are its important components. The prevalence of CAD in India is 14% in the adult urban population with the mortality rate of 16–20%. To be an Indian is itself a risk for CAD because the disease is premature, diffuse, 10 years earlier, extensive, three-vessel disease, poor distal run- off, has decreased ankle–brachial index, increased carotid intimal media thickness, higher coronary vulnerable plaques and emerging risk factors, etc. because of faulty lifestyle and genetic vulnerability due to Lpa. CVD mortality has decreased by 60% in Japan, Finland; 50% in Australia, Canada and the US; and 25% in W. Europe. The WHO projections are that there will be 100% rise in mortality from CVD in India by 2030.

The prevalence of hypertension in India varies from 35% to 44% in adult urban population and the prevalence rises with the rising age. It is 60% at the age of 60, 70% at the age of 70, and 80% at the age of 80. The prevalence of diabetes in India is 9–10% between the age group of 20 and 79 years, its prevalence increases with the advancement of age. The world prevalence of diabetes is 8–9%.

Out of various components of cardiometabolic syndrome, central obesity is the most powerful predictor of premature cardiac- and vascular-inflicted comorbidity and mortality. It is the cluster of abnormal variabilities in hypertension, dyslipidemia and diabetes mellitus with dominance of proinflammatory, proproliferative and vascular stiffness markers, such as HsCRP, interleukins, adinopectin, matrixins, abnormal oxidized LDL, which are highly correlated with cardio-diabetes. The prevalence of diabetes mellitus, all-cause mortality and, in particular, cardiovascular mortality, increases by 2–4 folds and mortality dramatically increases by presence of vasculopathy, micro- and macroangiopathy, diabetic nephropathy and stroke, etc. The projected mortality trend of CVD and stroke by the WHO Global Health Estimate was 63% in 2017 and is 72% in 2030.

The growing knowledge and understanding of interrelationship between diabetes and cardiovascular disease has been highlighted by recent guidelines for diabetes and CVD management. Indeed, primordial, primary, secondary and tertiary prevention of cardiovascular disease and diabetes needs a global strategy based on the knowledge of various risk factors—both conventional and emerging new risk factors. In fact, we are witnessing an emergence of new scientific discipline: *Cardiodiabetology,* which has a team of preventive, clinical, noninvasive, interventional cardiologist, along with endocrinologist, nephrologist, neurologist, lipidologist, peripheral vascular expert and ophthalmologist as a cardiodiabeto-metabolic team.

Various bioneuroendocrinal metabolic processes responsible for cardiodiabetes cluster also include insulin hypersensitivity, insulin resistance, altered hemorheology, endothelial dysfunction, inflammation, hypercoagulability and platelet abnormalities, which are predictors of premature acute and chronic vascular events following vascular injury, occult and overt atherosclerosis, vasculopathy and impaired glucose tolerance. Abnormal variability of blood pressure with abnormal glucose and lipid variability is the major cause of concern, which enhances vascular-inflicted comorbidity, responsible for premature CAD, CKD, strokes, retinopathy and peripheral vascular disease. Periodic biochemical evaluation along with ambulatory blood pressure and pulse monitoring is of paramount clinical relevance to understand the abnormal variability of blood pressure, such as nocturnal nondipper, extreme dipper, reverse dipper, morning surge, evening surge, persistent time elevation, hyperbaric index evaluation, and total systolic and diastolic blood pressure load along with double product is the need of the hour to understand the circadian, hormonal and autonomic influence. Carotid intima-media thickness, vascular stiffness evaluation and various echo variables, such as left atrial volume index, left ventricular myocardial performance index, left atrial, right atrial, left ventricular, right ventricular strain and strain rate and stiffness index evaluation along with intracardiac-filling pressures, such as LVEDP, LAP, and pulmonary capillary wedge pressure evaluation, are of great clinical implications to predict heart failure and atrial fibrillation. Prevalence of heart failure is more than 50% after the age of 70 years with annual mortality of 10%, and 5-year mortality 60% in men and 45% in women. Diastolic heart failure, including HFnEF, HFpEF, or HFrEF, is 40–55% amongst the patients with atrial fibrillation. The risk of heart failure increases with the age.

Atrial fibrillation is a major public health problem. Prevalence of AF in India varies from 2% to 10%—about 2% at the age of 40 years and 10% at the age of 80 years. About 95% of hypertensive, 62% of heart failure and 55% of stroke, are associated with atrial fibrillation in cardiodiabeto-metabolic syndromes.

Meticulous lifestyle intervention, including abstinence of smoking and trans fat, salt restriction, reduction of saturated fat, stress management, regular exercise and practice of yoga, including all the eight limbs, is of wide clinical applications. Timely effective drug intervention with beta blockers, calcium channel blockers, aspirin, statins, ACEIs, ARBs, especially azilsartan with thiazide-like diuretic, such as chlorthalidone and recently introduced cardiometabolic drugs, such as SGL2 inhibitors and meticulous control of diabetes, has definite impact by reducing cardiovascular-inflicted morbidity and mortality in cardiodiabetes besides various interventional modalities.

It gives us immense pleasure and great deal of satisfaction to present to you the enormous contribution by galaxy of eminent authors of international repute and experts in the field of cardiology, endocrinology, nephrology, neurology, critical care, pulmonology, dermatology, gynecology, imaging in this state-of-the-art *Cardiodiabetes Update: A Textbook of Cardiology*, despite their extremely busy schedule. We pay our tribute to all the authors from the bottom of our hearts and appreciate their enthusiasm and zeal for their contribution.

This book provides an insight into clinical spectrum, diagnostic methodology, management strategies, nutraceutical and obesity care, arrhythmia management, intervention, cardiac surgery, rehabilitation and future directions, including the future roadmap of cardiodiabetes care.

The book covers a wide range of topics from prevention to intervention and intervention to prevention, for reducing rising menace of cardiodiabetes.

We have made every possible effort to maintain the quality and standard of *Cardiodiabetes Update*. Despite our best efforts, there may be some unintentional errors. Kindly excuse us for the same. We are sure this book will serve as an important reference guide for the postgraduate students, fellows, internists, cardiologists, endocrinologists, nephrologists, neurologists, critical care physicians, pulmonologists, pediatricians, pediatric surgeons, cardiovascular surgeons, dermatologists, gynecologists, imaging experts and nutritionists, etc.

Bringing up *Cardiodiabetes Update* was a prodigious task and required well-structured team efforts with immense dedication, devotion and coordination.

We express our gratitude to all the eminent cardiologists, including M Khalilullah, Naresh Trehan, SC Manchanda, Amal Kumar Banerejee, Ashok Seth, C Venkata S Ram, SK Parashar, PK Deb, Santanu Guha, and Shirish (MS) Hiremath, for writing the Foreword for this book.

We also express our thanks to each and every member of the CSI, manuscript contributors, industry and our co-editors—Satyendra Tewari, PP Mohanan, Rakesh Gupta, Rajeev Gupta, Manish Bansal, NN Khanna, JPS Sawhney, Sameer Shrivastava, CK Ponde, Poonam Malhotra Kapoor, S Ramakrishnan, and Vidyut Jain, for their constant support.

We dedicate this state-of-the-art book to Cardiological Society of India, our teachers, all the members of CSI, our parents, our colleagues, patients, students and our family—Vinita, Karishma, Vikramjeet Singh, Parikshit, Nidhi, Kabir and Dhruv, for being supportive and encouraging throughout in bringing out this *Cardiodiabetes Update*.

We also express our thanks to Shri Jitendar P Vij (Group Chairman), Mr Ankit Vij (Group President), Ms Chetna Malhotra Vohra (Associate Director–Content Strategy), for publishing this book so well. We also thank Ms Sunita Katla (PA to Group Chairman and Publishing Manager), Mr KK Raman (Production Manager), Mr Ashutosh Srivastava (Asstt Editor), Ms Seema Dogra (Cover Visualizer), Mr Shravan Kumar Mishra (Proofreader), Mr Arvind Kumar (Typesetter), Mr Deepak Saxena, Mr Deep Dogra and Mr Gurvinder Singh of M/s Jaypee Brothers Medical Publishers (P) Ltd. New Delhi, India, for their help, guidance and timely active intervention in composing, designing and finalizing the book.

Our sincere thanks go to Mr Soban Singh, who worked really hard to keep the record of every minor and finer communication.

We hope that this book lives up to the expectations of everyone.

Albert Einstein once said–

"Try not to become a man of success, but rather try to become a man of value."

HK Chopra, Shashank R Joshi, GS Wander
Ravi R Kasliwal, Viveka Kumar, AK Pancholia

The Scientific Committee of Cardiodiabetes Update: A Textbook of Cardiology
Express their gratitude and thanks to

Platinum Academic Partners

USV Limited
Emcure Pharmaceutical Ltd.

Gold Academic Partners

Merck Limited
IPCA Laboratories Ltd.
Lupin Limited
Zydus Cadila Healthcare Ltd.
Dr. Reddy's Laboratories Limited
Sun Pharmaceutical Industries Ltd.
Sanofi India Limited
Ajanta Pharma Ltd.
Eris Lifesciences Pvt. Ltd.

Silver Academic Partners

Alkem Laboratories Ltd.

Bronze Academic Partners

Summous Healthcare Pvt. Ltd.
Intas Pharmaceuticals Ltd.
Nutrabuff Nutraceuticals

For rendering unrestricted education grant which made this book possible in its current enhanced form as "Global Education Initiative".

Contents

SECTION 1 CLINICAL SPECTRUM

SECTION 2 DIAGNOSIS

SECTION 3 MANAGEMENT STRATEGIES

SECTION 4 NUTRACEUTICAL AND OBESITY CARE

SECTION 5 ARRHYTHMIA MANAGEMENT

SECTION 6 INTERVENTION

SECTION 7 CARDIAC SURGERY

SECTION 8 REHABILITATION

SECTION 9 FUTURE DIRECTIONS

SECTION 1

Clinical Spectrum

CHAPTER 1

Clinical Spectrum of Cardiodiabetes: How Indians are Different

JPS Sawhney, Arjun Sreekumar, Saurabh Bagga

INTRODUCTION

India is a breeding ground for diabetes mellitus with the population living with it reaching epidemic proportions. The ICMR-INDIAB study calculated a diabetic population of 62.4 million people in the country way back in 2011,[1] while global predications have projected that figure to rise to 79.4 million by 2030.[2] A 2016 WHO report claimed that India has a diabetic prevalence of 7.8%, contributing to more than 200,000 deaths annually.[3] Diabetes is a well-known risk factor for cardiovascular disease, comprising coronary heart disease (CHD), peripheral vascular disease, and cerebrovascular disease. The disease in diabetics tends to be more severe. Multivessel CHD, silent myocardial ischemia, and cardiac event rates occur more frequently in them.[4] People of Asian Indian ethnicity, comprising of inhabitants of the Indian subcontinent and the diaspora living elsewhere tend to have excess visceral adiposity, and also more biochemical and metabolic abnormalities. These biochemical abnormalities comprise higher levels of insulin resistance, lower adiponectin, and higher C-reactive protein levels. The metabolic abnormalities include raised triglycerides and lower high-density lipoprotein (HDL). These factors render them with a predisposition to develop diabetes and premature CHD.[5] Various factors have been attributed to the higher cardiovascular burden in this population, such as genetic factors, environmental factors, and even intrauterine programming, predisposing to abnormal energy metabolism and visceral adipose accumulation.[6,7]

EPIDEMIOLOGY

The prevalence of diabetes in CHD patients from registry data internationally ranges around 15–21%. The same number reaches 39% in India as seen from the results of the OASIS registry of non-ST elevation acute coronary syndrome (ACS) patients.[8] Even the CREATE ACS registry had this figure at around 30%.[9] The OASIS registry data showed that long-standing diabetes is considered a CHD equivalent, as patients with diabetes without prior CHD were as prone to have future adverse cardiovascular events as nondiabetics with prior history of CHD. Diabetics tend to have a poorer prognosis after a clinical event.[8] Earlier considered as diseases of affluence, CHD, and diabetes are increasingly affecting lower socioeconomic groups. Moreover, healthcare-related disparities (rural–urban, public–private), lower awareness, and the asymptomatic nature of risk factors lead to delayed diagnoses, healthcare-seeking inertia and lack of effective self-management of risk factors.[10] The Chennai Urban Population Study, published in 2010, was a population-based study comprising adults aged 20 years and above, belonging to lower and middle income groups, inhabiting two residential areas in the city of Chennai, Tamil Nadu. The results showed a prevalence of diabetes of 12% overall and prediabetes of 5.9%. The overall prevalence of CHD, as assessed by electrocardiogram (ECG) changes and history was 11%. The figure rose to 21.4% among diabetics (25.3% in known diabetics, 13.1% in newly diagnosed diabetics). This was a much higher prevalence vis-a-vis prediabetics (14.9%) and nondiabetics (9.1%).

The same study also evaluated other atherosclerotic markers in the same population. The carotid intimal medial thickness was significantly higher in diabetics than the rest. Flow-mediated dilation, which is inversely related to endothelial dysfunction, was lower in diabetics and arterial stiffness, measured by the augmentation index was higher in diabetics. All these parameters suggested that Indian diabetic patients have an increased tendency to develop premature atherosclerosis compared to normal population. In fact, it was noted that prevalence of CHD directly correlated with fasting plasma glucose, even among nondiabetics. This implies that in Indian population, the risk for CHD is present even at prediabetic blood sugar levels.[11] This has also been proven in an earlier study from Bengaluru, Karnataka among acute myocardial infarction (MI) patients, where even after excluding diabetics, the test group had a higher fasting glucose as compared to controls, even in the euglycemic range. These patients also had a significantly higher fasting plasma insulin level than controls, a difference, which was abolished on excluding prediabetics from the analysis.[12]

Diabetes and Heart Failure

In an analysis by Center for Disease Control, New Delhi, the incidence of heart failure has been shown to increase from 2.3 per 1,000 person-years for a hemoglobin A1c (HbA1c) less than 6% to 11.9 per 1000 person-years for an HbA1c more than 11.9%. On considering projections from glucose control, it is estimated that annual incidence of heart failure due to diabetes can rise up to more than 160,000 by 2025 with an estimated 50% 5-year mortality. It is possible that these figures are underestimated due to conservative estimates of HbA1c.[13] The INTERnational Congestive Heart Failure Study (INTER-CHF) was prospective cohort study which studied mortality among clinically diagnosed heart failure patients from multiple centers worldwide. It was seen overall mortality rates from heart failure in India, at 23% out of 858 patients was second only to Africa (34%). This was despite the fact that Indians and Africans had the youngest mean age at baseline. In the study's analysis of cause-specific mortality, heart failure patients in India had the highest risk of cardiac death (hazard ratio 2.5). The prevalence of diabetes among the said population in India was 26%, more than other factors like hypertension, chronic kidney disease, and tobacco use.[14]

Association with Other Risk Factors

The landmark INTER-HEART study also revealed certain interesting data among South Asian population. The median age of first presentation of acute MI was 53 years among South Asians compared to China and Western Europe where it was 63 years. The first MI was reported to occur in 4.4% women and 9.7% men below the age of 40 years among Asians, which is 2–3.5 times higher than Western Europe. It was also seen that diabetes (Odds Ratio 2.48) had more severe effects on the South Asian population than the rest of the world.[15] Hyperlipidemia is also an important risk factor among Indians with diabetes. Indians tend to have lower HDL cholesterol and higher triglyceride levels.[16] In the INTER-HEART study, the highest population-attributable risk for CHD was abnormal lipids as measured by apolipoprotein B (ApoB)/ApoA1 ratio.[15]

Diabetic Dyslipidemia

Diabetic dyslipidemia is strongly related to cardiovascular diseases and outcomes. Even though patients may not have increased low-density lipoprotein (LDL) cholesterol levels, they still are prone to developing CHD.[17] Dyslipidemia in diabetics is characterized by reduced HDL cholesterol, increased triglycerides, and abnormalities in the composition of HDL, LDL, and triglyceride-rich lipoprotein particles. It is possible that many Indians due to high prevalence of hypertriglyceridemia may require fibrates along with statin therapy. Triglyceride-rich lipoproteins comprise very low-density lipoproteins (VLDL), VLDL metabolites, and chylomicron remnants. In diabetes, such particles are more in number and have higher levels especially postprandially.[18] The Indian diet too may play a role in higher levels seen in the population. Diabetics may not have higher LDL cholesterol concentrations compared to age-matched individuals without diabetes, but they tend to have smaller and denser LDL particles. These small LDL particles can be toxic to endothelial cells, cause greater production of procoagulant factors, be oxidized more readily, and be more readily immobilized by proteoglycans present in the arterial wall than the larger particles.[19] HDL cholesterol is also reduced in concentration and has compositional abnormalities, and impairing its antiatherogenic properties.[17]

Hypertension

The estimate for hypertension prevalence in Indian adult population is around 30% (34% in urban areas and 28% in rural areas) as per a study by Anchala et al.[20] In the Chennai Urban Population Study mentioned earlier, the overall prevalence of hypertension was 22.1% among the population studied. It was seen that the risk of developing CHD was significantly higher among subjects who both had diabetes and hypertension as compared to those with hypertension alone or normotensives.[12] The Screening

India's Twin Epidemic (SITE) study was a population-based cross-sectional study of over 15,000 patients from multiple centers in eight states of India. Out of the 7,212 hypertensives, diabetes was also present in 44.7% patients, while hypertension was prevalent in 59.5% of the 5,427 diabetics in this study.[21]

PATHOPHYSIOLOGY

The increased prevalence and mortality in Indians from CHD can be attributed to the higher prevalence to diabetes and higher levels of insulin resistance. The reasons for higher insulin resistance are mainly related to increased adiposity, central obesity, and intra-abdominal fat deposition. For the same body mass index (BMI), Indians have a higher body fat percentage, mostly deposited in the abdominal region. This translates into insulin resistance at a much lower level of BMI compared to other ethnic groups.[22] The role of high-glucose concentrations at molecular level is related to production of advanced glycation end products (AGEs), oxidative stress to the artery wall, and formation of several reactive oxygen species, which lead to LDL oxidation, leading to enhanced atherogenesis.[23]

Role of Inflammation

The role of inflammation has been well established in the pathogenesis of atherosclerosis. The endothelium responds to hyperglycemia and dyslipidemia by various means, like chemokine secretion, adhesion molecule expression, release of vasoactive mediators, and coagulation proteins. Inflammation and oxidative stress of adipose tissue also plays a part through fatty acid release, cytokines release, and through adipocyte-selective mediators like leptin.[24,25]

Role of Genetics

A 2008 publication expounded the potential mechanism for increased insulin resistance among Indians. During the early stages of human development, the genotype favoring visceral fat storage during periods of food abundance as a form of energy reserve had some survival benefits. But now, with food availability levels being higher and more consistent, the so-called "thrifty genotype" is seen to be detrimental.[26] The "thrifty phenotype" hypothesis suggests that intrauterine undernourishment causes a tendency to nutritional thrift and impaired fetal pancreatic beta-cell growth. Such individuals, if they have exposure to abundant food and less physical activity, can develop disturbances in glucose metabolism and a tendency toward adverse fat deposition.[27]

CONCLUSION

Diabetes is very important risk factor in the development of CHD. Indians in particular have higher levels of insulin resistance and abdominal adiposity. Among diabetic Indians, CHD tends to occur earlier, in a more severe form and with a higher rate of complications, and major adverse cardiovascular events. Importantly, even prediabetic levels of blood sugars can predispose to development of CHD. Therefore, the lifestyle modifications and control of blood sugar levels need to be initiated at an early age, as even intrauterine nutrition levels can possibly have a long-term effect on cardiovascular outcomes.

REFERENCES

1. Anjana RM, Pradeepa R, Deepa M, et al. Prevalence of diabetes and prediabetes (impaired fasting glucose and/or impaired glucose tolerance) in urban and rural India: phase I results of the Indian Council of Medical Research-INdia DIABetes (ICMR-INDIAB) study. Diabetologia. 2011;54:3022-7.
2. Wild S, Roglic G, Green A, et al. Global prevalence of diabetes-estimates for the year 2000 and projections for 2030. Diabetes Care. 2004;27:1047-53.
3. World Health Organisation. Global Report on Diabetes. Geneva: WHO Press; 2016.
4. Coutinho M, Gerstein HC, Wang Y, et al. The relationship between glucose and incident cardiovascular events. A meta-regression analysis of published data from 20 studies of 95,783 individuals followed for 12.4 years. Diabetes Care. 1999;22:233-40.
5. Mohan V, Sandeep S, Deepa R, et al. Epidemiology of type 2 diabetes: Indian scenario. Indian J Med Res. 2007;125:217-30.
6. Ramachandran A. Epidemiology of diabetes in India—three decades of research. J Assoc Physicians India. 2005;53:34-8.
7. Lev-Ran A. Human obesity: an evolutionary approach to understanding our bulging waistline. Diabetes Metab Res Rev. 2001;17:347-62.
8. Prabhakaran D, Yusuf S, Mehta S, et al. Two-year outcomes in patients admitted with non-ST elevation acute coronary syndrome: results of the OASIS registry 1 and 2. Indian Heart J. 2005;57: 217-25.
9. Xavier D, Pais P, Devereaux PJ, et al. Treatment and outcomes of acute coronary syndromes in India (CREATE): a prospective analysis of registry data. Lancet. 2008;371:1435-42.
10. Gupta R, Gupta VP, Sarna M, et al. Serial epidemiological surveys in an urban Indian population demonstrate increasing coronary risk factors among the lower socioeconomic strata. J Assoc Physicians India. 2003;51: 470-7.
11. Mohan V, Venkatraman JV, Pradeepa R. Epidemiology of cardiovascular disease in type 2 diabetes: The Indian Scenario. J Diabetes Sci Technol. 2010;4:158-70.
12. Anand SS, Yusuf S, Vuksan V, et al. Differences in risk factors, atherosclerosis, and cardiovascular disease between ethnic groups in Canada: the Study of Health Assessment and Risk in Ethnic groups. Lancet. 2000;356: 279-84.
13. Huffman MD, Prabhakaran N. Heart failure: Epidemiology and prevention in India. Nat Med J India. 2010;23: 283-8.
14. Dokainish H, Teo K, Zhu J, et al. Heart failure in low- and middle-income countries: background, rationale, and design of the INTERnational Congestive Heart Failure Study (INTER-CHF). Am Heart J. 2015;170:627-34.

15. Yusuf S, Hawken S, Ôunpuu S, et al. Effect of potentially modifiable risk factors associated with myocardial infarction in 52 countries (the INTERHEART study): case-control study. Lancet. 2004;364:937-52.
16. Goel PK, Bharat BB, Pandey CM, et al. A tertiary care hospital-based study of conventional risk factors including lipid profile in proven coronary artery disease. Indian Heart J. 2003;55:234-40.
17. Goldberg IJ. Diabetic dyslipidemia: causes and consequences. J Clin Endocrinol Metab. 2001;86:965-71.
18. Nordestgaard BB, Bebb M, Schnor P, et al. Nonfasting triglycerides and risk of myocardial infarction, ischemic heart disease, and death in men and women. JAMA 2007;298:299-308.
19. Sniderman AD, Scantlebury T, Cianflone K. Hypertriglyceridemic hyperapob: the unappreciated atherogenic dyslipoproteinemia in type 2 diabetes mellitus. Ann Intern Med. 2001;135:447-59.
20. Anchala R, Kannuri NK, Pant H, et al. Hypertension in India: a systematic review and meta-analysis of prevalence, awareness, and control of hypertension. J Hypertens. 2014;32:1170-7.
21. Joshi SJ, Saboo B, Vadivale M, et al, Prevalence of diagnosed and undiagnosed diabetes and hypertension in India—Results from the Screening India's Twin Epidemic (SITE) Study. Diabetes Technol Ther. 2012;14:8-15.
22. Ghosal N, Davies M, Patel K, et al. Type 2 diabetes and cardiovascular disease in South Asians. Primary Care Diabetes. 2011;5:45-56.
23. Piga R, Naito Y, Kokura S, et al. Short-term high glucose exposure induces monocyte endothelial cells adhesion and transmigration by increasing VCAM-1 and MCp-1 expression in human aortic endothelial cells. Atherosclerosis. 2007;193: 328-34.
24. Mazzone T, Chait A, Plutzky J. Cardiovascular disease risk in type 2 diabetes: insight from mechanistic studies. Lancet. 2008;371: 1800-9.
25. Hotamisligil GS. Inflammation and metabolic disorders. Nature. 2006;444:860-2.
26. Hall LML, Sattar N, Gill JMR. Risk of metabolic and vascular disease in South Asians: potential mechanisms for increased insulin resistance. Future Lipidol. 2008;3: 411-24.
27. Hales CN, Barker DJ. Type 2 (non-insulin-dependent) diabetes mellitus: the thrifty phenotype hypothesis. Diabetologia. 1992;35:595-601.

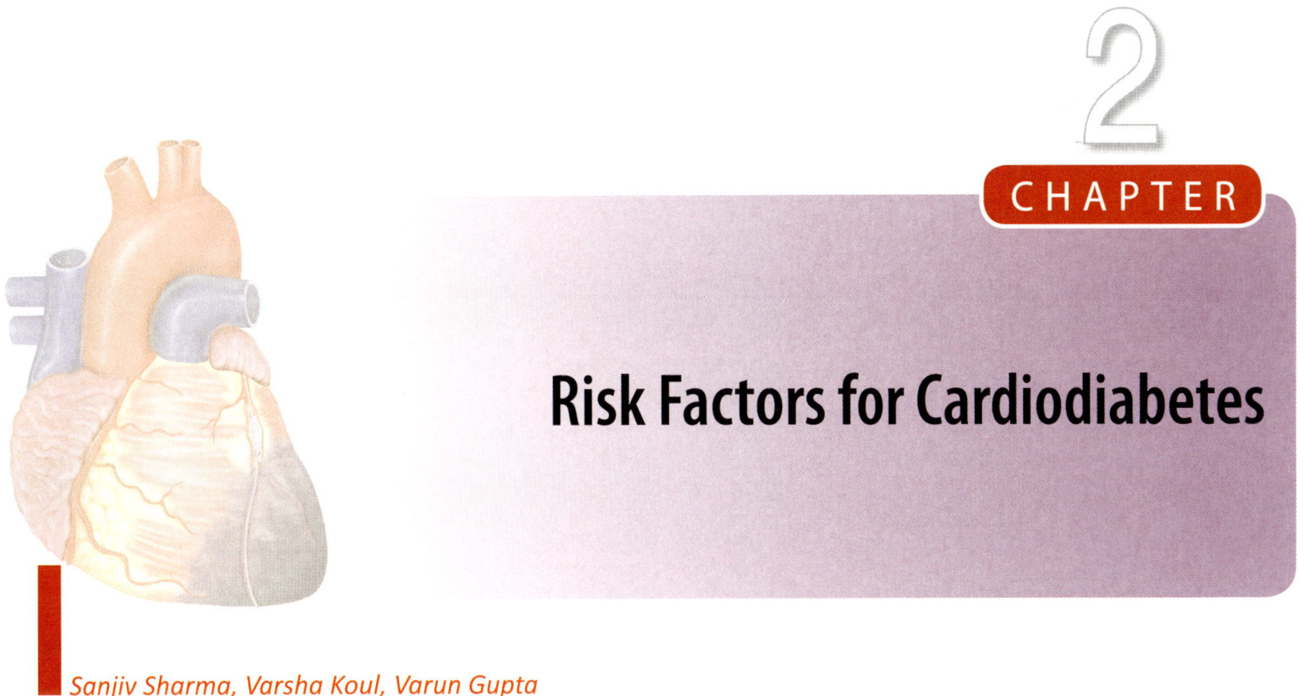

Risk Factors for Cardiodiabetes

Sanjiv Sharma, Varsha Koul, Varun Gupta

INTRODUCTION

Diabetes is a known independent risk factor for cardiovascular disease. Since diabetes and serious cardiovascular disease (CVD) are frequently observed together, researchers are increasingly using the term "cardiodiabetes" to describe the co-occurrence of diabetes and significant CVD.[1] People with cardiodiabetes have both diabetes and CVD, which may be subclinical and undiagnosed, but it is still present. In 2015, an estimated 415 million people had diabetes and this number is predicted to increase to 642 million by 2040, with type 2 diabetes mellitus (T2DM) accounting for the vast majority of cases.[2,3] India leads the world with 40.9 million people with diabetes in 2007. Moreover, it is projected that, by the year 2025, 80.9 million will have diabetes in India.[4,5] People with T2DM have a higher cardiovascular morbidity and mortality compared to nondiabetic subjects. The accelerated rate of atherosclerosis seen in diabetes mellitus leads to higher rates of coronary artery disease (CAD), stroke, peripheral vascular disease, and cardiovascular death.[6,7] The outcomes in patients with both diabetes and CVD are worse than those of other patients. Diabetic vascular disease is responsible for two- to fourfold rise in the occurrence of CAD and stroke, and two- to eightfold increase in the risk of heart failure.[8,9] Patients with T2DM and no previous history of CAD have similar risk for cardiac events as subjects with a prior myocardial infarction (MI).[10] Hence, diabetes is increasingly being considered as a coronary heart disease risk equivalent.[11,12] CVD is increased in T2DM subjects due to a complex combination of various traditional and nontraditional risk factors that have an important role to play in the beginning and the evolution of atherosclerosis over its long natural history from endothelial dysfunction to clinical events (Flow chart 1).[8]

The traditional risk factors include dyslipidemia, hypertension, obesity and abdominal obesity, physical exercise, and cigarette smoking, whereas the nontraditional risk factors include insulin resistance (IR) and hyperinsulinemia, postprandial hyperglycemia, microalbuminuria (MA), hematological and thrombogenic factors, inflammatory cascade, atherosclerosis and endothelial dysfunction, hyperhomocysteinemia (HHC) and vitamin D deficiency, erectile dysfunction (ED), genetics and epigenetics, and cardiovascular autonomic neuropathy (CAN).[8]

DYSLIPIDEMIA

Diabetic patients are at increased risk of developing dyslipidemia.[13,14] There is increased release of free-fatty acids (FFA) present in insulin-resistant fat cells, which promote triglyceride (TG) production, which in turn stimulates the secretion of apolipoprotein B (ApoB) and very low-density lipoproteins (VLDL) cholesterol. High levels of ApoB and VLDL have both been linked to increased risk of CVD.[15-18] Hyperglycemia is associated with low levels of high-density lipoprotein (HDL).[19] Hyperglycemia may also negatively impact lipoproteins through increased glycosylation and oxidation, decreasing vascular compliance and facilitating the development of aggressive atherosclerosis.[20]

Flow chart 1: Interactions of traditional and nontraditional risk factors in diabetes mellitus

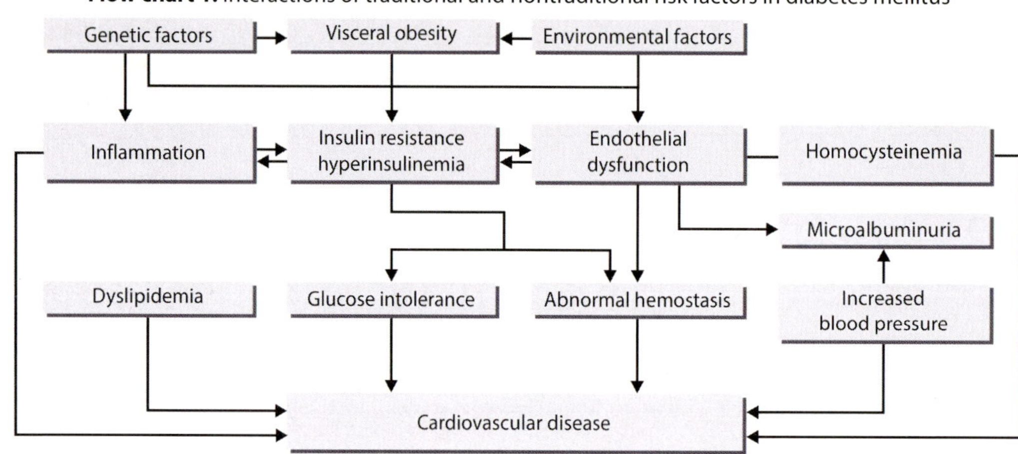

HYPERTENSION

Hypertension among diabetic patients is closely tied to the development of diabetic nephropathy (DN).[13,18,21] In DN, renal cells are stimulated by hyperglycemia, leading to the production of humoral mediators, cytokines, and growth factors. The production of these factors is responsible for structural alterations seen in the glomeruli of diabetic patients including hyaline arteriolosclerosis—primarily of the efferent arteriole, increased collagen deposition in the extracellular matrix, and increased permeability of the glomerular basement membrane.[22] These structural changes increase filtration pressure and lead to MA with a compensatory activation of the renin-angiotensin system (RAAS). If left untreated, DN can progress to a frank nephrotic syndrome, characterized by proteinuria, a hypercoagulable state (due to loss of antithrombin III) and hyperlipidemia.[23,24]

OBESITY AND ABDOMINAL OBESITY

Cardiodiabesity is a hybrid term used to define and describe the relationship between T2DM, obesity, metabolic syndrome, and CVD.[25] Generalized obesity assessed by the body mass index (BMI), and abdominal obesity determined by the waist circumference (WC), are related to a variety of CVD risk factors.[8,26,27] The impact of obesity on both atherogenesis and procoagulant and prothrombotic cardiovascular risk factors is of particular interest in diabetics, as they contribute to increased CVD mortality.[28-32] One possible mechanism linking DM and obesity with subsequent CVD is low-grade inflammation.[33] DM and IR are associated with overexpression of many cytokines by adipose tissue, which contributes to increased inflammation and lipid accumulation, causing endothelial dysfunction, MI, and cardiomyopathy.[11,34] Diabetic patients also have increased C-reactive protein (CRP) and decreased adiponectin levels, which also contribute to endothelial dysfunction.

PHYSICAL EXERCISE

Regular physical exercise correlates with a lower risk of cardiovascular morbidity and mortality, both in primary and secondary prevention. Exercise improves insulin sensitivity in diabetic patients.[35-37] Patients with diabetes have greater IR, which can be mediated by different defects in glucose metabolism, which include decreased number of insulin receptors and glucose transporters, reduction in the intracellular enzyme activity, and reduced oxygenation during exercise; some of which would improve with physical exercise. Aerobic exercises only or combined with resistance exercise improve glycemic control, blood pressure, and TG levels. But resistance exercise alone does not have a clear impact on cardiovascular risk factors.

CIGARETTE SMOKING

Smoking is linked with deterioration in metabolic control in diabetic patients, which is associated with an increased risk for development of macrovascular and microvascular complications and mortality in DM.[38,39] Administration of nicotine raises the circulating levels of insulin antagonistic hormones (growth hormone, catecholamines, and cortisol),[40-42] and affects the autonomic nervous system (ANS)[43] and decreases insulin sensitivity. Also, smoking increases circulating FFA levels,[41] which decrease insulin-mediated glucose uptake.[44] Smoking is an independent and significant risk factor for stroke[45] and peripheral vascular disease.[46]

INSULIN RESISTANCE AND HYPERINSULINEMIA

Insulin resistance is a principal characteristic of T2DM and it develops in multiple organs including skeletal muscles, liver, adipose tissue, and heart. IR is also associated with an elevation of plasma FFA's, leading to increase in muscle TG stores, hepatic glucose production, and hyperinsulinemia in patients with T2DM.[47] Although molecular mechanisms of IR are not yet entirely understood, abnormalities in insulin signaling have been postulated. Hyperinsulinemia can lead to a disproportionate proliferative signal, while the normal transport of glucose and glucose homeostasis are conserved. This stimulates an increased production of endothelin, plasminogen activator inhibitor-1 (PAI-1), proinflammatory cytokines, and augmented surface expression of adhesion molecules in vascular smooth muscle and endothelial cells.[48] There is endothelial dysfunction with a rise in the interaction between endothelial cells and leukocytes, increase in vascular tone and blood pressure and a prothrombotic state.[49] IR has also been linked to cardiomyopathy in diabetics via cardiomyocyte hypertrophy and contractile dysfunction.[47,50]

POSTPRANDIAL HYPERGLYCEMIA AND GLUCOSE VARIABILITY

Postprandial hyperglycemia leads to an augmented risk of cardiovascular events.[51,52] Postprandial glucose excursions, especially when accompanied by increased TG levels, are pathophysiologically related to systemic inflammation and endothelial dysfunction, which are associated with increase in atherosclerosis and cardiovascular events.[53]

Microalbuminuria

Microalbuminuria identifies people at increased risk of early cardiovascular death and progressive renal disease. MA is an early indicator of vascular damage to the glomerulus. MA is considered to be a renal symptom of generalized endothelial dysfunction.[54] MA also indicates ongoing low-level inflammatory process. Increasing MA is related to augmented levels of inflammatory markers, endothelial dysfunction, and platelet activation.[55] D-dimer is associated with MA in T2DM patients, which suggests that glomerular dysfunction is in part mediated by hypercoagulability.[56] MA is also independently linked with arterial stiffness and vascular inflammation in diabetic individuals. Also, patients with MA have more severe angiographically detected CAD than those without MA.[57]

HEMATOLOGICAL AND THROMBOGENIC FACTORS

Atherothrombosis is defined as the formation of thrombus on a pre-existing atherosclerotic plaque. Its major manifestations are sudden cardiac death, MI, stroke, and peripheral arterial ischemia. Diabetes is related to a hypercoagulable state, which is more pronounced during the postprandial period. Hyperactivated platelets at injured endothelial interfaces act together with an increased availability of thrombotic precursors, decreased coagulation inhibitors, and diminished fibrinolysis.[58] Atherosclerosis develops more quickly and aggressively in diabetes, and leads more frequently to thrombotic events due to the interaction between the vascular wall and hypercoagulability. The increased platelet activity signifies increased adhesion and aggregation in diabetic patients, in vascular smooth muscle and endothelial cells. There may also be a reduction in the tissue plasminogen activator levels, and increase in the PAI-1 and plasma fibrinogen levels, which have been implicated with an increase in cardiovascular morbidity and mortality.[59,60]

INFLAMMATORY CASCADE, ATHEROSCLEROSIS, ENDOTHELIAL DYSFUNCTION

Low-grade inflammation would be the causal common factor between diabetes, IR, obesity, and CVD. Accelerated atherosclerosis in diabetes may be explained by hyperglycemia, increased oxidative stress, advanced glycation end products (AGEs), dyslipidemia, autonomic imbalance, hyperinsulinemia, inflammatory markers excess, and genetic variables.[61,62] Endothelial vasodilation and vascular reactivity are impaired in diabetes,[63] which is associated with reduced action of nitric oxide (NO). Diabetes, obesity, and IR are associated with overexpression of cytokines produced by adipose tissue, activated macrophages, and other cells such as tumor necrosis factor-α, interleukin-1 (IL-1), IL-6, leptin, monocyte chemoattractant protein-1, PAI-1, CRP, fibrinogen, angiotensin, retinol-binding protein-4, and adiponectin.[64] These cytokines are involved in chronic inflammatory process in vessel walls promoting lipid accumulation leading to atherosclerosis and CVD.[65] Adipose tissue initiates obesity-induced inflammation leading to the recruitment of immune cells, which contributes to the maintenance of inflammatory response,[64] leading to endothelial dysfunction with increased expression of adhesion molecules, migration of monocytes, neutrophils, and T lymphocytes. IL-1 modulates vessel wall inflammation, leukocyte chemotaxis and adhesion, angiogenesis, upregulation of matrix metalloproteinases, and destabilization of atheromatous plaques that can lead to plaque rupture and thrombosis.[65] CRP is an acute-phase protein produced in the liver whose release is stimulated by IL-6 and TNF-α. Increased levels of CRP are related with the presence and severity of CAD.[66] CRP causes impaired endothelial production of NO and prostacyclin, increased production of endothelin-1 and other cell adhesion molecules, promotion of cell proliferation in vascular smooth muscle cells (VSMC) due to upregulation of the angiotensin type 1 receptor. CRP also increases the uptake of oxidized low-density lipoprotein (LDL) in coronary vasculature walls, contributing to endothelial dysfunction and development of atherosclerotic plaques.[8]

Adiponectin has many protective actions on the atherosclerotic process due to inhibition of LDL oxidation, reduction of adhesion molecules, inhibition of proliferation and migration of VSMC, and increased production of NO in endothelial cells. Hypoadiponectinemia is associated with an increase in CVD rates.[67] Leptin is secreted by adipose tissue and involved in the regulation of energy expenditure and food intake. It induces oxidative stress; cardiomyocyte hypertrophy; promoting migration, proliferation, hypertrophy of VSMC, and vascular cell wall calcification; stimulating platelet aggregation; attenuating cardiomyocyte contractility reduction of intracellular calcium, and decreased β-adrenergic response.[11,68]

HOMOCYSTEINE AND VITAMIN D

In T2DM subjects, elevated homocysteine (HC) levels have been associated with a rise in the CVD risk independent of other risk factors.[69] HC could play an etiologic role in the pathogenesis of T2DM, systemic inflammation, and endothelial dysfunction. HHC is considered as a risk factor for the development of peripheral arterial disease in T2DM individuals over 65 years of age.[70] Studies have shown that lower levels of vitamin D are related with a high incidence of cardiovascular events and mortality.[71] Vitamin D might protect against CVD, as the vitamin D receptor is also expressed in the vasculature. Increased production of NO, the inhibition of macrophage to foam-cell formation, or decreased expression of adhesion molecules in endothelial cells, might mediate the vascular-protective actions of vitamin D.[72]

CARDIOVASCULAR AUTONOMIC NEUROPATHY

Cardiovascular autonomic neuropathy is common among patients with diabetes and is correlated with increased mortality from CVD. The clinical manifestations of CAN are resting tachycardia, postural hypotension, exercise intolerance, abnormal coronary vasomotor regulation, increased QT interval, and perioperative instability. These are related to increased risk of renal disease, stroke, CVD, and sudden death.[73] The development and progression of CAN are likely related to dysregulation of the ANS with increased sympathetic activity and elevated inflammatory markers. ANS dysfunction can lead to arterial stiffness, left ventricular hypertrophy, and ventricular diastolic dysfunction.[13]

ERECTILE DYSFUNCTION

Men with DM have a higher prevalence of ED compared to the general population. ED might serve as a clinical marker for coronary, peripheral, or cerebrovascular diseases in these people. Several studies have found a positive correlation between ED and the risk of CVD.[8,74]

GENETICS AND EPIGENETICS

Epigenetic reactions could be an important mediator between diabetes, CVD, and chronic inflammatory response. Epigenetic factors could mediate the interplay between genes and environment resulting in activation or repression of genetic transcription. The most important epigenetic reactions affecting genetic transcription are acetylation and methylation, occurring mainly in the tail of histones.[11] Some comorbidities associated with diabetes have also been associated with epigenetics like hypertension and obesity.[75,76]

CONCLUSION

The term cardiodiabetes acknowledges the inter-relationship between diabetes and CVD, and creates a meaningful label for both physicians and patients. It also denotes a need to consider beyond traditional cardiovascular risk factors, glycemic control, and weight management.

REFERENCES

1. Robertson D. Cardiodiabetes—is a joint approach the way forward? Br J Cardiol. 2008;15:S8-10.
2. Ji L, Bonnet F, Charbonnel B, et al. Towards an improved global understanding of treatment and outcomes in people with type 2 diabetes: Rationale and methods of the DISCOVER observational study program. J Diabetes Complications. 2017;31:1188-96.
3. International Diabetes Federation. (2015). IDF Diabetes Atlas7th edition 2015. [online] Available from http://www.diabetesatlas.org/. [Accessed August 2017].
4. Mohan V, Venkatraman JV, Pradeepa R. Epidemiology of Cardiovascular Disease in Type 2 Diabetes: The Indian Scenario. J Diab Sci and Tech. 2010;4:158-70.

5. Sicree R, Shaw J, Zimmet P. Diabetes and impaired glucose tolerance. In: Gan D (Ed). Diabetes Atlas, 3rd edition. Belgium: International Diabetes Federation; 2006. pp.15-103.
6. Srilatha B. High Risk Factors of Cardiovascular Diseases in Type 2 Diabetes. J Diabetes Metab. 2011;2:164.
7. Li YW, Aronow WS. Diabetes Mellitus and Cardiovascular Disease. J Clinic Experiment Cardiol. 2011;2:114.
8. Martín-Timón I, Sevillano-Collantes C, Segura-Galindo A, et al. Type 2 diabetes and cardiovascular disease: Have all risk factors the same strength? World J Diabetes. 2014;5:444-70.
9. Prevalence of small vessel and large vessel disease in diabetic patients from 14 centres. The World Health Organisation Multinational Study of Vascular Disease in Diabetics. Diabetes Drafting Group. Diabetologia. 1985;28:615-40.
10. Haffner SM, Lehto S, Rönnemaa T, et al. Mortality from coronary heart disease in subjects with type 2 diabetes and in nondiabetic subjects with and without prior myocardial infarction. N Engl J Med. 1998;339:229-34.
11. Matheus AS, Tannus LR, Cobas RA, et al. Impact of diabetes on cardiovascular disease: an update. Int J Hypertens. 2013;2013:653789.
12. National Cholesterol Education Program (NCEP) Expert Panel on Detection, Evaluation, and Treatment of High Blood Cholesterol in Adults (Adult Treatment Panel III). Third report of the National Cholesterol Education Program (NCEP) expert panel on detection, evaluation, and treatment of high blood cholesterol in adults (Adult Treatment Panel III) final report. Circulation. 2002;106:3143-421.
13. Leon BM, Maddox TM. Diabetes and cardiovascular disease: Epidemiology, biological mechanisms, treatment recommendations and future research. World J Diabetes. 2015;6:1246-58.
14. Kannel WB. Lipids, diabetes, and coronary heart disease: insights from the Framingham Study. Am Heart J. 1985;110:1100-7.
15. Taskinen MR. Diabetic dyslipidaemia: from basic research to clinical practice. Diabetologia. 2003;46:733-49.
16. Krauss RM, Siri PW. Dyslipidemia in type 2 diabetes. Med Clin North Am. 2004;88:897-909.
17. Solano MP, Goldberg RB. Management of dyslipidemia in diabetes. Cardiol Rev. 2006;14:125-35.
18. Chahil TJ, Ginsberg HN. Diabetic dyslipidemia. Endocrinol Metab Clin North Am. 2006;35:491-510.
19. Mooradian AD, Albert SG, Haas MJ. Low serum high-density lipoprotein cholesterol in obese subjects with normal serum triglycerides: the role of insulin resistance and inflammatory cytokines. Diabetes Obes Metab. 2007;9:441-43.
20. Hamilton SJ, Watts GF. Endothelial dysfunction in diabetes: pathogenesis, significance, and treatment. Rev Diabet Stud. 2013;10:133-56.
21. The effect of intensive treatment of diabetes on the development and progression of long-term complications in insulin-dependent diabetes mellitus. The Diabetes Control and Complications Trial Research Group. N Engl J Med. 1993;329:977-86.
22. Schena FP, Gesualdo L. Pathogenetic mechanisms of diabetic nephropathy. J Am Soc Nephrol. 2005;16:S30-3.
23. Gesualdo L, Ranieri E, Monno R, et al. Angiotensin IV stimulates plasminogen activator inhibitor-1 expression in proximal tubular epithelial cells. Kidney Int. 1999;56:461-70.
24. Wolf G, Ziyadeh FN. The role of angiotensin II in diabetic nephropathy: emphasis on nonhemodynamic mechanisms. Am J Kidney Dis. 1997;29:153-63.
25. García-Fernández E, Rico-Cabanas L, Rosgaard N, et al. Mediterranean diet and cardiodiabesity: a review. Nutrients. 2014;6:3474-500.
26. Clinical Guidelines on the Identification, Evaluation, and Treatment of Overweight and Obesity in Adults—The Evidence Report. National Institutes of Health. Obes Res. 1998;6:S51-209.
27. Grundy SM, Cleeman JI, Daniels SR, et al. Diagnosis and management of the metabolic syndrome: an American Heart Association/National Heart, Lung, and Blood Institute Scientific Statement. Circulation. 2005;112:2735-52.
28. Sobel BE. Optimizing cardiovascular outcomes in diabetes mellitus. Am J Med. 2007;120:S3-11.
29. Sobel BE. Ancillary studies in the Bypass Angioplasty Revascularization Investigation 2 Diabetes (BARI 2D) Trial: Synergies and opportunities. Am J Cardiol. 2006;97:53G-58G.
30. Eckel RH. Mechanisms of the components of the metabolic syndrome that predispose to diabetes and atherosclerotic CVD. Proc Nutr Soc. 2007;66:82-95.
31. Van Gaal LF, Mertens IL, De Block CE. Mechanisms linking obesity with cardiovascular disease. Nature. 2006;444:875-80.
32. Després JP, Lemieux I. Abdominal obesity and metabolic syndrome. Nature. 2006;444:881-7.
33. Duncan BB, Schmidt MI, Pankow JS, et al. Atherosclerosis Risk in Communities Study. Low-grade systemic inflammation and the development of type 2 diabetes: the atherosclerosis risk in communities study. Diabetes. 2003;52:1799-805.
34. Vicenová B, Vopálenský V, Burýsek L, et al. Emerging role of interleukin-1 in cardiovascular diseases. Physiol Res. 2009;58: 481-98.
35. Phielix E, Meex R, Moonen-Kornips E, et al. Exercise training increases mitochondrial content and ex vivo mitochondrial function similarly in patients with type 2 diabetes and in control individuals. Diabetologia. 2010;53:1714-21.
36. Winnick JJ, Sherman WM, Habash DL, et al. Short-term aerobic exercise training in obese humans with type 2 diabetes mellitus improves whole-body insulin sensitivity through gains in peripheral, not hepatic insulin sensitivity. J Clin Endocrinol Metab. 2008;93:771-8.
37. Kirwan JP, Solomon TP, Wojta DM, et al. Effects of 7 days of exercise training on insulin sensitivity and responsiveness in type 2 diabetes mellitus. Am J Physiol Endocrinol Metab. 2009;297:E151-6.
38. Madsbad S, McNair P, Christensen MS, et al. Influence of smoking on insulin requirement and metabolic status in diabetes mellitus. Diabetes Care. 1980;3:41-3.
39. Chase HP, Garg SK, Marshall G, et al. Cigarette smoking increases the risk of albuminuria among subjects with type I diabetes. JAMA. 1991;265:614-7.
40. Cryer PE, Haymond MW, Santiago JV, et al. Norepinephrine and epinephrine release and adrenergic mediation of smoking associated hemodynamic and metabolic events. N Engl J Med. 1976;295:573-7.
41. Kershbaum A, Bellet S. Smoking as a factor in atherosclerosis. A review of epidemiological, pathological, and experimental studies. Geriatrics. 1966;21:155-70.
42. Wilkins JN, Carlson HE, Van Vunakis H, et al. Nicotine from cigarette smoking increases circulating levels of cortisol, growth hormone, and prolactin in male chronic smokers. Psychopharmacology (Berl). 1982;78:305-8.
43. Niedermaier ON, Smith ML, Beightol LA, et al. Influence of cigarette smoking on human autonomic function. Circulation. 1993;88:562-71.
44. Bergman RN, Ader M. Free fatty acids and pathogenesis of type 2 diabetes mellitus. Trends Endocrinol Metab. 2000;11:351-6.
45. Kothari V, Stevens RJ, Adler AI, et al. UKPDS 60: risk of stroke in type 2 diabetes estimated by the UK Prospective Diabetes Study risk engine. Stroke. 2002;33:1776-81.
46. Adler AI, Stevens RJ, Neil A, et al. UKPDS 59: hyperglycemia and other potentially modifiable risk factors for peripheral vascular disease in type 2 diabetes. Diabetes Care. 2002;25:894-9.
47. Leahy JL. Pathogenesis of type 2 diabetes mellitus. Arch Med Res. 2005;36:197-209.
48. Ridray S. Hyperinsulinemia and smooth muscle cell proliferation. Int J Obes Relat Metab Disord. 1995;19:S39-51.
49. Wang CC, Goalstone ML, Draznin B. Molecular mechanisms of insulin resistance that impact cardiovascular biology. Diabetes. 2004;53:2735-40.

50. Belke DD, Betuing S, Tuttle MJ, et al. Insulin signaling coordinately regulates cardiac size, metabolism, and contractile protein isoform expression. J Clin Invest. 2002;109:629-39.
51. Cavalot F, Petrelli A, Traversa M, et al. Postprandial blood glucose is a stronger predictor of cardiovascular events than fasting blood glucose in type 2 diabetes mellitus, particularly in women: lessons from the San Luigi Gonzaga Diabetes Study. J Clin Endocrinol Metab. 2006;91:813-9.
52. O'Keefe JH, Bell DS. Postprandial hyperglycemia/hyperlipidemia (postprandial dysmetabolism) is a cardiovascular risk factor. Am J Cardiol. 2007;100:899-904.
53. Monnier L, Mas E, Ginet C, et al. Activation of oxidative stress by acute glucose fluctuations compared with sustained chronic hyperglycemia in patients with type 2 diabetes. JAMA. 2006;295: 1681-7.
54. Monhart V. Microalbuminuria. From diabetes to cardiovascular risk. Vnitr Lek. 2011;57:293-8.
55. Kalaitzidis R, Bakris G. Pathogenesis and treatment of microalbuminuria in patients with diabetes: the road ahead. J Clin Hypertens. 2009;11:636-43.
56. Wakabayashi I, Masuda H. Association of D-dimer with microalbuminuria in patients with type 2 diabetes mellitus. J Thromb Thrombolysis. 2009;27:29-35.
57. Sukhija R, Aronow WS, Kakar P, et al. Relation of microalbuminuria and coronary artery disease in patients with and without diabetes mellitus. Am J Cardiol. 2006;98:279-81.
58. Colwell JA. Vascular thrombosis in type II diabetes mellitus. Diabetes. 1993;42:8-11.
59. Wood D, De Backer G, Faergeman O, et al. Prevention of coronary heart disease in clinical practice. Summary of recommendations of the Second Joint Task Force of European and other Societies on Coronary Prevention. J Hypertens. 1998;16:1407-14.
60. Saito I, Folsom AR, Brancati FL, et al. Nontraditional risk factors for coronary heart disease incidence among persons with diabetes: the Atherosclerosis Risk in Communities (ARIC) Study. Ann Intern Med. 2000;133:81-91.
61. Renard CB, Kramer F, Johansson F, et al. Diabetes and diabetes-associated lipid abnormalities have distinct effects on initiation and progression of atherosclerotic lesions. J Clin Invest. 2004;114:659-68.
62. Ait-Oufella H, Taleb S, Mallat Z, et al. Recent advances on the role of cytokines in atherosclerosis. Arteriosclerosis, thrombosis, and vascular biology. 2011;31:969-79.
63. Romano M, Pomilio M, Vigneri S, et al. Endothelial perturbation in children and adolescents with type 1 diabetes. Diabetes care. 2001;24:1674-8.
64. Hotamisligil GS. Inflammation and metabolic disorders. Nature. 2006;444:860-7.
65. Vicenová B, Vopálenský V, Burýsek L, et al. Emerging role of interleukin-1 in cardiovascular diseases. Physiological research. 2009;58:481.
66. Lu L, Pu LJ, Xu XW, et al. Association of serum levels of glycated albumin, C-reactive protein and tumor necrosis factor-alpha with the severity of coronary artery disease and renal impairment in patients with type 2 diabetes mellitus. Clin Biochem. 2007;40:810-16.
67. Yamauchi T, Kamon J, Minokoshi YA, et al. Adiponectin stimulates glucose utilization and fatty-acid oxidation by activating AMP-activated protein kinase. Nat Med. 2002;8:1288-95.
68. Yang R, Barouch LA. Leptin signaling and obesity. Circ Res. 2007;101:545-59.
69. Rudy A, Kowalska I, Straczkowski M, et al. Homocysteine concentrations and vascular complications in patients with type 2 diabetes. Diabetes Metab. 2005;31:112-7.
70. Kuswardhani RA, Suastika K. Age and homocystein were risk factor for peripheral arterial disease in elderly with type 2 diabetes mellitus. Acta Med Indones. 2010;42:94-9.
71. Pilz S, Kienreich K, Tomaschitz A, et al. Vitamin D and cardiovascular disease: update and outlook. Scand J Clin Lab Invest. 2012;243:83-91.
72. Brewer LC, Michos ED, Reis JP. Vitamin D in atherosclerosis, vascular disease, and endothelial function. Curr Drug Targets. 2011;12:54-60.
73. Rolim LC, Sá JR, Chacra AR, et al. Diabetic cardiovascular autonomic neuropathy: risk factors, clinical impact and early diagnosis. Arq Bras Cardiol. 2008;90:e24-31.
74. Thompson IM, Tangen CM, Goodman PJ, et al. Erectile dysfunction and subsequent cardiovascular disease. JAMA. 2005;294:2996-3002.
75. Millis RM. Epigenetics and hypertension. Curr Hypertens Rep. 2011;13:21-8.
76. Stöger R. Epigenetics and obesity. Pharmacogenomics. 2008;9: 1851-60.

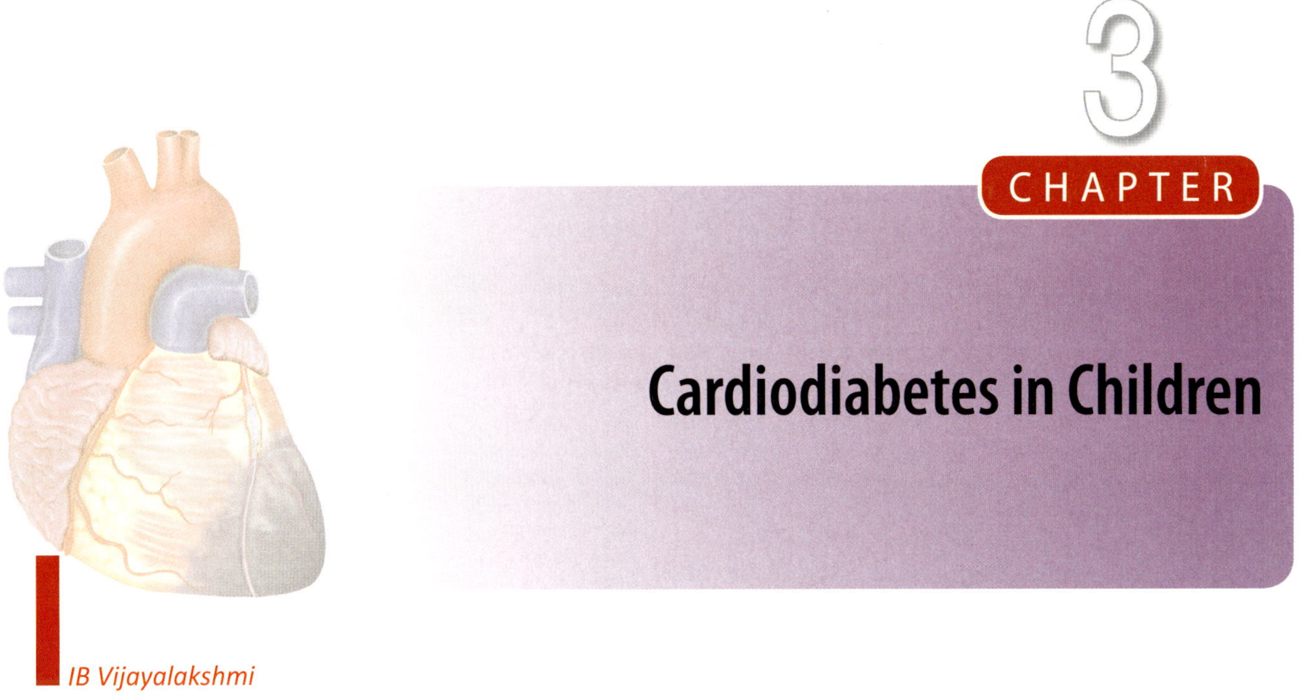

Cardiodiabetes in Children

IB Vijayalakshmi

INTRODUCTION

Metabolic syndrome (MetS) was first described by Reaven in the late-1980s.[1] Later, cardiometabolic syndrome (CMS), also known as insulin resistance syndrome or MetS X, a combination of metabolic disorders or risk factors that essentially includes a combination of diabetes mellitus, systemic arterial hypertension, central obesity, and hyperlipidemia gained recognition.[2] Now type 1 diabetes mellitus (T1DM) is one of the most prevalent autoimmune diseases in children.[3] Although insulin therapy has decreased the development of microvascular and macrovascular complications of diabetes to some extent,[4] however, it could promote weight gain and obesity-associated cardiovascular risk factors.[4-6] Despite the tight control with insulin, T1DM continues to carry a long-term burden of increased microvascular and macrovascular complications and increases the mortality risk by four- to eightfolds compared to nondiabetic age-matched children.[7]

PREVALENCE

Unfortunately, CMS has assumed a global epidemic proportion. Today, the menace of cardiodiabetes is not limited to adults, it has extended its tentacles to children also. T1DM is a common disease of childhood with a current prevalence of 1.7/1,000 among adolescents, according to the third National Health and Nutrition Examination Survey.[8] Four studies in Norway, Germany, Poland, and the Netherlands done to evaluate the prevalence of MetS in children with T1DM have shown that it ranges from 13 to 28% of children with T1DM in these European countries.[4,9-11]

DEFINITION

The metabolic syndrome cardiodiabetic syndrome is defined by many [WHO,[12,13] the National Cholesterol Education Program Adult Treatment Panel III (ATP III),[14] and the International Diabetes Federation (IDF)].[13] Modified criteria based on the same concept as in adults have been suggested in children.[15-18] Existing MetS definitions have shortcomings, especially for children. All definitions are based on dichotomization of the cardiovascular disease (CVD) risk factors and to be clinically diagnosed with the MetS the thresholds for at least three risk factors including obesity must be attained.[19] The cardiodiabetic syndrome is defined as a group of cardiovascular risk factors like abdominal obesity, insulin resistance, abnormal lipid profile, and hypertension, which are associated with increasing atherosclerosis in children with T1DM.[20] Other international organizations such as the IDF, European Group for study of Insulin Resistance (EGIR), and the American Association for Clinical Endocrinology (AACE) use slightly different diagnostic criteria to meet the definition of CMS. However, they all share the commonality of central obesity and insulin resistance, which are considered benchmarks for diagnosis.[21,22]

ETIOPATHOGENESIS

In diabetic patients, the insulin resistance-triggered common mechanism is occurrence of hypertension (BP), high triglycerides (TGs), glucose tolerance, and central obesity. This concept subsequently evolved to encompass a number of multiple risk factors like, dyslipidemia [elevated

TG, high apolipoprotein B, and depressed serum levels of high-density lipoprotein (HDL)], central obesity, systemic arterial hypertension, and hyperglycemia.[23] All these risk factors increase the incidence of various cardiovascular complications.

Cardiac Dysfunction

Patients with diabetes are at increased risk for heart failure independent of having an underlying ischemic heart disease. It has been postulated that long-standing hyperglycemia causes primary changes in the myocardium that lead to heart failure, although the exact molecular mechanism is still unclear. Echocardiography and Doppler studies have revealed presence of diastolic dysfunction in asymptomatic diabetics even in absence of systemic hypertension or coronary artery disease.[24,25] Similar to the findings in adults, adolescents with T1DM were also found to have cardiac functional abnormalities and females were more likely to be affected than males.[26] This is very important clinically, as it is known that women with diabetes have a fivefold increased risk of cardiac failure[27] compared to those without diabetes. In addition, the presence of cardiomyopathy makes the heart more susceptible to hypertension and ischemia-induced damage.[28,29]

PLASMA LIPIDS, LIPOPROTEINS, AND GLYCEMIC CONTROL

Dyslipidemia has been better characterized and more significantly associated with cardiovascular morbidity in persons with type 2 diabetes (T2D) compared to those with T1DM. The increased cardiovascular mortality seen in those with T1DM is only partly explained by abnormal lipid and lipoprotein profiles. Dyslipidemia is very strongly linked to glycemic status, and patients with poorly controlled diabetes show a worse lipid profile. Of interest, there appears to be a sex difference in lipid profiles—women who have T1DM have higher total cholesterol levels even after glycemic control is optimized. This may explain why women with T1DM have similar cardiovascular mortality as men, rather than their normal mortality advantage before menopause.[30]

Children with T1DM have also been shown to exhibit abnormal lipid profiles. The SEARCH for diabetes study examined the differing lipid abnormalities among children with T1DM and T2D.[31] Dyslipidemia was more frequent in youth with either T1DM or T2D compared with their nondiabetic counterparts. T2D patients had higher TG levels, while youth with T1DM had higher low-density lipoprotein cholesterol levels. Only a small proportion of the patients with dyslipidemia (1%) received pharmacologic

BOX 1: Management of dyslipidemia in children/adolescents with diabetes

Screening:
- After glycemic control is achieved
- Type 1:
  - Obtain lipid profile at diagnosis and then, if normal, every 5 years
  - Begin at age 12 years (or onset of puberty, if earlier)
  - Begin prior to age 12 years (if prepubertal) only if positive family history
- Type 2:
  - Obtain lipid profile at diagnosis and then every 2 years

Goals:
- LDL <100 mg/dL
- HDL >35 mg/dL
- TGs <150 mg/dL

Treatment strategies:
- Diet
- Maximize glycemic control
- Weight reduction, if indicated
- Medications:
  - Age >10 years
  - LDL ≥160 mg/dL
  - LDL 130–159 mg/dL: consider based on CVD risk profile
  - Statins ± resins
  - Fibric acid derivatives, if TGs >1,000 mg/dL
- Manage other CVD risk factors:
  - Blood pressure
  - Tobacco
  - Obesity
  - Inactivity

Abbreviations: CVD, cardiovascular disease; HDL, high-density lipoprotein; LDL, low-density lipoprotein; TGs, Triglycerides.
Source: American Diabetes Association Guidelines.

therapy, suggesting a discrepancy in identifying and appropriately addressing this important cardiovascular risk variable. In a recent consensus statement, the American Diabetes Association (ADA) defined optimal levels of each lipid class in children and adolescents with T1DM (Box 1).[32] However, the exact threshold at which pharmacologic treatment should be initiated is still unclear, especially since the safety of many lipid-lowering agents has not yet been established in children. Long-term randomized trials are therefore needed to examine the safety and efficacy of these agents in decreasing cardiovascular mortality in children with T1DM.

Multiple apolipoprotein abnormalities have been described to account for the increased cardiovascular mortality seen in patients with T1DM. These include elevated lipoprotein(a)[33] and apolipoprotein C III levels.[34] T1DM patients frequently have normal- to high-density lipoprotein cholesterol levels, but have inappropriately high-cardiovascular event rates. An abnormality in the distribution of lipoprotein subclasses has been postulated to explain this seemingly paradoxical finding. Some studies have shown an association between elevated lipoprotein(a) levels and cardiovascular mortality in T1DM,[35] while others have not found any such association.[36] Also, elevated apolipoprotein A levels have been suggested as a plausible mechanism behind the increased occurrence of macrovascular disease in T1DM patients with proteinuria.[37] A 15-year follow-up study in Switzerland showed apolipoprotein B to be a strong predictor of cardiovascular mortality in T1DM,[38] suggesting that measuring apolipoproteins may develop into a more useful clinical tool than assessing the fasting lipid profile, which is the current standard.

It is not yet resolved whether poor glycemic control or abnormal lipids and lipoproteins are more accountable for the accelerated atherogenesis seen in patients with T1DM. A recent review by Kanter and colleagues[39] examined the evidence supporting the contribution of each of these factors to the increased atherogenesis seen in diabetes. Studies on low-density lipoprotein receptor-deficient mice that have hyperglycemia but show no dyslipidemia have demonstrated an independent role of hyperglycemia on accelerating the formation of atherosclerotic lesions. The Diabetes Control and Complications Trial (DCCT) included participants aged 13–63 years with T1DM who were randomly assigned to intensive insulin therapy requiring multiple daily injections and frequent finger stick blood glucose monitoring or to the conventional regimen of fixed twice-a-day insulin. At the end of the study, it was unequivocally proven that patients receiving the intensive insulin regimen had less microvascular complications than patients receiving the conventional regimen.[40]

Obesity and Insulin Resistance in T1DM

With the obesity epidemic, there has been a growing interest in the presence of insulin resistance in T1DM patients, or what is sometimes referred to as double diabetes. Insulin resistance has been postulated not only to accelerate cardiovascular risk in T1DM but also to cause earlier β-cell dysfunction in individuals predisposed to autoimmunity, according to the accelerator hypothesis.[41] The Pittsburgh Epidemiology of Diabetes Complications Study[42] looked at the three separate definitions of the MetS and their components to compare the ability to predict the major outcomes of T1DM—coronary heart disease, renal failure, and diabetes-related death. The three definitions of the MetS used were those from the National Cholesterol Education Program Adult Treatment Panel III (NCEP ATP III), IDF, and the WHO. The NCEP ATP III considers patients to have MetS, if they have abnormalities in three out of the five following components—waist circumference, TGs, high-density lipoprotein cholesterol, systolic BP, and fasting glucose. The IDF considers abdominal obesity a mandatory component of the MetS. Patients must therefore have an enlarged waist circumference plus two of the other abnormalities, which include elevated TGs, decreased high-density lipoprotein cholesterol, elevated systolic or diastolic BP, and elevated fasting glucose. The WHO requires the presence of impaired glucose tolerance, diabetes, and/or insulin resistance for the diagnosis of the MetS and two other abnormalities of the following—elevated systolic or diastolic BP, elevated TGs and/or reduced high-density lipoprotein cholesterol levels, elevated waist-hip ratio, and microalbuminuria. The analysis by the Pittsburgh group revealed that the individual components of the MetS predicted major outcomes better than the separate definitions did, with hemoglobin A1c and microalbuminuria being the strongest predictors of major outcomes.[42] Thus in the clinical setting, it may be more prudent to pay attention to these individual factors than to the presence or absence of the MetS based on the current definitions. In the DCCT, insulin resistance, as measured by estimated glucose disposal rate, was associated with an increased risk of both microvascular and macrovascular complications. The estimated glucose disposal rate was based on clinical factors of the patient that showed a close relationship to insulin resistance when measured using the euglycemic hyperinsulinemic clamp method. Those clinical factors included waist-hip ratio, hypertension status, and hemoglobin A1c concentration. Although patients receiving an intensive regimen are tended to gain weight and develop the MetS compared with their counterparts receiving a conventional regimen, the improved glycemia is tended to provide protection against the cardiovascular complications of diabetes.[43]

Insulin resistance and obesity have also received attention in children with T1DM. Insulin dose per body surface area and insulin dose per ideal body weight seem to reflect the influence of overweight and hence insulin resistance in children with T1DM.[44] However, it has not yet been shown whether being overweight is associated with an adverse cardiovascular risk profile in children with T1DM. Further research is still needed in this area. If being overweight is associated with an adverse cardiovascular risk profile in children then the use of insulin sensitizers may be a useful option, though there is still no evidence that it would change the cardiovascular risk.

RECOMMENDATIONS

Guidelines for Treatment

The ADA has published a consensus statement on the care of children and adolescents with T1D.[45] The glycemic target for children varies with age due to the devastating effect that hypoglycemia can have on young children (Table 1). Recommendations on monitoring for

TABLE 1: Age-specific glycemic goals as recommended by the American Diabetes Association[45]

Age	Target hemoglobin A1c
<6 years	7.5–8.5%
6–12 years	≤8%
13–19 years	<7.5%

hypertension, microalbuminuria, and dyslipidemia are also available. Hypertension in children is defined as a BP value above the 95th percentile for age, sex, and height or more than 130/80 mm Hg. High-normal hypertension has been defined as a BP between the 90th and 95th percentile for age, sex, and height. Dietary intervention consisting of eliminating added salt in the diet and an increase in physical activity is recommended as the first line of treatment. If BP continues to be high-normal or elevated, the addition of a pharmacologic agent is advised, and using (as a first choice) an angiotensin-converting enzyme inhibitor, as this drug also protects against microalbuminuria. Annual screening for microalbuminuria should be performed starting at 10 years of age or earlier, if the child has had diabetes for more than or equal to 5 years. Suggested screening tests include spot urine microalbumin-creatinine ratio, timed overnight sample, or a 24-hour urine analysis. Diagnosis of microalbuminuria is based on two abnormal results out of three measurements on separate dates. As with treatment of hypertension, the recommended first line of therapy for microalbuminuria is an angiotensin-converting enzyme inhibitor. The patient is to be carefully educated on the importance of good glycemic control and cessation of smoking, if appropriate.[20]

Screening for dyslipidemia in children with T1DM has been recommended either at diagnosis if there is a positive family history or at age 12 if the family history is unremarkable. Positive family history includes a history of hypercholesterolemia, a cardiovascular event in anyone younger than 55 years, or an unknown family history. If lipid levels are normal, it is recommended to repeat screening at 5-year intervals.[20]

Treatment

Originally, the different CVD risk factors were mainly treated with drugs and it therefore seemed logical to use the cutoff point for each risk factor in the definition of the criteria for MetS. Criteria have been suggested by several organizations and researchers and have changed over time even if they all build on the same concept. Treatment of dyslipidemia is based on a target low-density lipoprotein cholesterol level of less than 100 mg/dL. Pharmacologic therapy is recommended, if low-density lipoprotein cholesterol is more than 160 mg/dL or if low-density lipoprotein cholesterol is consistently between 130 mg/dL and 159 mg/dL even after the institution of medical nutrition therapy. The preferred choice of pharmacologic agent is not stated and has been left to the discretion of the individual practitioner.[20] Despite advances in care, these data show that absolute and relative risks of CVD remain extremely high in patients with T1D. Women with T1D continue to experience greater relative risks of CVD than men compared with those without diabetes.[5]

RISK OF MAJOR CARDIOVASCULAR DISEASE BY AGE

The increased absolute risk for CVD in men and women with T1DM compared with control subjects was apparent across all current age bands. Heart rate for CVD was higher in younger women. T1DM men aged 45–55 years experienced absolute risks of CVD akin to nondiabetic men ~10–15 years older. In women, this difference was even greater. These high risks were seen for strokes, acute coronary events, and for coronary revascularizations. High-CVD incidence rates were reached in patients with T1DM at a much younger age compared with the general population, with large differences especially in women. Thus, CVD rates remain greatly elevated, despite improvements in treatment, notably since the St Vincent Declaration[46] and landmark findings of the Diabetes Control and Complications Trial that emphasized the need for intensive glycemic control based on efficacy in prevention of microvascular T1DM complications.[40] It is difficult to make any useful comparison with absolute risks of CVD morbidity in other cohorts of patients with T1DM, as these have not reported absolute risks by age bands and have widely varying estimates of overall risk, reflecting the small sample sizes in these cohorts and the differing age composition. [47-49] Estimates of coronary and cerebrovascular mortality (but not morbidity) reported by the large Diabetes UK cohort study are consistent with other study.[5,50] Relative risks for coronary heart disease mortality were reported of 8.8 [95% confidence interval (CI) 7.4–10.3] in women and 4.5 (3.9–5.1) in men with T1D, which compared with our relative risks reduction (RRR) of 9.6 (6.4–14.5) and 3.6 (2.8–4.6), respectively.[11] For stroke, the RRs were almost identical to Diabetes UK cohort data with 3.1 (2.2–4.3) in men and 4.4 (3.1–6.0) in women[22] compared with the General Practice Research Database (GPRD) with 3.7 (2.6–5.3) in men and 4.8 (3.0–7.9) in women.[5]

Fatal Cardiovascular Disease Risk

As the European Guidelines on CVD prevention are couched in terms of fatal CVD events only, with 10-year fatal CVD risks of 5% being considered high.[51] Typically,

T1DM patients reach a 10-year risk of fatal CVD of 5% near 50 years of age, 10–15 years before the general population typical risk reaches this level, a risk that is typically reached at age 60 in a nondiabetic population.

DISCUSSIONS

More than 6.2% of children had clustering of four or more CVD risk factors in T1DM in contrast to less than 1% in nondiabetic children, according to the IDF definition.[19] The British Diabetic Association Cohort Study showed that all-cause mortality was higher in patients with T1DM than in the general population at all ages.[8] T1DM narrows the sex gap for cardiovascular risk; whereas in the general population, women have lower risk of CVD, in patients with T1DM, cardiovascular risk is similar in men and women.[8,52] Young men and women with T1DM had a cumulative mortality rate of 35% from coronary artery disease by the age of 55 years, compared to only 4–8% in nondiabetic persons.[52] Collectively, these and other findings underscore the fact that medical management of T1DM should extend beyond blood glucose control to include reducing the cardiovascular risk that accompanies T1DM. Since T1DM appears predominantly during childhood, those with T1DN are at greater risk for coronary events early in life and face a lifetime requiring medical attention.[53] Thus, it is important that patient's, family members, and care providers understand the interaction of T1DM and cardiovascular risk. Traditional risk factors for CVD like an abnormal lipid profile (e.g. hypercholesterolemia and hypertriglyceridemia), hypertension, obesity, and insulin resistance accelerate atherosclerosis in young persons with T1DM. In a study of 27,000 German children and young adults (26 years) with T1DM, more than half had at least one atherogenic risk factor.[10] An additional 14% (range—6.2-21.7%) had two risk factors; the risk factor prevalence increased with age. Despite the presence of hypertension (8%) and dyslipidemia (29%), few of these patients were receiving antihypertensive or lipid-lowering medications. This study also demonstrated that the presence of cardiovascular risk factors increased with age, suggesting the need for early screening and counseling to prevent their occurrence and early treatment if present.

The implications of cardiovascular risk factors appearing among young persons with T1DM are becoming increasingly clear and should be of concern to patients and their healthcare providers. The presence of childhood cardiovascular risk factors has been unequivocally shown to be associated with accelerated atherosclerosis in the Bogalusa Heart Study and the Pathobiological Determinants of Atherosclerosis in Youth Study.[54,55] Several studies have reported that atherosclerosis is accelerated among T1DM patients using carotid intima-media thickness (CIMT) as their primary outcome measure,[56,57] while others have shown similar findings using radial artery tonometry[58] or measuring coronary artery calcification.[59]

The combined thickness of the carotid artery intimal and medial wall measured noninvasively by ultrasonography has been shown to be associated with the prevalence of adverse cardiovascular events. Increased CIMT has been shown to be associated with increasing prevalence of stroke and myocardial infarction later in life in both middle-aged men and women in the Atherosclerosis Risk in Communities study and in an elderly population in the Rotterdam study.[60,61] Results from the Epidemiology of Diabetes Interventions and Complications study, a long-term follow-up study of the DCCT, showed that adults with T1DM had increased CIMT compared with a healthy nondiabetic population 6 years into the study. The population that had received intensive treatment during the DCCT had much less progression in their CIMT compared with the cohort that had received conventional treatment. However, there was not a significant difference in their hemoglobin A1c concentration at that time, suggesting the presence of "metabolic memory".[56]

CONCLUSION

The morbidity and mortality due to CVD are dramatically increased in patients with T1DM. Both absolute and RRs of CVDs are more in T1DM, compared to those without diabetes. Cardiovascular mortality and morbidity continues to be high in patients with T1DM in spite of the great advances made in the field of insulin delivery and blood sugar management. A holistic approach is needed to address all the cardiovascular risk factors that are commonly seen in these patients instead of just focusing on glycemic control. Since T1DM is a disease of childhood, pediatric endocrinologists and pediatricians need to be aware of the high burden of CVD in this population. Further research is needed to elucidate the pathogenesis behind diabetic cardiomyopathy and to prevent its occurrence. The old adage "prevention is better than cure" rings true, especially in pediatric population.

REFERENCES

1. Reaven GM. Banting lecture 1988. Role of insulin resistance in human disease. Diabetes. 1988;37:1595-607.
2. Grundy SM, Cleeman JI, Daniels SR, et al. Diagnosis and management of the metabolic syndrome: an American Heart Association/National Heart, Lung, and Blood Institute Scientific Statement. Circulation. 2005;112:2735-52.
3. Patterson CC, Dahlquist GG, Gyürüs E, et al. Incidence trends for childhood type 1 diabetes in Europe during 1989–2003 and predicted new cases 2005–20: a multicentre prospective registration study. The Lancet. 2009;373:2027-33.

4. van Vliet M, Van der Heyden JC, Diamant M, et al. Overweight is highly prevalent in children with type 1 diabetes and associates with cardiometabolic risk. J Pediatr. 2010;156:923-9.
5. Soedamah-Muthu SS, Fuller JH, Mulnier HE, et al. High Risk of Cardiovascular Disease in Patients With Type 1 Diabetes in the U.K.: A cohort study using the General Practice Research Database. Diabetes Care. 2006;29:798-804.
6. Łuczy´nski W, Szypowska A, Głowi´nska-Olszewska B, et al. Overweight, obesity and features of metabolic syndrome in children with diabetes treated with insulin pump therapy. Euro J Ped. 2010;170:891-8.
7. Ingberg CM, Sarnblad S, Palmer M, et al. Body composition in adolescent girls with Type 1 diabetes. Diabet Med. 2003;20:1005-11.
8. Laing SP, Swerdlow AJ, Slater SD, et al. The British Diabetic Association Cohort Study, II: cause-specific mortality in patients with insulin-treated diabetes mellitus. Diabet Med. 1999;16:466-71.
9. Margeirsdottir HD, Larsen JR, Brunborg C, et al. High prevalence of cardiovascular risk factors in children and adolescents with type 1 diabetes: a population-based study. Diabetologia. 2008;51:554-61.
10. Schwab KO, Doerfer J, Hecker W, et al. Spectrum and prevalence of atherogenic risk factors in 27,358 children, adolescents, and young adults with type1 diabetes: cross-sectional data from the German diabetes documentation and quality management system (DPV). Diabetes Care. 2006;29:218-25.
11. Luczy´nski W, Szypowska A, Bossowski A, et al. Overweight, obesity and metabolic syndrome in children with type 1 diabetes melllitus [in Polish]. Pediatr Endocrinol Diabetes Metab. 2009;16:83-8.
12. Alberti K, Zimmet P. Definition, diagnosis and classification of diabetes mellitus and its complications. Part 1: diagnosis and classification of diabetes mellitus. Provisional report of a WHO Consultation. Diabet Med. 1998;15:539-53.
13. Alberti KG, Zimmet P, Shaw J. The metabolic syndrome—a new worldwide definition. Lancet. 2005:366:1059-62.
14. Grundy SM, Brewer HB Jr, Cleeman JI, et al. Definition of metabolic syndrome: Report of the National Heart, Lung, and Blood Institute/ American Heart Association conference on scientific issues related to definition. Circulation. 2004;109:433-8.
15. Zimmet P, Alberti KG, Kaufman F, et al. The metabolic syndrome in children and adolescents—an IDF consensus report. Pediatr Diabetes. 2007;8:299-306.
16. Weiss R, Dziura J, Burgert TS, et al. Obesity and the metabolic syndrome in children and adolescents. N Engl J Med. 2004;350:2362-74.
17. Cook S1, Weitzman M, Auinger P, et al. Prevalence of a metabolic syndrome phenotype in adolescents: findings from the third National Health and Nutrition Examination Survey, 1988-1994. Arch Pediatr Adolesc Med. 2003;157:821-7.
18. Jolliffe CJ, Janssen I. Development of age-specific adolescent metabolic syndrome criteria that are linked to the Adult Treatment Panel III and International Diabetes Federation criteria. J Am Coll Cardiol. 2007;49:891-8.
19. Andersen LB, Lauersen JB, Brønd JC, et al. A new approach to define and diagnose cardiometabolic disorder in children. J Diabetes Res. 2015;2015:539835:10 pages.
20. Krishnan S, Short KR. Prevalence and Significance of Cardiometabolic Risk Factors in Children with Type 1 Diabetes. J Cardio Metab Syndr. 2009;4:50-6.
21. Misra A, Khurana L. Obesity and the metabolic syndrome in developing countries. J Clin Endocrinol Metab. 2008;93:S9-30.
22. Grundy SM. Metabolic syndrome pandemic. Arterioscler Thromb Vasc Biol. 2008;28:629-36.
23. Irace C, Cortese C, Fiaschi E, et al. Components of the metabolic syndrome and carotid atherosclerosis: role of elevated blood pressure. Hypertension. 2005;45:597-601.
24. Albanna II, Eichelberger SM, Khoury PR, et al. Diastolic dysfunction in young patients with insulin-dependent diabetes mellitus as determined by automated border detection. J Am Soc Echocardiogr. 1998;11:349-55.
25. Schannwell CM, Schneppenheim M, Perings S, et al. Left ventricular diastolic dysfunction as an early manifestation of diabetic cardiomyopathy. Cardiology. 2002;98:33-9.
26. Suys BE, Katier N, Rooman RPA, et al. Female children and adolescents with type 1 diabetes have more pronounced early echocardiographic signs of diabetic cardiomyopathy. Diabetes Care. 2004;27:1947-53.
27. Kannel WB, Hjortland M, Castelli WP. Role of diabetes in congestive heart failure: the Framingham study. Am J Cardiol. 1974;34:29-34.
28. Factor SM, Minase T, Sonnenblick EH. Clinical and morphological features of human hypertensive-diabetic cardiomyopathy. Am Heart J. 1980;99:446-58.
29. Jaffe AS, Spadaro JJ, Schechtman K, et al. Increased congestive heart failure after myocardial infarction of modest extent in patients with diabetes mellitus. Am Heart J. 1984;108:31-7.
30. Perez A, Wagner AM, Carreras G, et al. Prevalence and phenotypic distribution of dyslipidemia in type 1 diabetes mellitus: effect of glycemic control. Arch Intern Med. 2000;160:2756-62.
31. Kershnar AK, Daniels SR, Imperatore G, et al. Lipid abnormalities are prevalent in youth with type 1 and type 2 diabetes: The search for diabetes in youth study. J Pediatr. 2006;149:314-9.
32. American Diabetes Association. Management of dyslipidemia in children and adolescents with diabetes. Diabetes Care. 2003;26:2194-7.
33. Torres-Tamayo M, Zamora-Gonzalez J, Bravo-Rios LE, et al. Lipoprotein a levels in children and adolescent with diabetes. Rev Invest Clin. 1997;49:437-43.
34. Klein RL, McHenry MB, Lok KH, et al. Apolipoprotein C-III protein concentrations and gene polymorphisms in type 1 diabetes: associations with microvascular disease complications in the DCCT/EDIC cohort. J Diabetes Complicat. 2005;19:18-25.
35. Labudovic DD, Toseska KN, Alabakovska SB, et al. Apolipoprotein a phenotypes and plasma lipoprotein a concentration in patients with diabetes mellitus. Clin Biochem. 2003;36:545-51.
36. Chaturvedi N, Fuller JH, Taskinen MR. Differing associations of lipid and lipoprotein disturbances with the macrovascular and microvascular complications of type 1 diabetes. Diabetes Care. 2001;24:2071-7.
37. Jenkins A, Steele JS, JS S, et al. Increased plasma apolipoprotein(a) levels in IDDM patients with microalbuminuria. Diabetes. 1991;40:787-90.
38. Stettler C, Suter Y, Allemann S, et al. Apolipoprotein B as a long-term predictor of mortality in type 1 diabetes mellitus: a 15-year follow up. J Intern Med. 2006;260:272-280.
39. Kanter JE, Johansson F, LeBoeuf RC, et al. Do glucose and lipids exert independent effects on atherosclerotic lesion initiation or progression to advanced plaques? Circ Res. 2007;100:769-81.
40. The Diabetes Control and Complications Trial Research Group. The effect of intensive treatment of diabetes on the development and progression of long-term complications in insulin-dependent diabetes mellitus. N Engl J Med. 1993;30:977-86.
41. Wilkin TJ. The accelerator hypothesis: weight gain as the missing link between type I and type II diabetes. Diabetologia. 2001;44:914-22.
42. Pambianco G, Costacou T, Orchard TJ. The prediction of major outcomes of type 1 diabetes: a 12-year prospective evaluation of three separate definitions of the metabolic syndrome and their components and estimated glucose disposal rate: the Pittsburgh Epidemiology of Diabetes Complications Study experience. Diabetes Care. 2007;30: 1248-54.
43. Kilpatrick ES, Rigby AS, Atkin SL. Insulin resistance, the metabolic syndrome, and complication risk in type 1 diabetes: "Double diabetes" in the Diabetes Control and Complications Trial. Diabetes Care. 2007; 30:707-12.

44. Reinehr T, Holl RW, Roth CL, et al. Insulin resistance in children and adolescents with type 1 diabetes mellitus: relation to obesity. Pediatr Diabetes. 2005;6:5-12.
45. Silverstein J, Klingensmith G, Copeland K, et al. Care of children and adolescents with type 1 diabetes: a statement of the American Diabetes Association. Diabetes Care. 2005;28:186-212.
46. Krans HMJ, Porta M, Keen H, et al. Diabetes Care and Research in Europe: the St. Vincent Declaration Action Programme. Implementation document. Copenhagen: World Health Organization Regional Office for Europe; 1995.
47. Soedamah-Muthu SS, Chaturvedi N, Toeller M, et al. The EURODIAB Prospective Complications Study Group: Risk factors for coronary heart disease in type 1 diabetic patients in Europe: the EURODIAB Prospective Complications Study (PCS). Diabetes Care. 2003;27: 530-7.
48. Orchard TJ, Olson JC, Erbey JR, et al. Insulin resistance-related factors, but not glycemia, predict coronary artery disease in type 1 diabetes: 10-year follow-up data from the Pittsburgh Epidemiology of Diabetes Complications study. Diabetes Care. 2003;26:1374-9.
49. Fuller JH, Stevens LK, Wang SL. Risk factors for cardiovascular mortality and morbidity: the WHO Multinational Study of Vascular Disease in Diabetes. Diabetologia. 2001;44:S54-64.
50. Laing SP, Swerdlow AJ, Slater SD, et al. Mortality from heart disease in a cohort of 23,000 patients with insulin-treated diabetes. Diabetologia. 2003;46:760-5.
51. De Backer G, Ambrosioni E, Borch-Johnsen K, et al. European guidelines on cardiovascular disease prevention in clinical practice: Third Joint Task Force of European and Other Societies on Cardiovascular Disease Prevention in Clinical Practice (constituted by representatives of eight societies and by invited experts). Atherosclerosis. 2004;173:381-91.
52. Libby P, Nathan DM, Abraham K, et al. Report of the National Heart, Lung, and Blood Institute-National Institute of Diabetes and Digestive and Kidney Diseases Working Group on Cardiovascular Complications of Type 1 Diabetes Mellitus. Circulation. 2005;111:3489-93.
53. Kavey REW, Allada V, Daniels SR, et al. Cardiovascular risk reduction in high-risk pediatric patients: a Scientific Statement From the American Heart Association Expert Panel on Population and Prevention Science; the Councils on Cardiovascular Disease in the Young, Epidemiology and Prevention, Nutrition, Physical Activity and Metabolism, High Blood Pressure Research, Cardiovascular Nursing, and the Kidney in Heart Disease; and the Interdisciplinary Working Group on Quality of Care and Outcomes Research: Endorsed by the American Academy of Pediatrics. Circulation. 2006;114:2710-38.
54. Katzmarzyk PT, Srinivasan SR, Wei C, et al. Body mass index, waist circumference, and clustering of cardiovascular disease risk factors in a biracial sample of children and adolescents. Pediatrics. 2004;114:e198-205.
55. McGill HC Jr, McMahan CA, Herderick EE, et al. Obesity accelerates the progression of coronary atherosclerosis in young men. Circulation. 2002;105:2712-8.
56. Nathan DM, Lachin J, Cleary P, et al. Intensive diabetes therapy and carotid intima-media thickness in type 1 diabetes mellitus. N Engl J Med. 2003;348:2294-303.
57. Distiller LA, Joffe BI, Melville V, et al. Carotid artery intima-media complex thickening in patients with relatively long-surviving type 1 diabetes mellitus. J Diabetes Complicat. 2006;20:280-4.
58. Haller MJ, Samyn M, Nichols WW, et al. Radial artery tonometry demonstrates arterial stiffness in children with type 1 diabetes. Diabetes Care. 2004;27:2911-7.
59. Maahs DM, Ogden LG, Kinney GL, et al. Low plasma adiponectin levels predict progression of coronary artery calcification. Circulation. 2005;111:747-53.
60. Bots ML, Hoes AW, Koudstaal PJ, et al. Common carotid intima-media thickness and risk of stroke and myocardial infarction: the Rotterdam Study. Circulation. 1997;96:1432-7.
61. Burke GL, Evans GW, Riley WA, et al. Arterial wall thickness is associated with prevalent cardiovascular disease in middle-aged adults: the Atherosclerosis Risk in Communities (ARIC) Study. Stroke. 1995;26:386-91.

CHAPTER

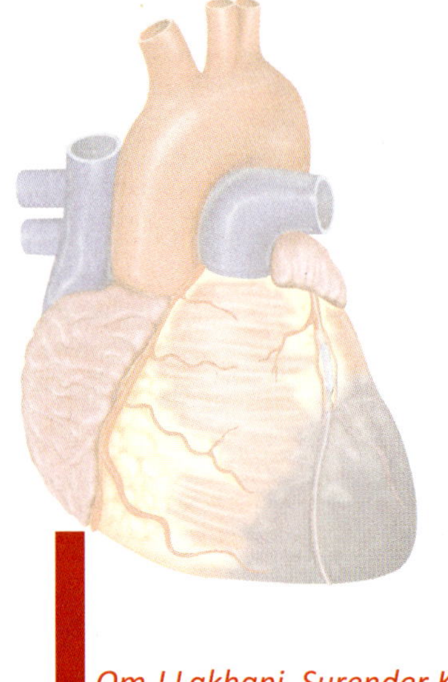

New Genes for Type 2 Diabetes: Indian Scenario

Om J Lakhani, Surender Kumar

INTRODUCTION

American Diabetes Association classifies diabetes into four major groups—(1) type 1 diabetes, (2) type 2 diabetes (T2D), (3) gestational diabetes mellitus, and (4) specific types of diabetes due to other causes.[1] In this chapter, we will discuss about the genetic studies amongst type 2 diabetics in India with special focus on newer data published in the last 10 years.

GENETICS OF TYPE 2 DIABETES

Type 2 diabetes is well known to be a disease caused by combination of genetic susceptibility and environmental factors. Barnett et al. conducted a study amongst 200 pairs of identical twins and found that if one twin had T2D, the chances of other twin developing diabetes was as high as 90%.[2] According to a study done by Klein et al. 39% of people with diabetes had at least one parent with the disease. The study also said that if both your parents were diabetics, the chances of developing diabetes in a person were 5 times that of regular population.[3] The genes implicated to cause T2D are classified into following categories—(1) genes involved in pancreatic development and β-cell function; (2) genes involved in insulin release and action; and (3) other genes.

TECHNIQUES USED FOR CONDUCTING GENETIC STUDIES IN A GIVEN POPULATION

To study which genes possibly cause T2D amongst a given population three types of studies are commonly conducted. The first is what is known as "Linkage analysis", the second is "candidate-gene approach", and finally "genome-wide association study" (GWAS). Linkage analysis is typically used to map genetic loci by use of observations of affected families.[4] *CAPN10* gene on chromosome 10 was the first gene to be identified to have association with T2D and this gene was identified via linkage analysis. However, this could not be replicated in subsequent studies.[5] Variants in *TCF7L2* (transcription factor 7 like 2) gene, well known as the "Prime-suspect" gene in T2D, was first identified by a linkage analysis conducted in Iceland.[6] Candidate-gene approach tries to answer the question that "is one allele of a candidate gene more frequently seen in subjects with the disease than in subjects without the disease?" A "case-control" study is often designed for using the candidate-gene approach.[7] For example, three specific single nucleotide polymorphisms (SNPs) in the *TCF7L2* gene were identified to have significant link with T2D in various Western studies.[8] Chandak et al. conducted a study whether these *TCF7L2* variants are associated with T2D amongst Indian population. The researchers studied the genotype of a number of T2D patients and looked for the presence or absence of these variants. Then, they compared the presence of these variants amongst the ethnically matched control population took see whether these variations are more common in the diseased population in comparison to the normal population.[9]

Another technique used by researchers in the field of genetic epidemiology is the "GWAS". In GWAS, the researchers scan the genome of the participants to look for common genetic variants called "SNP". SNP is the term used for "common" genetic variants seen in the population while the term mutation is used for "rare" genetic variants. For example a mutation in HNF4α leads to a form of monogenic diabetes called maturity onset of diabetes type 4 (MODY4). This change in the deoxyribonucleic acid (DNA) base pairs is relatively rare. On the other hand, a SNP titled as rs7903146 in the *TCF7L2* gene is a relatively common and has a strong link with T2D. This concept stems from a hypothesis called "common disease/common variant" (CD/CV) hypothesis. According to this hypothesis, genetic variations associated with common disorders (like T2D) are also more common in the population. On the other hand, genetic variations associated with rare disorders (like MODY) are also rare in the community.[10]

COMMON GENETIC VARIANTS ASSOCIATED WITH TYPE 2 DIABETES AMONGST INDIAN POPULATION

TCF7L2 Gene

The SNP, rs7903146 is currently the most significant genetic marker associated with T2D. This SNP has also been implicated in gestational diabetes.[11] The deCODE group in Iceland first identified this gene to have association with T2D.[12] A GWAS to look for candidate genes causing T2D amongst a French cohort, also identified this variant amongst those having T2D.[13] The relative risk of diabetes amongst those carrying this variant of the gene is 1.45 amongst heterozygotes and 2.41 amongst the homozygotes.[8] *TCF7L2* is a transcription factor, which is a part of Wnt/beta-catenin pathway.[11] Mutation in this gene leads to β-cell dysfunction, however, the exact mechanism by which mutation in this gene causes diabetes mellitus is not clear. In fact, the common SNP identified, rs7903146, actually resides in noncoding region.[14] The other possible mechanisms involved may be the influence of this gene on adipogenesis, myogenesis, development of the islets, and function of insulin secretory granules.[15] The Wnt signaling pathway also influences the glucagon-like peptide 1 (GLP-1) secretion.[16]

As far as Indian context is concerned, Uma Jyothi et al. conducted a study of SNP rs7903146 and two other common SNP amongst diabetic patients in Hyderabad and compared it with a control population. The frequency of these SNP was higher in the diabetic population compared to controls. Additionally, the highest risk was conferred by rs7903146, as also seen from studies conducted in the West.[16] Chandak et al. found a strong correlation of SNP rs12255372 with diabetes amongst Indian population.[9] Various other Indians studies have validated the role of *TCF7L2* gene in T2D across the various Indian subcommunities.[17,18] Tabassum et al. conducted a GWAS amongst Indian population and found that genetic variation in *TCF7L2* is associated with increased risk of T2D amongst Indian population with odds ratio of 1.56.[19]

TMEM163 Gene

The aforementioned study by Tabassum et al. identified a new potential locus as a marker for T2D amongst Indian population in the chromosome 2q21 involving the gene identified as *TMEM163*. Two SNPs identified in this region (rs6723108 and rs998451) were strongly associated with reduced fasting plasma insulin levels and HOMA-IR. Hence, it was proposed by the authors that the gene controls insulin secretion.[19] A GWAS done in the Mongolian population published in 2015 also identified SNP rs6723108 in the *TMEM163* gene to be strongly linked with diabetes mellitus.[20] However, using the candidate-gene approach, Sharma et al. studied the association between variants rs998451 and rs6723108 of gene *TMEM163* and T2D amongst the Northwest Indian population and found no significant correlation. This study brings out an important message that India being a population of heterogeneous ethnicity, the variations found to have link with diabetes in one set of population and may not be applicable to another set of population.[21]

FTO Gene

A GWAS done in UK to search for T2D-susceptibility genes identified a common variant of common variant in the *FTO* (fat mass and obesity-associated) gene, which was associated with higher body mass index (BMI). Those carrying the high-risk allele weight 3 kg more and had 1.67-fold higher odds of developing obesity compared to those not carrying the allele. This risk was not confined to adults and even children from age 7 and above had higher risk of obesity, if they were carrying the high-risk allele.[22] Yajnik et al. conducted a case-control study to study the significance of these variants in the *FTO* gene in the Indian population. They searched for two SNPs rs9939609 and rs7191344, in the *FTO* gene amongst more than a thousand patients with T2D and compared it with controls. They found a strong association of SNP rs9939609 with T2D with odds ratio of 1.26. However, interestingly, the variation was not associated increase BMI. The authors opined that the variation in *FTO* is certainly associated with T2D, however, the mechanism by which it operates amongst the Indian population may be other than increase in BMI.[23] Ramya et al. randomly selected type 2 diabetic patients from Chennai Urban Rural Epidemiological Study (CURES) and studied the presence of six variants of *FTO* gene in them. They found that amongst their south Indian cohort, SNPs rs9940128 A/G, rs11076023 A/T, and rs1588413 C/T amongst the *FTO* gene were associated with increased risk of T2D, while rs8050136 C/A variant of *FTO* gene was associated with obesity.[24]

HNF4A Gene

Mutation in *HNF4A* gene is well known to cause MODY1. Mutation in *HNF4A* in MODY1 is associated with pancreatic β-cell function and impaired insulin secretion.[25] However, common variants in this gene have also been found to be associated with T2D. Additionally, common variants of *HNF1A* (a mutation of which leads to MODY3) and variants in *KCNJ11* (mutation of which leads to permanent neonatal diabetes mellitus) have also been linked with T2D.[26,27] Kooner et al. conducted a GWAS amongst patients of South Asian ancestry from London, Pakistan, and Singapore. They identified common variants in six loci to be associated with T2D. These loci were *GRB14*, *ST6GAL1*, *VPS26A*, *HMG20A*, *AP3S2*, and *HNF4A*. A SNP rs4812829 in *HNF4A* was found to have a strong association with diabetes. A study done in North Indian patients found that *HNF4A* promoter P2 polymorphisms rs1884613 and rs2144908 had a strong association with T2D with an odds ratio of 1.37.[28]

IGF2BP2 Gene

As discussed above, the Indian population is genetically heterogeneous. Hence, it is quite likely that certain variants, which are associated with T2D amongst a certain population, may not be found in other population. This is classical illustrated by a study done amongst the Punjabi Sikh population by Saxena et al. The researchers found a SNP rs9552911 in the *SGCG* gene to be strongly associated with T2D. However, this could not find the variant amongst non-Sikh South Asian population having T2D.[29] This difference is also clearly illustrated by variations in *IGF2BP2* gene. Studies done by Saxena et al.[29] Chauhan et al.[17] and Sanghera et al.[30] amongst the North Indian population have found a clear association between T2D and variants in the *IGF2BP2* gene. However, studies done from South of India by Chidambaram M et al.[31] and Kommoju et al.[31] could not find these variants amongst their population.

ROLE OF OTHER GENES DISCOVERED TO BE ASSOCIATED WITH TYPE 2 DIABETES AMONGST INDIAN POPULATION

CAPN10 gene was the first gene to be identified to be associated with T2D.[32] A study done in Hyderabad replicated the role of SNP rs3792267 in the *CAPN10* gene amongst Indian population. The same study also found significant prevalence of SNP rs1801278 of the IRS1 in T2D.[33] rs1801282, also called P12A, is a common SNP in the peroxisome proliferator-activated receptor gamma (*PPARG*) gene. This was also one of the earliest genes discovered to be associated with T2D. A study done in the Sikh population confirmed the association of this variation with T2D amongst the given population.[30] However, a study done from South India could not replicate the role of this variant in T2D.[33] In 2003, the SNP rs5219 (E23K) in KCNJ11 gene was discovered to be associated with T2D. Phani et al. could not replicate the role of this variant amongst a study done in South Indian Population.[34]

Gupta et al. validated the role of 31 SNPs in 24 genes, which were known to be associated with T2D in Western Population, amongst a population of more than 3,000 patients from Lucknow, Nagpur, Hyderabad, and Bangalore. They found significant associations of *CXCR4* (rs932206), *TCF7L2* (rs7903146, rs12255372), and *CDKAL1* (rs7756992) with fasting glucose values. They also found *NOTCH2* (rs10923931), *HNF1B* (rs757210), *ADAM30* (rs2641348), and *CDKN2A/B* (rs10811661) were associated with higher fasting insulin values. Variants in *TCF-2*, *ADAM30*, and *CDKN2A/B* were associated with higher insulin resistance. *THADA* (rs7578597) was associated with T2D.[35]

CLINICAL IMPORTANCE OF KNOWING THE GENETIC VARIANTS ASSOCIATED WITH TYPE 2 DIABETES

Though the practical clinical utility of knowing the genetic variations which are associated with T2D are currently limited, especially in India, because of the cost constraints of genetic testing, if we look in the future we believe we would all be using the information obtained from these studies in our clinical practice. There are two important clinical utility of the use of this above mentioned importance in clinical practice.[36] The first clinical utility is to use the given information for prediction and screening of T2D. For example, if a patient has a strong family history of diabetes and wants to know his personal risk of developing the same, the presence or absence of these genetic variants in him can clarify the risk and can help to develop a plan for screening and take appropriate steps for prevention of T2D by controlling the environmental factors. Additionally, presence of a particular common variant found amongst a community can help us to screen for presence of these variants in other members of the same community. Another importance of screening for these genetic variants is to use personalized medicine for treating the patient. For example some genetic variants discussed above are associated with defective insulin secretion. Early use of insulin may be appropriate for management in such patients. Additionally, some studies have shown that those carrying *TCF7L2* allele are less likely to respond to sulfonylurea and more likely to have good response to metformin.[37] On the other hand, those harboring mutation in *KCNJ11* may have better response to sulfonylurea.[38] This field of study of development of personalized medicine based on genetic variation is what is known as "Pharmacogenetics".

CONCLUSION

Uncommon diseases (e.g. MODY) have uncommon variants in the gene which are called "mutations", while common diseases (e.g. T2D) have common variations which are called "SNP". Various studies conducted in the last one to two decades have revealed the role of variations in some specific loci to be strongly associated with T2D. Many of these genetic variations discovered in the west have been validated amongst Indian populations (e.g. *TCF7L2*). Additionally, some studies have revealed some novel loci to be associated with T2D amongst Indian population (e.g. *TMEM163*). Interestingly, considering the heterogeneous nature of Indian population, various studies have shown difference in importance of some of the genetic variations when compared in population from North India and South India (e.g. *IGF2BP2*). The study of these genetic variations which are associated with T2D is an exciting area in the field of endocrinology and is likely to be used commonly in clinical practice for risk prediction and personalized medicine.

REFERENCES

1. Cefalu WT, Bakris G, Boulton LBAJM, et al. Classification and Diagnosis of Diabetes. Diabetes Care. 2016.
2. Barnett AH, Eff C, Leslie RD, et al. Diabetes in identical twins. A study of 200 pairs. Diabetologia. 1981;20:87-93.
3. Klein BE, Klein R, Moss SE, et al. Parental history of diabetes in a population-based study. Diabetes Care. 1996;19:827-30.
4. Dawn Teare M, Barrett JH. Genetic linkage studies. The Lancet. 2005;366:1036-44.
5. Prasad R, Groop L. Genetics of Type 2 Diabetes—Pitfalls and Possibilities. Genes. 2015;6:87-123.
6. Reynisdottir I, Thorleifsson G, Benediktsson R, et al. Localization of a Susceptibility Gene for Type 2 Diabetes to Chromosome 5q34–q35.2. Am J Hum Genet. 2003;73:323-35.
7. Patnala R, Clements J, Batra J. Candidate gene association studies: a comprehensive guide to useful in silico tools. BMC Genetics. 2013;14:39.
8. Grant SF, Thorleifsson G, Reynisdottir I, et al. Variant of transcription factor 7-like 2 (TCF7L2) gene confers risk of type 2 diabetes. Nat Genet. 2006;38:320-3.
9. Chandak GR, Janipalli CS, Bhaskar S, et al. Common variants in the TCF7L2 gene are strongly associated with type 2 diabetes mellitus in the Indian population. Diabetologia. 2007;50:63-7.
10. Lewitter F, Bush WS, Moore JH, et al. Chapter 11: Genome-Wide Association Studies. PLoS Computational Biology. 2012;8:e1002822.
11. Vaquero AR, Ferreira NE, Omae SV, et al. Using gene-network landscape to dissect genotype effects of TCF7L2 genetic variant on diabetes and cardiovascular risk. Physiol Genomics. 2012;44: 903-14.
12. Hattersley AT. Prime suspect: the TCF7L2 gene and type 2 diabetes risk. J Clin Invest. 2007;117:2077-9.
13. Sladek R, Rocheleau G, Rung J, et al. A genome-wide association study identifies novel risk loci for type 2 diabetes. Nature. 2007;445:881-5.
14. Gloyn AL, Braun M, Rorsman P. Type 2 diabetes susceptibility gene TCF7L2 and its role in beta-cell function. Diabetes. 2009;58:800-2.
15. da Silva Xavier G, Loder MK, McDonald A, et al. TCF7L2 regulates late events in insulin secretion from pancreatic islet beta-cells. Diabetes. 2009;58:894-905.
16. Uma Jyothi K, Jayaraj M, Subburaj KS, et al. Association of TCF7L2 Gene Polymorphisms with T2DM in the Population of Hyderabad, India. PLoS ONE. 2013;8(4):e60212.
17. Chauhan G, Spurgeon CJ, Tabassum R, et al. Impact of common variants of PPARG, KCNJ11, TCF7L2, SLC30A8, HHEX, CDKN2A, IGF2BP2, and CDKAL1 on the risk of type 2 diabetes in 5,164 Indians. Diabetes. 2010;59:2068-74.
18. Sanghera DK, Nath SK, Ortega L, et al. TCF7L2 polymorphisms are associated with type 2 diabetes in Khatri Sikhs from North India: genetic variation affects lipid levels. Ann Hum Genet. 2008;72: 499-509.
19. Tabassum R, Chauhan G, Dwivedi OP, et al. Genome-wide association study for type 2 diabetes in Indians identifies a new susceptibility locus at 2q21. Diabetes. 2013;62:977-86.
20. Bai H, Liu H, Suyalatu S, et al. Association Analysis of Genetic Variants with Type 2 Diabetes in a Mongolian Population in China. J Diabetes Res. 2015;2015:613236.
21. Sharma V, Sharma I, Sethi I, et al. Replication of newly identified type 2 diabetes susceptible loci in Northwest Indian population. Diabetes Res Clin Pract. 2017;126:160-3.
22. Frayling TM, Timpson NJ, Weedon MN, et al. A common variant in the FTO gene is associated with body mass index and predisposes to childhood and adult obesity. Science. 2007;316:889-94.
23. Yajnik CS, Janipalli CS, Bhaskar S, et al. FTO gene variants are strongly associated with type 2 diabetes in South Asian Indians. Diabetologia. 2009;52:247-52.
24. Ramya K, Radha V, Ghosh S, et al. Genetic variations in the FTO gene are associated with type 2 diabetes and obesity in south Indians (CURES-79). Diabetes Technol Ther. 2011;13:33-42.
25. Yamagata K, Furuta H, Oda N, et al. Mutations in the hepatocyte nuclear factor-4α gene in maturity-onset diabetes of the young (MODY1). Nature. 1996;384:458-60.
26. Holmkvist J, Cervin C, Lyssenko V, et al. Common variants in HNF-1 α and risk of type 2 diabetes. Diabetologia. 2006;49:2882-91.
27. Florez JC, Jablonski KA, Kahn SE, et al. Type 2 Diabetes-Associated Missense Polymorphisms KCNJ11 E23K and ABCC8 A1369S Influence Progression to Diabetes and Response to Interventions in the Diabetes Prevention Program. Diabetes. 2007;56:531-6.
28. Chavali S, Mahajan A, Tabassum R, et al. Association of variants in genes involved in pancreatic β-cell development and function with type 2 diabetes in North Indians. Journal of Human Genetics. 2011;56:695-700.
29. Saxena R, Saleheen D, Been LF, et al. Genome-wide association study identifies a novel locus contributing to type 2 diabetes susceptibility in Sikhs of Punjabi origin from India. Diabetes. 2013;62:1746-55.
30. Sanghera DK, Ortega L, Han S, et al. Impact of nine common type 2 diabetes risk polymorphisms in Asian Indian Sikhs: PPARG2 (Pro12Ala), IGF2BP2, TCF7L2 and FTOvariants confer a significant risk. BMC Med Genet. 2008;9:59.
31. Chidambaram M, Radha V, Mohan V. Replication of recently described type 2 diabetes gene variants in a South Indian population. Metabolism. 2010;59:1760-6.

32. Lander ES, Altshuler D, Hirschhorn JN, et al. The common PPARgamma Pro12Ala polymorphism is associated with decreased risk of type 2 diabetes. Nat Genet. 2000;26:76-80.
33. Kommoju UJ, Maruda J, Kadarkarai Samy S, et al. Association of IRS1, CAPN10, and PPARG gene polymorphisms with type 2 diabetes mellitus in the high-risk population of Hyderabad, India. J Diabetes. 2014;6:564-73.
34. Phani NM, Guddattu V, Bellampalli R, et al. Population specific impact of genetic variants in KCNJ11 gene to type 2 diabetes: a case-control and meta-analysis study. PLoS ONE. 2014;9:e107021.
35. Gupta V, Vinay DG, Rafiq S, et al. Association analysis of 31 common polymorphisms with type 2 diabetes and its related traits in Indian sib pairs. Diabetologia. 2011;55:349-57.
36. Dorajoo R, Liu J, Boehm B. Genetics of Type 2 Diabetes and Clinical Utility. Genes. 2015;6:372-84.
37. Pearson ER, Donnelly LA, Kimber C, et al. Variation inTCF7L2 influences therapeutic response to sulfonylureas. Diabetes. 2007;56:2178-82.
38. Singh S, Usman K, Banerjee M. Pharmacogenetic studies update in type 2 diabetes mellitus. World J Diabetes. 2016;7:302-15.

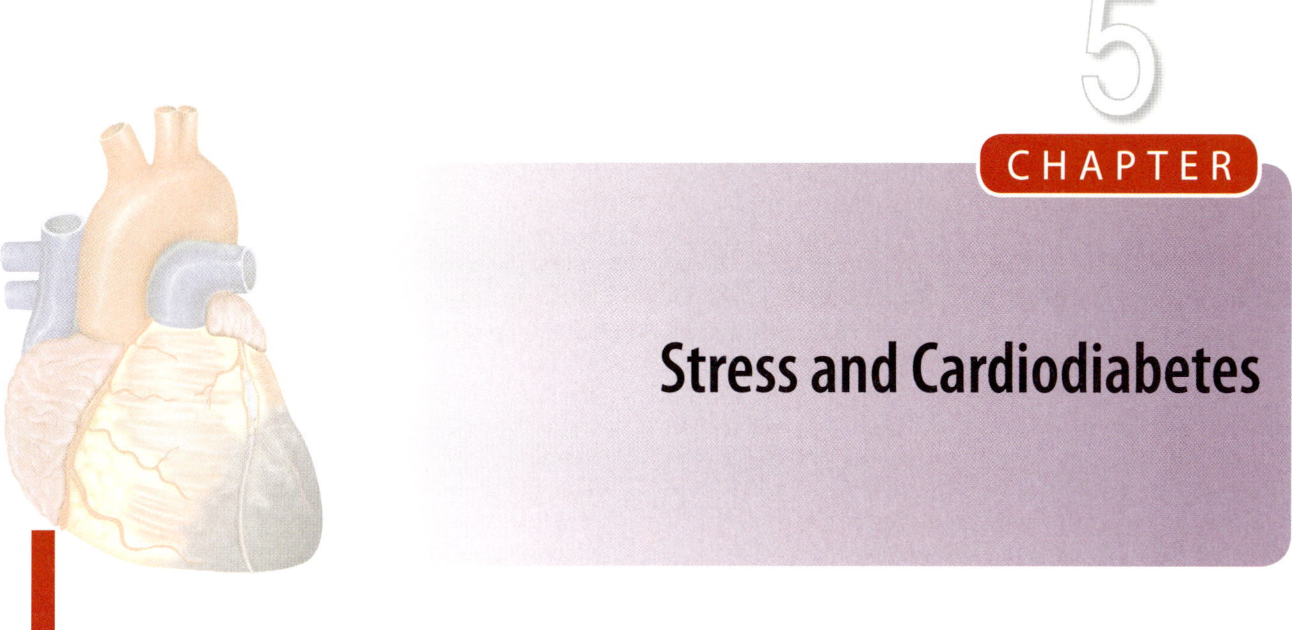

Stress and Cardiodiabetes

Satish Kr Gupta, Rahul Gupta

INTRODUCTION

Of all the possible complications of diabetes, the cardiac ones are the most lethal. Cardiovascular disease (CVD) is in fact the number one cause of death in patients with type 2 diabetes. At least 68% of the people age 65 or older with diabetes die from some form of CVD; and 16% of die of stroke, adults with diabetes are 2–4 times more likely die from CVD then adults without diabetes. American Heart Association considers diabetes to be one of the seven major conventional risk factors, e.g. hypertension, dyslipidemia, obesity, physical inactivity, smoking, etc. for CVD. The term "cardiodiabetes" acknowledges the strong correlationship between CVD and diabetes.[1] Clinical evidence that the patients with diabetes have multiple risk factors for CVD is undeniable and a need to consider risk factors beyond glycemic control and weight management for significantly decreasing morbidity and mortality due to CVD and diabetes.

Over 8% of the world population (415–420 million people) is currently suffering from diabetes as per International Diabetes Federation (IDF) and the World Health Organization (WHO) report. The prevalence is expected to rise to 10.4% (642 million) by 2040.[2,3] In the United States of America, an estimated 9.3% of the population (29.1 million people) have diabetes.[4] Worldwide, type 2 diabetes is the most common form of diabetes accounting for 90% of cases.[2,5] Diabetes is the fourth or fifth leading cause of mortality in most high-income countries and as such represents a significant burden to public health systems.[6] At present, around 366 million people globally are currently estimated to have diabetes according to IDF, of which 80% live in low- and middle-income countries.[7] The more worrisome fact is that about 50% of those with diabetes remain undiagnosed.[8,9] In 2015, health spending on diabetes represented 12% (USD 673 billion) of global health expenditure and it may account for up to 20% of national healthcare budgets in some countries.[2] Additionally, the indirect costs of diabetes such as a reduced labor force and lowered economic productivity are considerable.[10]

The European Society of Cardiology-European Association for the Study of Diabetes (ESC-EASD) Task Force guidelines of 2007 acknowledge the interrelationship between diabetes and CVD and call for an early, multidisciplinary approach to the reorganization, and intensive management of all cardiodiabetes risk factors. The evidence that diabetes is key factor[11] in CVD is also highlighted by the National Institute of Health and Clinical Excellence (NICE) clinical guidelines on lipid modification and type 2 diabetes, which recommends treatment of serum lipids in patients with type 2 diabetes mellitus and those with established CVD.[12,13]

"Prevention of CVD must focus equally on patients with established atherosclerosis disease and people with diabetes."

CARDIODIABETES: A LINK BEYOND CONVENTIONAL RISK FACTORS

Conventional risk factors (hypertension, diabetes, dyslipidemia, obesity, etc.); lifestyle risk factors (wrong diet, physical inactivity, smoking, and alcohol abuse); and psychosocial stress have been identified as modifiable risk factors for CVD development. In many reviews, clear and convincing evidence has been observed that psychosocial stress risk factors—negative emotional disorders (e.g. depression and anxiety), type A personality traits (e.g. anger, hostility, antagonistic interactions, cynicism, mistrust, etc.), external stressors (exposure to stressful conditions), social isolation, chronic life stress, etc. can significantly contribute to pathogenesis and expression of CVD.[14] Moreover, there is enough evidence that the link between CVD and diabetes is not fully accounted for by conventional risk factors and lifestyle risk factors. To understand the link between CVD and diabetes, it is necessary to look at the underlying biological und psychological pathways. Until today, research has identified several aspects of psychosocial stress, which might explain their relationship.

MECHANISMS LINKING PSYCHOSOCIAL STRESS WITH CARDIOVASCULAR DISEASE AND DIABETES

There is accumulating evidence that psychosocial stress plays a role in the pathogenesis of CVD.[15-17] Numerous systematic reviews and prospective analyses[18,19] are in agreement that chronic stressors and psychosocial factors predict future coronary heart disease in initially healthy populations independently of standard risk factors. Considering the strong links between CVD and diabetes, it is not surprising that there has been interest in investigating whether psychosocial stress plays a role in diabetes and whether this is related to CVD risk in this population. The following sections review evidence from prospective studies that have examined the links between different psychosocial stress factors and diabetes.

Psychosocial stress potentially affects diabetes and cardiovascular risk in several ways—(1) influencing behavioral/lifestyle risk factors for diabetes such as poor diet, physical inactivity, smoking, and excessive alcohol consumption; (2) affecting the development of diabetes directly through mechanisms such as glucose dysregulation and immune dysfunction (inflammation), central obesity, hypertension, dyslipidemia; and (3) shaping the processes through which diabetes stimulates cardiovascular complications (Flow chart 1).

Flow chart 1: Pathways linking psychosocial stress with diabetes and cardiovascular disease (CVD)

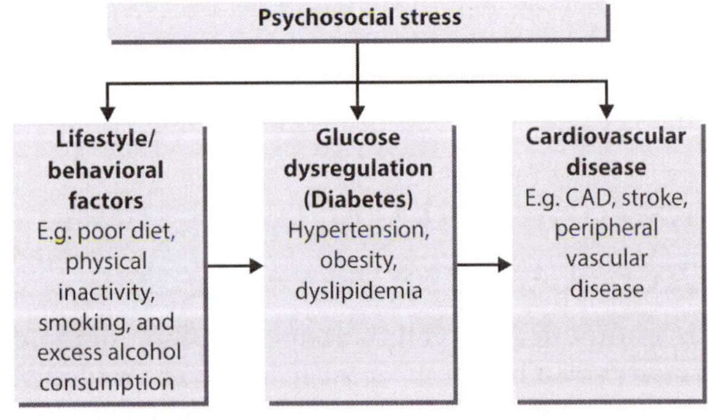

Abbreviation: CAD, coronary artery disease

These distinctions are important both in etiological understanding and because of their implications for disease management.

- Psychobiological mechanisms, including changes in the autonomic nervous, the hormonal, and the immune systems
- Behavioral mechanisms such as treatment adherence and health-related lifestyles, e.g. diet exercise, smoking, alcohol consumption, etc.

Psychobiological Mechanisms

Psychological diseases have their origin in mind and cognition, but they may affect many other systems of the human body. Dependent on their specific pathophysiology conditions of psychosocial stress for instance can provoke disturbances of the autonomic, hormonal, immune system balance, or elicit functional over-reactions of organs (Flow chart 2).

Autonomic Function

Numerous studies provide evidence that myocardial ischemia is associated with certain disorders of cardiac autonomic nervous system (ANS) function, in particular, with an autonomic neurocardiac imbalance characterized by increased sympathetic and decreased parasympathetic activity. Associated with this reaction are:

- A decreased heart rate variability (amount of fluctuation of the heartbeat-to-heartbeat differences), which increases risk of ventricular arrhythmias and sudden cardiac death from ventricular fibrillation[20,21]
- A low-frequency (LF) power of blood pressure variability that has been suggested to reflect changes of central sympathetic nervous system control. It has been shown that increased daytime systolic blood pressure variability is associated with increased risk of sudden cardiac death[22]
- Low baroreflex sensitivity that leads to high-blood pressure and predicts increased cardiovascular mortality.[23]

Hormone System

Psychosocial stress, depression, and anxiety could cause a hyperactivation of certain stress-related parts of the hormonal system (in particular the hypothalamic-pituitary-

Flow chart 2: Psychobiological and behavioral mechanisms linking psychosocial stress with cardiodiabetes

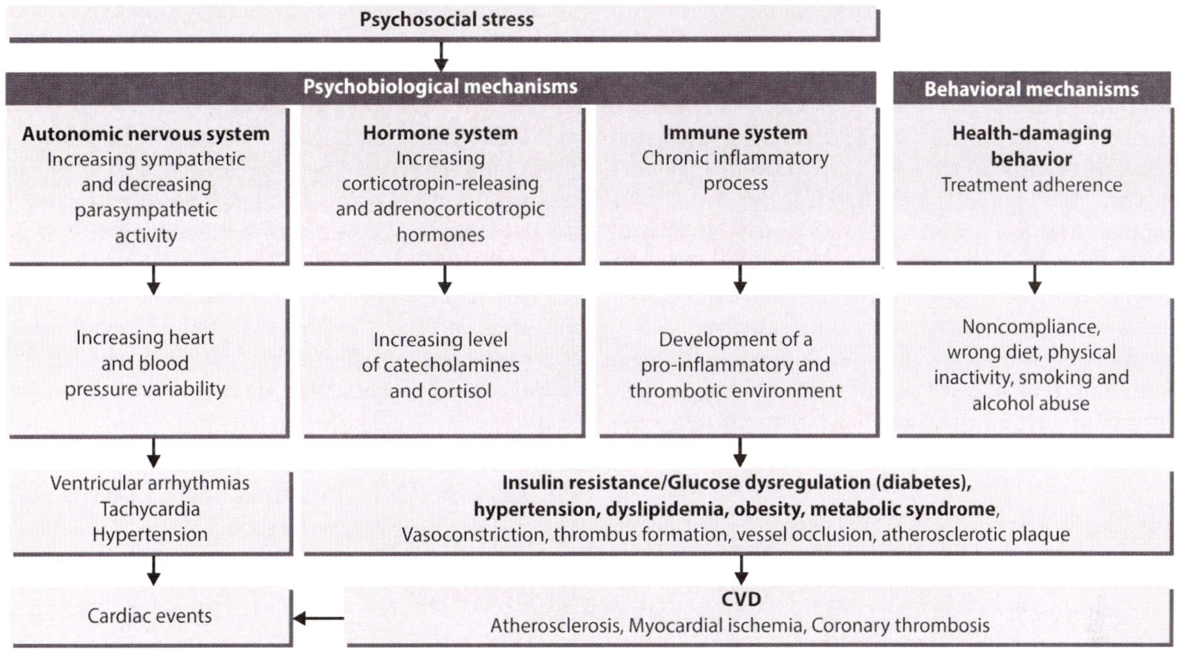

adrenocortical axis). Some of the involved stress hormones like *cortisol* and *catecholamines* can cause an elevation of blood pressure and a faster heart rate. Blood flow is decreased, which may then increase the risk of an acute angina attack. Corticosteroids mobilize glycogen from liver, free fatty acids, causing endothelial inflammation and excessive clotting, and are associated with insulin resistance/glucose dysregulation—a prestage of diabetes, hypertension, and hypercholesterolemia. Increased circulating lipids and endothelial shearing stress can lead to vascular damage and plaque formation. Increased level of catecholamines is also altering blood clotting and may lead to vessel occlusion. Moreover, increased insulin and cholesterol levels lead to increased risk of CVD in prediabetic and diabetic patients.

Immune System (Inflammation)

Psychosocial stress-induced immune dysfunction (inflammation) may mediate the relation between diabetes and CVD. It is known that the immune system has a central role in all stages of diabetes and atherosclerosis. Endothelial dysfunction caused by endothelial inflammation results in a breakdown in the anti-inflammatory and antithrombotic properties of the endothelium and could be one major step in the initiation of atherosclerosis. Consequent development of a proinflammatory and prothrombotic environment leads to increased recruitment of leukocytes, lipids, smooth muscle cells, fibroblasts, and platelets to the arterial wall. Repeated cycles of this process result in hyperplasia of the intima-medial layer of the vessel wall and the development of an atherosclerotic plaque. Particularly, C-reactive protein has emerged as a significant predictor of increased risk of atherosclerosis. Major depression also has been associated with elevated C-reactive protein levels. Thus, adverse cardiac outcomes in diabetics with depression could be linked through pathways with C-reactive protein or other markers.

Behavioral Mechanisms

The precise mechanisms linking psychosocial factors and diabetes remain to be elucidated. However, several potentially inter-related pathways that plausibly account for the link have been proposed. As noted in Flow chart 1, one possibility is that the adverse relationship between psychosocial factors and diabetes may be mediated via behavioral/lifestyle risk factors. Behavioral mechanisms include poor diet, physical inactivity, smoking, and excess alcohol consumption. Reduced adherence to self-care behaviors and cardioprotective medications such as blood pressure and lipid-lowering drugs could also play a role.

Several lines of research support this mechanism. Comorbid depression in diabetes increases nonadherence to a range of behaviors including diet, medication usage, and exercise.[24,25] For example, a study of 2,759 individuals with diabetes found that participants with persistent or increasing depression symptoms had significantly poorer adherence to dietary and exercise regimens than their counterparts without depression over a 5-year follow-up period.[25] A cross-sectional study with a similar sample size of 2,646 individuals with diabetes reported that physical inactivity doubled in the presence of depressive symptoms.[26] Considerably, less research has investigated the behavioral pathways linking other psychosocial factors and diabetes. The Copenhagen City Heart Study of 7,066 adults found that perceived stress was associated with physical inactivity and unsuccessful smoking cessation or alcohol reduction attempts over a 10-year follow-up as well as the development of overt diabetes among men.[27]

Negative psychosocial factors that are common in diabetes may also decrease motivation for healthy lifestyle choices that in turn affect CVD risk. However, the association between diabetes and CVD is not fully explained by behavioral risk factors,[28,29] and results from randomized controlled trials (RCTs) suggest that the modification of behavioral risk factors does not significantly lower CVD outcomes in people with diabetes, despite the fact that lifestyle change has a marked effect on diabetes incidence.[30] This offers the possibility that a direct psychobiological pathway could link psychosocial factors with CVD risk in people with diabetes.

Several different psychobiological mechanisms could link psychosocial stress with both CVD and diabetes. Depression, anxiety, and diabetes-related distress are associated with suboptimal glycemic control,[31-35] and there is evidence that the risk of CVD increases in line with the degree of hyperglycemia.[28,36] Long-term exposure to psychosocial stress factors can result in chronic allostatic load, which involves dysregulation of multiple biological systems including neuroendocrine, cardiovascular, metabolic, and inflammatory pathways.[37] Cross-sectional evidence suggests that people with diabetes demonstrate characteristics of high-allostatic load in response to a stressful experience.[38] Evidence from the same sample suggests that hostility (a psychosocial stress factor) can further exaggerate the disturbances in stress-related processes in people with diabetes.[39]

Many of the different pathways involved in stress-related allostatic load have been linked with both diabetes and CVD. Dysregulation of the stress hormone cortisol is associated with both acute and chronic stress factors,[40] and prospective evidence has linked changes in daily cortisol secretion with CVD mortality,[41] as well as new onset diabetes.[42] Another potential biological mechanism linking psychosocial factors to both CVD and diabetes is inflammation. Elevated inflammatory cytokine concentrations are observed in people reporting high levels of psychosocial stress.[43] Both diabetes[44] and CVD have been characterized as inflammatory conditions.[45] In initially healthy populations, heightened inflammatory cytokines levels have been associated with new onset CVD,[46] and it is plausible that raised cytokine levels could increase the risk of CVD in diabetes populations, too.

The complexity of the link between psychosocial factors and CVD risk in people with diabetes is reflected in the numerous pathways that may be involved. It is likely that the proposed behavioral and biological pathways do not act in isolation but rather that they are inter-related. For example, depression in diabetes might affect complications through poorer adherence to diet and exercise regimes. Future research in this area may benefit from investigating the synergies between behavioral and biological pathways in linking psychosocial factors to CVD risk in people with diabetes.

ROLE OF PSYCHOSOCIAL STRESSORS IN CARDIODIABETES

Depression

Depression is common in people with diabetes.[47-50] A meta-analysis of 10 studies with 51,331 individuals estimated the prevalence of depression to be almost doubled in people with diabetes compared to those without the condition [17.6 vs. 9.8%; odds ratio (OR) = 1.6; 95% confidence interval (CI) 1.2–2.0).[49] The vast majority of the studies have been conducted in Western countries, but a study of 213,797 people in 47 countries from around the world has shown that people with diabetes had a twofold greater prevalence of depressive symptoms than those without diabetes (OR 2.36; 95% CI 1.91–2.92).[47]

An increasing body of literature indicates that depression exacerbates the risk of macrovascular complications in people with diabetes. Prospective studies have found a relationship between comorbid depression and CVD in diabetes samples.[51,52] For instance, in the Pathways Epidemiological Follow-up Study of over 4,000 participants with diabetes, individuals with depression had a 24% increased risk of adverse macrovascular complications including myocardial infarction (MI), stroke, cardiovascular procedures, and cardiac death over 5 years of follow-up.[52] This association was independent of prior complications, sociodemographic characteristics, health behaviors, and diabetes self-care variables. Another study followed a cohort of 345,949 individuals who were free of CVD at baseline over a 7-year period. Results showed that participants with diabetes alone and those with major depression alone had a 30% increased risk of MI, whereas those with a double diagnosis (both diabetes and major depression) had an 82% excess risk of subsequent MI compared to participants without either condition.[53]

Another study published in 2016 examined the association between depressive symptoms or perceived stress at baseline and risk of CVD in 22,003 US adults.[54] Over almost 6 years of follow-up, people with diabetes who reported elevated depressive symptoms or perceived stress had a significantly increased incidence of stroke (HR 1.57; 95% CI 1.05–2.33) and acute CVD (HR 1.57; 95% CI 1.02–2.40). These associations were independent of demographics factors, but were attenuated when controlling for lifestyle factors. The majority of studies have focused on white samples in Western countries. To address this issue, Ting et al.[55] conducted a 7.4-year follow-up study in a sample of 7,835 Chinese patients with diabetes who were free of CVD at baseline. In this sample, diagnosed depression predicted CVD (HR = 2.18) and the majority of the risk appeared to be driven by stroke (HR = 3.55). The reported associations remained significant after adjustment for a wide range of conventional CVD risk factors. As might be expected from these findings, people with both depression and diabetes have greater CVD mortality as well as morbidity rates. An analysis of 16 prospective studies indicated that comorbid depression in diabetes is associated with a 39% increased risk of cardiovascular death and a 46% higher risk of all-cause mortality.[33]

Anxiety

In comparison with the research on comorbid depression, there is relatively little research on other psychosocial factors and their relationship to CVD risk in people with diabetes. However, there is some evidence that the prevalence of other psychosocial disorders is elevated in people with diabetes in comparison with the general population. Overviews of this research suggest that diabetes is associated with 20% increased odds of having an anxiety disorder and 48% increased odds of having elevated anxiety symptoms.[56] Comorbid anxiety is of clinical relevance to people with diabetes. An association between anxiety and glycemic control has also been reported in a number of studies,[33] but to our knowledge, only one study to date has investigated the prospective relationship between anxiety and diabetes complications such as retinopathy, neuropathy, or CVD, and no associations were found.[57] However, the number of cases of diabetes and anxiety was limited in this study, so it may have been unpowered to detect such effects.

Personality Traits

Personality factors are not well researched in relation to diabetes. Hostility is a trait that is typically conceptualized as a negative cynical attitude toward others, with a propensity for anger or aggression.[58] This trait has been associated prospectively with raised fasting glucose[59] and cross-sectionally with insulin resistance,[60,61] glycated hemoglobin (HbA1c),[61,62] and prevalent diabetes.[63] Additionally, angry temperament has been investigated in relation to diabetes development. In a cohort study of 11,615 individuals who were disease-free at baseline, individuals with an angry temperament had a 1.34 increased hazard of incident diabetes over the 6-year follow-up period.[64] This association has also been investigated in the Multi-Ethnic Study of Atherosclerosis (MESA) cohort[65] with a smaller sample size of 5,598 participants but a longer follow-up of 11.4 years. Participants reporting high levels of trait anger at baseline had a 48% greater risk of developing diabetes than those with low anger (HR 1.48; 95% CI 1.04–2.12) independent of demographic factors, exercise, diet, alcohol use, and smoking. However, the association was attenuated following adjustment for waist circumference.

So, although there have not been many studies investigating anger and hostility, the current evidence suggests that these characteristics may also be associated with an increased risk of diabetes in later life.

Psychological Distress and Diabetes-specific Distress

Psychological distress has been linked with CVD morbidity and increased mortality rates in people with diabetes. In a study of 1,533 individuals with diagnosed diabetes, distressed participants were found to have a 1.69 increased hazard of a CVD event and a 1.76-fold greater mortality rate compared to individuals without psychological distress over an average follow-up of 5.4 years.[66] This association was independent of CVD risk factors, and excluding participants who were receiving antidepressive treatment did not affect the results. It would be interesting in future studies to tease out what particular aspects of psychological distress are most strongly linked to CVD.

As well as depression, anxiety, and general psychological distress, diabetes-related emotional distress, a stress condition specifically resulting from concerns and worries about diabetes and its management, is common in people with diabetes.[67] According to estimates from a study of 8,596 adults with diabetes from 17 countries, 44.6% of patients suffer from significant diabetes-related distress.[68] Diabetes-related distress is of clinical significance, since several longitudinal studies suggest that it is associated with poor glycemic control independently of depression.[67,69,34] No studies to date have investigated the association between diabetes-distress and CVD.

POTENTIALLY PROTECTIVE PSYCHOSOCIAL FACTORS

The vast majority of work has investigated relationships between negative psychosocial stress factors and future diabetes. To our knowledge, only two studies have investigated associations with potentially protective positive factors. Crump et al. studied the relationship between resilience to stress in adolescence and diabetes in later life.[70] The study used an impressive sample of over 1.5 million Swedish military conscripts who were assessed for stress resilience during a semistructured interview at 18 years. The participants were followed up for an average of 25.7 years using national medical records. Participants with the lowest stress resilience had a 51% increased hazard of future diabetes compared to those with high levels of resilience (HR 1.51; 95% CI 1.46–1.57) independent of a range of diabetes risk factors. These findings suggest that personal resilience to stress might be an important factor in the development of diabetes. The other study looked at life satisfaction, emotional vitality, and optimism in 7,800 individuals from the Whitehall II cohort.[71] Over 13 years of follow-up, these well-being factors were not associated with incident diabetes as assessed by self-reported and glucose tolerance testing. The authors performed subanalyses to assess whether associations varied by type of diabetes diagnosis. Individuals with high life satisfaction (OR = 0.85; 95% CI = 0.76–0.95) and emotional vitality (OR = 0.86; 95% CI = 0.77–0.97) were less likely to report doctor-diagnosed diabetes. It is uncertain why associations differed for doctor-diagnosed and screen-detected diabetes.

ROLE OF SPIRITUALITY IN PSYCHOSOCIAL STRESS AND CARDIODIABETES

Spirituality is the sense of connection with life and other living beings. According to Banks,[72] spirituality acts as a unifying force that integrates the individual's physical, cognitive, emotional, and social experiences to create a sense of meaning and purpose in life. This creates a common bond amongst people, arising from awareness that each person has more in common with others than a directed focus on their uniqueness would suggest. Spirituality also reflects a faith in a higher power/Supreme being that cannot be visualized or easily described but may be felt.[72] The feeling of social connectedness and purpose that comes from a relationship with a Supreme being or God is a potent component of what we refer to as "spirituality" (as distinguished from religiosity, which we will use to refer to more objective measures such as church service attendance).[73] The conceptualization of spirituality as a relationship between an individual and God links this work with an extensive scientific literature on the effects of interpersonal connections on physiology, health, and well-being. Over a century ago, William James pointed to the need for psychophysical theory concerning the potential relation between spiritual values and "determinate sorts of physiological change". Some potential mediators of relations between spirituality and cardiovascular health, such as smoking, diet, or other health-related behaviors,[74] are transparent and may not require theoretical explication. Others, however, may benefit from a more theoretical grounding and conceptual modeling of the relevant physiological dimensions that underlie health relationships. This is the case for possible ANS mediators of potential relations between spirituality and cardiodiabetes and health. Certain spiritual or meditation practices have been reported to be associated with increased parasympathetic and decreased sympathetic cardiac control. Such a pattern of autonomic control could be a potential mediator of spirituality and health outcomes. High-sympathetic cardiac control, for example, is a known risk factor for uncontrolled diabetes and MI and for survival thereafter, and a hypersympathetic state appears to underlie human stress cardiomyopathy. Indeed, drugs that block sympathetic actions (primarily beta-adrenergic blockers) are a common treatment strategy after MI. In contrast, the parasympathetic system exerts antifibrillary actions, and low-parasympathetic activity is a predictor of negative outcomes after MI.[75]

The autonomic balance model continues to be represented in the contemporary literature, both as an individual difference characteristic and as a predictor of health outcomes. A current example is the proposed autonomic balance metric derived from measures of heart rate variability.[76] Specifically, high-frequency (HF) heart rate variability, in the respiratory frequency band, provides a relatively pure index of parasympathetic cardiac control, whereas LF variability reflects a combination of sympathetic and parasympathetic influences. Based on this and other empirical findings, Malliani et al. suggest that a ratio of LF to HF variability indexes the relative autonomic balance, along a continuum from sympathetic to parasympathetic predominance.

Low overall heart rate variability is not linked just with cardiovascular disorders and diabetes, but has been reported to be a risk factor for all-cause mortality and morbidity. Moreover, reduced "autonomic flexibility", reflected by low heart rate variability, has been reported under conditions as anxiety and dyspepsia.[77] These findings raise an additional or an alternative possibility to the sympathovagal balance model. A relevant health determinant may be the overall regulatory capacity, which supports flexible adjustments in the face of adaptive challenges.

THERAPEUTIC IMPLICATIONS

A confluence of pathophysiological and epidemiological studies establishes that both acute and chronic forms of psychosocial stress contribute to the pathogenesis of CVD and diabetes. These data establish an imperative role for enhancing behavioral interventions among diabetics with CVD at primary, secondary, tertiary level of prevention. Lifestyle interventions to prevent diabetes have been successful.[78-81] However, interventions to modify behavioral risk factors to prevent CVD in people with diabetes have been largely disappointing. This poses the question whether modifying psychosocial stress, another risk factor for CVD, would have a therapeutic impact. To date, the majority of research in this area has investigated whether the treatment of depression in diabetes is beneficial. A Cochrane review in 2012 included 19 RCTs investigating both psychological and pharmacological interventions for depression in patients with diabetes.[82] Psychological intervention studies showed a beneficial effect on short-, medium-, and long-term depression severity and had a good impact on depression remission compared to usual care.

However, the effect of psychological intervention on glycemic control was mixed and inconclusive. With regards to the pharmacological interventions, there was a moderate effect of antidepressant medication on short-term depression severity and depression remission, and interestingly, the pharmacological trials significantly improved glycemic control in the short-term as well. But no study to date has assessed the relationship between depression treatment and glycemic control in the longer term. Taking the evidence together, it appears that depression treatment is moderately effective in diabetes, but only pharmacological trials have shown a consistent improvement in glycemic control. Mindfulness-based interventions for modifying psychosocial stress factors have also been tested in people with diabetes.[83] They have been found in several studies to have psychological benefits, lowering depression, anxiety stress, and diabetes-distress symptoms in people with diabetes. However, the evidence for the effectiveness of these interventions on glycemic control is mixed. Out of the seven studies that assessed HbA1c as a marker of glycemic control, four interventions lowered HbA1c levels, but the three largest studies reported no change in HbA1c.[83] Mindfulness-based intervention in diabetes is a new field, and much of the research is exploratory. It may be that the short follow-up periods of many studies were not sufficient to observe significant changes in HbA1c.

In sum, there is little evidence as yet that the treatment of psychosocial factors in diabetes has a benefit on CVD outcomes. However, pharmacological interventions have been shown to improve glycemic outcomes in the short-term and hyperglycemia is linearly associated with increased CVD risk.[28,36] Additionally, both psychological and pharmacological treatments as well as mindfulness-based interventions appear to have beneficial effects on psychosocial factors in people with diabetes. Despite the limited effectiveness of these treatments on overt CVD outcomes, there have been calls that the psychological well-being in people with diabetes should be a priority for its own sake.[84] Since lifestyle interventions have been shown to be effective for preventing diabetes, perhaps targeting individuals before onset rather than after diagnosis might be the optimal strategy. Traditionally, cardiologists and diabetologists have played parallel roles in managing cardiovascular risks in their patients. There is no single model for the provision of care services to patients who fit the cardiodiabetes description and no real consensus on whether the care of such patients needs the creation of a cardiodiabetes specialists or specialist teams. Rather than developing a new specialty, more could be done to encourage experience sharing between specialists and to support primary care physician with a special interest in diabetes and CVD.

OUR EXPERIENCE

Evaluation of Brahmakumaris Rajyoga Meditation-based Lifestyle Intervention on Psychosocial Stressors in Diabetic and Nondiabetic angiographically documented Coronary Artery Disease (CAD) Patients.

Efficacy of unique user friendly *Brahmakumaris Rajyoga Meditation (BKRM)-based lifestyle intervention* [Three-dimensional (3D) Healthcare Model] was evaluated in two Multidisciplinary, Prospective, Open, and Randomized Controlled Studies, Mount Abu Open Heart Trial and Abu Healthy Heart Trial in 518 coronary artery disease (CAD) patients and was planned in 1995. The subjects were angiographically documented CAD patients who were also suffering from various other lifestyle-related disorders. Psychologists, physiologists, endocrinologists, cardiologists, clinicians, dietitians, fitness experts, and spiritualists worked hand-in-hand for more than 16 years. We, at J Watumull Global Hospital and Research Centre, Prajapita Brahma Kumari Ishwariya Vishwa Vidyalaya, Abu, collaborated with Defense Institute of Physiology and Allied sciences, New Delhi. This project was sponsored by Central Council for Research in Yoga and Naturopathy (CCRYN),

Ministry of Health and Family welfare, Government of India, New Delhi and Defense Research and Development Organization (DRDO), New Delhi.

Brahmakumaris Rajyoga Meditation-based Lifestyle Intervention

Three-dimensional Healthcare Model

The 3D Healthcare Model has evolved from the author's 37 years of clinical experience and 31 years of spiritual experience with BKRM. This included extensive literature reviews and intense research into the psychophysiology, psychoneuroendocrinology, and etiopathogenesis of various diseases. This model has been evaluated in more than 8,000 angiographically documented heart patients, from India and abroad. They were also suffering from other lifestyle-related illnesses, e.g. hypertension, obesity, diabetes, bronchial asthma, chronic obstructive pulmonary disease (COPD), cancer, generalized osteoporosis, autoimmune diseases, and mental health disorders. The present form of the 3D Healthcare Model represents a synthesis of psychological, physiological, endocrinological, clinical, and spiritual experiments with thousands of patients over 16 years.[85,86]

Brahmakumaris Rajyoga Meditation-based lifestyle intervention (3D healthcare) has the following principles to be sustained as far as possible in daily living:[85]

- *Self-responsibility through self-empowerment*: The word "healthy" is derived from two words; "heal" + "thy", i.e. to heal yourself. To heal oneself, one needs to be empowered by appropriate information about the mind-body connection, psychological and conventional risk factors, stress-management, diet, exercise, sleep, substance abuse, and usual medical care.
- *Self-awareness*: The Hindi word for healthy is "swasth", which consists of swa-, meaning "inner self", and -asth, meaning "conscious". The word "healthy" could also mean "inner self-conscious". Outer self-consciousness of the mortal body, or ever-changing role and material things, leads to instability and insecurity, which in turn leads to anger, anxiety, depression, type A behavior, isolation, and chronic life stresses. Conversely, inner self-consciousness of enduring and immortal spirit leads to stability and security, which in turn leads to peace, love, and happiness. A healthy lifestyle is an "inner self-conscious lifestyle".
- *Multidimensionality*: The current medical approach addresses only one dimension and the physical body. A new model of health, "3D healthcare" (soul-mind-body medicine) is called for. As per this new model, health is a dynamic process of harmony in flow of spiritual energy—knowledge of truth, purity, peace, love, happiness, and bliss:
  - *Power*—of discrimination, to judge, to withdraw, to pack up, to tolerate, to face, to accommodate, and to cooperate.
  - *Mental energy*—is positive thoughts, emotions, attitudes, and memories (TEAM), and *physical energy*—healthy diet, exercise, sleep, cessation of smoking and alcohol, proper adherence to prescribed treatment regimen, and medication.
- *Biological clock and circadian rhythm*: When activities are in rhythm with one's biological clock, energy expense, and stress are reduced, beneficial for the health of mind, intellect, and body.

During the study, largest data set of its kind was collected on various parameters of the human body [psychological, physiological {electroencephalography (EEG), heart rate variability}, hormonal, glycemic control, serum lipid profile, 2D-Echo (color Doppler) repeat coronary angiography, etc.]

Results from the present study suggest that CAD patients can be motivated to adopt BKRM-based lifestyle intervention (3D healthcare) for a fairly long period of 8 years of follow-up, while performing their routine activities outside the hospital framework. This program was found to be user-friendly, safe, flexible, and compatible with other treatments in the setting of advanced CAD, with a high degree of compliance. The primary endpoint of this study was change in percent diameter stenosis. In patients with most adherence, the average percent diameter stenosis decreased by 18.23 absolute percentage points (29.03% relative improvement), and in patients with medium adherence, it decreased by 11.85 absolute percentage points (19.10% relative improvement), but it progressed in patients with least adherence. Cardiac events were also markedly decreased in patients with most adherence compared to patients with least adherence. However, more than 50% adherence to the prescribed 3D Healthcare Model is essential to achieve significant regression in percent diameter stenosis and in the number of cardiac events. BKRM-based lifestyle intervention (3D healthcare) could modify psychosocial factors by significantly reducing anxiety, depression, anger, and type A behavior scores, improvement in healthy lifestyle and overall sense of well-being. The modification of psychosocial factors was reflected in better adherence to healthy lifestyle behavior like cessation of smoking, adherence to prescribed diet, and exercise schedules. Favorable highly significant changes were observed in New York Heart Association (NYHA) function class, angina severity and frequency, drug score, and exercise tolerance by day 7, which were further favorably modified at different stages of follow-up.

The long-term reduction in NYHA functional class, nitrate requirement, and increased exercise tolerance is at par with what is achieved following coronary angioplasty or bypass surgery.[86] The improvement in various metabolic parameters in these patients may be due to the low-cholesterol, high-fiber vegetarian diet, physical exercise, or BKRM independently, or due to the synergistic effect of all three.

The cardioprotective effects of BKRM may be mediated through an interaction between the ANS and the endocrine system.[87-89] In fact, in these CAD patients, the administration of BKRM-based lifestyle intervention (3D healthcare) also enhanced alpha activity of EEG and caused shift of autonomic balance toward relative parasympathetic predominance besides causing a marked reduction in secretion of stress hormones like epinephrine, norepinephrine, and cortisol.[89,90] BKRM is also a training in awareness, which produces definite changes in perception, attention, and cognition. During BKRM, the practitioner remains awake and vigilant but the body enters a state of deep-muscle relaxation. It also helps in building strong willpower for compliance to BKRM-based lifestyle intervention (3D healthcare); as it teaches a holistic lifestyle modification, the benefits of which the participants begin to experience, within 7 days of the intervention. Since Rajyoga Meditation also enhances inner strength to lead a stress-free and healthy life, it might have caused marked reduction in psychological stressors and favorably modified unhealthy behavioral patterns, which in turn may be responsible for regression in coronary atherosclerosis and reduction in coronary events. Reductions in coronary atherosclerosis and cardiac events were strongly reflected in program adherence in a "dose–response manner".

The results of univariate analysis in these patients indicate that the angiographic changes were attributable to the decrease in weight, triglycerides, diet, exercise schedule, and management of psychosocial stressors through Rajyoga Meditation. The multivariate analysis showed that the change in weight and lipid parameters is not independent predictors of CAD regression, but the management of psychosocial stressors through Rajyoga Meditation was an independent predictor of CAD regression. The Rajyoga Meditation also motivated CAD patients to adhere more to the diet, exercise, treatment schedules, and smoking cessation.

CONCLUSION

The current literature has amply shown that psychological stress factors play a role in the pathogenesis of diabetes. Various negative psychosocial factors have been shown to increase the risk of diabetes in initially healthy populations. There is less research on the involvement of psychosocial factors in CVD risk in people with existing diabetes. To date, most of the research in this area has been on depression, with evidence that a double diagnosis of diabetes and depression increases the risk of CVD in this population. Most of the studies are observational, so causal conclusions are difficult to draw. Therapeutic and lifestyle interventions have been shown to have a beneficial effect on psychosocial factors in people with diabetes, but the evidence for effects on glycemic control is mixed, and research on interventions affecting CVD outcomes in people with diabetes is lacking. Despite the limited evidence for effects on physiological outcomes, it can be argued that improving the psychological well-being of people with diabetes should be a priority in its own right for better outcome. The psychobiological and behavioral mechanisms contribute to the etiopathogenesis of insulin resistance, prediabetes, diabetes, hypertension, dyslipidemia, obesity, and CVD (CAD, stroke, and peripheral vascular disease). Hence, optimization of medication with spirituality/meditation-based lifestyle intervention can go a long way in managing the menace of epidemic of cardiodiabetes. The mechanisms through which psychosocial stress factors increase diabetes risk and affect outcomes in people with existing diabetes are yet to be fully understood. It is likely that both behavioral and biological pathways are involved.

REFERENCES

1. Robertson D. Cardiodiabetes—is a joint approach the way forward? Br J Cardiol. 2008;15:S8-10.
2. International Diabetes Federation. IDF Diabetes Atlas, 7th edition. Brussels: International Diabetes Federation; 2015.
3. World Health Organization. Global Report on Diabetes. Geneva: World Health Organization; 2016.
4. Centers for Disease Control and Prevention. National diabetes statistics report: estimates of diabetes and its burden in the United States, 2014. Atlanta: Department of Health and Human Services; 2014.
5. Holman N, Young B, Gadsby R. Current prevalence of type 1 and type 2 diabetes in adults and children in the UK. Diabet Med. 2015;32:1119-20.
6. WHO. Global status report on non-communicable disease 2010. Geneva: World Health Organization; 2011.
7. International Diabetes Federation. In: Unwin N, Whiting D, Guariguata L, Ghyoot G, Gan D (Eds). Diabetes Atlas, 5th edition. Brussels, Belgium: International Diabetes Federation; 2011. pp. 11-74.
8. Mohan D, Raj D, Shanthirani CS, et al. Awareness and knowledge of diabetes in Chennai—The Chennai Urban Rural Epidemiology Study [CURES-9]. J Assoc Physicians India. 2005;53:283-7.
9. Harris MI, Eastman RC. Early detection of undiagnosed diabetes mellitus: A US perspective. Diabetes Metab Res Rev. 2000;16:230-6.
10. Seuring T, Archangelidi O, Suhrcke M. The economic costs of type 2 diabetes: a global systematic review. Pharmaco Economics. 2015;33:811-31.
11. Ryden L, Standl E, Bartnik M, et al. Guidelines on diabetes, pre-diabetes, and cardiovascular diseases: executive summary. The Task

Force on Diabetes and Cardiovascular Diseases of the European Society of Cardiology (ESC) and of the European Association for the Study of Diabetes (EASD). Eur Heart J. 2007;28:88-136.
12. National Institute for Health and Clinical Excellence. Clinical Guideline 67. Lipid Modification. Cardiovascular risk assessment and the modification of blood lipids for the primary and secondary prevention of cardiovascular disease. May 2008.
13. National Institute for Health and Clinical Excellence. Clinical Guideline 66. Type 2 diabetes. May 2008.
14. Hackett RA, Steptoe A. Psychosocial Factors in Diabetes and Cardiovascular Risks. Curr Cardiol Rep. 2016;18:95.
15. Dimsdale JE. Psychological stress and cardiovascular disease. J Am Coll Cardiol. 2008;51:1237-46.
16. Hjemdahl P, Rosengren A, Steptoe A. Stress and cardiovascular. New York: Springer; 2012.
17. Steptoe A, Kivimäki M. Stress and cardiovascular disease: an update on current knowledge. Annu Rev Public Health. 2013;34:337-54.
18. Everson-Rose SA, Lewis TT. Psychosocial factors and cardiovascular diseases. Annu Rev Public Health. 2005;26:469-500.
19. Kuper H, Marmot M, Hemingway H. Systematic review of prospective cohort studies of psychosocial factors in the etiology and prognosis of coronary heart disease. Semin Vasc Med. 2002;2:267-314.
20. Kibler JL, Ma M. Depressive symptoms and cardiovascular reactivity to laboratory behavioral stress. Int J Behav Med. 2004;11:81-7.
21. Gorman JM, Sloan RP. Heart rate variability in depressive and anxiety disorders. Am Heart J. 2000;140:77-83.
22. Kikuya M, Hozawa A, Ohokubo T, et al. Prognostic significance of blood pressure and heart rate variabilities. Hypertension. 2000;36:901-6.
23. La Rovere MT, Bigger JT, Marcus FI, et al. Baroreflex sensitivity and heart-rate variability in prediction of total cardiac mortality after myocardial infarction. ATRAMI (Autonomic Tone and Reflexes after Myocardial Infarction) Investigators. The Lancet. 1998;351:478-84.
24. Gonzalez JS, Peyrot M, McCarl LA, et al. Depression and diabetes treatment nonadherence: a meta-analysis. Diabetes Care. 2008;31:2398-403.
25. Katon WJ, Russo JE, Heckbert SR, et al. The relationship between changes in depression symptoms and changes in health risk behaviors in patients with diabetes. Int J Geriatr Psychiatry. 2010;25:466-75.
26. Koopmans B, Pouwer F, de Bie RA, et al. Depressive symptoms are associated with physical inactivity in patients with type 2 diabetes. The DIAZOB Primary Care Diabetes study. Fam Pract. 2009;26:171-3.
27. Rod NH, Grønbæk M, Schnohr P, et al. Perceived stress as a risk factor for changes in health behaviour and cardiac risk profile: a longitudinal study. J Intern Med. 2009;266:467-75.
28. Emerging Risk Factors Collaboration, Sarwar N, Gao P, et al. Diabetes mellitus, fasting blood glucose concentration, and risk of vascular disease: a collaborative meta-analysis of 102 prospective studies. Lancet. 2010;375:2215-22.
29. Emerging Risk Factors Collaboration. Diabetes mellitus, fasting glucose, and risk of cause-specific death. N Engl J Med. 2011;364: 829-41.
30. Fox CS, Golden SH, Anderson C, et al. Update on prevention of cardiovascular disease in adults with type 2 diabetes mellitus in light of recent evidence: a scientific statement from the American Heart Association and the American Diabetes Association. Diabetes Care. 2015;38:1777-803.
31. Rush WA, Whitebird RR, Rush MR, et al. Depression in patients with diabetes: does it impact clinical goals? J Am Board Fam Med. 2008;21:392-7.
32. Lustman PJ, Anderson RJ, Freedland KE, et al. Depression and poor glycemic control: a metaanalytic review of the literature. Diabetes Care. 2000;23:934-42.
33. Anderson RJ, Grigsby AB, Freedland KE, et al. Anxiety and poor glycemic control: a metaanalytic review of the literature. Int J Psychiatry Med. 2002;32:235-47.
34. Fisher L, Mullan JT, Arean P, et al. Diabetes distress but not clinical depression or depressive symptoms is associated with glycemic control in both cross-sectional and longitudinal analyses. Diabetes Care. 2010;33:23-8.
35. Collins MM, Corcoran P, Perry IJ. Anxiety and depression symptoms in patients with diabetes. Diabet Med. 2009;26:153-61.
36. Goff DC, Gerstein HC, Ginsberg HN, et al. Prevention of cardiovascular disease in persons with type 2 diabetes mellitus: current knowledge and rationale for the Action to Control Cardiovascular Risk in Diabetes (ACCORD) trial. Am J Cardiol. 2007;99:4i-20i.
37. McEwen BS. Protective and damaging effects of stress mediators. N Engl J Med. 1998;338:171-9.
38. Steptoe A, Hackett RA, Lazzarino AI, et al. Disruption of multisystem responses to stress in type 2 diabetes: investigating the dynamics of allostatic load. Proc Natl Acad Sci U S A. 2014;111:15693-8.
39. Hackett RA, Lazzarino AI, Carvalho LA, et al. Hostility and physiological responses to acute stress in people with type 2 diabetes. Psychosom Med. 2015;77:458-66.
40. Adam EK, Hawkley LC, Kudielka BM, et al. Day-to-day dynamics of experience—cortisol associations in a population based sample of older adults. Proc Natl Acad Sci U S A. 2006;103:17058-63. Curr Cardiol Rep. 2016;18:95.
41. Kumari M, Shipley M, Stafford M, et al. Association of diurnal patterns in salivary cortisol with all-cause and cardiovascular mortality: findings from the Whitehall II study. J Clin Endocrinol Metab. 2011;96:1478-85.
42. Hackett RA, Kivimäki M, Kumari M, et al. Diurnal cortisol patterns, future diabetes, and impaired glucose metabolism in the Whitehall II cohort study. J Clin Endocrinol Metab. 2016;101:619-25.
43. Hänsel A, Hong S, Cámara RJA, et al. Inflammation as a psychophysiological biomarker in chronic psychosocial stress. Neurosci Biobehav Rev. 2010;35:115-21.
44. Akash MSH, Rehman K, Chen S. Role of inflammatory mechanisms in pathogenesis of type 2 diabetes mellitus. J Cell Biochem. 2013;114:525-31.
45. Hansson GK. Inflammation, atherosclerosis, and coronary artery disease. N Engl J Med. 2005;352:1685-95.
46. Libby P, Ridker PM, Hansson GK. Progress and challenges in translating the biology of atherosclerosis. Nature. 2011;473:317-25.
47. Mommersteeg PMC, Herr R, Pouwer F, et al. The association between diabetes and an episode of depressive symptoms in the 2002 World Health Survey: an analysis of 231, 797 individuals from 47 countries. Diabet Med. 2013;30:e208-14.
48. Anderson RJ, Freedland KE, Clouse RE, et al. The prevalence of comorbid depression in adults with diabetes: a metaanalysis. Diabetes Care. 2001;24:1069-78.
49. Ali S, Stone MA, Peters JL, et al. The prevalence of co-morbid depression in adults with type 2 diabetes: a systematic review and meta-analysis. Diabet Med. 2006;23:1165-73.
50. Roy T, Lloyd CE. Epidemiology of depression and diabetes: a systematic review. J Affect Disord. 2012;142:S8-21.
51. Black SA, Markides KS, Ray LA. Depression predicts increased incidence of adverse health outcomes in older Mexican Americans with type 2 diabetes. Diabetes Care. 2003;26:2822-8.
52. Lin EHB, Rutter CM, Katon W, et al. Depression and advanced complications of diabetes: a prospective cohort study. Diabetes Care. 2010;33:264-9.
53. Scherrer JF, Garfield LD, Chrusciel T, et al. Increased risk of myocardial infarction in depressed patients with type 2 diabetes. Diabetes Care. 2011;34:1729-34.

54. Cummings DM, Kirian K, Howard G, et al. Consequences of Comorbidity of Elevated Stress and/or Depressive Symptoms and Incident Cardiovascular Outcomes in Diabetes: results from the REasons for Geographic And Racial Differences in Stroke (REGARDS) study. Diabetes Care. 2016;39:101-9.
55. Ting RZW, Lau ESH, Ozaki R, et al. High risk for cardiovascular disease in Chinese type 2 diabetic patients with major depression—a 7-year prospective analysis of the Hong Kong Diabetes Registry. J Affect Disord. 2013;149:129-35.
56. Smith KJ, Béland M, Clyde M, et al. Association of diabetes with anxiety: a systematic review and meta-analysis. J Psychosom Res. 2013;74:89-99.
57. Edwards LE, Mezuk B. Anxiety and risk of type 2 diabetes: evidence from the Baltimore Epidemiologic Catchment Area Study. J Psychosom Res. 2012;73:418-23.
58. Cook WW, Medley DM. Proposed hostility and pharisaic-virtue scales for the MMPI. J Appl Psychol. 1954;38:414.
59. Shen BJ, Countryman AJ, Spiro A, et al. The prospective contribution of hostility characteristics to high fasting glucose levels. Diabetes Care. 2008;31:1293-8.
60. Suarez EC. Sex differences in the relation of depressive symptoms, hostility, and anger expression to indices of glucose metabolism in nondiabetic adults. Health Psychol. 2006;25:484-92.
61. Zhang J, Niaura R, Dyer JR, et al. Hostility and urine norepinephrine interact to predict insulin resistance: the VA normative aging study. Psychosom Med. 2006;68:718-26.
62. Kawakami N, Araki S, Ohtsu H, et al. Effects of mood states, smoking and urinary catecholamine excretion on hemoglobin A1c in male Japanese workers. Ind Health. 1995;33:153-62.
63. Williams ED, Steptoe A, Chambers JC, et al. Ethnic and gender differences in the relationship between hostility and metabolic and autonomic risk factors for coronary heart disease. Psychosom Med. 2011;73:53-8.
64. Golden SH, Williams JE, Ford DE, et al. Anger temperament is modestly associated with the risk of type 2 diabetes mellitus: the atheroslcerosis risk in communities study. Psychoneuroendocrinology. 2006;31:325-32.
65. Abraham S, Shah NG, Roux AD, et al. Trait anger but not anxiety predicts incident type 2 diabetes: the Multi-Ethnic Study of Atherosclerosis (MESA). Psychoneuroendocrinology. 2015;60: 105-13.
66. Dalsgaard EM, Vestergaard M, Skriver MV, et al. Psychological distress, cardiovascular complications and mortality among people with screen-detected type 2 diabetes: follow-up of the ADDITIONDenmark trial. Diabetologia. 2014;57:710-7.
67. Fisher L, Skaff MM, Mullan JT, et al. Clinical depression versus distress among patients with type 2 diabetes: not just a question of semantics. Diabetes Care. 2007;30:542-8.
68. Nicolucci A, Kovacs Burns K, Holt RIG, et al. Diabetes Attitudes, Wishes and Needs second study (DAWN2TM): cross-national benchmarking of diabetes related psychosocial outcomes for people with diabetes. Diabet Med. 2013;30:767-77.
69. Aikens JE. Prospective associations between emotional distress and poor outcomes in type 2 diabetes. Diabetes Care. 2012;35:2472-8.
70. Crump C, Sundquist J, Winkleby MA, et al. Stress resilience and subsequent risk of type 2 diabetes in 1.5 million young men. Diabetologia. 2016;59(4):728-33.
71. Boehm JK, Trudel-Fitzgerald C, Kivimaki M, et al. The prospective association between positive psychological well-being and diabetes. Health Psychol. 2015;34:1013-21.
72. Banks R. Health and spirituality dimension: Relationships and implications for professional preparation programs. J School Health. 1980;50:195-202.
73. Hill PC, Pargament KI. Advances in the conceptualization and measurement of religion and spirituality: implications for physical and mental health research. Am Psychol. 2003;58:64-74.
74. Rozanski A, Blumenthal JA, Davidson KW, et al. The epidemiology, pathophysiology, and management of psychosocial risk factors in cardiac practice: the emerging field of behavioral cardiology. J Am Coll Cardiol. 2005;45:637-51.
75. Manfrini O, Pizzi C, Trere D, et al. Parasympathetic failure and risk of subsequent coronary events in unstable angina and non-ST-segment elevation myocardial infarction. Eur Heart J. 2003;24:1560-6.
76. Malliani A. Heart rate variability: from bench to bedside. Eur J Int Med. 2005;16:12-20.
77. Friedman BH, Thayer JF. Anxiety and autonomic flexibility: a cardiovascular approach. Biol Psychol. 1998;49:303-23.
78. Knowler WC, Barrett-Connor E, Fowler SE, et al. Reduction in the incidence of type 2 diabetes with lifestyle intervention or metformin. N Engl J Med. 2002;346:393-403.
79. Uusitupa M, Peltonen M, Lindström J, et al. Ten-year mortality and cardiovascular morbidity in the Finnish Diabetes Prevention Study—secondary analysis of the randomized trial. PLoS One. 2009;4:e5656.
80. Li G, Zhang P, Wang J, et al. The long-term effect of lifestyle interventions to prevent diabetes in the China Da Qing Diabetes Prevention Study: a 20-year follow-up study. Lancet. 2008;371: 1783-9.
81. Look AHEAD Research Group, Wing RR, Bolin P, et al. Cardiovascular effects of intensive lifestyle intervention in type 2 diabetes. N Engl J Med. 2013;369:145-54.
82. Baumeister H, Hutter N, Bengel J. Psychological and pharmacological interventions for depression in patients with diabetes mellitus and depression. Cochrane Database Syst Rev. 2012;12:CD008381.
83. Noordali F, Cumming J, Thompson JL. Effectiveness of mindfulness-based interventions on physiological and psychological complications in adults with diabetes: a systematic review. J Health Psychol. 2017;22:965-83.
84. Jones A, Vallis M, Pouwer F. If it does not significantly change HbA1c levels why should we waste time on it? A plea for the prioritization of psychological well-being in people with diabetes. Diabet Med. 2015;32:155-63.
85. Gupta SK, Sawhney RC, Rai L, et al. Regression of Coronary Atherosclerosis through Healthy and Happy Lifestyle in Coronary Artery Disease Patients—Mount Abu Open Heart Trial. Indian Heart J. 2011;63:461-9.
86. Gupta SK. Three Dimensional Health care: Need of the Hour. Innovations in Healthcare Management. 2015;273-86.
87. Cunningham C, Brown S, Kaski J. Effects of transcendental meditation on symptoms and electrocardiographic changes in patients with cardiac syndrome X. AM J Cardiol. 2000; 85: 653-5.
88. Canter PH. The therapeutic effects of meditation. BMJ. 2003;326:1049-50.
89. Davidson RJ. Spirituality and Meditation: Science and Practice. Ann Fam Med. 2008;6:388-9.
90. Shakun S, Sawhney RC, Gupta SK. Impact of vegetarian diet, aerobic exercise and BKRM on hyperinsulemia, dyslipidaemia and hyperglycemia in coronary artery disease. ACBR Delhi University: PhD Thesis; 2005.

Hypothyroidism and Cardiodiabetes

M Somasundaram, C Elamaran

INTRODUCTION

Thyroid diseases and diabetes mellitus (DM) are the two most common endocrine disorders encountered in clinical practice, mutually influencing each other.[1] Diabetes is a major risk factor for cardiovascular disease (CVD). In patients with hypothyroidism and diabetes, CVD risk is increased through interrelationship with dyslipidemia, hypertension, insulin resistance (IR),[2] and vascular endothelial dysfunction. Diastolic hypertension, dyslipidemia, reduced left ventricular function, and increase in systemic vascular resistance can be reversed with thyroid hormone (TH) replacement[3] in hypothyroidism.

HYPOTHYROIDISM AND DIABETES

Thyroid dysfunction is more common in patients with DM than in the normal population. The prevalence of thyroid disorder in diabetic population was found to be 13.4% with the highest prevalence in females with type 1 DM (31.4%) and lowest prevalence in males with type 2 DM (6.9%).[4] Treatment of thyroid dysfunction in diabetic patients will benefit glycemic control and reduce cardiovascular risk. Clinical as well as subclinical hypothyroidism (SCH) can produce insulin resistant (IR) states.[5] DM influences thyroid function at the level of hypothalamic control of thyroid-stimulating hormone (TSH) release and at peripheral tissues by converting T_4 to T_3. The nocturnal TSH peak is blunted or abolished in diabetic patients and the TSH response to thyrotropin-releasing hormone (TRH) is also impaired. Decreased T_3 levels are seen in patients with uncontrolled diabetes. Impaired peripheral conversion of T_4 to T_3 is the reason for low T_3 state characterized by low serum total and free T_3 levels, increase in reverse T_3 but normal serum T_4 and TSH concentrations, which normalizes with improvement in glycemic control.

Subclinical Hypothyroidism and Diabetes

Type 2 diabetes mellitus patients are more likely to have SCH when compared with healthy population. SCH is seen in 5% of diabetic patients in the hospital outpatient setting[4] and 8.6% in community-based female diabetic patients.[6] Diabetic patients with SCH have more severe retinopathy than euthyroid patients with diabetes.[7] An increased risk of nephropathy was found in T2DM patients with SCH and treating hypothyroidism improves renal function.[8] Increased risk of nephropathy and retinopathy seen in diabetic patients with SCH provides justification of screening the patients with T2DM for thyroid dysfunction.

Hypothyroidism and Hypoglycemia

Hypoglycemia is seen in patients with hypothyroidism and diabetes. It is due to effects on glucose metabolism by reduced hepatic glucose output, gluconeogenesis, and peripheral glucose uptake which leads to hypoglycemia.[9] Frequent hypoglycemia is seen in children and adolescents with diabetes and SCH.

TABLE 1: Guidelines for thyroid screening in diabetes

	Guidelines	Type 2 diabetes	Comments
1.	American Thyroid Association Guidelines for detection of thyroid dysfunction[12]	Patients with diabetes may require more frequent testing	Recommends TSH from 35 years, and every 5 years thereafter in all adults; high-risk persons may require more frequent tests. Diabetes mentioned as high risk but does not distinguish between T1DM and T2DM
2.	American Association of Clinical Endocrinologists, Thyroid Disease Clinical Practice Guidelines, 2002[13]	Thyroid palpation and TSH at diagnosis and at regular intervals, especially if goiter or other autoimmune disease presents	No specific recommendation for T2DM
3.	British Thyroid Association and Association of Clinical Biochemistry Guidelines, 2006[14]	TFT a baseline but routine annual TFT is not recommended	TSH and antibodies are recommended in diabetic patients in pregnancy and postpartum
4.	American Diabetes Association. Standards of medical care in diabetes, 2009[15]	Not specifically mentioned	Thyroid palpation in all diabetic patients; TSH in adults >50 years, or patients with dyslipidemia

Insulin Resistance and Hypothyroidism

Insulin resistance (IR) is a condition in which there is a decreased sensitivity of muscles, adipose tissue, liver, and other body tissues to insulin, despite its normal or increased concentration in blood. In the study by Maratou et al., patients with overt hypothyroidism and SCH presented a reduced level of insulin-stimulated glucose transport in monocytes due to disrupted translocation of the GLUT4-glucose transporter in the plasma membrane.[5] Another important mechanism for IR in hypothyroidism is due to decreased blood flow in peripheral tissues. Hypothyroidism is associated with endothelial dysfunction.[10] A study in healthy euthyroid men found positive correlations between TSH, endothelial dysfunction, and IR[11] providing further evidence to the three-way relationship between thyroid status, IR, and CVD risk.

Diagnosis and Screening for Hypothyroidism in Diabetes

Highly sensitive immunoassay for serum TSH (detection limit of <0.1 mIU/mL) is the most reliable and sensitive screening test for hypothyroidism. Many studies show that yearly testing for thyroid dysfunction in T2DM patients is necessary, with baseline testing in newly diagnosed DM.

Guidelines for Thyroid Screening in Diabetes

The guidelines for thyroid screening in diabetes are given in Table 1.

Metformin and Thyroid Dysfunction

Metformin administration in diabetic patients with hypothyroidism associated with a significant reduction in the serum levels of TSH, with no change in free T_4. Re-evaluation of thyroid function within 6–12 months after starting metformin is necessary in diabetic patients with concomitant hypothyroidism.

HYPOTHYROIDISM AND CARDIOVASCULAR SYSTEM

Pathophysiology

The major cardiovascular changes that occur in hypothyroidism include: a decrease in cardiac output and cardiac contractility, a reduction in heart rate, and an increase in peripheral vascular resistance. There are also significant changes in modifiable atherosclerotic risk factors, including hypercholesterolemia, diastolic hypertension, carotid intimal media thickness, and endothelial-derived relaxation factor (Table 2, Box 1).[16]

TABLE 2: Cardiovascular hemodynamics in hypothyroidism

Systemic vascular resistance	↑	50–60% above normal
Systolic blood pressure	↓ or normal	Narrow pulse pressure
Diastolic blood pressure	↑ or normal	20% prevalence of diastolic hypertension
Heart rate	↓ or normal	
Cardiac contractility	↑ or normal	Both systolic and diastolic function impaired
Blood volume	↓	Decreased preload
Cardiac output	↓	30–50% below normal

BOX 1: Cardiovascular risks associated with hypothyroidism

- Impaired cardiac contractility and diastolic function
- Increased systemic vascular resistance
- Decreased endothelial-derived relaxation factor
- Increased serum cholesterol
- Increased C-reactive protein
- Increased homocysteine

Cardiac Contractility

Hypothyroidism is associated with systolic and diastolic dysfunctions and reduced cardiac output due to multifactorial causes such as increases in afterload, changes in expression of the genes for myocardial calcium regulatory proteins. Beta receptor expression is also decreased, resulting in a blunted response to catecholamine-mediated effects.

Vascular Resistance

Hypothyroidism causes a decrease in the release of endothelial-derived relaxation factor, which in turn, increases the peripheral vascular resistance which results in reduction in cardiac output.

Clinical Manifestations

Symptoms and signs of cardiovascular dysfunction are not prominent in patients with hypothyroidism. Following symptoms and signs may be seen—exertional dyspnea and exercise intolerance, although these symptoms are probably due to skeletal muscle dysfunction, bradycardia, diastolic hypertension, and left ventricular dysfunction with poor contractility.

Pericardial effusions are usually small but occasionally large. Cardiac tamponade is uncommon. Echocardiography demonstrates small to moderate effusions in up to 30% of hypothyroid patients.

Electrocardiography

Hypothyroidism is classically associated with sinus bradycardia. Atrial ectopy is rare but premature ventricular beats and occasional ventricular tachycardia can occur. The QT prolongation predisposes patients to ventricular arrhythmias, and some patients with acquired torsades de pointes have improved or completely resolved with TH replacement.[17] Low voltage and nonspecific ST changes also seen in hypothyroidism.

Blood Pressure

Diastolic blood pressure may vary directly with serum TSH levels over the entire spectrum of thyroid disease. About 20–40% of hypothyroid patients are hypertensive, primarily diastolic with reduced pulse pressure.

Coronary Artery Disease

Hypercholesterolemia, hypertension, and elevated levels of homocysteine may increase the risk for atherosclerosis and coronary artery disease.[17,18] Noninvasive studies like nuclear scans have demonstrated abnormalities in perfusion suggestive of myocardial ischemia, but these defects appear to resolve with TH treatment. Potential mechanisms in addition to lipid abnormalities and diastolic hypertension include elevated concentrations of C-reactive protein and endothelial dysfunction.

Laboratory Tests

Lipids

Dyslipidemia is common in hypothyroidism, and it increases both total and low-density lipoprotein (LDL) cholesterol in proportion to the rise in serum TSH levels.[17] The primary mechanism involves changes in LDL metabolism caused by decreases in LDL receptor number. Some patients have high serum very-low-density lipoprotein (VLDL) cholesterol concentrations, and a few have hypertriglyceridemia. A recent study reported that the liver selective TH agonist eprotirome has additive effect in lowering cholesterol levels in statin-treated patients.[19,20] If hypothyroidism is present, the patient should be treated for 3–4 months with TH (levothyroxine, T_4) to normalize serum TSH. If the serum lipid concentrations are not normal, then specific lipid-lowering therapy may be indicated. It should be noted that hypothyroidism may predispose to the development of statin-associated myopathy and that use of statins may "unmask" hypothyroid myopathy.

Homocysteine

Some patients with hypothyroidism have high serum homocysteine concentrations, which fall toward, if not to normal, with T_4 therapy.

Creatinine Kinase

Many hypothyroid patients have high serum creatinine kinase (CK) concentrations. The isoenzyme distribution is almost completely MM, with less than 4% constituting MB, indicating skeletal muscle, not myocardial origin. However, as many as 14% of patients with hypothyroidism have a raised serum concentration of CK-MB, which can be confusing in the evaluation of chest pain. This problem is obviated by measurement of serum troponin I, which is normal in hypothyroidism.

Thyroid Function Testing

Serum TSH level is the most widely used and sensitive measure for the diagnosis of hypothyroidism and hyperthyroidism. Serum TSH levels uniformly increase (>3.5 mIU/mL) in patients with primary hypothyroidism, the levels are low in hyperthyroidism (<0.1 mIU/mL). Measures of free T_4 can be useful when coexistent hepatic, nutritional, or genetic disease may alter thyroxin-binding globulin content. Autoimmune thyroid disease (Hashimoto and Graves) can be further diagnosed by using anti-thyroid antibodies, most specifically anti-thyroid peroxidase or anti-thyroglobulin antibodies.

Treatment

Dose and Monitoring

Initial dose: The average full replacement dose of T_4 in adults is approximately 1.6 µg/kg body weight per day but the range of required doses is wide, varying from 50 µg/day to ≥200 µg/day. The initial dose can be the full anticipated dose (1.6 µg/kg/day) in young, healthy patients, but older patients or those with coronary heart disease should be started on a lower dose (25–50 µg daily). The clearance of many drugs, including anticoagulant drugs, is decreased in hypothyroidism. In patients being treated with warfarin anticoagulation, the dose required to maintain a therapeutic prothrombin time increases during hypothyroidism, and this increase is reversed with restoration of a normal TSH (Table 3).

In all patients, TH replacement should be sufficient to restore the serum TSH level to normal so that they become clinically euthyroid. TH replacement should be accomplished with purified preparations of levothyroxine sodium.

TABLE 3: Initiating treatment

Patient population	*Thyroxine treatment*
In young patients without risk factors for CVD	Full replacement doses of levothyroxine (100–150 µg/day) can be given
Patients older than 50 years with known or suspected coronary artery disease	Decide whether to perform coronary artery revascularization before initiating TH replacement. If patients are not candidates for percutaneous intervention, CABG can be performed in those with unstable angina, left main coronary artery disease, or three-vessel disease with impaired left ventricular function even in the setting of overt hypothyroidism. TH replacement can be delayed until the postoperative period, then it can be administered in full doses parenterally or orally[20]
Patients with known stable cardiac disease in whom cardiac revascularization is not clinically indicated	Treatment can be started with low doses (12.5 µg) of levothyroxine and then stepwise increases (12.5–25 µg) every 6–8 weeks until the serum TSH level normalizes
Patients who are at risk for coronary artery disease, but without clinical signs or symptoms	TH replacement can be started at doses in the range of 25–50 µg/day, and then increased by 25 µg every 6–8 weeks until the serum TSH level is normal

Diagnosis

Hashimoto disease, radioiodine therapy for Graves' disease, and iodine deficiency are the leading causes of hypothyroidism. The finding of an elevated TSH level is sufficient to establish the diagnosis and form the basis for treatment. In routine practice, additional testing with a serum T_4 and T_3 assay is confirmatory. The prevalence of hypothyroidism is around 3–4% for overt disease and 7–10% for milder forms of disease and increases with advancing age.

TSH screening can be advised for all adults particularly in patients with hypertension, hypercholesterolemia, hypertriglyceridemia, coronary or peripheral vascular disease, unexplained pericardial effusions, pleural effusions, various musculoskeletal syndromes, and statin-associated myopathy.[21]

SUBCLINICAL HYPOTHYROIDISM

It is defined biochemically as a normal serum free thyroxine (T_4) concentration in the presence of an elevated serum TSH concentration. In SCH, the TSH levels are between 3 mIU/L and 20 mIU/L with normal T_4 and T_3 levels and it alters lipid metabolism, atherosclerosis, cardiac contractility, and systemic vascular resistance. Cholesterol levels rise in proportionate to the increase in TSH levels starting at 5 mIU/mL. Restoration of serum TSH levels to normal after TH replacement improves lipid levels, lowers systemic vascular resistance, improves cardiac contractility, and decreases carotid intimal-medial thickness.[22] Treatment of TSH levels between 5 mIU/mL and 10 mIU/mL lowered the incidence of ischemic heart disease events and cardiovascular mortality. TH replacement can be recommended for all patients with SCH.[23]

CONCLUSION

There is complex association between thyroid dysfunction, diabetes, and CVDs. Hypothyroidism increases cardiovascular disease risk in diabetic patients through interrelationships with dyslipidemia, IR, and vascular endothelial dysfunction. It is, therefore, important to diagnose thyroid dysfunction in diabetic and cardiac patients by regular screening and management of both clinical and SCH will reduce the morbidity.

REFERENCES

1. Gray RS, Irvine WJ, Clarke BF. Screening for thyroid dysfunction in diabetics. Br Med J. 1979;2:1439.
2. Danzi S, Klein I. Thyroid hormone and blood pressure regulation. Curr Hypertens Rep. 2013;5:513-20.

3. Palmieri EA, Fazio S, Lombardi G, et al. Subclinical hypothyroidism and cardiovascular risk: a reason to treat? Treat Endocrinol. 2004;3:233-44.
4. Perros P, McCrimmon RJ, Shaw G, et al. Frequency of thyroid dysfunction in diabetic patients: value of annual screening. Diabet Med. 1995;12:622-7.
5. Maratou E, Hadjidakis DJ, Kollias A, et al. Studies of insulin resistance in patients with clinical and subclinical hypothyroidism. Eur J Endocrinol. 2009;160:785-90.
6. Chubb SA, Davis WA, Inman Z, et al. Prevalence and progression of subclinical hypothyroidism in women with type 2 diabetes: the Fremantle Diabetes Study. Clin Endocrinol (Oxf). 2005;62:480-6.
7. Yang GR, Yang JK, Zhang L, et al. Association between subclinical hypothyroidism and proliferative diabetic retinopathy in type 2 diabetic patients: a case-control study. Tohoku J Exp Med. 2010;222:303-10.
8. den Hollander JG, Wulkan RW, Mantel MJ, et al. Correlation between severity of thyroid dysfunction and renal function. Clin Endocrinol (Oxf). 2005;62:423-7.
9. Mouradian M, Abourizk N. Diabetes mellitus and thyroid disease. Diabetes Care. 1983;6:512-20.
10. Owen PJ, Sabit R, Lazarus JH. Thyroid disease and vascular function. Thyroid. 2007;17:519-24.
11. Fernandez-Real JM, Lopez-Bermejo A, Castro A, et al. Thyroid function is intrinsically linked to insulin sensitivity and endothelium-dependent vasodilation in healthy euthyroid subjects. J Clin Endocrinol Metab. 2006;91:3337-43.
12. Ladenson PW, Singer PA, Ainetal KB. American Thyroid Association Guidelines for detection of thyroid dysfunction. Arch Intern Med. 2000;160:1573-5.
13. Baskin HJ, Cobin RH, Duicketal DS. American Association of Clinical Endocrinologists medical guidelines for clinical practice for the evaluation and treatment of hyperthyroidism and hypothyroidism. Endocr Pract. 2002;8:457-69.
14. British Thyroid Association. (2006). UK Guidelines for the Use of Thyroid Function Tests. [online] Available from *http://www.btf-thyroid.org/images/documents/tft_guideline_final_version_july_2006.pdf.* [Accessed August, 2017].
15. American Diabetes Association. Standards of medical care in diabetes-2009. Diabetes Care. 2009;32:S13-S61.
16. Klein I, Danzi S. Thyroid disease and the heart. Circulation. 2007;116:1725.
17. Hak AE, Pols HA, Visser TJ, et al. Subclinical hypothyroidism is an independent risk factor for atherosclerosis and myocardial infarction in elderly women: the Rotterdam Study. Ann Intern Med. 2000;132:270.
18. Walsh JP, Bremmer AP, Bulsara MK, et al. Subclinical thyroid dysfunction as a risk factor for cardiovascular disease. Arch Intern Med. 2005;165:2467.
19. Ladenson PW, Kristensen JD, Ridgway EC, et al. Use of the thyroid hormone analogue eprotirome in statin-treated dyslipidemia. N Engl J Med. 2010;362:906.
20. Garber JR, Cobin RH, Gharib H, et al. Clinical practice guidelines for hypothyroidism in adults: cosponsored by the American Association of Clinical Endocrinologists and the American Thyroid Association. Thyroid. 2012;22:1200-35.
21. Klein I, Danzi S. The cardiovascular system in hypothyroidism. In: Braverman LE, Cooper DS (Eds). Werner & Ingbar's The Thyroid: A Fundamental and Clinical Text, 10th edition. Philadelphia: Lippincott/Williams & Wilkins; 2012. pp. 575-81.
22. Kim SD, Kim SH, Park KS, et al. Regression of the increased common carotid artery-intima media thickness in subclinical hypothyroidism after thyroid hormone replacement. Endocr J. 2009; 56:753.
23. Razvi S, Weaver JU, Butler TJ, et al. Levothyroxine treatment of subclinical hypothyroidism, fatal and nonfatal cardiovascular events, and mortality. Arch Intern Med. 2012;172:811.

CHAPTER 7

Cardiodiabetes and Insulin Resistance in Obesity: Clinical Relevance

Ajay Kumar Sinha, Anand Gopal, Dinanath Kumar, Shaheen Ahmad, Asim Perwez, Vikas Singh

INTRODUCTION

Insulin resistance is not simply a problem of deficient glucose uptake in response to insulin, but a multifaceted syndrome that increases significantly the risk for cardiovascular disease. The links between insulin resistance and the associated dyslipidemia, hypertension, hypercoagulability, and atherosclerosis are numerous and complex. This complexity derives both from the almost certain multiple causes of the insulin resistance syndrome and from the interaction of genes predisposing to insulin resistance with other genes that have their own, independent impact on lipid metabolism, blood pressure regulation, coagulation, and artery wall biology.

BACKGROUND AND PATHOGENESIS

Advances over the last decade have expanded our understanding of the role of adipocytes in biology, and this has begun to provide mechanistic insights into the causal relationship between obesity and diabetes. It is now clear that adipocytes function as endocrine glands with wide-reaching effects on other organs including the brain. Yalow and Berson (1960)[1] were the first to point out that plasma immunoreactive insulin concentrations following an oral glucose challenge were as high, if not higher, in patients with what was then called "maturity-onset diabetes" than in a population with normal glucose tolerance. This led to the speculation that patients with maturity onset diabetes were probably "insulin resistant". Karam and colleagues[2] argued that plasma insulin concentrations were elevated in response to a glucose challenge only in patients with maturity-onset diabetes who were also obese. Based on these findings, they concluded that it was obesity, not maturity-onset diabetes, which was associated with insulin resistance. Rabinowitz and Zierler (1962),[3] used the perfused forearm technique to provide direct evidence that insulin-stimulated glucose disposal was impaired in obese individuals. Insulin resistance is a fundamental aspect of the etiology of type 2 diabetes and is also linked to a wide array of other pathophysiologic sequelae including hypertension, hyperlipidemia, atherosclerosis (i.e. the metabolic syndrome, or syndrome X), and polycystic ovarian disease.[4] There are also grounds for considering the related possibility that insulin resistance and hyperinsulinemia, in addition to being caused by obesity, can contribute to the development of obesity. Adipocytes are one of the most highly insulin-responsive cell types. Insulin promotes adipocyte triglyceride stores by a number of mechanisms, including fostering the differentiation of preadipocytes to adipocytes, and in mature adipocytes, stimulating glucose transport and triglyceride synthesis (lipogenesis), as well as inhibiting lipolysis (Fig. 1).

The term "insulin resistance" usually connotes resistance to the effects of insulin on glucose uptake, metabolism, or storage. Insulin resistance in obesity and type 2 diabetes is manifested by decreased insulin-stimulated glucose transport and metabolism in adipocytes and skeletal muscle and by impaired suppression of hepatic glucose output.[4] In all forms of obesity and diabetes, a major factor

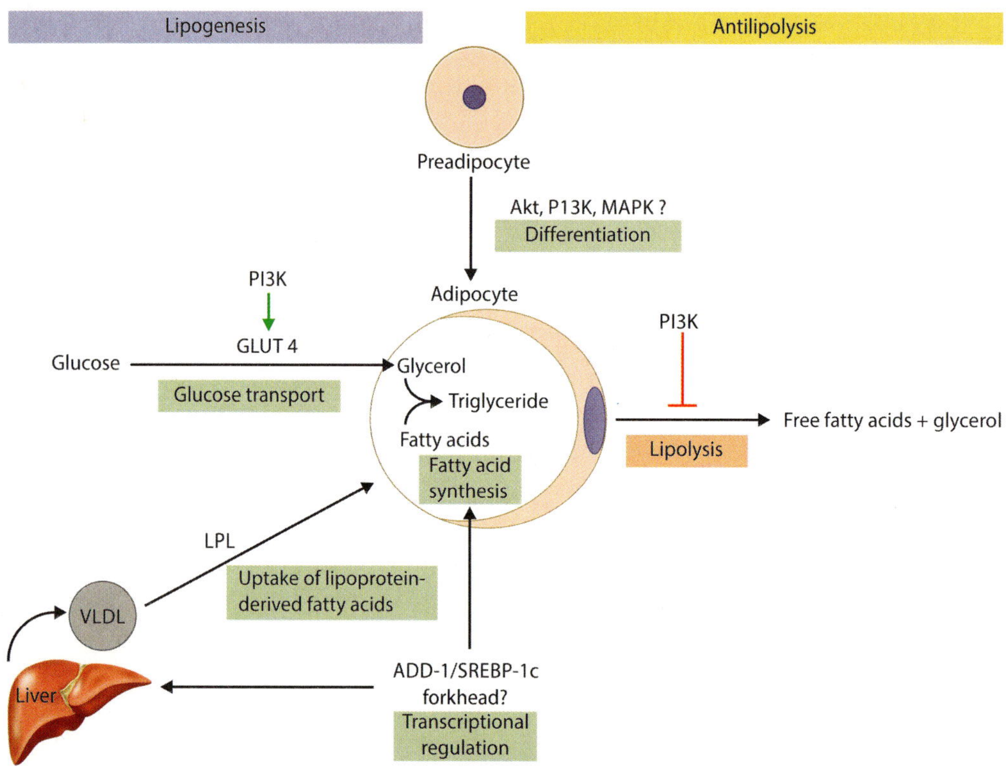

Fig. 1: Pleiotropic effects of insulin to promote adipose storage
Source: Kahn BB, Flier JS. Obesity and insulin resistance. J Clin Invest. 2000;106(4):473-81

contributing to the impaired insulin-stimulated glucose transport in adipocytes is the downregulation of GLUT4. However, in skeletal muscle of obese and diabetic humans, GLUT4 expression is normal[5] and defective glucose transport appears to be due to impaired translocation, docking, or fusion of GLUT4-containing vesicles with the plasma membrane.

Although insulin resistance is characteristic of obesity and type 2 diabetes, it is not established that all of insulin's actions are impaired in individuals with both conditions. It is possible that hepatic lipogenesis and lipid storage are being driven to excess in adipose tissue, whereas other insulin effects related to glucose homeostasis are impaired. The action of insulin to lower blood glucose levels results from suppression of hepatic glucose production and increased glucose uptake into muscle and fat. Muscle has long been considered the major site of insulin-stimulated glucose uptake in vivo, with adipose tissue contributing relatively little to total body glucose disposal [at least ten times more glucose per milligram of tissue goes into muscle than into white adipose tissue (WAT)]. Because muscle mass is considerably greater than WAT mass, at least in lean rodents and humans, this observation has been taken to indicate the prominent contribution of muscle to glucose disposal. Thus, it has been viewed as unlikely that diminished glucose uptake into fat could account for diminished whole body glucose uptake in obesity.

Further support for a potential direct role of adipocytes in regulating systemic glucose homeostasis comes from studies in which rodents or humans are treated with the β3 adrenergic agonist CL316,243.[6] β3 adrenergic receptors are expressed almost exclusively in fat and treatment with CL316,243 results in enhanced sensitivity of both whole body glucose uptake and suppression of hepatic glucose production.[6] Thus, increasing glucose uptake selectively in fat with β3 adrenergic receptor agonists may improve whole body glucose uptake, with the effects in fat indirectly resulting in increased insulin sensitivity in liver.

DOES LOCATION OF BODY FAT DETERMINE INSULIN RESISTANCE?

Large epidemiologic studies reveal that the risk for diabetes, and presumably insulin resistance, rises as body fat content [measured by body mass index (BMI)] increases from the very lean to the very obese, implying that the "dose" of body fat has an effect on insulin sensitivity across a broad range.[7] However, it is critical to realize that all sites of adiposity are not equal in this regard. Central (intra-abdominal) depots of fat are much more strongly linked to insulin resistance,

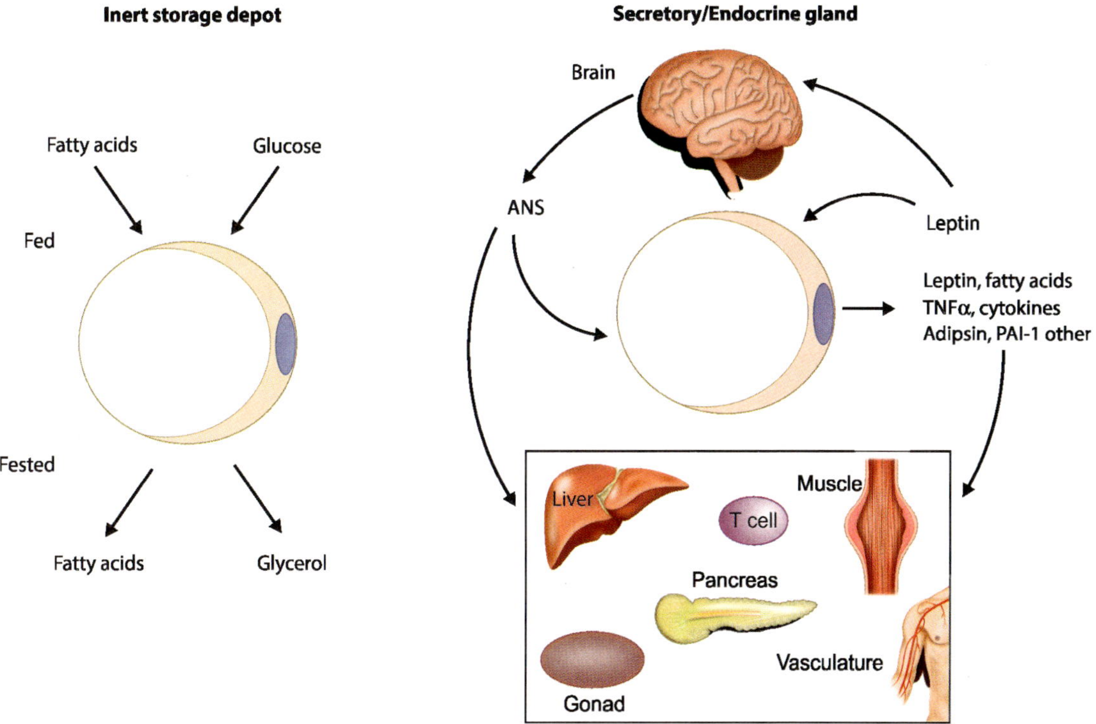

Fig. 2: Evolving view of the biological functions of the adipocyte

Source: Kahn BB, Flier JS. Obesity and insulin resistance. J Clin Invest. 2000;106(4):473-81

type 2 diabetes, and cardiovascular disease than are peripheral (gluteal/subcutaneous) fat depots.[8]

A leading hypothesis in this regard is that intra-abdominal adipocytes are more lipolytically active, in part due to their complement of adrenergic receptors. This would increase intraportal FFA levels and flux, which might inhibit insulin clearance and promote insulin resistance by mechanisms that are still uncertain. Hyperinsulinemia per se can cause insulin resistance by downregulating insulin receptors and desensitizing postreceptor pathways, as was confirmed by overexpression of insulin in livers of otherwise normal transgenic mice.[9] An alternate hypothesis is that since adipocytes are now known to secrete many factors that are capable of exerting systemic effects, the array of factors secreted by intra-abdominal adipocytes may be particularly harmful to systemic insulin sensitivity.

Adipocytes are well known for their essential role as energy storage depots for triglycerides. However, data emerging over the past several years have established an additional role for the adipocyte that of secretory cell (Fig. 2). Adipocytes express and secrete numerous peptide hormones and cytokines, including tumor necrosis factor alpha (TNF-α); plasminogen-activator inhibitor-1, which helps maintain hemostasis; angiotensinogen, whose proteolytic product regulates vascular tone; and leptin, which plays a central role in regulating energy balance. Adipose tissue can also produce active steroid hormones, including estrogen and cortisol.[10] Through such secreted products, adipocytes possess the capacity to influence local adipocyte biology, as well as systemic metabolism at sites as diverse as brain, liver, muscle, β cells, gonads, lymphoid organs, and systemic vasculature. This realization raises many possibilities for additional links between adipose function or mass and insulin resistance, independent of the adipocyte's roles in energy storage and release.

A great deal of interest has followed the discovery that adipocytes express and secrete the cytokine TNFα, and that enlarged adipocytes from obese animals and humans overexpress this factor.[11] However, not all studies have found TNF-α to be elevated in obesity and alternative approaches to assessing a role of TNF-α in systemic insulin resistance are therefore needed. Improvement of insulin resistance in response to loss of TNF signaling is at best partial, and the effect of TNF neutralization has not been seen in all experimental models. Thus, TNF-α may be a partial contributor to insulin resistance, but other factors must exist.

Leptin, the product of the *ob gene*, is an adipocyte-derived hormone and exerts pleiotropic effects, including profound effects on satiety, energy expenditure, and neuroendocrine function. Severe insulin resistance is a well-known feature of deficiency of leptin or its receptor in the ob/ob or db/db mouse strains, and these models were among the first to be investigated for the pathogenesis of insulin resistance in the early 1970s. Leptin's major site of action is the hypothalamus, especially in selected nuclei within the ventrobasal hypothalamus.[12] The fact that hyperinsulinemia and insulin resistance are produced by hypothalamic lesions affecting the ventromedial hypothalamic nucleus suggested a major role for the central nervous system (CNS) in regulation of insulin action or secretion. Our current understanding is that leptin exerts much of its effect on metabolism and satiety through actions within the ventrobasal hypothalamus.

Leptin has a clear insulin-sensitizing effect acutely and also after chronic administration to normal rodents.[13,14] The molecular basis for the insulin-sensitizing effect of leptin remains a topic of great interest. Two general views prevail. According to one, the metabolic actions of leptin are exerted predominantly through actions of leptin within the CNS, most likely within the hypothalamus. The second view of how leptin sensitizes to insulin involves direct effects at the level of insulin target tissues. Substantial data support the notion that leptin may have important effects through direct action on peripheral target cells, including β cells, liver, muscle, and fat. Some evidence suggests that in tissues including muscle and β cells, leptin promotes lipid oxidation and inhibits lipid synthesis, which would promote insulin sensitivity.[15] Since leptin fails to reverse insulin resistance and lipid accumulation in mice with ventromedial hypothalamic lesions, and low-dose central administration of leptin has major metabolic effects without changing blood leptin levels, it seems likely that central actions are required, and that without them, the peripheral actions are at best limited. Unlike rodents, the few humans with leptin or leptin receptor mutations and obesity do not appear to have extraordinary degrees of insulin resistance, as assessed by hyperinsulinemia, and none have as yet been described with diabetes.[16,17] This difference may be related to the fact that in humans, unlike mice, leptin has little effect on the HPA axis.

WHAT CAN BE DONE?

In order to prevent or reduce long-term risk for CVD, preventative interventions should be initiated with a focus on weight management to reduce excessive central fat accumulation. Starting treatment solely on the basis of large waist is perfectly reasonable. The severity of CHD could be estimated for individuals with additional risk factors. Management goal focuses on lifestyle changes such as daily intake of five portions of fruit and vegetables[18] and reduction in regular alcohol consumption to reverse modifiable risk factors for atherosclerotic disease and to prevent health complications including liver disease and cancer.[19] Maintaining BMI at 21–22 kg/m^2 is optimal for those at risk for genetic or for other reasons such as prevention of type 2 diabetes. However, a quite modest weight loss of 5–10% has been shown to substantially benefit in all metabolic risk factors for overweight individuals. Modest lifestyle interventions are also effective in reducing the risk of developing diabetes in individuals with glucose intolerance.[20,21] A number of drugs have been shown to improve insulin resistance and obesity, and may shed lights to the underlying biochemical disorders. The PPAR-gamma agonists thiazolidinediones act by shifting intra-abdominal fat to subcutaneous fat depot[22] with an associated improvement in glucose tolerance and lipid profile. The expanded mass of metabolically favorable subcutaneous adipose tissue appears to serve as a sump for glucose and lipid disposal. Biguanides, used to treat type 2 diabetes, have also been shown to improve lipid profile and regulate menstrual cycles and increase fertility in patients with polycystic ovary syndrome. However, biguanides have not been shown to alter body fat distribution.

Treatment with antiobesity drugs such as tetrahydrolipstatin (e.g. orlistat)[23] and serotonin-noradrenaline reuptake inhibitors (e.g. sibutramine)[24] leads to weight loss and, more importantly, reduction in long-term weight regain. These drugs have been shown to reverse or delay most components of the metabolic syndrome. Orlistat has been shown to reduce the incidence of metabolic syndrome and of diabetes by 30–40%[25] and sibutramine is expected to have similar properties, but their effects on CHD are unknown. Although sibutramine treatment is contraindicated in individuals with high cardiovascular risk factors, the Sibutramine Cardiovascular Outcome Trial (SCOUT) has shown that sibutramine treatment with weight management is well tolerated by the majority of high-risk individuals with CVD.[26] Medical treatment of obesity remains ineffective, particularly long-term weight loss, for a large number of people even when intensive lifestyle modification combined with the limited available pharmacological agents. Bariatric surgery offers an alternative, but it has never been shown that bariatric surgery works well in people who have failed with a formal drug and diet approach. Various surgical procedures are now available including gastric banding, sleeve gastrectomy and gastric bypass. Criteria for bariatric surgery require a BMI of above 40 or 35–40 kg/m^2 with other significant comorbidity (e.g. sleep apnea, type 2 diabetes or hypertension) that could be improved by weight loss. All bariatric surgical procedures have potential complications, therefore should be performed in a specialist center. If the aim is a more modest maintained weight loss of 15 kg (adequate to reverse type 2 diabetes) is the target, then low-energy liquid diet methods may be cheaper and safer than surgical option.[27]

CONCLUSION

The relationship of obesity to insulin resistance and type 2 diabetes is a long-recognized phenomenon with fundamentally important scientific and clinical implications. The paradox that either absence or excess of adipose tissue causes insulin resistance highlights the complexity of this relationship and underscores the fact that adipose tissue undoubtedly subserves multiple functions. The release of a wide variety of molecules including hormones such as leptin, cytokines such as TNF-α and substrates such as FFAs allows the adipose organ to play a major regulatory role in energy balance and glucose homeostasis. However, there is a need to deepen our understanding of the cellular and molecular mechanisms underlying insulin sensitivity and secretion, including previously unidentified pathways such as those mediated by nuclear receptors such as PPARγ. Most likely, the complex orchestration of the relationship between adipose tissue, insulin action, and glucose homeostasis evolved out of survival needs to maintain fuel supplies when food was scarce. The challenge to use the increasing repertoire of adipocyte functions to shift the equation of energy intake and utilization toward reduced fat storage holds great opportunities to alter the course of human disease.

REFERENCES

1. Yalow RS, Berson SA. Immunoassay of endogenous insulin in man. J Clin Invest. 1960;39:1157-75.
2. Karam JH, Pavlatos FC, Grodsky GM, et al. Critical factors in excessive serum insulin response to glucose. Lancet. 1965;1:286-9.
3. Rabinowitz D, Zierler KJ. Forearm metabolism in obesity and its response to intra-arterial insulin. Characterization of insulin resistance and evidence for adaptive hyperinsulinemia. J Clin Invest. 1962;41:2173-81.
4. Reaven GM. Pathophysiology of insulin resistance in human disease. Physiol Rev. 1995;75:473-86.
5. Shepherd PR, Kahn BB. Glucose transporters and insulin action: implications for insulin resistance and diabetes mellitus. N Engl J Med. 1999;341:248-57.
6. Weyer C, Tataranni PA, Snitker S, et al. Increase in insulin action and fat oxidation after treatment with CL 316,243, a highly selective beta3-adrenoceptor agonist in humans. Diabetes. 1998;47:1555-61.
7. Colditz GA, Willett WC, Stampfer MJ, et al. Weight as a risk factor for clinical diabetes in women. Am J Epidemiol. 1990;132:501-13. 28.
8. Kissebah AH, Krakower GR. Regional adiposity and morbidity. Physiol Rev. 1994;74:761-811.
9. Patti M, Kahn CR. Lessons from transgenic and knockout animals about noninsulin-dependent diabetes mellitus. Trends Endocrinol Metab. 1996;7:311-9.
10. Bujalska IJ, Kumar S, Stewart PM. Does central obesity reflect "Cushing's disease of the omentum"? Lancet. 1997;349: 1210-3.
11. Peraldi P, Spiegelman B. TNF-alpha and insulin resistance: summary and future prospects. Mol Cell Biochem. 1998;182:169-75.
12. Elmquist JK, Maratos-Flier E, Saper CB, et al. Unraveling the central nervous system pathways underlying responses to leptin. Nat Neurosci. 1998;1:445-450.
13. Halaas JL, Gajiwala KS, Maffei M, et al. Weight-reducing effects of the plasma protein encoded by the obese gene. Science. 1995;269:543-6.
14. Campfield LA, Smith FJ, Guisez Y, et al. Recombinant mouse OB protein: evidence for a peripheral signal linking adiposity and central neural networks. Science. 1995;269:546-9.
15. Shimabukuro M, Koyama K, Chen G, et al. Direct antidiabetic effect of leptin through triglyceride depletion of tissues. Proc Natl Acad Sci USA. 1997;94:4637-41.
16. Montague CT, Farooqi IS, Whitehead JP, et al. 1997. Congenital leptin deficiency is associated with severe early-onset obesity in humans. Nature. 1997;387:903-8.
17. Clement K, Vaisse C, Lahlou N, et al. A mutation in the human leptin receptor gene causes obesity and pituitary dysfunction. Nature. 1998;392:398-401.
18. Public Health Service. Healthy people 2000: national health promotion and disease prevention objectives [DHHS publication no. (PHS)90-50212]. Washington, DC: US Department of Health and Human Services, Public Health Service, 1990.
19. Department of Health. Alcohol Guidelines Review—report from the Guidelines development group to the UK Chief Medical Officers, January 2016. London: Produced by William Lea for the Department of Health; 2016.
20. Tuomilehto J, Lindstrom J, Eriksson JG, et al. Prevention of type 2 diabetes mellitus by changes in lifestyle among subjects with impaired glucose tolerance. N Engl J Med. 2001;344:1343-50.
21. Knowler WC, Barrett-Connor E, Fowler SE, et al. Reduction in the incidence of type 2 diabetes with lifestyle intervention or metformin. N Engl J Med. 2002;346:393-403.
22. Kelly IE, Han TS, Walsh K, et al. Effects of a thiazolidinedione compound on body fat and fat distribution of patients with type 2 diabetes. Diabetes Care. 2001;24:683-98.
23. Davidson MH, Hauptman J, DiGirolamo M, et al. Weight control and risk factor reduction in obese subjects treated for 2 years with orlistat: a randomized controlled trial. JAMA. 1999; 281:235-42.
24. Fujioka K, Seaton TB, Rowe E, et al. Sibutramine/Diabetes Clinical Study Group. Weight loss with sibutramine improves glycaemic control and other metabolic parameters in obese patients with type 2 diabetes mellitus. Diabetes Obes Metab. 2000;2:175-87.
25. Didangelos TP, Thanopoulou AK, Bousboulas SH, et al. TheORLIstat and CArdiovascular risk profile in patients with metabolic syndrome and type 2 DIAbetes (ORLICARDIA) Study. Curr Med Res Opin. 2004;20:1393-401.
26. Torp-Pedersen C, Caterson I, Coutinho W, et al. Investigators SCOUT. Cardiovascular responses to weight management and sibutramine in high-risk subjects: an analysis from the SCOUT trial. Eur Heart J. 2007;28:2915-23.
27. Lean M, Brosnahan N, McLoone P, et al. Feasibility and indicative results from a 12-month low-energy liquid diet treatment and maintenance programme for severe obesity. Br J Gen Pract. 2013;63:115-24.

Anemia and Cardiodiabetes: Management Strategies

RK Saran, Mahim Saran, Vasudha Jain

INTRODUCTION

Cardiovascular disease is a leading cause of mortality in patients with diabetes accounting for 68% of deaths in patients aged 65 years or more. Diabetic adults are two-to-four times more likely to die from heart disease than those without diabetes. The American Heart Association also considers diabetes as one of the major controllable risk factors for cardiovascular disease.[1] This strong correlation between cardiovascular disease and diabetes has led some researchers to use the term "cardiodiabetes" to define the convergence of these conditions. Anemia is independently associated with an increased mortality rate in patients with chronic heart failure, left ventricular hypertrophy, chronic kidney disease (CKD), diabetes mellitus, and acute coronary syndrome.[2-4] It goes beyond doubt that coexistence of anemia with cardiodiabetes will further increase the morbidity and mortality. In a pooled analysis of diabetic individuals by Vlagopoulos et al. anemia was found to be a risk factor for adverse cardiovascular events and all-cause mortality primarily in those who also have CKD.[5]

ANEMIA IN CARDIODIABETES: CAUSE OR EFFECT

Anemia in cardiodiabetes can be multifactorial. Antiplatelets and anticoagulants given for the underlying cardiac disease may cause anemia due to gastrointestinal (GI) and genitourinary blood loss. Iron deficiency may also occur in heart failure due to malabsorption (due to congestion and abnormal production of hepcidin),[6] and reduced intracellular uptake of iron.[7] The proinflammatory cytokine contributing to insulin resistance in diabetes can also account for anemia by increasing hepcidin and hence decreasing the availability of oral iron. Increase in interleukin (IL)-6 has an antierythropoietic effect by increasing the resistance to erythropoietin and causing apoptosis of immature erythrocytes. While oral antidiabetic drugs and underlying renal insufficiency can cause anemia in type 2 diabetes, anemia in type 1 diabetes may be autoimmune.[8] In routine practice, renal insufficiency and the underlying proinflammatory state remain the common causes of anemia in diabetes. The "Anemia Correction in Diabetes" (ACORD) trial demonstrated that correction of anemia prevented an additional increase in left ventricular mass, and was associated with a significant improvement in quality of life.[9] Anemia-associated decreased oxygen-carrying capacity is compensated by hyperdynamic circulation. The resultant volume overload leads to myocardial hypertrophy and increased sympathetic and neurohumoral activity. Vasopressin and endothelin levels are also increased. All these can worsen heart failure and cause adverse arrhythmogenic remodeling.[10]

ANEMIA MANAGEMENT: SETBACKS DUE TO UNDERLYING CARDIODIABETES

Although anemia is associated with adverse cardiovascular outcomes and correction of anemia is required to improve the associated morbidity and mortality, both anemia and blood transfusions are associated with increased mortality. The hemoglobin (Hb) levels below which the risk of anemia outweighs the risk of transfusion remains undetermined.[11] However, a few studies are in favor of transfusion if Hb less than or equal to 8 g/dL, and suggest a neutral or harmful effect if Hb more than or equal to 11 g/dL.[12-15] Goal-directed red blood cell (RBC) transfusion therapy may be more appropriate than targeting specific Hb level. This concept has shown benefit in patients with severe sepsis and septic shock where physiological target of central venous oxygen saturation ($ScvO_2$) more than 70% is used as a target. Currently, we do not have enough data to set physiological parameters for goal-directed transfusion therapy in cardiac patients. Deciding for or against blood transfusion becomes much more difficult, if the same patient has diabetic nephropathy, especially if the kidney disease is advanced as the risks of fluid overload, hyperkalemia, and alloimmunization to human leukocyte antigen (HLA) class I antigens on white blood cells (WBCs) (in a potential transplant recipient) also need to be considered. In view of the above considerations, with the exception of patients with severe anemia who require urgent correction, the dictum should be to replete the iron stores and correct the cause of anemia.

Iron Therapy: Oral or Parenteral

Iron deficiency is one of the comorbidities which usually go unnoticed, as its symptoms are nonspecific and only iron studies help in its diagnosis. In patients with heart disease, especially those with heart failure iron deficiency are one of the major reasons for exercise intolerance.[16] Numerous oral iron preparations are available, but all have poor GI tolerance. Theoretically, increased hepcidin associated with heart failure, renal insufficiency, and underlying proinflammatory state associated with insulin resistance should limit the absorption of oral iron. This is further backed up by Iron Repletion Effects on Oxygen Uptake in Heart Failure (IRONOUT-HF) trial, which found little effect of oral iron in repleting iron stores or improving exercise capacity in anemic heart failure patients.[17] Oral iron, when tolerated, can be given for treatment in patients with diabetes, with the exception of patients with advanced CKD or on hemodialysis where the amount of iron losses (5–6 mg/day) cannot be compensated by oral iron therapy. Further in a systematic review and meta-analysis, Hb response with intravenous (IV) iron was more than with oral iron. The effect was of a lower magnitude in nondialysis CKD patients than those on hemodialysis.[18,19] Parenteral iron-related hypotension and anaphylactoid reactions are considerably less with newer more stable preparations like ferric carboxymaltose. CONFIRM-HF and FAIR-HF trials showed significant improvement in functional class and quality of life with ferric carboxymaltose in patients with heart failure and iron deficiency with or without anemia.[20,21] The European Society of Cardiology (ESC), 2016, guidelines also consider only IV route for iron administration in patients with heart failure and iron deficiency (level of evidence—Class IIA-a). In conclusion, oral iron, when tolerated, may be considered for treatment of iron deficiency in cardiodiabetes with the exception of those with heart failure and those with CKD on hemodialysis.

Erythropoietin

Recombinant human erythropoietin has revolutionized the treatment of anemia in patients with CKD. Anemia and CKD are commonly associated with heart failure, collectively termed as cardiorenal anemia syndrome. Some studies have shown improvement of insulin resistance with erythropoietin in patients on hemodialysis.[22,23] But, hypertension and erythropoietin resistance are some of its potential side effects. Considering the fact that anemia is associated with poor prognosis in heart failure, correction of anemia with erythropoietin may be beneficial for these patients. But erythropoietin-associated hypertension and hyperviscosity may be detrimental for this condition. This is supported by various trials in CKD patients where treatment of patients to an Hb target of more than or equal to 13 g/dL increased mortality and adverse cardiovascular events.[24-26] A critical review of various randomized controlled trials and observational studies by Singh et al. concluded that no data supports the correction of Hb above 12 g/dL in patients on dialysis.[27]

Thus, the dictum should be to administer erythropoietin in patients of cardiodiabetes only if anemia is related to underlying CKD to maintain Hb between 11 g/dL and 12 g/dL.

CONCLUSION

Anemia in heart failure and diabetes can be multifactorial. It is associated with increased morbidity and mortality in cardiodiabetes. Identification and treatment of the cause of anemia should be the first priority. Blood transfusion should be reserved for patients with severe symptomatic anemia or Hb less than 8 g/dL. Oral iron, when tolerated, should be given with the exception of patients with heart failure and those on hemodialysis, where IV iron is recommended. Erythropoietin may be given in patients with CKD, but Hb should be maintained between 11 g/dL and 12 g/dL; and Hb target should not exceed 13 g/dL.

REFERENCES

1. American Heart Association. (2015). Cardiovascular disease and diabetes. [online] Available from http://www.heart.org/HEARTORG/Conditions/More/Diabetes/WhyDiabetesMatters/Cardiovascular-Disease-Diabetes_UCM_313865_Article.jsp/#.WVzhM_l942w. [Accessed August, 2017].
2. Horwich TB, Fonarow GC, Hamilton MA, et al. Anemia is associated with worse symptoms, greater impairment in functional capacity and a significant increase in mortality in patients with advanced heart failure. J Am Coll Cardiol. 2002;39:1780-6.
3. Muzzarelli S, Pfisterer M. Anemia as independent predictor of major events in elderly patients with chronic angina. Am Heart J. 2006;152:991-6.
4. Vaglio J, Safley DM, Rahman M, et al. Relation of anemia at discharge to survival after acute coronary syndromes. Am J Cardiol. 2005;96:496-9.
5. Vlagopoulos PT, Tighiouart H, Weiner DE, et al. Anemia as a risk factor for cardiovascular disease and all-cause mortality in diabetes: the impact of chronic kidney disease. J Am Soc Nephrol. 2005;16:3403-10.
6. Jankowska EA, von Haehling S, Anker SD, et al. Iron deficiency and heart failure: diagnostic dilemmas and therapeutic perspectives. Eur Heart J. 2013;34:816-29.
7. Maeder MT, Khammy O, dos Remedios C, et al. Myocardial and systemic iron depletion in heart failure implications for anemia accompanying heart failure. J Am Coll Cardiol. 2011;58:474-80.
8. Angelousi A, Larger E. Anaemia, a common but often unrecognized risk in diabetic patients: a review. Diabetes Metab. 2015;41:18-27.
9. Ritz E, Laville M, Bilous RW, et al. Target level for hemoglobin correction in patients with diabetes and CKD: primary results of the Anemia Correction in Diabetes (ACORD) Study. Am J Kidney Dis. 2007;49:194-207.
10. Xu D, Murakoshi N, Sairenchi T, et al. Anemia and reduced kidney function as risk factors for new onset of atrial fibrillation (from the Ibaraki prefectural health study). Am J Cardiol. 2015;115:328-33.
11. Du Pont-Thibodeau G, Harrington K, Lacroix J. Anemia and red blood cell transfusion in critically ill cardiac patients. Ann Intensive Care. 2014;4:16.
12. Alexander KP, Chen AY, Wang TY, et al. Transfusion practice and outcomes in non-ST-segment elevation acute coronary syndromes. Am Heart J. 2008;155:1047-53.
13. Aronson D, Dann EJ, Bonstein L, et al. Impact of red blood cell transfusion on clinical outcomes in patients with acute myocardial infarction. Am J Cardiol. 2008;102:115-9.
14. Wu WC, Rathore SS, Wang Y, et al. Blood transfusion in elderly patients with acute myocardial infarction. N Engl J Med. 2001;345:1230-6.
15. Garfinkle M, Lawler PR, Filion KB, et al. Red blood cell transfusion and mortality among patients hospitalized for acute coronary syndromes: a systematic review. Int J Cardiol. 2013;164:151-7.
16. Ponikowski P, Voors AA, Anker SD, et al. 2016 ESC Guidelines for the diagnosis and treatment of acute and chronic heart failure: The Task Force for the diagnosis and treatment of acute and chronic heart failure of the European Society of Cardiology (ESC). Developed with the special contribution of the Heart Failure Association (HFA) of the ESC. Eur Heart J. 2016;37:2129-200.
17. Lewis GD, Semigran MJ, Givertz MM, et al. Oral Iron Therapy for Heart Failure with Reduced Ejection Fraction. Circ Heart Fail. 2016;9(5): pii: e000345.
18. Rozen-Zvi B, Gafter-Gvili A, Paul M, et al. Intravenous versus oral iron supplementation for the treatment of anemia in CKD: systematic review and meta-analysis. Am J Kidney Dis. 2008;52:897-906.
19. Macdougall IC. Iron supRozen-Zvi B, Gafter-Gvili A, et al. Intravenous versus oral iron supplementation for the treatment of anemia in CKD: systematic review and meta-analysis. Am J Kidney Dis. 2008;52:897-906.
20. Ponikowski P, van Veldhuisen DJ, Comin-Colet J, et al. Beneficial effects of long-term intravenous iron therapy with ferric carboxymaltose in patients with symptomatic heart failure and iron deficiency. Eur Heart J. 2015;36:657-68.
21. Anker SD, Comin Colet J, Filippatos G, et al. Ferric carboxymaltose in patients with heart failure and iron deficiency. N Engl J Med. 2009;361:2436-48.
22. Mak RH. Correction of anemia by erythropoietin reverses insulin resistance and hyperinsulinemia in uremia. Am J Physiol. 1996;270:F839-44.
23. Spaia S, Pangalos M, Askepidis N, et al. Effect of short-term rHuEPO treatment on insulin resistance in haemodialysis patients. Nephron. 2000;84:320-5.
24. Besarab A, Bolton WK, Browne JK, et al. The effects of normal as compared with low hematocrit values in patients with cardiac disease who are receiving hemodialysis and epoetin. N Engl J Med. 1998;339:584-90.
25. Singh AK, Szczech L, Tang KL, et al. Correction of anemia with epoetin alfa in chronic kidney disease. N Engl J Med. 2006;355:2085-98.
26. Pfeffer MA, Burdmann EA, Chen CY, et al. A trial of darbepoetin alfa in type 2 diabetes and chronic kidney disease. N Engl J Med. 2009;361:2019-32.
27. Singh AK, Fishbane S. The optimal hemoglobin in dialysis patients—a critical review. Semin Dial. 2008;21:1-6.

CHAPTER 9

Endothelial Dysfunction in Atrial Fibrillation with Type 2 DM

Shishu Shankar Mishra, Biswaranjan Mishra, Satyanarayan Routray, Dipak Ranjan Das

INTRODUCTION

Diabetes mellitus is one of the most common chronic conditions and its prevalence is increasing. In 2014, the number of patients with diabetes was estimated at 387 millions people worldwide; of whom, around half were undiagnosed.[1] The projection for 2035 is that the number of patients with diabetes will have risen to 592 millions.[1] It is well known that cardiovascular and cerebrovascular diseases are substantially more frequent among patients with diabetes.[2] However, the mechanisms of this influence are still not completely understood. It is not known whether permanent hyperglycemia or wide fluctuations in glucose levels—from hypoglycemia to hyperglycemia, which is commonly seen in treated diabetics, is most responsible for cardiovascular damage. Atrial fibrillation (AF), the most frequent sustained cardiac arrhythmia, is associated with an increased risk of stroke, thromboembolism, heart failure, and recurrent hospital admissions.[3] The prevalence of AF is constantly increasing and it affects about 2.2 million individuals in America and 4.5 millions in Europe.[4,5] Studies have shown that diabetes is frequently associated with AF.[6] However, it is difficult to determine whether diabetes directly affects the atrial tissue or whether different pathways are involved, including hypertension, coronary artery disease (CAD), and abnormal activity of the autonomic nervous system. The number of diabetes patients are increasing in Indian subcontinent to extent that *India is said to be the capital of diabetes today*. The cardiovascular involvement in diabetes with AF can be studied early with detection of endothelial dysfunction (ED).

MECHANISM OF THE RELATIONSHIP BETWEEN DIABETES AND ATRIAL FIBRILLATION

Diabetes is associated with numerous metabolic defects including insulin resistance, impaired glucose tolerance, proinflammatory mediators, abnormalities of hemostasis, fibrinolysis, angiogenesis, and extracellular matrix turnover[7-9] (Fig. 1). All of these metabolic changes lead to ED, abnormal activation of the renin-angiotensin-aldosterone system (RAAS) and acceleration of atherogenesis, which could be responsible for AF occurrence.[2,7-9] Diabetes could also cause structural, electrical, electromechanical, and autonomic remodeling.[10] The possible mechanisms involved in AF are projected in Figure 1.

CLINICAL STUDIES ABOUT DIABETES AND ATRIAL FIBRILLATION

Many studies have correlated AF and diabetes. Studies like Swedish community study, ARIC study, CARAF study, NAVIGATOR investigators, Movahed et al. showed increased incidence of AF in diabetes. In this double jeopardy situation, the endothelium of whole body is at the risk of greater dysfunction.

ATRIAL FIBRILLATION AND ENDOTHELIAL DYSFUNCTION

Atrial fibrillation is the most common and clinically important arrhythmia.[11] Incidence of AF increases with age.

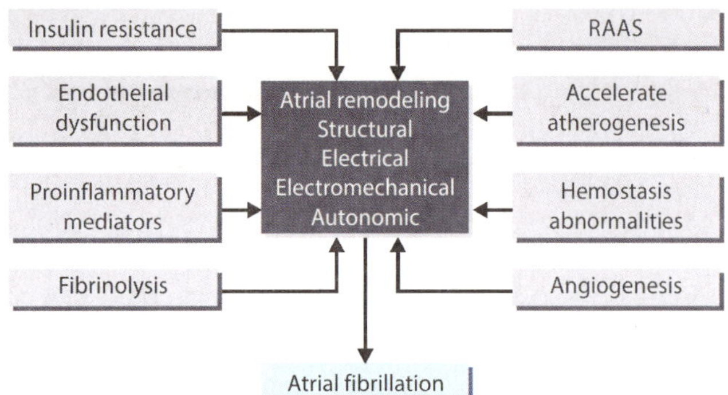

Fig. 1: Possible link of diabetes and atrial fibrillation
Abbreviations: RAAS, renin-angiotensin-aldosterone system

It is commonly associated with other structural heart diseases such as valvular heart disease, primary myocardial disease, CAD, pericardial disease, and grown up congenital heart diseases. It is also associated with other systemic diseases such as diabetes mellitus, hypertension, thyroid disorders, lung diseases, infection, and postcardiac surgery patients.[12] Although ED is associated with AF, the comorbid conditions associated with AF also have ED irrespective of presence or absence of AF. Several studies have identified left atrial ED in AF, even in cases of lone AF. Increased inflammatory and oxidative stress, platelet activation has been demonstrated in atrial endocardium in cases of AF.[13] Over the past decade, parameters of systemic ED such as brachial artery flow-mediated dilation (FMD) and other modalities have been demonstrated both experimentally and clinically in various subsets of AF patients.[14]

Dimethylarginines, the endogenous methylated derivatives of L-arginine, the precursor of nitric oxide (NO) are asymmetric dimethylarginine (ADMA), and symmetric dimethylarginine (SDMA). ADMA can inhibit NO synthase (NOS) and thus contribute to ED, inflammation, and oxidative stress in cardiovascular diseases.[15] ADMA also contributes to abnormal blood flow responses, ED, and atherogenesis in type 2 diabetics.[16] SDMA does not inhibit NOS directly but could interfere with the cellular uptake of L-arginine.[17] In patients with CAD, ADMA has shown to impair endothelium-dependent relaxation and is considered a circulating marker of ED.[18] ADMA is also implicated in cardiac dysfunction, reduced cardiac output, increased vascular resistance, and vascular injury in animal models.[19] Increased plasma level of ADMA has not only shown to be an independent risk factor for adverse cardiovascular events in CAD,[20] but also found to be increased in patients with AF and is an independent predictors of recurrence of AF after electrical cardioversion.[21] A recent study also confirmed that AF patients referred for a coronary angiogram had a higher level of ADMA than patients without AF, and they experienced more adverse cardiovascular events during follow-up independently of current risk scores.[22]

Takahashi et al. for the first time reported the association of systemic ED in AF by venous occlusion plethysmography in patients of AF.[23] He concluded that endothelium-dependent dilation is reduced. This landmark study generated interest for noninvasive evaluation of systemic endothelial function in AF. Publication of several trials subsequently established FMD technique as a reliable marker to assess endothelial function in AF.[24] These studies consistently showed impaired FMD in patients with AF as compared to healthy individuals.[25] In one of our cases, ED has been demonstrated in a patient with AF (Figs 2A and B). In the same patient, after 2 weeks of conversion to sinus rhythm, FMD normalized (Figs 3A and B). Improvement, in endothelial function after restoring sinus rhythm, was also demonstrated in a few trials.[26]

Nicolas Girerd et al. demonstrated association of periatrial epicardial adipose tissue (EAT) with increased levels of intercellular adhesion molecule 1 (ICAM-1) and von Willebrand factor (vWF), which are biomarkers of ED. These results suggest that local EAT rather than regional

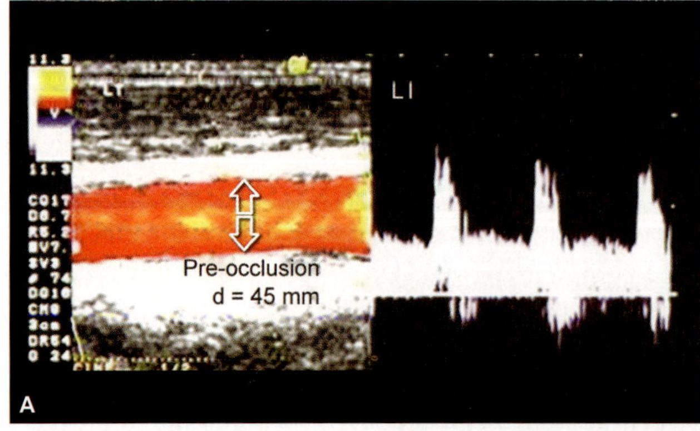

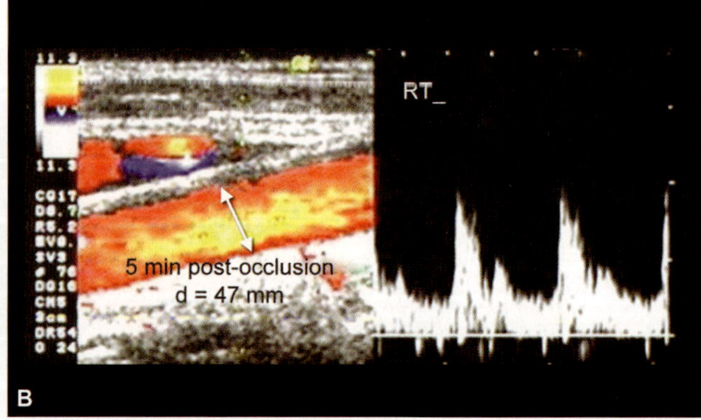

Figs 2A and B: (A) Pre-occlusion brachial artery dimension 45 mm; (B) post-occlusion dimension 47 mm, flow-mediated dilation (FMD) = 47 – 45/45 = 4% in a case of atrial fibrillation indicating severe endothelial dysfunction

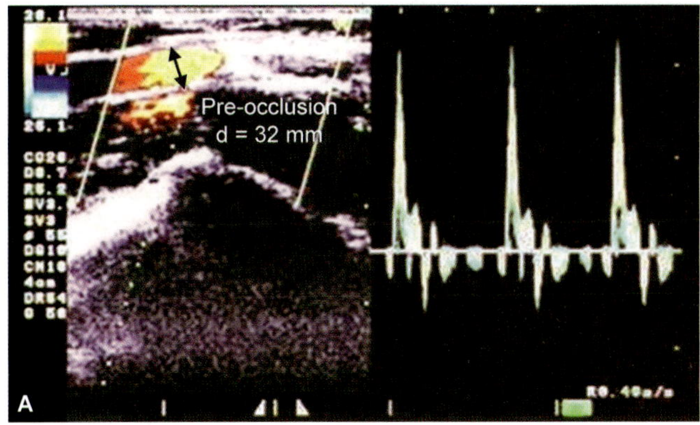

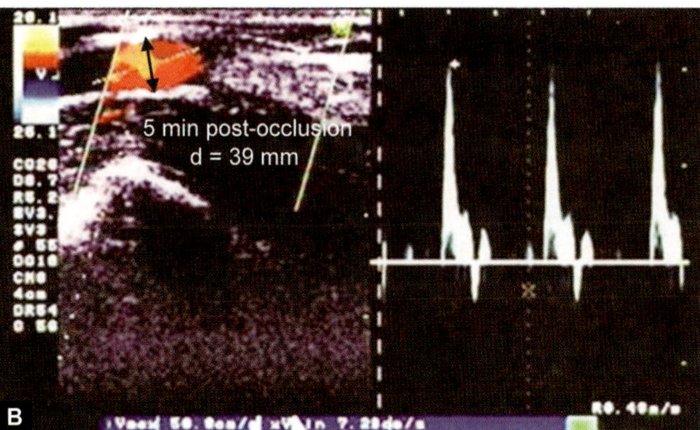

Figs 3A and B: Flow-mediated dilation (FMD) 2 weeks after conversion to sinus rhythm showing normalization of endothelial function: (A) Pre-occlusion brachial artery dimension 32 mm; (B) Post-occlusion dimension 39 mm, FMD = 39 – 32/32 = 21%

or total adiposity may modulate ED in patients with AF. These findings suggest that EAT may modulate ED possibly through a paracrine mechanism and this modulation might influence the prognosis of AF patients. These results suggest a potential role of EAT quantification to risk stratify these growing patient population.[27]

However, most of these trials included cases with AF, who have associated atherosclerotic risk factors such as aging, hypertension, CAD, and diabetes, which are known to be associated with ED. Keeping in view the known causes of ED, studies also demonstrated independent association of AF and ED after adjustments for various comorbidities.[28] ED has also been demonstrated in idiopathic AF and lone AF.[29]

PATHOPHYSIOLOGIC MECHANISM OF ENDOTHELIAL DYSFUNCTION AND ATRIAL FIBRILLATION

Endothelial dysfunction is maintained by a *regular rhythmic pulsatile movement of the whole cardiovascular tree*, irregular beats with variable stroke volume create a chaotic flow and pulsatility in the vascular system starting from the left atrium (LA) to the whole arterial tree; and, in the process, it stimulates the release of lots of endocrine and paracrine hormones that result in ED as a part of electrophysiological remodeling of the endothelium of the whole body.

Pathophysiologic mechanisms of ED in AF have not been fully understood. It is hypothesized that the pathophysiologic processes that give rise to remodeling of LA in AF may be similar to the mechanism of ED in systemic circulation. Shear stress by laminar blood flow controls NO production under different physiologic circumstances.[30] In AF, irregular cardiac cycles produce varying stroke volumes, and varying shear stress in systemic vessels, which *act as a negative stimulant for NO production and endothelial NOS expression,* which is further supported by findings of reduced plasma nitrite/nitrate levels in AF.[31] In some studies, heart rate is inversely related to FMD in the univariate analysis, possibly reflecting an unfavorable effect of changed hemodynamics in AF.[32] A causative link between oxidative stress and AF has been demonstrated with nicotinamide adenine dinucleotide phosphate (NADPH) oxidases as a source of reactive oxygen species (ROS).[33] Experimental data showed that AF causes a downregulation of NOS expression, with a fall in NO concentrations of 73% in the left atrial appendage, suggesting a positive feedback loop in the maintenance of AF.[34]

Other observations are that levels of ADMA, a marker of ED is found to be higher in patients with AF than those having sinus rhythm. ADMA levels are also higher in symptomatic AF when compared to silent AF. ADMA levels are associated with risk of developing AF beyond traditional risk factors. All these indicate pathophysiologic association between dimethylarginine and AF. SDMA competitively inhibits L-arginine uptake. It has also been reported the stimulating effects of SDMA on ROS production by monocytes.[34] Recent data shows that ADMA levels are higher in age-matched patients with AF than in control non-AF patients.[35] ADMA levels are elevated in acute and persistent tachyarrhythmia and after prolonged rapid atrial pacing.[36] When serum ADMA concentrations are increased, risk of recurrence of AF is more after radiofrequency catheter-based ablation or electrical cardioversion.[37] The mechanism postulated that ADMA may be responsible for increased oxidative stress by uncoupling of the electron transport between NOS and L-arginine, decreasing availability of NO.[38] ADMA has cytokine-like properties, which cause polymorphonuclear neutrophilic activation and significantly impair NO synthesis.[39] In human endothelial cell cultures, it has not been demonstrated that ADMA itself reduces NOS gene expression, but altered NO availability results in abnormal Ca^{2+} handling, fibrosis stimulation and development of AF.[40]

By reducing endothelial NO production, ADMA accumulation may result in ED in the LA, thus promoting thrombus formation and subsequent thromboembolic events.[41]

Another hypothesis proposes that AF-induced damage to the endocardium of the LA may contribute to systemic ED by *reducing circulating nitroso compounds* that serve as endogenous NO donors to systemic vessels.[42] These findings hypothesized that, though, AF involves the LA, ED as a systemic phenomenon is associated with it.

Several other pathophysiologic mechanisms are proposed, such as activation of renin–angiotensin–aldosterone axis,[43] and neurohumoral activation.[44] Heightened inflammatory and oxidative stress are also implicated in the development of systemic ED in AF. C-reactive protein (CRP) levels in AF patients are significantly higher than in healthy individuals reinforcing inflammation as one of the pathophysiologic mechanisms of ED. CRP is inversely related with FMD thereby reinforcing an independent association of CRP and FMD.[45]

ENDOTHELIAL DYSFUNCTION—A PROGNOSTIC INDICATOR IN ATRIAL FIBRILLATION

Long-term prognosis in AF is generally favorable when rate and rhythm control is adequately achieved. Although the prognostic implications of systemic ED determined by FMD in AF patients are not well elucidated, impaired endothelial function is definitely considered as an important risk factor for thrombosis and embolism.[46] Reduced NO availability and subsequent ED have recently been recognized as possible contributor to the worse prognosis in AF.[47] It is well known that incidence of heart failure and stroke is increased with increased indicators of ED.[48] Indicators of ED are also adversely associated with adverse vascular events in patients in sinus rhythm. The implication of these findings is that indicators of ED such as FMD may be considered as an indicator of increased risk of thrombosis and other adverse vascular event in AF patients. ADMA level, as a marker of ED and impaired NOS activity, provides additional prognostic information, complementary to left ventricular (LV) dysfunction or heart failure symptoms, which may be particularly relevant in these high-risk patients.

THERAPY IN ATRIAL FIBRILLATION DIRECTED TO ENDOTHELIAL DYSFUNCTION

Limitations in the current pharmacological and intervention-based therapies for AF have generated great interest in identification of various molecular pathways mediating structural and electrical atrial remodeling, including ED leading to AF. Considering the role of ED in genesis and maintenance of AF, correcting it is a challenge in therapy of AF.

Nitric oxide synthase inhibitors have emerged as a novel therapeutic target in AF.[49] An increased expression of adhesion molecules mediated by angiotensin II has been demonstrated in the fibrillating atria as an indicator of ED. Studies have shown that angiotensin-converting enzyme inhibitor (ACEIs) significantly reduce increased expression of adhesion molecules, supporting its role in correcting endothelial function. Aldosterone antagonists are therapeutic agents to handle the RAAS system.[50] The role of these agents becomes more important in AF, considering the evidence of intracardiac production of aldosterone. Further, data from trials investigating ACE and aldosterone inhibition as "upstream" therapies will yield useful information regarding the use of these agents possibly for prevention of AF.[51] Statins have an important role in the treatment of patients of AF with high level of high-sensitivity CRP. Research in the field of messenger ribonucleic acid (mRNA) is rapidly evolving and generates considerable interest in diagnostic and therapeutics in patients with AF. A better understanding of oxidative stress, ion channel remodeling, alterations of connexins may result in a definitive treatment of AF.[52]

CONCLUSION

Type 2 diabetes is one of the most common chronic conditions with increasing prevalence and AF is the most frequent sustained cardiac arrhythmia. The association of those two conditions is increasingly recognized with aging population. Diabetes mellitus is one of the major metabolic factors responsible for ED and when diabetes and AF are combined, it becomes a double jeopardy to the endothelium. Persistent AF is associated with ED and independent of associated risk factors. More the arrhythmia duration, more profound is the ED. Lower FMD and other makers of systemic ED are seen in patients with AF. Association of ADMA, a circulating marker of ED and oxidative stress has also been demonstrated in AF. Markers of ED have a role in risk stratifying AF, to those who have higher risk; which have important therapeutic implication. Newer therapeutic modalities for AF such as statins, ACEIs, angiotensin receptor blockers (ARBs), aldosterone antagonists, l-arginine, and targeted drugs for ion channels for improving endothelial function, particularly at molecular level, may not only prevent this dreadful arrhythmia, but also reduce the associated cardiovascular morbidity and mortality. Replenishing the endothelial progenitor cell may be another modality of future treatment for the endothelial derangement.

REFERENCES

1. International Diabetes Federation. (2014). Key findings. [online] Available from http://www.idf.org/diabetesatlas/update-2014. [Accessed August, 2017].
2. Martin-Timon I, Sevillano-Collantes C, Segura-Galindo A, et al. Type 2 diabetes and cardiovascular disease: have all risk factors the same strength? World J Diabetes. 2014;5:444-70.
3. Benjamin EJ, Levy D, Vaziri SM, et al. Independent risk factors for atrial fibrillation in a population-based cohort. The Framingham Heart Study. JAMA. 1994;271:840-4.
4. Camm AJ, Kirchhof P, Lip GY, et al. Guidelines for the management of atrial fibrillation: the Task Force for the management of atrial fibrillation of the European Society of Cardiology (ESC). Europace. 2010;12:1360-420.
5. Fuster V, Ryden LE, Cannom DS, et al. ACC/AHA/ESC 2006 guidelines for the management of patients with atrial fibrillation: full text: a report of the American College of Cardiology/American Heart Association Task Force on practice guidelines and the European Society of Cardiology Committee for Practice Guidelines (Writing Committee to Revise the 2001 guidelines for the management of patients with atrial fibrillation) developed in collaboration with the European Heart Rhythm Association and the Heart Rhythm Society. Europace. 2006;8:651-745.
6. Movahed MR, Hashemzadeh M, Jamal MM. Diabetes mellitus is a strong, independent risk for atrial fibrillation and flutter in addition to other cardiovascular disease. Int J Cardiol. 2005;105:315-8.
7. Sun Y, Hu D. The link between diabetes and atrial fibrillation: cause or correlation? J Cardiovasc Dis Res. 2010;1:10-1.
8. Tayebjee MH, Lim HS, MacFadyen RJ, et al. Matrix metalloproteinase-9 and tissue inhibitor of metalloproteinase-1 and -2 in type 2 diabetes: effect of 1 year's cardiovascular risk reduction therapy. Diabetes Care 2004;27:2049-51.
9. Lim HS, MacFadyen RJ, Lip GY. Diabetes mellitus, the renin-angiotensin-aldosterone system, and the heart. Arch Intern Med. 2004;164:1737-48.
10. Zhang Q, Liu T, Ng CY, et al. Diabetes mellitus and atrial remodeling: mechanisms and potential upstream therapies. Cardiovasc Ther. 2014;32:233-41.
11. Heeringa J, van der Kuip DA, Hofman A, et al. Prevalence, incidence and lifetime risk of atrial fibrillation: the Rotterdam study. Eur Heart J. 2006;27:949-53.
12. Schoonderwoerd BA, Smit MD, Pen L, et al. New risk factors for atrial fibrillation: causes of "not-so-lone atrial fibrillation". Europace. 2008;10:668-73.
13. Cai H, Li Z, Goette A, et al. Downregulation of endo-cardial nitric oxide synthase expression and nitric oxide production in atrial fibrillation. Circulation. 2002;106: 2854-8.
14. Mondillo S, Sabatini L, Agricola E, et al. Correlation between left atrial size, prothrombotic state and markers of endothelial dysfunction in patients with lone chronic nonrheumatic atrial fibrillation. Int J Cardiol. 2000;75:227-32.
15. Sibal L, Agarwal SC, Home PD, et al. The role of asymmetric dimethylarginine (ADMA) in endothelial dysfunction and cardiovascular disease. Curr Cardiol Rev. 2010;6:82-90.
16. Fard A, Tuck CH, Donis JA, et al. Acute Elevations of Plasma Asymmetric Dimethylarginine and Impaired Endothelial Function in Response to a High-Fat Meal in Patients With Type 2 Diabetes. Arterioscler Thromb Vasc Biol. 2000;20:2039-44.
17. Closs EI, Basha FZ, Habermeier A, et al. Interference of L-arginine analogues with L-arginine transport mediated by the y+ carrier hCAT-2B. Nitric Oxide. 1997;1:65-73.
18. Stuhlinger MC, Oka RK, Graf EE, et al. Endothelial dysfunction induced by hyperhomocyst(e)inemia: Role of asymmetric dimethylarginine. Circulation. 2003;108:933-8.
19. Schnabel R, Blankenberg S, Lubos E, et al. Asymmetric dimethylarginine and the risk of cardiovascular events and death in patients with coronary artery disease: Results from the atherogene study. Circ Res. 2005;97:e53-9.
20. Zeller M, Korandji C, Guilland JC, et al. Impact of asymmetric dimethylarginine on mortality after acute myocardial infarction. Arterioscler Thromb Vasc Biol. 2008;28:954-60.
21. Cengel A, Sahinarslan A, Biberoglu G, et al. Asymmetrical dimethylarginine level in atrial fibrillation. Acta cardiol. 2008;63: 33-7.
22. Chao TF, Lu TM, Lin YJ, et al. Plasma asymmetric dimethylarginine and adverse events in patients with atrial fibrillation referred for coronary angiogram. PloS one. 2013;8:e71675.
23. Takahashi N, Ishibashi Y, Shimada T, et al. Atrial fibrillation impairs endothelial function in forearm vessels in humans. J Cardiac Fail. 2001;7:45-54.
24. Freestone B, Chong A, Nuttall S, et al. Impaired flow mediated dilation as evidence of endothelial dysfunction in chronic atrial fibrillation: relationship to plasma von Willebrand factor and soluble E-selectin levels. Thromb Res. 2008;122:85-90.
25. Skalidis EI, Zacharis EA, Tsetis DK, et al. Endothelial cell function during atrial fibrillation and after restoration of sinus rhythm. Am J Cardiol. 2007;99:1258-62.
26. Guazzi M, Belletti S, Lenatti L, et al. Effects of cardioversion of atrial fibrillation on endothelial function in hypertension and diabetes. Eur J Clin Invest. 2007;37:26-34.
27. Nicolas G1, Alina S, Francis B, et al. Periatrial epicardial fat is associated with markers of endothelial dysfunction in patients with atrial fibrillation. Plos One. 2013;8:e77167.
28. Butt M, Dwivedi G, Blann A, et al. Endothelial dysfunction: methods of assessment & implications for cardiovascular disease. Curr Pharm Des. 2010;1:3442-54.
29. Potpara TS, Lyp GYH. Lone atrial fibrillation: what is known and what is to come. Int J Clin Pract. 2011;65:446-57.
30. Pan S. Molecular mechanisms responsible for the atheroprotective effects of laminar shear stress. Antioxid Redox Signal. 2009;11:1669-82.
31. Minamino T, Kitazake M, Sato H, et al. Plasma levels of nitrite/nitrate and platelet cGMP levels are decreased in patients with atrial fibrillation. Artherioscler Thromb Vasc Biol. 1997;17:3191-5.
32. Polovina M, Potpara T, Giga V, et al. Impaired endothelial function in lone atrial fibrillation. Vojnosanit Pregl. 2013;70:908-14.
33. Purohit A, Rokita AG, Guan X, et al. Oxidized Ca/calmodulin-dependent protein kinase ii triggers atrial fibrillation. Circulation. 2013;128:1748-57.
34. Schepers E, Glorieux G, Dhondt A, et al. Role of symmetric dimethylarginine in vascular damage by increasing ROS via store-operated calcium influx in monocytes. Nephrol Dial Transplant. 2009;24:1429-35.
35. Schulze F, Carter AM, Schwedhelm E, et al. Symmetric dimethylarginine predicts all-cause mortality following ischemic stroke. Atherosclerosis. 2010;208:518-23.
36. Goette A, Hammwohner M, Bukowska A, et al. The impact of rapid atrial pacing on ADMA and endothelial NOS. Int J Cardiol. 2012;154:141-6.
37. Xia W, Yin Z, Li J, et al. Effects of rosuvastatin on asymmetric dimethylarginine levels and early atrial fibrillation recurrence after electrical cardioversion. Pacing Clin Electrophysiol. 2009;32: 1562-6.
38. Usui M, Matsuoka H, Miyazaki H, et al. Increased endogenous nitric oxide synthase inhibitor in patients with congestive heart failure. Life Sci. 1998;62:2425-30.
39. Von Leitner EC, Klinke A, Atzler D, et al. Pathogenic cycle between the endogenous nitric oxide synthase inhibitor asymmetrical dimethylarginine and the leukocyte-derived hemoprotein myeloperoxidase. Circulation. 2011;124:2735-45.

40. Boos CJ, Anderson RA, Lip GY. Is atrial fibrillation an inflammatory disorder? Eur Heart J. 2006;27:136-49.
41. Liu H, Qu X, Liang Z, et al. Variance of DDAH/PRMT/ADMA pathway in atrial fibrillation dogs. Biochem Biophys Res Commun. 2008;377:884-8.
42. Guazzi M, Arena R. Endothelial dysfunction and pathophysiological correlates in atrial fibrillation. Heart. 2009;95:102-6.
43. Wachtell K, Lehto M, Gerdts E, et al. Angiotensin II receptor blockade reduces new-onset atrial fibrillation and subsequent stroke compared to atenolol: the Losartan Intervention for End Point Reduction in Hypertension (LIFE) Study. J Am Coll Cardiol. 2005;45:712-9.
44. Korantzopoulos P, Kolettis TM, Galarix D, et al. The role of oxidative stress in the pathogenesis and perpetuation of atrial fibrillation. Int J Cardiol. 2007;115:135-43.
45. Parthenakis FI, Patrianakos AP, Skalidis EI, et al. Atrial fibrillation is associated with increased neurohumoral activation and reduced exercise tolerance in patients with non-ischemic dilated cardiomyopathy. Int J Cardiol. 2007;118:206-14.
46. Freestone B, Chong AY, Nuttall S, et al. Soluble E-selectin, von Willebrand factor, soluble thrombomodulin, and total body nitrate/nitrite product as indices of endothelial damage/dysfunction in paroxysmal, persistent, and permanent atrial fibrillation. Chest 2007;132:1253-8.
47. Polovina MM, Lip GY, Potpara TS. Endothelial (dys)function in lone atrial fibrillation. Curr Pharm Des. 2015;21:622-45.
48. Yavuz BB, Yavuz B, Sener DD, et al. Advanced age is associated with endothelial dysfunction in healthy elderly subjects. Gerontology. 2008;54:153-6.
49. Rochette L, Lorin J, Zeller M, et al. Nitric oxide synthase inhibition and oxidative stress in cardiovascular diseases: Possible therapeutic targets? Pharmacol Ther. 2013;140:239-57.
50. Goette A, Schön N, Kirchhof P, et al. Angiotensin II-antagonist in paroxysmal atrial fibrillation (ANTIPAF) trial. Circ Arrhythm Electrophysiol. 2012;5:43-51.
51. Chen K, Mehta JL, Li D, et al. Transforming growth factor receptor endoglin is expressed in cardiac fibroblasts and modulates the profibrogenic actions of angiotensin II. Circ Res. 2004;95:1167-73.
52. Kanagaratnam P, Cherian A, Stanbridge RD, et al. Relationship between connexins and atrial activation during human atrial fibrillation. J Cardiovasc Electrophysiol. 2004;15:206-16.

CHAPTER

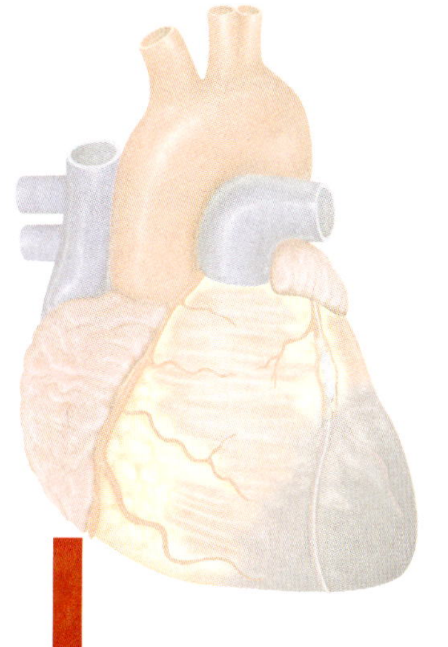

ACS, Cardiodiabetes, and Women

BP Singh, Ravi Vishnu Prasad, Nishant Tripathy, Nirav Kumar

INTRODUCTION

Cardiovascular diseases have become leading cause of death in women as well as in men worldwide. Each year, an estimated 4 million women develop new and recurrent myocardial infarction (MI) and/or coronary heart disease in the United States of America alone.[1,2] Women have worse outcomes after acute coronary syndromes (ACS) as compared to men. The reasons behind these differences remain unclear. These fundamental gaps in knowledge are compounded by the underrepresentation of women in cardiovascular clinical trials.[3]

RISK FACTORS OF ACUTE CORONARY SYNDROME IN CARDIODIABETES WOMEN

Women with ACS have long been described as older and sicker than their male counterparts. The GUSTO-IIb trial showed that women with ACS were older and had higher rates of traditional risk factors such as diabetes mellitus (DM), hypertension, and previous congestive heart failure as compared with men with ACS[4,5] (Fig. 1). Various other studies have also reported similar patterns.[6]

DIABETES MELLITUS—TRADITIONAL ATHEROSCLEROTIC CARDIOVASCULAR DISEASE RISK FACTOR IN WOMEN

Diabetes carries a differential risk of ACS between women and men. The increasing prevalence of DM is concerning because it is a potent risk factor for atherosclerotic cardiovascular disease (ASCVD) and has long been recognized for greater risk of ASCVD death in women as compared with men.[7] The INTER-HEART study, a global, case-control study in more than 27,000 participants, showed that women with diabetes were 4.3 times more likely to develop an MI than women without diabetes.[8] By contrast, in men with diabetes the risk of MI was 2.7 times higher than in men without diabetes. There is a three-fold excess fatal CAD risk in women with DM compared with nondiabetic women. In a meta-analysis of over 8,50,000 individuals, the relative risk for CVD was 44% greater in women with DM than in similarly affected men.[9] Thus, the presence of DM needs an aggressive CVD prevention strategy in women. Growing evidence suggests that these diabetic women have more impaired endothelium-dependent vasodilation, a hypercoagulable state and worse atherosclerotic progression.[10]

Other Risk Factors

Several lifestyle and psychosocial factors also carry a differential risk of ACS in women and men.

- Obesity is more common in young (aged <55 years) female patients with ACS than in their male counterparts, although this difference does not exist in older women.[11]
- Smoking is a stronger risk factor for MI in women than in men and the difference in risk is even greater in women aged less than 45. Also, smoking is the biggest risk factor for coronary plaque erosion, which is a particularly common mechanism of ACS in women.[12]

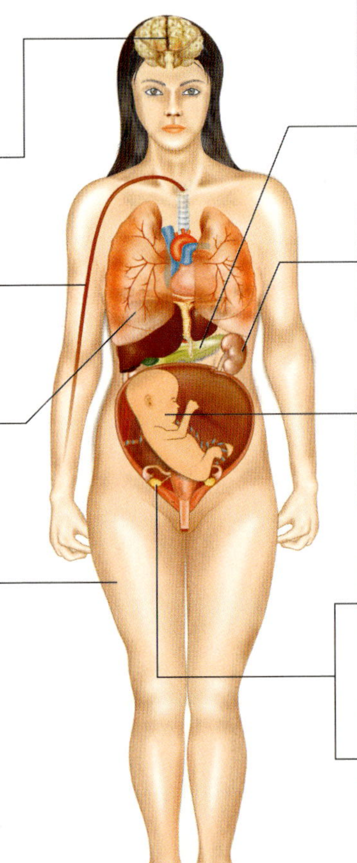

Common risk factors

Age
- Sex-specific differences in baseline risk factors vary by age
- Among patients with ACS, women generally are older than men

Depression
- More common in women with MI than in men
- This sex-specific difference is particularly pronounced at young ages (<55 years)

Hypertension
Women with ACS are more likely to have hypertension than men with ACS

Smoking
- Stronger risk factor for MI in women than in men
- The risk difference is even greater in women aged <45 years

Obesity
- In patients with ACS, the prevalence of obesity is higher in young women (aged <55 years) than in men in the same age group

Diabetes mellitus
- Among patients with ACS, diabetes is more common in women than in men
- The risk of MI and coronary heart disease is higher in women with diabetes than in men with diabetes

Chronic kidney disease
Approximately, two-fold more frequent in women than in men among patients with STEMI

Specific risk factors

Pregnancy
Women in peripartum period have a substantially increased risk of MI from spontaneous coronary artery dissection

Menopause
Incidence of acute MI rises sharply after menopause

Oral contraceptive therapy
The relative risk of ACS increases with higher doses of oestrogen, although the absolute risk is low

Fig. 1: Sex-specific differences in baseline risk factors for acute coronary syndrome (ACS). Women have higher rates than men of traditional risk factors such as diabetes mellitus, hypertension, and obesity, and have differential lifestyle and psychosocial determinants. In addition, women have sex-specific risk factors such as pregnancy and menopause

Abbreviations: MI, myocardial infarction; STEMI, non-ST-segment elevation myocardial infarction

- Psychosocial factors such as depression also influence the relationship between patient sex and likelihood of ACS. Among patients with MI, depression is more common in women than in men. This association is particularly pronounced in young women (aged <55 years), who are twice as likely to have depression compared with young men (prevalence 48% vs. 24%).[13]
- In patients with ST-segment elevation myocardial infarction (STEMI), chronic kidney disease is approximately two-fold more frequent in women than in men, and is associated with worse outcomes.[14]
- Menopause is thought to be an important risk factor in women because circulating estrogen has a protective role on the vascular endothelium. The incidence of acute MI rises sharply in women after menopause; however, the relationship between menopause, age, and cardiovascular events is difficult to unravel. Although endogenous estrogen seems to be protective, studies that examined the effect of exogenous estrogen therapy on women after menopause show that hormone replacement therapy precipitates acute coronary events.[15] Oral contraceptive therapy has long been associated with an increased risk of venous thromboembolic events.[16]

PRESENTATION OF ACUTE CORONARY SYNDROME

Acute coronary syndrome encompasses three types of conditions—(1) STEMI, which is characterized by complete thrombosis of a coronary artery and myocardial necrosis; (2) non-ST-segment elevation myocardial infarction (NSTEMI), which refers to partial thrombosis of a coronary artery and myocardial necrosis; and (3) unstable angina, in which the artery is partially occluded and myocardial necrosis has not yet occurred. An analysis of the GUSTO-IIb trial showed that STEMI was significantly less frequent in women than in men.[4] In the groups of patients with NSTEMI or unstable angina, women were more likely to have unstable angina than men.[4] The higher rate of STEMI in men than in women was later confirmed in a sample of 78,254 patients from the Get with the Guidelines—Coronary Artery Disease Registry.[17]

Symptoms

Symptom presentation in women with ACS is very different from that in men, and data from several large cohorts support this concept.[18] Specifically, the Global Registry of Acute Coronary Events (GRACE) registry indicated that women were more likely to have atypical symptoms such as nausea than men.[19] Similarly, a review of nine large cohort studies showed that the absence of chest pain was more common in women with ACS than in men (37% vs. 27%).[20] Women are also more likely to present with pain in the upper back, neck, arm, and jaw, and dyspnea, weakness, and a sense of dread.[21]

PATHOPHYSIOLOGY

Over the past 2 decades, mechanisms other than plaque rupture and thrombus formation have been increasingly recognized as the cause of a substantial proportion of ACS cases, especially in women (Fig. 2).[22] Different mechanisms of ACS that are more prevalent in women than in men include plaque erosion, coronary vasospasm, spontaneous coronary artery dissection (SCAD), and stress-related (Takotsubo) cardiomyopathy.

Plaque Erosion and Coronary Vasospasm

Acute coronary syndrome can be caused by coronary thrombosis with or without occlusion of the artery. Thrombosis, in turn, is caused most commonly by plaque rupture, but can also be caused by plaque erosion. In patients with MI, plaque rupture is considerably more common in men than in women.[23] The PROSPECT study showed that women had smaller coronary lumens, less plaque rupture, and differing coronary plaque characteristics (less necrotic core and calcium content) compared with men. Women were also more likely to have plaque erosions without true

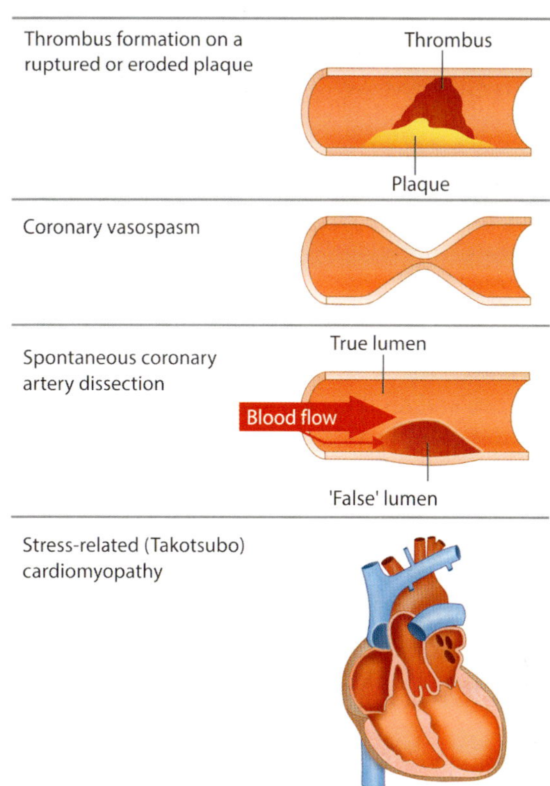

Fig. 2: Sex-specific differences in the pathophysiology of acute coronary syndrome. A substantial proportion of acute coronary syndrome cases, especially in women, is caused by mechanisms other than plaque rupture and thrombus formation. Plaque erosion, coronary vasospasm, spontaneous coronary artery dissection, and stress-related (Takotsubo) cardiomyopathy are more prevalent in women than in men

plaque rupture.[24] The pathophysiology of plaque erosion is postulated to be related to a multitude of mechanisms including endothelial dysfunction, leukocyte activation, and inflammation. Plaque erosion might also be related to coronary vasospasm. Vasospasm can lead to damage and erosions in the endothelium and this spasm probably occurs due to transient sympathovagal imbalance and decreased bioavailability of nitric oxide or other vasoactive substances.[25] Treatment of coronary vasospasm generally consists of therapy with calcium-channel blockers.[26]

Spontaneous Coronary Artery Dissection

Spontaneous coronary artery dissection is an uncommon, noniatrogenic, and nontraumatic cause of ACS. SCAD occurs when the layers of the coronary arterial wall separate leading to the formation of intramural hematoma, compression of the true lumen, and impairment of anterograde flow. It is often associated with systemic disease processes that predispose arterial beds to injury, such as fibromuscular dysplasia, systemic lupus erythematosus, and various connective tissue disorders. Overall, this condition is much more common in women than in men—approximately 70% of reported cases of SCAD to date have occurred in women.[27] SCAD is increasingly being recognized as an important cause of STEMI in women, accounting for 11% of cases. This dissection also seems to be associated with hormonal changes during pregnancy, leading to a substantial burden of disease in women in the peripartum period. In terms of management, no prospective and randomized data are available to address how to treat these patients. Overall, inhospital mortality for SCAD ranges from 1% to 5%. However, female patients particularly in the postpartum period have the worst prognosis.[28]

Stress-related (Takotsubo) Cardiomyopathy

Stress-related cardiomyopathy, also known as Takotsubo cardiomyopathy or transient apical ballooning syndrome, is a condition in which sudden, severe, reversible, left ventricular dysfunction is triggered by an acute emotional stress. Takotsubo cardiomyopathy has been shown to account for up to 3% of all ACS cases; however, this cardiomyopathy is far more common in women than in men and has a marked prevalence in postmenopausal women. Few data exist on treatment effectiveness because the heart failure usually resolves within weeks. Prognosis is generally good for patients who survive the initial acute phase of heart failure.[29]

EVALUATION AND MANAGEMENT

Diagnosis

Troponin levels in ACS presentation are on an average lower in women than in men. Lower cut-off values for troponin levels in women have been proposed for the new high-sensitivity assays for troponin, which might improve detection of MI in women.[30] Nevertheless, despite these new diagnostic tools and thresholds for troponin, the evidence suggests that diagnosis of ACS is missed more often in women than in men. In a study of 10,689 patients who presented to US emergency departments with ACS symptoms, women were slightly more likely to be discharged without hospitalization than men (3.4% vs. 1.4%; $p = 0.05$).[31] Additionally, data from the US National Registry of Myocardial Infarction indicated that young women (aged <60 years) were given a diagnosis other than ACS at the time of admission more frequently than young men.[32]

Delay in Presentation

Substantial evidence suggests that women present to the hospital for ACS treatment later than men.[33] The delay in presentation might contribute to poorer outcomes in women. The reasons for the greater delay in presentation in women than in men include lack of awareness, misinterpretation of symptoms, barriers to accessing care, fear, and embarrassment.[34]

TREATMENT

Overall, evidence-based medications and invasive procedures are similarly effective in women and men with ACS. However, women with ACS tend to receive fewer evidence-based medications and are less likely to have invasive interventions than their male counterparts.[35] The treatment strategies in both clinical trial and real-world settings are reviewed below.

Reperfusion Therapy

Results from clinical studies have shown that women and men with STEMI derive similar benefit from percutaneous coronary intervention (PCI) relative to fibrinolysis.[36] Multiple community-based studies show that women with ACS are significantly less likely to receive angiography and/or PCI than men with ACS.[37] Women with STEMI are also less likely to receive rapid reperfusion therapy compared with men with STEMI, either by fibrinolytic therapy (door-to-needle time <30 minutes; 28.3% vs. 35.2%; $p = 0.0005$) or with primary PCI (door-to-balloon time <90 minutes; 39.0% vs. 44.8%; $p < 0.0001$).[17] Among patients with NSTEMI aged less than or equal to 65 years, fewer women receive coronary intervention compared with their male counterparts, irrespective of angiographic findings.[38] Therefore, women with either STEMI or NSTEMI seem to receive less-aggressive invasive care than men.

Pharmacological Therapies

Most antiplatelet therapies have similar benefits in both women and men with ACS. Although the use of aspirin for primary prevention is of uncertain benefit in women, the use of aspirin at the time of ACS is of clear benefit in both sexes. Clopidogrel has also been shown to reduce adverse outcomes in both women and men with ACS who have undergone PCI.[39] By contrast, women and men might respond differently to glycoprotein IIb/IIIa inhibitors, an intravenous antiplatelet therapy. A large meta-analysis showed that men had a reduction in the risk of death or recurrent ACS events when taking glycoprotein IIb/IIIa inhibitors, but women did not.[40] The benefit of antiplatelet therapy in ACS must be weighed carefully against the risk of bleeding, which is higher in women than in men. This difference seems to be primarily attributable to sex-related differences in body surface area, drug metabolism, and pharmacokinetics.[41] Beyond antithrombotic therapy, a meta-analysis of β-blocker administration after MI showed similar benefits of these drugs in women and men.[42] Similarly, the long-term benefits of angiotensin-converting enzyme inhibition after MI seem similar in both women and men, with a similar risk reduction for the composite of death, heart failure, and MI in both sexes.[43] The use of statin therapy is also similarly beneficial for women and men.[44] Despite a clear role for the above medications in the treatment of ACS, women still seem to receive less-aggressive medical therapy than men. A study of the American College of Cardiology (ACC) database of patients with ACS undergoing PCI between 2004 and 2006 showed that during hospitalization, fewer women received aspirin [adjusted odds ratio (OR) 0.86, 95% confidence interval (CI) 0.83–0.88] and glycoprotein IIa/IIIb inhibitors (adjusted OR 0.90, 95% CI 0.88–0.92) compared with men.[45] Similar disparities in therapy have been shown with thienopyridines and heparin, β-blockers, and statins.[46]

OUTCOMES

A substantial body of evidence supports sex-related difference in short-term mortality after ACS, especially after STEMI. A meta-analysis including more than 136,000 patients from 11 randomized clinical trials of ACS showed that women with STEMI had worse 30-day outcomes than men, but women with NSTEMI or unstable angina had better outcomes.[47] The reasons for the differing short-term prognosis by ACS type in women and men are unknown. With regard to long-term outcomes, the evidence for a difference in mortality between female and male patients with ACS is conflicting. Some old studies suggest that no sex-based differences in long-term mortality exist, whereas other studies suggest that the crude death rates are different and this difference is attenuated after adjustment for baseline clinical factors.[48] A review including 39 studies published between 1966 and 2012 showed that, compared with men, women had a higher unadjusted death rate after MI at both 5 and 10 years.[49] However, these differences were largely explained by sex-related differences in age, comorbidities, and treatment use.[49]

A growing body of literature suggests that sex-related outcomes differ by age. Young women (aged <50 years) have a two-fold greater early risk of death after acute MI than similarly aged men. Young women (aged <65 years) with acute MI have a 22% higher risk of 30-day hospital readmission than young men, even after adjustment for confounders.[50] These differences persist over time such that the 2-year mortality after an ACS event is significantly higher in women than men among patients aged less than 60 years, but not among older patients (aged ≥70 years). The age dependence of the relationship between patient sex and outcomes after ACS seems to hold true for patients with STEMI and patients with NSTEMI in the short-term and in the long-term.[51] The VIRGO study, published in 2015, indicated that young women (aged <55 years) with STEMI received reperfusion therapy less frequently and were more likely to have reperfusion delays than similarly aged men.[52] Longer door-to-needle and door-to-balloon times, along with lower prescription rates of discharge medications (statins, angiotensin-converting enzyme inhibitors, and angiotensin-II receptor blockers), in women than in men were also found among patients aged less than 45 years included in the American Heart Association (AHA) Get with the Guidelines—Coronary Artery Disease registry.[53] Whether these differences in management contribute to the observed difference in outcomes between these two groups is unknown.

WOMEN IN CLINICAL TRIALS

Recommendations for ACS management in women are largely based on clinical trials that did not include an adequate number of women and that did not perform subgroup analyses by sex. In response to the widespread underrepresentation of women in clinical trials, both the National Institutes of Health (NIH) and the Food and Drug Administration (FDA) issued mandates in 1993 for the inclusion of women in clinical trials.[54] Since then, although the absolute number of women in clinical trials has increased, women remain markedly underrepresented, particularly in ACS trials.[55] The reasons for the underrepresentation of women in ACS trials are unknown, but are likely to be multifaceted. Possible reasons include concern about the safety of women of childbearing potential, for pregnant women, and for their fetuses, although this explanation cannot account for the low enrolment of old women in cardiovascular trials.[56] Further explanations might include a general unwillingness of women to volunteer to participate in studies, or a higher tendency for women to withdraw from studies before their completion compared with men. However, the adequate enrolment of women in hypertension trials discounts these claims, as does the enrolment of women in single-sex cardiovascular trials. Other barriers to enrolling an adequate number of women in mixed-sex trials must be present and further research is needed to elucidate these barriers and how they can be addressed.

URGENT RESEARCH QUESTIONS ABOUT SEX-BASED DIFFERENCES IN ACUTE CORONARY SYNDROME[5]

Presentation and Baseline Risk Factors

1. Are sex-based differences in the symptoms of ACS large enough to warrant a change in clinical practice?
2. Why does diabetes mellitus carry a greater relative risk of cardiovascular disease in women than in men?
3. Do psychological and behavioral risk factors such as depression have a larger role in the development of cardiovascular disease in women than in men?

Pathophysiology

1. Why is plaque erosion more common in women than in men and how can plaque erosion be prevented?
2. Does microvascular dysfunction have a major role in the development of coronary artery disease or ACS in women?
3. Does the different pathophysiology of ACS in women correlate with differences in symptoms at presentation?

Evaluation and Management

1. Why are young women with ACS more often misdiagnosed at the time of presentation than young men?
2. How should women with ACS and nonobstructive coronary artery disease on angiography be optimally managed?
3. How should spontaneous coronary artery dissection be managed medically; is there a role for revascularization?
4. What are the causes for women with ACS consistently receiving less aggressive invasive and pharmacological therapy than men?
5. How can treatment rates in women be increased when appropriate?

CONCLUSION

Though outcomes after ACS have improved over the years and women require special considerations because of varied pathophysiology, presentations, and risk factors. From very beginning, cardiovascular research has remained focus primarily on men leading to underrepresentation of women in various trials. Hence, it may be concluded that more trials should be designed with adequate power for gender-specific analysis, so that better understanding of pathophysiology, risk factors, and proper treatment of ACS in women could be achieved.

REFERENCES

1. US Centers for Disease Control and Prevention. (2013). Health, United States, 2013. [online] Available from http://www.cdc.gov/nchs/data/hus/hus13.pdf. [Accessed August, 2017].
2. Mozaffarian D, Benjamin EJ, Go AS, et al. Heart disease and stroke statistics—2015 update: a report from the American Heart Association. Circulation. 2015;131:e29-322.
3. Kannel WB, Sorlie P, McNamara PM. Prognosis after initial myocardial infarction: the Framingham Study. Am J Cardiol. 1979;44:53-9.
4. Hochman JS, Tamis JE, Thompson TD, et al. Sex, clinical presentation, and outcome in patients with acute coronary syndromes. N Engl J Med. 1999;341:226-32.
5. Pagidipati NJ, Peterson ED. Acute coronary syndromes in women and men. Nature Rev Cardiol. 2016;13:471-80.
6. Worrall-Carter L, McEvedy S, Wilson A, et al. Gender differences in presentation, coronary intervention, and outcomes of 28,985 acute coronary syndrome patients in Victoria, Australia. Womens Health Issues. 2016;26:14-20.
7. Peters SA, Huxley RR, Woodward M. Diabetes as risk factor for incident coronary heart disease in women compared with men: a systematic review and meta-analysis of 64 cohorts including 858,507 individuals and 28,203 coronary events. Diabetologia. 2014;57:1542-51.
8. Anand SS, Islam S, Rosengren A, et al. Risk factors for myocardial infarction in women and men: insights from the INTERHEART study. Eur Heart J. 2008;29:932-40.
9. van Dieren S, Beulens JW, van der Schouw YT, et al. The global burden of diabetes and its complications: an emerging pandemic. Eur J Cardiovasc Prev Rehabil. 2010;17:S3-8.
10. Tillin T, Hughes AD, Mayet J, et al. The relationship between metabolic risk factors and incident cardiovascular disease in Europeans, South Asians, and African Caribbeans: SABRE (Southall and Brent Revisited)—a prospective population-based study. J Am Coll Cardiol. 2013;61:1777-86.
11. Lopez-Jimenez F, Jacobsen SJ, Reeder GS, et al. Prevalence and secular trends of excess body weight and impact on outcomes after myocardial infarction in the community. Chest. 2004;125:1205-12.
12. Njolstad I, Arnesen E, Lund-Larsen PG. Smoking, serum lipids, blood pressure, and sex differences in myocardial infarction. A 12-year follow-up of the Finnmark Study. Circulation. 1996;93:450-6.
13. Smolderen KG, Strait KM, Dreyer RP, et al. Depressive symptoms in younger women and men with acute myocardial infarction: insights from the VIRGO study. J Am Heart Assoc. 2015;4:pii: e001424.
14. Sederholm Lawesson S, Alfredsson J, Szummer K, et al. Prevalence and prognostic impact of chronic kidney disease in STEMI from a gender perspective: data from the SWEDEHEART register, a large Swedish prospective cohort. BMJ Open. 2015;5:e008188.
15. Rossouw JE, Manson JE, Kaunitz AM, et al. Lessons learned from the Women's Health Initiative trials of menopausal hormone therapy. Obstet Gynecol. 2013;121: 172-6.
16. Schierbeck LL, Rejnmark L, Tofteng CL, et al. Effect of hormone replacement therapy on cardiovascular events in recently postmenopausal women: randomised trial. BMJ. 2012;345:e6409.
17. Jneid H, Fonarow GC, Cannon CP, et al. Sex differences in medical care and early death after acute myocardial infarction. Circulation. 2008;118:2803-10.

18. Canto JG, Goldberg RJ, Hand MM, et al. Symptom presentation of women with acute coronary syndromes: myth versus reality. Arch Intern Med. 2007;167:2405-13.
19. Dey S, Flather MD, Devlin G, et al. Sex-related differences in the presentation, treatment and outcomes among patients with acute coronary syndromes: the Global Registry of Acute Coronary Events. Heart. 2009;95:20-6.
20. Arslanian-Engoren C, Patel A, Fang J, et al. Symptoms of men and women presenting with acute coronary syndromes. Am J Cardiol. 2006;98:1177-81.
21. Coventry LL, Finn J, Bremner AP. Sex differences in symptom presentation in acute myocardial infarction: a systematic review and meta-analysis. Heart Lung. 2011;40:477-91.
22. Vaccarino V, Badimon L, Corti R, et al. Presentation, management, and outcomes of ischaemic heart disease in women. Nat Rev Cardiol. 2013;10:508-18.
23. Burke AP, Virmani R, Galis Z, et al. 34th Bethesda Conference: task force #2—what is the pathologic basis for new atherosclerosis imaging techniques? J Am Coll Cardiol. 2003;41:1874-86.
24. Lansky AJ, Ng VG, Maehara A, et al. Gender and the extent of coronary atherosclerosis, plaque composition, and clinical outcomes in acute coronary syndromes. JACC Cardiovasc Imaging. 2012;5:S62-72.
25. Falk E, Nakano M, Bentzon JF, et al. Update on acute coronary syndromes: the pathologists' view. Eur Heart J. 2013;34:719-28.
26. Walling A, Waters DD, Miller DD, et al. Long-term prognosis of patients with variant angina. Circulation. 1987;76:990-7.
27. Yip A, Saw J. Spontaneous coronary artery dissection—a review. Cardiovasc Diagn Ther. 2015;5:37-48.
28. Vanzetto G, Berger-Coz E, Barone-Rochette G, et al. Prevalence, therapeutic management and medium-term prognosis of spontaneous coronary artery dissection: results from a database of 11,605 patients. Eur J Cardiothorac Surg. 2009;35:250-4.
29. Akashi YJ, Nef HM, Mollmann H, et al. Stress cardiomyopathy. Annu Rev Med. 2010;61:271-86.
30. Daniels LB, Maisel AS. Cardiovascular biomarkers and sex: the case for women. Nat Rev Cardiol. 2015;12:588-96.
31. Pope JH, Aufderheide TP, Ruthazer R, et al. Missed diagnoses of acute cardiac ischemia in the emergency department. N Engl J Med. 2000;342:1163-70.
32. Vaccarino V, Parsons L, Every NR, et al. Sex-based differences in early mortality after myocardial infarction. N Engl J Med. 1999;341:217-25.
33. Nguyen HL, Gore JM, Saczynski JS, et al. Age and sex differences and 20-year trends in prehospital delay in patients hospitalized with acute myocardial infarction (1986 to 2005). Circ Cardiovasc Qual Outcomes. 2010;3: 590-8.
34. Kaur R, Lopez V, Thompson DR. Factors influencing Hong Kong Chinese patients' decision-making in seeking early treatment for acute myocardial infarction. Res Nurs Health. 2006;29:636-46.
35. Izadnegahdar M, Norris C, Kaul P, et al. Basis for sex-dependent outcomes in acute coronary syndrome. Can J Cardiol. 2014;30: 713-20.
36. Tamis-Holland JE, Palazzo A, Stebbins AL, et al. Benefits of direct angioplasty for women and men with acute myocardial infarction: results of the Global Use of Strategies to Open Occluded Arteries in Acute Coronary Syndromes Angioplasty (GUSTO II-B) substudy. Am Heart J. 2004;147:133-9.
37. Anand SS, Xie CC, Mehta S, et al. Differences in the management and prognosis of women and men who suffer from acute coronary syndromes. J Am Coll Cardiol. 2005;46:1845-51.
38. Tavris D, Shoaibi A, Chen AY, et al. Gender differences in the treatment of non-ST-segment elevation myocardial infarction. Clin Cardiol. 2010;33:99-103.
39. Mehta SR, Yusuf S, Peters RJ, et al. Effects of pretreatment with clopidogrel and aspirin followed by long-term therapy in patients undergoing percutaneous coronary intervention: the PCI-CURE study. Lancet. 2001;358:527-33.
40. Boersma E, Harrington RA, Moliterno DJ, et al. Platelet glycoprotein IIb/IIIa inhibitors in acute coronary syndromes. Lancet. 2002;360:342-3.
41. Mehran R, Pocock SJ, Nikolsky E, et al. A risk score to predict bleeding in patients with acute coronary syndromes. J Am Coll Cardiol. 2010;55:2556-66.
42. Bangalore S, Makani H, Radford M, et al. Clinical outcomes with β-blockers for myocardial infarction: a meta-analysis of randomized trials. Am J Med. 2014;127: 939-53.
43. Flather MD, Yusuf S, Køber L, et al. Long-term ACE-inhibitor therapy in patients with heart failure or left-ventricular dysfunction: a systematic overview of data from individual patients. Lancet. 2000;355:1575-81.
44. Cheung BM, Lauder IJ, Lau CP, et al. Meta-analysis of large randomized controlled trials to evaluate the impact of statins on cardiovascular outcomes. Br J Clin Pharmacol. 2004;57:640-51.
45. Akhter N, Milford-Beland S, Roe MT, et al. Gender differences among patients with acute coronary syndromes undergoing percutaneous coronary intervention in the American College of Cardiology-National Cardiovascular Data Registry (ACC-NCDR). Am Heart J. 2009;157:141-8.
46. Koopman C, Vaartjes I, Heintjes EM, et al. Persisting gender differences and attenuating age differences in cardiovascular drug use for prevention and treatment of coronary heart disease, 1998–2010. Eur Heart J. 2013;34:3198-205.
47. Berger JS, Elliott L, Gallup D, et al. Sex differences in mortality following acute coronary syndromes. JAMA. 2009;302:874-82.
48. Johansson S, Bergstrand R, Ulvenstam G, et al. Sex differences in preinfarction characteristics and long-term survival among patients with myocardial infarction. Am J Epidemiol. 1984;119: 610-23.
49. Bucholz EM, Butala NM, Rathore SS, et al. Sex differences in long-term mortality after myocardial infarction: a systematic review. Circulation. 2014;130:757-67.
50. Dreyer RP, Ranasinghe I, Wang Y, et al. Sex differences in the rate, timing, and principal diagnoses of 30-day readmissions in younger patients with acute myocardial infarction. Circulation. 2015;132:158-66.
51. Kumbhani DJ, Shishehbor MH, Willis JM, et al. Influence of gender on long-term mortality in patients presenting with non-ST-elevation acute coronary syndromes undergoing percutaneous coronary intervention. Am J Cardiol. 2012;109:1087-91.
52. D'Onofrio G, Safdar B, Lichtman JH, et al. Sex differences in reperfusion in young patients with ST-segment-elevation myocardial infarction: results from the VIRGO study. Circulation. 2015;131:1324-32.
53. Bangalore S, Fonarow GC, Peterson ED, et al. Age and gender differences in quality of care and outcomes for patients with ST-segment elevation myocardial infarction. Am J Med. 2012;125:1000-9.
54. US Food and Drug Administration. Guideline for the study and evaluation of gender differences in the clinical evaluation of drugs; notice. Fed Regist. 1993;58:39406-16.
55. GAO. United States General Accounting Office. (2001). Women sufficiently represented in new drug testing, but FDA oversight needs improvement. [online] Available from http://www.gao.gov/new.items/d01754.pdf. [Accessed August, 2017].
56. Harris DJ, Douglas PS. Enrollment of women in cardiovascular clinical trials funded by the National Heart, Lung, and Blood Institute. N Engl J Med. 2000;343:475-80.

CHAPTER

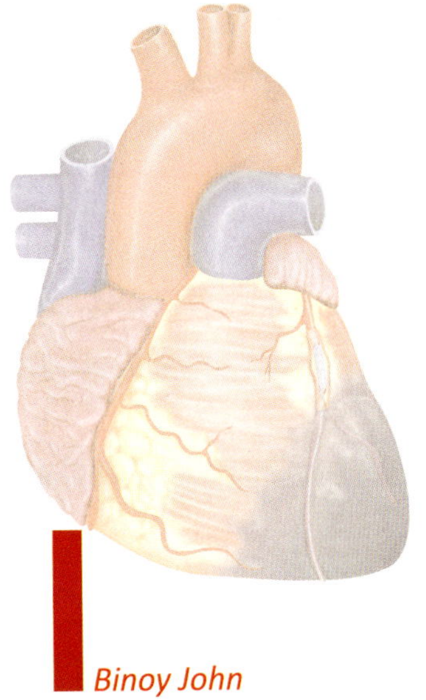

Coronary Artery Disease in Diabetes: How Different is It from Nondiabetics?

Binoy John

INTRODUCTION

With urbanization, sedentary lifestyle and obesity, the number of people affected with diabetes mellitus (DM) are on a rapid rise, already affecting an estimated 200 million people world over and the World Health Organization predicts that by the year 2030 that number would reach at least a staggering 366 million.[1] DM, when uncontrolled, is known to have devastating consequences in virtually all organ-systems of the human body. Coronary arteries are often the targets of this multisystem disorder. But, how different is coronary artery disease (CAD) in diabetics in contrast to nondiabetics?

DEFINITION AND PATHOPHYSIOLOGY

Diabetes mellitus refers to a group of common metabolic disorders that share the phenotype of hyperglycemia. Complications due to type 2 DM can be microvascular (ophthalmic, renal and neurologic involvement) or macrovascular (coronary, cerebrovascular and peripheral vascular involvement). Dyslipidemia, albuminuria and hypertension also play important roles in the macrovascular complications of DM. The pathophysiology of vascular disease in diabetic patients involves abnormalities of endothelial cells and vascular smooth muscle cells.[2] Diabetes causes increase in intracellular glucose, which leads to the formation of advanced glycosylation end-products (AGEs) by nonenzymatic glycosylation of extra- and intra-cellular proteins. Nonenzymatic glycosylation occurs due to interaction of glucose with the amino group of proteins. AGEs have the potential to cross-link proteins, accelerate atherosclerosis, reduce nitric oxide synthesis and induce endothelial dysfunction. Vascular calcification is also commoner in diabetic patients. High blood glucose levels were also associated with increased expression of Cbfal (transcription factor for bone formation) and bone morphogenetic protein factor (BMP)-2, which enhanced the calcification of vascular smooth muscle cells. High levels of BMP-2 induce proinflammatory and proatherogenic effects by inducing oxidative stress and endothelial dysfunction and promote plaque calcification by inducing an osteogenic phenotype in vascular smooth muscle cells.[3,4]

Diabetes mellitus has been shown to be an independent risk factor for cardiovascular disease (CVD) in various ethnic and racial groups in prospective studies like the Framingham, Honolulu and San Antonio Heart studies. The differences in CAD between diabetics and nondiabetics have been studied in various ethnic populations using modalities like computed tomography coronary angiography (CTCA) and conventional coronary angiography with notable differences. CTCA has been proven in various studies to be of benefit as a noninvasive imaging tool with high diagnostic performance in the detection and exclusion of CAD.[5,6]

How different was it? It has been observed in various studies that there were differences in the symptomatology of CAD, incidence, extent of disease, number of arteries involved, presence of obstructive disease, number of segments involved, severity of calcification, plaque characteristics, plaque distribution in the coronary arterial tree, morbidity, mortality and major adverse coronary events between patients with diabetes and those without.

Coronary artery disease is commoner in diabetics in comparison to nondiabetics. Patients with type 2 diabetes have a two to four times higher risk of CVDs, and CAD is the major cause of mortality in contrast to patients without diabetes.[7,8] These events also correlated with fasting and postprandial plasma glucose levels as well as with glycosylated hemoglobin levels.

PREVALENCE

In the coronary CT angiography evaluation for clinical outcomes (CONFIRM) registry,[9] of 10,110 patients who underwent CTCA with 3,370 diabetic patients and 6,740 propensity matched nondiabetic patients it was seen there were differences between the two groups in the prevalence, extent and severity of CAD. This study showed that diabetic patients exhibited lower prevalence of normal coronary arteries and higher rates of obstructive CAD. On a per-vessel basis, it was seen that patients with DM showed higher rates of obstructive one-vessel, two-vessel and three-vessel and left-main (LM) disease when compared with non-DM individuals. CONFIRM registry was the first prospective multicenter data to relate per-patient, per-vessel and per-segment prevalence, extent and severity of CAD findings by CTCA for DM and non-DM individuals who are similar to each other in age, sex and CAD risk factors. The increased prevalence, extent and severity of CAD for DM individuals were remarkably consistent across patient, vessel and segment based comparisons. Patients with DM had a 37% higher prevalence of obstructive CAD at a per-patient level which was consistent with the 36% and 29% increase in prevalence of obstructive one-vessel and two-vessel disease, respectively, at the per-vessel level.

In a single center study by Goncalves et al.[10] in 581 patients using CTCA for the evaluation of suspected CAD, it was seen that the prevalence of CAD based on any plaque was 74% in DM patients in contrast to 56% in non-DM patients ($p = 0.002$). The study also showed that the incidence of obstructive CAD (≥ 50% stenosis) was 31.8% vs 10.3% for DM vs non-DM individuals ($p < 0.001$) respectively, being significantly higher in individuals with DM.

SEGMENTAL AND MULTIVESSEL INVOLVEMENT AND OBSTRUCTIVE CAD

In the CONFIRM registry,[9] a segment involvement score (SIS) which reflected CAD distribution was calculated as the total number of coronary artery segments exhibiting plaque, irrespective of the degree of luminal stenosis within each segment (minimum = 0 and maximum = 16); and the segment stenosis score (SSS) which was used as a measure of overall coronary plaque burden with scores of 0–3 based on no to severe plaque based on the extent of obstruction of the coronary luminal diameter, with a summed up total score of all the 16 segments from 0–48 were used to assess the severity of CAD. It was seen that both SIS and SSS were similar for overall population. But, overall SSS for DM patients was higher than non-DM individuals (3 vs 2, $p < 0.0001$). Similarly, SIS was also higher for DM individuals than non-DM individuals (2 vs 1, $p < 0.0001$). On a per-segment basis, DM individuals possessed higher SSS compared with non-DM individuals for nearly every coronary segment and for all proximal and mid-coronary segments. Among segmental analyses for proximal and mid-portions of coronary arteries, stenosis scores ranged between 26% and 40% higher for patients with DM in contrast to matched non-DM individuals.

In a study by Yang et al.[11] 206 diabetics and 523 non-diabetics of age groups between 45 years and 75 years without history of CAD, were using CTCA for segmental CAD and then confirmed with coronary angiogram via Seldinger technique of all 16 segments of coronary arteries and side branches with luminal diameter ≥2.0 mm. Stenosis was classified as obstructive (>50% luminal diameter narrowing) or nonobstructive (≤50% luminal diameter narrowing). It was seen that diabetics demonstrated higher rates of abnormal CAD (76% vs 53% of patients; $p < 0.0001$) and fewer normal coronary arteries (24% vs 47%, $p < 0.0001$) compared with nondiabetics. Multivessel disease was seen more in diabetics (15%) than nondiabetics (7%) ($p < 0.0001$) The prevalence of the absence of any detectable CAD was 41% in nondiabetic patients and 19% in diabetic patients ($p < 0.0001$) and the presence of obstructive CAD was 19% and 38%, respectively ($p < 0.0001$). The number of segments with coronary plaque per patient seen on CTCA was nearly double as high in diabetic patients. So, also the number of segments with obstructive disease was twice higher in diabetic patients when compared to nondiabetic patients. In the study by Goncalves et al,[10] the coronary atherosclerotic burden indices evaluated (SIS, SSS) were also significantly higher in DM patients with SSS being 3–5-fold higher in diabetics. Some of these indices have been prognostically validated and demonstrated to have a good correlation with major cardiovascular events.[12,13] In the per-segment analysis, diabetics had a higher percentage of segments with plaque in every vessel (2.6/13.1/7.5/10.5% for DM patients vs 1.4/7.1/3.3/4.4% for non-DM patients in LM, left anterior descending (LAD) artery, left circumflex (LCx) artery, right coronary artery (RCA) respectively; $p < 0.001$ for all). This higher percentage of plaques in the LM and proximal locations in the coronary tree could explain the higher incidence of coronary events experienced by diabetic patients as seen in other studies too.[14]

SYMPTOMATOLOGY

The assessment of CAD in diabetic patients is especially challenging because classic anginal symptoms are absent in this subset of patients. In the study by Yang et al,[11] it was seen that atypical chest pain as a presenting symptom was common in diabetic patients than nondiabetic patients. (35% vs 12%, respectively p = 0.005) and so also typical angina (43% vs 29% respectively p = 0.076) and nonanginal symptoms or anginal equivalents patients (38% vs 18% respectively p = 0.007) were commoner in diabetic patients in contrast to nondiabetic patients. In another study by Diamond and Forrester et al.[15] it was seen that patients with typical angina had a higher likelihood of angiographic CAD than patients with atypical or nonanginal chest pain in both diabetic and nondiabetic patients.

CORONARY ARTERY CALCIFICATION

Coronary artery calcification scores are a sign of atherosclerosis and can be used to predict the likelihood of CAD and myocardial ischemia. It also indicates the total coronary artery atherosclerotic plaque burden.[16] In a study of 588 Chinese patients with 208 diabetic patients and 380 nondiabetic patients by Yang et al.[11,17] it was seen that in patients with and without diabetes, the diabetic patients had significantly higher CAC scores in LAD (155.03 ± 256.47 vs 92.78 ± 195.72 respectively; p = 0.003), LCx (39.11 ± 67.74 vs 22.97 ± 52.90 respectively; p = 0.003), RCA (88.82 ± 172.39 vs 32.38 ± 70.40, respectively; p < 0.001) and total CAC scores (309.00 ± 457.14 vs 180.09 ± 290.62 respectively, p < 0.001) than that in the non-diabetes group. However, no differences were found in the CAC levels in LM between the two groups.

PLAQUE CHARACTERISTICS AND DISTRIBUTION IN THE CORONARY ARTERIAL TREE

Diabetes mellitus has been associated with a variety of plaques like noncalcified plaque, mixed plaque and also with the extent of CAD. A study by Pundziute et al.[18] showed that diabetic patients had an increased number of mixed and obstructive plaque segments in contrast to patients without diabetes. Diabetic patients had more plaque burden and more extensive atherosclerosis when compared to nondiabetic patients. Also, it was seen that unstable noncalcified plaques and resultant acute coronary syndromes were more frequent in patients with diabetes. Intravascular ultrasound and magnetic resonance imaging have been used to identify the composition of plaque and mixed plaques were found by CTCA to be associated with higher-risk features.[18] It was seen that thin cap fibroatheromas occurred more commonly in mixed plaques than in calcified and noncalcified plaques. Scholte et al.[19] had shown that noncalcified plaques were the main subtype of plaque associated with asymptomatic diabetic patients in contrast to those without diabetes. The study by Yang et al.[17] showed the diabetes group had higher number of mixed plaque segments (2.72 ± 2.45 vs 1.69 ± 2.12 respectively, p < 0.001), noncalcified plaque segments (0.87 ± 1.36 vs 0.49 ± 0.97 respectively, p < 0.001) and total plaque segments (4.76 ± 3.10 vs 3.36 ± 2.58 respectively, p < 0.001) than the non-diabetes group, however no differences were observed in the levels of calcified plaque between the two groups. There were significantly higher number of obstructed vessels (1.00 ± 1.02 vs 0.54 ± 0.81 respectively, p < 0.001) and obstructed segments (1.92 ± 2.24 vs 0.77 ± 1.34 respectively, p < 0.001) in the diabetes group than in the non-diabetes group. In the study by Goncalves et al.[10] diabetics had higher percentage of both calcified (19.3 vs 9.2% p < 0.001) and noncalcified or mixed type plaques (14.4 vs 7.0%, p < 0.001). The study also showed that the ratio of proximal-to-distal relative plaque distribution (calculated as LM/proximal vs mid/distal/branches) was lower for DM patients (0.75 vs 1.04; p = 0.009). Thus, it was seen that diabetes was an independent predictor of CAD and was also associated with more advanced CAD as evaluated by the indices of coronary atherosclerotic burden.

MORBIDITY, MORTALITY AND MAJOR ADVERSE CARDIAC EVENTS

Survival in the CONFIRM registry[9] after a median follow-up of 2.2 years showed that patients with DM had a significantly higher rate of death compared with non-DM patients (3.2% vs 1.7%, p < 0.0001). Higher age and dyslipidemia were found to be the risk factors for both DM and non-DM individuals whereas male-sex, hypertension, current smoking or family history of CAD were not. This study also showed that when using a non-DM patient without DM as a reference, both presence of DM and increasing severity of CAD were associated with increased risk of mortality. In multi-variable analyses, when compared with a non-DM patient without CAD, it was seen that there was a "step-up" in risk of mortality, which increased for non-DM individuals with non-obstructive CAD (Hazard ratio (HR) 3.12 <95% CI 1.55–6.21, p = 0.0013), DM individuals with no CAD (3.63 <1.67 – 7.92> p = 0.001), DM individuals with non-obstructive CAD (5.25 <2.56 – 10.8> p < 0.0001), non-DM individuals with obstructive CAD (6.8 <3.52 – 13.1> p < 0.0001), and DM individuals with obstructive CAD (9.39 <4.85 – 18.2> p < 0.0001). When compared to non-DM patients without CAD, the risk of mortality was more than

5-fold higher for patients with DM with non-obstructive CAD and almost 10-fold higher for patients with DM and obstructive CAD. In the study by Yang et al.[11,17] according to multivariate analyses, it was seen that diabetes and CAC levels were independent predictors of cumulative major adverse cardiac events (MACE). The study also showed that diabetes is related to higher levels of CAC in outpatients with suspected CAD. It was observed that diabetes was related to mixed plaque, noncalcified plaque and extent of CAD. It was also seen that diabetes and CAC levels were significantly related to the incidence of MACE in these patients. Studies by Haffner et al.[20] and Scholte et al.[19] have all shown that CAD was a leading cause of morbidity and mortality among patients with DM. Another study by Seshasai et al.[21] showed that people with diabetes had nearly double the risk of CVD, even after adjusting for established cardiovascular risk factors.

TREATMENT

Most of these patients with diabetes have more extensive disease and management involves coronary artery by-pass surgery with multiple grafts or multivessel angioplasty with multiple stents or medical management where revascularization is not possible due to poor targets.

CONCLUSION

Thus, studies in various ethnic populations comparing CAD in diabetic patients and nondiabetic patients have shown numerous differences right from symptomatology to plaque characteristics, extent of disease, degree of obstruction and MACE. As the various diabetic associations currently recommend the use of widespread measures in the prevention of CVD and CAD, this information prompts for early investigation strategies in these diabetic patients and will aid in more aggressive preventive and treatment measures in them.

REFERENCES

1. Wild S, Roglic G, Green A, et al. Global prevalence of diabetes: estimates for the year 2000 and projections for 2030. Diabetes Care. 2004;27(5):1047-53.
2. Paneni F, Beckman JA, Creager MA, et al. Diabetes and vascular disease: pathophysiology, clinical consequences and medical therapy: part I. Eur Heart J. 2013;34:2436-43.
3. Willette RN, Gu JL, Lyska PG, et al. BMP-2 gene expression and effects on human vascular smooth muscle cells. J Vasc Res. 1999;36:120-5.
4. Li X, Tang HY, Giachelli CM. BMP-2 promotes phosphate uptake, phenotypic modulation and calcification of human vascular smooth muscle cells. Atherosclerosis. 2008;199:271-7.
5. Budoff MJ, Dowe D, Jollis JG, et al. Diagnostic performance of 64-multidetector row coronary computed tomographic angiography for evaluation of coronary artery stenosis in individuals without known coronary artery disease: results from the multicenter ACCURACY (Assessment by coronary computed tomography angiography of individuals undergoing invasive coronary angiography) trial. J Am Coll Cardiol 2008;52:1724-32.
6. Chow BJ, Small G, Yam Y, et al. CONFIRM investigators. Incremental prognostic value of cardiac computed tomography in coronary artery disease using CONFIRM: Coronary computed tomography angiography evaluation for clinical outcomes: an international multicenter registry. Circ Cardiovasc Imaging. 2011;4:463-72.
7. Beckman JA, Creager MA, Libby P. Diabetes and atherosclerosis: epidemiology, pathophysiology and management. JAMA. 2002;287:2570-81.
8. Elkeles RS. Coronary artery calcium and cardiovascular risk in diabetes. Atherosclerosis. 2010;210:331-6.
9. Min JK, Berman DS, Shaw LJ, et al. Differences in prevalence, extent, severity and prognosis of coronary artery disease among patients with and without diabetes undergoing coronary computed tomography angiography. Diabetes Care. 2012;35:1787-94.
10. Goncalves, Garcia HM, Carvalho MS, et al. Diabetes as an independent predictor of high atherosclerotic burden assessed by coronary computed tomography angiography: the coronary artery disease equivalent revisited. Int J Cardiovasc Imaging. 2013;29: 1105-14.
11. Yang H, Zheng H, Zhou Y, et al. Characteristics of coronary artery lesions in patients with and without diabetes mellitus. Ir J Med Sci. 2016;185:529-36.
12. Andreini D, Pontone G, Mushtaq S, et al. A long term prognostic value of coronary CT angiography in suspected coronary artery disease. JACC Cardiovasc Imaging. 2012;5(7):690-701.
13. Min JK, Dunning A, Lin FY, et al. Age and sex-related differences in all-cause mortality risk based on coronary computed tomography angiography findings results from the international multicenter CONFIRM (coronary CT angiography evaluation for clinical outcomes: an international multicenter registry) of 23,854 patients without known coronary artery disease. J Am Coll Cardiol. 2011;58(8):849-60.
14. Wang JC, Normand SL, Mauri L, et al. Coronary artery spatial distribution of acute myocardial infarction occlusions. Circulation. 2004;110(3):278-84.
15. Diamond GA, Forrester JS. Analysis of probability as an aid in clinical diagnosis of coronary artery disease. N Engl J Med. 1979;300:1350-8.
16. Rumberger JA, Simons DB, Fitzpatrick LA, et al. Coronary artery calcium area by electron beam computed tomography and coronary atherosclerotic plaque area. A histopathologic correlative study. Circulation. 1995;92:2157-62.
17. Zhu L, Liu J, Gao C, et al. Comparison of coronary plaque, coronary artery calcification and major adverse cardiac events in Chinese outpatients with and without type 2 diabetes. Springerplus. 2016;5:1678.
18. Pundziute G, Schuijf JD, Jukema JW, et al. Head to head comparison of plaque evaluation between multislice computed tomography and intravascular ultrasound radiofrequency data analysis. JACC Cardiovasc Interv. 2008;1:176-82.
19. Scholte AJ, Schuijf JD, Kharagjitsingh AV, et al. Prevalence of coronary artery disease and plaque morphology assessed by multi-slice computed tomography coronary angiography and calcium scoring in asymptomatic patients with type 2 diabetes. Heart. 2008;94:290-5.
20. Haffner SM, Lehto S, Ronnemaa T, et al. Mortality from coronary heart disease in subjects with type 2 diabetes and in nondiabetic subjects with and without prior myocardial infarction. N Engl J Med. 1998;339:229-34.
21. Seshasai SR, Kaptoge S, Thompson A, et al. Diabetes mellitus, fasting glucose, and risk of cause specific death. N Engl J Med. 2011;364: 829-41.

Cardiodiabetes and Heart Failure in the Elderly

Thachathodiyl Rajesh, Umesh C Samal

INTRODUCTION

The incidence of heart failure (HF) increases with age, with the highest rates occurring in those aged more than 65 years.[1,2] The diagnosis and management of HF in the elderly is complicated by unique pathophysiological features, multiple comorbidities, and polypharmacy. A consensus definition of elderly does not exist. Although traditionally, the age of 65 years has been the conventional threshold for older age, increased life expectancy may make this cut-off inappropriately low. Recent HF studies have classified elderly patients as those older than 70–80 years.[3,4]

Although major therapeutic advancements in HF have occurred in the last decade, and there is growing concern where trial patients are representative of patients encountered in daily clinical practice.[5] Elderly patients are underrepresented or often excluded in such large clinical trials. Limited data makes treatment decisions challenging for healthcare providers, as they need to extrapolate how to manage this special population. In this review, we highlight the importance of HF diagnosis and management in the older population. Pathophysiology of the aging heart and differential response to HF therapies in the elderly are also highlighted.

EPIDEMIOLOGY

Heart failure is a major public health problem worldwide with high morbidity and mortality as well as high costs. The median age of patients admitted to the hospital with HF is 75 years, and patients older than 65 years account for more than 75% of HF hospitalizations.[6] HF is the third leading cause of cardiovascular (CV) death in the elderly.[7] It is estimated that the number of hospitalizations in these patients will increase by approximately 50% in the next 20 years.[8] In India, approximately 43% of patients admitted with HF were aged 65 years or older.[9] The incidence of new HF events is higher in the elderly compared to their younger counterparts.[8]

Heart failure treatment is costly and generally has a poor prognosis, especially in the elderly. In developed countries, 2% of total healthcare spending is attributed to HF costs.[10] Although contemporary therapies have significantly improved HF outcomes, their benefit is less evident in older individuals. The median survival time after diagnosis of HF is 2.3–3.6 years in patients aged 67–74 years and 1.1–1.6 years in patients aged 85 years and older.[11]

RISK FACTORS

In elderly patients, the presence of multiple comorbidities makes the diagnosis and management of HF challenging. It has been reported that five or more noncardiac comorbidities were present in 39% of HF patients. Among all HF patients, patients with multiple comorbidities account for 81% of all hospital admission days.[12] The two most common HF comorbidities are hypertension and ischemic heart disease.[13] Other concomitant diseases such as atrial fibrillation, valvular heart disease, diabetes, chronic kidney disease, and obstructive airway disease substantially add to the complexity of HF care.

In addition, there is increasing evidence that geriatric conditions (cognitive impairment, frailty, falls, and incontinence) are common in older adults with HF and influence the disease progression and outcomes, including hospitalization and mortality, in these patients.[14] Several studies have found that cognitive impairment is independently associated with mortality in in HF.[15] It may affect outcomes by impeding HF self-care and making the hospital to home transition especially difficult. Frailty, defined as an increased physiologic vulnerability to stressors, has a complex relation between congestive HF. HF and its multiple therapies put additional stress on a frail patient, leading to disability, falls, hospitalizations, and death.[16]

PATHOPHYSIOLOGY OF AN AGING HEART

Aging lowers the threshold for the manifestation of HF by combining declining cardioprotective systems and increasing disease processes. As described by Lazzarini and colleagues (Flow chart 1), there are specific morphological and functional changes associated with cardiac aging that create a fertile ground for the development of HF.[5] Structurally, there is a decrease in number and in function of cardiomyocytes due to enhanced necrosis and apoptosis.[17] This loss is compensated by an increase in myocardial thickness and increase cardiomyocyte size.[18] These changes in thickness and shape of the left ventricular (LV) cavity have important implications with regards to cardiac wall stress and contractile efficiency. Impaired calcium regulation, morphological change in contractile proteins, and less-efficient adenosine triphosphate (ATP) utilization by heart contribute to the worsening cardiac function with age. In addition, a generalized increase in elastic and collagenous tissue with age results in a progressive decline in number of pacemaker cells leading to a lower resting heart rate. The incidence of atrial fibrillation (approximately 3–4%) in individuals greater than 60 years is strongly predictive of future cardiac morbidity and mortality.[19]

Flow chart 1: Pathophysiological mechanisms predisposing to the development of diastolic dysfunction and heart failure in otherwise healthy ageing hearts

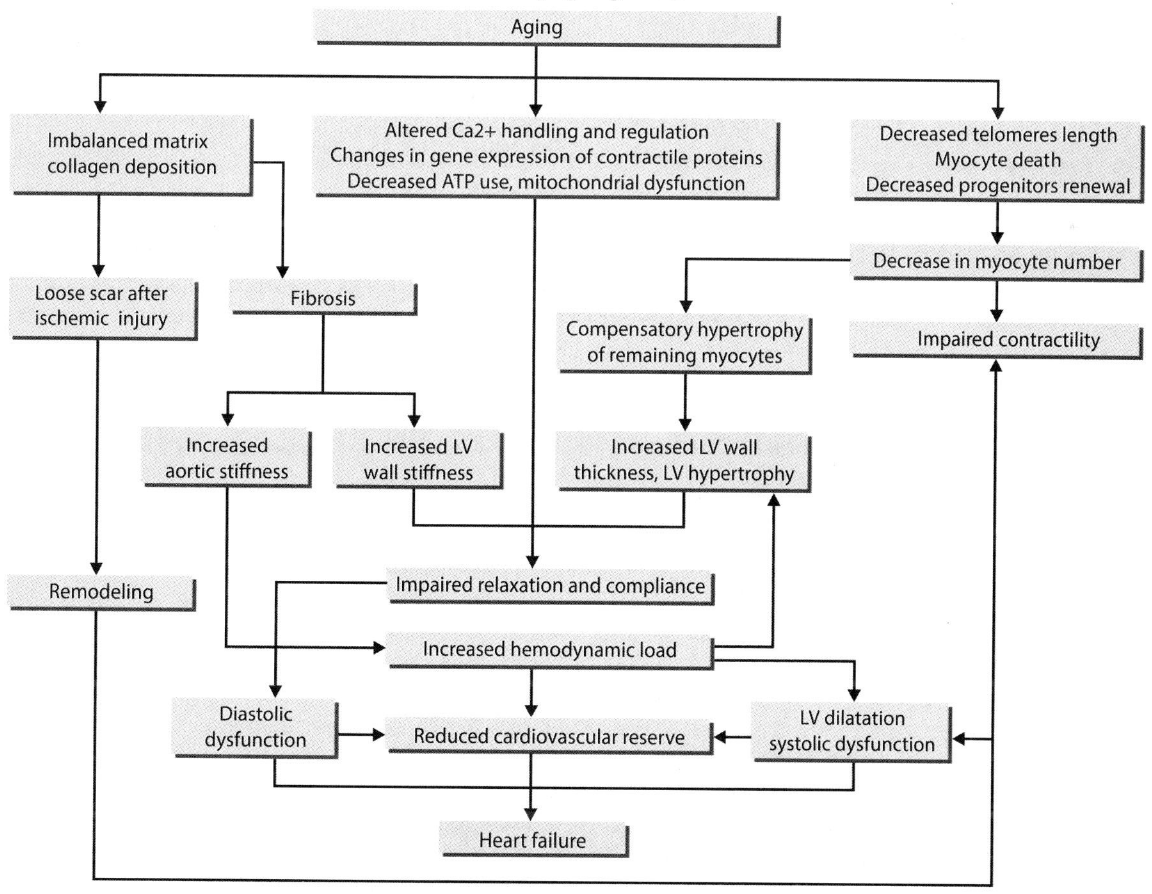

Abbreviation: LV, left ventricular

Source: Reproduced with permission from Lazzarini V, Mentz RJ, Fiuzat M, et al. Heart failure in elderly patients: distinctive features and unresolved issues. Eur J Heart Fail. 2013;15:717-23.

The effects of aging on the heart are most evident during exercise. Cardiac output falls almost 25% with aging and predominantly due to impaired heart rate acceleration.[20] The decline in cardiac reserve is a result a combination of factors including reduced intrinsic myocardial contractility, impaired autonomic regulation, and physical deconditioning. In addition, slowed relaxation, reduced beta-adrenergic responsiveness, and alternations in the pattern of diastolic relaxation have a negative impact on the cardiac functional reserve when an elderly individual is exposed to maximal exercise.[21] Blood vessels are dynamic structures that repair and remodel using complex signaling pathways in response to age. With age, increased collagen content and fraying of elastin fibrils occur in the media, which reduce arterial distensibility and increased stiffness.[22] An increased in aortic impedance can translate into increased end-diastolic pressure in a stiff ventricle, leading to pulmonary edema.[23] These mechanisms culminate in the development of the most common phenotype of HF in the elderly, HF with a preserved ejection fraction (HFpEF). Conditions such as atrial fibrillation that impair ventricular filling can trigger decompensation more easily in an aged heart. However with time and further deterioration, LV dilation and systolic dysfunction can occur as a final stage of HFpEF.[24]

CLINICAL CHARACTERISTICS AND ASSESSMENT

Among the geriatric population presenting with HF, patients tend be female and have a higher incidence of HFpEF.[3,4] As expected, they have increased prevalence of comorbidities including hypertension, atrial fibrillation, cerebrovascular disease, anemia, and chronic kidney disease.[25] With regards to clinical presentation, elderly patients with decompensated HF often present with acute pulmonary edema and hypertension. Orthopnea and paroxysmal nocturnal dyspnea are relatively specific symptoms for HF in older adults.[26] Atypical presentations are also common, including loss of appetite, fatigue, mental state changes, and decrease in body mass index.[27] Traditional HF symptoms, such as exertional dyspnea may be absent of difficult to interpret due to lack of specificity. In geriatric HF patients, bradycardia is more prevalent because of heart blocks or effects of medications such as β-blockers and digoxin. In thinner elderly patients, a visible palpable point of maximal impulse displacement can reveal the presence of cardiomegaly. It should be noted that evidence of long-standing volume overload and an S3 gallop are less likely in patients with preserved systolic function. Given the difficulty of accurately diagnosing older patients with suspected HF, utilization of investigations is crucial in management.[28]

Inadequacy in prediction of disease severity resulting in mismatch between risk stratification and intensity of therapy is a major challenge in management of elderly patients with HF. In addition, the presence of other comorbidities such as renal dysfunction, compromises the ability of biomarkers to accurately prognosticate short- and long-term outcomes in these patients. N-terminal pro b-type natriuretic peptide (NT-proBNP) is difficult for interpretation in the elderly partly because there are huge individual variations in particular when comorbidities are present, and partly because NT-proBNP levels increase dramatically with age. Several studies have demonstrated that NT-proBNP was a prognostic indicator for mortality only in univariate analysis but no in multivariate analysis in elderly HF populations.[29,30] Further research on the role of other biomarkers [red cell distribution width, cystatin C and midregional pro-atrial natriuretic peptide (MR-proANP)] in prognostication of outcomes in elderly HF patients is necessary.[31-33] In addition, there may be additional prognostic value of combined multiple biomarker models in the geriatric populations.

PROGNOSTIC FACTORS AND RISK STRATIFICATION

Although several risk stratification models have been developed to predict mortality risk of general HF patients, there is less conclusive evidence available for the elderly. Manzano and colleagues derived and validated a novel prediction model for risk stratification of elderly patients with HF. They identified five factors associated with increased risk of all-cause mortality or CV hospitalization, and all-cause mortality alone—(1) New York Heart Association (NYHA) class, (2) prior myocardial infarction (MI), (3) left atrial (LA) dimension, (4) uric acid, and (5) body mass index.[34] In a separate clinical model, Oudejans and colleagues suggested a diagnostic rule, consisting of six clinical variables (male sex, nocturnal dyspnea, absence of wheezing, loss of appetite, and lower BMI) and NT-proBNP showed good negative and positive predictive value for diagnosing HF in the elderly.[27] Significantly, prognostic models have shown that low ejection fraction (EF) may lose its prognostic value in elderly patients compared with young HF patients.[35] Therefore, the presence of HFpEF should not be considered benign. Although, several other studies have attempted to identify prognostic factors, the heterogeneity of the population studied limit the ability to draw conclusions.[27,34] As alluded to earlier, the presence of noncardiac conditions such as frailty and cognitive impairment should also be considered in a comprehensive risk assessment of elderly patients with HF.

PARTICIPATION OF ELDERLY PATIENTS IN CLINICAL TRIALS

While 50% of patients with HF are over 75 years of age and most clinical trials have included only younger patients with a mean age of 61 years. A gap still exists between patients enrolled in clinical trials and those treated in clinical practice. Reduced likelihood of elderly patients to be referred to a cardiologist during acute HF and fulfillment of additional enrolment criteria such as renal dysfunction, life expectancy, and cancer are reasons for the underrepresentation of the elderly in clinical trials.[36] Table 1 shows several landmark clinical trials that have focused on only the elderly population with HF. Inadequate data makes treatment decisions challenging for healthcare providers, as they need to extrapolate how best to treat this special population.[37]

TREATMENT

Unfortunately, elderly HF patients are underrepresented in clinical trials and as a result therapies recommended in the current guidelines are based largely on studies in a younger population with a different clinical profile. Data from recent trials focused on the elderly is limited (Table 1), and several gaps remain in evidence with regard to HF treatment in these patients.

Pharmacotherapy in elderly patients needs to be prudently selected and monitored for a multitude of reasons. Physiological age-related changes affect drug pharmacokinetics and pharmacodynamics. Aging is associated with a lower volume of distribution and higher plasma concentrations of hydrophilic drugs.[38,39] The presence of other comorbidities (e.g. renal, liver dysfunction) increases the risk of adverse effects of drug therapy. Polypharmacy, common in the elderly, increases the risk of drug-drug interaction.[40] Cognitive impairment, frailty, and caregiver burden are important considerations when choosing an appropriate management plan.

Evidence-based therapy for systolic HF involves the use of drugs that suppresses neurohormones (reninangiotensin-aldosterone system and sympathetic nervous system) and includes an angiotensin-converting enzyme (ACE) inhibitor or angiotensin receptor blocker (ARB) and a β-blocker, and in select patients, an aldosterone antagonist.[41] Diuretics are particularly useful in older patients with increased vascular stiffness presenting with acute HF, since significant reduction in pressure occur with relatively small changes in intravascular volume. Although, β-blockers have been shown to improve survival and other important CV outcomes, many older individuals with systolic HF are not receiving any or underdosed β-blocker therapy. ARB is usually a substitute for ACE inhibitor, especially in older woman with side effects of cough and stress incontinence. Subgroup analysis has shown that ARB can be a better first-line of therapy in the elderly.[42] Due to the risk of hyperkalemia, monitoring of serum potassium after initiating aldosterone antagonist is essential with recommended intervals of 1, 2, 3, 6, and 12 months and 6 months thereafter particularly in those over the age of 75. Gynecomastia occurs in 10% of men as the testosterone level declines with age.[43] Although, it does not impact survival and digoxin is indicated as an adjunct therapy for rate control of atrial fibrillation and for advanced HF. Symptoms of mild toxicity such as anorexia, confusion, and visual disturbances can be missed by the elderly and close monitoring of electrolyte abnormalities is crucial.[37] The evidence for drug therapy in patients with HFpEF, which are the most common phenotype of HF in the elderly, is very limited. The general guidelines are primarily directed toward managing hypertension, maintaining

TABLE 1: Heart failure trials focusing on the elderly

Trial	Year	Study treatment	Number of patients	Mean age (Years)	Age-related inclusion criteria
ELITE[51]	1997	Losartan	722	73	Age >65 years, EF <40%
SENIORS[52]	2004	Nebivolol	2135	76	Age >70 years, EF <35%
PEP-CHF[53]	2006	Perindopril	850	76	Age >70 years, EF >40%
I-PRESERVE[54]	2008	Irbesartan	4128	72	Age >60 years, EF >45%
CIBIS-ELD[55]	2011	Bisoprolol	883	73	Age >65 years

Abbreviations: ELITE, Evaluation of Losartan in the Elderly Study; SENIORS, Study of the Effects of Nebivolol Intervention on Outcomes and Rehospitalization in Seniors with Heart Failure; PEP-CHF, Perindopril in Elderly People with Chronic Heart Failure study; I-PRESERVE, Irbesartan in Heart Failure with Preserved Systolic Function; CIBIS-ELD, Cardiac Insufficiency Bisoprolol Study in Elderly; EF, ejection fraction

sinus rhythm, and controlling heart rate in atrial fibrillation.[38]

In terms of device therapy, the meta-analysis of primary prophylactic implantable cardioverter defibrillators (ICD) studies (post-MI, EF <35%) suggests that this therapy may be less beneficial for elderly patients with severe LV dysfunction than for younger patients.[44] Cardiac resynchronization therapy remains an excellent management in medically refractory patients with EF less than or equal to 35% with QRS more than 150 ms.[45,46] Elderly patients with end-stage HF may be ineligible for heart transplantation because of age and comorbidities.[47] Although, the available data is still limited, and LV-assist device (LVAD) as a destination therapy is a potential option for these patients.[48]

Early symptom recognition, advocating self-management, mediation compliance, and dietary restrictions are key elements in HF management in the elderly.[49,50] Depression and anxiety are common conditions in this subset and need to be diagnosed and treated adequately. Lastly, given the relatively low 5-year survival rate for HF patients, it is critical that healthcare providers discuss end-of-life care with HF patients and their families.

Vaccinations in Elderly Patients with Heart Failure[56] (Flow chart 2)

- Heart failure is a chronic syndrome characterized by acute exacerbations. There is significant overlap between respiratory infections and exacerbation of underlying HF. Vaccination against respiratory infections in patients with HF could serve as a potential cost-effective intervention to improve patients' quality-of-life and clinical outcomes (Tables 2 and 3).

Flow chart 2: Mechanism of actions of vaccinations in heart failure

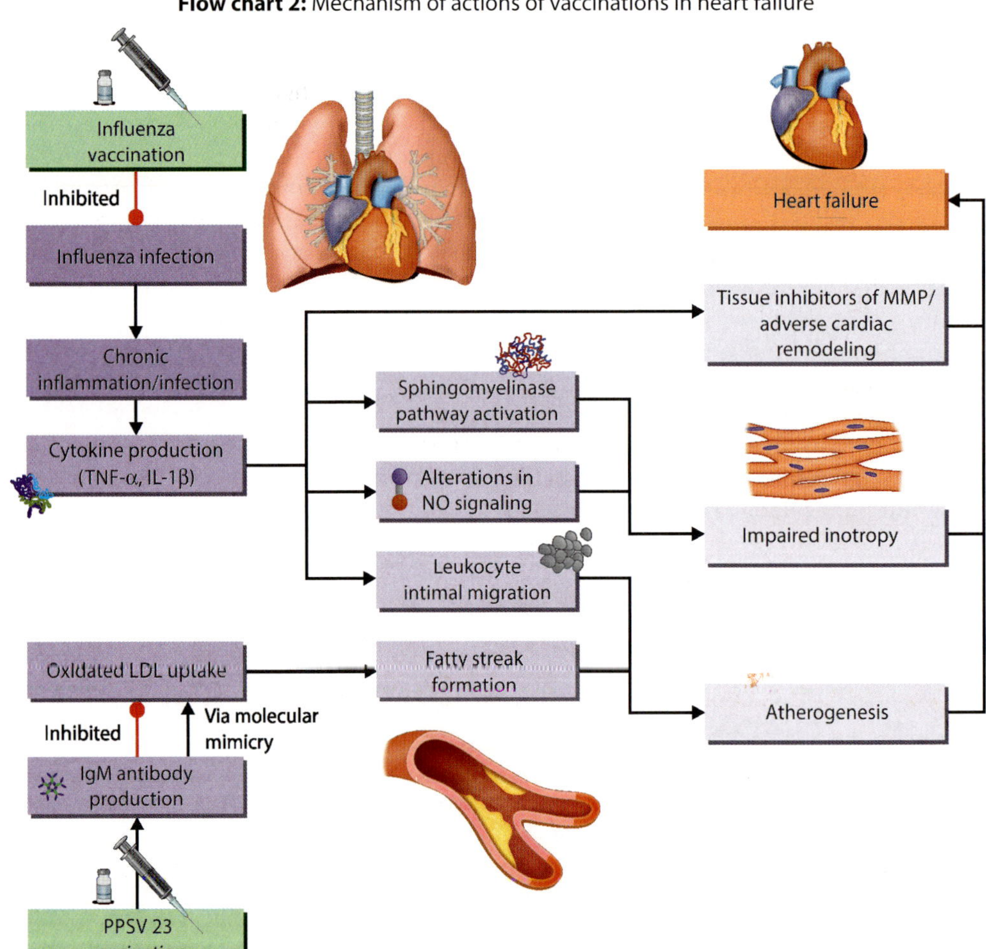

TABLE 2: Current guidelines recommendations on respiratory vaccination in cardiovascular (CV) disease

Society	Report	Recommendation
Centers for Disease Control (CDC)/ Advisory Committee on Immunization Practice (ACIP)	CDC website	Yearly vaccination with inactivated influenza vaccination for 'adults and children who have chronic disorders of the pulmonary or cardiovascular systems' Pneumococcal polysaccharide vaccination for all adults age >65 yrs and earlier in 'high risk immunocompetent patients such as those with chronic cardiovascular disease (except hypertension)'
American Heart Association/American College of Cardiology Foundation (AHA/ACCF)	2011 Secondary Prevention and Risk Reduction Therapy for Patients with Coronary and other Atherosclerotic Vascular Disease 2013 Guideline for the Management of HF	'Patients with cardiovascular disease should have an annual influenza vaccination' (Class I, Level of evidence: B) "Secondary prevention interventions (e.g., lipids, smoking cessation, influenza and pneumococcal vaccines)"
Heart Failure Society of America (HFSA)	2010 Comprehensive HF Practice Guideline	'Pneumococcal vaccine and annual influenza vaccination are recommended in all patients with HF in the absence of known contraindications' (Level of evidence B)
European Society of Cardiology	2012 European Guidelines on Cardiovascular Disease Prevention in Clinical Practice	"Annual influenza vaccinations are recommended for patients with established cardiovascular disease"

Abbreviation: HF, heart failure

TABLE 3: Randomized control efficacy trials evidence for respiratory vaccination in cardiovascular disease

Study/First author (year)	Total N	Country	Population	Intervention	Control	Primary Outcome Variable	Results
FLUVACS (2004)	301	Argentina	Inpatients: ACS or planned PCI	Trivalent, inactivated influenza vaccination	No vaccination	CV death (12 monts)	RR: 0.34 (95% CI: 0.17-0.71) P = 0.002
FLUCAD (2008)	658	Poland	Outpatients: angiography-confirmed CAD	Trivalent, inactivated influenza vaccination	No vaccination	CV death (12 months)	HR: 1.06 (95% CI: 0.15–7.56) P = 0.95
Phrommintikul et al. (2011)	439	Thailand	Inpatients: ACS within 8 weeks	Trivalent, inactivated influenza vaccination	No vaccination	Composite major CV events (death, hospitalization for ACS, HF and stroke) (12 months)	HR: 0.70 (95% CI: 0.57-0.86) P = 0.004
Van Ermen et al. (2013)	28	United States	Outpatients with HF	Double dose influenza vaccination	Standard dose influenza vaccination	Antibody production by hemagglutinin inhibition assay (2 and 4 weeks)	3.3 vs. 1.6 for A/H3N2 p < 0.001 1.9 vs 1.1. for A/H1N1 p = 0.009 1.7 vs 1 for B/H1N1 p = 0.02

Standard dose vaccination contains 15 μg of hemagglutinin/strain, and double dose contains 30 μg of hemagglutinin/strain.
Abbreviations: ACS, acute coronary syndrome; CAD, coronary artery disease; CI, confidence interval; FLUCAD, Influenza Vaccination in secondary prevention from coronary ischemic events in coronary artery disease; FLUVACS, Flu vaccination acute coronary syndromes; HR, hazard ratio; PCI, percutaneous coronary intervention; RR, risk ratio

- The 2005 Centers for Disease Control (CDC) report recommended routine yearly inactivated influenza vaccination in adults with chronic CV disease including HF. These recommendations are supported by major cardiology societies (Class I, Level of Evidence: B).
- The Heart Failure Society of America recommends yearly influenza vaccination specifically in patients with HF without contraindications (Level B), as does the European Society of Cardiology.

UNRESOLVED ISSUES/FUTURE DIRECTIONS

While elderly patients represent the majority of the HF population and have a worse prognosis, targeted treatment strategies have been insufficiently developed for them. Future trials need to address these issues by addressing specific enrolment goals for the elderly. Exercise capacity assessment in diagnosis and prognostication may need adjustment. Prognostic markers should be specifically studied in the elderly and risk stratification models need to be validated in prospective studies. Integrated, multispecialty management should be the goal of the future, and cost-effectiveness of these strategies should be evaluated.

CONCLUSION

Elderly patients with HF constitute the majority of patient with HF and their numbers are increasing. These patients have a complex clinical profile characterized by multiple comorbidities, polypharmacy, and social circumstances. Currently, only very limited evidence exists for management in these patients. A holistic, multidisciplinary, and comprehensive clinical evaluation is needed to ensure adequate and proportionate care. Continuous efforts to advance knowledge and to better understand this challenging clinical entity are necessary to improve care and prognosis of elderly patients with HF.

REFERENCES

1. McCullough PA, Philbin EF, Spertus JA, et al. Confirmation of a heart failure epidemic: findings from the Resource Utilization Among Congestive Heart Failure (REACH) study. J Am Coll Cardiol. 2002;39:60-9.
2. Lloyd-Jones D, Adams RJ, Brown TM, et al. Executive summary: heart disease and stroke statistics—2010 update: a report from the American Heart Association. Circulation. 2010;121:948-54.
3. Komajda M, Hanon O, Hochadel M, et al. Contemporary management of octogenarians hospitalized for heart failure in Europe: Euro Heart Failure Survey II. Eur Heart J. 2009;30:478-86.
4. Barsheshet A, Shotan A, Cohen E, et al. Predictors of long-term (4-year) mortality in elderly and young patients with acute heart failure. Eur J Heart Fail. 2010;12:833-40.
5. Lazzarini V, Mentz RJ, Fiuzat M, et al. Heart failure in elderly patients: distinctive features and unresolved issues. Eur J Heart Fail. 2013;15:717-23.
6. Samala RV, Navas V, Saluke E, et al. Heart failure in frail, older patients: we can do 'MORE'. Cleve Clin J Med. 2011;78:837-45.
7. Cleland JG, Swedberg K, Follath F, et al. The EuroHeart Failure survey programme— a survey on the quality of care among patients with heart failure in Europe. Part 1: patient characteristics and diagnosis. Eur Heart J. 2003;24:442-63.
8. Bleumink GS, Knetsch AM, Sturkenboom MC, et al. Quantifying the heart failure epidemic: prevalence, incidence rate, lifetime risk and prognosis of heart failure The Rotterdam Study. Eur Heart J. 2004;25:1614-9.
9. Harikrishnan S, Sanjay G, Anees T, et al. Clinical presentation, management, in-hospital and 90-day outcomes of heart failure patients in Trivandrum, Kerala, India: the Trivandrum Heart Failure Registry. Eur J Heart Fail. 2015;17:794-800.
10. Heidenreich PA, Albert NM, Allen LA, et al. Forecasting the impact of heart failure in the United States: a policy statement from the American Heart Association. Circ Heart Fail. 2013;6:606-19.
11. Croft JB, Giles WH, Pollard RA, et al. Heart failure survival among older adults in the United States: a poor prognosis for an emerging epidemic in the Medicare population. Arch Int Med. 1999;159: 505-10.
12. Braunstein JB, Anderson GF, Gerstenblith G, et al. Noncardiac comorbidity increases preventable hospitalizations and mortality among Medicare beneficiaries with chronic heart failure. J Am Coll Cardiol. 2003;42:1226-33.
13. Yancy CW, Jessup M, Bozkurt B, et al. 2013 ACCF/AHA guideline for the management of heart failure: a report of the American College of Cardiology Foundation/American Heart Association Task Force on Practice Guidelines. J Am Coll Cardiol. 2013;62:e147-239.
14. Dodson JA, Chaudhry SI. Geriatric conditions in heart failure. Curr Cardiovasc Risk Rep. 2012;6:404-10.
15. McLennan SN, Pearson SA, Cameron J, et al. Prognostic importance of cognitive impairment in chronic heart failure patients: does specialist management make a difference? Eur J Heart Fail. 2006;8:494-501.
16. Walston J, Hadley EC, Ferrucci L, et al. Research agenda for frailty in older adults: toward a better understanding of physiology and etiology: summary from the American Geriatrics Society/National Institute on Aging Research Conference on Frailty in Older Adults. J Am Geriatr Soc. 2006;54:991-1001.
17. Wong LS, van der Harst P, de Boer RA, et al. Aging, telomeres and heart failure. Heart Fail Rev. 2010;15:479-86.
18. Olivetti G, Melissari M, Capasso JM, et al. Cardiomyopathy of the aging human heart. Myocyte loss and reactive cellular hypertrophy. Circ Res. 1991;68:1560-8.
19. Strait JB, Lakatta EG. Aging-associated cardiovascular changes and their relationship to heart failure. Heart Fail Clin. 2012;8:143-64.
20. Fleg JL, Morrell CH, Bos AG, et al. Accelerated longitudinal decline of aerobic capacity in healthy older adults. Circulation. 2005;112:674-82.
21. Spina RJ, Turner MJ, Ehsani AA. Beta-adrenergic-mediated improvement in left ventricular function by exercise training in older men. Am J Physiol. 1998;274: H397-404.
22. Ungvari Z, Kaley G, de Cabo R, et al. Mechanisms of vascular aging: new perspectives. J Gerontol A Biol Sci Med Sci. 2010;65:1028-41.
23. Kawaguchi M, Hay I, Fetics B, et al. Combined ventricular systolic and arterial stiffening in patients with heart failure and preserved ejection fraction: implications for systolic and diastolic reserve limitations. Circulation. 2003;107:714-20.
24. Jelani A, Jugdutt BI. STEMI and heart failure in the elderly: role of adverse remodeling. Heart Fail Rev. 2010;15:513-21.
25. Mogensen UM, Ersboll M, Andersen M, et al. Clinical characteristics and major comorbidities in heart failure patients more than 85 years of age compared with younger age groups. Eur J Heart Fail. 2011;13:1216-23.
26. Wang CS, FitzGerald JM, Schulzer M, et al. Does this dyspneic patient in the emergency department have congestive heart failure? JAMA. 2005;294:1944-56.
27. Oudejans I, Mosterd A, Bloemen JA, et al. Clinical evaluation of geriatric outpatients with suspected heart failure: value of symptoms, signs, and additional tests. Eur J Heart Fail. 2011;13:518-27.
28. Najjar SS. Heart failure with preserved ejection fraction failure to preserve, failure of reserve, and failure on the compliance curve. J Am Coll Cardiol. 2009;54:419-21.
29. Neuhold S, Huelsmann M, Strunk G, et al. Comparison of copeptin, B-type natriuretic peptide, and amino-terminal pro-B-type natriuretic peptide in patients with chronic heart failure: prediction of death at different stages of the disease. J Am Coll Cardiol. 2008;52:266-72.
30. Aarones M, Gullestad L, Aakhus S, et al. Prognostic value of cardiac troponin T in patients with moderate to severe heart failure

scheduled for cardiac resynchronization therapy. Am Heart J. 2011;161:1031-7.
31. van Kimmenade RR, Mohammed AA, Uthamalingam S, et al. Red blood cell distribution width and 1-year mortality in acute heart failure. Eur J Heart Fail. 2010;12: 129-36.
32. von Haehling S, Jankowska EA, Morgenthaler NG, et al. Comparison of midregional pro-atrial natriuretic peptide with N-terminal pro-B-type natriuretic peptide in predicting survival in patients with chronic heart failure. J Am Coll Cardiol. 2007;50:1973-80.
33. Mohammed AA, van Kimmenade RR, Richards M, et al. Hyponatremia, natriuretic peptides, and outcomes in acutely decompensated heart failure: results from the International Collaborative of NT-proBNP Study. Circ Heart Fail. 2010;3:354-61.
34. Manzano L, Babalis D, Roughton M, et al. Predictors of clinical outcomes in elderly patients with heart failure. Eur J Heart Fail. 2011;13:528-36.
35. Satomura H, Wada H, Sakakura K, et al. Congestive heart failure in the elderly: comparison between reduced ejection fraction and preserved ejection fraction. J Cardiol. 2012;59:215-9.
36. Forman DE, Rich MW, Alexander KP, et al. Cardiac care for older adults. Time for a new paradigm. J Am Coll Cardiol. 2011;57:1801-10.
37. Azad N, Lemay G. Management of chronic heart failure in the older population. J Geriatr Cardiol. 2014;11:329-37.
38. Rich MW. Pharmacotherapy of heart failure in the elderly: adverse events. Heart Fail Rev. 2012;17:589-95.
39. Mangoni AA, Jackson SH. Age-related changes in pharmacokinetics and pharmacodynamics: basic principles and practical applications. Br J Clin Pharmacol. 2004; 57:6-14.
40. Gastelurrutia P, Benrimoj SI, Espejo J, et al. Negative clinical outcomes associated with drug-related problems in heart failure (HF) outpatients: impact of a pharmacist in a multidisciplinary HF clinic. J Cardiac Fail. 2011;17: 217-23.
41. Ahmed A. DEFEAT—Heart Failure: a guide to management of geriatric heart failure by generalist physicians. Minerva medica. 2009;100:39-50.
42. Pfeffer MA, Swedberg K, Granger CB, et al. Effects of candesartan on mortality and morbidity in patients with chronic heart failure: the CHARM-Overall programme. Lancet. 2003;362:759-66.
43. Braunstein GD. Clinical practice. Gynecomastia. N Eng J Med. 2007;357:1229-37.
44. Santangeli P, Di Biase L, Dello Russo A, et al. Meta-analysis: age and effectiveness of prophylactic implantable cardioverter-defibrillators. Ann Int Med. 2010;153: 592-9.
45. Jeevanantham V, Daubert JP, Zareba W. Cardiac resynchronization therapy in heart failure patients: an update. Cardiol J. 2009;16:197-209.
46. Veazie PJ, Noyes K, Li Q, et al. Cardiac resynchronization and quality of life in patients with minimally symptomatic heart failure. J Am Coll Cardiol. 2012;60:1940-4.
47. Mehra MR, Kobashigawa J, Starling R, et al. Listing criteria for heart transplantation: International Society for Heart and Lung Transplantation guidelines for the care of cardiac transplant candidates—2006. J Heart Lung Transplant. 2006;25:1024-42.
48. Butler CR, Jugdutt BI. Mechanical circulatory support for elderly heart failure patients. Heart Fail Rev. 2012;17:663-9.
49. Stromberg A. The crucial role of patient education in heart failure. Eur J Heart Fail. 2005;7:363-9.
50. Gwadry-Sridhar FH, Arnold JM, Zhang Y, et al. Pilot study to determine the impact of a multidisciplinary educational intervention in patients hospitalized with heart failure. Am Heart J. 2005;150:982.
51. Pitt B, Segal R, Martinez FA, et al. Randomised trial of losartan versus captopril in patients over 65 with heart failure (Evaluation of Losartan in the Elderly Study, ELITE). Lancet. 1997;349: 747-52.
52. Flather MD, Shibata MC, Coats AJ, et al. Randomized trial to determine the effect of nebivolol on mortality and cardiovascular hospital admission in elderly patients with heart failure (SENIORS). Eur Heart J. 2005;26:215-25.
53. Cleland JG, Tendera M, Adamus J, et al. The perindopril in elderly people with chronic heart failure (PEP-CHF) study. Eur Heart J. 2006;27:2338-45.
54. Massie BM, Carson PE, McMurray JJ, et al. Irbesartan in patients with heart failure and preserved ejection fraction. N Engl J Med. 2008;359:2456-67.
55. Dungen HD, Apostolovic S, Inkrot S, et al. Titration to target dose of bisoprolol vs. carvedilol in elderly patients with heart failure: the CIBIS-ELD trial. Eur J Heart Fail. 2011;13:670-80.
56. Bhatt AS, DeVore AD, Hernandez AF, et al. Can Vaccinations Improve Heart Failure Outcomes? Contemporary Data and Future Directions. JACC Heart Fail. 2017;5:194-203.

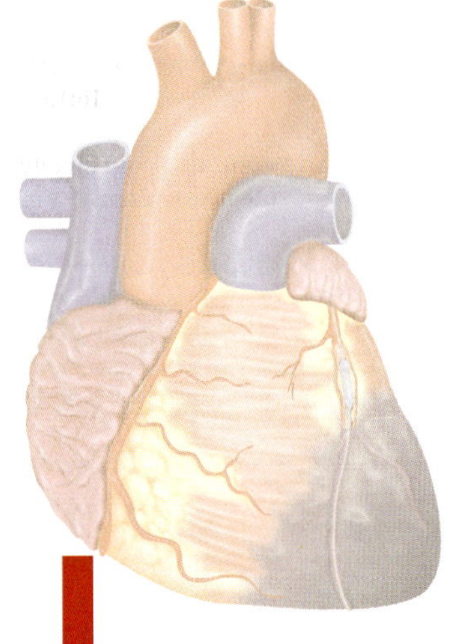

Prognosis of Heart Failure in Diabetes: Newer Perspectives

Jaideep C Menon, Umesh C Samal

INTRODUCTION

The prevalence of heart failure (HF) among the adult population is estimated at 1–2%, but there are reports as high as 10%, paralleling this scenario is a rapid rise in diabetes globally, with an estimated increase from 8.5% in 2011 to 9.8% in 2030.[1] Cardiovascular complications are frequent in type 2 diabetes (T2D), making this disease an important risk factor for subsequent HF, and, in addition, poor glucose control measured as glycated hemoglobin (HbA1c) predicts future development of HF. The true prevalence of this combination, as reported in clinical trials and registries, is inconsistent, varying between 13% and 47% (Table 1).[2]

The cardiac complications secondary to diabetes include:

- Secondary to coronary artery disease (CAD)
- Diabetic cardiomyopathy
- Sudden cardiac death (SCD).

PROGNOSIS OF PATIENTS WITH HEART FAILURE IN DIABETICS

Epidemiologic and clinical data from the last 2 decades have shown that the prevalence of HF in diabetes is very high, and the prognosis for patients with HF is worse in those with diabetes than in those without diabetes. Experimental data suggest that various mechanisms contribute to the impairment in systolic and diastolic function in patients with diabetes, and there is an increased recognition that these patients develop HF independent of the presence of CAD or its associated risk factors. In addition, current clinical data demonstrated that treatment with the sodium glucose co-transporter 2 inhibitor empagliflozin reduced hospitalization for HF in patients with type 2 diabetes mellitus (T2DM) and high cardiovascular risk. A retrospective cohort study analyzed data from the Kaiser Permanente Northwest database of 8,231 patients with diabetes, none of whom had HF at baseline, and 8,845 matched subjects without diabetes; the follow-up period was up to 6 years. Incident HF was 30.9 per 1,000 person-years in subjects with diabetes and 12.4 per 1,000 person-years in subjects without diabetes. Similar results were found in the Heart and Soul study, which showed a doubling of the risk of incident HF in patients with diabetes compared with subjects without diabetes in a population of 839 patients with stable CAD and no signs of HF at baseline (Fig. 1). However, neither study differentiated between HF with reduced ejection fraction (HFrEF) and heart failure with preserved ejection fraction (HFpEF).[3,4]

PROGNOSIS OF PATIENTS WITH DIABETES AND ESTABLISHED HEART FAILURE

The most meaningful clinical endpoints for prognosis in patients with HF are mortality and hospitalization for

TABLE 1: Reported prevalence of heart failure[2]

Study	Location	Overall prevalence rate	Prevalence rate in older age group
Surveys of treated patients			
RCGP (1958)	UK national data	3/1000	–
Gibson et al. (1966)	Rural cohort, USA	9–10/1000	65/1000 (>65 years)
RCGP (1986)	UK national data	11/1000	–
Parameshwar et al. (1992)	London, UK	4/1000	28/1000 (> 65 years)
Rodeheffer (1993)	Rochester, UK	3/1000 (< 75 years)	–
Mair et al. (1994)	Liverpool, UK	15/1000	80/1000 (> 65 years)
RCGP (1995)	UK national data	9/1000	74/1000 (65–74 years)
Clarke et al. (1995)	Nottinghamshire, UK	8–16/1000	40–60/1000 (> 70 years)
Population screening			
Droller and Pemberton (1953)	Sheffield, UK	–	30–50/1000 (> 62 years)
Garrison et al. (1966)	Georgia, USA	21/1000 (45–74 years)	35/1000 (65–74 years)
Framingham (1971)	Framingham, USA	3/1000 (< 63 years)	23/1000 (60–79 years)
Landahl et al. (1984)	Sweden (males only)	3/1000 (< 75 years)	80–170/1000 (> 67 years)
Eriksson et al. (1989)	Gothenburg, Sweden	–	130/1000 (> 67 years)
NHANES (1992)	USA national data	20/1000	80/1000 (> 65 years)
Cardiovascular Health Study (1993)	USA national data	20/1000	80/1000 (> 65 years)
RCGP (1995)	UK national data	9/1000 (25–74 years)	74/1000 (65–74 years)

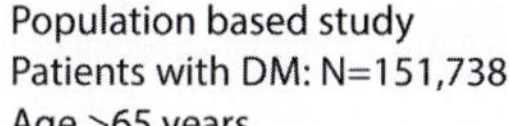

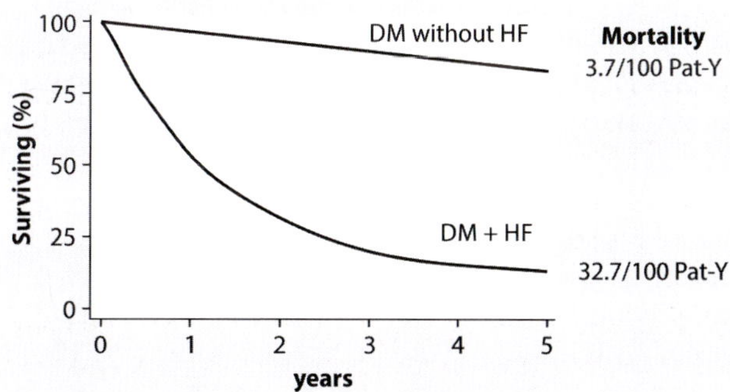

Fig. 1: In DM patients: HF predicts higher mortality. 151,738 diabetics were followed-up and it was seen that mortality was about nine times higher in diabetics with heart failure as compared with diabetics without heart failure

HF. The risk for these endpoints is markedly increased in subjects with diabetes compared with those without diabetes. The Danish Investigations of Arrhythmia and Mortality on Dofetilide (DIAMOND) study assessed the influence of diabetes on the risk of death in 5,491 patients hospitalized with congestive HF when followed up for 5–8 years. In this study population 16% of patients had diabetes at baseline, and approximately 50% had an ejection fraction less than 35%, suggesting that both HFrEF and HFpEF were present in this subpopulation. Crude mortality analyses suggested a one-year mortality of 31%, much higher than in subjects without diabetes, and 50% of all HF patients with diabetes died after 3 years (Fig. 2). Additional data on the prognosis of patients with diabetes and established HF came from large HF trials, such as the Survival and Ventricular Enlargement (SAVE) trial, the Valsartan in Acute Myocardial Infarction Trial (VALIANT), and the Candesartan in Heart Failure-Assessment of Reduction in Mortality and Morbidity (CHARM) trial. All of these trials showed an increased risk of death in men and women with diabetes. For example, in CHARM, which analyzed the effect of candesartan versus placebo in a population with HFrEF and HFpEF, it was shown that both men and women with diabetes exhibited a higher risk of cardiovascular death or hospitalization for HF compared with subjects without diabetes, with a cumulative incidence rate of approximately 40% over 3 years. Further, differentiated analyses in patients with or without diabetes and HFpEF or HFrEF showed that the highest mortality or hospitalization for HF risk occurred in patients with diabetes and low ejection fraction (i.e. HFrEF), followed by patients with diabetes and HFpEF. The cumulative incidence rate of cardiovascular death and HF hospitalization in subjects with diabetes plus HFpEF

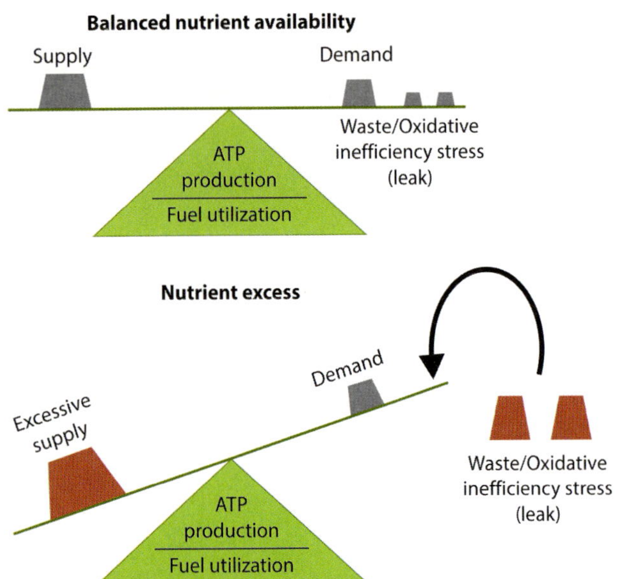

Fig. 2: Regulation of cellular bioenergetics efficiency under conditions of balance nutrient availability and under conditions of nutrient excess[6]

Abbreviation: ATP, adenosine triphosphate

Source: Adapted from Liea M, Shirihai OS. Mitochondrial dynamics in the regulation of nutrient utilization and energy expenditure. Cell Metab. 2013;17(4):491-506.

was similar to that in subjects without diabetes but with HFrEF. A similar trend was true for all-cause mortality. In patients with diabetes, cardiovascular mortality was 58.6 per 1,000 patient-years in those with HFpEF and 119.1 per 1,000 patient-years in those with a low ejection fraction (i.e. HFrEF). Similarly, in patients with diabetes, the risk for first hospital admission for HF was 116.6 per 1,000 patient-years for those with HFpEF, whereas the rate was 155.4 per 1,000 patient-years for those with HFrEF (Table 2). Compared with subjects without diabetes, the risk of hospitalization for HF was almost doubled in patients with diabetes independent of HFpEF or HFrEF. Consequently, among patients with HF, those with diabetes have a higher risk of mortality and hospitalization for HF than those without diabetes.[3,5-7]

PREDIABETES

Prevalence of prediabetes and diabetes is high among patients with HF and proves as a relevant predictor of prognosis. Data from Matsue et al. suggest that more than one-third of patients who are hospitalized for HF without a diagnosis of diabetes exhibit impaired fasting glucose or impaired glucose tolerance. As they discuss, more recent data from various registries show that the prevalence of

TABLE 2: In congestive heart failure (CHF): High prevalence of type 2 diabetes mellitus (DM)

CHF-trials	*T2DM prevalence*
CONSENSUS	23%
SOLVD	26%
CHARM	28%
EVEREST	40%
SENIORS	26%
SHIFT	30%
TOPCAT (HFpEF)	33%
EchoCRT	39%
PARADIGM-HF	35%
In healthy population	8–14%

diabetes in patients with HF ranges from approximately 25–40%, depending on the population studied. Again, none of these studies differentiated between HFrEF and HFpEF (Table 3).

The *Swedish Heart Failure Registry*[5] was an observational study in which patients with (n = 8,809) and without (n = 27,465) T2DM were included. The study was conducted in the period 2003–2011, wherein patients with a physician-based HF diagnosis were prospectively followed for long-term mortality (median follow-up time: 1.9 years, range 0–8.7 years). Left ventricular function expressed as EF did not differ between patients with and without T2DM. Survival was significantly shorter in patients with T2DM, who had a median survival time of 3.5 years compared with 4.6 years (P <0.0001). In subjects with T2DM unadjusted and adjusted odds ratios (ORs) for mortality were 1.37 [95% confidence interval (CI) 1.30–1.44] and 1.60 (95% CI 1.50–1.71), and T2DM predicted mortality in all age groups. Ischemic heart disease was an important predictor for mortality (OR 1.68, 95% CI 1.47–1.94), more abundant in patients with T2DM (59% vs 45%) among whom only 35% had been subjected to coronary angiography and 32% to revascularization. Evidence-based pharmacological HF treatment was somewhat more extensive in patients with T2DM.

Patients with T2DM compared with those without were somewhat younger, less frequently above the age of 80, and more often of male gender. Individuals with T2DM had a longer duration of HF and were more often in New York Heart Association (NYHA) class III–IV, while the EF was similar in the two groups. Patients with T2DM were heavier with a higher body mass index (BMI). Ischemic heart disease was more common in patients with T2DM (59% vs 45%). Similar proportions in both groups (35% vs 36%) had

TABLE 3: Mortality stratified by age grouped T2DM

Study name	Study population	Country	HF sample size	Definition of prediabetes	Prediabetes* (%)
Goode 2009	Prospective, stable HF clinic outpatients	UK	970	HbA1c > 6.0	50%
Suskin 2000 (Resolved study)	Baseline data of a multinational study; HF patients with NYHA II–IV and EF < 40%	Multi	487	FPG >6.1 mmol/L Fasting insulin resistance values ≥2.7	23% 33%
Matsue 2011	Patients admitted with a diagnosis of congestive HF	Japan	94	IGT: FPG < 126 mg/dL + OGTT 2-h glucose ≥ 140 mg/dL or FPG 110–125 mg/dL + OGTT 2-h glucose <140 mg/dL	39.4%
Witteles 2004	Clinic outpatients with stable HF and IDCM	US	43	IGT: OGTT 2-hour glucose level 140–199 mg/dL	27.9%
Egstrup 2011	Consecutive patients with SHF and EF ≤ 45% referred to a heart failure clinic	Denmark	227	IGT: FPG: <7.0 mmol/L + OGIT 2-h glucose 7.8–11.1 mmol/L	22.5%

*Prediabetes proportion reported amongst non-diabetic HF patients, i.e. the denominator does not include patients with HF + DM

Abbreviations: IDCM, idiopathic dilated cardiompathy; FPG, fasting plasma glucose; OGTT, oral glucose tolerance test; IGT, impaired glucose tolerance; HF, heart failure; EF, ejection fraction; SHF, systolic heart failure; NYHA, New York Heart Association

Source: Stefan anker, 2015

undergone coronary angiography, while more patients with T2DM had been subjected to revascularization (32 vs. 22%). Other comorbidities including hypertension (60% vs. 43%) and pulmonary disease (19% vs 17%) were more frequent in patients with T2DM, while atrial fibrillation (AF) (45% vs 49%) and idiopathic dilated cardiomyopathy (9% vs 12%) were more common among those without T2DM. Survival by time is shown in Figure 1. 1-year mortality was 23% in patients with and 19% in those without T2DM, whereas 5-year mortality was 59% and 52%, respectively. Table 3 presents 1-, and 5-year mortality stratified by age group and T2DM. Survival was significantly lower in those with compared with those without T2DM (median 3.5 vs 4.6 years; 95% CI 3.3–3.7 vs 4.5–4.7; *P* <0.0001). The mortality difference was most apparent below the age of 65 years in which quartile survival (95% CI) was 3.2 (2.8–3.5) years in patients with T2DM compared with 6 (6.2–7.6) years in those without (median survival time was not reached in the groups below 65 years of age). Median survival times (95% CI) in the age group 66–80 years were 4.0 (3.8–4.2) versus 6.1 (5.8–6.5) years, and at ages above 80 years they were 1.7 (1.6–1.8) and 2.1 (2.0–2.2) years, respectively.

Risks related to T2DM including unadjusted and adjusted ORs are outlined. Uni- and multivariate predictors for mortality in persons with T2DM are presented in Table 4. Important independent predictors for fatal outcome were creatinine clearance less than 30 mL (OR 4.43, 95% CI 3.41–5.75), ischemic heart disease (1.68, 95% CI 1.47–1.94), EF less than 30% (1.73, 95% CI 1.46–2.07), and presence of pulmonary disease (1.45, 95% CI 1.25–1.68), but not hypertension (0.81, 95% CI 0.72–0.92) (Fig. 3).

Indeed, few patients with T2DM and HF were alive after 8 years of follow-up. Importantly, T2DM was a strong independent risk factor for mortality in all age groups even after an extensive adjustment for other risk factors and differences in treatment (Tables 5 and 6).

The CHARM[6,8,9] investigators analyzed the outcomes in 7,599 patients with symptomatic HF and a broad range of ejection fractions. The prevalence of diabetes was 28.3% in patients with preserved EF (>40%) and 28.5% in those with low EF (≤40%). Diabetes was associated with a greater relative risk of CV death or HF hospitalization in patients with preserved EF [hazard ratio (HR) 2.0 (1.70–2.36)] than in patients with low EF [HR 1.60 (1.44–1.77); interaction test P = 0.0009]. For all-cause mortality, the risk conferred by diabetes was similar in both low and preserved EF groups. The effect of candesartan in reducing CV morbidity and mortality outcomes was not modified by having diabetes at baseline (P = 0.09 test for interaction).

The differences between diabetics and nondiabetics were amplified when EF category was considered—the most striking contrasts were between low EF HF patients with diabetes and preserved EF HF patients without diabetes. HF patients with diabetes were more often females and of non-European ethnicity than HF patients without diabetes.

TABLE 4: Baseline characteristics (n = number of observations)[1]

Variables	Type 2 diabetes					
	No			Yes		
	Missing[a] (n)	n=27465 (n)	(%)	Missing[a] (n)	n=8809 (n)	(%)
Demographics						
Age (mean ± SD)		75.1 ± 12.7			74.4 ± 0.5	
Male		72.9 ± 12.8			72.6 ± 10.5	
Female		78.5 ± 11.8			77.5 ± 9.8	
Age group (years)						
≤65		5835	21		1740	20
66–80		10393	38		4315	49
>80		11237	41		2754	31
Male gender		16459	60		5518	63
Weight (kg; mean ± SD)	1805	76 ± 18		477	84 ± 19	
Smoking habits (%; never/former/current)	7189	45/41/14		2349	41/46/13	
Duration of HF (%; below/above 6 months)	169	53/47		42	44/56	
NYHA	7320			2540		
I		2475	12		511	8
II		9310	46		2571	41
III		7397	37		2751	44
IV		963	5		436	7
Heart rate (bpm; mean ± SD)[b]	2211	74.7 ± 16.4		692	75.1 ± 15.5	
QRS duration (mean ± SD)	8520	110 ± 27		2799	112 ± 27	
QRS duration (%; below/above 120 ms)	8520	71/29		2799	68/32	
Blood pressure (mm Hg; mean ± SD)						
Systolic	315	127 ± 22		107	130 ± 22	
Diastolic	346	73 ± 13		117	73 ± 12	
Pulse pressure	357	54 ± 18		118	58 ± 19	
Previous or present disease[c]						
Ischemic heart disease	1154	11900	45	327	5034	59
Verified by coronary angiography		4232	36		1745	35
Hypertension	884	11474	43	277	5090	60
Atrial fibrillation	145	13438	49	79	3892	45
Pulmonary disease	623	4679	17	347	1633	19
Valvular heart disease	1363	5635	22	532	1485	18
Idiopathic dilated cardiomyopathy	1232	3104	12	464	754	9
Previous interventions						
Revascularization (CABG/PCI)	502	5871	22	232	2768	32
Valvular surgery[b]	306	1492	5	130	443	5

P-value <0.0001 unless otherwise stated.
Abbreviations: CABG, coronary artery bypass graft; HF, heart failure; T2DM, type 2 diabetes mellitus.
[a]Number of patients with missing information on variable.
[b]Not significant.
[c]One patient may have more than one diagnosis.

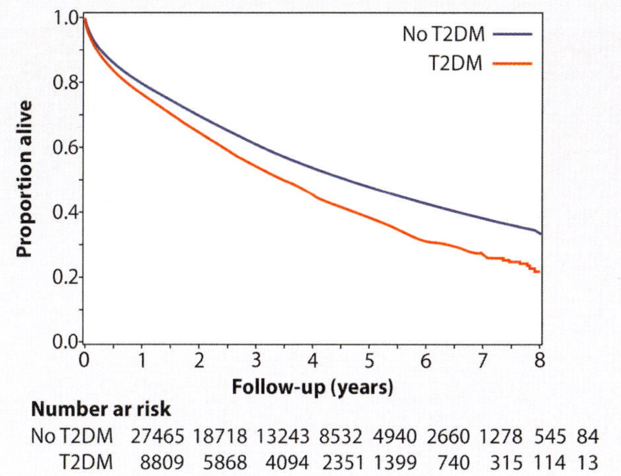

Fig. 3: Kaplan-Meier curves showing long-term survival in patients with HF with and without type 2diabetes mellitus (T2DM)[1]

Diabetic patients were more likely to be overweight or obese than nondiabetics. They were also less likely to be current smokers. They were more likely to have an investigator-designated ischemic or hypertensive etiology of HF than nondiabetics (and less likely to have idiopathic-dilated cardiomyopathy).

Functional Class, Signs, and Symptoms

Patients with diabetes had more signs and symptoms of HF and worse NYHA functional status than nondiabetics in both the low and preserved EF groups. The highest rates of symptoms and signs (and greatest proportion of III/IV vs II NYHA functional class) were seen in patients with a low EF and diabetes and the lowest rates (and proportion) in patients with preserved EF without diabetes.

Medical History

Regardless of EF, patients with diabetes had a higher prevalence of hypertension, myocardial infarction, coronary artery bypass grafting and stroke than patients without diabetes. The prevalence of hypertension in patients with preserved EF and diabetes (79%) was nearly double that in patients with low EF and no diabetes (44.0%).

Blood Chemistry, Hematology, and Renal Function

Diabetic patients had a slightly lower mean hemoglobin concentration and slightly lower eGFR than nondiabetics.

Treatment

Diabetic patients had higher rates of treatment with most CV drugs than nondiabetics, with the highest rates of use being in patients with a low EF and diabetes and the lowest rates in patients with preserved EF without diabetes (with the notable exception of calcium channel blockers).

About half of diabetic patients (50.7%) were treated with oral diabetic therapy and a third with insulin (32.7%).

Outcomes

The unadjusted rates of death and hospitalization from all causes were significantly higher in diabetic patients when compared with those in non-diabetics. After adjustment for 32 covariates, diabetes at baseline remained an independent predictor of the main primary and secondary outcomes, regardless of EF. The effect of diabetes on outcomes was not modified by sex or etiology of HF. Diabetes at baseline was associated with a higher risk of CV as well as non-CV death.[6] The risk of each of the major modes of CV death was also increased in diabetic compared to nondiabetic patients (Tables 7 and 8).

The same was true for CV hospitalizations. Of note, however, patients with preserved EF HF (which generally had better outcomes than those with reduced EF HF) and diabetes had a higher rate of CV hospitalization than patients with reduced EF HF, without diabetes (284.8 vs 229.2 admissions to hospital per 1,000 years of patient follow-up). This was also the case for hospitalization for HF and myocardial infarction separately.[9]

INTERACTION BETWEEN DIABETES AND LEFT VENTRICULAR EJECTION FRACTION

Cardiovascular Death and Heart Failure Hospitalization

Diabetes was associated with an increased risk of the combined primary outcome of CV death or HF hospitalization in patients with both low and preserved EF HF. In patients with low EF, diabetes was an independent predictor of CV death or HF hospitalization with an HR of 1.60 (1.44–1.77, $P < 0.0001$).The magnitude of the risk was even greater in patients with preserved EF, where diabetes was associated with a doubling of the risk of CV death or HF hospitalization [HR 2.0 (1.70–2.36, $P < 0.0001$)]. There was a statistically significant ($P = 0.0009$) interaction

TABLE 5: Laboratory variables and pharmacological and device treatment[1]

Variables	*Type 2 diabetes*					
	No			*Yes*		
	Missing[a] (n)	*n = 27465* (n)	(%)	*Missing[a]* (n)	*n = 8809* (n)	(%)
Biochemical						
Hb class (male, %; normal/mild anemia/severe anemia)		64/27/9			54/32/14	
Hb class (female, %; normal/mild anemia/severe anemia)		69/27/4			58/36/6	
Creatinine (μmol/L; mean ± SD)		108 ± 57			123 ± 71	
Creatinine clearance class (mL/min)[b]	1805			477		
<30		3464	14		1089	13
30–59		10809	42		3350	40
60–89		6668	26		2241	27
>90		4719	18		1652	20
Cholesterol (mmol/L)	22801	4.6 ±1.2		7263	4.2 ± 1.2	
Random plasma glucose[c] (mmol/L; mean ± SD)	20240	6.3 ±1.5		5926	8.7 ± 3.6	
HbA_{1c} (mmol/mol; mean ± SD)	26543	42 ± 9		7549	59 ± 17	
NT-proBNP (pg/mL; median, IQR)[b]	20397	2860 (1210–6290)		6621	2870 (1270–6448)	
Left ventricular function (echocardiography)[b]	*4255*			1322		
EF ≥50%		5047	22		1658	22
EF 40–49%		4921	21		1562	21
EF 30–39%		6316	27		2033	27
EF <30%		6926	30		2234	30
Pharmacological treatment						
RAS inhibition						
ACEi	185	17342	64	49	5324	61
ARB	576	4725	18	175	2190	25
ACE + ARB		426	1.6		256	2.9
MRA	212	7483	27	83	2816	32
Beta-blockers	154	22859	84	52	7501	86
ACEi/ARB + BB		18787	68		6416	73
ACEi/ARB + BB + MRA		5256	19		2143	24
Diuretics (loop/thiazide)	138	21643	79	28	7774	89
Digitalis	185	5050	19	55	1471	17
Statins	192	10121	37	46	4931	56
Nitrates (long-lasting)	227	4388	16	72	2083	24
Antithrombotic agents	198	9810	36	65	2872	33
ASA	216	13887	51	56	5268	60
Device treatment[b]	171			82		
Pacemaker		2499	9		812	9
CRT		516	1.9		190	2.2
Implantable cardioverter defibrillator		444	1.6		132	1.5

P-value <0.0001 unless otherwise stated.

Abbreviations: ACEi, ACE inhibitor; ASA, acetylsalicylic acid; Hb, hemoglobin; HbA1c, glycated haemoglobin; IQR, interquartile range; MRA, mineralocorticoid receptor antagonist; RAS, Renin–angiotensin system

[a]Number of patients with missing variables.

[b]Not significant.

[c]Variable excluded from case-report form since April 2010.

TABLE 6: One and five-years mortality stratified by type 2 diabetes mellitus[1]

Age group	*1-year mortality*		*5-year mortality*	
	No T2DM (%)	*T2DM (%)*	*No T2DM (%)*	*T2DM (%)*
All	19	23	52	59
≤65	5	10	52	59
66–80	13	19	43	58
>80	32	36	78	84

TABLE 7: Baseline characteristics[3]

Variable	*Overall (n = 7599)*		*PEF (n = 3023)*		*LEF (n = 4576)*	
	Diabetes mellitus (DM)	*No DM*	*DM*	*No DM*	*DM*	*No DM*
N	2163 (28.5%)	5436	857 (28.3%)	2166	1306 (28.5%)	3270
Demographics						
Age (years)	65.8 (10.0)	66.0 (11.4)	66.6 (10.0)	67.4 (11.5)	65.3 (9.9)	65.1 (11.4)
Male (%)	66.7	69.1	57.4	60.9	72.7	74.6
Female (%)	33.3	30.9	43.6	39.1	27.3	25.4
Non-European origin	329 (15.2%)	400 (7.4%)	131 (15.3%)	125 (5.8%)	198 (15.2%)	275 (8.4%)
Physiologic measure						
Body mass index (mean, kg/m²)	29.8 (5.9)	27.6 (5.1)	31.2 (6.3)	28.4 (5.3)	29.0 (5.5)	27.1 (4.9)
Underweight (<18.5)	12 (0.6%)	69 (1.3%)	3 (0.4%)	20 (0.9%)	9 (0.7%)	49 (1.5%)
Normal (18.5–24.9)	407 (18.8%)	1640 (30.2%)	115 (13.4%)	558 (25.8%)	292 (22.4%)	1082 (33.1%)
Overweight (25.0–29.9)	811 (37.5%)	2242 (41.2%)	302 (35.2%)	877 (40.5%)	509 (39.0%)	1365 (41.7%)
Obese (≥30.0)	923 (42.7%)	1464 (26.9%)	436 (50.9%)	699 (32.3%)	487 (37.3%)	765 (23.4%)
Heart rate (beats/min)	74.4 (12.5)	72.3 (13.2)	72.5 (11.7)	70.9 (12.7)	75.7 (12.8)	73.2 (13.4)
Systolic blood pressure (mm Hg)	131.9 (19.2)	130.5 (19.1)	137.4 (18.3)	135.7 (18.5)	128.3 (19.0)	127.0 (18.8)
Diastolic blood pressure (mm Hg)	75.7 (10.7)	77.0 (10.8)	76.3 (11.0)	78.4 (10.5)	75.3 (10.5)	76.1 (10.8)
Left ventricular ejection fraction (%)	38.6	39.0	53.9	54.1	28.5	29.0
Etiology of heart failure						
Ischemic heart disease	1426 (66.0%)	3255 (59.9%)	502 (58.6%)	1204 (55.6%)	924 (70.8)	2051 (62.7%)
Idiopathic dilated cardiomyopathy	294 (13.6%)	1033 (19.0%)	66 (7.7%)	197 (9.1%)	228 (17.5%)	836 (25.6%)
Hypertension	312 (14.4%)	669 (12.3%)	219 (25.6%)	465 (21.5%)	93 (7.1%)	204 (6.2%)
NYHA functional class						
NYHA (mean)	2.7 (0.5)	2.5 (0.5)	2.5 (0.6)	2.4 (0.5)	2.7 (0.5)	2.7 (0.5)
II	814 (37.6%)	2602 (47.9%)	428 (49.9%)	1408 (65.0%)	386 (29.6%)	1194 (36.5%)
III	1273 (58.9%)	2712 (49.9%)	405 (47.3%)	735 (33.9%)	868 (66.5%)	1977 (60.5%)
IV	76 (3.5%)	122 (2.2%)	24 (2.8%)	23 (1.1%)	52 (4.0%)	99 (3.0%)
Clinical features at baseline						
Peripheral edema	1467 (67.8%)	2977 (54.8%)	583 (68.0%)	1143 (52.8%)	884 (67.7%)	1834 (56.1%)
Orthopnea	1392 (64.4%)	2686 (49.4%)	512 (59.7%)	928 (42.8%)	880 (67.4%)	1758 (53.8%)
Paroxysmal nocturnal dyspnea	1150 (53.2%)	2269 (41.7%)	426 (49.7%)	741 (34.2%)	724 (55.4%)	1528 (46.7%)
Jugular venous pressure > 6 cm	765 (35.4%)	1509 (27.8%)	257 (30.0%)	451 (20.8%)	508 (38.9%)	1058 (32.4%)
Rest dyspnea	1259 (58.2%)	2708 (49.8%)	450 (52.5%)	909 (42.0%)	809 (61.9%)	1799 (55.0%)
Third heart sound	682 (31.5%)	1462 (26.9%)	186 (21.7%)	330 (15.2%)	496 (38.0%)	1132 (34.6%)
Pulmonary crackles-basilar	1463 (67.6%)	3252 (59.8%)	523 (61.0%)	1147 (53.0%)	940 (72.0%)	2105 (64.4%)
Medical history						
Hypertension	1481 (68.5%)	2705 (49.8%)	678 (79.1%)	1265 (58.4%)	803 (61.5%)	1440 (44.0%)
Prior myocardial infection	1215 (56.2%)	2789 (51.3%)	401 (46.8%)	939 (43.4%)	814 (62.3%)	1850 (56.6%)
Current angina pectoris	539 (24.9%)	1269 (23.3%)	250 (29.2%)	582 (26.9%)	289 (22.1%)	687 (21.0%)

Contd...

Contd...

Variable	Overall (n = 7599)		PEF (n = 3023)		LEF (n = 4576)	
	Diabetes mellitus (DM)	No DM	DM	No DM	DM	No DM
Prior coronary artery bypass grafting	624 (34.8%)	1167 (21.5%)	229 (26.7%)	425 (19.6%)	395 (30.2%)	742 (22.7%)
Stroke	237 (11.0%)	426 (7.8%)	101 (11.8%)	167 (7.7%)	136 (10.4%)	259 (7.9%)
Atrial fibrillation	562 (26.0%)	1521 (28.0%)	224 (26.1%)	657 (30.0%)	338 (25.9%)	864 (26.4%)
Cancer	139 (6.4%)	374 (6.9%)	65 (7.6%)	161 (7.4%)	74 (5.7%)	213 (6.5%)
Pacemaker	183 (8.5%)	454 (8.4%)	60 (7.0%)	161 (7.4%)	123 (9.4%)	293 (9.0%)
Implantable cardioverter defibrillator	44 (2.0%)	147 (2.7%)	6 (0.7%)	17 (0.8%)	38 (2.9%)	130 (4.0%)
Current smoker	264 (12.2%)	850 (15.6%)	91 (10.6%)	318 (14.7%)	173 (13.2%)	532 (16.3%)
Biochemistry and hematology						
Modification of diet in renal disease equation to estimate glomerular filtration rate (mL/mm/1.73 m²)	66.1 (26.4) (N = 996)	71.8 (25.6) (N = 1679)	67.2 (27.1) (N= 435)	72.9 (25.1) (N= 651)	65.3 (25.8) (N= 561)	71.2 (25.8) (N = 1028)
Hemoglobin (g/dL)	13.3 (1.7) (N = 992)	13.8 (1.6) (N = 1657)	13.1 (1.7) (N = 433)	13.6 (1.6) (N = 635)	13.4 (1.7) (N = 559)	13.8 (1.5) (N = 1022)
Cardiovascular medication						
Angiotensin-converting enzyme inhibitors	1019 (47.1%)	2106 (38.7%)	261 (30.5%)	315 (14.5%)	758 (58.0%)	1791 (54.8%)
Beta-blocker	1249 (57.7%)	2954 (54.3%)	490 (57.2%)	1194 (55.1%)	759 (58.1%)	1760 (53.8%)
Diuretics	1923 (88.9%)	4363 (80.3%)	717 (83.7%)	1542 (71.2%)	1206 (92.3%)	2821 (86.3%)
Long-acting nitrates	838 (38.7%)	1743 (32.1%)	316 (36.9%)	688 (31.8%)	522 (40.0%)	1055 (32.3%)
Spironolactone	398 (18.4%)	874 (16.1%)	117 (13.7%)	235 (10.8%)	281 (21.5%)	639 (19.5%)
Digitalis glycoside	1036 (47.9%)	2218 (40.8%)	269 (31.4%)	573 (26.5%)	767 (58.7%)	1645 (50.3%)
Calcium channel blocker	507 (23.4%)	1035 (19.0%)	304 (35.5%)	640 (29.5%)	203 (15.5%)	395 (12.1%)
Lipid-lowering drug	1046 (48.4%)	2107 (38.8%)	418 (48.8%)	844 (39.0%)	628 (48.1%)	1263 (38.6%)
Oral anticoagulant	634 (29.3%)	1704 (31.3%)	200 (23.3%)	548 (25.3%)	434 (33.2%)	1156 (35.4%)
Diabetes treatment						
Diet only	358 (16.6%)		151 (17.6%)		207 (15.8%)	
Insulin	707 (32.7%)		295 (34.4%)		412 (31.5%)	
Oral therapy	1096 (50.7%)		410 (47.8%)		686 (52.5%)	
Unknown	2 (0.1%)		1 (0.1%)		1 (0.1%)	
Age of diabetes onset (years)	54.1 (15.1)		54.6 (15.2)		53.7 (15.0)	

TABLE 8: Rates of death and admission to hospital per 100 patients years of follow-up diabetic status (P-values for univariate comparisons)[3]

Variable	All patients			Preserved EF			Low EF		
	Diabetes (n = 2163)	No diabetes (5436)	P-value	Diabetes (n = 857)	No diabetes (2166)	P-value	Diabetes (n = 1306)	No diabetes (3270)	P-value
Death									
Total	681	1150		185	296		496	854	
All causes	116.3	72.9	<0.001	77.4	46.0	<0.001	143.1	91.4	<0.001
Cardiovascular	94.4	57.5	<0.001	58.6	31.1	<0.001	119.1	75.7	<0.001
Heart failure	30.7	18.3	<0.001	16.3	9.8	0.011	40.7	24.2	<0.001
Sudden	40.0	25.9	<0.001	23.8	12.0	<0.001	51.1	35.5	<0.001
Myocardial infarction	8.0	4.1	<0.001	5.0	1.4	0.003	10.1	5.9	0.013
Stroke	6.1	3.4	0.005	5.9	3.0	0.048	6.3	3.6	0.046
Other cardiovascular	9.6	5.8	0.003	7.5	5.0	0.14	11.0	6.4	0.009
Non-cardiovascular	21.9	15.4	0.001	18.8	14.9	0.18	23.9	15.7	0.002

Contd...

Contd...

Variable	*All patients*			*Preserved EF*			*Low EF*		
	Diabetes (n = 2163)	*No diabetes (5436)*	*P-value*	*Diabetes (n = 857)*	*No diabetes (2166)*	*P-value*	*Diabetes (n = 1306)*	*No diabetes (3270)*	*P-value*
Hospital admissions (first)									
Total	1531	3266		606	1228		925	2038	
All causes	473.4	327.2	<0.001	466.6	296.3	<0.001	477.9	349.1	<0.001
Cardiovascular	306.5	207.4	<0.001	284.8	177.1	<0.001	321.8	229.2	<0.001
Heart failure	139.3	68.2	<0.001	116.6	45.9	<0.001	155.4	84.3	<0.001
Myocardial infarction	13.0	7.8	0.001	14.1	7.2	0.004	12.3	8.2	0.041
Stroke	14.0	9.2	0.002	15.7	9.4	0.014	12.9	9.0	0.058
Other cardiovascular	211.8	159.4	<0.001	200.5	137.1	<0.001	219.7	175.0	<0.001
Non-cardiovascular	222.9	152.7	<0.001	221.1	146.7	<0.001	224.2	156.8	<0.001
CV death or hospital admission for CV cause									
Total	1361	2708		492	924		869	1784	
	345.1	231.4	<0.001	302.6	189.4	<0.001	374.8	261.4	<0.001

between diabetes at baseline and EF with respect to this outcome. Diabetes was an independent risk factor for each component of this combined outcome in patients with both low and preserved EF HF. The adjusted HR for HF hospitalization in diabetics compared with non-diabetics was 1.64 (1.44–1.86, $p < 0.0001$) in patients with low EF and 2.04 (1.68–2.47, $p < 0.0001$) in patients with preserved EF HF.

That diabetes confers a greater risk for HF hospitalization in those with preserved EF than in those with low EF was confirmed by the interaction test ($p = 0.0029$). In absolute terms, patients with preserved EF and diabetes had a greater rate of HF hospitalization than those with low EF without diabetes (116.6 vs 84.3 admissions to hospital per 1,000 years of patient follow-up).

In the low EF group, the rates of CV death per 1000 years of patient follow-up were 119.1 and 75.7 for diabetics and non-diabetics, respectively [adjusted HR 1.54 (1.35–1.75, $p < 0.0001$)]. In those with preserved EF, the rates were 58.6 for diabetics and 31.1 for nondiabetics [adjusted HR 1.93 (1.52–2.45, $p < 0.0001$)]. The test for interaction was not, however, significant for this outcome.[6,8,9]

All-cause Mortality

In the low EF population, the absolute rates of death from any cause per 1,000 years of patient follow-up were 143.1 in diabetics and 91.4 in nondiabetics [adjusted HR 1.55 (1.38–1.74, $P < 0.0001$)]. In those with preserved EF, the rates were lower at 77.4 and 46.0 for diabetics and nondiabetics, respectively [adjusted HR 1.84 (1.51–2.26, $p < 0.0001$)]. Again, the test for interaction was not significant for this outcome.

Discussion

The CHARM study proved that diabetes is an independent predictor of morbidity and mortality in both low and preserved EF HF. The study also showed that diabetes conferred a greater increase in relative risk (and similar substantial increase in absolute risk) of the primary outcome of CV death or HF hospitalization in preserved EF HF when compared with low EF HF. Diabetes is not only an important independent predictor of morbidity and mortality in patients with low EF, but also in patients with preserved EF. In particular, we found that diabetes was associated with an increased risk of CV death or HF hospitalization in those with low and preserved EF HF. Furthermore, the relative risk conferred by diabetes was statistically significantly greater in patients with preserved EF than in those with low EF, and the increase in absolute risk was similarly large. The increase in events in patients with preserved EF and diabetes was primarily driven by an increased risk of HF hospitalization, with 27.8% hospitalized for HF compared with 12.9% of patients without diabetes. This risk related to diabetes in those with preserved EF was so marked that patients with preserved EF HF and diabetes had a greater rate of HF hospitalization than patients with low EF HF and no diabetes (27.8 vs 21.7%).

There are numerous pathophysiologic processes in diabetics that are thought to alter the myocardium resulting in inefficient, ineffective, contraction (e.g. collagen cross-linking secondary to advanced glycation end-products, disorders in calcium transport, and induction of the fetal gene program). It is possible that these processes have a more detrimental effect on cardiac function in a heart where the primary problem is impaired diastolic filling than

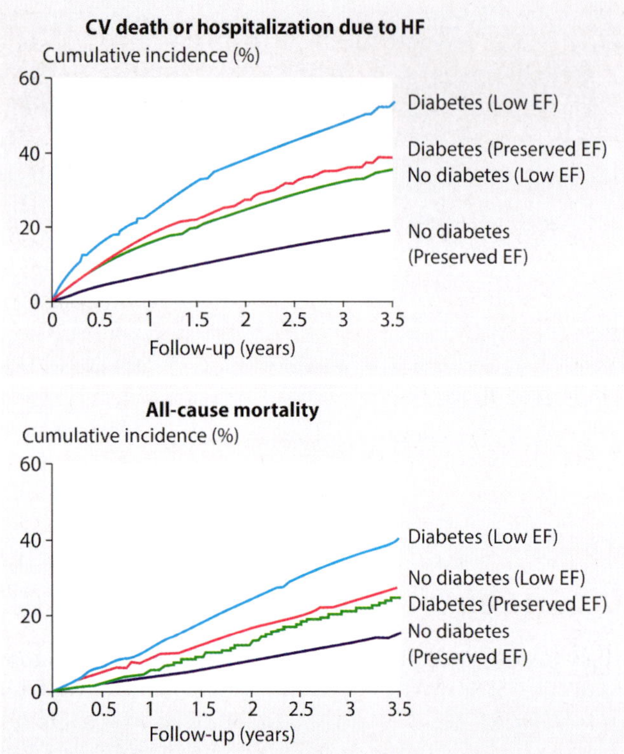

Fig. 4: Outcomes in diabetic and nondiabetic patients based on ejection fraction category (low vs preserved). The cumulative incidence of cardiovascular death or heart failure hospitalization and all-cause mortality in diabetic and nondiabetic patients based on ejection fraction category[3]

Abbreviations: CV, cardiovascular; EF, ejection fraction; HF, heart failure

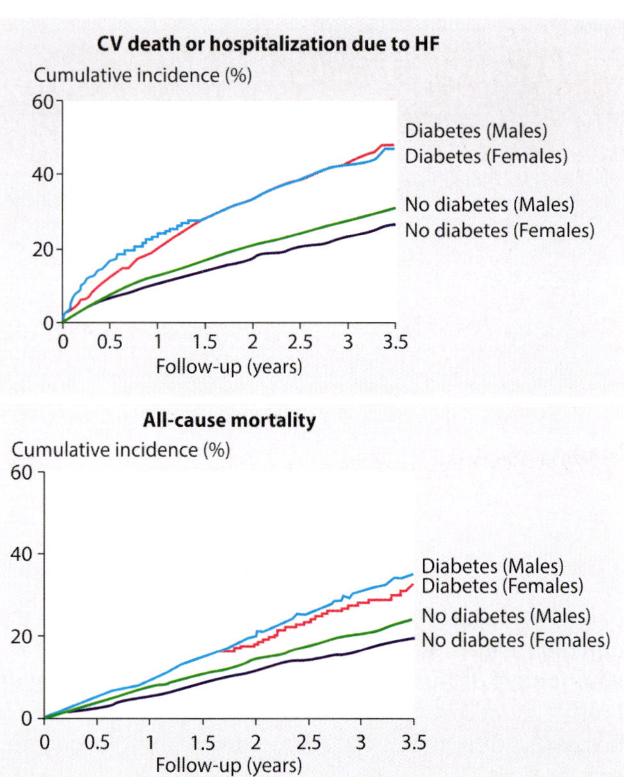

Fig. 5: Outcomes in diabetic and nondiabetic patients based on sex. The cumulative incidence of cardiovascular death or heart failure hospitalization and all-cause mortality in dieabetic and non-diabetic patient based on sex are shown here[3]

Abbreviations: CV, cardiovascular; HF, heart failure

in a heart where the main problem is systolic dysfunction. The other vascular and nonvascular effects of diabetes such as decreased arterial compliance, worse endothelial function, renal angiopathy, and autonomic dysfunction may also be relatively more important in patients with predominantly diastolic dysfunction. For example, these patients may be more sensitive to increases in preload and reductions in diastolic filling time due to increases in heart rate. Alternatively, diabetes has previously been identified as an independent predictor of the development of AF and a prior analysis from CHARM found that AF was associated with a greater increase in the risk of CV death and HF hospitalization in patients with preserved EF than in those with low EF HF. Development of AF and loss of atrial contribution to diastolic filling may result in a greater likelihood of cardiac decompensation in patients with diastolic than systolic dysfunction (Figs 4 to 8). Diabetes may also interact with other risk factors, e.g. hypertension, which is particularly prevalent in patients with preserved EF, to amplify risk.[6,8,9]

DIABETIC CARDIOMYOPATHY

The heart possesses a remarkable inherent capability to adapt itself to a wide array of genetic and extrinsic factors to maintain contractile function. Failure to sustain its compensatory responses results in cardiac dysfunction, leading to cardiomyopathy. Diabetic cardiomyopathy (DCM) is characterized by left ventricular hypertrophy and reduced diastolic function, with or without concurrent systolic dysfunction in the absence of hypertension and CAD. Changes in substrate metabolism, oxidative stress, endoplasmic reticulum stress, formation of extracellular matrix proteins, and advanced glycation end products constitute the early stage in DCM. These early events are followed by steatosis (accumulation of lipid droplets) in cardiomyocytes, which is followed by apoptosis, changes in *immune responses* with a consequent increase in fibrosis, remodeling of cardiomyocytes, and the resultant decrease in cardiac function. The heart is an omnivore, metabolically flexible, and consumes the highest amount of ATP in the

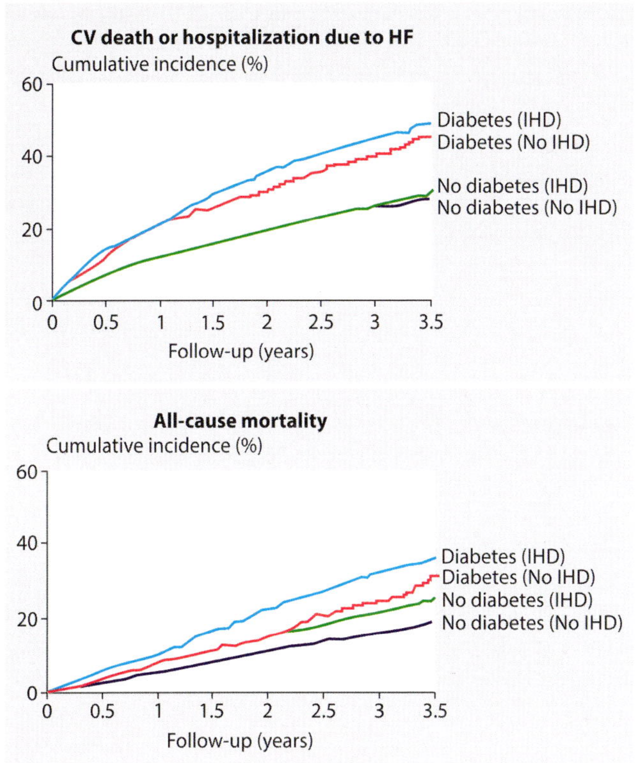

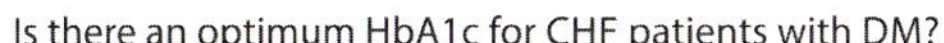

Fig. 6: Outcomes in diabetic and nondiabetic patients based on etiology (ischemic vs nonischemic). The cumulative incidence of cardiovascular death or heart failure hospitalization and all-cause mortality in diabetic and nondiabetic patient based on etiology heart failure are shown here[3]

Abbreviations: CV, cardiovascular; HF, heart failure; IHD, investigator designated ischemic heart disease etiology

body. Altered myocardial *substrate and energy metabolism* initiate the development of DCM. Diabetic hearts shift away from the utilization of glucose, rely almost completely on fatty acids (FAs) as the energy source, and become metabolically inflexible. Oxidation of FAs is metabolically inefficient as it consumes more energy. In addition to metabolic inflexibility and energy inefficiency, the diabetic heart suffers from impaired calcium handling with consequent alteration of relaxation-contraction dynamics leading to diastolic and systolic dysfunction. Sarcoplasmic reticulum (SR) plays a key role in excitation-contraction coupling as Ca^{2+} is transported into the SR by the SERCA2a (sarcoplasmic/endoplasmic reticulum calcium-ATPase 2a) during cardiac relaxation. Diabetic cardiomyocytes display decreased SERCA2a activity and leaky Ca^{2+} release channel resulting in reduced SR calcium load. The diabetic heart also suffers from marked downregulation of novel cardioprotective *microRNAs* (miRNAs) discovered recently.

The heart consumes about 6 kg of ATP, or approximately 20 times its own weight, per day that comes from the breakdown of fat, carbohydrate, protein, ketone bodies, or lactate. Of note, the amount of ATP in the heart is small (~10 mM, enough for only a few beats) compared with the demand (~10,000 times greater). About 95% of total energy is generated from oxidative phosphorylation of FAs and glucose. A dramatic metabolic shift takes place in diabetic heart, as they rely almost completely on FAs for their energy source. As for example, 46 atoms of oxygen are required to generate 105 molecules of ATP from oxidation of 1 molecule of palmitate. By contrast, oxidation of 1 molecule of glucose utilizes 12 atoms of oxygen to generate 31 molecules of

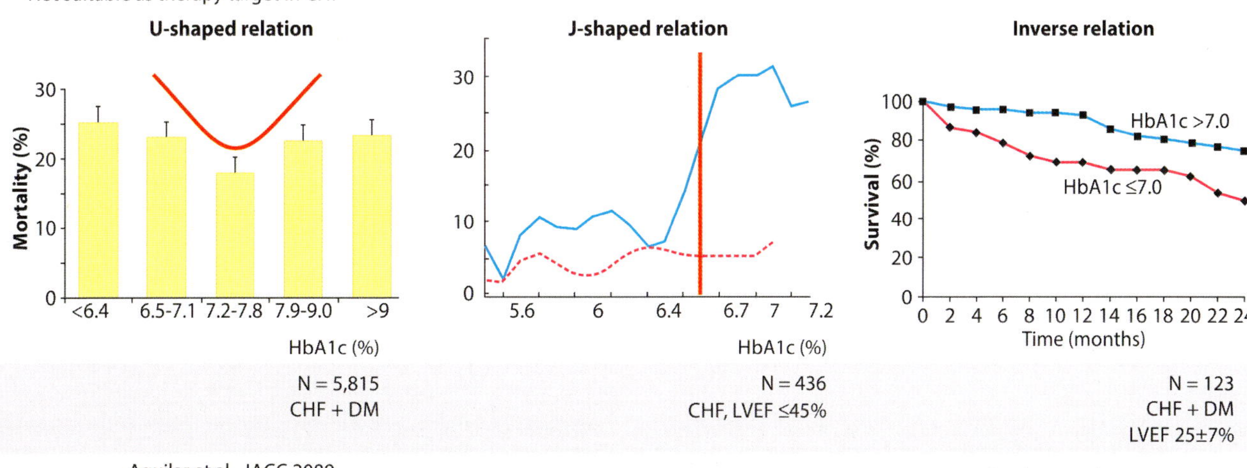

Fig. 7: Glycated hemoglobin (HbA1c) for outcome prediction in herat failure (HF)

Abbreviations: DM, diabetes mellitus; CHF, congestive heart failure; LVEF, left ventricular ejection fraction

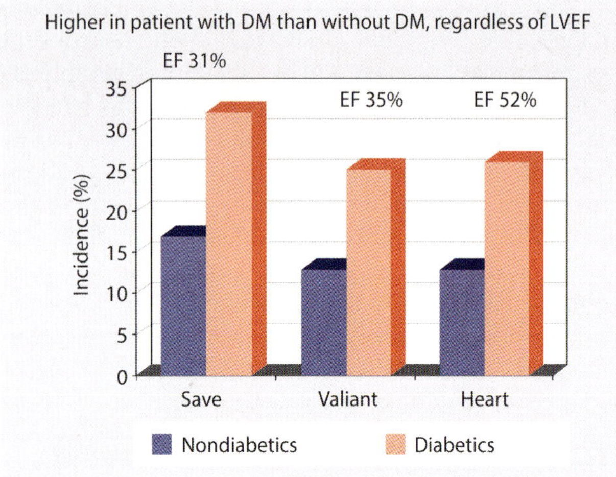

Fig. 8: Development of heart failure after myocardial infarction (MI)
Source: Stefan Anker, Aug 2016

ATP. Therefore, oxidation of FAs consumes approximately 0.3 oxygen molecules more than glucose to generate each molecule of ATP. Thus, the diabetic heart suffers from metabolic inflexibility due to its reliance on FAs. The lack of insulin production in T1DM patients causes a dramatic decrease in cardiac glucose uptake where hyperglycemia increases glucose oxidation and mitochondrial generation of superoxide. Increased production of superoxide damages DNA and activates poly (ADP ribose) polymerase 1 (PARP-1), which mediates inflammation and fibrosis in liver. PARP-1 inhibition improves cardiac function and prevents hyperglycemia-induced pathological processes. While decreased glucose transporter type 4 (Glut4) expression in T1DM animals causes decreased glucose uptake in cardiac and skeletal muscle.

miRnA inDiabetic Hearts: MicroRNAs are highly conserved endogenous small noncoding RNAs, approximately 22 nucleotides in length, that regulate gene expression by binding to partially complementary sequences of mRNA. The failing hearts consistently show chronic immune activation and aberrant miRNA expression. Thus, miR-155 plays an important role in the mammalian immune systems as well as during HF and is abundantly expressed in T-cells, B-cells, and monocytes. miRNAs are also differentially expressed during HF. STZ-induced diabetic heart expresses higher levels of miR-195 and silencing of miR-195 reduces DCM. Likewise, miR-141 is increased in diabetic heart and affects mitochondrial function and ATP generation. These miRNAs could be a potential target for developing a novel therapeutic strategy for the treatment of diabetic HF. Diabetes mellitus is a metabolic disease, and miRNAs play a crucial role in the regulation of metabolism. Increased levels of plasma cholesterol and triglyceride are common in diabetes, and liver specific ablation of miR-122, the most abundant miRNA in the liver, reduces plasma cholesterol and triglyceride levels (Figs 9 and 10).

DCM comprises several morphological and structural myocardial changes, which are induced through activation of various changes, with mechanical dysfunction as a fundamental change, consequent to unbalance between oxidants versus antioxidants, in favor of a pro-oxidative stress. Moreover, metabolic and functional alterations lead to a silent development of DCM, consisting of augmented free fatty acid (FFA) metabolism and modified intracellular signaling in cardiomyocytes, with consequent inefficient energy production and deficient cardiomyocyte contractility. The resulting diastolic and systolic dysfunction in DCM is also due to microvascular modifications with myocardial fibrosis and steatosis and also remodeling of the extracellular matrix Studies have highlighted that even when diastolic function is normal and left ventricle (LV) EF is preserved, there still exists a systolic LV strain alteration (MAPSE and longitudinal systolic LV strain), leading to the idea that diastolic dysfunction should not be considered the first sign of subclinical diabetic cardiomyopathy. This finding is also supported by the use of myocardial performance index (MPI) in order to evaluate global cardiac contractility, since it was demonstrated that an altered MPI is the earliest echocardiographic change in DCM, with recorded higher values in DCM patients compared with controls. Moreover, MPI might be useful in assessing the metabolic control or in indicating the necessity to early initiate pharmacologic therapy in T2DM, also offering the possibility to monitor the potential reversion of initial contractility dysfunction in DCM as response to optimal metabolic control. These stages comprise the following: stage 1 DCM (mixed hypertrophic and restrictive phenotype), stage 2 DCM (systolic dysfunction and dilatation), stage 3 DCM (systolic dysfunction to which microangiopathy and HTA have contributed), and stage 4 DCM (including dilatation, fibrosis, micro- and macroangiopathy). Assessing the cardiac function in diabetic patients can also be performed by cardiac magnetic resonance imaging (MRI), not only highlighting myocardial fibrosis as a first sign of left ventricular dysfunction, but also considering the possibility to distinguish the cardiac steatosis. This second metabolic landmark can be spotlighted through MRI as an early change in the course of DCM, considering that there is an increased uptake of FFA, with exceeding FFA oxidation, leading to enhanced accumulation of myocardial lipids and consequent altered intracellular signaling. The myocardial triglyceride content (but not perfusion reserve) is associated with LV diastolic dysfunction in T2DM, even after adjusting several parameters which could lead to

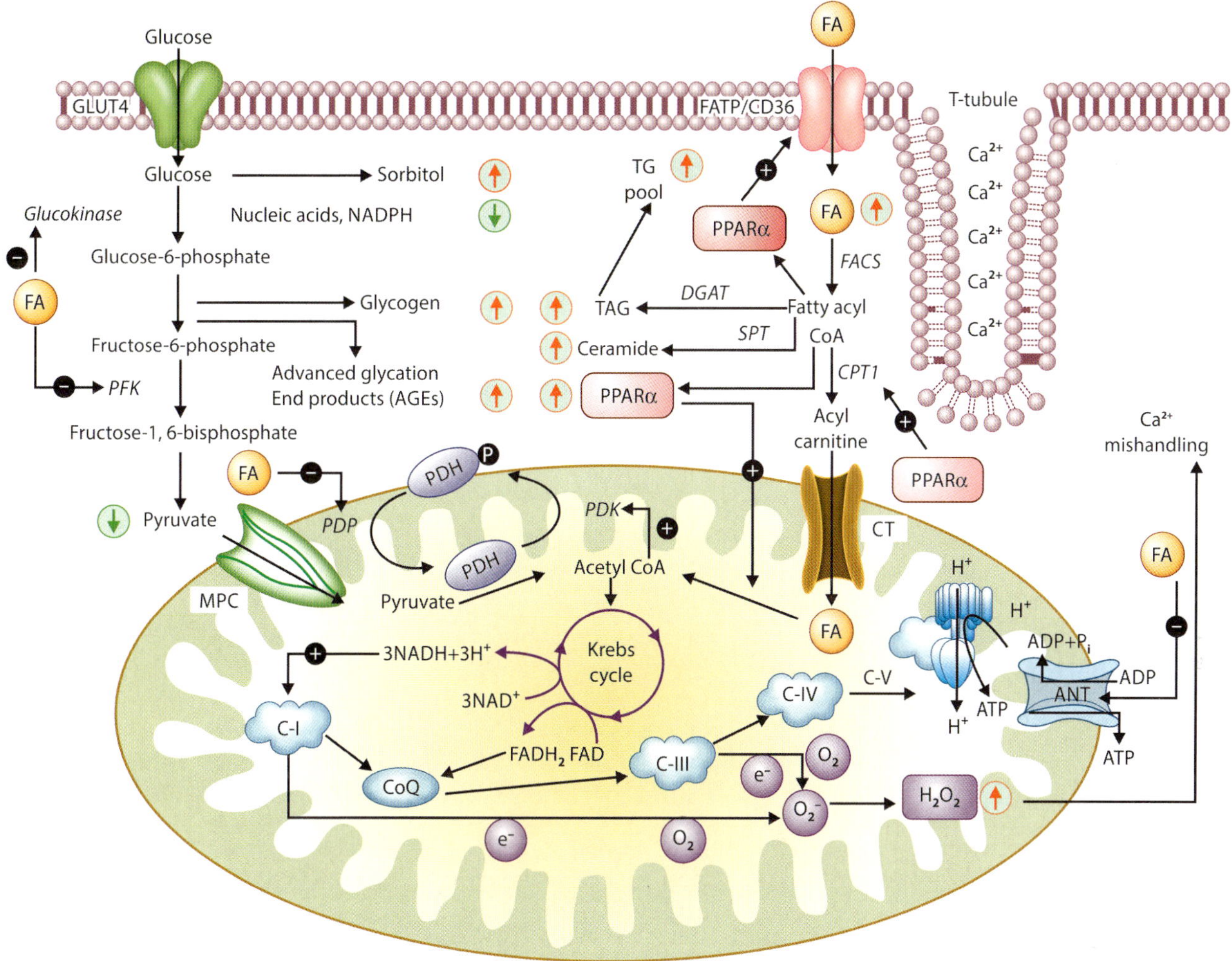

Fig. 9: Schematic diagram showing changes in cardiac metabolism in diabetic cardiomyopathy[4]

potential biases (such as duration of T2DM, blood pressure, or fasting blood glucose). As for biomarkers evaluating the risk for cardiovascular events in diabetic patients, MMP3, osteopontin and N-terminal prohormone of B-type natriuretic peptide (NTproBNP), and their combined value score are currently proposed to be introduced in evaluating diabetic patients, but first there is a need for more clear evidence that their use offers a more accurate risk stratification than the traditional risk factors.

Overview on Mechanisms involved in Diabetic Heart Disease and Potential Therapeutic Targets

Various metabolic changes are comprised during long time evolving DM—the cardiac uptake of albumin-fatty acid is augmented; the storage and catabolism of endogenous triglycerides are increased as well as the circulating lipoprotein levels, as a consequence of enhanced hepatic VLDL synthesis. In DCM, calcium signaling is altered; hence the contraction-relaxation dynamic is affected, with consequent alteration of structural components and activation of various signaling pathways, including NF-kB, c-Jun N-terminal kinases, and p38 mitogen-activated protein kinases through oxidative modifications. There is also impairment in protein folding, leading to toxicity and potential initiation of cardiomyocyte apoptosis.[10-13]

1. *Free fatty acid metabolism:* The FA metabolism is altered during DM, leading to lipotoxic cardiac injury; FAs enter the cell both via passive diffusion and facilitated transport, which can be mediated by various FA transport proteins, including fatty acid binding proteins (FABP). Once entered the cell, FAs can be used

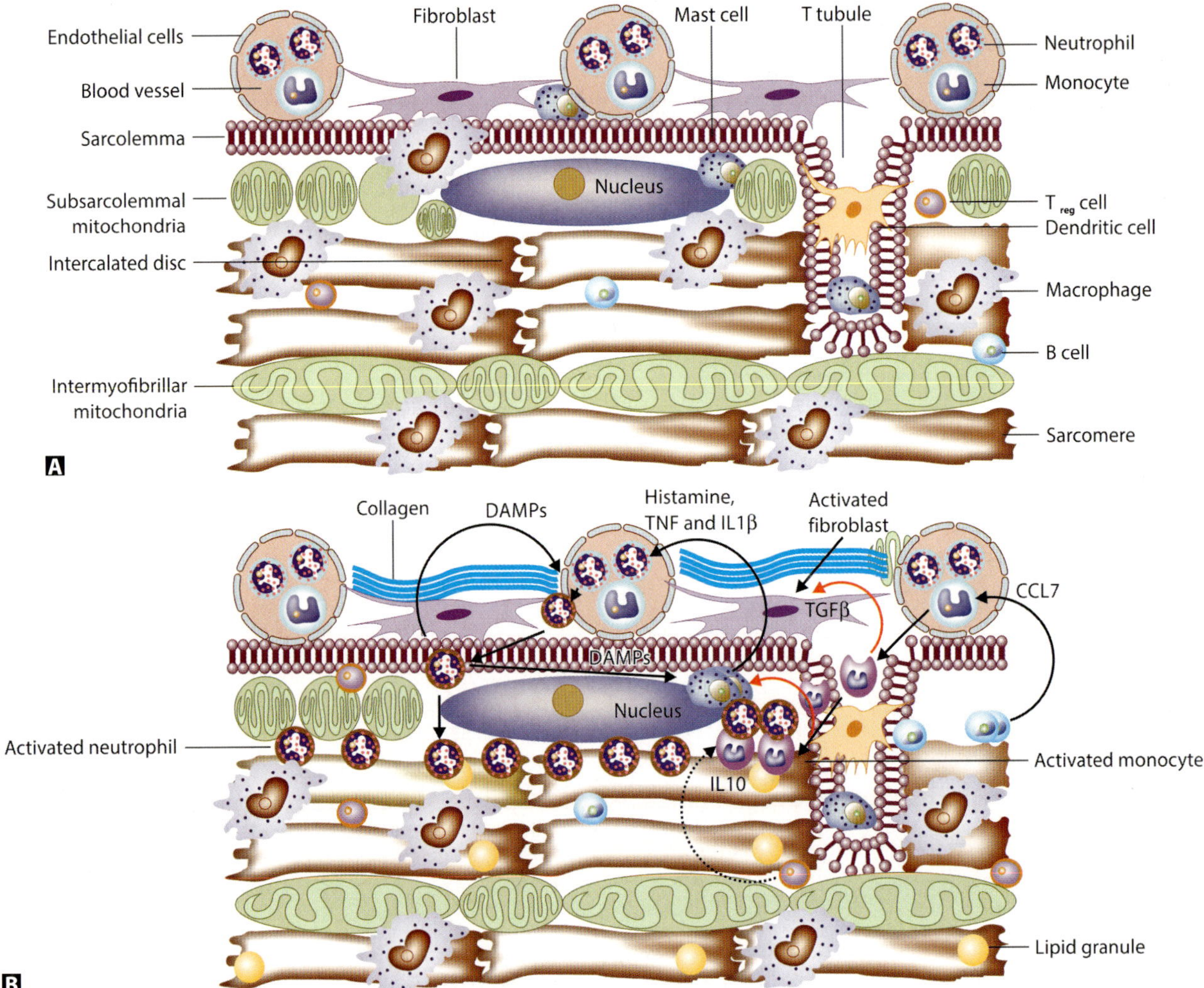

Figs 10A and B: (A) Schematic diagram showing immune cells in the healthy heart; (B) Schematic diagram showing infiltration of leukocytes[4]

as substrate by mitochondria to generate ATP, which can be temporarily stored after esterification or can activate PPAR, a class of nuclear mediators promoting transcription of genes coding proteins involved in FAs utilization. Overall, the myocardial FA build-up leads to decreased myocardial energy production, reduced myocyte contractility, and lipoapoptosis. Oxidative stress is also assumed to play a role in acceleration of apoptosis, through glycosylation and phosphorylation.

2. *Cardiac ubiquitin proteasome system (UPS):* Regarding cellular mechanisms, a pathogenic role has been recently attributed to the cardiac ubiquitin proteasome system (UPS), responsible for the maintenance of protein homeostasis by degrading the damaged proteins such as terminally misfolded proteins and oxidized proteins. In vitro and in vivo studies show that UPS dysfunction is an early event in diabetes and it triggers pathological remodeling in diabetic hearts.
3. *Deficiency in calcium handling:* In the development of cardiac contractility dysfunction, deficient calcium handling plays a key role, since it controls the excitation-contraction coupling. During contraction, calcium from the sarcoplasmic reticulum represents the major source of calcium, released from ryanodine receptor; the increased calcium cytoplasmic concentration triggers myofilament contraction. Abnormal function of RyR has been proved to contribute to various situations in which cardiac dysfunction is involved, such as cardiac

hypertrophy and ischemia-reperfusion lesions, but also in streptozotocin-induced type 1 diabetes, although the pathological significance is not well characterized. The reduced diastolic intracellular concentration may be due to AGE/RAGE interaction. Moreover, a reduced mitochondrial Ca uptake may significantly decrease ATP synthesis rate, leading to reduced contractility ability.[10-13]

Current Diagnosis of DCM

In the current clinical practice, the approach to diagnose DCM includes detecting structural and functional changes in the LV and adding proofs to exclude other cardiac disease as a potential etiology for the changes in a patient with diabetes. Most frequently, strain rate imaging and tissue Doppler imaging are used, offering the possibility to highlight the LV diastolic dysfunction during exercise stress, since the absence of echocardiographic changes at rest cannot exclude early DCM. However, there have been reports of systolic dysfunction (identified as abnormal systolic longitudinal strain rate) in the absence of diastolic dysfunction among diabetic patients. In order to early identify and evaluate cardiac dysfunction in diabetic patients, MR spectroscopy represents a potential novel diagnostic tool, considering its possibility to identify myocardial metabolic changes, such as quantifying myocardial triglycerides content. Since there is increasing evidence that the myocardial metabolism is altered during T2DM, with lipotoxic injury due to lipid oversupply, it has been demonstrated that myocardial triglyceride content is independently associated with biventricular changes in myocardial systolic and diastolic functions. In the early stages, there are only substructural changes in the cardiomyocytes, and the detection is possible only by very sensitive methods such as strain, strain rate, and myocardial tissue velocity. As for other novel techniques with potential to highlight early changes in heart metabolism, molecular MRI with specific labeling of free radicals might be a promising tool, with current use on animal models proving increased levels of free radicals in diabetic mice compared with controls. Considering myocardial fibrosis with increased extracellular matrix deposition, with consequent interstitial fibrosis, together with augmented free radical production as landmarks in the pathophysiology of DCM, in vivo imaging technique can prove to be useful in identifying the source and also the type of free radicals generated through oxidative stress during DCM. Assessment of interstitial fibrosis and steatosis by using delayed gadolinium enhancement cardiac MRI is possible but its diagnostic value has not been established. Since normal echocardiographic findings at rest cannot exclude DCM, left ventricular diastolic dysfunction detectable by TDI (and possible also by SRI) at exercise stress may be the earliest echocardiographic sign of diabetes induced LV dysfunction. As a consequence, there is a need to highlight earlier changes, for instance by assessing the level of interstitial fibrosis, using gadolinium-enhanced MRI. This method has not been confirmed as a valuable diagnostic tool and, consequently, the characterization of other metabolic changes in the cardiomyocyte is required; since there is evidence of reduced phosphocreatine/ATP ratio in the myocardium of diabetic patients, compared with control subjects, using magnetic resonance spectroscopy with ^{31}P or ^{1}H for determining it might represent a valuable tool. Using 1 H-MRS, it has been demonstrated that increased myocardial triglyceride content (i.e. myocardial steatosis) was associated with LV diastolic dysfunction in diabetic patients. In other study, myocardial steatosis was independently correlated with more pronounced impairment of ventricular contractility (evaluated by two-dimensional speckle tracking imaging) in patients with uncomplicated diabetes mellitus (Table 9).[10]

Future Directions for Diagnosis and Potential Treatment Targets for DCM

miRNA

The potential role of miRNAs in various pathologies has been recently emphasized, as a new perspective for diagnosis and treatment target has received considerable attention in biomedical research as a possible alternative for treatment of disease. Changes in the plasma level of cardiac biomarkers may reflect several myocardial metabolic changes. Although microribonucleic acids (miRNAs) are small noncoding RNA molecules, they play a key role in modulating gene expression and their altered level was found in the cardiomyocytes of experimental diabetes models. The expressions of several miRNAs are altered by matrix metalloproteinases (MMPs), which also play an important role in degrading extracellular matrix; the increased turnover of extracellular matrix proteins and alteration of MMPs levels are strongly correlated with active cardiac remodeling; furthermore, elevated level of MMP9 and reduced level of TIMPs are associated with myocardial fibrosis.

TABLE 9: DCM classification

Classification landmarks	*Stage 1 DCM (diastolic dysfunction, hypertrophy)*	*Stage 2 DCM systolic dysfunction and dilatation*	*Stage 3 DCM systolic dysfunction, dilatation, associated HTA*	*Stage 4 DCM including all confounders, also CAD*
Correspondence in NYHA classification	Asymptomatic	NYHA II	NYHA II-III	NYHA II–IV
Metabolic status	Impaired glucose tolerance; metabolic syndrome	Chronic hyperglycemia	Insulin resistance; DM with microangiopathic complications	DM with micro- and macroangiopathic complications
Echocardiographic features ± coronarography	Increased LV mass, diastolic dysfunction, decreased tissue velocities, normal EF	Increased LV mass and wall thickness, diastolic and systolic dysfunction (EF < 50%) mild cavity dilatation	Diastolic dysfunction and mild systolic dysfunction cavity dilatation	Moderate-severe systolic dysfunction cavity dilatation associated coronary artery disease
Other DM-related associated comorbidities			Microangiopathic complications; HTA	Macroangiopathic complications, including CAD
Serological markers to be monitored periodically regarding glycemic control, heart failure, and myocardial necrosis	NTproBNP, MMP-3, and osteopontin (according to van der Leeuw et al. 2016) Glc, lipid profile, HbA1c	MMP-3 and osteopontin (according to van der Leeuw et al. 2016) Glc, lipid profile, HbA1c, NTproBNP, BNP	MMP-3 and osteopontin (according to van der Leeuw et al. 2016) Glc, lipid profile, HbA1c, NTproBNP, BNP troponins increased in concurrent ischemia	Glc, lipid profile, HbA1c, NTproBNP, BNP troponins, increased in myocardial infarction or severe heart failure

Abbreviations: DDM, diabetes mellitus; EF, ejection fraction; Glc, glucose level; HTA, arterial hypertension, LV, left ventricle, MMP-3, metalloproteinase-3

Source: Adapted from Maisch, et al. 2011

Exosomes

Regarding DCM and the importance of miRNAs in this disease, exosomes emerge as potential biomarkers; although there is much to be elucidated regarding the role of these nanovesicles in DCM, it has been suggested that not only they represent the main vehicle for the plasmatic miRNAs, but also miRNAs are bound to complexes such as high density lipoproteins. Recently, it has been suggested that there is a strong relationship between nutrient sensing and exosome release. Under glucose deprivation conditions, there was an increased exosomes production from cardiomyocytes, with these nanovesicles containing glucose transporters and enzymes involved in glycolysis, consequently leading to an increase in glucose uptake and use with resulting pyruvate production in endothelial cells. Thus, cardiomyocyte-derived exosomes can regulate glucose transport in endothelial cells, the vesicle mechanism involving GTPases (guanosine triphosphatases) and several Rab (Ras-related proteins in brain) GTPases.

Mimetic Peptides Targeting Calcium Channels

There is intense experimental research on potential therapeutic approaches of DCM, and considering the essential role of intracellular calcium imbalance in contractile dysfunction, mimetic peptides (MP) targeting L-type calcium channels (LTCCs) have been tested.[1,14,15]

TREATMENT OF PATIENTS WITH DIABETES AND HFrEF

In patients with symptomatic NYHA class II-IV HF and reduced ejection fraction (LVEF <40%), treatment with angiotensin-converting enzyme (ACE) inhibitors [alternative: angiotensin receptor blockers (ARBs)] and beta-blockers is recommended, with titration to the maximum tolerated evidence-based dose. If patients are still symptomatic and exhibit an LVEF ≤35%, the addition of mineralocorticoid receptor antagonists is recommended. If still symptomatic, various therapeutic options exist for patients with NYHA II-IV HF. In patients who are able to tolerate ACE inhibitors or ARBs, angiotensin receptor neprilysin inhibitors should be used to replace ACE inhibitors or ARBs. In patients with sinus rhythm and a QRS duration more than 130 milliseconds, implantation of a cardiac resynchronization therapy device is recommended. Finally, patients with sinus rhythm and a heart rate more than 70 bpm should receive ivabradine; patients with symptoms and signs of congestion should receive diuretics. Moreover, patients with an LVEF ≤35% despite optimum medical therapy or a history of symptomatic ventricular tachycardia or ventricular fibrillation should receive an implantable cardioverter defibrillator. Similar recommendations were stated in a recent 2016 update of the American College of Cardiology/American Heart Association/Heart Failure Society of America HF guideline. Trials in patients with HFrEF are underway [e.g. EMPagliflozin outcomE tRial in Patients With chrOnic heaRt Failure With Reduced Ejection Fraction (EMPEROR-Reduced); NCT03057977]. These results, as well as those from future trials in patients with HFpEF, may inform future guidelines (Flow chart 1).[16-18]

TREATMENT OF PATIENTS WITH DIABETES AND HFpEF

Presently, treatment for HFpEF has not been shown to reduce mortality or morbidity; therefore, the guidelines recommend treatment of any comorbidities (e.g. hypertension, chronic kidney disease, chronic obstructive pulmonary disease). In addition, symptomatic therapy usually includes diuretics, especially in patients with congestion. The effect of various agents, including empagliflozin, on cardiovascular morbidity and mortality in patients with HFpEF will be determined by future trials

Flow chart 1: Therapeutic algorithm for a patient with symptomatic heart failure with reduced ejection fraction[6]

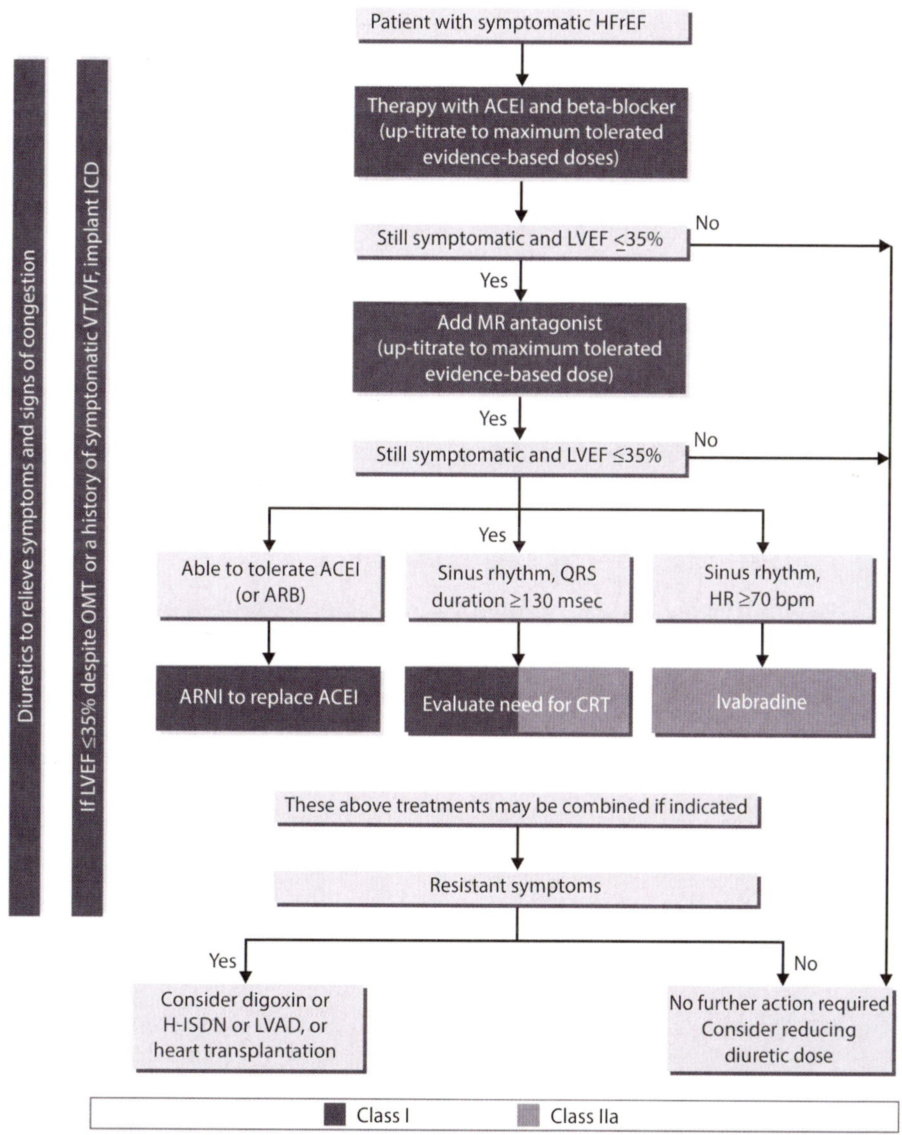

in HF [e.g. EMPagliflozin outcomE tRial in Patients With chrOnic heaRt Failure With Preserved Ejection Fraction (EMPEROR-Preserved; NCT03057951); and Dapagliflozin in T2D or Pre-diabetes, and PRESERVED Ejection Fraction Heart Failure (PRESERVED-HF; NCT03030235)]; however, thus far, symptom control is the major therapeutic goal.[19]

TREATMENT OF DIABETES IN PATIENTS WITH HEART FAILURE

Given the association of cardiac dysfunction with glucose metabolism, cardiac energy reserve, and steatosis, metabolic interventions aiming to improve glucose metabolism might have beneficial impact on cardiac function. Still, the optimal treatment strategy in patients with diabetes and HF remains controversial, and only some glucose-lowering medications have specifically been studied in patients with HF, which will be reviewed in the following sections.

Lifestyle

The efficacy of lifestyle intervention in comparison with standard of care was investigated in the Action for Health in Diabetes (Look-AHEAD) trial with 5,145 overweight or obese adults with T2DM. Despite significant weight loss in the intensive lifestyle intervention group (–8.6%) versus the control group (–0.7%) after 1 year, and initial improvement in physical fitness and HbA1c, intensive lifestyle intervention failed to improve cardiovascular outcomes during a mean follow-up of 9.6 years [hazard ratio (HR) 0.95; 95% confidence interval (CI), 0.83–1.09; P = 0.51]. HF events were numerically but not significantly reduced by intensive lifestyle intervention [HR 0.80; 95% CI, 0.61–1.04; P = 0.10). Interestingly, a recent posthoc analysis reported a significant reduction of cardiovascular events in patients who lost at least 10% of their body weight during the 1st year (21% of all individuals from both intervention arms; adjusted HR 0.79; 95% CI, 0.64–0.98; P = 0.034) in comparison with patients with stable body weight or weight gain. In addition, achievement of increased physical fitness (improvement by >2 metabolic equivalents reached by 13% of all individuals from both intervention arms) was associated with a significant reduction of the secondary composite endpoint that included HF (adjusted HR 0.77; 95% CI, 0.61–0.96; P = 0.023) but not of the original primary outcome of cardiovascular death, nonfatal myocardial infarction, or nonfatal stroke (adjusted HR 0.78; 95% CI, 0.60–1.03; P = 0.079). These results highlight the difficulty in performing lifestyle intervention trials, which largely depend on the motivation of individual study participants. Others have found that weight loss interventions reduce cardiac hypertrophy, decrease left atrial volume, and improve diastolic function in cohorts of obese individuals (approximately 30% of those experiencing weight loss had diabetes) with paroxysmal AF. Metabolically induced left ventricular dysfunction can consequently be reversed by lifestyle intervention. Importantly, both studies reported a potent reduction in AF as a primary endpoint, which gave weight loss management in obese patients a level IIa recommendation in the 2016 European Society of Cardiology (ESC) guidelines on AF.[11-13,20,21]

Glycemic Control

A variety of studies, including the UK Prospective Diabetes Study (UKPDS), the Action to Control Cardiovascular Risk in Diabetes (ACCORD) study, the Action in Diabetes and Vascular Disease Preterax and Diamicron Modified Release Controlled Evaluation (ADVANCE) study, and the Veterans Affairs Diabetes Trial (VADT), have aimed to reduce the cardiovascular risk of patients with diabetes by intensification of glycemic control. This led to a modest reduction in myocardial infarction but not cardiovascular mortality or HF hospitalization, and predisposed to more frequent hypoglycemia. Current guidelines suggest individualized, patient-centered HbA1c targets, which remain looser in patients with long-standing diabetes and established cardiovascular disease, but tighter in younger patients without manifest complications. More attention has since been given to drug-specific actions of diabetes medications on cardiovascular outcomes and HF, which will be discussed in the following sections.[21,22]

Metformin

Metformin is the first-line oral glucose-lowering drug for patients with diabetes. However, metformin therapy has long been avoided in patients with HF, attributable to its rare potential to cause lactic acidosis in unstable hemodynamic circumstances or renal impairment. Observational studies, however, suggest reduced mortality in metformin treated patients with HF. This led the US Food and Drug Administration (FDA) to remove congestive HF as a contraindication to metformin use in 2006, although acute or unstable HF remained a precaution. Metformin is now considered safe and the treatment of choice in patients with HF in the 2016 ESC guidelines. In 2016 new FDA recommendations now allow metformin use also in patients with mild to moderate kidney dysfunction, defined as an estimated glomerular filtration rate of 30–60 mL/min/1.73 m^2, but not in those with severe kidney dysfunction (estimated glomerular filtration rate <30 mL/min/1.73 m^2). A recent meta-analysis of 17 observational studies compared medical regimens that included metformin with those that did not in patients with diabetes and moderate impairment of kidney function, congestive HF, or chronic liver disease. Metformin use was associated with reduced all-cause mortality in all 3 patient groups and with fewer HF readmissions in patients with chronic kidney disease or congestive HF. Still, no reduction in HF events has been reported in a meta-analysis of randomized metformin intervention trials. Additional studies prospectively investigating the efficacy of metformin in patients with HF are consequently needed, as also pointed out by the American College of Cardiology Foundation/American Heart Association Guideline for the Management of Heart Failure 2013.

Sulfonylureas/Insulin

Limited data exist about the use of sulfonylureas or insulin and HF incidence. No difference in HF events was recorded in the UKPDS trial comparing sulfonylureas or insulin treatment with dietary intervention in 3,867 newly diagnosed patients with diabetes. A recent propensity score matched analysis of 10,089 patient pairs with diabetes treated with dipeptidyl peptidase-4 (DPP-4) inhibitors or sulfonylureas as add on to metformin reported DPP-4 inhibitors to be associated with a lower risk for all-cause mortality (HR 0.63; 95% CI, 0.55–0.72) and major adverse cardiac events (HR 0.68; 95% CI, 0.55–0.83) compared with sulfonylureas; however, no difference in HF hospitalization was reported. Nevertheless, others found sulfonylurea treatment to be associated with increased HF risk when compared with metformin in a retrospective cohort study. The impact of a glucose-lowering strategy with either an insulin-providing (sulfonylurea or insulin) or an insulin-sensitizing (metformin or thiazolidinedione) strategy was investigated in the Bypass Angioplasty Revascularization Investigation 2 Diabetes (BARI 2D) trial, which enrolled 2,368 patients with diabetes and CAD; among these, 141 had a history of HF. No difference for the primary endpoint of death, myocardial infarction, or stroke was found between both therapeutic strategies during a mean follow-up of 5.3 years. In addition, no difference in HF events was found in patients with or without HF at baseline. Still, a recent posthoc analysis reported older patients (>75 years; n = 182; 8% of the cohort) to have impaired cardiovascular outcome with the insulin-providing strategy (HR 1.65; 95% CI, 0.99-2.72; P = 0.050 by multivariate analysis), although no separate analysis for HF was reported. Other retrospective studies have suggested that insulin treatment worsens the prognosis of patients with diabetes and HF. Still, no increase in HF hospitalization or cardiovascular events was observed in the Outcome Reduction with an Initial Glargine Intervention (ORIGIN) trial. That study randomized 12,537 patients with impaired fasting glucose, impaired glucose tolerance, or T2DM to receive insulin glargine to target a fasting blood glucose level ≤95 mg/dL (5.3 mmol/L), which required approximately 30 units of insulin per day (0.31–0.40 units/kg). Whether higher daily doses of insulin could be considered safe was recently investigated in a cohort study of 6,072 patients with new insulin therapy added to preexisting metformin therapy. A requirement of more than 100 units of insulin per day was associated with increased cardiovascular mortality (HR 2.65; 95% CI, 1.65-4.25) when compared with a requirement of 25 units insulin per day or less. Still, no association of higher insulin doses was found with HF events. Further, adjustment to time-dependent variables, including HbA1c, body weight, and hypoglycemic/cardiovascular events, weakened the association of high insulin dose with cardiovascular mortality.

Thiazolidinediones

Thiazolidinediones (glitazones) have fluid retention potential, which leads to increased HF events. Thiazolidinediones are not recommended in patients with symptomatic HF, and initiation of therapy is contraindicated in patients with established NYHA III/IV HF.

DPP-4 Inhibitors

The DPP-4 inhibitors were the first class of diabetes agents for which trials were designed according to new requirements by the FDA and European Medicines Agency for cardiovascular safety. Cardiovascular safety sufficient to gain market approval is defined according to trial data showing that the upper bound of the 95% CI for the risk ratio of major adverse cardiovascular events compared with placebo is less than 1.3. Trial designs have typically aimed for glycemic equipoise in the drug and placebo groups; consequently, results are often independent of the HbA1c lowering efficacy of the tested drug. This also results in more intensive adjustment of background diabetes medications in subjects assigned to placebo. The DPP-4 inhibitors increase the bioavailability of the incretin hormones glucagon-like peptide 1 (GLP-1) and gastric inhibitory polypeptide (among other substrates), leading to glucose-dependent insulin secretion with no relevant effect on body weight. Three independent cardiovascular safety trials have been reported for the DPP-4 inhibitors.

Saxagliptin (Saxagliptin Assessment of Vascular Outcomes Recorded in Patients with Diabetes)

Mellitus-thrombolysis in myocardial infarction, alogliptin [Examination of Cardiovascular Outcomes with Alogliptin versus Standard of Care (EXAMINE)], and sitagliptin [Trial Evaluating Cardiovascular Outcomes with Sitagliptin (TECOS)]. These trials demonstrated cardiovascular safety in high-risk populations of patients with diabetes, although none of the substances proved superior to placebo on top of standard care. The secondary endpoint of HF hospitalization events was unexpectedly increased with saxagliptin in SAVOR-TIMI 53 (HR 1.27; 95% CI, 1.07–1.51; P = 0.007). A similar, albeit not significant, trend was found with alogliptin in the smaller EXAMINE trial [106 events (3.9%) vs 89 events (3.3%); HR 1.19; 95% CI, 0.90-1.58; P = 0.22], whereas no difference in HF hospitalization was found with sitagliptin in TECOS (HR 1.00; 95% CI, 0.83–1.20; P = 0.98). This suggests the absence of a class effect, which will be further evaluated in upcoming DPP-4 inhibitor trials. Retrospective propensity Score matched analysis of patients with HF and diabetes receiving DPP-4 inhibitors or other glucose lowering drugs found DPP-4 inhibitor treatment to be associated with reduced cardiac and all-cause mortality. Further, a large retrospective analysis including 78,553 new saxagliptin or 298,124 new sitagliptin users reported lower risk for HF hospitalization with DPP-4 inhibitor treatment in comparison with pioglitazone, sulfonylureas, or insulin treatment. In addition, neither DPP-4 inhibitors nor GLP-1 receptor agonists (GLP-1 RAs) were associated with increased HF hospitalization in a retrospective cohort analysis of 1,499,650 patients with diabetes, including 79,800 with a history of HF.

GLP-1 RAs

The GLP-1 RAs can be divided by their half-life as short and long-acting substances. Short-acting agonists more efficiently reduce postprandial glucose and have little effect on body weight, whereas long-acting substances primarily target fasting glucose levels and more efficiently cause weight loss. Fundamental differences have been found with respect to cardiovascular outcomes among these different agents. The short-acting lixisenatide (half-life 2–4 hours; administered once daily) proved safe, but not superior to placebo, in the Evaluation of Lixisenatide in Acute Coronary Syndrome (ELIXA) trial in patients with diabetes and acute coronary syndrome. In contrast, the long-acting liraglutide (half-life 13 hours; administered once daily) and the very long-acting semaglutide (half-life approximately 160 hours; administered once weekly) both significantly reduced cardiovascular events in high-risk patients with diabetes in the larger Liraglutide Effect and Action in Diabetes: Evaluation of Cardiovascular Outcome Results trial (LEADER; n = 9,340 patients) and the smaller Trial to Evaluate Cardiovascular and Other Long-term Outcomes with Semaglutide in Subjects with T2D (SUSTAIN-6; n = 3,297 patients). This was driven by a reduction in cardiovascular mortality in the LEADER trial (HR 0.78; 95% CI, 0.66–0.93; p = 0.007), which importantly translated to a reduction in total mortality (HR 0.85; 95% CI, 0.74–0.97; p = 0.02). In addition, nonsignificant reductions in nonfatal myocardial infarction, nonfatal stroke, and HF hospitalization were found. In contrast, semaglutide caused a significant reduction in nonfatal stroke (HR 0.61; 95% CI, 0.38–0.99; P = 0.04) and a nonsignificant reduction in nonfatal myocardial infarction (HR 0.74; 95% CI, 0.51–1.08; P = 0.12) with no difference in cardiovascular mortality or HF. These results demonstrate relevant differences among the different types of GLP-1 RAs. The reduction in cardiovascular mortality in the absence of HF improvement in LEADER suggests vasoprotective efficacy as a primary cardioprotective mechanism, which is supported by the SUSTAIN-6 results. Driven by favorable effects of GLP-1 and GLP-1 RAs in preclinical studies, a variety of smaller randomized trials have explored the efficacy of GLP-1 RAs for HF treatment in patients with or without diabetes. In the Functional Impact of GLP-1 for Heart Failure Treatment (FIGHT) trial, liraglutide did not improve cardiac function in 300 patients with advanced HF (LVEF ≤40%: 29% NYHA II and 68% NYHA III/IV; 60% with diabetes) during a period of 180 days. Unexpectedly, liraglutide numerically increased the combined endpoint of death and HF (HR 1.30; 95% CI, 0.92–1.83; log-rank p = 0.14), which became borderline significant in the subgroup of patients with diabetes (HR 1.54; 95% CI, 0.97-2.46; log-rank p = 0.07). No liraglutide-dependent increase of heart rate was observed in this trial, which has consistently been found in other studies using GLP-1 RAs. Further, liraglutide did not change LVEF in the Effect of Liraglutide on Left Ventricular Function in Chronic Heart Failure Patients With and Without T2DM (LIVE) trial, in which 241 patients with reduced LVEF (≤45%; among these 31% with diabetes) were randomly treated for 24 weeks. Heart rate increased in response to liraglutide by a mean of 7 beats per minute, whereas serious cardiac events occurred more often with liraglutide (n = 12; 10%) than with placebo (n = 3; 3%). Similarly, the GLP-1 RA albiglutide failed to improve LVEF of NYHA II/III HF patients without diabetes (LVEF <40%), while also leaving

6-minute walk distance, myocardial glucose uptake, or myocardial oxygen consumption unaffected. These data question the translatability of beneficial preclinical effects of GLP-1 in the context of manifest HF to the clinic.

SGLT2 Inhibitors

The SGLT2 inhibitors are a new class of antidiabetes drugs that block the SGLT2 receptor in the proximal tubule of the kidney, thus leading to increased urinary glucose excretion along with sodium. The first published cardiovascular outcomes trial to assess the effect of an SGLT2 inhibitor was Empagliflozin Cardiovascular Outcome Event Trial in T2DM Patients-Removing Excess Glucose (EMPA-REG OUTCOME), evaluating whether empagliflozin compared with placebo on top of standard-of-care treatment influences the incidence of cardiovascular events. The study in a high-risk population of 7,020 patients with T2DM and prior cardiovascular disease showed a significant 14% relative risk reduction in the primary endpoint of cardiovascular death, myocardial infarction, and stroke; a significant 38% relative risk reduction in cardiovascular death; as well as a significant 32% relative risk reduction in overall mortality, which translated into a number-needed-to-treat of 39 over 3 years to prevent 1 death. In addition, in a secondary analysis, empagliflozin led to a significant 35% relative risk reduction in hospitalization for HF (HR 0.65; 95% CI, 0.50–0.85; P <.002), with separation of the curves evident almost immediately during trial observation, suggesting a very early effect of the SGLT2 inhibitor on HF risk. The early effects of empagliflozin on cardiovascular mortality and hospitalization for HF suggest early hemodynamic effects of the drug. Furthermore, SGLT2 inhibition has been found to increase the concentration of circulating ketone bodies, which might provide an alternative energy source for the diabetic heart in the presence of insulin resistance. In addition, other potential mechanisms, such as weight loss, reduced blood pressure, sodium depletion, reduced oxidative stress, and arterial stiffness, as well as a reduction in sympathetic nerve activation, are currently being discussed. To date, prospective cardiovascular outcomes trial data for the SGLT2 inhibitor class are only available for empagliflozin. Because many of the potential mechanistic effects have also been described for other SGLT2 inhibitors, it will be interesting to see the results of the ongoing cardiovascular outcomes trials with dapagliflozin, canagliflozin, and ertugliflozin to determine whether the beneficial cardiovascular outcomes effects reported from the EMPA-REG OUTCOME trial are a class effect or unique to empagliflozin.[22,23]

CONCLUSION

Considering current trial results, patients with diabetes and HF may benefit most from glucose-lowering therapies with SGLT2 inhibition. This might relate to the elimination of glucose via the kidney, with net reduction of energetic substrate availability following SGLT2 inhibition, among other possible mechanisms. Reduced energetic substrate availability is also obtained with lifestyle intervention, which beneficially affects myocardial function in obese patients with and without diabetes. Further more limited evidence suggests beneficial effects with metformin, which reduces energetic substrate availability by decreasing endogenous glucose production, on HF in patients with diabetes. In contrast, no improvement in HF, or potential detrimental effects, have been reported for glucose-lowering strategies that directly or indirectly increase the availability of insulin. These considerations should be addressed in future study designs to optimize HF therapy in patients with diabetes.

REFERENCES

1. International Diabetes Federation (2011). IDF Diabetes Atlas. [online] Available from *http://www.idf.org/diabetesatlas.* [Accessed September, 2017].
2. McMurray JJ, Stewart S. Epidemiology, etiology and prognosis of heart failure. Heart. 2000;83:596-602.
3. Lehrke M. Diabetes and heart failure. Am J Med, 2017.
4. Kannel WB, Hjortland M, Castelli WP. Role of diabetes in congestive heart failure: the Framingham study. Am J Cardiol. 1974;34: 29-34.
5. Johansson I, Edner M, Dahlström U, et al. Is the prognosis in patients with Diabetes and Heart Failure a matter of unsatisfactory management? An observational study from the "Swedish Failure Heart Registry". Eur J Heart Fail. 2014;16(4):409-18.
6. MacDonald MR, Petrie MC, Varyani F, et al. Impact of diabetes on outcomes in patients with low and preserved ejection fraction heart failure (CHARM programme). Eur Heart J. 2008;29:1377-85.
7. Mishra PK, Ying W, Nandi SS, et al. Diabetic Cardiomyopathy: an immunometabolic perspective. Front Endocrinol, 2017.
8. Swedberg K, Pfeffer M, Granger C, et al. Candesartan in heart failure—assessment of reduction in mortality and morbidity (CHARM): rationale and design. Charm Programme Investigators. J Card Fail. 1999;5:276-82.
9. Pfeffer MA, Swedberg K, Granger CB, et al. Effects of candesartan on mortality and morbidity in patients with chronic heart failure: the CHARM-Overall programme. Lancet. 2003;362:759-66.
10. Gilca GE, Stefanescu G, Badulescu O, et al. Diabetic Cardiomyopathy: current approach and potential diagnostic and therapeutic targets. J Diabet Res. 2017:1310265.
11. Fitchett DH, Udell JA, Inzucchi SE, et al. Heart failure outcomes in clinical trials of glucose lowering agents in patients with diabetes. Eur J Heart Fail. 2017;19:43-53.
12. McMurray JJ, Adamopoulos S, Anker SD, et al. ESC guidelines for the diagnosis and treatment of acute and chronic heart failure 2012: the Task Force for the Diagnosis and Treatment of Acute and Chronic Heart Failure 2012 of the European Society of Cardiology. Developed

in collaboration with the Heart Failure Association (HFA) of the ESC. Eur J Heart Fail. 2012;14:803-69.
13. Lind M, Olsson M, Rosengren A, et al. The relationship between glycaemic control and heart failure in 83,021 patients with type 2 diabetes. Diabetologia. 2012;55:2946-53.
14. Erqou S, Lee CT, Suffoletto M, et al. Association between glycated haemoglobin and the risk of congestive heart failure in diabetes mellitus: systematic review and meta-analysis. Eur J Heart Fail. 2013;15:185-93.
15. Suskin N, McKelvie RS, Burns RJ, et al. Glucose and insulin abnormalities relate to functional capacity in patients with congestive heart failure. Eur Heart J. 2000;21:1368-75.
16. Domanski M, Krause-Steinrauf H, Deedwania P, et al. The effect of diabetes on outcomes of patients with advanced heart failure in the BEST trial. J Am Coll Cardiol. 2003;42:914-22.
17. Shindler DM, Kostis JB, Yusuf S, et al. Diabetes mellitus, a predictor of morbidity and mortality in the Studies of Left Ventricular Dysfunction (SOLVD) Trials and Registry. Am J Cardiol. 1996;77:1017-20.
18. Hogg K, Swedberg K, McMurray J. Heart failure with preserved left ventricular systolic unction: epidemiology, clinical characteristics, and prognosis. J Am Coll Cardiol. 2004;43:317-27.
19. Voors AA, van der Horst IC. Diabetes: a driver for heart failure. Heart. 2011;97:774-80.
20. Norhammar A, Malmberg K. Heart failure and glucose abnormalities: an increasing combination with poor functional capacity and outcome. Eur Heart J. 2000;21:1293-4.
21. Thrainsdottir IS, Aspelund T, Thorgeirsson G, et al. The association between glucose abnormalities and heart failure in the population based Reykjavik study. Diabetes Care. 2005;28:612-6.
22. Zinman B, Wanner C, Lachin JM, et al. Empagliflozin, cardiovascular outcomes and mortality in type 2 diabetes. NEJM. 2015;373:22.
23. Mosterd A, Hoes AW. Clinical epidemiology of heart failure. Heart. 2007;93:1137-46.

14 CHAPTER

Cardiodiabetes Management and STEMI: Prognostication

PB Jayagopal, T Kallarakkal Jain

INTRODUCTION

Coronary artery disease (CAD) is more common in diabetics and is more extensive and diffuse. Relative risk of acute myocardial infarction (AMI) is 50% higher in diabetic men and 150% more in diabetic women. Sudden death is 50% higher in diabetic men and 300% higher in diabetic women indicating higher prevalence and mortality. Thus diabetes mellitus (DM) is an important risk factor for mortality in patients with ST-segment elevation myocardial infarction (STEMI).[1]

STEMI IN DIABETES

Diabetic patients often present with the atypical presentation in unstable angina and myocardial infarction. That atypical presentation of acute coronary syndrome (ACS), more frequent in diabetic patients, includes anginal equivalents such as nausea, vomiting, diaphoresis, epigastric discomfort, dyspnea and an unexplained fatigue.[2] In a study, majority of nondiabetic STEMI patients who arrived early, experienced "moderate" and "severe" chest pain, whereas 51.7% of diabetic patients experienced "slight" or "no pain" which seemed equally indicative of serious disease as severe pain in nondiabetics. There were several important differences in pain perception between nondiabetic and diabetic patients. Analysis of individual pain qualities within the early arrival group showed a significantly higher frequency of anginal symptoms among nondiabetics and shortness of breath among diabetic patients. Shortness of breath was consistently more often reported in diabetics and that symptom seemed to be the main reason of their early hospital arrival, despite the lower intensity of pain or no pain at all.[3] DM patients have impaired microvascular structure and diffused endothelial dysfunction, which contributes to decreased blood perfusion in STEMI.[4] In the study, conducted by Marina Gradiser et al.,[3] the percentage of patients who achieved a Blush 3 score after the procedure was lower in the group with DM. Even with a thrombolysis in myocardial infarction (TIMI) flow grade 3 after primary percutaneous coronary intervention (PPCI), diabetic patients exhibit less complete resolution of the ST segment after stent implantation, which also indicates impaired microvascular flow.[5] These results corroborate the worse cardiovascular outcomes that DM patients exhibit after STEMI. DM is primarily associated with worse long-term outcomes in STEMI patients, whereas the increased cardiovascular risk was primarily due to hyperglycemia. It was observed that patients without DM and with admission hyperglycemia had a higher risk of in-hospital mortality, whereas DM patients with admission hyperglycemia had the worst long-term outcomes. In diabetic patients, plasma creatinine, glycated hemoglobin (HbA1c) and C-reactive protein (CRP) level are reportedly higher than in nondiabetic patients. Admission glucose was also higher in diabetic patients compared to nondiabetic patients. The complex pathophysiology in this subset of patients may include tissue inflammation, more reactive oxygen species production, endothelial dysfunction and increased activity of tissue renin-angiotensin-aldosterone system.

In-hospital mortality rate of diabetic patients suffering from myocardial infarction is 1.5–2 times higher than that of nondiabetic patients.[6] Diabetic women particularly have a poor prognosis, with mortality rates nearly two-fold higher than those of diabetic men. Oswald GA et al. showed no relation between the duration of known diabetes and in-hospital mortality after myocardial infarction.[7] It has been reported that serum CRP correlates with histological staining of CRP in fatal coronary artery lesions.[8] Biaseucci et al. found high-sensitivity (hs) CRP was the only predictor of events in nondiabetic patients but not in diabetic patients in 1-year follow-up. This points toward different pathophysiological mechanisms for cardiac events in unstable angina or AMI patients with or without diabetes. The excess short-term mortality of diabetic patients is primarily caused by an increased incidence of congestive heart failure (CHF).[9] Other possible mechanisms include increasing reinfarction rate, extension of infarction area and recurrent ischemia. Although survival after AMI is related to residual left ventricular function and the amount of damaged myocardium, several previous studies found no evidence that diabetic patients have more extensive infarctions than do nondiabetic patients, whether assessed by total creatine kinase (CK) activity,[10] radionuclide ventriculography or echocardiography.[11] But CHF and cardiogenic shock in patients with diabetes after AMI are more common and more severe than that would be predicted from infarction size.

As AMI can be silent or present atypically, all diabetic patients with atypical symptoms such as weakness, dyspnea on effort, sweating, giddiness, or restlessness should be considered as warning symptoms of AMI in diabetic patients. The management of AMI in a diabetic is the same as a nondiabetic with MI. Risk of bleeding complications with increased mortality has been reported in diabetic patients above 75 years of age. Thus, thrombolytic therapy should be applied with utmost caution in patients much more advanced in age. Invasive management should be considered for patients with ongoing ischemia or for symptomatic patients despite medical management. In the bypass angioplasty revascularization investigation trial (BARI) diabetics had a lower 5-year survival than nondiabetics in both the treatment groups. However, diabetics with bypass graft had 81% 5-year survival which was better than those treated with angioplasty who had a 66% survival. Angioplasty is less often successful due to extensive disease and is associated with higher rates of silent hazardous restenosis.

Although, perioperative mortality is higher in cases taken up for coronary artery bypass grafting (CABG) in diabetic compared to nondiabetic subjects (7.1% vs 9.5%), long-term graft patency may be similar in either group of the patients. Diabetic subjects are also more prone to restenosis following percutaneous transluminal coronary angioplasty (PTCA). Incidence of complications such as reinfarction, cardiogenic shock and CHF, malignant arrhythmias, conduction abnormalities and myocardial rupture are several-fold more common in diabetic patients compared to nondiabetic subjects with AMI. Congestive heart failure develops in 44% of women and 25% of men with diabetes leading to death in 22% and 6% respectively.[12] Overall, pump failure manifests CHF or cardiogenic shock, accounts for over 80% of in-hospital mortality.[13] High incidence of CHF in diabetic subjects, particularly in women, occur in spite of similar size of infarcts as compared to their nondiabetic counterparts. Arrhythmias and conduction defects account for over 10% of the mortality. Incidence of atrioventricular (AV) block and left bundle branch block (LBBB) detected in half of the dying patients are three times more common than in nondiabetic subjects. Overall mortality during the first week in hospital is three times higher in patients with diabetes or hyperglycemia. Relative risk of fatality is particularly higher in those with history of a previous attack, in women and in younger patients around 50 years of age.[14]

Autonomic neuropathy with impaired reflex induction of compensatory increase in heart rate and contractility may play some role in the poorer prognosis of AMI in diabetes. Raised levels of free fatty acids (FFA) in diabetic patients are detrimental for cardiac function as incidence of both arrhythmias and CHF are higher in such situations. Alterations in hemostatic mechanisms promoting more frequent thrombus formation and impairment of clot lysis due to raised levels of plasminogen activator inhibitor (PAI) that promotes extension of thrombus and reinfarction as well as retards the process of spontaneous recanalization. Prognostic variables that have been determined to be independent predictors of poor prognosis following AMI in diabetic subjects are—(1) Q-wave MI, (2) prior MI, (3) female gender, and (4) insulin treatment prior to hospitalization. Prompt control of both hyperglycemia and ketonemia are essential for improvement in the prognosis of AMI in patients with diabetes. Knowledge of the hypoglycemic agent used by patients with known diabetes may be helpful. In any case, it is desirable to institute therapy with highly purified soluble insulin administered in low doses through continuous intravenous infusion, so as to maintain glycemic levels between 100 mg/dL and 150 mg/dL.[15] Close monitoring is essential as episodes of hypoglycemia in the immediate postinfarction period are brought with risks of potentially fatal arrhythmias from bursts of catecholamine release working on the injured and irritable myocardium. In patients, where feeding of adequate calories poses problems, simultaneous infusion of 5–7.5 g of dextrose per hour may be necessary in order to normalize levels of plasma ketones as early as possible. This is required not only in patients with type I but in those with type II as well. Insulin treatment should be continued at least for a week in the latter group in the event of AMI.

CONCLUSION

Diabetes mellitus exerts a deleterious effect on the short and long-term course after AMI through various mechanisms, so application of intensive and effective preventive and therapeutic measures may result in a particularly large survival benefit. Diabetic patients are reported to have high levels of HbA1c and CRP levels than in nondiabetic patients. Poor outcome is associated with Q-wave MI, prior MI, female gender and insulin treatment prior to hospitalization. Complications such as reinfarction, cardiogenic shock, CHF, malignant arrhythmias, conduction abnormalities and myocardial rupture are significantly high in diabetic patients. Invasive management with newer generation of drug-eluting stents has significantly reduced the previous high rates of stent thrombosis and restenosis. Prompt control of hyperglycemia and ketonemia plays a significant role in the prognosis of AMI in patients with diabetes.

REFERENCES

1. Timmer JR, Ottervanger JP, Thomas K, et al. Long-term, cause-specific mortality after myocardial infarction in diabetes. Eur Heart J. 2004; 25:926-31.
2. Tbibiazar R, Edelman SV. Silent ischaemia in people with diabetes: A condition that must be heard. Clin Diabetes. 2003;21:5-9.
3. Marina G, Dario D, Jasna C, et al. Comparison of the hospital arrival time and differences in pain quality between diabetic and non-diabetic STEMI patients. Int J. Environ Res Public Health. 2015;12:1387-396.
4. Kawaguchi M, Techigawara M, Ishihata T, et al. A comparison of ultrastructural changes on endomyocardial biopsy specimens obtained from patients with diabetes mellitus with and without hypertension. Heart Vessels. 1997;12:267-74.
5. Angeja BG, de Lemos J, Murphy SA, et al. Impact of diabetes mellitus on epicardial and microvascular flow after fibrinolytic therapy. Am Heart J. 2002;144:649-56.
6. Stone PH, Muller JE, Hartwell T, et al. The effect of diabetes mellitus on prognosis and serial left ventricular function after acute myocardial infarction: contribution of both coronary disease and left ventricular dysfunction to the adverse prognosis. The MILIS Study Group. J Am Coll Cardiol. 1989;14:49-57.
7. Oswald GA, Corcoran S, Yudkin JS. Prevalence and risks of hyperglycemia and undiagnosed diabetes in patients with acute myocardial infarction. Lancet. 1984;1:1264-7.
8. Kjekshus J, Gilpin E, Cali G, et al. Diabetic patients and beta blockers after acute myocardial infarction. Eur Heart J. 1990;11: 43-50.
9. Best PJ, Lennon R, Ting HH, et al. The impact of renal insufficiency on clinical outcomes in patients undergoing percutaneous coronary intervention. J Am Coll Cardiol. 2002;39:1113-9.
10. Lehto S, Pyorala K, Miettinen H, et al. Myocardial infarct size and mortality in patients with non-insulin-dependent diabetes mellitus. J Intern Med. 1994;236:291-7.
11. Kouvaras G, Cokkinos D, Spyropoulou M. Increased mortality of diabetics after acute myocardial infarction attributed to diffusely impair left ventricular performance as assessed by echocardiography. Jpn Heart J. 1988;29:1-9.
12. Savage MP, Krolewski AS, Kenien GG, et al. Acute myocardial infarction in diabetes mellitus and significance of congestive heart failure as a prognostic factor. Am J Cardiol. 1988;62:665-9.
13. Gwilt DJ. Why do diabetic patients die after myocardial infarction? Practical Diabetes. 1984;1:36-9.
14. Czyzk A, Krolewski AS, Szablowska S, et al. Clinical course of myocardial infarction among diabetic patients. Diabetes Care. 1980;3:526-9.
15. Garber AJ. Myocardial infarction. In: Lebobitz HE (Ed). Therapy for Diabetes Mellitus and Related Disorder, 2nd edition. Alexandria: American Diabetic Association; 1994. pp. 338.

CHAPTER

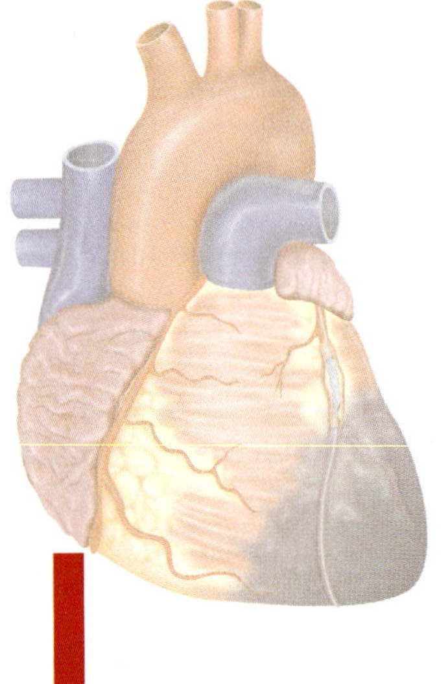

Small Vessel CAD in Cardiodiabetes

Arvind Sethi, Upendra Kaul

INTRODUCTION

Diabetes is a multisystem disease which has rapidly increasing global prevalence. Over long term, it results into various complications both at macrovascular and microvascular levels of which, cardiovascular disease (CVD) is the most common. CVD is by far the greatest cause of morbidity and mortality in individuals with diabetes.[1] Diabetes-associated risk factors including dyslipidemia, systemic hypertension and smoking account for most of this risk. However, uncontrolled diabetes has significant deleterious effects on vascular endothelial functioning and its associated vasoconstriction along with thrombosis. Increment of 1% of glycated hemoglobin is associated with 52.5% higher mortality risk in patients with type I diabetes which is much more as compared to 7.5% in those with type II diabetes.[2]

Cardiodiabetes, i.e. cardiovascular system involvement in diabetes occurs at both macrovascular level, i.e. obstructive epicardial coronary artery disease (CAD) and microvascular level which includes microvasculature as well as diabetic cardiomyopathy and its resultant manifestations.

Various possible mechanisms have been found to be responsible for causing complications, including polyol pathway, hexosamine pathway, protein kinase C (PKC) pathway and advanced glycation end-product (AGE) formation. All these have been shown to be activated by deleterious effects of overproduction of superoxide by the mitochondria as a result of hyperglycemia.[3]

Both these complications occur as a result of impaired endothelial function, neovascularization, vascular inflammation, apoptosis as well as procoagulant state.[4] Reactive oxygen species act as the final trigger for these complications in presence of other common associations of insulin resistance, dyslipidemia, smoking and systemic hypertension.

All these metabolic abnormalities result in myocardial fibrosis and/or hypertrophy and its consequent contractile dysfunction and left ventricular (LV) failure. At the microvascular level, these processes lead to endothelial swelling, and degradation as well as thickening of capillary basement membrane.[5] All these changes have been demonstrated by ultrastructural studies. [6] It has been shown that this mitochondrial degeneration, fatty infiltration along with basement membrane thickening of the capillaries may even lead to complete obliteration of the lumen. This constitutes the pathological hallmark of diabetic microangiopathy and has a characteristic patchy distribution.

PRESENTATION

Microvascular (small vessel) CAD can clinically produce symptoms on one hand related to myocardial hypertrophy, fibrosis and its resultant LV failure. On the other hand, coronary microvascular alterations lead to angina at the level of resistance coronary arteries. When this small vessel CAD (SVCAD) occurs in several cardiac and systemic diseases like cardiomyopathy, obstructive CAD and in patients who have undergone revascularization, it results in secondary microvascular angina (MVA). It, however, may occur as an independent entity resulting in primary microvascular angina.[7] For further discussions, SVCAD would be restricted to primary MVA.

It is thus a clinical syndrome where angina occurs in absence of significant epicardial coronary with less than 50% obstructions. It is an important entity as it remains a diagnostic and therapeutic challenge and even leads to significant economic, social and healthcare loss.[8]

Up to 30% of individuals undergoing coronary angiography for angina have insignificant CAD;[9] and of these, more than half are considered to be due to SVCAD.[10,11] It has been seen to occur more often in women around the age of 50–55 years. MVA can thus be defined as impaired vasodilation of arterioles and capillaries resulting in an inadequate increase in microcirculation from rest to stress. This may also be referred to as cardiac syndrome X.

DIAGNOSIS

Historically, invasive techniques like intracoronary Doppler or thermodilution were the only practical approaches to its diagnosis. However, the current gold standards for the clinical assessment of coronary microvascular function are invasive coronary flow reserve (CFR) as well as noninvasive myocardial perfusion reserve (MPR) by either positron-emission tomography (PET) or cardiac MRI, respectively. Variable thresholds of 1.5–2.3 have been used to define cut off values in various prognostic studies.[12] PET imaging is now accepted as gold standard as it gives highly accurate myocardial blood flow (MBF) analysis. It shows linear relationship between MBF and isotope intensity.[13] Most commonly used isotopes for the purpose are ^{13}N, H^{3}, ^{85}Pb and ^{15}O. However, choice of technique can significantly affect MPR value.[14]

Cardiovascular magnetic resonance (CMR), on the other hand, has some potential advantages as superior spatial and temporal resolution, avoidance of ionizing radiation and wider availability. However, semiquantitative analysis underestimates MPR and lengthy offline postprocessing limits its applicability.[15] Considerable heterogeneity has been described as its possible mechanism which includes derangement of the smooth muscle relaxation in response to vasodilator agents.[16] Impaired flow-mediated vasodilation, i.e. endothelial dysfunction.[17] Further, accelerated response to vasoconstrictor stimuli also has significant contribution.[18] Even the causative factors are also heterogeneous. Traditional risk factors associated with diabetes do play a definite role in its causation. However these may not be able to explain a lot of cases.[19] Several other factors which may have a significant role in its causation have been proposed including low grade inflammation of the microvasculature,[20] increased sympathetic activity,[21] insulin resistance[22] and estrogen deficiency especially in perimenopausal females.[23]

PROGNOSIS

Prospective studies in the past have consistently shown good overall long-term outcome.[24] Recent studies have however, challenged this opinion and have suggested that the patients with SVCAD, especially when documented may be a relatively higher risk of CV events.[25] Nevertheless, SVCAD is associated with significant long-term morbidity despite good overall prognosis. Up to one-third of the patients report worsening of symptoms (both intensity and frequency) resulting in compromised quality of life.[26] Worsening of complaints possibly indicate either progression of the small vessel disease and/or reduction in pain perception threshold.

TREATMENT

Medical treatment is the cornerstone in the management of this condition as the main purpose of treatment is the control of distressing symptoms and the consequent improvement in the quality of life of the patient. Studies reported in literature have shown emphasis on soft endpoints rather than hard endpoints. Similar factors in disease causation as for obstructive CAD, suggest that standard anti-ischemic medication is possibly the first-line medication for the treatment of SVCAD, however, with limited efficacy. Thus, other alternative forms of therapy have been utilized with variable effects.

Standard Treatment Options

β-blockers

These help by reducing myocardial oxygen consumption. These are more appropriate, especially in situations of increased sympathetic activity. They also help in increasing diastolic perfusion time and thus have a compelling role in the management of this condition. Of the available β-blockers, atenolol in tolerable doses has been consistently found to have beneficial effect in the amelioration of symptoms.[27] It has, however, not been shown that other β-blocking agents would be as efficacious in similar situations.

Calcium Channel Antagonists

These agents might improve the symptoms by helping in relaxation of the diseased microvasculature as also by the reduction in afterload. Non-dihydropyridine derivatives especially may improve the symptoms by their negative chronotropic properties.[28] Similar effects have been shown with respect to exercise-induced symptoms. However, these effects have not been consistent in all the studies.[29] Inconsistencies have also been reported regarding the effect of diltiazem on coronary flow reserve.[30]

Nitrates

These agents show their effect mainly by smooth muscle relaxation and resultant vasodilation, thus, reducing the preload. These effects are, however, limited in coronary microvasculature.[31] Short-acting nitrates may relieve acute angina attacks in SVCAD, whereas chronic oral nitrates have failed to produce significant relief even in short-term studies.[32] Nitrates are thus not recommended as first-line treatment; these may, however, be added to β-blockers empirically.

Additional Treatment Options

Ranolazine

It inhibits the late inward Na^+ current and thus leads to reduction in intramyocardial calcium transfer resulting in improved myocardial relaxation and improvement in diastolic function. It has also been suggested to improve endothelial function and its resultant vasorelaxation. It has been shown to improve anginal symptoms in patients with reduced MPR.[33]

Ivabradine

It is a novel anti-ischemic drug, which shows its effect by reducing the heart rate and prolonging the diastolic filling period. Thus results in reduced myocardial oxygen consumption and consequent improvement in angina symptoms in SVCAD[34] similar to that in obstructive CAD.

Xanthine Derivatives

Small studies have shown improvement in exercise-induced and/or stress-induced electrocardiogram (ECG) changes with these drugs.[35] When administered intravenously, these drugs (aminophylline) may reduce exercise-induced myocardial ischemia by redistribution of coronary flow, facilitating it more towards ischemic regions through specific effects over adenosine and norepinephrine. Further, by its adenosine antagonism, it may also exert its analgesic effect.[36] However, oral administration over long term has not shown any significant benefit[37] and requires further evaluation.

Angiotensin-converting Enzyme Inhibitors

These drugs have potentially favorable effects on coronary microvasculature and thus facilitate vasodilation by increased availability of nitric oxide (NO) and also by reduction of angiotensin II and its resultant sympathetic inhibition. These drugs have been reported to have beneficial effects both alone as well as in combination with statins.[38]

α-antagonists

These drugs have been considered due to their α-mediated sympathetic blocking effect on coronary microvasculature. However, neither doxazocin nor prazosin has been demonstrated to be effective in improving CFR in controlled studies.[39] Another major limiting factor of drug tolerance makes it unfit for being recommended for the purpose.

Nicorandil

This produces nitrate like effect by opening of adenosine triphosphate/potassium channel (ATP/K^+) on coronary resistance vessels. It has been shown to reduce angina and improve MBF in SVCAD.[40,41] This offers a suitable alternative to nitrates especially those intolerant to them.

Trimetazidine

This drug acts by metabolic modulation of the microvasculature, i.e. shifting of cell metabolism from free fatty acids (FFA) to glucose utilization. Although a novel concept, however, mixed response has been reported in patients with SVCAD.[42,43]

Statins

Apart from cholesterol-lowering effects, these drugs are known to improve endothelial function by their pleiotropic effects, including antioxidant and anti-inflammatory actions. Alone as well as in combination with ACE inhibitors, these drugs have been shown to have a favorable effect on exercise-induced angina in SVCAD.[38,44]

Estrogen

Perimenopausal women constitute a major group of patients with SVACD suggesting estrogen deficiency as a possible pathogenic mechanism in its causation. Estrogen replacement therapy has also been shown to be effective in controlled studies in improving exercise-induced symptoms.[45] Although initial benefits may reduce over long-term treatment.[46] These also have some safety concerns over prolonged administration.

Imipramine

It works on the principle of inhibition of transmission and perception of visceral pain. The drug is especially effective for patients with SVCAD who are resistant to anti-ischemic measures. It has been found to reduce angina by 50% over short term although with no significant improvement in quality of life due to occurrence of distressing side effects.[47] Hence, it is of limited applicability.

Nonpharmacological Measures

Not all cases of SVCAD respond favorably to the medication available. Those refractory to pharmacotherapy may be offered other therapies, including—

Spinal Cord Stimulation

Dorsal horns of spinal cord at the level of C7-T1 are stimulated electrically by multipolar electrodes through a programmable device. This again works on the principle of modulation of pain perception and transmission along with modification of sympathetic activity.[48] Various studies have shown significant benefit in reduction to angina intensity, and improvement in exercise tolerance.[49]

Enhanced External Counterpulsation

Sequential beat-to-beat programmed inflation and deflation of pneumatic cuffs over patient's limbs has shown to improve diastolic perfusion and also endothelial function.[50] It needs to be further evaluated in controlled long-term studies. Applicability is again limited by intolerable side effects.

Other Supportive Measures

Psychological counseling and relaxation techniques are especially helpful in those refractory to medication. It helps significantly to overcome the reactive component as well as those individuals suffering from psychological illnesses.[51]

Graded exercise-customized programs have also been shown to be helpful in the reduction of pain perception as well as improvement in tolerance to pain in patients with SVCAD.[52] Heterogeneous nature of the disease entity makes it difficult to manage the condition. Treatment is mainly empirical and may often be unpredictable, thus requiring customization according to individual requirement. European Society of Cardiology (ESC) guidelines 2013 recommend β-blockers as first-line therapy along with other preventive measures including aspirin and statins.[53] Calcium channel antagonists can be utilized in those whom β-blockers are ineffective. Ivabradine has specific advantages in those intolerant to β-blockers. Other drugs and nonpharmacological measures can also be utilized depending on individual responsiveness. Close physician-patient interaction and reassurance are also crucial in achieving the goal.

ONGOING RESEARCH

"Coronary microvascular disease and endothelial function in women and men", is an open-label, early phase I interventional study by a single group at Cedar-Sinai Medical Centre. It is currently recruiting patients with the aim of establishing prevalence of microvascular disease (Syndrome X), to assess the utility of noninvasive testing like peripheral artery tonometry and cardiac magnetic resonance (CMR) in diagnosing Syndrome X, to assess its prognosis as well as to further elucidate risk factors, clinical features, diagnosis and treatment of this heterogeneous condition.

REFERENCES

1. Haffner SM, Lehto S, Rönnemaa T, et al. Mortality from coronary heart disease in subjects with type 2 diabetes and in nondiabetic subjects with and without prior myocardial infarction. N Engl J Med. 1998;339:229-34.
2. Juutilainen A, Lehto S, Rönnemaa T, et al. Similarity of the impact of type 1 and type 2 diabetes on cardiovascular mortality in middle-aged subjects. Diabetes Care. 2008;31:714-9.
3. Brownlee M. The pathobiology of diabetic complications: a unifying mechanism. Diabetes. 2005;54:1615-25.
4. Herrmann J, Lerman LO, Rodriguez-Porcel M, et al. Coronary vasa vasorum neovascularization precedes epicardial endothelial dysfunction in experimental hypercholesterolemia. Cardiovasc Res. 2001;51:762-6.
5. Asghar O, Al-Sunni A, Khavandi K, et al. Diabetic cardiomyopathy. Clin Sci (Lond). 2009;116:741-60.
6. Fischer VW, Barner HB, Larose LS. Pathomorphologic aspects of muscular tissue in diabetes mellitus. Hum Pathol. 1984;15:1127-136.
7. Camici PG, Crea F. Coronary microvascular dysfunction. N Engl J Med. 2007;356:830-40.
8. Shaw LJ, Merz CNB, Pepine CJ, et al. The economic burden of angina in women with suspected ischemic heart disease: results from the National Institutes of Health-National Heart, Lung, and Blood Institute-sponsored Women's Ischemia Syndrome Evaluation. Circulation 2006;114:894-904.
9. Farrehi PM, Bernstein SJ, Rasak M, et al. Frequency of negative coronary arteriographic findings in patients with chest pain is related to community practice patterns. Am J Manag Care. 2002;8:643-8.
10. Geltman EM, Henes CG, Senneff MJ, et al. Increased myocardial perfusion at rest and diminished perfusion reserve in patients with angina and angiographically normal coronary arteries. J Am Coll Cardiol. 1990;16:586-95.
11. Graf S, Khorsand A, Gwechenberger M, et al. Typical chest pain and normal coronary angiogram: cardiac risk factor analysis versus PET for detection of microvascular disease. J Nucl Med. 2007;48:175-81.
12. Murthy VL, Naya M, Foster CR, et al. Improved cardiac risk assessment with noninvasive measures of coronary flow reserve. Circulation. 2011;124:2215-24.
13. Saraste A, Kajander S, Han C, et al. PET: is myocardial flow quantification a clinical reality? J Nucl Cardiol. 2012;19:1044-59.

14. Murthy VL, Lee BC, Sitek A, et al. Comparison and prognostic validation of multiple methods of quantification of myocardial blood flow with 82Rb PET. J Nucl Med. 2014;55:1952-8.
15. Pärkkä JP, Niemi P, Saraste A, et al. Comparison of MRI and positron emission tomography for measuring myocardial perfusion reserve in healthy humans. Magn Reson Med. 2006;55:772-9.
16. Opherk D, Zebe H, Weihe E, et al. Reduced coronary dilatory capacity and ultrastructural changes of the myocardium in patients with angina pectoris but normal coronary arteriograms. Circulation. 1981;63:817-25.
17. Chauhan A, Mullins PA, Taylor G, et al. Both endothelium-dependent and endothelium-independent function is impaired in patients with angina pectoris and normal coronary angiograms. Eur Heart J. 1997;18:60-8.
18. Ong P, Athanasiadis A, Mahrholdt H, et al. Increased coronary vasoconstrictor response to acetylcholine in women with chest pain and normal coronary arteriograms (cardiac syndrome X). Clin Res Cardiol. 2012;101:673-81.
19. Sestito A, Lanza GA, Di Monaco A, et al. Relation between cardiovascular risk factors and coronary microvascular dysfunction in cardiac syndrome X. J Cardiovasc Med. 2011;12:322-7.
20. Lanza GA, Sestito A, Cammarota G, et al. Assessment of systemic inflammation and infective pathogen burden in patients with cardiac syndrome X. Am J Cardiol. 2004;94:40-4.
21. Lanza GA, Giordano A, Pristipino C, et al. Abnormal cardiac adrenergic nerve function in patients with syndrome X detected by [123I] metaiodobenzylguanidine myocardial scintigraphy. Circulation. 1997;96:821-6.
22. Dean JD, Jones CJ, Hutchison SJ, et al. Hyperinsulinaemia and microvascular angina (''syndrome X''). Lancet. 1991;337:456-7.
23. Rosano GM, Collins P, Kaski JC, et al. Syndrome X in women is associated with oestrogen deficiency. Eur Heart J. 1995;16:610-4.
24. Kaski JC, Rosano GMC, Collins P, et al. Cardiac syndrome X: clinical characteristics and left ventricular function: long-term follow-up study. J Am Coll Cardiol. 1995;25:807-14.
25. Pepine CJ, Anderson RD, Sharaf BL, et al. Coronary microvascular reactivity to adenosine predicts adverse outcome in women evaluated for suspected ischemia results from the National Heart, Lung and Blood Institute WISE (Women's Ischemia Syndrome Evaluation) study. J Am Coll Cardiol. 2010;55:2825-32.
26. Lamendola P, Lanza GA, Spinelli A, et al. Long-term prognosis of patients with cardiac syndrome X. Int J Cardiol. 2010;15:197-9.
27. Fragasso G, Chierchia SL, Pizzetti G, et al. Impaired left ventricular filling dynamics in patients with angina and angiographically normal coronary arteries: effect of beta adrenergic blockade. Heart. 1997;77:32-9.
28. Ferrini D, Bugiardini R, Galvani M, et al. Opposing effects of propranolol and diltiazem on the angina threshold during an exercise test in patients with syndrome X. G Italian Cardiol. 1986;16:224-31.
29. Li L, Gu Y, Liu T, et al. A randomized, single-center double blinded trial on the effects of diltiazem sustained-release capsules in patients with coronary slow flow phenomenon at 6-month follow-up. PLoS One. 2012;7:e38851.
30. Sütsch G, Oechslin E, Mayer I, et al. Effect of diltiazem on coronary flow reserve in patients with microvascular angina. Int J Cardiol. 1995;52:135-43.
31. Harrison DG, Bates JN. The nitrovasodilators: new ideas about old drugs. Circulation. 1993;87:1461-7.
32. Lamendola P, Nerla R, Pitocco D, et al. Effect of ranolazine on arterial endothelial function in patients with type 2 diabetes mellitus. Atherosclerosis. 2013;226:157-60.
33. Mehta PK, Goykhman P, Thomson LE, et al. Ranolazine improves angina in women with evidence of myocardial ischemia but no obstructive coronary artery disease. JACC Cardiovasc Imaging. 2011;4:514-22.
34. Villano A, Di Franco A, Nerla R, et al. Effects of ivabradine and ranolazine in patients with microvascular angina pectoris. Am J Cardiol. 2013;1:8-13.
35. Radice M, Giudici V, Pusineri E, et al. Different effects of acute administration of aminophylline and nitroglycerin on exercise capacity in patients with syndrome X. Am J Cardiol. 1996;78:88-90.
36. Crea F, Pupita G, Galassi AR, et al. Role of adenosine in pathogenesis of anginal pain. Circulation. 1990;81:164-72.
37. Elliott PM, Krzyzowska-Dickinson K, Calvino R, et al. Effect of oral aminophylline in patients with angina and normal coronary arteriograms (syndrome X). Heart. 1997;77:523-6.
38. Pizzi C, Manfrini O, Fontana F, et al. Angiotensin-converting enzyme inhibitors and 3-hydroxy-3-methylglutaryl coenzyme A reductase in cardiac syndrome X: role of superoxide dismutase activity. Circulation. 2004;109:53-8.
39. Rosen SD, Lorenzoni R, Kaski JC, et al. Effect of alpha1-adrenoceptor blockade on coronary vasodilator reserve in cardiac syndrome X. J Cardiovasc Pharmacol. 1999;34:554-60.
40. Chen JW, Lee WL, Hsu NW, et al. Effects of short-term treatment of nicorandil on exercise-induced myocardial ischemia and abnormal cardiac autonomic activity in microvascular angina. Am J Cardiol. 1997;80:32-8.
41. Yamabe H, Namura H, Yano T, et al. Effect of nicorandil on abnormal coronary flow reserve assessed by exercise 201Tl scintigraphy in patients with angina pectoris and nearly normal coronary arteriograms. Cardiovasc Drugs Ther. 1995;9:755-61.
42. Nalbantgil S, Altinti A, Yilmaz H, et al. The effect of trimetazidine in the treatment of microvascular angina. Int J Angiol. 1999;8:40-3.
43. Leonardo F, Fragasso G, Rossetti E, et al. Comparison of trimetazidine with atenolol in patients with syndrome X: effects on diastolic function and exercise tolerance. Cardiologia. 1999;44:1065-9.
44. Kayikcioglu M, Payzin S, Yavuzgil O, et al. Benefits of statin treatment in cardiac syndrome-X. Eur Heart J. 2003;24:1999–2005.
45. Rosano GMC, Peters NS, Lefroy D, et al. Symptomatic response to 17β-estradiol in women with syndrome X. J Am Coll Cardiol. 1996;28:1500-5.
46. Jhund PS, Dawson N, Davie AP, et al. Attenuation of endothelin-1 induced vasoconstriction by 17beta estradiol is not sustained during long-term therapy in postmenopausal women with coronary heart disease. J Am Coll Cardiol. 2001;37:1367-73.
47. Cox ID, Hann CM, Kaski JC. Low dose imipramine improves chest pain but not quality of life in patients with angina and normal coronary angiograms. Eur Heart J. 1998;19:250-4.
48. Norrsell H, Eliasson T, Mannheimer C, et al. Effects of pacing-induced myocardial stress and spinal cord stimulation on whole body and cardiac norepinephrine spillover. Eur Heart J. 1997;18:1890-6.
49. Lanza GA, Sestito A, Sgueglia GA, et al. Effect of spinal cord stimulation on spontaneous and stress-induced angina and "ischemia-like" ST-segment depression in patients with cardiac syndrome X. Eur Heart J. 2005;26:983-9.
50. Kronhaus KD, Lawson WE. Enhanced external counterpulsation is an effective treatment for syndrome X. Int J Cardiol. 2009;135:256-7.
51. Bass C, Wade C. Chest pain with normal coronary arteries: a comparative study of psychiatric and social morbidity. Psychol Med. 1984;14:51-61
52. Asbury EA, Slattery C, Grant A, et al. Cardiac rehabilitation for the treatment of women with chest pain and normal coronary arteries. Menopause. 2008;15:454-60.
53. Montalescot G, Sechtem U, Achenbach S, et al. 2013 ESC guidelines on the management of stable coronary artery disease: the Task Force on the management of stable coronary artery disease of the European Society of Cardiology. Eur Heart J. 2013;34:2949-3003.

16

CHAPTER

Cardiodiabetes and Deep Venous Thrombosis

Nagesh S Waghmare, Anil Kumar

INTRODUCTION

The incidence of venous thromboembolism (VTE) is approximately 1.5 cases per 1,000 person-years as described in Western literature.[1] The deep venous thrombosis (DVT) cases are approximately twice as common as pulmonary embolism (PE). In the past, it was considered that the incidence of DVT in Indian population is rare, but various studies have found that it is not that rare and is increasing significantly, as our country is experiencing increasing urbanization and associated lifestyle-related noncommunicable diseases. The prospective registry on venous thromboembolic events (PROVE) conducted in 19 countries, 2,33,526 patients with symptomatic DVT were enrolled; out of which 667 were from India.[2] Compared with the overall PROVE population, the prevalence of previous DVT, PE, or superficial leg thrombosis was similar in Indian patients. In a retrospective study done by Vijayraghawan et al.[3] the incidence of DVT in India was found to be significant (1.79 per thousand general population). These findings suggest that the DVT incidence and related consequences are similar in Indian population and the problem was initially underestimated may be because of lack of studies. As a result of lack of awareness in our country, the rate of prophylaxis to eligible patients to prevent DVT is low.

RISK FACTORS—PROVOKED AND UNPROVOKED DVT

The Virchow's triad stood the test of time in describing the possible mechanisms leading to development of DVT. These factors were abnormality of flow, abnormal vessel wall and abnormal blood constituents. A contemporary viewpoint of Virchow's triad should consider: inflammation, endothelial dysfunction, and atherosclerosis (i.e. abnormal vessel wall), abnormalities of hemorheology and turbulence at bifurcations and stenotic regions (i.e. abnormal blood flow), and finally, abnormalities in platelet function, coagulation, fibrinolysis, and metabolic or hormonal factors (i.e. abnormal blood constituents).[4] The disease conditions leading to one of these three components are considered the risk factors/triggers for development of DVT. DVT occurring as a result of these triggers is labeled as provoked DVT.[5] In many studies, it was found that at least half of the cases of DVT are without any identifiable triggers,[1] these are labeled as idiopathic or unprovoked DVT. The results of PROVE study[2] showed that in Indian patients the DVT was idiopathic in 43%, following a precipitating event in 52%, and recurrent in 6% (44%, 49%, and 9% for the overall PROVE population, respectively).

Provoking factors may be temporary or persistent. The well-recognized temporary provoking factors are trauma, lower limb fractures, major surgery, immobilization, long-distance travel, pregnancy and estrogen containing contraceptive pills. The examples of persistent provoking risk factors are cancer, inflammatory bowel disease, nephrotic syndrome or other chronic medical diseases, increasing age, genetic abnormalities, coagulation factor like factor V Leiden. Presence of provoking factors significantly increases the risk of DVT.[6]

Atherosclerosis and DVT

Inflammation, systemic and local hypercoagulability, and endothelial injury play an integral mechanistic role

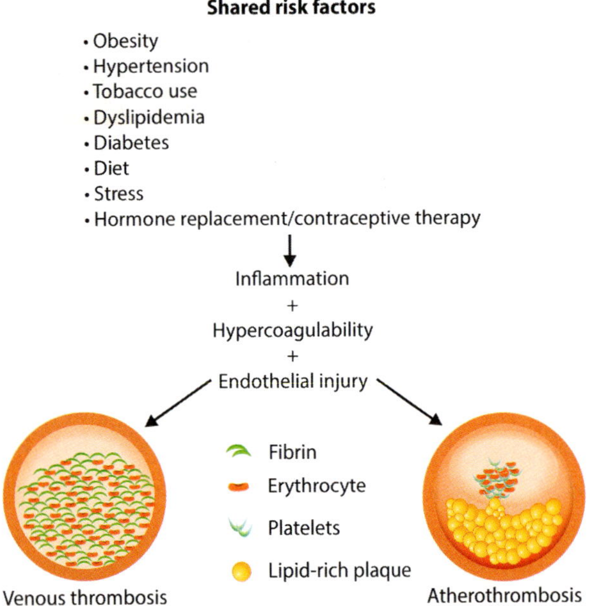

Fig. 1: Common risk factors shared by the two groups of diseases

in the pathophysiology of atherothrombosis (Fig.1). An improved understanding of VTE integrates these same pathophysiological processes.[7] The association between atherosclerosis and DVT is biologically plausible as atherosclerosis is associated with activation of platelets and blood coagulation as well as an increase in fibrin turnover, which can lead to thrombotic complications.[8] Also the initial case-control and prospective studies have found an association between venous thromboembolic disorders and chronic peripheral arterial disease, hyperlipidemia, or hypertension. Prandoni and colleagues[8] assessed the relation between atherosclerosis in the form of carotid artery plaques and diagnosed cases of DVT. They compared the results between three groups of patients namely unprovoked DVT, provoked DVT and control subjects, and found that the odds ratios for carotid plaques in patients with unprovoked DVT, as compared with patients with provoked DVT and with controls, were 2.3 and 1.8, respectively. They concluded that there is an association between atherosclerotic disease and unprovoked DVT, but it was not clear whether the association is causal or temporal with common risk factors. In a prospective clinical outcome, study of patients with acute pulmonary embolism, Becattini et al.[9] found that cardiovascular events are more common in patients with unprovoked VTE than in patients with provoked VTE. Cardiovascular events were the major cause of death in patients with idiopathic pulmonary embolism. In this study, they had excluded patients having cancer. Ageno et al.[10] conducted a meta-analysis of 21 case control and cohort studies comparing the association between cardiovascular risk factors and VTE. They found that cardiovascular risk factors were associated with increased VTE. The risk of VTE was 2.33 for obesity, 1.51 for hypertension, 1.42 for diabetes mellitus, 1.18 for smoking, and 1.16 for hypercholesterolemia. But the study suffered many limitations like the distinct possibility exists that the strength of association may be weaker with a multifactorial regression analysis. In this meta-analysis, it was not possible to adjust or stratify for potential confounders. Till now many longitudinal studies and meta-analysis have shown a relation between the two diseases but a causal relation of atherosclerosis with DVT, remains to be proven. If causally related, then treatment of atherosclerosis should positively affect VTE.

Heart Failure and DVT

Congestive heart failure (CHF) is now a well-established risk factor for VTE. In one of the earlier studies, the frequency of PE in patients with CHF ranges from 0.9% to 39%, and the frequency of DVT varies from 10% to 59%.[11] Another study reported that the incidence of VTE in decompensated heart failure patients ranges from 4% to 26% in Western countries.[12] The incidence of PE with congestive heart failure at autopsy ranges from 28% to 48%. A research in Japan reported that the incidence of DVT in heart failure patients was 11.2%, and the incidence is highest in patients classified as NYHA IV (NYHA II: 4.4%, NYHA III: 4.8%, NYHA IV: 25.5%, $p < 0.01$).[13] The genesis of the prothrombotic tendency in CHF can be described in the background of Virchow's classic triad[14] (Fig. 2). The first constituent, "abnormal blood flow," or stasis, is a consequence of both depressed cardiac output and patient immobility. "Abnormalities in the vessel wall" are reflected in CHF-associated endothelial dysfunction. For example, endothelium-derived nitric oxide release is impaired and von Willebrand factor (vWf) levels are elevated in heart failure. Finally, the hemostatic abnormalities of CHF fulfill the third component of the triad, "abnormalities in blood constituents." For instance, in a cross-sectional analysis of 120 patients with stable CHF (median ejection fraction, 30%), both plasma viscosity ($p = 0.001$) and fibrinogen ($p = 0.02$) were significantly elevated compared to healthy controls. The elevated risk of VTE with CHF is classically associated with left ventricular systolic impairment.[13] Several studies have documented an inverse relationship between ejection fraction and risk of VTE (Table 1).[15] Reduced heart failure patients have increased risk of VTE. In addition, immobilization, infections, central venous catheters and leads from implantable cardiac defibrillators and pacemakers are related to VTE and are

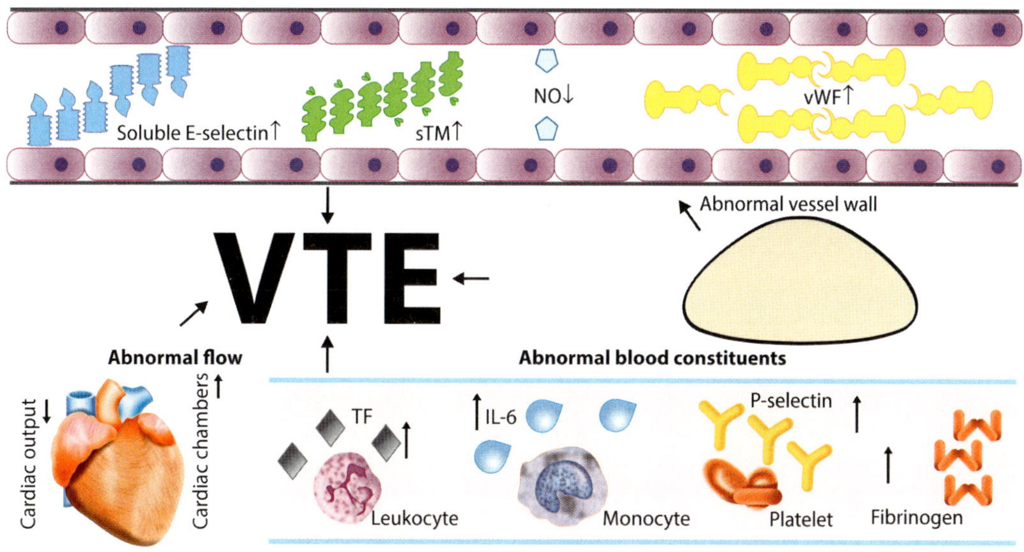

Fig. 2: Pathophysiology of thromboembolism in heart failure patients

TABLE 1: Logistic regression model evaluating LVEF and risk of VTE[15]

LVEF (%)	Odds ratio (95% confidence interval)
<20%	38.3 (9.6–152.5)
20–44%	2.8 (1.4–5.7)
>45%	1.7 (1.03–2.9)

Abbreviations: LVEF, left ventricular ejection fraction; VTE, venous thromboembolism
Source: Adapted from Howell MD, Geraci JM, Knowlton AA. Congestive heart failure and outpatient risk of venous thromboembolism: a retrospective, case-control study. J Clin Epidemiol. 2001; 54:810-6

common among heart failure patients.[16] Also heart failure and VTE patients both tend to be older.[17] Moreover, in return, acute PE deteriorates the right ventricular (RV) function, which makes the condition complicated and leads to high mortality rates in heart failure patients with VTE. In a landmark population-based cohort study of 14,629 person-years follow up, Heit et al.[18] reported that the survival to be significantly less after VTE than expected survival. The pulmonary embolism was an independent predictor of reduced survival for up to 3 months after onset as compared to DVT alone. 7-day, 30 days and 1-year VTE survival rates were 74.8% (DVT—96.2%, PE—59.1%), 72.0% (DVT—94.5%, PE—55.6%) and 63.6% (DVT—85.4%, PE—47.7%), respectively.

Metabolic Syndrome and DVT

A number of longitudinal studies have confirmed that individuals with the metabolic syndrome are at increased risk of cardiovascular events and death,[19] and that this risk increases linearly with the number of features of the syndrome. Because the metabolic syndrome is characterized by an inflammatory and a hypercoagulable state, Walter Ageno et al. in a case-control study explored the hypothesis that this syndrome may also increase the risk of VTE. In a case-control study, they compared the incidence of the metabolic syndrome in a group of 93 patients with a first episode of unprovoked DVT and in 107 controls. In this study, the metabolic syndrome was significantly more prevalent in patients with unprovoked DVT than in controls, with an adjusted odds ratio (OR) of 2.16. This observation has been confirmed subsequently by the results of three other case-control studies.[20] But many subsequent longitudinal studies did not confirm this finding and showed that only obesity, abdominal obesity associated strongly with increased risk of unprovoked DVT (Post-hoc analysis of HOPE trial,[21] TROMSO,[22] and LITE[23] studies). Obesity, in particular, central and abdominal obesity, is associated with increased thrombin formation and decreased fibrinolysis.[24,25] Obesity is also associated with immobility and is another risk factor for thrombosis.[26]

Diabetes and DVT

Diabetes mellitus (DM) is one of the risk factors for DVT and pulmonary embolism (PE).[27] Although some investigators have suggested that the risk of DVT is markedly increased in patients with diabetes, this risk is generally considered to be far less than that attributed to the classical DVT provoking risk factors. Moreover, other investigators have suggested that diabetes is not an independent risk factor for venous thromboembolism.[27] However, in keeping with the Virchow's triad, hyperglycemia is associated with stasis, endothelial injury resulting in damage to blood vessel walls and hypercoagulation,[28,29] thereby increasing the risk of VTE. Clinically, some patients who received standard anti-coagulation therapy still have a high risk of recurrence and post-thrombotic syndrome (PTS). In a recently published meta-analysis by Mi et al.[30] including 9 case-control and 6 cohort studies with 44,809 subjects with thrombosis and 83,207 controls. The study included data on subjects with diabetes mellitus. As shown in Figure 3, the prevalence of VTE was significantly higher among participants with diabetes than in those without diabetes [case-control studies —OR = 1.78; cohort studies—relative risk (RR) = 1.41]. Though, diabetes mellitus is considered

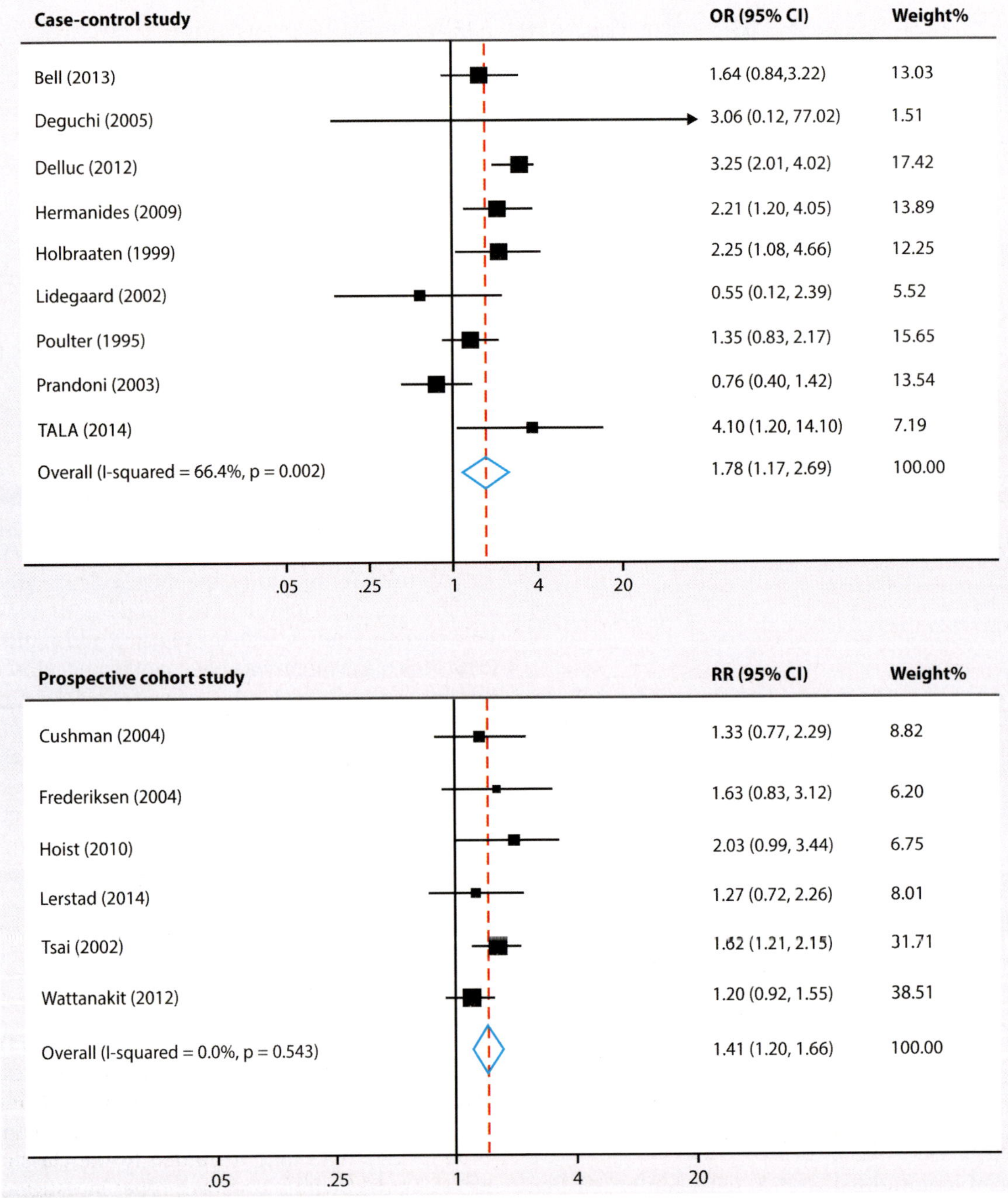

Fig. 3: Meta-analysis of the effect of diabetes mellitus on venous thromboembolism (based on 9 case-control and 6 cohort studies). Squares represent point estimates for effective size expressed as an OR/RR with the size proportional to the inverse variance of the estimate. Diamond represents pooled estimate. Lines represent 95% CIs

a risk factor for unprovoked DVT, a population-based case-control study conducted by Heit et al.[31] found contradictory results. They tested diabetes and diabetes complications (retinopathy, nephropathy or neuropathy, and ketoacidosis) as potential VTE risk factors, both alone and after adjusting for VTE risk factors. Univariately, diabetes by clinical diagnosis or by stricter criteria (fasting ambulatory blood glucose 140 mg/dL drug therapy), and diabetes complications were associated with overall incident VTE (OR = 1.32). However, after controlling for hospitalization for major surgery or medical illness and nursing home confinement, diabetes was no longer associated with VTE (p = 0.68) (Table 2). Diabetes mellitus has alterations in metabolism leading to presence of all the factors described in Virchow's triad for the development of venous thrombosis. Logically, all the patients with diabetes are at increased risk of DVT but we do not see diabetes patients being treated in outpatient department, commonly developing unprovoked DVT. It is difficult to believe that diabetes is a pathological mechanism for DVT/VTE. Simultaneously, it is important to notice that diabetes is associated with increased rate of obesity and recurrent hospitalization for various morbidities and these may be the reasons for increased risk of DVT. The findings in the study done by Heit et al.[31] suggest that the more direct path to reducing VTE incidence is to reduce the need for surgery, hospitalization for acute medical illness, or nursing home confinement among persons with diabetes. There is one more aspect of diabetic patients with DVT that diabetics more commonly have post-thrombotic syndrome and

TABLE 2: Odds ratio (OR) and 95% confidence intervals (CI) for an association of diabetes mellitus by clinical diagnosis with incident venous thromboembolism, 1976 to 2000

Models	*Adjusting Risk Factor Variable*	*Adjusting Risk Factor OR*			*Diabetes by Clinical Diagnosis OR*		
		OR	*95% CI*	*P-Value*	*OR*	*95% CI*	*P-Value*
Diabetes alone					1.32	1.07, 1.63	0.009
Diabetes adjusted for each indicated independent risk factor, individually	Age	1.00	0.92, 1.08	0.992	1.32	1.07, 1.63	0.009
	BMI	1.02	1.01, 1.03	0.001	1.26	1.03, 1.56	0.028
	Hospitalization with major surgery	14.59	10.29, 20.68	0.001	1.30	1.03, 1.64	0.028
	Hospitalization for acute medical illness	4.60	3.65, 5.79	0.001	1.25	1.00, 1.56	0.052
	Nursing home confinement	2.30	1.80, 2.95	0.001	1.24	1.01, 1.54	0.044
	Active cancer	8.45	6.32, 11.30	0.001	1.39	1.11, 1.74	0.004
	Trauma/fracture	6.02	4.40, 8.22	0.001	1.32	1.07, 1.64	0.011
	Neurological disease with leg paresis	5.59	3.67, 8.50	0.001	1.28	1.04, 1.59	0.022
	Prior superficial vein thrombosis	3.06	2.39, 3.91	0.001	1.35	1.09, 1.68	0.005
	Varicose veins	1.34	1.16, 1.56	0.001	1.32	1.07, 1.63	0.009
Diabetes adjusted for hospitalization† surgery and nursing home confinement, jointly	Hospitalization with major surgery	24.72	16.98, 36.01	0.001	0.94	0.72, 1.24	0.68
	Hospitalization for acute medical illness	9.06	6.88, 11.94	0.001			
	Nursing home confinement	6.33	4.63, 8.66	0.001			
Diabetes adjusted for all indicated risk factors, jointly	Age	1.06	0.94, 1.19	0.34	0.92	0.68, 1.25	0.59
	BMI	1.05	1.03, 1.06	0.001			
	Hospitalization with major surgery	17.05	11.43, 25.43	0.001			
	Hospitalization for acute medical illness	7.12	5.21, 9.73	0.001			
	Nursing home confinement	5.64	3.96, 8.05	0.001			
	Active cancer	7.14	5.00, 10.18	0.001			
	Trauma/fracture	3.86	2.61, 5.73	0.001			
	Neurological disease with leg paresis	4.05	2.37, 6.94	0.001			
	Prior superficial vein thrombosis	3.09	2.23, 4.28	0.001			
	Varicose veins	1.12	0.90, 1.39	0.33			

†Models also adjusted for age

recurrent DVT than nondiabetic patients. In a study of 2,488 patients of VTE, Piazza et al.[32] found that patients with diabetes were more likely to have a complicated course after venous thromboembolism than nondiabetic patients. Patients with diabetes were more likely to suffer recurrent deep vein thrombosis (14.9% vs 10.7%) and long-term major bleeding complications (16.4% vs 11.7%) (All p = 0.01) than patients without diabetes. Diabetes was associated with a significant increase in the risk of recurrent DVT [adjusted odds ratio (AOR) 1.74; 95% confidence interval (CI), 1.21–2.51].

SPECIAL ISSUES IN DIAGNOSIS AND MANAGEMENT OF PATIENTS OF DVT WITH CARDIODIABETES

All the routine protocols for diagnosis and treatment as well as prophylaxis of DVT/VTE are applicable in these groups of patients except those with heart failure. The diagnosis of DVT/VTE in presence of acutely decompensated heart failure is challenging and needs special attention. Pulmonary embolism in existing heart failure cases is likely to go undiagnosed. Indeed, it is often misdiagnosed as worsening heart failure because of the overlapping signs and symptoms and the lack of specific laboratory markers, like dyspnea and d-dimer. Dyspnea occurs both in heart failure and PE patients. The d-dimer laboratory marker is used to help diagnose PE, but it is also elevated in heart failure patients.[14] Strong clinical suspicion of diagnosis is required if a known patient of heart failure remains persistently symptomatic with elevated jugular venous pulse and relatively clear lung fields on auscultation. Routine imaging examinations such as X-ray, electrocardiogram and echocardiogram also have specificity problems for the diagnosis of PE. Contrast-enhanced chest computerized tomography (CT) is accurate in the diagnosis of PE.

Role of Rosuvastatin and Metformin in DVT Prevention

Rosuvastatin

In substudy of large randomized JUPITER trial,[33] it was noticed that treatment with 20 mg of rosuvastatin daily was associated with a significant reduction in the occurrence of VTE. The investigators could not elaborate the exact mechanism of action but they argued that statins inhibit isoprenylation of signaling proteins, with several potential antithrombotic consequences, such as reduced tissue factor expression and thrombin generation, attenuated fibrinogen cleavage, and activation of factors V and VII. Statins also augment the activity of the transcription factor Kruppel-like factor 2 (KLF-2), promoting thrombomodulin expression on endothelial cells, thereby enhancing the activity of the protein C anticoagulant pathway. Many observational studies showed that there is no association between other lipid-lowering drugs and VTE. JUPITER trial showed that rosuvastatin reduces cardiovascular events in significantly less number of hospitalizations in rosuvastatin group, and with less chance of VTE. But the benefits of Rosuvastatin extend beyond this factor.

Metformin

Lu et al.[34] studied the effectiveness of metformin in type 2 DM in reducing the risk of DVT and found that subjects with metformin experienced a 0.427-fold (p = 0.004) changes of risk reduction in development of DVT, which was independent of age, sex and comorbidities. Although the mechanism is still not clear, metformin may help to restore endothelial function via modulation of insulin resistance. In addition to the antihyperglycemic effects, metformin provides additional cardioprotective effects beyond sugar lowering, which may be related to the actions of metformin on lipid metabolism, vascular smooth muscle and cardiomyocyte intracellular calcium handling, endothelial function, hypercoagulation and platelet hyperactivity.

CONCLUSION

Cardiodiabetes patients are highly vulnerable to have DVT and VTE. Therefore, meticulous management and DVT prophylaxis is the need of the hour in all patients of cardiodiabetes to reduce the mortality and morbidity.

REFERENCES

1. Mann DL, Zipes DP, Libby Peter et al. Pulmonary Embolism. In: Braunwald's heart disease—a textbook of cardiovascular medicine, 10th edition. Philadelphia: Elsevier/Saunders; 2014. pp. 1668-9.
2. Pinjala RK, Agarwal MB, Turpie AGG. A characterization of patients with symptomatic DVT in India; for PROVE investigators. J Thromb Haemost. 2005;3:1043.
3. Vijayraghwan KS, Sharma S, Pai VM et al. DVT in South Indian Population. Ind J Surg. 2001;63:199-201.
4. Jerjes-Sanchez C. Venous and arterial thrombosis: a continuous spectrum of the same disease? Eur Heart J. 2005;26:3-4.
5. Kearon C. Duration of anticoagulation for venous thromboembolism. J Thromb Haemost. 2001;12:59-65.
6. White RH. Identifying risk factors for venous thromboembolism. Circulation. 2012;125:2051-3.
7. Piazza G, Goldhaber SZ. Venous thromboembolism and atherothrombosis. Circulation. 2010;121:2146-50.
8. Prandoni P, Bilora F, Marchiori A. An Association between Atherosclerosis and Venous Thrombosis. N Engl J Med. 2003;348:1435-41.

9. Becattini C, Agnelli G, Prandoni P et al. A prospective study on cardiovascular events after acute pulmonary embolism. Eur Heart J. 2005;26:77-83.
10. Ageno W, Dentali F, Grandi AM. New evidence on the potential role of the metabolic syndrome as a risk factor for venous thromboembolism. J Thromb Haemost. 2009;7:736-8.
11. Dean SM, Abraham W. Venous thromboembolic disease in congestive heart failure. Congest Heart Fail. 2010;16:164-9.
12. Piovella F, D'Armini AM, Barone M, et al. Chronic thromboembolic pulmonary hypertension. Semin Thromb Hemost. 2006;32:848-55.
13. Ota S, Yamada N, Tsuji A, et al. Incidence and clinical predictors of deep vein thrombosis in patients hospitalized with heart failure in Japan. Circ J. 2009;73:1513-7.
14. Zhu R, Hu Y, Tang L. Reduced cardiac function and risk of venous thromboembolism in Asian countries. Thrombosis J. 2017;15:12.
15. Howell MD, Geraci JM, Knowlton AA. Congestive heart failure and outpatient risk of venous thromboembolism: a retrospective, case-control study. J Clin Epidemiol. 2001;54:810-6.
16. Piazza G, Goldhaber SZ. Pulmonary embolism in heart failure. Circulation. 2008;118:1598-601.
17. Piazza G, Seddighzadeh A, Goldhaber SZ. Deep vein thrombosis in the elderly. Clin Appl Thromb Hemost. 2008;14:393-8.
18. Heit JA, Silverstein MD, Mohr DN, et al. Predictors of survival after deep vein thrombosis and pulmonary embolism. Arch Intern Med. 1999;159:445-53.
19. Ageno W, Prandoni P, Romualdi E, et al. The Metabolic Syndrome and the Risk of Venous Thrombosis. A Case-control study. J Thromb Haemost. 2006;4:1914-8.
20. Ageno W, Dentali F, Grandi AM. New Evidence on the Potential Role of the Metabolic Syndrome as a Risk Factor for Venous Thromboembolism. J Thromb Haemost. 2009;7:736-8.
21. Ray JG, Lonn E, Yi Q, et al. HOPE-2 Investigators. Venous thromboembolism in association with features of the metabolic syndrome. Q J Med. 2007;100:679-84.
22. Borch KH, Braekken SK, Mathiesen EB, et al. Abdominal obesity is essential for the risk of venous thromboembolism in the metabolic syndrome-the Tromso Study. J Thromb Haemost. 2009;7: 739-45.
23. Steffen LM, Cushman M, Peacock JM, et al. Metabolic syndrome and risk of venous thromboembolism: longitudinal investigation of thromboembolism etiology (LITE). J Thromb Haemost. 2009; 7:746.
24. Sundell B, Nilsson TK, Råndy M, et al. Fibrinolytic variables are related to age, sex, blood pressure, and body build measurements: a cross-sectional study in Norsjö, Sweden. J Clin Epidemiol. 1989;42:719-23.
25. Landin K, Stigendal L, Eriksson E, et al. Abdominal obesity is associated with an impaired fibrinolytic activity and elevated plasminogen activator inhibitor-1. Metabolism. 1990;39: 1044-8.
26. Ageno W, Becattini C, Brighton T, et al. Cardiovascular risk Factors and Venous Thromboembolism - A Meta-analysis. Circulation. 2008;117:93-102.
27. Zhang Y, Shi Y, Ye R, et al. Diabetes mellitus-associated hyperglycemia is a risk factor for recurring deep vein thrombosis and post-thrombotic syndrome-cohort study. Int J Clin Exp Med. 2016;9:17739-49.
28. Aso Y, Matsumoto S, Fujiwara Y, et al. Impaired fibrinolytic compensation for hypercoagulability in obese patients with type 2 diabetes: association with increased plasminogen activator inhibitor-1. Metabolism. 2002;51:471-6.
29. Murakami H, Okazaki M, Amagasa H, et al. Increase in hepatic mRNA expression of coagulant factors in type 2 diabetic model mice. Thromb Res. 2003;111:81-7.
30. Mi Y, Yan S, Lu Y, et al. Venous thromboembolism has the same risk factors as atherosclerosis-a PRISMA-compliant systemic review and meta-analysis. Medicine. 2016;95:e4495.
31. Heit JA, Leibson CL, Ashrani AA, et al. Is Diabetes Mellitus an Independent Risk Factor for Venous Thromboembolism? A population-based case-control study. Arterioscler Thromb Vasc Biol. 2009;29:1399-405.
32. Piazza G, Goldhaber S, Kroll A, et al. Venous thromboembolism in patients with diabetes mellitus. Am J Med. 2012;125:709-16.
33. Glynn RJ, Danielson E, Fonseca FAH, et al. A Randomized trial of rosuvastatin in the prevention of venous thromboembolism. N Engl J Med. 2009;360:1851-61.
34. Lu DY, Huang CC, Huang PH, et al. Metformin use in patients with type 2 diabetes mellitus is associated with reduced risk of deep vein thrombosis: a non-randomized, pair-matched cohort study. BMC Cardiovascular Disorders. 2014;14:187.

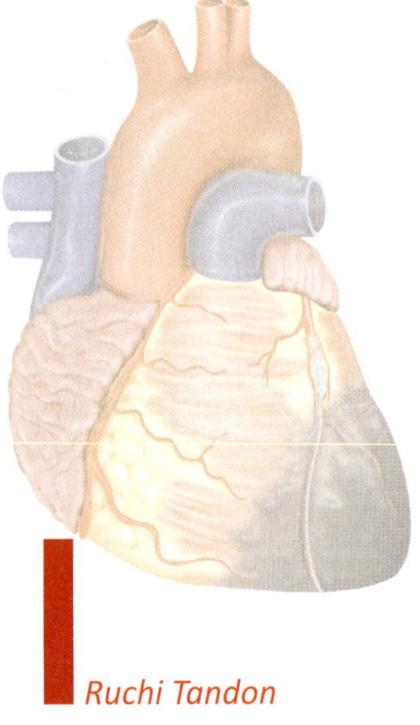

Pregnancy and Cardiodiabetes

Ruchi Tandon

INTRODUCTION

Gestational diabetes mellitus (GDM) is a condition of glucose intolerance with onset or first recognition in pregnancy that is not clearly overt diabetes. Normal pregnancy is characterized by pancreatic β-cell hyperplasia resulting in higher fasting and postprandial insulin levels. Increased secretion of placental hormones leads to increasing insulin resistance, especially throughout the third trimester. GDM occurs when β-cell function is insufficient to overcome this insulin resistance. GDM affects approximately 6% of pregnancies in the United States, and it is increasing in prevalence. Pregnant women without known diabetes mellitus should be screened for GDM after 24 weeks of gestation. GDM is defined as glucose intolerance of variable degree with onset or first recognition during pregnancy.

A study by Stuebe et al. found this condition to be associated with persistent metabolic dysfunction in women at 3 years after delivery, separate from other clinical risk factors.[1] Infants of mothers with pre-existing diabetes mellitus experience double the risk of serious injury at birth, triple the likelihood of cesarean delivery, and quadruple the incidence of newborn intensive care unit (NICU) admission. GDM accounts for 90% of cases of diabetes mellitus in pregnancy, while preexisting type 2 diabetes accounts for 8% of such cases.

SCREENING FOR DIABETES MELLITUS DURING PREGNANCY

Gestational Diabetes

The following 2-step screening system for gestational diabetes is currently recommended in the United States:

1. 50 g, 1-hour glucose challenge test (GCT)
2. 100 g, 3-hour oral glucose tolerance test (OGTT)—for patients with an abnormal GCT result.

Alternatively, for high-risk women or in areas in which the prevalence of insulin resistance is 5% or higher (e.g. the southwestern and southeastern United States), a 1-step approach can be used by proceeding directly to the 100 g, 3-hour OGTT. Some clinicians may use a 1-step approach and administer only a 75 g 2-hour fasting OGTT. The optimal screening approach is controversial. Although women with elevated glucose levels on the 75 g test have an increased risk of adverse pregnancy outcomes, no trials have demonstrated that treatment of GDM in these women improves outcomes. Most, but not all, US guidelines favor a 2-step approach. The US Preventive Services Task Force (USPSTF) recommends screening for GDM after 24 weeks of pregnancy. The recommendation applies to asymptomatic women with no previous diagnosis of type 1 or type 2 diabetes mellitus.[2,3] The recommendation does not specify whether the 1-step or 2-step screening approach would be preferable.

Type 1 Diabetes

- The disease is typically diagnosed during an episode of hyperglycemia, ketosis, and dehydration.
- It is most commonly diagnosed in childhood or adolescence; the disease is rarely diagnosed during pregnancy.
- Patients diagnosed during pregnancy most often present with unexpected coma—early pregnancy may provoke diet and glycemic control instability in patients with occult diabetes.

Type 2 Diabetes

According to the American Diabetes Association's "Standards of Medical Care in Diabetes—2010",[4,5] the presence of any one of the following criteria supports the diagnosis of diabetes mellitus:

1. Hemoglobin A1c (HbA1c) = 6.5%
2. Fasting plasma glucose = Greater than 126 mg/dL (7.0 mmol/L)
3. A 2-hour plasma glucose level = 200 mg/dL (11.1 mmol/L) during a 75 g OGTT
4. A random plasma glucose level = 200 mg/dL (11.1 mmol/L) in a patient with classic symptoms of hyperglycemia or hyperglycemic crisis.

In the absence of unequivocal hyperglycemia, a diagnosis based on any of the first three criteria should be confirmed by repeat testing on a different day.

Risk factors for GDM have been shown in Table 1.

Prediabetes

Women with prediabetes identified before pregnancy should be considered at extremely high risk for developing GDM during pregnancy. As such, they should receive early (first trimester) diabetic screening.

Postdiagnostic Testing

Once the diagnosis of diabetes is established in a pregnant woman, continued testing for glycemic control and diabetic complications is indicated for the remainder of the pregnancy.

Complications of GDM have been shown in Table 2.

First-trimester laboratory studies: Hemoglobin A1c, blood urea nitrogen (BUN), serum creatinine, thyroid-stimulating hormone, free-thyroxine levels, spot urine protein-to-creatinine ratio, capillary blood sugar levels.

Second-trimester laboratory studies: Spot urine protein-to-creatinine study in women with elevated value in first trimester, repeat HbA1c, capillary blood sugar levels.

Ultrasonography: First trimester—ultrasonographic assessment for pregnancy dating and viability; second trimester—detailed anatomic ultrasonogram at 18–20 weeks and a fetal echocardiogram if the maternal glycohemoglobin value was elevated in the first trimester; third trimester—growth ultrasonogram to assess fetal size every 4–6 weeks from 26 weeks to 36 weeks in women with

TABLE 1: Risk factors for gestational diabetes mellitus

Risk factors	*Adjusted odds ratio or relative risk*
Gestational diabetes mellitus in previous pregnancy	OR = 13.2
Body mass index > 25 kg/m^2	OR = 3.2
Ethnicity	
Asian	RR = 2.3
Native American	RR = 2.1
Pacific Islander	RR = 2.1
Black	RR = 1.8
Hispanic	RR = 1.5
Diabetes in first-degree relative	RR = 1.7
Weight gain of more than 11 lb (5 kg) since 18 years of age	RR = 1.7
Maternal age older than 35 years	OR = 1.6
Gestational weight gain in excess of Institute of Medicine guidelines	OR = 1.4
Macrosomia in previous pregnancy	OR = 1.4

Abbreviations: OR, odds ratio; RR, relative risk.

TABLE 2: Adverse outcomes associated with gestational diabetes mellitus

Outcome	*Relative risk*
Maternal	
Subsequent development of type 2 diabetes mellitus	7.4
Gestational hypertension	1.6
Preeclampsia	1.5
Cesarean delivery	1.3
Fetal	
Shoulder dystocia/birth trauma	2.9
Macrosomia	1.6
Subsequent adolescent and childhood overweight	1.5
Birth defects	1.2
Hyperbilirubinemia	*
Hypoglycemia	*

* Study heterogeneity precludes reliable estimate of increased risk of metabolic complications.

TABLE 3: Screening and diagnostic criteria for gestational diabetes mellitus

Two-step screening:				
Administer a nonfasting 50 g oral glucose challenge test.				
If the value meets or exceeds the thresholds below and is ≤ 200 mg/dL (11.1 mmol/L), administer a 100 g oral glucose tolerance test.				
Diagnose GDM if two or more values on a 100 g test meet or exceed the thresholds below.				
The American Diabetes Association does not consider a value >200 mg/dL on a 50 g oral glucose challenge test to be necessarily diagnostic of GDM; however, it is reasonable to treat these patients empirically as if they have GDM (without performing a 100 g oral glucose tolerance test) because they require insulin during pregnancy more often than patients with GDM diagnosed using the 100 g test.				
Test	*Time*	*Threshold for abnormal result*	*Comments*	
50 g oral glucose challenge test	1 hour	130 mg/dL (7.2 mmol/L)	Use of any threshold value is acceptable.	
		or	A cutoff of 130 mg/dL is more sensitive (99% vs. 85%) but less specific (77% vs. 86%) compared with a cutoff of 140 mg/dL.	
		135 mg/dL (7.5 mmol/L)		
		or		
		140 mg/dL (7.8 mmol/L)		
		Threshold for abnormal result		
		Carpenter and Coustan criteria15	*National Diabetes Data Group criteria16*	
100 g oral glucose tolerance test	Fasting	95 mg/dL (5.3 mmol/L)	105 mg/dL (5.8 mmol/L)	Use of either set of criteria is acceptable.
	1 hour	180 mg/dL (10.0 mmol/L)	190 mg/dL (10.5 mmol/L)	
	2 hours	155 mg/dL (8.6 mmol/L)	165 mg/dL (9.2 mmol/L)	
	3 hours	140 mg/dL (7.8 mmol/L)	145 mg/dL (8.1 mmol/L)	
One-step screening:				
Administer a fasting 75 g oral glucose tolerance test.				
Diagnose GDM if one or more thresholds are met or exceeded.				
Test	*Time*	*Threshold for abnormal result*	*Comments*	
75 g oral glucose tolerance test	Fasting	92 mg/dL (5.1 mmol/L)	Compared with the two-step approach, the one-step approach results in a higher prevalence of GDM (6% vs 15–20%).	
	1 hour	180 mg/dL (10.0 mmol/L)		
	2 hours	153 mg/dL (8.5 mmol/L)		

Abbreviation: GDM, gestational diabetes mellitus

overt preexisting diabetes; perform a growth ultrasonogram for fetal size at least once at 36–37 weeks for women with GDM.

Electrocardiography: If maternal diabetes is long-standing or associated with known microvascular disease, obtain a baseline maternal electrocardiogram (ECG) and echocardiogram.

Screening and diagnostic criteria for GDM have been shown in Table 3.

Management

In the largest single trial of GDM treatment, investigators randomized 1,000 women with GDM to no treatment or to intervention with lifestyle modifications, blood glucose self-monitoring, and insulin therapy, if needed. Adverse perinatal outcomes—defined as infant death, shoulder dystocia, bone fracture, and/or nerve palsy—were 4% in the no treatment group compared with 1% in the intervention group ($p = 0.01$). A more recent systematic review and

Flow chart 1: Managing gestational diabetes

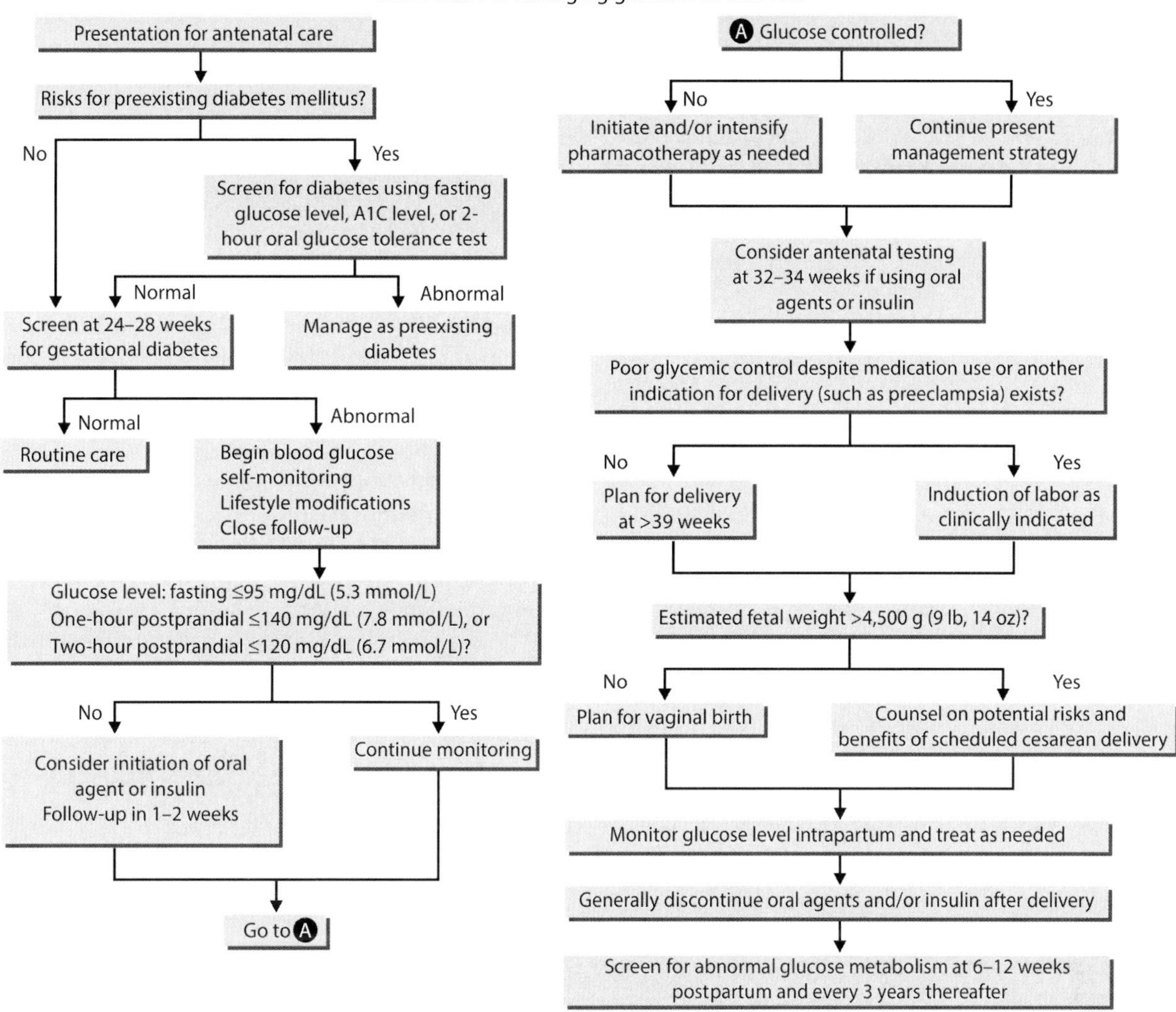

meta-analysis that included five randomized controlled trials and six cohort studies found that treating GDM results in a statistically significant decrease in the incidence of preeclampsia, shoulder dystocia, and macrosomia (Flow chart 1).

Gestational diabetes is diagnosed during pregnancy when the body cannot cope with the extra demand for insulin production resulting in high blood glucose levels. Gestational diabetes is managed by monitoring blood glucose levels, adopting a healthy eating plan and performing regular physical activity. Effective management of gestational diabetes will reduce the risk of complications during pregnancy and the birth of fetus. The healthcare team including your doctor, specialist, dietitian, and credential diabetes educator can help with blood glucose monitoring, healthy eating and physical activity.

There are three basic components in effectively managing gestational diabetes: (1) monitoring blood glucose levels, (2) adopting a healthy eating pattern, and (3) physical activity.

Gestational diabetes can often initially be managed with healthy eating and regular physical activity. However, for some women with gestational diabetes, insulin injections will be necessary for the rest of the pregnancy. Approximately, 10–20% of women will need insulin; however, once the baby is born, insulin is no longer needed. After the baby is born, gestational diabetes usually disappears. A special blood glucose test (OGTT) is performed 6 weeks after delivery to ensure that blood glucose levels have returned to normal. However, women who have had gestational diabetes have an increased risk of developing type 2 diabetes later in life and should be tested for diabetes at least every 2–3 years.

Lifestyle Changes

Initial treatment for GDM involves diet and activity modification. Women with GDM should receive individualized nutrition counseling from a registered dietitian, which commonly includes a recommendation to limit carbohydrate intake to 33–40% of calories. No high-quality data exist on the optimal diet for women with GDM. A Cochrane review of nine small trials comparing different types of dietary advice did not demonstrate any significant differences in perinatal outcomes. Some, but not all, trials suggest that a low glycemic index diet may result in improved glycemic control. Although the few trials evaluating the effects of exercise on women with GDM have yielded inconsistent results, aerobic exercise and resistance training clearly improve glycemic control in patients with diabetes. Exercise for 30 minutes most days of the week is a reasonable goal for most patients with GDM. Attention to maternal weight gain is also important in minimizing the risk of fetal macrosomia. Maternal obesity, excess gestational weight gain, and GDM are independent and additive risk factors for macrosomia. For example, among women with obesity, GDM, and gestational weight gain greater than 40 lb (18.1 kg), the risk of fetal macrosomia is nearly 40%. The goal of dietary therapy is to avoid single large meals and foods with a large percentage of simple carbohydrates. The diet should include foods with complex carbohydrates and cellulose, such as whole grain breads and legumes.

Insulin

The goal of insulin therapy during pregnancy is to achieve glucose profiles similar to those of nondiabetic pregnant women. In gestational diabetes, early intervention with insulin or an oral agent is key to achieving a good outcome when diet therapy fails to provide adequate glycemic control.

Insulin is required in women who have uncontrolled blood glucose levels despite lifestyle changes and use of oral medications, and in women who elect to avoid a trial of oral medications. Insulin does not cross the placenta; rapid , intermediate-, and long-acting insulins are considered safe for use in pregnancy. One approach to starting insulin therapy is to calculate a total daily dosage of 0.7–1.0 units/kg. Half of the total daily requirement is administered as a single dose of long-acting insulin [e.g. glargine (Lantus), detemir (Levemir)], and the other half is administered in three divided doses at mealtimes as rapid-acting insulin [e.g. lispro (Humalog), aspart (Novolog)]. Insulin dosing should be individualized and adjusted as needed.

Glyburide and Metformin

The efficacy and safety of insulin have made it the standard for treatment of diabetes during pregnancy. Diabetic therapy with the oral agents like glyburide and metformin, however, has been gaining in popularity. Trials have shown these two drugs to be effective, and no evidence of harm to the fetus has been found, although the potential for long-term adverse effects remains a concern.[6]

An elevated blood glucose level despite lifestyle modifications is an indication for pharmacologic therapy. Although insulin has historically been the standard therapy for women with uncontrolled GDM, oral medications are now appropriate first-line therapies as well.[7] Options for oral medications include metformin (Glucophage) and glyburide. Although neither glyburide nor metformin has been approved by the US Food and Drug Administration for the treatment of GDM, both are pregnancy category B. Metformin and glyburide cross the placenta but have not been associated with birth defects or short-term adverse neonatal outcomes.[8,9] However, data on long-term metabolic effects on children with in utero exposure are limited. Clinicians may consider counseling patients on the lack of long-term safety data for these medications.

No consensus exists on the threshold values above which medications should be prescribed; therefore, clinicians can consider gestational age, frequency and severity of blood glucose elevations, fetal growth, and patient preference. One approach is to begin pharmacologic therapy if more than two values at the same meal during a 2-week period are above target by more than 10 mg/dL (0.6 mmol/L).[6] Another approach is to initiate medications if 50% of the values in a given week are elevated. Glycemic control, maternal and neonatal outcomes, and adverse effects are similar among patients treated with oral hypoglycemic medications versus insulin, although glyburide may be associated with a lower failure rate (i.e. need for insulin therapy) than metformin. Metformin is typically started at 500 mg once daily with food, and titrated to a maximum dosage of 2,500 mg/day (given in divided doses with meals). Glyburide is initiated at 2.5 mg once per day 1 hour before eating, and increased to a maximum of 10 mg twice per day, as needed. Between 15% and 40% of women initially prescribed oral medications for GDM, ultimately require insulin.

FETAL ASSESSMENT

There is no consensus on the optimal approach to fetal surveillance in pregnancies complicated by GDM. Antenatal testing in women who have GDM that is well controlled without medications is not beneficial, because the risk of stillbirth is not increased in this population. Antenatal testing is commonly performed in women who require medication for GDM, although data supporting this practice are limited to older observational studies. The American College of Obstetricians and Gynecologists (ACOG) recommend that clinicians perform antenatal testing in accordance with local practice patterns. Such testing could include twice weekly nonstress tests or weekly modified biophysical profiles beginning at 32–34 weeks of gestation. The role of ultrasonography in pregnancies complicated by GDM varies among clinicians and institutions. Some physicians obtain serial ultrasonography (separated by at least 4 weeks) to monitor fetal growth in patients with GDM. Several small trials have found that instituting tighter glycemic control for women with accelerated fetal growth may result in a lower incidence of large-for-gestational-age infants. However, larger studies are needed before routine use of ultrasonography to guide management of GDM can be recommended, especially because undergoing third-trimester ultrasonography may be an independent risk factor for cesarean delivery.

Other physicians perform ultrasonography near the end of pregnancy to assess the risk of fetal macrosomia. However, a sonographically estimated fetal weight of greater than 4,000 g (8 lb, 13 oz) is only modestly predictive of an actual fetal weight greater than 4,000 g, with a positive likelihood ratio of 5.7 [95% confidence interval (CI), 4.3–7.6] and a negative likelihood ratio of 0.48 (95% CI, 0.38–0.60). Among fetuses weighing more than 4,000 g, clinical estimates (using Leopold maneuvers and fundal height measurements) are as predictive of macrosomia as ultrasonography, and appear comparable to the estimates of parous women of their baby's size. ACOG recommends that clinicians assess fetal growth in patients with GDM late in the third trimester, stating that ultrasonography or clinical examination is appropriate.

TIMING AND ROUTE OF DELIVERY

The optimal timing of delivery in pregnancies complicated by GDM is unclear. Given the neonatal risks associated with early term births, induction of labor before 39 weeks should occur only if glycemic control remains poor despite medication use, or if another indication for delivery is present. Limited evidence suggests that induction of women with GDM at 39 weeks, compared with further expectant management, is associated with a lower risk of macrosomia and shoulder dystocia, without increasing the risk of cesarean delivery. Expectant management beyond 39 weeks is also associated with an increased risk of stillbirth (relative risk = 1.8; 95% CI, 1.2–2.6), although the absolute risk remains low (5.7/10,000 deliveries). Although ACOG has not made an evidence-based recommendation on the ideal timing of delivery for patients with GDM, many physicians offer induction between 39 weeks and 40 weeks, particularly for patients with other risks of stillbirth. For women with GDM and an estimated fetal weight greater than 4,500 g (9 lb, 14 oz), scheduled cesarean delivery, compared with vaginal birth, reduces the risk of permanent brachial plexus injury, although the number needed to treat may be as high as 588. It is reasonable to offer a scheduled cesarean delivery to these patients, although they should be counseled on the difficulty of accurately estimating fetal weight and the risks associated with cesarean delivery in the index pregnancy and future pregnancies.

INTRAPARTUM AND POSTPARTUM MANAGEMENT

Maintaining euglycemia during labor and delivery can minimize risks of neonatal hypoglycemia and acidosis. Women with diet-controlled GDM rarely require intrapartum insulin. A variety of protocols exist to guide intrapartum management of blood glucose among women receiving insulin, but in general, glucose levels should be monitored every 1–2 hours during active labor, and 5% dextrose or insulin infused as needed to maintain glucose levels between 70 mg/dL and 110 mg/dL (3.9 mmol/L and 6.1 mmol/L). It may be reasonable to have women with GDM use only one-half of their usual dose of long-acting insulin up to the day of delivery. Clinicians should prepare to manage shoulder dystocia at the time of delivery and exercise caution when considering an operative vaginal delivery.

CONCLUSION

Women with GDM rarely need oral agents or insulin immediately after delivery. Before discharge, it is reasonable to confirm that fasting glucose values are normal. However, short- and long-term follow-up is critical. Women with GDM should undergo screening at 6–12 weeks postpartum with a fasting glucose measurement or 75 g 2-hour glucose tolerance test; up to 36% of women with GDM may have persistently abnormal glucose tolerance. GDM is a significant risk factor for subsequent development of diabetes. In high-risk populations, diabetes develops in up to 50% of women with GDM. Women with a history of GDM should be screened every 3 years for overt diabetes. Breastfeeding may reduce the subsequent risk of developing type 2 diabetes in women who had GDM. Any form of contraception that is otherwise medically appropriate can be used by women with a history of GDM.

REFERENCES

1. Stuebe AM, Mantzoros C, Kleinman K, et al. Gestational glucose tolerance and maternal metabolic profile at 3 years postpartum. Obstet Gynecol. 2011;118(5):1065-73.
2. Busko M. US Task Force: screen for diabetes after 24 weeks' gestation. Medscape Medical News. 2014.
3. Moyer VA. Screening for gestational diabetes mellitus: US Preventive Services Task Force recommendation statement. Ann Intern Med. 2014;160(6):414-20.
4. American Diabetes Association. Standards of medical care in diabetes—2010. Diabetes Care. 2010;33(Suppl 1):S11-61.
5. American Diabetes Association. Standards of medical care in diabetes—2013. Diabetes Care. 2013;36(Suppl 1):S11-66.
6. Moore LE, Clokey D, Rappaport VJ, et al. Metformin compared with glyburide in gestational diabetes: a randomized controlled trial. Obstet Gynecol. 2010;115(1):55-9.
7. Committee on Practice Bulletins—Obstetrics. Practice Bulletin No. 137: gestational diabetes mellitus. Obstet Gynecol. 2013;122(2 Pt 1):406-16.
8. Gilbert C, Valois M, Koren G. Pregnancy outcome after first-trimester exposure to metformin: a meta-analysis. Fertil Steril. 2006;86(3):658-63.
9. Hebert MF, Ma X, Naraharisetti SB, et al. Obstetric-Fetal Pharmacology Research Unit Network. Are we optimizing gestational diabetes treatment with glyburide? The pharmacologic basis for better clinical practice. Clin Pharmacol Ther. 2009;85(6):607-14.

18

CHAPTER

Cardiodiabetes and Autonomic Insufficiency

Ankit Bansal, Vivek Chaturvedi

INTRODUCTION

The first description of cardiovascular autonomic neuropathy (CAN) in diabetes was given in 1975 by Low et al. after determining that diabetic neuropathy also compromised autonomic control of the cardiovascular system, as evidenced by orthostatic hypotension (OH) and abnormal autonomic responses to different stimuli.[1] CAN is caused by damage to the autonomic nerve fibers that innervate the heart and blood vessels and leads to abnormalities in cardiovascular hemodynamics.[2] Hyperglycemia and hyperinsulinemia induce metabolic alterations that lead to oxidative stress and demyelination.[3] Good glycemic control, control of cardiovascular disease (CVD) risk factors and pharmacologic modulation of oxidative stress, and autonomic dysregulation reduce its progression and its adverse consequences.[3]

EPIDEMIOLOGY

Diabetes mellitus (DM) is a chronic noncommunicable disease of high public health impact in all countries irrespective of their income level with a high global burden that has escalated into an epidemic. The International Diabetes Federation (IDF) has estimated a global prevalence of 8.8% (415 million people), with an expected increase to 10.4% (642 million people) in 2040.[4] Ageing of population, sedentary lifestyle, unhealthy habits, and obesity are responsible for this exponential growth. Complications of DM include involvement of both macro [stroke, coronary artery disease (CAD), peripheral artery disease, and cerebrovascular disease] and micro (retinopathy, nephropathy, and neuropathy) vasculature. CAN is a very common and often overlooked consequence of DM and yet has a major impact on mortality and morbidity. The CAN Subcommittee of the Toronto Consensus Panel on Diabetic Neuropathy,[5] defines it as 'the impairment of cardiovascular autonomic control in patients with established DM following the exclusion of other causes'. CAN may be subclinical in the early stages but as the disease progresses, it becomes clinically evident. Its prevalence is up to 17% of patients with type 1 DM (T1DM) and 22% of those with type 2 DM (T2DM), increasing to 40% in those with insulin dependence.[3,6] Moreover, the duration of diabetes is an independent factor for developing CAN irrespective of diabetes type.[5] It is estimated that the risk for developing CAN increases annually by approximately 6% and 2% in patients with T1DM and T2DM, respectively. There is a strong association between CAN and mortality and in patients with advanced autonomic denervation and OH, the mortality rates increase to 16–35% in 5 years.[3,6]

PATHOPHYSIOLOGY

Diabetic CAN is caused by complex interactions among a number of pathogenic pathways. Hyperglycemia is the leading cause of the initiation of this pathogenic process.[7] Hyperglycemia leads to sympathetic denervation, changes in myocardial autonomic neurotransmitter levels, altered expression of neuropeptides and their signaling pathways,

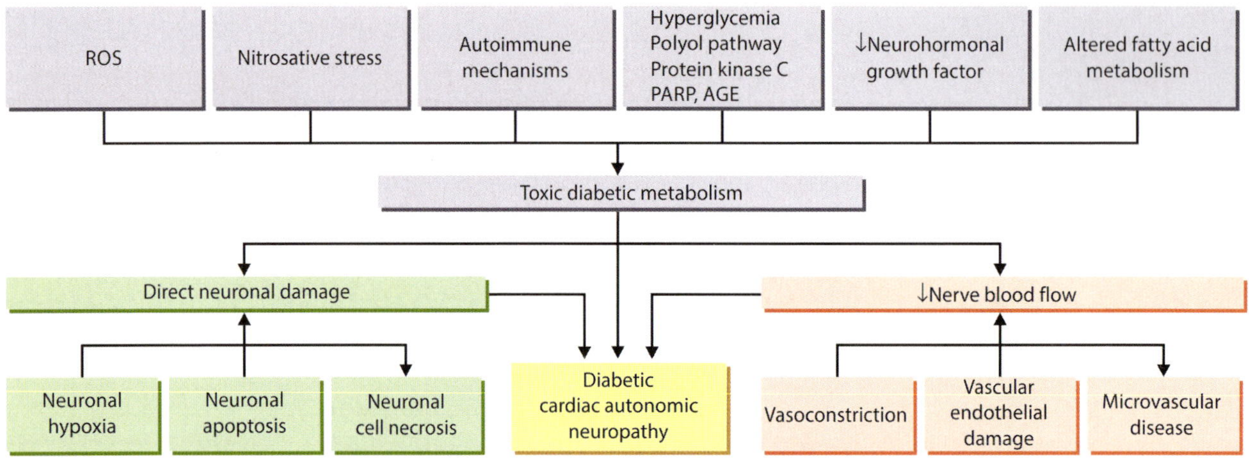

Fig. 1: Pathogenesis of diabetic cardiac autonomic neuropathy

Abbreviations: AGE, advanced glycation end products; PARP, poly(ADP-ribose) polymerase; ROS, reactive oxygen species

together with an altered beta-receptor density. It causes an increase in intracellular sorbitol leading to accumulation of intracellular osmotic particles, reduction of levels of nicotinamide adenine dinucleotide phosphate (NADPH) and formation of advanced glycation end-products. This leads to oxidative stress, activation of endoproteases [protein kinase C and mitogen-activated protein kinase (PKC and MAPK)], and altered endoneural and perineural blood flow resulting in nerve hypoxia, ischemia and axonal degeneration, together with demyelination.[3] Insulin resistance impairs myocardial contractility via reduced Ca^{2+} influx through L-type Ca^{2+} channels, reverse mode Na^{2+}/Ca^{2+} exchange and impairment of the PI3-kinase/Akt pathway.[3,6] These molecular changes lead to diastolic dysfunction, left ventricular hypertrophy (LVH), cardiac remodeling secondary to interstitial myocardial fibrosis, and ultimately to left ventricle (LV) systolic dysfunction.[3,6,7] The relative predominance of sympathetic activity at the onset of CAN stimulates the renin-angiotensin-aldosterone system (RAAS), which not only increases the hemodynamic stresses and energy requirements of the LV by sodium retention and peripheral vasoconstriction, but may also exert direct noxious effects on cardiomyocytes that cause more impairment of LV performance.[3,6,7] Autonomic dysfunction has also been associated with an impaired response to hypoglycemia with potentially lethal consequences (Fig.1).

CLINICAL MANIFESTATIONS

Clinical manifestations of diabetic CAN include: resting heart rate (HR) disorders, exercise intolerance, intraoperative cardiovascular lability, orthostatic alterations in HR and blood pressure (BP), QTc prolongation, abnormal diurnal and nocturnal BP variations, silent myocardial ischemia (SMI), and diabetic cardiomyopathy.

Impaired Heart Rate Variability

Heart rate variability (HRV) is a physiological variation in the interval between heartbeats (R-R interval) and is regulated by the interaction of the sympathetic and parasympathetic tone.[3,7] A wide variability reflects the heart's ability to adapt to the body's metabolic needs. One of the initial manifestations of CAN is a decrease in HRV which is apparent at the subclinical stage and can be detected during deep respiration.

Resting Tachycardia

Resting tachycardia is a common manifestation of CAN that occurs at a relatively early stage of the disease. A HR of 90–130 beats per minute (bpm) can be observed and is associated with a reduction in parasympathetic tone followed by increased sympathetic activity as diabetic CAN progresses. As the disease progresses and involves both parasympathetic and sympathetic nerves, the HR tends to return to the normal range but remains higher than in healthy individuals.[3,6] Resting HR is independently associated with CAN and has a high predictive value in predicting CAN in the general population.[8] A steady HR less responsive to exercise, stress or sleep is suggestive of almost total cardiac denervation, which indicates severe CAN.

Exercise Intolerance

Autonomic dysfunction impairs exercise tolerance, reduces reflex changes in HR and BP, and blunts increases in cardiac output (CO) in response to exercise due to limited adjustability of HR and BP to conditions of increased work demand.[3,6,7] Concomitant CAD, diastolic and systolic LV dysfunction may also contribute to exercise intolerance.[3,7]

Orthostatic Hypotension

On assuming standing from supine posture, individuals with diabetic CAN may have abnormal responses, such as hypotension, tachycardia, or even bradycardia.[3,6,7] OH is defined as a decrease in systolic BP (SBP) of at least 20 mm Hg (atleast 30 mm Hg in patients with hypertension) or diastolic BP (DBP)of 10 mm Hg within 2 minutes of standing from supine position. Blood volume depletion due to diuretic therapy, sweating, diarrhea or polyuria, and concomitant medications like antihypertensives, insulin, tricyclic antidepressants, and phenothiazines can also contribute to development of OH.[3,6,7] It usually presents as dizziness, fatigue, visual disturbances, and syncope but may also remain asymptomatic. Postural orthostatic tachycardia syndrome (POTS) is diagnosed when the HR increases by more than 30 bpm from baseline, or an absolute value of 120 bpm is documented within 12 minutes of transition from the supine to the upright position during tilt test. It is an independent prognostic factor for CVD and all-cause mortality.[3,6,7]

Abnormal Blood Pressure Regulation

In normal individuals BP has diurnal variations due to predominance of vagal tone and decreased sympathetic tone at night leading to reduction in nocturnal BP. In CAN, this pattern is altered, resulting in nocturnal sympathetic predominance during sleep and subsequent nocturnal hypertension also known as nondipping (lack of or a less than 10% reduction in nocturnal BP) and reverse dipping.[3,6,7] These are associated with a higher frequency of LVH, poor CV and renal outcomes.

QT Interval Prolongation

The electrocardiography (ECG) QT interval is the elapsed time between the start of the depolarization (QRS complex) and the end of the T wave. This interval should be corrected by the HR (QTc), and its measure is inversely proportional to the HR. The QTc interval is considered prolonged if more than 450 ms in men and more than 460 ms in women. The pathogenesis of QTc prolongation is multifactorial and includes imbalance in cardiac sympathetic innervation, intrinsic metabolic and electrolytic changes, LVH, CAD, and genetic factors.[3,6,7] Reversible QTc prolongation may be induced by hyperinsulinemia, hyperglycemia and acute hypoglycemia. Night time hypoglycemic episodes and reactive increase in sympathetic activity frequently leads to QTc prolongation and is associated with malignant ventricular arrhythmia.

Perioperative and Intraoperative Complications

Patients with CAN exhibit a two to three-fold increase in perioperative morbidity and mortality are more likely to require vasopressor support in the operation room and are susceptible to reductions in HR and BP during the induction of anesthesia as well as prone to severe intraoperative hypothermia.[3,6,7] These findings can be explained by an impairment or absence of the normal vasoconstrictive response.[3,6,7]

Silent Myocardial Ischemia

Silent myocardial ischemia is defined as the objective documentation of myocardial ischemia without angina or its equivalents. Upshift in anginal perceptual threshold, atypical presentation of acute coronary events and/or asymptomatic course of myocardial infarction can be facets of SMI. In patients with CAN, silent ischemia is due to impairment of pain transmission caused by dysfunction of the afferent fibers of the autonomic nervous system.[3,6,7] Patients with diabetic CAN show delayed onset of angina symptoms after the appearance of ECG ischemic changes during exercise testing or very often develop atypical symptoms such as unexplained fatigue, confusion, nausea, vomiting, sweating, coughing, and dyspnea.[3,6,7] Therefore, presence of atypical symptoms should be regarded as of myocardial origin unless proven otherwise.[3,6,7]

Sudden Death

Severe asymptomatic ischemia leading to fatal arrhythmias has been postulated as the main cause of sudden death in CAN. Other mechanisms include QTc interval prolongation, increased sympathetic activity, and oxidative stress.

Diabetic Cardiomyopathy

Diabetic cardiomyopathy is defined as structural and functional myocardial abnormalities without coronary artery disease, hypertension or valvular heart disease.[9] It is characterized by diastolic dysfunction.[9] The responsible mechanisms are LVH (increased LV mass and concentric remodeling), myocardial lipotoxicity, increased oxidative stress, cell death, interstitial and perivascular fibrosis, impaired contractile reserve, changes in myocardial substrate and energy metabolism, altered substrate utilization, and mitochondrial dysfunction.[9] In patients with CAN, the initial augmentation in cardiac sympathetic activity stimulates the RAAS and increases heart rate, stroke volume, and peripheral vascular resistance.[9] In addition, the combination of sympathetic hyperactivity and regional myocardial sympathetic denervation cause reduced coronary blood flow and diastolic dysfunction which may lead to impairment of systolic function.

SCREENING

The majority of diabetes patients with CAN have subclinical or asymptomatic disease and once the symptoms appears, the disease might have reached an advanced level and management becomes more difficult. Screening for early CAN is therefore considered good clinical practice, several reasons as summarized in Box 1.

According to the 2011 recommendations of the expert panel of Toronto[5] and the 2016 recommendations of the American Diabetes Association,[10] CAN screening is advised for following conditions in Box 2.

DIAGNOSIS

Early detection and early treatment of CAN is necessary to achieve survival benefit.[3,5-7] The most commonly employed methods for diagnosing CAN are based on assessing HRV and on the physiological changes in BP in response to specific stimuli. These tests are non-invasive, safe, clinically relevant, easy to perform, standardized, reproducible, and have high diagnostic accuracy. During the 1970s, Ewing et al. described five tests that are still being used today as the basis for diagnosing CAN:[11,12] HR response to respiration, HR response to standing, HR and BP behavior during the valsalva maneuver, BP changes during standing, and BP changes during isometric exercise. Cardiovascular autonomic reflex tests for assessing autonomic function can be classified as Table 1.

BOX 1: Significance of screening for cardiovascular autonomic neuropathy (CAN)

- It enables the accurate and clinical relevant diagnosis of various CAN forms
- It assists in the appropriate detection and subsequently the tailored treatment of CAN, multiple clinical manifestations as described in the previous section
- It provides a clinical tool for the risk stratification for diabetic complications as well as the cardiovascular morbidity and mortality
- It can be used for the modulation of targets of diabetes treatment

BOX 2: Indications for cardiovascular autonomic neuropathy (CAN) screening

- Type 2 DM at the time of diagnosis
- Type 1 DM in the first 5 years of the diagnosis
- In the presence of compatible symptoms or microvascular complications
- As part of the preoperative assessment
- Before starting an intensive physical activity program
- The annual reassessment of symptoms and the use of diagnostic tests for detection in the subclinical phase are also recommended

TABLE 1: Classification of cardiovascular autonomic reflex tests

System	Relevant test
Parasympathetic	HR response to breathing
	HR response to standing
	Spectral analysis of HRV high-frequency domain
	Total spectral power of HRV
Sympathetic	SBP response to standing
	DBP response to handgrip
	QTc prolongation
	Spectral analysis of HRV low-frequency domain
	[123] MIBG, [11C]-HED cardiac imaging
	Microneurography
	Catecholamine levels
Both parasympathetic and sympathetic	Resting HR
	Valsalva ratio
	Nocturnal BP dipping
	Baroreflex sensitivity

Abbreviations: HR, heart rate; HRV, heart rate variability; SBP, systolic blood pressure; DBP, diastolic blood pressure; MIBG, metaiodobenylguanide; BP, blood pressure

HEART RATE VARIABILITY

Heart rate variability testing is non-invasive and objective in the evaluation of cardiac autonomic function and can be performed by recording electrocardiograms during deep breathing, standing, and valsalva maneuvers. HRV analysis enables the independent measurement of the sympathetic and parasympathetic components of the autonomic nervous system.

Heart Rate Variability Beat-to-Beat

- *Technique:* In supine position, HR is monitored with the ECG while the patient breathes deeply at a rate of 6 breaths per minute
- *Response:* Evaluates the parasympathetic system
- *Normal:* Increased HR during inspiration and decreased HR during expiration. The difference in HR during inspiration and expiration should be more than 15 bpm
- *Abnormal:* Difference less than 10 bpm.

The R-R interval ratio in expiration or inspiration decreases with age:

20–24 years: ≥1.17; 25–29: ≥1.15; 30–34: ≥1.13; 35–39: ≥1.12; 40–44: ≥1.10; 45–49: ≥1.08; 50–54: ≥1.07; 55–59: ≥1.06; 60–64: ≥1.04; 65–69: ≥1.03; 70–75: ≥1.02.

Hear Rate Response to Standing

- *Technique:* While being monitored with ECG, the individual is made to stand from sitting position. The shortest RR interval (between beats 5 and 25) and the longest RR interval (between beats 20 and 40) is calculated. This is the ratio 30:15
- *Response:* Evaluates the parasympathetic system. Physiological response to standing is tachycardia followed by HR reduction. Normal value: R-R ratio 30:15 more than equal to 1.03.

Heart Rate Response to the Valsalva Maneuver

- *Technique:* The patient blows with a pressure gauge to 40 mm Hg for 15 seconds while monitored. The shortest R-R interval in the pressure phase and longest in the relaxation phase are measured
- *Response:* Evaluates both sympathetic and parasympathetic system.

Physiological Response

Tachycardia and vasoconstriction during the pressure phase and bradycardia in the relaxation phase. Normal value: greater R-R or lesser R-R interval more than equal to 1.12.

Systolic Blood Pressure Response to Standing

- *Technique:* BP is measured in supine position and within 3 minutes of standing
- *Response:* Evaluates the sympathetic system.

Physiological Response

Reduction in SBP less than equal to10 mm Hg when standing.

Orthostatic hypotension is a sustained reduction of SBP more than equal to 20 mm Hg (at least 30 mm Hg in patients with hypertension) or DBP 10 mm Hg within 3 minutes of standing.

Diastolic Blood Pressure Response to Isometric Exercise

- *Technique:* The patient squeezes a dynamometer as hard as possible. The patient then maintains a force of 30% of the maximum force exerted for 5 minutes. The DBP is measured before and after the exercise
- *Response:* Evaluates the sympathetic system. Normal response: increase in DBP more than equal to 16 mm Hg in the contralateral arm
- *Positive test:* Increase in DBP less than equal to10 mm Hg in the contralateral arm.

Apart from above mentioned simple and non-invasive tests, there are more sophisticated, sensitive, and specific methods that are particularly employed in research settings. These include:

- Heart rate variability analysis using the domains of time and frequency: Time domain analysis is a useful tool in the assessment of parasympathetic activity by measuring the normal R-R intervals, whereas the frequency domain is based on the spectral analysis of R-R interval and other cardiovascular and respiratory signals based on short-term ECG recordings (2–5 minutes).
- Scintigraphy assessment of cardiac sympathetic innervation: The use of single-photon emission computed tomography (SPECT) and/or positron emission tomography (PET) and sympathetic neurotransmitter analogues such as the 123I-metaiodobenylguanide (123I-MIBG) (SPECT), the 11C-metahydroxyephedrine (11C-HED) (PET), and 11 C-epinephrine has enabled the quantitative scintigraphic evaluation of cardiac sympathetic innervation.[6]
- Baroreflex sensitivity (BRS): It assesses the reflex ability to increase parasympathetic activity in response to a sudden increase in BP. A reduction in BP induces opposite responses. The test can be performed either with the use of pharmacological methods (intravenous bolus injection of epinephrine) or nonpharmacological techniques (physical maneuvers such as postural change).

Baroreflex sensitivity can be used for detecting subclinical CAN in diabetes, as it can be abnormal before the demonstration of any clinical signs or conventional autonomic function tests.[6] BRS is also a strong independent risk factor for mortality.

- Muscle nerve sympathetic nerve activity (MNSA): It records the efferent sympathetic nerve signals in the skeletal muscles either at rest or in response to physiological stimuli with the use of microelectrodes into a fascicle or a distal sympathetic nerve of the skin or muscle (microneurography)—usually the peronealnerve. MSNA is the most direct measure of peripheral sympathetic activity and therefore a useful research tool.

8th International Symposium on Diabetic Neuropathy in 2010 suggested the following criteria for the diagnosis and staging of CAN which is summarized in Table 2 and Figure 2.

TABLE 2: Criteria for the diagnosis and staging of cardiovascular autonomic neuropathy (CAN)

Single abnormal CART result	Possible or early CAN
Two abnormal test among the seven autonomic cardiovascular indices (5 CARTS, time-domain and frequency-domain HRV tests)	Definite or confirmed CAN
Orthostatic hypotension in addition to the above criteria	Severe advanced CAN

Abbreviations: CART, combined antiretroviral treatment; CAN, cardiovascular autonomic neuropathy

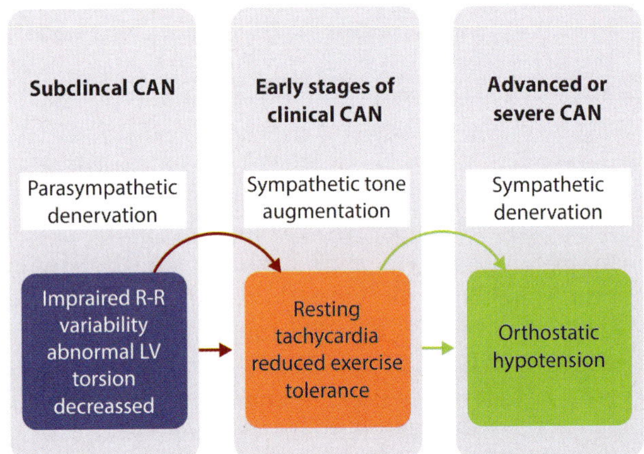

Fig. 2: Stages of cardiovascular autonomic neuropathy (CAN) and correlation with clinical signs and symptoms

THERAPEUTIC APPROACHES

Early determination of CAN is significant for the success of therapeutic strategies as cardiovascular denervation seems to be reversible at onset. In less affected patients, lifestyle changes including graded supervised exercise leading to weight loss and improve HRV.

Optimization of Glycemic Control and Management of Cardiovascular Risk Factors

A good glycemic and CV risk factor control avoiding glycemic variability and hypoglycemia seems the most important therapeutic approach for prevention of CAN. In the Diabetes Control and Complications Trial (DCCT), intensive glycemic control in T1DM reduced the CAN incidence by 50% over 6.5 years follow-up compared with conventional therapy (7% vs. 14%, respectively).[13] The benefit of intensive glycemic control in the prevention and progression of CAN is less apparent in T2DM. In the Steno-2 study done among patients with T2DM and microalbuminuria, intensive multifactorial therapy (control of glycemia, hypertension and dyslipidemia, and lifestyle changes) lowered the incident rate of CAN by approximately 60%.[14]

Exercise has favorable effect on the functioning of the autonomic nervous system; however, it should be introduced in graded manner to allow the patients' cardiovascular system to adapt.

TREATMENT OF ORTHOSTATIC HYPOTENSION

Because OH is a relatively late complication of CAN, the treatment is challenging due to advanced nature of disease. Treatment utilizes both nonpharmacological (Box 3) and pharmacological methods.

Drug Treatment

The main objective of drug treatment is to increase plasma volume using a mineralocorticoid agent (fludrocortisone at a starting dosage of 0.1 mg/day in the morning, with weekly increases to a maximum of 0.3 mg/day depending on the response). The treatment can promote hypertension and peripheral edema. Potassium levels should be monitored a week after each dosage adjustment. Midodrine, a selective alpha-1 agonist is a second-choice drug in the event of intolerance or lack of response to fludrocortisone. The dosage should be titrated from 2.5 to 10 mg 3 times a day.

Other agents undergoing research include fluoxetine, oral or intranasal desmopressin, subcutaneous octreotide, yohimbine, somatostatin, and dihydroergotamine.

TREATMENT OF ORTHOSTATIC TACHYCARDIA

Triggers should be avoided, and physical activity and hydration should be encouraged. Increased salt intake in the absence of hypertension is recommended. Drugs such

BOX 3: Nonpharmacological treatments for orthostatic hypotension

- Increase the fluid intake
- Compression stockings
- Avoidance of sudden postural changes to standing up
- Avoidance of medicines such as vasodilators, diuretics, phenothiazines, and tricyclic antidepressants that provoke hypotension
- Eating frequent, small meals to prevent postprandial hypotension
- Avoidance of exercises and maneuvers that increase intra-abdominal and intrathoracic pressure resulting in decrease of venous return
- Use of physical preventive maneuvers, such as crossing of the legs and squatting may counter decreases in blood pressure

as fludrocortisone and midodrine and in more severe cases, beta-blockers and ivabradine[15] may be used, although none of them have been specifically studied in the diabetic population.

CONCLUSION

Cardiovascular autonomic neuropathy is a frequently overlooked and underdiagnosed microvascular complication of DM. With strong causal links to intraoperative and perioperative cardiovascular instability, abnormal BP profile, OH , SMI, arrhythmias, diabetic cardiomyopathy, and stroke, CAN is associated with significant increases in morbidity and mortality. Patients may have subclinical CAN for several years before it becomes clinically apparent. Diagnosis is simple but requires time and skills for making and interpreting autonomic reflex tests. Tailored and individualized management with avoidance of hypoglycemia and OH is important in these patients. It is imperative to begin recognizing CAN early to accomplish a better prognosis and reduce CVD mortality among people with long-standing DM.

REFERENCES

1. Low PA, Walsh JC, Huang CY, et al. The sympathetic nervous system in diabetic neuropathy. A clinical and pathological study. Brain. 1975;98(3):341-56.
2. Vinik AI, Erbas T. Diabetic autonomic neuropathy. Handb Clin Neurol. 2013;117:279-94.
3. Karayannis G, Giamouzis G, Cokkinos DV, et al. Diabetic cardiovascular autonomic neuropathy: clinical implications. Expert Rev Cardiovasc Ther. 2012;10(6):747-65.
4. International Diabetes Federation. IDF Diabetes Atlas, 7th edition. Belgium: IDF; 2015.
5. Spallone V, Ziegler D, Freeman R, et al. Cardiovascular autonomic neuropathy in diabetes: clinical impact, assessment, diagnosis, and management. Diabetes Metab Res Rev. 2011;27(7):639-53.
6. Dimitropoulos G, Tahrani AA, Stevens MJ. Cardiac autonomic neuropathy in patients with diabetes mellitus. World J Diabetes. 2014;5(1):17-39.
7. Balcıoğlu AS, Müderrisoğlu H. Diabetes and cardiac autonomic neuropathy: Clinical manifestations, cardiovascular consequences, diagnosis and treatment. World J Diabetes. 2015;6(1):80-91.
8. Tang ZH, Zeng F, Li Z, et al. Association and predictive value analysis for resting heart rate and diabetes mellitus on cardiovascular autonomic neuropathy in general population. J Diabetes Res 2014;2014:215473.
9. Boudina S, Abel ED. Diabetic cardiomyopathy, causes and effects. Rev Endocr Metab Disord. 2010;11(1):31-9.
10. American Diabetes Association. Microvascular complications and foot care. Diabetes Care. 2016;39(suppl 1):S72-80.
11. Ewing DJ, Martyn CN, Young RJ, et al. The value of cardiovascular autonomic function tests: 10 years experience in diabetes. Diabetes Care. 1985;8(5):491-8.
12. Tesfaye S, Boulton AJ, Dyck PJ, et al. Diabetic neuropathies: update on definitions, diagnostic criteria, estimation of severity, and treatments. Diabetes Care. 2010;33(10):2285-93.
13. The effect of intensive diabetes therapy on measures of autonomic nervous system function in the Diabetes Control and Complications Trial (DCCT). Diabetologia. 1998;41:416-23.
14. Gaede P, Vedel P, Larsen N, et al. Multifactorial intervention and cardiovascular disease in patients with type 2 diabetes. N Engl J Med. 2003;348(5):383-93.
15. McDonald C, Frith J, Newton JL. Single centre experience of ivabradine in postural orthostatic tachycardia syndrome. Europace. 2011;13(3):427-30.

19

CHAPTER

Cardiodiabetes and Pulmonary Embolism: Is the Outcome Different?

Mrinal Kanti Das, Tapan Sinha

INTRODUCTION

Pulmonary embolism (PE) associated with diabetes mellitus (DM) is a sparsely discussed topic, though the combination is potentially dangerous. In a landmark study in 2005, prevalence of PE was studied in patients with type II diabetes mellitus (T2DM).[1] PE was present in 2,011 patients with DM (0.7%) versus 2,759 patients (0.5%) in the control group. Using multivariate analysis, DM remained independently associated with PE [odds ratio (OR), 1.27; 95% confidence interval (CI), 1.19–1.35; $p < 0.001$] and with PHT (OR, 1.53; 95% CI, 1.45–1.60; $p < 0.001$). In the United States, from 1990 to 2010, in T2DM patients, there has been 67.85% decrease in incidences of complications of myocardial infarction and 51.4% fall in major vascular events.[2] Only a few cases of PE were reported in that study. Lifestyle modifications, better glycemic control, and concomitant therapeutic interventions for endothelial stability and vascular rheology, all had their positive contributions.[3,4] As there is considerable overlap in pathophysiological mechanism of both, there are substantial reasons for extrapolation of data to figure out an adverse relationship. Though Indian data are limited, in a retrospective registry, it was found that majority (53%) of patients had comorbid cardiovascular disease, including DM. Hypertension (25%) was the most common comorbidity followed by DM (19%) in this patient population. In addition, obesity (11%) was a common risk factor in deep vein thrombosis (DVT) complicated by PE. There was no discussion on the outcome results.[5] In the absence of Indian data, discussion in the chapter will depend on mostly the western publications.

EPIDEMIOLOGY

Pulmonary embolism is an underdiagnosed, potentially life-threatening cardiopulmonary disease. The mortality rate associated with PE is 15% in the first 3 months of diagnosis and nearly 25% cases present with sudden death.[6] The annual incidence of venous thromboembolism (VTE) and embolization from right ventricle (RV) is estimated at 1.2 cases per 1,000 adults.[7] PE usually occurs 3–7 days after the onset of DVT after RV dysfunction.[7,8] Blacks have three-fold higher incidence for PE than whites, blacks and Hispanics, suffer fatal PE at a significantly younger age than whites, and they also have higher incidences on T2DM.[9] In 2002, India had 31.7 million diabetic population. Taking these figures on board and generally sedentary lifestyle of Indian population, there is enough reason to believe in large number of fatal and nonfatal PEs among Indian population. Relative risk for vascular events is higher in female patients with type 2 diabetes than in male patients with type 2 diabetes. The reason for the sex difference is largely unknown but could be at least in part explained by a heavier risk-factor burden and a greater effect of blood pressure and atherogenic dyslipidemia (AD) on the risk of cardiovascular disease (CVD) in diabetic women than in diabetic men.[10]

PATHOPHYSIOLOGY

Pathophysiology of PE in patients with T2DM is for lipids, altered homeostasis for coagulation derangements and platelet dysfunctions, glycemic control, endothelial damages, and right ventricular dysfunction (RVD). All these are inseparably interlinked with each other.

Cholesterols

Total and low-density lipoprotein (LDL) cholesterol levels are usually normal in type 2 diabetic individuals, but compositional changes in LDL particles occur (small dense LDL, high triglyceride content, and oxidative modification of LDL particles), and the number of LDL particles are increased.[11] Because each LDL particle contains one apolipoprotein B molecule, patients with type 2 diabetes also have increased levels of apolipoprotein B. An increased number of LDL particles might contribute to atherogenesis.[12] Small dense LDL particles rapidly enter the arterial wall and can be toxic to endothelial cells, cause greater production of procoagulant factors, and can be oxidized more readily than the large buoyant particles. Very low-density lipoprotein 1 (VLDL1) triglyceride level is the major predictor of LDL size in individuals with or without type 2 diabetes.

Diabetes Mellitus II, Coagulation, Endothelium Dysfunction, and Pulmonary Embolism

Hyperglycemia directly contributes to endothelial injury through irreversible glycation of collagen and other subendothelial structural proteins of the vessel, forming advanced glycation end products (AGEPs).[13] AGEPs accumulate in the subendothelium over time influenced by increases in blood sugar levels and are directly related to atherosclerosis and renal failure.[14] AGEPs cause changes in structure and biophysical properties of the basement membrane causing changes in permeability and vasodilation of blood vessels.[15] One method to assess vascular integrity is by the measurement of plasma thrombomodulin (TM) since this is essentially a membrane protein.[16] Thus, increased plasma TM levels may provide laboratory evidence of endothelial injury and indirectly, a reduction in the effectiveness of the protein C anticoagulant pathway. Particularly in T2DM patients, increased levels of TM appear to be associated with a diffuse vascular injury. Long-term DM is characterized by widespread alterations of basal lamina (BL). All parts of the lung are equally affected by DM. The thickening of BL is of the same magnitude in lung and kidney. This is associated with asymmetrical concentration of dimethylarginine. There is no relationship between the thickening of the lung BL and the known duration and type of DM.[17] Thickening of BL is associated with endothelial dysfunction which results in rapid transformation of partial occlusion (25–30% occlusion) to total or subtotally (50–70% or more) occluding PE. Another marker of endothelial injury is the von Willebrand factor (vWF). In some conditions such as hypertension and hyperinsulinemia, vWF levels are elevated. The vWF levels drop in coronary artery disease patients when they start the treatment to reduce hypercholesterolemia. Intervention studies have shown that treatment of hypercholesterolemia, hypertension, diabetes, and hyperhomocysteinemia reduces vWF levels as does smoking cessation. An increase in vWF has been observed preceding T2DM, and there is a positive association between increased vWF and progression to microvascular and macrovascular dysfunction in diabetes. Insulin resistance and diabetes are associated with prothrombotic risk (coagulation factors VII, XII, and fibrinogen) and with suppression of fibrinolysis due to elevated concentrations of the fibrinolytic inhibitor plasminogen activator inhibitor-1 (PAI-1). In insulin-resistant states, impaired endothelial function suppresses nitrogen oxide (NO) production and prostacyclin synthesis and platelets tend to aggregate. Hyperglycemia and glycation contribute to the generation of clot that is resistant to fibrinolysis. Elevated levels of PAI-1 have been shown to be associated with insulin resistance and type 2 diabetes and are independent of obesity and poor glycemic control.

Type 2 Diabetes Mellitus, Right Ventricle Dysfunction, and Pulmonary Embolism

Diabetic cardiomyopathy has a complex and multifactorial pathogenesis. Atherosclerosis, subclinical microinfarctions, mitochondrial dysfunction, and lipotoxicity—all have been proposed as contributors to diabetic cardiomyopathy. Furthermore, it has been recognized that deposition of AGEPs caused by long-standing hyperglycemia affects ventricular stiffness. The formation of AGEPs yields fibrosis by cross-linking collagen, thus increasing myocardial stiffness. RV involvement in diabetic cardiomyopathy might be of importance because the RV has a substantial contribution to overall myocardial contractility. RV function has proven to be of importance for patient risk stratification in heart failure and for prediction of development of atrial fibrillation. In general, RVD and fibrosis are associated with lethal ventricular arrhythmias, sudden death, exercise limitation, and impaired RV cardiac output. In addition, the prevalence of cardiac conduction abnormalities is increased in diabetic patients.[18] RVD was the single most important predictor of in-hospital death in the international registry of 2,454 patients with

PE. Therefore, echocardiography has emerged as an important diagnostic tool for assessing the degree of RVD in patients with acute PE. However, associations of cardiac troponins I and II and RV dysfunction are less clear.[19] N-terminal pro b-type natriuretic peptide (NT-proBNP) below 300 pg/mL appears to be a good risk stratification marker in identifying low-risk patients with nonmassive PE with T2DM who could be treated in an outpatient setting.[20] Cardiac troponin (cTnI) was elevated (≥0.07 ng/mL) in 45% of patients and elevated serum myoglobin was found very early after symptoms (<4 h) in 55% of T2DM patients with PE. Elevated serum cTnI and myoglobin were significantly associated with electrocardiogram (ECG) signs of right ventricular strain and echocardiographic evidence of RVD. The results of previous studies strongly support the integration of troponin and myoglobin testing into the risk stratification and management of patients with established acute PE.[21] Heart-type fatty acid binding protein (H-FABP) is a promising early indicator in T2DM patients of right ventricular injury and dysfunction in acute PE. It may help optimize risk stratification algorithms and treatment strategies. Over 14% cases with PE with T2DM confirmed by pulmonary CT angiography and with echocardiography proved that RVD and NT-proBNP/troponin I serum level measurements showed significantly higher RV/LV ratios and NT-proBNP/troponin I levels compared to those without RVD. A combination of RV/LV volume with NT-proBNP or troponin I measurements improves the diagnostic accuracy of either test alone.[22] Cardiovascular risk factors may contribute to unprovoked venous thromboembolism (VTE). VTE may be an early symptomatic event in patients at high cardiovascular risk, including diabetic patients. Compelling evidences suggest that T2DM is associated with a higher risk of development and progression of atrial fibrillation (AF). Furthermore, in AF patients with a coexisting T2DM, the risk of cardioembolic stroke and systemic thromboembolism appeared increased. Thus, T2DM has been included as one of the items of the $CHADS_2$ score and of the subsequent CHA_2DS_2-VASc score that have been developed to assess the arterial thromboembolic risk of AF patients. Such a high incidence of thromboembolic events observed in these clinical subsets may be attributable to the DM-related prothrombotic state due to a number of changes in primary and secondary hemostasis. Thus, analytes such as von Willebrand factor, factor VIII, fibrinogen, and D-dimer are markers that should be interpreted differently in diabetic patients. Laboratory evidence of hemostatic abnormalities in diabetic patients supports clinical observations that diabetes is a state of hypercoagulability and hypofibrinolysis. Strategies for clinical intervention and medications are not well established considering the results of the hemostatic markers. There are two major groups of natural anticoagulants: (1) serine protease inhibitors [antithrombin (AT), heparin cofactor II, and tissue factor pathway inhibitor (TFPI)] and (2) inhibitors of activated protein C (PC) and its cofactor protein S (PS). These mechanisms limit fibrin formation to the area where there is endothelial injury. Deficiencies of PC, PS, and AT in T2DM are considered risk factors for thrombotic events. Although hyperglycemia, dyslipidemia, and hypertension may independently cause vascular damage, endothelial dysfunction may be intrinsic to T2DM. This condition can lead to an activated state characterized, in part, by platelet adhesion and increased aggregation. Moreover, the osmotic effect of glucose consists of a mechanism by which hyperglycemia increases the propensity of platelets to aggregate and degranulate. As hypercoagulability and hypofibrinolysis states are present in diabetic patients, the expression of markers such as D-dimer may be underestimated. Moreover, one should take into account that more rigid fibrin from glycated fibrinogen may also contribute to relatively low values, as this fibrin is more difficult to break down. The clinical utility of D-dimer is currently limited to excluding DVT and pulmonary thromboembolism from the diagnosis with the finding of low values due to the negative predictive value of this marker. However, we cannot ignore the increased levels of D-dimer that are not directly associated with DVT and pulmonary thromboembolism.

Pulmonary Embolism and Diabetes Mellitus

The annual incidence rate of VTE among diabetic patients in the population was 432 per 100,000 individuals (95% CI 375–496). In nondiabetic individuals, it was 78 (95% CI 68–88). The age-adjusted incidence rate among the diabetic population was 274 (95% CI 262–286). The annual incidence rate of VTE was elevated in T1DM (type 1 diabetes mellitus) and T2DM patients and the incidence rates were 704 (95% CI 314–1,566) and 412 (95% CI 312–544), respectively. The overall standardized morbidity ratio was 2.27 (95% CI 1.75–2.95), i.e. diabetic patients were more prone to VTE after adjustment for age differences and had higher incidences for PE.[23]

THERAPEUTIC CONSIDERATIONS

Therapeutic considerations are multifactorial:

- Thrombolysis
- Anticoagulants for PE
- Antithrombotic for platelet dysfunction
- Treatment for RV dysfunction

- Treatment outcome for T2DM
- Treatment by statins, both as lipid-lowering agent and for their vascular endothelial anti-inflammatory properties.

Detailed review of each is beyond scope of this chapter. However, in absence of any large study comparing outcome of PE in T2DM and patients without DM, we shall have to rely on surrogated interpretation of results of treatment modalities for confounding factors.

Thrombolysis in Pulmonary Embolism

Thrombolytic agents accelerate clot lysis by converting plasminogen to its active form, plasmin, dissolving intrapulmonary clot, and clot that is at risk for subsequent embolization from the deep veins. At present, there are three agents (streptokinase, urokinase, and tissue plasminogen activator) approved by the Food and Drug Administration (FDA) for thrombolysis of pulmonary emboli. All are administered intravenously or angiographically for direct clot lysis in patients without contraindications. Results are adversely affected in T2DM. Streptokinase, urokinase, and recombinant tissue plasminogen activator (rtPA) all are recommended in ESC 2014 Guideline, with recommendations strongest for rtPA.[24] Table 1 shows the different types and dosage of thrombolytics as adopted from the guideline.

While no large individual trial has demonstrated a statistically significant mortality, benefit from lytic therapy compared with heparinization alone in patients with PE, lysis does lead to a more rapid reduction in angiographic clot burden and pulmonary hypertension, restores RV function, and reduces the risk of recurrent pulmonary emboli. However, lytic therapy must be weighed against the 9–22% risk of major bleeding, including 1–5% risk of intracranial hemorrhage. Meta-analyses of lytic therapy trials have shown that the majority of benefit from thrombolytic therapy is limited to PE patients with hemodynamic instability. While normotensive patients with evidence of RV dysfunction have increased mortality, and thrombolytic therapy has been shown to improve RV dysfunction; definitive data demonstrating a significant morbidity and/ or mortality benefit from lytic therapy in this population are lacking. Several studies have examined the efficacy of lytic therapy in normotensive patients with RV dysfunction and PE, but they lack uniform tools [transthoracic echocardiograms (TTE) vs electrocardiogram (ECG)] and uniform terminology for defining RV dysfunction and/or fail to state how outcome criteria for PE-related mortality was assessed, fail to confirm the diagnosis of PE, or have potential patient selection biases. Despite the high specificity of TTE, the positive predictive value of the modality in predicting in-hospital mortality is low (4–5%), potentially subjecting an unnecessarily large number of patients to lytic therapy. This is more significant in presence of T2DM. Further, studies that limit data to normotensive patients with PE-related RV dysfunction reveal lower short-term mortality differences (4–5%) than trials examining mortality differences (4–14%) in all PE patients with RV dysfunction and presence of T2DM. Thus, further studies are needed to determine which hemodynamically stable patients will benefit from lytic therapy in the setting of RV dysfunction.[24,25]

TABLE 1: Approved thrombolytic regimens for pulmonary embolism

Streptokinase	250,000 IU as a loading dose over 30 minutes, followed by 100,000 IU/h over 12–24 hours
	Accelerated regimen: 1.5 million IU over 2 hours
Urokinase	4400 IU/kg as a loading dose over 10 minutes followed by 4400 IU/kg per hour over 12–24 hours
	Accelerated regimen: 3 million IU over 2 hours
rtPA	100 mg over 2 hours or
	0.6 mg/kg over 15 minutes (maximum dose 50 mg)

Source: 2014 ESC guideline

Anticoagulants for Pulmonary Embolism

Once daily, unmonitored, subcutaneous administration of fondaparinux was not inferior to the use of unfractionated heparin for the initial treatment of hemodynamically stable PE, and rates of adverse events were similar with the two therapies. However, because of its simplicity, once daily subcutaneous administration of fondaparinux without anticoagulation monitoring could replace intravenous administration of unfractionated heparin in most patients with this disorder.[26] Head-on study between enoxaparin and fondaparinux placese the latter marginally ahead.[27] The reduction in arterial thrombotic events observed with apixaban raises the possibility that such events are part of the continuing risk of thrombosis in patients with VTE.[28] While heparin reduces the morbidity and mortality from recurrent PEs, it does not affect the clot(s) causing the initial hemodynamic insult.

Antiplatelets for Pulmonary Embolism

Antiplatelets are no more recommended for treatment or secondary prevention for PE. For primary prevention, the data are inconclusive.

Treatment Outcome for Right Ventricular Dysfunction

In patients with symptomatic and asymptomatic RVD and shock, T2DM has its faltering contributions. While cardiogenic shock occurs in less than 5% of patients with PE, the mortality of patients with cardiogenic shock ranges from 25% to 40%, and is as high as 65–95% in patients requiring cardiopulmonary resuscitation. The majority of patients who sustain massive PEs (defined as >50% occlusion of the pulmonary vasculature) do not have clinical cardiogenic shock and, therefore, have a much lower mortality than those patients with shock. Anatomically, massive PEs account for only 50% of the mortality in PE with the remaining fatalities occurring in patients with submassive or recurrent pulmonary emboli. Presence of T2DM adversely influences outcome of all cases of shock. Patients presenting with PE in cardiogenic shock should immediately receive vasopressor support, anticoagulation, and then be considered for thrombolysis and or embolectomy where available. Unstable patients with pulmonary emboli who have failed maximal medical management with vasopressor resistant hypotension or cardiac arrest, or who have contraindications to thrombolytic therapy can be considered for percutaneous or surgical embolectomy. Catheter-based embolectomies include clot aspiration, clot fragmentation, and rheolytic thrombectomy. The percutaneous techniques, however, are limited by the size of clot that can be removed through a small catheter lumen. In Indian scenario, this might be a wishful approach as the availability of catheterization laboratories is only in the city-based hospitals. Same is with the surgical embolectomy which is also not widely available but offers the ability to extract larger clots while providing cardiopulmonary bypass support. The current data available on embolectomy are from case reports or trials with small numbers of patients. But, mortality varies from 16% to 46%, with the higher mortality found in older studies and in studies that included patients with cardiac arrest with T2DM. Antecedent lytic therapy has not been cited as a contraindication to surgical embolectomy, but an increase in complications should be anticipated.

Finally, in patients presenting with RV failure, a differentiation between acute and chronic PE is required as management strategies, follow-up, and prognosis differ. Patients with acute PE should have close follow-up after discharge to ensure that chronic thromboembolic pulmonary hypertension does not develop. Treated patients with dyspnea that persists in the outpatient setting should provoke concern for the development of chronic pulmonary embolic hypertension, and radiologic imaging (contrast-enhanced computed tomography or ventilation-perfusion scanning) should be employed. These patients should be referred to a pulmonary arterial hypertension (PAH) specialist for consideration of thromboendarterectomy, vasodilator therapy, or lung transplantation as appropriate.[25]

Treatment Outcome for T2DM and Statins

American Diabetic Association Guidelines over the years were first to advocate use of statins in all cases of diabetic patients regardless of level of pretreatment cholesterol levels. Their conclusions were based on lesser number of vascular and cardiac complications associated with statin, which remained independent of glycemic control. Subsequent studies attributed this to pleiotropic effect of statins on vascular endothelium. Justification for the Use of Statins in Prevention: an Intervention Trial Evaluating Rosuvastatin (JUPITER) examined the question of whether treatment with 20 mg of rosuvastatin daily, as compared with placebo, would reduce the rate of first major cardiovascular events. The occurrence of VTE was a protocol-specified secondary end point of the trial.[29]

CONCLUSION

2014 ESC Guidelines on the diagnosis and management of acute PE place DM as weak risk factor (odds ratio <2). Whereas the same guideline places previous MI within 3 months and previous VTE as strong risk factors for PE (odds ratio >10). On the other hand, from our discussion above it is apparent that DM is an important risk factor for both MI and VTE. This becomes contradictory from pathophysiological aspect. We believe the guideline is suboptimal in this regard. In absence of focused studies on PE in DM patients, the outcome results are not supported by hard-core data. We also observed that DM with PE with right ventricular failure and cardiogenic shock had poorer outcome in terms of mortality and morbidity and this group warrants utmost care.

REFERENCES

1. Movahed MR, Hashemzadeh M, Jamal MM. The prevalence of pulmonary embolism and pulmonary hypertension in patients with type ii diabetes mellitus. Chest. 2005;128(5):3568-71.
2. Gregg EW, Li Y, Wang J, et al. Changes in diabetes-related complications in the United States, 1990-2010. N Engl J Med. 2014;370(16):1514-23.
3. Li G, Zhang P, Wang J, et al. Cardiovascular mortality, all-cause mortality, and diabetes incidence after lifestyle intervention for people with impaired glucose tolerance in the Da Qing Diabetes Prevention Study: a 23-year follow-up study. Lancet Diabetes Endocrinol. 2014;2(6):474-80.

4. Markku Laakso. Cardiovascular disease in type 2 diabetes from population to man to mechanisms: The Kelly West Award Lecture 2008. Diabetes Care. 2010;33(2):442-9.
5. Kamerkar DR, John MJ, Desai SC, et al. Arrive: a retrospective registry of Indian patients with venous thromboembolism. Indian J Crit Care Med. 2016;20(3):150-8.
6. Piazza G, Goldhaber SZ. Acute pulmonary embolism: part 1. Epidemiology and diagnosis. Circulation. 2006;114:e28-32.
7. Heit JA. The epidemiology of venous thromboembolism in the community. Arterioscler Thromb Vasc Biol. 2008;28:370-2.
8. Torbicki A, Perrier A, Konstantinides S, et al. Guidelines on the diagnosis and management of acute pulmonary embolism: The Task Force for the diagnosis and management of acute pulmonary embolism of the European Society of Cardiology (ESC). Eur Heart J. 2008;29:227-315.
9. Tang Y, Perrier A, Konstantinides S, et al. Ethnic differences in out-of-hospital fatal pulmonary embolism. Circulation. 2011;123:2219-25.
10. Juutilainen A, Kortelainen S, Lehto S, et al. Gender difference in the impact of type 2 diabetes on coronary heart disease risk. Diabetes Care. 2004;27:2898-904.
11. Mazzone T, Chait A, Plutzky J. Cardiovascular disease risk in type 2 diabetes mellitus: insights from mechanistic studies. Lancet. 2008;371:1800- 9.
12. Austin MA, King MC, Vranizan KM, et al. Atherogenic lipoprotein phenotype: a proposed genetic marker for coronary heart disease risk. Circulation. 1990;82:495-506.
13. Anna LS, Marinez de OS, Ana PS, et al. Hemostatic changes in patients with type 2 diabetes mellitus. Revista Brasileira de Hematologia e Hemoterapia. 2010;32:482-8
14. Grant PJ. Diabetes mellitus as a prothrombotic condition. J Int Med. 2007;262:157-72.
15. Natali A, Toschi E, Baldeweg S, et al. Clustering of insulin resistance with vascular dysfunction and low-grade inflammation in type 2 diabetes. Diabetes. 2006;55:1133-40.
16. Ralph L. Rutger W, Johannes WAS, et al. Right ventricular involvement in diabetic cardiomyopathy. Diabetes Care. 2013;36:457-62.
17. Weynand B, Jonckheere A, Frans A, et al. Diabetes mellitus induces a thickening of the pulmonary basal lamina. Respiration. 1999;66:14-9.
18. Kucher N, Wallmann D, Carone A, et al. Incremental prognostic value of troponin I and echocardiography in patients with acute pulmonary embolism. Eur Heart J. 2003;24(18):1651-6.
19. Nyberg K. The promise of cardiac biomarkers in type 2 diabetes. Diabetes Management Resource Center. [online] Medpage Today website. Available from *https://www.medpagetoday.com/resource-center/diabetes-management-resource-center/cardiac-biomarkers-in-diabetes/a/54328* [Accessed Sep 2017].
20. Arram EO, Fathy A, Abdelsamad AA, et al. Value of cardiac biomarkers in patients with acute pulmonary embolism. Egyptian J Chest Dis Tuberc. 2014;63(1):247-52.
21. Puls M, Dellas C, Lankeit M, et al. Heart-type fatty acid-binding protein permits early risk stratification of pulmonary embolism. Eur Heart J. 2007;28(2):224-9.
22. Henzler T, Roeger S, Meyer M, et al. Pulmonary embolism: CT signs and cardiac biomarkers for predicting right ventricular dysfunction. Eur Respi J. 2012;39:919-26.
23. Petrauskiene V, Falk M, Waernbaum I, et al. The risk of venous thromboembolism is markedly elevated in patients with diabetes. Diabetologia. 2005;48(5):1017-21.
24. Konstantinides S, Torbicki A, Agnelli G, et al. 2014 ESC Guidelines on the diagnosis and management of acute pulmonary embolism - web addenda. The Task Force for the Diagnosis and Management of Acute Pulmonary Embolism of the European Society of Cardiology (ESC). Endorsed by the European Respiratory Society (ERS). Eur Heart J. 2014;35:3033-80.
25. Matthews JC, McLaughlin V. Acute right ventricular failure in the setting of acute pulmonary embolism or chronic pulmonary hypertension: a detailed review of the pathophysiology, diagnosis, and management. Curr Cardiol Rev. 2008;4(1):49-59.
26. Harry RB, Davidson BL, Decousus BL, et al. Fondaparinux or enoxaparin for the initial treatment of symptomatic deep venous thrombosis: a randomized trial. Ann Int Med. 2004;140(11): 867-73.
27. Subcutaneous Fondaparinux versus Intravenous Unfractionated Heparin in the Initial Treatment of Pulmonary Embolism. The Matisse Investigators. N Engl J Med. 2003;349:1695-702.
28. Giancarlo A, Harry RB, Alexander C, et al. Apixaban for extended treatment of venous thromboembolism. N Engl J Med. 2013;368: 699-708.
29. Ridker PM, Danielson E, Fonseca FAH, et al. Rosuvastatin to prevent vascular events in men and women with elevated C-reactive protein. N Engl J Med. 2008;359(21):2195-207.

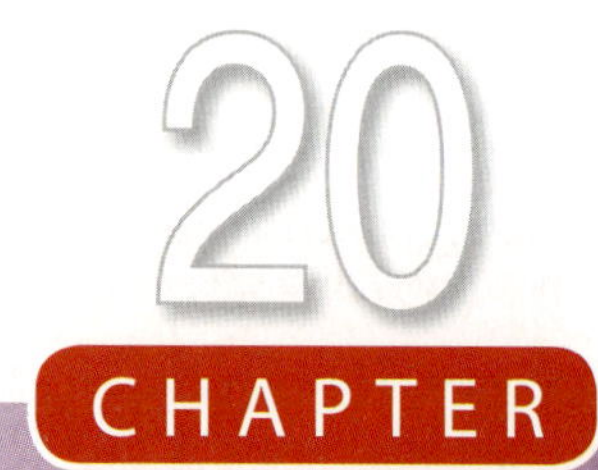

CHAPTER

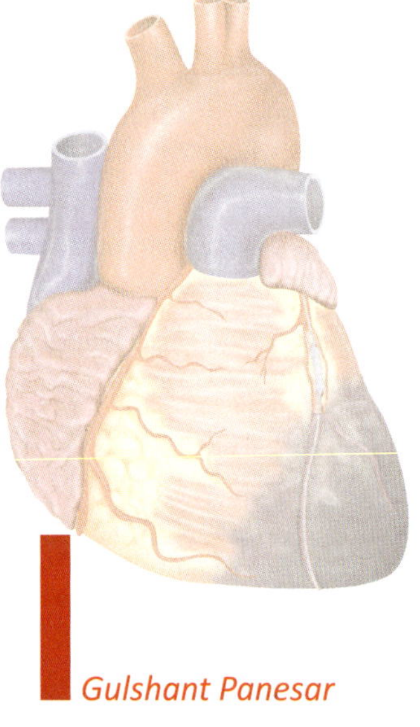

Cardiodiabetes and Cutaneous Manifestations

Gulshant Panesar

INTRODUCTION

Diabetes mellitus (DM) and coronary artery disease (CAD) are the common diseases which can be prevented by modification of lifestyle. In 2015, CAD affected 110 million people and resulted in 8.9 million deaths. It makes up 15.9% of all deaths making it the most common cause of death globally.[1] Globally, an estimated 422 million adults were living with diabetes in 2014, compared to 108 million in 1980. The global prevalence (age-standardized) of diabetes has nearly doubled since 1980, rising from 4.7 to 8.5% in the adult population. This reflects an increase in associated risk factors such as being overweight or obese. Over the past decade, diabetes prevalence has risen faster in low- and middle-income countries than in high-income countries.[2] DM and the prediabetic state are associated with a number of skin manifestations. Cutaneous manifestations are seen in a minimum of 30% of diabetics during the course of their illness, and some may even appear before the diagnosis of DM is confirmed.[3,4] Acanthosis nigricans (AN), skin tags (STs), diabetic dermopathy (DD), rubeosis faciei (RF), pruritus (PR), granuloma annulare (GA), necrobiosis lipoidica (NL), scleredema diabeticorum (SD), bullosis diabeticorum (BD), and xanthelasma/xanthoma are most commonly seen cutaneous manifestations associated with DM.[4]

ACANTHOSIS NIGRICANS

Acanthosis nigricans is a skin disorder characterized by darkening (hyperpigmentation) and thickening (hyperkeratosis) of the skin occurring mainly in the folds of the skin, back of the neck, the axilla and/or groin, knuckles, elbows, and face (Figs 1 and 2). If is now recognized as a cutaneous sign indicating insulin resistance, diabetes, metabolic syndrome, Cushing's syndrome, internal malignancy, polycystic ovarian syndrome, etc.[5] It is linked to increased levels of insulin which stimulates keratinocytes and dermal fibroblasts through insulin-like growth factor (IGF) which incites epidermal cell propagation.[6,7] At high concentrations, insulin may exert potent proliferative effects via high affinity binding to IGF-1 receptors. In addition, free IGF-1 levels may be elevated in obese patients with hyperinsulinemia leading to accelerated cell growth and differentiation. As a consequence, thickened and hyperpigmented velvety skin develops in body folds, mostly the axillae and flexural areas of the posterior neck. The literature supports a higher frequency of AN among the darker-skin colored populations.[7,8,9] Since AN is often seen in cases of hyperinsulinemia, therefore it may also be considered as a cutaneous manifestation of the prediabetic state.[8,10] In an Indian study, the prevalence of AN correlated positively with female gender, obesity, high triglyceride levels, and presence of diabetes. The presence of AN was significantly associated with higher fasting insulin levels.[11]

Weight-loss along with increased physical activity alleviates the condition by reducing the circulating insulin level.[6,17] Screening for AN is a noninvasive procedure, and suggested optimal screening is initiated at the age of five and repeated every second year for individuals with multiple risk factors such as a family history of T2DM, ethnicity and obesity.[13]

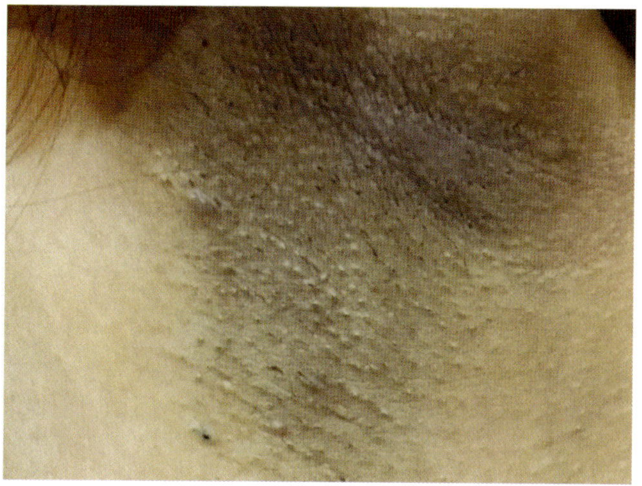

Fig. 1: Acanthosis nigricans, axilla

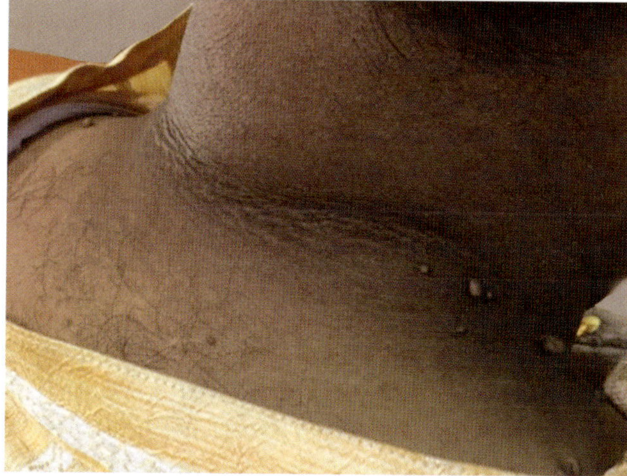

Fig. 2: Skin tags and acanthosis nigricans

SKIN TAGS

Acrochordons or fibroepithelial polyps, ST, and soft fibromas are pedunculated outgrowths of normal skin on a narrow stalk, most commonly located on the eyelids, neck, axilla, and groin (Fig. 2). They are found in ~25% of adults, and their number and prevalence increases with age.[14] Familial history of obesity and AN have been related to acrochordons; the relationship between hyperinsulinemia and skin tags has been well-established.[13] In a study by Erdog an et al.[15] comprising 36 patients with STs and 22 healthy controls, it was found that the mean body mass index (BMI), homeostasis model assessment of insulin resistance, and total cholesterol were significantly higher in patients showing STs than in controls.

A positive correlation has been found between the total number of ST and mean fasting plasma glucose. Patients with more than 30 STs are at an increased risk of developing DM, and females with ST beneath their breasts are particularly prone to developing DM.[16] It is important to stress that hypertension, hyperlipidemia, atherosclerosis, and AN appear at a much higher rate in the ST population.[17-20] Treatment is usually cosmetic or for cases involving irritation, excision may be performed with forceps, fine-grade scissors, cryosurgery with liquid nitrogen, or electrodesiccation or radiofrequency ablation.

DIABETIC DERMOPATHY

Diabetic dermopathy, also named shin spots, is the most common cutaneous manifestation of DM and it is almost considered pathognomonic.[21] It has been reported in up to 55% of patients with DM.[22] It is observed on the pretibial skin as asymmetric, bilateral atrophic and hyperpigmented round-to-oval macules, and is diagnosed clinically (Fig. 3). Studies suggest that DD has a microangiopathic origin,[22] which should alert physicians to investigate for other diabetic complications related to the microvasculature including retinopathy and peripheral neuropathy. Additionally, neuropathy may be an etiologic factor and it has been postulated that patients with peripheral neuropathy are more prone to trauma leading to the development of DD lesions.[23]

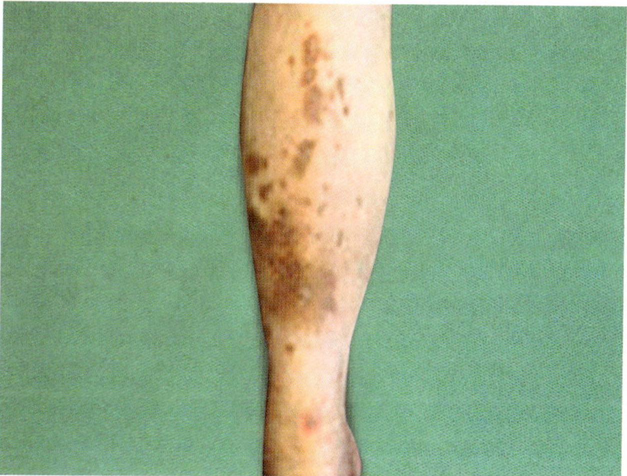

Fig. 3: Diabetic dermopathy

RUBEOSIS FACIEI

In a recent study, the prevalence of RF was found to be 7% in patients with type 1 DM (T1DM).[24] The condition can be exacerbated by hypertension, and the underlying mechanism is suggested to be diabetic microangiopathy which results in dilatation of superficial veins. The degree of RF reflects the incidence of DM, and also the severity of microangiopathy.

PRURITUS

Pruritus presents itself as localized or generalized itching without visible primary skin lesions. Generalized PR has been reported in upto 50% of patients with DM[25] and can be an initial symptom of DM. Many diabetics have involvement of the genital and truncal areas. There seems to be a correlation between postprandial glucose and generalized PR in patients with DM; diabetic smokers are predisposed to developing PR to a higher degree than non-diabetic smokers.[26] Additionally, PR is a marker for polyneuropathy as it appears among patients who lack the Achilles tendon reflex or patients who present with numbness of their soles and palms.[26]

GRANULOMA ANNULARE

Granuloma annulare may be generalized or localized and the generalized distribution seems to be more prevalent in diabetics. The skin lesions of GA are typically symmetrically distributed along the distal region of the extremities and sun exposed skin areas. The papular eruption gradually expands with skin-colored or red borders creating a central involuted crater (Figs 4A and B). It was found to be more prevalent among adult females.[27]

Though several studies have failed to show an association between GA and DM, it has been recommended that all individuals presenting with GA should be screened for DM, and it was also suggested that individuals above the age of 30 years with generalized GA should be screened annually.[28]

NECROBIOSIS LIPOIDICA

The typical lesion is a sharply defined atrophic telangiectatic plaque with a glazed content of yellow-brown color. It is most commonly located pretibially, and in 80% of cases it will have a bilateral distribution. Usually diabetics develop lesions in their fourth decade of life. The prevalence of NL among diabetics is 0.3% and the condition is more frequent among women.[4] Pathogenesis is explained by microangiopathic changes and hypoxia,[4] although an antibody-mediated vasculitis has also been suggested. The lesions exhibit the Koebner phenomenon and are usually painless although some patients may experience itching or pain especially if the skin lesions ulcerate (Fig. 5).

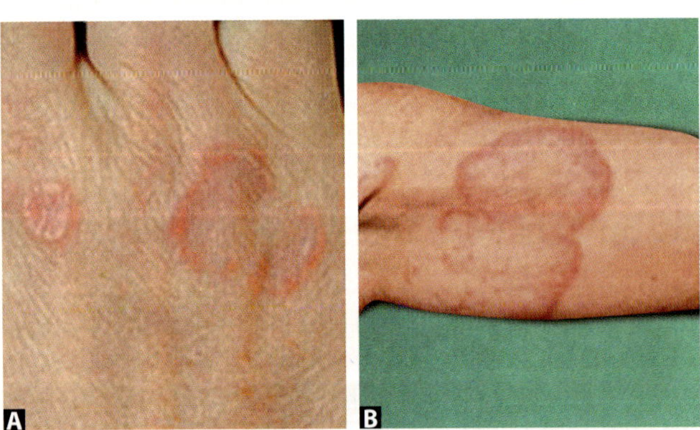

Figs 4A and B: Granuloma annulare

SCLEREDEMA DIABETICORUM

Scleredema diabeticorum manifests by severe permanent thickening of the skin of the posterior neck and upper back. Typically the skin thickening develops over years and presents like peau d'orange resulting in decreased sensation to pain (Fig. 6). It is primarily seen in individuals

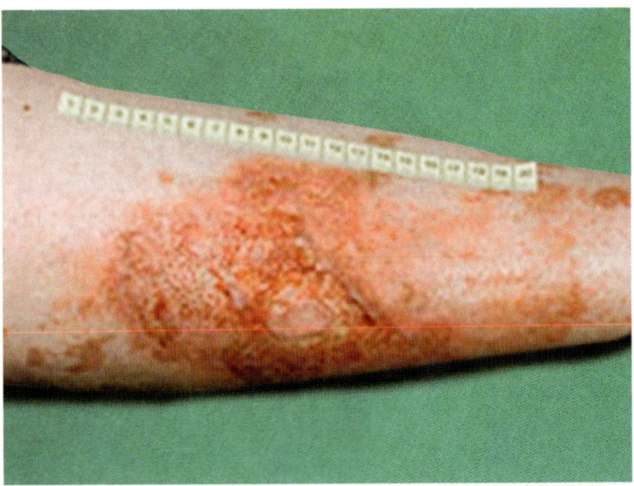

Fig. 5: Necrobiosis lipoidica ulcerative type

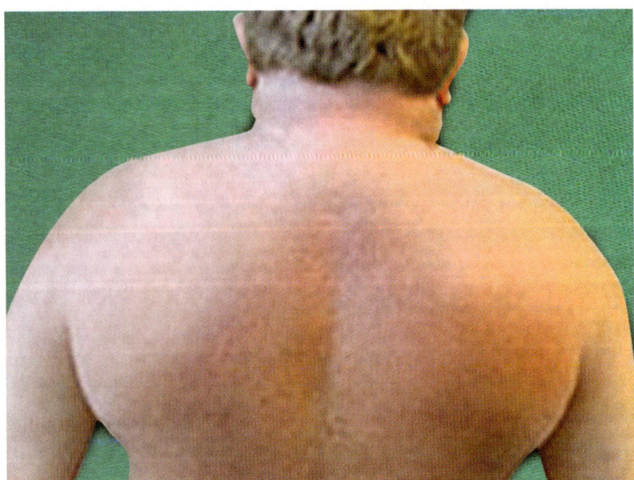

Fig. 6: Scleredema diabeticorum

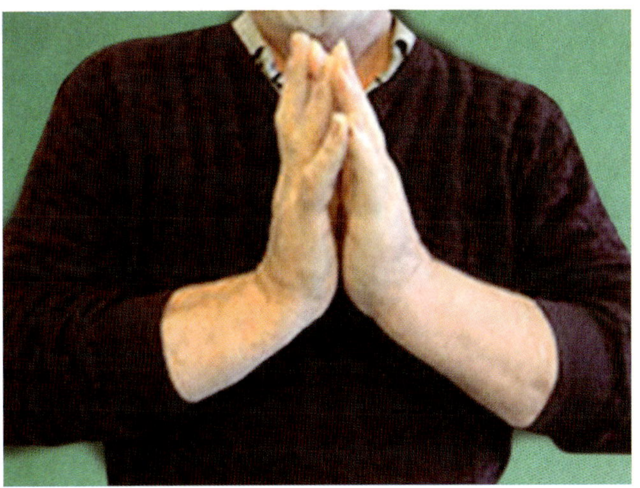

Fig. 7: Prayer sign

with long-standing DM. The prevalence of SD among T2DM patients is approximately 2.5%.[29] On the other hand more than 90% of those with this lesion have DM. A suggested mechanism is the effect of hyperglycemia on collagen in the skin where skin biopsies of diabetics show skin thickening with swollen collagen.[4] Others are particularly affected on their hands and fingers. In these patients, the condition can easily be demonstrated by the 'prayer sign', where patients are asked to oppose the two hands firmly (Fig. 7) and they are unable to do so.[30]

BULLOSIS DIABETICORUM

Bullosis diabeticorum is described as resembling a blister secondary to a burn without the erythematous surrounding. The condition usually appears spontaneously overnight excluding minor trauma as the causative mechanism and the bullae vary in size from 0.5 cm^2 to 10 cm^2 containing sterile fluid (Figs 8A and B).[31] BD is considered a benign lesion with total remission within 5–10 weeks. Most frequently it is observed as a unilateral lesion involving the foot. The prevalence is 0.16% in tertiary care centers and there is a higher prevalence among males with a median age of 65 years.[31] Typically patients have long-standing T1DM. It has also been recognized as a prediabetic manifestation.

XANTHELASMA/XANTHOMA

These are yellow plaques that occur most commonly near the inner canthus of the eyelid, more often on the upper lid than the lower lid. Xanthelasma palpebrarum is the most common cutaneous xanthoma. It can be soft, semisolid or calcareous. Frequently they are symmetrical; often all four lids are involved (Fig. 9). They have a tendency to progress, coalesce and become permanent.[5]

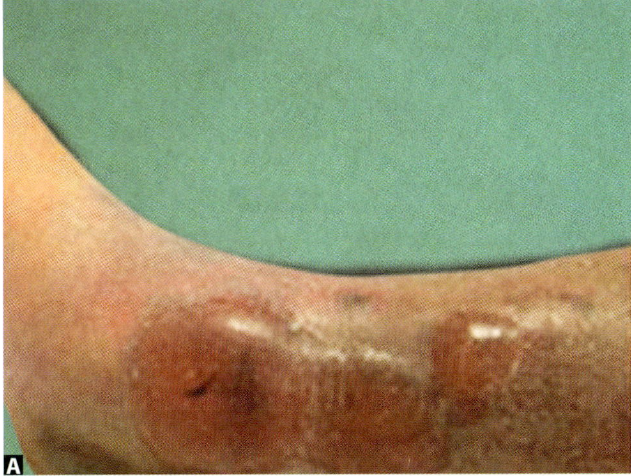

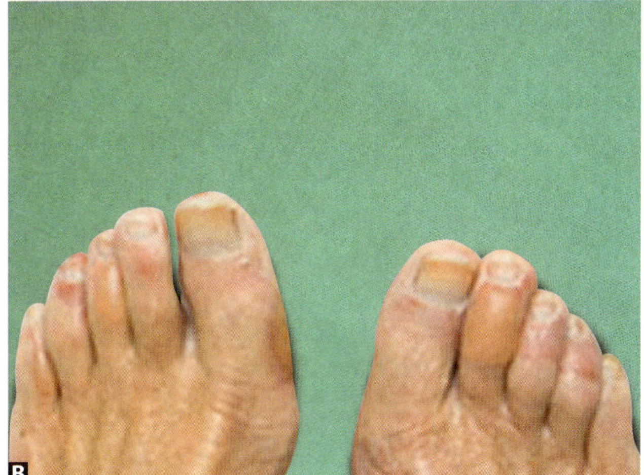

Figs 8A and B: Diabetic bulla

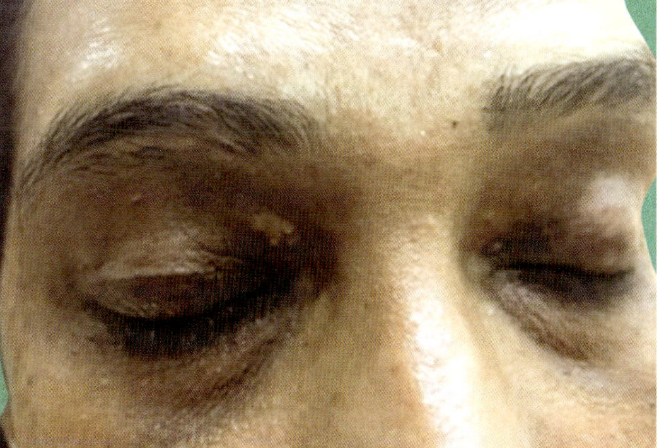

Fig. 9: Xanthelasma palpebrarum

Xanthomas (Fig. 10) usually are associated with a disturbance of lipid metabolism. The mechanism of accumulation of lipids in skin lesions involves the role of modified low-density lipoprotein (LDL) and

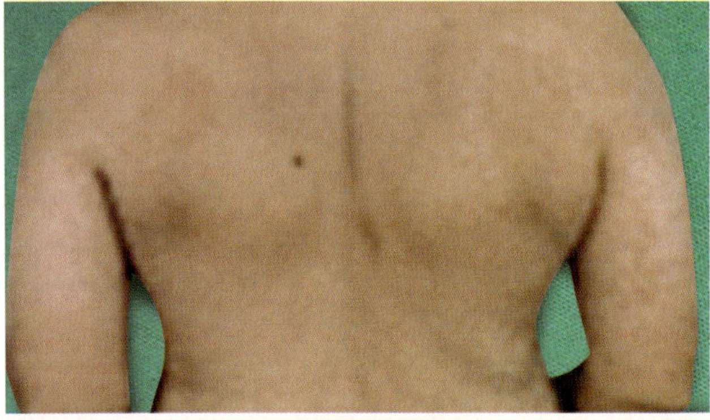

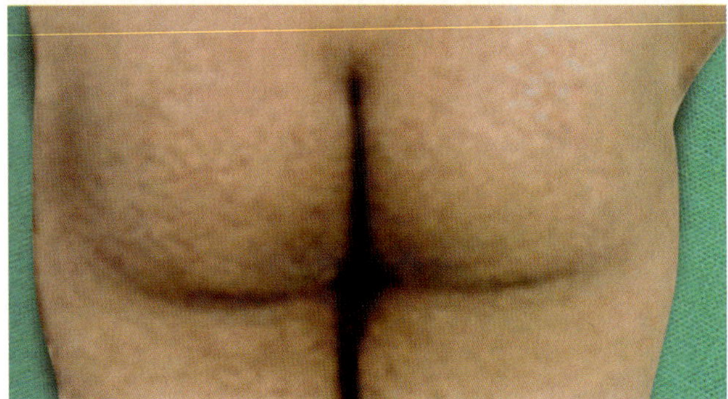

Fig. 10: Xanthomas spread over the back and gluteal region

accumulation of lipids in macrophages. One-half of these lesions are associated with elevated plasma lipid levels. They frequently occur in patients with type II and type IV hyperlipidemia.

Types

Xanthomas are of many types including xanthelasma palpebrarum, tuberous xanthoma, tendinous eruptive xanthomas, plane xanthomas, diffuse plane xanthomatosis, xanthoma disseminatum, and giant gluteal xanthoma. Tuberous and tendinous xanthomas are typical of familial hypercholesterolemia and are common symptoms of homozygous familial hypercholesterolemia.

Therapy

Therapy focuses on adjustment of diet (elimination of dietary fat and concentrated saccharides); in the long run patients have to strictly observe their dietary regime based on the type of hyperlipoproteinemia. As regards drug therapy, fibrates and atorvastatin are the drugs of choice. It is very important not to focus on symptoms, i.e. xanthoma or xanthelasma but to correct the associated dyslipidemia or the disease that underlies hyperlipoproteinemia (e.g. type 2 DM or metabolic syndrome). Xanthelasma palpebrarum can be removed by radiofrequency ablation.

Other markers

Many studies have also associated ear lobe crease, premature balding and greying, and psoriasis with CAD.

CONCLUSION

Recognizing above dermal conditions by thorough physical examination and relevant investigations in cardiodiabetes, the disease burden and complications due to timely management can be significantly reduced.

REFERENCES

1. GBD 2015 Mortality and Causes of Death, Collaborators. Global, regional, and national life expectancy, all-cause mortality, and cause-specific mortality for 249 causes of death, 1980-2015: a systematic analysis for the Global Burden of Disease Study 2015. Lancet. 2016;388(10053):1459-544.
2. World Health Organization. (2016). Global report on diabetes. [online] Available from http://apps.who.int/iris/bitstream/10665/204874/1/WHO_NMH_NVI_16.3_eng.pdf[Accessed August, 2017].
3. Nathan DM. Long-term complications of diabetes mellitus. N Engl J Med. 1993;328(23):1676-85.
4. Bustan RWS, Wasim D, Yderstraede KB, et al. Specific skin signs as a cutaneous marker of diabetes mellitus and the prediabetic state–a systematic review. Dan Med J. 2017;64(1):A5316.
5. Dwivedi S, Jhamb R. Cutaneous markers of Coronary artery disease. World J Cardiol. 2010;2(9):262-9.
6. Brickman WJ, Binns HJ, Jovanovic BD, et al. Acanthosis nigricans: a common finding in overweight youth. Pediatr Dermatol. 2007;24(6):601-6.
7. Grandhe NP, Bhansali A, Dogra S, et al. Acanthosis nigricans: relation with type 2 diabetes mellitus, anthropometric variables, and body mass in Indians. Postgrad Med J. 2005;81:541-4.
8. Kong AS, Williams RL, Rhyne R, et al. Acanthosis nigricans: high prevalence and association with diabetes in a practice-based research network consortium–a primary care multi-ethnic network (PRIME net) study. J Am Board Fam Med. 2010;23(4):476-85.
9. Bahadursingh S, Mungalsingh C, Seemungal T, et al. Acanthosis nigricans in type 2 diabetes: prevalence, correlates and potential as a simple clinical screening tool–a cross-sectional study in the Caribbean. Diabetol Metab Syndr. 2014;96:77.
10. Stoddart ML, Blevins KS, Lee ET, et al. Cherokee diabetes study. Association of acanthosis nigricans with hyperinsulinemia compared with other selected risk factors for type 2 diabetes in Cherokee Indians: The Cherokee Diabetes Study. Diab Care. 2002;25(6):1009-14.
11. Kumar KV, Gilchrist A, Sundaram KR, et al. Acanthosis nigricans and insulin levels in a south Indian population (ADEPS paper 2). Obes Res Clin Pract. 2008;2:43-50.
12. Demir S, Demir Y. Acrochordon and impaired carbohydrate metabolism. Acta Diabet. 2002;39(3):57-9.
13. Kahana M, Grossman E, Feinstein A, et al. Skin tags: a cutaneous marker for diabetes mellitus. Acta Dermato-Venereologica. 1987;67(2):175-7.
14. Banik R, Lubach D. Skin tags: localization and frequencies according to sex and age. Dermatologica. 1987;174(4):180-3.
15. Erdogan BS, Aktan S, Rota S, et al. Skin tags and atherosclerotic risk factors. J Dermatol. 2005;32(5):371-5.
16. Rasi A, Soltani-Arabshahi R, Shahbazi N. Skin tag as a cutaneous marker for impaired carbohydrate metabolism: A case-control study. Int J Dermatol. 2007;46(11):1155-9.

17. Sari R, Akman A, Alpsoy E, et al. The metabolic profile in patients with skin tags. Clin Exp Med. 2010;10(3):193-7.
18. Shah R, Jindal A, Patel N. Acrochordons as a cutaneous sign of metabolic syndrome: a case control study. Ann Med Health Sci Res. 2014;4(2):202-5.
19. Norman A. Dermal manifestations of diabetes. Norman R (Ed). Geriatric Dermatology. New York: Parthenon Publishing; 2001. pp. 143-54.
20. Morgan AJ, Schwartz RA. Diabetic dermopathy: a subtle sign with grave implications. J Am Acad Dermatol. 2008;58(3):447-5.
21. Wigington G, Ngo B, Rendell M. Skin blood flow in diabetic dermopathy. Arch Dermatol. 2004;140:1248-50.
22. Brugler A, Thompson S, Turner S, et al. Skin blood flow abnormalities in diabetic dermopathy. J Am Acad Dermatol. 2011;65(3):559-63.
23. Pavlovic MD, Milenkovic T, Dinic M, et al. The prevalence of cutaneous manifestations in young patients with type 1 diabetes. Diab Care. 2007;30(8):1964-7.
24. Al-Mutairi N, Zaki A, Sharma AK, et al. Cutaneous manifestations of diabetes mellitus. Study from Farwaniya hospital, Kuwait. Med Princ Pract. 2006;15(6):427-30.
25. Yamaoka H, Sasaki H, Yamasaki H, et al. Truncal pruritus of unknown origin may be a symptom of diabetic polyneuropathy. Diab Care. 2009;33(1):150-5.
26. Muhlemann MF, Williams DR. Localized granuloma annulare is associated with insulin-dependent diabetes mellitus. Br J Dermatol. 1984;111(3):325-9.
27. Kidd GS, Graff GE, Davies BF, et al. Glucose tolerance in granuloma annulare. Diab Care. 1985;(4):380-4.
28. Cole GW, Headley J, Skowsky R. Scleredema diabeticorum: a common and distinct cutaneous manifestation of diabetes mellitus. Diab Care. 1983;(2):189-92.
29. Yosipovitsch G, Hodak E, Vardi P, et al. The prevalence of cutaneous manifestations in IDDM patients and their association with diabetes risk factors and microvascular complications. Diab Care. 1998;21:506-9.
30. Sawatkar GU, Kanwar AJ, Dogra S, et al. Spectrum of cutaneous manifestations of type 1 diabetes mellitus in 500 South Asian patients. Br J Dermatol. 2014;171(6):1402-6.
31. Zhang AJ, Garret M, Miller S. Bullosis diabeticorum: case report and review. NZ Med J. 2013;126:91-4.

21

CHAPTER

Benidipine for Hypertension in Chronic Kidney Disease with Cardiodiabetes

DS Rana

INTRODUCTION

Chronic kidney disease (CKD) has always been considered as an important risk factor for cardiovascular disease. Various guidelines propose strict blood pressure (BP) control in hypertensive patients with renal dysfunction.[1] It is believed that mild renal dysfunction and proteinuria may exacerbate hypertension through progression of renal disease, and this exacerbation of hypertension can further impair renal function.[1] Hypertension associated with diabetes will further worsen the problem.

Proteinuria and albuminuria are risk factors for both end-stage renal disease and cardiovascular disease (CVD) in CKD patients. Hence, reductions in proteinuria and albuminuria are associated with a reducing trend in renal death and cardiovascular events. These findings extend the novel concept that high albuminuria/proteinuria alone should be a target for reducing hard endpoints, as in established treatments for high BP, high blood glucose, and high LDL-cholesterol. Thus, albuminuria/proteinuria reduction is one of the most important surrogate goals of hypertension treatment as it reduces both renal death and CVD in diabetic or nondiabetic patients[2] (Abe et al. BMC Nephrology 2013).

It has been suggested that albuminuria not only reflects glomerular damage, but also serves as a sensitive indicator of generalized endothelial dysfunction and capillary vasculopathy that leads to penetration of atherosclerotic lipoproteins into the arterial wall. Studies have shown that albuminuria is associated with endothelial dysfunction in the systemic circulation. As endothelial and vascular damage become advanced, more and more glomeruli are injured, resulting in a substantial amount of albuminuria and reduced glomerular filtration rate (GFR). Therefore, albuminuria, which indicates the presence of advanced glomerular as well as systemic vascular lesions, is a very high risk factor for both renal and cardiovascular events in subjects with CKD and the risk will be higher in diabetic patients.[2]

Proteinuria is further detrimental to the kidney because ultrafiltration of proteins across the glomerular basement membrane brings about mesangial and tubular protein overload, which provokes inflammation and ultimately results in glomerulosclerosis and tubulointerstitial fibrosis.[3] According to the hyperfiltration theory, an increase in glomerular capillary pressure (that is, glomerular hypertension) has an important role in the progression of diabetic and nondiabetic kidney disease. Intraglomerular capillary pressure is dependent on the tone of the glomerular arterioles as well as the level of systemic arterial pressure.[3]

Renin-angiotensin system (RAS) inhibitors and calcium channel antagonists [calcium channel blockers (CCBs)] are useful for controlling BP in hypertensive patients with chronic kidney disease. However, RAS inhibitors should be administered with caution to new patients with incompletely documented medical histories because drugs of this class are contraindicated in patients with bilateral renal artery stenosis or renal dysfunction.[1]

BENEFICIAL EFFECTS OF BENIDIPINE IN HYPERTENSIVE CHRONIC KIDNEY DISEASE PATIENTS WITH OR WITHOUT DIABETES

Reduction of Albuminuria/Proteinuria

Efferent arteriolar dilation followed by attenuation of glomerular hypertension: There are three types of calcium channels: (1) L-type calcium channels, which are distributed widely in smooth muscle cells of peripheral resistance arteries; (2) N-type channels, which are located in the cells of the brain; and (3) T-type channels, which are localized to the sinus node and the brain. In renal tissues, the L-type calcium channels are present only in the afferent arterioles, whereas the N-type and T-type calcium channels are localized in both efferent and afferent arterioles benidipine, another dual L-/T-type CCB, dilates both efferent and afferent arterioles and reduces glomerular pressure. Therefore, benidipine also may exert renoprotective effects.[4]

As per Abe et al., the respective add-on effects of benidipine and amlodipine on albuminuria reduction were demonstrated in 100 CKD patients on top of the angiotensin-receptor blockers (ARBs), telmisartan and olmesartan where 47 patients were diabetic hypertensives with CKD, greater albuminuria reduction was obtained with benidipine combined with ARB. Moreover, benidipine reduced albuminuria while maintaining the eGFR.[2]

This post-hoc analysis showed that compared to amlodipine, an L-type CCB, benidipine, an L- and T-type CCB, results in a greater reduction in albuminuria and improved composite ranking of relative risk according to the 2009 KDIGO CKD severity classification in patients with CKD (Figs 1 and 2). These effects of benidipine seem to make the drug more advantageous in terms of the progression of renal outcome and prevention of cardiovascular events in patients with hypertensive CKD.[2]

When the renal protective activity of amlodipine and benidipine was compared where 32% of the patients were diabetic and 40% were with kidney disease, there was a significant reduction in UAE in amlodipine recipients with less than 20 mm Hg decrease in morning systolic blood pressure (SBP) compared with those with less than 20 mm Hg decrease in morning SBP (-112.4–127.6 vs 1.3–3.8 mg/g creatinine; $p < 0.001$). In contrast, no significant differences in change in UAE were observed between benidipine recipients with less than 20 mm Hg decrease and less than 20 mm Hg decrease in morning SBP (-67.6–74.4 and -112.4–127.6 mg/g creatinine, respectively). With significant reduction in blood pressure in CKD patients, benidipine successfully maintained eGFR for 1 year, whereas eGFR significantly decreased in patients taking amlodipine over the same period (Figs 3A to D).[1]

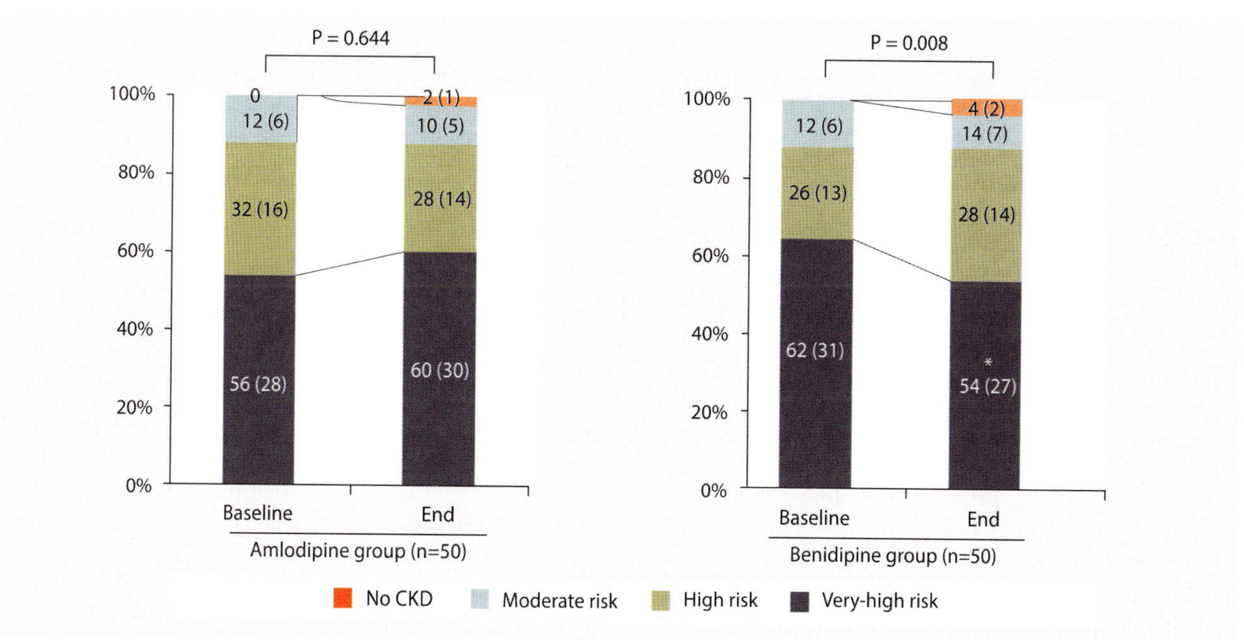

Fig. 1: Changes in CKD severity according to Kidney Disease: Improving Global Outcomes (KDIGO) 2009 categories between baseline and after CCB treatment in the two treatment groups. Numbers in bars indicate % (n)

*$P < 0.05$ versus at baseline.

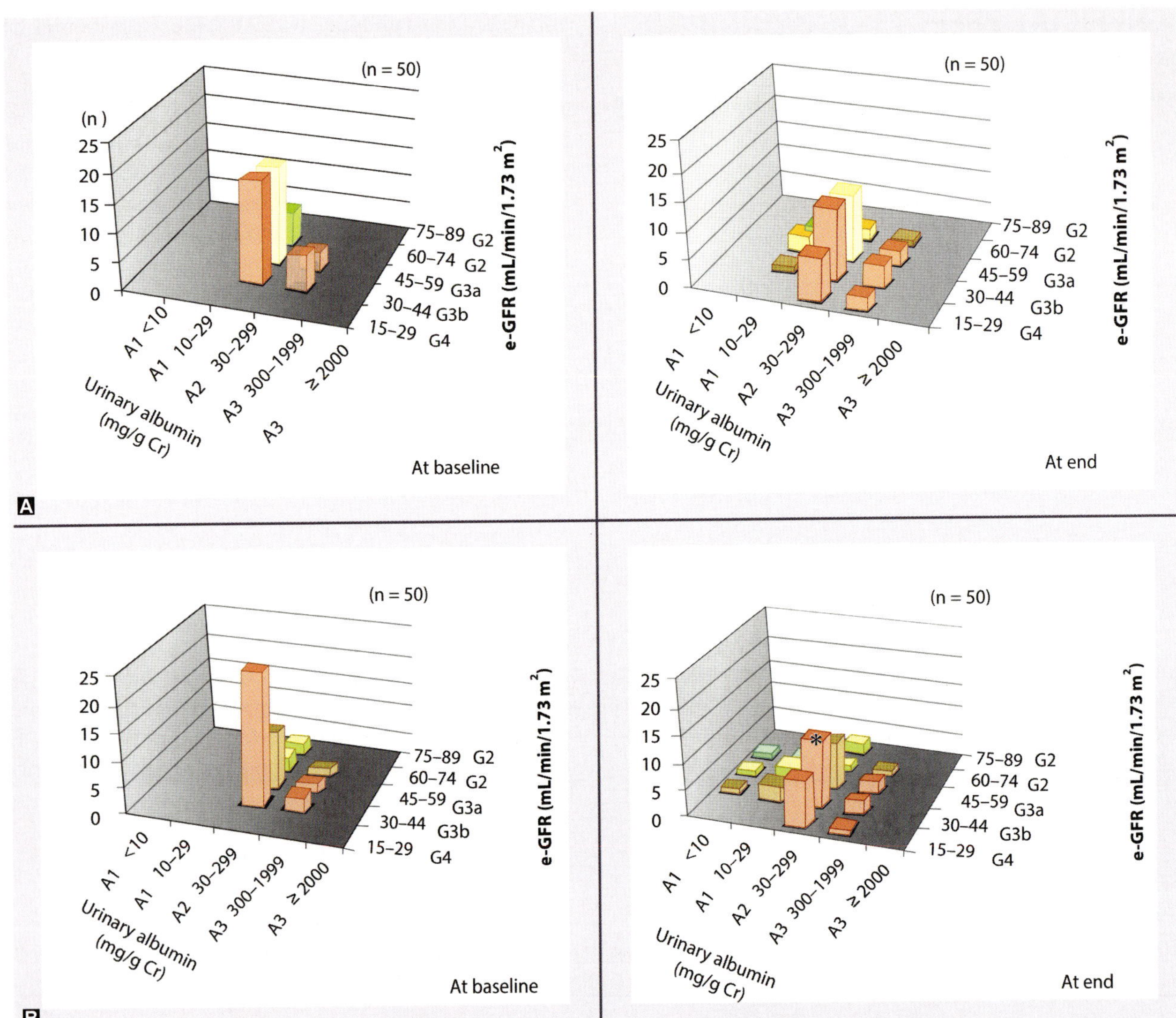

Figs 2A and B: Changes in details of the Kidney Disease: Improving Global Outcomes (KDIGO) 2009 categories at baseline and after CCB treatment. In (A) the amlodipine group and (B) the benidipine group

* P < 0.001 versus at baseline.

Benidipine in hypertensive diabetics with stage 3–5 CKD[4]: As per the data published Hypertension Research (2009), a 6-months' study was conducted to determine the effects of benidipine on BP and renoprotection in Japanese hypertensive patients with moderate-to-advanced stages of CKD (stages 3–5) and who are already being treated with a maximum recommended dose of ARBs where 22 patients were having diabetes. The final doses were 7.6 ± 0.56 mg day_1 of amlodipine and 11.7 ± 0.87 mg day_1 of benidipine in the A and B groups, respectively (Fig. 4).

Study showed that benidipine is more beneficial than amlodipine as an additional medication for hypertensive patients with moderate-to-advanced stage CKD associated with significant proteinuria (urinary protein–Cr ratio 4,300 mg/g Cr), and who are under treatment with the current maximum recommended dose of ARBs.

In another study, it was reported that a higher urinary protein excretion ($P < 0.0001$), lower GFR ($P = 0.0011$) and the presence of diabetes ($P = 0.0284$) correlated with the reduction of urinary proteins when the treatment with amlodipine was replaced with treatment with benidipine (Fig. 5).

The intraglomerular pressure is higher in patients with diabetic nephropathy than in patients with chronic glomerulonephritis or hypertensive nephroscleréosis, and

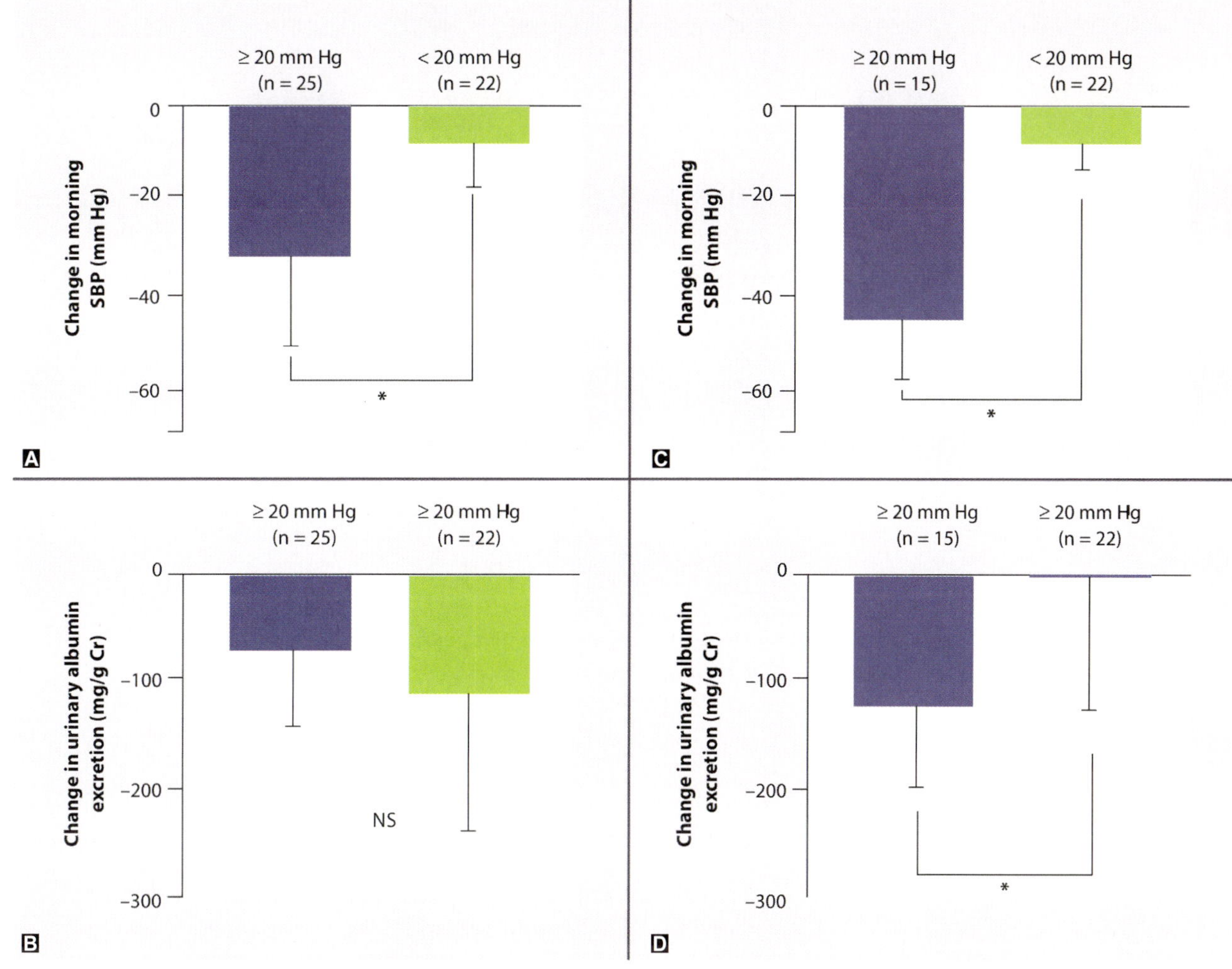

Figs 3A to D: Correlation between change in urinary albumin excretion and reduction in morning systolic blood pressure (SBP) from pretreatment values following (A, B) benidipine or (C, D) amlodipine treatment. Values shown are means – SD

Abbreviations: Cr, creatinine; NS, not significant
* p < 0.001.

the number of patients with diabetic nephropathy in this study was high.[4]

Hence, it was considered that benidipine was more effective than amlodipine in the case of diabetic patients. Hence benidipine proved to be beneficial for hypertensive diabetic patients with stage 3–5 CKD to ameliorate urinary protein excretion in hypertensive patients with moderate-to-advanced-stage CKD who are already being treated with ARBs. Therefore, a combination therapy with benidipine and ARBs even for patients with advanced-stage CKD can be considered. Moreover, the administration of this combination therapy might lead to the delay of the initiation of renal replacement therapy.[4]

Reduction in Albuminuria in Mild-to-Moderate Stage Chronic Kidney Disease with Albuminuria[3]

As per the data published in Hypertension Research (2011) hypertensive patients with mild-to-moderate CKD and diabetes were treated benidipine (52) and amlodipine (52) where 44% patients were diabetes heart rate at the end of the study was significantly reduced in the benidipine group compared with baseline, (benidipine group: from 75.1 ± 1.4 to 73.7 ± 1.3 beats/min. Blood pressure reduction was comparable.

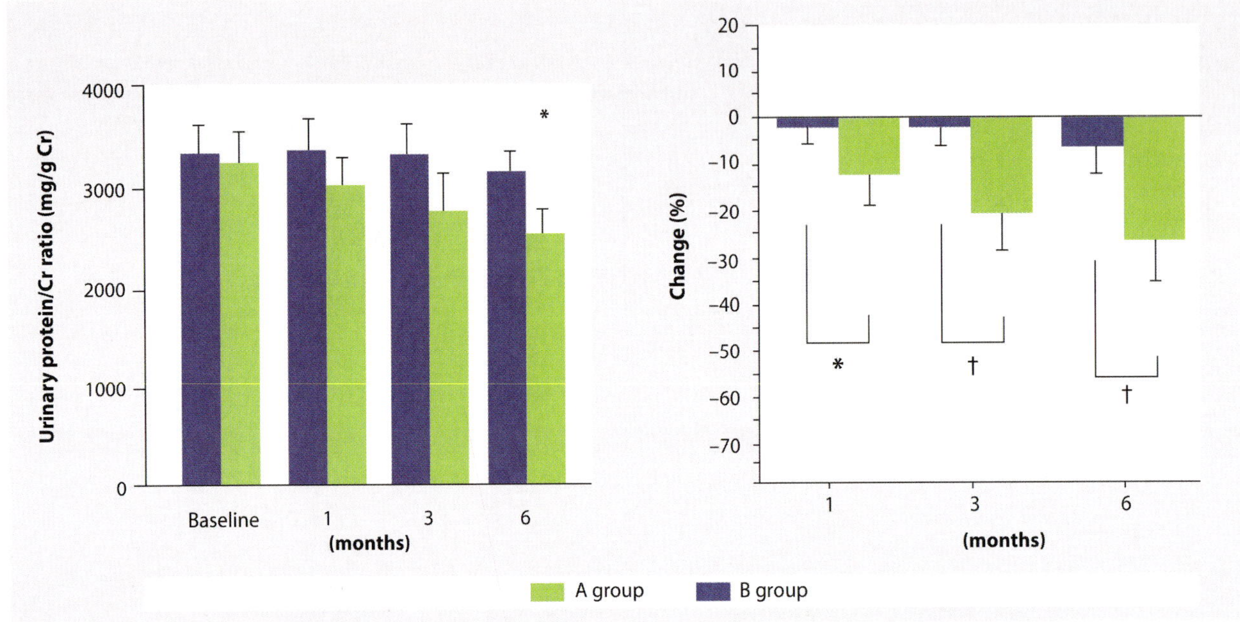

Fig. 4: Changes in the urinary protein–Cr ratio and the respective percent changes from baseline

*P < 0.05, †P < 0.01, A group versus B group.

Abbreviation: Cr, creatinine

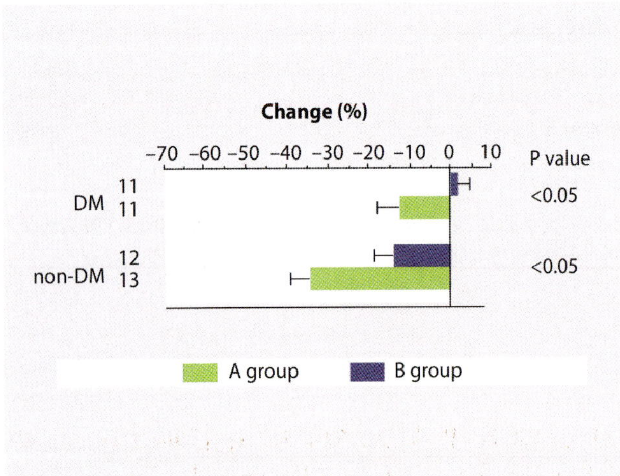

Fig. 5: Percentage changes in the urinary protein–Cr ratio after 6 months of treatment in diabetic and nondiabetic patients with different baseline characteristics

Abbreviations: Cr, creatinine; DM, diabetes mellitus; non-DM, nondiabetes mellitus

Although the urinary albumin/Cr ratio did not change significantly in the amlodipine group throughout the study period, it did decrease significantly in the benidipine group from 3 months of treatment compared with the baseline value. Furthermore, the urinary albumin/Cr ratio in the last month was significantly lower in the benidipine group than in the amlodipine group (benidipine group: 120 ± 14 mg/g Cr; amlodipine group: 163 ± 34 mg/g Cr, P < 0.01). When the percent change from baseline was calculated, there was a significant difference between the two groups from 3 months of treatment (24.8 ± 4.6% vs 0.5 ± 0.1%, P < 0.0001) (Fig. 6).

Effect on plasma renin activity in mild-to-moderate stage chronic kidney disease with albuminuria[3]—plasma aldosterone levels were decreased in the benidipine group, and there was a significant difference between the two groups at the end of study (71.9 ± 5.0 vs 90.4 ± 5.0 pg mL_1, P < 0.05). Urinary K/Cr ratio was significantly decreased and the Na/K ratio was significantly increased in the benidipine group compared with the baseline value. Adverse reactions were not observed in the benidipine group. Therefore, benidipine, an L-/T-type CCB, should offer additive benefits over CCB-inhibiting L-type Ca channels, but not T-type Ca channels.

Effect on aldosterone levels in mild-to-moderate stage chronic kidney disease with albuminuria—Aldosterone can directly damage various organs, including the heart and blood vessels, via mineralocorticoid receptors, independent of changes in BP. It has been suggested that hypertensive incidents and organ damage in humans may occur even at plasma aldosterone levels within the normal physiological range. Therefore, targeting aldosterone

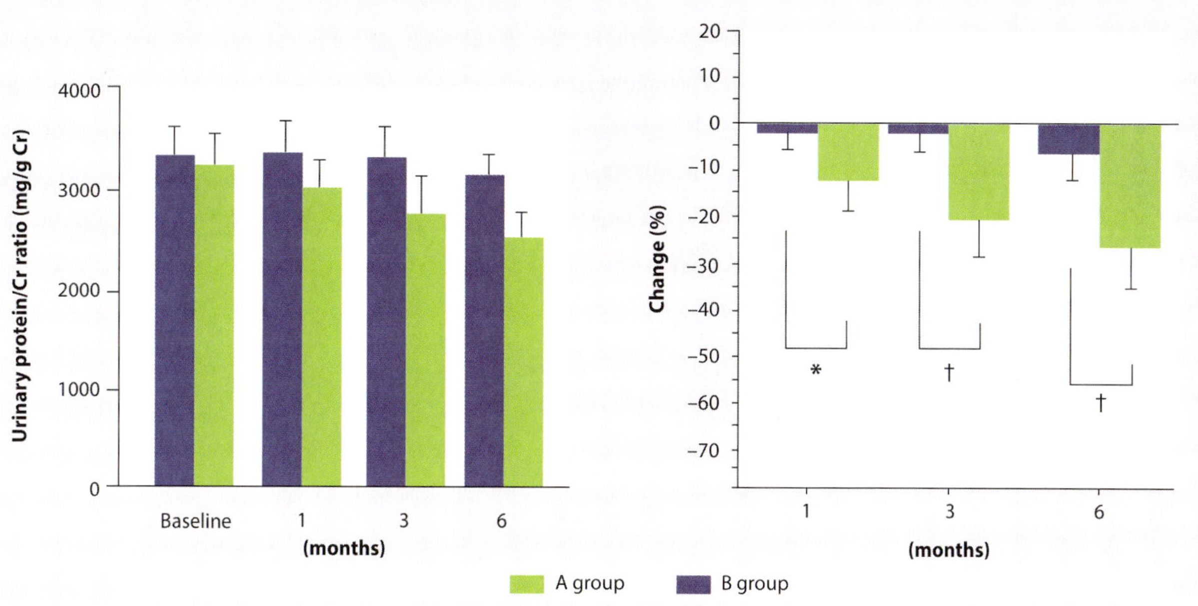

Fig. 6: Changes in the urinary albumin/Cr ratio and the respective percent changes from baseline

Abbreviation: Cr, creatinine

*P < 0.01, †P < 0.0001 versus amlodipine group.

synthesis and release may be clinically important in preventing cardiovascular disease. T-type CCBs have a dual effect on plasma renin activity and renin messenger RNA expression in vivo, with low concentrations stimulating and high concentrations inhibiting the renin system. Benidipine may have a direct inhibitory effect on of aldosterone secretion. As per the study published in *Hypertension Research (2011) serum* Na and K levels were not changed after treatment with either CCB (amlodipine and benidipine), urinary K/Cr and Na/K ratios were decreased in the benidipine group without any decrease in eGFR. These findings suggest that benidipine decreased plasma aldosterone levels without any effect on serum Na and K levels when administered to patients with mild-to-moderate stage CKD (Fig. 7).

Thus, in addition to lowering blood pressure, benidipine would be expected to provide renoprotection in diabetic and nondiabetics by inhibiting aldosterone production. Long-term treatment with ACE inhibitors or ARBs can cause escape or rebound of plasma aldosterone levels. In such a situation; aT-type CCB benidipine might be a suitable addition for the purpose of inhibiting aldosterone production and managing aldosterone escape.

Delay in initiation of RRT[5]: As per the data published in Journal of Pharmacological Sciences 2006, in a prospective randomized comparison between benidipine and nifedipine for 3 years; the time course of blood pressure was similar in both the benidipine treatment group and the nifedipine treatment group. The percentage of patients who reached the primary endpoint (a 1.5-fold rise in the serum creatinine level from the baseline, requiring hemodialysis or kidney transplantation, eventually leading to death) was significantly lower in the benidipine treatment group than in the nifedipine treatment group (Fig. 8).[5]

Improvement in endothelial dysfunction:[5] Since benidipine has vasculo protective effects on both the coronary artery and the glomerulus through improvements in vascular endothelial function, it is expected to reduce both renal events and cardiovascular disease.[1] In a study using cultured endothelial cells, benidipine was shown to suppress endothelial damage induced by lysophosphatidylcholine [one of the lipids constituting oxidized low density lipoprotein (LDL)] more potently than nifedipine and amlodipine. Benidipine suppresses the formation of oxygen radicals. Since oxidized LDL is a factor responsible for the onset and progression of atherosclerosis, this finding suggests that benidipine may suppress the onset of atherosclerosis.[5]

Effect on nitric oxide (NO): Benidipine is reported to stimulate NO production in the kidney and decrease intraglomerular pressure by dilating the efferent.[1] In the model of intimal thickening in the carotid artery of mice, benidipine elevated the endothelial nitric oxide

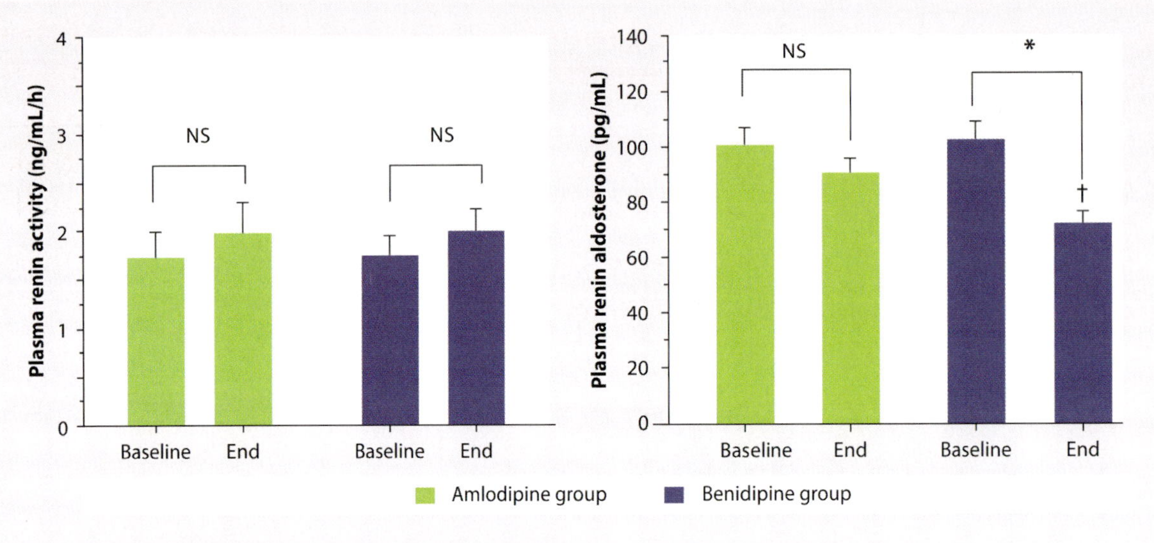

Fig. 7: Changes in plasma renin activity and plasma aldosterone levels in the two groups

Abbreviations: NS, not significant

*P < 0.01 versus baseline; †P < 0.05 versus amlodipine group.

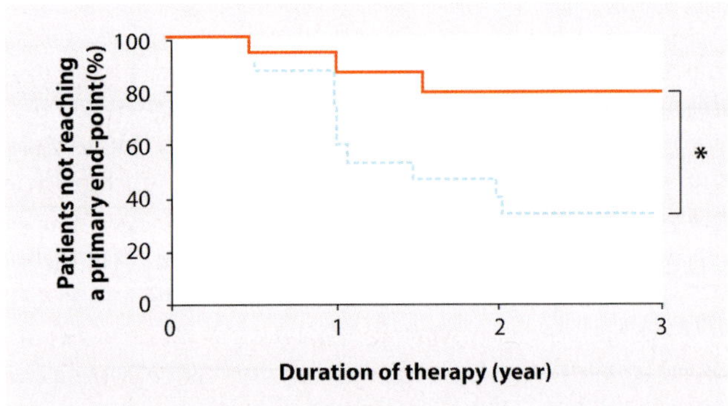

Fig. 8: Renal survival in hypertensive patients with renal impairment administered (—) benidipine or (—) nifedipine retard

*P < 0.05 (log-rank test: P = 0.014, Wilcoxon's test: P = 0.022), n = 15 for each of the benidipine- and nifedipine-treated groups.

synthase (eNOS) levels in vascular endothelial cells, and the increased NO improved vascular remodeling. NO suppresses damage to the endothelial cells induced by oxidized LDL in addition to exerting direct protective effects on the cells that constitute the vascular wall. Therefore, benidipine is expected to suppress the progression of atherosclerosis by stimulating the formation of NO by its direct action on vascular endothelial cells in addition to exerting antioxidative effects.[5]

CONCLUSION

Therefore, because of the antiproteinuric effect, protective effect on endothelium, antioxidant effect benidipine would seem to be more advantageous than an L-type CCB, not only by slowing the progression of renal tissue injuries but also by reducing the incidence of cardiovascular events in hypertensive diabetic patients with CKD.

REFERENCES

1. Ohta M, Sugawara S, Sato N, et al. Effects of benidipine, a long-acting T-type calcium channel blocker,on home blood pressure and renal function in patients with essential hypertension a retrospective, 'real-world' comparison with amlodipine. Clin Drug Investig. 2009;29(11):739-46.
2. Abe M, Okada K, Suzuki H, et al. T/L-type calcium channel blocker reduces the composite ranking of relative risk according to new KDIGO guidelines in patients with chronic kidney disease. BMC Nephrol. 2013;14:135.
3. Abe M, Okada K, Maruyama N, et al. Benidipine reduces albuminuria and plasma aldosterone in mild-to moderate stage chronic kidney disease with albuminuria. Hypertens Res. 2011;34:268-73.
4. Abe M, Okada K, Maruyama T, et al. Comparison of the antiproteinuric effects of the calcium channel blockers benidipine and amlodipine administered in combination with angiotensin receptor blockers to hypertensive patients with stage 3-5 chronic kidney disease. Hypertens Res. 2009;32:270-5.
5. Yao K, Nagashima K, Miki H. Pharmacological, pharmacokinetic, and clinical properties of benidipine hydrochloride, a novel, long-acting calcium channel blocker. J Pharmacol Sci. 2006;100:243-61.

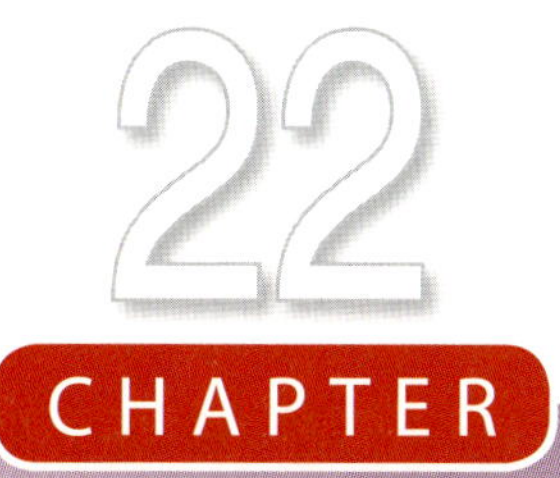

CHAPTER

Cardiorenal Diabetes: Triple Jeopardy

Ramesh Hotchandani, Nikhil Bhat, Neelam Bisht, Abhimanyu Bhatia

INTRODUCTION

Diabetes is best viewed as a vascular disease which causes serious microvascular (retinopathy, nephropathy, neuropathy) or macrovascular problems (stroke, renovascular disease, limb ischemia, and above all heart disease). Hence, hyperglycemia is one aspect of a far reaching metabolic derangement and it can bring about a danger of loss or harsh (jeopardy) to kidneys and heart. Diabetes is the leading cause of kidney disease. About 25% of the patients with diabetes have kidney disease. Renal failure is a global health issue and the incidence of renal failure has increased over the past decades. Between 8% and 10% of the adult population have some form of kidney damage, and every year millions die prematurely of complications related to chronic kidney diseases (CKD). Diabetes is also seen as an independent risk factor for cardiovascular diseases (CVD)[2,5,6] and these patients sustain a worse prognosis for survival than CVD patients without diabetes. A close link exits between diabetes and CVD. Cardiovascular risk factors such as obesity, hypertension, and dyslipidemia are common in patients with diabetes placing them at increased risk for cardiac events. CVD is the cause of death in around 65% of the patients with diabetes. Heart and kidney have close interaction with each other. Maintenance of blood volume, vascular tone, and hemodynamic stability depends on a set of elegant interaction between heart and kidney. If kidney failure and heart failure coexist, morbidity and mortality are negatively affected. CVD is the leading cause of mortality, consisting of 43.6% of all deaths in patients with end stage renal disease. Clinical and epidemiological observations have shown that both kidney failure and heart failure are associated with a high incidence of the failure of the other organ. The single most important intervention in the long-term care of diabetes mellitus (DM) is the control of BP, to protect the heart, the kidney, and the brain. Example of target in DM if no proteinuria: 130/80 mm Hg; if microalbuminuria/proteinuria is present, aim: 125/75 mm Hg.[1]

Cardiorenal syndrome (CRS) is a complication that is closely related to diabetes and is defined as bidirectional pathological impairment of either heart or the kidney due to acute or chronic primary dysfunction in either organ.[2] At a consensus conference of the Acute Dialysis Quality Initiative (ADQI), the CRS was classified into five subtypes primarily based upon the organ that initiated the insult as well as the activity of the disease (Table 1).[3,4]

PATHOGENESIS

In the diabetic state, progressive sclerosis/fibrosis and proteinuria occur in the kidney most likely due to the over reactivity of the transforming growth factor—beta system and to some extent the vascular endothelial growth factor system. The pathogenesis of CVD in diabetes is multifactorial, involving hemodynamic forces, hormonal/metabolic factors, and oxidative stress (Fig. 1). Additionally, it has been suggested that endothelial dysfunction may lead to simultaneous development and progression of renal and cardiac pathology in diabetes.[5]

TABLE 1: Acute Dialysis Quality Initiative classification system of the cardiorenal syndrome

	Inciting event	*Secondary disturbance*
CRS type 1	Acute decompensated heart failure	Acute kidney injury
CRS type 2	Chromic heart failure	Chronic kidney disease
CRS type 3	Acute kidney injury	Acute heart failure
CRS type 4	Chronic kidney disease	Chronic heart failure
CRS type 5	Codevelopment of heart failure and kidney disease	Codevelopment of heart failure and kidney disease

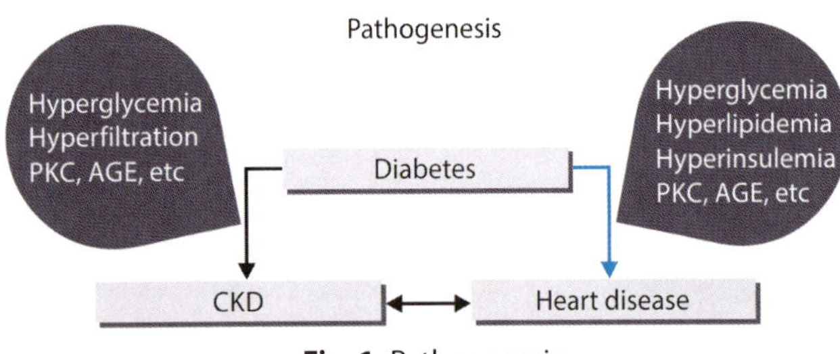

Fig. 1: Pathogenesis

Abbreviation: CKD, chronic kidney disease

Source: Richard J, Feehally J, Floege J. Pathogenesis, clinical manifestations, and natural history of diabetic nephropathy. Comprehensive Clin Nephrol.[7]

Flow chart 1: Pathophysiology of cardiorenal syndrome

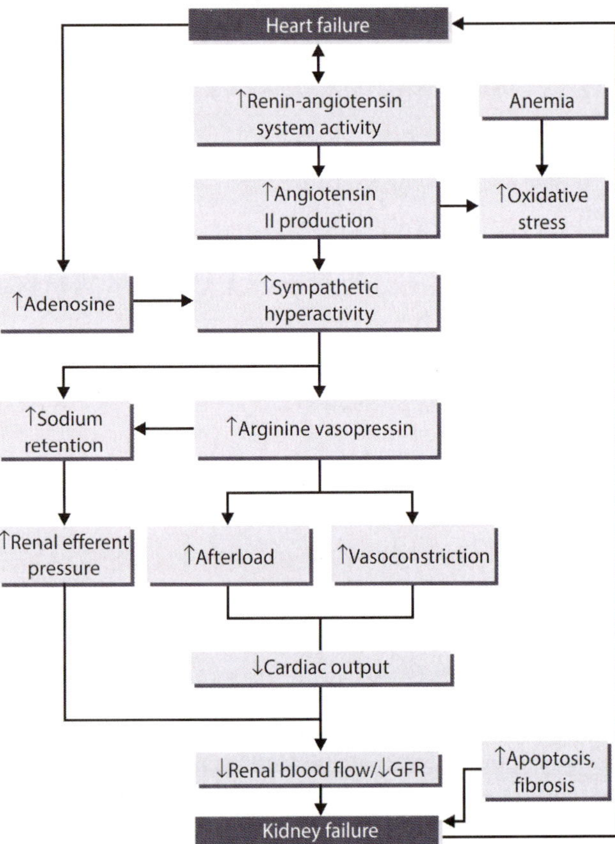

Source: Song MK, Davies NM, Roufogali BD, et al. Management of cardiorenal metabolic syndrome in diabetes mellitus: A phytotherapeutic perspective. J Diabetes Res. 2014(2014). Article ID 313718. http://dx.doi.org/10.1155/2014/313718.

OVERVIEW OF MAJOR ESTABLISHED AND PROPOSED MECHANISMS OF CVD IN PATIENTS WITH DM AND CKD (FIG. 2)

A cross-sectional study found strong association between diabetes and type 2 CRS, researches have found that diabetes and CVD independently have an impact on CKD. According to this study after controlling for CVD—related risk factors in a multi ethnic population, individuals who have CVD and diabetes have a 125% higher likelihood of developing CKD than those who do not have CVD.[2,6,7] Consequently diabetes needs to be addressed and monitored closely in patients with type 2 CRS (Flow chart 1).[8]

RISK FACTORS FOR CARDIOVASCULAR DISEASE IN CHRONIC KIDNEY DISEASE (FIG. 3)

Traditional Risk Factors

- Age
- Male sex
- Hypertension
- Smoking
- Left ventricular hypertrophy
- Diabetes
- Dyslipidemia.

Novel- and Uremic-related Risk Factors

- Oxidative stress
- Inflammation
- Endothelial dysfunction
- Anemia
- Vascular calcification
- Coagulation disorders
- Atherosclerotic plaque
- Sympathetic activation
- Subclinical hypothyroidism
- Uremic bone disease
- Volume overload
- Protein energy wasting
- Insulin resistance
- Uremic toxins

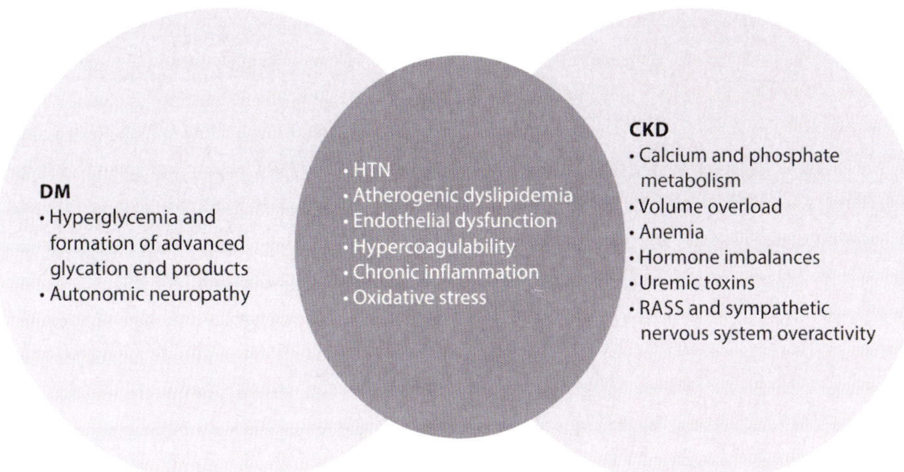

Fig. 2: Review of major established and proposed mechanisms of CVD in patient with DM and CKD

Abbreviations: DM, diabetes mellitus; CVD, cardiovascular diseases; CKD, chronic kidney disease

- Fat mass; adipokinase imbalance
- Genetics/epigenetics.

PREVALENCE

The prevalence of DM in the United States has grown steeply over the past few decades. Diabetes was recently estimates to affect 11.3% of the adult population. Globally, the number of people with diabetes is increasing as well and is expected to exceed 430 million by 2030. Patients with diabetes are more than twice as likely to die from vascular causes as those without diabetics and CVD accounts for approximately 60% of the life years lost from diabetes. It appears to be caused not only by a higher incidence of cardiovascular events, but also by higher CVD outcomes among those with diabetes. Patients with diabetes but no prior history of myocardial infarction (MI) appear as likely to die from coronary artery disease as patients without diabetes who have established coronary artery disease. Accordingly, diabetes have been considered to be a coronary artery disease equivalent by many as a result clinical guidelines have placed strong emphasis on primary and secondary presentation of CVD among patient with diabetes.[9-12]

MANAGEMENT OF TRIPLE THREAT

As from the word itself all the three aspects—heart, kidney, and diabetes have to be taken care simultaneously. Here, the primary aim should be prevention of heart failure, increase cardiac output, increase perfusion to the kidneys, and a tight glycemic control. The pathogenesis of CVD in diabetes is multifactorial, involving hemodynamic force, hormonal/metabolic factors, and oxidative stress. Additionally, it has been suggested that endothelial dysfunction may lead to simultaneous development and progression of renal and cardiac pathology in diabetes. The risk of microvascular complications can be reduced by intensive glycemic control in patients with type I and type II DM whereas benefits to the cardiovascular system is less clear. However, intensified intervention involving other CVD risk factor like hypertension and dyslipidemia and interception of the rennin-angiotensin-aldosterone system in patients with type II diabetes has been shown to be associated with significant reduction in the risk for the renal disease progression that was paralleled by a significant reduction in CVD burden.[13,14]

Nutrition

- Diabetic diet, decreased sodium, decreased potassium, decreased phosphate, and decreased oral fluids.

Strict Glycemic Control

- Monitoring of HbA1c
- Use of oral hypoglycemic agents—metformin, sulfonylureas, and glitazones.

Prevention of Heart Failure

- Restrict fluid and sodium intake
- Diuretics—use loop diuretics furosemides, thiazides, or metolazone can be added.

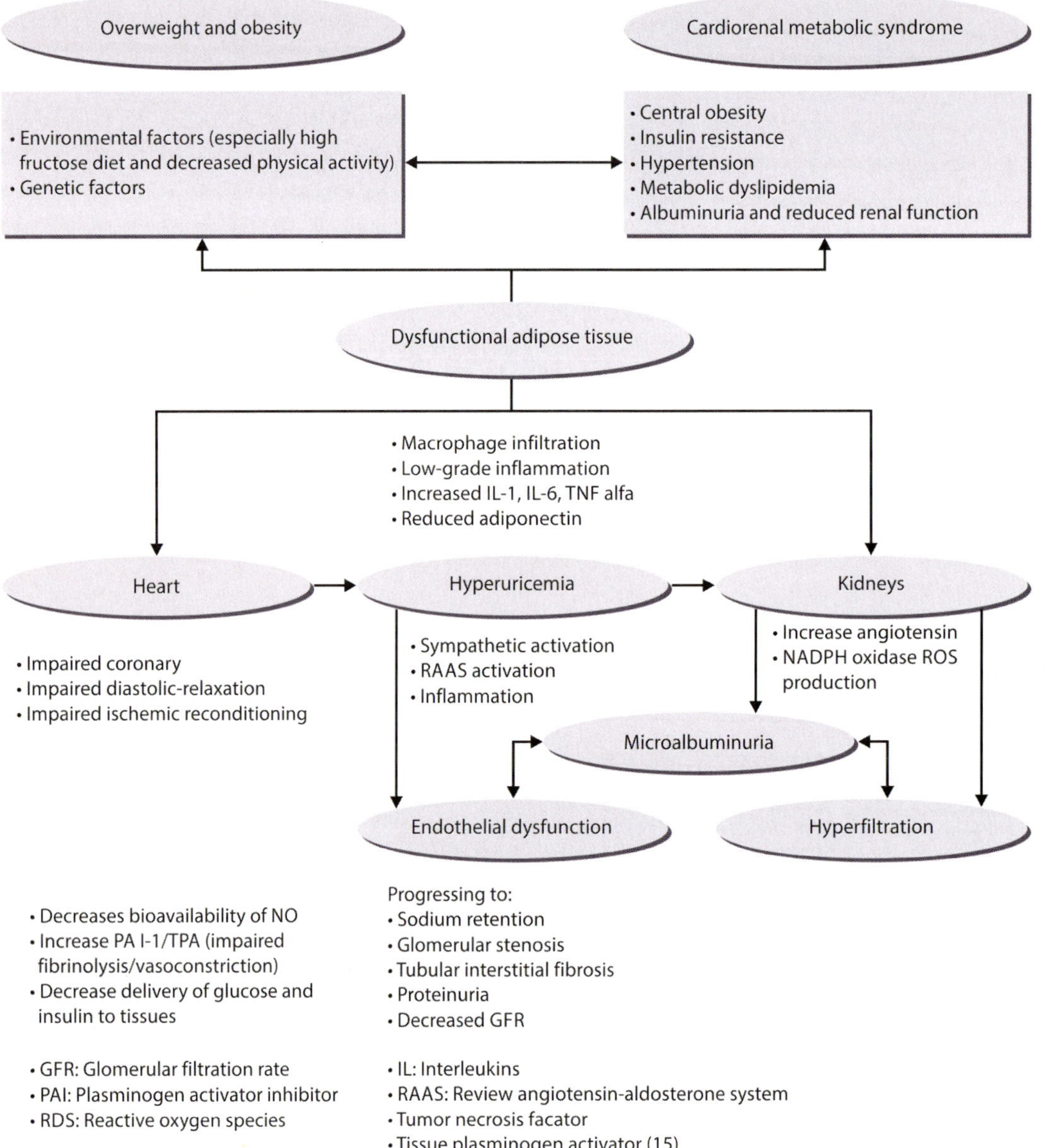

Fig. 3: The interrelationship between adiposity and maladaptive changes in the heart and kidney in cardiorenal syndrome

Antiarrhythmic Drugs

- Low-dose dopamine/dobutamine in order to increase cardiac contractility
- Insert intraaortic balloon pump in cardiogenic shock
- Management of hypertension— angiotensin-converting enzyme (ACE) inhibitors, angiotensin receptor blockers (ARBs), and diuretics.

Prevention of Arrhythmias

- Amiodarone, dilzem, beta blockers, and lidocaine.

Renal Prevention

- Monitoring of kidney functions
- Monitoring of urine output—adequate.

To Avoid Nephrotoxic Drugs

- Drugs to be given as per renal clearance
- Fluid and electrolyte balance
- Preparation for renal replacement therapy—hemodialysis, home, or in-hospital dialysis, ultrafiltrate as per volume status

- Renal transplant
- Calcium, phosphorous, vit D, hyperparathyroidism, serum sodium, serum potassium, regular check, and maintenance of electrolyte balance.

Coronary Artery Disease Prevention/ Management

- Use of antiplatelet drugs, statins
- Lipid management.

Anemia—Correction of Anemia—Chronic Kidney Diseases

- Patients have low hemoglobin levels due to lack of erythropoietin. Low hemoglobin levels decrease cardiac perfusion, thus increasing its demand.

Preventive Cardiology

- Balanced diet
- Sedentary lifestyle to be avoided
- Maintaining BMI ratio
- Tobacco cessation.

REFERENCES

1. Wilkinson IB, Raine T, Wiles K, et al. Oxford Handbook of Clinical Medicine, 10th edition. England, UK: OUP Oxford; 2017.
2. Banerjee S, Panas R. Diabetes and cardiorenal syndrome: Understanding the triple threat. Hellenic J Cardiol. 2017. [Epub ahead of print]
3. Renco C, Mc Collough P, Anker SD, et al. Cardiorenal symdromes report from the conference of the acute dialysis journal, quality initiative. Eur Heart J. 2010;31(6):7013-711.
4. Vishwanathan G, Gilbert S. The cardiorenal syndrome: Making the connection. Int J Nephrol. 2011;2011:1-10.
5. Karnib HH, Zujadeh FN. The cardiorenal syndrome in diabetes mellitus. Diabetes Re Clin Pract. 2010;89(3):201-8.
6. Schiffrin EL, Lipman ML, Mann JFE. Chronic kidney disease. Circulation. 2007;116(1):87-97.
7. Wolf G, Sharma K. Chapter 30: Pathogenesis, clinical manifestations and natural history of diabetes nephropathy. In: Johnson RJ, Feehally J, Florge J (Eds). Comprehensive Clinical Nephrology. Philadelphia, PA: Elsevier Saunders; 2010. pp. 354-71.
8. Andrassy KM. Comments on 'K1DGO 2012 Clinical Practice Guideline for the Evaluation and Management of Chronic Kidney Disease'. Kidney Int. 2013;84(3):622-3.
9. Centers for Disease Control and Prevention. (2011). National diabetes fact sheet: national estimates and general information on diabetes and prediabetes in the United States, 2011. Centers for Disease Control and Prevention. Atlanta, GA: U.S. Department of Health and Human Services. [online] Available from http://www.cdc.gov/diabetes/pubs/pdf/ndfs [Accessed Oct. 2017]
10. Kannel WB, McGee DL. Diabetes and cardiovascular disease. The Framingham Study. JAMA. 1979;241(19):2035-8.
11. Huxley R, Barzi F, Woodward M. Excess risk of fatal coronary artery disease associated with diabetes in men n women. Metaanalysis of 37 prospective cohort studies. BMJ. 2006;332(7533):13-8.
12. Fox CS, Motsushta K, Woodward M, et al. Associations of kidney disease measures with mortality and end stage renal disease in individuals with and without diabetes: a meta analysis level. 2012;380(9854):1662-73.
13. Karnib HH, Zujadesh FN. The cardiorenal syndrome in diabetes. Diabetes Res Clin Pract. 2010;89(3)201-8.
14. The Journal of Pediatr 2009;155:049. copyright@2011 karger publisher.basels:t2erlar

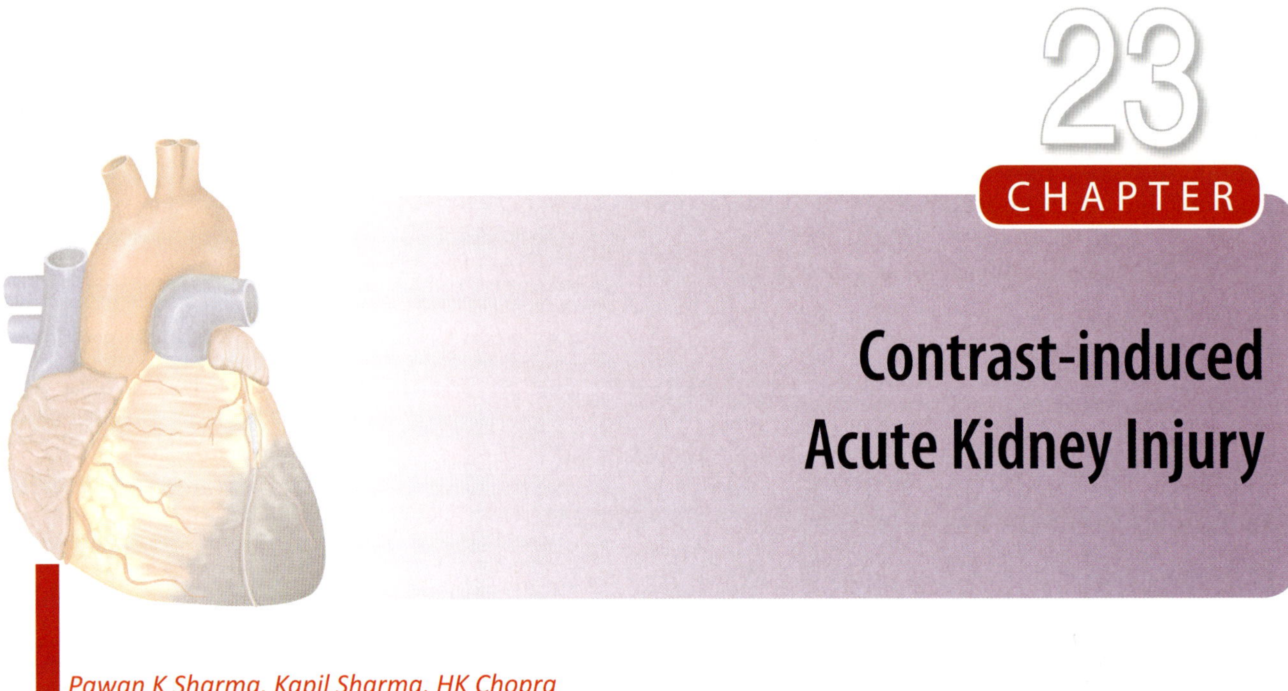

Contrast-induced Acute Kidney Injury

Pawan K Sharma, Kapil Sharma, HK Chopra

INTRODUCTION

Contrast-induced acute kidney injury (CI-AKI) is the new onset or exacerbation of renal dysfunction after contrast administration in the absence of other causes. It is defined as an increase in serum creatinine (sCr) concentration of greater than 0.5 mg/dL (44.2 μmol/L) or 25% above baseline within 48 hours of contrast administration. The contrast-induced nephropathy consensus panel recommends using relative increase in sCr to define CI-AKI, independent of baseline renal function.[1] The CI-AKI typically develops 24–48 hours postcontrast exposure, with creatinine peaking at 5–7 days. The Kidney Disease International Global Outcomes Guidelines suggested definition of CI-AKI as a rise in sCr greater than or equal to 0.3 mg/dL or a greater than or equal to 50% elevation from baseline. The overall incidence of CI-AKI in general population is less than 2%. However, in high risk patients such as those with chronic renal insufficiency, diabetes mellitus, congestive heart failure, anemia, and older age, CI-AKI occurs up to 50%.[2,3] Preexisting renal disease is the most important risk factor for developing CI-AKI. Other risk factors for CI-AKI include diminished left ventricular function, dehydration, hypotension, and the use of intra-aortic balloon pump (Box 1). The use of agents such as antibiotics, furosemide, and nonsteroidal anti-inflammatory drugs (NSAIDs) is also a prognostic factor for CI-AKI.[2,3]

BOX 1: Risk factors for developing contrast-induced acute kidney injury (CI-AKI)

- Renal insufficiency
- ST-elevation myocardial infarction (STEMI)
- Cardiogenic shock
- Older age
- Anemia
- Contrast volume
- Need for intra-aortic balloon pump (IABP)
- Diabetes mellitus
- Advanced congestive heart failure
- Diminished left ventricular (LV) systolic function
- Dehydration
- Hypotension
- Drugs such as certain antibiotics, diuretics (furosemide), nonsteroidal anti-inflammatory drugs (NSAIDs)

EPIDEMIOLOGY

Despite the increase in number of patients undergoing cardiac catheterization procedures, the incidence of CI-AKI, and AKI overall, has declined over the past decade. However, among those undergoing cardiac surgery after coronary angiography, AKI, and AKI requiring dialysis (AKI-D) may be increasing. A study involving 31,532 patients[4] with acute myocardial infarction (AMI) showed that the rate of AKI declined from 26.6% in 2000 to 19.7% in 2008. This reduction of 26% was based on a definition per the Kidney Disease International Global Outcomes Guidelines of a rise in sCr greater than or equal to 0.3 mg/dL or a greater than or equal to 50% elevation from baseline over the course of hospitalization. The National Cardiovascular Data Registry Cath-percutaneous coronary intervention (PCI) considers CI-AKI as sCr rise greater than or equal to 0.3 mg/dL. In a report involving 985,737 patients who underwent elective and urgent PCI, there were 69,658 (7.1%) cases of CI-AKI and 3,005 (0.3%) cases of AKI-D.[5] The normal estimated glomerular filtration rate (eGFR) is greater than 60 mL/min/1.73 m^2. As chronic kidney disease (CKD) progresses and eGFR worsens, there is a sharp increase in the rates of both CI-AKI and AKI-D (Table 1). The most important factors associated with a more than doubling in the rates of CI-AKI and significant increases in the risk of AKI-D were STEMI, eGFR less than 30 mL/min/1.73 m^2, and cardiogenic shock. Mean contrast volumes among those with CI-AKI was 140–260 mL which is similar to those without CI-AKI (140–245 mL). Thus, although rates of CI-AKI may have trended down over the past decade, the risk is still significant in the patients with the greatest need for urgent PCI, including those with STEMI and those developing cardiogenic shock. The overall age in this report from the Cath-PCI registry is 64.8 ± 12.2 years and is not reflective of the growing numbers of the elderly patients undergoing PCI currently. A comprehensive risk prediction score, which includes age, hemoglobin, preexisting CKD, contrast volume, need for intra-aortic balloon counter pulsations, and other variables, has been developed which could help predict the risk of developing CI-AKI, and the need for renal replacement therapy.[6] But this score is not helpful before the procedure because it incorporates variables that can only be known after the case is completed in the catheterization laboratory. For preprocedural counseling, the most useful parameters are the eGFR and presence of diabetes. In general, eGFR less than 60 mL/min/1.73 m^2 with diabetes increases the risk of CI-AKI sufficiently above the baseline of ~5% to ~10%. Thus, appropriate counseling and preventive measures are important to minimize this potential adverse consequence of angiography.

TABLE 1: Incidence of contrast-induced acute kidney injury (CI-AKI) and new end-stage renal disease (ESRD) requiring dialysis according to baseline glomerular filtration rate (GFR) from the American College of Cardiology (ACC) Cath-percutaneous coronary intervention (PCI) Registry[5]

GFR	Severity	CI-AKI	AKI-D
>60	Normal	5.2%	0.07%
45–60	Mild	8.0%	0.3%
30–45	Moderate	12.9%	0.7%
<30	Severe	26.6%	4.3%

TYPES OF IODINATED CONTRAST MEDIA

Contrast media (CM) have four categories based on whether they are ionic or nonionic and monomeric or dimeric (Table 2).[7] All forms of iodinated contrast are highly water-soluble carbon-based benzene rings that exist as monomers with three iodine atoms attached or as dimers with six iodine atoms attached. The iodine concentration varies between 270 mg/dL and 400 mg/dL, which is sufficient to provide adequate radiographic opacification.[8] The first generation agents (diatrizoate meglumine, and iothalamate) were hyperosmolar ionic monomers with osmolality 5–6 times that of plasma. These high-osmolar contrast media (HOCM) have osmolality 1,200 mOsm/kg or higher and are no longer used for cardiac catheterization. The next generation of contrast agents were nonionic monomers, referred to as low-osmolality contrast media (LOCM). They had lower osmolality than the first generation HOCM agents but still hyperosmolar relative to plasma. These agents include iohexol (Omnipaque), iomeprol (Iomeron), iopamidol (Isovue), ioversol (Optiray), and iopromide (Ultravist), ioxilan (Oxilan). One LOCM, ionic dimer, ioxaglate (Hexabrix) was also developed. The iso-osmolar contrast medium (IOCM) is nonionic, dimer

TABLE 2: Iodinated contrast media (CM)

Generic name (CM)	Trade name (CM)	Ionicity	Chemical structure	Class	Osmolality (mOsm/kg)
Diatrizoate	Renografin	Ionic	Monomer	HOCM	1,500–1,860
Iothalamate	Conray				
Ioxitalamate	Telebrix				
Ioxaglate	Hexabrix	Ionic	Dimer	LOCM	600
Iohexol	Omnipaque	Nonionic	Monomer	LOCM	521–695
Iomeprol	Lomeron				
Iopamidol	Isovue				
Ioversol	Optiray				
Iopromide	Ultravist				
Ioxilan	Oxilan				
Iodixanol	Visipaque	Nonionic	Dimer	IOCM	290–320

iodixanol (Visipaque). The most common types of contrast agents used today for intravascular injection are either iso-osmolar (approximately 290 mOsm/kg) iodixanol, or low-osmolar (700–850 mOsm/kg) nonionic monomers (iohexol, iomeprol, iopamidol, iopromide, ioversol, and ioxilan).[9] In general, nonionic CM are better tolerated than ionic CM.[10] There is no difference between nonionic and ionic when comparing LOCM with IOCM in the incidence of emergent bypass surgery, MI, and cardiac death.[8]

PATHOPHYSIOLOGY/MECHANISM OF CONTRAST-INDUCED ACUTE KIDNEY INJURY

Although, the iodine concentration of various CM is similar, however, when administered in the blood at 37°C, the iodixanol has viscosity of 11.8 centipoise (cps) which is significantly higher than that of iohexol, at 6.3 cps, the lowest in the low-osmolar category. The higher the osmolality or the particle concentration in solution, the greater the vascular symptoms of warmth and pain during injection, as well as CI-AKI.[11] Possible mechanism for development of CI-AKI is described as follows. When iodinated contrast is injected into the systemic arterial system, it causes transient endothelium-dependent vasodilation mediated by release of nitric oxide. This is followed by arteriolar vasoconstriction lasting for several seconds to minutes in the peripheral circulation.[12] In the afferent glomerular arteriole, efferent arteriole, peritubular network, and the vasa recta, this transient dilation can be followed by a period of sustained vasoconstriction that lasts for several hours.[12] Patients with CKD and diabetes may have reduced renal parenchymal mass and fewer nephrons leading to reduction in renal blood flow. This reduced renal blood flow can be sufficiently sustained to impair oxygenation to the outer medulla, resulting in ischemia to the proximal and distal tubules. Iodinated contrast does not injure the glomerulus, therefore, no hematuria is seen. Contrast is water soluble and freely filtered, which allows its easy reabsorption by the proximal tubular cells.[13] Tubular cells undergo swelling and apoptosis. As a result, there is stasis of contrast within the kidneys where it causes cellular damage.[13] Due to stasis of high concentrations of contrast within and surrounding renal tubular cells, there is direct cellular toxicity with loss of the tubular brush border, breakdown of desmosomes, loss of cell membrane integrity, and sloughing of material into the urinary tubular space (Tamm–Horsfall protein). The combination of both ischemic and chemotoxic injury to the proximal tubules triggers a process called tubuloglomerular feedback, which signals the glomerulus to reduce filtration, and hence the rise in the plasma concentration of creatinine (Cr) is seen approximately 24–48 hour after there has been a significant reduction in filtration.[14] Within few hours of tubular injury, some new urine markers can be elevated which represent tubular damage (neutrophil gelatinase-associated lipocalin, fatty-acid binding protein) and cell-cycle arrest (insulin-like growth factor binding protein-7, tissue inhibitor of metalloproteinase-2).[15] These markers may prove to be useful for the detection of subclinical CI-AKI, and early detection of more severe cases. This information in turn could be beneficial for development of future treatments before there is complete cessation of renal function (Box 2).

BOX 2: Markers of contrast-induced acute kidney injury (CI-AKI)

- Urine markers of tubular damage
  - Neutrophil gelatinase-associated lipocalin (NGAL)
  - Fatty acid binding protein
- Cell cycle arrest markers
  - Insulin-like growth factor binding protein-7 (IGFBP-7)
  - Tissue inhibitor of metalloproteinase-2 (TIMP-2)

There is also evidence to suggest that as renal tubular cells are damaged, the mitochondria release intracellular catalytic or unbound iron, which serves as the catalyst to drive oxidative stress and the production of the dangerous hydroxyl radical.[16] A similar process is accentuated by exposure of iron-rich myoglobin in the setting of rhabdomyolysis, as well as heme in the setting of cardiac surgery.[17] Of interest, the three ways of reducing these oxidative stress reactions are: (1) reduce temperature (as is done during cardiac surgery); (2) alkalinize the environment; or (3) remove the substrate and or catalyst.[16] Additionally, alkalinization reduces the precipitation of Tamm–Horsfall protein in the tubular lumen.[18] Subclinical CI-AKI may occur in every patient exposed to iodinated contrast. Since healthy subjects have tubular repair capability, this process may not have any clinical consequences.[19] However, in patients with CKD and diabetes mellitus, who have a reduced number of functioning nephrons and an impaired ability to regenerate tubular epithelial cells, routine cardiac procedures using average doses of iodinated contrast can cause CI-AKI that is clinically important. The natural history of acute tubular injury follows a time course of approximately 8–10 days, with recovery and regeneration of tubular cells from within the tubule structure. However, with each exposure of contrast, there may be significant destruction of some nephrons that recovery is not possible, and ultimately, there is fibrosis and loss of the functional unit. Thus, in those with few functioning nephron units and advanced CKD (eGFR <30 mL/min/1.73 m^2), CI-AKI can result in reduction of renal filtration leading to azotemia, volume overload, and hyperkalemia warranting renal replacement therapy. In approximately one-half of these cases, there is permanent end-stage renal disease (ESRD), whereas in the other one-half, there can be eventual recovery that allows some period of dialysis-free survival.

Intra-arterial versus Intravenous Contrast Administration

With catheter administration of intra-arterial contrast, there could be microshowers of atheroembolic material to the renal and systemic circulation. The renal atheroemboli may also lead to CI-AKI after transcatheter aortic valve replacement (TAVR). The proportion of cases that result in severe acute kidney injury appears to be higher in TAVR than reported with PCI. However, a pooled analysis has suggested that TAVR is associated with a lower risk of AKI compared with surgical valve replacement.[20] Additionally, acute coronary syndrome (ACS) and, in particular, STEMI patients have been observed to have nearly double the rates of CI-AKI. This may be due to neurohormonal activation, release of catalytic iron from the heart, inadequate opportunity for volume expansion, and greater rates of hemodynamic instability. In studies of patients with similar levels of renal function and contrast doses given in the venous system, there are consistently lower rates of CI-AKI, largely because there is no opportunity for atheroembolism and possibly because of a greater admixture of contrast in the blood pool before the kidneys are exposed.

PROGNOSIS

Contrast-induced acute kidney injury is associated with higher rates of complication after PCI. The CI-AKI may lead to volume overload and hyperkalemia requiring urgent dialysis, development of ESRD, and death. In the report from the Cath-PCI registry, the rates of recurrent MI, major bleeding and death in those not on dialysis, and with no evidence of CI-AKI after contrast administration were 2.1% MI, 1.4% bleeding, and 0.5% death. These outcomes were all significantly higher in those with CI-AKI (3.8% MI, 6.4% bleeding, and 9.7% death) and considerably greater in those with AKI-D (7.9% MI, 15.8% bleeding, and 34.3% death). The development of CI-AKI is a clinical marker for individuals who are more frail, and susceptible to medical and procedural complications. The factors such as older age, female sex, diabetes, severity of coronary disease, left ventricular dysfunction, presentation as non-STEMI, STEMI, cardiogenic shock, or cardiac arrest also increase the risk of CI-AKI.

MANAGEMENT

Principles of management include using volumes of contrast that are as low as reasonably achievable (ALARA) and selection of the least-toxic iodinated contrast agent in the highest-risk patients. Low-osmolar contrast agents are reasonable for moderate-risk patients and iso-osmolar contrast is indicated for the highest-risk patients. In patients with high-risk profiles [eGFR <30 mL/min/1.73 m^2 with diabetes, heart failure (HF), or urgent PCI for ACS], there is no absolutely safe limit of contrast dose; hence, the most reasonable approach is to maximize the benefit to risk balance of the procedure by performing revascularization and then expectantly manage the CI-AKI to follow. Contrast minimization can be achieved using in-line devices in the contrast tubing manifold system that work to reduce injection overshoot by the operator (AVERT Plus System, Osprey Medical, Minnetonka, MN, United States).[21] Avoiding left ventriculography and aortography are additional strategies commonly used to reduce the overall contrast dose. Because iodinated contrast is water soluble, it is amenable to prevention strategies that expand intravascular volume and increase renal filtration and tubular flow of urine into collecting ducts, and on into the ureters and bladder. CI-AKI is responsive to intravascular administration of isotonic crystalloid solutions to enhance renal elimination of contrast via the urine.

TREATMENT MODALITIES

Following treatment modalities have been studied for prevention of CI-AKI.

Intravenous Sodium Bicarbonate versus Intravenous Saline

Hypothesis for using sodium bicarbonate to prevent contrast-induced nephropathy (CIN) is that the alkalinization of tubular fluid diminishes the production of free oxygen radicals, which may cause CIN. The meta-analysis of 19 randomized controlled trials (RCTs) showed that intravenous (IV) sodium bicarbonate did not have a clinically important effect on CIN risk when compared with IV saline. Intravenous sodium bicarbonate showed clinically important reduction in CIN that was not statistically significant when compared with IV saline in patients receiving LOCM and did not lead to reduction in CIN in patients receiving IOCM. The strength of evidence (SOE) was low for all comparisons of IV sodium bicarbonate. The overall analysis did not suggest that IV sodium bicarbonate was superior to IV saline.[22] There have been numerous randomized trials *comparing isotonic bicarbonate solutions to intravenous saline*, and in the largest trials, there have been no differences in the rates of renal outcomes.[23,24] Hence, either isotonic crystalloid solution is recommended, with some guidance on the quantity of fluid according to patient factors.

N-acetylcysteine Plus Intravenous Saline versus Intravenous Saline

N-acetylcysteine is a direct scavenger of free radicals and improves blood flow through nitric oxide-mediated pathways, which results in vasodilatation. Both these antioxidant and vasodilatory properties of *N*-acetylcysteine are believed to protect against CIN. High-dose *N*-acetylcysteine plus IV saline had small effect on reducing CIN risk that was clinically unimportant and not statistically significant, and low-dose *N*-acetylcysteine plus IV saline had a borderline clinically important effect on preventing CIN. Overall analysis did not suggest that any intervention was superior and the SOE was low or insufficient.[22]

N-acetylcysteine Plus Intravenous Saline versus Sodium Bicarbonate

Analysis of seven RCTs showed no clinically important benefit in reducing CIN risk when *N*-acetylcysteine plus IV saline was compared to sodium bicarbonate. The SOE was insufficient to draw any conclusion.[22]

Role of Left Ventricular End-diastolic Pressure

The POSEIDON (Prevention of Contrast Renal Injury with Different Hydration Strategies) trial randomized 396 patients with eGFR less than 60 mL/min/1.73 m^2 and 1 additional risk factor to a strategy of measurement of left ventricular end-diastolic pressure (LVEDP) and expanding plasma volume versus usual care. Each group had standard-of-care of normal saline 3 mL/kg for 1 hour before cardiac catheterization. The LVEDP-guided approach was associated with more intensive fluid administration during and after the procedure, and was associated with a reduction in CI-AKI (6.7%) compared with the control group (16.3%; $p = 0.005$).

Intravenous Crystalloid with Forced Diuresis

Even more intensive management with intravenous crystalloid with forced diuresis has been tested in a series of randomized trials using a fluid balance system that measures and controls intravenous crystalloid volume with urine output (RenalGuard System, PLC Medical Systems, Milford, Massachusetts, United States). All of these trials have demonstrated that elevation of urine output to greater than 150 mL/hr before and during the procedure reduces rates of CI-AKI.[25] In a single-center trial, 112 consecutive patients undergoing TAVR were randomly assigned to normal saline controlled by the RenalGuard system with urine flow initially augmented by furosemide (RenalGuard group) or normal saline-based usual care (control group). The primary endpoint was the incidence of CI-AKI (Cr rise ≥0.3 mg/dL or ≥50%) in the first 72 hour after the procedure. The AKI rate was lower in the RenalGuard group than in the control group (5.4% vs 25.0%, respectively; $p = 0.014$). No case of in-hospital AKI-D was reported. No significant differences in terms of mortality, cerebrovascular events, bleeding, and hospitalization for HF were noted in either group at 30 days.

To date, no adjunctive pharmaceutical has been demonstrated to effectively prevent or treat CI-AKI. There has been a pattern of small, randomized trials, and meta-analyses of these trials showing benefit with a specific agent such as *N*-acetylcysteine, ascorbic acid, aminophylline, trimetazidine, and fenoldopam.[22,26] When subjected to large randomized clinical trials, every agent tested to date has failed to prevent and/or treat CI-AKI. Thus, large clinical trials have an important role in this field.

At the present time, however, two chronic therapies may have an influence on CI-AKI, despite being used for other reasons, statins and renin-angiotensin system inhibitors (RASi): angiotensin-converting enzyme inhibitors (ACEI) and angiotensin-receptor blockers (ARB).

Statins

In observational and randomized studies, statins appear to protect against the development of CI-AKI. Possible renoprotective mechanisms of statins include inhibition of uptake of contrast into renal tubular cells, attenuation of endothelial dysfunction and oxidative stress, anti-inflammation, antiproliferation of mesangial cells, and protection of podocytes (Box 3). A meta-analysis which included 7 studies and 1,399 patients looked at the benefit of short-term, high-dose statins in the prevention of CI-AKI.[27] It showed a significant improvement in the incidence of CI-AKI, but no benefit in AKI-D. Leoncini et al. analyzed the

BOX 3: Renoprotective mechanism of statins

- Inhibition of uptake of contrast into renal tubular cells
- Attenuation of endothelial dysfunction and oxidative stress
- Anti-inflammation, antiproliferation of mesangial cells, and protection of podocytes

role of rosuvastatin in statin-naive patients for preventing CI-AKI.[28] They randomized 504 statin-naive non-STEMI ACS patients undergoing PCI to statin or no statin therapy. Statin group received rosuvastatin 40 mg on admission, then 20 mg daily, whereas the control patients did not receive statins during the hospitalization. At discharge, the statin group continued treatment with 20 mg/day rosuvastatin (10 mg/day for patients with GFR <30 mL/min/m^2), whereas controls received 40 mg/day atorvastatin. CI-AKI was defined as a rise in sCr by 0.5 mL/dL or 25% above baseline within 72 hour of receiving contrast. The study found the statin group had a significantly lower rate of CI-AKI than the no statin group (6.7% vs 15.1%, $p = 0.003$). In addition to the primary endpoint, multiple positive secondary endpoints were noted. There was a decrease in 30-day composite death, dialysis, MI, stroke, or persistent renal damage in the statin group (3.6% vs 7.9%, respectively; $p = 0.036$), as well as a trend toward a decrease in death or MI at 6 months (3.6% vs 7.2%, respectively; $p = 0.07$). Another study[29] tested rosuvastatin in prevention of CI-AKI in 2,998 patients with diabetes and CKD who were undergoing coronary or peripheral angiography with or without intervention. Patients who were on statins previously were asked to hold their statin for 14 days before the procedure. Patients were randomized to statin therapy or standard of care (no statin). The statin group received rosuvastatin 10 mg daily starting 2 days before the procedure and continuing for 5 days. The standard of care group and statin group resumed statin therapy 3 days after intervention. CI-AKI was defined as an increase of sCr concentration greater than or equal to 0.5 mg/dL or 25% above baseline at 72 hour. The statin group had a significantly lower incidence of CI-AKI (2.3% vs 3.9%; $p = 0.01$). Additionally, a significantly lower rate of HF was noted in the statin group at the 30-day follow-up (2.6% vs 4.3%; $p = 0.02$).[30] The proposed mechanism related to CIN prevention is that statins acted as stabilizers of the endothelium and free radical scavengers in a model of ischemic nephropathy.[30]

Five studies compared statins added to *N*-acetylcysteine and IV saline with *N*-acetylcysteine plus IV saline or sodium bicarbonate. The SOE was insufficient.

Ascorbic Acid

It is an antioxidant which acts as a scavenger of reactive oxygen species, reducing oxidative stress and possibly preventing CIN. In a meta-analysis of six RCT, ascorbic acid was compared with IV saline and patients received intervention with IA administration of LOCM or IOCM.[31-36] The studies comparing ascorbic acid with IV saline showed clinically important and statistically insignificant reduced risk for CIN. Similarly, comparison of ascorbic acid with *N*-acetylcysteine showed clinically unimportant and statistically insignificant difference.

Renin-angiotensin System Inhibitors

Renin-angiotensin system inhibitors are useful for treatment of hypertension, HF and are indicated to reduce the progression of diabetic nephropathy. The chronic beneficial effect of RASi on the kidney is mediated, in part, by reduction of intraglomerular pressure due to efferent glomerular arteriolar dilation. This mechanism, however, may be deleterious to the kidneys in the setting of acute illness or in the setting of iodinated contrast, where the ability to raise intraglomerular pressure/filtration via tubuloglomerular feedback may be beneficial in maintaining glomerular filtration and forward flow of urine through the proximal tubules and the remainder of the nephron. The trial to address this issue was the CAPTAIN (Angiotensin Converting Enzyme Inhibitor/Angiotensin Receptor Blocker and Contrast Induced Nephropathy in Patients Receiving Cardiac Catheterization) trial, which randomly assigned 208 patients with Cr greater than or equal to 1.7 mg/dL within 3 months or greater than or equal to 1.5 mg/dL within 1 week before coronary angiography to hold RASi (ACEI 72.1% or ARB 27.9%) greater than or equal to 24 hour preprocedure or continue RASi. The primary outcome was the incidence of CI-AKI, defined as an absolute rise in sCr greater than or equal to 0.5 mg/dL from baseline and/or a relative rise in sCr greater than or equal to 25%. At 48–96 hour, CI-AKI occurred in 10.9% of RASi-held compared to 18.4% of RASi-continued patients ($p = 0.16$). In a prespecified secondary outcome, there was a lower rise in mean sCr after the procedure in patients who held ACEI/ARB (0.3 ± 0.5 mg/dL vs 0.1 ± 0.3 mg/dL; $p = 0.03$). A clinical composite of death, MI, ischemic stroke, congestive HF, rehospitalization for cardiovascular cause, or need for dialysis periprocedural occurred in none of the RASi-held and 3.9% of the RASi-continued groups ($p = 0.06$). These data, combined with reports from CKD trials, suggest that although RASi are beneficial chronically, either too intensive RASi (ACEI + ARB) or direct renin inhibition appears to have excessive toxicity in the setting of hospitalization, and probably in the setting of cardiac catheterization and PCI as well.[37-39] Thus, it appears to be reasonable to hold RASi before coronary angiography in moderate and high-risk patients.

DISCUSSION

Many strategies have been used to prevent CIN. They include oral hydration, volume expansion with sodium chloride or bicarbonate or both; administration of *N*-acetylcysteine;

withdrawal of metformin, ACEI, angiotensin II-receptor blockers, or NSAIDs; hemofiltration or hemodialysis, statins, use of LOCM, IOCM, on nonionic contrast media; and reducing the volume of contrast media administered. Despite these varied strategies, no clear consensus exists in clinical practice about the most effective intervention to prevent or reduce CIN. The HOCM is no longer used in clinical practice in the United States.

Following studies showed clinically important and statistically significant benefit:

- Low-dose *N*-acetylcysteine plus IV saline versus IV saline (low SOE)
- *N*-acetylcysteine plus IV saline versus IV saline in patients receiving LOCM (moderate SOE)
- Statins plus *N*-acetylcysteine versus *N*-acetylcysteine (low SOE).

Following studies showed clinically important but statistically insignificant benefit:

- Sodium bicarbonate versus IV saline in patients receiving LOCM (low SOE)
- Statins plus IV saline versus IV saline alone (low SOE)
- Ascorbic acid plus IV saline versus IV saline (low SOE).

The joint American College of Cardiology/American Heart Association 2012 guideline recommends against the use of *N*-acetylcysteine for patients receiving IA contrast media in cardiac procedures. The 2012 Kidney Disease Improving Global Outcomes Clinical Practice Guideline for Acute Kidney Injury suggests using oral *N*-acetylcysteine with IV fluids in patients with increased CIN risk, acknowledging low SOE.[40] Although, *N*-acetylcysteine is inexpensive and safe, the evidence is not strong enough to support routine use.

FUTURE GOALS

Cineangiography and complex interventional procedures remain an important part of invasive cardiology. Technology to minimize contrast by avoiding overinjection and accurately recording contrast volumes will provide some help as our procedures become even more complicated.[41] Novel forms of nontoxic radiopaque contrast would be ideal; however, there are no such new contrast media in development. Agent like cyclodextrin makes contrast stay in the urinary space and less likely to penetrate the kidney tissue and cause damage. This action may render the iodine-based radiocontrast less toxic.[42] Finally, the development of cellular protectants continues to be an area of interest and, despite the disappointing results with *n*-acetyl cysteine, sodium bicarbonate, prostaglandins, fenoldopam, and other agents, there is hope that an adjunctive agent could be administered that would render the kidneys less susceptible to damage, and possibly protect the heart and other organs as well.

CONCLUSION

Contrast-induced acute kidney injury remains a serious problem for patients undergoing procedures utilizing intravascular iodinated contrast. Minimizing contrast by use of ALARA principles and strategies to maximize the benefit of contrast exposure are reasonable. Although there is no consensus but statin use appears to reduce the incidence and severity of CI-AKI, whereas continuation of RASi appears to increase the risk for CI-AKI. Based on the eGFR, McCullough et al.[43] have proposed the following scheme for management of CI-AKI.

- If the eGFR greater than or equal to 60 mL/min/1.73 m^2
  - Discontinue metformin, nephrotoxic drugs, and renin-angiotensin-aldosterone system (RAAS) inhibitors
  - Maintain good hydration and intravenous volume
- If the eGFR 30–59 mL/min/1.73 m^2
  - Discontinue metformin, nephrotoxic drugs, and RAAS inhibitors
  - Use statins preprocedure
  - Intravenous isotonic crystalloid 3 mL/kg/hr for 1 hour before procedure
    - Initial LVEDP-guided isotonic crystalloid:
      - Left ventricular end-diastolic pressure less than 13 mm Hg → 5 mL/kg/hr × 4 hour
      - Left ventricular end-diastolic pressure 13–18 mm Hg → 3 mL/kg/hr × 4 hour
      - Left ventricular end-diastolic pressure greater than 18 mm Hg → 1.5 mL/kg/hr × 4 hour
  - Use low-osmolar contrast (LOCM)
  - Use iso-osmolar contrast (iodixanol) if ACS, CKD, DM, HF, TAVR (IOCM)
  - Contrast volume ALARA
  - Continue statin postprocedure.
- If the eGFR less than 30 mL/min/1.73 m^2
  - Discontinue metformin, nephrotoxic drugs, and RAAS inhibitors
  - Use statins preprocedure
  - Consider hospital admission, nephrology consultation, and dialysis planning
  - IV isotonic crystalloid 3 mL/kg/hr for 1 hour before procedure
  - Use iso-osmolar contrast (iodixanol) during procedure
  - Daily serum creatinine and measure renal damage markers.

REFERENCES

1. Solomon R, Deray G. How to prevent contrast-induced nephropathy and manage risk patients: practical recommendations. Kidney Int Suppl. 2006;100:S51-3.
2. Goldenberg I, Matetzky S. Nephropathy induced by contrast media: Pathogenesis, risk factors and preventive strategies. CMAJ. 2005;172:1461-71
3. Nikolsky E, Aymong ED, Halkin A, et al. Impact of anemia in patients with acute myocardial infarction undergoing primary percutaneous coronary intervention: analysis from the Controlled Abciximab and Device Investigation to Lower Late Angioplasty Complications (CADILLAC) Trial. J Am Coll Cardiol. 2004;44(3):547-53.
4. Amin AP, Salisbury AC, McCullough PA, et al. Trends in the incidence of acute kidney injury in patients hospitalized with acute myocardial infarction. Arch Intern Med. 2012;172(3):246-53.
5. Tsai TT, Patel UD, Chang TI, et al. Contemporary incidence, predictors, and outcomes of acute kidney injury in patients undergoing percutaneous coronary interventions: insights from the NCDR Cath-PCI registry. JACC Cardiovasc Interv. 2014;7(1):1-9.
6. Mehran R, Aymong ED, Nikolsky E, et al. A simple risk score for prediction of contrast-induced nephropathy after percutaneous coronary intervention: development and initial validation. J Am Coll Cardiol. 2004;44(7):1393-9.
7. Sharma SK. Iodinated contrast media and contrast-induced nephropathy: Is there a preferred cost-effective agent? J Invasive Cardiol. 2008;20(5):245-8.
8. Schrader R. Contrast media selection in interventional cardiology. J Clin Basic Cardiol. 2002;4(4):245-8.
9. McCullough PA. Radiocontrast-induced acute kidney injury. Nephron Physiol. 2008;109:61-72.
10. Lasser EC, Lyon SG, Berry CC. Reports on contrast media reactions: analysis of data from reports to the US Food and Drug Administration. Radiology. 1997;203(3):605-10.
11. McCullough PA, Capasso P. Patient discomfort associated with the use of intra-arterial iodinated contrast media: a meta-analysis of comparative randomized controlled trials. BMC Med Imaging. 2011;11:12.
12. Liu ZZ, Viegas VU, Perlewitz A, et al. Iodinated contrast media differentially affect afferent and efferent arteriolar tone and reactivity in mice: a possible explanation for reduced glomerular filtration rate. Radiology. 2012;265(3):762-71.
13. Tervahartiala P, Kivisaari L, Kivisaari R, et al. Structural changes in the renal proximal tubular cells induced by iodinated contrast media. Nephron. 1997;76(1):96-102.
14. Guitterez NV, Diaz A, Timmis GC, et al. Determinants of serum creatinine trajectory in acute contrast nephropathy. J Interv Cardiol. 2002;15(5):349-54.
15. McCullough PA, Bouchard J, Waikar SS, et al. Implementation of novel biomarkers in the diagnosis, prognosis, and management of acute kidney injury: executive summary from the tenth consensus conference of the Acute Dialysis Quality Initiative (ADQI). Contrib Nephrol. 2013;182:5-12.
16. Kell DB. Iron behaving badly: inappropriate iron chelation as a major contributor to the aetiology of vascular and other progressive inflammatory and degenerative diseases. BMC Med Genomics. 2009;2:2.
17. Haase M, Bellomo R, Haase-Fielitz A. Novel biomarkers, oxidative stress, and the role of labile iron toxicity in cardiopulmonary bypass-associated acute kidney injury. J Am Coll Cardiol. 2010;55:2024-33.
18. Stahl F, Lepple-Wienhues A, Kuppinger M, et al. Electrogenic sodium-bicarbonate cotransport in human ciliary muscle cells. Am J Physiol 1992;262:C427-35.
19. Akrawinthawong K, Ricci J, Cannon L, et al. Subclinical and clinical contrast-induced acute kidney injury: data from a novel blood marker for determining the risk of developing contrast-induced nephropathy (ENCINO), a prospective study. Ren Fail. 2015;37(2):187-91.
20. Thongprayoon C, Cheungpasitporn W, Srivali N, et al. Acute kidney injury after transcatheter aortic valve replacement: a systematic review and meta-analysis. Am J Nephrol. 2015;41(4-5):372-82.
21. Osprey Medical. (2015). AVERT Clinical Trial for Contrast Media Volume Reduction and Incidence of CIN (AVERT) (ClinicalTrials.gov). [online] Available from: https://clinicaltrials.gov/ct2/show/NCT01976299?term=osprey&rank=3. [Accessed August, 2017].
22. Subramaniam RM, Suarez-Cuervo C, Wilson RF, et al. Effectiveness of prevention strategies for contrast-induced nephropathy: a systematic review and meta-analysis. Ann Intern Med. 2016;164(6):406-16.
23. Solomon R, Gordon P, Manoukian SV, et al. Randomized trial of bicarbonate or saline study for the prevention of contrast-induced nephropathy in patients with CKD. Clin J Am Soc Nephrol. 2015;10(9):1519-24.
24. Brar SS, Shen AY, Jorgensen MB, et al. Sodium bicarbonate vs sodium chloride for the prevention of contrast medium-induced nephropathy in patients undergoing coronary angiography: a randomized trial. 2008. JAMA;300(9):1038-46.
25. Solomon R. Forced diuresis with the RenalGuard system: impact on contrast induced acute kidney injury. J Cardiol. 2014;63(1):9-13.
26. Sadat U, Usman A, Gillard JH, et al. Does ascorbic acid protect against contrast-induced acute kidney injury in patients undergoing coronary angiography: a systematic review with meta-analysis of randomized, controlled trials. J Am Coll Cardiol. 2013;62(23):2167-75.
27. Li Y, Liu Y, Fu L, et al. Efficacy of short-term high-dose statin in preventing contrast-induced nephropathy: a meta-analysis of seven randomized controlled trials. PLoS One. 2012;7(4):e34450.
28. Leoncini M, Toso A, Maioli M, et al. Early high-dose rosuvastatin for contrast-induced nephropathy prevention in acute coronary syndrome: results from the PRATO-ACS Study (Protective Effect of Rosuvastatin and Antiplatelet Therapy on contrast-induced acute kidney injury and myocardial damage in patients with Acute Coronary Syndrome). J Am Coll Cardiol. 2014;63(1):71-9.
29. Han Y, Zhu G, Han L, et al. Short-term rosuvastatin therapy for prevention of contrast-induced acute kidney injury in patients with diabetes and chronic kidney disease. J Am Coll Cardiol. 2014;63(1):62-70.
30. Gueler F, Rong S, Park JK, et al. Postischemic acute renal failure is reduced by short-term statin treatment in a rat model. J Am Soc Nephrol. 2002;13(9):2288-98.
31. Brueck M, Cengiz H, Hoeltgen R, et al. Usefulness of N-acetylcysteine or ascorbic acid versus placebo to prevent contrast-induced acute kidney injury in patients undergoing elective cardiac catheterization: a single-center, prospective, randomized, double-blind, placebo-controlled trial. J Invasive Cardiol. 2013;25(6):276-83.
32. Boscheri A, Weinbrenner C, Botzek B, et al. Failure of ascorbic acid to prevent contrast-media induced nephropathy in patients with renal dysfunction. Clin Nephrol. 2007;68(5):279-86.
33. Dvorsak B, Kanic V, Ekart R, et al. Ascorbic acid for the prevention of contrast-induced nephropathy after coronary angiography in patients with chronic renal impairment: a randomized controlled trial. Ther Apher Dial. 2013;17(4):384-90.
34. Spargias K, Alexopoulos E, Kyrzopoulos S, et al. Ascorbic acid prevents contrast-mediated nephropathy in patients with renal dysfunction undergoing coronary angiography or intervention. Circulation, 2004;110(18):2837-42.
35. Zhou L, Chen H. Prevention of contrast-induced nephropathy with ascorbic acid. Intern Med. 2012;51(6): 531-5.
36. Albabtain MA, Almasood A, Alshurafah H, et al. Efficacy of ascorbic acid, N-acetylcysteine, or combination of both on top of saline

hydration versus saline hydration alone on prevention of contrast-induced nephropathy: a prospective randomized study. J Interv Cardiol. 2013;26(1):90-6.
37. Fried LF, Duckworth W, Zhang JH, et al. Design of combination angiotensin receptor blocker and angiotensin-converting enzyme inhibitor for treatment of diabetic nephropathy (VA NEPHRON-D). 2009. Clin J Am Soc Nephrol. 4(2):361-8.
38. Parving HH, Brenner BM, McMurray JJ, et al. Cardiorenal end points in a trial of aliskiren for type 2 diabetes. N Engl J Med. 2012;367(23):2204-13.
39. Levine GN, Bates ER, Blankenship JC, et al. 2011 ACCF/AHA/SCAI Guideline for Percutaneous Coronary Intervention: executive summary: a report of the American College of Cardiology Foundation/American Heart Association task Force on Practice Guidelines and the Society for Cardiovascular Angiography and Interventions. Catheter Cardiovasc Interv. 2012;79(3):453-95.
40. Kidney Disease Improving Global Outcomes (KDIGO), Acute Kidney Injury Work Group. KDIGO clinical practice guideline for acute kidney injury. Kidney Int Suppl. 2012;2:1-138.
41. Prasad A, Ortiz-Lopez C, Kaye DM, et al. The use of the AVERT system to limit contrast volume administration during peripheral angiography and intervention. Catheter Cardiovasc Interv. 2015;86(7):1228-33.
42. Biswas S, Rowe ES, Mosher G, et al. TCT 138: veropaque, a novel contrast formulation, mitigates contrast induced acute kidney injury. J Am Coll Cardiol. 2012;60(17S).
43. McCullough PA, Choi JP, Feghali GA, et al. Contrast-Induced Acute Kidney Injury. J Am Coll Cardiol. 2016;68(13):1465-73.

CHAPTER 24

Cardiodiabetes and Hypertension: Double Jeopardy

Praveen Jain, Mohammad Jibran

INTRODUCTION

The presence of hypertension (HT) causes a 7.2-fold increase in mortality in diabetic patients. In India, about 50% of diabetic individuals have HT. In the Screening India's Twin Epidemic (SITE) cross-sectional study conducted in 10 Indian states, diabetes mellitus (DM) and HT were coexistent in 20.6% patients, which demonstrate that the substantial burden of DM and HT is on the rise in India. The macrovascular complications, which are well recognized in patients with long-standing diabetes or HT, include stable coronary artery disease, myocardial infarction, stroke, congestive heart failure, and peripheral vascular diseases. Although microvascular complications (retinopathy, nephropathy, and neuropathy) are conventionally linked to hyperglycemia, studies have shown that HT constitutes an important risk factor, especially for nephropathy. Several studies conducted in different ethnic groups show a close association between HT and DM, where the prevalence of HT is significantly higher in the patients with noninsulin-dependent DM (NIDDM or type 2 DM). Both systolic and diastolic HT has been reported and conclusive evidence indicated that the link between DM and essential HT is hyperinsulinemia. HT is often present as part of the metabolic syndrome of insulin resistance, also including central obesity and dyslipidemia. In recent years, adequate data from well-designed randomized clinical trials have demonstrated the effectiveness of aggressive treatment of HT in reducing diabetes complications on both types.

DIABETIC PATIENT WITH HYPERTENSION

Among the complications of diabetes, cardiovascular and renal vascular diseases are among the most costly in terms of human suffering and national healthcare costs. Over the past several years, a number of controlled multicenter clinical trials have demonstrated the safety and efficacy of specific antihypertensive therapeutic programs that can significantly alter the outcomes of these cardiovascular and renal complications. In a recent large prospective cohort study that included 12,550 adults, the development of type 2 diabetes was almost 2.5 times as likely in persons with HT than in their normotensive counterparts.[1] This, in conjunction with considerable evidence of the increased prevalence of HT in diabetic persons,[2,3] suggests that these two common chronic diseases frequently coexist. Moreover, each pathophysiological disease entity, although independent in its own natural history, serves to exacerbate the other.[2,3] In a report of Gress et al.,[1] hypertensive patients, who were taking β-blockers had a 28% higher risk of diabetes than those taking no medication. In contrast, patients with HT, who received thiazide diuretics, angiotensin-converting enzyme (ACE) inhibitors, or Ca^{2+} antagonists, were found not to be at greater risk for subsequent diabetes than were patients who were not receiving any antihypertensive medications. However, that study was not prospective or randomized,[1] and other randomized prospective trials have not shown an increase in the development of diabetes with β-blocker or low-dose diuretic treatment of HT.[4-6] Other studies have reported that ACE inhibitor therapy reduced the propensity of hypertensive patients to develop type 2 diabetes by 11%[7] and 34%[8] in trials extending for 6 and 4 years, respectively, suggesting that antihypertensive treatment may have a significant impact on the propensity for the development of diabetes in this population.[9] These observations are in contrast to a report[1] in which no reduction in progression to diabetes on ACE inhibition therapy was observed. There is an increasing body of data from controlled clinical trials indicating that rigorous control of arterial pressure to levels less than 140/90 mm Hg markedly reduces cardiovascular and renal morbidity and mortality in persons with type 2 diabetes.[6-13] In the Systolic Hypertension in the Elderly Program (SHEP) study,[4] elderly persons with type 2 diabetes derived more benefit from aggressive systolic blood pressure lowering in reduction of cardiovascular disease (CVD) than did those without diabetes. Baseline therapy in the SHEP study used a low-dose diuretic, which is often a necessary component of the antihypertensive regimen because of the sodium sensitivity and expanded plasma volume that is often present in diabetic patients.[14] Data from the subset analysis of type 2 diabetes in the Hypertension Optimal Treatment (HOT) trial[10] suggest that reduction in diastolic pressures from less than 90 mm Hg to values less than 85 mm Hg is beneficial in reducing CVD events. The initial drug therapy in HOT was with a dihydropyridine Ca^{2+} antagonist, but more than 70% of diabetic patients required at least three drugs to control the diastolic pressure to levels less than 85 mm Hg. Special benefits of aggressive blood pressure lowering in the diabetic population was observed in a subanalysis of this cohort in the Systolic Hypertension in Europe (Syst-Eur) trial.[11] In that trial, although systolic pressure was reduced by a comparable amount in each group [22.0 ± 16 mm Hg (nondiabetic group) vs 22.1 ± 14 mm Hg (diabetic group)], the risk reduction in mortality from CVD was 13% in nondiabetic patients versus 76% for the diabetic patients.[11] Again, diabetic patients required more antihypertensive treatment to achieve goal blood pressures, with up to two-thirds requiring more than or equal to two medications as previously observed.[4,10] Moreover, the benefit confirmed per mm Hg blood pressure reduction was greater in diabetic patients than in those patients with HT but without concomitant DM, providing further evidence for rigorous reduction of arterial pressure in diabetic patient.

UNITED KINGDOM PROSPECTIVE DIABETES STUDY GROUP

In the United Kingdom Prospective Diabetes Study (UKPDS) group,[12,13] blood pressure lowering was similarly effective for captopril and atenolol-based regimens in reducing the incidence of both microvascular and macrovascular diabetic complications. Many of these type 2 diabetic patients required both drugs plus a diuretic for "tight control" of pressure (i.e. 144/82 mm Hg). The necessity for use of at least three drugs for tight control was also observed in the diabetic cohorts of the HOT and Syst-Eur studies as well.[10,11] In the UKPDS, reductions in risk in the group assigned to tight control were 24% in diabetes-related endpoints, 32% in death-related endpoints to diabetes, 44% in strokes, and 37% in microvascular endpoints, especially diabetic retinopathy. Moreover, in the UKPDS trial, the relative benefit on CVD risk reduction was conferred in a far more powerful fashion by intensive blood pressure reduction rather than by tight glucose control.[12] ACE inhibitors are currently recognized as first-line antihypertensive therapy in diabetic persons with proteinuria,[2,15,16] and these agents afford unique benefits in modifying the progression and severity of CVD as well as of diabetic nephropathy (Flow chart 1). Indeed, a cardioprotective effect of ACE inhibitors has been suggested from results of the Fosinopril versus Amlodipine Cardiovascular Events Trial (FACET),[17] the Captopril Prevention Project (CAPPP),[7] the Heart Outcomes Prevention Evaluation (HOPE) trial,[8] and the

Flow chart 1: Algorithm for antihypertensive therapy in the diabetic individual

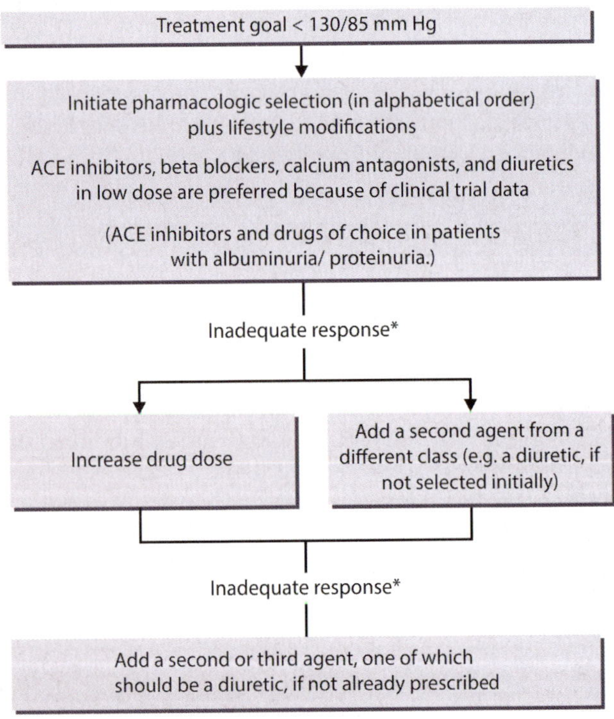

Abbreviation: ACE, angiotensin-converting enzyme
*An adequate response indicates that goal blood pressure is achieved or considerable progress is made.

Shunt Thrombotic Occlusion Prevention by Picotamide (STOP)-2 hypertensive trial.[6] FACET[16] was an open-label single-center trial designed to compare the effects of fosinopril and amlodipine on serum lipids and glycemic control. Patients were assigned to treatment with either amlodipine or fosinopril; if blood pressure was not controlled, the other drug was added. The incidence of CVD events was less in the fosinopril-treated group than in the amlodipine-treated group, but the incidence was least in the group that received both antihypertensive agents.[18] Furthermore, it should be noted that there was no placebo group in the FACET study, so that the impact of Ca^{2+} antagonists alone could not be ascertained. These results, as well as those of the Syst-Eur[11] and HOT[10] studies, suggest that the combination of a dihydropyridine Ca^{2+} antagonist (such as amlodipine or nitrendipine) and an ACE inhibitor is an acceptable approach to the treatment of this high-risk population. It is clear from these recent studies that reaching goal blood pressure in diabetic patients, especially if they have renal disease, will require treatment with several antihypertensive agents. Results of the SHEP[8] and the UKPDS[12] trials suggest that diuretics and β-blockers as well as ACE inhibitors are also useful therapeutic agents in diabetic hypertensive patients who often require more than or equal to two drugs to control blood pressure adequately (Flow chart 1).[19]

CAPTOPRIL PREVENTION PROJECT TRIAL

The Captopril Prevention Project[7] was an unblinded prospective trial that enrolled 10,985 patients aged 25–66 years with diastolic pressure of 100 mm Hg or more. Patients were randomized to receive either captopril (in one or two doses up to 100 mg/d), with a thiazide diuretic added if necessary or the clinician's choice of a thiazide diuretic or β-blocker, with the alternative agent as add-on therapy if necessary. Over a follow-up period of approximately 6.1 years, in part because of inadequate randomization for baseline blood pressure, there was a small increase in stroke in the captopril group and a slight reduction in myocardial infarction and other cardiovascular deaths in this treatment group for the nondiabetic cohort. However, the risk of developing new diabetes was 11% less in the captopril-treated group. In diabetic patients (n = 572), there was a reduction in the CVD endpoints (P = 0.02) in the group receiving captopril. In the diabetic cohort, there was a better outcome with regard to all outcomes in patients randomized to captopril.[7] The study suggested that although overall events may be similar to β-blocker/diuretic treatment compared with an ACE/diuretic regimen, there appears to be an advantage to the latter regimen in diabetic persons.

HEART OUTCOMES PREVENTION EVALUATION TRIAL

The Heart Outcomes Prevention Evaluation was a randomized double-blind evaluation of the ACE inhibitor ramipril in patients at high risk for vascular disease complications but without clinically evident heart failure.[8] The HOPE trial tested the hypothesis that ACE inhibitors in general, and ramipril in particular, have beneficial effects on vascular disease complications above and beyond their effects on blood pressure. However, the small reduction in blood pressure with ramipril may have contributed to its beneficial effects.[8] All patients enrolled in the HOPE trial had documented vascular disease, i.e. a history of coronary artery disease, stroke, peripheral vascular disease, or diabetes, with one additional cardiovascular risk factor. A total of 9,297 patients were randomized to either ramipril or matching placebo and were followed for a mean duration of 5 years. The primary endpoints were myocardial infarction, stroke, or death from a cardiovascular cause. Secondary outcomes were death from all causes, need for coronary artery revascularization, hospitalization for unstable angina, heart failure, and complications related to diabetes. The 3,577 diabetic patients enrolled in the HOPE trial were also examined separately in a substudy of microalbuminuria and cardiovascular and renal outcomes (MICRO-HOPE).[20] In keeping with the findings of the major trial, the primary outcome (a composite of myocardial infarction, stroke, or death from a cardiovascular cause) was reduced by 25% [95% confidence interval (CI) 12–36%, P < 0.0004] in diabetic patients treated with ramipril compared with diabetic patients receiving placebo. Secondary outcomes of total mortality and need for revascularization were also significantly lower among diabetic patients receiving ramipril. Admissions to the hospital for unstable angina or heart failure did not differ between patients receiving ramipril and those receiving placebo. However, there was a significant 16% reduction in progression to overt nephropathy (95% CI 1–29%, P = 0.036), and there were nonsignificant trends toward less laser therapy for retinopathy and less progression to end-stage renal disease in the ramipril group as well. One of the most striking observations from the HOPE trial is that relatively large reductions in risk were achieved in the face of comparatively small reductions in blood pressure. Patients enrolled in the HOPE trial were not required to be hypertensive, and the average blood pressure on admission was 139/79 mm Hg. By 2 years, when the trends in endpoints first reached statistical significance, the average reduction in blood pressure was only 3/2 mm Hg. This striking finding points toward possible direct effects of ramipril (and ACE inhibitors as a class) on the heart and vasculature in addition to their additional effect on blood pressure. In the HOPE trial, diabetic patients derived an even greater reduction in CVD than did the rest of the high-risk population.[8]

The HOPE study also showed a 34% reduction in the development of diabetes in those patients without diabetes at the onset of the study. Furthermore, in another study, the ACE inhibitor perindopril was reported to reduce insulin resistance in obese hypertensive patients without diabetes.[21] Thus, the lessons learned from these three studies suggest that ACE inhibitor therapy can improve insulin sensitivity and also delay the development of diabetes in patients at high risk for the development of this disease. The mechanism whereby ACE inhibitors improve glucose metabolism and protect against the development of clinical diabetes may involve the improvement of blood flow through the microcirculation to fat and skeletal muscle tissue and/or the improvement of insulin action at the cellular level [by interfering with the angiotensin II (Ang II) antagonism of insulin signaling] (Fig. 1). The fact that ACE inhibitors, but not Ang II receptor antagonists, improve insulin resistance[21] suggests that their action on glucose metabolism may be mediated via (at least in part) bradykinin metabolism. Significant improvement of insulin responsiveness, which was achieved by the addition of an ACE inhibitor to a tissue culture,[22] indicated that the protective effect of ACE inhibition on diabetes is not (or is not solely) related to changes in blood flow. This improvement is also likely mediated at a cellular level, as shown by increase in glucose transporter type-4 (GLUT-4) protein and the activity of hexokinase, one of the major enzymes of glucose metabolism, in skeletal muscle of obese rats treated with an ACE inhibitor (Fig. 1).

Interrupting the effects of the renin-angiotensin system (RAS) may improve the cellular actions of insulin by several mechanisms. Ang II in vascular and heart tissue interferes with insulin stimulation of phosphatidylinositol 3-kinase (PI3-kinase) activation, a major pathway for insulin signal transduction (Fig. 1).[23-25] The relationship between the RAS and insulin is complex and includes several intracellular mechanisms and signaling pathways. Normally, insulin binds to its receptor [insulin receptor (IR)] on the surface of the insulin-sensitive cell and triggers autophosphorylation of the IR β-subunit, which, in turn, phosphorylates tyrosine in the IR substrate (IRS) molecules. This allows the regulating p85 subunit of PI3-kinase to connect to the IRS-1 and form an IRS-1/PI3-kinase complex, which is involved in many of the actions of insulin, including chemotaxis, translocation of cellular elements, and glucose transport.[26] This pathway has also been implicated in mediating the activation of nitric oxide (NO) synthase and the Na^{2+} pump activity in vascular tissue[26,27] and in facilitating vascular relaxation. Ang II, acting via an Ang II type 1 G-protein–linked receptor, phosphorylates a number of proteins, including IRS-1 and -2. Such phosphorylation leads to the activation of catalytic activity of the p110 subunit of

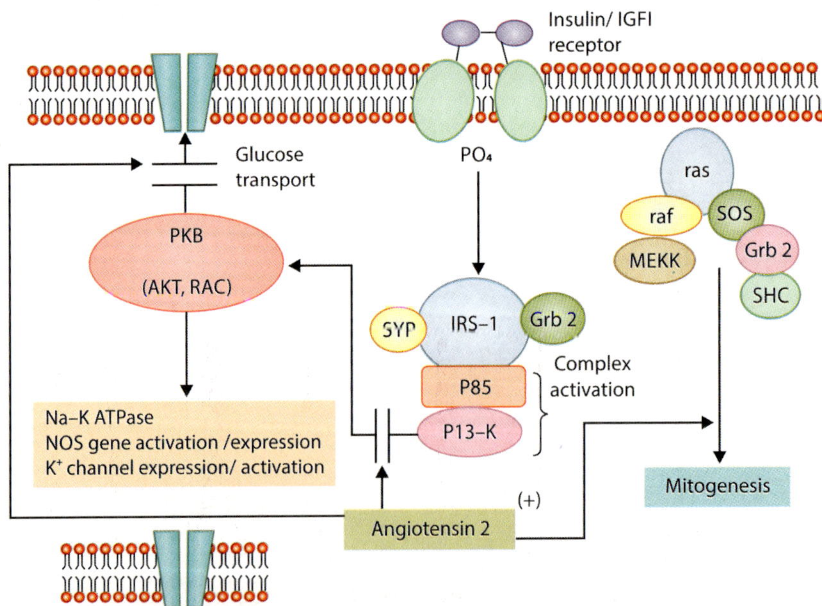

Fig. 1: Intracellular signaling pathways of insulin/IGF-1

Abbreviations: IGF-1, insulin-like growth factor-1; IRS-1, insulin receptor substrate-1; NOS, nitric oxide synthase; PKB, protein kinase B

PI3-kinase, the same enzyme that belongs to the insulin-signaling pathway. Paradoxically, this process interferes with insulin-dependent activation of PI3-kinase and, therefore, inhibits this major pathway of insulin signaling and decreases the ability of the cell to consume glucose in response to insulin.[12] Precise mechanisms of such inhibition remain unclear, but it has been shown that Ang II inhibits the insulin-stimulated association between IRS-1 and the regulatory p85 subunit of PI3-kinase by 30–50% in a dose-dependent manner,[23,24] interrupts the insulin-signaling cascade, and, therefore, contributes to the development of insulin resistance. This insulin resistance can be manifested as diminished glucose transport in skeletal muscle tissues and adipocytes and impaired vascular relaxation.[27]

Even though they are not completely understood, the cellular actions of ACE inhibitors on glucose metabolism lead to increase in GLUT-4 concentration and activation of one of the major enzymes of glucose pathway, hexokinase.[27] These changes are probably secondary to activation of the PI3-kinase signaling pathway by the enhancement of tyrosine phosphorylation of IRS-1 and the improvement of PI3-kinase/IRS-1 complexing.[28] ACE inhibitors are also able to facilitate blood flow through the microcirculation in skeletal muscles.[29] This effect is bradykinin dependent and occurs through the activation of cell surface β2-adrenergic receptors.[29] ACE inhibitors prolong the action of bradykinin by blocking its enzymatic breakdown and facilitating its action.[29] Facilitation of blood flow to insulin-sensitive tissues, such as skeletal muscle, would lead to an increase in glucose delivery to these tissues. In turn, bradykinin not only causes vasodilation but also independently increases the basal and insulin-stimulated rate of glucose uptake in skeletal muscle in insulin-resistant obese Zuckerrats[30] by improving postreceptor insulin signaling and enhancing GLUT-4 translocation to the cell membrane.[30] Thus, in addition to blocking the negative effect of Ang II on PI3-kinase signaling, there are additional mechanisms by which ACE inhibitor therapy may improve the insulin sensitivity associated with HT.[31]

OTHER FACTORS CONTRIBUTING TO INCREASED CARDIOVASCULAR DISEASE IN DIABETIC PATIENTS

Cardiovascular disease accounts for up to 80% of the deaths in persons with type 2 diabetes (Fig. 2).[31] Indeed, age-adjusted relative risk of death due to cardiovascular events in persons with type 2 diabetes is threefold higher than in the general population.[14,31] A recent population-based study showed that CVD mortality was 7.5 times greater among persons with type 2 diabetes without a previous

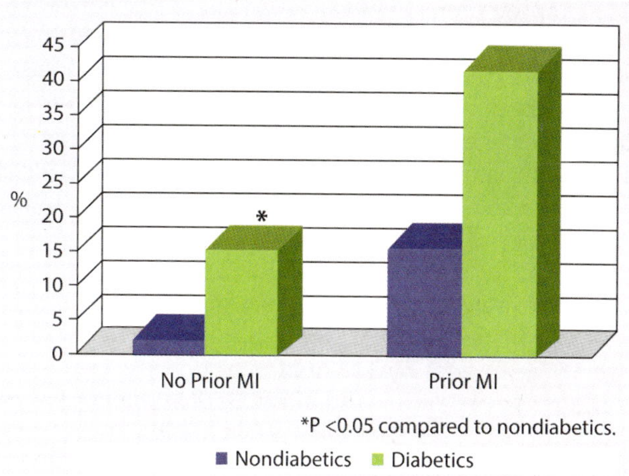

Fig. 2: Incidence of death from cardiovascular causes in diabetic and nondiabetic individuals after a 7-year follow-up

Abbreviation: MI, myocardial infarction

myocardial infarction than in those without diabetes (Fig. 2).[31] Furthermore, the incidence of CVD mortality was threefold higher among individuals with diabetes who had suffered a myocardial infarction than among nondiabetic individuals.[31] Diabetes is associated with a relatively greater risk for CVD in women than in men.[32] Moreover, diabetes negates the normal gender differences in the prevalence of CVD, and when adjusted for other risk factors, the risk rate for increased mortality is 2.4 times greater for diabetic men and 3.5 times greater for diabetic women.[32,33]

A number of factors, in addition to HT, contribute to the high prevalence of CVD in type 2 diabetic persons. Within the Multiple Risk Factor Intervention Trial (MRFIT),[34] more than 5,000 diabetic patients were followed for 12 years and were compared with more than 350,000 persons without diabetes. The occurrence of CVD death at the 12-year follow-up was approximately three times more in diabetic men than in their nondiabetic controls, regardless of systolic pressure, age, cholesterol, ethnic group, or use of tobacco. This study also confirmed that systolic HT, elevated cholesterol, and cigarette smoking were independent predictors of mortality and that the presence of more than or equal to one of these risk factors had a greater impact on increasing CVD mortality in persons with diabetes than in those without diabetes.

Other risk factors that are involved in the cardiometabolic syndrome include the following: Obesity, hyperlipidemia, hyperuricemia, and albuminuria.[15,16,25] The hyperuricemia that occurs in essential HT (when not ascribed to gout, diuretic therapy, or other factors known to produce hyperuricemia) is related to reduced renal blood flow and increased renal vascular resistance.[25] This elevation in serum uric acid not only accompanies the vascular alterations associated with nephrosclerosis but also follows the development of left ventricular hypertrophy (echocardiographically) and accompanies the foregoing renal hemodynamic involvement in patients with the early stages of essential HT, even before the development of proteinuria or impaired renal excretory function.[25] On the other hand, microalbuminuria has been reported to develop before any clinical evidence of coronary heart disease (CHD) (e.g. myocardial infarction and cardiac failure) or intrarenal vascular disease in patients having diabetes with or without HT.[15,16] Nephrosclerosis associated with HT and renal diabetic vascular disease affects the intrarenal arterioles, whereas CHD, associated with occlusive epicardial coronary artery disease, as manifested by myocardial infarction, is an arterial disease. In the case of the latter, both HT and diabetes exacerbate the atherosclerotic occlusive disease.

DIABETIC CARDIOMYOPATHY

Diabetic cardiomyopathy, a diabetes-related myopathic state, is characterized mainly by impaired diastolic function.[35-38] In experimental diabetes, the mechanical properties of the myocardium and cardiomyocytes in vitro involve prolongation of contraction and relaxation as well as considerable slowing in relaxation velocity.[36-38] Diabetic cardiomyopathy is observed in chemically induced insulinopenic[36,37] as well as in genetically predisposed insulin-resistant[38] rodent models. Potential abnormalities underlying this cardiomyopathic state include altered K^+ channel function,[39-41] alterations in Na^+ pump function,[42] alterations in sarcoplasmic (endoplasmic) reticulum Ca^{2+}-ATPase,[43,44] Na^+-Ca^{2+} exchanger[45] function, and abnormalities of protein kinase C metabolism.[46] Diabetic cardiomyopathy may be associated with a balance between the cardiac RAS and the autocrine/paracrine actions of insulin-like growth factor-1 (IGF-1). The peptides, Ang II, and IGF are generated by cardiomyocytes and exert pleiotropic effects in an autocrine/paracrine fashion.[27,47] IGF-1 also has been demonstrated to increase myocardial contractility by increasing (Ca^{2+}) ion and cardiomyocyte myofilament Ca^{2+} sensitivity.[47] IGF-1 is synthesized by cardiomyocytes under the control of insulin, Ang II, mechanical stress, and increased total peripheral resistance.[47] IGF-1 and Ang II have opposing actions on key signaling pathways of the heart but work synergistically in promoting growth.[47] One of the major pathways of IGF-1 signaling involves the activation of the PI3-kinase/IRS-1 complex.[48,49] The PI3-kinase pathway is known to mediate many insulin/IGF-1 actions, including receptor trafficking, glucose transport, cytoskeletal reorganization, the Na^+, K^+-ATPase and K^+ channel expression/activity, and myofilament-Ca^{2+} sensitivity.[23,24,27] Ang II, acting via its G-protein–linked receptor, also induces tyrosine phosphorylation of IRS-1.[23,24] In cardiac tissue in contrast to insulin/IGF-1, Ang II acutely inhibits basal as well as insulin/IGF-1–stimulated PI3-kinase activity (Fig. 1).[23,47] Thus, it has been proposed that overexpression of the RAS, as occurs in the diabetic heart, would predispose one to a resistance to the actions of insulin/IGF-1 on the PI3-kinase–mediated activation of K^+ channel and Na^+ pump expression/activation as well as myofilament-$Ca2^+$ sensitivity.[47] Indeed, reduced cardiomyocyte glucose transport and attenuated PI3-kinase response to insulin IGF-1 have been observed in insulin-resistant rodent models.[36,50] These abnormalities are associated with decreased expression/activation of the K^+ channel and Na^+ pump in both type 1 and type 2 diabetic states.[36,47,51] Resistance to the PI3-kinase–mediated actions of IGF-1 and insulin (Fig. 1)[50] could explain the abnormalities of both diastolic and systolic function and left ventricular hypertrophy,[52] which characterize "diabetic cardiomyopathy". However, unabated action of both IGF-1 and Ang II could help explain why patients with diabetes appear to have greater left ventricular mass than do nondiabetic cohorts with comparable blood pressures.[52]

MICROALBUMINURIA AND CARDIOVASCULAR DISEASE IN DIABETES

There is considerable evidence that the presence of HT in type 1 diabetes is a consequence rather than a cause of renal disease. For example, with low levels of microalbuminuria, the arterial pressure remains normal, a finding that suggests that nephropathy precedes the raise in blood pressure.[2,14] Regardless of whether HT in type 1 diabetes is the etiologic factor of nephropathy or a complication of it, it is clear that a genetic predisposition to HT is important in the development of nephropathy in those 30% of type 1 diabetics who develop this complication and that nephropathy and HT exacerbate each other.[53] On the other hand, microalbuminuria is an independent risk factor for the development of CVD and a predictor of cardiovascular mortality in the diabetic population. It is associated with insulin resistance,[54] atherogenic dyslipidemia,[54] central obesity,[54] and the absence of nocturnal drop in both systolic and diastolic pressures[55,56] and is a part of the metabolic cardiovascular syndrome associated with HT (Box 1).[55,57] Because microalbuminuria is part of the cardiometabolic syndrome[54,57] and is related to endothelial dysfunction and increased oxidative stress, it is not surprising that diabetic glomerulosclerosis parallels diabetic atherosclerosis and is

BOX 1: Cardiovascular risk factors that cluster with microalbuminuria

- Central obesity
- Insulin resistance
- Low high-density lipoprotein (HDL) cholesterol levels
- High triglyceride levels
- Systolic hypertension
- Absent nocturnal drop in blood pressure
- Salt sensitivity
- Male sex
- Increased cardiovascular oxidative stress
- Impaired endothelial function
- Abnormal coagulation/fibrinolytic profiles.

a very powerful risk factor for CHD and stroke in diabetic persons.[15,16,57]

THERAPEUTIC IMPLICATIONS

It is clear from the foregoing review of newer information concerning the CVD complications of DM and their interaction with HT and its complications that the recent national recommendations concerning the treatment of patients with HT[19] are all the more important. Thus, although there is a necessity for risk stratification of patients with HT according to the stage of blood pressure elevation, it is apparent that the inclusion of all patients with HT whose systolic and diastolic pressures exceed 130 and/or 85 mm Hg, respectively, should probably receive antihypertensive drug therapy. Although a goal blood pressure of 130/85 mm Hg is relatively arbitrary, it is also recognized by other organizations, such as the Canadian Hypertension Society,[58] as a reasonable goal to maximally preserve function and reduce CVD morbidity and mortality. Clearly, lifestyle modifications are important for all patients with diabetes, but in those with even high normal levels of blood pressure elevation, pharmacotherapy of HT is particularly important. It is further evident from these Joint National Committee-6 recommendations and recent clinical trial data cited in the present report that the first choice in antihypertensive agents is the selection of an ACE inhibitor. Indeed, ACE inhibitor therapy has been shown to reduce the progression of renal disease[20,59] and CVD[8] in diabetic persons with "normal blood pressure".

Although it is clearly not our purpose to review the pharmacological treatment of diabetes and HT, a few compelling observations are in order. A review of recently completed clinical trials indicates that more than 65% of people with diabetes and HT will require more than or equal to two different antihypertensive medications to achieve the new suggested target blood pressure of less than 130/85 mm Hg.[19] ACE inhibitor therapy should be an integral component of any antihypertensive regime in patients with diabetes, in as much as these agents have been demonstrated to reduce CVD[7,8] and renal disease[53] in this population. Not every patient with diabetes and HT can take an ACE inhibitor either because of specific side effects from therapy or because of absolute contraindications. Thus, if a persistent cough secondary to the ACE is intolerable and precludes its further use, then selection of an Ang II (type 1) receptor antagonist appears appropriate. A number of multicenter trials are ongoing and are directed to support this recommendation. However, because results supporting their use are not yet available, it is not unreasonable to conclude that Ang II receptor antagonists are appropriate choices. Other complications of ACE inhibitor therapy, particularly in patients with diabetes, may be the progression of renal functional impairment and/or hyperkalemia. In these patients, a number of studies have supported the use of Ca^{2+} antagonists.[19] Finally, the use of ACE inhibitors or Ang II antagonists in any pregnant woman (including one with diabetes) is definitely contraindicated.

CONCLUSION

Over and above the foregoing therapeutic recommendations, it is also important to assess the status of the diabetic patient's serum concentration of low-density lipoprotein (LDL) cholesterol and glycated hemoglobin.[1,2,10,19,59-61] Thus, in those patients with an LDL cholesterol of 100 mg/dL and glycated hemoglobin of more than or equal to 6.5, more vigorous control of both lipids and of glycated hemoglobin levels is particularly indicated. Finally, all diabetic patients should receive aspirin unless there is absolute contraindication.[60,61]

REFERENCES

1. Gress TW, Nieto FJ, Shahar E, et al. Hypertension and antihypertensive therapy as risk factors for type 2 diabetes mellitus. Atherosclerosis Risk in Communities Study. N Engl J Med. 2000;342(13):905-12.
2. National High Blood Pressure Education Program Working Group report on hypertension in diabetes. Hypertension. 1994;23(2):145-58.
3. Sowers JR, Epstein M. Diabetes mellitus and associated hypertension, vascular disease, and nephropathy. An update. Hypertension. 1995;26(6 Pt 1):869-79.
4. Curb JD, Pressel SL, Cutler JA, et al. Effect of diuretic-based antihypertensive treatment on cardiovascular disease risk in older diabetic patients with isolated systolic hypertension. Systolic Hypertension in the Elderly Program Cooperative Research Group. JAMA. 1996;276(23):1886-92.
5. Grimm RH, Flack JM, Grandits GA, et al. Long-term effects on plasma lipids of diet and drugs to treat hypertension. Treatment of Mild Hypertension Study (TOMHS) Research Group. JAMA. 1996;275(20):1549-56.
6. Lindholm LH. The outcome of STOP-Hypertension-2 in relation to the 1999 WHO/ISH hypertension guidelines. Blood Pressure. 2000;2 Suppl:21-4.

7. Hansson L, Lindholm LH, Niskanen L, et al. Effect of angiotensin-converting-enzyme inhibition compared with conventional therapy on cardiovascular morbidity and mortality in hypertension: the Captopril Prevention Project (CAPPP) randomised trial. Lancet. 1999;353(9153):611-6.
8. Heart Outcomes Prevention Evaluation Study Investigators, Yusuf S, Sleight P, et al. Effects of an angiotensin-converting-enzyme inhibitor, ramipril, on cardiovascular events in high-risk patients. N Engl J Med. 2000;342(3):145-53.
9. Sowers JR, Bakris GL. Antihypertensive therapy and the risk of type 2 diabetes mellitus. N Engl J Med. 2000;342(13):969-70.
10. Hansson L, Zanchetti A, Carruthers SG, et al. Effects of intensive blood-pressure lowering and low-dose aspirin in patients with hypertension: principal results of the Hypertension Optimal Treatment (HOT) randomised trial. HOT Study Group. Lancet. 1998;351(9118):1755-62.
11. Tuomilehto J, Rastenyte D, Birkenhäger WH, et al. Effects of calcium-channel blockade in older patients with diabetes and systolic hypertension. Systolic Hypertension in Europe Trial Investigators. N Engl J Med. 1999;340(9):677-84.
12. Tight blood pressure control and risk of macrovascular and microvascular complications in type 2 diabetes: UKPDS 38. UK Prospective Diabetes Study Group. BMJ. 1998;317(7160):703-13.
13. Efficacy of atenolol and captopril in reducing risk of macrovascular and microvascular complications in type 2 diabetes: UKPDS 39. UK Prospective Diabetes Study Group. BMJ. 1998;317(7160):713-20.
14. Sowers JR, Epstein M. Risk factors for arterial disease in diabetes: hypertension. In: Tooke JE (Ed). Diabetic Angiopathy. London: Arnold Publishers; 1999. pp. 45-63.
15. Kuusisto J, Mykkänen L, Pyörälä K, et al. Hyperinsulinemic microalbuminuria. A new risk indicator for coronary heart disease. Circulation. 1995;91(3):831-7.
16. Dinneen SF, Gerstein HC. The association of microalbuminuria and mortality in non-insulin-dependent diabetes mellitus. A systematic overview of the literature. Arch Intern Med. 1997;157(13):1413-8.
17. Tatti P, Pahor M, Byington RP, et al. Outcome results of the Fosinopril versus Amlodipine Cardiovascular Events Randomized Trial (FACET) in patients with hypertension and NIDDM. Diabetes Care. 1998;21(4):579-603.
18. Sowers JR. Comorbidity of hypertension and diabetes: the fosinopril versus amlodipine cardiovascular events trial (FACET). Am J Cardiol. 1998;82(9B):15R-19.
19. Sowers JR, Reed J. 1999 Clinical Advisory Treatment of Hypertension and Diabetes. J Clin Hypertens (Greenwich). 2000;2(2):132-3.
20. Effects of ramipril on cardiovascular and microvascular outcomes in peoples with diabetes mellitus: results of the HOPE study and MICRO-HOPE substudy. Heart Outcomes Prevention Evaluation Study Investigators. Lancet. 2000;355(9200):253-9.
21. Fogari R, Zoppi A, Lazzari P, et al. ACE inhibition but not angiotensin II antagonism reduces plasma fibrinogen and insulin resistance in overweight hypertensive patients. J Cardiovasc Pharmacol. 1998;32(4):616-20.
22. Caldiz CI, de Cingolani GE. Insulin resistance in adipocytes from spontaneously hypertensive rats: effect of long-term treatment with enalapril and losartan. Metabolism. 1999;48(8):1041-6.
23. Folli F, Kahn CR, Hansen H, et al. Angiotensin II inhibits insulin signaling in aortic smooth muscle cell at multiple levels. A potential role for serine phosphorylation in insulin/angiotensin II crosstalk. J Clin Invest. 1997;100(9):2158-69.
24. Velloso LA, Folli F, Sun XJ, et al. Cross-talk between the insulin and angiotensin signaling systems. Proc Natl Acad Sci USA. 1996;93(22):12490-5.
25. Richey JM, Ader M, Moore D, et al. Angiotensin II induces insulin resistance independent of changes in interstitial insulin. Am J Physiol. 1999;277(5):E920-6.
26. Somwar R, Sumitani S, Taha C, et al. Temporal activation of p70 S6 kinase and Akt1 by insulin: PI 3-kinase-dependent and -independent mechanisms. Am J Physiol. 1998;275(4 Pt 1):E618-25.
27. Li D, Sweeney G, Wang Q, et al. Participation of PI3K and atypical PKC in Na^+ -K^+-pump stimulation by IGF-1 in VSMC. Am J Physiol. 1999;276(6):H2109-16.
28. Nawano M, Anai M, Funaki M, et al. Imidapril, an angiotensin-converting enzyme inhibitor, improves insulin sensitivity by enhancing signal transduction via insulin receptor substrate proteins and improving vascular resistance in the Zucker fatty rat. Metabolism. 1999;48(10):1248-55.
29. Erdös EG, Deddish PA, Marcic BM. Potentiation of Bradykinin Actions by ACE Inhibitors. Trends Endocrinol Metab. 1999;10(6):223-9.
30. Henriksen EJ, Jacob S, Kinnick TR, et al. ACE inhibition and glucose transport in insulinresistant muscle: roles of bradykinin and nitric oxide. Am J Physiol. 1999;277(1 Pt 2):R332-6.
31. Haffner SM, Lehto S, Rönnemaa T, et al. Mortality from coronary heart disease in subjects with type 2 diabetes and in nondiabetic subjects with and without myocardial infarction. N Engl J Med. 1998;339(4):229-34.
32. Sowers JR. Diabetes mellitus and cardiovascular disease in women. Arch Intern Med. 1998;158(6):617-21.
33. Garcia MJ, McNamara PM, Gordon T, et al. Morbidity and mortality in diabetes in the Framingham population. Sixteen year follow-up study. Diabetes. 1974;23(2):105-11.
34. Stamler J, Vaccaro O, Neaton JD, et al. Diabetes, other risk factors, and 12-yr cardiovascular mortality for men screened in the Multiple Risk Factor Intervention Trial. Diabetes Care. 1993;16(2):434-44.
35. Frohlich ED. Uric acid: a risk factor for coronary artery disease. JAMA. 1993;270:354-9.
36. Brown RA, Filipovich P, Walsh MF, et al. Influence of sex, diabetes and ethanol on intrinsic contractile performance of isolated rat myocardium. Basic Res Cardiol. 1996;91(5):353-60.
37. Ren J, Dominguez LJ, Sowers JR, et al. Troglitazone attenuates high-glucose-induced abnormalities in relaxation and intracellular calcium in rat ventricular myocytes. Diabetes. 1996;45(12):1822-5.
38. Ren J, Sowers JR, Walsh MF, et al. Reduced contractile response to insulin and IGF-1 in ventricular myocytes from genetically obese Zucker rats. Am J Physiol. 2000;279(4):H1708-14.
39. Wong DW, Kiyosue T, Shigematsu S, et al. Abnormalities of K^+ and Ca^{2+} currents in ventricular myocytes from rats with chronic diabetes. Am J Physiol. 1998;269(4 Pt 2):H1288-96.
40. Shimoni Y, Ewart HS, Severson D. Insulin stimulation of rat ventricular K^+ currents depends on the integrity of the cytoskeleton. J Physiol (Lond). 1999;514(Pt 3):735-45.
41. Casis O, Gallego M, Iriarte M, et al. Effects of diabetic cardiomyopathy on regional electrophysiologic characteristics of rat ventricle. Diabetologia. 2000;43(1):101-9.
42. Golfman L, Dixon IM, Takeda N, et al. Cardiac sarcolemmal Na^+-Ca^{2+} exchange and Na^+-K^+ ATPase activities and gene expression in alloxan-induced diabetes in rats. Mol Cell Biochem. 1998;188(1-2):91-101.
43. Ziegelhöffer A, Ravingerová T, Styk J, et al. Mechanisms that may be involved in calcium tolerance of the diabetic heart. Mol Cell Biochem. 1997;176(1-2):191-8.
44. Matsubara H, Kanasaki M, Murasawa S, et al. Differential gene expression and regulation of angiotensin II receptor subtypes in rat cardiac fibroblasts and cardiomyocytes in culture. J Clin Invest. 1994;93(4):1592-601.
45. Schaffer SW, Ballard-Croft C, Boerth S, et al. Mechanisms underlying depressed Na^+/Ca^{2+} exchanger activity in the diabetic heart. Cardiovasc Res. 1997;34(1):129-36.
46. Giles TD, Ouyang J, Kerut K, et al. Changes in protein kinase C in early cardiomyopathy and in gracilis muscle in the BB/W or diabetic rat. Am J Physiol. 1998;274(1):H295-307.

47. Ren J, Samson WK, Sowers JR. Insulin-like growth factor I as a cardiac hormone: physiological and pathophysiological implications in heart disease. J Mol Cell Cardiol. 1999;31(11): 2049-61.
48. Cittadini A, Ishiguro Y, Strömer H, et al. Insulin-like growth factor-1 but not growth hormone augments mammalian myocardial contractility by sensitizing the myofilament to Ca^{2+} through a wortmannin-sensitive pathway: studies in rat and ferret isolated muscles. Circ Res. 1998;83(1):50-9.
49. LeRoith D. Insulin-like growth factors. N Engl J Med. 1998;336: 633-40.
50. Kolter T, Uphues I, Eckel J. Molecular analysis of insulin resistance in isolated ventricular cardiomyocytes of obese Zucker rats. Am J Physiol. 1997;273(1):E59-67.
51. Guo W, Kada K, Kamiya K, et al. IGF-1 regulates K(+)-channel expression of cultured neonatal rat ventricular myocytes. Am J Physiol. 1997;272(6):H2599-606.
52. Grossman E, Shemesh J, Shamiss A, et al. Left ventricular mass in diabetes-hypertension. Arch Intern Med. 1992;152(5): 1001-4.
53. Taal MW, Brenner BM. Renoprotective benefits of RAS inhibition: from ACEI to angiotensin II antagonists. Kidney Int. 2000;57(5): 1803-17.
54. Bianchi S, Bigazzi R, Quiñones Galvan A, et al. Insulin resistance in microalbuminuric hypertension. Sites and mechanisms. Hypertension. 1995;26(5):789-95.
55. Pinkney JH, Foyle WJ, Denver AE, et al. The relationship of urinary albumin excretion rate to ambulatory blood pressure and erythrocyte sodium-lithium countertransport in NIDDM. Diabetologia. 1995;38(3):356-62.
56. Mitchell TH, Nolan B, Henry M, et al. Microalbuminuria in patients with non-insulin-dependent diabetes mellitus relates to nocturnal systolic blood pressure. Am J Med. 1997;102(6):531-5.
57. Sowers JR, Lester M. Diabetes and cardiovascular disease. Diabetes Care. 1999;22(Suppl 3):C14-20.
58. Feldman RD. The Canadian recommendations for the management of hypertension: on behalf of the Task Force for the Development of the 1999 Canadian Recommendations for the Management of Hypertension. Can J Cardiol. 1999;15:S57G-64.
59. Ravid M, Lang R, Rachmani R, et al. Long-term renoprotective effect of angiotensin-converting enzyme inhibition in non-insulin-dependent diabetes mellitus: A 7-year follow-up study. Arch Intern Med. 1996;156(3):286-9.
60. Colwell JA. Aspirin therapy in diabetes. Diabetes Care. 1997;20:1767-71.
61. Sowers JR, Epstein M, Frohlich ED. Diabetes, hypertension, and cardiovascular disease: an update. Hypertension. 2001;37(4):1053-9.

CHAPTER

Cardiodiabetes and Obstructive Sleep Apnea

Avi Kumar, Tanu Satija, HK Chopra

INTRODUCTION

Global prevalence of obesity has been increasingly exponentially, creating a global health crisis. About 500 million adults have been suffering from obesity worldwide, with prevalence rates constantly increasing in young and adolescents.[1] Obesity has been associated with lot of chronic diseases, notably cardiovascular diseases (CVD), diabetes, and sleep-disordered breathing (SDB).[2] Peppard PE et al. observed that 20% of the adult population aged 30–70 years and approximately one-third of those aged between 50 years and 70 years had SDB with an apnea-hypopnea index (AHI) of ≥15/h.[3] Obstructive sleep apnea (OSA) is most common form of SDB in general population, which leads to collapse of pharynx during sleep with consequent upper airway obstruction. In 2000, large prospective epidemiological study reported that a 10% weight gain led to a six-fold increase in the odds of developing moderate-to-severe OSA, independent of confounding factors.[4] Significant relationship has been found between OSA and most forms of cardiovascular disease,[5,6] cancer, chronic obstructive pulmonary disease (COPD),[7] stroke,[8] and type II diabetes mellitus (DM).[9] Although obesity occupies a central position in causation and has been notifiable risk factor for OSA, insulin resistance (IR) and particularly CVD, current evidence suggests that OSA itself is an independent risk factor for both IR and CVD (Table 1).[2]

OBSTRUCTIVE SLEEP APNEA AND CARDIOVASCULAR DISEASES: AN INTERTWISTING TALE

The entire spectrum of CVD notably coronary artery disease (CAD), arterial hypertension, congestive heart failure (HF), and arrhythmias are strongly associated with OSA. Intermittent hypoxia with fragmentation of normal sleep contributes to significant autonomic dysfunction plus proinflammatory and procoagulopathy states, leading to IR and CVD, as has been described in Table 2.[2] Repetitive hypoxia due to airway obstruction, concomitant activation of sympathetic neural activity (SNA), hemodynamic disturbances, and sleep disruption are the known pathogenic mechanisms leading to cardiovascular consequences.[10-14] OSA induces pan inflammatory response with increased levels of key inflammatory mediators such as tumor necrosis factor-alpha, C-reactive protein, and chemokines. Figure 1[15] shows the possible mechanisms involved in OSA and the associated cardiovascular adverse effects.

Obstructive Sleep Apnea and Coronary Artery Disease

Danzi Soares NJ et al.[16] documented OSA in 87% of CAD patients referred for coronary artery bypass graft surgery.

TABLE 1: Summary of cross-sectional prevalence and prospective incidence epidemiological trials that show an independent link between severe obstructive sleep apnea and cardiovascular risk[2]

	Cross-sectional prevalence	*Prospective incidence*	*Interventional*
Hypertension	Yes	Yes (not in elderly)	Yes, but small
Insulin resistance	Yes	Conflicting data	Yes, nondiabetic
Ischemic heart disease	Yes	Yes	Not available
Atrial fibrillation	Yes	Not available	Not available
Heart failure	Yes	Yes	Yes
Stroke	Yes	Yes	Not available
Mortality	Yes	Yes (uncertain in elderly)	Not available

TABLE 2: Schematic summary of precipitating factors towards obstructive sleep apnea with physiological consequences and downstream cardiovascular consequences

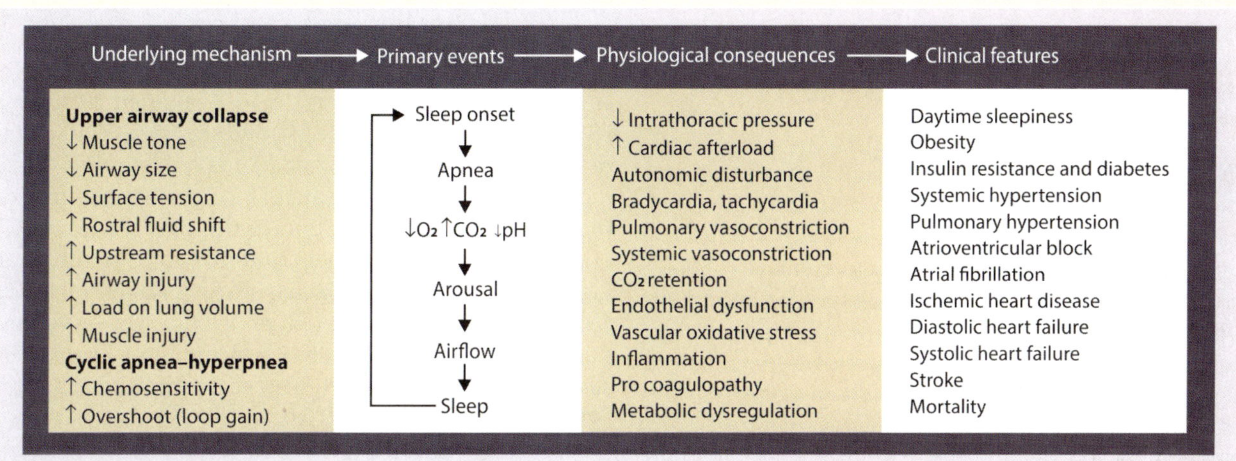

Underlying mechanism →	Primary events →	Physiological consequences →	Clinical features
Upper airway collapse ↓ Muscle tone ↓ Airway size ↓ Surface tension ↑ Rostral fluid shift ↑ Upstream resistance ↑ Airway injury ↑ Load on lung volume ↑ Muscle injury **Cyclic apnea–hyperpnea** ↑ Chemosensitivity ↑ Overshoot (loop gain)	Sleep onset ↓ Apnea ↓ ↓O_2 ↑CO_2 ↓pH ↓ Arousal ↓ Airflow ↓ Sleep	↓ Intrathoracic pressure ↑ Cardiac afterload Autonomic disturbance Bradycardia, tachycardia Pulmonary vasoconstriction Systemic vasoconstriction CO_2 retention Endothelial dysfunction Vascular oxidative stress Inflammation Pro coagulopathy Metabolic dysregulation	Daytime sleepiness Obesity Insulin resistance and diabetes Systemic hypertension Pulmonary hypertension Atrioventricular block Atrial fibrillation Ischemic heart disease Diastolic heart failure Systolic heart failure Stroke Mortality

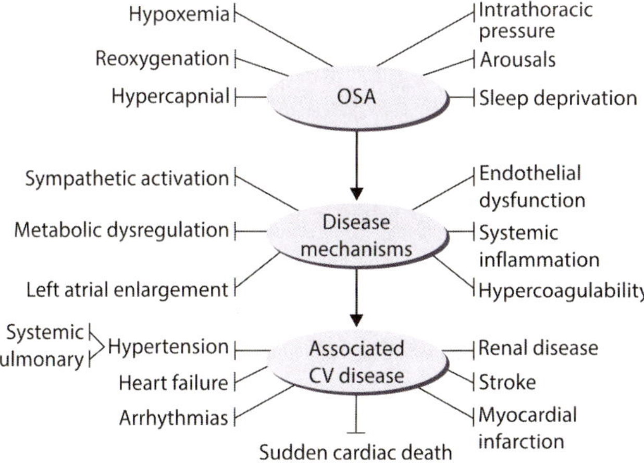

Fig. 1: Pathophysiological components of obstructive sleep apnea (OSA), activation of cardiovascular disease mechanisms, and consequent cardiovascular disease

In revascularized CAD cohort group, Glanzt H, et al.[17] observed higher prevalence of OSA than that of obesity hypertension, diabetes, and atrial fibrillation (AF). Peker Y et al.[18] conducted 7-year follow-up of the Gothenburg Sleep Cohort, and observed CAD in 16% patients with SDB (defined as ≥30 oxygen desaturation events per hour) compared with 5.4% of patients without SDB, with reduced rates of CAD among those with SDB who used CPAP. A Spanish observational study[19] profounded that patients with untreated severe SDB had a 2.9-fold increased risk of fatal and 3.2-fold increased risk of nonfatal cardiovascular events compared with healthy participants. The Sleep Heart Health Study[5] showed that men aged 40–70 years with an AHI of more than or equal to 30/hr had 68% higher propensity to develop CAD compared with those who had an AHI of less than 5/hr. The prevalence of moderate-to-severe sleep apnea (AHI ≥15/hr) was as high as 55% in one

German center, first few days after an acute myocardial infarction (MI).[20] In longer-term studies, SDB in patients with CAD was associated with a significant increase in the composite endpoint of death, MI, and cerebrovascular events at a 5-year median follow-up interval. This composite endpoint occurred in 28% of men with SDB and in 16% of men without SDB. The corresponding percentages for women were 20% and 14 %.[21]

Milleron O et al. observed decrease in the occurrence of new cardiovascular events on treatment of OSA, in patients with combined OSA and CAD.[22] However, McEvoy RD et al. conducted a randomized trial of CPAP therapy in 2,717 men with moderate-to-severe sleep apnea with cardiovascular disease. The Sleep Apnea Cardiovascular Endpoints (SAVE) trial reported no significant reduction in cardiovascular events.[23]

Obstructive Sleep Apnea and Hypertension

International guidelines have profounded the role of OSA in the pathogenesis of hypertension.[15] An estimated 30% of hypertensive patients have OSA and about half-OSA patients have been reported to be hypertensive.[24] Logan MG et al. have found OSA in 80% of severely refractory hypertensive patients.[25] OSA has been implicated in preceding and predicting the onset of hypertension. Longitudinal data from Wisconsin Sleep Cohort Study, propagated consistent linear OSA-blood pressure (OSA-BP) dose-response relationship, even after controlling for age, sex, body mass index (BMI), and antihypertensive medications.[26] There have been plenty of cross-sectional studies supporting directly proportional relationship between sleep-disordered breathing and hypertension independent of obesity.[27]

Nondippers having attenuated nocturnal BP decline, may be more likely to have coexisting OSA.[28] The most common mechanism for attenuation of nocturnal dipping of BP has been activation of nocturnal sympathetic system.[29] Repetitive upper airway obstruction, intermittent negative intrathoracic pressure swings, sleep deprivation, and recurrent episodes of hypoxemia and hypercapnia, have been implicated in chronically elevated BP even during nonsleep periods.[20] Increased aldosterone has been suggested as a possible contributor to resistant hypertension in sleep apnea.

Recently, Fava C et al. had a meta-analysis of 32 randomized controlled trials (RCTs), and found significant mean reduction in daytime and night-time systolic and diastolic BP with CPAP. They found relationship between baseline OSA severity and the beneficial effects of CPAP on BP, with the greatest reductions seen in those with more severe OSA ($\beta \pm$ standard error, 0.08 ± 0.04).[30] In patients with OSA and refractory hypertension Liu L et al. reported pooled reductions of 4.78 and 2.95 mm Hg in 24-hour ambulatory systolic and diastolic BP, respectively.[31] Schwarz EI found significant relationship between OSA severity and the extent of BP increase in response to CPAP withdrawal.[32]

Obstructive Sleep Apnea and Heart Failure

The Sleep Heart Health Study propagated OSA as an independent risk factor for the development of HF. The prevalence of OSA in HF was greater in men (38% versus 31%; $p<0.005$).[20] The prevalence of SDB in patients with HF with preserved or reduced ejection fraction is around 75% and about 50% of these patients have moderate-to-severe sleep apnea.[33] Chan J et al. evaluated 20 subjects with symptomatic diastolic HF and reported SDB, mainly obstructive apneas in 55% of patients.[34]

Several pathologic mechanisms have been implicated that shows OSA contribution to the progression of HF: (1) by eliciting greater sympathetic traffic to the heart, kidney, and resistance vessels during wakefulness and sleep[35]; (2) by increasing left ventricular (LV) afterload, both acutely and chronically; (3) by inducing hypoxia and secondary increases in right ventricular afterload; and (4) by increasing the risk of MI.

Recent randomized trials reported significant improvements in LV ejection fraction (LVEF) after 1 month and 3 months and improved quality of life, exercise capacity and autonomic control, after CPAP therapy in patients with OSA and HF.[36] The 2010 HF Society of America Comprehensive HF guidelines and the 2013 American College of Cardiology Foundation (ACCF)/American Heart Association (AHA) guidelines recommended that HF patients with OSA should receive treatment for sleep apnea to improve their HF status.[15] Recent observational data by Wang et al. suggested lower mortality rate in HF patients with CPAP-treated OSA as compared with untreated OSA.[37]

Obstructive Sleep Apnea and Arrhythmias

Prevalence of sleep apnea is high in arrhythmias, especially AF. Bitter T et al. reported SDB in nearly half of the patients with paroxysmal or persistent AF.[38] About 75% of AF patients presenting for electrical cardioversion had been reported to have SDB.[40] The Sleep Heart Health Study analyzed

228 subjects with sleep-disordered breathing (respiratory disturbance index ≥ 30) and 338 subjects without sleep-disordered breathing (respiratory disturbance index <5). Sleep-disordered breathing had a higher incidence of arrhythmias as compared with those without sleep-disordered breathing, namely, 4.8 versus 0.9% (p = 0.003) for AF; 5.3 versus 1.2% (p = 0.004) for nonsustained ventricular tachycardia; 25.0 versus 14.5% (p = 0.002) for complex ventricular ectopy. The study reported 4 times the odds of AF (odds ratio [OR], 4.02; 95% confidence interval [CI], 1.03–15.74), 3 times the odds of nonsustained ventricular tachycardia (OR, 3.40; 95% CI, 1.03–11.20), and almost twice the odds of complex ventricular ectopy (OR, 1.74; 95% CI, 1.11–2.74) in patients with SDB.[40]

Hypoxemia, sympathetic activation, pressor surges, transmural pressure changes, and systemic inflammation commonly seen in OSA, have also been implicated in the development of AF.[15] Stevenson IH et al. reported an OR of 3 for having AF in moderate OSA patients. Recently, Ng CY et al. meta-analysis of six studies with a total of 3,995 patients and reported 25% greater risk of AF recurrence after catheter ablation in OSA patients (risk ratio 1.25, 95% CI 1.08–1.45, p = 0.003).[41] The relationship between OSA and AF has been highlighted by AF management guidelines.[42] Screening for sleep apnea in such patients is reasonable, and in OSA patients, treatment with CPAP may maximize the effectiveness of other rhythm-control strategies.

Ventricular arrhythmias, primarily premature ventricular contractions, have been reported in upto 66% of patients with sleep apnea.[43] In most OSA patients, ventricular arrhythmias have been reported mostly during sleep, especially during apneic periods.[44] Hypoxemia, bradyarrhythmias, and sympathetic activation induced by apneic events have been implicated as possible mechanisms in causation of ventricular arrhythmias in OSA. Treatment of OSA may decrease the incidence and severity of ventricular arrhythmias. Recently published RCT reported 58% reduction in the frequency of ventricular premature complexes during sleep as well as reduction in nocturnal urinary norepinephrine concentrations on treatment of OSA by CPAP.[45]

OBSTRUCTIVE SLEEP APNEA AND DIABETES

Sleep-disordered breathing has been commonly linked with IR and type 2 DM. Atleast two-third of type 2 diabetes patients had been reported to have mild OSA. A cross-sectional study from 1,387 participants in the Wisconsin Sleep Cohort identified greater prevalence of diabetes (14.7%) in subjects with an AHI of 15 or greater as compared with subjects with an AHI of less than 5 (2.8%). The OR for having physician-diagnosed DM in patients with an AHI of 15 versus an AHI of less than 5 was 4.75 (95% CI, 2.62–8.63; p < 0.0001) when adjusted for age and sex. They also found that the OR for developing DM with an AHI of 15 or greater compared with an AHI of less than 5 was 4.06.[46] Several cross-sectional studies have indicated that increasing levels of AHI are independently associated with worsened IR and glucose intolerance. In a cross-sectional study conducted by Meslier N on 595 male patients, type-2 diabetes was present in 30.1% of OSA syndrome (OSAS) patients and 13.9% of nonapneic snorers. They also reported impaired glucose intolerance (IGT) in 20.0% of OSAS patients and 13.9% of nonapneic snorers.[47]

A number of pathophysiological mechanisms had been implicated in causation of IR in OSA patients. The common culprits of the physiologic stress involved in pathogenesis of IR had been identified as intermittent hypoxia and/or sleep fragmentation. Sympathetic nervous system activation due to nocturnal hypoxia as well as sleep fragmentation had been involved in glucose and fat metabolism, further contributing to IR and type 2 DM. Stamatakis K et al. had reported decreased insulin sensitivity and impaired glucose tolerance due to sleep deprivation and intermittent hypoxia. Hypothalamic-pituitary-adrenal (HPA) axis alterations leading to elevation of cortisol levels due to nocturnal hypoxia, had been known to influence insulin sensitivity and insulin secretion. Activation of inflammatory markers as well as changes in adipokine profiles seen in OSA has been known to add to IR and glucose intolerance.[48] Figure 2 shows the possible mechanisms linking sleep apnea with glucose intolerance.

A lot of studies had been conducted to determine improvement of glycemic control with treatment of OSA with CPAP. Iftikhar IH et al. recently did meta-analysis of five RCTs (four with crossover design), and reported improved IR on CPAP treatment in subjects with OSA without diabetes.[49] In 2015, an updated meta-analysis of RCTs was conducted on the effect of continuous CPAP on IR, as measured by homeostasis model assessment of IR (HOMA-IR), visceral abdominal fat (VAF), and adiponectin. They suggested significant difference in HOMA-IR (-0.43 [95% CIs: -0.75--0.11], p = 0.008), and no significant difference in VAF or adiponectin between CPAP treated and non-CPAP treated participants.[50] There was clear evidence of favorable effect of CPAP on IR. Some studies suggest the variable effects of CPAP on glucose control may relate to duration of CPAP treatment (potentially >3 months) and that the effects may be greatest in patients who are less obese.

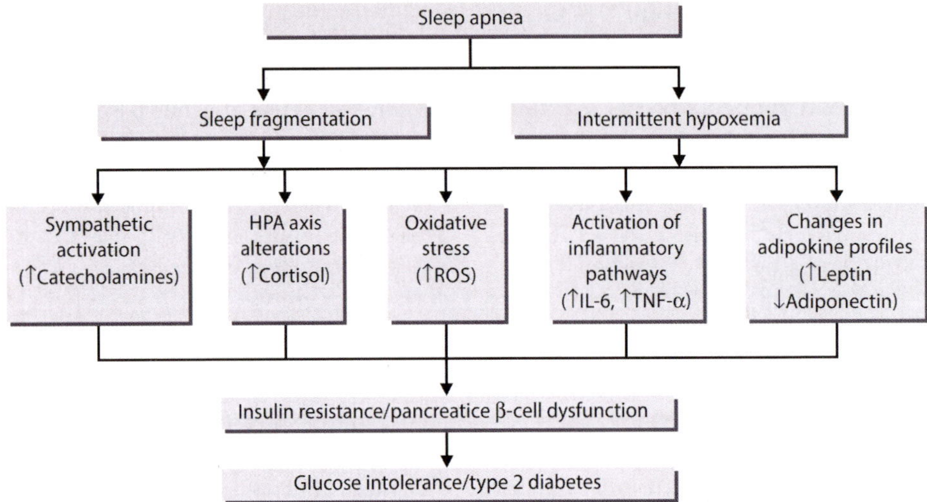

Fig. 2: Potential mechanisms linking obstructive sleep apnea (OSA) and glucose intolerance

Abbreviations: ROS, reactive oxygen species; TNF, tumor necrosis factor

CONCLUSION

The high prevalence of OSA, and its direct intertwisting link with a lot of chronic conditions, which adds to considerable morbidity and mortality, suggests early recognition and treatment of OSA. With the advent of CPAP and its positive impact on the disease itself and quality of life, provides a new opportunity to reduce the severity of OSA and its allied diseases. Timely therapeutic intervention for OSA in cardiodiabetes has a huge impact in morbidity and mortality reduction.

REFERENCES

1. Finucane MM, Stevens GA, Cowan MJ, et al. National, regional, and global trends in body-mass index since 1980: systematic analysis of health examination surveys and epidemiological studies with 960 country-years and 9.1 million participants. Lancet. 2011;377(9765):557-67.
2. Hamilton GS, Naughton MT. Impact of obstructive sleep apnea on diabetes and cardiovascular disease. Med J Aust. 2013;199(8): S27-30.
3. Peppard PE, Young T, Barnet JH, et al. Increased prevalence of sleep disordered breathing in adults. Am J Epidemiol. 2013;177(9):1006-14.
4. Peppard PE, Young T, Palta M, et al. Longitudinal study of moderate weight change and sleep-disordered breathing. JAMA. 2000;284(23):3015-21.
5. Gottlieb DJ, Yenokyan G, Newman AB, et al. Prospective study of obstructive sleep apnea and incident coronary heart disease and heart failure: the Sleep Heart Health Study. Circulation. 2010;122(4):352-60.
6. Lee CH, Sethi R, Li R, et al. Obstructive sleep apnea and cardiovascular events after percutaneous coronary intervention. Circulation. 2016;133(21):2008-17.
7. Shawon MS, Perret JL, Senaratna CV, et al. Current evidence on prevalence and clinical outcomes of comorbid obstructive sleep apnea and chronic obstructive pulmonary disease: a systematic review. Sleep Med Rev. 2017;32:58-68.
8. Dziewas R, Humpert M, Hopmann B, et al. Increased prevalence of sleep apnea in patients with recurring ischemic stroke compared with first stroke victims. J Neurol. 2005;252(11):1394-8.
9. Punjabi NM, Shahar E, Redline S, et al. Sleep-disordered breathing, glucose intolerance, and insulin resistance: the Sleep Heart Health Study. Am J Epidemiol. 2004;160(6):521-30.
10. Bagai K. Obstructive sleep apnea, stroke, and cardiovascular diseases. Neurologist. 2010;16(6):329-39.
11. Bradley TD, Floras JS. Obstructive sleep apnoea and its cardiovascular consequences. Lancet. 2009;373(9657):82-93.
12. Leung RS, Comondore VR, Ryan CM, et al. Mechanisms of sleep-disordered breathing: causes and consequences. Pflugers Arch. 2012;463(1):213-30.
13. Sharma S, Kavuru M. Sleep and metabolism: an overview. Int J Endocrinol.2010;2010:270832.
14. Tasali E, Ip MS. Obstructive sleep apnea and metabolic syndrome: alterations in glucose metabolism and inflammation. Proc Am Thorac Soc. 2008;5(2):207-17.
15. Somers VK, Amin R, Abraham WT, et al. AHA/ACCF scientific statement sleep apnea and cardiovascular disease. Circulation. 2008;118:1080-111.
16. Danzi-Soares NJ, Genta PR, Nerbass FB, et al. Obstructive sleep apnea is common among patients referred for coronary artery bypass grafting and can be diagnosed by portable monitoring. Coron Artery Dis. 2012;23(1):31-8.
17. Glantz H, Thunstrom E, Herlitz J, et al. Occurrence and predictors of obstructive sleep apnea in a revascularized coronary artery disease cohort. Ann Am Thorac Soc. 2013;10(4):350-6.
18. Peker Y, Hedner J, Kraiczi H, et al. Respiratory disturbance index: an independent predictor of mortality in coronary artery disease. Am J Respir Crit Care Med. 2000;162(1):81-6.
19. Marin JM, Carrizo SJ, Vicente E, et al. Long-term cardiovascular outcomes in men with obstructive sleep apnoea-hypopnoea with or without treatment with continuous positive airway pressure: an observational study. Lancet. 2005;365(9464):1046-53.
20. Cowie MR. Sleep apnea: state of art. Trends Cardiovasc Med. 2017;27(4):280-9.

21. Mooe T, Franklin KA, Holmstrom K, et al. Sleep disordered breathing and coronary artery disease: long-term prognosis. Am J Respir Crit Care Med. 2001;164(10 pt 1):1910-3.
22. Milleron O, Pilliere R, Foucher A, et al. Benefits of obstructive sleep apnoea treatment in coronary artery disease: a long-term follow-up study. Eur Heart J. 2004;25(9):728-34.
23. McEvoy RD, Antic NA, Heeley E, et al. CPAP for prevention of cardiovascular events in obstructive sleep apnea. N Engl J Med. 2016;375(10):919-31.
24. Somers VK, White DP, Amin R, et al. Sleep apnea and cardiovascular disease: an American Heart Association/American College of Cardiology Foundation Scientific Statement from the American Heart Association Council for High Blood Pressure Research Professional Education Committee, Council on Clinical Cardiology, Stroke Council, and Council on Cardiovascular Nursing. J Am Coll Cardiol. 2008;52(8):686-717.
25. Logan AG, Tkacova R, Perlikowski SM, et al. Refractory hypertension and sleep apnoea: effect of CPAP on blood pressure and baroreflex. Eur Respir J. 2003;21(2):241-7.
26. Peppard PE, Young T, Palta M, et al. Prospective study of the association between sleep-disordered breathing and hypertension. N Engl J Med. 2000;342:1378-84.
27. Harrington RA, Narula J, Eapen ZJ, et al. Sleep-disordered breathing and cardiac disease. In: Cowie MR, Fuster V, Harrington R (Eds). Hurst's the Heart, 14th edition. New York, USA: McGraw-Hill; 2017.
28. Portaluppi F, Provini F, Cortelli P, et al. Undiagnosed sleep-disordered breathing among male nondippers with essential hypertension. J Hypertens. 1997;15(11):1227-33.
29. Somers VK, Dyken ME, Clary MP, et al. Sympathetic neural mechanisms in obstructive sleep apnea. J Clin Invest. 1995;96(4):1897-904.
30. Fava C, Dorigoni S, DalleVedove F, et al. Effect of CPAP on blood pressure in patients with OSA/hypopnea a systematic review and meta- analysis. Chest. 2014;145:762-71.
31. Liu L, Cao Q, Guo Z, et al. Continuous positive airway pressure in patients with obstructive sleep apnea and resistant hypertension: a meta-analysis of randomized controlled trials. J Clin Hypertens (Greenwich). 2016;18(2):153-8.
32. Schwarz EI, Schlatzer C, Rossi VA, et al. Effect of CPAP withdrawal on blood pressure in OSA: data from three randomized controlled trials. Chest. 2016;150:1202-10.
33. Oldenburg O, Lamp B, Faber L, et al. Sleep-disordered breathing in patients with symptomatic heart failure: a contemporary study of prevalence in and characteristics of 700 patients. Eur J Heart Fail. 2007;9(3):251-7.
34. Chan J, Sanderson J, Chan W, et al. Prevalence of sleep-disordered breathing in diastolic heart failure. Chest. 1997;111(6):1488-93.
35. Spaak J, Egri ZJ, Kubo T, et al. Muscle sympathetic nerve activity during wakefulness in heart failure patients with and without sleep apnea. Hypertension. 2005;46(6):1327-32.
36. Mansfield DR, Gollogly NC, Kaye DM, et al. Controlled trial of continuous positive airway pressure in obstructive sleep apnea and heart failure. Am J Respir Crit Care Med. 2004;169(3):361-6.
37. Wang H, Parker JD, Newton GE, et al. Influence of obstructive sleep apnea on mortality in patients with heart failure. J Am Coll Cardiol. 2007;49(15):1625-31.
38. Bitter T, Westerheide N, Faber L, et al. Adaptive servoventilation in diastolic heart failure and Cheyne-Stokes respiration. Eur Respir J. 2010;36(2):385-92.
39. Bitter T, Faber L, Hering D, et al. Sleep-disordered breathing in heart failure with normal left ventricular ejection fraction. Eur J Heart Fail. 2009;11(6):602-8.
40. Mehra R, Benjamin EJ, Shahar E, et al. Association of nocturnal arrhythmias with sleep-disordered breathing: The Sleep Heart Health Study. Am J Respir Crit Care Med. 2006;173:910-6.
41. Ng CY, Liu T, Shehata M, et al. Meta-analysis of obstructive sleep apnea as predictor of atrial fibrillation recurrence after catheter ablation. Am J Cardiol. 2011;108(1):47-51.
42. Calkins H, Kuck KH, Cappato R, et al. Heart Rhythm Society Task Force on Catheter and Surgical Ablation of Atrial Fibrillation: 2012 HRS /EHRA /ECAS expert consensus statement on catheter and surgical ablation of atrial fibrillation: recommendations for patient selection, procedural techniques, patient management and follow-up, definitions, endpoints, and research trial design: a report of the Heart Rhythm Society (HRS) Task Force on Catheter and Surgical Ablation of Atrial Fibrillation. Developed in partnership with the European Heart Rhythm Association (EHRA), a registered branch of the European Society of Cardiology (ESC) and the European Cardiac Arrhythmia Society (ECAS); and in collaboration with the American College of Cardiology (ACC), American Heart Association (AHA), the Asia Pacific Heart Rhythm Society (APHRS), and the Society of Thoracic Surgeons (STS). Endorsed by the governing bodies of the American College of Cardiology Foundation, the American Heart Association, the European Cardiac Arrhythmia Society, the European Heart Rhythm Association, the Society of Thoracic Surgeons, the Asia Pacific Heart Rhythm Society, and the Heart Rhythm Society. Heart Rhythm. 2012;9(4):632-96.
43. Hoffstein V, Mateika S. Cardiac arrhythmias, snoring, and sleep apnea. Chest. 1994;106(2):466-71.
44. Harbison J, O'Reilly P, McNicholas WT. Cardiac rhythm disturbances in the obstructive sleep apnea syndrome: effects of nasal continuous positive airway pressure therapy. Chest. 2000;118(3): 591-5.
45. Ryan CM, Usui K, Floras JS, et al. Effect of continuous positive airway pressure on ventricular ectopy in heart failure patients with obstructive sleep apnoea. Thorax. 2005;60(9):781-5.
46. Reichmuth KJ, Austin D, Skatrud JB, et al. Association of sleep apnea and type II diabetes: a population-based study. Am J Respir Crit Care Med. 2005;172(12):1590-5.
47. Meslier N, Gagnadoux P Giraud, Person C, et al. Impaired glucose insulin metabolism in males with obstructive sleep apnea syndrome. Eur Respir J. 2003;22(1):156-60.
48. Shaw JE, Punjabi NM, Wilding JP, et al. Sleep-disordered breathing and type 2 diabetes A report from the International Diabetes Federation Taskforce on Epidemiology and Prevention. Diabetes Res Clin Pract. 2008;81(1):2-12.
49. Iftikhar IH, Khan MF, Magalang UJ, et al. Meta-analysis: continuous positive airway pressure improves insulin resistance in patients with sleep apnea without diabetes. Ann Am Thorac Soc. 2013;10(2): 115-20.
50. Iftikhar Ih, Hoyos CM, Philips CL et al. Meta-analyses of the Association of Sleep Apnea with Insulin Resistance, and the Effects of CPAP on HOMA-IR, Adiponectin, and Visceral Adipose Fat. J Clin Sleep Med. 2015;11(4):475-85.

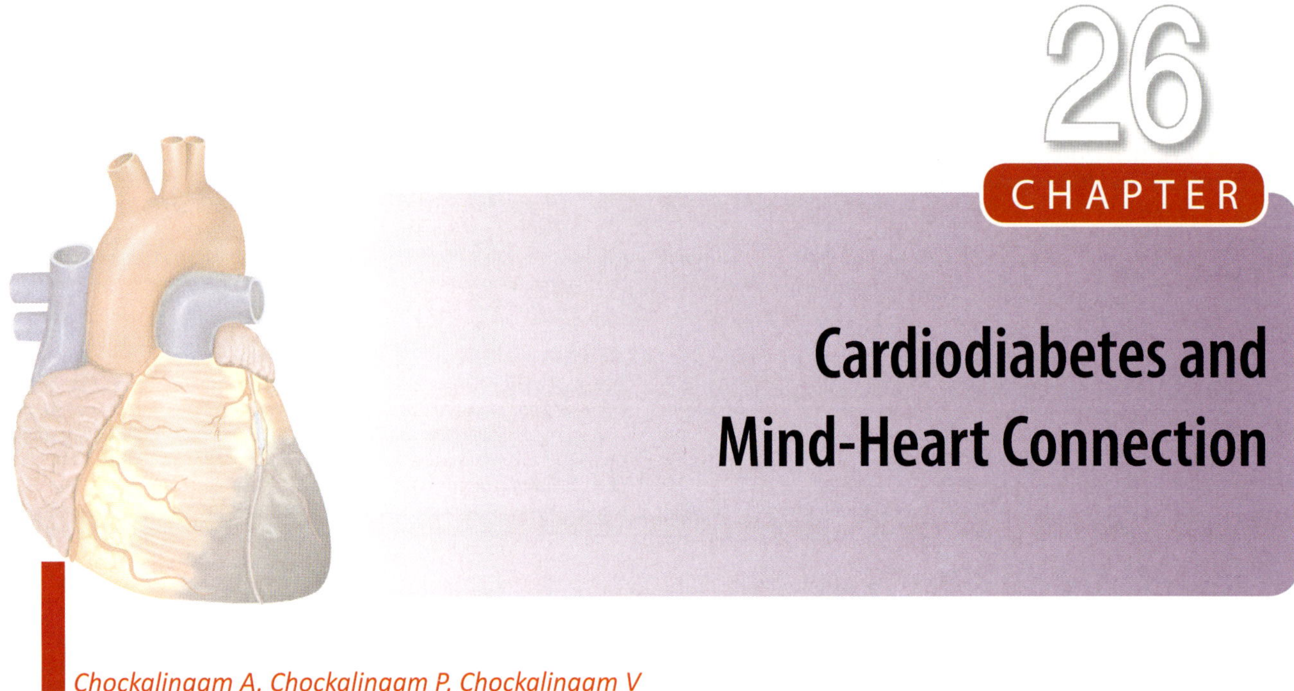

Cardiodiabetes and Mind-Heart Connection

Chockalingam A, Chockalingam P, Chockalingam V

INTRODUCTION

Cardiovascular diseases (CVDs) and diabetes claim about 20 million lives per year worldwide.[1] Currently the leading cause of death globally, CVD, is a lifestyle disease. This means that 90% of CVD can be prevented by lifestyle changes.[2] In India, CVD and diabetes have increased dramatically accounting for about 30% of all deaths.[3] South Asians succumb to CVD at a much younger age than in the West.[4,5] The crucial contribution of the mind-heart connection is increasingly recognized in both causing and treating CVD.

ROLE OF MIND IN CVD CAUSATION

Psychological stressors may be acute, such as natural disasters or bereavement, or chronic, owing to work stress, marital conflict, financial issues, or lack of social support. The emotional factors associated with CVDs are depression, anger, hostility, anxiety and pessimism.[6,7] We have demonstrated the association between subjective stress and acute coronary events.[8] The association between childhood psychosocial wellbeing and its influence on cardiovascular outcomes in adulthood has been recently established.[9,10] Depression is a key risk factor and may cause a twofold increase of CVD.[11] It is believed to affect the heart through inflammatory processes, autonomic nervous system dysfunction, and impaired coronary flow reserve. Bidirectional influences and feedback loops such as physical inactivity lead to an increase in inflammation and depressive symptoms, which are challenging to quantify. There is clear evidence that mindset can cause illness or promote health (Fig. 1).[11]

In stable coronary artery disease (CAD) patients, mental stress-induced myocardial ischemia (MSIMI) is a known entity that is associated with abnormal wall motion and reduced left ventricular ejection fraction, independent of conventional risk factors.[12] Both negative health behaviors

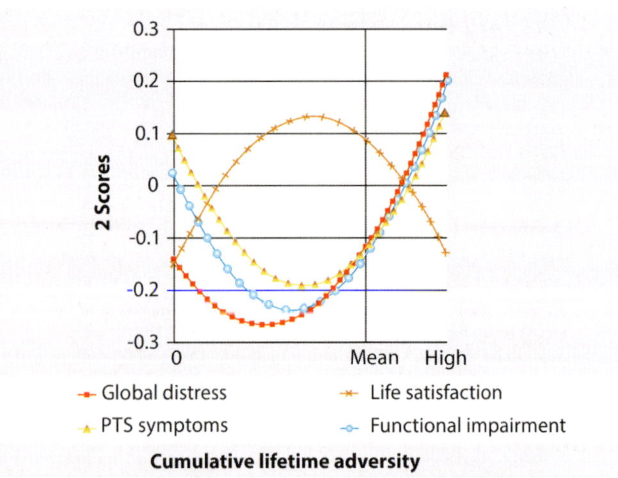

Fig. 1: Behavioral and psychosocial factors are related to CHD. The continuum ranging from positive factors that promote health to negative factors which promote disease are shown here

Source: Rozanski A. Behavioral cardiology: current advances and future directions. J Am Coll Cardiol. 2014;64:100-10.

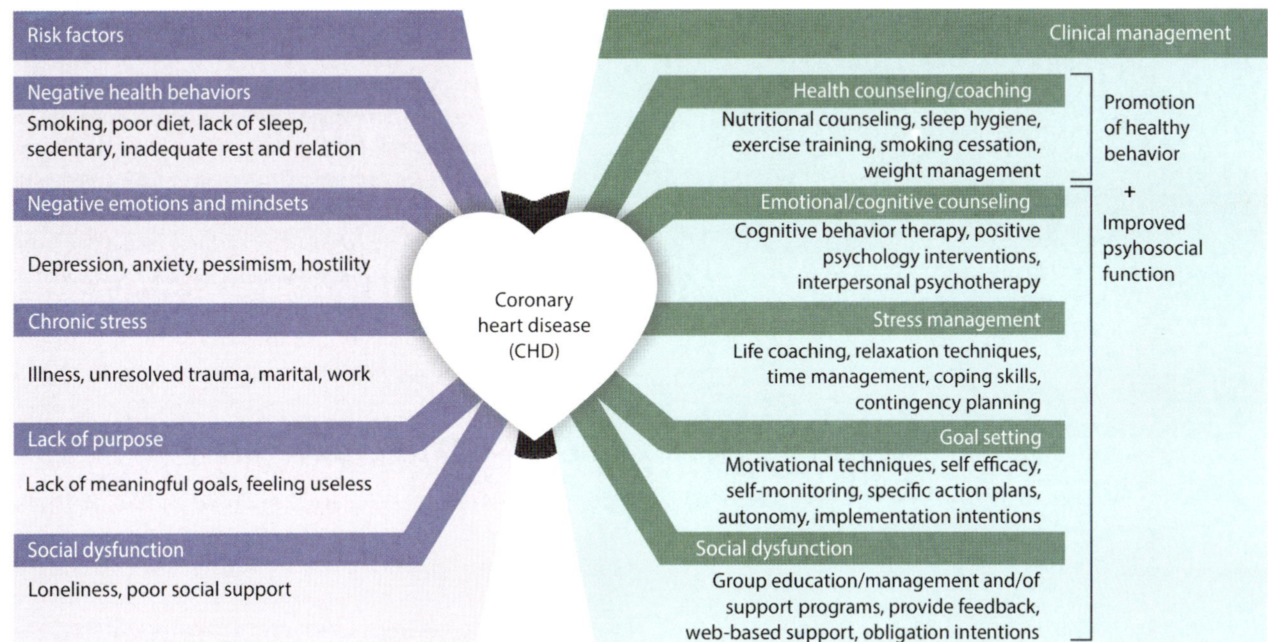

Fig. 2: The clinical basis for behavioral cardiology. While negative health behaviors and a variety of psychosocial risk factors increase the risk for CHD, often in synergistic fashion, evidence-based techniques are promoting healthy behaviors and psychosocial wellbeing

Source: Rozanski A. Behavioral cardiology: current advances and future directions. J Am Coll Cardiol. 2014;64:100-10.

and psychosocial factors increase CAD risk through atherosclerosis progression and triggering either plaque erosion or rupture, leading to acute coronary events. Acute psychological factors may lead to acute coronary syndrome by triggering coronary atherothrombosis or coronary artery spasm; this can occur rapidly even in normal coronaries. Rozanski outlined the main psychological factors contributing to CAD and the key steps to improve health in his diagram, "the clinical basis for behavioral cardiology" (Fig. 2).[11]

MIND-HEART CONNECTION IN MANAGING CVD

The authors have emphasized the key role of addressing stress and developing a positive mindset to improve CVD outcomes for several decades. Both optimism and positive mindset improve physical activity and healthy eating in a bidirectional manner.[13] The role of addressing emotional aspects in the management of individuals with CAD and their families cannot be overemphasized. This is why comprehensive cardiac rehabilitation programs, incorporating exercise, nutritional education and psychosocial counseling, are replacing exercise-only programs worldwide. Positive lifestyle plays a crucial role in the management of a wide spectrum of CVD including heart failure, arrhythmia, hypertension, stroke and peripheral artery disease. The authors have spearheaded a multidisciplinary preventive cardiology program for the South Indian population and have witnessed the negative impact of chronic stress and the benefits of appropriate stress management on CAD.[14] The Department of Veterans Affairs in the USA is recognizing the crucial importance of holistic health. Figure 3 illustrates the emphasis on prevention and complementary approaches while spirituality and mindfulness have become central to overall health. One of the authors has been leading this effort, training local physicians and healthcare providers towards developing whole health programs for CVD reduction.

DIVERGENCE FROM OUR HISTORIC LIFESTYLE

Our hunter-gatherer ancestors relied on their fright-fight-flight response to survive close encounters with predators and unexpected natural calamities. They ran and walked about 10 miles in search of food daily and rested by nightfall. Our evolution to an agricultural society occurred around 10,000 years ago, and the dramatic changes of modern life have only emerged within the last few generations. Science and technology have reduced the need for physical exertion for survival. While we no longer encounter the adrenergic surge of near-death situations, chronic stress has increased significantly. From childhood onwards, humans in the

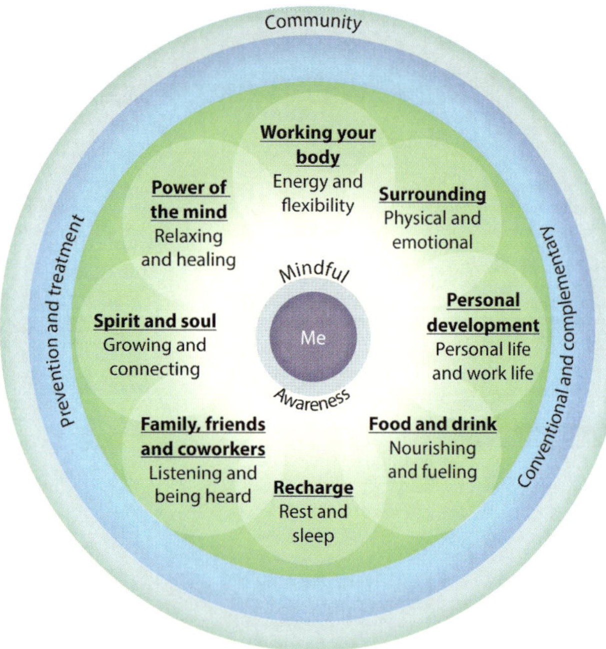

Fig. 3: Novel whole health program now offered by the Department of Veterans Affairs. Mindfulness and self-awareness are central to implementing holistic lifestyle and wellness

world over have to deal with numerous challenges, time constraints, financial pressures and artificial targets. The sympathetic hyperactivation that was meant to cope with acute dangers has become a chronic new baseline state of existence. While we are wired as social beings, this is the first time in human history that a majority of the adult population is choosing to live alone. Technology has succeeded in drastically reducing our reliance on family and friends and is expected to change our lifestyle further over the next 20–30 years. Yet, biologically we are still very close to our ancestors, and therefore we see the discrepancy in terms of physical and mental health. Understanding our origins, these unnatural challenges and coping mechanisms are central to dealing with modern stress and lifestyle pressures.

YOGA AND MEDITATION

India has the pride of giving birth to the oldest religious traditions, meditative techniques and yoga practices. Yoga is safe and can be practiced at all ages. The true goal of yoga is self-realization through meditation. Cardiac patients will significantly benefit from the healthy and natural diet, stretching exercises, meditation and all the basic tenets of yoga. Several studies have demonstrated the benefits of yoga in reducing cardiovascular events (CVE), summarized well in recent publications.[15,16] Vegetarian diet, smoking cessation, meditation, relaxation methods, exercise techniques from yoga and effective stress management have been the focus of majority of the trials in the US and India demonstrating benefit for CAD patients. Recent evidence shows that adopting a healthier lifestyle arrests progression and may even reverse CAD.[17,18] The power of the human mind has helped us achieve tremendous success, but at a cost—we have moved farther away from our instinctual, natural way of life. Yoga in essence is the science of calming the mind so we may rediscover healthy food, exercise and meaningful pursuits suitable to our true nature. Yoga moves us, with little conscious effort, towards our center or inner self thereby helping us attain and sustain a healthy lifestyle.

SLEEP AND RELAXATION

Our awareness about sleep disorders has increased significantly in the last few decades. With normal healthy adults requiring 6–8 hours of sound sleep every day, insufficient sleep as well as excessive sleep may increase CAD.[19] The clustering of obesity, sedentary lifestyle and unhealthy diets increases the risk for obstructive sleep apnea (OSA). In turn, OSA increases sympathetic activation and perpetuates the risk factors through more anxiety, hypertension and poorer lifestyle choices. The feedback accentuation of OSA with CAD risk factors and lifestyle should be recognized by healthcare providers.[20]

The direct benefits of treating OSA are better control of blood pressure, pulmonary pressures, and atrial and ventricular arrhythmias. Better sleep improves autonomic balance and can benefit endothelial function. Once patients recognize that underlying obesity is often the basis of OSA, they are motivated to take the necessary action to optimize their weight. Treating OSA with continuous positive airway pressure (CPAP) or surgery gives symptom relief, but providers can educate and encourage towards really curing the condition with lifestyle modification and weight management.[21]

Relaxation is the state when the mind and body are free from tension and anxiety. It is more of a necessity than a luxury to stay relaxed in this fast-paced life. Taking time off from daily chores and indulging in a hobby or acquiring a new skill, more so active hobbies and skills that require physical exercise and mental agility and coordination, is a key component in improving heart health. Leisure activities like gardening and exergaming (video games to improve physical exercise) have been proven to have beneficial effects on the mind and heart.[22,23]

STRESS MANAGEMENT

Only in the recent years, time pressure has taken center stage in society. Today, we are able to accomplish more complex and intricate tasks faster. However, the trade-off has been sleepless nights to meet deadlines, loss of quality time with family, inability to connect with nature and a nagging urge to race ahead in life. Effective time management is really about recognizing our priorities. The most productive people are rarely rushed. Our physical and emotional resources have to be reconciled with realistic goals. At every level and sphere of life, we can actively explore options to outsource work to other people or to novel technologies. *We are most productive when we specialize in what inspires us.* This universal phenomenon can be capitalized to determine the right balance of productivity without burnout, enthusiastic participation without boredom, and creativity without time pressure.

Cognitive behavioral therapy makes use of techniques such as progressive muscle relaxation, visual imagery and other strategies to train individuals in prioritizing, managing time, establishing personal values, and avoiding stressful situations. A recent study clearly demonstrates the superior clinical outcomes of adding a 12 week stress management training (SMT) program to a comprehensive cardiac rehabilitation (CR) program.[24]

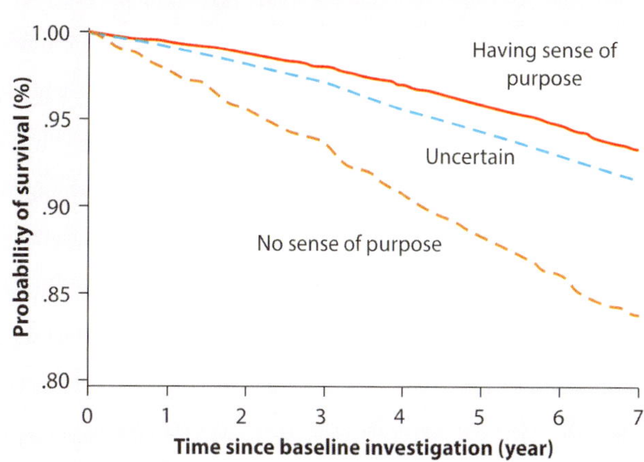

Fig. 4: Sense of purpose and mortality risk. Kaplan-Meier curve of all-cause mortality associated with a high, uncertain, and low sense of life purpose

Source: 1. Rozanski A. Behavioral cardiology: current advances and future directions. J Am Coll Cardiol. 2014;64:100-10.
2. Adapted with permission from Sone T, Nakaya N, Ohmori K, et al. Sense of life worth living (ikigai) and mortality in Japan: Ohsaki Study. Psychosom Med. 2008;70: 709-15.

MEANINGFUL LIFE

At the core of our existence is a sense of belonging and meaning in life that arises from positive interaction with people around us. For some, it is family; for others, it may be friends and neighbors. Purpose in life derives from a sense of helping others grow and thrive. Older age still means continued active participation and leadership in many societies. Health metrics and longevity are surprisingly better despite lesser resources and technology when this is true culturally. Figure 4 illustrates the key role that a sense of purpose plays in survival over 70 years. In a study involving 43,391 subjects, the adjusted hazard ratio for all-cause mortality among those reporting a low versus high sense of purpose in life was 1.5 (95% confidence interval [CI]: 1.3–1.7).[11,25]

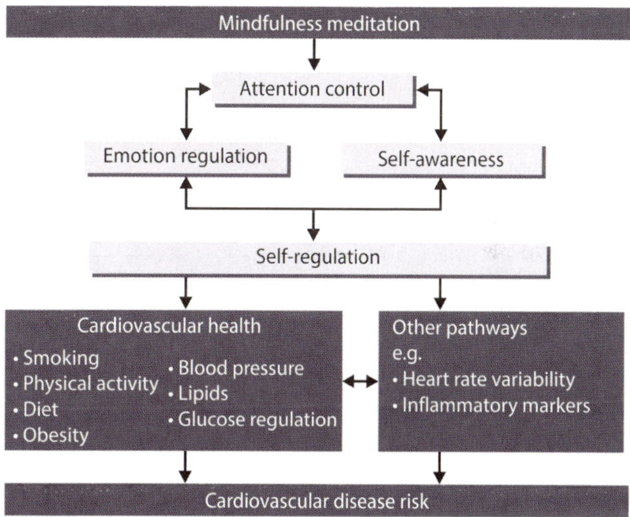

Fig. 5: Plausible mechanisms by which mindfulness meditation may influence CVD risk

Source: Loucks EB, Schuman-Olivier Z, Britton WB, et al. Mindfulness and Cardiovascular Disease Risk: State of the Evidence, Plausible Mechanisms, and Theoretical Framework. Curr Cardiol Rep. 2015;17:112.

MINDFULNESS

Mindfulness reduces mental stress and anxiety as well as CAD risk factors.[26] These techniques from India and Tibet have spread across the Western world over the last 3 decades. Mindfulness and meditation have overcome political, religious and cultural boundaries. Mindfulness is the opposite of multitasking and enhances our mind's awareness and capacity to remain in the moment.

Mindfulness can be learned and practiced at all ages. Physical disabilities and illness do not limit its scope; in fact, mindfulness helps manage diseases better and with fewer medications. Large corporations and health insurance providers are realizing the potential to increase productivity and reduce healthcare costs of employees. Incentivized stress reduction and weight control programs are increasingly offered based on mindfulness practice.[27] Smoking cessation and de-addiction, chronic pain control, palliative care and anxiety disorders are only a few of the ever-increasing areas where mindfulness can be helpful. Figure 5 from a recent review illustrates how mindfulness meditation may influence CVD risk.[28] The research and literature about mindfulness has grown exponentially. Mindfulness trains the mind to be aware of our surroundings, our thoughts and our self. Mindfulness overcomes the numbing routines of life, painful memories of the past as well as anxieties about the future. Mindfulness opens our consciousness to draw strength from our inner true nature.

Transcendental meditation has shown significant benefit in improving stress and reducing cardiovascular risk factors and coronary events.[29] Combined together with mindfulness and yoga, it is a powerful mind-body technique. While the positive effects of mind-body practices on the cardiovascular system have been established,[30] only regular pursuit of these techniques will enable freeing the mind of thoughts and developing a deeper awareness of self.

FUTURE DIRECTIONS

With research into behavioral cardiology and neurocardiology gaining ground, our understanding of the mind-heart connection is bound to evolve.[11,31] High quality scientific studies are the need of the hour, especially in evaluating the role of behavioral interventions in preventing CVD.[32] Authors' words of wisdom for heart healthy living have been compiled recently.[33] There is a huge opportunity for a multidisciplinary team approach involving physicians, psychologists, geneticists, paramedical staff, technologists and medical educators to bring about new scientific evidence in this exciting field of medicine. An empathetic approach addressing the physiological, psychosocial and spiritual needs of patients is the foundation for sustained improvements in health parameters.

CONCLUSION

This chapter addresses some of the key aspects of mind-heart connection and how this interplay can cause as well as help control heart disease. The role of a systematic approach to understand emotional and psychosocial triggers and the need for an empathetic approach to altering these risk factors using holistic mind-body methods cannot be overstressed. With medical advances adding more years to life, we have to work to add more life to the years of our patients.

REFERENCES

1. World Health Organization. (2012). Deaths from cardiovascular diseases and diabetes. [online] Available from: http://www.who.int/gho/ncd/mortality_morbidity/cvd/en/ [Accessed August, 2017].
2. Yusuf S, Hawken S, Ounpuu S, et al. Effect of potentially modifiable risk factors associated with myocardial infarction in 52 countries (the INTERHEART study): case-control study. Lancet. 2004;364:937-52.
3. World Health Organization. (2014). Noncommunicable diseases country profiles 2014. [online] Available from: http://apps.who.int/iris/bitstream/10665/128038/1/9789241507509_eng.pdf?ua=1 [Accessed August, 2017].
4. Joshi P, Islam S, Pais P, et al. Risk factors for early myocardial infarction in South Asians compared with individuals in other countries. JAMA. 2007;297:286-94.
5. Pillai HS, Ganapathi S. Heart failure in South Asia. Curr Cardiol Rev. 2013;9:102-11.
6. Chockalingam P, Chockalingam A, Chockalingam V. Role of Psychosocial Factors and Relaxation Techniques in the Etiology and Prevention of Cardiovascular Diseases. Cardiology Update 2014. New Delhi: Jaypee Brothers Medical Publishers Pvt Ltd; 2015.
7. Steptoe A, Kivimaki M. Stress and cardiovascular disease: an update on current knowledge. Annu Rev Public Health. 2013;34:337-54.
8. Chockalingam A, Venkatesan S, Dorairajan S, et al. Estimation of subjective stress in acute myocardial infarction. Journal of postgraduate medicine. 2003;49:207-10.
9. Appleton AA, Buka SL, Loucks EB, et al. A prospective study of positive early-life psychosocial factors and favorable cardiovascular risk in adulthood. Circulation. 2013;127:905-12.
10. Juonala M, Pulkki-Råback L, Elovainio M, et al. Childhood Psychosocial Factors and Coronary Artery Calcification in Adulthood: The Cardiovascular Risk in Young Finns Study. JAMA Pediatr. 2016;170:466-72.
11. Rozanski A. Behavioral cardiology: current advances and future directions. J Am Coll Cardiol. 2014;64:100-10.
12. Jiang W, Samad Z, Boyle S, et al. Prevalence and clinical characteristics of mental stress-induced myocardial ischemia in patients with coronary heart disease. J Am Coll Cardiol. 2013;61:714-22.
13. Huffman JC, DuBois CM, Mastromauro CA, et al. Positive psychological states and health behaviors in acute coronary syndrome patients: A qualitative study. J Health Psychol. 2016;21:1026-36.
14. Chockalingam P, Sakthi Vinayagam N, Ezhil Vani N, et al. Outcomes of a multidisciplinary coronary heart disease prevention programme in southern India. Heart Asia. 2016;8:39-44.
15. Chu P, Gotink RA, Yeh GY, et al. The effectiveness of yoga in modifying risk factors for cardiovascular disease and metabolic syndrome: A systematic review and meta-analysis of randomized controlled trials. Eur J Prev Cardiol. 2016;23:291-307.
16. Manchanda SC. Yoga–a promising technique to control cardiovascular disease. Indian Heart J. 2014;66:487-9.
17. Chockalingam P, Vinayagam NS, Chockalingam V, et al. Remarkable regression of coronary atherosclerosis: An interplay of pharmacotherapeutic and lifestyle factors. Indian Heart J. 2016;68:188-9.
18. Esselstyn CB Jr. We Can Prevent and Even Reverse Coronary Artery Heart Disease. MedGenMed. 2007;9:46.
19. Cappuccio FP, Cooper D, D'Elia L, et al. Sleep duration predicts cardiovascular outcomes: a systematic review and meta-analysis of prospective studies. Eur Heart J. 2011;32:1484-92.
20. Somers VK, White DP, Amin R, et al. Sleep apnea and cardiovascular disease: an American Heart Association/American College Of Cardiology Foundation Scientific Statement from the American Heart Association Council for High Blood Pressure Research Professional Education Committee, Council on Clinical Cardiology, Stroke Council, and Council On Cardiovascular Nursing. In collaboration with the National Heart, Lung, and Blood Institute National Center on Sleep Disorders Research (National Institutes of Health). Circulation. 2008;118:1080-111.

21. Araghi MH, Chen YF, Jagielski A, et al. Effectiveness of lifestyle interventions on obstructive sleep apnea (OSA): systematic review and meta-analysis. Sleep. 2013;36:1553-62, 62a-62e.
22. Shiue I. Gardening is beneficial for adult mental health: Scottish Health Survey, 2012-2013. Scand J Occup Ther. 2016;23:320-5.
23. Klompstra L, Jaarsma T, Strömberg A. Exergaming to increase the exercise capacity and daily physical activity in heart failure patients: a pilot study. BMC Geriatr. 2014;14:119.
24. Blumenthal JA, Sherwood A, Smith PJ, et al. Enhancing Cardiac Rehabilitation with Stress Management Training: A Randomized, Clinical Efficacy Trial. Circulation. 2016;133:1341-50.
25. Sone T, Nakaya N, Ohmori K, et al. Sense of life worth living (ikigai) and mortality in Japan: Ohsaki Study. Psychosom Med. 2008;70:709-15.
26. Parswani MJ, Sharma MP, Iyengar S. Mindfulness-based stress reduction program in coronary heart disease: A randomized control trial. Int J Yoga. 2013;6:111-7.
27. Olson KL, Emery CF. Mindfulness and weight loss: a systematic review. Psychosom Med. 2015;77:59-67.
28. Loucks EB, Schuman-Olivier Z, Britton WB, et al. Mindfulness and Cardiovascular Disease Risk: State of the Evidence, Plausible Mechanisms, and Theoretical Framework. Curr Cardiol Rep. 2015;17:112.
29. Ray IB, Menezes AR, Malur P, et al. Meditation and coronary heart disease: a review of the current clinical evidence. Ochsner J. 2014;14:696-703.
30. Younge JO, Gotink RA, Baena CP, et al. Mind-body practices for patients with cardiac disease: a systematic review and meta-analysis. Eur J Prev Cardiol. 2015;22:1385-98.
31. Shivkumar K, Ajijola OA, Anand I, et al. Clinical neurocardiology defining the value of neuroscience-based cardiovascular therapeutics. J Physiol. 2016;594:3911-54.
32. Gardner B, Broström A, Nilsen P, et al. From does it work? To what makes it work?: The importance of making assumptions explicit when designing and evaluating behavioural interventions. Eur J Cardiovasc Nurs. 2014;13:292-4.
33. Chockalingam V, Chockalingam A, Chockalingam P. Mind your heart: Healthy heart for hearty health. J Clin Prev Cardiol. 2017;6:78-80.

27

CHAPTER

Aortic Aneurysm Surgery in Cardiodiabetes: Is the Outcome Different?

Jayesh Suresh, Anita Dhar, Anil Bhan

INTRODUCTION

Diabetes is a known risk factor for atherosclerosis and peripheral arterial disease. Atherosclerosis in turn is a risk factor for aortic aneurysm formation. Surprisingly, diabetes has an inverse relationship with aortic aneurysm. Aortic aneurysm defined as a localized dilatation of aorta is a significant cause of morbidity and mortality in aging populations. The prevalence of abdominal aortic aneurysm (AAA) estimated from ultrasound screening in adults aged greater than or equal to 65 years ranged from 1.7% to 12.9% among men and from 0.6% to 1.7% among women in the western world. Mortality of ruptured AAA is as high as 70% for patients reaching the hospital and 35% for those undergoing emergency surgery.[1]

RISK FACTORS

Age, gender, smoking, and family history are the most significant risk factors for developing an AAA. Other risk factors include cardiovascular disease and its associated complicating factors like hypertension, hyperlipidemia, and atherosclerosis. Hypertension is associated both with increased risk of rupture as well as increased prevalence of AAA. It is hemodynamics that can weaken the aortic wall. Hyperlipidemia and atherosclerosis generally increase the risk of complications within the cardiovascular system, and increase the risk of AAA. Chronic obstructive pulmonary disease (COPD), trauma, infectious and inflammatory conditions, autoimmune diseases, vasculitis like Takayasu's arteritis and Marfan syndrome can cause cystic medial necrosis and can result in aortic aneurysm. In the case of inflammatory AAA, 10–47% of patients have been reported to have arterial occlusive disease. Diabetes has been shown to have a significant negative association with aortic aneurysm compared to nondiabetics in most studies. Shanti Kumar et al. published in 2009 a meta-analysis which suggested a reduced prevalence of diabetes in patients with AAA (OR = 0.81, 0.66–0.99, p = 0.038).[2] Evidence for an inverse association between diabetes mellitus and AAA was shown in a large case–control study including 73,451 veterans in which the odds ratio was 0.54 for the presence of diabetes mellitus and AAA.[3] Rango et al. conducted a meta-analysis of 17 population prevalence studies in which they concluded that there was significant inverse association between diabetes and AAA.[4] In a retrospective case–control study conducted by Prakash et al. based on nationwide inpatient sample data, they observed that diabetes remained significantly and negatively associated with thoracic aortic aneurysms and dissections.[5] In a meta-analysis conducted by Xiong et al. comprising of 49 studies on prevalence of AAA in diabetics and 13 studies on the effect of diabetes in growth rate of AAA; a strongly negative association was found between diabetes and AAA. The annual mean effect of diabetes on AAA growth rate was –0.60 mm/year.[6] These two above mentioned studies show that not only diabetes has a negative association with aortic aneurysm but also it has an effect on the expansion of the aneurysm and the dissection which can occur as a result of aneurysm. AAA growth was shown to be decreased substantially in patients with diabetes mellitus as compared to those without diabetes mellitus.[7] Takagi and Umemoto performed a

TABLE 1: Diabetes mellitus and abdominal aortic aneurysm[9]

Variable	Diabetes mellitus	
	No	Yes
Patients with AAA > 4.0 cm	19%	12%
Growth of AAA (mm/year)	2.21 (all subjects)	1.70
Patients with AAA among those with >50% carotid stenosis	10.2%	2.8%

meta-analysis of 19 studies including 9,777 patients and compared the growth of small AAAs in patients with and without diabetes. The result of the study was that diabetes is associated with reduced abdominal aortic aneurysmal growth.[8] Gertz et al. conducted an epidemiologic study and observed that those with diabetes mellitus had a decreased overall prevalence and slower rate of progression of AAA than those without diabetes mellitus (Table 1).[9]

POTENTIAL MECHANISM FOR THE PROTECTIVE EFFECT OF DIABETES

Diabetes actually decreases the risk for aortic aneurysm, even though it increases the risk for atherosclerosis and peripheral vascular disease. This is contrary to the logic. Macrophages and matrix-digesting metallo proteinases (MMPs) may play a key role in such an association. With enhanced glycation (as in diabetes mellitus), more glycated collagen may be formed, with effects on matrix metalloproteinase secretion. There is marked reduction of MMP-9, MMP-2, and interleukin-6 (IL-6) secretion by activated monocytes. The hyperglycemic stage leads to the reduction of the proteolysis of the aortic walls of diabetics. The glycation end products will form crosslinks with the collagen and elastin of the arterial walls, promote smooth muscle proliferation and thereby increase matrix stiffness which is resistant to proteolysis.[2,10] Therefore, the metabolic milieu of diabetes may impart a degree of resistance to aneurismal disease by creating a stiffened aortic wall less prone to degeneration.

DIABETIC MEDICINES AND AORTIC ANEURYSM

Medication taken by diabetes patients may contribute to the protective effect of aortic disease. Metformin has cardiovascular protection effect independent of its hypoglycemic effects.[11,12] In a retrospective study by Hsu et al. in a total of 4,468 patients, diagnosed with aortic aneurysm and 4,468 matched controls, metformin use, sulfonylurea use, and thiazolidinedione were associated with lower risk of developing aortic aneurysm.[13] Angiotensin Converting Enzyme (ACE) inhibitors prevent aortic expansion and rupture.

DIABETES AND AORTIC DISEASE COMPLICATIONS

Diabetes has been shown to be protective against complications and mortality due to aortic aneurysms. In a hospital-based case-control study conducted in Chinese population, the prevalence of diabetes was lower in aortic dissection cases than that of control subjects, and diabetes was found to be associated with lower aortic dissection risk (odds ratio, 0.2).[14] Theivacumar et al. did a study on the mortality due to aortic rupture in diabetic patients with aortic aneurysms and found that they are significantly less likely to present with rupture or to die from aneurysm rupture when compared with nondiabetic patients with aortic aneurysms (Table 2).[15]

PROGNOSIS OF DIABETICS AFTER AORTIC SURGERY FOR AORTIC ANEURYSM SURGERY

The prognosis of diabetics after surgery for aortic aneurysm remains controversial. There are multiple studies for and against in this regard. Hughes et al. did a study in 2010 American College of Surgeons' National Surgical Quality Improvement Program patients who underwent an open, elective, nonruptured AAA repair. Of these patients, 245

TABLE 2: Ten-year mortality data of patients with abdominal aortic aneurysm and total aortic aneurysm with regard to diabetes[15]

	Total	Died due to rupture	Died with intact aneurysm	Odds ratio (CI)	P
Patients with diabetes who died with AAA	75	6 (8%)	69 (92%)	0.37 (0.15–0.88)	0.03
Nondiabetic patients died with AAA	397	76 (19%)	321 (81%)		
Patients with diabetes who died with aortic aneurysm (TAA + TAAA + AAA)	79	7 (8.9%)	72 (91.1%)	0.31 (0.13–0.69)	0.004
Nondiabetic patients died with aortic aneurysm (TAA + TAAA + AAA)	446	107 (24%)	339 (76%)		

Abbreviations: AAA, abdominal aortic aneurysm; CI, confidence interval; TAA, thoracic aortic aneurysm; TAAA, thoracoabdominal aortic aneurysm

TABLE 3: Comparison of postoperative complications in diabetics versus nondiabetics in open abdominal aortic aneurismal repair[17]

Postoperative complications	Diabetics (n) (%)	Nondiabetics (n) (%)	P
Mortality	13 (5.3)	66 (3.5)	0.171
Pneumonia	20 (8.2)	183 (9.8)	0.411
Stroke/cerebrovascular accident	3 (1.2)	16 (0.9)	0.568
Surgical site infections	11 (4.5)	30 (1.2)	0.002
Urinary tract infection	6 (2.5)	69 (3.4)	0.419

(11.6%) had diabetes mellitus. The overall mortality rate was 3.7% (5.3% for diabetics and 3.5% for nondiabetics). Postoperatively, there was no significant difference in mortality or in cardiac, pulmonary, or renal complications. Diabetics were more likely to develop superficial surgical site infections (4.5% versus 1.6%) (Table 3).[16] Rayan et al. have also suggested that diabetics may have a trend toward higher operative morbidity and mortality rates compared with nondiabetics undergoing elective AAA repair.[17]

INFLUENCE OF DIABETES MELLITUS ON THE ENDOVASCULAR TREATMENT

Leurs et al. in 2005 have observed significantly higher risk of device-related complications in diabetic patients undergoing endovascular repair (8% vs 6%). Mortality was significantly higher in the diabetic population (13%) compared to the nondiabetic patients (10%, p, 0.039; OR 1.27) which occurred at a higher frequency within the 30-day perioperative period in diabetic patients, which were primarily due to cardiac complications. The cumulative survival after 48 months did not differ significantly: 74% in diabetics and 79% in the population without diabetes.[18]

CONCLUSION

There is evidence in literature that diabetes has an inverse relationship with aortic aneurysm. Postoperatively, there was no significant difference in mortality or in cardiac, pulmonary, or renal complications. Diabetics were more likely to develop superficial surgical site infections (4.5% vs 1.6%). The cumulative survival after 48 months did not differ significantly: 74% in diabetics and 79% in the population without diabetes after endovascular treatment.

REFERENCES

1. Wang L, Zhang X, Song Y. Paradoxical Association of Diabetes and obesity with abdominal aortic aneurysms. North Am J Med Sci. 2017;10(2):83-7.
2. Shantikumar S, Ajjan R, Porter KE, et al. Diabetes and the abdominal aortic aneurysm. Eur J Vasc Endovasc Surg. 2010;39(2):200-7.
3. Lederle FA, Johnson GR, Wilson SE. Prevalence and associations of abdominal aortic aneurysm detected through screening. Aneurysm Detection and Management (ADAM) Veterans Affairs Cooperative Study Group. Ann Intern Med. 2000;160:1425-30.
4. De Rango P, Farchioni L, Fiorucci B, et al. Diabetes and abdominal aortic aneurysms. Eur J Vasc Endovasc Surg. 2014;47:243-61.
5. Prakash SK, Pedroza C, Khalil YA, et al. Diabetes and reduced risk for thoracic aortic aneurysms and dissections—nationwide case-control study. J Am Heart Assoc. 2012;1:e000323.
6. Xiong J, Wu Z, Chen C, et al. Association between diabetes and prevalence and growth rate of abdominal aortic aneurysms: a meta-analysis. Int J Cardio. 2016;221:484-95.
7. De Rango P, Cao P, Cieri E. Effects of diabetes on small aortic aneurysms under surveillance according to a subgroup analysis from a randomized trial. J Vasc Surg. 2012;56:1555-63.
8. Takagi H, Umemoto T. Diabetes and abdominal aortic aneurysm growth. Angiology. 2015;67:513-25.
9. Gertz SD, Gavish L, Mintz Y, et al. Contradictory effects of hypercholesterolemia and diabetes mellitus on the progression of abdominal aortic aneurysm. Am J Cardiol. 2015;115:399e401.
10. Nienaber CA. Diabetes mellitus and thoracic aortic disease: are people with diabetes mellitus protected from acute aortic dissection? J Am Heart Assoc. 2012;1:e001404.
11. Xie Z, Lau K, Eby B, et al. Improvement of cardiac functions by chronic metformin treatment is associated with enhanced cardiac autophagy in diabetic OVE26 mice. Diabetes. 2011;60:1770-8.
12. He C, Zhu H, Li H, et al. Dissociation of Bcl-2-Beclin1complex by activated AMPK enhances cardiac autophagy and protects against cardiomyocyte apoptosis in diabetes. Diabetes. 2013;62:1270-81.
13. Golledge J, Cooper ME, Chai Z. Diabetes and Aortic Aneurysm. Angiology. 2016;67(6):510-2.
14. Xingwei H, Xintian L, Wanjun L, et al. Association between diabetes and risk of aortic dissection: a case-control study in a Chinese population. PLoS One. 2015;10:e0142697.
15. Theivacumar NS, Stephenson MA, Mistry H, et al. Diabetes mellitus and aortic aneurysm rupture. a favorable association? Vasc Endovascular Surg. 2014;48(1):45-50.
16. Hughes K, Jackson JD, Prendergast TI, et al. Diabetes mellitus is not associated with major morbidity following open abdominal aortic aneurysm repair. J Surg Res. 2013;184:751-4.
17. Rayan SS, Campbell DR, Akbari CM. Is Diabetes a risk factor for patients undergoing open abdominal aortic aneurysm repair? Vasc Endovascular Surg. 2002;36:33.
18. Leurs LJ, Laheij RJ, Buth J. Influence of diabetes mellitus on the endovascular treatment of abdominal aortic aneurysms. J Endovasc Ther. 2005;12:288.

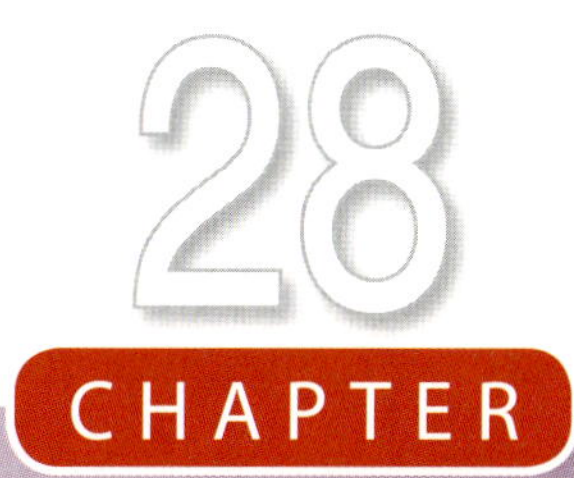

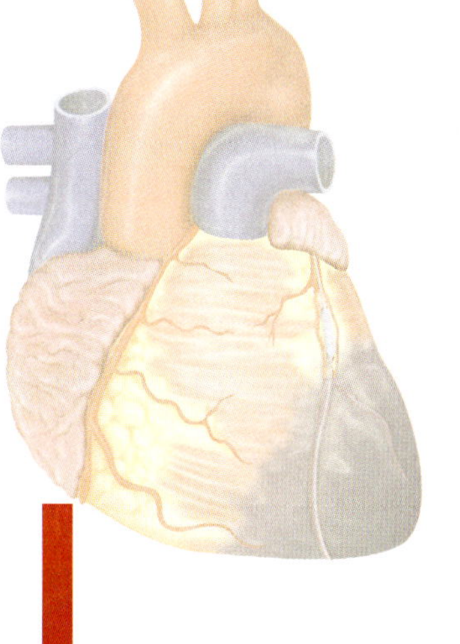

Cardiodiabetes and Syncope

Rakesh Varma, Rajat Jain

INTRODUCTION

Of all the possible complications of diabetes, the cardiac ones are the most lethal. Cardiovascular disease is in fact the number one cause of death in patients with type 2 diabetes. Researchers are using the term *"cardiodiabetes"* to describe the co-occurrence of diabetes and significant cardiovascular disease (CVD). Diabetes is a known, independent, risk factor for cardiovascular disease. Since diabetes and serious CVD are frequently observed together, the term *"cardiodiabetes"* is increasingly applied to describe the convergence of these conditions. People with cardiodiabetes do have both diabetes and CVD. The CVD may be subclinical and undiagnosed. Traditionally, cardiologists and diabetologists have played parallel roles in managing cardiovascular risks in their patient populations. A number of terms are used to describe the convergence of CVD and type 2 diabetes in a patient. While there is an increasingly prevalent view that diabetes should be viewed from the outset as a vascular disease, The European Society of Cardiology-European Association for the Study of Diabetes (ESC-EASD) Task Force guidelines of 2007 acknowledge the inter-relationship between diabetes and CVD and call for an early, multidisciplinary approach to the recognition and intensive management of all cardio-diabetes risk factors. The consensus view of the group was that use of hybrid terms to acknowledge the concurrent diseases and risks at play is useful for both clinicians and for patients. Prevention of CVD must focus equally on patients with established atherosclerotic disease and on people with diabetes. In recognition that many patients with diabetes and CVD may be obese, *"cardiodiabesity"* was suggested as an appropriate catch all term. Further, the high risk for renal complications in patients with convergent diabetes and CVD led to the suggestion of *"cardiorenal diabetes"* as another descriptor. The term cardiodiabetes was viewed as most useful for clinicians, serving to remind diabetologists of the need to assess blood pressure and lipid parameters in addition to weight and glucose management, and similarly serving to prompt cardiologists to consider diabetes-related risk factors in patient assessment and management. For patients too, the combined term is meaningful, and the addition of the "cardio" prefix to diabetes adds impact to the overall descriptor. Despite improvements in CVD morbidity and mortality, diabetes mellitus (DM) continues to elevate CVD risk. DM is an established independent risk factor for CVD development. Longitudinal data from the Framingham Heart Study suggest that the risk factor adjusted risk ratio of CVD is 1.38 times [95% confidence interval (CI), 0.99–1.92] higher, and the risk for CVD death is 1.86 times (95% CI, 1.17–2.93) higher for each 10-year increase in the duration of DM. A number of studies have demonstrated that the increased prevalence of DM is being followed by an increasing prevalence of CVD morbidity and mortality.

SYNCOPE

Syncope is a temporary loss of consciousness usually related to insufficient blood flow to the brain. It is also called fainting or passing out. It usually occurs when blood pressure is too low (hypotension) and the heart does not pump enough oxygen to the brain. Syncope is a symptom that can be due to several causes ranging from benign to life-threatening conditions. Many non-life-threatening factors such as overheating, dehydration, heavy sweating, exhaustion or the pooling of blood in the legs due to sudden changes in body position, can trigger syncope. It is important to determine the cause of syncope and any underlying conditions. Several serious heart conditions such as bradyarrhythmias, tachyarrhythmias, obstructive valvular lesion and cardiomyopathies can also cause syncope and has to be treated differently from more common benign causes of syncope.

Neurally-mediated Syncope

Neurally-mediated syncope (NMS) is the most common form of fainting and a frequent reason for emergency department visits. It is also called reflex, neurocardiogenic, vasovagal or vasodepressor syncope (VVS). It is benign and rarely requires medical treatment. Situational syncope, which is a type of NMS, is related to certain physical functions, such as violent coughing (especially in men), laughing or swallowing. Other disorders can cause syncope, which also can be a side effect of some medicines. Some types of syncope suggest a serious disorder such as those occurring with exercise, associated with palpitations or irregularities of the heart and with family history of recurrent syncope or sudden death.

Cardiac Syncope

Cardiac or cardiovascular syncope caused by various heart conditions, particularly tachyarrhythmias and bradyarrhythmias, are the second most common cause of syncope, accounting for 10–20% of syncopal episodes.[1] It can increase the risk of sudden cardiac death (SCD). 1-year mortality of syncope patients underlying cardiac causes has been consistently high, ranging between 18% and 33%. Mortality is higher than those in patients with a noncardiac cause (0–12%) or in patients with unknown cause (6%)[2] per annum. People suspected of having cardiac syncope but who do not have serious medical conditions may be managed as outpatients. Further, inpatient evaluation is needed if serious medical conditions are present. Conditions that may warrant hospital evaluation and treatment include various cardiac arrhythmic conditions, cardiac ischemia, severe aortic stenosis and pulmonary embolism. If evaluation suggests arrhythmias, an ambulatory external or implantable cardiac monitor may be required. Heart failure (HF), atrial fibrillation and other serious cardiac conditions can cause recurrent syncope in older adults, with a sharp increase after the age of 70.[3]

RISK FACTORS FOR SYNCOPE

Syncope is common, but adults over the age of 80 are at greater risk of hospitalization and death. Younger people without cardiac disease but who have experienced syncope while standing or have specific stress or situational triggers are not as likely to experience cardiac syncope. Causes of syncope are enumerated in Box 1 and Table 1. Syncope due to cardiac causes is more likely in people older than 60 years, men, in presence of known heart disease, brief palpitations or sudden loss of consciousness, fainting during exertion, fainting while supine, an abnormal cardiac examination or family history of inheritable conditions. Other evaluation of comorbid conditions and medications used are particularly important in older patients.

BOX 1: Causes of syncope

Vascular
- Anatomic
  - Vascular steal syndromes (subclavian steal syndrome)
- Orthostatic
  - Autonomic insufficiency
  - Idiopathic
  - Volume depletion
  - Drug and alcohol induced
- Reflex mediated
  - Carotid sinus hypersensitivity
  - Neurally-mediated syncope (common faint, vasodepressor, neurocardiogenic, vasovagal)
  - Glossopharyngeal syncope
- Situational (acute hemorrhage, cough, defecation, laugh, micturition, sneeze, swallow, postprandial)

Cardiac
- Anatomic
  - Obstructive cardiac valve disease
  - Aortic dissection
  - Atrial myxoma
  - Pericardial disease, tamponade
  - Hypertrophic obstructive cardiomyopathy
  - Myocardial ischemia, infarction
  - Pulmonary embolism
  - Pulmonary hypertension
- Arrhythmias
  - Bradyarrhythmias
  - Atrioventricular block
- Sinus node dysfunction, bradycardia
  - Tachyarrhythmias
  - Supraventricular tachycardia
  - Atrial fibrillation
  - Paroxysmal supraventricular tachycardia (AVNRT, WPW)
  - Other
- Ventricular tachycardia
  - Structural heart disease
  - Inherited syndromes (ARVD, HCM, Brugada syndrome, long-QT syndrome)
  - Drug-induced proarrhythmia
- Implanted pacemaker or ICD malfunction

TABLE 1: Common causes of syncope by age

Younger patients	*Older patients*
Vasovagal Situational Psychiatric	Cardiac • Structural • Arrhythmic
Long QT syndrome	Orthostatic hypotension
Brugada syndrome	Drug induced
WPW syndrome	Neurally mediated
RV dysplasia	Multifactorial
Hypertrophic cardiomyopathy	
Catecholaminergic VT	

Abbreviations: VT, ventricular tachycardia; RV, right ventricle

CARDIOVASCULAR AUTONOMIC NEUROPATHY AND SYNCOPE

Cardiovascular autonomic neuropathy (CAN) is a common form of autonomic neuropathy, causing abnormalities in heart rate control and central and peripheral vascular dynamics. CAN has been linked to postural hypotension, exercise intolerance, enhanced intraoperative cardiovascular lability, and increased incidence of asymptomatic ischemia, myocardial infarction (MI), and decreased likelihood of survival after MI. Cardiovascular autonomic neuropathy occurs in approximately 17% of patients with type 1 diabetes and 22% of those with type 2. An additional 9% of type 1 patients and 12% of type 2 patients have borderline dysfunction.[4] In a review of several epidemiological studies among individuals with diabetes, the 5-year mortality rate is five times higher for individuals with cardiovascular autonomic neuropathy than for individuals without cardiovascular autonomic involvement.[5] The stronger association observed in studies defining CAN by the presence of two or more abnormalities may be due to more severe autonomic dysfunction in these patients or a higher frequency of other comorbid complications that contributed to their higher mortality risk. An increased resting heart rate is observed frequently in diabetic patients most likely due to the vagal cardiac neuropathy that results in unopposed cardiac sympathetic activity. The tachycardia may be followed by a decrease in heart rate and, ultimately, a fixed heart rate due to progressive dysfunction of the cardiac sympathetic nervous system. Heart rate variability is considered the earliest indicator and most frequent finding in symptomatic cardiovascular autonomic dysfunction. CAN leads to a reduced cardiac ejection fraction and systolic dysfunction and decreased diastolic filling. Limited exercise tolerance is due to impaired sympathetic and parasympathetic responses that normally augments cardiac output and redirect peripheral blood flow to skeletal muscles. Exercise tolerance is also reduced by a reduced ejection fraction, systolic dysfunction, and decreased diastolic filling. A prolonged corrected QT interval and QT dispersion (the difference between the longest and shortest QT interval) indicates an imbalance between right and left sympathetic innervation. Diabetic patients with a regional sympathetic imbalance and QT interval prolongation may be at greater risk for arrhythmias. Regional myocardial autonomic denervation and altered vascular responsiveness in diabetic autonomic neuropathy may predispose to malignant arrhythmogenesis and SCD.

Diabetic patients have a high rate of coronary heart disease, which may be asymptomatic owing to autonomic neuropathy. Silent ischemia is significantly more frequent in patients with than in those without autonomic neuropathy (38% versus 5%).[6] The cause of silent myocardial ischemia in diabetic patients is controversial. It is clear, however, that a reduced appreciation for ischemic pain can impair timely recognition of myocardial ischemia or infarction and thereby delay appropriate therapy. In nondiabetic patients, acute MI has a circadian variation with a significant morning peak. The characteristic diurnal variation in the onset of myocardial infarction is altered in diabetic patients, with a lower morning peak and a higher percentage of infarction during evening hours. The blunted morning surge of incidence of myocardial infarction results from altered sympathovagal balance in patients with CAN. Mortality rates after a MI are also higher for diabetic patients than for nondiabetic patients. This may be due to autonomic insufficiency, increasing the tendency for development of ventricular arrhythmia and cardiovascular events after infarction.

Orthostatic hypotension is defined as a decrease in systolic blood pressure of 20 mm Hg or a decrease in diastolic blood pressure of 10 mm Hg within 3 minutes of standing when compared with blood pressure from the sitting or supine position.[7] In patients with diabetes, orthostatic hypotension is usually due to damage to the efferent sympathetic vasomotor fibers, particularly in the splanchnic vasculature. In addition, there is a decrease in cutaneous, splanchnic, and total vascular resistance that occurs in the pathogenesis of this disorder. Normally, in response to postural change there is an increase in plasma norepinephrine. For individuals with orthostatic hypotension, there may be a reduction in this response relative to the fall in blood pressure. Diminished cardiac acceleration and cardiac output, particularly in association with exercise, may also be important in the presentation of this disorder. Patients with orthostatic hypotension typically present with lightheadedness and presyncopal symptoms. Symptoms such as dizziness, weakness, fatigue, visual blurring, and neck pain may be due to orthostatic hypotension. Many patients, however, remain asymptomatic despite significant fall in blood pressure.

Cardiovascular Autonomic Function Tests

In the early 1970s, Ewing et al. proposed five simple noninvasive cardiovascular reflex tests (Valsalva maneuver, heart rate response to deep breathing, heart rate response to standing up, blood pressure response to standing up, and blood pressure response to sustained handgrip) that have been applied successfully. Today, sensitive and early assessment of CAN is possible by means of noninvasive autonomic function tests, including power spectral analysis of a series of successive R-R intervals (frequency domain analysis). This can be performed on short R-R sequences (e.g. 7 minute) or on 24-hour electrocardiogram recordings. The heart rate power spectrum is typically divided into two frequency bands: low (0.04–0.15 Hz) and high (0.15–0.4 Hz). The high-frequency region is generally considered a marker of vagal activity, whereas the low-frequency component is influenced by both sympathetic and vagal activity.[8] The association of mortality and cardiovascular autonomic dysfunction indicates that individuals with abnormal autonomic function tests are candidates for close surveillance. Thus, it has been recommended that a baseline determination of cardiovascular autonomic function be performed upon diagnosis in type 2 diabetes and within 5 years of diagnosis for those with type 1 diabetes, followed by an yearly repeat test. In addition, the presence of autonomic dysfunction should alert the healthcare professionals to search for associated risk factors of cardiovascular disease and implementation of an intense program to reduce these factors and thereby reduce the risk of mortality.

SYNCOPE AND SUDDEN CARDIAC DEATH

Sudden cardiac death is an event that can occur in asymptomatic individuals, as well as in those with advanced cardiovascular (CV) disease. SCD typically manifests as a structural abnormality coupled with a disturbance in cardiac electrical activity that leads to fatal arrhythmias. However, in 5–10% of SCD cases, no definable structural cardiac abnormality exists. Patients may either be asymptomatic or experience symptoms including palpitations, chest pain or discomfort, dyspnea, fatigue, or syncope. Sudden cardiac arrest (SCA), in which an electrical malfunction causes the heart to stop abruptly, may occur in these patients; if the heart is not quickly shocked back into rhythm, SCD ensues. At least 90–95% of SCA cases in the community setting end in death before the patient receive medical assistance. SCD has been associated with diabetes, although it is unclear whether diabetes is a risk factor for SCD or not. Diabetes is a risk factor for common preventable comorbidities associated with SCD, including coronary artery disease (CAD), MI, and HF. Researchers are seeking ways to measure susceptibility to SCD, but because of SCD's multifactorial development, most likely no single test will be able to identify at-risk individuals. Until tests with proven predictive value are available, preventive efforts should focus on slowing the progression or development of CVD that frequently cause SCD. This can be accomplished by promptly initiating angiotensin-converting enzyme (ACE) inhibitors, angiotensin receptor blockers, beta-blockers, antiplatelet agents (aspirin), and possibly statin therapy for CAD, hypertension, and/or hypercholesterolemia. SCD prevention strategies for the general population are the same as those for patients with diabetes. In the United States, the annual number of SCDs is estimated to be between 250,000 and 300,000, with predominance in males and an increased incidence with age for both the genders.[9] SCD is the first cardiac event in approximately 55% of men and 68% of women, while in other cases SCD follows multiple cardiac events. Unfortunately, the prevalence of SCD is difficult to determine since previously there was no unified definition of the condition. In general, SCD is defined as unexpected death occurring within a specific time frame after initial onset of cardiac symptoms. Depending upon the study being reviewed for SCD, the time frame between symptom onset and death varies greatly, from less than 1 hour up to 24 hours. SCA occurs in the setting of abnormalities of the coronary arteries, myocardium, and electrogenesis and propagation in the heart. Of particular relevance to this review, type 2 diabetes is associated with a set of interrelated determinants of SCA risk, including—(1) the presence and extent of atherosclerotic coronary artery disease that results in clinical coronary heart disease (CHD); (2) patchy areas of myocardial fibrosis that results in impaired left ventricular (LV) filling (diastolic dysfunction) and/or LV systolic HF; and, (3) abnormalities of electrical propagation in the myocardium that is reflected in electrocardiographic repolarization and conduction abnormalities, e.g. prolongation of the QT interval and QRS interval. These characteristics are known to be associated with an increased risk of SCA in the community.[10]

The most common and preventable comorbidities associated with SCD include CAD, MI, and HF.[11] Since diabetes is a risk factor for these comorbidities, it has been deemed to have an association with SCD. The association between diabetes and SCD may involve a combination of macrovascular and microvascular complications that can affect the electrical system controlling cardiac rhythm, thus increasing the propensity for SCD.[12,13] With the number of diabetes patients growing in epidemic proportions (approximately 29.9 million in the US), there is an urgent need to determine whether having diabetes increases one's risk for SCD. It is difficult to ascertain whether diabetes is a direct risk factor for SCD. The notion that diabetes results in enhanced susceptibility to SCD is generally accepted, but is not evidence based. Although diabetes is recognized as a clinical risk marker for SCD, it is not currently used for risk stratification. If the incidence of SCD is greater in patients with diabetes, the root cause remains unclear. Overall, mortality remains high, most likely owing to the unexpectedness of the event and failure to recognize warning symptoms in a timely manner. Thus, it is critically important to develop prediction and prevention strategies for SCD.

SYNCOPE AND HYPOGLYCEMIA

Hypoglycemic syncope is uncommon, affecting 1.9% of diabetic patients using insulin therapy.[14] It is characterized clinically by brief periods of unconsciousness with slow recovery and without loss of postural muscle tone. The difficulty in correlating loss of consciousness to hypoglycemia arises from mismatching symptoms, that is, there may be mental symptoms such as confusion, loss of memory or consciousness, in the absence of autonomic manifestations such as sweating or blurred vision. There are currently no established glucose values that define the level of hypoglycemia that causes loss of consciousness. So, hypoglycemic syncope should be suspected in older diabetic patients with preserved postural tone, usually but not always using insulin therapy, who show a slow recovery from transient loss of consciousness with persisting neurological impairment and low blood glucose levels. However, hypoglycemia is not a true cause of syncope, and impaired mental status due to hypoglycemia should not be defined as syncope.

CONCLUSION

Adults with diabetes are two to four times more likely to die from heart disease than adults without diabetes. The American Heart Association considers diabetes to be one of the seven major controllable risk factors for CVD. Diabetes is treatable, but even when glucose levels are under control it greatly increases the risk of heart disease and stroke. However, by managing their risk factors, patients with diabetes may avoid or delay the development of heart and blood vessel disease. People with diabetes can work with their health care team to develop and use an action plan to reach their ABC goals. An action plan can help people to reach and stay at a healthy weight. Being overweight or obese is a risk factor for heart attack and stroke. Get at least 30–60 minutes of physical activity. Brisk walking or a similar activity most days of the week can help with weight loss and lower blood pressure. Eat foods that are low in saturated fats, trans fats, cholesterol, salt (sodium), and added sugars; choose lean meats, poultry, fish, nuts (in small amounts), fat free or low fat milk, and milk products. Eat more fiber, whole grains, fruits, vegetables, and dry peas and beans. Stop smoking or ask their healthcare team for help to quit. Smoking is one of the major risk factors associated with heart attack and stroke. Take medications as directed and ask their doctor about taking daily aspirin.

REFERENCES

1. Calkins GC, Zipes DP. Hypotension and syncope. In: Mann DL, Zipes DP, Libby P (Eds). Braunwald's Heart Disease: A Textbook of Cardiovascular Medicine, 10th edition. Philadelphia: Elsevier; 2014. pp. 864.
2. Farwell DJ, Sulke AN. Does the use of a syncope diagnostic protocol improve the investigation and management of syncope? Heart. 2004;90:52-8.
3. Fox CS, Sullivan L, D'Agostino RB, et al. The significant effect of diabetes duration on coronary heart disease morality: The Framingham Heart Study. Diabetes Care. 2004;27:704-8.
4. Ziegler D, Gries FA, Muhlen H, et al. Prevalence and clinical correlates of cardiovascular autonomic and peripheral diabetic neuropathy in patients attending diabetes center. The DiaCAN Multicenter Study Group. Diabetes Metab. 1993;19:143-51.
5. Balcıoğlu AS, Müderrisoğlu H. Diabetes and cardiac autonomic neuropathy: Clinical manifestations, cardiovascular consequences, diagnosis and treatment. World J Diabetes. 2015;6:80-91.
6. Johnston SC, Easton JD. Are patients with acutely recovered cerebral ischemia more unstable? Stroke. 2003;4:2446.
7. Lanier JB Mote MB, Clay EC. Evaluation and management of orthostatic hypotension. Am Fam Physician. 2011;84:527-36.
8. Freeman R, Saul P, Roberts M, et al. Spectral analysis of heart rate in diabetic autonomic neuropathy. Arch Neurol. 1991;48:185-90.
9. State-specific mortality from sudden cardiac death–United States, 1999. MMWR Morb Mortal Wkly Rep. 2002;51:123-6.
10. Siscovick DS, Sotoodehnia N, Rea TD, et al. Type 2 diabetes mellitus and the risk of sudden cardiac arrest in the community. Rev Endocr Metab Disord. 2010;11:53-9.
11. Spooner PM. Sudden cardiac death: influence of diabetes. Diabetes Obes Metab. 2008;10:523-32.
12. El-Atat FA, McFarlane SI, Sowers JR, et al. Sudden cardiac death in patients with diabetes. Curr Diab Rep. 2004;4:187-93.
13. El-Menyar AA. Dysrhythmia and electrocardiographic changes in diabetes mellitus: pathophysiology and impact on the incidence of sudden cardiac death. J Cardiovasc Med (Hagerstown). 2006;7: 580-5.
14. Lagi A. Syncope and hypoglycemia. Int J Clin Med. 2011;2:129-32.

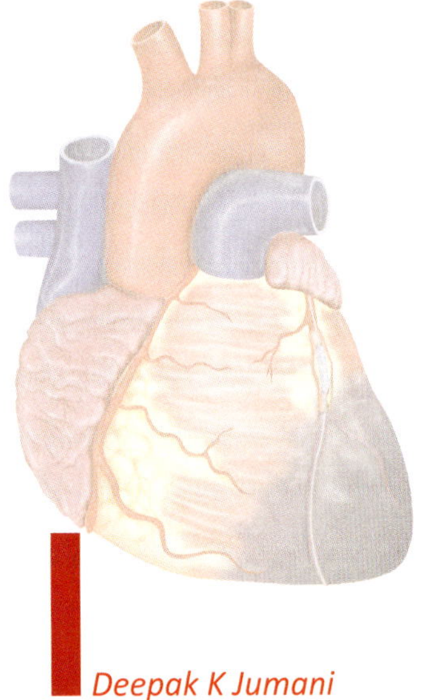

Cardiodiabetes and Sexual Dysfunction

Deepak K Jumani

INTRODUCTION

Diabetes is the biggest sexual health tsunami of 21st Century. According to IDF (International Diabetes Federation) in every 6 seconds one person dies of diabetes and in the same 6 seconds two patients develop diabetes. Of the 417 million diabetics across the globe, one-third of these diabetics are in India either in diabetic or prediabetic state, in fact India is the diabetes capital of the world and is closely competing with China, so China and India (Chindia) are the diabetes capital of the world. The most common complication of type 2 diabetic men is erectile dysfunction (ED). So Chindia are the ED capital of the world. Diabetes also is a prime risk factor for cardiovascular disease (CVD). Hyperglycemia which is the hallmark of diabetes results in myocardial damage after ischemic events. CVD accounted for 52% of the deaths among patients with diabetes in the World Health Organization (WHO) multinational study,[1] while data from the National Health and Nutrition Examination Survey (NHANES) showed a rate of 69.5%.[2] In fact, the risk of an acute coronary event in a patient with diabetes mellitus (DM) (type 1 or type 2), with no prior cardiac history, is similar to that of patients without diabetes but with established coronary artery disease (CAD).[3,4] It means that the diagnosis of DM alone places a patient in a high-risk category alongside patients with established CAD. In fact has been recognized by the American Heart Association, which established diabetes as a major cardiovascular risk factor in addition to other traditional risk factors[5]is effect of DM is not limited to the incidence of CAD but persists following an acute coronary event as well.

In both type 1 (Diabetes Control and Complications Trial)[6] and type 2 diabetes (United Kingdom Prospective Diabetes Study),[7] intensive glucose control affected macrovascular disease less than microvascular disease. Huxley and colleagues[8] in a meta-analysis of 37 studies of type 2 diabetes and fatal coronary heart disease among a total of 447,064 patients reported a 50% higher relative risk (RR) for fatal CAD in diabetic women than men. A recent Finnish study of more than 1,000 patients showed a considerably higher diabetes-related RR for a major CAD event in diabetic women (hazard ratio [HR], 14.7) than in men (HR, 3.8).[9] DM seems to eliminate the normal advantage that women have with regard to cardiovascular morbidity and mortality.

The duration of DM is of important clinical relevance. In 20 years of follow-up of more than 120,000 patients, Hu and colleagues[10] showed that the RR of death increased from 2.75 in women with DM for 5 years to 11.9 in patients with DM for 25 years, compared with non-diabetic women. A recent study showed that diabetes increased the risk of CAD to an equivalent degree as aging 10–15 years.[11,12] For each decade of life, DM increases the 10-year risk of CAD mortality by 86%.[6,13] In the presence of prior CAD, diabetes is associated with a 30-fold increased risk of fatal CAD.[10]

Healthcare providers are now focused on decreasing cardiovascular risk in patients with diabetes by treating dyslipidemia and hypertension and by improving glycemic control.[14] Moreover, the American Diabetes Association/ American College of Cardiology "Make the Link" public awareness campaign has improved knowledge related to CVD in patients with diabetes.

Today there is enough scientific wisdom in this field, from defects in the large blood vessels (macrovasculature) and the small blood vessel (microvasculature) to the less well understood cellular and molecular mechanisms of CVD in patients with diabetes. Atherosclerosis is the major threat to the macrovasculature for patients with and without diabetes. Clinically, dyslipidemia is highly correlated with atherosclerosis, and up to 97% of patients with diabetes have raised triglycerides, reduced high-density lipoprotein (HDL) and raised low-density lipoprotein (LDL).[15,16] In diabetes, the predominant form of LDL cholesterol is the small and dense form. Small LDL particles are more atherogenic than large LDL particles because they can more easily penetrate and form stronger attachments to the arterial wall and they are more susceptible to oxidation. The oxidized LDL is proatherogenic and initiates several abnormal biological responses, such as attracting leukocytes to the intima of the vessel, improving the ability of the leukocytes to ingest lipids and differentiate into foam cells, and stimulating the proliferation of leukocytes, endothelial cells, and smooth muscle cells, all of which are steps in the formation of atherosclerotic plaque. Also glycation of LDL particles lengthens its half-life and increases the ability of LDL to promote more atherogenesis and paradoxically glycation of HDL shortens its half-life making it less protective against atherogenesis. Hypertriglyceridemia can lead to increased production of the small, dense form of LDL and to decreased HDL transport of cholesterol back to the liver.[17]

However, small vessels throughout the body are affected by diabetes, including those in the brain, heart, and peripheral vasculature. This small vessel damage is typically not related to atherosclerosis and is not predicted by lipid levels. Whereas atherosclerosis is the major threat to the macrovasculature, a variety of cellular and molecular mechanisms contribute to microvascular disease in diabetes. The microvascular complications are due to central autonomic nervous system which includes sympathetic and parasympathetic nerves which reach the vascular smooth muscles and local regulation is carried out by substances produced by endothelial cells and the local products of metabolism. The endothelium produces both vasodilators and vasoconstrictors. Normally, the vascular smooth muscle receives continuous regulatory nerve signals and a continual supply of vasodilating nitric oxide (NO) from the endothelium, as well as a continuous flow of metabolic products. These regulatory mechanisms adjust microvascular flow instantaneously to meet the metabolic needs of the tissue.[18] Diabetes contributes to defects in the autonomic nervous system, the endothelium, and local metabolism, all of which can result in microvascular disease. Patients with diabetic autonomic neuropathy (DAN) have increased rates of sudden cardiac death as well as a higher overall cardiovascular mortality rate.[19,20] In addition to the dysregulation of vascular tone caused by DAN, subjects with diabetes have been found to have decreased bioavailability of NO, a potent vasodilator, as well as increased secretion of the vasoconstrictor endothelin-1. This resulting state of vasoconstriction has been found in subjects with the metabolic syndrome as well as those with diabetes. In this situation, the vasculature is in a hyperconstricted state. Not only do hypertension and its concomitant complications result from vasoconstriction, but blood flow is limited to respective tissues. Diabetes decreases NO bioavailability because of either insulin deficiency or defective insulin signaling (insulin resistance) in endothelial cells.[21,22] Hyperglycemia also acutely inhibits the production of NO in arterial endothelial cells.[23-24] Capillary basement membrane thickening associated with prolonged hyperglycemia is a structural hallmark of diabetic microvascular disease. Thickening of the basement membrane impairs the amount and selectivity of transport of metabolic products and nutrients between the circulation and the tissue. In fact, in skeletal muscle of patients with type 2 diabetes, exercise-stimulated oxygen delivery from the capillaries is delayed, which may account in part for the poor exercise tolerance found in people with type 2 diabetes.[25-26] The basement membrane thickening increases microvascular permeability because of alterations in the physical dimensions of the meshwork and changes in the normal electrical charge surrounding the pores between endothelial cells. These abnormalities allow for the transport of large molecules normally excluded from passage across the microvasculature. In clinical terms, transcapillary leak of albumin in the kidney provides an important indicator of microvascular disease.[27]

Diabetes has long been considered a state of chronic, low-level inflammation, and there is some evidence to suggest that this immune activation may precede insulin resistance in diabetic and prediabetic states and ultimately may be the factor that initially increases cardiovascular risk in these disease processes.[28]

Researchers have found a reduced production of the potent vasodilator NO and an increased secretion of the vasoconstrictor and growth factor endothelin-1 in subjects with the metabolic syndrome, and these abnormalities not only enhance vasoconstriction, but are associated with the release of proinflammatory cytokines. Proinflammatory cytokines cause or exacerbate injury by a variety of mechanisms including enhanced vascular permeability, programmed cell death (apoptosis), recruitment of invasive leukocytes, and the promotion of reactive oxygen species (ROS) production.[29] Pickup and Mattock found serum sialic acid, a marker of low-grade inflammation, to be strongly predictive of type 2 diabetes in 128 patients from the United Kingdom who were followed for a mean of 12.8 years. In addition to predicting type 2 diabetes, this marker also predicted cardiovascular mortality independent of other known risk factors for CVD, including preexisting CVD.[30,31] In addition to diabetes, obesity is associated with increased levels of a number of adipokines (cytokines released from adipose tissue), including tumor necrosis factor, interleukin 1, interleukin 6, and plasminogen activator inhibitor 1 (PAI-1), all linked to the inflammatory response.[32] However one anti-inflammatory adipokine, adiponectin which is also seen to be reduced thus exacerbating the chronic inflammatory state.

All the above proinflammatory cytokines also increase the oxidative stress by enhancing the production of ROS. The term ROS refers to a subset of molecules called "free radicals". This term refers to any molecule that contains an unpaired electron in the outer orbital. This unpaired electron makes the molecule highly reactive, seeking to either donate an electron to another compound or take up protons from another compound to obtain a stable electron pair. This high reactivity leads to the formation of bonds between the ROS and other compounds, altering the structure and function of the tissue. Because of the reactive propensity of these molecules, ROS can directly damage a number of cell components, such as plasma membranes and organelles.

According to Brownlee, there are four mechanisms by which chronic hyperglycemia causes diabetes complications: (1) activation of the polyol pathway; (2) increased formation of advanced glycosylation end products; (3) activation of protein kinase C, an enzyme involved in numerous molecular signaling pathways; (4) and activation of the hexosamine pathway. Through decades of research, Brownlee and his colleagues found that hyperglycemia-induced mitochondrial ROS production activates each of the four major pathways of hyperglycemic damage.[33-35] Moreover, blocking ROS production or interfering with ROS signaling attenuated the activity of all four pathways. Thus, oxidative stress is a crucially important concept in the pathophysiology of the cardiovascular complications in diabetes. Oxidative stress occurs when the cellular production of ROS exceeds the capacity of anti-oxidant defenses within cells. Numerous studies have demonstrated chronic oxidative stress in diabetic humans and animals, purportedly related to the metabolism of excess substrates (glucose and fatty acids) present in the hyperglycemic state, as well as to the mitochondrial dysfunction associated with insulin resistance. For example, plasma levels of hydroperoxides (one ROS) are higher in subjects with type 2 diabetes compared to nondiabetic subjects.[36]

The inflammatory response appears to be over-activated in insulin resistance and in diabetes. Leukocytes are major mediators of inflammation. They also contribute to the oxidative stress associated with diabetes. ROS are generated not only from the mitochondria, but also from activated leukocytes. Hokama et al. found that the expression of adhesion proteins on the surface of neutrophils, which suggests activation and ROS production, was significantly increased in diabetes.[37] The excess chronic oxidative stress produced in the hyperglycemic state by the mitochondria, as well as the additional acute stress mediated by accumulated leukocytes, may largely explain the mechanism of increased oxidative injury associated with ischemic heart disease in diabetes.

In addition to affecting the leukocytes in the blood, diabetes is also related to a hypercoagulable state. The coagulability of the blood is crucially important in ischemic cardiovascular events because the majority of myocardial infarction (MI) and stroke events are caused by the rupture of atherosclerotic plaque and the resulting occlusion of a major artery by a blood clot (thrombus). Up to 80% of patients with diabetes die a thrombotic death. Seventy-five percent of these deaths are the result of an MI, and the remainders are the result of cerebrovascular events and complications related to peripheral vascular disease (PVD).[38]

The first defense against a thrombotic event is the vascular endothelium. Diabetes contributes to widespread endothelial dysfunction. Patients with diabetes exhibit enhanced activation of platelets and clotting factors in the blood. Increased circulating platelet aggregates, increased platelet aggregation in response to platelet agonists, and the presence of higher plasma levels of platelet coagulation products, such as beta-thromboglobulin, platelet factor 4, and thromboxane B, demonstrate platelet hyperactivity in diabetes.

Coagulation activation markers, such as prothrombin activation fragment 1+2 and thrombin–antithrombin complexes are also elevated in diabetes. In addition, patients with diabetes have elevated levels of many clotting factors including fibrinogen, factor VII, factor VIII, factor XI, factor XII, kallikrein, and von Willebrand factor. Conversely, anticoagulant mechanisms are diminished in diabetes. The fibrinolytic system, the primary means of removing clots, is relatively inhibited in diabetes because of abnormal clot structures that are more resistant to degradation, and also because of an increase in PAI-1.[39,40] Myocardial damage in the absence of CAD (macrovascular) is most likely related to microvascular dysfunction. Microvascular damage in the diabetic heart may lead to the myocardial injury, fibrosis, and hypertrophy found in diabetic cardiomyopathy.[41] In type 1 diabetic patients without CAD, impaired coronary flow reserve (dependent on the microvasculature) predicts diastolic dysfunction and may be related to autonomic neuropathy.[42] Microvascular disease, including endothelial dysfunction caused by DAN and decreased NO bioavailability is of crucial importance.

Diabetes has been associated with sexual dysfunction both in men[43] and in women. Diabetes is an established risk factor for sexual dysfunction in men; a three-fold increased risk of ED was documented in diabetic compared with nondiabetic men. Among women, the evidence regarding the association between diabetes and sexual dysfunction is less conclusive, although most studies have reported a higher prevalence of female sexual dysfunction (FSD) in diabetic women as compared with nondiabetic women.[42-45]

ERECTILE DYSFUNCTION

Erectile dysfunction is defined as the persistent inability to achieve or maintain penile erection for successful sexual intercourse, causing decreased quality of life in men.[46-49] In the Massachusetts Male Aging Study,[44] diabetic men showed a three-fold probability of having ED than men without diabetes. Moreover, the age-adjusted risk of ED was doubled in diabetic men compared with those without diabetes. In addition, it has been estimated that the worldwide prevalence of ED will rise to 322 million cases by the year 2025.[49-51] ED is a marker of significantly increased risk of CVD, CHD, stroke, and all-cause mortality.[52-54] Advanced age and longer duration of diabetes have been associated with an increased risk of ED in diabetic patients but the occurrence of ED is 10–15 years earlier in men with diabetes.[44]

Pathogenesis of Erectile Dysfunction

The pathogenesis of ED in diabetes is multifactorial, as it depends on both psychological and organic factors (which play major roles in ED), mostly diabetic vasculopathy which includes microangiopathy, macroangiopathy and endothelial dysfunction, autonomic neuropathy, insulin resistance, visceral adiposity and hypogonadism. Macrovascular disease in diabetes corresponds to the atherosclerotic damage in the blood vessels, which limits blood flow to the penis. The chronic insult of hyperglycemia on the endothelium results in endothelial dysfunction. Endothelial dysfunction in diabetes is manifested as the decreased bioavailability of NO, resulting in insufficient relaxation of the vascular smooth muscle of the corpora cavernosa. The potential mechanisms involved in endothelial dysfunction include the accumulation of advanced glycation end products; increased levels of oxygen free radicals that reduce the bioavailability of NO; impaired endothelial and neuronal NO synthesis, expression, and activity; and an imbalance between the vasoconstrictive and vasorelaxant intracellular pathways favoring increased vasoconstriction. Esposito et al. observed an increase in circulating endothelial microparticles—an emergent marker of endothelial dysfunction in diabetic men with ED, as compared with nondiabetic men.[55] Microvascular disease determines ischemic damage in the distal circulation and autonomic and peripheral neuropathy. Both somatic and autonomic neuropathies may contribute to diabetes-induced ED due to the impairment of sensory impulses from the penis to the reflexogenic erectile center, and reduced or absent parasympathetic activity necessary for relaxation of the smooth muscle of the corpus cavernosum.[56-57] Insulin resistance and visceral adiposity, which are both distinctive clinical traits of type 2 diabetes, are associated with a proinflammatory state that results in the decreased availability and activity of NO, leading to ED in overweight and obese diabetic men.[58-61] Subnormal testosterone concentrations have been found in 25% of men with type 2 diabetes in association with inappropriately low luteinizing hormone (LH) and follicle-stimulating hormone (FSH) concentrations. Testosterone regulates nearly every component of erectile function, from pelvic ganglions to smooth muscle, and to the endothelial cells of the corpora cavernosa. It also modulates the timing of the erectile process, which occurs as a function of sexual desire, coordinating penile erection with sex. The mechanisms involved in testosterone deficiency in diabetes include low levels of the sex hormone-binding globulin due to insulin resistance, increased aromatase activity in visceral adipose tissue leading to an augmented conversion of testosterone in estradiol, leptin resistance causing reduced secretion of LH and testosterone, and increased levels of inflammatory mediators, which may suppress the secretion of gonadotropin-releasing hormone and LH.[62-64] Bellastella et al.[65] suggested a possible autoimmune pathogenesis of hypogonadotropic hypogonadism in type 2 diabetic patients, as indicated by the presence of antipituitary antibodies at high titers, as compared with age-matched controls.

Treatment of Erectile Dysfunction

To understand the treatment of ED one must understand that a normal vascular and neuronal endothelium produces endothelial nitric oxide synthase (eNOS) and neuronal nitric oxide synthase (nNOS). eNOS and nNos initiate the NO to enter in the corpora cavernosa spongy tissue and converts guanosine monophosphate to cyclic guanosine monophosphate with the help of an enzyme guanylate cyclase. This cyclic GMP is the main chemical which relaxes

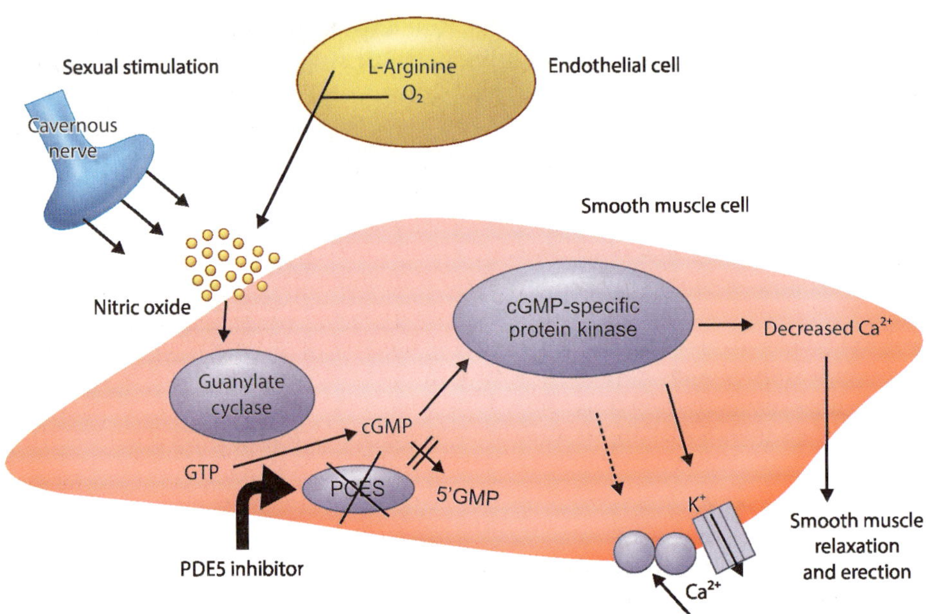

Fig. 1: Pathophysiology of erectile dysfunction

TABLE 1: Various drugs and their parameters

Parameter	*Sildenafil*	*Tadalafil*	*Udenafil*
Doses available	25 mg, 50 mg, 100 mg	5 mg, 20 mg	100 mg
Administration	Taken 90–120 min prior the act	Taken at least 120 min prior to act	Taken at least 60 min prior to act
Food interaction	Avoid fatty meals	None	None
Mean time to peak concentration (C_{max})	60 min	120 min	60 min
T1/2	3–5 hours	17.5 hours	10–12 hours

the smooth muscle cell of the corpora and allows the blood to flow in penile vasculature. This cGMP also decreases the calcium influx through specific protein kinases and allows the smooth muscle relaxation and erections. But soon cGMP gets hydrolyzed to 5-guanosine monophosphate with the help of an enzyme phosphodiesterase-5 (Fig. 1).

So for a good enough erection one has to see that the endothelium has to be normal functional, adequate NO, guanylate cyclase activators and stimulators, and cGMP to be present in more bioavailable form to maintain tumusence and lastly something to block the PDE5 enzyme.

The first-line of treatment is oral drugs and counseling. The second-line of treatment is intracavernous injection of papaverine and largactil and prostaglandin, vacuum therapy and intraurethral drugs like prostaglandin, along with counseling. The third-line of therapy is surgical treatment with implants and counseling.

So, counseling forms the mainstay for the treatment of ED. The oral drugs are phosphodiesterase-5 inhibitors (PDE5 inhibitors). These drugs block the conversion of cyclic guanosine monophosphate (cGMP) to 5-guanosine monophosphate and make cGMP more bioavailable which relaxes the smooth muscles and allows the blood to flow in the intracavernosal vasculature. The three PDE5 inhibitors available in our country are sildenafil citrate, tadalafil, and udenafil (Table 1).

Side Effects of PDE5 Inhibitors

It include facial flushing, headache, nasal congestion, dizziness, dyspepsia, visual disturbance (blue halo), central serous chorioretinopathy following oral tadalafil intake,[16] non-arteritic ischemic optic neuropathy (NAION), priapism.

Contraindications of PDE5 Inhibitors

Contraindications include recent cardiovascular event, nitrates, hypotension, anatomical deformity (angulation, cavernosal fibrosis, peyronie's disease), predisposition to prolonged erection, sickle cell disease, multiple myeloma, leukemia. PDE6 enzyme inhibition is less with udenafil compared to sildenafil—no visual abnormality, PDE11 enzyme inhibition with udenafil is less than tadalafil—no myalgia. Now we also have mouth dissolving films of sildenafil and tadalafil which have faster onset of action and lesser side effects. The newer oral drugs which shall soon be available are avanafil, mirodenafil, lodenafil carbonate and SLX-2101. The second-line of treatment is intracavernosal injection of papaverine and largactil with or without prostaglandin available as Bimix or Trimix self-filled injection. Always caution the patient of priapism. The site of injections which should be avoided are 12 o'clock position as it can damage the neurovascular bundle and 6 o'clock position of the shaft of the penis as this can damage the urethra.

Vacuum devices can be advised to patients who have undergone prostatectomy or elderly diabetics. Though this devise is noninvasive drug free and cost-effective; it is cumbersome. Sometimes patients complain of pain and numbness and delayed ejaculations. MUSE is medicated urethral insertion of drugs with the help of a device and prostaglandin pellets are introduced in the urethra. The other noninvasive treatment available is low-intensity extracorporeal shockwave therapy improves ED through angiogenesis.

The surgical treatment of ED is insertion of penile prosthesis or implants. The cheapest implant is made by Dr Rupin Shah, which is noninflatable and has a differential rigidity. Today we have 2 piece implants and 3 piece implants and the most widely recommended is 3 piece implant as these are totally concealed in body. Device is inflated to provide rigidity and deflated for concealment, erection longevity is controllable. When deflated, the cylinders are soft and flaccid and they do expand the penis in girth. The other surgical interventions include penile revascularization which is achieved by arterio-arterial anastomosis, which is needed during hip fractures and pudendal nerve and internal pudendal artery, or arterio-venous anastomosis by mobilizing deep dorsal vein and anastomosing it with internal epigastric artery. In case of venous leak from the dorsal vein, venous ligation is tried. According to Masters and Johnson's male sexual response, one has to have a desire to get a proper arousal and if the desire is inadequate (Figs 2A and B).

We have only focused on erection and ignored the desire which is the first to be in a male sexual response. So there exists a therapeutic gap in treatment of hypoactive sexual desire disorders in men with diabetes. But we now have a novel nutraceutical which has a tremendous effect of improving the sexual desires of our diabetic men. These nutraceuticals have L-arginine which is a proven NO donor and ingredients combined with it are saponised Fenugreek which has been studied to improve free testosterone levels to almost double and do not have any adverse side effects like synthetic testosterone. These nutraceuticals also have zinc which helps in spermatogenesis and also magnesium which has a relaxing effect and pyridoxine which helps in absorption of zinc and magnesium. There are many phyto-nutraceuticals which have L-arginine combined with Pycnogenol, Safed Musli, Terrestris Trichuris, Asparagus adscendens,Withania somnifera, Mucuna pruriens, Ginesing and Ginkgo biloba. These combinations with L-arginine help in improving the sexual desire and not give any side effects like synthetic testosterone. We have an ongoing study of this nutraceutical and it has been showing us a promising future.

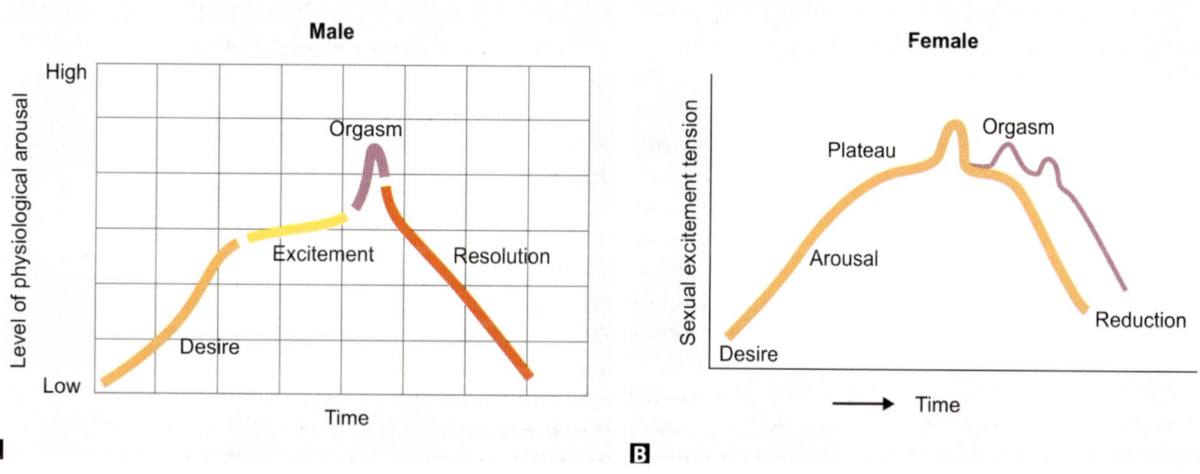

Figs 2A and B: (A) Male sexual response; (B) Female sexual response

Newer Therapies (Regenerative Therapies)

The newer therapies are regenerative therapies which include (Table 2):

- *Guanalyl cyclase activators and stimulators* as these increase the cellular cGMP concentration via the direct activation of sGC, which results in both vasorelaxation and inhibition of platelet aggregation.
- *Rho-Kinase inhibitors*: Inhibition of the calcium sensitization pathway with Rho-kinase inhibitors offers a therapeutic option for the treatment of ED that does not involve the direct targeting of the NO/sGC/cGMP pathway.
- *Gene therapy*: An adenoviral vector constructed to introduce a gene coding for a protein has been useful for improving ED.
- *Mesenchymal stem cell therapy*: Increasing evidences suggest the presence of penile endogenous stem cells, with the regenerative potential that rely on endogenous stem cells/progenitor cells thus offer new insights into ED therapy.
- *Nano technology*: Primarily this technology applies for topical delivery of drugs for on demand erectile function, injectable gels into the penis to prevent morphology changes post-prostatectomy, hydrogels to promote CN regeneration/neuroprotection and encapsulation of drugs to increase erectile function (primarily of PDE5i).

FEMALE SEXUAL DYSFUNCTION

The diagnostic and statistical manual of mental disorders, 5th edition (DSM-5)[66] released newer and revised definitions, in which sexual desire and arousal disorders have been combined into the "female sexual interest/arousal disorder" category, and vaginismus and dyspareunia have been grouped into the "genito-pelvic pain/penetration disorder" category. Moreover, all of the sexual dysfunctions outlined in the DSM-5 require a minimum duration of approximately 6 months, and more precise severity criteria must be met in order to provide useful thresholds for making a diagnosis and for distinguishing transient sexual difficulties from more persistent sexual dysfunction. Due to complex nature of female sexuality, the sexual dysfunctions are characterized by disturbances in the psychophysiological changes associated with the sexual response cycle in women, and it includes disorders of sexual desire, arousal, orgasm, and pain. There are common risk factor categories associated with sexual dysfunction in women; these include aging, DM, CVD, hypertension, concurrence of genitourinary disease, psychiatric/psychological disorders, cancer, and other chronic diseases. Moreover, limited social relations, financial difficulties, employment status, religious beliefs, educational background, and lack of exercise represent the sociocultural risk factors of FSD.[67-68]

Female sexual dysfunction have been described in diabetic women since the early 1980s. Sexual disorders reported in women with diabetes include the reduction or loss of sexual interest or desire, arousal or lubrication difficulties, dyspareunia, and loss of the ability to reach orgasm.[69-70] FSD has been associated with both type 1 and type 2 diabetes. A recent meta-analysis[70] that included 26 studies, 3,168 diabetic women, and 2,823 controls showed that FSD is more frequent, and is associated with a lower Female Sexual Function Index (FSFI) score in diabetic women than in controls. An increased risk of FSD was found in premenopausal women with "any diabetes", but not in

TABLE 2: Summary of the behavioral and pharmacological therapies of erectile dysfunction in diabetes

Therapy	*Mechanism of action*	*Indication*
Lifestyle changes (weight reduction, smoking cessation, physical exercise)	Risk factor modification	Obesity and associated cardiovascular risk factors
PDE5 inhibitors	They inhibit the PDE5 enzyme, prolonging the activity of cGMP in the cavernous smooth muscle, resulting in increased vasorelaxation and rigid penile erection	First-line pharmacological therapy (contraindicated in nitrate users)
Intracavernosal or transurethral vasoactive substances:		Second-line pharmacological therapy, unresponsive to PDE5 inhibitors
– PGE1	It increases the concentration of cAMP, causing smooth muscle relaxation	
– Phentolamine	Alpha adrenoreceptor blocker	
– Papaverine	Nonspecific PDE inhibitor	
Testosterone	It replaces normal testosterone levels	Diabetes-associated hypogonadism

Abbreviations: PDE5, phosphodiesterase-5; cGMP, cyclic guanosine monophosphate; PGE1, prostaglandin E1; cAMP, cyclic adenosine monophosphate; PDE, phosphodiesterase

postmenopausal women. Results from a large prospective study of 625 women with type 1 diabetes[43] showed that depression was the major predictor of sexual dysfunction. In one large study[71] that evaluated 613 diabetic women and 524 controls, it was found that the longer duration of diabetes, older age, higher BMI, the presence of CVD, and the presence of diabetic complications was significantly associated with worse sexual function.

The Pathogenesis of FSD in Diabetes

Diabetes may affect the integrity sensory and autonomic nervous systems, vascular supply to clitoris and external genitalia, smooth muscle relaxation of the genitalia erectile tissue, enhancement of genital blood flow which are dependent upon the action of nonadrenergic/noncholinergic neurotransmitters, such as vasoactive intestinal polypeptide (VIP) and NO. NO and PDE5 have been identified in human clitoral smooth muscle, indicating a key role of NO in female sexual function and normal levels of various hormones leading to diminished response to erotic stimuli leading to sexual dysfunction. So the mechanisms involved include hyperglycemia, infections, vascular and neurological damage, and hormonal disorders.[72]

Hyperglycemia reduces the hydration of the vaginal mucous membranes, producing poor vaginal lubrication and dyspareunia. Moreover, hyperglycemia increases the risk of genitourinary infections which, in turn, may lead to vaginal discomfort and dyspareunia.[73-74] Diabetes may affect arousal and orgasmic sexual responses by inducing impaired relaxation responses of the vaginal tissue to almost all transmitter systems,[75] decreasing nerve-stimulated clitoral and vaginal blood flow, producing diffuse fibrosis of the clitoris and vaginal tissues, and reducing the muscular layer and epithelial thickness in the vagina. Vascular abnormalities,[76] including atherosclerotic damage and diabetes-induced endothelial dysfunction, may be responsible for reducing the engorgement of the clitoris and for reducing lubrication of the vagina, leading to decreased arousal and dyspareunia during sexual intercourse. Diabetic neuropathy may further contribute to the pathogenesis of sexual dysfunctions by altering both the normal transduction of sexual stimuli and the triggered sexual response.[77] Epidemiological studies show a correlation between alterations in the levels of androgens, estrogens, as well as sex hormone-binding globulin and sexual problems in diabetic women.[78] Certain endocrine disorders of thyroid, hypothalamic-pituitary dysfunctions, hyperprolactinemia and polycystic ovarian syndrome, may further contribute to sexual dysfunctions in these women.[79]

Depression is strongly associated with diabetes in both type 1 and type 2 diabetes and is the principally established determinant of sexual dysfunction in women with diabetes.[80-81] To sum up FSD pathogenesis in diabetes is complex, and current studies have not yet clarified all of the pathological pathways involved; these studies are limited by small sample sizes, lack of standardized definitions of sexual dysfunction, and inadequate characterization of diabetes with regard to glycemic control, the presence of complications, and the presence of depression.

Treatment of FSD

At present, no specific guidelines are currently available for the treatment of FSD in diabetes; therefore, therapeutic possibilities for sexual dysfunction in diabetic women refer to lifestyle changes, optimal diabetic control, selected hormone replacement therapy and resolution of psychological issues, psychotherapy and the treatment of depression with specific medical therapy. In women tablet dehydroepiandrosterone (DHEA) 25 mg once a day for 6 weeks increases the sexual desire. For hypothyroid women correction of thyroid improves the desire. For high prolactin levels, tablet Bromocriptine 2.5 mg once at bed time for 6 weeks has been tried also tablet Cabergoline 0.5 mg once a week for 6 weeks shows promising results. Flibanserin is a new kid in the block for treatment of hypoactive sexual desire disorders in females. Flibanserin acts as a full agonist of the 5-HT1A receptor (Ki = 1 nM) and, with lower affinity, as an antagonist of the 5-HT2A receptor (Ki = 49 nM) and antagonist or very weak partial agonist of the D4 receptor (Ki = 4–24 nM).[82] Flibanserin preferentially activates 5-HT1A receptors in the prefrontal cortex, demonstrating regional selectivity, and has been found to increase dopamine and norepinephrine levels and decrease serotonin levels in the rat prefrontal cortex, actions that were determined to be mediated by activation of the 5-HT1A receptor. As such, flibanserin has been described as a norepinephrine-dopamine disinhibitor (NDDI). Flibanserin is given in the dose of 100 mg at bed time and the commonest side effects include dizziness, nausea, fatigue, sleepiness, and trouble sleeping.

Phosphodiesterase-5 inhibitors might theoretically improve vaginal lubrication and vulvar engorgement, this is likely due to the inconsistencies observed between the physiological and psychological factors on sexual response, or the low PDE5 levels noted in the female reproductive system. The adoption of healthy lifestyles may reduce insulin resistance, endothelial dysfunction, and oxidative stress, all of which are desirable achievements for diabetic patients. The resulting improved well-being may further help reduce and prevent sexual dysfunction in women.[83-84]

CONCLUSION

Diabetes mellitus is a growing public health concern, leading to cardiovascular, psychological, and sexual dysfunctions. Diabetes is a well-known cause of ED, moreover, ED is an independent risk factor for the new onset of CVD, and it is an important predictor of the development of major cardiovascular events in diabetic patients with known CAD. Sexual function and dysfunction in India, with special reference to the long-neglected issue of female sexuality, require to be systematically investigated if this branch of medicine is to become relevant to the needs of the population. Until recently, there has been limited clinical or scientific research in the field of FSD. Although some progress has been made, additional research is needed to assess treatment efficacy and establish national treatment guidelines. Because many patients are reluctant to initiate discussion of their sex lives, physicians should address this topic directly to elicit a history of sexual dysfunction. Population based surveys of sexual health can provide evidence to characterize normative, diverse, and evolving aspects of various domains of sexual health to inform community health priorities. In addition, such data can contribute to the development of effective policy actions, age-appropriate and culturally sensitive services and prevention programs, and resource allocation for optimizing public health activities. Lastly certain issues which affect sexual functions are that Indian studies show that resistance to inter-religious and inter-caste marriage typically comes from the girl's family, who risk losing respect or "honor" in their communities since their daughter making her own choices and this shows her family's apparent lack of control over her. The choices, freedom, attitudes and experiences of today's youth are radically different from everything that has preceded them and today's young Indians have a very different set of experiences than their parents, grandparents, and generations before them. India is at the first stage of this revolution. In India's case, the emancipation of women, the redefinition of sexual mores, the shift from arranged marriage to love marriage, is all happening at the very same time, and relationships between men and women in this country have changed more in the past 10 years than they have in the previous 3,000 years.

However, in India we see men at a higher risk of CAD after 40 years of life and a strong link between ED and CAD has been established. Indian women are more sedentary, gain weight soon after marriage and birth of first child and are not erotically intelligent as they often dress unattractively when at home and these biological and behavioral issues reduce their sexual appeal and also becomes a turn off for the husbands. The modern Indian girl is empowered today meets all the challenges of life and are self-reliant and this professional status translates into their aggression with their spouses and Indian men are not attuned to this and these issues become a relationship troubles and leads to sexual dysfunctions in men and some couples have a different work pattern and timings as they have to work to meet up the challenges of surviving and they meet only on weekends and they hardly have any time to be intimate as they are busy solving other errands of life. These real facts of today's couples are the reasons for increased incidences of sexual dysfunctions.

REFERENCES

1. Morrish NJ, Wang SL, Stevens LK, et al. Mortality and causes of death in the WHO Multinational Study of Vascular Disease in Diabetes. Diabetologia. 2001;44(Suppl 2): S14-21.
2. Gu K, Cowie CC, Harris MI. Mortality in adults with and without diabetes in a national cohort of the U.S. population, 1971–1993. Diabetes Care. 1998;21:1138-45.
3. Malmberg K, Yusuf S, Gerstein HC, et al. Impact of diabetes on long-term prognosis in patients with unstable angina and non-Q-wave myocardial infarction: results of the OASIS (Organization to Assess Strategies for Ischemic Syndromes) Registry. Circulation. 2000;102:1014-9.
4. Haffner SM, Lehto S, Ronnemaa T, et al. Mortality from coronary heart disease in subjects with type 2 diabetes and in nondiabetic subjects with and without prior myocardial infarction. N Engl J Med. 1998;339:229-34.
5. Grundy SM, Benjamin IJ, Burke GL, et al. Diabetes and cardiovascular disease: a statement for healthcare professionals from the American Heart Association. Circulation. 2000;101:1629-31.
6. Huxley R, Barzi F, Woodward M. Excess risk of fatal coronary heart disease associated with diabetes in men and women: meta-analysis of 37 prospective cohort studies. BMJ. 2006;332:73-8.
7. Juutilainen A, Kortelainen S, Lehto S, et al. Gender difference in the impact of type 2 diabetes on coronary heart disease risk. Diabetes Care. 2004;27:2898-904.
8. Booth GL, Kapral MK, Fung K, et al. Relation between age and cardiovascular disease in men and women with diabetes compared with non- diabetic people: a population-based retrospective cohort study. Lancet. 2006;368:29-36.
9. Fox CS, Sullivan L, D'Agostino RB Sr, et al. The significant effect of diabetes duration on coronary heart disease mortality: the Framingham Heart Study. Diabetes Care. 2004;27:704-8.
10. Hu FB, Stampfer MJ, Solomon CG, et al. The impact of diabetes mellitus on mortality from all causes and coronary heart disease in women: 20 years of follow-up. Arch Intern Med. 2001;161:1717-23.
11. Thomas JE, MD, Foody JM. Pathophysiology of Cardiovascular Disease in Diabetes Mellitus and the Future of Therapy. New Haven, CT: Department of Cardiology, Yale School of Medicine.
12. Abouma G, Mannirfasha C. Potentials of Phtyto therapeutic treatment of Erectile Dysfunction. South Africa: Department of Biomedical Sciences, Faculty of health and wellness. pp. 57172-4.
13. Lu Z, Lin G, Reed-Maldonado A. Can Low-Intensity Extracorporeal Shock Wave Therapy Improve Erectile Dysfunction: A Systematic Review and Meta-analysis. Eur Urol. 2010;58:241-9.
14. Garber AJ. Attenuating cardiovascular risk factors in patients with type 2 diabetes. Am Fam Phys. 2002;62:2633-42, 2645-6.
15. Fagot-Campagna A, Rolka DB, Beckles GL, et al. Prevalence of lipid abnormalities, awareness, and treatment in US adults with diabetes. Diabetes. 2000;49 (Suppl 1):A78.
16. Shen GX. Lipid disorders in diabetes mellitus and current management. Curr Pharm Analysis. 2007;3:17-24.

17. Duell PB, Oram JF, Bierman EL. Nonenzymatic glycosylation of HDL and impaired HDL-receptor-mediated cholesterol efflux. Diabetes. 1991;40:377-84.
18. Lewis DH. The effect of trauma on the regulation of the microcirculation [Abstract]. Pathophysiol. 1998;5 (Suppl 1):191.
19. Ewing DJ, Campbell D, Clarke BF. The natural history of diabetic autonomic neuropathy. Q J Med. 1980;49:95-108.
20. Taskiran M, Fritz-Hansen T, Rasmussen V, et al. Decreased myocardial perfusion reserve in diabetic autonomic neuropathy. Diabetes. 2002;51:3306-10.
21. Diabetes Control and Complications Trial Research Group. The effect of intensive treatment of diabetes on the development and progression of long-term complications in insulin-dependent diabetes mellitus. N Engl J Med. 1993;329:977-86.
22. UK Prospective Diabetes Study (UKPDS) Group. Intensive blood-glucose control with sulphonylureas or insulin compared with conventional treatment and risk of complications in patients with type 2 diabetes (UKPDS 33). Lancet. 1998;352:837-53.
23. Brownlee M: Biochemistry and molecular cell biology of diabetic complications. Nature. 2001;414:813-20.
24. Williams SB, Goldfine AB, Timimi FK, et al. Acute hyperglycemia attenuates endothelium-dependent vasodilation in humans in vivo. Circulation. 1998;97:1695-701.
25. Hayden MR, Sowers JR, Tyagi SC. The central role of vascular extracellular matrix and basement membrane remodeling in metabolic syndrome and type 2 diabetes: the matrix preloaded. Cardiovasc Diabetol. 2005;4:9-29.
26. Bauer TA, Reusch JEB, Levi M, et al. Skeletal muscle deoxygenation after the onset of moderate exercise suggests slowed microvascular blood flow kinetics in type 2 diabetes. Diabetes Care. 2007;30:2880-5.
27. Tooke JE. Microcirculation and diabetes. British Med Bull. 1989;45:206-23.
28. Festa A, D'Agostino Jr R, Howard G, et al. Chronic subclinical inflammation as part of the insulin resistance syndrome. Circulation. 2000;102:42-7.
29. Woods M, Mitchell JA, Wood EG, et al. Endothelin-1 is induced by cytokines in human vascular smooth muscle cells: evidence for intracellular endothelin-converting enzyme. Mol Pharmacol. 1999;55:902-9.
30. Pickup JC, Mattock MB. Activation of the innate immune system as a predictor of cardiovascular mortality in type 2 diabetes mellitus. Diabet Med. 2003;20:723-6.
31. Pickup JC, Mattock MB, Chusney GD, et al. NIDDM as a disease of the innate immune system: association of acute-phase reactants and interleukin-6 with metabolic syndrome X. Diabetologia. 1997;40:1286-92.
32. Trayhurn P, Wood IS. Signaling role of adipose tissue: adipokines and inflammation in obesity. Biochem Soc Trans. 2005;33:1078-81.
33. Testa CM. Mitochondria in movement disorders. In: Watts RL, Koller WC (Eds.) Movement Disorders, 2nd edition. New York: McGraw Hill; 2004. pp. 61-86.
34. Nourooz-Zadeh J, Rahimi A, Tajaddini-Sarmadi J, et al. Relationships between plasma measures of oxidative stress and metabolic control in NIDDM. Diabetologia. 1997;40:647-53.
35. Brownlee M. The pathobiology of diabetic complications: a unifying mechanism. Diabetes. 2005;54:1615-25.
36. Petersen KF, Dufour S, Befroy D, et al. Impaired mitochondrial activity in the insulin-resistant offspring of patients with type 2 diabetes. N Engl J Med. 2004;350:664-71.
37. Hokama J, Ritter LS, Davis-Gorman G, et al. Diabetes enhances leukocyte accumulation in the coronary microcirculation early in reperfusion following ischemia [Abstract]. J Diabetes Comp. 2000;14:96-107.
38. Gu K, Cowie CC, Harris ML. Mortality in adults with and without diabetes in a national cohort of the US population, 1971–1993. Diabetes Care. 1998;21:1138-45.
39. Weyrich AS, Prescott SM, Zimmerman GA. Platelets, endothelial cells, inflammatory chemokines, and restenosis: signaling in the vascular play book. Circulation. 2002;106:1433-5.
40. Carr ME. Diabetes: a hypercoagulable state. J Diabetes Comp. 2001;15:44-54.
41. Kawaguchi M, Techigawara M, Ishihata T, et al. A comparison of ultrastructural changes on endomyocardial biopsy specimens obtained from patients with diabetes mellitus with and without hypertension. Heart Ves. 1997;12:267-74.
42. Pop-Busui R, Kirkwood I, Schmid H, et al. Sympathetic dysfunction in type 1 diabetes: association with impaired myocardial blood flow reserve and diastolic dysfunction. J Am Coll Cardiol. 2004;44:2368-74
43. Enzlin P, Rosen R, Wiegel M, et al. DCCT/EDIC Research Group. Sexual dysfunction in women with type 1 diabetes: long-term findings from the DCCT/EDIC study cohort. Diabetes Care. 2009;32(5):780-5.
44. Feldman HA, Goldstein I, Hatzichristou DG, et al. Impotence and its medical and psychosocial correlates: results of the Massachusetts Male Aging Study. J Urol. 1994;151(1):54-61.
45. Giugliano F, Maiorino M, Bellastella G, et al. Determinants of erectile dysfunction in type 2 diabetes. Int J Impot Res. 2010;22(3):204-9.
46. NIH Consensus Conference. Impotence. NIH Consensus Development Panel on Impotence. JAMA. 1993;270(1):83-90.
47. Laumann EO, Paik A, Rosen RC. Sexual dysfunction in the United States: prevalence and predictors. JAMA. 1999;281(6):537-44.
48. De Berardis G, Franciosi M, Belfiglio M, et al. Quality of Care and Outcomes in Type 2 Diabetes (QuED) Study Group. Erectile dysfunction and quality of life in type 2 diabetic patients: a serious problem too often overlooked. Diabetes Care. 2002;25(2):284-91.
49. Johannes CB, Araujo AB, Feldman HA, et al. Incidence of erectile dysfunction in men 40 to 69 years old: longitudinal results from the Massachusetts male aging study. J Urol. 2000;163(2):460-3.
50. Bacon CG, Mittleman MA, Kawachi I, et al. Sexual function in men older than 50 years of age: results from the health professionals follow-up study. Ann Intern Med. 2003;139(3):161-8.
51. Ayta IA, McKinlay JB, Krane RJ. The likely worldwide increase in erectile dysfunction between 1995 and 2025 and some possible policy consequences. BJU Int. 1999;84(1):50-6.
52. Dong JY, Zhang YH, Qin LQ. Erectile dysfunction and risk of cardiovascular disease: meta-analysis of prospective cohort studies. J Am Coll Cardiol. 2011;58(13):1378-5.
53. Ponholzer A, Temml C, Obermayr R, et al. Is erectile dysfunction an indicator for increased risk of coronary heart dis- ease and stroke? Eur Urol. 2005;48(3):512-8; discussion 517-8.
54. Araujo AB, Travison TG, Ganz P, et al. Erectile dysfunction and mortality. J Sex Med. 2009;6(9):2445-54.
55. Esposito K, Ciotola M, Giugliano F, et al. Endothelial microparticles correlate with erectile dysfunction in diabetic men. Int J Impot Res. 2007;19(2):161-6.
56. Nehra A, Moreland RB. Neurologic erectile dysfunction. Urol Clin North Am. 2001;28(2):289-308.
57. 65. Sáenz de Tejada I, Angulo J, Cellek S, et al. Pathophysiology of erectile dysfunction. J Sex Med. 2005;2(1):26-39.
58. Esposito K, Giugliano D. Obesity, the metabolic syndrome, and sexual dysfunction in men. Clin Pharmacol Ther. 2011;90(1):169-73.
59. Dhindsa S, Prabhakar S, Sethi M, et al. Frequent occurrence of hypogonadotropic hypogonadism in type 2 diabetes. J Clin Endocrinol Metab. 2004;89(11):5462-8.
60. Kapoor D, Aldred H, Clark S, et al. Clinical and biochemical assessment of hypogonadism in men with type 2 diabetes: correlations with bioavailable testosterone and visceral adiposity. Diabetes Care. 2007;30(4):911-7.
61. Shabsigh R, Rajfer J, Aversa A, et al. The evolving role of testosterone in the treatment of erectile dysfunction. Int J Clin Pract. 2006;60(9):1087-92.

62. Isidori AM, Buvat J, Corona G, et al. A critical analysis of the role of testosterone in erectile function: from pathophysiology to treatment–a systematic review. Eur Urol. 2014;65(1):99-112.
63. Dandona P, Dhindsa S. Update: Hypogonadotropic hypogonadism in type 2 diabetes and obesity. J Clin Endocrinol Metab. 2011;96(9): 2643-51
64. Bellastella G, Maiorino MI, Olita L, et al. Anti-pituitary antibodies and hypogonadotropic hypogonadism in type 2 diabetes: in search of a role. Diabetes Care. 2013;36(8):e116-7.
65. American Psychiatric Association. Appendix. Highlights of changes from DSM-IV to DSM-5. In: Diagnostic and Statistical Manual of Mental Disorders, 5th edition. Arlington, VA: American Psychiatric Association; 2013.
66. Doumas M, Tsiodras S, Tsakiris A, et al. Female sexual dysfunction in essential hypertension: a common problem being uncovered. J Hypertens. 2006;24(12):2387-92.
67. Krychman M, Millheiser LS. Sexual health issues in women with cancer. J Sex Med. 2013;10 (Suppl 1):5-15.
68. Enzlin P, Mathieu C, Vanderschueren D, et al. Diabetes mellitus and female sexuality: a review of 25 years' research. Diabet Med. 1998;15(10):809-15.
69. Pontiroli AE, Cortelazzi D, Morabito A. Female sexual dysfunction and diabetes: a systematic review and meta-analysis. J Sex Med. 2013;10(4):1044-51.
70. Abu Ali RM, Al Hajeri RM, Khader YS, et al. Sexual dysfunction in Jordanian diabetic women. Diabetes Care. 2008;31(8):1580-1.
71. Bargiota A, Dimitropoulos K, Tzortzis V, et al. Sexual dysfunction in diabetic women. Hormones (Athens). 2011;10(3):196-206.
72. Meeking DR, Fosbury JA, Cummings MH. Sexual dysfunction and sexual health concerns in women with diabetes. Practical Diabetes. 2013;30(8):327-31.
73. Muniyappa R, Norton M, Dunn ME, et al. Diabetes and female sexual dysfunction: moving beyond "benign neglect". Curr Diab Rep. 2005;5(3):230-6.
74. GiraldiA, PerssonK, WerkströmV, et al. Effects of diabetes on neurotransmission in rat vaginal smooth muscle. Int J Impot Res. 2001;13(2):58-66.
75. Park K, Ahn K, Chang JS, et al. Diabetes induced alteration of clitoral hemodynamics and structure in the rabbit. J Urol. 2002;168(3): 1269-72.
76. Duby JJ, Campbell RK, Setter SM, et al. Diabetic neuropathy: an intensive review. Am J Health Syst Pharm. 2004;61(2):160-73; quiz 175.
77. Feldhaus-Dahir M. The causes and prevalence of hypoactive sexual desire disorder: part I. Urol Nurs. 2009;29(4):259-60, 263.
78. Bhasin S, Enzlin P, Coviello A, et al. Sexual dysfunction in men and women with endocrine disorders. Lancet. 2007;369(9561): 597-611.
79. Schram MT, Baan CA, Pouwer F. Depression and quality of life in patients with diabetes: a systematic review from the European depression in diabetes (EDID) research consortium. Curr Diabetes Rev. 2009;5(2):112-9.
80. Rockliffe-Fidler C, Kiemle G. Sexual function in diabetic women: a psychological perspective. Sex Relation Ther. 2003;18(2): 143-59.
81. Chivers ML, Rosen RC. Phosphodiesterase type 5 inhibitors and female sexual response: faulty protocols or paradigms? J Sex Med. 2010;7(2 Pt 2):858-72.
82. Maiorino MI, Bellastella G, Esposito K. Diabetes and sexual dysfunction: current perspectives. Diabetes Metab Syndr Obes. 2014;7:95-105.
83. Uckert S, Ellinghaus P, Albrecht K, et al. Expression of messenger ribonucleic acid encoding for phosphodiesterase isoenzymes in human female genital tissues. J Sex Med. 2007;4(6):1604-9.
84. Goldfischer E, Cotton D, Mikl J, et al. Efficacy of continued Flibanserin treatment on sexual functioning in premenopausal women with HSDD: Results from the ROSE Study. J Sex Med, 2008.

CHAPTER

Cardiodiabetes and Erectile Dysfunction

Naveen Garg, KK Kapur, HK Chopra

INTRODUCTION

Diabetes as a lifestyle disease has emerged as a prime cause of erectile dysfunction in men. Erectile dysfunction (ED) means repeated inability to achieve or sustain an erection sufficient enough for satisfactory sexual intercourse. Over the past decade, there have been several studies and surveys in the literature as regards the causes and treatment of erectile dysfunction. It has been estimated that one in ten males are suffering from erectile dysfunction and diabetes directly or indirectly account for 50% of these cases. Erectile dysfunction is common with increasing age. There is 77.5% likelihood of having ED at age above 70 years whereas in younger age group (20–30 years) this is less than 6.5%. Erectile dysfunction is one of the most important factors leading to breakdown of interpersonal relationships. Erectile dysfunction has adverse psychological impacts which further aggravate the problem. Several years ago ED was considered to be mainly psychological but over the last few years several organic causes have been elucidated. The pathophysiology of erectile dysfunction involves vasculogenic, neurogenic, and myogenic etiologies which interact with several molecular factors.[1-3]

IMPACT OF DIABETES ON ERECTILE DYSFUNCTION

Diabetes contributes about 50% to its causation (Fig. 1). In a landmark Massachusetts male aging study, it was observed that diabetic men (especially type 2) had three times chances of having ED when compared with counterparts without diabetes. The Boston University Medical Center study concluded that about half of men who are diagnosed with type 2 diabetes will develop ED within 5–10 years of their diagnosis. If these men also had heart disease, their odds of becoming impotent are even greater.[4-6] Both type-1 and type 2 diabetes have been found to be important in the etiology of ED. In METRO study (Management and Technology for Transition) involving 211 subjects in the age group of 18–35 years, it was observed that 37% (57 of 151) patients with type 1 diabetes had ED versus only 6% (4 of 60) of those without diabetes. Since these participants were in the younger age group (18–35 years), this study shows that in type 1 diabetes, ED occurs rather early in life.[7-8] In diabetics ED occur 10–15 years earlier than in nondiabetics. It is also more severe in nature, difficult to treat and less likely to be responsive to pharmacotherapy. It, thus, adversely affects quality of life and could lead to depression. The pathophysiological factors in diabetic patient leading to ED are endothelial dysfunction, atherosclerotic obstruction and autonomic neuropathy. These are depicted as in Figure 2.

PATHOPHYSIOLOGY OF ERECTILE DYSFUNCTION IN DIABETES

The penile erection is a complex phenomenon that involves neurogenic, hormonal, vascular and molecular pathways.[9-10] The somatic stimulation from dorsal nerve of penis triggers responses in spinal cord, cerebrum and efferent massages through pudendal nerve leads to dilatation of cavernosal arteries and increased the blood flow into the cavernosal

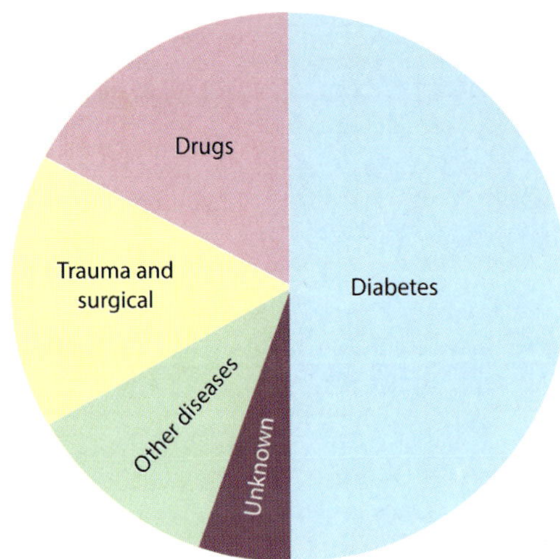

Fig. 1: Etiology of erectile dysfunction (ED)

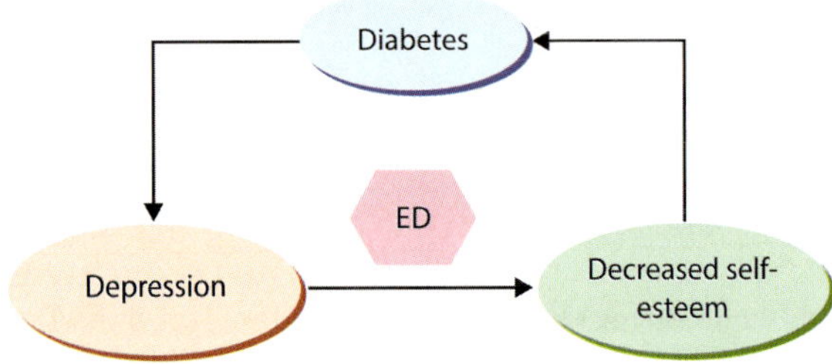

Fig. 2: Vicious circle of erectile dysfunction (ED) in diabetics

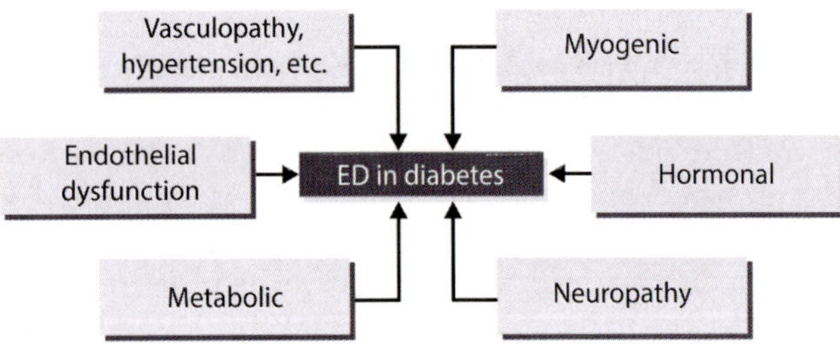

Fig. 3: Factors causing erectile dysfunction (ED) in diabetics

muscles. This increased arterial flow in cavernosal arteries leads to cavernosal venoconstriction and thus entraps the blood within the penile tissue. Therefore, the hemodynamics involving increased cavernosal inflow and practically no outflow (veno-occlusive mechanism) maintains penile erection. During detumescence sympathetic nerves cause constriction of arteries and opening up of the +cavernosal venules. This results in emptying of cavernosal sinusoids into venouses. The effects of diabetes on pathophysiology of penile erection are summarized as (Fig. 3).

- *Vascular effects*
  - Diabetes is known to cause increased *atherosclerosis* in the arteries. The increased plaque formation hampers the perfusion to the distal tissues. The plaques formation in pudendal arteries results in decreased blood flow to the penile tissues during the erectile phase especially with the abnormal blood pressure variations which can be deducted by ambulatory blood pressure monitoring.
  - The *size of the arteries* in diabetic patients is often small than of their counterparts. These result due to long-standing hyperglycemia associated with hyperlipidemia and hyperinsulinemia. This results in the genesis of various mediators like advanced glycation end products (AGEs) as well as reactive oxygen species (ROS). This then leads to reduced calcium influx and sequestration; thereby causing impairment in arterial wall relaxation. These mediators also cause abnormalities in cross linkages in collagen and elastin proteins which also increase arterial stiffness and further compromise arterial relaxation.
  - *Microvascular ischemia*: Hyperglycemia, lipid abnormalities and smoking cause oxidative stress on the vascular endothelium leading to decreased production of nitric oxide (NO). This adversely affects vasa-vasorum of the arteries and results in ischemic damage and perivascular fibrosis.
  - *Endothelial dysfunction*: The decreased sheer stress of blood flow further decreases the production of NO. The release of acetylcholine presents in the nerve endings in decreased as a result of diabetic neuropathy and thus adversely aggravates the vascular dilation process.
- *Neurogenic effects*
  - *Neuronal ischemia* results from atherosclerosis and endothelial dysfunction of vasa-nervosum, is a well-established cause of diabetic neuropathy. Small blood vessel dysfunction results in progression of neural dysfunction.
  - *Polyol pathway hyperactivity*: Hyperglycemia in diabetic patients induces alternative metabolic pathway which ultimately results in increased intracellular sorbitol accumulation and decreased amounts of oxidative stress scavengers like glutathione. This results in nerve damage.
  - *Oxidative stress*: Autoxidation of glucose, increased intracellular formation of AGEs, altered mitochondrial function and overactivity of the hexosamine pathway; all results in increased oxidative stress in neuronal tissues. Enhanced free radical formation and deficiency in antioxidants play a major role among the pathogenesis of diabetic neuropathy.[11-12]
- *Hormonal effects*
  - *Low testosterone* levels in both type 1 and type 2 diabetic patients cause decrease in libido.

- Diabetes has been linked to decreased levels of *dopamine* in brain and increased level of depression and anxiety.[13-15]
- *Myogenic effects*
  - Animal experimental studies had revealed a decrease in *cavernosal muscle density* and increased fibrosis in diabetic subjects. This change in cavernosal tissue impacts the blood flow and tissue resistance and, hence adversely affects penile erections.[16-18]
  - *Peyronie's disease* is common in diabetics. In fact diabetes is thought to exaggerate the fibrotic process in this condition and therefore, Peyronie's disease could be a silent consequence of diabetes.[19-20]

Other Associated Factors which Contribute to Erectile Dysfunction in Diabetics

Other associated factors which contribute to ED in diabetics are summarized in Table 1.

DIAGNOSIS OF ERECTILE DYSFUNCTION

Approach to a patient with ED needs a proper history taking and psychological evaluation. Following stepwise approach may help in evaluating ED in men.[21-23]

1. Step-1: History taking and knowing psychological impact
2. Step-2: Undergoing blood analysis to rule out associated pathologies
3. Step-3: IIEF-5 or IIEF-15 questionaries' to know the severity of symptoms
4. Step-4: Penile erection studies—ultrasonography and Doppler assessment of peak systolic velocity of penile arteries (including pharmacological response—Figs 4A and B, Table 2), tumescence (rigidity) studies, neurological studies including bulbocavernous reflex, somatosensorial evoked potential and perineal electromyography.

TABLE 1: Other factors that may play role in ED in association with diabetes

Increased blood cholesterol	***Insomnia***	*Drugs (β-blockers digoxin diuretics, etc.)*
Uncontrolled blood pressure	Obstructive sleep apnea	
Obesity	Alcohol intake	
Sedentary lifestyle	Cardiovascular events	
Smoking	Depression	

TREATMENT STRATEGIES[24-25]

- *Counseling and lifestyle changes*
- *Pharmacotherapies*
  - PDE-5 inhibitors—Sildenafil, Tadalafil
  - Alfa-2-antagonist—Yohimbine

TABLE 2: Doppler assessment of erectile dysfunction (ED)

Peak systolic velocity after injecting intracavernosal vasodilator agent	***End-diastolic velocity***	***Interpretation***
<25 cm/sec		Arteriogenic plaque or obstruction
25–35		Endothelial dysfunction
>35	<5	Normal
>35	<5	Myogenic if hardness is less
>35	>10	Venous leak

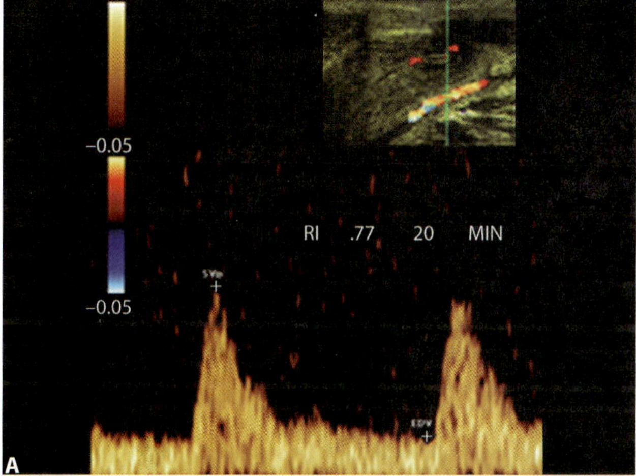

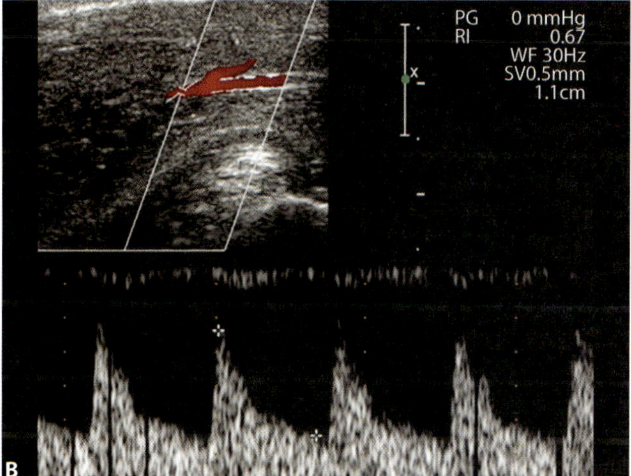

Figs 4A and B: Ultrasonographic/Doppler assessment. (A) Showing PSV 55.7 cm/s, EDV 12.7 cm/s and RI 0.77 at 20 minutes highly suggestive of anatomical venous leak; (B) Showing PSV 23.1 cm/s is consistent with arteriogenic etiology of ED

  - Prostaglandin E1 (PGE1)—Alprostadil
  - Papaverine
- *Mechanical devices*
  - Vacuum erection devices
  - Constriction band/rings
  - Implants.

CONCLUSION

Meticulous control of diabetes, hypertension by lifestyle optimization and timely effective medicalization will prevent erectile dysfunction in cardiodiabetes. Therefore, need for primordial, primary, secondary and tertiary preventive strategies are of paramount importance. The future treatment of ED lies on stem cell or gene therapies that will enhance the cavernosal muscle activity and increase the endothelial performance by augmenting the production of nitric oxide.

REFERENCES

1. UK Health Centre. Erectile dysfunction statistics. [online] Available at *www.healthcentre.org.uk*. [Accessed Oct. 2017].
2. Prins J, Blanker MH, Bohnen AM, et al. Prevalence of erectile dysfunction: a systematic review of population-based studies. Int J Impot Res. 2002;14:422-32.
3. Kubin M, Wagner G, Fugl-Meyer AR. Epidemiology of erectile dysfunction. Int J Impot Res. 2003;15:63-71.
4. Feldman HA, Goldstein I, Hatzichristou DG, et al. Impotence and its medical and psychosocial correlates: results of the Massachusetts Male Aging Study. J Urol. 1994;151(1):54-61.
5. O'Donnell AB, Araujo AB, McKinlay JB. The health of normally aging men: The Massachusetts Male Aging Study (1987-2004). Exp Gerontol. 2004;39(7):975-84.
6. Boston University. Epidemiology of ED. 2002 [online] Available at *www.bumc.bu.edu*. [Accessed Oct., 2017].
7. Maiorino MI, Bellastella G, Della Volpe E, et al. Erectile dysfunction in young men with type 1 diabetes. Int J Impot Res. 2017;29:17-22.
8. Chitaley K. Type 1 and Type 2 diabetic-erectile dysfunction: same diagnosis (ICD-9), different disease? J Sex Med. 2009;6(Suppl 3):262-8.
9. Dean RC, Lue TF. Physiology of penile erection and pathophysiology of erectile dysfunction. Urol Clin North Am. 2005;32(4):379-95, v.
10. Giuliano, F. Neurophysiology of erection and ejaculation. J Sex Med. 2011;8:310-5.
11. Schreiber AK, Nones CF, Reis RC, et al. Diabetic neuropathic pain: Physiopathology and treatment. World J Diabetes. 2015;6(3):432-44.
12. Yagihashi S, Mizukami H, Sugimoto K. Mechanism of diabetic neuropathy: Where are we now and where to go? J Diabetes Investig. 2011;2(1):18-32.
13. Salminen M, Vahlberg T, Räihä I, et al. Sex hormones and the risk of type 2 diabetes mellitus: A 9-year follow up among elderly men in Finland. Geriatr Gerontol Int. 2015;15(5):559-64.
14. Grossmann M, Thomas MC, Panagiotopoulos S, et al. Low testosterone levels are common and associated with insulin resistance in men with diabetes. J Clin Endocrinol Metab. 2008;93:1834-40.
15. Kleinridders A, Cai W, Cappellucci L, et al. Insulin resistance in brain alters dopamine turnover and causes behavioral disorders. Proc Natl Acad Sci. 2015;112(11):3463-8.
16. Burchardt T, Burchardt M, Karden J, et al. Reduction of endothelial and smooth muscle density in the corpora cavernosa of the streptozotocin induced diabetic rat. J Urol. 2000;164(5):1807-11.
17. Abidu-Figueiredo M, Ribeiro IC, Chagas MA, et al. The penis in diabetes: structural analysis of connective tissue and smooth muscle alterations in a rabbit model. BJU Int. 2011;108(3):400-4.
18. Wei AY, He SH, Zhao JF, et al. Characterization of corpus cavernosum smooth muscle cell phenotype in diabetic rats with erectile dysfunction. Int J Impot Res. 2012;24(5):196-201.
19. Kendirci M, Trost L, Sikka SC, et al. Diabetes mellitus is associated with severe Peyronie's disease. BJU Int. 2007;99(2):383-6.
20. Tefekli A, Kandirali E, Erol B, et al. Peyronie's disease: a silent consequence of diabetes mellitus. Asian J Androl. 2006;8(1):75-9.
21. Garg N, Kapur KK. Chapter 30: Penile Doppler Study. In: khanna NN, Henry M (Eds). Handbook of Interventions for Structural Heart and Periopheral Vascular Diseases. New Delhi: Jaypee Brothers Medical Publishers (P) Ltd, 2015.
22. Patel DV, Halls J, Patel U. Investigation of erectile dysfunction. Br J Radiol. 2012;85:S69-S78.
23. Ghanem H, Shamloul R. An evidence-based perspective to commonly performed erectile dysfunction investigations. J Sex Med.2008;5(7):1582-9.
24. Handelsman DJ, Conway AJ. The management of erectile dysfunction. Aust Prescr. 1998;21:46-8.
25. Gareri P, Castagna A, Francomano D, et al. Erectile dysfunction in the elderly: an old widespread issue with novel treatment perspectives. Int J Endocrinol. 2014, Article ID 878670, 15 pages.

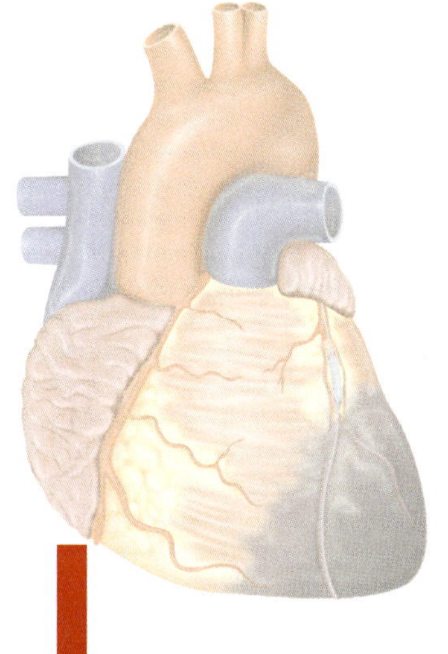

Endothelial Cell Dysfunction in DM, HT and CAD, and Its Pathophysiology

GS Sainani, Manisha Sawhney, Nitin Joshi, Aneesa Kapadia, Rajesh Sainani

INTRODUCTION

Over last few decades, endothelium has assumed a vital role. Earlier endothelium was thought to be a smooth, intact nonthrombogenic lining of the arterial walls. But now it is clear that endothelium produces several vasoactive substances which regulate vascular tone and structure. As a matter of fact, with its total mass of approximate five normal hearts weighing about 1,800 g, the endothelium is considered as the largest endocrine organ. Total vascular surface area is equivalent to six tennis courts in an adult weighing 70 kg. The vascular endothelium that lines the luminal surface of the coronary arteries is a physiologically active organ that plays an important role in the regulation of coronary arteries vasomotion as well as in the prevention of platelet, neutrophil and monocyte activation and adhesion to the lumen surface.[1]

The endothelial factors that help to regulate vasomotion are divided into two groups—(1) endothelial derived relaxing factors (EDRFs) and (2) endothelial derived constricting factors (EDCFs). EDRFs include nitric oxide (NO) and prostacyclin (PG2) and EDCFs include endothelin-1 (ET1) and thromboxane A2 (TXA2). These factors balance the effects of vascular tone and vascular structure as shown in Figure 1. All factors work together in the normal coronary vascular endothelium to regulate vasomotion and to preserve a smooth nonthrombotic luminal surface (Fig. 2). The alterations in these factors, if allowed to become chronic, are responsible for changes in vascular structure and growth and adhesiveness to platelets and leukocytes leading to atherosclerosis.[2,3] Our aim should be to maintain smooth endothelial lining by proper diet and lifestyle that will ensure the integrity of vascular structure of our body (Fig. 3). The most important vasculatures are coronary, cerebral and peripheral blood vessels.

The functions of endothelium are: Maintenance of normal vascular tone and growth by a balanced secretion of vasoconstrictor growth promoting (ET1, TXA2) as well as vasorelaxant and antiproliferative (NO, PG2) factors, regulate transport of macromolecules from the blood stream into the vessel wall, and prevent circulating blood cells (monocytes, platelets) from adhering to the vessel wall. NO has been the most important molecule. It has multifaceted role in the vessel wall (Fig. 4). It inhibits platelet aggregation, neutrophil adhesion, adhesion cell molecules, causes vasodilatation and it prevents smooth muscle proliferation. Thus NO is very vital agent as it protects against vasoconstriction and atherosclerosis.[4-6]

Endothelin-1 is the most potent endogenous vasoconstrictor and growth promoting factor. It stimulates the release of oxygen free radicals from leukocytes. Oxygen free radicals cause destruction of cell membrane and stimulate atherosclerosis. In healthy individuals, very small amount of ET-1 is released and the effects of NO and ET-1 are well balanced. But NO release is impaired in case of endothelial dysfunction, the predominant actin of ET-1 leads to vasoconstriction and atherosclerosis.[7] One may surmise that a healthy endothelium is not leaky, not sticky and able to mediate relaxation through NO release. Endothelial cell dysfunction (ECD) is triggered by risk factors such as hypertension (HTN), hyperlipidemia, hyperglycemia and smoking.[8] This results in reduction of NO activity, increase in ET-1 activity, increase in endothelial cell permeability. Macromolecules such as LDL as well as monocytes secrete

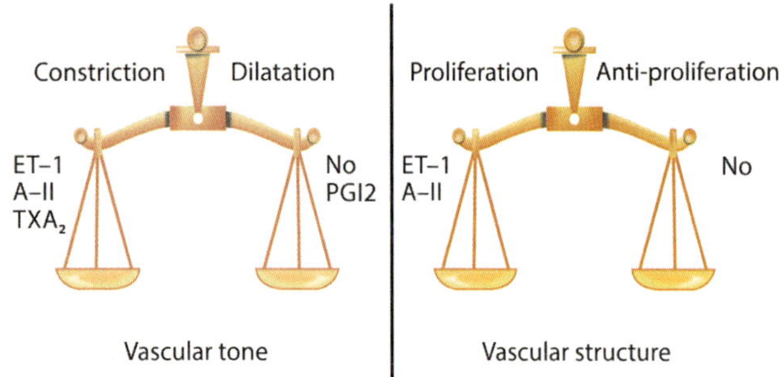

Fig. 1: Factors produced by the endothelium balancing in healthy person

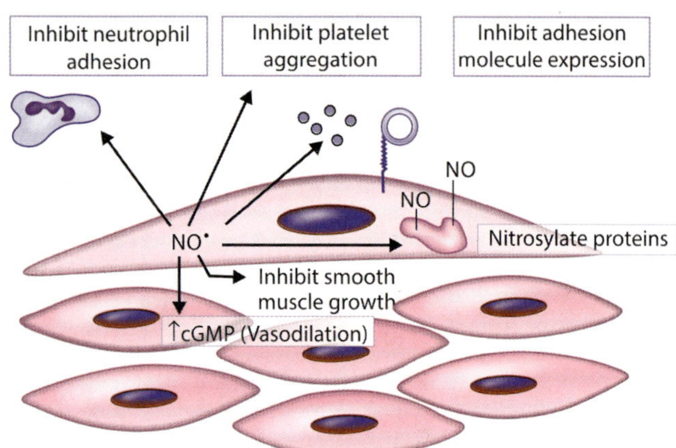

Fig. 4: Multifaceted role of nitric oxide in the vessel wall

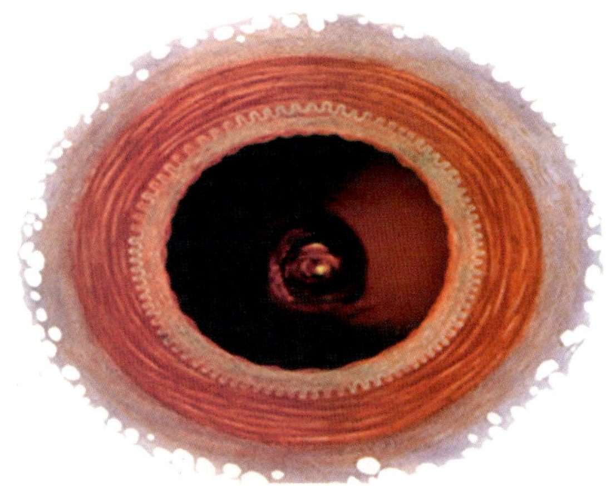

Fig. 2: Normal vascular endothelium with smooth nonthrombotic luminal surface

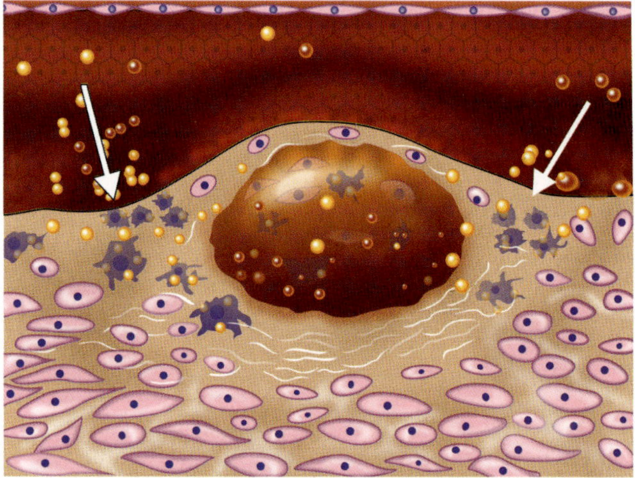

Fig. 5: The vulnerable plaque-consisting of lipid core covered by smooth muscle cells, thin-collagen cap, and plenty of macrophages and neutrophils at the periphery

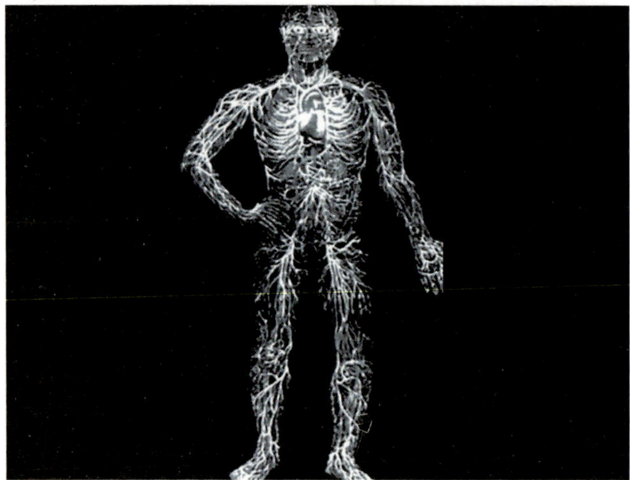

Fig. 3: Vasculature of human body

adhesion cell molecules. Monocytes and platelets stick to the endothelium. Monocytes penetrate in the vessel wall and change into macrophages which pick up oxidized LDL (Ox-LDL) and get transformed into foam cells leading to formation of fatty streak. At the same time, thrombogenic factors such as platelets, factors VII and fibrinogen come into play and lead to formation of atheromatous plaque.[9] Amongst the atheromatous plaques, it is the vulnerable (unstable) plaque which has tendency to rupture resulting in acute coronary syndromes such as unstable angina, acute myocardial infarction (AMI) and sudden cardiac death. The vulnerable plaque (Fig. 5) consists of central lipid core which is covered by smooth muscle cells and thin-collagen cap and at the periphery of the plaque, there are plenty of cells (macrophages and neutrophils). Interplay between plaque vulnerability and hemodynamic stresses determine the moment and point of plaque rupture resulting in acute coronary syndromes.[5,6]

Endothelin-1, angiotensin II (AII) and TxA2 cause vasoconstriction whereas NO and PG2 cause vasodilation. ET-1 and AII cause proliferation of smooth muscle whereas NO has antiproliferative action. Endothelial cells regulate the homeostasis of the arterial wall. Healthy endothelium is not leaky, not sticky and is able to relax (Fig. 6). Risk factors such

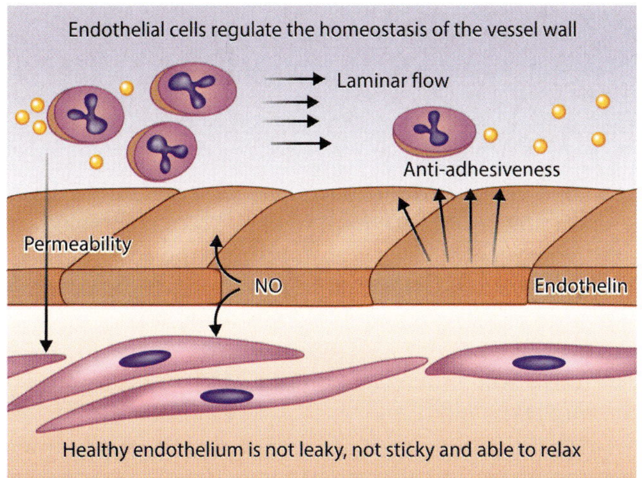

Fig. 6: Healthy endothelium is not leaky, not sticky and able to relax. Regulation of homeostasis of the vessel wall regulated by the endothelial cells

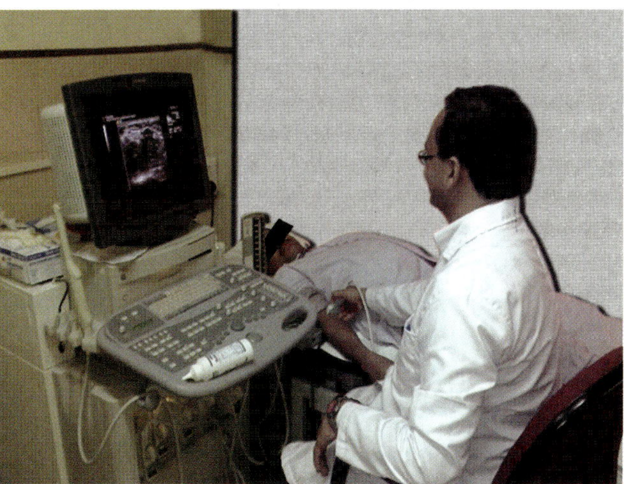

Fig. 8: FMD being measured using 6.0 MHZ phased array linear transducer attached to Acuson Sequoia machine

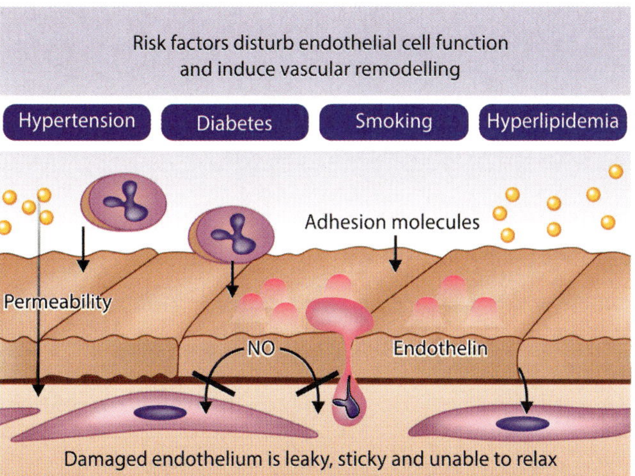

Fig. 7: Damages endothelium due to various risk factors is leaky, sticky and unable to relax

as HTN, diabetes mellitus (DM), smoking and hyperlipidemia cause ECD and induce vascular remodeling. Damaged endothelium is leaky, sticky and unable to relax (Fig. 7).[10]

ASSESSMENT OF ENDOTHELIAL CELL DYSFUNCTION BY BRACHIAL ARTERY FLOW MEDIATED VASODILATATION IN PATIENTS WITH DM WITHOUT CAD AND CAD WITHOUT DM

Material and Methods

We studied 50 adult patients in the age group (37–75 years) drawn from both sexes (males 32 and females 18). These patients were divided into 2 groups. Since DM is now considered as coronary artery disease (CAD) risk equivalent, we therefore aimed to determine whether similar degree of ECD occurs in DM and CAD.

Group 1: Documented cases of DM as per World Health Organization (WHO) criteria but no CAD.

Group 2: Documented cases of CAD (H/o AMI or confirmation on coronary angiography) but without DM.

Technique for Assessing ECD

Celermajer et al. (1992),[11] described the technique of assessing brachial artery flow-mediated dilatation (FMD) as follows: brachial artery imaging with high-resolution ultrasound during reactive hyperemia following release of cuff inflated to suprasystolic pressure is used in assessing endothelial cell function. The magnitude of change in vessel diameter from baseline period to the peaked observed during reactive hyperemia is indicative of endothelial cell function.

Brachial Artery Flow-Mediated Dilatation

It was done in all patients using 6.0 MHZ phased array linear transducer attached to Acuson Sequoia machine. The test was done in morning hours. All vasoactive drugs were withheld for 24 hours. With patient in supine position, sphygmomanometer cuff was tied over right arm. With brachial artery imaged in antecubital fossa, its diameter was measured 1.5 cm above the midpoint of antecubital fossa (brachial artery diameter at baseline) (Fig. 8).

Measurements

The systolic and diastolic VTI (velocity time integrals) were recorded using pulsed wave Doppler. The brachial artery was occluded with the cuff inflated to suprasystolic BP for 5 minutes and then released. Reactive hyperemia occurs due to NO release. The brachial artery diameter was measured immediately within 15 seconds of the release of cuff. The brachial artery diameter was again measured at peak (1 minute of cuff release) to assess FMD.

Calculation of FMD

The difference between the peak value at 1 minute and the baseline diameter gives the assessment of FMD. The baseline flow in the brachial artery, reactive hyperemia flow and FMD were calculated by standard complex formulas.

Results

The results for the assessment are given in Figures 9 to 12.

Discussion

In our study we found almost similar degree of FMD impairment in DM without CAD and CAD patients without DM. Dogra et al.,[12] YUHI et al.[13] and Clarkson et al.[14] showed FMD significantly impaired in DM compared to controls and degree of impairment was directly related to duration of DM. Bhargava et al.[15] found similar degree of FMD impairment in diabetes without CAD and CAD patients without DM.

Clinical utility of FMD shows that it can provide prognostic value independent of that provided by assessment of traditional risk factors. Suwaidi et al.[16] and

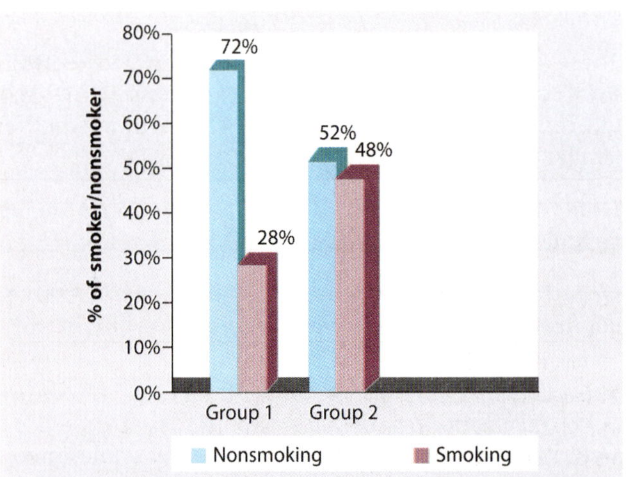

Fig. 9: Comparison of FMD% in nonsmokers and smokers/ tobacco chewers

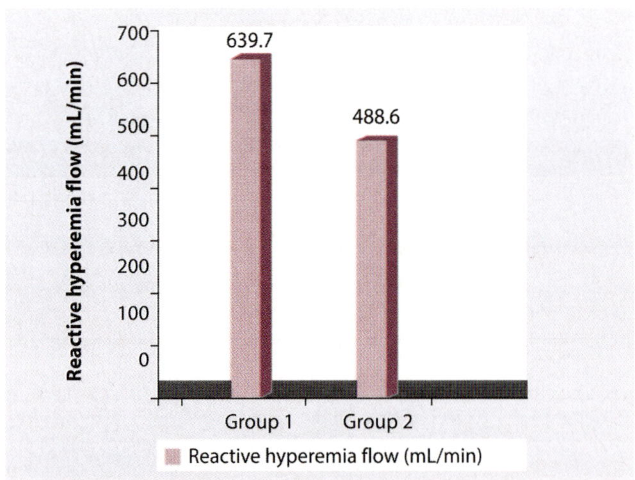

Fig. 11: Reactive hyperemia flow was better in DM group compared to CAD group but it was statistically insignificant

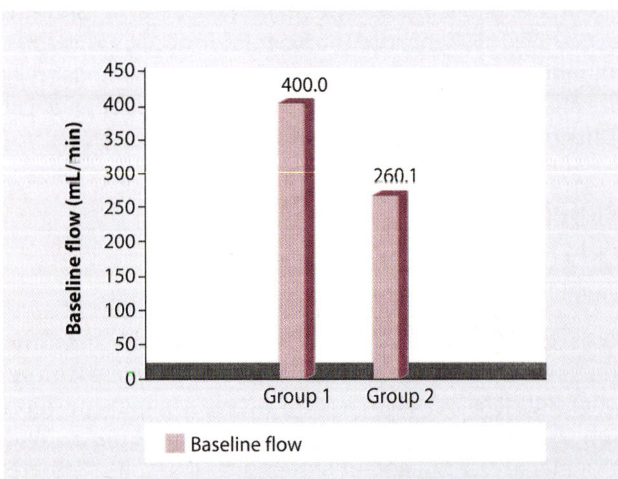

Fig. 10: The baseline flow was better in DM group compared to CAD group but it was statistically insignificant

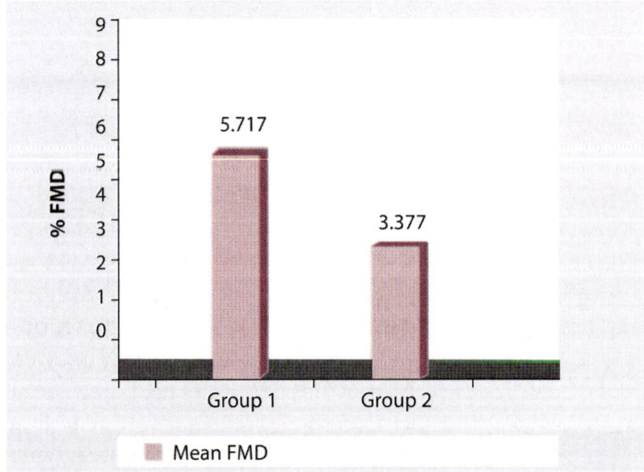

Fig. 12: FMD was better in DM group compared to CAD group but it was statistically insignificant

Schachinger et al.[17] showed that there were significantly more coronary events over a 2–3 year follow-up period in post coronary artery bypass surgery (CABG) patients with ECD than in those with normal ECD. ECD predicted an increase in cardiovascular events even in patients with angiographically normal coronary arteries.

Jeffery et al.[18] showed that presence of well-preserved brachial artery vasoreactivity predicts the absence of CAD. Jadhav et al.[19] in their study showed that FMD less than 4.5% was associated with CAD. Neunteufl et al.[20] showed that degree of impairment of FMD in CAD was correlated to the severity of CAD. We also found that FMD less than 4.5% was seen in all patients having documented CAD by coronary angiography. Thus brachial artery FMD is a useful noninvasive test to predict the presence and severity of CAD.

Conclusion

Assessment of endothelial dysfunction by brachial artery flow-mediated vasodilatation is a simple noninvasive test. The flow-mediated vasodilatation (FMD%) in response to ischemia induced in the forearm is directly proportional to the severity of ECD. DM affects normal endothelial function to a great extent nearing as that of proven CAD. Patients with CAD have significantly reduced FMD% in response to inducible ischemia and can predict the severity of the disease in a given patient. Smokers have significantly reduced FMD%.

ASSESSMENT OF ENDOTHELIAL DYSFUNCTION BY BRACHIAL ARTERY FLOW-MEDIATED DILATATION IN CONTROLS, HYPERTENSION WITHOUT CORONARY ARTERY DISEASE AND CORONARY ARTERY DISEASE WITHOUT HYPERTENSION

Hypertension and Endothelial Cell Dysfunction

Essential hypertension (EHTN) is the most common cardiovascular disorder. It is associated with functional and morphological alterations of the endothelium. Due to its position between blood stream and smooth muscle cells (responsible for peripheral resistance), the endothelium is thought to be both target and mediator of arterial HTN. The endothelial dysfunction could facilitate the maintenance of elevated peripheral resistance, which would favor the occurrence of complications such as atherosclerosis.

Material and Methods

We studied a total of 100 patients. Patients in the age group between 37 years to 75 years were selected from HTN clinic, out patients and indoor patients. Patients with history of HTN on treatment or newly diagnosed with systolic blood pressure (SBP) greater than 140 mm Hg and diastolic blood pressure (DBP) greater than 90 mm Hg and patients with documented CAD with either a history of documented myocardial infarction or confirmed by coronary angiography.

We assessed endothelial dysfunction, an important early event in the atherogenic process, by a noninvasive test (brachial artery FMD) and tried to compare the FMD amongst 3 groups:

1. Patients who had neither HTN nor coronary artery disease nor any risk factors for the same (controls)
2. Patients with HTN without coronary artery disease
3. Patients with coronary artery disease without HTN.

Results

The results for the assessment are mentioned in Figures 13 to 16.

Discussion

In our study we found significant impairment in FMD% in the HTN group as compared to the control group.

In the CAD group the degree of impairment in FMD% was even greater. The baseline parameters (i.e. baseline diameter and baseline flow) were also significantly reduced in both HTN and CAD groups.

Hamburg et al.[21] showed that FMD was found to correlate with higher SBP, advancing age and higher body

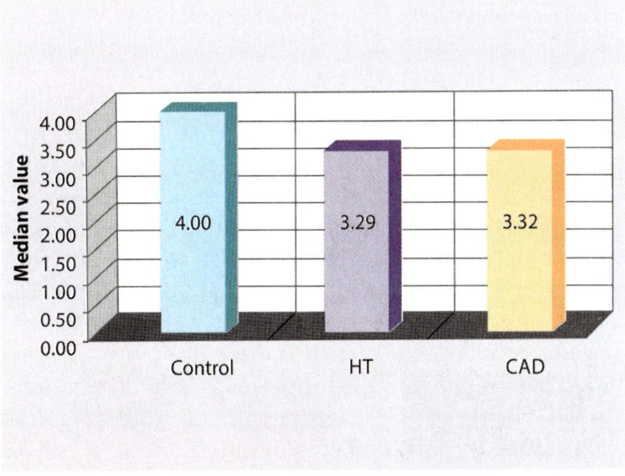

Fig. 13: Comparison of baseline diameter

Note: The baseline diameter was significantly reduced in both HTN and CAD groups.

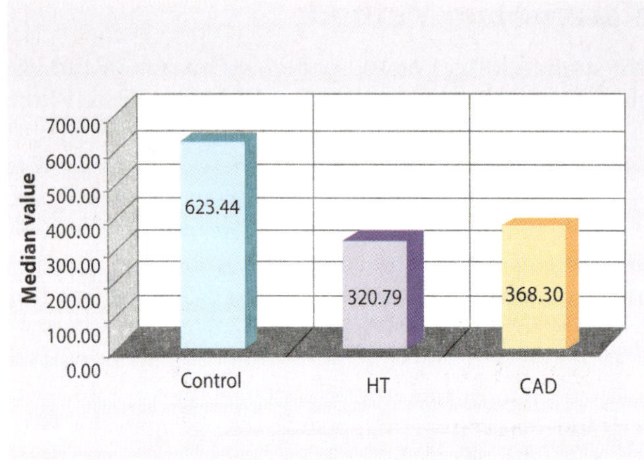

Fig. 14: Comparison of baseline flow

Note: The baseline flow was significantly reduced in both HTN and CAD groups

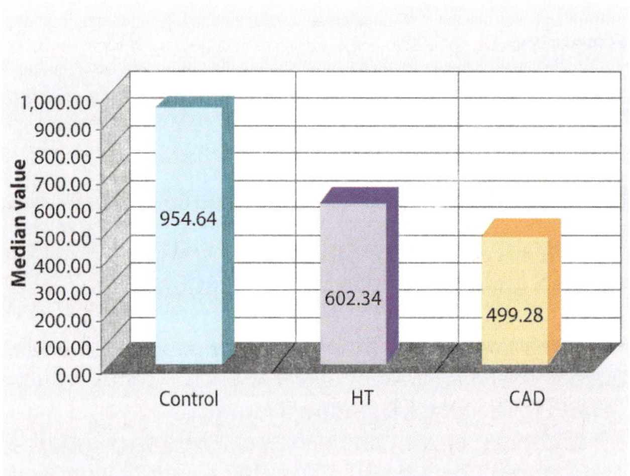

Fig. 15: Comparison of reactive hyperemia flow (at 15 sec)

Note: Reactive hyperemia was significantly reduced in both HTN and CAD groups.

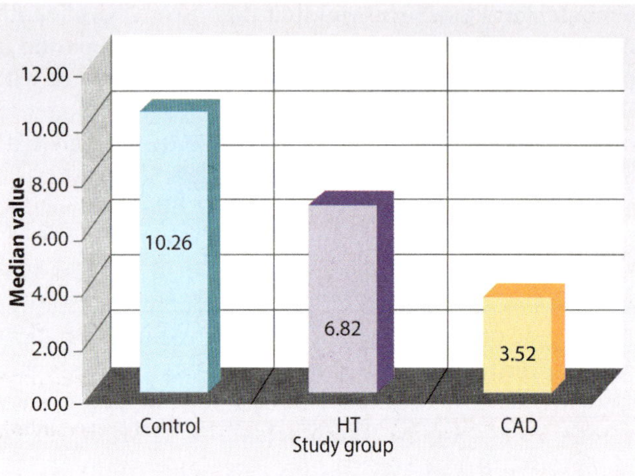

Fig. 16: Comparison of FMD% (at 1 min)

Note: FMD% is significantly reduced in both HTN and CAD groups but much more in CAD group.

mass index (BMI) in the Framingham Heart Study. Antony et al.[22] showed that FMD was impaired in hypertensive in both peripheral (brachial) as well as coronary circulation and serves as a good prognostic test. Muiesan et al.[23] showed that assessment of endothelial dysfunction in hypertensive identifies patients at risk of cardiovascular events. Park et al.[24] studied FMD in brachial artery in HTN and found a generalized impairment. Kimura et al.[25] showed significantly impaired FMD in the elderly hypertensive group versus the control group. Deng[26] also carried out a similar study in elderly hypertensive with similar results.

Lazdam et al.[27] studied 47 subjects over a 10-year period and showed that those with low average FMD had significant increase in mean arterial pressure (MAP). They concluded that persistently reduced or declining endothelial function during adolescence is a sensitive early marker associated with subclinical changes in HTN and thus future CAD. Therefore this can be used to implement primary prevention strategies for HTN as early as adolescence. Clinical utility of FMD shows that it can provide prognostic value independent of that provided by assessment of traditional risk factors showed that degree of impaired FMD in CAD was correlated to the severity of CAD. We also found that the mean FMD of less than 4.5% was seen in patients having documented CAD on coronary angiography. Thus brachial artery FMD is a useful noninvasive test to predict the presence and severity of CAD.

Assessment of endothelial dysfunction by brachial artery FMD is a simple noninvasive test. The FMD (FMD%) in response to ischemia induced in the forearm is directly proportional to the severity of endothelial dysfunction. HTN affects normal endothelial function to a great extent nearing as that of proven CAD. Patients with CAD have significantly reduced FMD% in response to inducible ischemia and can predict the severity of the disease in a given patient.

CONCLUSION

- Given the paucity of facilities for invasive evaluation of CAD in India, assessment of endothelial dysfunction by this method should be included in the routine work-up of patients with conventional risk factors for CAD.
- Since brachial artery FMD is noninvasive, nonradioactive and cost-effective, not time consuming and can be performed on an OPD basis in USG department, it should be used in clinical practice by physicians in cases of DM, HTN, suspected cases and/or

preangiographic evaluation of CAD in prognosticating and evaluating morbidity and mortality.

REFERENCES

1. Kaiser L, Sparks HV. Endothelial cells: not just a cellophane wrapper. Arch Intern Med. 1987;147:569-73.
2. Petty PG, Pearson JD. Endothelium the axis of vascular health and disease. Jr Royal Coll Physicians. 1989;23:92-101.
3. Celermajor DS. Endothelial dysfunction. Does it matter? It is reversible? Am Col Cardiology. 1997;30:325-33.
4. Kelly RA, Smith IW. Nitric oxides and nitrovasodilators-similarities, differences and interactions. A J Cardiol. 1996;2C-7C.
5. Dinerman JL, Mehta JL. Endothelial platelet and leukocyte interactions in ischaemic heart disease insights into potential mechanism and their clinical relevance. J Am Coll Cardiol. 1990;16:207-22.
6. Shah PK. New insights into the pathogenesis and prevention of acute coronary syndromes. Am J Cardiol. 1997;79(12B):17-23.
7. Masaki T. The discovery, the present state and the future prospects of endothelin. J Cardio Vas Pharmacol. 1989;13 Suppl 5:S1-4.
8. Sainani GS, Manisha SB, Rajesh S. Endothelial cell dysfunction-key factor in atherogenesis and its reversal (laboratory and clinical study). Kluwer Academic Publisher; 2003. pp. 27-48.
9. Awiram M, Dankner G, Grook JG. Platelet secretory products increases LDL oxidation, enhance its uptake by macrophages and reduces its fluidity. Arteriosclerosis. 1990;10:559-63.
10. Shah PK. Pathophysiology of plaque rapture and concept of plaque stabilization. Cardiol Clin. 1996;14:17-29.
11. Celemajer DS, Sorenzen K, Gooch VM, et al. Non-invasive detection of endothelial dysfunction in children and adults at risk of atherosclerosis. Lancet. 1992;340:1111-5.
12. Dogra G, Rich L, Stanton K, et al. Endothelium-dependent and independent vasodilatation studies at normoglycemia in type 1 diabetes mellitus with or without microalbuminuria. Diabetologica. 2001;44:593-601.
13. Yu HI, Sheu WH, Lai CJ, et al. Endothelial dysfunction in type 2 diabetes mellitus subjects with peripheral artery disease. Int J Cardiol. 2001;78:19-25.
14. Clarkson P, Celermajer DS, Donald AE, et al. Impaired vascular reactivity in insulin dependent diabetes is related to disease duration and low-density lipoprotein cholesterol levels. J Am Coll Cardiol. 1996;28:573-9.
15. Bhargava K, Hansa G, Bansal M, et al. Endothelium Dependent Brachial Artery Flow Mediated Vasodilatation in Patients with Diabetes Mellitus with and without coronary artery disease. JAPI. 2003;51:355-58.
16. Suwaidi J, Hamasaki S, Higano S. Long-term follow-up patients with mild coronary artery disease and endothelial dysfunction. Circulation. 2000;101:948-54.
17. Schachinger V, Britten M, Zeiher A. Prognostic impact of coronary vasodilator dysfunction on adverse long-term outcome of coronary heart disease. Circulation. 2000;101:1899-906.
18. Kuvin JT, Patel R, Sliney K. Peripheral vascular endothelial function testing as a non-invasive indicator of coronary artery disease. J Am Coll Cardiol. 2001;38:1843-9.
19. Jadhav UM, Anand S, Kadam NN. Noninvasive assessment of Endothelial Dysfunction by Brachial Artery Flow Mediated Dilatation in prediction of coronary artery disease in Indian Subjects. Indian Heart J. 2003;55:44-8.
20. Neunteufl T, Heher S, Kostner K. Contribution of nicotine to acute endothelial dysfunction in long-term smokers. J Am Coll Cardiol. 2002;39:251-156.
21. Hamburg NM, Palmisano J, Larson MG. Relation of Brachial and Digital Measures of Vascular Function in the Community: The Framingham Heart Study. Hypertension. 2011;57: 390-6.
22. Antony I, Lerebours G, Nitenberg A. Angiotensin-converting enzyme inhibition restores flow-dependent and cold pressor test-induced dilations in coronary arteries of hypertensive patients. Circulation. 1996;94:3115-22.
23. Muiesan ML, Salvetti M, Paini A. Prognostic role of flow-mediated dilatation of the brachial artery in hypertensive patients. J Hypertens. 2008;26(8):1612-8.
24. Park JB, Charbonneau F, Schiffrin EL. Correlation of endothelial function in large and small arteries in human essential hypertension. 2001;19(3):415-20.
25. Kimura Y, Matsumoto M, Den YB. Impaired endothelial function in hypertensive elderly patients evaluated by high resolution ultrasonography. Can J Cardiol. 1999;15(5):563-8.
26. Deng YB, Wang XF, Le GR. Evaluation of endothelial function in hypertensive elderly patients by high-resolution ultrasonography. Clin Cardiol. 1999;22(11):705-10.
27. Lazdam M, Lewandowski AJ, Kylintireas I. Impaired endothelial responses in apparently healthy young people associated with subclinical variation in blood pressure and cardiovascular phenotype. Am J Hypertens. 2012;25(1):46-53.

SECTION 2

Diagnosis

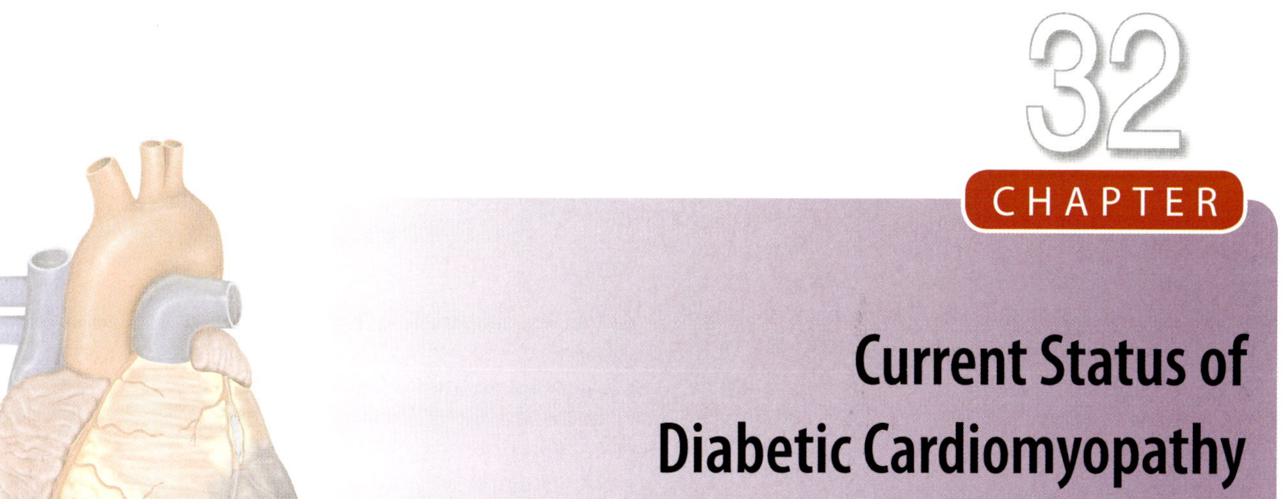

Current Status of Diabetic Cardiomyopathy

PC Mondal, Manotosh Panja, Madhumanti Panja

INTRODUCTION

A twin pandemic of obesity and diabetes mellitus has recently been described, with 1.46 billion overweight adults [body mass index (BMI) $\geq$ 25 kg/m^2] in 2008, including 500 million who were obese (BMI $\geq$ 30 kg/m^2).[1] Diabetes mellitus has reached an epidemic level worldwide, with a prevalence of 4% in 1995 and an anticipated prevalence of 5.4% in 2025, corresponding to 300 million adults with diabetes worldwide.[2] Diabetes mellitus is a complex metabolic disorder that includes insulin resistance (in type 2), often associated with hypertension and obesity.[3] All those conditions are associated with a high risk of coronary artery disease but may also exert a direct negative effect on the myocardium, leading to diabetic cardiomyopathy (DCM). Cardiovascular diseases represent the primary cause of death in this population.

DEFINITION OF DIABETIC CARDIOMYOPATHY

Diabetic cardiomyopathy (DCM) was first described 40 years ago, based on postmortem observations in four diabetic patients with heart failure but no coronary artery disease or other etiological conditions explaining heart failure.[4] The authors observed left ventricular (LV) hypertrophy associated with myocardial fibrosis in those patients and introduced for the first time the concept of DCM. Five years later, Regan et al.[5] confirmed those results and described cases of heart failure in familial diabetes without coronary artery disease, hypertension, or obesity. A higher myocardial collagen and lipid content was also reported in those cases compared with control subjects. Since those initial studies, DCM has been defined as the existence of LV dysfunction in diabetic patients without coronary artery disease, hypertension, or other potential etiological conditions.

EXPERIMENTAL EVIDENCES FOR DIABETIC CARDIOMYOPATHY

Numerous experimental studies, mainly based on rodent models, have demonstrated a direct negative effect of diabetes mellitus on the myocardium.[6] Pathophysiological mechanisms include metabolic alterations with impaired calcium homeostasis, alteration of substrate utilization (increase in lipid use and decrease in glucose oxidation), lipotoxicity, glucotoxicity with intervention of advanced glycation end products, mitochondrial dysfunction, increase in oxidative stress, renin-angiotensin-aldosterone system activation, and cardiac dysautonomia. All these mechanisms lead to an increase in myocardial cellular death (necrosis and apoptosis) and to myocardial fibrosis, with the consequent development of myocardial dysfunction and overt heart failure.[7]

EPIDEMIOLOGICAL EVIDENCES FOR DIABETIC CARDIOMYOPATHY

The Framingham Heart Study investigators demonstrated that diabetes mellitus was an independent risk factor for heart failure.[8] Risk of heart failure was 2.4-fold and 5-fold higher in diabetic men and women, respectively, than in nondiabetic subjects. The increased incidence of heart failure in diabetic patients persisted even after adjustment for age, hypertension, obesity, coronary artery disease, or dyslipidemia. The Cardiovascular Health Study, including 5,888 subjects aged more than 65 years with a mean delay of 5.5 years follow-up, reported an incidence rate for heart failure of 19.3/1,000 person-years, with a substantially higher incidence (approximately two-fold) associated with diabetes mellitus.[9] In a large case–control study, Bertoni et al.[10] tested the hypothesis that diabetes mellitus was independently associated with idiopathic cardiomyopathy. In the French EPICAL study, prevalence of diabetes mellitus among patients with nonischemic advanced heart failure was 19.7%.[13] In the Reykjavik study, Thrainsdottir et al.[11] explored the associations between heart failure and abnormal glucose regulation (impaired glucose tolerance or impaired fasting glucose) or type 2 diabetes mellitus in a population-based cohort of 19,381 participants. The odds ratio was 2.8 [95% confidence interval (CI) 2.2–3.6] for the association between type 2 diabetes mellitus and heart failure and 1.7 (95% CI 1.4–2.1) for the association between abnormal glucose regulation and heart failure. Finally, the Strong Heart Study recently confirmed diabetes mellitus as an independent risk factor of heart failure.[13] In a population-based cohort of 1,204 subjects, the authors showed a 1.5-fold higher risk of heart failure in patients with diabetes mellitus after adjustment for multiple cofactors (age, sex, obesity, central fat distribution, antihypertensive medications, atrial fibrillation, urinary albumin/creatinine ratio, plasma cholesterol, Hb1Ac, smoking habit, alcohol use, educational level, and physical activity). Interestingly, for the first time, intercurrent myocardial infarction was censored in this analysis.[12] In diabetic patients the prevalence of DCM is 12% and reaches 22% in people over 64 years old[13] In the United Kingdom Prospective Diabetes Study (UKPDS),[14] an increased prevalence of heart failure was recorded in patients with diabetes mellitus type 2, correlating with levels of glycosylated hemoglobin (HbA1c). The incidence of heart failure is 2.3 cases per 1,000 person-years in patients with HbA1c < 6% in contrast to 11.9 per 1,000 person-years in patients with significantly high HbA1c (>10%). There are identifiable risk factors for developing DCM, such as increased HbA1c, high BMI, advanced age, use of insulin, proteinuria, the coexistence of coronary artery disease and/or peripheral target organ diseases such as retinopathy and nephropathy.

STRUCTURAL MYOCARDIAL ABNORMALITIES ASSOCIATED WITH DIABETES

Myocardial Fibrosis

Myocardial fibrosis as initially described by Rubler et al.[15] and confirmed in both histological studies in humans and experimental studies is a major consequence of the adverse effects of diabetes mellitus on the heart. Backscatter is an ultrasound tissue characterization technique based on the measurement of myocardial tissue echoreflectivity, which is related to myocardial collagen content.[16] Di Bello et al.[17] showed an increase in myocardial echodensity as assessed by the integrated backscatter index in 26 insulin-dependent diabetic normotensive patients compared with 17 age- and sex-matched control subjects. Fang et al.[18] confirmed these results using calibrated integrated backscatter in a larger study. Biomarkers of collagen synthesis [carboxyterminal propeptide of procollagen type I (PICP); aminoterminal propeptide of procollagen type I (PINP); carboxyterminal propeptide of procollagen type III (PIIICP); aminoterminal propeptide of procollagen type III (PIIINP)] or collagen degradation [carboxyterminal telopeptide of collagen type I (CITP)] have been showed to be of clinical interest in detecting myocardial fibrosis.[19] In addition, markers of extracellular matrix turnover [such as matrix metalloproteinase (MMP)] and their inhibitors [tissue inhibitors of MMP (TIMP)] might also be useful.[20] However, few studies have used these biomarkers in diabetic patients. An increase in CITP was recently described in type 2 diabetic patients compared with control subjects and was correlated with diastolic function (mitral A duration minus pulmonary vein atrial reversal velocity duration).[21] MMP-7 has also been shown to be associated with diastolic dysfunction with microvascular complications (nephropathy).[22] Patients with diastolic dysfunction demonstrated an increase in MMP-9 and a decrease in TIMP-1/MMP-9. Finally, in a small group of diabetic patients, correlation was found between PICP and LV systolic variables (fractional shortening and midwall fractional shortening).[23]

Myocardial Steatosis

An increase in myocardial lipid content (myocardial steatosis) has been demonstrated in diabetic patients using magnetic resonance spectroscopy. McGavock et al.[24,25] showed an increase in myocardial triglyceride content in glucose intolerant patients and in patients with type 2 diabetes mellitus compared with controls. Myocardial triglyceride content was associated with diastolic function variables (E/A ratio and E wave deceleration time).[25] In a group of 42 men with type 2 diabetes mellitus, patients with high myocardial triglyceride content (superior to the median of the population) presented a decrease in systolic strain and strain rate whereas LV ejection fraction was similar in the two groups.[26]

MORPHOLOGICAL AND FUNCTIONAL ABNORMALITIES

Concentric Remodeling and Left Ventricular Hypertrophy

Concentric remodeling is defined as an increase in relative wall thickness [(2 × posterior wall thickness)/end-diastolic diameter] with normal LV mass index values, whereas LV hypertrophy is defined as abnormal LV mass index values.[27] Concentric remodeling and LV hypertrophy, known to be of adverse prognostic value,[28] are the most frequently described morphological abnormalities associated with diabetes mellitus. In the Framingham Heart Study, Galderisi et al.[29] showed an increase in LV mass and wall thickness independently associated with diabetes mellitus, but in multivariable analysis, statistical significance was reached only in women. In the Cardiovascular Health Study, an increase in LV mass was independently associated with diabetes mellitus even after adjustment for body weight, blood pressure, heart rate, and prevalent coronary or cerebrovascular disease. However, in contrast to previous findings, this association was significant in both men and women. The Strong Heart Study also revealed similar results in a large cohort of American Indians (1,810 patients with diabetes and 944 nondiabetic subjects). In this population, increases in wall thickness and LV mass were associated with a slight decrease in LV fractional shortening and midwall fractional shortening in diabetic patients compared with glucose-tolerant subjects.[30] However, the Northern Manhattan Study (NOMAS) described diabetes mellitus as an independent determinant of LV mass but in addition to central obesity as assessed by waist circumference.[31]

Impact of Diabetes on Left Ventricular Remodeling

The Framingham Heart Study investigators showed, in a first report, an increase in LV mass in diabetic subjects during a 16-year follow-up.[32] Diabetic subjects (without heart failure or previous myocardial infarction) experienced a steeper increase in LV mass with advancing age than nondiabetic subjects. In a second report, Cheng et al.[33] demonstrated an increase in wall thickness with advancing age associated with a decrease in LV diameter and a concomitant increase in fractional shortening. This study pointed out the influence of diabetes mellitus, in addition to sex and hypertension, on LV remodeling over life. Indeed, diabetes mellitus was associated with a greater increase in wall thickness coupled with a smaller decrease in LV diameter.[34] Finally, Markus et al.[33,35] also reported the influence of diabetes mellitus on LV remodeling. During a 10-year follow-up in a population-based cohort of 1,005 subjects, the authors observed a greater increase in LV mass in patients with prevalent diabetes mellitus associated with an increase in LV end-diastolic diameter, whereas this last variable remained stable over time in euglycemic subjects,[36] this was associated with a decrease in LV ejection fraction in prevalent diabetic subjects whereas an increase was observed in euglycemic subjects.[37]

FUNCTIONAL ABNORMALITIES

Longitudinal Systolic Impairment

Myocardial strain imaging, such as tissue Doppler imaging (TDI) and speckle-tracking imaging (STI), is useful for detecting ischemia[38] and facilitate demonstration of subclinical impairment of systolic function in asymptomatic diabetic patients without overt heart disease and a normal standard echocardiography.[39] Whereas conventional methods such as LV ejection fraction and fractional shortening were insensitive in terms of detecting early preclinical abnormalities, longitudinal dysfunction was demonstrated in many studies using both TDI and STI. For some authors, longitudinal strain decrease was correlated with diabetes imbalance (glycated hemoglobin) or microvascular complications (microalbuminuria).[39] However, longitudinal alteration is independently associated with diabetes mellitus, regardless of LV hypertrophy or other conventional risk factors.

Radial Systolic Impairment

Radial systolic function[39] was increased or preserved to compensate for longitudinal function alteration. These finding were based on TDI and its derived velocity and strain rate measurements that depend on Doppler angle. The TDI measurements are limited to the segments in which motion and deformation are aligned with the ultrasound beam and hence do not provide an optimal evaluation of radial function. STI is an angle-independent method and allows a more robust and extensive evaluation of radial function.[40] Among reports based on STI, the study by Ng et al.[38] described preserved radial function compared with euglycemic subjects (radial strain 40.6 ± 11.1% vs 42.7 ± 12.1%, respectively; p not significant). However, this study was based on a highly selected population that included uncomplicated patients and only men with a short duration of diabetes mellitus (4 years) and a strictly controlled HbA1c concentration (6.4 ± 0.7%).

Contractile Reserve

Whether diabetes mellitus is also responsible for a decrease in contractile reserve in asymptomatic patients without overt heart disease is a controversial issue.[39] Galderisi et al.[41] demonstrated an impaired inotropic response to dobutamine in 24 diabetic patients compared with 16 controls. With dobutamine, myocardial strain assessed by TDI increased by 36.4 ± 15.9% in diabetic patients versus 57.1 ± 22.1% in controls (p = 0.0001). Ha et al.[42] showed impairment of longitudinal function reserve (as assessed by mitral annular systolic velocity) during exercise. However, Fang et al.[43] reported a normal response to dobutamine stress, suggesting that ischemia due to small vessel disease might not be important in early diabetic heart muscle disease.[44]

Diastolic Dysfunction

Prevalence of diastolic dysfunction is high in diabetic patients, ranging from 21% to 75% and based on populations enrolled and methodological issues regarding the assessment of diastolic function. Indeed, it is not true if based on one single abnormal variable using mitral inflow pattern, its variation with the Valsalva maneuvre or combined indices derived from mitral inflow pattern and pulmonary venous flow.[45] TDI-based diastolic velocities and derived indices are better reflectors. In the study of Poulsen et al.,[46] including a population of patients with type 2 diabetes mellitus, 9% presented a LV ejection fraction less or equal than 50% and 30% of patients presented perfusion abnormalities assessed by scintigraphy. Kiencke et al.[47] included 100 patients with type 2 diabetes mellitus and explored diastolic function using a comprehensive algorithm close to the current recommendations; they found a prevalence of diastolic dysfunction of 48%. Diastolic dysfunction has been traditionally considered as the first marker of DCM. In contrast to systolic impairment in diabetic patients, diastolic variables are mainly associated with other factors (including age, rate pressure product, history of hypertension, and BMI) and that some of the most frequently used diastolic variables (E/A ratio, é velocity) are not independently associated with diabetes mellitus.[48] In addition, standard LV systolic variables are mostly insensitive to detecting systolic impairment. Diastolic variables are related to prognosis in diabetic patients without evident heart disease.[47] In a first retrospective study, including 486 diabetic patients, From et al.[46] demonstrated that the E/é ratio was associated with an increase in global mortality after adjustment for age, sex, coronary artery disease, hypertension, LV ejection fraction, left atrial volume, and delay between diabetes diagnosis and echocardiography. Kiencke et al.[45] confirmed that patients with diastolic dysfunction had a lower overall event-free survival rate than patients without diastolic dysfunction (54% vs 87%; p = 0.001).

MICROVASCULAR ALTERATION

Alteration of microvessels associated with endothelial dysfunction has been described in both experimental models of diabetes[49] and humans.[50] Those abnormalities result in a decrease in myocardial blood flow reserve that has been described using myocardial contrast echocardiography (with dipyridamole and exercise), technetium 99 m sestamibi scintigraphy (with dipyridamole),[51] or positron emission tomography (with dipyridamole or cold pressor test).[52]

The Right Ventricle

Right ventricle (RV) dysfunction is associated with a worse prognosis in a variety of cardiovascular diseases, including acute myocardial infarction and heart failure. The effect of diabetes on the functionality and geometry of the RV is equally detrimental. In patients with DCM, RV is influenced by both the LV, via a biventricular interaction mechanism, and the diabetes mellitus *per se*. Interestingly, it has been demonstrated that in diabetic patients both the systolic and diastolic function of the RV are affected. Van den Brom et al. have shown that in diabetic mice the changes caused by diabetes in the functionality of the RV are in line with those observed in the LV, but the changes in geometry and remodeling are not similar. More specifically, LV changes are characterized by hypertrophy of myocardial cells without dilation, while the opposite was observed in the RV.

Mechanisms of Heart Failure in Diabetes Mellitus

Many pathophysiological mechanisms are involved in the stepwise progression from diabetes mellitus to heart failure. These include direct myocardial injury (e.g. in myocardial ischemia or cardiomyopathy), volume overload (e.g. in aortic valve insufficiency), and pressure overload (e.g. in arterial hypertension). Diabetes not only intensifies the process of atherosclerosis in epicardial coronary arteries, but also promotes the appearance of structural and functional disorders in smaller vessels, resulting in an increased ischemic burden for the myocardium.

Furthermore, DCM aggravates hypertension, resulting in increased afterload and pressure overload, and, by contributing to the occurrence of renal failure (diabetic nephropathy), it leads to fluid retention and eventually volume overload.[53] From the pathophysiological point of view, in diabetes, because of the lack of insulin or because of insulin resistance in the tissues, the body does not use glucose but instead uses fatty acids as fuel. Although the heart tissue of normoglycemic people prefers free fatty acids as fuel rather than glucose, in diabetic patients this phenomenon is accentuated even further. On the other hand, myocardial cells of normoglycemic patients with heart failure or patients who have suffered a myocardial infarction use glucose as an energy source rather than fatty acids. It seems that in this case glucose exerts a protective role against ischemia. The almost exclusive use of fatty acids in diabetes patients leads to their accumulation into the heart muscle, which is followed by the appearance of lipotoxicity. Of particular note is palmitic acid, the accumulation of which influences myocardial contractility and also induces apoptosis of myocardial cells. It has been found that persistent hyperglycemia in the myocardium of diabetic rats stimulates the expression of muscle carnitine palmitoyltransferase enzyme 1. On the other hand, the main feature of diabetes, hyperglycemia, can cause damage to the myocardium via modified proteins [advanced glycation end products (AGEs)] and free oxygen radicals [reactive oxygen species (ROS)]. The AGEs, for example, produced by glycation of collagen lead to its accumulation in the extracellular matrix and eventually in fibrosis of the heart, resulting in diastolic dysfunction. Furthermore, soluble AGEs connected in related receptors [receptors for AGEs (RAGEs)], trigger nicotinamide adenine dinucleotide phosphate (NADPH) oxidase, leading to the production of peroxide and ultimately of free oxygen radicals. These in turn cause direct damage to myocyte deoxyribonucleic acid (DNA).[54]

THERAPEUTIC PERSPECTIVES

Diabetes cardiomyopathy has a long latent phase which is asymptomatic followed by overt signs of congestive heart failure. At the stage of heart failure, treatment of DCM is currently based on common heart failure guidelines.[55] However, the main challenge in this pathology is to develop preventive therapeutic options in order to avoid or delay the progression of early myocardial dysfunction associated with diabetes. Effects of diabetes mellitus on the myocardium at a very early preclinical stage need to be defined in order to develop a preventive strategy for patients at high-risk.

Lifestyle

Smoking cessation, healthy eating habits, reduction in body weight, and aerobic exercise are the cornerstones in terms of lifestyle change. It has been shown in people with diabetes mellitus type 2 that following reduction of their body weight and increased aerobic activity, the incidence of DCM decreased significantly.

Glycemic Control

Poor glycemic control increases the risk of developing heart failure in diabetes. Evidence suggests that good glycemic control is beneficial in the early stages of myocardial dysfunction. Strong recommendations regarding the choice of current glucose-lowering therapies in patients with DCM cannot be made because of lack of evidence. In general, the choice of antidiabetic therapy in DCM should be dictated by clinical characteristics, such as the presence or absence of renal dysfunction, risk of hypoglycemia, age, volume status, and concomitant drug therapy.

Neurohormonal Antagonism

The important role of the renin-angiotensin-aldosterone system in the pathogenesis of complications in diabetic patients is well described. Evidence supports the use of angiotensin-converting enzyme inhibitors in preventing myocardial fibrosis, cardiac hypertrophy, and myocardial mechanical dysfunction associated with DCM.[56] Evidence suggests a beneficial effect of aldosterone-antagonism in diastolic heart failure by virtue of their beneficial effects on cardiac hypertrophy and fibrosis.[57]

Beta-blockers

Beta-blockers are the standard of care in patients with systolic heart failure. A subgroup analysis of the Metoprolol CR/XL Randomised Intervention Trial in Congestive Heart Failure (MERIT-HF) showed that beta-blockers reduce mortality, hospital admissions, and improve symptoms, without significant differences between diabetes mellitus type 2 and nondiabetic patients. Beta-blockers recommended in heart failure and diabetes mellitus type 2 are metoprolol succinate in the slow release form (MERIT-HF), bisoprolol [Cardiac Insufficiency Bisoprolol Study (CIBIS II)], and Carvedilol [Carvedilol Prospective Randomized Cumulative Survival (COPERNICUS) and Carvedilol or Metoprolol European Trial (COMET)].[58-61] Adverse effects of beta-blockers in patients with diabetes mellitus type 2 and heart failure include: (a) hypoglycemia especially with noncardioselective regimens and (b) negative metabolic effects (hypoglycemia, dyslipidemia, and decreased insulin sensitivity).[62]

CARDIAC RESYNCHRONIZATION THERAPY

Presence of diabetes mellitus is not a contraindication for cardiac resynchronization therapy and/or cardiac transplantation in patients with advanced systolic heart failure.

CONCLUSION

Cardiovascular disease remains the leading cause of morbidity and mortality in diabetes mellitus which needs intervention at multiple levels for prevention. Cardiovascular mortality is solely not due to atherosclerosis and its complications. Increased risk of congestive heart failure irrespective of other risk factors is a major way leading to both morbidity and mortality. Arrhythmic death is also high in diabetes mellitus which got heightened with coexistent DCM.

REFERENCES

1. Anand SS, Yusuf S. Stemming the global tsunami of cardiovascular disease. Lancet. 2011;377: 529-32.
2. King H, Aubert RE, Herman WH. Global burden of diabetes, 1995–2025: prevalence, numerical estimates, and projections. Diabetes Care. 1998;21:1414-31.
3. Barthelemy O, Jacqueminet S, Rouzet F, et al. Intensive cardiovascular risk factors therapy and prevalence of silent myocardial ischemia in patients with type 2 diabetes. Arch Cardiovasc Dis. 2008;101:539-46.
4. Cohen A, Ederhy S, Boccara F. Left ventricular diastolic (dys) function in type 2 diabetes: time for a critical reappraisal. Diabetes Metab. 2007;33:1-2.
5. Regan TJ, Lyons MM, Ahmed SS, et al. Evidence for cardiomyopathy in familial diabetes mellitus. J Clin Invest. 1977;60:884-99.
6. Boudina S, Abel ED. Diabetic cardiomyopathy revisited. Circulation. 2007;115:3213-23.
7. Boudina S, Abel ED. Diabetic cardiomyopathy, causes and effects. Rev Endocr Metab Disord. 2010;11:31-9
8. Kannel WB, Hjortland M, Castelli WP. Role of diabetes in congestive heart failure: the Framingham study. Am J Cardiol. 1974;34:29-34.
9. Gottdiener JS, Arnold AM, Aurigemma GP, et al. Predictors of congestive heart failure in the elderly: the Cardiovascular Health Study. J Am Coll Cardiol. 2000;35:1628-37.
10. Bertoni AG, Tsai A, Kasper EK, et al. Diabetes and idiopathic cardiomyopathy: a nationwide case-control study. Diabetes Care. 2003;26(10):2791-5.
11. Thrainsdottir IS, Aspelund T, Thorgeirsson G, et al. The association between glucose abnormalities and heart failure in the population-based Reykjavik study. Diabetes Care. 2005;28:612-6.
12. Simone G de, Devereux RB, Chinali M, et al. Diabetes and incident heart failure in hypertensive and normotensive participants of the Strong Heart Study. J Hypertens. 2010;28:353-60.
13. Zannad F, Briancon S, Juilliere Y, et al. Incidence, clinical and etiologic features, and outcomes of advanced chronic heart failure: the EPICAL Study. Épidemiologie de l'Insuffisance Cardiaque Avancee en Lorraine. J Am Coll Cardiol. 1999;33:734-42.
14. Stratton IM, Adler AI, Neil HA, et al. Association of glycaemian with macrovascular and microvascular complications of type 2 Diabetes (UKPDS 35): prospective observational study. Brit Med J. 2000; 321:405-12.
15. Rubler S, Dlugash J, Yuceoglu YZ, et al. New type of cardiomyopathy associated with diabetic glomerulosclerosis. Am J Cardiol. 1972;30:595-602.
16. Van Hoeven KH, Factor SM. A comparison of the pathological spectrum of hypertensive, diabetic, and hypertensive-diabetic heart disease. Circulation. 1990;82:848-55.
17. Mizushige K, Yao L, Noma T, et al. Alteration in left ventricular diastolic filling and accumulation of myocardial collagen at insulin-resistant prediabetic stage of a type II diabetic rat model. Circulation. 2000;101:899-907.
18. Hoyt RH, Collins SM, Skorton DJ, et al. Assessment of fibrosis in infarcted human hearts by analysis of ultrasonic backscatter. Circulation. 1985;71:740-4.
19. Di Bello V, Talarico L, Picano E, et al. Increased echodensity of myocardial wall in the diabetic heart: an ultrasound tissue characterization study. J Am Coll Cardiol. 1995;25:1408-15.
20. Fang ZY, Yuda S, Anderson V, et al. Echocardiographic detection of early diabetic myocardial disease. J Am Coll Cardiol. 2003;41:611-7.
21. Lopez B, Gonzalez A, Diez J. Circulating biomarkers of collagen metabolism in cardiac diseases. Circulation. 2010;121:1645-54.
22. Ihm SH, Youn HJ, Shin DI, et al. Serum carboxy-terminal propeptide of type I procollagen (PIP) is a marker of diastolic dysfunction in patients with early type 2 diabetes mellitus. Int J Cardiol. 2007;122:e36-8.
23. Ban CR, Twigg SM, Franjic B, et al. Serum MMP-7 is increased in diabetic renal disease and diabetic diastolic dysfunction. Diabetes Res Clin Pract. 2010;87:335-41.
24. Gonzalez-Vilchez F, Ayuela J, Ares M, et al. Oxidative stress and fibrosis in incipient myocardial dysfunction in type 2 diabetic patients. Int J Cardiol. 2005;101:53-8.
25. McGavock JM, Lingvay I, Zib I, et al. Cardiac steatosis in diabetes mellitus: a 1H-magnetic resonance spectroscopy study. Circulation. 2007;116:1170-5.
26. Rijzewijk LJ, van der Meer RW, Smit JW, et al. Myocardial steatosis is an independent predictor of diastolic dysfunction in type 2 diabetes mellitus. J Am Coll Cardiol. 2008;52:1793-9.
27. Ng AC, Delgado V, Bertini M, et al. Myocardial steatosis and biventricular strain and strain rate imaging in patients with type 2 diabetes mellitus. Circulation. 2010;122:2538-44.
28. Devereux RB, Roman MJ, Paranicas M, et al. Impact of diabetes on cardiac structure and function: the strong heart study. Circulation. 2000;101:2271-6.
29. Galderisi M, Anderson KM, Wilson PW, et al. Echocardiographic evidence for the existence of a distinct diabetic cardiomyopathy (the Framingham Heart Study). Am J Cardiol. 1991;68:85-9.
30. Lee M, Gardin JM, Lynch JC, et al. Diabetes mellitus and echocardiographic left ventricular function in free-living elderly men and women: the Cardiovascular Health Study. Am Heart J. 1997;133:36-43.
31. Lieb W, Xanthakis V, Sullivan LM, et al. Longitudinal tracking of left ventricular mass over the adult life course: clinical correlates of short- and long-term change in the Framingham offspring study. Circulation. 2009;119:3085-92.
32. Cheng S, Xanthakis V, Sullivan LM, et al. Correlates of echocardiographic indices of cardiac remodeling over the adult life course: longitudinal observations from the Framingham Heart Study. Circulation. 2010;122:570-8.

33. Markus MR, Stritzke J, Wellmann J, et al. Implications of prevalent and incident diabetes mellitus on left ventricular geometry and function in the ageing heart: the MONICA/KORA Augsburg cohort study. Nutr Metab Cardiovasc Dis. 2011;21:189-96.
34. Thibault H, Derumeaux G. Assessment of myocardial ischemia and viability using tissue Doppler and deformation imaging: the lessons from the experimental studies. Arch Cardiovasc Dis. 2008;101: 61-8.
35. Andersen NH, Poulsen SH, Eiskjaer H, et al. Decreased left ventricular longitudinal contraction in normotensive and normoalbuminuric patients with Type II diabetes mellitus: a Doppler tissue tracking and strain rate echocardiography study. Clin Sci (Lond). 2003;105: 59-66.
36. Ernande L, Rietzschel ER, Bergerot C, et al. Impaired myocardial radial function in asymptomatic patients with type 2 diabetes mellitus: a speckle tracking imaging study. J Am Soc Echocardiogr. 2010;23:1266-72.
37. Mogelvang R, Sogaard P, Pedersen SA, et al. Tissue Doppler echocardiography in persons with hypertension, diabetes, or ischaemic heart disease: the Copenhagen City Heart Study. Eur Heart J. 2009;30:731-9.
38. Ng AC, Delgado V, Bertini M, et al. Findings from left ventricular strain and strain rate imaging in asymptomatic patients with type 2 diabetes mellitus. Am J Cardiol. 2009;104:1398-401.
39. Stefanidis A, Bousboulas S, Kalafatis J, et al. Left ventricular anatomical and functional changes with ageing in type 2 diabetic adults. Eur J Echocardiogr. 2009;10:647-53.
40. Leitman M, Lysyansky P, Sidenko S, et al. Two-dimensional strain a novel software for real-time quantitative echocardiographic assessment of myocardial function. J Am Soc Echocardiogr. 2004;17:1021-9.
41. Galderisi M, de Simone G, Innelli P, et al. Impaired inotropic response in type 2 diabetes mellitus: a strain rate imaging study. Am J Hypertens. 2007;20:548-55. 2003;42:446-53.
42. Ha JW, Lee HC, Kang ES, et al. Abnormal left ventricular longitudinal functional reserve in patients with diabetes mellitus: implication for detecting subclinical myocardial dysfunction using exercise tissue Doppler echocardiography. Heart. 2007;93:1571-6.
43. Fang ZY, Najos-Valencia O, Leano R, et al. Patients with early diabetic heart disease demonstrate a normal myocardial response to dobutamine. J Am Coll Cardiol.
44. From AM, Scott CG, Chen HH. Changes in diastolic dysfunction in diabetes mellitus over time. Am J Cardiol. 2009;103:1463-6.
45. Poirier P, Bogaty P, Garneau C, et al. Diastolic dysfunction in normotensive men with well-controlled type 2 diabetes: importance of maneuvers in echocardiographic screening for preclinical diabetic cardiomyopathy. Diabetes Care. 2001;24: 5-10.
46. Poulsen MK, Henriksen JE, Dahl J, et al. Left ventricular diastolic function in type 2 diabetes mellitus: prevalence and association with myocardial and vascular disease. Circ Cardiovasc Imaging. 2010;3:24-31.
47. Kiencke S, Handschin R, von Dahlen R, et al. Preclinical diabetic cardiomyopathy: prevalence, screening, and outcome. Eur J Heart Fail. 2010;12:951-7.
48. Ernande L, Bergerot C, Rietzschel ER, et al. Diastolic dysfunction in patients with type 2 diabetes mellitus: is it really the first marker of diabetic cardiomyopathy? J Am Soc Echocardiogr. 2011;24:1268-75.
49. Thompson EW. Structural manifestations of diabetic cardiomyopathy in the rat and its reversal by insulin treatment. Am J Anat. 1988;182:270-82.
50. Gherasim L, Tasca C, Havriliuc C, et al. A morphological quantitative study of small vessels in diabetic cardiomyopathy. Morphol Embryol (Bucur). 1985;31:191-5.
51. Storto G, Pellegrino T, Sorrentino AR, et al. Estimation of coronary flow reserve by sestamibi imaging in type 2 diabetic patients with normal coronary arteries. J Nucl Cardiol. 2007;14:194-9.
52. Yokoyama I, Momomura S, Ohtake T, et al. Reduced myocardial flow reserve in non-insulin-dependent diabetes mellitus. J Am Coll Cardiol. 1997;30:1472-7.
53. Voulgari C, Papadogiannis D, Tentolouris N. Diabetic cardiomyopathy: from the pathophysiology of the cardiac myocytes to current diagnosis and management strategies. Vasc Health Risk Manag. 2010; 6:883-903.
54. Bodiga VL, Eda SR, Bodiga S. Advanced glycation end products: role in pathology of diabetic cardiomyopathy. Heart Fail Rev. 2014;19: 49-63.
55. Raimondi L, De Paoli P, Mannucci E, et al. Restoration of cardiomyocyte functional properties by angiotensin II receptor blockade in diabetic rats. Diabetes. 2004;53:1927-33.
56. Rajesh M, Mukhopadhyay P, Batkai S, et al. Cannabidiol attenuates cardiac dysfunction, oxidative stress, fibrosis, and inflammatory and cell death signaling pathways in diabetic cardiomyopathy. J Am Coll Cardiol. 2010;56:2115-25.
57. Ye G, Metreveli NS, Donthi RV, et al. Catalase protects cardiomyocyte function in models of type 1 and type 2 diabetes. Diabetes. 2004;53:1336-43.
58. Deedwania PC, Giles TD, Klibaner M, et al. Efficacy, safety and tolerability of metoprolol CR/XL in patients with diabetes and chronic heart failure: experiences from MERIT-HF. Am Heart J. 2005;149:159-67.
59. The Cardiac Insufficiency Bisoprolol Study II (CIBIS-II): a randomised trial. Lancet. 1999;353:9-13.
60. Packer M, Coats AJ, Fowler MB, et al. Effect of Carvedilol on survival in severe chronic heart failure. N Engl J Med. 2001;344:1651-8.
61. Hjalmarson A, Goldstein S, Fagerberg B, et al. Effects of controlled-release metoprolol on total mortality, hospitalizations, and well-being in patients with heart failure: the Metoprolol CR/XL Randomized Intervention Trial in congestive heart failure (MERIT-HF). MERIT-HF Study Group. JAMA. 2000;283:1295-302.
62. Poole-Wilson PA, Swedberg K, Cleland JG, et al. Comparison of Carvedilol and metoprolol on clinical outcomes in patients with chronic heart failure in the Carvedilol or Metoprolol European Trial (COMET): randomised controlled trial. Lancet. 2003;362:7-13.

CHAPTER

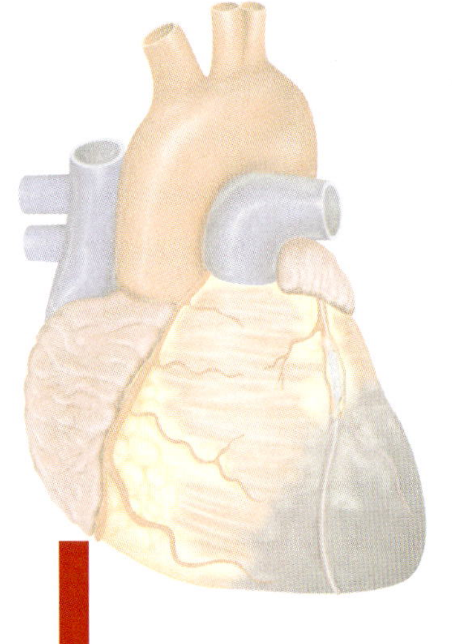

Insulin Therapy and Cardiodiabetes

Vitull K Gupta, Meghna Gupta, Varun Gupta

INTRODUCTION

Cardiovascular diseases (CVDs) are leading cause of death worldwide and along with diabetes mellitus (DM) it causes increased morbidity and mortality especially in the Indian Asian population. CVDs account for 21.9% of total deaths and are projected to increase to 26.3% by 2030.[1] The incidence of DM is increasing worldwide such that global burden has increased from 30 million in 1985 to 382 million in 2014 and it is predicted to increase further[2] so much so that by 2035, 592 million people worldwide will be diabetics.[3] DM and CVD are closely linked as they share common risk factors and CVD is the most prevalent cause of mortality and morbidity in diabetic populations. DM type 2 (T2DM) has a close association with coronary heart disease (CHD) such that patients with diabetes have two to fourfold higher risk of developing CHD than people without DM, and CVD accounts for an overwhelming 65–75% of deaths in people with DM.[4]

Diabetes mellitus is a complex metabolic disorder characterized by insulin resistance and progressive deterioration of beta-cell function leading to hyperglycemia. Evidence shows that the pancreatic beta-cell function drops to approximately 50% by the time DM is diagnosed and gradually declines at the rate of approximately 5% per year indicating deterioration of glycemic control over time as the disease progresses requiring multiple treatment interventions and most patients will ultimately require insulin. Early and timely initiation of insulin can help to reverse glucotoxicity and preserve beta-cell function for longer time as compared to oral antidiabetic drugs (OADs) alone.[5,6] UK Prospective Diabetes Study (UKPDS) demonstrated that intensive glycemic control was associated with substantial reductions in the risk of both microvascular and macrovascular complications. Each 1% reduction in glycated hemoglobin (HbA1c) is associated with a 14% reduction in myocardial infarction (MI), 37% reduction in microvascular complications, 21% reduction for any endpoint related to DM, and 21% reduction of deaths related to diabetes.[7]

INDIA-SPECIFIC GUIDELINES

A number of country-specific guidelines such as those from American Diabetes Association (ADA), American College of Cardiology Foundation or American Heart Association, National Institute of Health and Clinical Excellence, Scottish Intercollegiate Guidelines Network from UK, Canadian Diabetes Association and Australian Diabetes Society focus on diagnosis and management of diabetes in patients of their respective regions. The Indian population with wide ethnogeographic differences and a higher-than-normal genetic predisposition to diabetes has Indian-specific guidelines issued by Research Society for the Study of Diabetes in India (RSSDI) and Journal of Association of Physicians of India (JAPI) for optimal practices for diagnosis and management of hyperglycemia in different clinical situations.

THERAPEUTIC STRATEGIES FOR CARDIODIABETES

Oral antidiabetic drugs have different mechanisms of action and most of them require some degree of endogenous insulin for their action. So these agents will ultimately become ineffective even in combination with progression of DM because beta-cell function declines with increasing duration of diabetes and will require insulin to achieve their glycemic targets. Insulin is the best antidiabetic agent since 1920s with proven safety profile in renal, hepatic, and cardiac diseases and in pregnancy, which can bring any level of elevated A1C to target levels.[8] Therapeutic strategies to reduce glycemic burden are plentiful and number of available antihyperglycemic agents are ever expanding, requiring the clinician to consider many of the following factors when choosing medications—degree of hyperglycemia, risk of hypoglycemia, medication effectiveness at reducing diabetes complications (microvascular and/or macrovascular), medication effects on body weight, medication side effects, concomitant medical conditions, ability to adhere to regimen, cost, and patient preferences. Lifestyle modification, including nutritional therapy and physical activity, should form an integral part of diabetes management. Although oral drugs show antihyperglycemic efficacy either as monotherapy or in combination, their utility is often limited owing to their frequent side effects, contraindications, and the loss of efficacy over time, particularly in patients with severe beta-cell dysfunction and then insulin treatment becomes mandatory.[9]

CARDIOPROTECTIVE EFFECTS OF INSULIN

Insulin exerts cardioprotective effects via glucose-dependent and glucose-independent mechanisms, including aversion of glucose toxicity, positive inotropy, the interrelated modulation of oxidative stress, inflammation and apoptosis and regulation of blood flow,[10] decreased plasminogen activator inhibitor-1 (PAI-1), improved platelet function, decreased circulating free fatty acids (FFA), decreased myocardial oxygen consumption, and stimulate nitric oxide formation by vascular endothelium.[11] Insulin is an anabolic hormone that influences vascular tone in both large caliber conductance vessels and small caliber exchange vessels such as the capillary microcirculation.[12,13]

INSULIN THERAPY IN CARDIODIABETES

Glycemic control is the cornerstone of the management of T2DM. Insulin is the oldest and the best available treatment for maintaining normal glycemic levels and managing T2DM. Unlike OADs, insulin has potential to reduce blood glucose from any level to the recommended blood glucose targets. In view of the increased burden of CVD in patients with DM, insulin therapy has the potential to improve CVD prognosis by modulating both metabolic and vascular functions. Insulin has been shown to achieve optimal glycemic control as initial therapy, in both lean and obese patients.[14] Evidence has proved that early in the natural history of DM, tight glycemic control can have lasting benefits on both microvascular and macrovascular complications, popularly termed as "metabolic memory" or "Legacy effect".[15] Almost all international and national guidelines suggest insulin as second-line therapy for patients with uncontrolled diabetes treated with metformin alone. The benefits of intensified insulin therapy (IIT) in achieving good glycemic control and reducing the risk of complications have been confirmed by Diabetes Control and Complications Trial (DCCT).[16,17]

INDICATIONS OF INSULIN THERAPY[16]

Indications of insulin in T2DM in newly detected patient:

- Those patients, who at the time of diagnosis are symptomatic and have one of the following:
  - Hemoglobin A1c more than 9%
  - Fasting hyperglycemia in excess of 250 mg/dL
  - Postprandial hyperglycemia in excess of 300 mg/dL
  - In catabolic stage
  - Ketone positive
- When patient presents with acute stress like infection, dehydration or acute CVD such as acute coronary syndrome or acute MI, insulin has the advantage of being effective where other agents may not be. Insulin should be considered as part of any combination regimen:
  - In these cases insulin may be started as monotherapy or with metformin if not contraindicated.
  - As the patient's glucose toxicity resolves, the regimen can, potentially, be subsequently simplified and a switch over to only oral agents may be considered.

Indications of insulin in T2DM in patients with already established diagnosis:

- If a trial of adequate doses of three non-insulin agents for 6–9 months fails to achieve HbA1c to target levels, addition of insulin may be justified as the landmark studies suggest that achieving intensive glycemic control (if not contraindicated) in initial few years of diagnosis is of profound benefit.
- It has to be understood that during first year of diagnosis, as we do not expect complete insulinopenia and as sulfonylurea is still considered to be the most potent and the cheapest of all oral drugs, one of these three (or more) medicines should be sulfonylurea.
- Lifestyle changes including medical nutrition therapy, exercise, smoking cessation, etc. must be

continued vigorously and education at all stages will be complimentary to the management.
- While initiating insulin, doses of sulfonylurea should be reduced and a strict watch must be kept on occurrence of hypoglycemia.
- Hemoglobin A1c targets must be determined as per criteria set for individualized therapy and efficacy of each agent of reducing HbA1c as combination therapy must be considered.[18]

GLYCATED HEMOGLOBIN AND GLYCEMIC TARGETS[17]

Numerous aspects must be considered when setting glycemic targets. The ADA proposes optimal targets, but each target must be individualized to the needs of each patient and his or her disease factors. The glycemic recommendations for many nonpregnant adults with diabetes are:
- Glycated hemoglobin of less than 7.0%
- Preprandial capillary plasma glucose 80–130 mg/dL
- Peak postprandial capillary plasma glucose less than 180 mg/dL.

More or less stringent glycemic goals may be appropriate for individual patients. Goals should be individualized based on duration of diabetes, age per life expectancy, etc.

TYPES OF INSULIN

Various types of insulin are as follows:
- *Rapid-acting insulin*: The onset of action is about 15 minutes after injection, peaks in about 1 hour, and duration of action is 2–4 hours.
  Types: Insulin glulisine, insulin lispro, and insulin aspart.
- *Regular or short-acting insulin*: It usually reaches the bloodstream within 30 minutes after injection, peaks anywhere from 2 hours to 3 hours after injection, and is effective for approximately 3–6 hours.
  Types: Human regular insulin.
- *Intermediate-acting insulin*: It generally reaches the bloodstream about 2–4 hours after injection, peaks 4–12 hours later, and is effective for about -18 hours.
  Types: Human neutral protamine hagedorn (NPH).
- *Long-acting insulin*: It reaches the bloodstream several hours after injection and tends to lower glucose levels fairly evenly over a 24-hour period.
  Types: Insulin detemir, insulin glargine, and insulin degludec.
- *Premixed insulin products*: Regular insulin and NPH insulin are available in a premixed formulation with 30:70, 50:50, and 25:75 proportions.

Premixed preparations are available with protamine insulin with the same insulin analog like lispro or aspart. These preparations are available in 25:75, 30:70, and 50:50 proportions.

THE CHOICE OF INSULIN REGIMEN

The choice of insulin regimen depends on several factors such as type of diabetes, duration of diabetes, baseline and current A1C levels, age, existing comorbidities, ability to adhere to medical instructions, number of injections, hypoglycemia, weight gain, and frequency of monitoring,[19,20] assessment of the patient's risk for hyperglycemia and related complications versus the risks of therapy, assessment of psychological status, capacity for self-care, economic considerations, and family and social support systems.

Insulin Regimes[17,21]

Common insulin regimes include basal insulin regime, basal-bolus regime, premix insulin regime, and combination injectable regime, which may involve human insulins or insulin analogs.

Insulin Initiation with Basal Insulin

In T2DM patients poorly controlled on oral drug therapy, addition of basal analog insulin (insulin glargine, insulin detemir, and insulin degludec) over basal human insulin (NPH) is recommended to achieve guideline-recommended A1C with reduced hypoglycemia and lesser weight gain. Addition of insulin degludec is preferred over glargine to achieve similar glycemic control with lower risk of overall and nocturnal hypoglycemia with lower glycemic variability and flexibility in the time of administration.

Basal Insulin

Basal insulin alone is the most convenient initial insulin regimen, beginning at 10 units/day or 0.1–0.2 units/kg/day, depending on the degree of hyperglycemia. Basal insulin is usually prescribed in conjunction with metformin and sometimes one additional noninsulin agent. While there is evidence for reduced risk of hypoglycemia with newer, longer-acting basal insulin analogs, people with T2DM without a history of hypoglycemia may use NPH insulin safely and at much lower cost.

Insulin Intensification with Basal Bolus

Despite comparable glycemic control in T2DM patients, all analog basal-bolus regimen may be considered over all human basal-bolus regimen for reduced risk of nocturnal hypoglycemia, less weight gain, and lower day-to-day within-person variation in fasting plasma glucose (FPG). Insulin degludec shows significantly lower rates of both overall and nocturnal confirmed hypoglycemia in T2DM with comparable glycemic control as compared with insulin glargine as part of basal bolus therapy.

Bolus Insulin

Many individuals with T2DM may require mealtime bolus insulin dosing in addition to basal insulin. Rapid-acting analogs are preferred due to their prompt onset of action after dosing. The recommended starting dose of mealtime insulin is 4 units, 0.1 U/kg, or 10% of the basal dose. If A1C is 8% when starting mealtime bolus insulin, consideration should be given to decreasing the basal insulin dose.

Insulin Initiation with Premixed Insulins

Both premixed insulin and basal insulin can be considered as starting insulin in patients with T2DM. When FPG is elevated consider initiating insulin therapy with basal insulin. When both FPG and postprandial plasma glucose (PPG) are high, consider initiating insulin therapy with premixed insulin or insulin coformulation of degludec plus (IDegAsp) which is a soluble coformulation of insulin degludec (70%) and insulin aspart (30%). For patients who have high FPG and high PPG, once daily IDegAsp can be considered for initiation over basal insulin for superior glycemic control and higher chances of reaching glycemic target without hypoglycemia. Since, PPG response to a meal is more pronounced in ethnic Asian communities, premixed insulin that improves PPG should be the preferred method of insulin initiation in this population.

Premixed Insulin

Premixed insulin products contain both basal and prandial components, allowing coverage of both basal and prandial needs with a single injection. NPH/regular 70/30 insulin, for example, is composed of 70% NPH insulin and 30% regular insulin.

Insulin Intensification with Premixed Insulins

When intensifying premix insulin therapy from OD to BID, split the OD dose into equal breakfast and dinner doses (50:50) and titrate further. When intensifying premixed insulin therapy from BID to TID, consider adding 2–6 U or 10% of total daily premixed insulin dose before lunch which may require down-titration of morning dose (2–4 U). For patients on previous treatment with premixed/basal insulin failing to achieve A1C target, twice daily IDegAsp can be recommended over premixed insulin analogs for intensification. For patients requiring further intensification of basal or premixed insulin twice daily, IDegAsp can be considered as a reasonable option ahead of basal-bolus therapy, for simplicity of regimen.

Combination Injectable Therapy

If basal insulin has been titrated to an acceptable FPG level (or if the dose is 0.5 units/kg/day) and A1C remains above target, consider advancing to combination injectable therapy. When initiating combination injectable therapy, metformin therapy should be maintained while other oral agents may be discontinued on an individual basis to avoid unnecessary complex or costly regimens (i.e. adding a fourth antihyperglycemic agent). Once an insulin regimen is initiated, dose titration is important with adjustments made in both mealtime and basal insulins based on the blood glucose levels and an understanding of the pharmacodynamic profile of each formulation (pattern control). Other options for treatment intensification include adding a single injection of rapid-acting insulin analog (lispro, aspart, or glulisine) before the largest meal or stopping the basal insulin and initiating a premixed (or biphasic) insulin NPH/regular 70/30, 70/30 aspart mix, 75/25 or 50/50 lispro mix, twice daily, usually before breakfast and before dinner. Each approach has its advantages and disadvantages. Regular human insulin (RHI) and human NPH/regular premixed formulations (70/30) are less costly alternatives to rapid-acting insulin analogs and premixed insulin analogs, respectively, but their pharmacodynamic profiles may make them less optimal. If a patient is still above the A1C target on premixed insulin twice daily, consider switching to premixed analog insulin three times daily (70/30 aspart mix, 75/25 or 50/50 lispro mix). In general, three times daily premixed analog insulins have been found to be noninferior to basal-bolus regimens with similar rates of hypoglycemia.[22] If a patient is still above the A1C target on basal insulin, one single injection of rapid-acting insulin before the largest meal, advance to a basal-bolus regimen injections of rapid-acting insulin before meals. Consider switching patients from one regimen to another (i.e. premixed analog insulin three times daily to basal-bolus regimen or vice-versa) if A1C targets are not being met and/or depending on other patient considerations (Flow chart 1).[23,24]

Continuous Subcutaneous Insulin Infusion[25]

Continuous subcutaneous insulin infusion (CSII) by insulin pump is the most sophisticated and precise insulin delivery method aims to mimic endogenous insulin delivery profile

Flow chart 1: Combination injectable therapy for type 2 diabetes[17]

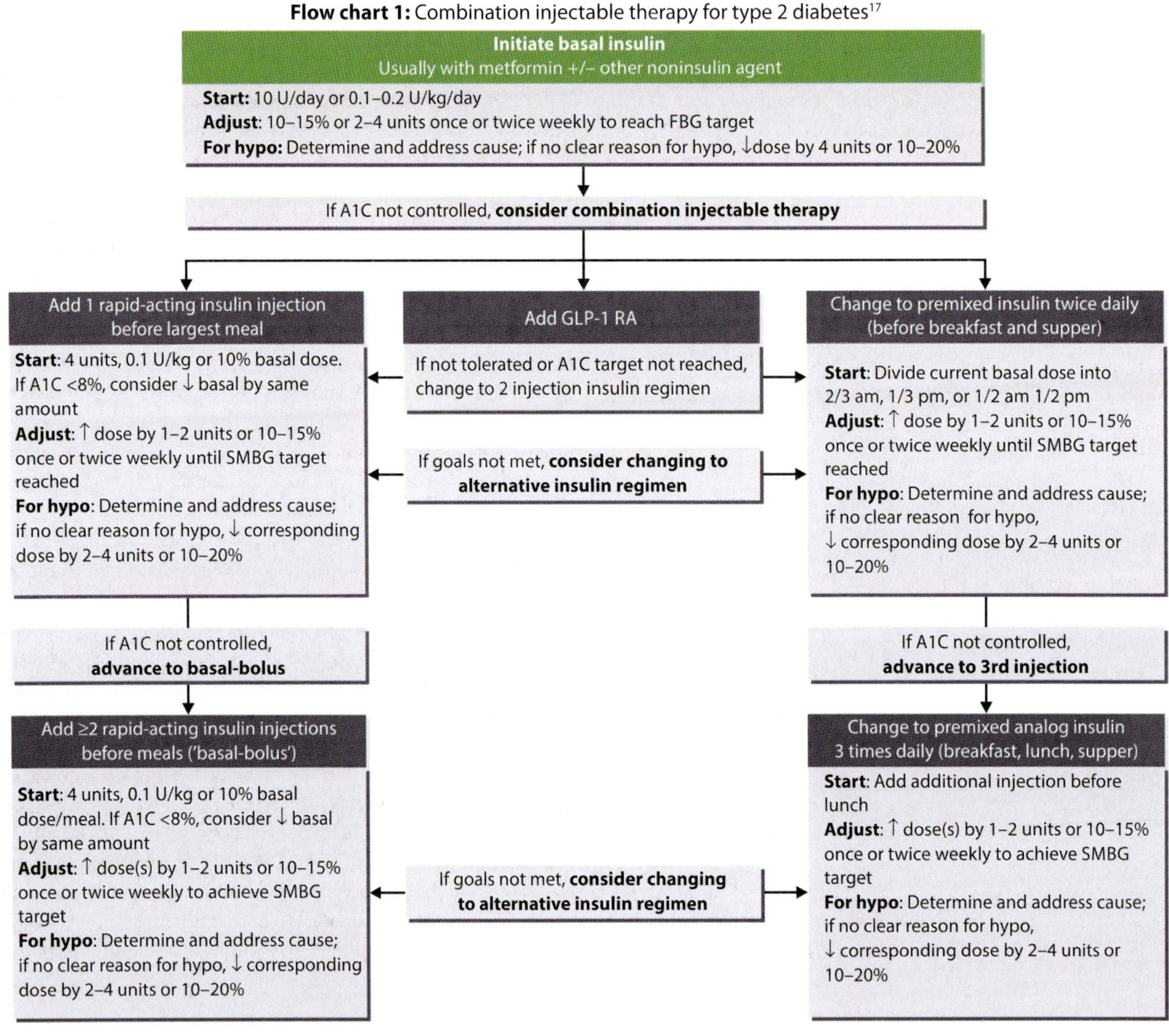

Abbreviations: FBG, fasting blood glucose; SMBG, self-monitoring of blood glucose

Source: Adapted from American Diabetes Association. Standards of Medical Care in Diabetes 2017. Diabetes Care. 2017;40(Suppl 1):S64-74.

more closely to the pattern of insulin delivery from pancreas, by providing continuously infused, low-volume basal insulin for fasting periods and delivery of increased rate boluses to cover meals. Most pumps use rapid-acting insulin analogs (RAIAs), i.e. lispro, aspart, and glulisine, as they have a rapid onset and shorter duration than RHI. Evidences from several studies indicate that CSII provides equal or better glycemic control, lower hypoglycemic episodes, better quality of life, improved psychosocial functioning, and more flexibility with lifestyle when compared to multiple daily injections (MDIs) therapy (Flow chart 2).

Rapid-acting insulin analogs should be preferred over RHI for use in insulin pumps. Currently, OADs do not have a role as an adjunct along with insulin pump. Wherever required metformin or insulin sensitizers may be considered when encountering high insulin resistance. However, it is emphasized that there is no role for OADs like sulphonylureas, dipeptidyl peptidase-4 inhibitors, meglitinides, and others.

Indications for CSII include any patient with T1DM or T2DM on insulin therapy who can afford and is seeking improved quality of life, patients with diabetic complications, e.g. nephropathy, neuropathy, high insulin requirement, frequent episodes of severe hypoglycemia with MDI, any patient requiring exogenous insulin therapy but not controlled with optimal MDI therapy.

Contraindications include, psychiatric illness, unwillingness to self-monitor, lack of time and motive, cannot be trained on essential technical aspect of insulin pump therapy, etc.

Flow chart 2: Algorithm for initiation, optimization, and continuation of insulin therapy in patients with type 2 diabetes mellitus[30]

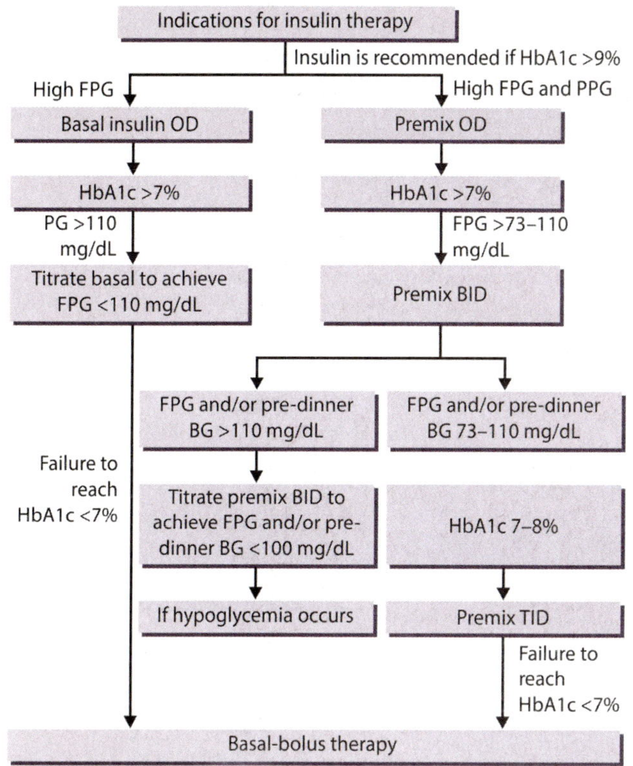

Abbreviations: HbA1c, hemoglobin A1c; FPG, fasting plasma glucose; PPG, postprandial plasma glucose

MANAGEMENT

Management of hyperglycemia in patients undergoing coronary artery bypass grafting in patients with diabetes in India.[26] A glycemic target of 120–180 mg/dL should be considered if the patient is on parenteral feed and 140–180 mg/dL should be considered for patients on oral feed with diabetes undergoing coronary artery bypass grafting (CABG). Known diabetes patients on OADs with an A1C less than 7.5% undergoing CABG or percutaneous coronary intervention (PCI) should be continued on insulin therapy up to 6 weeks from discharge and the patient should be reassessed for continuation of insulin and in absence of any contraindications to OADs, can be switched from insulin to OADs. Continuous intravenous insulin infusion (CIII) should be used as the mainstay of perioperative glycemic management in patients with diabetes undergoing CABG. CIII should be initiated in patients if the blood glucose (BG) level is more than 180 mg/dL for two (1 hourly) consecutive readings. CIII should be continued up to 24 hours or till the last four values are between 120 mg/dL and 180 mg/dL and the patient starts oral feeding, then the patient can be switched to subcutaneous (SC) insulin with basal-bolus regimen. For diabetic patients undergoing CABG, CIII should be initiated during the surgical procedure and continued till the third postoperative day. Monitoring must be done once hourly, until BG of 125–175 mg/dL is reached or if a change in BG is less than 15 mg/dL is observed while the infusion rate is unchanged for 4 hours. Subsequently a two-hourly monitoring is sufficient, which can be stopped on the third day postoperatively. However, when patients are being weaned off vasopressors, a half hourly rate of monitoring is recommended. Due to the lack of sufficient evidence pointing to significant benefits in using OADs for perioperative glycemic management during CABG in patients with diabetes, the use of OADs even as adjunct therapy is not recommended. Known diabetes patients well controlled on OADs with an HbA1c less than 7% and without any intervention can be shifted to OADs after 7 days or at the time of discharge.

HUMAN INSULIN VERSUS ANALOGS

Human insulin is synthetic insulin manufactured from recombinant DNA technology and is identical to insulin produced by the human pancreas. Analog insulins are molecular-engineered formulations designed to improve the pharmacokinetics, absorption profile, and duration of action of human insulin. The escalating cost of diabetes care and the advent of new quality and economic initiatives worldwide have favored resurgence in the use of human insulins. The introduction of modern insulin analogs has contributed to improvements in patient outcomes with better glucose control and convenience to patients and lower risk of hypoglycemia. A meta-analysis showed that insulin aspart, compared with RHI, was associated with minor improvements in A1C and postprandial glucose, with no change in FPG with significant reductions in nocturnal hypoglycemic episodes.[27] Another meta-analysis comparing long-acting analogs (glargine or detemir, used once daily) and NPH insulin showed no significant differences in A1C outcomes.[28] Two separate systematic reviews comparing long-acting insulin analogs with NPH insulin have reported no significant glycemic efficacy benefits, but indicate a reduced risk of nocturnal and symptomatic hypoglycemia with basal analogs.[29] During occurrence of hypoglycemic events, analog insulins appear to have statistically significant advantages as compared to RHIs, but these advantages are not consistent across types of insulin (rapid or long-acting) or types of diabetes, and the clinical importance of these differences is not clear. It is observed that trials assessing analog insulins are of relatively low quality and linked to the pharmaceutical industry with resultant potential for bias with patient-reported outcomes (i.e. hypoglycemia) as well as some degree of publication bias. Given the lack of clear benefits, the current evidence does not indicate a strong advantage for analog insulins compared to RHI for both T1DM and T2DM.

CONCLUSION

Cardiodiabetes is leading cause of death worldwide. Glycemic control is the cornerstone of the management of T2DM and to reduce complications. OADs will ultimately become ineffective even in combination with progression of DM and will require insulin to achieve their glycemic targets. Almost all international and national guidelines suggest insulin as second-line therapy for patients with uncontrolled diabetes treated with metformin alone. Insulin exerts cardioprotective effects via glucose-dependent and glucose-independent mechanisms. The choice of insulin regimen depends on several factors and common insulin regimes include basal insulin regime, basal-bolus regime, premixed insulin regime, and combination injectable regime, which may involve human insulins or insulin analogs and CSII by insulin pumps. Each approach has its advantages and disadvantages and current evidence does not indicate a strong advantage for analog insulins compared to RHI for both T1DM and T2DM. Evidence shows that tight glycemic control early in the natural history of DM can have lasting benefits on both microvascular and macrovascular complications and almost all international and national guidelines suggest insulin as second-line therapy for patients with uncontrolled diabetes treated with metformin alone.

REFERENCES

1. World Health Organization. World Health Statistics. Department of Measurement & Health Information Systems of the Information, Evidence and Research Cluster. Geneva: WHO Press; 2008. p. 29-31.
2. Wild S, Roglic G, Green A, et al. Global prevalence of diabetes: estimates for the year 2000 and projections for 2030. Diabetes Care. 2004;27(5):1047-53.
3. Aguiree F, Brown A, Cho NH, et al. IDF Diabetes Atlas. 2013.
4. Matheus AS, Tannus LR, Cobas RA, et al. Impact of diabetes on cardiovascular disease: an update. Int J Hypertens. 2013;2013:653789.
5. UKPDS Group. UK prospective diabetes study 16. Overview of 6 years' therapy of type 2 diabetes: A progressive disease. Diabetes. 1995;44(11):1249-58.
6. Nathan DM, Buse JB, Davidson MB, et al. Medical management of hyperglycaemia in type 2 diabetes mellitus: a consensus algorithm for the initiation and adjustment of therapy: a consensus statement from the American Diabetes Association and the European Association for the Study of Diabetes. Diabetologia. 2009,52(1):17-30.
7. Stratton IM, Adler AI, Neil HA, et al. Association of glycemia with macrovascular and microvascular complications of type 2 diabetes (UKPDS 35): prospective observational study. BMJ. 2000;321:405-12.
8. Ranjit Unnikrishnan I, Anjana RM, Mohan V. Importance of controlling diabetes early– the concept of metabolic memory, legacy effect and the case for early insulinisation. J Assoc Physicians India. 2011;59 Suppl:8-12.
9. Indian National Consensus Group. Premix Insulin: Initiation and Continuation Guidelines for Management of Diabetes in Primary Care. J Assoc Physicians India. 2009;57(Suppl):42-6.
10. Ng KW, Allen ML, Desai A, et al. Cardioprotective effects of insulin: how intensive insulin therapy may benefit cardiac surgery patients. Circulation. 2012;125(5):721-8.
11. Nicasio J, McFarlane SI. Early insulin therapy and the risk of cardiovascular disease in Type 2 diabetes. Therapy. 2005;2(5):685-8.
12. Baron AD. Hemodynamic actions of insulin. Am J Physiol. 1994;267(2 Pt 1):E187-202.
13. Sydow K, Mondon CE, Cooke JP. Insulin resistance: potential role of the endogenous nitric oxide synthase inhibitor ADMA. Vasc Med. 2005;10(Suppl 1):S35-43.
14. Palumbo PJ. The case for insulin treatment early in type 2 diabetes. Cleve Clin J Med. 2004;71(5):385-6,391-2,394.
15. Nathan DM, Cleary PA, Backlund JY, et al. Intensive diabetes treatment and cardiovascular disease in patients with type 1 diabetes. N Engl J Med. 2005;353(25):2643-53.
16. Madhu SV, Saboo B, Makkar BM, et al. RSSDI Clinical Practice Recommendations for Management of Type 2 diabetes Mellitus, 2015. Intl J Diabetes Developing Countries. 2015;35(Suppl 1):1-71.
17. American Diabetes Association. Standards of Medical Care in Diabetes 2017. Diabetes Care. 2017;40(Suppl 1):S64-74.
18. Inzucchi SE, Bergenstal RM, Buse JB, et al. Management of hyperglycemia in type 2 diabetes, 2015: a patient-centered approach: update to a position statement of the American Diabetes Association and the European Association for the Study of Diabetes. Diabetes Care. 2015;38(1):140-9.
19. Mooradian AD, Bernbaum M, Albert SG. Narrative review: a rational approach to starting insulin therapy. Ann Intern Med. 2006;145(2):125-34.
20. Nathan DM, Buse JB, Davidson MB, et al. Medical management of hyperglycemia in type 2 diabetes: a consensus algorithm for the initiation and adjustment of therapy. A consensus statement of the American Diabetes Association and the European Association for the Study of Diabetes. Diabetes Care. 2009;32(1):193-203.
21. Kesavadev J, Rajput R, John M, et al. Consensus statement on Choice of Insulin Therapy in Type 2 diabetes. J Assoc Physicians India. 2016;Suppl.
22. Giugliano D, Chiodini P, Maiorino MI, et al. Intensification of insulin therapy with basal-bolus or premixed insulin regimens in type 2 diabetes: a systematic review and meta-analysis of randomized controlled trials. Endocrine. 2016;51:417-28.
23. Dieuzeide G, Chuang L-M, Almaghamsi A, et al. Safety and effectiveness of biphasic insulin aspart 30 in people with type 2 diabetes switching from basal-bolus insulin regimens in the A1chieve study. Prim Care Diabetes. 2014;8(2):111-7.
24. Mathieu C, Storms F, Tits J, et al. Switching from premixed insulin to basal-bolus insulin glargine plus rapid-acting insulin: the ATLANTIC study. Acta Clin Belg. 2013;68(1):28-33.
25. Kesavadev J, Jain SM, Muruganathan A, et al. Consensus evidence-based guidelines for use of insulin pump therapy in the management of diabetes as per Indian clinical practice. J Assoc Physicians India. 2014;62(7 Suppl):34-41.
26. Ahluwalia A, Baliarsinha AK, Gupta SB, et al. Consensus evidence-based guidelines for management of hyperglycaemia in patients undergoing coronary artery bypass grafting in patients with diabetes in India. J Assoc Physicians India. 2014;62(7 Suppl):42-8.
27. Rys P, Pankiewicz O, Łach K, et al. Efficacy and safety comparison of rapid-acting insulin aspart and regular human insulin in the treatment of type 1 and type 2 diabetes mellitus: a systematic review. Diabetes Metab. 2011;37(3):190-200.
28. Sanches AC, Correr CJ, Venson R, et al. Insulin analogues versus human insulin in type 1 diabetes: direct and indirect meta-analyses of efficacy and safety. Brazi J Pharma Sci. 2013;49:501-9.
29. Monami M, Marchionni N, Mannucci E. Long-acting insulin analogues versus NPH human insulin in type 2 diabetes: a meta-analysis. Diabetes Res Clin Pract. 2008;81(2):184-9.
30. Shah S, Sharma SK, Singh P, et al. Consensus evidence-based guidelines for insulin initiation, optimization and continuation in type 2 diabetes mellitus. J Assoc Physicians India. 2014;62(7 Suppl):49-54.

CHAPTER

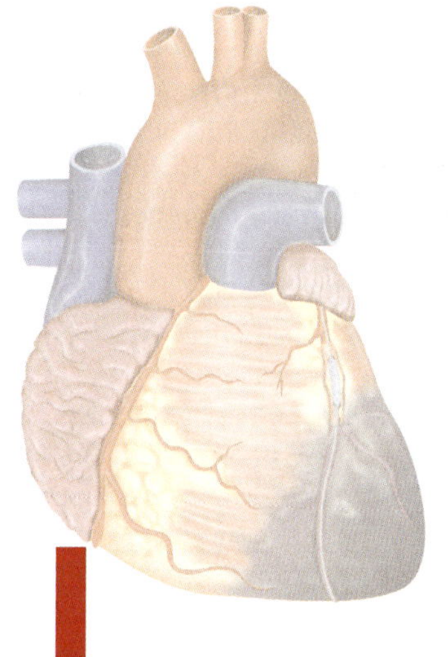

Echo-guided CRT in Cardiodiabetes

Rahul Mehrotra, Raj Kumar Dahiya, Meeta Maheshwari

INTRODUCTION

Heart failure (HF) is a complex clinical entity and has been variously defined in the past. The most recent and comprehensive definition states that it is a clinical syndrome characterized by typical symptoms (e.g. breathlessness, ankle swelling, and fatigue) that may be accompanied by signs (e.g. elevated jugular venous pressure, pulmonary crackles, and peripheral edema) caused by a structural and/or functional cardiac abnormality, resulting in a reduced cardiac output state and/or elevated intracardiac pressures at rest or during stress.[1]

Heart failure has a prevalence of more than 23 million worldwide and is a major public health problem, associated with significant mortality, morbidity, and healthcare expenditure.[2] Apart from the problems related to impairment of quality of life, a major issue faced by the patients is the need of frequent hospitalizations for HF-related morbidity. The treatment of HF is aimed at reducing the risk of sudden death, frequent hospitalizations, and overall improvement in the quality of life. Pharmacological treatment of HF has evolved considerably with drugs like beta-blockers, some diuretics, angiotensin-converting enzyme inhibitors (ACEIs), angiotensin receptor blockers (ARBs), and several anti-arrhythmic agents showing significant benefits in large-scale randomized clinical trials. Besides, several new drugs are under evaluation—Valsartan-Sacubitril combination being the latest addition to the armamentarium. Another aspect of the HF treatment is device therapy in the form of cardiac resynchronization therapy (CRT) or implantable cardioverter defibrillator (ICD), or a combination of both, in suitable patients. The combination of effective pharmacological therapy with CRT and ICD devices has led to positive outcomes for patients with HF by reducing both—HF hospitalization and mortality. Heart transplant and left ventricular-assist devices (LVAD) are the high-end therapies for these patients, limited in scope due to cost, availability of donors, and expertise for the surgery, but are also being increasingly used in India and have resulted in marked improvement in quality of life and survival of these patients.

DIABETES AND HEART FAILURE

Type 2 diabetes mellitus (DM) affects more than 100 million persons worldwide and its prevalence is increasing in both developed and developing countries.[3] The prevalence of DM in patients with HF approaches approximately 30%. Also, the patients with type 2 DM develop CHF more frequently than patients without diabetes. The strong association of DM and HF has been well recognized for several decades now. DM contributes to the development and progression of HF and worsens the prognosis as type 2 DM patients have substantially higher lifetime risk of mortality from HF. HF in the diabetic patients may develop regardless of typical risk factors such as hypertension and coronary artery disease.[4] These observations are further supported by evidence from experimental studies demonstrating development of structural and functional abnormalities in the myocardium of the diabetic subjects.[5]

The pathophysiologic mechanisms linking type 2 diabetes and HF include the adverse effects of hyperglycemia on endothelial function and redox state, effects of excess circulating glucose and fatty acids on cardiomyocyte ultrastructure, intracellular signaling and gene expression, and the possibility that diabetes may impair recruitment of the myocardial insulin-responsive glucose transport system in response to ischemia.[3]

In this chapter, we discuss the role of echocardiography-guided CRT in patients with HF and diabetes.

INDICATIONS FOR CARDIAC RESYNCHRONIZATION THERAPY

Not all patients of HF benefit from CRT and there is a significant proportion of non-responders. Clinical trials have brought out the patients who are likely to respond with this expensive and invasive therapy. Currently, the patients of HF with reduced ejection fraction only are considered candidates for this therapy. The current recommendations for use of CRT in patients with HF are as follows:[6]

- For symptomatic patients with HF in sinus rhythm with a QRS duration more than or equal to 150 ms and left bundle branch block (LBBB) QRS morphology and with left ventricular ejection fraction (LVEF) less than or equal to 35%, despite optimal medical treatment (OMT) to improve symptoms and reduce morbidity and mortality (Class I, Level A).
- For symptomatic patients with HF in sinus rhythm with a QRS duration of 130–149 ms and LBBB QRS morphology and with LVEF less than or equal to 35% despite OMT to improve symptoms and reduce morbidity and mortality (Class I, Level B). CRT rather than right ventricular (RV) pacing alone is recommended for patients with HF with reduced ejection fraction (EF) (HFrEF) regardless of New York Heart Association (NYHA) class, who have an indication for ventricular pacing and high-degree AV block, in order to reduce morbidity. This includes patients with atrial fibrillation (AF) (Class I, Level A).
- For symptomatic patients with HF in sinus rhythm with a QRS duration more than or equal to 150 ms, non-LBBB QRS morphology and with LVEF less than or equal to 35% despite OMT, in order to improve symptoms and reduce morbidity and mortality (Class IIa, Level B).
- For symptomatic patients with HF in sinus rhythm with a QRS duration of 130–149 ms and non-LBBB QRS morphology and with LVEF less than or equal to 35% despite OMT in order to improve symptoms and reduce morbidity and mortality (Class IIb, Level B).
- For patients with LVEF less than or equal to 35% in NYHA Class III–IV despite OMT in order to improve symptoms and reduce morbidity and mortality, if they are in AF and have a QRS duration more than or equal to 130 ms provided a strategy to ensure biventricular capture is in place or the patient is expected to return to sinus rhythm (Class IIa, Level B).
- Patients of HF with reduced EF, who have received a conventional pacemaker or an ICD and subsequently develop worsening HF despite OMT, and who have a high proportion of RV pacing may be considered for upgrade to CRT. This does not apply to patients with stable HF (Class IIb, Level B).
- Cardiac resynchronization therapy is *contraindicated* in patients with a QRS duration less than 130 ms (Class III, Level A).

As evident, the indications for CRT in HF, encompass all the patients of HFrEF, including those with presence of DM. The presence of diabetes does not thus alter the indication for CRT in any way whatsoever. The most important factors remain the severity of LV systolic dysfunction determined by echocardiography, symptomatic status in spite of the use of guideline-determined optimal medical therapy and electrocardiography (ECG) pattern. The blood sugar levels do not have any bearing on the decision to use CRT in these patients.

ROLE OF ECHOCARDIOGRAPHY IN CRT

Cardiac resynchronization therapy is an interventional technique for patients with HF, refractory to medical therapy, who are likely to benefit most with this technique. Although, not apparent in the indications mentioned, echocardiography has a key role to play in the whole scenario of use of CRT for patients of HF. Echocardiography with its various modalities is an inexpensive, safe, and versatile tool, used for decision making in various stages of use of CRT in patients with HF. It provides valuable information for patient selection, optimization of device settings, and deciding about the response and outcome.[7]

Before Cardiac Resynchronization Therapy

At the very outset, echocardiography is necessary to determine whether the symptomatic patients suspected of having HF have any cardiac structural or functional disorder. Echocardiography, safely and easily categorizes the patients of HF into those with reduced EF from those with preserved (HFpEF) or mid-range EF (HFmrEF). This difference is fundamental first step as the treatment approach of patients of HFpEF is completely different and CRT is not indicated in these patients. The next step in patients with reduced EF is the accurate assessment of EF for assessment of suitability for CRT in patients of HFrEF. A variety of echocardiographic techniques are currently available to assess the extent of LV systolic dysfunction and

EF and a comprehensive echocardiac assessment is made by using the different modalities at the first instance. The various modalities used are:

- Biplane Simpson's method can be used to determine LV end-diastolic and systolic volumes, and calculate LVEF.[8] It is the method of choice while using two-dimensional echocardiography, for calculation of these parameters. Apart from EF, end-diastolic volume, end-systolic volume, and stroke volume recorded at the baseline serve as the basis for assessment of response after CRT implantation. A visual estimate of regional wall motion abnormalities, presence and location of scarring along with estimation of EF can also be accurately made by experienced echocardiographers and is quite reliable, but volumes cannot be estimated by this method. Three-dimensional echocardiography (3DE) is an accurate, reliable, and reproducible method for assessment of LV volumes and systolic functions. It should be used wherever available for this purpose.
- Pulsed-wave (PW) Doppler, continuous wave Doppler, and tissue Doppler are used to measure stroke volume and cardiac output, assess LV diastolic function, calculate diastolic filling time (DFT), detect the presence of diastolic mitral regurgitation and estimate RV systolic and diastolic pressures.
- Color flow imaging is used to evaluate the severity of mitral regurgitation and detect the presence of other regurgitant lesions. RV systolic function is also assessed using M-mode echocardiography.

After confirming the presence of LV systolic dysfunction along with a comprehensive evaluation by echocardiography, the next step is to look for evidence of cardiac mechanical dyssynchrony. The three types of cardiac dyssynchrony that have been described are—atrioventricular (AV), interventricular (VV), and intraventricular dyssynchrony. Several approaches have been used and different cutoffs are proposed for them. Although the presence of mechanical dyssynchrony by echocardiography is not a prerequisite for use of CRT, its use may further help in careful selection of patients who are very likely to respond and is paramount for assessment of response to CRT later on as discussed later.

Atrioventricular Dyssynchrony

Atrioventricular dyssynchrony can be measured by dividing DFT (time from onset of "E" wave to end of "A" wave measured by pulse wave Doppler at the tips of mitral leaflets in the apical four-chamber view in diastole), from R-R interval (measured on the screen from the ECG). This is also known as the diastolic filling fraction (DFF) (Fig. 1). DFF value of less than 0.40 (less than 40% of cardiac cycle) is considered to signify presence of AV dyssynchrony.

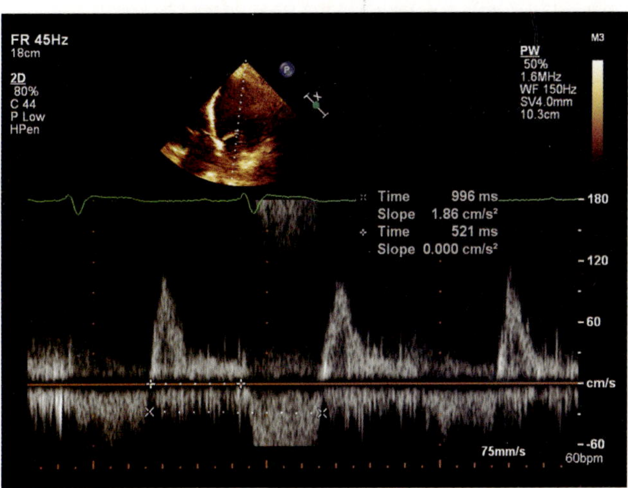

Fig. 1: Pulse wave Doppler measurement of mitral inflow velocity at mitral leaflet tips for assessment of AV dyssynchrony. DFF is 0.52 suggestive of no significant AV dyssynchrony

Abbreviations: AV, atrioventricular; DFF, diastolic filling fraction.

Interventricular Dyssynchrony

Interventricular dyssynchrony represents the temporal discordance between right ventricle and left ventricular contraction. Firstly, the right and left ventricular pre-ejection periods are determined. These are calculated by using the PW cursor at the RV outflow and the LV outflow in different views. The intervals from the onset of Q wave on the ECG trace to the onset of RV and LV outflow track Doppler traces (Figs 2A and B) are the right and left pre-ejection periods, respectively. The difference between RV and LV pre-ejection periods is normally less than 40 ms.[8] A difference of greater than 40 ms is considered abnormal. If LV pre-ejection period is greater than 140 ms, it is considered prolonged.[9]

Intraventricular Dyssynchrony

This is one of the most important parameters to look for in assessment of dyssynchrony as it denotes the difference in contraction times of different areas within the LV. The presence and extent of intraventricular dyssynchrony can be measured using different techniques.

A septal and posterior wall contraction delay longer than 130 ms measured by M-mode echocardiography in parasternal long-axis view is considered to represent significant intraventricular dyssynchrony.

Tissue Doppler imaging (TDI) can be used to determine the regional electromechanical delay in the LV by measuring the time interval from onset of QRS to the time of peak longitudinal systolic strain of different LV segments in apical four-chamber, two-chamber, and three-chamber views. It has been shown that if positioned at the site of

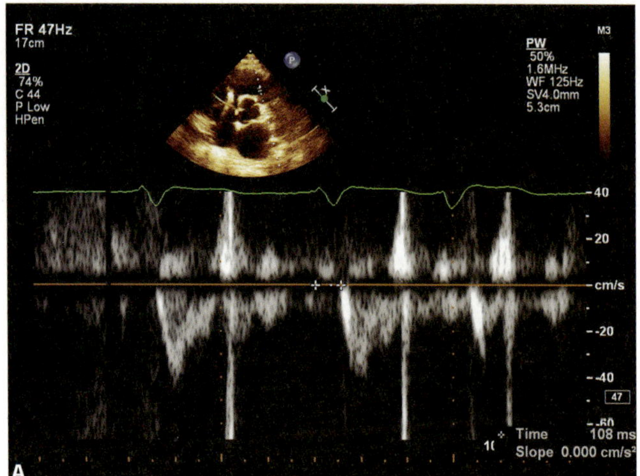

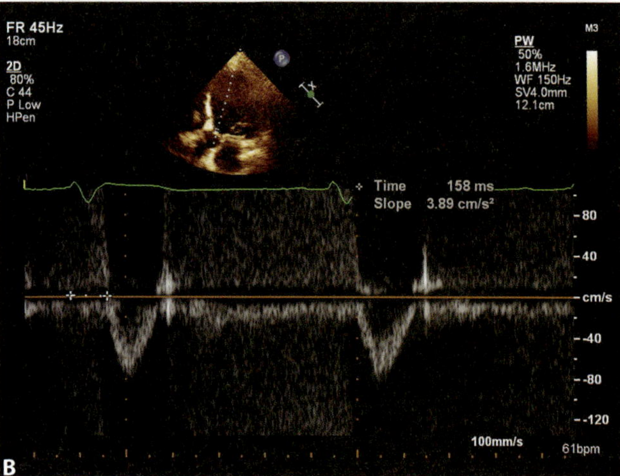

Figs 2A and B: Pulse wave spectral Doppler display at (A) right ventricular outflow tract showing pulmonary pre-ejection period, and (B) left ventricular outflow tract showing aortic pre-ejection period. The difference between the aortic and pulmonary pre-ejection period is 50 ms suggestive of significant interventricular dyssynchrony

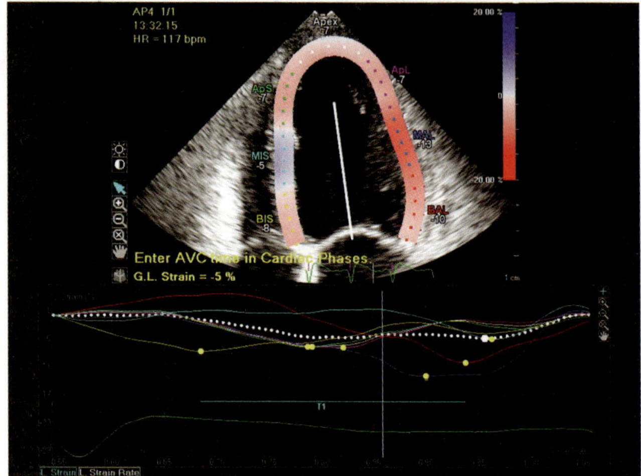

Fig. 3: Two-dimensional speckle tracking method for measurement of longitudinal strain in four-chamber view at basal ventricular level showing asynchronous contraction of basal segments. Basal anterolateral wall (red curve) is significantly delayed (>200 ms) as compared to basal inferoseptum (yellow curve)

longest electromechanical delay, the benefit of LV pacing is maximal.[10] However, significant delay in the timing of regional contraction among LV segments may not always be present in patients with a prolonged QRS interval.

Three-dimensional echocardiography also plays an important role in the assessment of intraventricular dyssynchrony. It enables the comparison of synchrony in all segments in the same cardiac cycle. The data can be represented in the form of global and regional volume curves, parametric maps, and the calculated systolic dyssynchrony index (SDI). Quantification of mechanical dyssynchrony with real-time 3-dimensional echocardiography (RT3DE) takes all myocardial segments into account by examining the composite effect of radial, circumferential, and longitudinal contraction and has been found to be quite reproducible.[11]

Strain imaging is increasingly being evaluated for assessment of dyssynchrony. Several studies have utilized circumferential, radial, and longitudinal strain measured by TDI and Speckle tracking method (Fig. 3) and have shown encouraging results. The angle dependency with pulse TDI-based strain, availability, and vendor dependency on software for strain are some limiting factors preventing its widespread use.

Table 1 summarizes the different parameters and commonly used cutoffs for assessment of mechanical dyssynchrony by echocardiography.[12] It should be emphasized again that rather than relying on these parameters alone, the decision should be made taking into account the overall impression—the shape of LV, presence and location of scarring, mitral regurgitation, etc.

Echocardiographic Assessment after CRT Device Implantation

At the time of device implantation, optimal parameters are set in the catheterization laboratory after appropriate placement of the leads, using the device programmer to address the different dyssynchrony present, using the pacing parameters. However, after CRT, echocardiography is again very helpful in fine-tuning and adjusting the AV delay and interventricular (VV) delay to achieve maximal cardiac filling (DFT) and cardiac output.[7] This is done using different parameters by the iterative method.

TABLE 1: Parameters used to assess cardiac dyssynchrony with their reference values[17]

S. No	Dyssynchrony type	Parameters	Reference value
1.	Atrioventricular dyssynchrony	DFF	40%
2.	Interventricular dyssynchrony	Difference between aortic pre-ejection and pulmonary pre-ejection time	>40 ms
3.	Intraventricular dyssynchrony	Strain difference in opposing segments	>65 ms
		Strain difference between any two segments	>100 ms
		M-mode echocardiography measuring septal posterior wall delay	>130 ms

Abbreviation: DFF, diastolic filling fraction

Atrioventricular Delay

Proper AV delay should ensure sufficient time for LV filling. The mitral inflow pattern with the E and A waves should be broad enough and the waves as separate as possible. An optimal AV interval should place the end of the atrial filling wave (A wave) at the onset of isovolumic contraction, and can be achieved by the pulsed Doppler mitral inflow method using Ritter formula or the aortic velocity time integral method.[13] The aortic velocity time integral method may provide a better determinant of the optimal AV delay for CRT, because it represents the direct systolic performance rather than the diastolic filling alone.

Interventricular Delay

It is believed that sequential biventricular pacing provides greater synchrony than simultaneous biventricular pacing.[8] LV before RV pacing with optimal VV delay may result in maximal hemodynamic improvement. The stroke volume assessment at the left ventricular outflow tract (LVOT) by echocardiography is the most common way to evaluate VV optimization. The average interval of the VV delay is kept around 20–40 ms but this varies from patient to patient.[14]

The patient is left on the best AV and VV delay settings and cardiac output. These parameters are readjusted on follow-up if the symptomatic status of the patient requires re-evaluation.

CRT IN DIABETES MELLITUS

As discussed earlier, diabetic patients are more prone to develop HF as compared to nondiabetic individuals. Besides, patients with both DM and HF have a 1.5- to 2-fold higher risk of death than nondiabetic patients with HF.[15] The medical therapy of HF in presence of DM remains the same along with the indications for CRT as described earlier. The role of echocardiography in CRT is also similar, with no difference for diabetic and nondiabetic individuals. There are, however, minor differences related to the CRT procedure and its complications which will be discussed elsewhere. In a study of diabetic patients with HF receiving CRT with ICD, DM was independently associated with greater risks of death and rehospitalization, but similar risks of procedural complications.[16] In a meta-analysis, it was concluded that CRT may reduce mortality from progressive HF in patients with or without DM, but mortality may be higher for patients with diabetes than without diabetes after CRT for HF.[17] There has been, however, no separate study related to the role of echocardiography and the parameters used as predictors of response in HF patients with co-existing diabetes.

CONCLUSION

Cardiac resynchronization therapy is helpful in improving symptoms and quality of life in patients of diabetes in association with HF and reduced LVEF. Despite the development of effective pharmacological and nonpharmacological treatments in recent years, the quality of life of many patients with HF is considerably impaired because of the frequent worsening of symptoms, hospitalizations, and considerably poor survival with sudden cardiac death being a major cause. Patients of HFrEF with DM treated by CRT when indicated, continue to have higher mortality rates than those without DM. The hospital readmission rates among patients with DM are also higher than among those without DM. Currently, echocardiography continues to play a critical role in the patients who have HF and are candidates for CRT, including those who have diabetes. Further studies are required to study the role of echocardiography and its tools in the diabetic patients to enumerate any difference in approach required in this very vital subset.

REFERENCES

1. Roger VL. Epidemiology of heart failure. Circ Res. 2013;113(6):646-59.
2. Ponikowski P, Voors AA, Anker SD, et al. 2016 ESC Guidelines for the diagnosis and treatment of acute and chronic heart failure The Task Force for the diagnosis and treatment of acute and chronic heart failure of the European Society of Cardiology (ESC) developed with the special contribution of the Heart Failure Association (HFA) of the ESC. Eur Heart J. 2016;37(27):2129-200.
3. Jagasia D, McNulty PH. Diabetes mellitus and heart failure. Congest Heart Fail. 2003;9(3):133-9.

4. Bell DS. Diabetic cardiomyopathy: a unique entity or a complication of coronary artery disease? Diabetes Care. 1995;18(5):708-14.
5. Cowie MR, Mosterd A, Wood DA, et al. The epidemiology of heart failure. Eur Heart J. 1997;18(2):208-25.
6. Ponikowski P, Voors AA, Anker SD, et al. 2016 ESC Guidelines for the diagnosis and treatment of acute and chronic heart failure: The Task Force for the diagnosis and treatment of acute and chronic heart failure of the European Society of Cardiology (ESC). Developed with the special contribution of the Heart Failure Association (HFA) of the ESC. Eur J Heart Fail. 2016;18(8):891-975.
7. Mazur W, Chung ES. The role of echocardiography in cardiac resynchronization therapy. Curr Heart Fail Rep. 2009;6(1):37-43.
8. Chen CH, Ko WC, Chin CH, et al. The role of echocardiography in cardiac resynchronization therapy. J Med Ultrasound. 2008;16(1):1-6.
9. Cazeau S, Bordachar P, Jauvert G, et al. Echocardiographic modeling of cardiac dyssynchrony before and during multisite stimulation: a prospective study. Pacing Clin Electrophysiol. 2003;26(1 Pt 2):137-43.
10. Ansalone G, Giannantoni P, Ricci R, et al. Doppler myocardial imaging to evaluate the effectiveness of pacing sites in patients receiving biventricular pacing. J Am Coll Cardiol. 2002;39(3): 489-99.
11. Kapetanakis S, Kearney MT, Siva A, et al. Real-time three-dimensional echocardiography: a novel technique to quantify global left ventricular mechanical dyssynchrony. Circulation. 2005;112:992-1000.
12. Mehrotra R, Bansal M, Chopra HK, et al. Echocardiography for assessment of electromechanical dyssynchrony. Indian Heart J. 2009;61(2):218-22.
13. Faddis MN, Waggoner AD, Garhwal S, et al. AV delay optimization by aortic VTI is superior to the pulsed Doppler mitral inflow method for cardiac resynchronization therapy. Pacing Clin Electrophysiol. 2003;26:1042.
14. Agler DA, Adams DB, Waggoner AD. Cardiac resynchronization therapy and the emerging role of echocardiography (part 2): the comprehensive examination. J Am Soc Echocardiogr. 2007;20:76-90.
15. Sun H, Guan Y, Wang L, et al. Influence of diabetes on cardiac resynchronization therapy in heart failure patients: a meta-analysis. BMC Cardiovasc Disord. 2015;15:25.
16. Echouffo-Tcheugui JB, Masoudi FA, Bao H, et al. Diabetes mellitus and outcomes of cardiac resynchronization with implantable cardioverter-defibrillator therapy in older patients with heart failure. Circ Arrhythm Electrophysiol. 2016;9:8.
17. Mangiavacchi M, Gasparini M, Genovese S et al. Insulin treated type 2 diabetes is associated with a decreased survival in heart failure patients after cardiac resynchronization therapy. Pacing Clin Electrophysiol. 2008;31(11):1425-32.

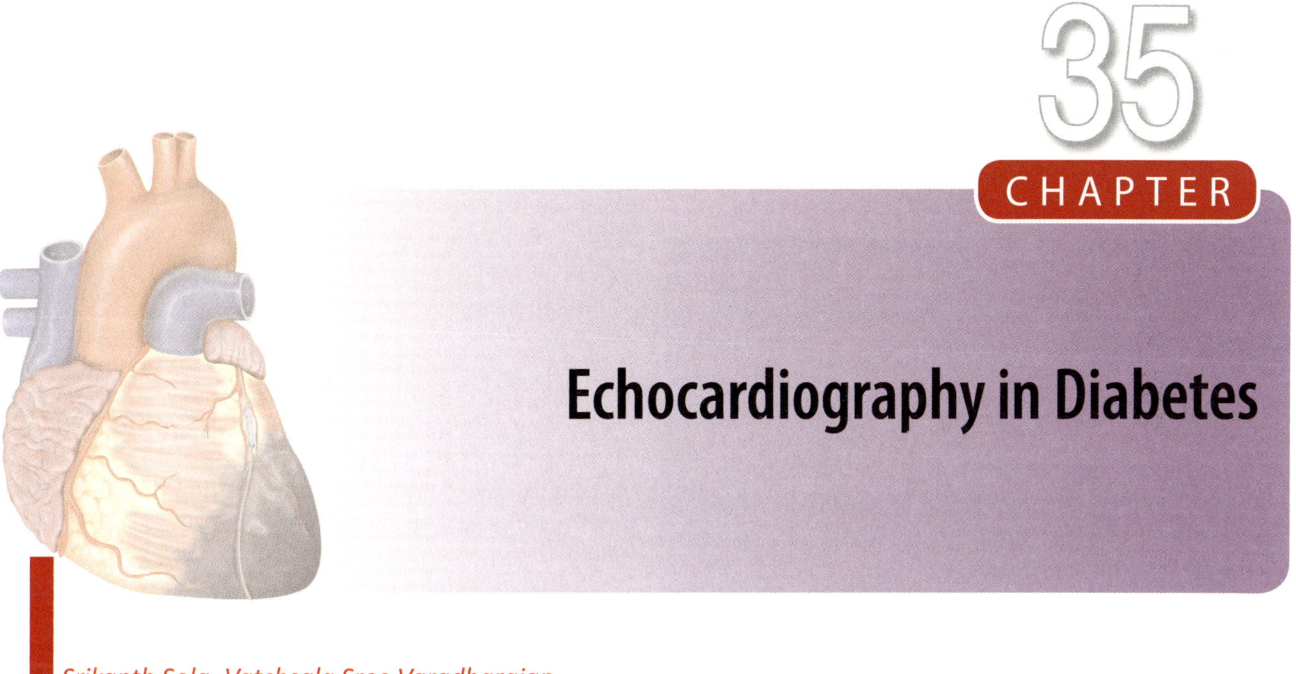

Echocardiography in Diabetes

Srikanth Sola, Vatchsala Sree Varadharajan

INTRODUCTION

Echocardiography is an essential tool in the evaluation of patients with suspected heart disease. It is noninvasive, portable, relatively inexpensive, and safe, with no exposure to ionizing radiation. Newer echo-based techniques such as three-dimensional (3D) echocardiography and strain imaging provide incremental value that is useful in patients with diabetes, particularly in high-risk patients or when subclinical disease is a concern. This chapter focuses on the use of transthoracic echocardiography (TTE) in patients with diabetes, particularly in the evaluation of coronary artery disease (CAD), diastolic dysfunction, and diabetic cardiomyopathy.

ECHOCARDIOGRAPHIC ASSESSMENT OF CORONARY ARTERY DISEASE

Coronary artery disease is the most common cause of mortality and morbidity in diabetes. Echocardiographic assessment helps in the diagnosis (TTE, stress echo, and speckle tracking echo), evaluation of the extent and severity (TTE and stress echo), and the hemodynamic complications of CAD (Doppler and color flow) in both stable ischemic heart disease and acute coronary syndromes.

Assessment of Left Ventricular Volume and Global Systolic Function

The size (dimensions and volume) and function of the left ventricle (LV) are the most important echocardiographic data in patients with suspected CAD. LV ejection fraction (LVEF) is one of the strongest predictors of all-cause mortality and major adverse cardiac events in patients with CAD. Current guidelines of the Indian Academy of Echocardiography for two-dimensional (2D) echo-based assessment of left ventricular size and ejection fraction (LVEF) recommend the Biplane Simpson's method of discs summation.[1] This method uses data from images acquired during end-diastole and end-systole from apical four-chamber and apical two-chamber views. For accurate measurements, care must be taken to avoid foreshortening of the LV and to carefully delineate the endocardial border, tracing only the compacted myocardium. Three-dimensional echo-based measurements of LVEF provide superior accuracy compared to 2D echo. Foreshortening of the LV is avoided, and the entire ventricle is traced (Fig. 1), unlike the 2D biplane method, where the LV is measured from only two planes. When available, 3D echo for assessment of LV function, particularly in patients with reduced ejection fraction, is preferred. Modern echo machines allow rapid calculation of not only LV volumes and ejection fraction but also the right ventricle as well as left and right atrial dimensions. In patients with suboptimal image quality (defined as ≥2 or more myocardial segments not seen), LV contrast agents should be encouraged to obtain an optimal image for both 3D and 2D techniques.

Depending upon the values of the LVEF, LV systolic function can be classified as follows, with mild variations based on gender and ethnicity. Mortality increases linearly with worsening LV function.

- *Hyperdynamic*: LVEF is greater than 70%
- *Normal*: LVEF 56–70% (midpoint 60%)

- *Mild dysfunction*: LVEF 40–56% (midpoint 45%)
- *Moderate dysfunction*: LVEF 30–39% (midpoint 35%)
- *Severe dysfunction*: LVEF is less than 30%.

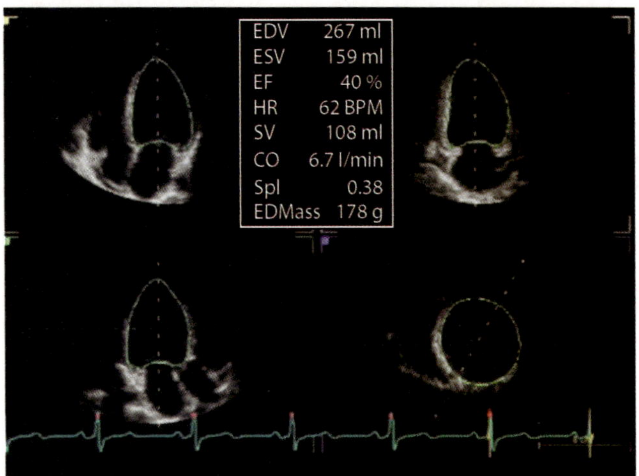

Fig. 1: Three-dimensional evaluation of left ventricular ejection fraction. Example of quantification of left ventricular size and quantification using three-dimensional echocardiography. The left ventricular endocardial borders are traced (green lines) during end diastole (shown here) and end systole from the three-dimensional volumes. The software automatically calculates a number of volumetric parameters, most important of which are—end diastolic volume (for size) and ejection fraction (center rectangle)

Abbreviations: EDV, end-diastolic volume; ESV, end-systolic volume; EF, ejection fraction; HR, heart rate; SV, stroke volume; CO, cardiac output)

Assessment of Regional Left Ventricle Systolic Function Using 2D Echo

As global function provides information on overall LV systolic function, regional impairment of systolic function occurs in various diseases (Table 1). If regional dysfunction occurs in a specific coronary artery territory, CAD should be suspected. When ischemia is mild, reversible, and sometimes, transient impairment of regional myocardial contraction occur. However, when ischemia is persistent and severe (e.g., after myocardial infarction), the myocardium develops necrosis followed by scarring, LV remodeling, and permanent damage to the myocardial contractility in a region subtended by the coronary artery involved. Visual or qualitative assessment of regional myocardial function uses a combination of three factors: myocardial contraction; the echogenicity of the myocardium; and end-diastolic wall thickness. A common semiquantitative practice is to grade myocardial contraction based on the amount of increased wall thickness during systole. *Normal contraction* is defined as greater than 40% increase in wall thickness during systole in a particular segment. *Hypokinesis* is present when there is only a 10–40% increase in thickness during systole, whereas a segment is defined as *akinetic* when there is less than 10% increase in all thickness. A segment is considered *dyskinetic* when it exhibits outward motion during systole (away from the ventricular cavity). Myocardium that is very bright in appearance is called *echogenic*. When echogenic myocardium occurs in a segment with decreased wall

TABLE 1: Advanced techniques for assessment of left ventricular systolic function by echocardiography

Parameters	*Stroke volume*	*Myocardial performance index (Tei index)*	*dp/dt*
Technique	Pulse wave Doppler across the LVOT, and two-dimensional measurement of the LVOT diameter from the parasternal long-axis view.	Pulse wave Doppler or tissue Doppler imaging (the latter is preferred due to superior image quality). Measured from the mitral annulus.	Continuous wave Doppler. Used as a surrogate of global systolic function
Principle of measurement	Amount of blood ejected from the left ventricle with each heartbeat. Provides a noninvasive estimate of cardiac output (calculated as stroke volume × heart rate).[22]	Doppler index of combined systolic and diastolic myocardial performance in patients with systolic dysfunction. Based on the principle that when there is LV systolic dysfunction the isovolumic contraction time (IVCT) and the isovolumic relaxation time (IVRT) are prolonged whereas the ejection time (ET) is shortened.[23]	Change in pressure over time as measured from continuous wave Doppler flow across the mitral valve. Reflects LV contractility. At least mild mitral regurgitation is required for measurement.[24]
Formula	SV = LVOT VTI × LVOT area	MPI = (IVCT + IVRT)/ET	dp/dt = 32/time interval of the MR jet between 1 m/s and 3 m/s. These times are chosen as this is the period when left atrial pressure is constant.
Normal value	60–120 mL	0.39 ± 0.05 ms	1000–1200 mmHg/s

Abbreviations: LVOT, left ventricular outflow tract; VTI, velocity-time integral; MR, mitral regurgitation

thickness, the myocardium is said to be thinned and scarred—a finding that is seen in ventricular remodeling after myocardial infarction. Thinned myocardium—that is myocardium that has an end-diastolic wall thickness is less than 5.5 mm—is a sensitive but not specific sign of nonviable myocardium—tissue that has been damaged by CAD and is unlikely to recover contractile function after revascularization. The wall motion score index (WMSI) is a quantitative assessment of overall LV myocardial contraction which incorporates each segment separately. Each visualized segment is assigned a specific number of points as follows, using the definitions just described:

- Normal or hyperkinetic
- Hypokinetic (reduced thickening)
- Akinetic (absent or negligible thickening)
- Dyskinetic (systolic thinning or stretching or aneurysm).

An aneurysmal segment is one that is thinned with focal dilatation which is either akinetic or dyskinetic. Usually the ventricle is arbitrarily divided into 16 or 17 segments, and the standard method applied to categorize the myocardial segments. Depending upon the number of segments visualized and the score of the myocardial contraction, a WMSI can be calculated which is equal to the sum of all segmental scores divided by the number of visualized segments.[2] A WMSI of 1 is normal. A higher WMSI indicates regional wall motion abnormalities, a globally worsened LV systolic function, and an overall worse prognosis.

Tissue Doppler Imaging

Tissue Doppler imaging (TDI) is an echocardiographic technique which uses Doppler principles to measure velocities of tissue movement. In contemporary clinical practice, TDI is most commonly used to estimate the velocities of the mitral annulus (Sa) as part of diastolic function measurement, and occasionally the myocardial segments (Sm). The peak systolic velocity of the mitral annulus is a sensitive marker of mildly reduced LV systolic function, even when global LV function appears normal, such as in diabetic subjects without overt heart disease. Reduced TDI velocities can be used to predict later development of impaired LVEF,[3] and is an independent predictor of mortality. The major limitation of TDI is that it is angle-dependent, which limits its use to the apical windows.

Myocardial Deformation

The LV myocardium undergoes deformation (change in length and direction in all three dimensions) during ventricular contraction that enables it to effectively fill and eject blood from the LV cavity. The deformation is described by three mechanisms: strain, rotation, and twist. Strain is the lengthening (relaxation) and shortening (contraction) of the myocardial fibers and can be measured in the longitudinal, circumferential, or radial directions. Of all these strain parameters, longitudinal strain is the most important as it is more reproducible and easily measured than radial strain, circumferential strain, rotation, or twist. Extending this further, global longitudinal strain (GLS), which measures the myocardial deformation of the entire LV, provides important information on global LV function beyond that of LVEF. Although there are marked variations in the normal range of the GLS between different published literatures, as a general, a value less than (more negative than) –20% is considered to be normal.[4] In patients with diabetes, however, normal GLS values are lower, typically from –15% to –18%, due to underlying microvascular disease and endothelial dysfunction, even in the absence of hemodynamically significant CAD (Figs 2A and B).[5] The main clinical application of longitudinal strain assessment is to detect subclinical myocardial dysfunction (normal LVEF, but reduced GLS) before such dysfunction can be detected using routine visual assessment. GLS is reduced in patients with CAD. Longitudinal strain will be typically reduced in the coronary segments subtended by the stenosed artery, while segments remote from the stenosis have normal strain (Figs 3A to C). Both longitudinal and circumferential strain can be used to diagnose the presence of CAD, its severity, and coronary distribution. Subclinical LV dysfunction is common, and indicates a worse prognosis. In one study of 101 patients with diabetes mellitus (DM), strain analysis found reduced LV systolic function as measured by GLS in 24% of the study group who otherwise had normal systolic function using conventional 2D echo-based measurements of LVEF.[6] A number of studies have demonstrated that reduced longitudinal systolic strain is associated with increased risk of major adverse cardiovascular events and provides incremental prognostic value beyond that of routine echocardiographic parameters.[7,8] The major limitation of strain analysis is substantial inter-vendor variability in measurements, although significant progress is being made in this area.

DIAGNOSIS OF CORONARY ARTERY DISEASE USING STRESS ECHOCARDIOGRAPHY

Stress echocardiography (SE) can be used to diagnose ischemia in patients with suspected CAD. It provides information on the functional significance of any coronary artery stenosis that may be present by assessing changes in myocardial contractility during stress. SE can be performed using a pharmacological agent (dobutamine) or using exercise such as a treadmill or a reclined stationary bicycle at

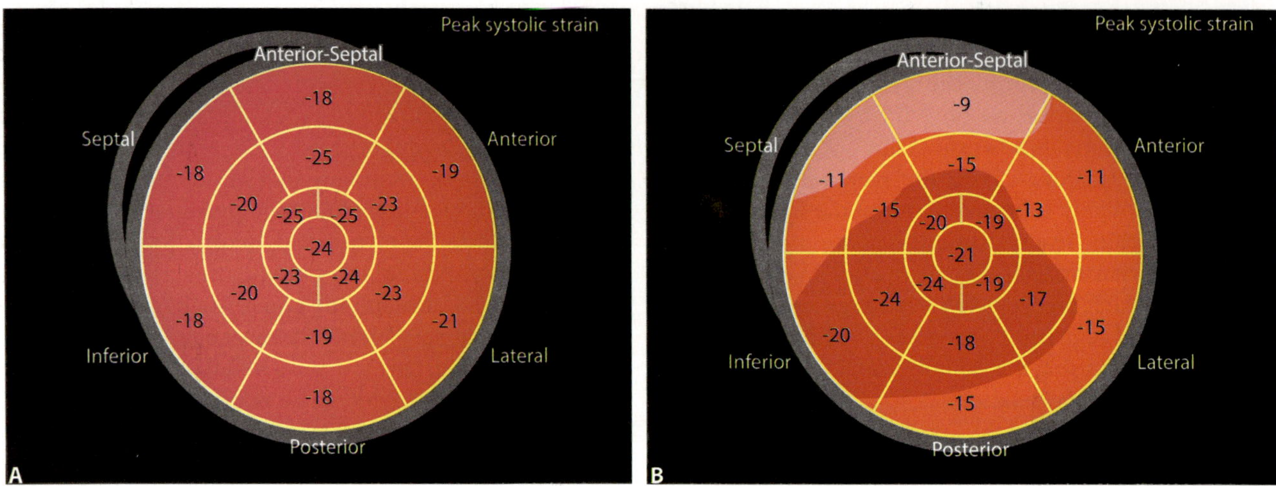

Figs 2A and B: Reduced global longitudinal strain in diabetes mellitus. (A) Bulls-eye map of longitudinal strain in a normal healthy patient without diabetes and normal left ventricular systolic function. Global longitudinal strain is normal in this patient. (B) Similar Bulls-eye map in a patient with diabetes, normal left ventricular systolic function, and no coronary artery disease. The lighter pink shaded segments show reduced segmental strain, but in a noncoronary distribution that typical for diseases such as diabetes. Global longitudinal strain is at the lower end of normal

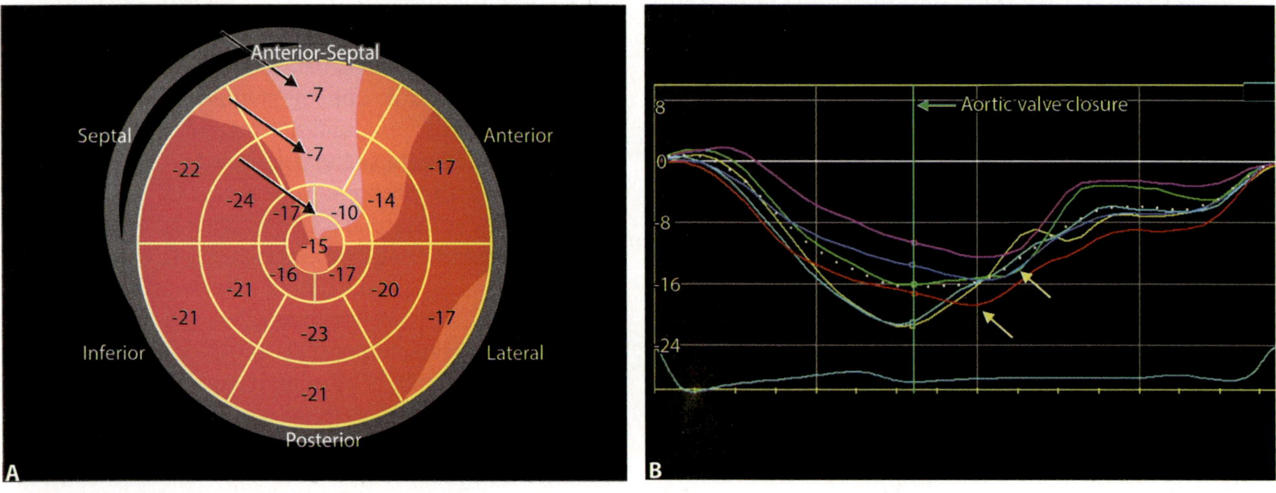

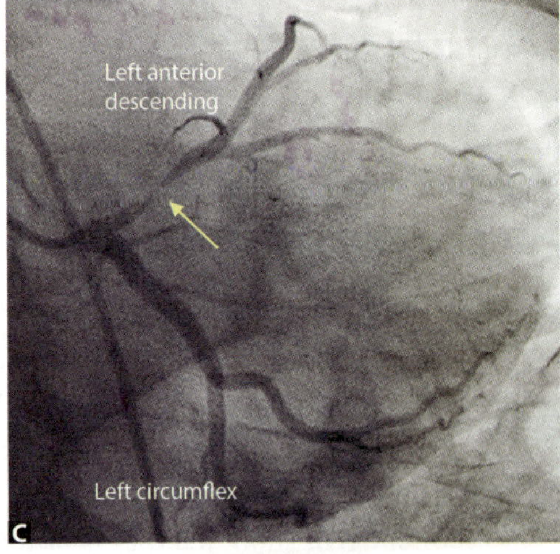

Figs 3A to C: Strain in coronary artery disease. A diabetic patient presented with chronic stable angina. Both resting electrocardiogram and left ventricular ejection fraction by two-dimensional echo were normal. Strain analysis showed reduced global longitudinal strain. (A) Bulls-eye map demonstrated reduced segmental strain in the segments supplied by the left anterior descending coronary artery (arrows). (B) Strain tracings from the apical 2-chamber view demonstrate postsystolic shortening, defined as a peak systolic strain excursion after aortic valve closure (green arrow), in this example in segments supplied by the left anterior descending artery (red, blue, and purple lines in this view, corresponding to the basal-, mid-, and distal-anterior segments; yellow arrows). (C) Subsequent invasive coronary angiography demonstrated an 80% stenosis in the proximal left anterior descending coronary artery (arrow).

progressively increasing speed and/or resistance. Exercise SE is generally preferred, as the functional information on a patient's exercise capacity provides important prognostic information. Patients who exercise to less than 6 METS (equivalent to sweeping the floor) have a poor prognosis, whereas patients who can exercise greater than 10 METS have an excellent prognosis, even when hemodynamically significant CAD is present. Exercise SE has a sensitivity and specificity in the range of 74–97% and 64–86%, respectively, depending on the image quality obtained.[9] Pharmacologic SE is best suited to patients with significant LV dysfunction or who are unable to exercise due to orthopedic, neurologic, or other limitations. It also has better specificity than exercise SE for the diagnosis of CAD when a left bundle branch block is present on electrocardiogram (ECG), due to the tendency to develop wall motion abnormalities in the interventricular septum in the latter. Dobutamine SE has 80% sensitivity and 86% specificity in detecting CAD compared with invasive coronary angiography. Regardless of whether exercise or pharmacologic agents are used as a stressor, SE is cost-effective, widely available, and avoids radiation exposure when compared to CT coronary angiography or nuclear medicine techniques such as radionuclide single photon emission computed tomography (SPECT) or cardiac PET. SE is contraindicated in patients with active cardiac chest pain, unstable cardiac arrhythmias, uncontrolled hypertension, decompensated heart failure, mobile LV thrombus, aortic dissection, or symptomatic aortic aneurysm.[10] The main limitation is poor echo windows, which can occur in 10–20% of patients, depending on the population being studied. Echo contrast can be used to provide high-quality diagnostic studies in such circumstances, albeit at an increased financial cost. Exercise or pharmacologic stress myocardial perfusion imaging has been recommended by the American Heart Association for the evaluation of CAD in patients with diabetes. Nearly 25–50% of asymptomatic adult patients with diabetes will have an abnormal stress echocardiogram study, suggesting underlying CAD. A substantial proportion of these patients will present with major adverse cardiac events within 3–5 years.[11] Patients who have an abnormal SE test have a worse prognosis, even when significant CAD is absent, likely due to the development of microvascular disease or endothelial dysfunction. In a study of 563 patients with type II diabetes who underwent SE and were followed for a median of 3 years, event rates were higher in patients with an abnormal stress test but no disease on invasive coronary angiography as compared with those with a normal SE test. The highest event rate (death or nonfatal myocardial infarction) was seen in those patients with evidence of multivessel disease on SE.[10]

Assessment of Diastolic Dysfunction by Echocardiography

Diastolic dysfunction refers to abnormal relaxation of the myocardium. Patients with diastolic dysfunction on echocardiography have an increased risk of all-cause mortality, heart failure, and myocardial infarction. Diastolic dysfunction is common in both impaired glucose tolerance and overt DM type II. The overall prevalence of diastolic dysfunction is estimated to be 50% in patients with DM type II alone and increases to 70% when CAD is present. Isolated diastolic dysfunction accounts for 50% of all admissions for acute decompensated heart failure (heart failure with preserved ejection fraction).[12] The diastolic dysfunction in diabetes can occur in the absence of CAD, valvular pathology, and hypertension. It can also happen in conjunction with CAD.[13] Diastolic dysfunction is generally quantified by a combination of echocardiography techniques, including pulse wave Doppler, tissue Doppler imaging, and 2D measurements of left atrial volumes (Figs 4A to C).[14] While no single technique by itself is used for the diagnosis of diastolic dysfunction, taken together they are well validated, sensitive, reproducible, user-friendly, and readily available. Although a detailed description of diastolic function is beyond the scope of this chapter, the most commonly accepted parameters are mitral E/A ratio, E/E′ ratio (which provides an estimate of LV end diastolic pressure), pulse wave Doppler evaluation of pulmonary venous inflow, and left atrial volume index.[15]

Assessment of Diabetic Cardiomyopathy by Echocardiography

The term diabetic cardiomyopathy was coined by Ruber et al in 1972 to describe a condition in patients with DM that includes LV diastolic dysfunction and/or reduced LVEF, pathological left ventricular hypertrophy (LVH), and interstitial fibrosis. These changes can develop regardless of the presence or absence of CAD, valvular heart disease, or hypertension. This LV remodeling presents most commonly as either a dilated LV with LV systolic dysfunction or as a normal-sized LV with normal systolic function but with concentric hypertrophy and diastolic dysfunction. Diabetic cardiomyopathy develops in 12% of adult patients with DM type II and increases in prevalence to 22% in those over 64 years of age. Echocardiography is the frontline test to diagnose diabetic cardiomyopathy. In addition, noninvasive testing (exercise treadmill test, SE, SPECT, CT coronary angiography) or invasive coronary angiography is frequently done to rule out concomitant CAD. In patients with suspected diabetic cardiomyopathy, conventional 2D

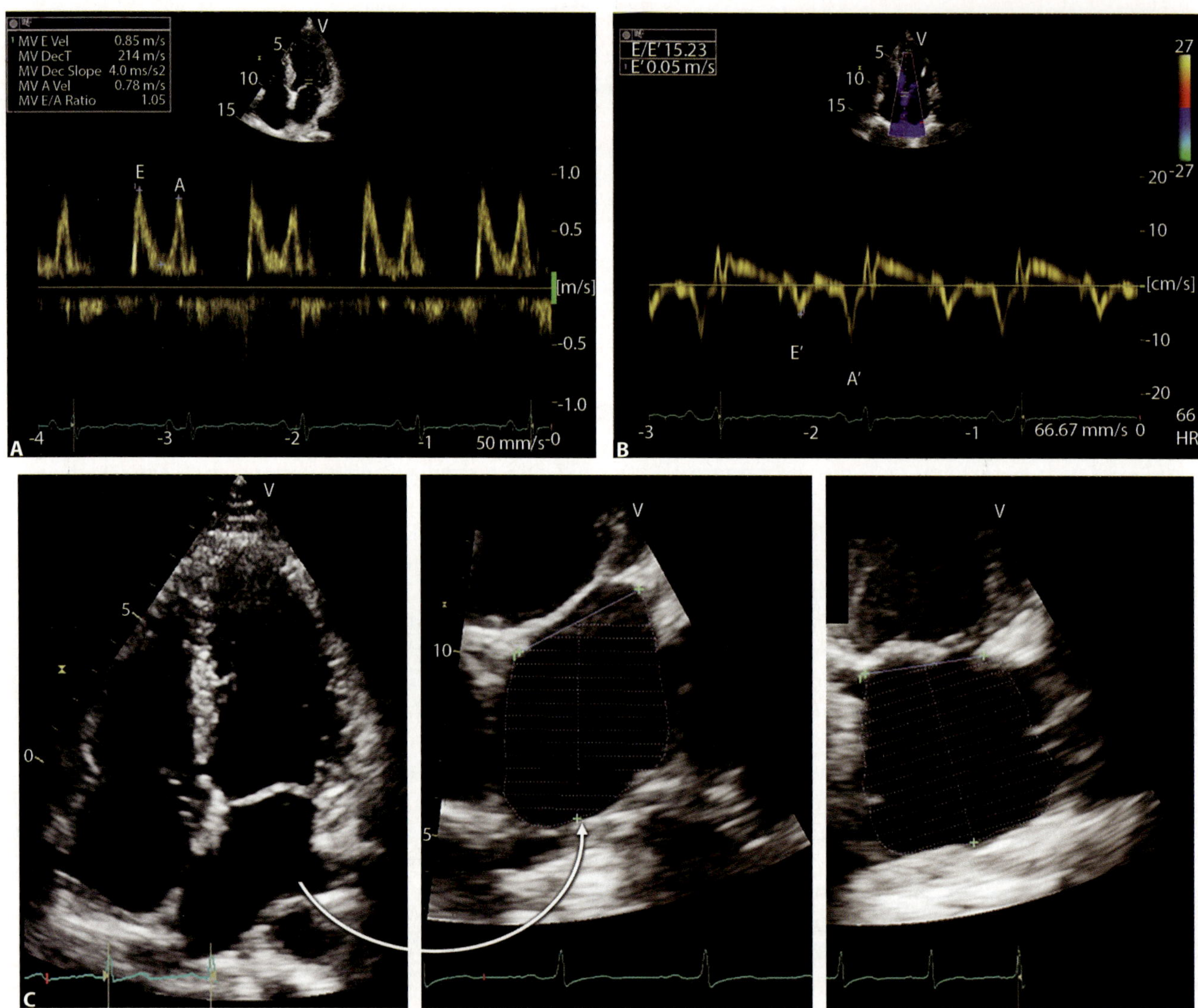

Figs 4A to C: Diastolic assessment. Diastolic dysfunction in a diabetic patient. (A) Pulse wave Doppler of mitral inflow at the level of the mitral leaflet tips. Mitral E/A ratio is 1, consistent with a stage 1 diastolic dysfunction. (B) Tissue Doppler imaging of the septal mitral annulus. The E' velocity from this view is combined with the mitral E-wave velocity across the mitral valve to calculate the E/E' ratio, which estimates left atrial pressure. E/E' ratio was 15.2; greater than 15 is consistent with elevated left atrial pressure. (C) In the absence of mitral valve disease, left atrial volume index is a good assessment of chronic left ventricular diastolic dysfunction, as it reflects the effects of elevated left ventricular-filling pressures over time. The left panel shows an apical 4-chamber view, which was zoomed to measure the left atrial area and length (middle panel). Similar measurements were made from the apical 2-chamber view (right panel). Left atrial volume index was 40 mL/m^2 (normal < 34 mL/m^2), suggestive of diastolic dysfunction. Together, these indices suggest an increased risk of adverse cardiac outcomes, including all-cause mortality, heart failure, atrial fibrillation, and stroke.

echocardiographic techniques provide information on left ventricular size and systolic function, presence and severity of LVH, regional wall motion abnormalities (that may indicted CAD), and valvular pathology. Echocardiographic Doppler techniques provide information on diastolic dysfunction and estimates LV-filling pressures. Strain analysis can diagnose subclinical LV-dysfunction when LVEF is grossly normal, and can diagnose underlying CAD when regional impairment of longitudinal strain or post-systolic shortening is present.[16]

Assessment of Right Ventricular Function

Diabetes induces subclinical impairment in right ventricular (RV) systolic and diastolic function. The basal and apical segments of the RV free wall are most commonly affected which is manifested as reduced strain in the RV free wall.[17] Diabetes increases the occurrence of RV dysfunction post-myocardial infarction by three-fold and is an independent predictor of mortality.[18]

AORTIC VALVE DISEASE IN DIABETES

Echocardiography is the primary modality used to quantify severity of disease in patients with valvular aortic stenosis. Patients with diabetes have a higher incidence of degenerative calcific aortic stenosis compared with age and gender-matched patients without diabetes. In a study that compared patients with AS with and without DM over time, there was greater decline in aortic valve area in the diabetes group compared with the nondiabetes group (0.25 cm^2/year vs 0.14 cm^2/year, $p = 0.0016$).[19] In addition to its relationship with aortic valve calcification, diabetes also exacerbates LVH produced by pressure overload of a stenotic aortic valve. Increased LV mass, concentric LVH, LV dilatation, and reduced systolic strain are seen more often in aortic stenosis and diabetes compared to patients with aortic stenosis but no diabetes.[20]

OTHER INDICATIONS FOR ECHOCARDIOGRAPHY IN DIABETES MELLITUS

Echocardiography can be a useful tool in the research setting to assess the effectiveness of antidiabetic medications on the heart (e.g. empagliflozin, liraglutide, and other medicines with beneficial effects on cardiovascular outcomes). Metformin has been shown to have a positive effect on cardiac remodeling.[21]

CONCLUSION

Diabetes is predicted to be the seventh leading cause of death by 2030. Diagnosis of cardiac involvement at a preclinical state can help to optimize medical therapy, and recognition of clinical disease can be the basis for further medical, percutaneous, or surgical therapy. Echocardiography is widely available and cost-effective, and has an important role to play in patients with diabetes. Newly developed echocardiographic techniques such as 3D echo and strain imaging should be encouraged and incorporated into routine clinical practice wherever available.

REFERENCES

1. Burkule N, Bansal M, Mehrotra R, et al. Indian academy of echocardiography performance standards and recommendations for a comprehensive transthoracic echocardiographic study in adults. J Indian Acad Echocardiogr Cardiovasc Imaging. 2017;1(1):1-17.
2. Votavová R, Linhartová A, Kořínek J, et al. Echocardiography in coronary artery disease. Cor Vasa. 2015;57(6):e408-e418.
3. Marwick TH. Diabetic heart disease. Heart. 2006;92(3):296-300.
4. Collier P, Phelan D, Klein A. A test in context: myocardial strain measured by Speckle-tracking echocardiography. J Am Coll Cardiol. 2017;69(8):1043-56.
5. Bansal M, Kasliwal RR. How do I do it? Speckle-tracking echocardiography. Indian Heart J. 2013;65(1):117-23.
6. Fang ZY, Schull-Meade R, Leano R, et al. Screening for heart disease in diabetic subjects. Am Heart J. 2005;149(2):349-54.
7. Ernande L, Bergerot C, Girerd N, et al. Longitudinal myocardial strain alteration is associated with left ventricular remodeling in asymptomatic patients with type 2 diabetes mellitus. J Am Soc Echocardiogr. 2014;27(5):479-88.
8. Holland DJ, Marwick TH, Haluska BA, et al. Subclinical LV dysfunction and 10-year outcomes in type 2 diabetes mellitus. Heart. 2015;101(13):1061-6.
9. Marwick TH. Stress echocardiography. Heart. 2003;89(1):113-8.
10. Senior R, Monaghan M, Becher H, et al. Stress echocardiography for the diagnosis and risk stratification of patients with suspected or known coronary artery disease: a critical appraisal. Supported by the British Society of Echocardiography. Heart. 2005;91(4):427-36.
11. Cortigiani L, Picano E. Stress echocardiography in diabetes. In: Picano E (Ed). Stress Echocardiography. Cham: Springer International Publishing; 2015. pp. 521-9.
12. von Bibra H, St John Sutton M. Diastolic dysfunction in diabetes and the metabolic syndrome: promising potential for diagnosis and prognosis. Diabetologia. 2010;53(6):1033-45.
13. Rubler S, Dlugash J, Yuceoglu YZ, et al. New type of cardiomyopathy associated with diabetic glomerulosclerosis. Am J Cardiol. 1972;30(6):595-602.
14. Bess RL, Khan S, Rosman HS, et al. Technical aspects of diastology: why mitral inflow and tissue Doppler imaging are the preferred parameters? Echocardiography. 2006;23(4):332-9.
15. Yu CM, Sanderson JE, Marwick TH, et al. Tissue Doppler imaging a new prognosticator for cardiovascular diseases. J Am Coll Cardiol. 2007;49(19):1903-14.
16. Lorenzo-Almorós A, Tuñón J, Orejas M, et al. Diagnostic approaches for diabetic cardiomyopathy. Cardiovasc Diabetol. 2017;16(1):28.
17. Kosmala W, Przewlocka-Kosmala M, Mazurek W. Subclinical right ventricular dysfunction in diabetes mellitus—an ultrasonic strain/strain rate study. Diabet Med. 2007;24(6):656-63.
18. Roifman I, Ghugre N, Zia MI, et al. Diabetes is an independent predictor of right ventricular dysfunction post-ST-elevation myocardial infarction. Cardiovasc Diabetol. 2016;15(1):34.
19. Kamalesh M, Ng C, El Masry H, et al. Does diabetes accelerate progression of calcific aortic stenosis? Eur J Echocardiogr. 2009;10(6):723-5.

20. Lindman BR, Arnold SV, Madrazo JA, et al. The adverse impact of diabetes mellitus on left ventricular remodeling and function in patients with severe aortic stenosis. Circ Heart Fail. 2011;4(3):286-92.
21. Andersson C, Sogaard P, Hoffmann S, et al. Metformin is associated with improved left ventricular diastolic function measured by tissue Doppler imaging in patients with diabetes. Eur J Endocrinol. 2010;163(4):593-9.
22. Huntsman LL, Stewart DK, Barnes SR, et al. Noninvasive Doppler determination of cardiac output in man. Clinical validation. Circulation. 1983;67(3):593-602.
23. Tei C, Ling LH, Hodge DO, et al. New index of combined systolic and diastolic myocardial performance: a simple and reproducible measure of cardiac function—a study in normals and dilated cardiomyopathy. J Cardiol. 1995;26(6):357-66.
24. Chen C, Rodriguez L, Lethor JP, et al. Continuous wave Doppler echocardiography for noninvasive assessment of left ventricular dP/dt and relaxation time constant from mitral regurgitant spectra in patients. J Am Coll Cardiol. 1994;23(4):970-6.

CHAPTER

Echo/Doppler Assessment of Increased Left-sided Filling Pressures and Diastolic Heart Failure in Patients with Normal Systolic Function in Cardiodiabetes

Omar Tageldin, Ahmed Abdelhaleem, Mohammed J Arisha, Ayman Battisha, Swetha Srialluri, Adel A Farhoud, Mohamed S Mahmoud, Hassan Kamel, HK Chopra, Navin C Nanda

INTRODUCTION

Two-dimensional transthoracic echocardiography (2DTTE) has been used to assess increased left-sided filling pressures and left ventricular (LV) diastolic heart failure in patients with normal or near-normal systolic function.[1] Guidelines have also been published and updated recently. In this chapter, we summarize the recent guidelines which have been recommended for assessment of LV diastolic function together with several caveats and pitfalls inherent in its evaluation.[2] In a patient with normal (LV ejection fraction ≥ 55%) or near-normal (LVEF 45–54%) systolic ventricular function by 2DTTE, the presence of clinical signs of heart failure indicates that the heart failure is on the basis of diastolic dysfunction. In our opinion, this is the best way to diagnose this entity. In cases where it is difficult to assess the presence of heart failure clinically, 2DTTE takes on importance as a useful modality to assess increased left-sided filling pressures. In day-to-day clinical practice, the main cause of increased left-sided filling pressures is systemic hypertension. A dilated inferior or superior vena cava especially with minimal or no collapse on 2DTTE suggests increased right atrial pressure and therefore most likely right-sided heart failure if other causes of a dilated vena cava can be excluded.[3] A common cause of right-sided heart failure is left-sided heart failure and, therefore, a dilated vena cava may be a helpful finding in assessing this entity.[4]

The echo or Doppler parameters used to assess left-sided filling pressures in patients with normal or near-normal LV ejection fraction as well as caveats and pitfalls in using them are summarized in Boxes 1 and 2 (Figs 1 to 6). These are reported to be more reliable in patients with cardiac disease and hence should be applicable in those with diabetes mellitus which is a known important risk factor for atherosclerotic heart disease. The reliability of these findings further increases when other clinical and echocardiographic findings suggest high left-sided filling pressures.

Although most patients with a ratio of early mitral diastolic inflow velocity wave (E) to late diastolic mitral inflow wave (A) of less than or equal to 0.8 (so called grade I diastolic dysfunction) have delayed relaxation but normal left atrial filling pressure and normal LV end-diastolic pressure (LVEDP), a subset may have high LVEDP (>16 mm Hg) and therefore left-sided heart failure without elevated left atrial filling pressure (≤12 mm Hg). These can be identified if the pulmonary vein reversal velocity duration (Ar) is greater than mitral A wave duration (high sensitivity and specificity) or increased mitral M-mode A-C duration which presents with a localized bulge on the A-C slope often called the B-point or B-bump. The presence of B-point has a high specificity but much lower sensitivity in assessing increased LVEDP. A B-bump can also occur with first degree A:V block and one needs to be aware of this pitfall before making a diagnosis of increased LVEDP (Fig. 7).

CONCLUSION

Echo or Doppler techniques represent valuable noninvasive modalities in the armamentarium of physicians and cardiologists for assessment and confirmation of high left-sided filling pressures or diastolic heart failure in patients with normal systolic LV function especially in cardio-diabetes.

BOX 1: Echo or Doppler assessment of left-sided filling pressures in patients with cardiac disease and normal left ventricular systolic function

A. Four important parameters to be considered
   1. Maximum (max) early diastolic mitral annulus velocity (E′) septal (<7 cm/s) or lateral (< 10 cm/s)
   2. Early diastolic mitral inflow velocity (E)/early diastolic mitral annulus velocity (E′). Average of both mitral annuli > 14, only lateral annulus >13, only medial annulus > 15.
   3. Maximum tricuspid regurgitation velocity (>2.8 m/s)
   4. Left atrial volume index by biplane method of disks, modified Simpson's rule (>34 mL/m^2)

   The presence of at least three of above parameters indicates high left-sided filling pressures.

B. Mitral E/late diastolic velocity (A) ratio ≥ 2 also indicates high left-sided filling pressures after taking into account clinical findings (e.g. shortness of breath and pulmonary rales) and other echo data (e.g. mitral valve E wave deceleration time < 150 ms, maximum pulmonary vein systolic velocity/maximum diastolic pulmonary vein velocity < 1, pulmonary vein atrial reversal velocity, Ar, minus mitral A velocity duration > 30 ms).

C. Mitral E/A ratio ≤ 0.8 but E > 50 cm/s or E/A ratio between 0.8 and 2, plus presence of two of last three parameters in (A) also indicate increased left-sided filling pressures.

D. Mitral E/A ratio ≤ 0.8 and E ≤ 50 cm/s indicate normal left-sided filling pressures.

BOX 2: Pitfalls in evaluating increased left-sided filling pressures by echo or Doppler

1. Use apical four-chamber view. Place pulsed wave Doppler sample volume (5–10 mm) at or 1 cm below the mitral annulus on either side.[1]
2. Do not use poor quality echo or incomplete Doppler waveforms to avoid false results.
3. Mitral E, E′, and E/E′ unreliable in patients with (a) significant mitral annular calcification (MAC, subjectively assessed) and moderate or severe mitral regurgitation. Both increase mitral E. E′ decreases with MAC, (b) mitral valve prosthesis and rings, CAD with WMA in basal segments and constrictive pericarditis (lateral E′ may be lower), (c) atrial fibrillation, atrial flutter, HCM, arrhythmias, tachycardia (E and A may fuse), and first degree A:V block, and (d) perioperative settings and children.
4. LA volume index may be unreliable in bradycardia, heart transplant patients (with biatrial technique), atrial fibrillation, atrial flutter, significant MV disease, and athletes (LA can be dilated). LA volume may be reduced if LA foreshortened.
5. Parameters are more reliable if the patient has clinical heart disease and other clinical or echocardiographic findings (see under B in Box 1).

Abbreviations: A:V, atrio-ventricular; CAD, coronary artery disease; HCM, hypertrophic cardiomyopathy; LA, left atrium; WMA, wall motion abnormality

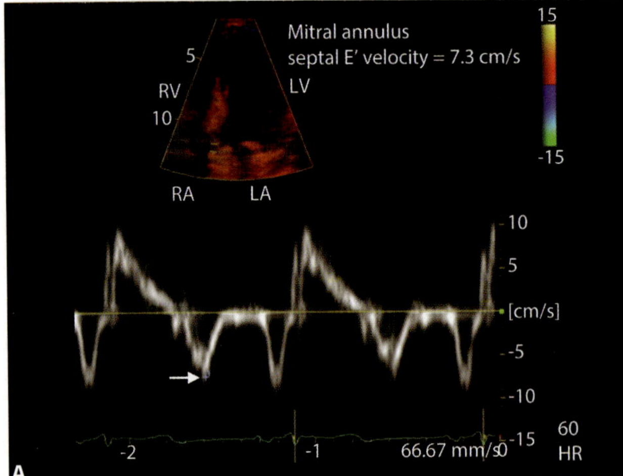

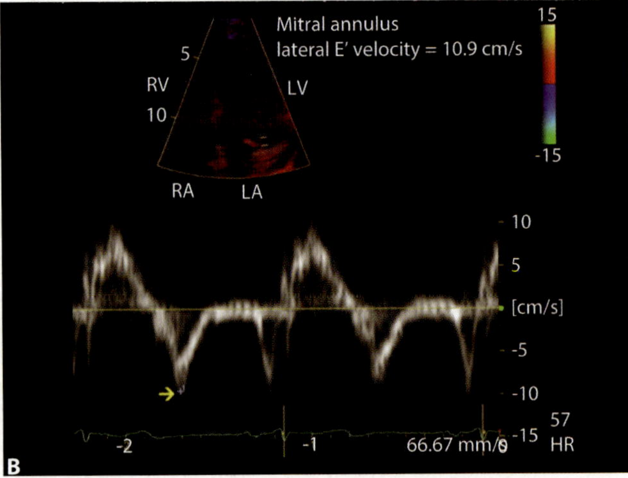

Figs 1A and B: Tissue Doppler imaging in a 60-year-old male with end-stage renal disease. Both maximum (A) septal and (B) lateral mitral annulus velocities are normal measuring 7.3 cm/s and 10.9 cm/s (arrow), respectively. Lower velocities may represent increased left-sided filling pressures when associated with other echo or Doppler parameters

Abbreviations: LA, left atrium; LV, left ventricle; RA, right atrium; RV, right ventricle

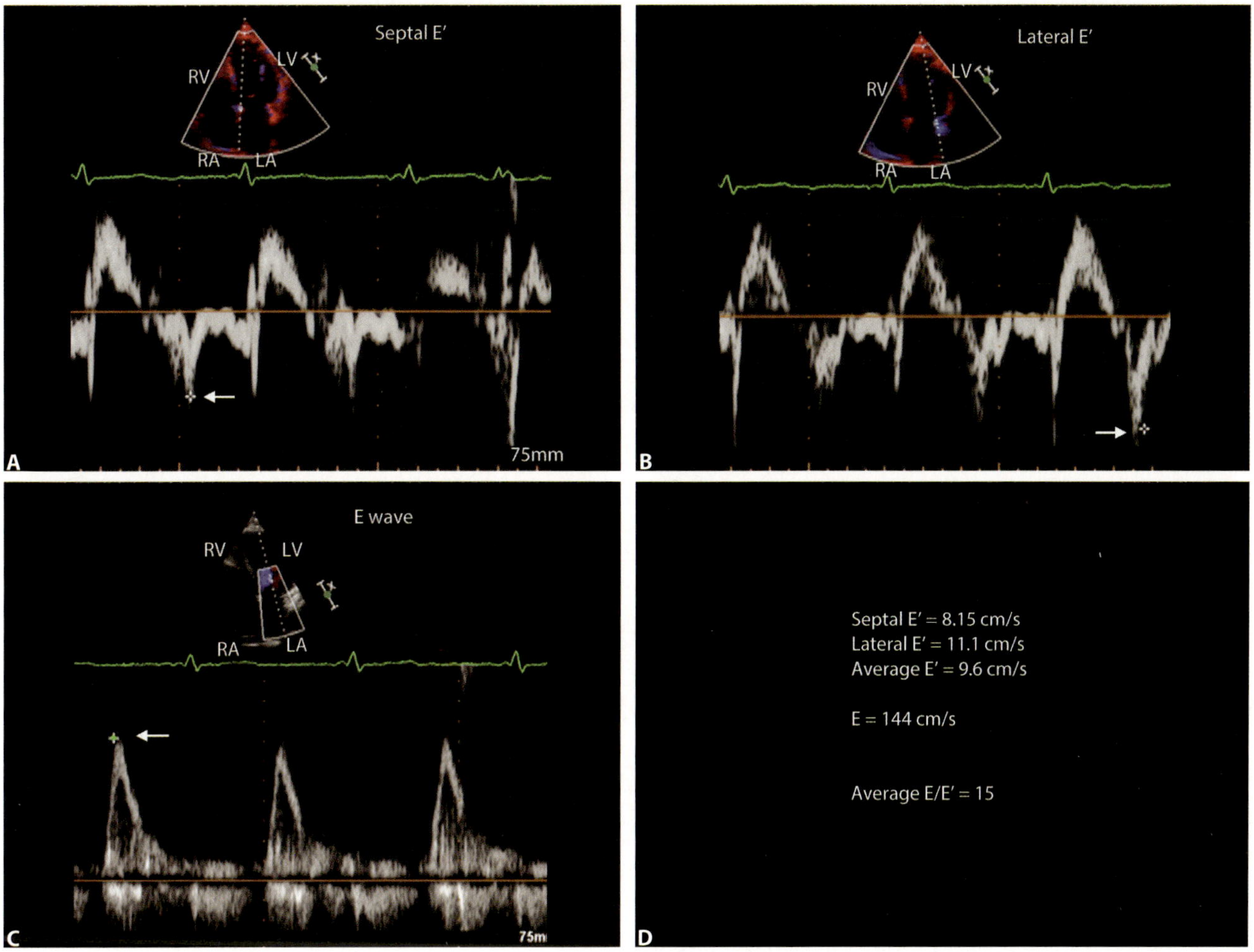

Septal E′ = 8.15 cm/s
Lateral E′ = 11.1 cm/s
Average E′ = 9.6 cm/s

E = 144 cm/s

Average E/E′ = 15

Figs 2A to D: Mitral inflow and annulus velocities in a 42-year-old male status post-heart transplant. Arrows point to (A) maximal septal and (B) maximal lateral mitral annulus velocities by tissue Doppler imaging and (C) maximal mitral inflow E velocity by pulsed Doppler. (D) The average mitral E/E′ ratio is high at 15 suggesting increased left-sided filling pressure

Abbreviations: LA, left atrium; LV, left ventricle; RA, right atrium; RV, right ventricle

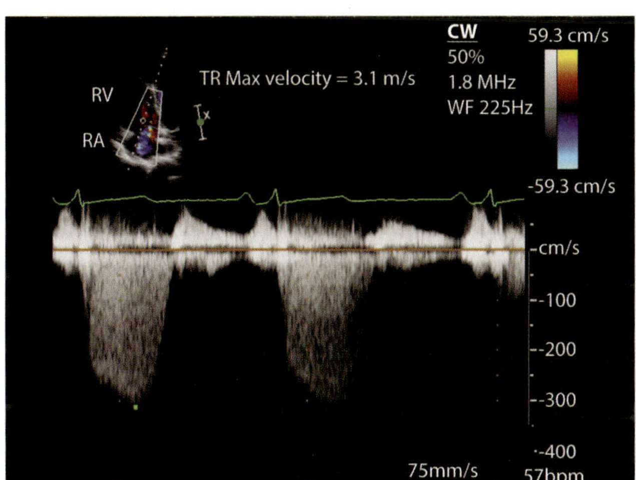

Fig. 3: Tricuspid regurgitation velocity in a 57-year-old female with a murmur. Arrow points to maximal velocity of 3.1 m/s obtained by continuous wave Doppler. A velocity of more than 2.8 m/s is one of the Doppler parameters used in the evaluation of increased left-sided filling pressures

Abbreviations: RA, right atrium; RV, right ventricle

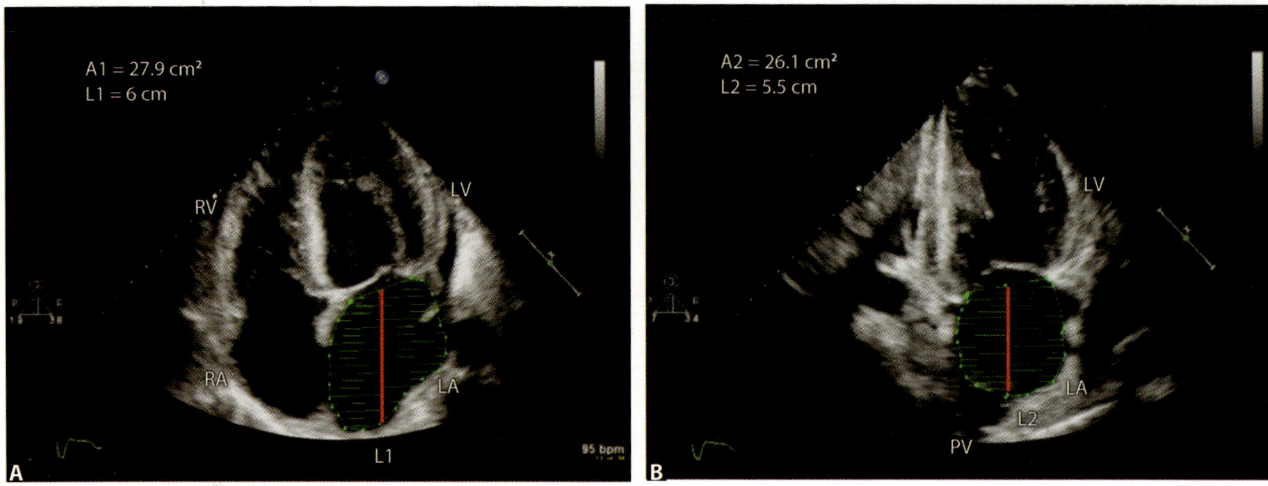

Figs 4A and B: Left atrial volume measurement in a 36-year-old male with chronic kidney disease. Left atrial (LA) areas in (A) apical four-chamber (A1) and (B) apical two-chamber (A2) views are planimetered one to two frames before mitral valve opening excluding LA appendage and pulmonary veins (PV). The shorter of the two vertical lengths (L1 and L2) is taken for LA volume calculation using the biplane area–length method as follows: $8/3\pi \times (A1 \times A2/L2) = 112.5$ mL, 51.2 mL/m^2 indexed to body surface area (BSA) of 2.2 m^2 (normal LA volume $\leq$ 34 mL/m^2)

Abbreviations: LA, left atrium; LV, left ventricle; RA, right atrium; RV, right ventricle

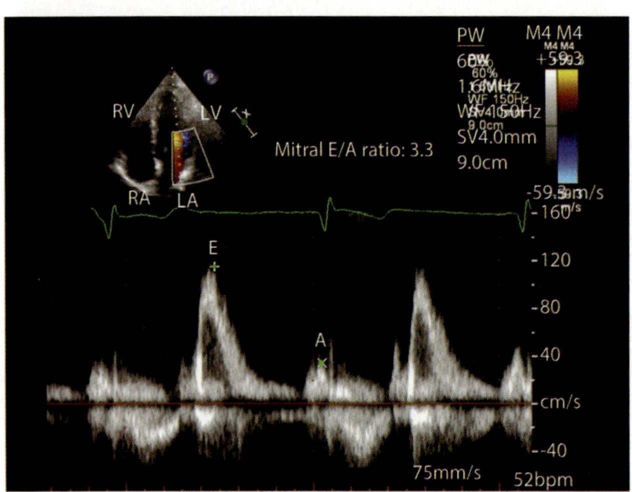

Fig. 5: Mitral E/A ratio in a 26-year-old male suspected of having aortic root dilatation. The ratio in this patient is high at 3.3 (normal < 2) and this has been noted in patients with high left-sided filling pressure. Left ventricular systolic function was normal and the aortic root and aorta were normal in size. Clinically, he has no symptoms or signs of heart failure

Abbreviations: LA, left atrium; LV, left ventricle; RA, right atrium; RV, right ventricle

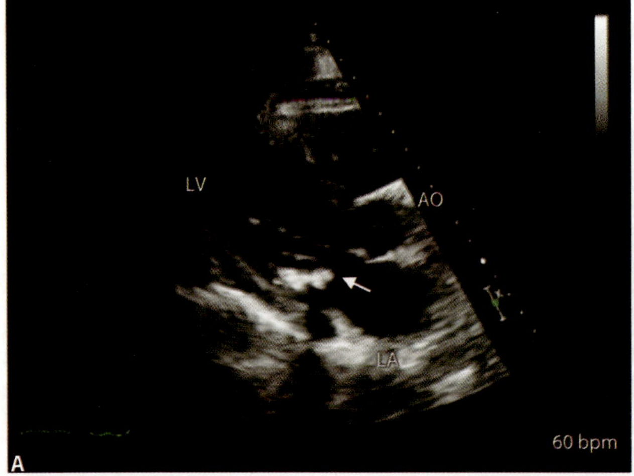

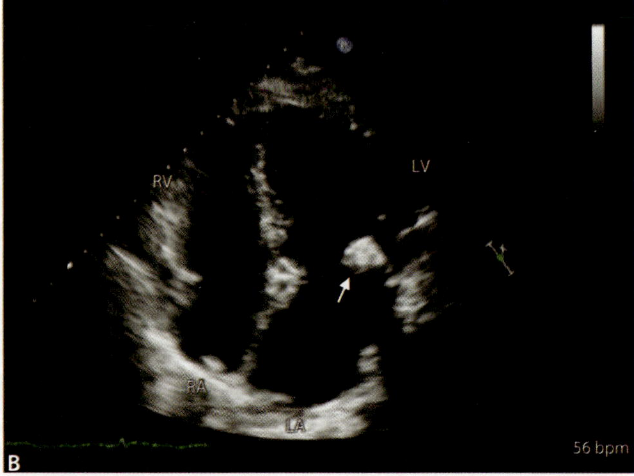

Figs 6A and B

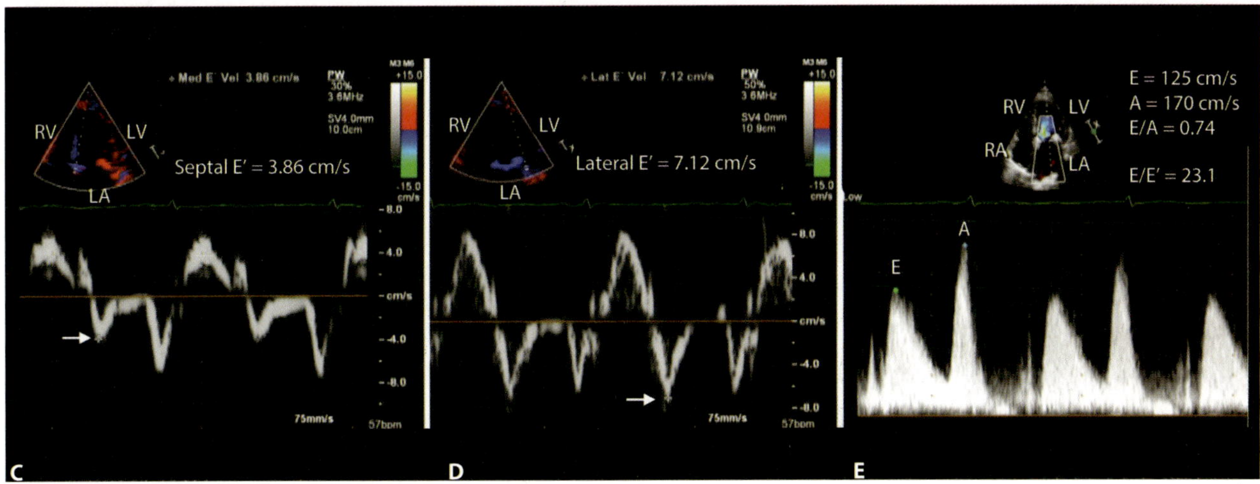

Figs 6C to E

Figs 6A to E: Limitation of using mitral E/E ratio to diagnose high left-sided filling pressures. This 66-year-old elderly female has significant mitral annular calcification visualized in (A) parasternal long axis (arrow) and (B) apical four chamber (arrow) views. This may result in low (C) septal (3.86 cm/s) and (D) lateral (7.12 cm/s) mitral annular velocities and a (E) high mitral E velocity (125 cm/s) as well as a high mitral E/E ratio (23.1) mimicking high left-sided filling pressures. Average of septal and lateral annulus velocities was used, and normal value of mitral E/E ratio is less than or equal to 14

Abbreviations: AO, aorta; LA, left atrium; LV, left ventricle; RA, right atrium; RV, right ventricle

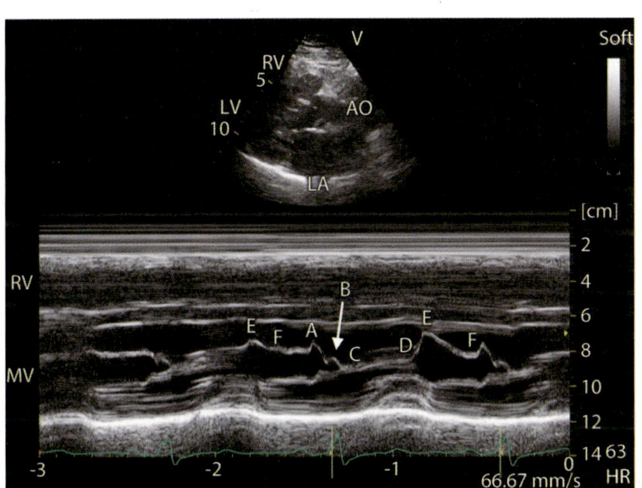

Fig. 7: M-mode of the mitral valve in an adult patient with the first degree A:V block. Note the prominent B–point or bump

Abbreviations: A, atrial wave; C, closure point; D, opening point; E, maximum early opening; F, early diastolic slope; LA, left atrium; LV, left ventricle; RA, right atrium; RV, right ventricle

REFERENCES

1. Nagueh SF, Appleton CP, Gillebert TC, et al. Recommendations for the evaluation of left ventricular diastolic function by echocardiography. Eur J Echocardiogr. 2009;10(2): 165-93.
2. Nagueh SF, Smiseth OA, Appleton CP, et al. Recommendations for the evaluation of left ventricular diastolic function by echocardiography: An update from the American Society of Echocardiography and the European Association of Cardiovascular Imaging. Eur Heart J Cardiovasc Imaging. 2016;17(12): 1321-60.
3. Rudski LG, Lai WW, Afilalo J, et al. Guidelines for the echocardiographic assessment of the right heart in adults: a report from the American Society of Echocardiography endorsed by the European Association of Echocardiography, a registered branch of the European Society of Cardiology, and the Canadian Society of Echocardiography. J Am Soc Echocardiogr. 2010;23(7): 685-713.
4. Voelkel NF, Quaife RA, Leinwand LA, et al. Right ventricular function and failure: report of a National Heart, Lung, and Blood Institute working group on cellular and molecular mechanisms of right heart failure. Circulation. 2006;114(17): 1883-91.

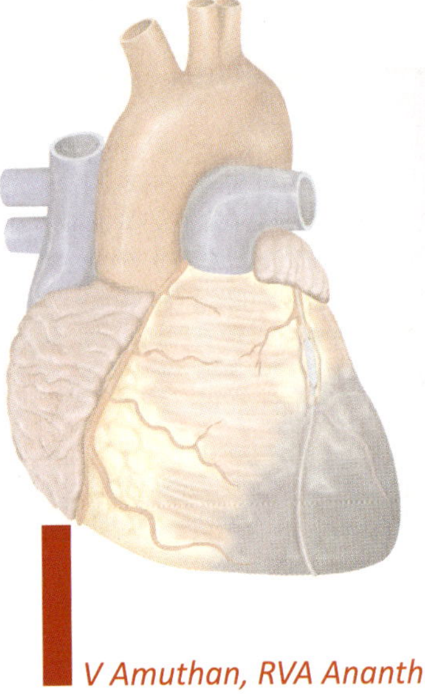

3D Echo and Cardiodiabetes

V Amuthan, RVA Ananth

INTRODUCTION

Cardiac problems develop in concert with development of Diabetes.[1] The 2011 estimate of 360 million people with diabetes globally is estimated to increase to 552 million by 2030.[2] This epidemic proportion of diabetes in the context of the fact that India is the diabetic capital of the world has necessitated the early diagnosis of cardiac problems in diabetes. Although the conventional two-dimensional (2D) echocardiography and Doppler studies remain the sheet anchor of diagnosis, early diagnosis is missed by these technologies. Three-dimensional echocardiography and the use of speckle tracking echocardiographic analysis of longitudinal, circumferential, radial strain and left ventricular (LV) torsional deformation analysis score over the earlier techniques (Fig. 1).[3,4]

DIABETIC CARDIOMYOPATHY

The observation of frequent association of heart failure and diabetes was made by Leyden et al. in 1881.[5] However, it was Rubler in 1972, who introduced the term diabetic cardiomyopathy.[6] The minimal criteria to diagnose diabetic cardiomyopathy include

- Concentric LV hypertrophy with left ventricular diastolic dysfunction (LVDD) and interstitial fibrosis
- Eccentric dilated cardiomyopathy (DCM) with reduced LV systolic function independent of coronary artery disease, systemic hypertension or valvular heart disease.[7]

THREE-DIMENSIONAL ECHOCARDIOGRAPHY

The advantages of 3D/4D echocardiography in the evaluation of diabetic patients include—(1) the evaluation of cardiac chamber volumes and mass, which avoids geometric assumptions. (2) The assessment of regional LV wall motion and quantification of systolic dyssynchrony. (3) Presentation of realistic views of heart valves. (4) Volumetric evaluation of regurgitant lesions and with 3D echocardiographic color Doppler imaging and (5) 3D echocardiographic stress imaging.[8]

DIASTOLIC FUNCTION IN DIABETIC CARDIOMYOPATHY

Abnormal E/A and Deceleration Time

Abnormal relaxation characterized by decreased E/A ratio and prolonged deceleration time and restrictive pattern with increased E/A ratio and decreased deceleration time are well described in early studies (Fig. 2).[8]

Abnormal E/e' Ratio

The ratio of early diastolic flow velocity of mitral inflow (E) to early diastolic mitral annular velocity (E/e') has been shown to be the most accurate noninvasive marker of elevated LV filling pressure.[9,10] In particular, echocardiographic indices of elevated LV filling pressure are clearly associated with

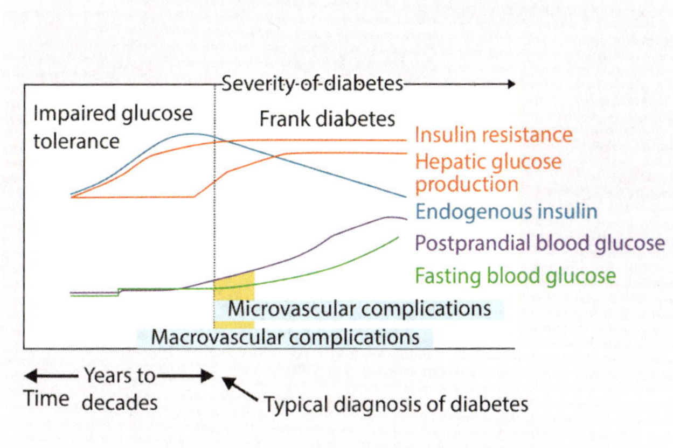

	Early	*Middle*	*Late*	*Advantages/disadvantages*
Conventional 2D echo and Doppler		Diastolic dysfunction 1.↑ E/A 2.↑ LV mass 3.↓ Cavity size 4.↑ Deceleration time	Systolic dysfunction ↓ LV ejection fraction	Universally available Interobserver variability
Tissue Doppler imaging		E/e' > 14	Abnormal strain	Quantification of myocardial velocities Angle dependent
3D echo and strain by speckle tracking	Abnormal longitudinal and circumferential strain	Diastolic strain abnormalities	Systolic strain abnormalities GLS < −14	Technique is available in only high-end machines and requires expertise
3D echo and myocardial mechanics by LV torsion	Higher peak and time to peak twist and untwist angle	Attenuated and delayed LV twist and untwist angle		Technique is available in only high-end machines and requires expertise

Fig. 1: Evaluation of Cardiodiabetes by echocardiography in relation to severity

Abbreviations: GLS, global longitudinal strain; LV, left ventricular

poor cardiac functional and clinical outcome. E/e' more than 15 is the strongest predictor of cardiac death and readmission for heart failure (Figs 2A to D).

3D LV Mass Assessment

Calculation of LV mass by M-mode (cube formula) and 2D echocardiography (area length or truncated ellipse) is cumbersome geometrical assessment that is not applicable when there is LV distortion or foreshortening, asymmetric LV hypertrophy, DCM and in patients with regional wall motion abnormalities.[11-13] The LV mass calculation is based on converting volume to mass using multiplication of volume by myocardial density of 1.05 g/mL and is normalized for the body surface area as LV mass index. LV hypertrophy is defined as LV mass index of more than 115 g/m^2 and more than 95 g/m^2 for women.[14] 3D echocardiographic quantification of LV mass correlates better with cardiovascular magnetic resonance (CMR) measurements.[15,16] The methodology of 3D LV mass assessment is shown in Figure 3A and Box 1.

3D Evaluation of Left Atrium

Left atrial size is a powerful marker of prognosis in diabetes under a variety of clinical situations and is a strong predictor of mortality and morbidity.[17] Because, 3D volume calculation of left atrium is devoid of geometrical assumptions, it correlates better with cardiac magnetic resonance imaging (MRI).[18] Normal left atrial maximal volume and total emptying fraction have been published (Fig. 3B).[19] Regional assessment of left atrial function by speckle tracking echocardiography (STE) has also evolved to be a novel echocardiographic technique (Fig. 4).[20]

3D Echocardiographic Assessment of Systolic Dysfunction

Left Ventricular Ejection Fraction

The cornerstone of the prognostication and treatment schedule for echocardiographic evaluation of diabetic cardiomyopathy starts with evaluation of left ventricular

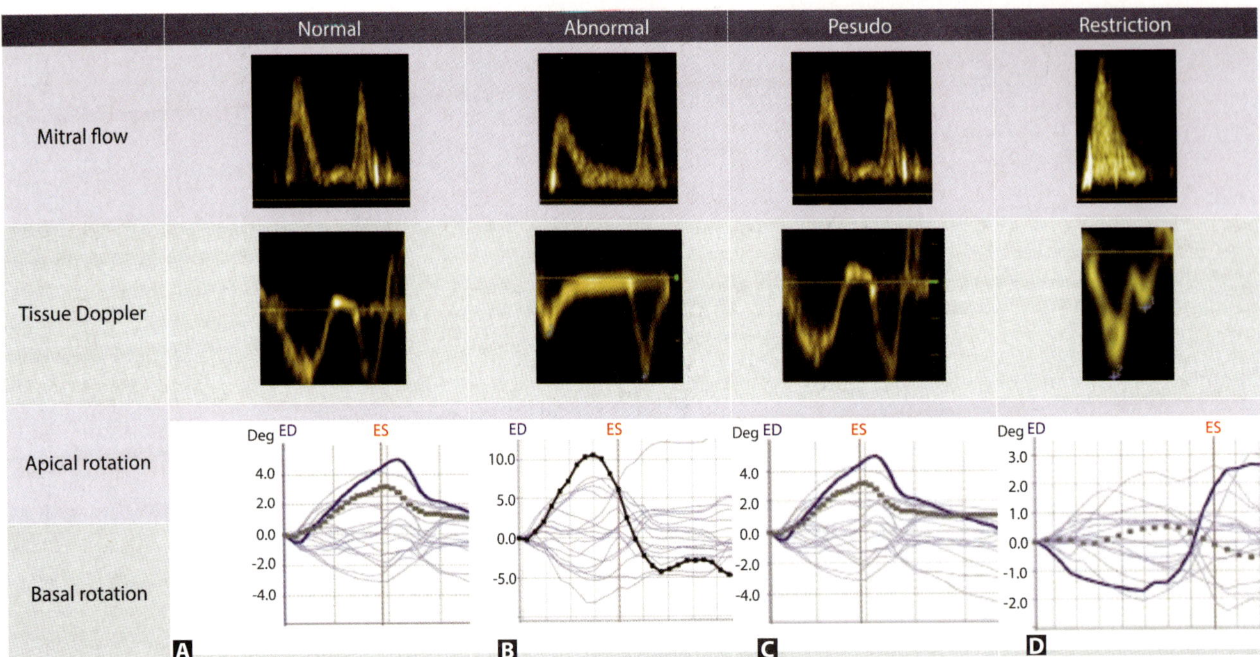

Figs 2A to D: Mitral flow spectral Doppler, tissue Doppler medial mitral annular movement, and left ventricular (LV) basal and apical rotation (negative and positive waves) during one cardiac cycle. (A) *Normal subject*—Normal values for LV rotation and net twist angle in a recent study of a large group of healthy volunteers reported a mean value of peak LV twist angle as 7.7 ± 3.5°. (B) A patient with *diabetes without LV hypertrophy*—Note less prominent initial clockwise twist, higher peak twist, delayed time to peak, and lower untwisting during early diastole in the patient with diabetes compared with the normal subject. (C) In a patient with *advanced diabetes and left ventricular hypertrophy* and normal ejection fraction—Note the relatively preserved LV twist mechanics, although LV twisting and untwisting velocities, are both attenuated and delayed. (D) In a patient with advanced *diabetic cardiomyopathy and reduced ejection fraction*

ejection fraction (LVEF). The evidence base for modern cardiology is so heavily based on this simple measurement that it is unlikely to disappear. The problems in calculating ejection fraction (EF) as the ratio between stroke volume and end-diastolic volume are geometry dependence, load dependence, the effect of high and low heart rate due to heart blocks, tachycardia (especially atrial fibrillation), and insensitivity to minor change when close to 50%.[21] 3D imaging is now available with echocardiography and its results are comparable to cardiac MRI.[22] The main attraction and advantage of 3D imaging is to avoid geometric assumptions when calculating LV volumes, and reducing errors created by cutting a 3D structure in two dimensions. The current software for 3D evaluation of LVEF is much easier and can be performed within minutes in the setting of emergency room. The sphericity index derived from 3D echocardiography [left ventricular end-diastolic volume (LVEDV) divided by the volume of a sphere whose diameter is the LV end-diastolic long axis] is an added by product and is the best predictor for LV dilatation.

STRAIN IMAGING IN DECISION MAKING IN DIABETIC CARDIOMYOPATHY

Global Longitudinal Strain

Global longitudinal strain (GLS) has evolved as one of the most robust parameter, and this has been shown to identify subclinical LV dysfunction. GLS is calculated using a variety of proprietary software (EchoPAC, GE Medical Systems, Milwaukee, Wisconsin, USA; Syngo velocity vector imaging, Siemens, Mountain View, California, USA; LV analysis, TomTec GmbH, Unterschlessheim, Germany). GLS is well validated as a marker for the measurement of LV longitudinal deformation, which has emerged as a sensitive and specific marker to detect early and subtle myocardial dysfunction. In one of the recent meta-analysis, Kalam et al., have shown the independent prognostic significance of GLS in patients with mild LV global impairment. The

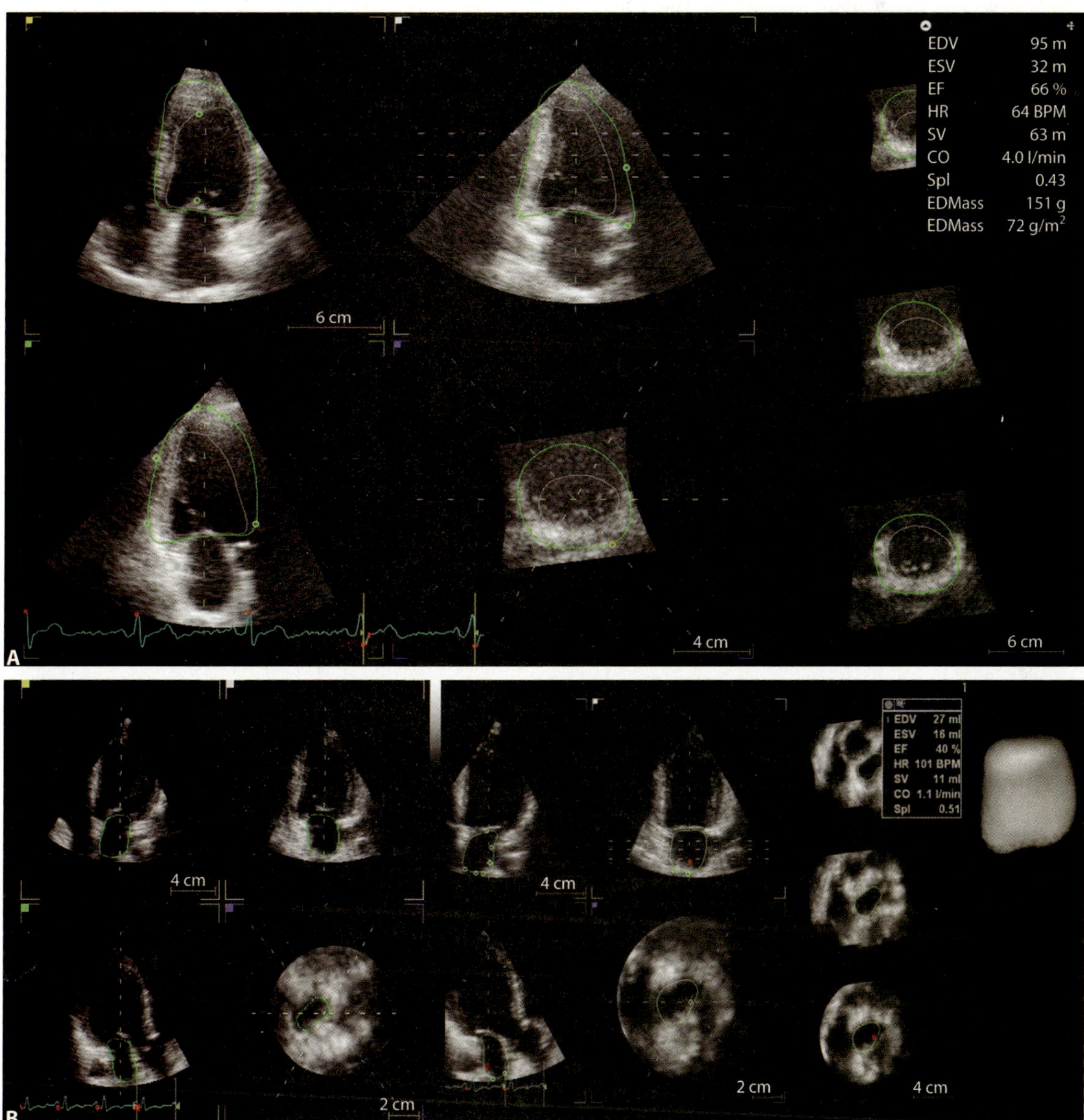

Figs 3A and B: (A) Calculation of left ventricular (LV) mass. (B) Three-dimensional calculation of maximal LA volume and total emptying fraction

BOX 1: Steps in three-dimensional (3D) speckle tracking echocardiography and estimation of myocardial deformation

1. *Step 1:* It is essential to acquire multi-gated images from the left ventricular apex with electrocardiographic (ECG) gating and at a frame rate of more than 40 frames/s in end diastole and end systole and endocardial borders are marked.
2. *Step 2:* Identification of the left ventricular myocardium—Left ventricular mass and marking of region of interest (ROI).
3. *Step 3:* 3D speckle tracking is done and the results are displayed as (A) strain curves from different segments and (B) Bull's eye plot or automated functional images for longitudinal strain, circumferential strain, area strain, and radial strain.
4. *Step 4:* In addition, left ventricular deformation imaging as viewed from the LV apex can be plotted as left ventricular twist and torsion.

prognostic value of this information seems likely to be superior to that provided by LVEF.[23]

Current Status of 3D Myocardial Strain Estimation

With developments in 3D transducer technology and improvements in hardware and software, 3D datasets with adequate temporal and spatial resolution are now possible and these 3D approaches can measure 3D strain from a multi-beat acquisition with a frame rate set above 40 frames/s. The ability to estimate true 3D myocardial motion and deformation using various 3D STE approaches

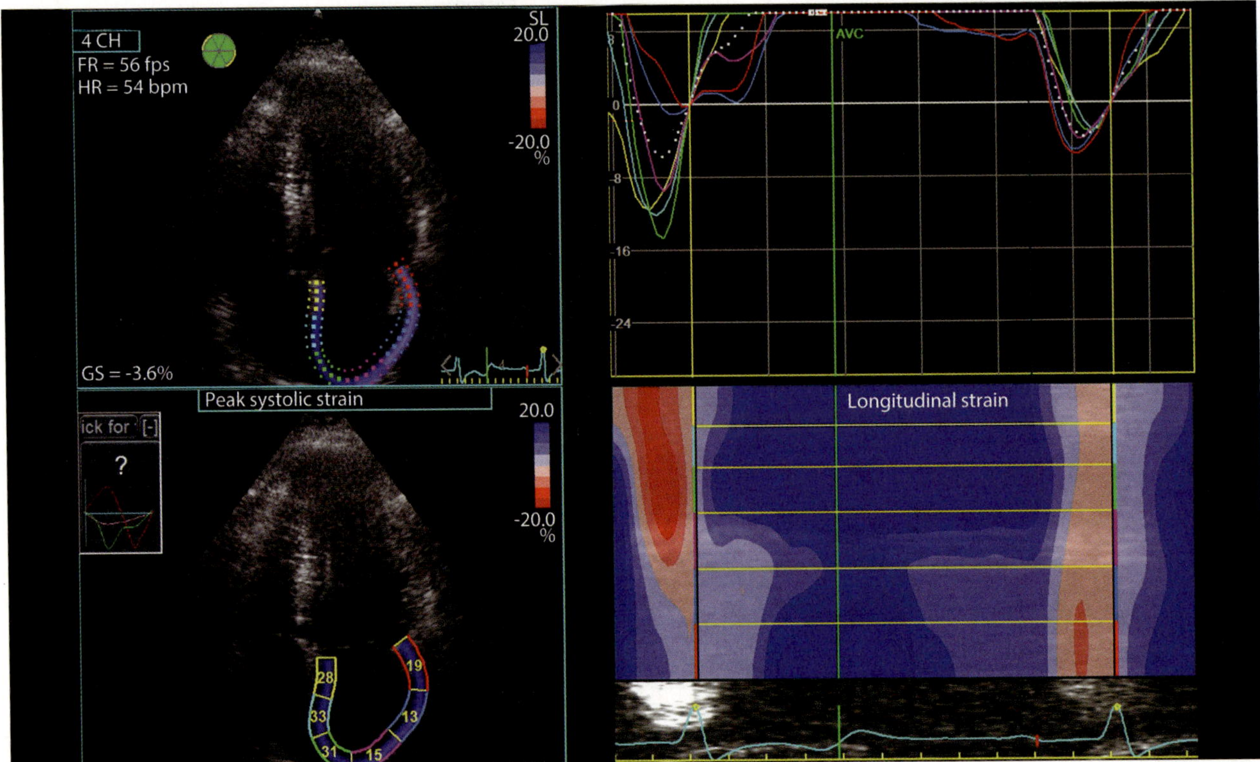

Fig. 4: Assessment of left atrial function by speckle tracking echocardiography

may provide cardiologists with a better view of regional myocardial mechanics, which may be important for diagnosis, prognosis, and therapy.

LV Torsional Deformation and 3D Speckle-tracking Echocardiography

Shortening and lengthening which are the basic functions of the myocardial fibers result in a systolic twist followed by a diastolic untwisting of the left ventricle due to helical orientation of the fibers. In systole, the LV apex undergoes a counter clockwise rotation about its longitudinal axis as viewed from the apex. Rotation of the LV base in systole is opposite in direction compared to apical rotation. This motion has been compared with that used to squeeze water out of a wet towel. The main determinant of the LV twist is the apical rotation. 3D STE has emerged as an alternative noninvasive technique to assess LV rotation. The problems with 2D STE are the lower values for apical rotation and LV twist, due to difficulties in selection of optimal imaging planes for computation, as the images are acquired separately from entirely different cardiac cycles and rotation at each level peaks at a different time in the cardiac cycle. A recent study by Muhammad Ashraf et al., to compute LV twist from 3D echocardiography concluded despite lower spatiotemporal resolution of 3D echocardiography, LV twist and torsion can be computed accurately.[23-25] LV twist is reduced in DCM due to cardiac fibrosis resulting in alteration of myocardial fiber orientation.[26] Figure 2 shows abnormally reduced twist and torsion in a normal individual, a patient with early diabetes without left ventricular hypertrophy (LVH), in a patient with severe LVH and finally in a patient with diabetic cardiomyopathy and LV dysfunction. A decreased and delayed systolic LV torsion as well as depressed, delayed, and disorganized LV untwisting have been previously reported in patients with DCM.[27] Moreover, paradoxical reversal of LV rotation, with the base rotating counter clockwise and the apex clockwise, with subsequent reduction or even loss of LV twist was observed in some patients with DCM.

CASE EXAMPLES

1. *Normal subject*: Echo evaluation from a control nondiabetic nonhypertensive 50 years individual. Note the normal E/A ratio, deceleration time, E/e' ratio, and

apical counter clockwise and basal clockwise rotation. Normal values for LV rotation and net twist angle in a recent study of a large group of healthy volunteers reported a mean value of peak LV twist angle as 7.7 ± 3.5.

2. A patient with 3 years of *diabetes without LV hypertrophy*. Note the attenuation of E wave or early filling wave, prolongation of the deceleration time and accentuation of A wave or atrial filling velocities. There is also alteration of E/e′ ratio. Note less prominent initial clockwise twist, higher peak twist, delayed time to peak, and lower untwisting during early diastole in this patient, compared with the normal subject.
3. In a patient with *advanced diabetes and left ventricular hypertrophy* and normal EF. Note the pseudo-normalization with normal E/A ratio, deceleration time, and abnormal E/e′. Note the relatively preserved LV twist mechanics, although LV twisting and untwisting velocities are both attenuated and delayed.
4. In a patient with advanced *diabetic cardiomyopathy and reduced ejection fraction*: Note the abnormally increased E/A ratio, decreased deceleration time, and E/e′. There is marked reduction in amplitude of apical counter clockwise and basal clockwise rotation.

CONCLUSION

Evaluation of all diabetic patients with 3D echocardiography for the presence of diabetic cardiomyopathy leads to detection of early and preventable changes. Thus, the treatment approaches may be changed in these conditions to include the cardio protective drugs, for example DPP4 inhibitors and statins.

REFERENCES

1. Lorenzo-Almorós A, Tuñón J, Orejas M, et al. Diagnostic approaches for diabetic cardiomyopathy. Cardiovasc Diabetol. 2017; 16(1):28.
2. Rydén L, Grant PJ, Anker SD, et al. ESC Guidelines on diabetes, pre-diabetes, and cardiovascular diseases developed in collaboration with the EASD: The Task Force on diabetes, pre-diabetes, and cardiovascular diseases of the European Society of Cardiology (ESC) and developed in collaboration with the European Association for the Study of Diabetes (EASD). Eur Heart J. 2013;34(39): 3035-87.
3. Smiseth OA, Torp H, Opdahl A, et al. Myocardial strain imaging: how useful is it in clinical decision making? Eur Heart J. 2016;37(15):1196-207.
4. Sorrentino R, Esposito R, Pezzullo E, et al. Realtime three dimensional speckle tracking echocardiography: technical aspects and clinical applications. Res Rep Clin Cardiol. 2016;7:147-58.
5. Asghar O, AlSunni A, Khavandi K, et al. Diabetic cardiomyopathy. Clin Sci Lond Engl. 1979;2009(116):741-60.
6. Rubler S, Dlugash J, Yuceoglu YZ, et al. New type of cardiomyopathy associated with diabetic glomerulosclerosis. Am J Cardiol. 1972;30(6):595-602.
7. Seferović PM, Paulus WJ. Clinical diabetic cardiomyopathy: a twofaced disease with restrictive and dilated phenotypes. Eur Heart J. 2015;36(27):1718-27, 1727a-c.
8. Lang RM, Bierig M, Devereux RB, et al. Recommendations for chamber quantification: a report from the American Society of Echocardiography's Guidelines and Standards Committee and the Chamber Quantification Writing Group, developed in conjunction with the European Association of Echocardiography, a branch of the European Society of Cardiology. J Am Soc Echocardiogr. 2005;18(12):1440-63.
9. Galderisi M. Diastolic dysfunction and diabetic cardiomyopathy: evaluation by Doppler echocardiography. J Am Coll Cardiol. 2006;48(8):1548-51.
10. Bouchard A, Sanz N, Botvinick EH, et al. Noninvasive assessment of cardiomyopathy in normotensive diabetic patients between 20 and 50 years old. Am J Med. 1989;87(2):160-6.
11. Pérez JE, McGill JB, Santiago JV, et al. Abnormal myocardial acoustic properties in diabetic patients and their correlation with the severity of disease. J Am Coll Cardiol. 1992;19(6):1154-62.
12. Kinno M, Waller AH, Gardin JM. Approaches to echocardiographic assessment of left ventricular mass. What does the echocardiography add? Expert analysis. Am Coll Cardiol. 2016.
13. Lang RM, Badano LP, Mor-Avi V, et al. Recommendations for cardiac chamber quantification by echocardiography in adults: an update from the American Society of Echocardiography and the European Association of Cardiovascular Imaging. J Am Soc Echocardiogr. 2015;28(1):1-39.e14.
14. Koren MJ, Devereux RB, Casale PN, et al. Relation of left ventricular mass and geometry to morbidity and mortality in uncomplicated essential hypertension. Ann Intern Med. 1991;114(5):345-52.
15. Chuang ML, Beaudin RA, Riley MF, et al. Three-dimensional echocardiographic measurement of left ventricular mass: comparison with magnetic resonance imaging and two-dimensional echocardiographic determinations in man. Int J Card Imaging 2000;16(5):347-57.
16. Mor-Avi V, Sugeng L, Weinert L, et al. Fast measurement of left ventricular mass with real-time three-dimensional echocardiography: comparison with magnetic resonance imaging. Circulation. 2004;110(13):1814-8.
17. Leung DY, Boyd A, Ng AA, et al. Echocardiographic evaluation of left atrial size and function: current understanding, pathophysiologic correlates, and prognostic implications. Am Heart J. 2008;156(6):1056-64.
18. Mor-Avi V, Yodwut C, Jenkins C, et al. Real-time 3D Echocardiographic quantification of left atrial volume: multicenter study for validation with CMR. JACC Cardiovasc Imaging. 2012;5(8): 769-77.
19. Badano LP, Miglioranza MH, Mihăilă S, et al. Left atrial volumes and function by three-dimensional echocardiography reference values, accuracy, reproducibility, and comparison with two-dimensional echocardiographic measurements. Circ Cardiovasc Imaging. 2016;9(7):e004229.
20. Cameli M, Lisi M, Righini FM, et al. Novel echocardiographic techniques to assess left atrial size, anatomy and function. Cardiovasc Ultrasound. 2012;10:4.
21. Marwick TH. Methods used for the assessment of LV systolic function: common currency or tower of Babel? Heart. 2013;99(15):1078-86.
22. Jenkins C, Bricknell K, Hanekom L, et al. Reproducibility and accuracy of echocardiographic measurements of left ventricular

parameters using real-time three-dimensional echocardiography. J Am Coll Cardiol. 2004;44(4):878-86.
23. Kalam K, Otahal P, Marwick TH. Prognostic implications of global LV dysfunction: a systematic review and meta-analysis of global longitudinal strain and ejection fraction. Heart. 2014;100(21):1673-80.
24. Ashraf M, Myronenko A, Nguyen T, et al. Defining Left Ventricular Apex-to-Base Twist Mechanics Computed From High-Resolution 3D Echocardiography Validation Against Sonomicrometry. JACC Cardiovasc Imaging. 2010;3(3):227-34.
25. Beladan CC, Călin A, Roşca M, et al. Left ventricular twist dynamics: principles and applications. Heart. 2014;100(9):731-40.
26. Helle-Valle T, Crosby J, Edvardsen T, et al. New noninvasive method for assessment of left ventricular rotation: speckle tracking echocardiography. Circulation. 2005;112(20):3149-56.
27. Kauer F, Geleijnse ML, van Dalen BM. Role of left ventricular twist mechanics in cardiomyopathies, dance of the helices. World J Cardiol. 2015;7(8):476-82.

CHAPTER

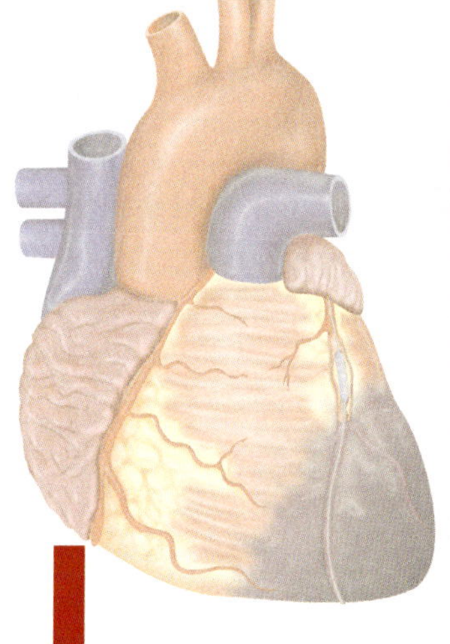

Emergency Echocardiography in Cardiodiabetes

Rekha Mishra, Sanjeev Asotra, Krishna CK, Manish Bansal, HK Chopra

INTRODUCTION

India has come up as a diabetic capital of the world with 62 million diabetics and the number is expected to rise to 70 million by 2025.[1,2] Studies in different parts of India have demonstrated an ever-increasing prevalence of diabetes in both urban and rural population. More than 65% of patients with diabetes die of cardiovascular diseases (CVD) and coronary artery diseases (CAD) tend to develop a decade or two earlier and triple-vessel disease is more common. Mortality after an acute coronary event is also 40% higher in Asian-Indian patients.[3-5] The economic burden of diabetes, involving care of diabetics, escalates manyfold once vascular complication develops. High rates of CVD have been reported in India. The prevalence of hypertension and coronary heart diseases is very high. Wide disparities in socioeconomic levels, educational background, and availability of diabetes care pose major challenges in management of disease and its complications. The causes of mortality in diabetes continue to be infections, renal failure, CAD, and CVD. Management of diabetes, presenting in emergency care facilities, poses a fair challenge for healthcare professionals due to highly variable symptom complexes, and multisystem involvement. Echocardiography has emerged as an important noninvasive tool in diabetic patients presenting with hemodynamic instability.

EMERGENCIES IN DIABETES

- Infections and sepsis
- Endocrine emergencies
- Cardiovascular
  - Acute coronary syndrome
  - Heart failure (HF)
  - Arrhythmias
  - Stroke

Indications of Emergency Echocardiography in Diabetics

The indications have been listed in Box 1.

ROLE OF ECHOCARDIOGRAPHY IN ACUTE CHEST PAIN

Acute Coronary Syndrome

Acute coronary syndrome (ACS) consists of a spectrum of illnesses ranging from unstable angina, non-ST elevation myocardial infarction (N-STEMI), ST elevation MI and sudden death. Diabetic patients can present with atypical symptoms and even can have silent infarctions. Mortality is two-to-three times higher as compared to nondiabetics. So, an early diagnosis and appropriate therapeutic approach is lifesaving in the golden hour. Echo plays a pivotal role in the diagnosis and management of patients presenting with ACS:

- Assessment of presence and location of regional wall motion abnormality
- Estimation of infarct size
- Assessment of ventricular systolic and diastolic function
- Evaluation of complications
- Assessment of reperfusion.

BOX 1: Indications of emergency echocardiography in diabetics

- Acute chest pain
- Acute dyspnea
- Hemodynamic instability or shock
- New onset of murmur
- Stroke
- Syncope

Assessment of Presence and Location of Regional Wall Motion Abnormality

Normal systolic contraction consists of both myocardial thickening and inward excursion of the endocardium. Immediately after the onset of ischemia, myocardial thickening ceases and depending on the severity of ischemia, the wall motion becomes hypokinetic, akinetic or dyskinetic. The wall motion abnormality helps to predict the location of the culprit coronary artery.

The American Society of Echocardiography advocates the use of 17-segment model, dividing the left ventricle (LV) into three levels (basal, mid, and apical) with further subdivision into six segments at the basal and mid-level and four segments at the apical level and a single segment at the apex to produce 17 segments. Each segment is assigned a score based on its contractility: 1 = normal, 2 = hypokinesis, 3 = akinesis, 4 = dyskinesis, and 5 = aneurysm.

Based on the wall motion analysis, a wall motion score index (WMSI) can be derived to calculate the extent of segmental dysfunction severity:

$$\text{WMSI} = \frac{\text{Sum of wall motion scores}}{\text{Number of segments visualized}}$$

A normally contracting LV has a WMSI of 1. The larger the infarct size, the greater the WMSI because wall motion abnormalities become more severe.[6]

Estimation of Infarct Size

Size of infarct is estimated by the extent of regional wall motion abnormality and its quantification is done using wall motion score index. Higher the score, the more severe is the ventricular dysfunction.

Assessment of Ventricular Systolic and Diastolic Function

In clinical practice, systolic function is usually assessed using ejection fraction. Lower the ejection fraction (EF), greater the complications such as HF, arrhythmias, and death. Left ventricular ejection fraction (LVEF), fractional shortening and E-point septal separation assessments are good indicators of systolic functions.[7,8]

Diastolic function can be assessed by mitral inflow, mitral annular velocities and LA volume index.

Assessment of LV diastolic dysfunction grade in normal LVEF: According to the latest guidelines from the American Society of Echocardiography and the European Association of Cardiovascular imaging, only four variables need to be evaluated in determining the diastolic function if LV systolic function is normal.[9] LV diastolic function is normal if more than half of the available variables do not meet the cut-off values for identifying abnormal function.

These four variables and their abnormal variables are:
- Annular e' velocity (septal e' velocity < 7.0 cm/second, lateral e' < 10 cm/second)
- An average E/e' ratio of more than 14
- Left atrium (LA) maximum volume index more than or equal to 34 mL/m^2
- Peak tricuspid regurgitation (TR) velocity of more than 2.8 m/sec.

At times, only the medial or lateral e' velocity is available and in these circumstances a medial E/e' ratio more than 15 or a lateral E/e' more than 13 is considered abnormal.

Assessment of LV diastolic dysfunction grade in reduced LVEF (Figs 1A to D): In patients with reduced LV systolic function, evaluation of LV diastolic function is slightly variable.[10]
- Transmitral inflow pattern is the first variable to be assessed. If the ratio of mitral E/A is less than 0.8 and mitral E wave velocity is less than 50 cm/second, then usually the LV filling pressure is normal.
- If E/A is more than 2.0, then it indicates significantly increased LA pressure. In case of indeterminate values, the three other parameters to be evaluated are:
    i. Average E/e' more than 14
    ii. TR velocity more than 2.8 cm/sec
    iii. LA volume index more than or equal to 34 mL/m^2.

Pulmonary vein systolic and diastolic velocity (S/D) ratio may be used if one of the above parameters is not available. A ratio less than 1 is consistent with increased LAP.

Since diabetes is associated with diastolic dysfunction very frequently, comments on LV filling pressure and grade of LV diastolic dysfunction should always be included.

Diastolic dysfunction is seen early in the course of ischemia or infarction. The greater the degree of diastolic dysfunction, the worse is the prognosis.

Evaluation of Complications (Figs 2A to G)

Complications detected by echo are:[11]
- Pericardial effusion
- Infarct expansion
- Aneurysm formation and thrombus formation
- *Myocardial rupture*: Free wall, ventricular septal defect, and papillary muscle
- Right ventricular (RV) infarct
- Ischemic acute mitral regurgitation (MR).

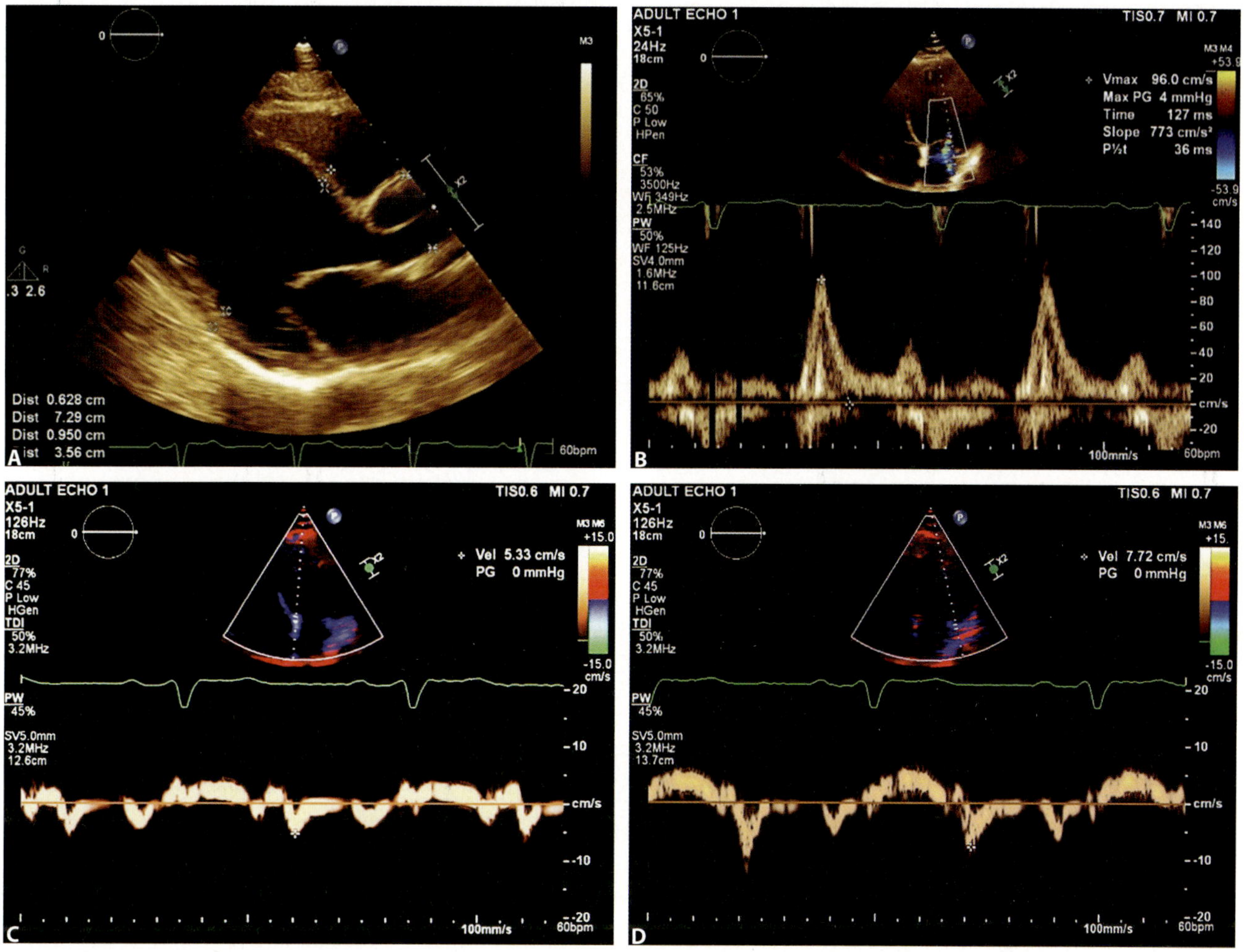

Figs 1A to D: (A) Dilated LV with akinetic and thin anterior IVS in a PLAX view: (B) Mitral inflow showing E/A > 2 with short deceleration Time consistent with restrictive pattern; (C) and (D) Septal and lateral tissue Doppler early (e') diastolic velocities are reduced consistent with severely impaired LV relaxation, Average E/e' ratio = 14.7, consistent with elevated mean LAP

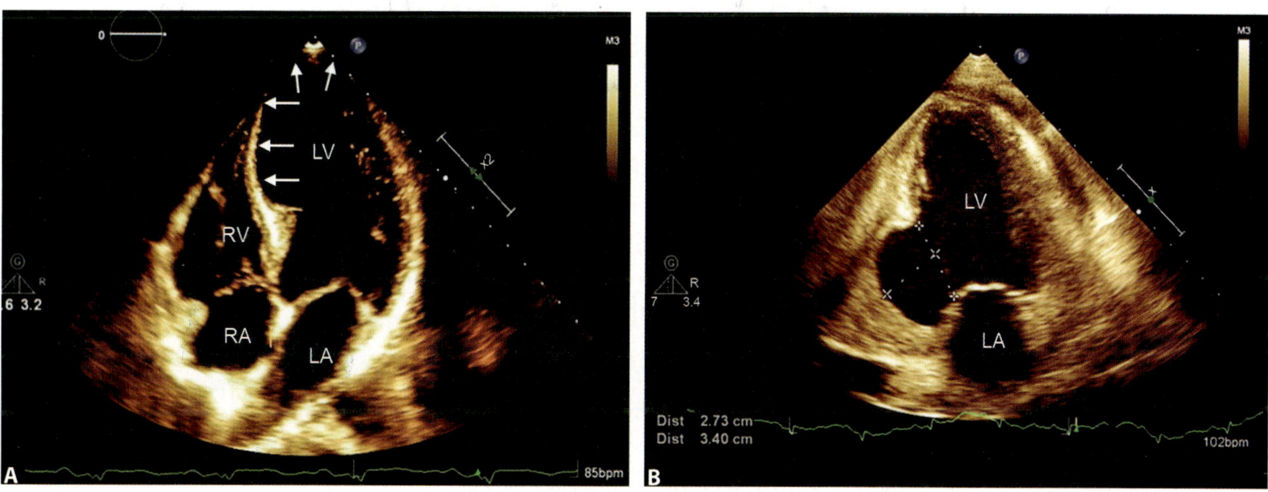

Figs 2A and B

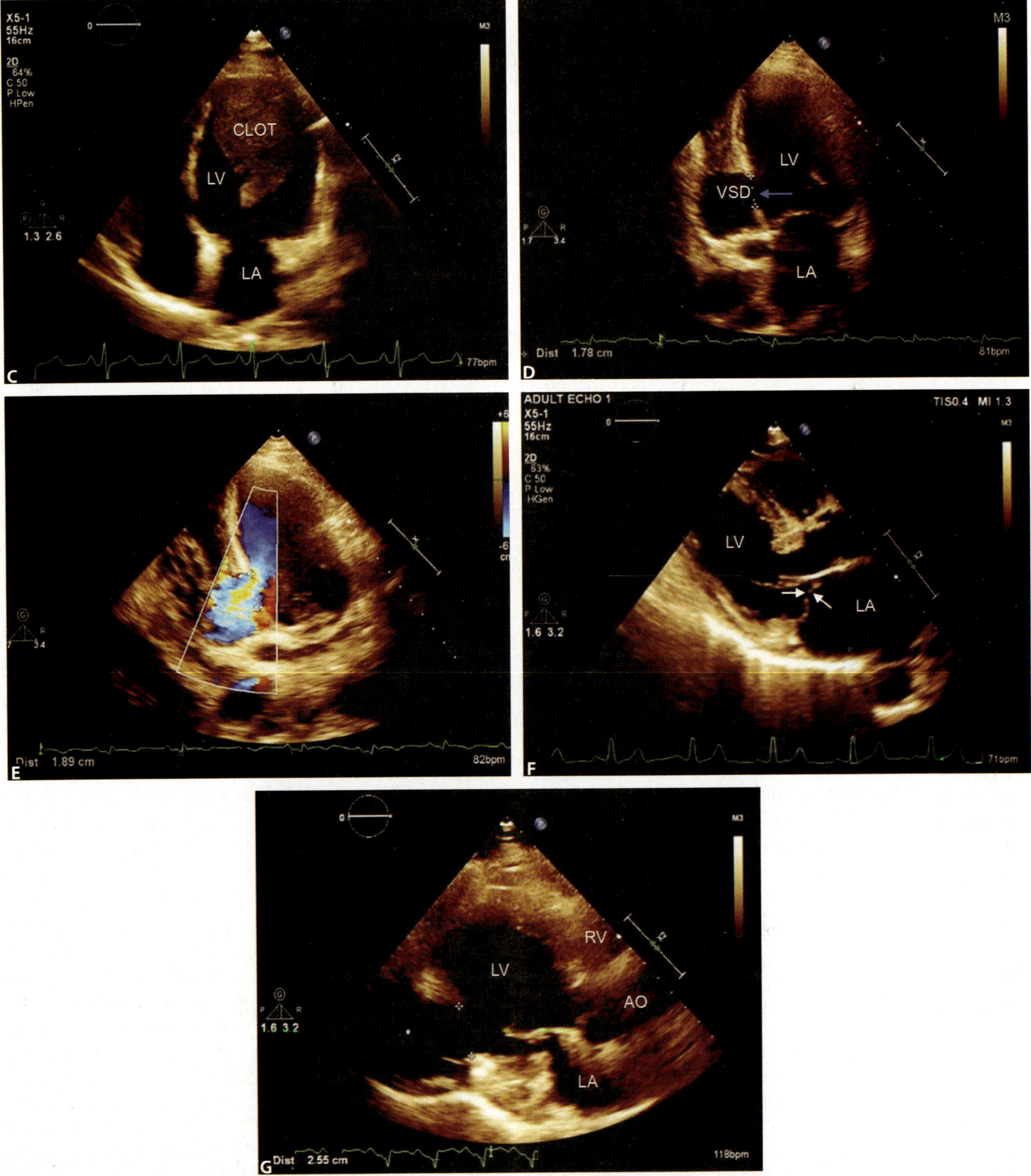

Figs 2A to G: (A) Apical 4-C view showing thin and akinetic IVS and apex; (B) Apical 2-C view showing a large inferior basal aneurysm with a wide neck; (C) Apical 4-C view in a patient with extensive anteroapical infarct with a large thrombus occupying more than half of LV; (D) Apical 2-C view showing a large inferoventricular septal defect (arrow); (E) Color flow imaging shows a shunt from the left to right ventricle via the ventricular septal defect; (F) PLAX view in a patient of inferoposterior MI showing flail posterior mitral leaflet due to chordal rupture (arrows); (G) PLAX view shows a large pseudoaneurysm in the posterior aspect of LV in a patient of inferoposterior MI

Assessment of Reperfusion

After successful reperfusion, the wall motion may resolve and echo helps in assessing the improvement in regional wall motion abnormalities.

ROLE OF ECHO IN ACUTE DYSPNEA

Heart Failure

Heart failure is the most common cardiac cause of acute dyspnea in diabetic patients, which can be either due to worsening of preexisting HF or a new onset HF.[12] Patients may present with HF complicating an ACS, acute pulmonary edema, cardiogenic shock, or isolated RV dysfunction. Dyspnea may be a presenting symptom of ACS. Echocardiography helps in rapid evaluation of functional and structural changes associated with HF as well as underlying cause and differentiate between HF due to systolic and isolated diastolic dysfunction.[13]

Echocardiography allows the physician to identify the etiology, the precipitants and to assess the heart from the physiological perspective (Table 1).

Three step-by-step sonographic assessments can help differentiate acute HF from other causes of dyspnea by assessing for pulmonary edema, central venous congestion, and elevated LV end-diastolic pressure (LVEDP) (Fig. 3).

Step 1: Pulmonary ultrasound has shown to be accurate in detecting acute HF with sensitivities of 86–100% and specificity of 95–98%.[14] Increased interstitial edema produces characteristic sonographic comet tail artifacts known as B lines that arise from visceral-parietal lung interface, extend to the bottom of the viewing field, move with respiration and are less than 7 mm apart. Three or more B lines per viewing field are pathological and constitute alveolar interstitial syndrome, which can be focal or diffuse as in pneumonias or diffuse and bilateral as in pulmonary edema.[15,16]

Step 2: Assessment of inferior vena cava (IVC) and collapsibility of the patient in supine position in end expiration and during deep inspiration. IVC size and collapsibility index are shown to correlate with right atrial pressure.[17] The important limitations of these two parameters are patients with moderate-to-severe TR and acute RV dilatation from pulmonary embolism or RV infarction.

Step 3: Doppler assessment of left-sided filling pressure. Early diastolic tissue Doppler velocity (e') measured and averaged at septal and lateral portion of the mitral annulus used in combination with peak early diastolic (E) flow velocities across mitral valve can be used to assess the raised LVEDP. The ratio of E /e' correlates closely with LV filling pressure. There is a strong correlation in patients with preserved ejection fraction and moderate correlation in HF with reduced ejection fraction when septal E/e' more than 15.[10]

TABLE 1: Echocardiographic signs suggestive of the cause of acute heart failure

Systolic heart failure	*Diastolic heart failure*
• Left ventricular ejection fraction (LVEF) < 45–50%	• LVEF ≥ 50%
• Left ventricular end-diastolic volume (LVEDV) > 97 mL/m²	• LVEDV < 97 mL/m²
• Left ventricular end systolic volume (LVESV) > 43 mL/m²	• LVESV < 43 mL/m²
• Abnormal wall motion	• Left atrial (LA) volume ≥ 34 mL/m²
• Functional mitral regurgitation (MR) and/or tricuspid regurgitation (TR)	• Peak tricuspid velocity > 3 m/s
• Peak tricuspid velocity > 3 m/s.	

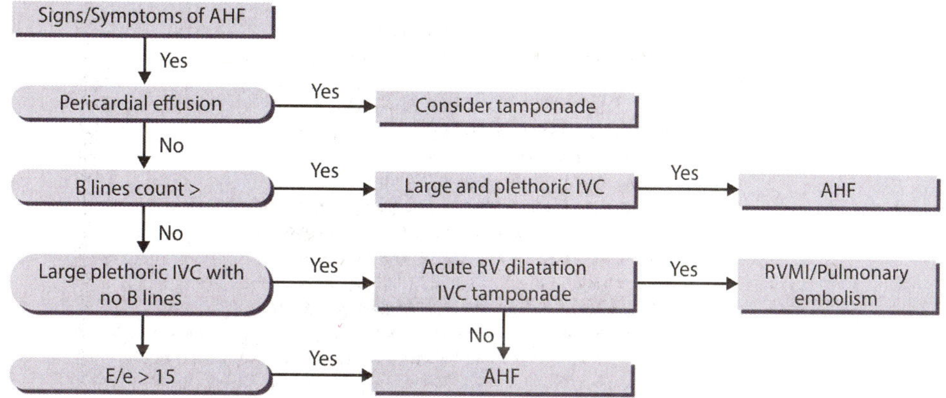

Fig. 3: Algorithm for determining signs of acute heart failure (AHF) and heart failure with reduced or preserved ejection fraction in dyspneic emergency department patients

Step 4: Differentiating between the preserved and reduced left ventricular ejection by E point septal separation, mitral annular plane excursion, fractional shortening and visual estimation of EF can place the patient into normal, moderately reduced and severely reduced EF.

ECHOCARDIOGRAPHY IN SHOCK

Echocardiography plays a very important role in management of shock in diabetic patients. No other bedside tool can offer a similar diagnostic capability. Diabetic patient can present with all four core causes of shock namely cardiogenic, hypovolemic, obstructive or vasoplegic. Shock may be multifactorial in a given individual. Basic hemodynamic assessment by echocardiography helps in differentiating four major categories of circulatory shock and enables proper and immediate hemodynamic support (Table 2).

Cardiogenic Shock

Cardiogenic shock is the extreme end of deteriorating HF spectrum and it carries very high mortality. Although cardiogenic shock relates to underlying coronary artery pathology but a large number of etiologies may result into severe HF.

The primary focus is to assess the systolic function, cardiac performance, assessing valvular pathology and LV diastolic function.

Left ventricular ejection fraction is most often used to assess the LV systolic function and is evaluated by modified Simpson's multidisk method or by eyeballing. The interpretation of EF needs to take into account the effect of inotropes, vasopressors and afterload agents. dp/dt can be calculated in the presence of mitral regurgitation and the value less than 800 mm Hg is considered abnormal.[17] Using tissue Doppler imaging (TDI), myocardial systolic velocity (S') measured from multiple segments correlates with LVEF. S′ value of 5.4 cm averaged from multiple segments correlate with an LVEF more than 50%.[18] Myocardial performance index, left ventricular outflow tract (LVOT) view, velocity time integral (VTI), and mitral annular plane systolic excursion (MAPSE) can be used to assess the cardiac performance. The LVOT-VTI as a single parameter is reliable to assess the stroke volume. A value more than 18 cm implies normal stroke volume.

Assessing the structural integrity of valves is important. Peri-infarction rupture of papillary muscle can result into severe MR.

Assessment of diastolic function using spectral Doppler of mitral inflow, the ratio of E/A more than 2 and E wave deceleration time of less than 120 ms predicts LAP more than 20 mm Hg. Using TDI, the mitral annulus offers a quick guide to know the presence of LV diastolic dysfunction. The lateral e' less than 10 and medial e' less than 7 cm/s is highly suggestive of diastolic dysfunction and raised left atrial pressure (LAP).

Hypovolemic Shock

Assessment of intravascular volume is important step in these patients. When hypovolemia is severe, the two-dimensional (2D) imaging shows the collapse of LV walls in the end systole so called the kissing walls (Fig. 4).[19,20] IVC diameter less than 21 mm that collapses on sniff, caval or collapsibility index ($D_{max} - D_{min})/D_{max} \times 100\%$) indicates right atrial pressure (RAP) of 3 mm Hg, whereas IVC diameter more than 21 mm that collapses less than 50 with a sniff indicates RAP more than 15 mm Hg (Fig. 4).[21] The fixed bowing of left atrial septum into right atrium throughout the cardiac cycle may imply raised LAP and lesser need of fluids. Administration of a bolus of IV fluid and passive leg raising causing on an average more than 15% of stroke volume (SV) or cardiac output (CO) are good indicators of fluid responsiveness.[22]

TABLE 2: Hemodynamics of shock

	CVP	*PCWP*	*Cardiac output*	*SVR*
Hypovolemic	Decreased	Decreased	Increased	Increased
Cardiogenic	Increased	Increased	Decreased	Increased
Septic	Decreased	Decreased	Increased	Decreased
Obstructive	Either	Increased	Decreased	Increased

Abbreviations: CVP, central venous pressure; PCPW, pulmonary capillary wedge pressure; SVR, systemic vascular resistance

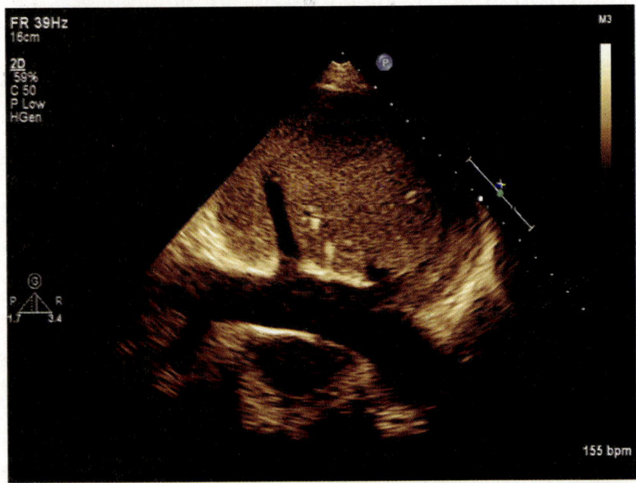

Fig. 4: Subcostal view showing marked dilatation of inferior vena cava (IVC) consistent with elevated right atrial pressure (RAP)

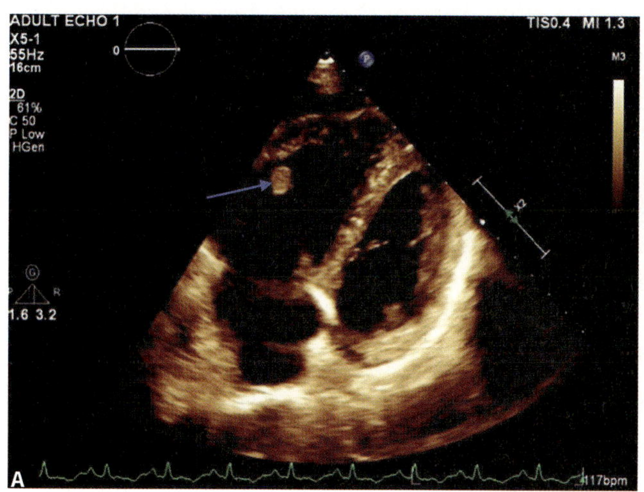

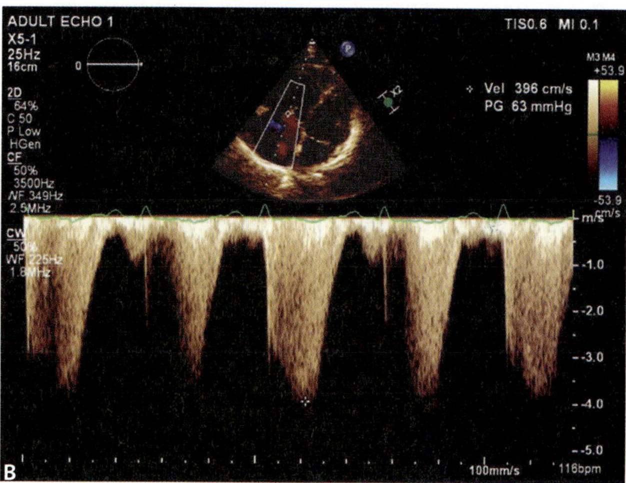

Figs 5A and B: (A) Apical 4-C view showing marked dilatation of right atrium (RA) and right ventricle (RV) with a clot (*arrow*) attached to lateral wall of RV in a patient with pulmonary embolism; (B) Continuous wave Doppler of tricuspid regurgitation, markedly increased trans-tricuspid pressure gradient indicating severe pulmonary hypertension

Obstructive Shock

The most common mechanisms in patients with diabetes having obstructive shock are acute pulmonary embolism, pericardial tamponade or LVOT obstruction. Dilated right heart chambers, changes in right ventricular contraction, elevated pulmonary artery pressure, decreased cardiac output and uncommonly presence of intracavitary thrombi can lead to diagnosis of pulmonary thromboembolism.[23] Dilatation of RV can be assessed in apical four-chamber view with RV/LV ratio of more than 0.6 (Fig. 5A). Tricuspid annular plane systolic excursion (TAPSE) is reliable and easily obtainable parameter with a normal value of more than 16 mm.[24] Lateral tricuspid annular S′ velocity less than 11.5 cm/s predicts RV dysfunction on TDI (Fig. 5B). The McConnell sign showing good apical but poor free wall contraction is an important sign.[25] The pulmonary artery pressures can be assessed in the presence of TR or pulmonary regurgitation (PR). In absence of them, the acceleration time of pulmonary ejection signal (PAcT) can be used. Value of 70–90 ms indicates pulmonary artery systolic pressure of more than 70 mm Hg.[26] The classical 2D sign of pulmonary hypertension resulting in a marked increase in RV pressures is paradoxical septal motion and a D-shaped LV may be seen on the parasternal short axis and M mode.[23]

Presence of pericardial effusion is easily identified on echo. Right atrial wall collapse for longer than one-third of cardiac cycle, right ventricular diastolic collapse and dilated IVC are signs of tamponade. Increase in peak tricuspid velocity more than 25% and peak mitral velocity more than 15% is present in tamponade (Fig. 6).[27]

Patients of hypertrophic cardiomyopathy, hypertension with LV hypertrophy which can be easily identified by echo, in the presence of tachycardia, hypovolemia and inotropes can develop dynamic LVOT obstruction (Fig. 7A).[28] 2D examination reveals hyperdynamic LV and systolic anterior motion of the anterior mitral leaflet. Color Doppler reveals turbulent flow through the LVOT with continuous wave Doppler picking up high velocities across the LVOT with a classical “Dagger “shape of LVOT flow (Fig. 7B).

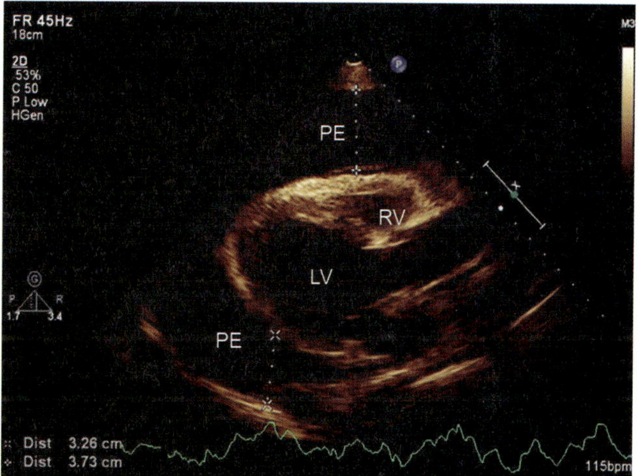

Fig. 6: Parasternal long-axis (PLAX) view showing a large pericardial effusion with compressed RV consistent with cardiac tamponade

Septic Shock

Variety of cardiac changes in the form of abnormal LV systolic, diastolic, and RV function have been described, although a normal study also is not unusual. Left ventricular dilatation with/without global hypokinesia, LV segmental

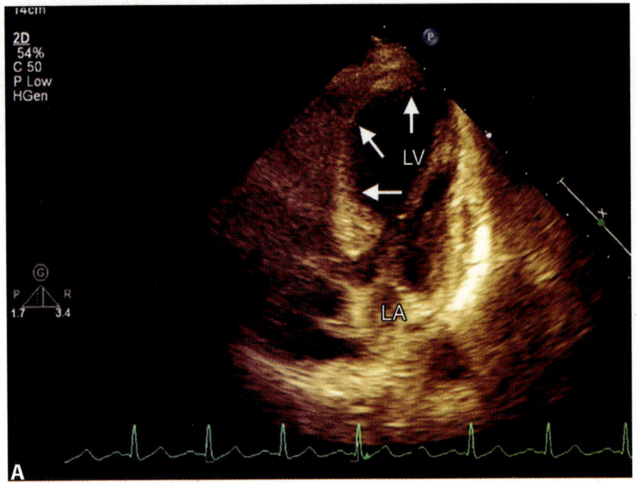

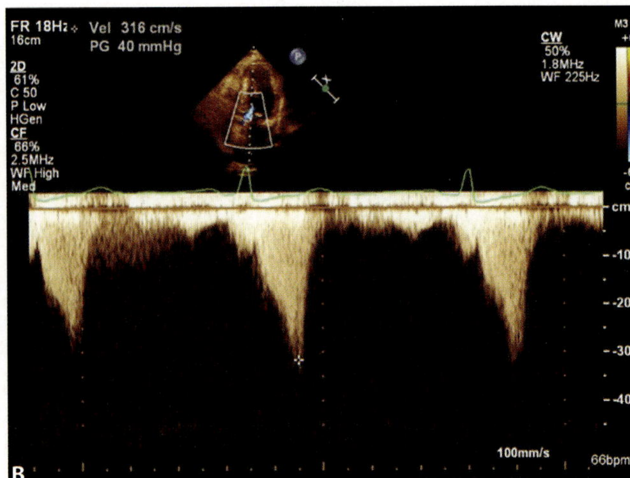

Figs 7A and B: (A) Apical 4-C view in a patient of Takotsubo cardiomyopathy with apical ballooning and left ventricular outflow tract obstruction (LVOTO) due to hypercontractile basal left ventricle (LV) and systolic anterior motion (SAM); (B) Continuous wave Doppler across LVOT showing a typical late peaking configuration resembling a dagger shape

wall motion defect pattern, dilated RV with impaired functions can be seen and is almost always reversible over days.[29] Contractile impairment presenting in the form of Takotsubo cardiomyopathy may be documented.[30] Hemodynamic assessment is important for fluid management of the patients. Endocarditis or perivalvular abscess may be the cause of septic shock (Table 2).

Echocardiography is perhaps the single most useful tool in diagnosis and management of shock in diabetic patients where the etiology is generally undifferentiated or multifactorial. It is the golden standard in the initial hemodynamic assessment and has extremely powerful role for the cardiac abnormalities as a cause for hemodynamic instability.

ROLE OF ECHO IN NEW MURMUR

A new murmur in a diabetic patient with acute cardio-respiratory symptoms suggesting structural heart disease is a strong indication for echocardiography. It provides valuable information regarding etiology, valvular morphology and function, quantification of valvular lesions, chamber size and ventricular function and pulmonary artery pressures.

Acute Mitral Regurgitation

Acute mitral regurgitation is a potentially life-threatening complication of MI. It can be secondary to LV dysfunction without structural valvular abnormalities resulting from increased leaflet tethering or can result from acute papillary muscle dysfunction or rupture.[31]

Ventricular septal defect occurs in around 2% in MI and they have high mortality rate.[32] Echocardiography shows the site and size of the shunt by 2D echo and color Doppler. TR may appear in patients with pulmonary embolism or RV infarction and TR is used to calculate pulmonary artery (PA) systolic pressure differentiating pulmonary embolism from RV infarct. TR is generally of low pressure in RV infarct until and unless preexisting pulmonary artery hypertension.

The other differential diagnoses of a new murmur in patients with acute MI are free wall rupture and LVOT obstruction.

ROLE OF ECHO IN STROKE

Epidemiological studies have shown that DM is a well-established independent modifiable risk factor for stroke. Emerging risk factor collaboration study showed that adjusted hazards ratio was 2.27 (1.9–2.65) for ischemic stroke, 1.54 (1.19–2.05) for hemorrhagic stroke and 1.84 (1.59–2.13) for unclassified stroke.[33] Cardioembolism stroke accounts for 14–30% of all cerebral infarcts.[34] Atrial fibrillation (AF), dilated cardiomyopathy, and MI are common causes of cardioembolism in DM. The incidence of AF in DM is reported to be 14.9%.[35] The link between AF and DM is much more mutual and reciprocal.[36] A recent meta-analysis published by Huxley et al. revealed that patients with DM had a 40% greater risk of developing AF compared to patients without diabetes.[37]

The primary role of echocardiography is to establish the existence of a source of embolism, guide therapy and prevention of cardiac source of embolism in an individual. Echocardiography should be considered in all patients with suspected cardiac source of embolism, especially in patients where therapeutic decisions like anticoagulation and cardioversion depend on echocardiographic

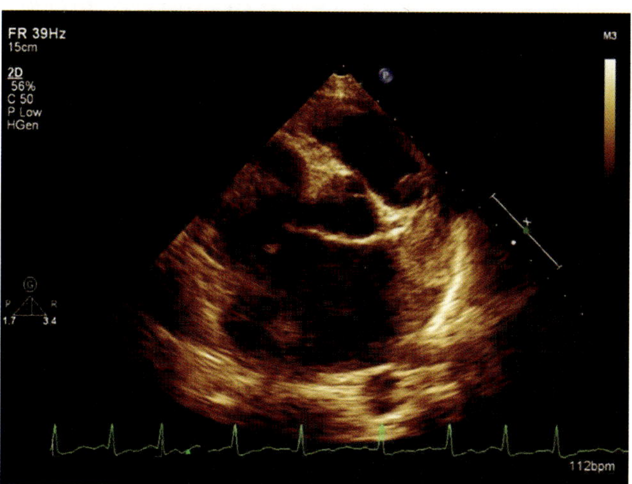

Fig. 8: Short-axis (SAX) view showing a large clot in left atrial appendage (LAA) in a patient with atrial fibrillation

BOX 2: Echocardiographic findings known to be associated with syncope

- Left ventricular systolic dysfunction
- Hypertrophic obstructive cardiomyopathy
- Myxomatous mitral valve
- Mitral stenosis
- Aortic stenosis
- Pulmonary hypertension
- Intracardiac mass
- Pericardial effusion

findings. Cardiac sources of emboli include thrombus, tumor fragments, vegetations, calcified particles, and atherosclerotic debris.[38] A thrombus located in the left atrial appendage (LAA) is the most prevalent source of cardioembolic events and is mostly associated with atrial fibrillation. TEE is the modality of choice for the evaluation of LAA anatomy and function (Fig. 8).

ROLE OF ECHO IN SYNCOPE (BOX 2)

Syncope evaluation in diabetes is a difficult clinical problem. Causes may be neural, cardiac, metabolic, and orthostatic hypotension.[39] Metabolic syncope comprises about 5% of all syncope. Hypoglycemic syncope is the most common metabolic syncope, with a reported incidence of 0.6% in diabetic patients.[40] Cardiac cause of syncope includes arrhythmias, structural heart disease, MI and LV dysfunction.

Echocardiography is useful in the diagnostic evaluation of diabetic patients with syncope through its ability to diagnose, quantitate the severity of the cardiac lesion thus helping in risk stratification.[41,42]

CONCLUSION

Timely echocardiographic navigation in cardiodiabetes is of tremendous clinical relevance in taking decision for emergency cardiac management in cardiodiabetes. It has huge impact in reducing cardiodiabetes-inflicted morbidity and mortality.

REFERENCES

1. Joshi SR, Parikh RM. India—diabetes capital of the world: now heading towards hypertension. J Assoc Physicians India. 2007;55:323-4.
2. Kumar A, Goel MK, Jain RB, et al. India towards diabetes control: Key issues. Australas Med J. 2013;6(10):524-31.
3. Ali MK, Narayan KM, Tandon N. Diabetes and coronary heart disease: current perspectives. Indian J Med Res. 2010;132: 584-97.
4. Enas EA, Singh V, Munjal YP, et al. Reducing the burden of coronary artery disease in India: challenges and opportunities. Indian Heart J. 2008;60(2):161-75.
5. Mohan V, Venkatraman JV, Pradeepa R. Epidemiology of cardiovascular disease in Type 2 DM: Indian Scenario. J Diabetes Sci Technol. 2010;4(1):158-70.
6. Moller JE, Hillis GS, Oh JK, et al. Wall motion score index and ejection fraction for risk stratification after acute myocardial infarction. Am Heart J. 2006;151(2):419-25.
7. Stammn RB, Carlitto BA, Mayas DL, et al. Two-dimensional echocardiographic measurement of left ventricular ejection fraction: prospective analysis of what constitutes an adequate determination. Am Heart J. 1982;104(1):136-44.
8. Lang RM, Badano LP, Mor-Avi V. Recommendations for cardiac chamber quantification by echocardiography in adults: an update from the American Society of Echocardiography and the European Association of Cardiovascular Imaging. Eur Heart J Cardiovasc Imaging. 2015;16(3):233-71.
9. Nagueh SF, Smiseth OA, Appleton CP, et al. Recommendations for the evaluation of left ventricular diastolic function by echocardiography: An update from American Society of Echocardiography and the European Association of Cardiovascular Imaging. J Am Soc Echocardiogr. 2016;29(4):277-314.
10. Dokainish H, Nguyen JS, Bobek J, et al. Assessment of the American Society of Echocardiography-European Society of Echocardiography guidelines for diastolic function in patients with depressed ejection fraction: an echocardiography and invasive hemodynamic study. Eur J Echocardiogr. 2011;12(11):857-64.
11. Neskovic AN, Hagendorff A, Lancellotti P, et al. Emergency echocardiography: the European Association of Cardiovascular Imaging recommendations. Euro Heart J Cardiovasc Imaging. 2013;14:1-11.
12. Metra M, Brutsaert D, Dei Cas L, et al. Acute heart failure: epidemiology, classification and pathophysiology. In: Tubaro M, Danchin N, Filippatos G, Goldstein P, Vranckx P, Zagher D (eds). The ESC Textbook of Intensive and Acute Cardiac Care. Oxford: Oxford University Press; 2010. pp. 471-82.
13. Lancellotti P, Price S, Edvardsen T, et al. The use of echocardiography in acute cardiovascular care: Recommendations of the European Association of Cardiovascular Imaging and the Acute Cardiovascular Care Association. Eur Heart J Cardiovasc Imaging. 2015;16(2): 119-46.
14. Volpicelli G, Mussa A, Garofalo G, et al. Bedside lung ultrasound in assessment of alveolar-interstitial syndrome. Am J Emerg Med. 2006;24:689-96.

15. Lichtenstien DA, Meziere GA. Relevance of lung ultrasound in diagnosis of acute respiratory failure: the blue protocol. Chest. 2008;134(1):117-25.
16. Volpicelli G, Cardinale L, Garofalo G, et al. Usefulness of lung ultrasound in bedside difference between pulmonary edema and exacerbation of COPD. Emerg Radiol. 2008;15(3):145-51.
17. Nishimura RA, Tajik AJ. Quantitative hemodynamics by Doppler echocardiography: a noninvasive alternative to cardiac catheterization. Prog Cardiovasc Dis. 1994;36(4):332.
18. Gulati VK, Katz WE, Follansbee WP, et al. Mitral annular descent velocity by tissue Doppler echocardiography as an index of global left ventricular function. Am J Cardiol. 1996;77(11):979-84.
19. Brennam JM, Blair JE, Goonewardena S, et al. A comparison by medicine residents of physical examination versus hand-carried ultrasound for estimate; on of right atrial pressure. Am J Cardiol. 2007;99(11):1614-6.
20. Goonewardena SN, Gemignani A, Ronan A, et al. Comparison of hand-carried ultrasound assessment of inferior vena cava and N-terminal pro-brain natriuretic peptide for predicting readmission after hospitalization for acute decompensated heart failure. JACC Cardiovasc Imaging. 2008;1:595-601.
21. Rudski LG, Lai WW, Afilalo J, et al. Guidelines for echocardiographic assessment of right heart in adults: a report from the American Society of Echocardiography. J Am Soc Echo. 2010;23(7):685-713.
22. Nagdev AD, Merchant R, Tirado-Gonzalez A, et al. Emergency department bedside ultrasonographic measurement of caval index for non-invasive determination of a low central venous pressure. Ann Emerg Med. 2010;55(3):290-5.
23. Jardin F, Dubourg O, Bourdarias JP. Echocardiographic pattern of acute cor pulmonale. Chest. 1997;111(1):209-17.
24. Meluzin J, Spinarova L, Bakala J, et al. Pulsed Doppler tissue imaging of the velocity of tricuspid annular systolic motion; a new rapid and non-invasive method of evaluating right ventricular systolic function. Eur Heart J. 2001;22(4):340-8.
25. Chan CM, Woods C, Sharr AF. The validation and reproducibility of pulmonary embolism severity index. J Thromb Haemost. 2010;8(7):1509-14.
26. Tossavainen E, Soderrberg S, Gronlund C, et al. Pulmonary acceleration time in identifying pulmonary hypertension patients with raised pulmonary vasacular resistance. Eur Heart J (Cardiovasc Imag). 2013;14(9):890-7.
27. Lapostolle F, Petrovic T, Lenoir G, et al. Usefulness of hand-held ultrasound devices in out of hospital diagnosis performed by emergency physicians. Am J Emrg Med. 2006;24 (2):237-42.
28. Roldan FJ, Vargas-Barron J, Espinola-Zavaleta N, et al. Severe dynamic obstruction of the left ventricular outflow tract induced by Dobutamine Echocardiography. 2000;17(1):37-40.
29. Pulido JN, Afessa B, Masaki M, et al. Clinical spectrum frequency and significance of myocardial dysfunction in severe sepsis and septic shock. Mayo Clinc Proc. 2012;87(7):620-8.
30. Kawaji T, Shiomi H Morimoto T, et al. Clinical impact of left ventricular outflow tract obstruction in Takotsubo cardiomyopathy. Circ J. 2015;79(4):839-46.
31. Engstrom A, Vis M, Bouma B, et al. Mitral regurgitation is an independent predictor of 1-year mortality in ST-elevation myocardial infarction patients presenting in cardiogenic shock on admission. Acute Card Care. 2010;12(2):51-7.
32. Reeder GS. Identification and treatment of complications of myocardial infarction. Mayo Clinic Proceedings. 1995;70: 880-4.
33. Collaboration TERF Diabetes Mellitus, fasting blood sugar concentration and risk of vascular disease: a collaborative meta-analysis of 102 prospective studies. Lancet. 2010;375(9733):2215-22.
34. Cui R, Iso H, Yamagishi K, et al. Diabetes mellitus and risk of stroke and its subtypes among Japanese men and women. Diabetologia. 2004;47:2137-4.
35. Jonghorbani M, Hu FB, Willette WC, et al. Prospective study of type 1 and type 2 diabetes and risk of stroke subtypes. The nurses' health study. Diabetes Care. 2007;30(7):1730-3.
36. Movehed MR, Hashemzudeh M, Jamel MM. Diabetes Mellitus is a strong independent risk factor for atrial fibrillation and atrial flutter in addition to other cardiovasacular disease. Int J Cardiol. 2005;105(3):315-8.
37. Huxley RR, Filion KB, Konety S, et al. Meta-analysis of cohort & case control studies of Type 2 diabetes mellitus & risk of atrial fibrillation. Am J Cardiol. 2011;108(1):56-62.
38. Saric M, Armour A, Amout S, et al. Guidelines for the use of Echocardiography in the evaluation of a cardiac source of Embolism. ASE guidelines and standard. J Am Soc Echocardiograph. 2016;29(1):1-42.
39. Patel PR, Quinn J. Syncope: a review of emergency department management and disposition. Clin Exp Emerg Med. 2015;2(2): 67-74.
40. Bingham EM, Dunn JT, Smith D, et al. "Differential changes in brain glucose metabolism during hypoglycemia accompany loss of hypoglycemia unawareness in men with type 1 Diabetes Mellitus: An [11C]-3-O-methyl-D-glucose PET Study", Diabetologia. 2005;48(10):2080-9.
41. Sarasin FP, Junod AF, Carballo D, et al. Role of echocardiography in the evaluation of syncope: a prospective study. Heart. 2002;88(4):363-7.
42. Panther R, Mahmood S, Gal R. Echocardiography in the diagnostic evaluation of syncope. J Am Soc Echocardiograph. 1998;11(3): 294-8.

CHAPTER 39

Diabetic Cardiomyopathy: Studies on Global Longitudinal Strain in Asymptomatic Diabetic Subjects

G Vijayaraghavan

INTRODUCTION

Is diabetes mellitus a cardiovascular disease? Does microangiopathy of islets of Langerhans result in destruction of beta cells and cause hyperinsulinism followed by insulin resistance and finally insulin deficiency and changes in carbohydrate metabolism? We have enough evidence to show that the long-term morbidity and mortality of diabetes mellitus is often determined by the micro- and macroangiopathic changes. As every tissue in the human body gets altered in a diabetic, so also the heart. The changes in the heart can be classified as primary or secondary due to systemic hypertension and atherosclerotic vascular disease. Limitations in our knowledge are mainly in the realm of cardiomyopathy primarily due to diabetes mellitus. The concept of "diabetic cardiomyopathy" is still controversial and a specific strategy to investigate, prevent, and treat heart disease due to diabetes is still lacking.[1] Although type I diabetes mellitus and type II diabetes mellitus differ in etiology and metabolic profiles, the two types share many features of diabetic cardiomyopathy.[1] Diabetic patients have increased incidence of cardiac failure even after controlling coronary artery disease and hypertension. Rubler et al. introduced the term "diabetic cardiomyopathy" in 1972.[2] They found four autopsied subjects with heart failure without diabetic glomerulosclerosis and without the background of systemic hypertension and coronary artery disease. The current definition of diabetic cardiomyopathy comprises structural and functional abnormalities of the myocardium in diabetic patients without coronary artery disease or hypertension. Interstitial and perivascular fibrosis is a histological hallmark of diabetic cardiomyopathy and the extent of fibrosis correlates with the heart weight.[2,3] Human myocardium biopsied at the time of coronary artery bypass surgery showed an increase in cross-sectional area of cardiomyocytes with interstitial fibrosis in diabetic patients compared with nondiabetics.[4] Miki et al. speculate that long-standing metabolic derangements and modifications of microcirculation by diabetes induce different levels of hypertrophy, atrophy, and loss of myocytes in the myocardium depending on the duration of diabetes and/or comorbidities such as hypertension. In many patients, particularly those with type 2 diabetes (T2DM), diabetes associated changes are amplified by the existence of comorbidities like hypertension and coronary artery disease, which will augment the development of left ventricular hypertrophy, increase the susceptibility of the heart to ischemic injury and increase the overall likelihood of developing heart failure.[5]

ECHOCARDIOGRAPHY

Conventional transthoracic echocardiography could image the cardiac chambers and assess the systolic and diastolic dysfunction only when it becomes clinically evident. It is a poor clinical tool to demonstrate early changes in the myocardium and its impact on the diastolic and systolic function. Left ventricular mass had been found to be increased in diabetic women but not in men in the Framingham heart study.[6] In a recent study, magnetic resonance imaging demonstrated significant association between insulin resistance and hyperglycemia with increase in left ventricular muscle mass regardless of age and gender.[7] Interstitial fibrosis in diabetic hearts can be assessed by integrated backscatter—myocardial ultrasound reflectivity in two-dimensional echocardiography, as well as by late gadolinium enhancement by cardiac magnetic resonance imaging.[8] Transthoracic echocardiography has shown that T2DM is associated with left ventricular hypertrophy or concentric remodeling in females more often than in men. Few studies in type I diabetes have shown an increase in left ventricular mass possibly due to the younger age and lower incidence of hypertension in this disease.[6] Hypertrophied ventricles often show diastolic relaxation abnormalities very early in its natural history. In obese and elderly diabetic subjects, transthoracic echocardiography is not the ideal investigation to demonstrate anatomic and pathophysiological changes and we may have to resort to cardiac magnetic resonance imaging.

DIASTOLIC DYSFUNCTION

Left ventricular diastolic dysfunction is noticed early in asymptomatic diabetic subjects on routine echocardiographic examination. Increasing content of myocardial interstitial collagen and fibrosis results in impaired myocardial relaxation and compliance. Increased cardiac lipid accumulation and altered calcium homeostasis have also been observed in diabetic subjects. The mitral diastolic flow and mitral annular tissue Doppler techniques suggest a prevalence of diastolic dysfunction in 40–75% of individuals with type 1 and type 2 diabetes without overt coronary artery disease.[9,10] Indeed, indices for diastolic dysfunction such as E/E′ and E/A ratios (where E and A are the mitral peak velocity of early and late ventricular filling respectively and E′ is the early diastolic mitral annular velocity) were impaired in type 2 diabetic patients.[9,11] Liu et al. in a study of 247 subjects with type 2 diabetes without any obvious cardiovascular disease observed that diastolic dysfunction is detectable in diabetic hearts without hypertrophy indicating that hypertrophy is not the cause of ventricular diastolic dysfunction. Diastolic dysfunction is closely associated with the state of insulin resistance, impaired fasting glucose and medical history of coronary microvascular disease.[12-14] Diastolic dysfunction as assessed by the E/E′ ratio of more than 15 has been shown to be associated with 1.08–1.61-fold increased risk of cardiovascular events.[15] Liu et al. noticed that only a small fraction of patients with diabetes without heart disease will reach an E/E′ ratio of more than 15. He noticed that the E/E′ ratio was only mildly elevated and only 14 (5.7%) patients had an E/E′ ratio of more than 15. Nonetheless, E/E′ ratio remains significantly associated with cardiovascular events in the present, in his patients with no history of cardiovascular complications. Further, ROC curve demonstrated that a cutoff value of 13.6 for E/E′ provides a reasonable sensitivity to predict cardiovascular events. This finding thus supports the assessment of diastolic dysfunction to improve risk stratification, even in patients who have not developed cardiovascular complication.

SYSTOLIC DYSFUNCTION

Systolic dysfunction accompanies myocardial hypertrophy. Interstitial collagen and fibrosis produces impaired contraction. This will be evident clinically as well as in routine echocardiographic measurements like left ventricular ejection fraction and other systolic indices. Using tissue Doppler strain analysis and measurements of peak systolic velocity, subtle abnormalities in systolic function have been described in up to 24% of randomly selected patients with diabetes mellitus after excluding subjects with coronary artery disease or left ventricular hypertrophy.[16,17] Strain is nothing but shortening fraction in percentage of a given myocardial segment. Tissue Doppler-based strain measurement is angle dependent and can sample only few segments of left ventricular myocardium reliably. Speckle tracking allows segmental and global measurement of strain with much ease as we use only apical views. Strain analysis derived from speckle tracking enables detection of subclinical myocardial systolic dysfunction beyond conventional assessment of left ventricular ejection fraction. Studies have demonstrated that impaired global left ventricular stain was observed in T2DM patients with no history of cardiovascular complications but also in asymptomatic T2DM patients even when they were normotensive.[18-20] Similar findings are common in patients with diabetic complications, like hypertension, hypertriglyceridemia, overweight, or obesity resulting in further damage to myocardial contractility.[21-23]

Very few workers evaluated the prognostic value of global longitudinal strain in patients with T2DM. In a recent study by Blomstrand and colleagues involving 406 patients, global longitudinal strain did not demonstrate independent prognostic value.[15] Even though Holland et al. in their study included only patients who had no history of cardiovascular complication and global longitudinal strain was able to predict cardiovascular events,[23] Liu et al. were the first one to demonstrate the incremental prognostic value of global longitudinal strain beyond clinical data, HbA1c and diastolic function. In particular, a global longitudinal strain of more than or equal to 17.9% provides a sensitivity of 77.8%. This finding thus highlights the usefulness of global longitudinal strain assessment in patients with T2DM.

Their demonstration of E/E' ratio of more than 13.6 and global longitudinal strain more than or equal to 17.9%, and its association of cardiovascular events in diabetes added additional methods to improve risk stratification of diabetic patients. They stressed the fact that E/E' ratio more than 15 indicated definite diastolic dysfunction which was present only in 5.7% of their patients. What is important in risk stratification is the detection of even mild forms of diastolic dysfunction with abnormalities in global longitudinal strain in diabetic subjects? Even when you analyze the strain values, one may take less than or equal to17.9 as normal, even though at its lower limits. But the combination of subtle diastolic and systolic dysfunction could risk stratify diabetic patients. Another important study was published by Jensen and coworkers[24] after studying 1065 type I diabetic patients without known heart disease using global longitudinal strain values and compared the same from 198 age and sex-matched controls. There was no significant difference between the two groups. It was values interesting to note that global longitudinal strain values were significantly different when patients with albuminuria and controls were compared. Of course, there was no difference when controls and normoalbuminuric (<30 mg/24 hours) patients were compared. But controls and patients with microalbuminuria (30–300 mg/24 hours) or macroalbuminura (>300 mg/24 hours) differed significantly in their strain values.

Global longitudinal strain values and the significant difference to control population (p values):

Normoalbuminuria (<30 mg/24 hours): 18.5 ± 2.5% NS

Microalbuminuria (30–300 mg/24 hours): 17.9 ± 2.7%; $p > 0.001$

Macroalbuminuria (>300 mg/24 hours): 17.4 ± 2.9%; $p < 0.001$.

Inclusion of diastolic dysfunction in the multivariate models did not change the relationship between albuminuria and reduced global strain values. The association between albuminuria and the risk of cardiovascular disease and mortality has been shown in several population studies and albuminuria has been shown to be one of the most important prognostic factors in diabetes.[15,21,23] Connelly et al.[25], in an experimental study, have shown that hyperglycemia and the presence of kidney disease or changes in the RAAS seem instrumental in the development of diabetic cardiomyopathy. Albuminuria is a marker of general vascular damage and the treatment could be focused on inhibition of RAAS system. What do these subtle systolic strain abnormalities portend? Roos and colleagues[26] demonstrated progression in left ventricular systolic and diastolic abnormalities in asymptomatic diabetic subjects. They could demonstrate worsening impairment of circumferential strain, longitudinal strain and peak diastolic inflow strain rate, despite the patients remaining symptom free.[27]

CONCLUSION

Speckle tracking and strain imaging are rather new innovations in echocardiography and its implication in clinical scenario is only being appreciated in the recent past. Its role in unraveling subtle abnormalities in systolic function is being utilized in ischemic heart disease and its usefulness in diabetes mellitus is still a research tool. However, our limited knowledge has thrown some light in the direction of detection of subclinical myocardial changes and this information may help us to adopt preventive strategies in the near future.

REFERENCES

1. Miki T, Yuda S, Kouzu H, et al. Diabetic cardiomyopathy: Pathophysiology and clinical features. Heart Fail Rev. 2013;18(2):149-66.
2. Rubler S, Dlugash J, Yuceoglu YZ, et al. New type of cardiomyopathy associated with diabetic glomerulosclerosis. Am J Cardiol. 1972;30(6):595-602.
3. Van Hoeven KH, Factor SM. A comparison of the pathological spectrum of hypertensive, diabetic, and hypertensive-diabetic heart disease. Circulation. 1990;82(3):848-55.
4. Fischer VW, Barner HB, Larose LS. Pathomorphologic aspects of muscular tissue in diabetes mellitus. Human Pathol. 1984;15(12):1127-36.
5. Boudina S, Abel ED. Diabetic cardiomyopathy, causes and effects. Rev Endocr Metab Disord. 2010;11(1):31-9.
6. Galderisi M, Anderson KM, Wilson PF, et al. Echocardiographic evidence for the existence of a distinct diabetic cardiomyopathy (The Framingham Heart Study). Am J Cardiol. 1991;68(1):85-9.
7. Heckbert SR, Post W, Pearson GD, et al. Traditional cardiovascular risk factors in relation to left ventricular mass, volume, and systolic function by cardiac magnetic resonance imaging: the Multiethnic Study of Atherosclerosis. J Am Coll Cardiol. 2006;48(11):2285-92.
8. Kwong RY, Sattar H, Wu H, et al. Incidence and prognostic implication of unrecognized myocardial scar characterized by cardiac magnetic resonance in diabetic patients without clinical evidence of myocardial infarction. Circulation. 2008;118(10):1011-20.
9. Brooks BA, Franjic B, Ban CR, et al. Diastolic dysfunction and abnormalities of the microcirculation in type 2 diabetes. Diabetes Obes Metab. 2008;10(9):739-46.
10. Shivalkar B, Dhondt D, Goovaerts I, et al. Flow mediated dilatation and cardiac function in type 1 diabetes mellitus. Am J Cardiol. 2006;97(1):77-82.
11. Muranaka A, Yuda S, Tsuchihashi K, et al. Quantitative assessment of left ventricular and left atrial functions by strain rate imaging in diabetic patients with and without hypertension. Echocardiography. 2009;26(3):262-71.
12. Boonman-de Winter LJ, Rutten FH, Cramer MJ, et al. High prevalence of previously unknown heart failure and left ventricular dysfunction in patients with type 2 diabetes. Diabetologia. 2012;55(8):2154-64.

13. Fontes-Carvalho R, Ladeiras-Lopes R, Bettencourt P, et al. Diastolic dysfunction in the diabetic continuum: association with insulin resistance, metabolic syndrome and type 2 diabetes. Cardiovasc Diabetol. 2015;14:4.
14. Milwidsky A, Maor E, Kivity S, et al. Impaired fasting glucose and left ventricular diastolic dysfunction in middle-age adults: a retrospective cross-sectional analysis of 2971 subjects. Cardiovasc Diabetol. 2015;14:119.
15. Blomstrand P, Engvall M, Festin K, et al. Left ventricular diastolic function, assessed by echocardiography and tissue Doppler imaging, is a strong predictor of cardiovascular events, superior to global left ventricular longitudinal strain, in patients with type 2 diabetes. Eur Heart J Cardiovasc Imaging. 2015;16: 1000-7.
16. Lacombe VA, Viatchenko-Karpinski S, Terentyev D, et al. Mechanisms of impaired calcium handling underlying subclinical diastolic dysfunction in diabetes. Am J Physiol Regul Integr Comp Physiol. 2007;293(5):R1787-97.
17. Gallego M, Alday A, Urrutia J, et al. Transient outward potassium channel regulation in healthy and diabetic hearts. Can J Physiol Pharmacol. 2009;87(2):77-83.
18. Liu JH, Chen Y, Yuen M, et al.. Incremental prognostic value of global longitudinal strain in patients with type 2 diabetes mellitus. Cardiovasc Diabetol. 2016;15:22.
19. Enomoto M, Ishizu T, Seo Y, et al. Subendocardial Systolic Dysfunction in Asymptomatic Normotensive Diabetic Patients Circ J. 2015;79(8):1749-55.
20. Mochizuki Y, Tanaka H, Matsumoto K, et al. Clinical features of subclinical left ventricular systolic dysfunction in patients with diabetes mellitus. Cardiovasc Diabetol. 2015;14:37.
21. Wang Q, Gao Y, Tan K, et al. Subclinical impairment of left ventricular function in diabetic patients with or without obesity: a study based on three-dimensional speckle tracking echocardiography. Herz. 2015;40(Suppl 3):260-8.
22. Wang Q, Gao Y, Tan K, et al. Assessment of left ventricular function by three-dimensional speckle-tracking echocardiography in well-treated type 2 diabetes patients with or without hypertension. J Clin Ultrasound. 2015;43(8):502-11.
23. Holland DJ, Marwick TH, Haluska BA, et al. Subclinical LV dysfunction and 10-year outcomes in type 2 diabetes mellitus. Heart. 2015;10(13)1:1061-6.
24. Jensen MT, Sogaard P, Andersen HU, et al. Global longitudinal strain is not impaired in Type 1 patients without albuminuria. JACC: CV Imaging. 2015;8(4):400-10.
25. Connelly KA, KJolly DJ, Zhang Y, et al. Functional, structural and molecular aspects of diastolic heart failure in the diabetic (mRen-2)27 rat. Cardiovasc Res. 2007;76(2):280-91.
26. Roos JC, Scholte AJ, Kharjithsingh AV, et al. Changes in multidirectional LV strain in asymptomatic patients with type 2 diabetes mellitus: A 2-year follow-up study. EHJ–CV Imaging. 2014;15(1);41-7.
27. Ng AC, Delgado V, Bertini M, et al. Findings from left ventricular strain and strain rate imaging in asymptomatic patients with type 2 diabetes mellitus. Am J Cardiol. 2009;104(10):1398-401.

CHAPTER

Strain and Strain Rate Imaging in Cardiodiabetes

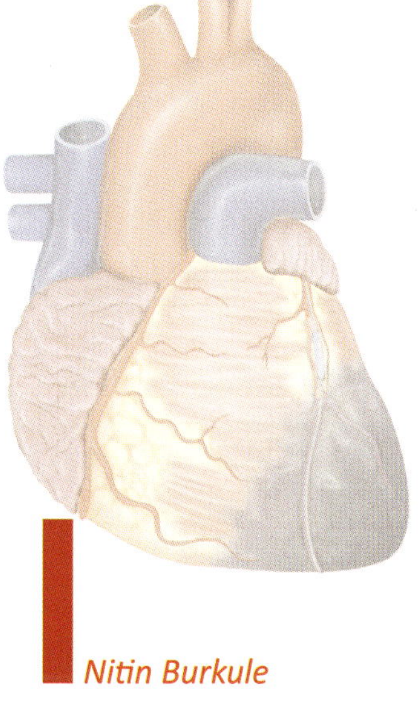

Nitin Burkule

INTRODUCTION

In the patients with prediabetes or overt diabetes mellitus (DM), the myocardial remodeling process goes through a clinically silent phase. The clinical heart failure manifests once these myocardial ultrastructural changes are sufficiently advanced. There is a window of opportunity to detect the diabetic cardiomyopathy in the silent phase and to prevent its further progression to heart failure by instituting pharmacotherapy and intensive life style management. The strain (S) and strain rate (SR) imaging by echocardiography holds a big promise for early detection of myocardial remodeling associated with diabetes with good sensitivity and cost efficacy.

PATHOPHYSIOLOGY OF DIABETIC CARDIOMYOPATHY

In prediabetic and diabetic patients, subtle or overt myocardial dysfunction is observed even in absence of hypertension and coronary artery disease. Several mechanisms are proposed to explain the pathogenesis of diabetic cardiomyopathy.[1-15]

Hyperinsulinemia leads to sympathetic and renin angiotensin activation resulting in myocardial hypertrophy and dysfunction. The hyperglycemia associated with diabetes leads to advanced glycation products of myocardial and vascular interstitial molecules like collagen causing increased stiffness of left ventricular (LV) and aorta. The hypertriglyceridemia associated with diabetes leads to accumulation of fatty acids in the myocytes. There is altered substrate handling in the intracellular metabolism. The fatty acids are preferentially used for energy generation over glucose. There is intracellular accumulation of intermediate metabolites of nonoxidative metabolism of fatty acids like ceramide. These toxic metabolites cause cellular dysfunction by interfering with cellular signal pathways, myocardial calcium homeostasis, mitochondrial damage and lead to apoptosis. The hyperglycemic, hyperadrenergic and the systemic inflammatory environment associated with diabetes and the free oxygen radicles generation in the myocardium ultimately leads to cellular dysfunction, apoptosis and replacement fibrosis. Earlier in the natural course of diabetic cardiomyopathy, the ischemia due to diabetic microangiopathy and the metabolic damage of the myocytes affects the myocardial subendocardial region first.

DETECTION OF EARLY LEFT VENTRICULAR REMODELING IN SILENT PHASE OF DIABETIC CARDIOMYOPATHY

The speckle-tracking echocardiography (STE) detects the LV myocardial deformation in longitudinal, radial and circumferential direction in systole and diastole. Similarly, the STE can detect longitudinal myocardial deformation in the thin-walled chambers like left atrium (LA), right atrium (RA) and the right ventricle (RV). The ultrastructural changes in the myocardium associated with DM, as described earlier, lead to reduction and delaying of the myocardial deformation (strain) or rate of deformation (strain rate) in systole and diastole. Therefore, the S and SR imaging by STE is very useful to detect diabetic cardiomyopathy during its silent phase.

LEFT VENTRICULAR SYSTOLIC STRAIN/ STRAIN RATE DEFORMATION IN THREE DIMENSIONS IN DIABETES

Since the subendocardial fibers are affected at the earlier stage, the LV systolic global longitudinal strain (GLS) declines earliest in the progress of diabetic cardiomyopathy (Fig. 1). The fall in left ventricular global longitudinal strain (LV GLS) less than 18% is associated with higher LV end systolic volume and higher relative wall thickness at baseline and LV adverse remodeling in long-term follow-up.[16] The LV deformation in other directions and LV twist and torsion tries to compensate for the loss of longitudinal function. However, the diabetic cardiomyopathy eventually progresses to reduce the global radial strain (GRS) and global circumferential strain (GCS), global area strain (GAS) and LV torsion. The magnitude of reduction in LV GLS, GRS, GAS and GCS is directly proportional to the glycemic control as measured by HbA1c value. In a study[17] of 31 patients with HbA1c less than 7 and 37 patients with HbA1c greater than 7 and 63 matched controls, the three-dimensional (3-D) STE strain parameters were measured, and compared with the glycemic control. Patients with uncontrolled DM (HbA1c greater than 7) had decreased GLS, GCS, GAS, and GRS as compared with healthy controls and patients with controlled DM (HbA1c less than 7). GLS, GCS, GAS, and GRS values in uncontrolled DM compared with controls (16.2 ± 2.4 vs 19.1 ± 3.4, 16.2 ± 2.7 vs 18.5 ± 3.1, 28.8 ± 3.6 vs 32.9 ± 4.8, and 45.2 ± 8.3 vs 54.4 ± 11.3) respectively and in uncontrolled DM compared with controlled DM group (16.2 ± 2.4 vs 17.7 ± 2.6, 16.2 ± 2.7 vs 18.1 ± 2.9, 28.8 ± 3.6 vs 31.7 ± 4.5, and 45.2 ± 8.3 vs 51.5 ± 10.6) respectively. The level of HbA1c was independently associated with the values of GLS, GCS, and GAS. Compared to healthy controls, only GLS was reduced in the controlled DM patients while all the strain parameters like GLS, GCS, GAS, and GRS were reduced in uncontrolled DM.

In yet another study[18] the risk of clinical heart failure was 1.56 times in the patients with uncontrolled DM (HbA1c greater than10) compared to the patients with controlled DM (HbA1c less than 7). In a STE study[19] of 100 male subjects (47 with and 53 without DM) the LV GLS and LV systolic SR were significantly reduced as compared to controls. (LV GLS: DM patients –18.3 ± 2.2 vs control –19.9 ± 1.9, LV systolic SR: DM patients –0.99 ± 0.17 vs control –1.07 ± 0.13). However, the S and SR in circumferential and radial directions remained normal. In early diabetic cardiomyopathy, various segments of LV myocardium may reach peak longitudinal strain at different time intervals causing dispersion or dyssynchrony of strain curves (Fig. 2). The strain dispersion appears to be an earliest subclinical manifestation of diabetic cardiomyopathy as assessed by 3-D echocardiography. In a strain imaging study[20] 3-D STE strain dispersion was 46.5 ± 6.4 ms in patients with DM, 52.2 ± 7.9 ms in patients with DM and heart failure and 23.72 ± 1.45 ms in healthy control. Statistically, strain dispersion values in patients with DM and patients with DM and congestive cardiac failure (CCF) were not significantly different. Although, LV longitudinal

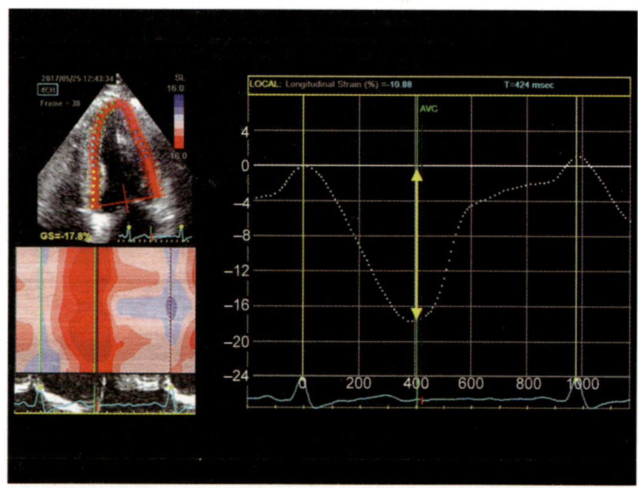

Fig. 1: LV global longitudinal systolic strain in an uncontrolled diabetic patient (yellow arrow) by speckle-tracking echocardiography

Abbreviations: GS, global strain; AVC, aortic valve calcification.

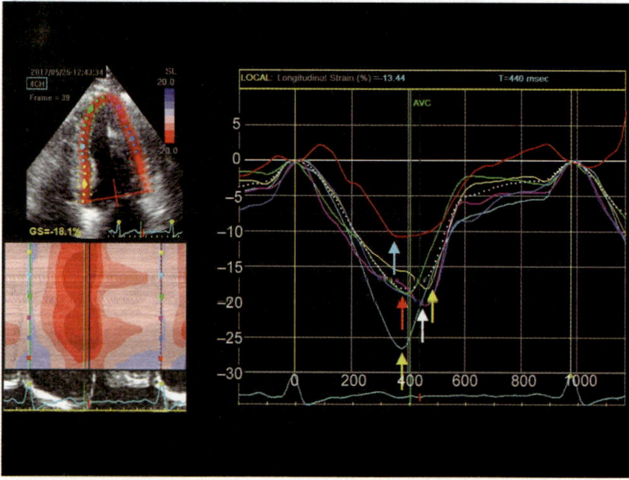

Fig. 2: LV strain dispersion. LV longitudinal strain curves by speckle-tracking echocardiography derived from 6 segments in 4-chamber view in an asymptomatic diabetic patient. The different strain curves reach peak values at different time intervals (multicolored arrows)

Abbreviations: GS, global strain; AVC, aortic valve calcification.

function reduces very early in diabetes, the LV radial function also gets affected later with the silent preclinical progress of diabetic cardiomyopathy. An imaging study[21] using STE evaluated both longitudinal and radial strain in 114 type 2 diabetic patients and 88 age-matched controls. In patients with DM compared to controls, the LV mid-wall fractional shortening (18% ± 3% vs 20% ± 3%), LV GLS (-19% ± 3% vs -22% ± 2%), and LV GRS (50% ± 16% vs 56% ± 12%) were significantly reduced. In another study[22] of 114 patients with type II DM and 88 age-matched healthy volunteers, only factors associated with a significant decrease in strain in the DM group were DM and male gender for GLS and only DM for GRS, suggesting that the S and SR are robust parameters.

The LV diastolic dysfunction indices like reduced mitral flow E/A, prolonged E deceleration time and isovolumic relaxation time and increased "E/e" are regarded as the hall mark of early diabetic cardiomyopathy and are seen in 47% diabetic patients without clinical heart disease.[23] The LV GLS and GRS are reduced in 32% and 38% of diabetic patients without clinical heart disease, respectively. However, GLS and GRS reduction is seen in 28% of patients with DM and normal diastolic function and in 35% of patients with DM and diastolic dysfunction. This underlines the fact that the LV systolic strain dysfunction precedes or occurs concurrently with diastolic dysfunction. In addition, the diastolic parameters are affected by age, rate pressure product, hypertension, and obesity while the systolic strain parameters are more reliable as they are affected only by glycemic control and gender. The intramyocyte accumulation of triglyceride (TG), called myocardial steatosis is presumed to be one of the causes of diabetic cardiomyopathy. A study[24] of 42 men with type 2 DM, directly correlated the intramyocardial TG content, measured by magnetic resonance spectroscopy (high TG greater than 0.76%, low TG less than 0.76%), with the STE-derived LV and RV systolic and diastolic S and SR. Patients with high TG content had greater reduction in LV myocardial strain and strain rate. (LV GLS: Low TG -19.3 (18.5–20.1), High TG -17.1 (16.3–17.7) ; LV Systolic SR: Low TG -1.02 (0.96–1.14) , High TG - 0.87 (0.82–0.98))

LEFT VENTRICULAR DIASTOLIC STRAIN/STRAIN RATE IN EARLY AND LATE DIASTOLE IN DIABETES

Diastolic dysfunction is considered as the hall mark of diabetic cardiomyopathy. In patients with DM, tissue Doppler and STE-derived LV early diastolic strain rate is decreased and the mitral E/e' is raised significantly suggesting impaired LV relaxation and elevation in mean LA pressure (Figs 3 and 4).

A study[25] of tissue Doppler-derived strain rate included 48 patients with impaired fasting glucose (IFG), 44 patients with both impaired fasting glucose and impaired glucose tolerance (IFG+IGT) and 48 patients with type 2 DM, and 60 age-matched healthy volunteers. The LV early diastolic strain rate was significantly reduced in IFG+IGT and DM compared to control. (IFG+IGT 1.77 ± 0.7, DM 1.68 ± 0.66, control 2.20 ± 0.73). Similarly, e' was reduced (IFG+IGT 6.9 ± 1.8, DM 6.9 ± 1.7, control 7.9 ± 1.8) and E/e' was elevated (IFG+IGT 11.1 ± 2.6, DM 11.5 ± 3, control 9.8 ± 2.2). However, all tissue Doppler SR and e' parameters were comparable in

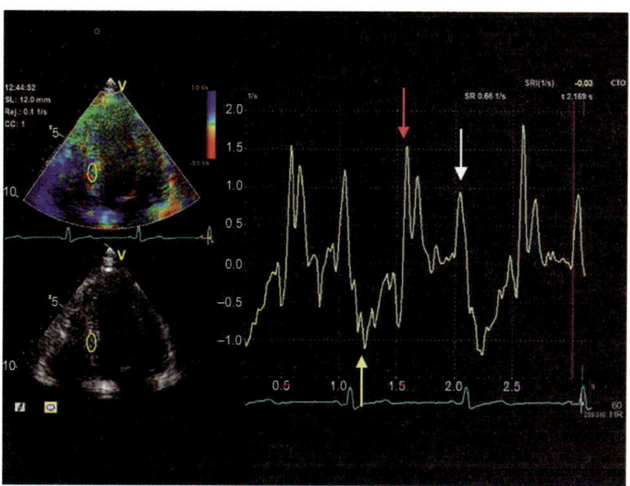

Fig. 3: LV strain rate in an asymptomatic diabetic patient derived from tissue Doppler imaging shows LV systolic strain rate (yellow arrow), LV early diastolic strain rate (red arrow), and LV late diastolic strain rate (white arrow)

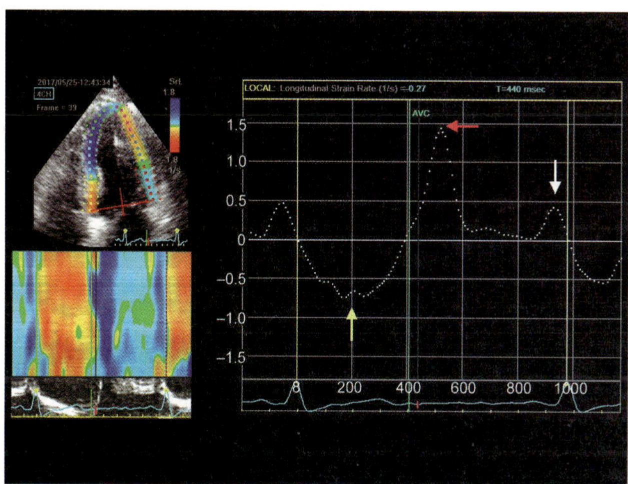

Fig. 4: LV strain rate in an asymptomatic diabetic patient derived from speckle-tracking echocardiography shows LV systolic strain rate (yellow arrow), LV early diastolic strain rate (red arrow) and LV late diastolic strain rate (white arrow)

Abbreviation: AVC, aortic valve calcification.

the IFG and control group. In a STE study[26] of 338 subjects stratified into lean (112), obese (121), and DM (105) groups, the presence of DM was strongly associated with LV early diastolic strain abnormalities beyond that predicted by CV risk factors alone. In the study[24] described earlier, correlating myocardial TG content with STE parameters, patients with high TG content had greater impairment of LV myocardial early diastolic SR compared to patients with low TG content. (LV early diastolic SR: Low TG 1.11 (1.05–1.23), High TG 0.93 (0.77–1.11).

LEFT VENTRICULAR APICAL ROTATIONAL FUNCTION IN DIABETES

In early diabetic cardiomyopathy, as the LV longitudinal function deteriorates progressively, the LV ejection function is preserved by compensatory increase in LV torsional function (LV apical twist per unit LV long axis length). In a study[27] of 33 asymptomatic Type 1 DM subjects and 32 age-matched healthy controls the LV torsion on STE and myocardial perfusion reserve (index of microangiopathy) on cardiac magnetic resonance imaging were directly compared. Peak LV torsion was significantly increased in the patients with Type 1 DM as compared to healthy controls (1.9 ± 0.6 vs 1.4 ± 0.7). A significant increase in LV torsion was identified in patients with longer duration of DM (2 ± 0.7/cm vs 1.4 ± 0.7/cm) and patients with diabetic retinopathy (1.9 ± 0.7/cm vs 1.4 ± 0.7/cm) as compared to healthy controls. Though LV torsion increases in DM, the LV untwisting rate goes down suggesting reduced LV elastic recoil and LV myocardial relaxation. In a study[28] of LV apical rotation by STE in 17 patients with DM, 16 patients with DM + hypertension (HT) and 20 patients with DM + HT + LV hypertrophy, the apical untwisting velocity reduced by 20% in all these groups compared to 12 normal subjects. The fall in untwisting velocity preceded the increase in E/e' ratio and LA volume suggesting that it is a marker of early diastolic dysfunction in DM.

LEFT VENTRICULAR DEFORMATION IN DIABETES AND ISCHEMIC HEART DISEASE

The impairment of LV strain in DM gets further aggravated in presence of ischemia due to epicardial coronary artery disease (CAD). FACTOR-64 study[29] was designed to evaluate the effect of computed tomography (CT) screening for CAD in asymptomatic diabetic patients on future cardiovascular events. A cohort of 82 consecutive patients was evaluated by STE for circumferential strain and early diastolic strain from LV short axis images. Abnormal strain was defined as circumferential strain less than 10%. About 35.9% of subjects with left main (LM) or multivessel disease (MVD) had abnormal strain compared to 11.6% of the subjects with nonsignificant or one vessel CAD. After adjusting for other variables, circumferential strain less than 10% predicted LM [odds ratio (OR)=8.6], and LM or MVD disease (OR=2.4). Diabetic patients with myocardial infarction (MI), show reduced circumferential strain not only in the infarcted segments but also in the remote segments due to subclinical diabetic cardiomyopathy, leading to adverse LV remodeling and heart failure. A cardiac MRI study[30] evaluated circumferential and longitudinal LV strains in 27 DM and 32 non-DM patients within one week of MI. DM patients had significantly reduced circumferential strain in nondiseased areas compared to nondiseased areas in non-DM patients. This explains higher incidence of post-MI heart failure in diabetic patients compared to nondiabetic patients.

LEFT ATRIUM STRAIN DURING RESERVOIR, CONDUIT AND BOOSTER FUNCTION IN DIABETES

The LA reservoir function, conduit function and LA booster pump function correlate with the LA peak positive atrial longitudinal strain (PALS) during ventricular systole, LA negative longitudinal strain during early ventricular diastole (ALS_{early}) and LA negative longitudinal strain during late ventricular diastole (ALS_{late}) respectively (Fig. 5). In early diabetic cardiomyopathy, the PALS, ALS_{early}, ALS_{late}, and the atrial SR during reservoir and conduit

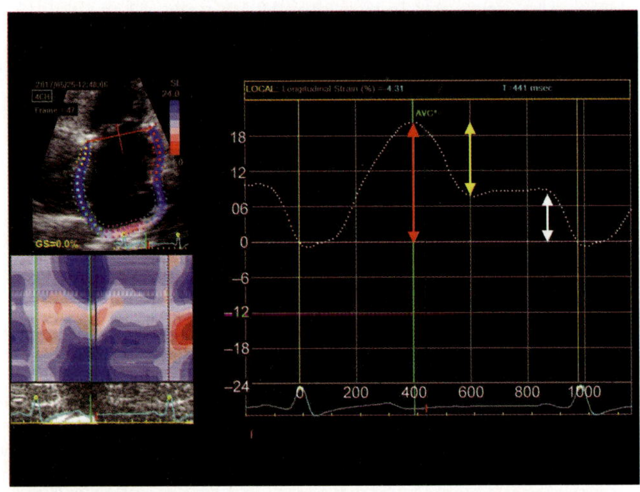

Fig. 5: LA strain curve by speckle-tracking echocardiography in an asymptomatic diabetic patient shows: 1) LA peak longitudinal strain (red arrow) corresponding to LA reservoir function, 2) LA early diastolic strain (yellow arrow) corresponding to LA conduit function, 3) LA late diastolic strain (white arrow) corresponding to LA booster pump function

Abbreviation: GS, global strain

function are uniformly reduced even before increase in the LA volume. A study[31] of S and SR evaluation of LA function by STE included 83 patients with hypertension, 34 patients with diabetes, and 38 patients with both diabetes and hypertension and 36 age-matched controls, with normal LA volumes. PALS was reduced in patients with hypertension (29.0 ± 6.5%) and patient with diabetes (24.7 ± 6.4%) and patients with diabetes and hypertension (18.3 ± 5.0%) compared to controls (39.6 ± 7.8%). Similar reduction was observed for ALS_{early} (controls, 19.1 ± 7.3%; patients with hypertension, 12.5 ± 6.1%; patients with diabetes, 8.8% ± 6.0%; patients with diabetes and hypertension, 5.2 ± 3.8%) and ALS_{late} (controls, 20.4 ± 5.0%; patients with hypertension, 16.6 ± 3.3%; patients with diabetes, 15.9% ± 3.5%; patients with diabetes and hypertension, 13.1 ± 3.1%). The time to PALS (percentage of RR interval) was prolonged in patients with diabetes and hypertension (controls, 44.5 ± 5.8%; patients with hypertension, 49.3 ± 9.1%; patients with diabetes, 51.2 ± 7.9%; patients with diabetes and hypertension, 53.7 ± 9.8%). In the same study, the strain rate for reservoir function ($ALSR_{syst}$) was reduced in patients with hypertension (1.0 ± 0.4 sec) and patients with diabetes (1.0 ± 0.4 sec) and in patients with diabetes and hypertension (0.6 ± 0.3 sec) compared with the controls (1.3 ± 0.5 sec). Similar reduction was observed for strain rate during LA conduit function ($ALSR_{early}$).(controls, 1.8 ± 0.7 sec; patients with hypertension, 1.3 ± 0.4 sec; patients with diabetes, 1.3 ± 0.3 sec; patients with diabetes and hypertension, 0.9 ± 0.4 sec). However, the strain rate during atrial systole was preserved in diabetic and hypertensive patients (Fig. 6).

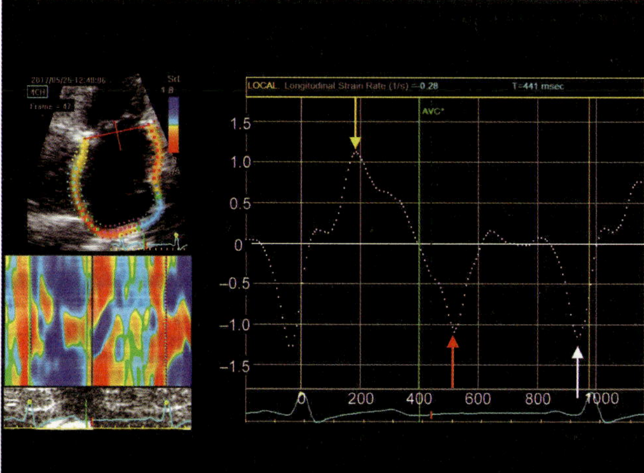

Fig. 6: LA strain rate in an asymptomatic diabetic patient derived from speckle-tracking echocardiography shows LA systolic strain rate (yellow arrow), LA early diastolic strain rate (red arrow), and LA late diastolic strain rate (white arrow)

Abbreviation: AVC, aortic valve calcification

RIGHT VENTRICULAR SYSTOLIC LONGITUDINAL DEFORMATION AND RIGHT ATRIUM RESERVOIR FUNCTION IN DIABETES

The deleterious effect of prediabetic or diabetic metabolic status reduces both RV and RA systolic and early diastolic function, in similar magnitude and direction, independent of LV function, but preserving the compensatory late diastolic atrial booster function. In a 2D and 3D strain and volume evaluation study[32] of RV and RA function 47 untreated normotensive subjects with prediabetes, 57 recently diagnosed normotensive patients with diabetes, and 54 healthy controls were included. There was no difference in 3D echocardiographic RV ejection fraction among the three groups. RV volumes assessed by 3D echocardiography progressively decreased from healthy subjects through patients with prediabetes to those with diabetes. In the same study RV and RA global strains and systolic, early diastolic strain rates were significantly decreased in patients with prediabetes and in those with DM compared with controls (RV strain: control -27 ± 5, prediabetic -25 ± 4, DM -24 ± 4; RA strain: control 43 ± 5, prediabetic 39 ± 4, DM 37 ± 4; RV systolic strain rate: control -1.73 ± 0.33, prediabetic -1.55 ± 0.27, DM 1.42 ± 0.33; RA systolic strain rate: control 2.05 ± 0.36, prediabetic 1.86 ± 0.32, DM 1.7 ± 0.29; RV early diastolic SR: control 1.83 ± 0.38, prediabetic 1.67 ± 0.35, DM 1.54 ± 0.32; RA early diastolic SR: control -2.13 ± 0.32, prediabetic -1.92 ± 0.28, DM -1.83 ± 0.25). However, RV and RA late diastolic strain rates were increased in prediabetic and DM patients probably as compensatory mechanism.

In the study[24] described earlier, correlating myocardial TG content with STE parameters, patients with high TG content had greater reduction of RV free wall myocardial systolic S and SR, and RV diastolic SR compared to patients with low TG content (Figs 7 and 8). [RV free wall systolic S: Low TG -27.7 (25.1–40.2) , High TG -24.5 (19.0–27.7); RV free wall systolic SR: Low TG -2.11 (1.77–2.46), High TG -1.74 (1.44–1.85); RV free wall early diastolic SR: Low TG 2.10 (1.75-2.61), High TG 1.65 (1.12–1.86)].

CONCLUSION

In diabetic and prediabetic patients, the ventricular and atrial myocardial mechanics are altered very early in the disease process. This subtle myocardial dysfunction can be detected by strain and strain rate imaging using speckle-tracking echocardiography. The STE is a robust technique to detect early silent diabetic cardiomyopathy, before it progresses to clinical heart failure syndrome. This imaging technique gives us a window of opportunity to institute preventive pharmacotherapy.

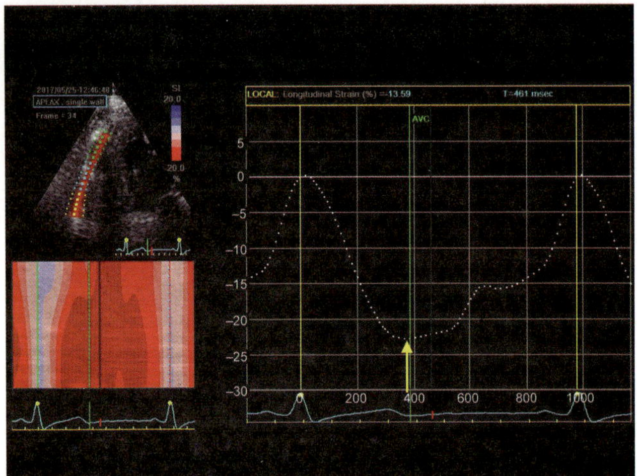

Fig. 7: RV free wall longitudinal systolic strain in an uncontrolled diabetic patient (yellow arrow) by speckle-tracking echocardiography

Abbreviation: AVC, aortic valve calcification

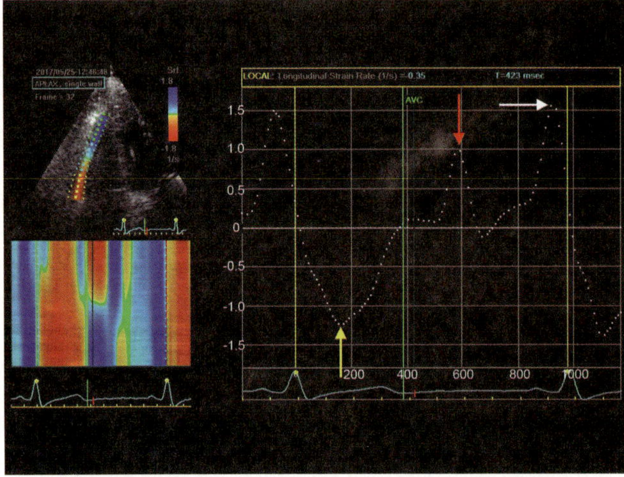

Fig. 8: RV free wall strain rate in an asymptomatic diabetic patient derived from speckle-tracking echocardiography shows RV systolic strain rate (yellow arrow), RV early diastolic strain rate (red arrow) and RV late diastolic strain rate (white arrow)

Abbreviation: AVC, aortic valve calcification

REFERENCES

1. Rodrigues B, Cam MC, McNeill JH. Metabolic disturbances in diabetic cardiomyopathy. Mol Cell Biochem. 1998;180(1-2):53-7.
2. Mizushige K, Yao L, Noma T, et al. Alteration in left ventricular diastolic filling and accumulation of myocardial collagen at insulin-resistant prediabetic stage of a type II diabetic rat model. Circulation. 2000;101(8):899-907.
3. van Hoeven K, Factor SM. A comparison of the pathological spectrum of hypertensive, diabetic, and hypertensive-diabetic heart disease. Circulation. 1990;82(3):848-55.
4. Frustaci A, Kajstura J, Chimenti C, et al. Myocardial cell death in human diabetes. Circ Res. 2000;87(12):1123-32.
5. Cai L, Wang Y, Zhou G, et al. Attenuation by metallothionein of early cardiac cell death via suppression of mitochondrial oxidative stress results in a prevention of diabetic cardiomyopathy. J Am Coll Cardiol. 2006;48(8):1688-97.
6. Taegtmeyer H, McNulty P, Young ME. Adaptation and maladaptation of the heart in diabetes, part I. Circulation. 2002;105:1727-33.
7. An D, Rodrigues B. Role of changes in cardiac metabolism in development of diabetic cardiomyopathy. Am J Physiol Heart Circ Physiol. 2006;291(4): H1489-506.
8. Candido R, Forbes JM, Thomas MC, et al. A breaker of advanced glycation end products attenuates diabetes-induced myocardial structural changes. Circ Res. 2003;92(7):785-92.
9. Cai L, Li W, Wang G, et al. Hyperglycemia-induced apoptosis in mouse myocardium: mitochondrial cytochrome C-mediated caspase-3 activation pathway. Diabetes. 2002;51(6):1938-48.
10. Bojunga J, Nowak D, Mitrou PS, et al. Antioxidative treatment prevents activation of death-receptor- and mitochondrion-dependent apoptosis in the hearts of diabetic rats. Diabetologia 2004;47(12):2072-80.
11. Holmang A, Yoshida N, Jennische E, et al. The effects of hyperinsulinaemia on myocardial mass, blood pressure regulation and central haemodynamics in rats. Eur J Clin Invest. 1996; 26(11):973-8.
12. Anderson EA, Hoffman RP, Balon TW, et al. Hyperinsulinemia produces both sympathetic neural activation and vasodilation in normal humans. J Clin Invest. 1991;87:2246-52.
13. Ingelsson E, Sundstrom J, Arnlov J, et al. Insulin resistance and risk of congestive heart failure. JAMA. 2005;294(3):334-41.
14. Kern W, Peters A, Born J, et al. Changes in blood pressure and plasma catecholamine levels during prolonged hyperinsulinemia. Metabolism. 2005;54(3):391-6.
15. Tarquini R, Lazzeri C, Pala L, et al. The diabetic cardiomyopathy. Acta Diabetol. 2011;48(3):173-81.
16. Ernande L, Bergerot C, Girerd N, et al. Longitudinal myocardial strain alteration is associated with left ventricular remodeling in asymptomatic patients with type 2 diabetes mellitus. J Am Soc Echocardiogr. 2014;27(5):479-88.
17. Zhang X, Wei X, Liang Y, et al. Differential changes of left ventricular myocardial deformation in diabetic patients with controlled and uncontrolled blood glucose: a three-dimensional speckle-tracking echocardiography based study. J Am Soc Echocardiogr. 2013;26(5):499-506.
18. Iribarren C, Karter AJ, Go AS, et al. Glycemic control and heart failure among adult patients with diabetes. Circulation. 2001;103(22):2668-73.
19. Ng AC, Delgado V, van der Meer RW, et al. Left ventricular strain and strain rate imaging in asymptomatic patients with type 2 diabetes mellitus. Circulation. 2009;120:S328.
20. Upton R, Levelt E, Gamble J, et al. Strain dispersion is an early subclinical manifestation of diabetic cardiomyopathy assessed by 3D echocardiography. Circulation. 2014;130:A12183.
21. Ernande L, Rietzschel ER, Bergerot C, et al. Impaired myocardial radial function in asymptomatic patients with type 2 diabetes mellitus: a speckle-Tracking Imaging Study. J Am Soc Echocardiogr. 2010;23:1266-72.
22. Ernande L, Bergerot C, Rietzschel ER, et al. Speckle Tracking Imaging Detects Sub-Clinical Myocardial Dysfunction in Asymptomatic Patients with Type 2 Diabetes Mellitus. Circulation. 2008;118:S_851.
23. Ernande L, Bergerot C, Rietzschel ER, et al. Diastolic Dysfunction in Patients with Type 2 Diabetes Mellitus: Is It Really the First Marker of Diabetic Cardiomyopathy? J Am Soc Echocardiogr. 2011;24:1268-75.
24. Ng AC, Delgado V, Bertini M, et al. Myocardial Steatosis and Biventricular Strain and Strain Rate Imaging in Patients With Type 2 Diabetes Mellitus. Circulation. 2010;122(24):2538-44.
25. Ceyhan K, Kadi H, Koc F, et al. Longitudinal left ventricular function in normotensive prediabetics: a tissue doppler and strain/strain rate echocardiography study. J Am Soc Echocardiogr. 2012;25(3):349-56.

26. Madsen NL, Khoury PR, Gao Z, et al. Abnormalities in cardiac strain are found in young adults with type 2 diabetes mellitus. circulation. 2014;130:A13187.
27. Shivu GN, Phan T, Abozguia K, et al. The Role of Coronary Microvascular Function and Rotational Deformation Delay in the Development of Increased Left Ventricular Torsion in Uncomplicated Type 1 Diabetes. Circulation. 2009;120:S758.
28. Zhao W, Li P, Hong G, et al. Torsional and Reverse Rotational Mechanics of the Left Ventricular Apex Is Abnormal in Patients with Type 2 Diabetes Mellitus Independent of Presence of Hypertension, Left Ventricular Hypertrophy, Elevated Filling Pressures and Left Atrial Volume. Circulation. 2007;116:II_548.
29. Rosen B, Horton KD, Balling KD, et al. Lower Global Strain Predicts Left Main and Multi-Vessel Coronary Artery Disease in Asymptomatic Diabetic Patients. Factor 64 Study. Circulation. 2012;126:A10852.
30. Seibert AM, Gladden JD, Butler M, et al. Diseased Myocardial Segments Following Myocardial Infarction in Patients With Type-2 Diabetes Mellitus. Circulation. 2009;120:S762.
31. Mondillo S, Cameli M, Caputo ML, et al. Early detection of left atrial strain abnormalities by speckle-tracking in hypertensive and diabetic patients with normal left atrial size. J Am Soc Echocardiogr. 2011;24(8):898–908.
32. Tadic M, Celic V, Cuspidi C, et al. Right heart mechanics in untreated normotensive patients with prediabetes and type 2 diabetes mellitus: a two- and three-dimensional echocardiographic study. J Am Soc Echocardiogr. 2015;28:317–27.

Dobutamine Stress Echo for Coronary Artery Disease Evaluation in Diabetics

Naveen Garg, KK Kapur

INTRODUCTION

World Health Organization (WHO) had projected that by 2030 more than 439 million adults will have diabetes. However, considering the increasing rate of prevalence (4.7% in 1980 to 8.5% in 2014—measuring 422 million in 2014), this figure is likely to be an underestimate. In epidemiological terms, diabetes is potentially devastatingly lethal disease with approximately 1.5 million deaths every year being attributed to this condition. Cardiovascular complications account for a vast majority of these deaths. As per the WHO data, diabetes is projected to be one of the leading causes of deaths after by 2030 [after myocardial infarction (MI), stroke, and cancer].[1,2] Increase in the prevalence of diabetes has been observed mainly in middle and low-income countries and India is considered to be "diabetic capital of the world", harboring about one-fourth of world diabetics populations (50 million vs 200 million).[3]

A large body of epidemiological and pathological data documents that diabetes is an independent risk factor for cardiovascular disease (CVD) in both men and women. Patients with diabetes have two to four times increased risk of having coronary artery disease (CAD), ischemic stroke, and other associated vascular events. Owing to higher mortality (about 1.5–3.6 times) than in nondiabetics, the expected life expectancy in diabetics is reduced by about 4–8 years.[4-6] Because of its earlier onset, type 1 diabetes leads to cardiovascular complications at a relatively younger age (3rd–4th decades) than in type 2 diabetes, where these complications occur by 4th–6th decades. Diabetic patients have a higher prevalence of silent myocardial ischemia and thus are more likely to have atypical presentations or remain undiagnosed. In premenopausal (estrogen positive) diabetic women, the hormonal protection is largely lost and these women has the same cardiovascular risk as their male counterparts, (relative risk of 2.5 vs 1.85 of men).[7-9]

Owing to this high prevalence of CVD in diabetics and silent myocardial ischemia, it is imperative that an early diagnosis of CAD is made in these patients, so that secondary prevention and treatment interventions can be instituted.

CORONARY ARTERIES IN DIABETIC PATIENTS

In diabetics, the coronary arteries and their branches have been shown to have smaller diameters than in normal subjects. The CAD in diabetic patients is more severe, extensive, diffuse, and rapidly progressive. These types of coronary lesions usually have an unfavorable angiographic anatomy thus limiting the possibility of achieving a complete revascularization. The higher prevalence of complex coronary lesions, such as multivessel, multilesion, extensive, small vessel involvement, higher incidence of left main stem disease, and complex type C lesions may explain the poor prognosis of CAD in diabetic patients. The reasons for this trend are because patients with diabetes have a greater burden of progressively increasing atherosclerotic disease, and exaggerated neointimal hyperplasia.[10,11]

TABLE 1: Cardiovascular risk factors associated with diabetes

Traditional	*Nontraditional*
• Hypertension	• Insulin resistance
• Dyslipidemia	• Hyperglycemia
• Obesity	• Wide glucose fluctuations
• Sedentary lifestyle	• Microalbuminuria
• Smoking	• C-reactive protein
	• Thrombogenic factors
	• Erectile dysfunction
	• Hematological factors
	• Genetics

Diabetes mellitus (DM) (especially type 2) is associated with a host of traditional and nontraditional other cardiovascular risk factors which promote the development of CAD. These risk factors have been summarized in Table 1.

DIABETIC CARDIOMYOPATHY

Diabetic cardiomyopathy (DbCM)[12-14] was first described by Rubler et al.[15] in 1972 based on autopsy data on four diabetic patients with congestive heart failure and normal coronary arteries.[16] This entity could be defined as myocardial dysfunction occurring in diabetic patients in the absence of CAD, hypertension, or valvular heart disease. The reported prevalence of DbCM is variable depending upon the patient selection criteria as well as the imaging modalities utilized in evaluating diabetic patients (systolic and diastolic function have been reported in 30–60% of diabetic patients). Furthermore, the presence of microvascular CAD with normal epicardial coronaries as well as associated cardiac autonomic neuropathy interacts with hyperglycemia-induced myocardial dysfunction. The general consensus among experts is that metabolic abnormalities including chronic hyperglycemia, hyperlipidemia, and inflammation play a pivotal role in the etiopathogenesis of DbCM (Table 2).

Combined Diabetic Cardiomyopathy with Hypertension and Coronary Artery Disease

Although DbCM is diagnosed by exclusion of CAD and hypertension, it is likely to be associated with latter two entities in many patients. A combination of these conditions could result in rapid progression and heart failure. This association is very likely because 50–80% patients with type 2 diabetes and a smaller percentage (30%) of type 1 diabetes have coexisting hypertension. Moreover about 60% of patients have CAD.[17-22]

Cardiac Remodeling in Diabetic Cardiomyopathy

As a result of structural abnormalities in the myocardium different modes of remodeling can occur in patients with DbCM. In patients with predominantly left ventricular hypertrophy (LVH) and diastolic dysfunction (DD) there is concentric remodeling with maintained LV size, LV ejection fraction (LVEF) with increased filling pressures, and left atrial (LA) dimensions. In some patients there is eccentric remodeling (LV dilatation as well as hypertrophy) with reduced LVEF as well as elevated filling pressures. Eccentric remodeling can occur subsequent to concentric remodeling and therefore represents a more advanced myocardial involvement in patients with DbCM together with associated CAD and hypertension. However, less commonly eccentric remodeling can occur independently.[23-28] *The earlier changes in DbCM are depicted in Figure 1.*

Diabetic Cardiomyopathy in Type 1 versus Type 2 Diabetes Mellitus

Diabetic cardiomyopathy as classically described in the literature occurs in type 2 diabetes (usually associated with hyperlipidemia, hyperinsulinemia, and insulin resistance). The hyperinsulinemia promotes cardiac myocyte hypertrophy and myocardial fibrosis. In addition there is impairment of myocardial flow reserve which may be due to perivascular and interstitial fibrosis as well as endothelial dysfunction.[29]

The association of DbCM in type 1 DM is less well established. Data from Swedish Diabetes national registry[30,31] show that heart failures (HFs) per 1,000 patient years (pt-year) in type 1 DM shows an inverse relationship with the glycemic control. For every 1% increase of hemoglobin A1c (HbA1c) there is 30% increase in risk of HF. Wilhelmsen L et al.[32] had shown that incidence of HF in men with type 1 DM of age group of 40–45 years DM type 1 was 2.4 per 1,000 pt-year and similar to the risk of HF in

TABLE 2: Risk factors for diabetic cardiomyopathy

Hyperglycemia	*IR*	*Lipotoxicity*	*Obesity*	*CAN*	*RAS*	*AGEs*	*ROS*	*ED*	*Genetic*

Abbreviations: AGEs, advanced glycation end products; CAN, cardiac autonomic neuropathy; ED, endothelial dysfunction; IR, insulin resistance; RAS, renin-angiotensin system; ROS, reactive oxygen species.

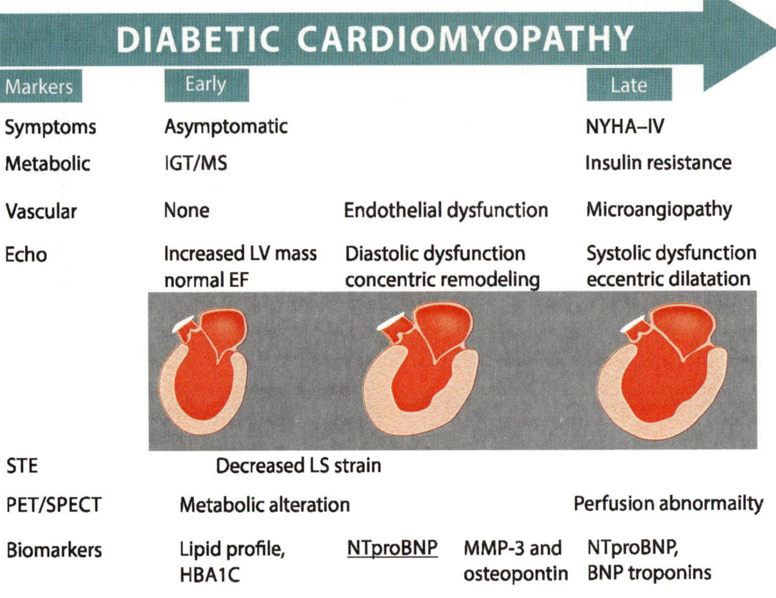

Fig. 1: Diabetic cardiomyopathy in time line

Abbreviations: HBA1c, hemoglobin A1c; EF, ejection fraction; IGT, impaired glucose tolerance; LV, left ventricular; MS, metabolic syndrome; MMP-3, metalloproteinase 3; NTproBNP, N-terminal prohormone of B-type natriuretic peptide; PET/SPECT, positron emission tomography/single-photon emission computed tomography; STE, speckle tracking echocardiography

no diabetics who are in age group of 55–65 years (15 years older than type 1 DM).[33]

Several studies using transmitral Doppler and tissue Doppler have shown that diastolic dysfunction in type 1 DM occurs several decade earlier than in the healthy controls.[34-36]

However, a few studies have shown that in metabolically well-controlled patients with long-standing type 1DM have similar echocardiographic and Doppler parameters as compared to the age-matched healthy control group. This could indicate that appropriate treatment with insulin could normalize the metabolically derangements induced by insulin deficiency and thus prevent impairment of myocardial dysfunction. In general, DD in type 1 DM is more likely to be due to coexisting hypertension, CAD, autonomic dysfunction, and microangiopathy rather than due to direct diabetic involvement of myocardium (which usually occurs in type 2 DM).[37,38]

NONINVASIVE TESTS IN DIABETICS FOR CORONARY ARTERY DISEASE (WHICH TESTS)

The exercise stress testing has been a time honored tool for risk stratification in asymptomatic and symptomatic diabetes patients. Some of widely used noninvasive tests are of following:

- *Exercise electrocardiogram test (treadmill test)*—Treadmill and bicycle testing is used as first-line test in the assessment of future cardiac events in ambulatory patients. These tests are useful to identify the ECG changes during exercise. Exercise-induced ischemic ST-T changes help in diagnosing and stratifying CAD in both symptomatic and asymptomatic diabetics. However, these tests lack sensitivity and specificity and are highly dependent on patient's capacity to exercise to the point ischemia.
  However, exercise stress test is limited by the presence of preexisting ST-T changes in ECG, bundle branch blocks, drugs usage (digoxin, beta-blockers, and calcium channel-blockers), and could be nondiagnostic in female population. Its sensitivity is lower than imaging stress modalities and it also does not accurately localize the site and extent of ischemia and thus the need for revascularization.[39-41]
- *Exercise echocardiographic testing:* Stress echocardiography is a well-established imaging modality to evaluate wall motion abnormality for the purpose of diagnosing and risk stratification of CAD. Exercise stress echocardiography has a superior diagnostic accuracy as compared to standard stress ECG. Moreover this test provides incremental prognostic information as compared to clinical and exercise ECG variables. Many studies had shown that diabetics are at higher risk of cardiac events than nondiabetics.[42,43]
  Abdou Elhendy et al.[44,45] performed ex-echocardiography study on 563 diabetic patients follow-up for a median of 3 years, were assessed for new or worsening wall motion

abnormality. Cardiac events occurred in 50 patients (cardiac death in 23 and nonfatal MI in 27). The event rate was significantly lower in patients who had normal exercise echocardiograms compared to those with abnormal exercise echocardiogram at 1 year (0% vs 1.9%), at 3 years (1.8% vs 11.9%), and at 5 years (7.6% vs 23.3%), respectively.

- *Pharmacological stress echocardiography:* Pharmacologic stress testing is generally instituted when there are contraindications to exercise stress test or when the patient is unable to exercise because of debilitating conditions. The following includes general indications to pharmacological stress testing: Elderly patients with decreased functional capacity, patients with chronic debilitation, younger patients with functional impairment due to injury, orthopedic, vascular, or neurological problems, and unstable angina. In other words any physical limitation that prevents a patient from exercising maximally is an indication for pharmacological stress testing.
- *Myocardial perfusion imaging test*: Two types of noninvasive, nonechocardiographic nuclear techniques are currently used to evaluating occlusive CAD either by detecting regional myocardial hypoperfusion [perfusion heterogeneity/perfusion defect single-photon emission computed tomography (SPECT)] or by assessing myocardial metabolism during hypoperfusion [positron emission tomography (PET)]. An inducible perfusion abnormality indicates decreased coronary flow reserve that usually implies obstruction in the corresponding epicardial artery.

  The overall sensitivity, specificity, and diagnostic accuracy of myocardial nuclear perfusion imaging are quite similar to that of exercise echocardiography although costly but are less operator dependent.[46-48]

  In a large cohort study by Rory Hachamovitch et al.[49] evaluated 7,376 consecutive patients with normal exercise or adenosine myocardial perfusion imaging (MPI)-SPECT and concluded that the "warranty period" of a normal scan may be limited to only 2 years in high-risk diabetic patients.
- *Calcium scoring computed tomography scan:* Coronary calcium scoring involves estimation of calcium deposition in the medial layers of coronary arteries. This deposition tends to increase with age as well as with the degree of atherosclerosis. Several studies had indicated that the extent of coronary calcium (or calcium score) could predict the probability of CAD and to some extent the degree of coronary artery narrowing. However, there have been no observational or randomized studies particularly for diabetic patients. Therefore, routine use of calcium scoring in symptomatic or asymptomatic diabetic patients for the assessment of CAD is controversial and probably of no incremental benefit.[49-56]

VARIOUS GROUP OF PATIENTS TO BE INVESTIGATED BY STRESS ECHOCARDIOGRAPHY (BOTH EXERCISE OR PHARMACOLOGICAL)

Diabetic patients may be grouped into:

- Asymptomatic without cardiovascular risk factors
- Asymptomatic with cardiovascular risk factors
- Symptomatic with no prior revascularization [after acute coronary syndrome (ACS)]
- Diabetics after revascularization.

Asymptomatic without Cardiovascular Risk Factors

Some of the earlier studies [DECODE, Detection of Ischemia in Asymptomatic Diabetics (DIAD)] suggest that hyperglycemia independently increases the risk for cardiac mortality and nonfatal cardiac events in diabetes and prediabetes (DECODE trial) and that many asymptomatic diabetic patients with no risk factors could have occult CAD. In addition the DIAD study revealed that approximately 22% of diabetic patients (aged 50–75 years) have silent MIs. Thus, both the type 1 and type 2 diabetes are both considered as coronary risk equivalent.[57-59]

The general consensus is that asymptomatic diabetic patients have at least an intermediate probability of CAD, a prevalence that may justify screening by noninvasive testing including stress echocardiography (The NECP-ATPIII 2001 guidelines).[60] However, subsequent large epidemiological studies[61-63] over a long follow-up period has shown cardiac event risk was much lower in diabetics without CAD than in patients with CAD without diabetes.

Therefore, the ADA in its latest recommendation (2013) states that "in asymptomatic patients, routine screening for CAD is not recommended as it does not improve outcomes as long as atherosclerotic cardiovascular disease risk factors are treated" evidence level-A.[64]

Asymptomatic with Cardiovascular Risk Factors

In asymptomatic diabetic patients without overt evidence of CAD, certain clinical features and risk factors could indicate a high likelihood of cardiac involvement. These features (clinical, electrocardiographic, and biochemical) and as well as presence of cardiac risk factors include:[65]

High-risk Asymptomatic Diabetics that must be Screened for Coronary Artery Disease

(1) Typical or atypical cardiac symptoms, (2) Resting electrocardiograph suggestive of ischemia or infarction,

(3) Peripheral or carotid occlusive arterial disease, (4) Sedentary lifestyle, age more than 35 years, and plans to begin a vigorous exercise program, and (5) Two or more of the risk factors listed here (A to E) in addition to diabetes.

(A) Total cholesterol more than 240 mg/dL, low-density lipoprotein (LDL) cholesterol more than 160 mg/dL, or high-density lipoprotein (HDL) cholesterol less than 35 mg/dL, (B) Blood pressure more than 140/90 mm Hg, (C) Smoking, (D) Family history of premature CAD, and (E) Positive micro/macroalbuminuria test.

The European Society of Cardiology (ESC) gives the following appropriate guidelines that are given in Table 3.[66]

Symptomatic Patients with no Revascularization (after Acute Coronary Syndrome)

Diabetic patients who had experienced myocardial damage (after ACS and have breathlessness, or angina on exertion) have a high probability of underlying CAD and thus these patients should be subjected to stress echocardiography. This facilitates risk assessment for subsequent cardiac events and helps to plan further management (interventional vs optimum medical therapy). The goals of the noninvasive evaluation after ACS include an assessment of: (1) LV systolic function, (2) The presence of multivessel CAD, (3) The presence or absence of provocable ischemia and myocardial viability, and (4) The risk of reinfarction and death.

In an elegant study, Ming-Jui Hung et al. determined the prognostic value of dobutamine stress echocardiography (DSE) in diabetic (116) and nondiabetic patients (222), who had known acute myocardial infarctions (AMIs) and were not revascularized. Over a mean follow-up of 21 ± 9 months for hard events, the authors concluded "in diabetics, prognostic value of positive DSE test in predicting future cardiovascular events was high but not as good as in nondiabetic patients". Diabetics with very high future cardiac events had very short dobutamine induced ischemia time (time from the infusion of dobutamine to the development of obvious abnormality).[67,68]

Satyendra Giri et al. in their large multicenter study followed a large cohort of symptomatic diabetics who underwent SPECT-MPI for a period of 2.5 ± 1.5 years. This study concluded that stress imaging could independently stratify symptomatic diabetics and the so called warranty period after a negative test was only 2 years.[69,70]

Jors N Van Der Sijde et al. in a landmark prospective study with 13-years follow-up of diabetic population which also included patients with history of MI, concluded that DSE provided optimal risk stratification up to 7 years after initial testing (the so called warranty period). However, this population comprised low-risk category of patients (<1% annual chance of cardiac events).[71]

TABLE 3: ESC guidelines: Cardiovascular risk assessment in diabetes—2012

Recommendations	Class of recommendation	Level of evidence
It should be considered to classify patients with DM as at very high or high risk for CVD depending on the presence of concomitant risk factor and target organ damage	IIa	C
It is not recommended to assess the risk for CVD in patients with DM based on risk scores developed for the general population	III	C
It is indicated to estimate the urinary albumin excretion rate when performing risk stratification in patients with diabetes	I	B
Screening for silent myocardial ischemia may be considered in selected high-risk patients with DM	IIb	C

Abbreviations: CVD, cardiovascular disease; ESC, European Society of Cardiology; DM, diabetes mellitus

Diabetics after Revascularization

Several angiographic-based studies have confirmed a high degree of restenosis rate in asymptomatic patients after single vessel or multivessel stenting. The restenosis rate in these studies was higher in diabetics versus nondiabetics (BARI study—35% in nondiabetic vs 61% in insulin-dependent diabetics).[72,73] Similar results were also observed in another study which showed that in nonrandomized patients after revascularization the restenosis rate after type 1, type 2, and nondiabetics were 35% versus 25% versus 16%, respectively.[74] Therefore, it is reasonable to conclude that stress echocardiographic studies would be useful in detecting myocardial ischemia as well as regional and global systolic LV function in these patients. However, there is paucity of data on the routine use of stress echocardiography in diabetic and nondiabetic population after revascularization.[75,76]

Some studies have used stress SPECT-MPI after myocardial revascularization in asymptomatic diabetic and nondiabetic patients and had concluded a significant number of patients with positive test despite absence of any symptom.[77]

However, none of these studies have directly compared diabetic patients versus nondiabetic patients, both as regards stress test positivity as well as cardiovascular events.

The overall take away message from all earlier studies is that so called warranty period in asymptomatic diabetic patients after revascularization is approximately 2–3 years. Thus, in our opinion stress echocardiography either exercise or pharmacological should be performed in all asymptomatic diabetic patients after revascularization within 2–5 years. However, good prospective randomized studies are required to document our opinion.

PHARMACOLOGICAL STRESS ECHOCARDIOGRAPHY PROTOCOL

Instituting pharmacological agent as a stressor in symptomatic patients is useful alternative in whom there are contraindications to exercise echocardiography.[78]

The commonly used pharmacological stressors for detecting myocardial perfusion and/or contractile dysfunction are dipyridamole, adenosine, and dobutamine.

These can be classified as:

- *Inotropic stressors*—such as dobutamine, cause an increase in myocardial oxygen demand.
- *Vasodilator stressors*—e.g. dipyridamole, adenosine, and regadenoson, acts by causing perfusion heterogeneity (coronary steal phenomenon).
- *Inodilators stressors*—e.g. enoximone, cause both inotropic and vasodilatory stress.

These agents are infused in staged incremental dose protocol so as to increase the heart rate to target levels. During this infusion echocardiography is performed to assess global and regional LV systolic function and to detect any resting or induced wall motion abnormalities. Wall motion scoring is performed as shown here in Table 4.

Wall motion score index (WMSI) is derived as a ratio of the total wall motion score to the number of visualized LV segments. The results are interpretation as shown in Table 5.[78]

TABLE 4: Wall motion scoring

1	Normal
2	Hypokinesis
3	Akinesis
4	Dyskinesis
5	Aneurysmal

TABLE 5: Interpretation of results of pharmacological stress echocardiography

Rest	Low dose	High dose	Interpretation	Intervention
N	N	N	No coronary artery disease (CAD)	None
N	H	H	CAD	Revascularization
H	N	N	No CAD	None
H	N	H	CAD	Revascularization
A	D	D	Scarred myocardium No intervention needed	
D	A	A		

PHARMACOLOGICAL STRESSORS

Dobutamine

Dobutamine is a synthetic catecholamine, with strong inotropic (increases contractility), good chronotropic agent (increases heart rate) as well as a powerful vasodilator of the systemic arterial circulation. Therefore, it acts primarily by increasing the myocardial oxygen demand and thus leads to significant ischemia if coronary blood flow is impaired. A standard well-equipped DSE laboratory with infusion and resuscitative facilities also requires a well-trained support staff together with an expert echocardiographer.

The patient is advised for at least 4 hours of fasting and should be "off" β-blockers and nitrates. Patient should lie in a left lateral decubitus position and ECG electrodes appropriately placed. After digital acquisition of baseline echocardiogram using DSE package, dobutamine infusion is started and acquisitions of various corresponding echo planes (PLAX, SAX, AP-4C, AP-2C, and AP-long axis) is performed at low dose, high dose, and recovery. Simultaneous with the dobutamine infusion, handgrip exercise is also instituted which further helps in attaining the target heart rates and at a relatively lower infusion rates.

The standard dobutamine infusion protocol involves a graded increase in dobutamine dose beginning at ultra-low dose of 2.5 μg/kg/min (for viability assessment) and then increased at 3 minutes intervals to 20 μg/kg/min (low-dose infusion) and then at intervals of 3 minutes up to 30–40 μg/kg/min (high-dose study for inducing ischemia). Accelerated protocols using 2 minutes staged protocols of 10, 20, 30, and 40 μg/kg/min can also be used in laboratories having a high work load burden.

Small bolus doses of atropine of 0.2 mg are used if the required target heart rate is not attained despite high-dose dobutamine infusion.

The various parameters to assess the LV wall motion and global as well as regional systolic function include resting and stress wall motion score index, percentage of normal myocardium, LVEF, number of ischemic segments as well as total number of abnormal segments (Figs 2A to D). On low-dose dobutamine echo, the prime objective is to assess viable myocardium which is potentially salvageable with revascularization.

The low-dose DSE is useful to assess for viable myocardium which can be salvaged after revascularization. On DSE the dysfunctional myocardium can be categorised as:

- *Viable—if it exhibits increased contractility (systolic thickening) at low-dose dobutamine when compared to the resting.*
- *Viable and ischemic—if it demonstrate increased contractility at low dose and followed by reduced contractility at high dose. This response is also termed*

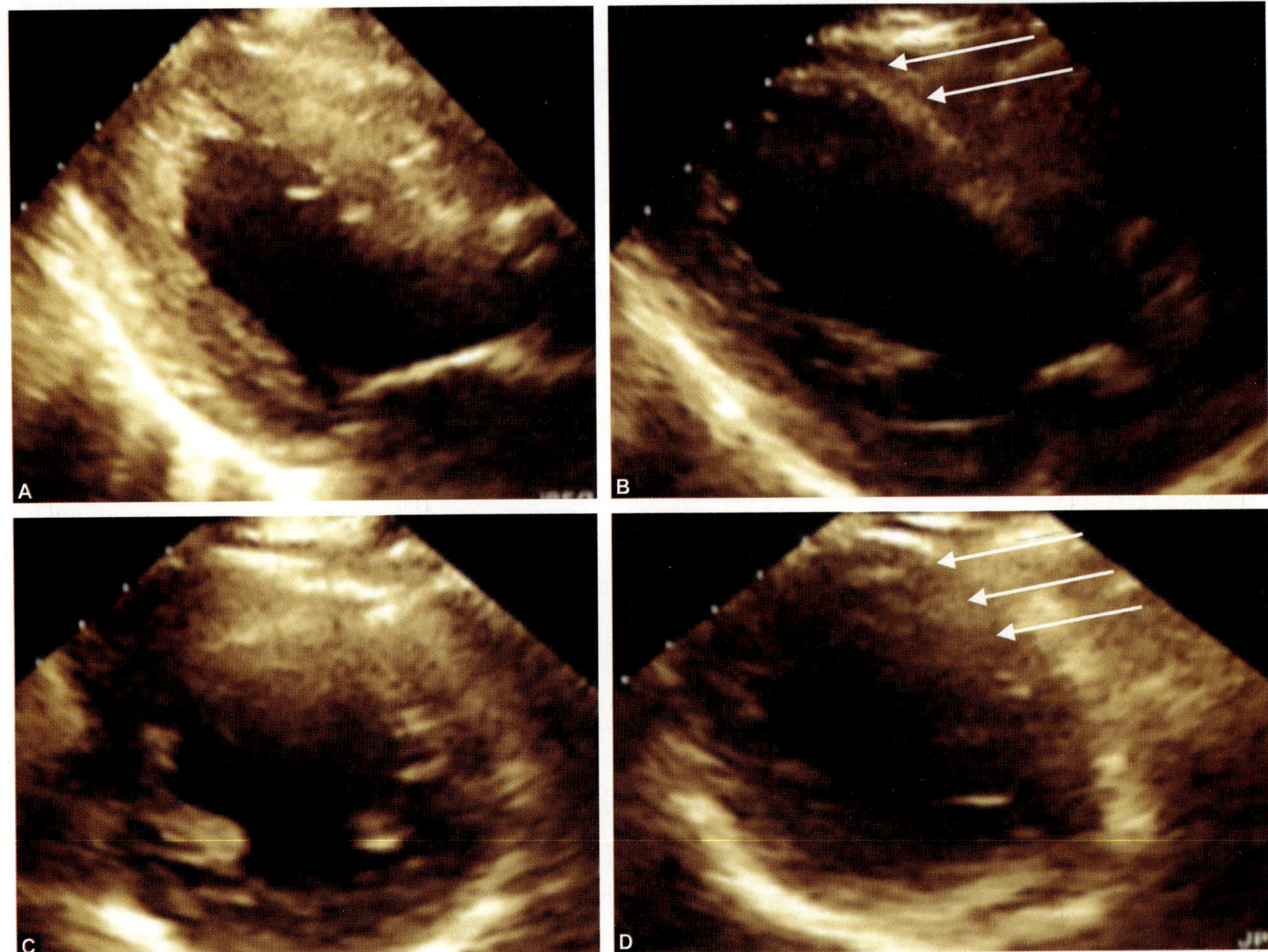

Figs 2A to D: Anteroseptal regional wall motion abnormality on dobutamine stress echocardiography (DSE) (arrows) in parasternal long axis (B) and short axis (D) views

as biphasic and is most predictive of functional recovery following revascularization.

- *Nonviable or necrotic/scarred—if it fails to shows increased contractility at low dose or at high dose.*

Dobutamine Stress Echocardiography Terminating Endpoints

Target heart rate achieved, new wall motion abnormality, arrhythmias, alterations in blood pressure (increase in systolic BP above 200 mm Hg or diastolic more than 110 mm Hg or decrease more than 20 mm Hg),and intolerable symptoms.

There are several limitations in the use of DSE:

- *Technical:*
  - *A poor acoustic window will result in suboptimal images and inadequate visualization of myocardial segments. This leads to an improper assessment of wall motion and therefore an erroneous assessment of presence or absence of viability.*
  - *Operator dependence—The performance and interpretation of DSE is operator dependent requiring a high degree of technical and interpretative expertise. Adequately trained personal may not be available in many centers.*[79,80]
- *Feasibility of revascularization and incomplete revascularization—in extremely small arteries, with long segment stenosis, calcified vessels and microvascular thrombosis;it is difficult to revascularize the myocardium by either CABG or PCI. Therefore, in these patients correctly assessed dysfunctional but viable myocardial segments may not show improvement after attempted revascularization.*
- *Admixture of viable myocardium and scar tissue—in this setting the dysfunctional myocardial segments will not show any significant improvement even after adequate restoration of myocardial blood flow.*

Dobutamine Stress Echocardiography in Diabetic Cardiomyopathy

Diabetic involvement of the heart could be either due to CAD or based on myocardial dysfunction with normal epicardial arteries (DbCM). The assessment of DbCM by DSE should be performed using the standard protocol to assess for improvement in myocardial contractility (contractile reserve). A significant improvement in myocardial function (a 10% relative increase in global EF) indicates good long-term prognosis with a strong probability of recovery of myocardial function after adequate control of hyperglycemia and hyperlipidemia. On the other hand a poor contractile reserve (<5% increase) could indicate a less favorable prognosis.

A combination of both epicardial CAD and DbCM is a more common occurrence and DSE is the investigation of choice to assess for both regional dyssynergy as well as impaired contractile reserve out of proportion to the epicardial coronary involvement.

Recent innovative techniques incorporated into dobutamine stress echo:

- *Contrast echocardiography*—The use of fluorinated hydrocarbon transpulmonary contrast agents has been major advance in the accurate assessment of wall motion abnormalities as well as in abnormalities of myocardial perfusion. Both LV opacification (LVO) and myocardial contrast echo (MCE) modalities are used. The LVO mode allows excellent endocardial delineation and therefore improves the diagnostic value of echocardiogram in patients with poor acoustic window. The MCE mode on the other hand assesses myocardial perfusion subsequent to the LVO phase.
  - Myocardial perfusion defects are common in diabetes due to macrovascular (CAD) as well as microvasculature involvement (which results in low capillary area and small diameter compared with nondiabetics).[81,82] The use of MCE improves CAD detection rate when used during dobutamine stress test. The perfusion pattern provides a specificity of 87% in detecting multivessel CAD in diabetic patients. These findings suggest that MCE is a promising technique for to analyze the extent or multivessel CAD in diabetic patients.[83,84] The use of stress MCE demonstrating CAD is shown in Figure 3.

  Myocardial contrast echo is a novel approach for detecting myocardial perfusion defects. This technique is in its evaluation, needs expertise to interpret the results. The results of MCE are comparable to nuclear scans.
- *Speckle tracking echocardiography*—The tracking of myocardial speckles by two-dimensional (2D) echo and more recently by three-dimensional (3D) echo has been a quantum leap in the objective, operator independent assessment of regional myocardial function. This technique has been applied in both DbCM as well as in CAD in diabetics. Though there is a paucity of data on the role of speckle strain imaging during DSE in patients with DbCM, Karina Wierzbowska-Drabik et al. have shown a decrease in peak systolic LS in diabetic patients during the recovery phase of DSE (17.3 + 4.0% at rest to 15.3 + 3.2%, p < 0.01 at recovery) versus nondiabetic patients (18.7 + 3.3% at rest to 17.2 + 3.3% p = ns, at

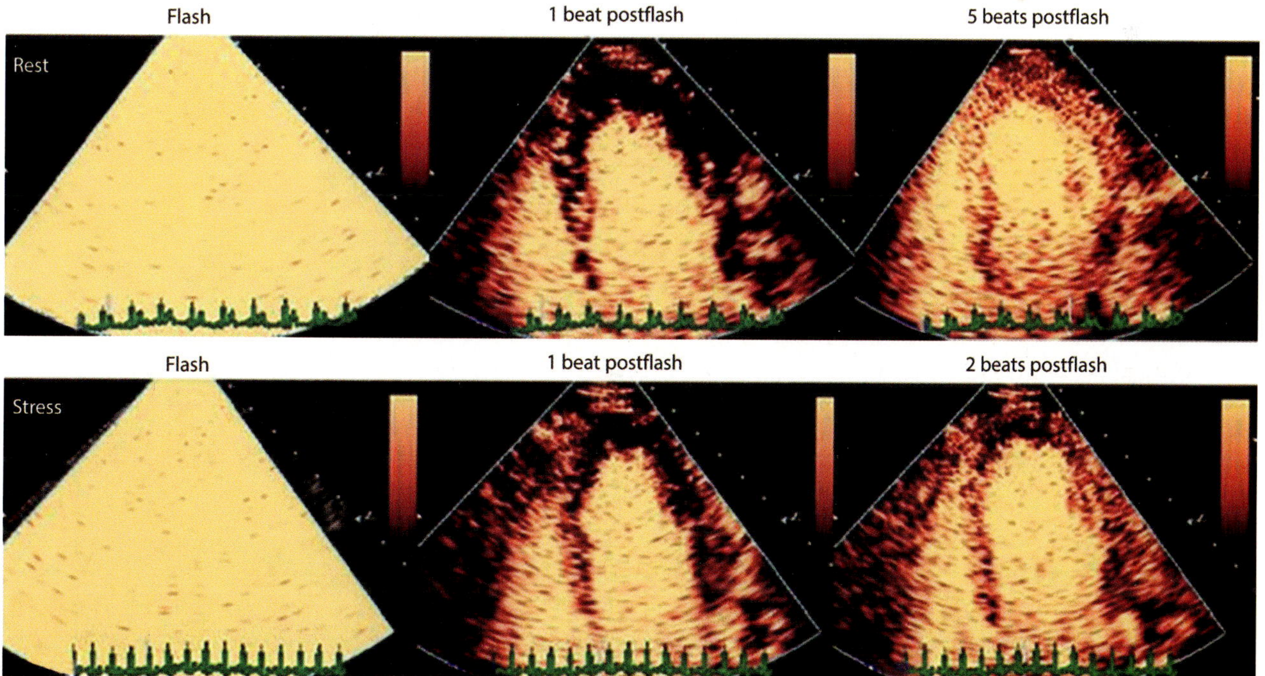

Fig. 3: Use of myocardial contrast echo (MCE) in depicting perfusion defect on stress in LAD territory

recovery).[85-90] On the other hand Thomas Cognet et al. (using dipyridamole stress) had shown an increase in the peak systolic LS during dipyridamole infusion and therefore an increase in LS reserve and LS rate reserve in diabetic patients versus nondiabetic controls.[91] Therefore, the utility of pharmacological (dobutamine vs dipyridamole) stress speckle tracking imaging in the detection of early diabetic myocardial involvement is at present uncertain.

Many studies have shown that speckle tracking derived LS had high diagnostic accuracy for angiographically significant CAD that is comparable with visualized wall motion analysis.[92-94] Thus, the STE during DSE could be an additional method for CAD assessment[95] as shown in Figures 4A and B. Many studies had also shown the prognostic implications of resting GLS after cardiac insult or therapy in patients with and without diabetes.[96-98]

However, there are several limitations in use of STE during DSE including good acoustic window with clear endocardial delineation and fast heart rates.

Dobutamine Stress Echocardiography and Other Noninvasive Modalities

Over the last decade there has been proliferation of various noninvasive modalities to detect myocardial function. Broadly speaking these techniques can be divided into those which assess the contractile reserve and those which assess myocardial perfusion or myocardial metabolism as shown in Table 6.

TABLE 6: Dobutamine stress echocardiography and other noninvasive modalities

Contractile reserve	*Perfusion defect*	*Metabolism*	*Scar tissue*
DSE	SPECT-Thallium	PET	MSCT-DSE
DS-CMR	SPECT-Tech-99		LGE contrast MRI

Abbreviations: DSE, dobutamine stress echocardiography; LGE-CMR, late-gadolinium enhancement CMR MRI, magnetic resonance imaging; MSCT, multislice computed tomography; PET, positron emission tomography; SPECT, single-photon emission computed tomography.

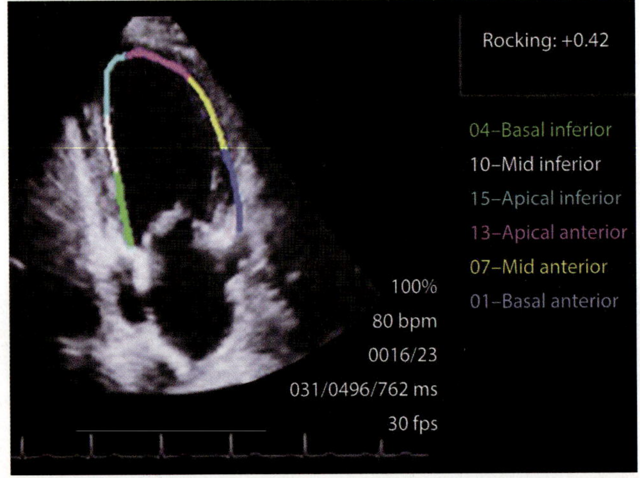

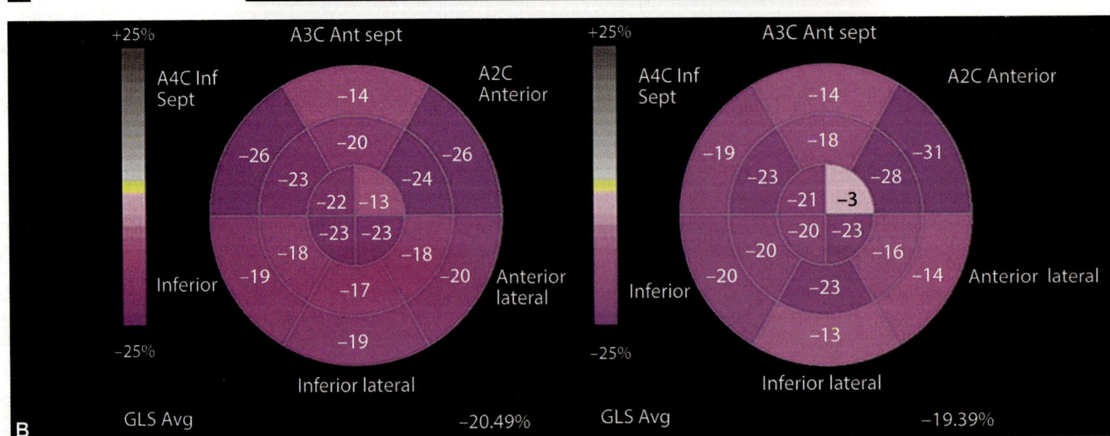

Figs 4A and B: (A) Speckle strain at different regions of left ventricular (LV); (B) Bulls eye pictorial diagram of regional strains depicting stress-induced ischemia evidenced by decreased speckle strains. Though there is negligible change in global strain values

The diagnostic accuracy of these various noninvasive technologies including their sensitivity, specificity, positive predictive value (PPV), and negative predictive value (NPV) are shown in Table 7, while their relative merits and demerits are depicted in Table 8.[99-102]

Safety

Dobutamine stress has been found to be extremely safe technique. The life-threatening complications of DSE are less than 0.01% which includes cardiac rupture. Ventricular arrhythmias are more common especially in patients with low LVEF (<35%) and those having ischemic cardiomyopathy. It is estimated that ventricular fibrillation or MI occurs in 1 of 2,000 studies. Mild side effects include palpitations, nausea, headache, chills, urinary urgency, and anxiety. Atropine is relatively safe but may cause urinary retention, increased intraocular pressure, delirium, flushing, constipation, nausea, and dry mouth due to its anticholinergic properties.

Contraindications to Dobutamine Stress Echocardiography

Although DSE is extremely safe in most clinical scenarios post-ST-elevation myocardial infarction (STEMI), there are several situations in which risk-benefit ratio for the use of DSE is unfavorable. In such instances DSE is relatively contraindicated: Known case of ventricular arrhythmias, complications of MI (myocardial rupture, papillary muscle rupture, and cardiogenic shock), unstable angina/ACS (up to 48 hours), significant left ventricular outflow obstruction, aortic dissection, high-grade blood pressure systolic more than 200 mm Hg, diastolic more than 110 mm Hg, intracranial aneurysms or history of recent stroke, or transient ischemic attack.

TABLE 7: Diagnostic accuracy

Myocardial perfusion images	*Sensitivity (%)*	*Specificity (%)*	*PPV*	*NPV*
PET	92	63	74	87
Contrast MRI-LGE	95	51	69	90
MSCT	57	73	90	83
DSE	81	78	75	83
DSE-CMR	81	91	93	75
SPECT Tech-99	83	65	74	76
SPECT Thallium-201	87	54	67	79

Abbreviations: DSE, dobutamine stress echocardiography; LGE-CMR, late-gadolinium enhancement CMR; MRI, magnetic resonance imaging; MSCT, multislice computed tomography; NPV, negative predictive value; PET, positron emission tomography; PPV, positive predictive value; SPECT, single-photon emission computed tomography.

OTHER PHARMACOLOGICAL STRESSORS

Dipyridamole

It was the first pharmacological stress agent used for the diagnosis of CAD. It provokes vasodilatation in coronary arteries and cause hyperemic response but it also induces ischemia by coronary steal phenomenon in myocardial regions supplied by moderately or critically stenosed arteries. Being a powerful dilator this molecule facilitates the application of coronary flow reserve (CFR) after the left anterior descending (LAD) is optimally imaged. Minor self-limiting side effects such as flushing and headache, occur due to systemic vasodilatory effect of the drug are seen in about two-third of patients undergoing dipyridamole stress echo. Major complications such as MI, arrhythmias, conduction blocks, or death were found to be quite rare (less 1/10,000). In case, prolonged angina occurs. Aminophylline and/or nitrates are effective antidotes.

Adenosine

It is a powerful endogenous vasodilator and is routinely used for termination of paroxysmal supraventricular tachycardias. However, it is also used as a pharmacological stressor owing to its vasodilatory properties causing a myocardial steal and thus leading to ischemia, similar to dipyridamole. Angina or bronchospasm could be provoked. However, owing to the short half-life these side effects are self limiting and do not require an antidote. Some of the side effects are depicted in Table 9.

TABLE 8: Merits and demerits

Technologies	*Cost of equipment*	*Floor space*	*Maintenance cost*	*Time taken to study*	*Operator dependence*	*Portability*	*Characteristics of viability*
DSE	Low	Less	Less	Less	High	Yes	Contractile reserve
MRI	High	More	More	More	Low	No	Perfusion
PET	High	More	More	More	Low	No	Cell metabolism
MSCT	High	More	More	More	Low	No	Scar tissue

Abbreviations: DSE, dobutamine stress echocardiography; MRI, magnetic resonance imaging; PET, positron emission tomography; MSCT, multislice computed tomography.

TABLE 9: Other side effects of adenosine [incidence in percentage (%)]

Side effects	Percentage
AV block 1st degree	7.6%
Second degree AV block	4%
Complete heart block	<1%
ST-segment depression of 1 mm or greater	5%–7%
Myocardial infarction	Extremely rare

Abbreviation: AV, atrioventricular

Regadenoson

The pharmacological profile of this stressor agent is similar to adenosine with a slightly longer half-life (2–4 minutes). This agent is administered intravenously as a rapid bolus of 5 mL (0.4 mg regadenoson) into a peripheral vein lasting approximately 10 seconds. Owing to the technical ease of administration, it could be a promising agent in future for pharmacological stress echocardiography. A relatively recent review involving 2,015 patients has shown that regadenoson is no inferior to adenosine for the detection of inducible myocardial ischemia.[103,104]

DIAGNOSTIC ACCURACY AND PREDICTIVE VALUE

Although vasodilator stressors either dipyridamole or adenosine have been shown to have a lower sensitivity (55–70%), a lower diagnostic accuracy, and a higher specificity (95–100%) as compared to dobutamine stress echo, these agents have a potential utility in evaluating patients on β-blockers. However, DSE is the mainstay in detecting both viability and reversible ischemia and is the dominant pharmacological agent used worldwide.[105-107] *Comparative sensitivity and specificity of exercise and various pharmacological stressors is shown in Table 10.*

Although DSE has a good sensitivity, specificity, and diagnostic accuracy in evaluating patients having CAD and contractile reserve, false positive and false negative results do occur. The various potential factors which could cause inaccurate results are shown in Table 11.

TABLE 10: Comparative sensitivity and specificity

Stressors	Sensitivity (%)	Specificity (%)
Exercise	83	84
Dobutamine	81	84
Dipyridamole	72	95
Adenosine	79	91

TABLE 11: Causes of false results after stress echocardiography

False negative	False positive
• Inadequate stress	• Interpreter bias
• Antianginal drugs	• Inferior wall abnormalities
• Mild artery stenosis	• Conduction defects left bundle branch block (LBBB)
• Left circumflex disease	• Cardiomyopathies
• Poor echocardiographic window	• Hypertensive responses to stress

Coronary Flow Velocity Reserve

The assessment of coronary flow velocity reserve (CFVR) in the LAD coronary artery in parasternal long-axis view is used to assess the coronary artery stenosis; sometimes in conjunction to pharmacology stress echocardiography. Patients showing normal myocardial contractility and normal CFVR in the LAD have mortality lower than 1% per year, while those with impaired contractility and abnormal CFVR have mortality greater than 10% per year.

The LAD is visualized based on acquisition from the low parasternal long-axis, two-chamber, or modified three-chamber view. At low color flow Nyquist limit of about 20 cm/s, LAD can be visualized and a colored-guided Doppler flow with diastolic predominance is noted. Resting and peak flows are obtained and the Doppler spectrums are planimeter for velocity time integral (VTI). CFVR is obtained as ratio of peak flow VTI to resting flow VTI. The CFVR value more than 2 is considered normal and whereas value less than 2 is indicative of low myocardial perfusion. Thus, a CFVR less than 2.0 is an additional parameter to assess the severity of inducible ischemia especially if the wall motion study is negative, CFVR more than 2.0 during pharmacological stress echocardiography could imply a favorable prognosis.

Even in the absence of significant epicardial coronary artery stenosis CFVR can be used to assess microvascular dysfunction in diabetic patients.[108] Some of the published guidelines recommend that CFVR should be routinely performed in diabetics undergoing pharmacological stress test especially with dipyridamole/adenosine as the stressors.[109-111]

Takayuki Kawata et al.[112] evaluated 111 consecutive asymptomatic patients with type 2 diabetes without a history of CAD with follow-up of 79 months. The pharmacological stressor agent used in this study was adenosine and CFVR was assessed. Patients with CFVR less than 2.5 had a worse long-term outcome as shown in Table 12.

TABLE 12: Percentage of cardiac events in relation to coronary flow velocity reserve (CFVR) in asymptomatic type 2 diabetes

	CFVR > 2.5	CFVR <2.5
All cause death (%)	2.4	10.3
Acute coronary syndrome (%)	3.6	13.8
Revascularization (%)	3.6	17.2

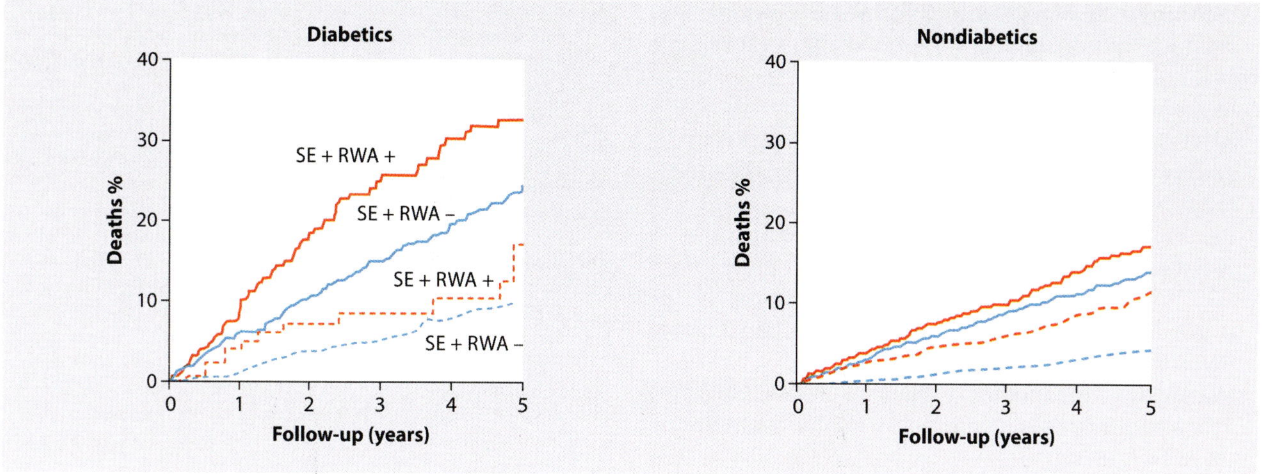

Fig. 5: Increased mortality in diabetics versus nondiabetics. Patients with regional wall motion abnormalities (RWAs) after positive stress test (SE) have increased death rates than their counterparts in both groups

The limitations to noninvasive assessment of CFVR include its technical difficult in visualizing LAD. Moreover, LAD is the only artery that has been assessed. It should also be noted that CFVR cannot distinguish between microvascular versus macrovascular or both micro and macrovascular CAD. In some studies, when LAD is visualized, the sensitivity and specificity for the cutoff value of less than two CFVR to detect significant LAD stenosis are both more than 90%.[113]

Dobutamine Stress Echocardiography in Diabetic versus Nondiabetic Patients on Antianginal Medication

Although DSE performed in patients on antianginal medications reduces the sensitivity of the test, it has been shown that in the diabetic population myocardial ischemia could still be induced despite the use of antianginal drugs (other than β-blockers). Thus, DSE performed in diabetic population retains its diagnostic accuracy and prognostic power as regards outcomes, despite the patients being on prescribed medication.[107-111]

RISK STRATIFICATION FOR CORONARY ARTERY DISEASE IN DIABETIC PATIENTS

Stress echocardiography both exercise and pharmacological are excellent technique for risk stratifying diabetic and nondiabetic patients with CAD. Diabetics have a 2–3 times higher cardiovascular mortality as compared to nondiabetic counterparts in the various stress echocardiographic positive and negative profiles with or without resting wall motion abnormality. This *is clearly depicted in an elegant study by Lauro Cortigiani et al. (Fig. 5).*[114]

TABLE 13: Various parameters for risk stratification in diabetes

	Very low < 0.5%/year	*Low < 1%/ year*	*Intermediate*	*High > 3%*
Resting LVEF	>50	<50	<50 –>50	<40–50
WMSI	1	1–1.3	1.3–1.6	>1.6
Baseline dyssynergy	Absent	Homozonal	Hetrozonal	Heterozonal
CRVF	>2.5	>2	<2	<2
Stressor dose	High	High	Low	Low
Recovery	Fast	Fast	Fast	Slow

Abbreviations: CRVF, coronary flow velocity reserve; LVEF, left ventricular ejection fraction; WMSI, wall motion score index

The various parameters used to prognosticate and risk stratify diabetic and nondiabetic patients with and without CAD using DSE are given here. A high poststress WMSI, resting dyssynergy, resting LVEF, and stressor dose are important prognostic parameters. The coronary flow reserves CRVF although a useful parameter is not widely used and for that an additional vasodilator stress protocol is required (Table 13).[74,108,115]

Low risk of hard events generally considered as less than 1% per year and high risk are considered diabetics having chances of more than 3% hard events per year after DSE. All other variable results of DSE are considered as of intermediate risk of 1–3% per year.

CONCLUSION AND FUTURE DIRECTIONS

- Myocardial involvement occurs in approximately two-thirds of diabetic patients due to CAD, DbCM, or both. Resting and stress echocardiography is an excellent technique to detect abnormalities of systolic and diastolic dysfunction as well as to diagnose reversible ischemia.

- In patients who are unable to exercise or exercise is contraindicated, pharmacological stress echocardiography has emerged as a major noninvasive diagnostic tool in evaluating such a patients.
- Resting wall motion abnormality, abnormalities of diastolic function, myocardial hypertrophy, and global and regional systolic dysfunction are some of the major parameters used to assess diabetic myocardial involvement.
- Stress echocardiography provides an incremental value over and above the resting studies for both systolic and diastolic function.
- Of the various pharmacological stressors, dobutamine is most widely used and has stood the test of time. It has a good sensitivity, specificity, and diagnostic accuracy especially when performed and interpreted by experts.
- Although regional dyssynergy, WMSI, and LVEF are the mainstay major parameters utilized in stress echocardiography of diabetic patients, there have been several newer innovations which have been incorporated into this technology. These include contrast echo (both LVO and MCE), myocardial flow reserve, STE, and 3D stress echo. While most of these innovations have been increasingly applied, their incremental value and cost effectiveness is yet to be evaluated.
- With further refinements in technology, some of these emerging innovations are likely to provide greater objectivity as well as time saving and in addition a higher accuracy, and reproducibility in the evaluation of diabetic patients for cardiac involvement. This would simplify risk stratification of diabetic patients and facilitate evaluation after interventions.

REFERENCES

1. World Health Organization (WHO). (2017). Introduction. [online] Available from www.who.int. [Accessed October, 2017].
2. World Health Organization (WHO). (2017). Global report on diabetes. [online] Available from www.who.int/diabetes/global-report/en/. [Accessed October, 2017].
3. Diabetes Foundation. (2013). Introduction. [online] Available from www.diabetesfoundationindia.org. [Accessed October, 2017].
4. Prem S, Singh K, Zafar S, et al. Risk of cardiovascular disease among diabetic patients in rural population of Central India. Int J Res Med Sci. 2017;5(4):1563-70.
5. Ali MK, Narayan KM, Tandon N. Diabetes & coronary heart disease: Current perspectives. Indian J Med Res. 2010;132(5):584-97.
6. Prabhakaran D, Jeemon P, Roy A. Cardiovascular Diseases in India: Current Epidemiology and Future Directions. Circulation. 2016;133(16):1605-20.
7. Soedamah-Muthu SS, Fuller JH, Mulnier HE, et al. High risk of cardiovascular disease in patients with type 1 diabetes in the U.K.: a cohort study using the general practice research database. Diabetes Care. 2006;29(4):798-804.
8. Booth GL, Kapral MK, Fung K, et al. Relation between age and cardiovascular disease in men and women with diabetes compared with non-diabetic people: a population-based retrospective cohort study. Lancet. 2006;368(9529):29-36.
9. Anagnostis P, Majeed A, Johnston DG, et al. Cardiovascular risk in women with type 2 diabetes mellitus and prediabetes: is it indeed higher than men? Eur J Endocrinol. 2014;171(6):R245-55.
10. Wu TG, Wang L. Angiographic characteristics of the coronary artery in patients with type 2 diabetes. Exp Clin Cardiol. 2002;7(4):199-200.
11. Hegde SS, Mallesh P, Yeli SM, et al. Comparitive Angiographic Profile in Diabetic and Non-Diabetic Patients with Acute Coronary Syndrome. J Clin Diagn Res. 2014;8(9):MC07-10.
12. Burke AP, Kolodgie FD, Zieske A, et al. Morphologic findings of coronary atherosclerotic plaques in diabetics: a postmortem study. Arterioscler Thromb Vasc Biol. 2004;24(7):1266-71.
13. Kato K, Yonetsu T, Kim SJ, et al. Comparison of nonculprit coronary plaque characteristics between patients with and without diabetes: a 3-vessel optical coherence tomography study. JACC Cardiovasc Interv. 2012;5(11):1150-8.
14. Burgmaier M, Hellmich M, Marx N, et al. A score to quantify coronary plaque vulnerability in high-risk patients with type 2 diabetes: an optical coherence tomography study. Cardiovasc Diabetol. 2014;13:117.
15. Rubler S, Dlugash J, Yuceoglu YZ, et al. New type of cardiomyopathy associated with diabetic glomerulosclerosis. Am J Cardiol. 1972;30(6):595-602.
16. Yilmaz S, Canpolat U, Aydogdu S, et al. Diabetic Cardiomyopathy; Summary of 41 Years. Korean Circ J. 2015;45(4):266-72.
17. Pappachan JM, Varughese GI, Sriraman R, et al. Diabetic cardiomyopathy: Pathophysiology, diagnostic evaluation and management. World J Diabetes. 2013;4(5):177-89.
18. Hayat SA, Patel B, Khattar RS, et al. Diabetic cardiomyopathy: mechanisms, diagnosis and treatment. Clin Sci (Lond). 2004;107(6):539-57.
19. Seferovic PM, Paulus WJ. Clinical diabetic cardiomyopathy: a two-faced disease with restrictive and dilated phenotypes. Eur Heart J. 2015;36(27):1718-27.
20. Fuentes-Antrás J, Picatoste B, Gómez-Hernández A, et al. Updating experimental models of diabetic cardiomyopathy. J Diabetes Res. 2015;2015:656795.
21. van Hoeven KH, Factor SM. A comparison of the pathological spectrum of hypertensive, diabetic, and hypertensive-diabetic heart disease. Circulation. 1990;82(3):848-55.
22. Cheung BM, Li C. Diabetes and hypertension: is there a common metabolic pathway? Curr Atheroscler Rep. 2012;14(2):160-6.
23. Matshela MR. Second in a series on diabetes and the heart: diabetic cardiomyopathy-mechanisms and mode of diagnosis. Eur Soc Cardiol. 2016.
24. Lorenzo-Almorós A, Tuñón J, Orejas M, et al. Diagnostic approaches for diabetic cardiomyopathy. Cardiovasc Diabetol. 2017;16:28.
25. Gilca GE, Stefanescu G, Badulescu O, et al. Diabetic Cardiomyopathy: Current Approach and Potential Diagnostic and Therapeutic Targets. J Diabetes Res. 2017;2017:1310265.
26. Miki T, Yuda S, Kouza H, et al. Diabetic cardiomyopathy: pathophysiology and clinical features. Heart Fail Rev. 2013;18(2):149-66.
27. Maisch B, Alter P, Pankuweit S. Diabetic cardiomyopathy–fact or fiction? Herz. 2011;36(2):102-15.
28. Francis GS. Diabetic cardiomyopathy: fact or fiction? Heart. 2001;85(3):247-8.

29. Hölscher ME, Bode C, Bugger H. Diabetic Cardiomyopathy: Does the Type of Diabetes Matter? Int J Mol Sci. 2016;17(12):2136.
30. Lind M, Bounias I, Olsson M, et al. Glycaemic control and incidence of heart failure in 20,985 patients with type 1 diabetes: an observational study. Lancet. 2011;378(9786):140-6.
31. Johansson I, Edner M, Dahlström U, et al. Is the prognosis in patients with diabetes and heart failure a matter of unsatisfactory management? An observational study from the Swedish Heart Failure Registry. Eur J Heart Fail. 2014;16(4):409-18.
32. Wilhelmsen L, Rosengren A, Eriksson H, et al. Heart failure in the general population of men—morbidity, risk factors and prognosis. J Intern Med. 2001;249(3):253-61.
33. Livingstone SJ, Levin D, Looker HC, et al. Estimated life expectancy in a Scottish cohort with type 1 diabetes, 2008-2010. JAMA. 2015;313(1):37-44.
34. Raev DC. Which left ventricular function is impaired earlier in the evolution of diabetic cardiomyopathy? An echocardiographic study of young type I diabetic patients. Diabetes Care. 1994;17(7):633-9.
35. Berková M, Opavsky J, Berka Z, et al. Left ventricular diastolic filling in young persons with type 1 diabetes mellitus. Biomed Pap Med Fac Univ Palacky Olomouc Czech Repub. 2003;147(1):57-61.
36. Labombarda, F, Leport M, Morello R, et al. Longitudinal left ventricular strain impairment in type 1 diabetes children and adolescents: a 2D speckle strain imaging study. Diabetes Metab. 2014;40(4):292-8.
37. Romanens M, Fankhauser S, Saner B, et al. No evidence for systolic or diastolic left ventricular dysfunction at rest in selected patients with long-term type I diabetes mellitus. Eur J Heart Fail. 1999;1(2):169-75.
38. Litwin SE. Diabetes and the heart: is there objective evidence of a human diabetic cardiomyopathy? Diabetes. 2013;62(10):3329-30.
39. Detrano R, Gianrossi R, Froelicher V. The diagnostic accuracy of the exercise electrocardiogram: a meta-analysis of 22 years of research. Prog Cardiovas Dis. 1989;32(3):173-206.
40. Lee DP, Fearon WF, Froelicher VF. Clinical utility of the exercise ECG in patients with diabetes and chest pain. Chest. 2001;119(5):1576-81.
41. Albers AR, Krichavsky MZ, Balady GJ. Stress testing in patients with diabetes mellitus: diagnostic and prognostic value. Circulation. 2006;113(4):583-92.
42. Kamalesh M, Matorin R, Sawada S. Prognostic value of a negative stress echocardiographic study in diabetic patients. Am Heart J. 2002;143(1):163-8.
43. Kamalesh M, Feigenbaum H, Sawada S. Assessing prognosis in patients with diabetes mellitus—the Achilles' heel of cardiac stress imaging tests? Am J Cardiol. 2007;99(7):1016-9.
44. Elhendy A, Arruda AM, Mahoney DW, et al. Prognostic stratification of diabetic patients by exercise echocardiography. J Am Coll Cardiol. 2001;37(6):1551-7.
45. Oliveira JL, Barreto-Filho JA, Oliveira CR, et al. Prognostic value of exercise echocardiography in diabetic patients. Cardiovasc Ultrasound. 2009;7:24.
46. Kostkiewicz M. Myocardial perfusion imaging in coronary artery disease. Cor et Vasa. 2015;57(6):e446-52.
47. Sultan A, Piot C, Mariano-Goulart D, et al. Myocardial perfusion imaging and cardiac events in a cohort of asymptomatic patients with diabetes living in southern France. Diabet Med. 2006;23(4):410-8.
48. Boiten HJ, van Domburg RT, Valkema R, et al. Dobutamine stress myocardial perfusion imaging: 8-year outcomes in patients with diabetes mellitus. Eur Heart J Cardiovasc Imaging. 2016;17(8):871-6.
49. Hachamovitch R, Hayes S, Friedman JD, et al. Determinants of risk and its temporal variation in patients with normal stress myocardial perfusion scans: what is the warranty period of a normal scan? J Am Coll Cardiol. 2003;41(8):1329-40.
50. Agarwal S, Morgan T, Herrington DM, et al. Coronary calcium score and prediction of all-cause mortality in diabetes: the diabetes heart study. Diabetes Care. 2011;34(5):1219-24.
51. Valenti V, Hartaigh BO, Cho I, et al. Absence of Coronary Artery Calcium Identifies Asymptomatic Diabetic Individuals at Low Near-Term But Not Long-Term Risk of Mortality: A 15-Year Follow-up Study of 9715 Patients. Circ Cardiovasc Imaging. 2016;9(2):e003528.
52. Kuhn MJ, Chen N, Sahani DV, et al. The PREDICT study: a randomized double-blind comparison of contrast-induced nephropathy after low- or isoosmolar contrast agent exposure. AJR Am J Roentgenol. 2008;191(1):151-7.
53. Tehrani DM, Malik S, Wong ND. Coronary Artery Calcium Screening in Persons with Metabolic Syndrome and Diabetes: Implications for Prevention. Metab Syndr Relat Disord. 2013;11(3):143-8.
54. Qu W, Le TT, Azen SP, et al. Value of coronary artery calcium scanning by computed tomography for predicting coronary heart disease in diabetic subjects. Diabetes Care. 2003;26(3):905-10.
55. Saremi F, Achenbach S. Coronary plaque characterization using CT. Am J Roentgenol. 2015;204(3):W249-60.
56. Bax JJ, Inzucchi SE, Bonow RO, et al. Cardiac imaging for risk stratification in diabetes. Diabetes Care. 2007;30(5):1295-304.
57. Balkau B. The DECODE study. Diabetes epidemiology: collaborative analysis of diagnostic criteria in Europe. Diabetes Metab. 2000;26(4):282-6.
58. Glucose tolerance and mortality: comparison of WHO and American Diabetes Association diagnostic criteria. The DECODE Study group. European Diabetes Epidemiology Group. Diabetes Epidemiology: Collaborative analysis of Diagnostic criteria in Europe. Lancet. 1999;354(9179):617-21.
59. Wackers FJ, Young LH, Inzucchi SE, et al. Detection of silent myocardial ischemia in asymptomatic diabetic subjects: the DIAD study. Diabetes Care. 2004;27(8):1954-61.
60. Expert Panel on Detection, Evaluation, and Treatment of High Blood Cholesterol in Adults. Executive Summary of The Third Report of The National Cholesterol Education Program (NCEP) Expert Panel on Detection, Evaluation, and Treatment of High Blood Cholesterol in Adults (Adult Treatment Panel III). JAMA. 2001;285(19):2486-97.
61. Rana JS, Liu JY, Moffet HH, et al. Diabetes and Prior Coronary Heart Disease are Not Necessarily Risk Equivalent for Future Coronary Heart Disease Events. J Gen Intern Med. 2016;31(4):387-93.
62. Rana JS. Is Diabetes Really a CHD Risk Equivalent? Expert Analysis. Am Coll Cardiol. 2016.
63. Bulugahapitiya U, Siyambalapitiya S, Sithole J, et al. Is diabetes a coronary risk equivalent? Systematic review and meta-analysis. Diabet Med. 2009;26(2):142-8.
64. American Diabetes Association. Cardiovascular Disease and Risk Management. Diabetes Care. 2016;39(Suppl 1):S60-71.
65. American Diabetes Association. Standards of medical care in diabetes. Diabetes Care. 2007;30:S4-41.
66. Authors/Task Force Members, Rydén L, Grant PJ, et al. ESC Guidelines on diabetes, pre-diabetes, and cardiovascular diseases developed in collaboration with the EASD: the Task Force on diabetes, pre-diabetes, and cardiovascular diseases of the European Society of Cardiology (ESC) and developed in collaboration with the European Association for the Study of Diabetes (EASD). Eur Heart J. 2013;34(39):3035-87.
67. Hung MJ, Wang CH, Cherng WJ. Can Dobutamine Stress Echocardiography Predict Cardiac Events in Nonrevascularized Diabetic Patients Following Acute Myocardial Infarction? Chest. 1999;116(5):1224-32.
68. Panza JA, Curiel RV, Laurienzo JM, et al. Relation between ischemic threshold measured during dobutamine stress echocardiography and known indices of poor prognosis in patients with coronary artery disease. Circulation. 1995;92(8):2095-101.
69. Bigi R, Desideri A, Cortigiani L, et al. Stress Echocardiography for Risk Stratification of Diabetic Patients With Known or Suspected Coronary Artery Disease. Diabetes Care. 2001;24(9):1596-601.

70. Giri S, Shaw LJ, Murthy DR, et al. Impact of diabetes on the risk stratification using stress single-photon emission computed tomography myocardial perfusion imaging in patients with symptoms suggestive of coronary artery disease. Circulation. 2002;105(1):32-40.
71. van der Sijde JN, Boiten HJ, Sozzi FB, et al. Long-term prognostic value of dobutamine stress echocardiography in diabetic patients with limited exercise capability. a 13-year follow-up study. Diabetes Care. 2012;35(3):634-9.
72. Chaitman BR, Rosen AD, Williams DO, et al. Myocardial infarction and cardiac mortality in the Bypass Angioplasty Revascularization Investigation (BARI) randomized trial. Circulation. 1997;96(7):2162-70.
73. BARI Investigators. The final 10-year follow-up results from the BARI randomized trial. J Am Coll Cardiol. 2007;49(15):1600-6.
74. Mehran R, Dangas GD, Kobayashi Y, et al. Short- and long-term results after multivessel stenting in diabetic patients. J Am Coll Cardiol. 2004;43(8):1348-54.
75. Harb SC, Cook T, Jaber WA, et al. Exercise testing in asymptomatic patients after revascularization: are outcomes altered? Arch Intern Med. 2012;172(11):854-61.
76. Coma-Canella I, Daza NS, Orbe LC. Detection of restenosis with dobutamine stress test after coronary angioplasty. Am Heart J. 1992;124(5):1196-204.
77. Elhendy A, Schinkel AF, van Domburg RT, et al. Risk stratification of patients after myocardial revascularization by stress Tc-99m tetrofosmin myocardial perfusion tomography. J Nucl Cardiol. 2003;10(6):615-22.
78. Garg N. Dobutamine Stress Echocardiography after ST-elevation Myocardial Infarction. New Delhi: Jaypee Brothers Medical Publishers (P) Ltd; 2015.
79. Gilstrap LG, Bhatia RS, Weiner RB, et al. Dobutamine stress echocardiography: a review and update. Dovepress. 2014;5(1):69-81.
80. Picano E, Lattanzi F, Orlandini A, et al. Stress echocardiography and the human factor: the importance of being expert. J Am Coll Cardiol. 1991;17(3):666-9.
81. Abdelmoneim SS, Basu A, Bernier M, et al. Detection of myocardial microvascular disease using contrast echocardiography during adenosine stress in type 2 diabetes mellitus: prospective comparison with single-photon emission computed tomography. Diab Vasc Dis Res. 2011;8(4):254-61.
82. Cosyns B, Droogmans S, Hernot S, et al. Effect of streptozotocin-induced diabetes on myocardial blood flow reserve assessed by myocardial contrast echocardiography in rats. Cardiovasc Diabetol. 2008;7:26.
83. Elhendy A, Tsutsui JM, O'Leary EL, et al. Noninvasive diagnosis of coronary artery disease in patients with diabetes by dobutamine stress real-time myocardial contrast perfusion imaging. Diabetes Care. 2005;28(7):1662-7.
84. Moir S, Marwick TH. Combination of contrast with stress echocardiography: A practical guide to methods and interpretation. Cardiovasc Ultrasound. 2004;2:15.
85. Moir S, Haluska B, Jenkins C, et al. Comparison of specificity of quantitative myocardial contrast echocardiography for diagnosis of coronary artery disease in patients with versus without diabetes mellitus. Am J Cardiol. 2005;96(2):187-92.
86. Nakai H, Takeuchi M, Nishikage T, et al. Subclinical left ventricular dysfunction in asymptomatic diabetic patients assessed by two-dimensional speckle tracking echocardiography: correlation with diabetic duration. Eur J Echocardiogr. 2009;10(8):926-32.
87. Enomoto M, Ishizu T, Seo Y, et al. Myocardial dysfunction identified by three-dimensional speckle tracking echocardiography in type 2 diabetes patients relates to complications of microangiopathy. J Cardiol. 2016;68(4):282-7.
88. Bakhoum SW, Habeeb HA, Elebrashy IN, et al. Assessment of left ventricular function in young type 1 diabetes mellitus patients by two-dimensional speckle tracking echocardiography: Relation to duration and control of diabetes. Egyptian Heart J. 2016; 68(4):217-25.
89. Li RJ, Yang J, Yang Y, et al. Speckle tracking echocardiography in the diagnosis of early left ventricular systolic dysfunction in type II diabetic mice. BMC Cardiovasc Disord. 2014;14:141.
90. Wierzbowska-Drabik K, Hamala P, Kasprzak JD. Delayed longitudinal myocardial function recovery after dobutamine challenge as a novel presentation of myocardial dysfunction in type 2 diabetic patients without angiographic coronary artery disease. Eur Heart J Cardiovasc Imaging. 2015;16(6):676-83.
91. Cognet T, Vervueren PL, Dercle L, et al. New concept of myocardial longitudinal strain reserve assessed by a dipyridamole infusion using 2D-strain echocardiography: the impact of diabetes and age, and the prognostic value. Cardiovasc Diabetol. 2013;12:84.
92. Ingul CB, Stoylen A, Slordahl SA, et al. Automated analysis of myocardial deformation at dobutamine stress echocardiography: an angiographic validation. J Am Coll Cardiol. 2007;49(15):1651-9.
93. Hanekom L, Cho GY, Leano R, et al. Comparison of two-dimensional speckle and tissue Doppler strain measurement during dobutamine stress echocardiography: an angiographic correlation. Eur Heart J. 2007;28(14):1765-72.
94. Uusitalo V, Luotolahti M, Pietilä M, et al. Two-Dimensional Speckle-Tracking during Dobutamine Stress Echocardiography in the Detection of Myocardial Ischemia in Patients with Suspected Coronary Artery Disease. J Am Soc Echocardiogr. 2016;29(5): 470-9.e3.
95. Aggeli C, Lagoudakou S, Felekos I, et al. Two-dimensional speckle tracking for the assessment of coronary artery disease during dobutamine stress echo: clinical tool or merely research method. Cardiovasc Ultrasound. 2015;13:43.
96. Rifqi S, Sungkar S, Sobirin MA, et al. Early recovery of left ventricular function after revascularization of coronary artery disease detected by myocardial strain. Biomed Res. 2016.
97. Ismail AM, Samy W, Aly R, et al. Speckle Tracking Echocardiography in Diabetic Patients with STEMI. Med J Cairo Univ. 2016;84(1): 1579-85.
98. Hoogslag GE, Abou R, Joyce E, et al. Comparison of Changes in Global Longitudinal Peak Systolic Strain After ST-Segment Elevation Myocardial Infarction in Patients With Versus Without Diabetes Mellitus. Am J Cardiol. 2015;116(9):1334-9.
99. Harb SC, Marwick TH. Prognostic value of stress imaging after revascularization: a systematic review of stress echocardiography and stress nuclear imaging. Am Heart J. 2014;167(1):77-85.
100. Dagianti A, Penco M, Agati L, et al. Stress echocardiography: comparison of exercise, dipyridamole and dobutamine in detecting and predicting the extent of coronary artery disease. J Am Coll Cardiol. 1995;26(1):18-25.
101. Nixdorff U, Küfner C, Achenbach S, et al. Head-to-head comparison of dobutamine stress echocardiography and cardiac computed tomography for the detection of significant coronary artery disease. Cardiology. 2008;110(2):81-6.
102. Nedeljkovic I, Ostojic M, Beleslin B, et al. Comparison of exercise, dobutamine-atropine and dipyridamole-atropine stress echocardiography in detecting coronary artery disease. Cardiovasc Ultrasound. 2006;4:22.
103. Sicari R, Ripoli A, Picano E, et al. The prognostic value of myocardial viability recognized by low dose dipyridamole echocardiography in patients with chronic ischaemic left ventricular dysfunction. Eur Heart J. 2001;22(10):837-44.
104. Cerqueira MD, Nguyen P, Staehr P, et al. Effects of age, gender, obesity, and diabetes on the efficacy and safety of the selective A2A agonist regadenoson versus adenosine in myocardial perfusion imaging integrated ADVANCE-MPI trial results. JACC Cardiovasc Imaging. 2008;1(3):307-16.

105. Picano E, Molinaro S, Pasanisi E. The diagnostic accuracy of pharmacological stress echocardiography for the assessment of coronary artery disease: a meta-analysis. Cardiovasc Ultrasound. 2008;6:30.
106. Sicari R, Cortigiani L. The clinical use of stress echocardiography in ischemic heart disease. Cardiovasc Ultrasound. 2017;15:7.
107. Severi S, Picano E, Michelassi C, et al. Diagnostic and prognostic value of dipyridamole echocardiography in patients with suspected coronary artery disease. Comparison with exercise electrocardiography. Circulation. 1994;89(3):1160-73.
108. Cortigiani L, Rigo F, Gherardi S, et al. Prognostic meaning of coronary microvascular disease in type 2 diabetes mellitus: a transthoracic Doppler echocardiographic study. J Am Soc Echocardiogr. 2014;27(7):742-8.
109. Sicari R, Nihoyannopoulos P, Evangelista A, et al. Stress Echocardiography Expert Consensus Statement—Executive Summary: European Association of Echocardiography (EAE) (a registered branch of the ESC). Eur Heart J. 2009;30(3):278-89.
110. Lowenstein JA, Caniggia C, Rousse G, et al. Coronary flow velocity reserve during pharmacologic stress echocardiography with normal contractility adds important prognostic value in diabetic and nondiabetic patients. J Am Soc Echocardiogr. 2014;27(10):1113-9.
111. Cortigiani L, Gherardi S, Faggioni M, et al. Dual-imaging Stress Echocardiography for Prognostic Assessment of High-Risk Asymptomatic Patients with Diabetes Mellitus. J Am Soc Echocardiogr. 2017;30(2):149-58.
112. Kawata T, Daimon M, Hasegawa R, et al. Prognostic value of coronary flow reserve assessed by transthoracic Doppler echocardiography on long-term outcome in asymptomatic patients with type 2 diabetes without overt coronary artery disease. Cardiovasc Diabetol. 2013;12:121.
113. Simova I. Coronary Flow Velocity Reserve Assessment With Transthoracic Doppler Echocardiography. ECR. 2015.
114. Cortigiani L, Borelli L, Raciti M, et al. Prediction of mortality by stress echocardiography in 2,835 diabetic and 11,305 nondiabetic patients. Circ Cardiovasc Imaging. 2015;8(5):e002757.
115. Chaowalit N, Arruda AL, McCully RB, et al. Dobutamine stress echocardiography in patients with diabetes mellitus: enhanced prognostic prediction using a simple risk score. J Am Coll Cardiol. 2006;47(5):1029-36.

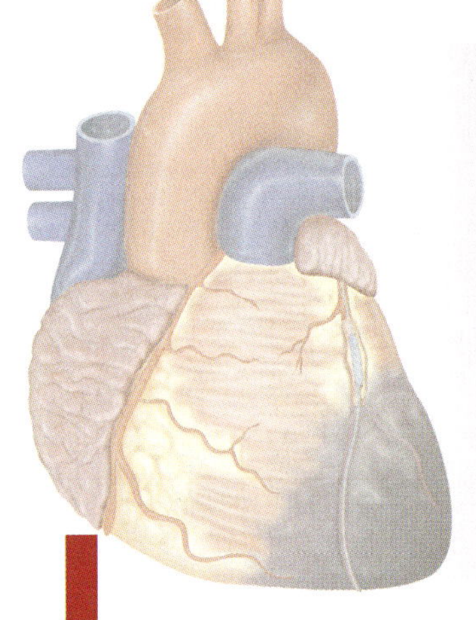

Noninvasive Cardiovascular Imaging for Risk Assessment in Asymptomatic Diabetic Patients

Pawan K Sharma, HK Chopra

INTRODUCTION

Worldwide, there are currently 515 million adults aged 20–79 who have diabetes and 318 million adults have impaired glucose tolerance. The number of people with diabetes would rise to 642 million by the year 2040. China, India, and USA are the top three countries with the highest number of diabetics. India is second highest in the world (after China), with 69.2 million adults with diabetes which will increase to 123.5 million in 2040.[1] Diabetes is associated with at least two-fold increased risk of coronary heart disease (CHD) and two- to four-fold increased risk of CHD and stroke mortality as compared with patients without diabetes.[2-4] About two-thirds of death among diabetics is related to cardiovascular disease (CVD).[4] Formerly, diabetes was regarded as a "coronary risk equivalent" implying a 10-year cardiovascular risk of greater than 20% for every diabetes patient.[5] This was based on an observational Finnish study by Haffner et al.,[5] which showed that people with diabetes without prior myocardial infarction (MI) had a similar risk of CHD to those with MI but without diabetes. In a systemic review and meta-analysis, Bulugahapitiya et al.[6] included 13 studies involving 45,108 patients. The mean duration of follow-up was 13.4 years (range 5–25 years). Patients with diabetes without prior MI had a 43% lower risk of developing CHD compared with patients without diabetes with previous MI. The results showed that patients with diabetes were at lower risk of developing total CHD events compared with patients without diabetes with established CHD.[6] It is now acknowledged that diabetic patients are not always at the highest risk.[6,7] Guidelines have suggested that further risk stratification in patients with diabetes is warranted and selective diagnostic testing may be more useful in high-risk asymptomatic diabetic patients rather than routine testing in all diabetics.[8,9] We review the role of gender and chronic renal insufficiency (CRI) along with the evidence regarding the use of noninvasive testing to stratify asymptomatic patients with diabetes with regard to CHD risk.

ROLE OF GENDER IN PATIENTS WITH DIABETES MELLITUS

Diabetes mellitus is a major risk factor for adverse coronary events in both men and women. Diabetic women in particular are at an increased risk of cardiovascular events. The highest risk group with increased risk of death includes patients with a combination of DM above 15 years and prior coronary artery disease (CAD).[10] The presence of the metabolic syndrome appears to increase the risk of cardiovascular events in women.[11] In the Women's Ischemia Syndrome Evaluation (WISE) study, women with angiographically significant CAD and the metabolic syndrome had significantly higher risk of cardiovascular events than those with normal metabolic status.[12] An increased prevalence of other cardiovascular risk factors such as lipid disorders, hypertension, obesity, physical inactivity and endothelial dysfunction[13] may contribute to this increased risk in women with diabetes and metabolic syndrome. The metabolic syndrome and diabetes are also associated with systemic inflammation and a hypercoagulable state.[12] Women whether diabetic or nondiabetic tend to present with less obstructive coronary disease compared with their male counterparts. The Bypass Angioplasty Revascularization Investigation (BARI) 2D trial showed that there were no sex differences in death, MI, or cerebrovascular accident among patients enrolled in the trial.[14] Studies involving cardiac imaging in women have illustrated the role of gender in diabetic patients and in those with metabolic syndrome. An echocardiographic study involving women with metabolic syndrome showed higher posterior wall thickness, relative wall thickness, concentric LV hypertrophy, and more advanced diastolic abnormalities. Such differences were not seen in men with or without metabolic syndrome.[15] Stress testing studies with cardiac imaging in symptomatic and asymptomatic diabetic women have demonstrated less extensive ischemia compared with men.[16,17] The prognosis for women with DM is worse as compared with men despite smaller perfusion defects and similar summed stress scores on adenosine perfusion single-photon emission computed tomography (SPECT) imaging.[17] In summary, the risk of cardiovascular events is significantly increased in women with DM and with metabolic syndrome.[18] Similar to nondiabetic women, women with DM have a lesser burden of coronary atherosclerosis, thus leading to less ischemia on stress testing. Despite the smaller burden of disease, the symptoms and prognosis are worse in females than in matched male counterparts.

ROLE OF CHRONIC RENAL INSUFFICIENCY IN PATIENTS WITH DIABETES MELLITUS

Diabetes mellitus and chronic renal insufficiency (CRI), both are contributors to the development of CVD. Among individuals with end-stage renal disease, coronary artery calcium (CAC) is highly prevalent, progresses rapidly, and is associated with an increased risk of death.[19-23] Coronary artery calcium is due to the accumulation of calcification in the media of the vessel wall with resultant increased arterial stiffness, increased pulse wave velocity, and LV hypertrophy,[24] as well as intimal calcification, more directly related to atherosclerosis as in the general population.[25] The CRIC (Chronic Renal Insufficiency Cohort) study showed a direct relationship between severity of CRI and CAC, independent of traditional risk factors. Among traditional risk factors, patients with CRI and with DM had more than a three-fold odds of having a high (greater than 100) CAC score compared with those with CRI but without DM.[26,27] Similarly, analyses from the Dallas Heart Study, demonstrated that patients with diabetes and CRI had a nine-fold greater odds of having a CAC score greater than 10 than patients with diabetes but without CRI.[28] The data from Multi-Ethnic Study of Atherosclerosis (MESA) study showed that incident CAC developed at a rate of 14.8%/year in men and 6.1%/year in women. CAC progression in CRI patients in this study was strongly associated with the presence of diabetes.[29,30] Both baseline and progression of CAC in patients with CRI have been shown in observational and randomized trials to be associated with increased mortality. Because DM is among the most frequent etiologies of end-stage renal disease and it is associated with rapid progression of CAC, this may become an important marker of risk in patients with advanced stages of CRI.[31-33]

NONINVASIVE IMAGING TO ASSESS CHD RISK IN ASYMPTOMATIC DIABETICS

An important clinical question remains whether asymptomatic diabetic patients need routine screening for CHD, and if so, how? Role of various noninvasive studies to stratify asymptomatic patients with diabetes with regard to CHD risk (Box 1) is discussed herewith.

Role of Exercise Stress Testing

Curtis, et al.[34] sought to determine the prevalence and correlates of exercise-induced cardiac abnormalities on exercise test in 5,783 overweight/obese asymptomatic middle-aged patients with type 2 diabetes.[34] They found that exercise-induced abnormalities were present in 1,303 (22.5%) participants, of which 693 (12.0%) consisted of impaired exercise capacity. ST-segment depression occurred in 440 (7.6%) and abnormal heart rate recovery in 206 (5.0%). Among the potential predictors, only older age was associated with increased prevalence of all abnormalities. In the DADDY-D (Does coronary Atherosclerosis Deserve to be Diagnosed and treated early in Diabetics?) trial involving 520 moderate-to-high-risk asymptomatic diabetic patients in an open-label randomized trial, one-half of the patients were randomized to undergo an exercise stress test

BOX 1: Imaging for risk assessment in asymptomatic diabetic patients

- Exercise stress test
- Carotid intima-media thickness (CIMT)
- Coronary artery calcium (CAC)
- Echocardiography
- SPECT myocardial perfusion imaging (SPECT-MPI)
- Positron-emission tomography (PET)
- Coronary computed tomography angiography (Coronary CTA)
- Cardiac magnetic resonance imaging (Cardiac MRI)

aimed at identifying obstructive-CAD, and the other one-half were managed with pharmacological and behavioral therapy.[35] It showed silent ischemia in 7.6% of patients and concluded that screening and revascularization of silent CAD in patients with diabetics failed to demonstrate a significant reduction in cardiac events and heart failure episodes.[36] Subjects with diabetes also have a delayed heart rate recovery at 1 minute after exercise completion due to autonomic dysfunction.[37,38] Heart rate recovery has been shown to be an independent prognostic indicator for CVD and all-cause mortality in 2,333 men with documented diabetes.[39] The prevalence of silent myocardial ischemia is 2.2 times higher in patients with DM than in nondiabetic control subjects. Diabetic patients who received insulin had a 2.6 times higher prevalence of silent myocardial ischemia, and patients with diabetic retinopathy had a 2.5 times higher prevalence of silent myocardial ischemia.[40] Thus, exercise stress testing can identify diabetic patients with silent myocardial ischemia, however, it has not been demonstrated whether exercise testing results in improved outcomes in patients with diabetes.

Carotid Intima-Media Thickness

Carotid intima-media thickness (CIMT) is considered a surrogate marker of atherosclerosis, and is associated with incident coronary heart disease.[41-44] In an analysis of MESA study participants with metabolic syndrome and diabetes, Malik et al.[45] showed that diabetic patients with a CIMT in the fourth quartile had no significant increase in cardiovascular events compared to those in the first quartile. CIMT is not deemed reasonable for cardiovascular risk assessment in asymptomatic adults who are at intermediate risk as per the 2013 ACC/AHA (American College of Cardiology/American Heart Association) guidelines due to results from several studies showing lack of a significant relationship with CHD events.[9,46-49]

Coronary Artery Calcium

The extent of coronary artery calcium (CAC) is closely associated with total coronary atherosclerotic plaque burden[50] and CAC scores predict incident CAD in the general population.[51,52] Type 2 DM patients have larger amounts of CAC than nondiabetic patients of a similar age,[53] additionally the extent and prevalence of CAC in patients with type 2 diabetes asymptomatic for CAD is similar to that of patients with established CAD but without diabetes.[54-56] Unlike the general population, women and men with type 2 DM have a similar extent of CAC, confirming that women with diabetes do not have any advantage over men with diabetes in prevalence and extent of atherosclerosis.[54,56] In nondiabetic patients, the prevalence of ischemia, noted by single-photon emission computed tomography myocardial perfusion imaging (SPECT-MPI), increases when CAC score is above 400.[57,58] However, in diabetic patients this threshold has been reported to be lower and studies have demonstrated that increased CAC in persons with metabolic syndrome and diabetes is associated with increased prevalence of ischemia.[59] CAC is a better predictor of incident cardiovascular events[60] compared with the Framingham risk score and the United Kingdom Prospective Diabetes Study (UKPDS). CAC also allows identification of patients at lower risk for whom aspirin preventive treatment might not be beneficial.[61] A large number of adults with diabetes have a CAC score of 0 or below 10 and have an excellent prognosis with very low mortality rate (approximately 1% at 5 years) suggesting that diabetes *per se* is not a CHD equivalent. Raggi et al.[62] noted that 39% of asymptomatic DM patients have CAC of 0 or below 10. In MESA study, 38% of DM patients were reported to have CAC score of 0 and this study also showed that DM had a stronger association with CAC in blacks than in other races.[60,63,64] Rapid progression of CAC identifies patients at higher risk for CHD events and future MI.[64-67] In summary, CAC provides strong risk stratification of patients with diabetes, with an increase in mortality for each increase in CAC score category. The mortality risk is higher for each CAC category in the patients with diabetes than in the patients without diabetes. The overall evidence supports the use of CAC scanning for risk stratification and to guide management in the asymptomatic DM patient, as recommended with a Class IIa indication in the 2010 AHA/ACC guidelines.[9]

Echocardiography in Patients with DM

Higher prevalence of diastolic dysfunction between 43% and 78% has been reported in diabetic patients than in normal individuals.[68-70] Marwick et al.[71] studied 937 DM patients with known or suspected CAD who underwent stress echocardiography or dobutamine stress echocardiogram (DSE). This study showed that the presence and extent of resting LV dysfunction and ischemia were predictive of death. The strongest predictor of death was referral for DSE rather than exercise. The total mortality of persons with DM with a negative test was approximately 4%/year, which is higher than 1%/year previously reported for unselected patients. Most of the excess in mortality was seen in the patients undergoing DSE, possibly due to higher comorbidities and risk factor burden in patients referred for pharmacological stress testing. The risk of death in patients with ischemia correlated with the extent of ischemia.[71]

Similarly, Cortigiani et al.[72] evaluated 5,456 patients (749 diabetic) who underwent dipyridamole or dobutamine stress echocardiography. After a median of 31 months, stress-induced ischemia, resting wall motion score index, and age were noted to be independent predictors of death and hard events in both diabetics and nondiabetic patients. However, diabetic patients with a normal stress test had a two-fold greater annual event rate during follow up compared with nondiabetic patients.[72] This study illustrates the short warranty period for DM in the setting of a normal stress test. Newer echocardiographic tools such as strain and strain rate allow the detection of systolic and diastolic dysfunction at the subclinical level. Both pharmacological and exercise stress echocardiography provide excellent prognostic information in the diabetic population. However, the late event rate is higher in diabetics than the nondiabetic population even in those with a normal stress test, which serves as a reminder of the rapid progression and high-risk nature of diabetic CAD.

Radionuclide Imaging of the High-Risk Asymptomatic Diabetic Patient

The gated SPECT-MPI can provide prognostic value for screening asymptomatic DM patients.[73] A normal myocardial perfusion scan in DM patients is associated with a slightly higher risk of adverse cardiac events (1.6%/year) compared with nondiabetic patients (greater than 1%/year). Thus, the SPECT-MPI can help assess the elevated cardiovascular risk in the DM patient.[74] Also, the warranty period of a normal MPI is lower in the DM patient, with event-free survival curves beginning to diverge from nondiabetic populations in the second year after the index normal scan.[75,76]

The prospective Detection of Ischemia in Asymptomatic Diabetics (DIAD) study, involving asymptomatic patients, reported a prevalence of any perfusion defect or LV function abnormality (22%) or moderate-to-large ischemia (6%), and may represent the true prevalence of asymptomatic myocardial ischemia in DM patients.[16] An analysis of 1,354 patients (302 with diabetes) without angina or dyspnea who underwent clinically indicated stress testing revealed a low prevalence of any myocardial ischemia (7.2%) or prognostically significant ischemia (4.4%) in the overall study population. The prevalence of asymptomatic ischemia was significantly higher in patients with diabetes (12.5% versus 5.6%) compared with those without.[77] The yield of stress testing in asymptomatic DM patients can be improved by selecting patients based on the pretest clinical risk of CAD. The retrospective studies that showed a high prevalence of stress test abnormalities included patients with abnormal electrocardiograms (ECGs) (43% with Q waves) and vascular disease (28%). A high CAC score is predictive of moderate-to-severe silent myocardial ischemia on SPECT in diabetic patients (48% and 71% ischemia, if CAC score is greater than 400 and greater than 1,000, respectively).[75] It is noteworthy that depending on age and duration of diabetes, between one-third and one-half of asymptomatic DM patients have no or minimal (less than10 AU) CAC.[75] In summary, analogous to the general population, the data in DM suggest that routine screening with MPI of all asymptomatic patients is likely to have a low yield and have a limited effect on patient outcome. The yield of MPI can be improved by selecting a higher-risk group of patients with symptoms, peripheral vascular disease, CKD, an abnormal ECG, or a high CAC score (e.g. greater than 400).[78,79] Whether coronary revascularization offers additive prognostic benefit to medical therapy when the ischemic burden exceeds any particular threshold is still unclear for the asymptomatic diabetic population.

Role of Positron-Emission Tomography in Diabetes

The assessment of coronary flow reserve (CFR) using positron-emission tomography (PET) is very useful in assessing the effects of focal stenosis, diffuse disease, and coronary microvascular function. Murthy et al.[80] studied its prognostic value in patients with diabetes. They found low cardiac mortality risk amongst diabetic patients without known CAD (prior revascularization or MI) but with CFR above 1.6 and those without diabetes. In contrast, the subgroup of diabetic patients without known CAD but with CFR below 1.6 had essentially the same risk as patients without diabetes but with CAD.

Coronary Computed Tomography Angiography for Risk Stratification of the Asymptomatic Diabetic Patient

The studies involving use of coronary computed tomography angiography (coronary CTA) in asymptomatic diabetic patients have shown that patients with diabetes have a high prevalence of coronary atherosclerosis and obstructive CAD, as well as a higher prevalence of plaques with features of instability compared with nondiabetic subjects. Approximately, 25–30% of asymptomatic diabetic patients have no demonstrable plaque on coronary CTA. The proportion of patients having greater than 50% stenosis generally ranged from 24% to 32%. These findings further support the concept that diabetes by itself is not a CHD equivalent, because one-third of patients have no demonstrable coronary atherosclerosis.[62,75] At the same time, the prevalence of obstructive CAD is nearly 25%, much higher in diabetics than would be expected in the nondiabetic population.[81-83] A study involving 427 asymptomatic diabetic patients found coronary plaques in 77% of them and greater than 50% stenosis in 1 or more vessels in 23%.[82] Despite a prevalence of atherosclerotic plaques in nearly 70% of diabetic patients, the event rate in diabetic patients with no or minimal plaque burden is very low. Min et al.[84] reported the occurrence of all-cause mortality, nonfatal MI, or late revascularization among 400 asymptomatic diabetic patients in the CONFIRM (Coronary CT Angiography Evaluation For Clinical Outcomes: An International Multicenter Registry) registry. After a mean follow-up of 2.4 ± 1.1 years, 33 events occurred (3.4% annualized event rate). On multivariable analysis, the presence of obstructive disease on coronary CTA added to the CAC score and age in prediction of adverse events. In the FACTOR-64 randomized trial, 900 asymptomatic diabetic patients were randomized to routine coronary CTA versus guideline-directed diabetes care.[85] CTA showed no CAD in 31%, mild stenosis in 46%, moderate in 12%, and severe stenosis in 11% of the patients. Coronary CTA prompted a stress test in 14% of the cases, and angiography in 8%, of whom 53% underwent subsequent percutaneous coronary intervention (PCI) and 19% underwent coronary artery bypass grafting (CABG). There was 20% lower rate of events in the CTA group—for the primary endpoint of all-cause death, nonfatal MI, and hospitalization for unstable angina, the rate was 6.2% in the CTA arm versus 7.6% in the standard-care group. The authors concluded that coronary CTA screening led to more aggressive risk factor modification in 70% of patients, including improvements in statin use and more aggressive treatment of serum lipids and systemic blood pressure; however, there was no significant reduction in CHD events. Coronary CTA is currently not recommended and is not considered appropriate as a risk stratification tool in the asymptomatic diabetic population.[39,86]

Cardiac Magnetic Resonance Imaging

Diabetic patients are at risk of developing severe cardiomyopathy due to CAD and metabolic deregulations even in the absence of CAD. Cardiovascular magnetic resonance (CMR) provides an accurate means to assess myocardial structure and function. With steady-state free precession sequences, investigators have been able to show substantial aberrations of LV volume, mass, and function in patients with insulin resistance and type 2 and type 1 DM.[87,88] The presence of late gadolinium hyperenhancement as a marker of prior MI in diabetic patients with unsuspected CAD has been linked with a four-fold increased risk of major adverse cardiovascular events and a seven-fold increased risk of mortality.[89] Late gadolinium hyperenhancement was demonstrated in 4.3% of asymptomatic type 1 diabetic patients in the DCCT (Diabetes Control and Complications Trial)/EDIC (Epidemiology of Diabetes Interventions and Complications) trial[88] and in 17% of asymptomatic older diabetic patients.[90,91] The newer technique of T1 mapping has the advantage of enhanced T1 relaxation times induced by gadolinium accumulated in the extracellular space. This allows an assessment of interstitial fibrosis, also described as extracellular volume (ECV) fraction. Employing T1-mapping, Wong et al.[92] demonstrated a higher short-term mortality in patients with increased ECV. Although similar outcome data are not available for diabetic patients, but it has been noted that ECV is increased in these patients[93,94] and is inversely related to diastolic function.[94] Although magnetic resonance spectroscopy (MRS) is still investigational, it can provide useful insights into the pathophysiology of diabetic cardiomyopathy. Using ^{1}H spectroscopy, Rijzewijk et al.[95] demonstrated a higher myocardial content of triglycerides in type 2 diabetic patients asymptomatic for CAD than in age-, sex-, and BMI-matched healthy volunteers. The increase in triglycerides content was directly correlated with abnormalities of LV diastolic function.[95] An association between myocardial triglyceride content in healthy diabetic patients and myocardial strain assessed by echocardiography has also been demonstrated.[96] Adenosine stress magnetic resonance myocardial perfusion index (MR-MPI) is an excellent test for the detection of obstructive CAD (greater than 70% luminal stenosis) in the general population and in diabetic patients.[97,98] Since a small number of diabetic patients were enrolled in the stress MR studies,[97,98] therefore, no definitive conclusions can be drawn based on these small studies.

GUIDELINES AND APPROPRIATE USE CRITERIA

Current guidelines[8,9,99,100] support risk factor assessment (Class I), CAC scanning (Class IIa), and hemoglobin A_{1c} for risk assessment (Class IIb), but not CIMT (Class III) or routine functional testing (Class III) in the asymptomatic DM population. Exercise ECG is rated appropriate in asymptomatic patients with diabetes who are considered to be in the high global CAD risk category. Stress radionuclide imaging, stress echocardiography, stress cardiac magnetic resonance, calcium scoring, and coronary CTA are considered "may be appropriate" (Box 2). The physician's judgment must finally adjudicate the need, or lack thereof, for diagnostic testing.[101]

CONCLUSION

There is great heterogeneity in the global CHD risk of patients with DM. Since 25–30% of patients with DM can now be considered as low risk on the basis of absence

BOX 2: Proposed noninvasive assessment of asymptomatic diabetics

- *Appropriate:*
  - Risk assessment
  - Echocardiogram
  - Exercise treadmill test.
- *May be appropriate:*
  - Coronary artery calcium score
  - If CAC is greater than 400, SPECT, stress echo, stress cardiovascular magnetic resonance (CMR), coronary computed tomography angiography (coronary CTA) may be appropriate.
- *Inappropriate: (if patient is asymptomatic):*
  - Carotid intima-media thickness (CIMT)
  - Routine testing such as SPECT, stress echo, stress CMR, coronary CTA.

BOX 3: High-risk factors for coronary heart disease in diabetics

- Female gender
- Advanced age
- Obesity
- Physical inactivity
- Known coronary artery disease (CAD)
- Longer duration of diabetes (greater than 15 years)
- Peripheral vascular disease
- Clinical symptoms
- Chronic kidney disease
- Metabolic syndrome
- Abnormal ECG at baseline
- High calcium score greater than 400
- Hypertension
- Smoking
- Dyslipidemia.

of coronary atherosclerosis, it is clear that DM by itself is not a CHD risk equivalent. The risk of patients with DM ranges from very low in one-third of asymptomatic diabetic patients with no or minimal coronary calcium to high observed in diabetic patients, particularly women, with advanced atherosclerosis (i.e. CAC greater than 400), symptoms, multiple risk factors, and/or CKD, compared with their nondiabetic counterparts (Box 3). The CAC screening is the most sensitive noninvasive risk stratification tool among asymptomatic persons with DM. As per the AHA/ACC guidelines, CAC imaging currently has a Class IIa recommendation for screening in this population.[9] Functional stress testing may further refine risk estimation in asymptomatic patients with DM who have a high CAC. The available data suggest that this might result in a future recommendation for CAC screening in type 2 diabetes, followed by functional testing for ischemia in patients with a pre-determined CAC threshold. However, although this approach has been shown to improve the stratification of persons with DM, it has not yet been shown to result in improved outcomes. Further clinical trials are needed to address this issue.

REFERENCES

1. International Diabetes Federation (2017). IDF Diabetes Atlas. [online] Available from *http://www.diabetesatlas.org* [Accessed February 2017].
2. Sarwar N, Gao P, Seshasai S.R, et al. Diabetes mellitus, fasting blood glucose concentration, and risk of vascular disease: a collaborative meta-analysis of 102 prospective studies. Lancet. 2010;375:2215-22.
3. Kannel WB, McGee DL. Diabetes and glucose tolerance as risk factors for cardiovascular disease: the Framingham study. Diabetes Care. 1979;2:120-6.
4. Gu K, Cowie CC, Harris MI. Mortality in adults with and without diabetes in a national cohort of the US population, 1971–1993. Diabetes Care. 1998;21:1138-45.
5. Haffner SM, Lehto S, Rönnemaa T, et al. Mortality from coronary heart disease in subjects with type 2 diabetes and in nondiabetic subjects with and without prior myocardial infarction. N Engl J Med. 1998;339:229-34.
6. Bulugahapitiya U, Siyambalapitiya S, Sithole J, et al. Is diabetes a coronary risk equivalent? Systematic review and meta-analysis. Diabet Med. 2009;26:142-8.
7. Rana JS, Liu JY, Moffet HH, et al. Diabetes and prior coronary heart disease are not necessarily risk equivalent for future coronary heart disease events. J Gen Intern Med. 2016;31:387-93.
8. Greenland P, Bonow RO, Brundage BH, et al. ACCF/AHA 2007 clinical expert consensus document on coronary artery calcium scoring by computed tomography in global cardiovascular risk assessment and in evaluation of patients with chest pain: a report of the American College of Cardiology Foundation Clinical Expert Consensus Task Force (ACCF/AHA Writing Committee to Update the 2000 Expert Consensus Document on Electron Beam Computed Tomography) developed in collaboration with the Society of Atherosclerosis Imaging and Prevention and the Society of Cardiovascular Computed Tomography. J Am Coll Cardiol. 2007;49:378-402.
9. Greenland P, Alpert JS, Beller GA, et al. 2010 ACCF/AHA guideline for assessment of cardiovascular risk in asymptomatic adults: a report of the American College of Cardiology Foundation/American Heart Association Task Force on Practice Guidelines. J Am Coll Cardiol. 2010;56:50-103.
10. Hu FB, Stampfer MJ, Solomon CG, et al. The impact of diabetes mellitus on mortality from all causes and coronary heart disease mortality in women: 20 years of follow-up. Arch Intern Med. 2001;161:1717-23.
11. Kannel WB. Metabolic risk factors for coronary heart disease in women: perspectives from the Framingham study. Am Heart J. 1987;114:413-29.
12. Marroquin OC, Kip KE, Kelley DE, et al. Metabolic syndrome modifies the cardiovascular risk associated with angiographic coronary artery disease in women. Circulation. 2004;109:714-21.
13. Helmut HO, Paradisi G, Cronin J, et al. Type II diabetes abrogates sex differences in endothelial function in premenopausal women. Circulation 2000;101:2040-6.
14. Tamis-Holland JE, Lu J, Korykowski M, et al. Sex differences in presentation and outcome among patients with type 2 diabetes and coronary artery disease treated with contemporary medical therapy with or without prompt revascularization: a report from the BARI 2D Trial (Bypass Angioplasty Revascularization Investigation 2 Diabetes). J Am Coll Cardiol. 2013;61:1767-76.
15. Nicolini E, Martegani G, Maresca AM, et al. Left ventricular remodeling in patients with metabolic syndrome: influence of gender. Nutr Metab Cardiovasc Dis. 2013;23:771-5.
16. Wackers FJ, Young LH, Inzucchi SE, et al., for the Detection of Ischemia in Asymptomatic Diabetics Investigators. Detection of silent myocardial ischemia in asymptomatic diabetic subjects: the DIAD study. Diabetes Care. 2004;27:1954-61.

17. Berman DS, Kang X, Hayes SW, et al. Adenosine myocardial perfusion single-photon emission computed tomography in women compared to men. Impact of diabetes mellitus on incremental prognostic value and effect on patient management. J Am Coll Cardiol. 2003;41:1125-33.
18. Budoff MJ, Achenbach S, Blumenthal RS, et al. Assessment of coronary artery disease by cardiac computed tomography, a scientific statement from the American Heart Association Committee on Cardiovascular Imaging and Intervention, Council on Cardiovascular Radiology and Intervention, and Committee on Cardiac Imaging, Council on Clinical Cardiology. Circulation. 2006;114:1761-91.
19. Blacher J, Guerin AP, Pannier B, et al. Arterial calcifications, arterial stiffness, and cardiovascular risk in end-stage renal disease. Hypertension. 2001;38:938-42.
20. Raggi P, Boulay A, Chasan-Taber S, et al. Cardiac calcification in adult hemodialysis patients: a link between end-stage renal disease and cardiovascular disease? J Am Coll Cardiol. 2002;39:695-701.
21. Block GA, Spiegel DM, Ehrlich J, et al. Effects of sevelamer and calcium on coronary artery calcification in patients new to hemodialysis. Kidney Int. 2005;68:1815-24.
22. Qunibi WY, Abouzahr F, Mizani MR, et al. Cardiovascular calcification in Hispanic Americans (HA) with chronic kidney disease (CKD) due to type 2 diabetes. Kidney Int. 2005;68:271-7.
23. Russo D, Palmiero G, De Blasio AP, et al. Coronary artery calcification in patients with CRF not undergoing dialysis. Am J Kidney Dis. 2004; 44:1024-30.
24. London GM, Guerin AP, Marchais SJ, et al. Arterial media calcification in end-stage renal disease: impact on all-cause and cardiovascular mortality. Nephrol Dial Transplant. 2003;18: 1731-40.
25. Nakamura S, Ishibashi-Ueda H, Niizuma S, et al. Coronary calcification in patients with chronic kidney disease and coronary artery disease. Clin J Am Soc Nephrol. 2009;4:1892-900.
26. Budoff MJ, Rader DJ, Reilly MP, et al. Relationship of estimated GFR and coronary artery calcification in the CRIC (Chronic Renal Insufficiency Cohort) Study. Am J Kidney Dis. 2011;58:519-26.
27. He J, Reilly M, Yang W, et al.CRIC Investigators. Risk factors for coronary artery calcium among patients with chronic kidney disease (from the Chronic Renal Insufficiency Cohort Study). Am J Cardiol. 2012;110:1735-41.
28. Kramer H, Toto R, Peshock R, et al. Association between chronic kidney disease and coronary artery calcification: the Dallas Heart Study. J Am Soc Nephrol. 2005;16:507-13.
29. Kestenbaum B, Adeney K, de Boer IH,et al. Incidence and progression of coronary calcification in chronic kidney disease: the Multi-Ethnic Study of Atherosclerosis. Kidney International. 2009;76:991-8.
30. Adeseun GA, Xie D, Wang X, et al. Carotid plaque, carotid intima-media thickness, and coronary calcification equally discriminate prevalent cardiovascular disease in kidney disease. Am J Nephrol. 2012;36:342-7.
31. Shantouf RS, Budoff MJ, Ahmadi N, et al. Total and individual coronary artery calcium scores as independent predictors of mortality in hemodialysis patients. Am J Nephrol. 2010;31:419-25.
32. Block GA, Raggi P, Bellasi A, et al. Mortality effect of coronary calcification and phosphate binder choice in incident hemodialysis patients. Kidney Int. 2007;71:438-41.
33. Di Iorio B, Bellasi A, Russo D, et al., INDEPENDENT Study Investigators. Mortality in kidney disease patients treated with phosphate binders: a randomized study. Clin J Am Soc Nephrol. 2012;7:487-93.
34. Curtis JM, Horton ES, Bahnson J, et al. Prevalence and predictors of abnormal cardiovascular responses to exercise testing among individuals with type 2 diabetes: the Look AHEAD (Action for Health in Diabetes) study. Diabetes Care. 2010;33:901-7.
35. Turrini F, Messora R, Giovanardi P, et al. Screening asymptomatic patients with diabetes for unknown coronary artery disease: does it reduce risk? An open-label randomized trial comparing a strategy based on exercise testing aimed at revascularization with management based on pharmacological/behavioural treatment of traditional risk factors. DADDY-D Trial (Does coronary Atherosclerosis Deserve to be Diagnosed and treated early in Diabetics?). Trials. 2009;10:119.
36. Turrini F, Scarlini S, Mannucci C, et al. Does coronary atherosclerosis deserve to be diagnosed and treated early in diabetic patients? The DADDY-D Trial. Screening diabetic patients for unknown coronary disease. Eur J Intern Med. 2015;26:407-13.
37. Banthia S, Bergner DW, Chicos AB, et al. Detection of cardiovascular autonomic neuropathy using exercise testing in patients with type 2 diabetes mellitus. J Diabetes Complications. 2013;27:64-9.
38. Georgoulias P, Demakopoulos N, Orfanakis A, et al. Evaluation of abnormal heart-rate recovery after exercise testing in patients with diabetes mellitus: correlation with myocardial SPECT and chronotropic parameters. Nucl Med Commun. 2007; 28:165-71.
39. Cheng YJ, Lauer MS, Earnest CP, et al. Heart rate recovery following maximal exercise testing as a predictor of cardiovascular disease and all-cause mortality in men with diabetes. Diabetes Care. 2003;26:2052-7.
40. Naka M, Hiramatsu K, Aizawa T, et al. Silent myocardial ischemia in patients with non-insulin-dependent diabetes mellitus as judged by treadmill exercise testing and coronary angiography. Am Heart J. 1992;123:46-53.
41. Chambless LE, Heiss G, Folsom AR, et al. Association of coronary heart disease incidence with carotid arterial wall thickness and major risk factors: the Atherosclerosis Risk in Communities (ARIC) Study, 1987–1993. Am J Epidemiol. 1997;146:483-94.
42. Taylor AJ, Kent SM, Flaherty PJ, et al. ARBITER: Arterial Biology for the Investigation of the Treatment Effects of Reducing Cholesterol: a randomized trial comparing the effects of atorvastatin and pravastatin on carotid intima medial thickness. Circulation. 2002;106:2055-60.
43. Chambless LE, Folsom AR, Davis V, et al. Risk factors for progression of common carotid atherosclerosis: the Atherosclerosis Risk in Communities Study, 1987–1998. Am J Epidemiol. 2002;155:38-47.
44. Burke GL, Evans GW, Riley WA, et al. Arterial wall thickness is associated with prevalent cardiovascular disease in middle-aged adults. The Atherosclerosis Risk in Communities (ARIC) Study. Stroke. 1995;26:386-91.
45. Malik S, Budoff MJ, Katz R, et al. Impact of subclinical atherosclerosis on cardiovascular disease events in individuals with metabolic syndrome and diabetes: the Multi-Ethnic Study of Atherosclerosis. Diabetes Care. 2011;34:2285-90.
46. Perk J, De Backer G, Gohlke H, et al. European Guidelines on Cardiovascular Disease Prevention in Clinical Practice (version 2012): The Fifth Joint Task Force of the European Society of Cardiology and Other Societies on Cardiovascular Disease Prevention in Clinical Practice. Eur Heart J. 2012;33:1635-1701.
47. Goff DC, Lloyd-Jones DM, Bennett G, et al. 2013 ACC/AHA guideline on the assessment of cardiovascular risk: a report of the American College of Cardiology/American Heart Association Task Force on Practice Guidelines. J Am Coll Cardiol. 2014; 63(25 Pt B):2935-59.
48. Yeboah J, McClelland RL, Polonsky TS, et al. Comparison of novel risk markers for improvement in cardiovascular risk assessment in intermediate-risk individuals. JAMA. 2012;308:788-95.
49. Den Ruijter HM, Peters SA, Anderson TJ, et al. Common carotid intima-media thickness measurements in cardiovascular risk prediction: a meta-analysis. JAMA. 2012;308:796-803.
50. Rumberger JA, Simons DB, Fitzpatrick LA, et al. Coronary artery calcium area by electron beam computed tomography and coronary atherosclerotic plaque area: a histopathologic correlative study. Circulation. 1995;92:2157-62.

51. Detrano R, Guerci AD, Carr JJ, et al. Coronary calcium as a predictor of coronary events in four racial or ethnic groups. N Engl J Med. 2008;358:1336-45.
52. Budoff MJ, Möhlenkamp S, McClelland R, et al. A comparison of outcomes with coronary artery calcium scanning in unselected populations: the Multi-Ethnic Study of Atherosclerosis (MESA) and Heinz Nixdorf RECALL (HNR) study. J Cardiovasc Comput Tomogr. 2013;7:182-91.
53. Wong ND, Sciammarella MG, Polk D, et al. The metabolic syndrome, diabetes, and subclinical atherosclerosis assessed by coronary calcium. J Am Coll Cardiol. 2003;41:1547-53.
54. Mielke CH, Shields JP, Broemeling LD. Coronary artery calcium, coronary artery disease, and diabetes. Diabetes Res Clin Pract. 2001; 53:55-61.
55. Schurgin S, Rich S, Mazzone T. Increased prevalence of significant coronary artery calcification in patients with diabetes. Diabetes Care. 2001;24:335-8.
56. Khaleeli E, Peters SR, Bobrowsky K, et al. Diabetes and the associated incidence of subclinical atherosclerosis and coronary artery disease: implications for management. Am Heart J. 2001;141:637-44.
57. Berman DS, Wong ND, Gransar H, et al. Relationship between stress-induced myocardial ischemia and atherosclerosis measured by coronary calcium tomography. J Am Coll Cardiol. 2004;44:923-30.
58. He ZX, Hedrick TD, Pratt CM, et al. Severity of coronary artery calcification by electron beam computed tomography predicts silent myocardial ischemia. Circulation. 2000;101:244-51.
59. Wong ND, Rozanski A, Gransar H, et al. Metabolic syndrome and diabetes are associated with an increased likelihood of inducible myocardial ischemia among patients with subclinical atherosclerosis. Diabetes Care. 2005;28:1445-50.
60. Yeboah J, Erbel R, Delaney JC, et al. Development of a new diabetes risk prediction tool for incident coronary heart disease events: The Multi-Ethnic Study of Atherosclerosis and the Heinz Nixdorf Recall Study. Atherosclerosis. 2014;236:411-7.
61. Silverman MG, Blaha MJ, Budoff MJ, et al. Potential implications of coronary artery calcium testing for guiding aspirin use among asymptomatic individuals with diabetes. Diabetes Care. 2012;35:624-6.
62. Raggi P, Shaw LJ, Berman DS, et al. Prognostic value of coronary artery calcium screening in subjects with and without diabetes. J Am Coll Cardiol. 2004;43:1663-9.
63. Lehmann N, Möhlenkamp S, Mahabadi AA, et al. Effect of smoking and other traditional risk factors on the onset of coronary artery calcification: results of the Heinz Nixdorf Recall study. Atherosclerosis.2014;232:339-45.
64. Pandey AK, Blaha MJ, Sharma K, et al. Family history of coronary heart disease and the incidence and progression of coronary artery calcification: Multi-Ethnic Study of Atherosclerosis (MESA). Atherosclerosis. 2014;232:369-76.
65. Budoff MJ, Hokanson JE, Nasir K, et al. Progression of coronary artery calcium predicts all-cause mortality. J Am Coll Cardiol Img. 2010;3:1229-36.
66. Raggi P, Cooil B, Ratti C, et al. Progression of coronary calcification and occurrence of myocardial infarction in patients with and without diabetes mellitus. Hypertension. 2005;46:238-43.
67. Kiramijyan S, Ahmadi N, Isma'eel H, et al. Impact of coronary artery calcium progression and statin therapy on clinical outcome in subjects with and without diabetes mellitus. Am J Cardiol. 2013; 111:356-61.
68. Boyer JK, Thanigaraj S, Schechtman KB, et al. Prevalence of ventricular diastolic dysfunction in asymptomatic, normotensive patients with diabetes mellitus. Am J Cardiol. 2004;93:870-75.
69. Zabalgoitia M, Ismaeil MF, Anderson L, et al. Prevalence of diastolic dysfunction in normotensive, asymptomatic patients with well controlled type 2 diabetes mellitus. Am J Cardiol. 2001;87:320-23.
70. Kadappu KK, Boyd A, Eshoo S, et al. Changes in left atrial volume in diabetes mellitus: more than diastolic dysfunction? Eur Heart J Cardiovasc Imaging. 2012;13:1016-23.
71. Marwick TH, Case C, Sawada S, et al. Use of stress echocardiography to predict mortality in patients with diabetes and known or suspected coronary artery disease. Diabetes Care. 2002;25:1042-8.
72. Cortigiani L, Bigi R, Sicari R, et al. Prognostic value of pharmacological stress echocardiography in diabetic and nondiabetic patients with known or suspected coronary artery disease. J Am Coll Cardiol. 2006; 47:605-10.
73. Hachamovitch R, Kang X, Amanullah AM, et al. Prognostic implications of myocardial perfusion single-photon emission computed tomography in the elderly. Circulation. 2009;120: 2197-206.
74. Acampa W, Cantoni V, Green R, et al. Prognostic value of normal stress myocardial perfusion imaging in diabetic patients: a meta-analysis. J Nucl Cardiol. 2014; 21:893-902.
75. Anand DV, Lim E, Hopkins D, et al. Risk stratification in uncomplicated type 2 diabetes: prospective evaluation of the combined use of coronary artery calcium imaging and selective myocardial perfusion scintigraphy. Eur Heart J. 2006;27:713-21.
76. Giri S, Shaw LJ, Murthy DR, et al. Impact of diabetes on the risk stratification using stress single-photon emission computed tomography myocardial perfusion imaging in patients with symptoms suggestive of coronary artery disease. Circulation. 2002;105:32-40.
77. Malhotra S, Sharma R, Kliner DE, et al. Relationship between silent myocardial ischemia and coronary artery disease risk factors. J Nucl Cardiol. 2013;20:731-8.
78. Hachamovitch R, Rozanski A, Shaw LJ, et al. Impact of ischaemia and scar on the therapeutic benefit derived from myocardial revascularization vs. medical therapy among patients undergoing stress-rest myocardial perfusion scintigraphy. Eur Heart J. 2011;32:1012-24.
79. Navare SM, Mather JF, Shaw LJ, et al. Comparison of risk stratification with pharmacologic and exercise stress myocardial perfusion imaging: a meta-analysis. J Nucl Cardiol. 2004;11:551-61.
80. Murthy VL, Masano N, Foster CR, et al. Association between coronary vascular dysfunction and cardiac mortality in patients with and without diabetes mellitus. Circulation. 2012;126:1858-68.
81. Sassa S, Shimada K, Yoshida K, et al. Comparison of 64-slice multi-detector computed tomography coronary angiography between asymptomatic, type 2 diabetes mellitus and impaired glucose tolerance patients. J Cardiol. 2008;52:133-9.
82. Halon DA, Dobrecky-Mery I, Gaspar T, et al. Pulse pressure and coronary atherosclerosis in asymptomatic type 2 diabetes mellitus: a 64-channel cardiac computed tomography analysis. Int J Cardiol. 2010;143:63-71.
83. Jeong HC, Kim I, Park KH, et al. New strategy for detection of subclinical coronary atherosclerosis in asymptomatic patients with type 2 diabetes based on cardiac multi-detector computed tomography and treadmill test. Circ J. 2014; 78:671-8.
84. Min JK, Dunning A, Lin FY, et al. CONFIRM Investigators. Age- and sex-related differences in all-cause mortality risk based on coronary computed tomography angiography findings results from the international multicenter CONFIRM (Coronary CT Angiography Evaluation for Clinical Outcomes: An International Multicenter Registry) of 23,854 patients without known coronary artery disease. J Am Coll Cardiol. 2011;58:849-60.
85. Muhlestein JB, Lappe DL, Lima JA, et al. Effect of screening for coronary artery disease using CT angiography on mortality and cardiac events in high-risk patients with diabetes: the FACTOR-64 randomized clinical trial. JAMA. 2014;312:2234-43.
86. Taylor AJ, Cerqueira M, Hodgson JM, et al. ACCF/SCCT/ACR/AHA/ASE/ASNC/NASCI/SCAI/SCMR 2010 appropriate use criteria for

cardiac computed tomography: a report of the American College of Cardiology Foundation Appropriate Use Criteria Task Force, the Society of Cardiovascular Computed Tomography, the American College of Radiology, the American Heart Association, the American Society of Echocardiography, the American Society of Nuclear Cardiology, the North American Society for Cardiovascular Imaging, the Society for Cardiovascular Angiography and Interventions, and the Society for Cardiovascular Magnetic Resonance. J Am Coll Cardiol. 2010;56:1864-94.

87. Velagaleti RS, Gona P, Chuang ML, et al. Relations of insulin resistance and glycemic abnormalities to cardiovascular magnetic resonance measures of cardiac structure and function: the Framingham Heart Study. Circ Cardiovasc Imaging. 2010;3:257-63.
88. Turkbey EB, Backlund JY, Genuth S, et al. Myocardial structure, function, and scar in patients with type 1 diabetes mellitus. Circulation. 2011;124:1737-46.
89. Manfrini O, Russo V, Ciavarella A, et al. Coronary plaque quantification and composition in asymptomatic patients with type II diabetes mellitus. J Cardiovasc Med. 2012;13:423-31.
90. Kwong RY, Sattar H, Wu H, et al. Incidence and prognostic implication of unrecognized myocardial scar characterized by cardiac magnetic resonance in diabetic patients without clinical evidence of myocardial infarction. Circulation. 2008;118:1011-20.
91. Schelbert EB, Cao JJ, Sigurdsson S, et al. Prevalence and prognosis of unrecognized myocardial infarction determined by cardiac magnetic resonance in older adults. JAMA. 2012;308:890-6.
92. Wong TC, Piehler K, Meier CG, et al. Association between extracellular matrix expansion quantified by cardiovascular magnetic resonance and short-term mortality. Circulation. 2012;126:1206-16.
93. Ng AC, Auger D, Delgado V, et al. Association between diffuse myocardial fibrosis by cardiac magnetic resonance contrast-enhanced T(1) mapping and subclinical myocardial dysfunction in diabetic patients: a pilot study. Circ Cardiovasc Imaging. 2012; 5:51-59.
94. Jellis C, Wright J, Kennedy D, et al. Association of imaging markers of myocardial fibrosis with metabolic and functional disturbances in early diabetic cardiomyopathy. Circ Cardiovasc Imaging. 2011;4:693-702.
95. Rijzewijk LJ, van der Meer RW, Smit JW, et al. Myocardial steatosis is an independent predictor of diastolic dysfunction in type 2 diabetes mellitus. J Am Coll Cardiol. 2008;52:1793-9.
96. Ng AC, Delgado V, Bertini M, et al. Myocardial steatosis and biventricular strain and strain rate imaging in patients with type 2 diabetes mellitus. Circulation. 2010;122:2538-44.
97. Plein S, Radjenovic A, Ridgway JP, et al. Coronary artery disease: myocardial perfusion MR imaging with sensitivity encoding versus conventional angiography. Radiology. 2005;235:423-30.
98. Greenwood JP, Maredia N, Younger JF, et al. Cardiovascular magnetic resonance and single-photon emission computed tomography for diagnosis of coronary heart disease (CE-MARC): a prospective trial. Lancet. 2012;379:453-60.
99. Hendel RC, Berman DS, Di Carli MF, et al. ACCF/ASNC/ACR/AHA/ASE/SCCT/SCMR/SNM 2009 appropriate use criteria for cardiac radionuclide imaging: a report of the American College of Cardiology Foundation Appropriate Use Criteria Task Force, the American Society of Nuclear Cardiology, the American College of Radiology, the American Heart Association, the American Society of Echocardiography, the Society of Cardiovascular Computed Tomography, the Society for Cardiovascular Magnetic Resonance, and the Society of Nuclear Medicine. J Am Coll Cardiol. 2009;53:2201-29.
100. Stone NJ, Robinson JG, Lichtenstein AH, et al. 2013 ACC/AHA guideline on the treatment of blood cholesterol to reduce atherosclerotic cardiovascular risk in adults: a report of the American College of Cardiology/American Heart Association Task Force on Practice Guidelines. J Am Coll Cardiol. 2014; 63(25 Pt B):2889-934.
101. Wolk MJ, Bailey SR, Doherty JU, et al. ACCF/AHA/ASE/ASNC/HFSA/HRS/SCAI/SCCT/SCMR/STS 2013 multimodality appropriate use criteria for the detection and risk assessment of stable ischemic heart disease: a report of the American College of Cardiology Foundation Appropriate Use Criteria Task Force, American Heart Association, American Society of Echocardiography, American Society of Nuclear Cardiology, Heart Failure Society of America, Heart Rhythm Society, Society for Cardiovascular Angiography and Interventions, Society of Cardiovascular Computed Tomography, Society for Cardiovascular Magnetic Resonance, and Society of Thoracic Surgeons. J Am Coll Cardiol. 2014;63:380-406.

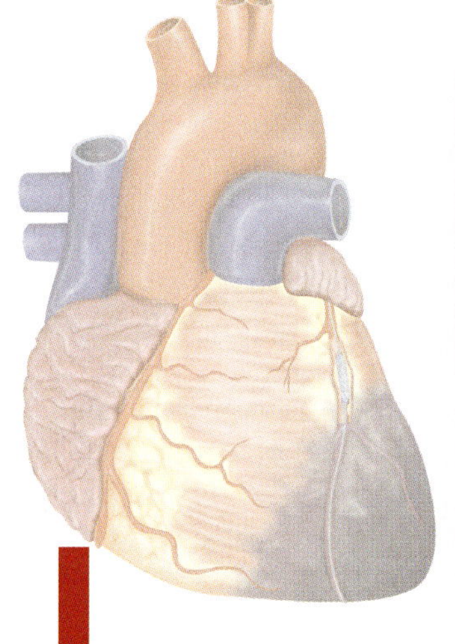

CHAPTER 43

Value of Ankle–Brachial Index in Cardiodiabetes

Shraddha Ranjan, Manish Bansal, Ravi R Kasliwal, HK Chopra

INTRODUCTION

Peripheral arterial disease (PAD) affects approximately 200 million people worldwide.[1] It is a major cause of morbidity and disability. However, even greater importance lies in the fact that the patients with PAD are also at substantially higher risk of developing myocardial infarction and stroke, resulting in increased mortality.[2] Accordingly, timely recognition of PAD is important not only for limb salvage but also for reducing overall cardiovascular (CV) mortality. Unfortunately, most of the patients with PAD are asymptomatic, resulting in delay in recognition of the disease. Ankle-brachial index (ABI) is a simple noninvasive tool that permits recognition of the asymptomatic occlusive PAD and can allow timely institution of the corrective measures. Given the high prevalence of asymptomatic and unrecognized PAD and the high rate of CV events in PAD, the American Heart Association (AHA) and the American College of Cardiology (ACC) recommend screening high-risk groups (such as those with age >70 years and those with age 50–69 with history of diabetes or smoking) with the ABI.[3] Apart of being a diagnostic tool, ABI values reflect also the severity of PAD, making it a widely used marker for the presence and progression of PAD in major CV trials.[4-6] Recent studies have also suggested that low ABI was modestly but independently associated with increased risk of incident diabetes in the general population.[7] Diabetes is a proven risk factor for PAD which in turn is responsible for a substantial proportion of morbidity and hospitalization of diabetic patients.[8]

ANKLE–BRACHIAL INDEX: WHAT IS IT?

Ankle-brachial index is the ratio of the systolic blood pressure (SBP) measured at the ankle to that measured at the brachial artery. This index, also known as Winsor's index was initially described by Winsor in 1950[9] and was supported by some other researchers to be a valuable tool for the noninvasive diagnosis of lower-extremity PAD.[10,11] The term ABI was proposed by AHA proceeding on atherosclerotic peripheral vascular disease in 2008, recognizing its widespread use.[12]

Physiology

The blood pressure (BP) waveform amplifies as it travels away from the heart, resulting in a gradual increase in SBP along with a decrease in diastolic BP. This is due to two predominant mechanisms—retrograde wave reflection from resistant distal arterioles, and changes in vessel wall thickness causing stiffness.[13] Significant arterial occlusive disease anywhere between the heart and the BP cuff will cause a decrease in systolic pressure at cuff level and hence decrease in ABI. Age, height, ethnicity, and even the order of measurement can affect the ABI. Arterial stiffening and sclerosis associated with aging is expected to cause decrease in ABI.[14] Taller people have higher ABIs than shorter people as a consequence of the progressive SBP increase with greater distance from the heart.[15] Black PAD-free participants in a study were found to have slightly lower ABI than non-Hispanic white counterparts in the Multi-ethnic Study on Atherosclerosis (MESA) and Atherosclerosis Risk in Communities (ARIC) studies.[16,17]

Post-exercise ABI

Systolic blood pressure, as measured in the arm, increases with exercise physiologically, due to increase in left ventricular systolic pressure. If the patient is doing leg exercise, peripheral vasoconstriction occurs in nonexercising limbs and other organs, whereas vasodilatation occurs in the exercising muscles. This leads to a mild decrease in the ABI in healthy patients when measured immediately after exercise which reaches its normal value quickly (1–2 minutes). However, in cases of significant PAD, the ankle pressure decreases more during treadmill exercise compared with healthy patients, and the recovery time to the pre-exercise value is also prolonged, proportional to the severity of PAD which is of diagnostic value in subclinical cases.[18,19]

Measurement of ABI

Technique

The resting SBP at the ankle is compared with the arm SBP and the ratio of the two pressures defines the ankle-brachial (or ankle-arm) index. The patients must rest for 15–30 minutes prior to and should not smoke atleast 2 hours before the ABI measurement. The cuff should be chosen adequately according to the limb size and width should be at least 40% of the limb circumference. An 8–10-MHz Doppler probe with Doppler gel is commonly used which should be placed in the area of the pulse at a 45–60° angle to the surface of the skin and moved around until the clearest signal is heard. To obtain the ankle pressure, BP cuff is placed just above the ankle. Then, while listening to either the dorsalis pedis or posterior tibial artery signal with a continuous wave Doppler, cuff is inflated to a pressure above which the audible Doppler signal disappears and then slowly released until the pedal signal returns and this systolic pressure is noted. This process is then repeated for contralateral side, followed by measurement of brachial artery pressure bilaterally in a similar fashion with the BP cuff placed around the upper arm. The goal is to detect occlusive disease by identifying pressure drop between the proximal aorta and distal circulation (ankle). The ABI is then calculated by dividing the higher ankle pressure (dorsalis pedis or posterior tibial artery) in each lower extremity by the higher of the two brachial artery systolic pressures.[19] There are several other methods that are used for measuring ABI including plethysmography, photoplethysmography, applanation tonometry, and oscillometry; but due to suboptimal reproducibility and high intra/interobserver variability these methods are not recommended as the preferred options. However, the ease of performing ABI measurement using these automated methods in comparison to time and training needed for Doppler-based measurements makes the former methods more popular at most of the centers.[20] The automated plethysmography technique involves measuring blood flow in the legs by first inflating a cuff on the upper thigh to inhibit venous return flow, and then measuring the increase in leg volume via strain gauges. This method is faster and easier, while maintaining accuracy as clinical results comparing alternative ABI methods to Doppler ABI have shown concordance above 90%.[21-23] More recently, oscillometry has been used for automated BP measurement and for estimation of ABI. In this method, four BP cuffs are tied around both arms and legs simultaneously. The cuffs are then automatically inflated and deflated at the same time and the respective limb pulse waveforms are recorded using the oscillometric sensors present in the BP cuffs. From this data, ABI can be easily calculated (Fig. 1).

Interpretation of Results

Table 1 provides normal range of ABI as well as partition values for various grades of PAD severity as recognized by ABI. The ABI values between 0.9 and 1.3 are generally considered to be normal.[19]

Abnormally High ABI

In some cases, the ankle artery is incompressible and the systolic pressure measured there is much higher than the brachial artery systolic pressure, leading to an ABI that exceeds the normal range. This is usually seen in presence of the calcification of the arterial wall and may occur in patients with medial calcinosis, diabetes mellitus, or end-stage renal disease. When vascular calcification is present, it can be assumed that lumen is narrow but actually the stenotic disease cannot be detected by ABI. Measurement of the toe-brachial index is useful in such circumstances because the digital vessels rarely develop calcification.[24]

Diagnostic Value in Diabetic Subjects

The sensitivity of ABI for detection of PAD is known to be suboptimal in diabetic patients as falsely high ABI values (>1.3–1.4) are particularly frequent in them, more specifically when diabetes is concomitant to kidney disease, neuropathy or foot lesions, and severe medial artery calcification.[25] Chung et al. showed that the most influential factor affecting the validity of ABI was diabetes, with high false negative results

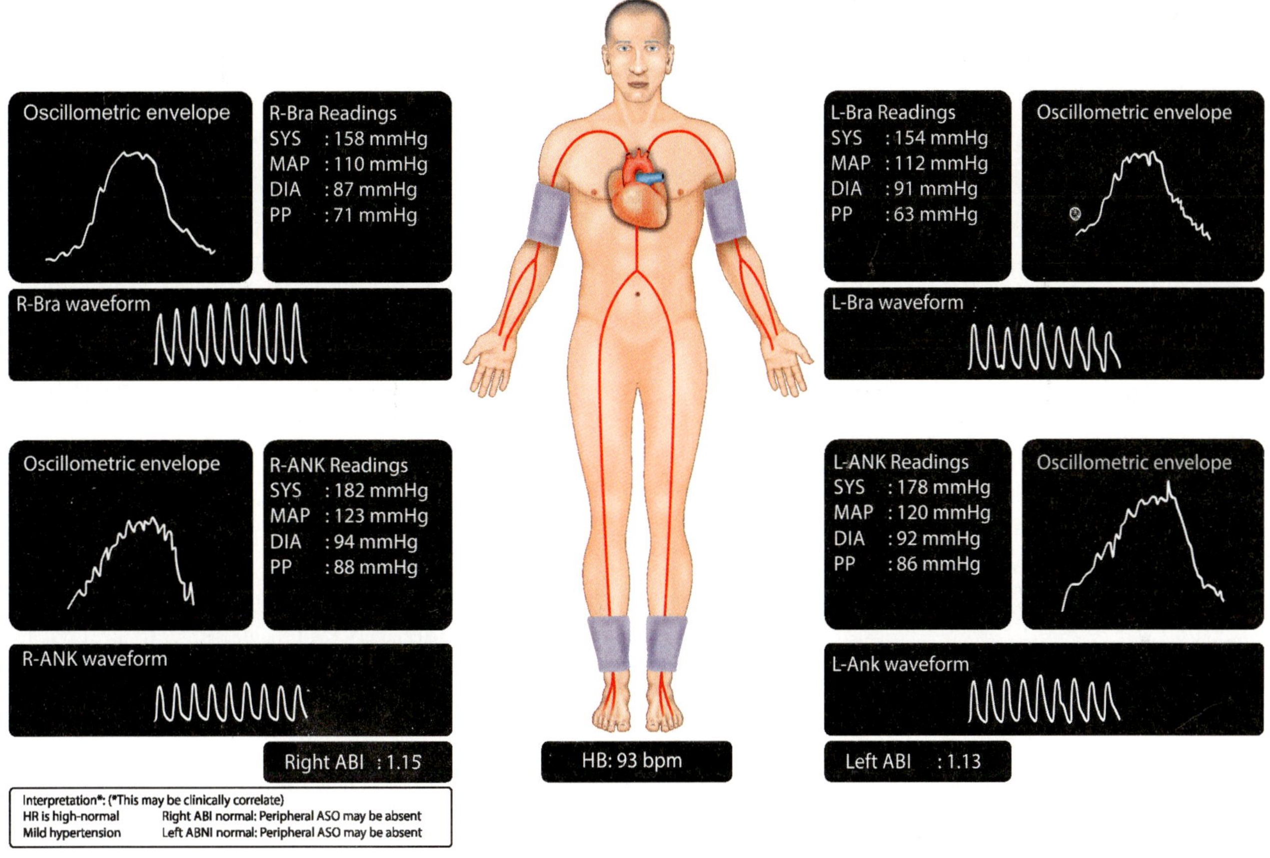

Fig. 1: Oscillometric method for automated measurement of ankle–brachial index

TABLE 1: Normal range of ankle–brachial index (ABI) and partition values for various grades of peripheral arterial disease (PAD) severity

ABI value	Interpretation	Comments
0.9–1.3	Normal	Usually excludes arterial occlusive disease but false negative results can occur. If symptoms strongly suggest claudication, exercise testing should be performed
<0.9	Occlusive arterial disease	If symptomatic (claudication) 95% sensitivity and 99% specificity for detecting arteriogram positive disease
<0.4	Severe occlusive disease	Often associated with multilevel disease (iliac, femoral or tibial vessel disease) and may be associated with nonhealing ulcerations, ischemic rest pain or pedal gangrene
>1.3	Suggests calcified vessels	Other diagnostic modalities are required for diagnosis

observed.[26] This observation is supported by several studies which showed that the decrease of the diagnostic efficiency of ABI is related to certain clinical situations related to diabetes such as neuropathy or foot wounds.[27,28] One way to improve the diagnostic efficiency of ABI might be to use a higher threshold, around 1–1.1, or to use the lowest value of ankle systolic pressure for calculating it. However, in these cases, a better method is to perform toe-pressure measurement as toe-brachial index is more sensitive than ABI, as mentioned earlier.[19]

Prognostic Value of ABI

The ABI is useful for diagnosing and evaluating the severity of PAD and plays an important role in the management of the same. It has a good prognostic value in patients of PAD as ABI values more than 0.5 are infrequently associated with progression to critical ischemia over next 6 years. More importantly, however, it is now a proven fact that ABI has an independent and important value in estimating global vascular prognosis.

CARDIOVASCULAR MORBIDITY AND MORTALITY

The ABI is a measure of the severity of atherosclerosis in the legs but is also an independent indicator of the risk of subsequent atherothrombotic events elsewhere in the vascular system. The ABI may be used as a risk marker both in the general population free of clinical CV disease (CVD) and in patients with established CVD. The ABI has been investigated as a risk predictor in several population-based cohort studies, mostly in the western world.[29-31] These studies have consistently found that a low ABI is associated with an increased risk for myocardial infarction, stroke, and both total and CVD-related mortality. Furthermore, as this association is independent of established CVD and CVD risk factors, incorporation of ABI can potentially enhance the accuracy of risk scoring systems like Framingham risk score.[2] A large international registry of patients found that among established PAD patients, 5.4% had a major CV event [CV death, myocardial infarction (MI), or stroke] at 1 year which was comparable to patients who had diagnosed coronary artery disease (CAD) or cerebrovascular disease.[32] 11-year follow-up in the Cardiovascular Health Study found an almost twofold increased risk for mortality in participants with ABI 0.71–0.9 compared to those with ABI 1.1–1.2.[33] A meta-analysis of nine studies evaluating ABI and subsequent CV outcomes in patients with ABI 0.8–0.9 also reached the same conclusion. Importantly, half of these patients with low ABI were asymptomatic and were identified through screening only.[34] A meta-analysis of 16 cohort studies comparing CV risk predicted by the Framingham risk score (FRS) compared to the risk predicted by ABI found that inclusion of the ABI in the CV risk stratification would lead to reclassification of the risk and a change in the treatment recommendations in around 20% of the patients. Thus, a low or high ABI is associated with increased CV risk, and the risk prediction extends beyond that of the FRS alone. The post-exercise ABI is also predictive of risk. In the case of a normal ABI at rest, the presence of an abnormal ABI after exercise is associated with increased mortality.[2]

Patients with established CVD who also have a low ABI are at higher risk compared with the patients who have CVD but have a normal ABI. In the Heart Outcomes Prevention Evaluation (HOPE) study of the patients with CAD, stroke, or diabetes mellitus, ABI values in the range of 0.60–0.90 were associated with a risk ratio for future nonfatal MI of 1.4, nonfatal stroke of 1.2, and CV mortality of 1.6 compared with higher ABI values.[35]

DIABETIC POPULATION

It has been shown that diabetes is the main risk factor for the occurrence of PAD. With every 1% increase in the glycosylated hemoglobin (HbA1c), there was a 28% increase in the risk of PAD in the United Kingdom Prospective Diabetes Study (UKPDS).[36] Unfortunately, despite increased prevalence of PAD, ABI has suboptimal sensitivity for diagnosing PAD in diabetic population due to the factors already discussed. Nonetheless, ABI is a valid prognostic factor for diabetic patients also, as it predicts the course of PAD as well as concomitant CAD and nephropathy in these patients. The Fremantle diabetes study showed that in type 2 diabetic population, an ABI less than 0.9 increased the risk of cardiac death by 67% and was an independent risk factor for amputation with a relative risk of 2.21.[37] A Chinese study and a Swedish study done with a longer follow-up came to the same conclusion and showed significantly higher risk of CV morbidity and mortality in diabetic patients with low ABI.[38,39] High ABI values (above the normal range) could also be an indicator of CV system damage. In a recent sub-analysis of the Strong Heart Study, Resnick et al. showed that any increase of ABI above 1.4 was an independent CV risk factor. The adjusted risk for CV mortality was 2.52 with an ABI below 0.9 and 2.09 with an ABI above 1.4. This association was positive in diabetic patients also, who represented 67.8% of the patients with a high ABI (i.e. >1.4).[40] Thus, not only low, but also high ABI values are prognostic of CV risk as well as the risk of occurrence of foot-related injuries and amputations, especially in diabetic patients. In a recent analysis of the National Health and Examination Survey, Wu et al. studied the relationship between PAD, defined as an ABI less than 0.9 or more than 1.4, and renal failure and/or microalbuminuria in 7,068 subjects of whom 1,156 were diabetics. The presence of abnormal renal function [glomerular filtration rate (GFR) < 60 mL/min/1.73 m^2] was strongly associated with PAD in the diabetic patients, whereas there was no significant association in the nondiabetic patients.[41] However, this observation could not be translated into a beneficial change in the treatment protocol because most of these patients already qualified for statin as per the existing AHA guideline which recommends statins for all patients with PAD and most people with diabetes.

In the recently published data from the ARIC study, done in more than 12,000 patients with a median follow-up of 21 years, the investigators found that low or borderline low ABI (≤1.0) was associated with a moderately increased risk for diabetes.[7] The association was independent of other atherosclerotic CVD, physical activity, and other potential confounders.

SCREENING—IS IT NEEDED?

There is now enough literature which suggests that screening for PAD in asymptomatic individuals should be considered in terms of CV, and not just limb-related outcomes. The goal should be to identify patients at high risk for CAD or other CVD and aggressively treat the risk factors to prevent CV events. Widespread ABI screening could be particularly useful if it identified a large number of individuals with a low ABI who would otherwise not qualify for cholesterol-lowering therapy. It can be argued that because majority of the patients with PAD are asymptomatic, measurement of ABI only when prompted by symptoms will result in most cases of PAD going unrecognized, whereas the patients who present with symptomatic PAD are already likely to have clinically established CVD in whom the preventive strategies will be of much less benefit. For example, in the PAD Awareness, Risk, and Treatment: New Resources for Survival (PARTNERS) study, 44% of those found to have an ABI below 0.90 had no prior diagnosis of PAD.[27]

RECOMMENDATIONS

- *The Trans-Atlantic Inter-Society (TASC) II report (2007)*: The TASC-II consensus document on management of PAD[42] recommends screening for PAD by ABI measurement in primary care for:
  - Patients with exertional leg symptoms
  - Patients aged 50–69 with CV risk factors
  - All patients 70 years of age or older
  - Subjects with a 10-year risk of a CV event between 10% and 20%, as determined by SCORE or Framingham risk score.
- *The ACC/AHA recommendations*: The 2011 update of 2005 guideline from the ACC/AHA states that individuals with asymptomatic lower extremity PAD should be identified by examination and/or measurement of the ABI specially in the following high-risk groups:[43]
  - Less than 50 years with diabetes and an additional CVD risk factor
  - More than or equal to 50 years with a history of smoking or diabetes
  - More than or equal to 65 years

Additionally, AHA (2013) and European Society of Cardiology (2016) both recommend (II B) in latest guidelines that if, after quantitative risk assessment, a risk-based treatment decision is uncertain, assessment of ABI may be considered to inform treatment decision.[44,45]

CONCLUSION

The ABI is a simple noninvasive tool for detection of asymptomatic PAD. Given the strong association between PAD and atherosclerotic CVD involving other vascular beds, detection of asymptomatic PAD by ABI provides an excellent opportunity to institute aggressive risk reduction strategies to prevent development of CV events in the affected individuals. Apart from this, ABI is also a useful tool for monitoring disease progression and treatment response in PAD patients. Finally, ABI may also be used as a predictor for future development of diabetes among those who are at risk for developing diabetes.

REFERENCES

1. Fowkes FG, Rudan D, Rudan I, et al. Comparison of global estimates of prevalence and risk factors for peripheral artery disease in 2000 and 2010: a systematic review and analysis. Lancet. 2013;382(9901):1329-40.
2. Ankle Brachial Index Collaboration, Fowkes FG, Murray GD, et al. Ankle brachial index combined with Framingham Risk Score to predict cardiovascular events and mortality: a meta-analysis. JAMA. 2008;300(2):197-208.
3. Hirsch AT, Haskal ZJ, Hertzer NR, et al. ACC/AHA 2005 guidelines for the management of patients with peripheral arterial disease (lower extremity, renal, mesenteric, and abdominal aortic): executive summary a collaborative report from the American Association for Vascular Surgery/Society for Vascular Surgery, Society for Cardiovascular Angiography and Interventions, Society for Vascular Medicine and Biology, Society of Interventional Radiology, and the ACC/AHA Task Force on Practice Guidelines (Writing Committee to Develop Guidelines for the Management of Patients With Peripheral Arterial Disease) endorsed by the American Association of Cardiovascular and Pulmonary Rehabilitation; National Heart, Lung, and Blood Institute; Society for Vascular Nursing; TransAtlantic Inter-Society Consensus; and Vascular Disease Foundation. J Am Coll Cardiol. 2006;47(6):1239-312.
4. Belch J, MacCuish A, Campbell I, et al. The prevention of progression of arterial disease and diabetes (POPADAD) trial: factorial randomised placebo controlled trial of aspirin and antioxidants in patients with diabetes and asymptomatic peripheral arterial disease. BMJ. 2008;337:a1840.
5. CAPRIE Steering Committee. A randomised, blinded, trial of clopidogrel versus aspirin in patients at risk of ischaemic events (CAPRIE). CAPRIE Steering Committee. Lancet. 1996;348(9038):1329-39.
6. Feringa HH, Karagiannis SE, van Waning VH, et al. The effect of intensified lipid-lowering therapy on long-term prognosis in patients with peripheral arterial disease. J Vasc Surg. 2007;45(5):936-43.
7. Hua S, Loehr LR, Tanaka H, et al. Ankle-brachial index and incident diabetes mellitus: the atherosclerosis risk in communities (ARIC) study. Cardiovasc Diabetol. 2016;15(1):163.
8. American Diabetes Association. Peripheral arterial disease in people with diabetes. Diabetes Care. 2003;26(12):3333-41.
9. Winsor T. Influence of arterial disease on the systolic blood pressure gradients of the extremity. Am J Med Sci. 1950;220(2):117-26.

10. Carter SA. Indirect systolic pressures and pulse waves in arterial occlusive diseases of the lower extremities. Circulation. 1968;37(4):624-37.
11. Yao ST, Hobbs JT, Irvine WT. Ankle systolic pressure measurements in arterial disease affecting the lower extremities. Brit J Surg. 1969;56(9):676-9.
12. Hiatt WR, Goldstone J, Smith SC, et al. Atherosclerotic Peripheral Vascular Disease Symposium II: nomenclature for vascular diseases. Circulation. 2008;118(25):2826-9.
13. Safar ME, Protogerou AD, Blacher J. Statins, central blood pressure, and blood pressure amplification. Circulation. 2009;119(1):9-12.
14. Katz S, Globerman A, Avitzour M, et al. The ankle-brachial index in normal neonates and infants is significantly lower than in older children and adults. J Pediatr Surg. 1997;32(2):269-71.
15. London GM, Guerin AP, Pannier B, et al. Influence of sex on arterial hemodynamics and blood pressure. Role of body height. Hypertension. 1995;26(3):514-9.
16. Aboyans V, Criqui MH, McClelland RL, et al. Intrinsic contribution of gender and ethnicity to normal ankle-brachial index values: the Multi-Ethnic Study of Atherosclerosis (MESA). J Vasc Surg. 2007;45(2):319-27.
17. Zheng ZJ, Rosamond WD, Chambless LE, et al. Lower extremity arterial disease assessed by ankle-brachial index in a middle-aged population of African Americans and whites: the Atherosclerosis Risk in Communities (ARIC) Study. Am J Prev Med. 2005;29(5 Suppl 1):42-9.
18. Carter SA. Response of ankle systolic pressure to leg exercise in mild or questionable arterial disease. N Engl J Med. 1972;287(12): 578-82.
19. Aboyans V, Criqui MH, Abraham P, et al. Measurement and interpretation of the ankle-brachial index: a scientific statement from the American Heart Association. Circulation. 2012;126(24):2890-909.
20. Diage TR, Johnson G, Ravipati G. Digital ankle-brachial index technology used in primary care settings to detect flow obstruction: a population based registry study. BMC Res Notes. 2013;6:404.
21. Jonsson B, Laurent C, Eneling M, et al. Automatic ankle pressure measurements using PPG in ankle-brachial pressure index determination. Eur J Vasc Endovasc Surg. 2005;30(4):395-401.
22. Khandanpour N, Armon MP, Jennings B, et al. Photoplethysmography, an easy and accurate method for measuring ankle brachial pressure index: can photoplethysmography replace Doppler? Vasc Endovasc Surg. 2009;43(6):578-82.
23. Whiteley MS, Fox AD, Horrocks M. Photoplethysmography can replace hand-held Doppler in the measurement of ankle/brachial indices. Ann R Coll Surg Engl. 1998;80(2):96-8.
24. Aboyans V, Ho E, Denenberg JO, et al. The association between elevated ankle systolic pressures and peripheral occlusive arterial disease in diabetic and nondiabetic subjects. J Vasc Surg. 2008;48(5):1197-203.
25. Potier L, Abi Khalil C, Mohammedi K, et al. Use and utility of ankle brachial index in patients with diabetes. Eur J Vasc Endovasc Surg. 2011;41(1):110-6.
26. Chung CM, Tseng YH, Lin YS, et al. Association of brachial-ankle pulse wave velocity with atherosclerosis and presence of coronary artery disease in older patients. Clin Interv Aging. 2015;10: 1369-75.
27. Hirsch AT, Hiatt WR, PARTNERS Steering Committee. PAD awareness, risk, and treatment: new resources for survival--the USA PARTNERS program. Vasc Med. 2001;6(3 Suppl):9-12.
28. Davis WA, Norman PE, Bruce DG, et al. Predictors, consequences and costs of diabetes-related lower extremity amputation complicating type 2 diabetes: the Fremantle Diabetes Study. Diabetologia. 2006;49(11):2634-41.
29. Leng GC, Fowkes FG, Lee AJ, et al. Use of ankle brachial pressure index to predict cardiovascular events and death: a cohort study. BMJ. 1996;313(7070):1440-4.
30. Hooi JD, Kester AD, Stoffers HE, et al. Asymptomatic peripheral arterial occlusive disease predicted cardiovascular morbidity and mortality in a 7-year follow-up study. J Clin Epidemiol. 2004;57(3):294-300.
31. van der Meer IM, Bots ML, Hofman A, et al. Predictive value of noninvasive measures of atherosclerosis for incident myocardial infarction: the Rotterdam Study. Circulation. 2004;109(9):1089-94.
32. Steg PG, Bhatt DL, Wilson PW, et al. One-year cardiovascular event rates in outpatients with atherothrombosis. JAMA. 2007;297(11):1197-206.
33. O'Hare AM, Katz R, Shlipak MG, et al. Mortality and cardiovascular risk across the ankle-arm index spectrum: results from the Cardiovascular Health Study. Circulation. 2006;113(3):388-93.
34. Doobay AV, Anand SS. Sensitivity and specificity of the ankle-brachial index to predict future cardiovascular outcomes: a systematic review. Arterioscler Thromb Vasc Biol. 2005;25(7):1463-9.
35. Duprez D. HOPE brings hope for the use of the ankle-brachial index as cardiovascular risk marker. Eur Heart J. 2004;25(1):1-2.
36. Adler AI, Stevens RJ, Neil A, et al. UKPDS 59: hyperglycemia and other potentially modifiable risk factors for peripheral vascular disease in type 2 diabetes. Diabetes Care. 2002;25(5):894-9.
37. Norman PE, Davis WA, Bruce DG, et al. Peripheral arterial disease and risk of cardiac death in type 2 diabetes: the Fremantle Diabetes Study. Diabetes Care. 2006;29(3):575-80.
38. Li J, Luo Y, Xu Y, et al. Risk factors of peripheral arterial disease and relationship between low ankle - brachial index and mortality from all-cause and cardiovascular disease in Chinese patients with type 2 diabetes. Circ J. 2007;71(3):377-81.
39. Ogren M, Hedblad B, Engstrom G, et al. Prevalence and prognostic significance of asymptomatic peripheral arterial disease in 68-year-old men with diabetes. Results from the population study 'Men born in 1914' from Malmo, Sweden. Eur J Vasc Endovasc Surg. 2005;29(2):182-9.
40. Resnick HE, Lindsay RS, McDermott MM, et al. Relationship of high and low ankle brachial index to all-cause and cardiovascular disease mortality: the Strong Heart Study. Circulation. 2004;109(6):733-9.
41. Wu CK, Yang CY, Tsai CT, et al. Association of low glomerular filtration rate and albuminuria with peripheral arterial disease: the National Health and Nutrition Examination Survey, 1999-2004. Atherosclerosis. 2010;209(1):230-4.
42. Norgren L, Hiatt WR, Dormandy JA, et al. Inter-Society Consensus for the Management of Peripheral Arterial Disease (TASC II). J Vasc Surg. 2007;45 Suppl S:S5-67.
43. Rooke TW, Hirsch AT, Misra S, et al. 2011 ACCF/AHA Focused Update of the Guideline for the Management of Patients With Peripheral Artery Disease (updating the 2005 guideline): a report of the American College of Cardiology Foundation/American Heart Association Task Force on Practice Guidelines. J Am Coll Cardiol. 2011;58(19):2020-45.
44. Goff DC, Lloyd-Jones DM, Bennett G, et al. 2013 ACC/AHA guideline on the assessment of cardiovascular risk: a report of the American College of Cardiology/American Heart Association Task Force on Practice Guidelines. J Am Coll Cardiol. 2014;63(25 Pt B):2935-59.
45. Piepoli MF, Hoes AW, Agewall S, et al. 2016 European Guidelines on cardiovascular disease prevention in clinical practice: The Sixth Joint Task Force of the European Society of Cardiology and Other Societies on Cardiovascular Disease Prevention in Clinical Practice (constituted by representatives of 10 societies and by invited experts) Developed with the special contribution of the European Association for Cardiovascular Prevention & Rehabilitation (EACPR). Eur Heart J. 2016;37(29):2315-81.

CHAPTER 44

Computed Tomography Evaluation of Abdominal Arterial Wall Calcification in Patients with Type 2 Diabetes Mellitus

Charu Paruthi, Shivya Tucker, HK Chopra, Reeta Kanaujiya, Gauri Gupta

INTRODUCTION

The incidence and prevalence of type 2 diabetes is continuously increasing and by 2025, more than 380 million people worldwide are estimated to be diabetics.[1] Arterial wall calcification is a common finding in diabetic patients. Calcification of the tunica media is found pathologically, a process called Monckeberg's sclerosis or arteriosclerosis, which is nonocclusive and is seen as concentric calcifications in the arterial wall on computed tomography (CT) or ultrasound. Intimal calcification also occurs and presents as eccentric occlusive calcific foci in the arterial wall. These are related to atherosclerotic plaques. The former is more common in diabetes and has been related to greater incidence of cardiovascular morbidity, disease progression, and poor prognosis. Diffuse arterial wall calcification has been described in literature, and the coronary arteries, aorta, and limb vessels are most commonly studied.[2,3] Information regarding involvement of abdominal artery calcification in diabetes is scanty and there is no data about any particular artery being more commonly involved than the others. This study was conducted to look for pattern and distribution of abdominal arterial calcification in diabetic patients and find out if any particular artery is more commonly involved than the others.

MATERIALS AND METHODS

This cross-sectional study was conducted in the radiology department at our hospital. A total of 61 patients aged more than 50 years, who underwent CT scan of the abdomen over a 2 month period, were included in the study. Noncontrast scans were reviewed by two radiologists and the site and extent of abdominal arterial wall calcification was recorded. History of type 2 diabetes and chronic kidney disease (CKD) was obtained from hospital records. The different sites of arterial wall calcifications in diabetic patients were noted and compared with nondiabetics using chi-square test. Presence of coexistent diabetes and CKD was also noted and its correlation was done for arterial sites showing significantly greater calcification in diabetics. A p-value of greater than 0.5 was considered to be significant.

OBSERVATIONS AND RESULTS

A total of 61 patients with an average age of 65.1 ± 1.2 years and age range of 50–98 years were included in the study. Male to female ratio was approximately 2:1.18 patients (29.5%) were type 2 diabetics and 43 patients (30.5%) were nondiabetics. 13 patients (23.1%) in the study group had hypertension, out of which seven had coexistent type 2 diabetes. CKD details were available only for 32 patients. Seven patients had CKD, out of which five had coexistent type 2 diabetes. Distribution of wall calcification in various abdominal arteries in the study population is shown in Table 1.

Overall, most of the patients showed wall calcifications in the aorta, followed by common iliac arteries and proximal internal iliac arteries. The arterial sites showing significantly greater calcification in diabetics include symmetrical circumferential wall calcifications in bilateral distal internal

TABLE 1: Wall calcification in various abdominal arteries.

Artery	Total	Diabetics	Nondiabetics	p-value*
Aorta	51	17	34	0.26
Aorta—eccentric	45	13	32	0.55
Aorta—circumferential	11	5	6	0.28
Splenic artery	7	6	1	0.002
CIA	34	11	23	0.39
Proximal IIA	25	6	19	0.57
Distal IIA circumferential	15	12	3	0.00
Coeliac artery	5	4	1	0.02
SMA	10	7	3	0.005
IMA	4	4	0	0.006
Renal artery	8	3	5	0.44

Abbreviations: CIA, common iliac artery; IMA, inferior mesenteric artery; IIA, internal iliac artery; SMA, superior mesenteric artery

**chi-square*

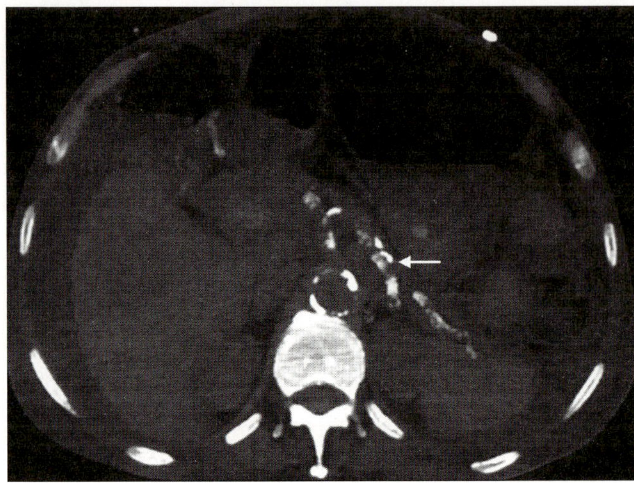

Fig. 2: Noncontrast computed tomography (NCCT) scan of abdomen showing circumferential wall calcification in splenic artery (arrow)

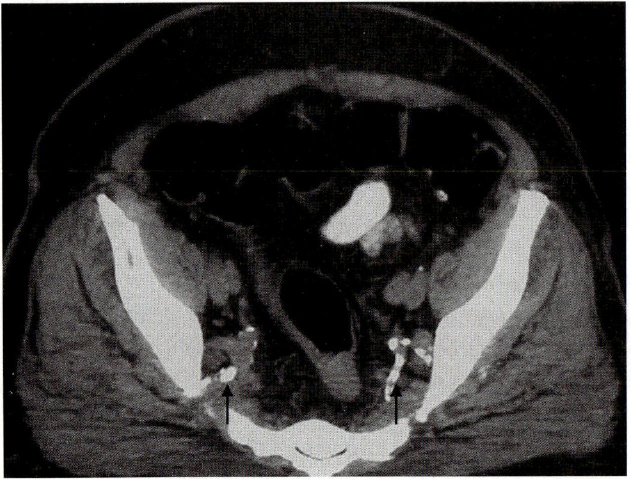

Fig. 1: Noncontrast computed tomography (NCCT) section of pelvis showing bilaterally symmetrical circumferential calcification in bilateral distal internal iliac arteries (arrows)

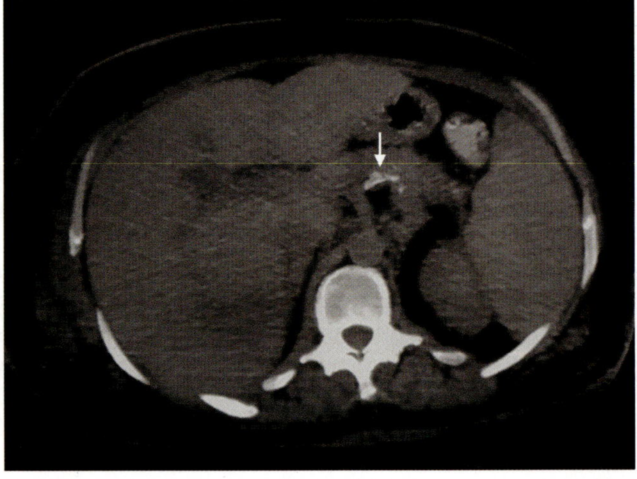

Fig. 3: Noncontrast computed tomography (NCCT) abdomen showing eccentric wall calcification in proximal splenic artery (arrow)

iliac arteries and splenic artery (Figs 1 and 2). Five out of six diabetic patients with splenic artery calcification showed circumferential calcifications involving greater than 50% of the arterial circumference. One patient showed eccentric long segment calcification involving less than half of arterial circumference (Fig. 3). Coeliac artery, superior mesenteric artery (SMA), and inferior mesenteric artery (IMA) also showed significantly greater calcification in diabetics than nondiabetics. These were either circumferential or eccentric and no significant pattern was observed. Most of these were a part of diffuse calcifications in the entire arterial tree (Figs 4A and B). For diabetics having calcifications in distal internal iliac artery (IIA), coeliac artery, SMA, and IMA, no significant correlation was seen with CKD. However, four out of six diabetic patients with splenic artery calcification had concomitant CKD. In the study population, a total of six patients showed extensive circumferential wall calcifications involving most of the visualized arteries. Out of these, four had concomitant type 2 diabetes and CKD, one had only diabetes, and one had only CKD.

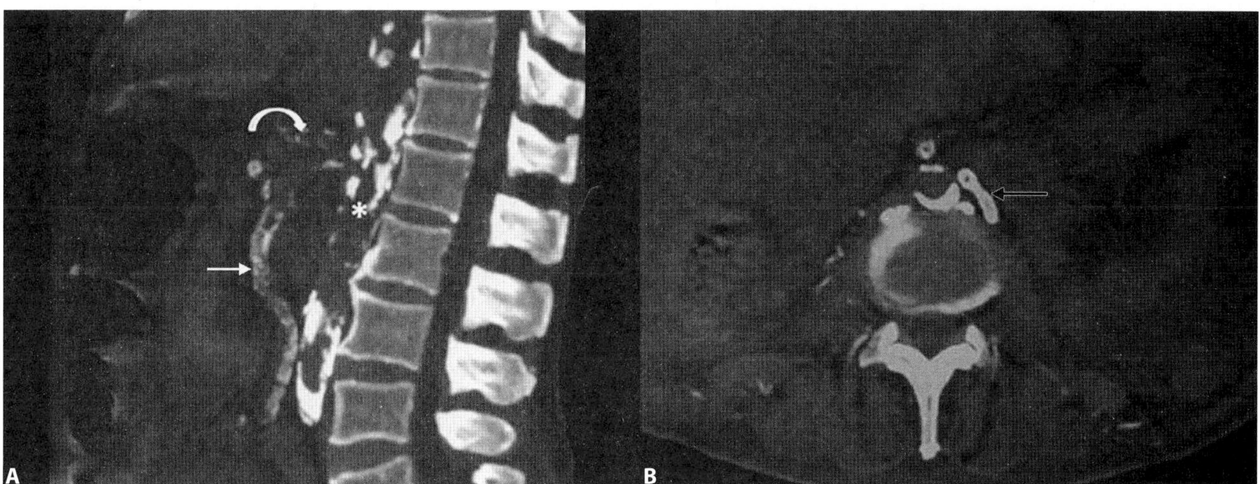

Figs 4A and B: (A) NCCT abdomen in sagittal; and (B) Axial planes showing diffuse wall calcification of the arterial tree involving the aorta (asterisk), coeliac artery (curved arrow), SMA (white straight arrow), and IMA (black arrow)

Abbreviations: IMA, inferior mesenteric artery; NCCT, noncontrast computed tomography; SMA, superior mesenteric artery

DISCUSSION

Vascular wall calcification is a common phenomenon in diabetes. This calcification includes intimal layer calcification, which is associated with atherosclerosis, and medial layer calcification, which is associated with arteriosclerosis. Newer studies dismiss the notion of these two being separate entities and consider them to be a continuum.[4,5] Arterial wall calcification in diabetes is considered to be an active and complex cell-mediated process, involving various metabolic, cytokine, and inflammatory factors. Multiple factors associated with bone homeostasis are now believed to be regulating it, similar to end-stage renal disease. This is further potentiated by hyperglycemia and hypoxia.[6] Vascular wall calcification is considered to be an independent risk factor for cardiovascular mortality and disease progression.[2,3] Wall calcification leads to decreased arterial compliance and its impaired function, leading to distal organ dysfunction and symptoms.[7] Studies have found a link between peripheral vascular calcification and bilaterally symmetrical distal peripheral neuropathy in diabetics. Also, osteopenia is often coexistent in diabetics with arterial calcification.[8]

Peripheral and coronary arterial calcifications are most commonly studied in diabetics. Diabetes is a systemic disease and involves arteries in all parts of the body, including abdominal arteries. We found that abdominal aorta was the most common artery showing calcifications, irrespective of the diabetic status. This is because being a large-sized vessel with multiple branches, aorta is a common site for atherosclerotic plaque due to high shear and stress. A large number of other conditions like dyslipidemia, old age, etc. also lead to aortic calcifications.[9,10] An interesting finding was that a significantly greater number of diabetic patients had circumferential and symmetrical wall calcification in bilateral distal internal iliac arteries. Distal distribution of arterial calcification in limb vessels in diabetic patients is a known phenomenon and has recently been linked to peripheral neuropathy.[8] Though peripheral neuropathy is typically the "glove and stocking" neuropathy or distal symmetric polyneuropathy involving the limbs, neuropathy involving the inguinal and perineal regions is also common in diabetics.[11,12] As these regions are supplied by the distal and cutaneous branches of IIAs, calcification in distal IIA found in diabetics could be related to neuropathy in these regions in diabetic patients.

Splenic artery calcifications were also significantly greater in diabetics in our study. Some of them were a spectrum of diffuse arterial tree calcifications involving most of the visualized arteries, and majority were found to have coexistent CKD. Preferential involvement of splenic artery in diabetics can be explained by the fact that pancreatic arterial supply is derived from splenic artery. Pathological studies have shown arteriolar changes and sclerosis within the pancreatic parenchyma in diabetics, with some of the arterioles showing intimal hyalinization and luminal occlusion. Pancreatic parenchymal fibrosis and atrophy increases with the duration of diabetes and so does the arteriolar changes. Thus, increased inflammatory mediators in parenchymal vessels would lead to their increase in the parent vessel, the splenic artery, as well, which would explain its greater involvement in diabetics.[13,14] This could also lead to a greater involvement of coeliac axis in diabetics. This finding was observed in our study. However, most of the cases were a part of diffuse wall calcification of the arterial tree. Some of the pitfalls of the study were that the sample size was small and renal function details of all patients were not available. Further studies with a population of a larger size and different ethnicity may bring more information on this topic.

CONCLUSION

Abdominal arterial calcification is common in type 2 diabetics. Circumferential symmetric calcification in bilateral IIAs and calcifications in splenic artery is significantly greater in diabetics than nondiabetics. Study of distribution of arterial calcification may help in further understanding the pathophysiology of related symptoms in patients and may be useful in planning treatment for disease control and complication prevention, as arterial calcifications are independent risk factors for disease progression and related morbidity. Further studies are required to confirm and validate our findings.

REFERENCES

1. Scholte AJ, Schuijf JD, Kharagjitsingh AV, et al. Prevalence of coronary artery disease and plaque morphology assessed by multislice computed tomography coronary angiography and calcium scoring in asymptomatic patients with type 2 diabetes. Heart. 2008;94(3):290-5.
2. Kovacic JC, Fuster V. Vascular Calcification, Diabetes and Cardiovascular Disease - Connecting the Dots. JACC Cardiovasc Imaging. 2012;5(4):367-9.
3. Liu KH, Chu WC, Kong AP, et al. US assessment of medial arterial calcification: a sensitive marker of diabetes-related microvascular and macrovascular complications. Radiology. 2012;265(1):294-302.
4. Chistiakov DA, Sobenin IA, Orekhov AN, et al. Mechanisms of medial arterial calcification in diabetes. Curr Pharm Des. 2014;20(37):5870-83.
5. Chen NX, Moe SM. Arterial calcification in diabetes. Curr Diab Rep. 2003;3(1):28-32.
6. Rogers MA, Aikawa E. Modifying Vascular Calcification in Diabetes: Contribution of O-GlcNAcylation. Circ Res. 2014;114(7):1074-6.
7. Stabley JN, Towler DA. Arterial Calcification in Diabetes Mellitus: Preclinical Models and Translational Implications. Arterioscler Thromb Vasc Biol. 2017;37(2):205-17.
8. Jeffcoate WJ, Rasmussen LM, Hofbauer LC, et al. Medial arterial calcification in diabetes and its relationship to neuropathy. Diabetologia. 2009;52(12):2478-88.
9. Kim ED, Kim JS, Kim SS, et al. Association of abdominal aortic calcification with lifestyle and risk factors of cardiovascular disease. Korean J Fam Med. 2013;34(3):213-20.
10. Jayalath RW, Mangan SH, Golledge J. Aortic calcification. Eur J Vasc Endovasc Surg. 2005;30(5):476-88.
11. Aring AM, Jones DE, Falko JM. Evaluation and prevention of diabetic neuropathy. Am Fam Physician. 2005;71(11):2123-8.
12. Boulton AJ. Management of Diabetic Peripheral Neuropathy. Clin Diabetes. 2005;23(1):9-15.
13. Volk BW, Wellmann KF. The Diabetic Pancreas, 1st edition. New York: Plenum Press; 1977.
14. Patil PV, Patil MG, Patil AM. Isolated intrasplenic vascular calcifications in a child with type 1 diabetes mellitus---A case report. J Clin Ultrasound. 2017;45(7):438-40.

CHAPTER

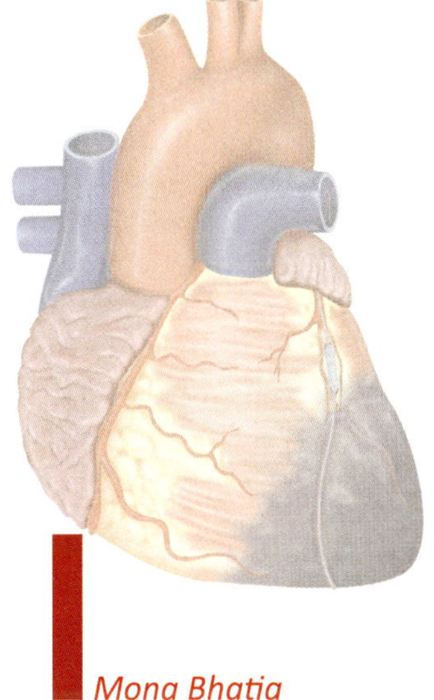

Cardiac MRI: A Promise, Hope or Hype in Cardiodiabetes

Mona Bhatia

INTRODUCTION

Diabetes mellitus is one of the major risk factors of cardiovascular disease[1-4] and is growing exponentially globally.[2] Leyden et al. in 1881, first established the relationship between diabetes and heart disease.[5] The resultant diabetic cardiomyopathy (DCM) encompasses diabetes-related structural and functional myocardial dysfunction. This is independent of other traditional risk factors as hypertension, valvular heart disease, and coronary artery disease (CAD).[6-9] Associations of DCM include left ventricular diastolic dysfunction and/or reduced left ventricular ejection fraction (EF), pathological left ventricle hypertrophy, and interstitial fibrosis.[10] The left ventricular remodeling may be eccentric with left ventricular systolic dysfunction or concentric with left ventricular diastolic dysfunction.[11] Two phenotypes of DCM are described. The first being restrictive or heart failure with preserved left ventricular ejection fraction (HFPEF) more often seen in diabetes mellitus-induced metabolic derangements prevalent in obesity and dilated or heart failure with impaired or reduced left ventricular ejection fraction (HFREF) more often seen with autoimmunity in type 1 DM.[12] Vascular pathologies including macroangiopathic and microangiopathic complications are known to frequently coexist with DCM. Besides accelerated atherosclerosis and obstructive coronary disease,[13] complications of macroangiopathy include heart disease, stroke, and peripheral arterial disease,[14] while complications related to microangiopathy encompass retinopathy,[15] neuropathy,[16] and nephropathy.[16]

DIAGNOSTIC MODALITIES

The availability of multiple noninvasive and invasive diagnostic modalities as echocardiography, nuclear medicine, computed tomography (CT), magnetic resonance imaging (MRI), and endocardial biopsy, today offer a wide range of techniques available for evaluation of diabetic heart disease. Standard echocardiographic and nuclear techniques have limitations of suboptimal imaging windows, obesity and increased dose of ionizing radiation, multivessel coronary disease, with challenges from balanced ischemia. The current state-of-the-art cardiac magnetic resonance (CMR) imaging is emerging as the promise and hope in cardiodiabetes. Cardiac MRI provides a very high spatial and temporal resolution that rivals echocardiography. CMR is the gold standard to quantify cardiac function and structure. It further has the advantage of being less operator-dependent, and free of ionizing radiation. CMR today provides highly accurate assessment of myocardial function and morphology including myocardial edema, perfusion, energetics, and fibrosis assessment.[17-21] Hence, the role of CMR is fast growing in diabetic heart disease, from evaluating subclinical to clinical myocardial ischemia to nonischemic remodeling.

Cardiac MRI in Assessment of Cardiodiabetes

The sequences commonly used are gradient echo MRI for cine display of the cardiac chambers through the entire cardiac cycle with high spatial and temporal resolution.[22] This sequence is extremely useful in characterization of ventricular dimensions, function, and contractility.[23] Tagging sequences further assist in assessment of cardiac deformation along cardiac cycles,[24] myocardial strain,[25] and subclinical systolic and diastolic function.[26] Direction and velocity of flow assessment is possible with phase contrast imaging.[27]

Post-gadolinium-enhanced CMR imaging can assess presence, extent, and location of perfusion defects, fibrosis, and scars within the heart, which bear a prognostic importance particularly in subclinical or clinically unrecognized myocardial infarction (MI) or ischemia. Stress CMR using stress vasodilators as regadenoson or adenosine or adrenergic agents as dobutamine and more recently exercise agents enable accurate evaluation of stress rest first-pass myocardial perfusion.[28,29] Myocardial scar detection, extent, and localization is possible with post-gadolinium early and delayed imaging with high spatial resolution.

Cardiac magnetic resonance is extremely accurate in detection of subendocardial scars with an in-plane spatial resolution of 1–2 mm.[30] Scar transmurality also has a prognostic value.

Recent techniques include T1 mapping with T1 time estimation and sequential T1 mapping to map cardiac extracellular matrix remodeling, which is a hallmark of DCM.[31] Patients with type 2 diabetes have a significantly shorter myocardial T1 time.[31] A shorter myocardial T1 time is associated with poorer diastolic function, more impaired exercise capacity and more insulin resistance.[32] Advance spectroscopic techniques as 31P-CMR spectroscopy and 1H-CMR spectroscopy have emerged as research tools to investigate physiology and therapeutic effects by measuring myocardial energetics and myocardial lipid contents, respectively.[33,34] In total, CMR provides a unique comprehensive assessment of clinically validated measures of LV mass, structure, and function, myocardial perfusion, fibrosis, and energetics.

Limitation of Cardiac MRI

However, MRI has its limitations including challenges faced with claustrophobic patients, incompatibility with some pacemakers, implantable defibrillators, and underestimation of diastolic dysfunction.[35]

Role of Cardiac MRI in CAD in Diabetics

Diabetes is an important risk factor for CAD. Diabetics are at an increased risk of subclinical and clinical MI and post-MI complications. Impaired collateralization, ischemic preconditioning, and atypical or absence of chest pain from ischemia lead to missed or delayed diagnosis and treatment. CMR has an important role in assessment of CAD and its complications (e.g., MI, HF, and sudden cardiac death) which are the most common cause of morbidity and mortality in patients with diabetics.[36] In the evaluation of ischemic cardiac disease CMR has an established role to accurately evaluate ventricular structure, function, degree, and extent of ischemia and myocardial scar. Subclinical or clinically unrecognized MI detected by LGE is associated with long-term risk of mortality identical to clinical MI patients. Besides unrecognized MI is often undertreated.[37] Stress perfusion CMR is an impressive single modality to identify prognostically important myocardial indices. Stress perfusion defects and stress-induced wall motion abnormalities contribute independently to major adverse cardiac events (MACE).[38-42] In detection of angiographically significant coronary stenosis, CMR has 86.5% sensitivity and 83.4% specificity.[43] Thus CMR has an important diagnostic and prognostic role and can impact clinical outcomes with revascularization of ischemic myocardium.

CONCLUSION

Cardiac MRI is an extremely robust and comprehensive tool with a wide range of sequences to accurately detect, localize, and quantitate myocardial function, structure, perfusion, fibrosis, scar, remodeling, energetics, lipid metabolism, and diffuse extracellular matrix expansion to evaluate the entire spectrum of diabetic cardiovascular disease encompassing ischemic myocardial disease and nonischemic remodeling. With the exponential growth in diabetic numbers, and increasing promise and availability of cardiac MRI, an exponential usage of cardiac MRI in DCM is most definite.

REFERENCES

1. Bertoni AG, Hundley WG, Massing MW, et al. Heart failure prevalence, incidence, and mortality in the elderly with diabetes. Diabetes Care. 2004;27(3):699-703.
2. Kannel W, Hjortland M, Castelli WP. Role of diabetes in congestive heart failure: the Framingham Study. Am J Cardiol. 1974;34(1):29-34.
3. de Simone G, Devereux RB, Chinali M, et al. Diabetes and incident heart failure in hypertensive and normotensive participants of the Strong Heart Study. J Hypertens. 2010;28(2):353-60.

4. Burchfiel CM, Reed DM, Marcus EB, et al. Association of diabetes mellitus with coronary atherosclerosis and myocardial lesions: an autopsy study from the Honolulu Heart Program. Am J Epidemiol. 1993;137(12):1328-40.
5. Asghar O, Al-Sunni A, Khavandi K, et al. Diabetic cardiomyopathy. Clin Sci Lond Engl. 1979;2009(116):741-60.
6. Liu Q, Wang S, Cai L. Diabetic cardiomyopathy and its mechanisms: Role of oxidative stress and damage. J Diabetes Investig. 2014;5(6):623-34.
7. Boudina S, Abel ED. Diabetic cardiomyopathy revisited. Circulation. 2007;115(25):3213-23.
8. Miki T, Yuda S, Kouzu H, et al. Diabetic cardiomyopathy: pathophysiology and clinical features. Heart Fail Rev. 2013;18(2):149-66.
9. Rubler S, Dlugash J, Yuceoglu YZ, et al. New type of cardiomyopathy associated with diabetic glomerulosclerosis. Am J Cardiol. 1972;30(6):595-602.
10. Fontes-Carvalho R, Ladeiras-Lopes R, Bettencourt P, et al. Diastolic dysfunction in the diabetic continuum: association with insulin resistance, metabolic syndrome and type 2 diabetes. Cardiovasc Diabetol. 2015;14:4.
11. Seferović PM, Paulus WJ. Clinical diabetic cardiomyopathy: a two-faced disease with restrictive and dilated phenotypes. Eur Heart J. 2015;36(27):1718-27, 1727a-c.
12. Matshela MR. Diabetic cardiomyopathy: Mechanisms and mode of Diagnosis. J Cardiol Pract. 2016;14:15-28.
13. Fang ZY, Prins JB, Marwick TH. Diabetic cardiomyopathy: evidence, mechanisms, and therapeutic implications. Endocr Rev. 2004;25(4):543-67.
14. Franconi F, Campesi I, Occhioni S, et al. Sex-gender differences in diabetes vascular complications and treatment. Endocr Metab Immune Disord Drug Targets. 2012;12(2):179-96.
15. Kurioka S, Ose H, Fukuma K, et al. Severity of diabetic retinopathy is associated with left ventricular diastolic dysfunction in patients with type 2 diabetes. Diabetes Res Clin Pract. 2013;99(3):287-91.
16. Mochizuki Y, Tanaka H, Matsumoto K, et al. Clinical features of subclinical left ventricular systolic dysfunction in patients with diabetes mellitus. Cardiovasc Diabetol. 2015;14:37.
17. American College of Cardiology Foundation Task Force on Expert Consensus Documents, Hundley WG, Bluemke DA, et al. ACCF/ACR/AHA/NASCI/SCMR 2010 expert consensus document on cardiovascular magnetic resonance: a report of the American College of Cardiology Foundation Task Force on Expert Consensus Documents. J Am Coll Cardiol. 2010;55(23):2614-62.
18. Al-Saadi N, Nagel E, Gross M, et al. Noninvasive detection of myocardial ischemia from perfusion reserve based on cardiovascular magnetic resonance. Circulation. 2000;101(12):1379-83.
19. Raman SV, Simonetti OP, Winner MW, et al. Cardiac magnetic resonance with edema imaging identifies myocardium at risk and predicts worse outcome in patients with non-ST-segment elevation acute coronary syndrome. J Am Coll Cardiol. 2010;55(22):2480-8.
20. Assomull RG, Prasad SK, Lyne J, et al. Cardiovascular magnetic resonance, fibrosis, and prognosis in dilated cardiomyopathy. J Am Coll Cardiol. 2006;48(10):1977-85.
21. Hudsmith LE, Tyler DJ, Emmanuel Y, et al. (31)P cardiac magnetic resonance spectroscopy during leg exercise at 3 Tesla. Int J Cardiovasc Imaging. 2009;25(8):819-26.
22. Tillquist MN, Maddox TM. Update on diabetic cardiomyopathy: inches forward, miles to go. Curr Diab Rep. 2012;12(3):305-13.
23. Korosoglou G, Humpert PM. Non-invasive diagnostic imaging techniques as a window into the diabetic heart: a review of experimental and clinical data. Exp Clin Endocrinol Diabetes. 2007;115(4):211-20.
24. Fischer SE, McKinnon GC, Maier SE, et al. Improved myocardial tagging contrast. Magn Reson Med. 1993;30(2):191-200.
25. Ng AC, Delgado V, Bertini M, et al. Myocardial steatosis and biventricular strain and strain rate imaging in patients with type 2 diabetes mellitus. Circulation. 2010;122(24):2538-44.
26. Rosen BD, Saad MF, Shea S, et al. Hypertension and smoking are associated with reduced regional left ventricular function in asymptomatic: individuals the Multi-Ethnic Study of Atherosclerosis. J Am Coll Cardiol. 2006;47(6):1150-8.
27. Diamant M, Lamb HJ, Groeneveld Y, et al. Diastolic dysfunction is associated with altered myocardial metabolism in asymptomatic normotensive patients with well-controlled type 2 diabetes mellitus. J Am Coll Cardiol. 2003;42(2):328-35.
28. Paetsch I, Jahnke C, Wahl A, et al. Comparison of dobutamine stress magnetic resonance, adenosine stress magnetic resonance, and adenosine stress magnetic resonance perfusion. Circulation. 2004;110(7):835-42.
29. Gebker R, Jahnke C, Paetsch I, et al. MR myocardial perfusion imaging with k-space and time broad-use linear acquisition speed-up technique: feasibility study. Radiology. 2007;245(3):863-71.
30. Schwitter J, Nanz D, Kneifel S, et al. Assessment of myocardial perfusion in coronary artery disease by magnetic resonance: a comparison with positron emission tomography and coronary angiography. Circulation. 2001;103(18):2230-5.
31. Ng AC, Auger D, Delgado V, et al. Association between diffuse myocardial fibrosis by cardiac magnetic resonance contrast-enhanced T(1) mapping and subclinical myocardial dysfunction in diabetic patients: a pilot study. Circ Cardiovasc Imaging. 2012;5(1):51-9.
32. Jellis C, Wright J, Kennedy D, et al. Association of imaging markers of myocardial fibrosis with metabolic and functional disturbances in early diabetic cardiomyopathy. Circ Cardiovasc Imaging. 2011;4(6):693-702.
33. Rijzewijk LJ, van der Meer RW, Lamb HJ, et al. Altered myocardial substrate metabolism and decreased diastolic function in nonischemic human diabetic cardiomyopathy: studies with cardiac positron emission tomography and magnetic resonance imaging. J Am Coll Cardiol. 2009;54(16):1524-32.
34. Rijzewijk LJ, van der Meer RW, Smit JW, et al. Myocardial steatosis is an independent predictor of diastolic dysfunction in type 2 diabetes mellitus. J Am Coll Cardiol. 2008;52(22):1793-9.
35. Severson DL. Diabetic cardiomyopathy: recent evidence from mouse models of type 1 and type 2 diabetes. Can J Physiol Pharmacol. 2004;82(10):813-23.
36. Gu K, Cowie CC, Harris MI. Mortality in adults with and without diabetes in a national cohort of the U.S. population, 1971–1993. Diabetes Care. 1998;21(7):1138-45.
37. Turkbey EB, Backlund JY, Genuth S, et al. Myocardial structure, function, and scar in patients with type 1 diabetes mellitus. Circulation. 2011;124(16):1737-46.
38. Jahnke C, Nagel E, Gebker R, et al. Prognostic value of cardiac magnetic resonance stress tests: adenosine stress perfusion and dobutamine stress wall motion imaging. Circulation. 2007;115(13):1769-76.
39. Buckert D, Dewes P, Walcher T, et al. Intermediate-term prognostic value of reversible perfusion deficit diagnosed by adenosine CMR: a prospective follow-up study in a consecutive patient population. JACC Cardiovasc Imaging. 2013;6(1):56-63.

40. Korosoglou G, Elhmidi Y, Steen H, et al. Prognostic value of high-dose dobutamine stress magnetic resonance imaging in 1,493 consecutive patients: assessment of myocardial wall motion and perfusion. J Am Coll Cardiol. 2010;56(15):1225-34.
41. Bingham SE, Hachamovitch R. Incremental prognostic significance of combined cardiac magnetic resonance imaging, adenosine stress perfusion, delayed enhancement, and left ventricular function over preimaging information for the prediction of adverse events. Circulation. 2011;123(14):1509-18.
42. Steel K, Broderick R, Gandla V, et al. Complementary prognostic values of stress myocardial perfusion and late gadolinium enhancement imaging by cardiac magnetic resonance in patients with known or suspected coronary artery disease. Circulation. 2009;120(14):1390-400.
43. Greenwood JP, Maredia N, Younger JF, et al. Cardiovascular magnetic resonance and single-photon emission computed tomography for diagnosis of coronary heart disease (CE-MARC): a prospective trial. Lancet. 2012;379(9814):453-60.

CHAPTER

CT for CVD Evaluation in Cardiodiabetes

Priya Jagia, Arun Sharma, Kartik Ganga, Pankaj Kumar

INTRODUCTION

Diabetes mellitus (DM) is quite common with recent statistics suggesting that there are approximately 347 million people living with this condition and it constitutes one of the most important risk factor for cardiovascular disease (CVD).[1,2] India reportedly has the largest population of diabetic subjects in the world earning the disturbing distinction of being termed as the "diabetes capital of the world". This can have long lasting adverse effects on nation's health and economy.[3]

Cardiovascular disease is the most important cause of morbidity and mortality among individuals with type 2 diabetes mellitus[4,5] and diabetics have a higher risk of CVD as compared to nondiabetics with similar risk factors. Moreover, myocardial ischemia due to coronary atherosclerosis is usually asymptomatic in these patients and hence they present with multi-vessel disease and consequently have a worse prognosis.[6-8] Myocardial dysfunction in diabetics is a consequence of multiple pathological processes including coronary artery disease (CAD), altered metabolism, interstitial fibrosis, endothelial dysfunction, autonomic dysfunction and microvascular disease.[9] Multimodality imaging can demonstrate these pathophysiological processes, and their multitude of effects on myocardial function. CT plays a major role in early detection and characterization of CAD whereas magnetic resonance imaging (MRI) is the investigation of choice for myocardial abnormalities.

ROLE OF COMPUTED TOMOGRAPHY

Early identification of asymptomatic CAD may allow for more aggressive lifestyle changes or pharmacological interventions to prevent its progression and clinical manifestations of overt clinical event. Because CAD can present in a silent fashion and symptomatic disease is associated with worse clinical outcomes in DM, the detection of disease before occurrence of acute coronary events is all the more vital in these patients.

Multidetector computed tomography (MDCT) evaluation is of paramount importance for mapping of arterial tree and the diagnosis of concomitant carotid, coronary, renal and peripheral arterial disease. It is noninvasive, rapid and low cost modality which is usually available round the clock and provides multiplanar images. The newer third generation dual source computed tomography (CT) scanners provide excellent image quality over a wide range of body sizes and heart rates at lower radiation doses than the previous generation CT scanners. Faster gantry rotation time combined with larger z-axis volume coverage per rotation allow for single-heartbeat acquisitions in most patients with heart rates up to 75–80 beats per minute. Low contrast protocols described in various studies[10] result in significant reduction in contrast medium requirements (around 30–40 mL with newer scanners), without any difficulties in contrast medium timing or unsatisfactory vessel enhancement.

Moreover, volumetric acquisition enables extensive image postprocessing, including multiplanar reformatted and maximum intensity projection images to create an arterial map. With optimized timing of the acquisition, collaterals and arteries distal to occlusions can also be seen with greater accuracy which may not appear on arteriogram images. Computed tomography angiography (CTA) has good soft-tissue contrast and thus shows

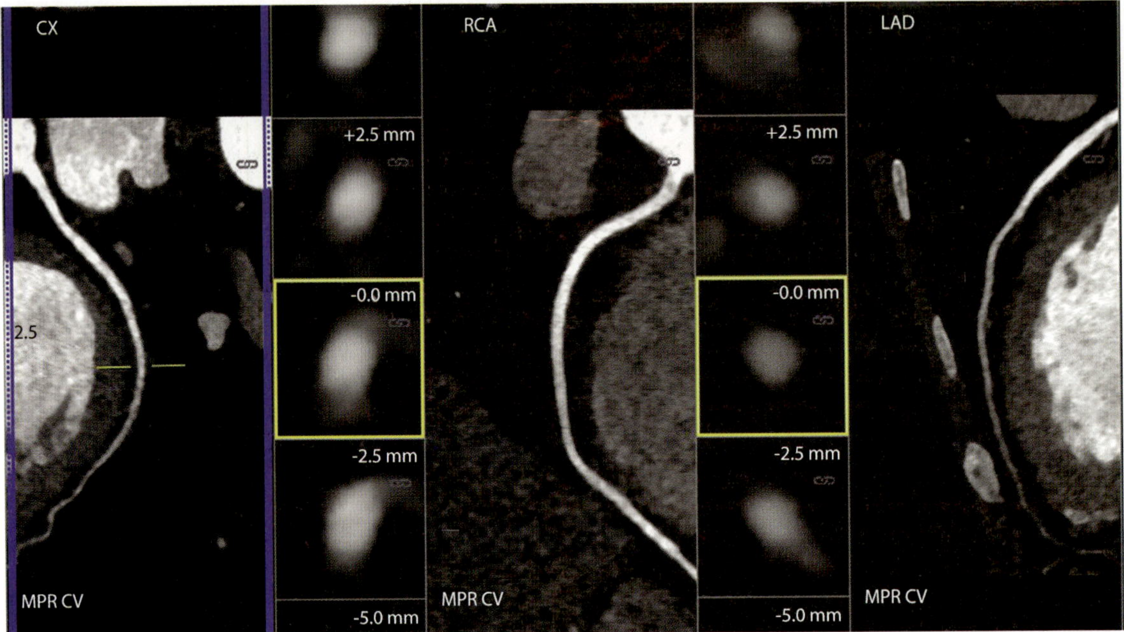

Fig. 1: Curved multiplanar coronary CTA images depicting normal coronary arteries. The side panel allows quantification of cross sectional diameter or area reduction

Abbreviations: CTA, computed tomography angiography; RCA, right coronary artery; CX, left circumflex artery; LAD, left anterior descending artery

nonvascular findings as well as vascular lesions associated with aneurysms and cystic adventitial disease that are not detected with the lumen imaging inherent to catheter arteriography. However, heavily calcified atheromatous disease that can occur in these patients, may limit the ability to interpret CT images.

At present, CT techniques, such as coronary artery calcium (CAC) scoring and coronary CTA, are considered the most robust imaging techniques for noninvasive visualization of coronary atherosclerosis. CAC scoring detects calcium present within atherosclerotic plaques. As a marker of atherosclerosis, CAC scores predict cardiac event risks in both diabetic and nondiabetic patients.[11] CTA can provide detailed information on coronary artery anatomy (Fig. 1), and assess both coronary artery atherosclerosis as well as luminal stenosis (Fig. 2). Advances in CT technology have led to significant improvements in the diagnostic accuracy of coronary CTA (Figs 3A and B) for the detection of coronary artery stenosis (sensitivity: 86–99%, specificity: 92–98%, negative predictive value: 92–100%). Most importantly, it detects early nonobstructive disease which allows for the early institution of medical therapy and lifestyle modifications.

Coronary Artery Calcium Scoring

Coronary artery calcium score can characterize the location as well as the burden of CAD by detecting calcium within atherosclerotic plaques. Image acquisition for CAC scoring typically involves acquiring non-contrast gated images of the entire heart. Using a cutoff value of greater than 130 Hounsfield unit (HU) density to define calcium, coronary calcifications can be identified as bright white areas on the CT images, which are usually automatically color coded according to each coronary artery. Semi-quantification of coronary calcium is commonly expressed by the Agatston score, which uses the plaque size, density, and a weighting

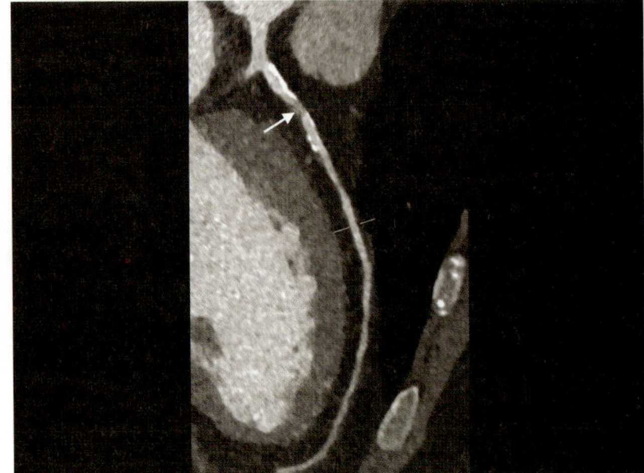

Fig. 2: CTA image showing diffused significant proximal-to-mid left anterior descending disease with mixed calcific plaques

Abbreviation: CTA, computed tomography angiography

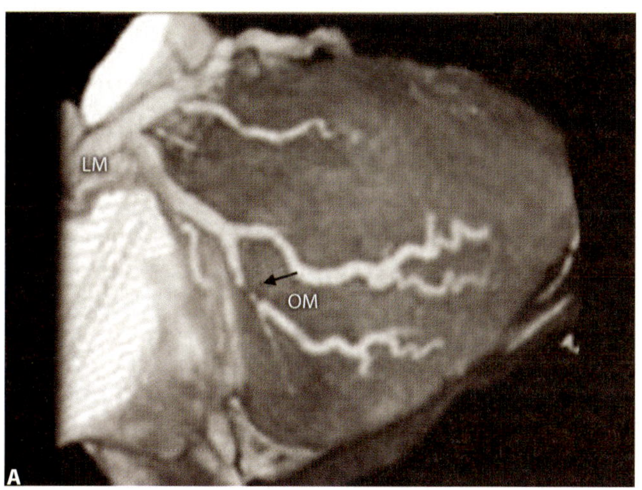

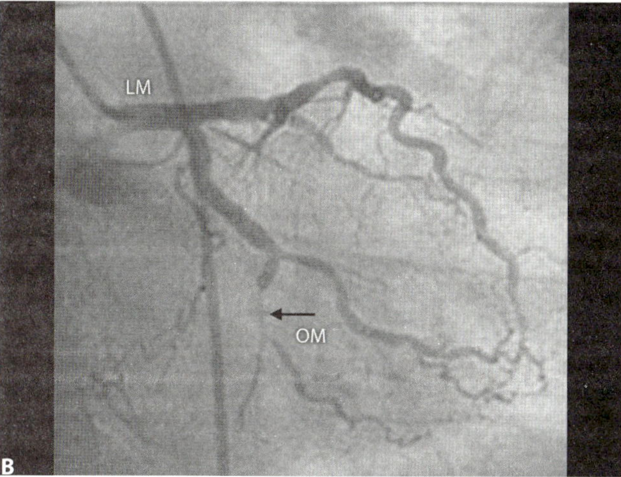

Figs 3A and B: Volume rendered CT image showing tight stenosis in obtuse marginal branch of left circumflex artery with corresponding catheter angiogram

Abbreviations: CT, computed tomography; OM, obtuse marginal; LM, left main

factor to calculate a value ranging from 0 (absence of detectable calcium) to over 1000 (indicating extensive coronary calcification). Importantly, there is a relationship between the CAC score and the extent of coronary atherosclerosis, as well as the presence of significant coronary stenosis.[12] However, the association between CAC score and extent of coronary atherosclerosis is not linear as severe coronary stenosis can occur at sites with limited calcium deposition and vice versa. Thus, rather than being a diagnostic test for obstructive coronary artery disease, *CAC scoring is used as a risk stratification tool to identify high-risk patients who might benefit from further investigations.*

An elevated CAC score has consistently been associated with increased mortality and adverse cardiovascular events, independent of other risk factors. Similar findings have also been observed in diabetic patients.[11] Some studies have indicated that a linear relationship exists between CAC and clinical CVD events among diabetics. Also, patients with diabetes mellitus have a greater prevalence and extent of CAC than those without diabetes mellitus and the prognostic significance of elevated CAC in predicting adverse events are greater in patients with diabetes mellitus than in those without DM.[11,13,14] It has been demonstrated that in diabetic patients, CAC scores of less than 10 were associated with very low clinical cardiac event rates. More importantly, the absence of coronary calcium portends a remarkably favorable prognosis, with none of patients experiencing adverse cardiac events during 5 years of follow-up.[11] CAC score has been found to be superior to well-established cardiovascular risk factor models for predicting silent myocardial ischemia and short- term outcomes.[15] For these reasons, *ACC/AHA guidelines (2010) consider CAC scoring a reasonable modality for cardiovascular risk assessment in asymptomatic patients with diabetes mellitus who are greater than 40 years of age.*[16]

Coronary CT Angiography

Detailed information on the coronary anatomy can be derived from coronary CTA. Importantly, CT retains high sensitivity and specificity for diagnosing stenosis in diabetic patients.[17,18] The advantage of this technique is that its high negative-predictive value approaches almost 100%. Coronary CTA is also unlikely to miss severe coronary artery diseases such as left main or triple-vessel disease which is known to occur in diabetics, without clinically manifest symptoms. CT also allows identification of coronary atherosclerotic plaques in the absence of calcium or stenosis, thus permitting visualization of early subclinical atherosclerosis. *Vulnerable plaques (plaques with low attenuation core, spotty calcium and positive remodeling), which account for acute coronary syndromes, are identified with greater accuracy on CTA in both symptomatic and asymptomatic diabetic patients* (Fig. 4). This may help in early institution of optimal medical therapy in asymptomatic patients to avoid an overt clinical event.

Coronary artery disease is the cause of mortality in greater than fifty percent of all diabetics, while others have symptoms of congestive heart failure or angina. Patients with diabetes but without other conventional risk factors for atherosclerosis have a risk of death from CAD which is 2–4 times more than that of age-matched controls.[19,20] Diabetics with CAD usually fare worse than patients without diabetes. And those who present with a myocardial infarction are at increased risk of dying from it. They also, benefit less from thrombolysis in the setting of an acute

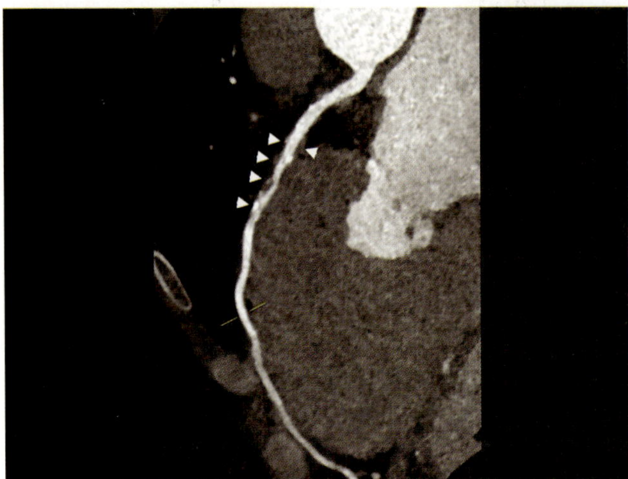

Fig. 4: CTA image from an adult diabetic patient showing vulnerable plaque (low attenuation core, spotty calcium, ulceration and positive remodeling) in mid left anterior descending artery (arrowheads)

Abbreviation: CTA, computed tomography angiography

myocardial infarction.[21-23] Coronary artery bypass surgery and percutaneous transluminal coronary angioplasty are associated with greater long-term mortality in diabetic patients than in those without diabetes.[23-25] Silent ischemia is of particular concern in diabetic patients. Clinically, patients with diabetes are more likely to be without chest pain in the setting of myocardial infarction, and thus late presentation contributes to a higher mortality in these patients.

Using coronary CTA, it was recently demonstrated that diabetic patients have more extensive, diffuse coronary atherosclerosis (Fig. 2) compared with matched nondiabetic patients.[26] Interestingly, this increased plaque burden was mainly attributable to an increased number of nonobstructive lesions. These observations were later confirmed using CT as well as invasive plaque imaging with gray scale and virtual histology as depicted by intravascular ultrasound.[27] In another study, researchers compared CAC scoring and CTA and demonstrated that CTA may reveal substantial plaque burden even in patients with zero CAC scores.[28] Thus, coronary CTA may be more accurate in evaluating the presence and extent of coronary atherosclerosis in diabetic patients compared with CAC scoring. Preliminary results suggest that CTA has incremental prognostic information over baseline clinical variables in both diabetic and nondiabetic patients. Recent advancements in CT technology make coronary CTA a very useful modality in imaging the coronaries with reduced radiation dose (1–4 mSv as compared to 6–9 mSv in standard coronary angiogram) and low contrast load, which is of paramount importance in diabetic patients with reduced renal function.[29]

Diabetic Heart Disease

Diabetic cardiomyopathy is defined as myocardial dysfunction that occurs independently of CAD and hypertension. This dysfunction may be subclinical but indicates that patient has a higher risk of developing clinical heart failure.[30,31] Myocardial structural changes in diabetic myocardium results in increased left ventricular stiffness and impairment of diastolic and eventually systolic performance. Although it is not a prerequisite for patients to have preexisting cardiomyopathy to develop heart failure, the presence of diabetic cardiomyopathy increases the risk for subsequent development of secondary heart failure. Thus, early detection of diabetic heart disease may permit early treatment and prevention of heart failure progression.

Currently, diagnosis of diabetic heart disease requires the demonstration of myocardial dysfunction that is independent of other causes, such as significant coronary stenosis or hypertension. Often, echocardiography is used to demonstrate left ventricular diastolic and systolic dysfunction in diabetic heart disease. Though MRI remains the gold standard technique for functional assessment, but functional assessment can be done using software with data already acquired during coronary CTA using current generation scanners (Figs 5A and B). Systolic and diastolic functional assessment by CT is accurate and can be used as a reference, with minimal inter and intraobserver variability. These allow earlier detection of subclinical functional abnormalities in these patients.

Carotid Artery Disease and Role of Carotid Intima-Medial Thickness (CIMT)

Increasing age, hyperglycemia, duration of diabetes, hypertension, cholesterol and inflammatory markers have previously been determined as independent factors for carotid atherosclerosis in diabetes. Early diagnosis of carotid artery disease in patients with modifiable risk factors like diabetes may play an important role in the prevention of a consequent stroke.

Various studies have shown that diabetic subjects have higher CIMT values than nondiabetics.[32-34] In asymptomatic patients with diabetes, CIMT has also been shown to be a significant predictor of CVD.[35] CIMT assessment using carotid Doppler is quite simple, noninvasive, convenient and highly reproducible. CTA is helpful in precise assessment of disease severity (Fig. 6) and simultaneous mapping of intracranial circulation, thereby helping in treatment planning and follow-up.

Modest correlations between CIMT and CAD as detected by CT, demonstrated by various studies,[36] indicate

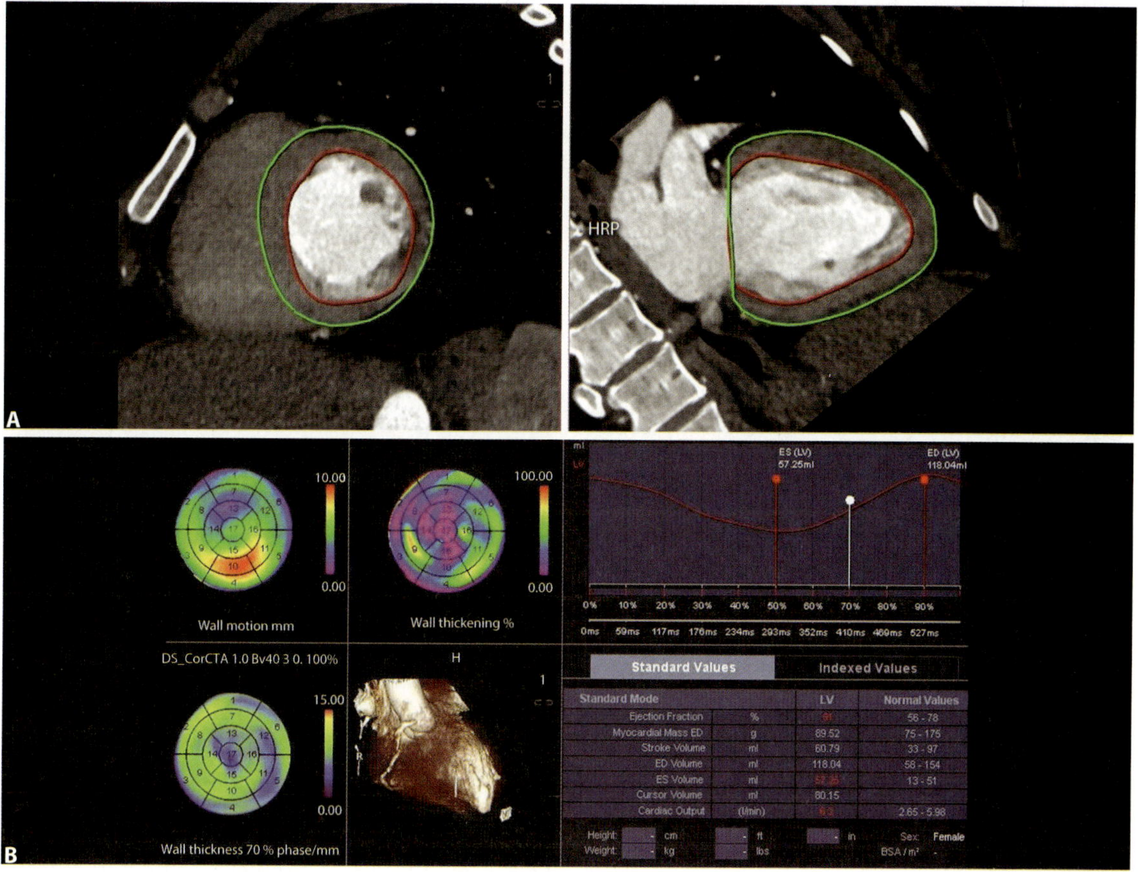

Figs 5A and B: Functional assessment using CTA. (A) Automated left ventricular contours with (B) Cardiac function parameters as displayed

Abbreviation: CTA, computed tomography angiography

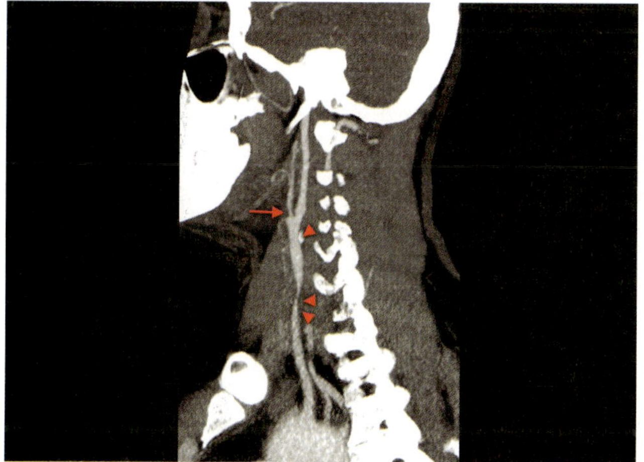

Fig. 6: CTA reformatted sagittal image from an adult diabetic patient showing diffuse left common carotid artery disease with mixed plaques (arrowheads) and significant stenosis of left common carotid artery. Note is also made of mild disease of cervical internal carotid artery with significant ostial stenosis of external carotid artery (arrow).

Abbreviation: CTA, computed tomography angiography

that atherosclerosis has a heterogeneous distribution. This relationship may be affected by risk factor profile. Studies have found that CIMT was more closely related to diabetes, and CAC was more closely related to hypertension.[37] However, because of modest correlations between the modalities, the selection of an imaging modality should be guided by patient profile. As more studies continue to evaluate CIMT with the combination of plaque metrics (including composition and stenosis measures), it is possible that CIMT will be readdressed as an important tool for risk in intermediate to high-risk asymptomatic patients with diabetes.

ROLE OF COMPUTED TOMOGRAPHY IN RENAL ARTERY EVALUATION

Increased prevalence (17–30%) of atherosclerotic renal artery stenosis has been documented in patients with DM and hypertension as compared to general hypertensive population.[38, 39]

Initially, contrast enhanced magnetic resonance angiography (MRA) was perceived as a safe noninvasive

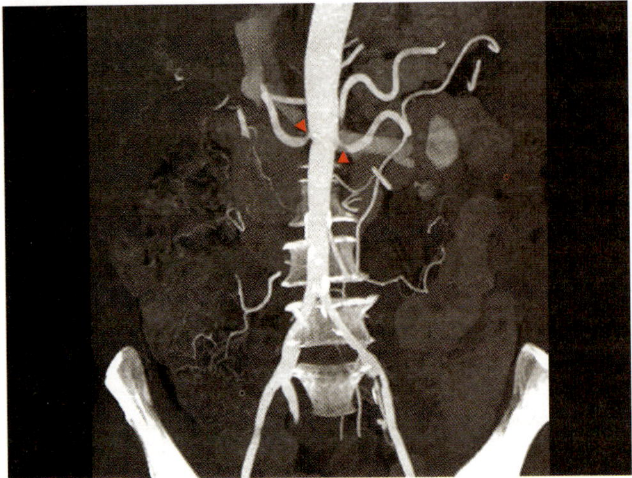

Fig. 7: CTA image showing bilateral significant ostial renal artery stenosis (left greater than right) in a diabetic adult male with mild diffuse aortoiliac disease

Abbreviation: CTA, computed tomography angiography

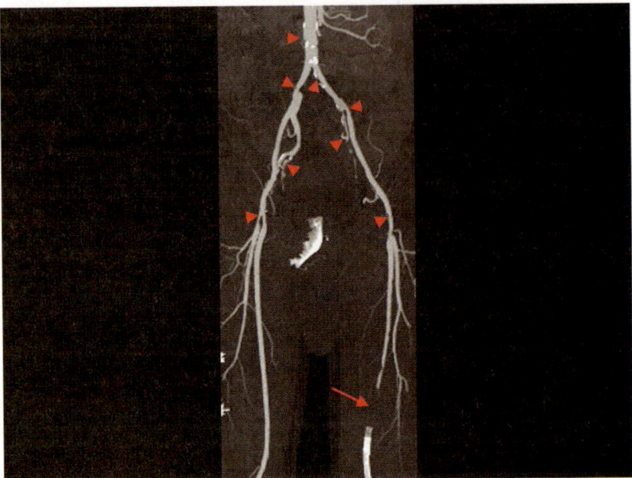

Fig. 8: CTA reformatted coronal image showing diffused aortoiliac, common femoral and profunda femoris artery disease (arrowheads) with occluded mid left SFA proximal to the stent, which was placed previously for symptomatic significant diffuse distal SFA disease

Abbreviations: CTA, computed tomography angiography; SFA, superficial femoral artery

technique to image the renal arteries. However, gadolinium, used in MRA, has been implicated in the development of a serious complication: nephrogenic systemic fibrosis, especially in patients with a glomerular filtration rate (GFR) of less than 30 mL/min/1.73 m^2.

Contrast-enhanced CTA also provides accurate anatomic images of the renal arteries with isotropic data sets that enable the reconstruction of high-resolution images (Fig. 7). Moreover, it is noninvasive with faster acquisition and offers multi-planar evaluation. The disadvantages of CT are its ionizing radiation and use of nephrotoxic contrast material. A high sensitivity and specificity of 100% and 98% respectively have been shown using CTA for renal artery stenosis evaluation by various studies.[40]

CTA can also be used to assess the patency of renal stents. Steinwender, et al. described CTA evaluation of 95 renal artery stents in which 98% of the stents were assessable on CTA, and there was 100% sensitivity and 99% specificity for detecting in-stent stenosis.[41]

Peripheral Vascular Disease

Peripheral vascular disease (PVD) in diabetic patients is associated with a particularly high-rate of cardiovascular mortality.[42,43] Lower extremity PVD is an independent risk factor for mortality in diabetic patients with similar degrees of CAD. These patients also have higher rate of morbidity and mortality after surgery.[44] They are likely to be asymptomatic even in the presence of significant CAD due to limitation of activity by lower extremity PVD. In a study in PVD patients without known CAD, 57% had evidence of myocardial ischemia or infarct on radioisotope perfusion scanning.[45] Patients with diabetes and PVD by history or on exam should be considered to be at high-risk for CAD and should undergo stress testing.

When compared to catheter arteriography, CTA for lower limb arterial evaluation offers volumetric as opposed to planar images and generally requires less radiation exposure with comparable or lower iodine loads. In proximal ileofemoral disease, CTA or preferably MRA (in calcified arteries) are the investigation of choice for demonstration of distal run off. This is because proximal disease or occlusion precludes selective limb injection during digital subtraction angiography (DSA). Lesion morphology is well seen on CTA images which can be reconstructed in any plane for better delineation of a stenosis (Fig. 8). The sensitivity and specificity of CTA for detection of stenosis greater than 50% diameter is 90–100%, making CTA an important tool in the assessment of PVD.[46]

PRECAUTIONS WHILE PERFORMING CONTRAST ENHANCED CT IN DIABETIC PATIENTS (TABLE 1)

There are certain issues with the diabetic patient: fasting, renal failure, and ongoing medication (insulin, oral antidiabetics especially metformin). Fasting can cause hypoglycemic incidents and renal failure could be worsened by the injection of a contrast agent while metformin exposes

TABLE 1: Checklist in diabetic patients scheduled for computed tomography examination

- Prior to CT evaluation:
  - Renal function assessment
  - Antidiabetic drug therapy, especially metformin use
  - Instructions regarding fasting and hydration.
- On the day of CT:
  - Checking all pertinent case records
  - Minimal optimal fasting
  - Good hydration
  - Isoosmolar iodinated contrast usage

Stop metformin based on eGFR status.

- Post-CT evaluation:
  - Renal function assessment before restarting metformin
  - Good hydration.

Abbreviations: CT, computed tomography; eGFR, estimated glomerular filtration rate

patient to the risk of lactic acidosis by diminution of renal clearance in cases of contrast induced nephropathy. General measures to reduce these complications would include: having a recent creatinine report (less than 3 months) and good hydration. If the patient is on insulin, it should not be discontinued. Fasting for longer periods is not recommended and the examination should be performed as soon as possible, with four hours fasting. As per ACR guidelines[47] on contrast media use in patients on metformin, there is no need to discontinue metformin either prior to or following the intravenous administration of iodinated contrast media, if there is no evidence of acute kidney injury (AKI) and estimated glomerular filtration rate (eGFR) is greater than or equal to 30 mL/min/1.73m^2. *In patients taking metformin* and in those with eGFR less than 30, metformin should be temporarily discontinued at the time of or prior to the procedure, and withheld for 48 hours subsequent to the procedure and reinstituted only after renal function has been reevaluated and found to be normal. Oral antidiabetic medications other than metformin can be continued regardless of contrast media use.

CONCLUSION

Coronary artery disease may be asymptomatic in diabetic patients, thus mandating imaging for early detection of coronary atherosclerosis, vulnerable plaques and coronary stenosis, which tends to be multivessel and diffused in these patients. Precautions must be exercised during CTA in these patients, if patient has concomitant renal dysfunction or is on metformin. Coronary CTA and CAC scoring help in early identification and quantification of coronary stenosis, besides documenting the myocardial dysfunction, thus paving the path for early intervention. Concomitant renal, carotid and peripheral arterial disease too, can be accurately assessed using CTA.

REFERENCES

1. McGavock JM, Victor RG, Unger RH, et al. Adiposity of the heart, revisited. Ann Intern Med. 2006;144(7):517-24.
2. Perk J, De Backer G, Gohlke H, et al. European Guidelines on cardiovascular disease prevention in clinical practice (version 2012). The Fifth Joint Task Force of the European Society of Cardiology and Other Societies on Cardiovascular Disease Prevention in Clinical Practice (constituted by representatives of nine societies and by invited experts). Eur Heart J. 2012;33(13):1635-701.
3. Mohan V, Sandeep S, Deepa R, et al. Epidemiology of type 2 diabetes: Indian scenario. Indian J Med Res. 2007;125(3):217-30.
4. Morrish NJ, Wang SL, Stevens LK, et al. Mortality and causes of death in the WHO Multinational Study of Vascular Disease in Diabetes. Diabetologia. 2001;44(Suppl 2):S14-21.
5. Redberg RF, Greenland P, Fuster V, et al. Prevention Conference VI: Diabetes and Cardiovascular Disease: Writing Group III: risk assessment in persons with diabetes. Circulation. 2002;105(18):e144-52.
6. Mellbin LG, Malmberg K, Ryden L, et al. The relationship between glycaemic variability and cardiovascular complications in patients with acute myocardial infarction and type 2 diabetes: a report from the DIGAMI 2 trial. Eur Heart J. 2013;34(5):374-9.
7. Donnan PT, Donnelly L, New JP, et al. Derivation and validation of a prediction score for major coronary heart disease events in a U.K. type 2 diabetic population. Diabetes Care. 2006;29(6):1231-6.
8. Herlitz J, Malmberg K, Karlson BW, et al. Mortality and morbidity during a five-year follow-up of diabetics with myocardial infarction. Acta Med Scand. 1988;224(1):31-8.
9. Marwick TH. The diabetic myocardium. Curr Diab Rep. 2006;6(1):36-41.
10. Meyer M, Haubenreisser H, Schoepf UJ, et al. Closing in on the K edge: coronary CT angiography at 100, 80, and 70 kV-initial comparison of a second- versus a third-generation dual-source CT system. Radiology. 2014;273(2):373-82.
11. Raggi P, Shaw LJ, Berman DS, et al. Prognostic value of coronary artery calcium screening in subjects with and without diabetes. J Am Coll Cardiol. 2004;43(9):1663-9.
12. Sarwar A, Shaw LJ, Shapiro MD, et al. Diagnostic and prognostic value of absence of coronary artery calcification. JACC Cardiovasc Imaging. 2009;2(6):675-88.
13. Elkeles RS, Godsland IF, Feher MD, et al. Coronary calcium measurement improves prediction of cardiovascular events in asymptomatic patients with type 2 diabetes: the PREDICT study. Eur Heart J. 2008;29(18):2244-51.
14. Nasir K, Rubin J, Blaha MJ, et al. Interplay of coronary artery calcification and traditional risk factors for the prediction of all-cause mortality in asymptomatic individuals. Circ Cardiovasc Imaging. 2012;5(4):467-73.
15. Anand DV, Lim E, Hopkins D, et al. Risk stratification in uncomplicated type 2 diabetes: prospective evaluation of the combined use of coronary artery calcium imaging and selective myocardial perfusion scintigraphy. Eur Heart J. 2006;27(6): 713-21.
16. Greenland P, Alpert JS, Beller GA, et al. 2010 ACCF/AHA guideline for assessment of cardiovascular risk in asymptomatic adults: executive summary: a report of the American College of Cardiology Foundation/American Heart Association Task Force on Practice Guidelines. Circulation. 2010;122(25):2748-64.
17. Burgstahler C, Beck T, Reimann A, et al. Diagnostic accuracy of multislice computed tomography for the detection of coronary artery disease in diabetic patients. J Diabetes Complications. 2007;21(2):69-74.
18. Schuijf JD, Bax JJ, Jukema JW, et al. Noninvasive angiography and assessment of left ventricular function using multislice computed

tomography in patients with type 2 diabetes. Diabetes Care. 2004;27(12):2905-10.
19. DeStefano F, Ford ES, Newman J, et al. Risk factors for coronary heart disease mortality among persons with diabetes. Ann Epidemiol. 1993;3(1):27-34.
20. Stamler J, Vaccaro O, Neaton JD, et al. Diabetes, other risk factors, and 12-yr cardiovascular mortality for men screened in the Multiple Risk Factor Intervention Trial. Diabetes Care. 1993;16(2):434-44.
21. Zuanetti G, Latini R, Maggioni AP, et al. Influence of diabetes on mortality in acute myocardial infarction: data from the GISSI-2 study. J Am Coll Cardiol. 1993;22(7):1788-94.
22. Fava S, Azzopardi J, Muscat HA, et al. Factors that influence outcome in diabetic subjects with myocardial infarction. Diabetes Care. 1993;16(12):1615-8.
23. Orlander PR, Goff DC, Morrissey M, et al. The relation of diabetes to the severity of acute myocardial infarction and post-myocardial infarction survival in Mexican-Americans and non-Hispanic whites. The Corpus Christi Heart Project. Diabetes. 1994;43(7):897-902.
24. Influence of diabetes on 5-year mortality and morbidity in a randomized trial comparing CABG and PTCA in patients with multivessel disease: the Bypass Angioplasty Revascularization Investigation (BARI). Circulation. 1997;96(6):1761-9.
25. Stein B, Weintraub WS, Gebhart SP, et al. Influence of diabetes mellitus on early and late outcome after percutaneous transluminal coronary angioplasty. Circulation. 1995;91(4):979-89.
26. Pundziute G, Schuijf JD, Jukema JW, et al. Noninvasive assessment of plaque characteristics with multislice computed tomography coronary angiography in symptomatic diabetic patients. Diabetes Care. 2007;30(5):1113-9.
27. Pundziute G, Schuijf JD, Jukema JW, et al. Type 2 diabetes is associated with more advanced coronary atherosclerosis on multislice computed tomography and virtual histology intravascular ultrasound. J Nucl Cardiol. 2009;16(3):376-83.
28. Scholte AJ, Schuijf JD, Kharagjitsingh AV, et al. Prevalence of coronary artery disease and plaque morphology assessed by multi-slice computed tomography coronary angiography and calcium scoring in asymptomatic patients with type 2 diabetes. Heart. 2008;94(3):290-5.
29. Bastarrika G, Lee YS, Huda W, et al. CT of coronary artery disease. Radiology. 2009;253(2):317-38.
30. From AM, Scott CG, Chen HH. The development of heart failure in patients with diabetes mellitus and pre-clinical diastolic dysfunction a population-based study. J Am Coll Cardiol. 2010;55(4):300-5.
31. Bell DS. Heart failure: the frequent, forgotten, and often fatal complication of diabetes. Diabetes Care. 2003;26(8):2433-41.
32. Suzuki M, Shinozaki K, Kanazawa A, et al. Insulin resistance as an independent risk factor for carotid wall thickening. Hypertension. 1996;28(4):593-8.
33. Abdelghaffar S, El Amir M, El Hadidi A, et al. Carotid intima-media thickness: an index for subclinical atherosclerosis in type 1 diabetes. J Trop Pediatr. 2006;52(1):39-45.
34. Golden SH, Folsom AR, Coresh J, et al. Risk factor groupings related to insulin resistance and their synergistic effects on subclinical atherosclerosis: the atherosclerosis risk in communities study. Diabetes. 2002;51(10):3069-76.
35. Yoshida M, Mita T, Yamamoto R, et al. Combination of the Framingham risk score and carotid intima-media thickness improves the prediction of cardiovascular events in patients with type 2 diabetes. Diabetes Care. 2012;35(1):178-80.
36. Cohen GI, Aboufakher R, Bess R, et al. Relationship between carotid disease on ultrasound and coronary disease on CT angiography. JACC Cardiovasc Imaging. 2013;6(11):1160-7.
37. Bauer M, Mohlenkamp S, Lehmann N, et al. The effect of age and risk factors on coronary and carotid artery atherosclerotic burden in males-Results of the Heinz Nixdorf Recall Study. Atherosclerosis. 2009;205(2):595-602.
38. Sawicki PT, Kaiser S, Heinemann L, et al. Prevalence of renal artery stenosis in diabetes mellitus--an autopsy study. J Intern Med. 1991;229(6):489-92.
39. Postma CT, Klappe EM, Dekker HM, et al. The prevalence of renal artery stenosis among patients with diabetes mellitus. Eur J Intern Med. 2012;23(7):639-42.
40. Farres MT, Lammer J, Schima W, et al. Spiral computed tomographic angiography of the renal arteries: a prospective comparison with intravenous and intraarterial digital subtraction angiography. Cardiovasc Intervent Radiol. 1996;19(2):101-6.
41. Steinwender C, Schutzenberger W, Fellner F, et al. 64-Detector CT angiography in renal artery stent evaluation: prospective comparison with selective catheter angiography. Radiology. 2009;252(1):299-305.
42. Consensus development conference on the diagnosis of coronary heart disease in people with diabetes: 10-11 February 1998, Miami, Florida. American Diabetes Association. Diabetes Care. 1998;21(9):1551-9.
43. Janka HU. Increased cardiovascular morbidity and mortality in diabetes mellitus: identification of the high risk patient. Diabetes Res Clin Pract. 1996;30(Suppl):85-8.
44. Brown KA, Rowen M. Prognostic value of a normal exercise myocardial perfusion imaging study in patients with angiographically significant coronary artery disease. Am J Cardiol. 1993;71(10):865-7.
45. Nesto RW, Phillips RT, Kett KG, et al. Angina and exertional myocardial ischemia in diabetic and nondiabetic patients: assessment by exercise thallium scintigraphy. Ann Intern Med. 1988;108(2):170-5.
46. Heijenbrok-Kal MH, Kock MC, Hunink MG. Lower extremity arterial disease: multidetector CT angiography meta-analysis. Radiology. 2007;245(2):433–9.
47. Goergen SK, Rumbold G, Compton G, et al. Systematic review of current guidelines, and their evidence base, on risk of lactic acidosis after administration of contrast medium for patients receiving metformin. Radiology. 2010;254(1):261-9.

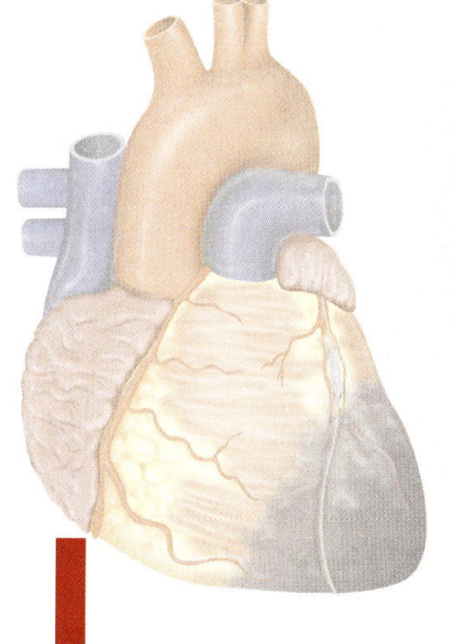

Recent Advances in Nuclear Cardiology and Cardiodiabetes

GN Mahapatra, Mary Anne Joseph

INTRODUCTION

Coronary artery disease (CAD) is the leading cause of morbidity and mortality in patients with diabetes worldwide. In 2000, global estimates indicated 200 million individuals currently have diabetes and projections by the World Health Organization and others suggest that its prevalence will exceed 300 million by 2025 and 360 million by 2030. More than 90% of these individuals will have type 2 diabetes. Management guidelines in Europe and the US consider type 2 diabetes to be a cardiovascular disease equivalent. These patients have a two to fourfold higher risk of a cardiovascular event than nondiabetic patients. Importantly cardiovascular death is the most common cause of mortality in the type 2 diabetic population. It has been estimated that after myocardial infarction, 79% of diabetic patients die of cardiac complications. Accordingly accurate cardiovascular risk stratification of patients with type 2 diabetes is needed, as CAD is often asymptomatic in these patients until the onset of myocardial infarction or sudden cardiac death. Consequently, proper screening and diagnosis of CAD is crucial for the prevention and early treatment of coronary events. The patient with diabetes experience more diffused, calcified and extensive CAD, more often have left ventricular dysfunction often have more advanced coronary disease at the time of diagnosis and more often experience silent ischemia. In addition, diabetic patients generally have a less favorable response to revascularization, as they require frequent need for repeat percutaneous coronary intervention or coronary artery bypass grafting and a reduced long time survival. Accordingly, early accurate diagnosis of CAD in patients with diabetes is needed and reliable prognostication is mandatory. The American Diabetes Association has recommended an algorithm whereby symptomatic diabetic patients would be referred for either stress myocardial perfusion imaging (stress MPI) or stress echo or evaluation by a cardiologist. The exception would be individuals with atypical chest pain and a normal electrocardiogram who might undergo a simple exercise stress test followed by stress MPI study unless they have multiple other cardiovascular risk factors in which case, imaging studies would be preferred.

In association with the elevated prevalence, morbidity, mortality of CAD worldwide, there has been a steady increase in the use of cardiac imaging techniques, including those based on nuclear medicine. In fact cardiac studies have outgrown nuclear medicine and have constituted an individual subspecialty of nuclear cardiology. The most popular commonly available nuclear imaging, i.e. myocardial perfusion imaging (MPI) which by its turn means the evaluation of myocardial perfusion after stress versus at rest using a variety of tracers and stressor agents in different protocols including metabolic imaging and innervation imaging.

MYOCARDIAL PERFUSION IMAGING

Nuclear cardiology is an established subspecialty that has grown significantly in recent years due to the fact that functional information provided by nuclear techniques can play a significant role in cardiodiabetology for the last two decades, MPI has been an essential part of the diagnostic and prognostic assessment of patients for known or suspected CAD. However, as time went by and new demand and technologies have been developed, other changes in the technology of MPI have emerged, e.g. in the 1980's, planar and then tomographic [single photon emission computed tomography (SPECT)] perfusion imaging was found to reliably diagnose CAD. In 1990's, the prognostic value of MPI was defined and later with the advent of gating, left ventricular ejection fraction, wall motion and end-systolic wall thickening thus providing additional diagnostic and prognostic information (Figs 1 and 2).

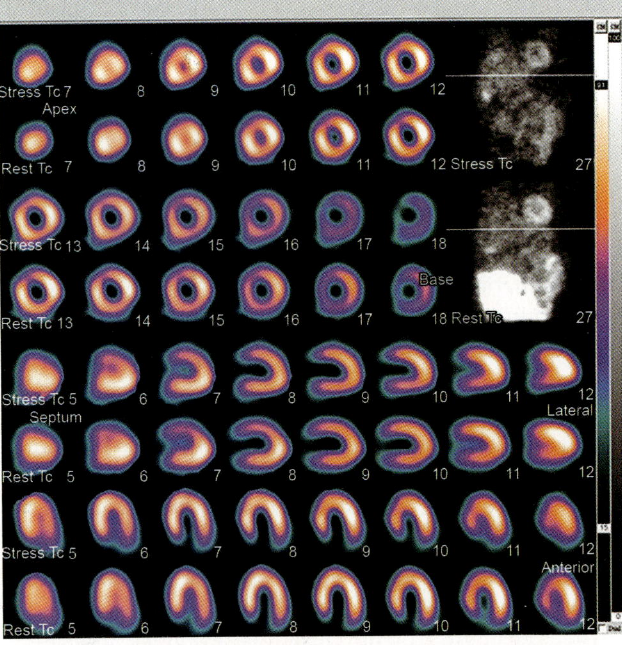

Fig. 1: Normal stress sestamibi myocardial perfusion scan

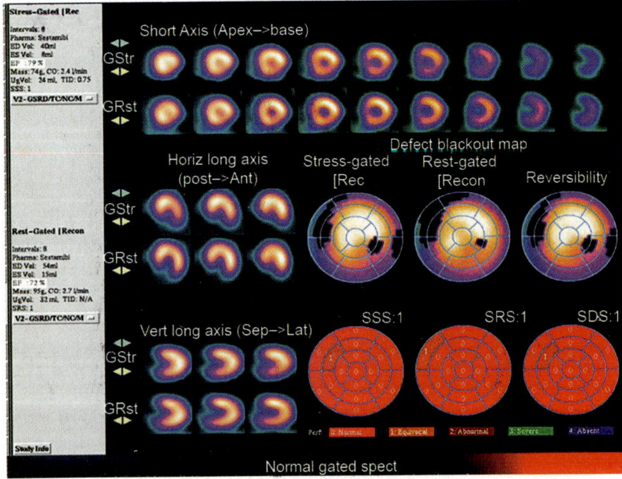

Fig. 2: Normal-gated SPECT

Diagnostic Assessment

Myocardial perfusion imaging is useful tool for the diagnosis of CAD. It is most effective when used in patients with an intermediate pretest likelihood of CAD. Even in lower likelihood of CAD, a normal stress MPI scan rules out the presence of CAD, similarly in patients with high likelihood of CAD, MPI can still be used for risk stratification (Fig. 3).

Prognostic Assessment

Myocardial perfusion imaging may be applied for prognostic evaluation both for patients with known or suspected CAD. It relies on two principles: first, a normal MPI study indicates as low as 1% cardiac events in the future; second, there is a relationship between myocardial ischemia such that the risk of events increases exponentially as ischemia increases. Even in patients with a high likelihood of CAD or definite CAD, a normal stress MPI defines those who have a less than 1% risk of cardiac events in the next 1–3 years as there have been developments of sufficient collaterals thereby reducing the cardiac event rate. This defines a group in which conservative management (i.e., avoiding myocardial revascularization) is appropriate. When some conditions are present, like diabetes, inability to exercise leading to the use of pharmacologic stress (IV adenosine or IV dobutamine), abnormal rest ECG or exercise-induced ST segment depression, a normal stress-gated MPI study still delineates low risk, but somewhat increased compared with patients with normal MPI and none of those. For patients with abnormal finding in MPI study with or without lung uptake, the risk of events is associated with the magnitude of ischemia. This subset of the patients is the strongest determinant of the referral to coronary angiography and also the strongest predictor of benefit with revascularization. Besides that, a number of other findings obtained from MPI studies, such as abnormal lung uptake or transient left ventricular dilatation, have consistently been associated with increased risk (Figs 4A and B).

Therapeutic Assessment/ Myocardial Perfusion Imaging as a "Gatekeeper"

An increasingly used application of nuclear cardiology is to evaluate the anti-ischemic effects of various therapies by means of identifying changes in left ventricular perfusion defect size by sequential MPI and thereby track patient risk for subsequent cardiac events on the basis of ischemic areas suppression. An example is the COURAGE trial, which evaluated percutaneous coronary intervention (PCI) plus optimal medical therapy (OMT) vs OMT alone in stable CAD patients. The results basing on nuclear substudy, the results showed that ischemia reduction was greater with PCI

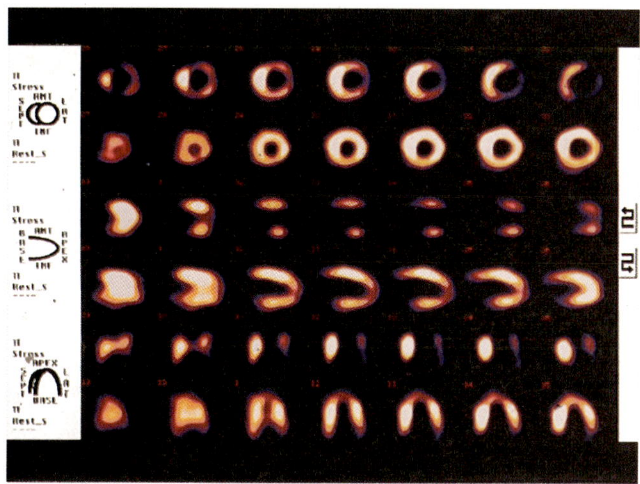

Fig. 3: Stress thallium myocardial perfusion scan showing a large area of stress perfusion defect involving anterolateral myocardial segments which shows fair amount of reperfusion in resting image suggestive of anterolateral myocardial ischemia

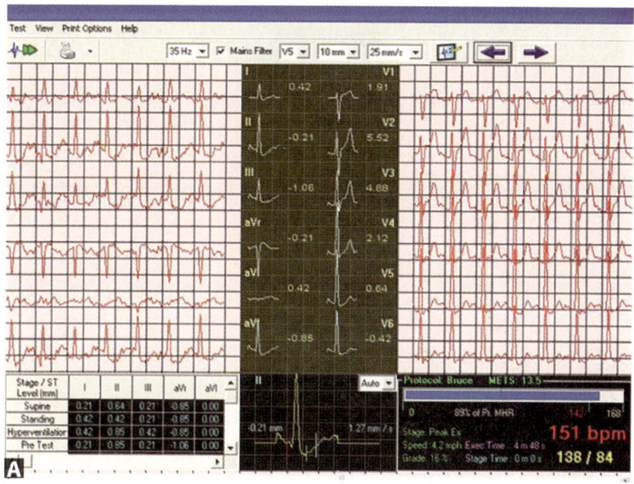

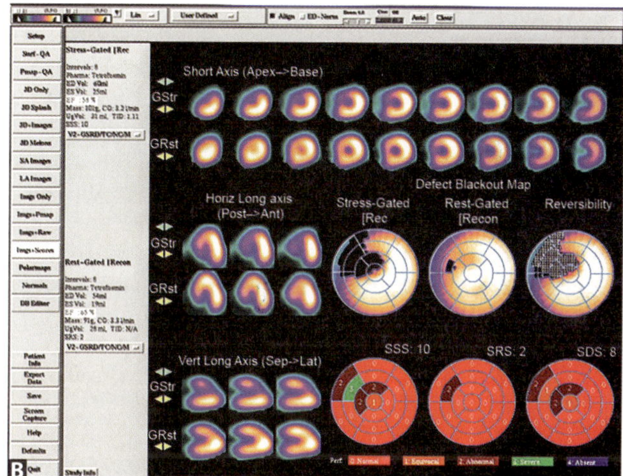

Figs 4A and B: (A) Treadmill stress test shows no significant ST-T depression in any of the chest leads; (B) Stress gated SPECT tetrofosmin myocardial perfusion scan involving anteroseptal segment with evidence of significant reversible ischaemia

+ OMT than with OMT alone (33.3% vs 19.8%). This study indicated that, for stable CAD patients, having knowledge of the ischemic burden is helpful in decision-making with respect to selecting initial therapy, and regardless of the therapeutic modality used, assessment of the response to therapy, which is related to long-term outcome, is also important. Another aspect of this same application of MPI is the identification of revascularization candidates according to the amount of jeopardized myocardium and the survival benefit that a patient may obtain from a specific therapy as a function of MPI results. MPI has been able to discriminate (as a "gatekeeper") which patients will likely benefit from invasive coronary angiography followed by coronary revascularization and who may be well suited with medical therapy. Additionally, quantitative analysis of MPI studies on the demonstration of a threshold value of ischemia which will lead to each type of management (Figs 5 and 6).

Screening Asymptomatic Population for CAD

The noninvasive detection of silent CAD is an important clinical goal in certain high-risk asymptomatic populations. Occult CAD precedes the onset of clinically manifested CAD which too often presents as sudden death or acute myocardial infarction. Detection of occult CAD in a preclinical stage might lead to risk factor modification and institution of treatment, which would prevent or delay the onset of clinical diseases, since there is now good evidence that aggressive risk factor modification can slow the progression of atherosclerosis. Screening may not be

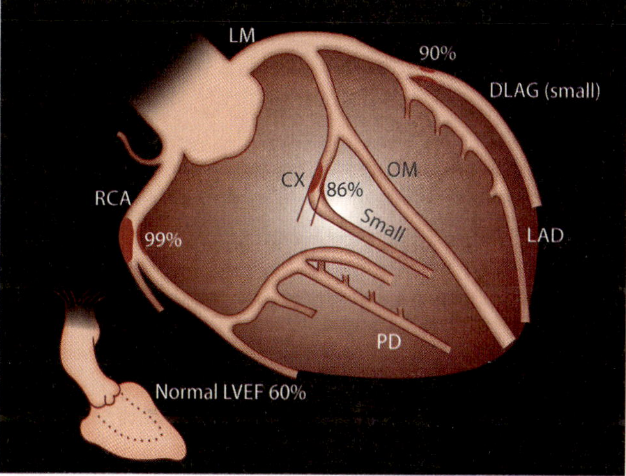

Fig. 5: Coronary angiography shows multiple significant lesions in LAD, circumplex and right coronary arteries

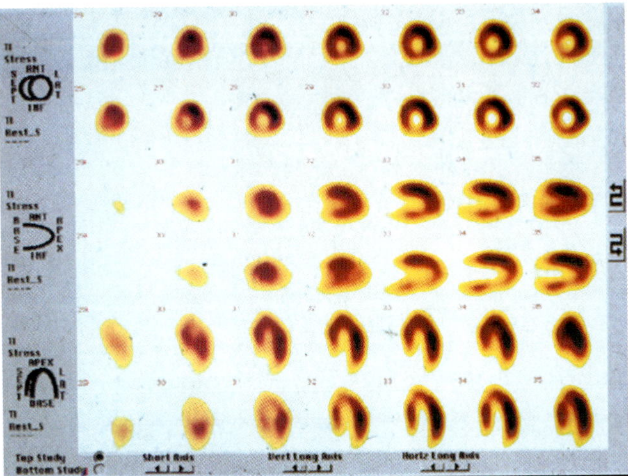

Fig. 6: Stress sestamibi myocardial perfusion scan shows almost uniform perfusion pattern seen involving anteroseptal, anterolateral, posterolateral myocardial segments with a small area of reduced perfusion pattern seen involving inferior segment

considered appropriate for the general population, given the sensitivity and specificity of even the best noninvasive test. Screening seems more suitable for selected, high-risk groups, such as patients with chronic renal failure, metabolic syndrome, and diabetes; in the latter, several studies have demonstrated a high prevalence of silent CAD detected with MPI.

Myocardial Viability

Noninvasive imaging to determine the presence and extent of dysfunctional but viable myocardium has become an important component of the diagnostic assessment of patients with CAD and depressed left ventricular function. It is now well-established that left ventricular dysfunction in patients with CAD is not always an irreversible process related to previous myocardial infarction because left ventricular function may improve substantially after revascularization procedures in patients with chronic CAD, and this may translate into an improvement in survival. The differentiation of viable from nonviable myocardium is highly relevant in patients with left ventricular dysfunction considered for revascularization, because these procedures often have high morbidity and mortality rates in this subset of patients, even though this is the population that ultimately benefits the most from revascularization.

Therefore, accurate methods to detect viable myocardium are essential. In SPECT, there are various imaging protocols, the most frequently used being the thallium-201 protocols (rest/redistribution and reinjection studies). According to the hypothesis of resting hypoperfusion (hibernation) rest images demonstrate thallium uptake early after injection, which represents regional myocardial blood flow, whereas delayed uptake reflects cell membrane integrity, since 3–4 hour redistribution images may underestimate the presence of viable myocardium. Reinjection of thallium at rest after redistribution imaging may improve the assessment of myocardial ischemia and viability in up to 49% of apparently irreversible defects 3–4 hours. As technetium-99m tracers are widely used due to favorable imaging properties compared to thallium, the use of these tracers for the assessment of viability has been studied, and quantitative measures of regional technetium-99m sestamibi activity have been shown to correlate with estimates of viability with other techniques. Glucose metabolism assessment with F-18 fluorodeoxyglucose (FDG) positron emission tomography (PET) also allows the identification of viable myocardium, with higher sensitivity, a perfusion metabolism mismatch (reduced blood flow associated with preserved or enhanced FDG uptake) identifies potentially reversible myocardial dysfunction. PET, the gold standard modality of investigation in the assessment of myocardial viability has several advantages over SPECT for cardiac imaging including better spatial resolution, higher sensitivity and the ability to measure tracer distribution in absolute terms, PET can also assess myocardial perfusion as well as metabolism (Figs 7 and 8).

Myocardial Innervation Imaging

I-123 metaiodobenzylguanidine (MIBG) has been used as a potential neuronal imaging agent and has been shown with reduced localization and delayed wash out in denervated region of the myocardium, after myocardial infarction, in diabetes and dilated cardiomyopathy. In addition MIBG imaging evaluate the sympathetic nervous system distribution in the myocardium and is an important prognosticator in patients with heart failure.

POSITRON EMISSION TOMOGRAPHY

In the present day clinical practice with the wide spread availability of positron emission tomography (PET) cameras and the radiotracer has changed the present scenario of the assessment of myocardial viability in dysfunctional myocardium in chronic stable angina/chronic CAD patients. This leads to real benefit, since PET has several technical advantages over SPECT, including higher spatial resolution, accurate attenuation correction, higher temporal resolution quantitative myocardial blood flow imaging capability that affords measurement of rapidly changing radiotracer activity concentration in blood and myocardium. All of these parameters have clinical advantages over SPECT, which often uncovers only the

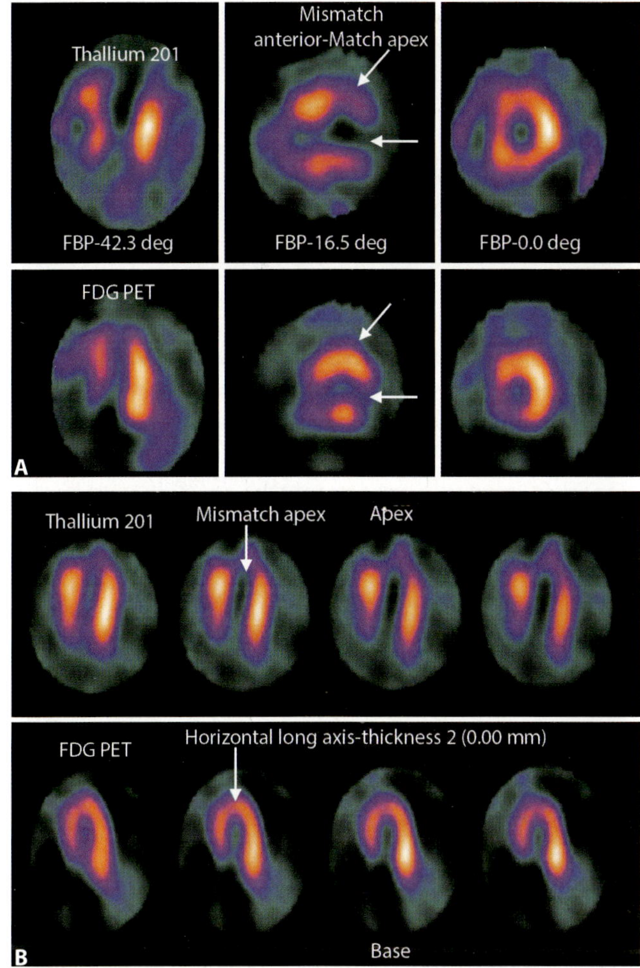

Figs 7A and B: (A) Dual isotope myocardial imaging shows a stress defect involving part of anterior and apical myocardial segments which shows adequate metabolism involving anterior segments only. However apical seems to have no metabolism suggesting scarred myocardium as evidenced from F-18 FDG metabolism study; (B) Stress myocardial perfusion imaging with Thallium-201 perfusion showing an apical defect which shows adequate metabolism with F-18 FDG metabolism study as evidenced from the bottom row segments of images

territory supplied by the most severe stenosis and therefore may underestimate the significance of coronary lesions, in this regard PET has superior capability to detect multivessel CAD.

The Association with Computed Tomography: SPECT-CT/PET-CT

Computed tomography of the coronary arteries (CTA) has gained enormous popularity in a short time period and has been taken by some as a "threat" for nuclear cardiology. CTA and MPI differ in what each evaluates anatomy for

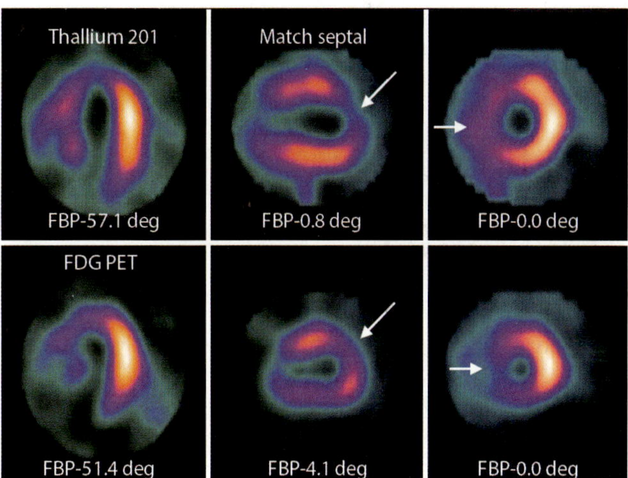

Fig. 8: Stress thallium myocardial perfusion study shows a perfusion defect involving anteroseptal segments which seems to have absent metabolism using F-18 FDG metabolic study

one and physiology for the other. Hybrid systems are now available allowing the combined assessment of anatomy and function, linking and anatomic richness of CTA and the functional importance of perfusion either from SPECT or PET, MPI and CTA are most likely complementary imaging modalities.

FATTY ACID IMAGING

β-methyl-p-123I-Iodophenyl-Pentadecanoic Acid (BMIPP) is a fatty acid analog which allows metabolic imaging since most of the energy requirement of the normal myocardium under aerobic status is derived from the metabolism of fatty acids. Since under ischemia or in heart failure, beta -oxidation of fatty acids in mitochondria is reduced, early washout of BMIPP from the myocardium occurs and the uptake detected by SPECT is reduced. BMIPP imaging may be used in unstable angina, vasospastic angina and cardiomyopathies, among other indications. In particular, BMIPP metabolic imaging may be used to reveal "ischemic memory". Since even after resolution of chest pain, metabolic abnormalities may persist, and BMIPP images may be abnormal, with sensitivity of nearly70–80% and specificity of nearly 90% (Fig. 9).

MOLECULAR IMAGING/PLAQUE IMAGING

The management of CAD in the context of diabetes mellitus has almost always been based on demonstration of the severity of luminal stenosis, such an approach however, does not characterize the plaque morphology that

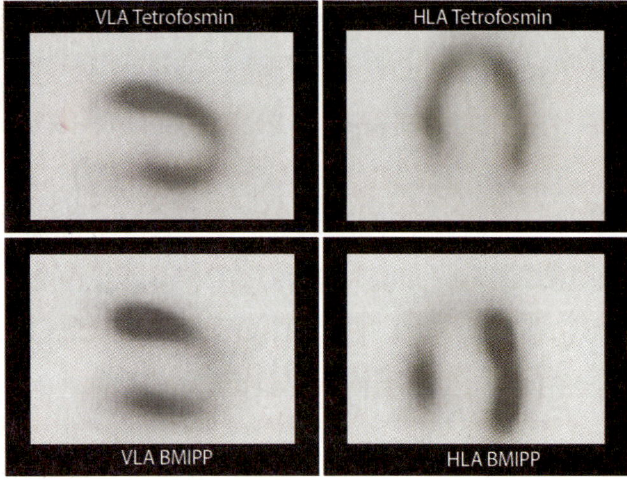

Fig. 9: BMIPP fatty acid I metabolism and Tc99m labeled tetrofosmin MPI studies show reduced metabolism showing anteroseptal and apical myocardial segments as compared to almost uniform perfusion pattern seen involving anteroseptal and apical myocardial segments

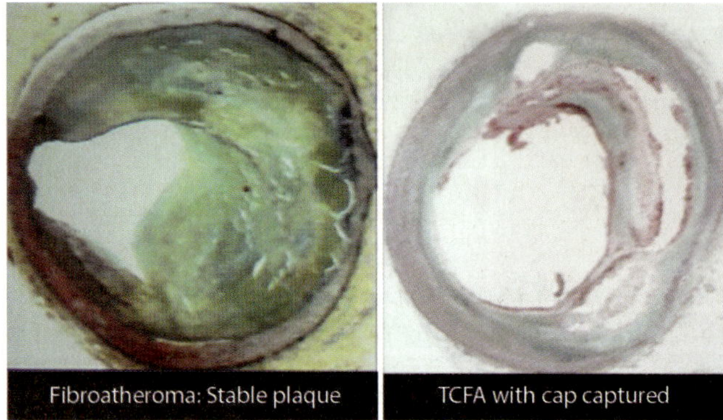

Fig. 10: Left side of the image shows a stable plaque as compared to unstable plaque seen in the lumen of the artery

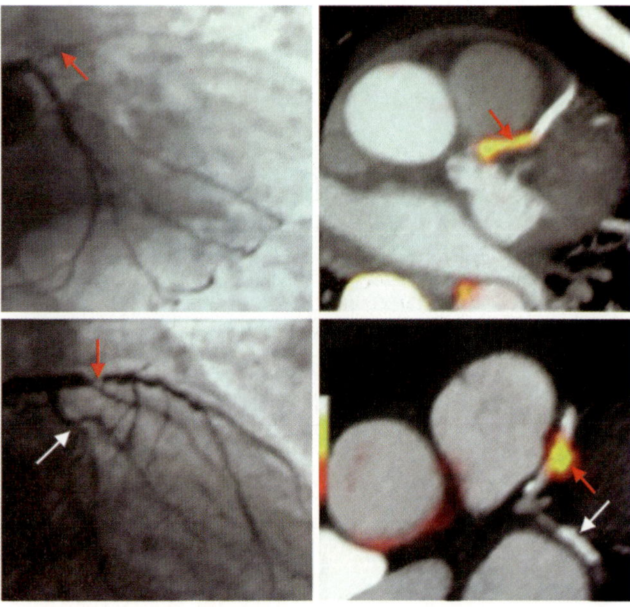

Fig. 11: Significant F-18 Na F tracer uptake seen in the proximal part of left anterior descending artery suggesting unstable atheromatous plaque

happens to be the major determinant of clinical outcome. Appropriate targeting strategies with radionuclide imaging techniques (using F-18 FDG/ F-18 NaF) may identify the predominant cellular population in the atherosclerotic plaque and help to predict the likelihood of clinical events: It is now well understood that progressive luminal stenosis of the coronary artery is generally not associated with an acute event and that thrombotic occlusion usually occurs as a result of plaque rupture particularly in silent myocardial ischemia in type 2 diabetes mellitus. The plaques that are vulnerable to rupture have large lipid cores, attenuated fibrous cap and intense infiltration of macrophages, which release metalloproteinase that digests matrix and induces fibrous cap rupture. Plaque rupture exposes thrombogenic lipid core leading to thrombotic luminal obstruction (Figs 10 and 11).

CONCLUSION

Noninvasive imaging techniques have been shown to be extremely useful in diagnostic and prognostic assessment to coronary disease in individuals with diabetes mellitus. An exercise treadmill test (TMT) can be safe and effective in initial screening test in patients who can exercise and have normal base line ECG. If a baseline ECG on a positive tread mill stress testing or be contradiction and false positivity to TMT, a functional study such as nuclear stress MPI or stress echocardiography may be strongly recommended to assess the presence of ischemia. However, nuclear cardiology has grown and it keeps moving. Many advances have increased its applications and many more regarding novel instrumentation techniques and new tracers including emerging one of labeling the unstable plaque are on their way to clinical practice. The greatest potential for the future of nuclear cardiology lies in molecular imaging and nuclear cardiology and it may hopefully achieve one of the most difficult goals in cardiology to identify the vulnerable rupture prone coronary plaque particularly in the subset of asymptomatic type 2 diabetes mellitus patients.

BIBLIOGRAPHY

1. Berman DS, Hachamovitch R, Kiat H, et al. Incremental value of prognostic testing in patients with known or suspected ischemic heart disease: a basis for optimal utilization of exercise technetium-99m sestamibi myocardial perfusion single-photon emission computed tomography. J Am coll cardiol. 1995;26:639–47.
2. Botvinick EH, Taradash MR, Shames DM, et al. Thallium-201 myocardial perfusion Scintigraphy for the clinical clarification of normal, abnormal & equivocal electrocardiographic stress tests. Am J Cardiol. 1978;41:43–51.
3. Boucher CA, Zir LM, Beller GA, et al. Increased lung uptake of thallium-201 during exercise myocardial imaging: Clinical, hemodynamic and angiographic implications in patients with coronary artery disease. Am J Cardiol. 1980;46:189–96.
4. Boyne TS, Koplan BA, Parsons WJ, et al. Predicting adverse outcome with exercise SPECT technetium-99m sestamibi imaging in patients with suspected or known coronary artery disease. Am J Cardiol. 1997;79:270–4.
5. Brown KA. Prognostic value of myocardial perfusion imaging: State of the art and new developments. J Nucl Cardiol. 1996;3:516–37.
6. Brown KA. Prognostic value of thallium-201 myocardial perfusion imaging. A diagnostic tool comes of age. Circulation. 1991;83:363–81.
7. Chouraqui P, Rodrigues EA, Berman DS, et al. Significance of dipyridamole-induced transient dilation of the left ventricle during thallium-201 scintigraphy in suspected coronary artery disease. Am J Cardiol. 1990;66:689–94.
8. Hachamovitch R, Hayes S, Friedman JD, et al. Comparison of the short-term survival benefits associated with revascularization compared with medical therapy in patients with no prior coronary artery disease undergoing stress myocardial perfusion single photon emission computed tomography. Circulation. 2003;107:2900–7.
9. Hachamovitch R, Hayes S, Friedman JD, et al. Determinants of risk and its temporal variation in patients with normal stress myocardial perfusion scans: what is the warranty period of a normal scan? J Am Coll Cardiol. 2003;41:1329–40.
10. Hachamovitch R, Hayes S, Friedman JD, et al. Stress myocardial perfusion SPECT is clinically effective & cost-effective in risk stratification of patients with a high likelihood of coronary artery disease (CAD) but no known CAD. J Am coll cardiol. 2004;43:200–8.
11. Kang X, Berman DS, Lewin H, et al. Incremental prognostic value of myocardial perfusion single photon emission computed tomography in patients with diabetes mellitus. Am Heart J. 1999;138:1025–32.
12. Klocke FJ, Baird MG, Lorell BH, et al. ACC/AHA/ASNC Guidelines for the clinical use of Cardiac Radionuclide Imaging Executive Summary. A Report of the American College of Cardiology/American Heart Association Task Force on Practice Guidelines (ACC/AHA/ASNC Committee to Revise the 1995 Guidelines for the Clinical Use of Cardiac Radionuclide Imaging). Circulation. 2003;108:1404–18.
13. Sharir T, Germano G, Kang X, et al. Prediction of myocardial infraction versus cardiac death by gated myocardial perfusion SPECT: risk stratification by the amount of stress-induced ischemia and the poststress ejection fraction. J Nucl Med. 2001;42:831–7.
14. Sharir T, Germano G, Kavanagh PB, et al. Incremental prognostic value of post-stress left ventricular ejection fraction & volume by gated myocardial perfusion single-photon emission computed tomography. Circulation. 1999;79:270–4.
15. Shaw LJ, Berman DS, Maron DJ, et al. Optimal medical therapy with or without percutaneous coronary intervention to reduce ischemic burden: results from the Clinical Outcomes Utilizing Revascularization and Aggressive Drug Evaluation (COURAGE) trial nuclear substudy. Circulation. 2008;117:1283–91.
16. Shaw LJ, Iskandrian AE. Prognostic value of gated myocardial perfusion SPECT. J Nucl Cardiol. 2004;11:171–85.

Blood Pressure Variability in Cardiodiabetes

Rajan Joseph Manjuran, Sulthan Raslin Salih

INTRODUCTION

Elevated blood pressure (BP) has been recognized as a major risk factor for atherosclerosis-related complications.[1] Systolic hypertension and diabetes can mutually aggravate the risk of cardiovascular (CV) diseases. An increase of every 20 mm Hg systolic BP above 115 mm Hg can double the risk of stroke.[2] Almost 50% of the type 2 diabetic patients are having systemic hypertension.[3] Systolic BP variability is being more and more recognized as a risk factor for stroke.[4]

BLOOD PRESSURE VARIABILITY

Variability of BP is calculated as standard deviation (sd) and coefficient of variation (sd/mean BP) of BP measured at intervals.[5] Blood pressure variability (BPV) is often associated with other CV risk factors like diabetes, systemic hypertension, and increasing age. Since BPV occurs in patients with preexisting risk factors, the most important question to analyze is whether BPV is in itself a risk factor or has just additive value to existing risk. Hsieh et al.[5] found that the systolic BPV is independently correlated with CV events. However, BPV occurred in patients with several risk factors and hence its relevance as an individual risk factor is not strong. Even in patients with controlled BP, the BPV indicated CV risk implying that treating BPV may be beneficial.[5] These patients had type 2 diabetes, hypercholesterolemia or hyperhomocysteinemia, and hence reducing the relevance of BPV alone.

BLOOD PRESSURE VARIABILITY AND TYPE 2 DIABETES

The lack of normal variability of BP, the nocturnal dipping, has been reported in diabetics.[6] The failure of sympathetic tone to decrease at night is postulated as the mechanism for nondipping. The nondipping of nocturnal BP is correlated with diabetic complications.[7] Visit to visit (VTV) BPV has been shown to be a risk factor for stroke. This is independent of systolic BP.[4] VTV BPV is strongly correlated with CV risk and mortality in type 2 diabetes.[5] This also was independent of systolic BP. The authors also found that VTV variability of pulse pressure also predicted future CV events.[5] Increase in arterial stiffness in patients of type 2 diabetes predisposes for increase and variability in pulse pressure.[8] VTV BPV can be considered as a therapeutic target to prevent future CV events. Mokhtar et al.[9] reported reduced small arterial compliance in type 2 diabetes patients which is an independent predictor of CV events. BPV also was observed in these patients.[9] Both these indicate that in diabetes, most likely hyperglycemia can affect the compliance of the arterial system thereby causing the BP variation. BPV has been shown to cause end-organ damage in diabetes mellitus patients. Hyperglycemia by reducing the compliance of the arterial system can lead to BPV.[9]

In the Action in Diabetes and Vascular Disease: Preterax and Diamicron Modified Release Controlled Evaluation (ADVANCE) trial, the VTV systolic BPV was a predictor of major macrovascular and microvascular complications in type 2 diabetes.[10] In the ADVANCE trial, VTV BPV predicted future myocardial infarction and risk of CV death,[10] while Rothwell et al.[4] observed greater risk for both stroke and coronary artery disease in patients with VTV BPV. In a Japanese study, the Ohasama study, systolic BPV increased the risk for stroke mortality but not cardiac mortality.[11] It may be thought from the above observation that BPV in Asian population predisposes for stroke. In the Ohasama study,[11] home BP was recorded, while in other studies, it was clinic or hospital BP recording in which whitecoat effect can also play a part. In ADVANCE trial,[10] VTV systolic BPV was a risk factor for microvascular complications of type 2 diabetes mellitus. In a Japanese study on type 2 diabetes patients, systolic BP was associated with microalbuminuria suggestive of microvasculopathy.[12] Hence, it is logical to conclude that VTV systolic BPV is a risk factor for microvascular complications among type 2 diabetes mellitus patients. Hata et al.[10] found that mean systolic BP was a predictor of future CV risk than systolic BPV. However, the impact of systolic BPV on CV risk was independent of systolic BP and hence systolic BPV can be a therapeutic target. The proposed mechanisms for VTV BPV in type 2 diabetes mellitus are:

- As a sequelae to arterial stiffness leading to reduced vascular compliance,[13]
- Increased sympathetic activity which can cause vascular events[1] and/or BP-lowering medication defaulting.[14-16]

Blood pressure variability can cause endothelial damage and renin–angiotensin system stimulation which leads to end-organ damage.[17] The Diabetic Control and Complication trial also reported that variability of systolic and diastolic BP predicted future nephropathy in type I diabetic patients.[18] Okada et al.[17] studied BPV in 354 patients with type 2 diabetes mellitus and concluded that VTV systolic BPV is a risk factor for diabetic nephropathy. Rothwell et al. observed that coefficient of variation of systolic BP predisposes to diabetic nephropathy. The mechanism of vascular or organ damage secondary to BPV is not clear. According to Kawai et al.[18] VTV BPV can cause renal vascular resistance which can lead to albuminuria. Diaz et al.[19] proposed that BPV correlated with endothelial dysfunction and resulted in impaired vascular smooth muscle response to nitric oxide. Wang et al.[20] in a meta-analysis concluded that VTV BPV is a risk factor for all-cause mortality, CV mortality, and stroke and coronary artery disease. Sohn et al.[21] reported that VTV BPV had strongest correlation with microvascular complications, especially nephropathy in diabetic population. The authors also observed that the patients with the highest variability are more likely to have associated retinopathy and neuropathy. In the ADVANCE-ON (ADVANCE Observational) study,[22] increased VTV BPV was correlated with higher risk of major macrovascular events, major renal damage and all-cause mortality in patients of type 2 diabetes mellitus over a follow-up period of 8 years. Wang et al.[20] in a systematic review concluded that VTV BPV can more likely predispose for cardiac events in Asians while stroke is more frequent in whites. However, this has not been confirmed in other studies where stroke was more frequent in Asians.[10,11]

CONCLUSION

Blood pressure variability and antihypertensives: The class of antihypertensives and their regular usage can determine the BPV in hypertensive population. In a review and meta-analysis Webb, et al. comparing various classes of antihypertensives concluded that calcium channel blockers had the minimum VTV BPV followed by diuretics. On the contrary, angiotensin-converting enzyme inhibitors, angiotensin II receptor blockers, beta blockers, and alpha blockers had greater BPV.[23] However, this observation has not been confirmed by others.[24]

REFERENCES

1. Lawes CM, Vander Hoorn S, Rodgers A. International Society of Hypertension. Global burden of blood-pressure-related disease, 2001. Lancet. 2008;371:1513-8.
2. Kengne AP, Patel A, Barzi F, et al. Systolic blood pressure, diabetes and the risk of cardiovascular diseases in the Asia-Pacific region. J Hypertens. 2007;25:1205-13.
3. Turner R, Holman R, Stratton I, et al. Tight blood pressure control and risk of macrovascular and microvascular complications in type 2 diabetes: UKPDS 38. UK prospective diabetes study group. BMJ. 1998;317:703-13.
4. Rothwell PM, Howard SC, Dolan E, et al. Prognostic significance of visit-to-visit variability, maximum systolic blood pressure, and episodic hypertension. Lancet. 2010;375:895-905.
5. Hsieh YT, Tu ST, Cho TJ, et al. Visit-to-visit variability in blood pressure strongly predicts all-cause mortality in patients with type 2 diabetes: a 5·5-year prospective analysis. Eur J Clin Invest. 2012;42:245-53.
6. Tóth L, Vörös P, Lengyel Z, et al. Diurnal blood pressure variations in incipient and end-stage diabetic renal disease. Diabetes Res Clin Pract. 2000;49:1-6.
7. Kaplan NM. Ambulatory blood pressure monitoring: valuable in diabetic subjects?. Diabetes Rev Int. 1996;5:11-4.
8. Stehouwer CD, Henry RM, Ferreira I. Arterial stiffness in diabetes and the metabolic syndrome: a pathway to cardiovascular disease. Diabetologia. 2008;51:527-39.
9. Mokhtar RH, Ayob A, Noor NM. Blood pressure variability in patients with diabetes mellitus. Asian Cardiovasc Thorac Ann. 2010;18:344-8.
10. Hata J, Arima H, Rothwell PM, et al. Effects of visit-to-visit variability in systolic blood pressure on macrovascular and microvascular complications in patients with type 2 diabetes mellitus: the ADVANCE trial. Circulation. 2013;128:1325-34.
11. Kikuya M, Ohkubo T, Metoki H, et al. Day-by-day variability of blood pressure and heart rate at home as a novel predictor of prognosis: the Ohasama study. Hypertension. 2008;52:1045-50.
12. Okada H, Fukui M, Tanaka M, et al. Visit-to-visit variability in systolic blood pressure is correlated with diabetic nephropathy and

atherosclerosis in patients with type 2 diabetes. Atherosclerosis. 2012;220:155-9.
13. Imai Y, Aihara A, Ohkubo T, et al. Factors that affect blood pressure variability. A community-based study in Ohasama, Japan. Am J Hypertens. 1997;10:1281-9.
14. Palatini P, Julius S. The role of cardiac autonomic function in hypertension and cardiovascular disease. Curr Hypertens Rep. 2009;11:199-205.
15. Su DF. Treatment of hypertension based on measurement of blood pressure variability: lessons from animal studies. Curr Opin Cardiol. 2006;21:486-91.
16. Kilpatrick ES, Rigby AS, Atkin SL. The role of blood pressure variability in the development of nephropathy in type 1 diabetes. Diabetes Care. 2010;33:2442-7.
17. Okada H, Nakanishi N, Fukui M, et al. Visit-to-visit blood pressure variability is a novel risk factor for the development and progression of diabetic nephropathy in patients with type 2 diabetes. Diabetes Care. 2013;36:1908-12.
18. Kawai T, Ohishi M, Kamide K, et al. The impact of visit-to-visit variability in blood pressure on renal function. Hypertens Res. 2012;35:239-43.
19. Diaz KM, Veerabhadrappa P, Kashem MA, et al. Relationship of visit-to-visit and ambulatory blood pressure variability to vascular function in African Americans. Hypertens Res. 2012;35:55-61.
20. Wang J, Shi X, Ma C, et al. Visit-to-visit blood pressure variability is a risk factor for all-cause mortality and cardiovascular disease: a systematic review and meta-analysis. J Hypertens. 2017;35:10-7.
21. Sohn MW, Epstein N, Huang ES, et al. Visit-to-visit systolic blood pressure variability and microvascular complications among patients with diabetes. J Diabetes Complications. 2017;31:195-201.
22. Ohkuma T, Woodward M, Jun M, et al. Prognostic value of variability in systolic blood pressure related to vascular events and premature death in type 2 diabetes mellitus: The ADVANCE-ON study. Hypertension. 2017;70:461-8.
23. Webb AJ, Fischer U, Mehta Z, et al. Effects of antihypertensive-drug class on interindividual variation in blood pressure and risk of stroke: a systematic review and meta-analysis. Lancet. 2010;375:906-15.
24. Blacher J, Safar ME, Ly C, et al. Blood pressure variability: cardiovascular risk integrator or independent risk factor? J Hum Hypertens. 2015;29:122-6.

CHAPTER

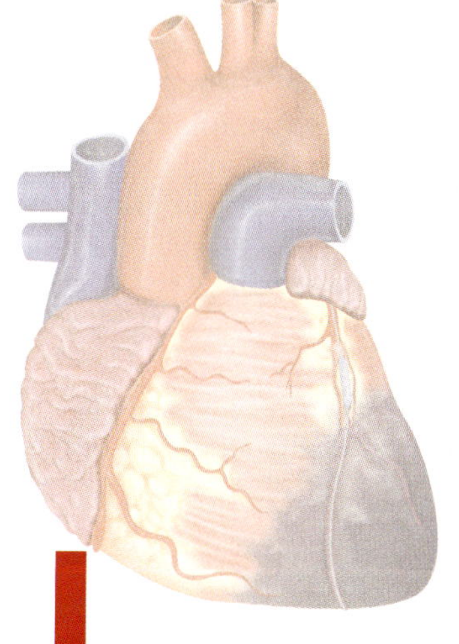

Central Aortic Blood Pressure Evaluation for Hypertension in Cardiodiabetics

Bahekar Anurag D, George Koshy, K Venugopal

INTRODUCTION

Central aortic pressure (CAP) is defined as "systolic pressure at the aortic root". It is now considered that CAP may correlate better with cardiovascular events than conventional blood pressure (BP) measured in the extremities.

WHY IS IT RELEVANT TODAY?

Dr Scipione Riva-Rocci published a report in Gazzetta medica di Torino in December 1886 on "a new sphygmomanometer". Our understanding of BP and its role in cardiology has come a long way since then. How relevant is it today? Are we measuring the right value? This debate was sparked by the marked differences in the pulse pressure (PP) between the central aorta and peripheral limbs.[1] The left ventricle encounters the aortic systolic pressure as afterload during systole while the aortic diastolic pressure fuels the coronary perfusion. Systemic diseases such as hypertension, diabetes, and aging significantly change these dynamics in the central arteries. However, the muscular peripheral arteries are much less influenced by these changes. The BP readings give an estimate of the pressure load on various organs. As the distance from heart increases the arteries become progressively smaller and stiffer with increase in wall tension. As a result, systolic blood pressure (SBP) in the distal vasculature is generally higher than that in the central arteries. Diastolic BP is roughly similar between the central and peripheral arteries. However, PP may differ substantially. Consequently, BP readings only give a rough idea of the true BP experienced by organs.

Brachial BP (BrBP) is thus a composite measure of both the CAP and the degree of amplification of the central pressure. The relationship between CAP and BrBP is not fixed, as it depends on a number of factors including arterial wall distensibility and arterial pressure, and the ratio between the two BPs has been termed the amplification ratio. Systolic pressure amplification is the ratio between brachial and central SBP. Pulse pressure amplification (PPA) is the ratio of brachial to central PP. In healthy individuals, PPA is approximately 1.5 and varies from 1.7 at less than 20 years of age to 1.2 at more than 80 years of age. CAP, increases with age as large arteries become stiffer, is reduced by low heart rate and shorter body height (reflecting reducing aortic length and volume), and is reduced with low diastolic pressure. Female gender on average is associated with a lower CAP in comparison with males. PPA is generally lower in females indicative of a higher central relative to brachial pressure.[2] CAP at the aortic root is regarded as an index of aortic stiffness and represents the true load imposed on heart, brain, kidney, and large arteries. Central BP can be a very useful additional clinical tool as studies have shown: (1) major discrepancies in central BP among people with similar brachial BP; (2) independent relationship of central BP with end-organ damage; (3) independent relationship of central BP with cardiovascular events and mortality; (4) differential central and brachial BP responses to antihypertensive medications; and (5) improvements in end-organ damage after therapy more strongly relate to central than brachial BP.[3] In the Anglo-Cardiff collaborative trial by McEniery et al.[4] in more than 10,000 subjects, it was demonstrated that approximately 32% of men and 10% of women with normal brachial SBP could have been classified as having stage 1 hypertension based on equivalent central aortic SBP. Central PP has also been shown to be superior to ambulatory BP in the prediction of all-cause and cardiovascular mortality.[5]

HOW TO MEASURE CENTRAL AORTIC BLOOD PRESSURE?

Central blood pressure (CBP) cannot be directly measured noninvasively. It has to be estimated from peripheral pressure waveforms. Advances in knowledge and technology such as pulse wave analysis (PWA), pressure transfer function-based waveform estimation, and precise applanation tonometry of the radial artery are needed for measuring central BP.

Following instruments are currently available:

- SphygmoCor® (AtCor Medical, Australia) or HEM-9000AI® (Omron Healthcare, Japan) was used to estimate CBP in various recent studies. "Suprasystolic" or "stop-flow" recordings are made with a cuff pressure above SBP so that the brachial artery is totally occluded. These devices can measure CBP as well as ambulatory blood pressure monitoring (ABPM) at one time. The SphygmoCor®, using this method, was used in a large clinical trial (CAFE study)[6] after extensive validation studies. It is considered as standard for CBP estimation.
- Mobil-O-Graph® (APC Cardiovascular, United Kingdom) and BPLab® + Vasotens® software (OOO Petr Telegin, Russia), uses ordinary oscillometric pulse volume recording data which is fed into a certain transfer function to estimate a CAP waveform.
- Arteriograph® (MedExpert, Hungary) and BPPlus CardioScope® + VasomonR® software (PulseCor, New Zealand), uses oscillometric technique that has been modified to acquire suprasystolic recordings of oscillometric brachial pulse waves to estimate CBP parameters.[7]

HOW IS HYPERTENSION DIFFERENT IN DIABETICS?

Patients with diabetes have increased pulse wave velocities compared with age-matched patients without diabetes.[8] Most recently, among 872 adults with normal glucose tolerance, insulin resistance was independently associated with increased brachial-ankle pulse wave velocity (PWV).[9] In another study of 232 previously healthy Japanese adults, brachial-ankle PWV was shown to increase linearly with increasing fasting blood glucose and hemoglobin A1c (HbA1c). It increased stepwise in patients with normal, impaired fasting glucose (IFG), and diabetes mellitus (DM), respectively.[10] This suggests that even early insulin resistance is associated with arterial stiffness. In a longitudinal study, Tomiyama et al. followed 2,080 Japanese men for 3 years. They noted that in patients with metabolic syndrome, PWV was higher even after adjusting for BP. Regression of metabolic syndrome parameters was associated with slowing of arterial stiffness.[11]

Type 1 Diabetes Mellitus

Sweitzer et al. measured aortic PWV and pulsatile hemodynamics in 17 patients with type 1 DM (average length of DM was 15 years) and compared them to age- and sex-matched controls. Compared to controls without DM, patients with type 1 DM had elevated central and peripheral PP, despite having similar mean BP. Aortic characteristic impedance was increased in the group with DM, even when PWV was not different. Aortic impedance was specially increased in patients with albuminuria.[12]

Type 2 Diabetes Mellitus

Taniwaki et al. compared carotid intimal-medial thickness (IMT) and carotid-femoral PWV between populations with and without DM. They showed a positive correlation between measures of arterial thickness and stiffness. Both were increased in patients with DM. They also showed that PWV increased with age, and that this slope was steeper in patients with type 2 DM than in controls.[13] The Asklepios study has evaluated the basis for an increased PP in type 2 DM using comprehensive assessments of arterial hemodynamics.[14] It was shown to be due to increased aortic stiffness and a lower total arterial compliance (most of which is normally provided by the aorta), rather than increased wave reflections. Similar findings were obtained in a previous study, which included over 10,000 subjects from large population-based cohorts around the world. In patients with type 2 DM, augmentation index (AIx) was significantly reduced.[15] The Hoorn study, a large population based-cohort study of nearly 2,500 subjects in the Netherlands, showed that after adjusting for age and BP, IFG was associated with increased arterial stiffness that was intermediate between that of normal controls and patients with type 2 DM.[8] DM may lead to preferential increase in large artery stiffness. This may reduce the impedance mismatch with more distal muscular arteries, resulting in a lower reflection magnitude. The impedance matching at the interface between the aorta and medium-sized muscular arteries may also result in increased penetration of pulsatile energy to distal vascular beds, which may contribute to the microvascular complications of DM.

PATHOPHYSIOLOGY OF AORTIC STIFFNESS AND INCREASED CENTRAL AORTIC PRESSURE IN DIABETICS

The role of advanced glycation end products is described in Flow chart 1.[16-19]

The role of nitric oxide (NO)-mediated vasodilatation—NO has vasodilatory, antiplatelet, anti-inflammatory, and antioxidant properties is described in Flow chart 2.[20]

While initial increase in NO levels may be compensatory with early insulin resistance, there is baseline abnormal response to vasodilation agents.[21,22]

More recently, Semba et al. demonstrated that in a community-dwelling population, higher serum advanced glycation end (AGE) product levels were significantly associated with carotid-femoral PWV even after adjusting for age, BP, and the presence of DM.[2]

Flow chart 1: Role of advanced glycation end products

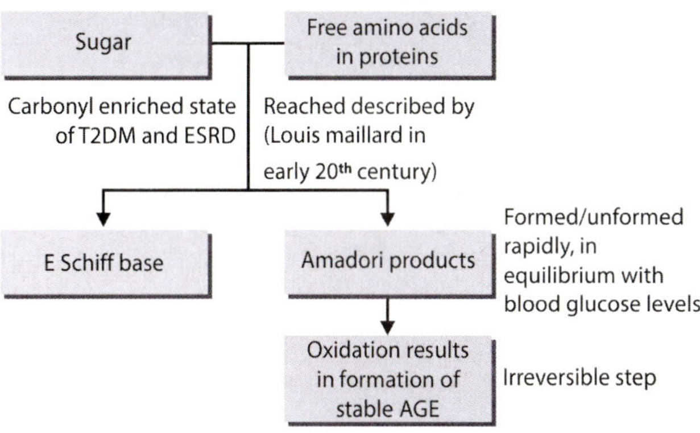

Abbreviations: T2DM, type 2 diabetes mellitus; ESRD, end stage renal disease; AGE, advanced glycation end product

Flow chart 2: Role of nitric oxide (NO)-mediated vasodilatation

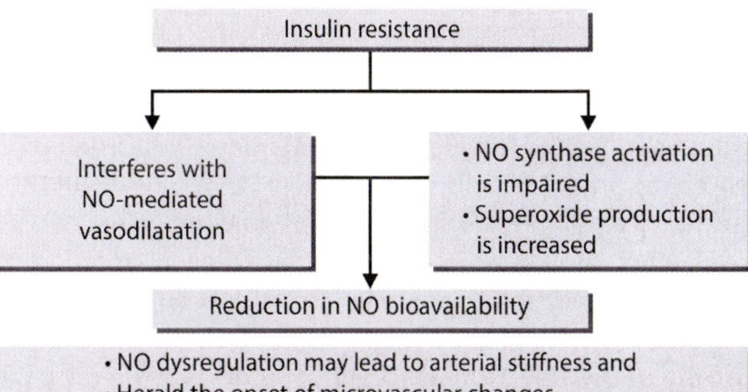

In DM, glucose dysregulation leads to arterial stiffness, however arterial stiffness itself may beget abnormal glucose metabolism. The propagation of increased pressure and flow pulsations to small blood vessels that supply target organs, such as the brain and kidneys, may over time lead to target organ dysfunction, such as albuminuria and stroke.[23,24] Arterial stiffness and elevated PP identify subjects at risk for developing type 2 DM. Whether hemodynamic changes related to increased arterial pulsatility play a direct role in the development of DM requires further investigation.

WHAT IS THE DATA ON CARDIOVASCULAR OUTCOMES?

Landmark BP Guide study:[25] This was a prospective, open-label, blinded-end point study in 286 patients with hypertension randomized to treatment decisions guided by best-practice usual care (n = 142; using office, home, and 24-hour ambulatory BP) or, in addition, by central BP intervention (n = 144; using SphygmoCor). Therapy was reviewed every 3 months for 12 months. Outcome measures were—medication quantity (daily defined dose), quality of life, and left ventricular mass (three-dimensional echocardiography). The principal findings of this study was that guidance of hypertension management with central BP results in a significantly different therapeutic pathway than conventional cuff BP, with less use of medication to achieve BP control and no adverse effects on left ventricular mass, aortic stiffness, or quality of life. One issue in this trial is the effect of heart rate on the relationship between central and radial PP as was seen in the studies assessing the effects of β-adrenergic blockade (atenolol) as a hypertensive treatment, where central aortic systolic pressure was shown to be relatively higher than the amlodipine group for similar brachial systolic pressure. However, this was not a significant concern in the study by Sharman et al. because only approximately 7% of subjects in the whole cohort were on β-blockers (BBs), and there was no difference in heart rate among the groups. The study also showed that a reduced defined daily dose (DDD) in the central aortic BP group was associated with a trend for reduced left ventricular (LV) mass index. Another important meta-analysis in this subject is the meta-analysis of prediction of cardiovascular events and all-cause mortality with central hemodynamics. The meta-analysis included 11 longitudinal studies that had employed measures of central hemodynamics and had followed 5,648 subjects for a mean follow-up of 45 months. The age-and risk-factor-adjusted pooled relative risk (RR) of total cardiovascular (CV) events was 1.088 for a 10 mm Hg increase of central systolic pressure, 1.137 for a 10 mm Hg increase of central pulse pressure (PP), and 1.318 for a 10% absolute increase of central AIx.

Furthermore, they found that a 10% increase of central AIx was associated with a RR of 1.384 for all-cause mortality. When compared with brachial PP, central PP was associated with marginally but not significantly higher RR of clinical events ($p < 0.057$).

The meta-analysis concluded that central pressure components and indices predict independently future clinical events. For central PP, this ability is marginally but not significantly better compared with peripheral pressures. AIx predicts clinical events independently of peripheral pressures. Superiority of vasodilating drugs with regards to outcome may be partly due to their differential effects on central pressure despite similar effects on brachial pressure. Central hemodynamics shows the potential to be implemented in clinical practice.[26] Data from the Conduit Artery Function Evaluation (CAFE) trial[6] shows that agents that reduce central aortic as well as peripheral pressures are associated with a lower CV risk profile compared with agents that lower only peripheral pressures.

Drug Data in Diabetics

In the EFFORT study, the effect of addition of nebivolol in predominantly African American patients with type 2 diabetes already receiving maximally tolerated doses of renin-angiotensin system (RAS) blockers was assessed. Patients with type 2 diabetes and hypertension on maximal RAS blockade (n = 70) were randomized to nebivolol or metoprolol succinate daily. Doses were titrated until SBP was less than 130 mm Hg. Radial artery applanation tonometry and PWV analysis were used to derive CAPs and hemodynamic indices at repeated visits at intervals during a 6-month period. Both metoprolol succinate and nebivolol groups demonstrated reductions in brachial SBP ([-8.2 ± 4.3 mm Hg (P = .01) and -7.8 ± 3.7 (P = .002), respectively] and aortic diastolic blood pressure (DBP) [-2.4 ± 1.8 (P = .039) and -4.0 ± 2.9 mm Hg (P = .013), respectively]. Aortic SBP decreased in the nebivolol group only (125.3 ± 8 to 121.6 ± 8.2, P = 0.025). There were no between group differences in aortic SBP, DBP, AIx, or PWV reduction. A significant increase in HbA1c was observed only in the metoprolol group. In patients with well-controlled type 2 DM and hypertension treated with maximally tolerated RAS blockade, nebivolol did not offer significant reductions in aortic BP over metoprolol succinate but maintained a stable metabolic profile. The role of maximally tolerated RAS blockers improving vascular compliance must not be overlooked as a confounding factor. Angiotensin-converting enzyme inhibitors (ACEIs) are known to improve arterial compliance and central pressure in people with diabetes and arterial stiffness.[27] A review article by Protogerou (2009) summarized the effects of different classes of antihypertensive drugs on CAP beyond peripheral BP. It reported that newer antihypertensive drugs [ACEIs, angiotensin receptor blockers (ARBs), and calcium-channel blockers (CCBs)] as well as nitrates have a more beneficial effect on pressure amplification than older drugs (diuretics and BBs). It also showed the relative detrimental effect of BBs (mainly atenolol) on CAP and convincing evidence that ACEIs increase pressure amplification. PARAMETER trial showed that sacubitril/valsartan, reduces CAP and central aortic pulse pressure (CAPP) more effectively than an ARB in high-risk older patients with systolic hypertension and an increased PP. The beneficial effects on central aortic hemodynamics and function could provide a therapeutic advantage beyond those observed with RAS blockade alone. In a meta-analysis, in diabetic patients the pooled estimate demonstrated statistically significant reduction in ankle-brachial PWV with thiazolidinediones (TZDs) (either pioglitazone or rosiglitazone). However, only one trial consisting of 30 patients demonstrated independent reduction in arterial stiffness with TZD therapy.[28]

WHAT DOES THE FUTURE HAVE IN STORE?

Two large studies TRANS (TRanscend Arterial stiffNess Substudy), and ONTARGET (Ongoing Telmisartan Alone and in Combination with Ramipril Global Endpoint Trial) are ongoing to evaluate the effects of BP lowering drugs on arterial stiffness. TRANS study would assess the beneficial effects of telmisartan on CV outcome and its relation to improvement in arterial stiffness.

WHAT IS THE CURRENT ROLE?

The 2013 European Society of Hypertension/European Society of Cardiology Guidelines for the management of arterial hypertension state that although the measurement of central aortic BP is of interest in terms of analyses for elucidating mechanisms related to pathophysiology, pharmacology, and therapeutics, further investigations are needed before central aortic BP can be recommended for routine clinical use (with the only possible exception being isolated systolic hypertension in youth). Indeed, trials are required to assess hard end points, where subjects are followed-up for a longer period (of the order of 5 years, similar to many other intervention studies). In addition, the design should be expanded where central aortic BP is measured in all subjects, but where one group is assessed by measurements of brachial cuff pressure but blind to the results of central BP and the other groups guided by the results of central BP but blind to the results of brachial BP.

CONCLUSION

As our knowledge of pathophysiology of diabetes, role of arterial stiffness, CAP and its effect on blood vessels grows; we face an ever-increasing number of questions. Is there a role of diabetes control in decreasing arterial stiffness and so BPs? Will targeting AGE and NO effectively decrease CAPs and improve CV outcomes? How do the currently available drugs affect these variables? Will improving dynamics of aortic stiffness improve the various microvascular complications of diabetes? Are we targeting the right marker? Standardization of CAP across various age groups using a clinically friendly device will open up new horizons to explore. Will CAP become the next big thing in assessing hemodynamics? Will CAP estimation replace current arm BP techniques? Only time will tell.

REFERENCES

1. Rowell LB, Brengelmann GL, Blackmon JR, et al. Disparities between aortic and peripheral pulse pressures induced by upright exercise and vasomotor changes in man. Circulation. 1968;37(6):954-64.
2. Williams B, Brunel PC, Lacy P, et.al. Application of non-invasive central aortic pressure assessment in clinical trials: clinical experience and value. Art Res. 2017;17:1-15.
3. Sherman JE, Laurent S. Central blood pressure in the management of hypertension: soon reaching the goal? J Hum Hypertens. 2013;27(7):405-11.
4. McEniery CM, Yasmin, McDonnell B, et al. Central pressure: variability and impact of cardiovascular risk factors: the Anglo-Cardiff Collaborative Trial II. Hypertension. 2008;51(6):1476-82.
5. Huang CM, Wang KL, Cheng HM, et al. Central versus ambulatory blood pressure in the prediction of all-cause and cardiovascular mortalities. J Hypertens. 2011;29(3):454-9.
6. Miyashita H. Clinical assessment of central blood pressure. Curr Hypertens Rev. 2012;8(2):80-90.
7. Williams B, Lacy PS, Thom SM, et al. Differential impact of blood pressure-lowering drugs on central aortic pressure and clinical outcomes: principal results of the Conduit Artery Function Evaluation (CAFE) study. Circulation. 2006;113(9):1213-25.
8. Schram MT, Henry RM, van Dijk RA, et al. Increased central artery stiffness in impaired glucose metabolism and type 2 diabetes: the Hoorn Study. Hypertension. 2004;43(2):176-81.
9. Fang FS, Liu MY, Cheng XL, et al. Insulin resistance correlates with the arterial stiffness before glucose intolerance. Intern Med. 2014;53(3):189-94.
10. Ohnishi H, Saitoh S, Takagi S, et al. Pulse wave velocity as an indicator of atherosclerosis in impaired fasting glucose: the Tanno and Sobetsu study. Diabetes Care. 2003;26(2):437-40.
11. Tomiyama H, Hirayama Y, Hashimoto H, et al. The effects of changes in the metabolic syndrome detection status on arterial stiffening: a prospective study. Hypertens Res. 2006;29(9):673-8.
12. Sweitzer NK, Shenoy M, Stein JH, et al. Increases in central aortic impedance precede alterations in arterial stiffness measures in type 1 diabetes. Diabetes Care. 2007;30(11):2886-91.
13. Taniwaki H, Kawagishi T, Emoto M, et al. Correlation between the intima-media thickness of the carotid artery and aortic pulse-wave velocity in patients with type 2 diabetes. Vessel wall properties in type 2 diabetes. Diabetes Care. 1999;22(11):1851-7.
14. Chirinos JA, Segers P, Gillebert TC, et al. Central pulse pressure and its hemodynamic determinants in middle-aged adults with impaired fasting glucose and diabetes: the Asklepios study. Diabetes Care. 2013;36(8):2359-65.
15. Chirinos JA, Kips JG, Roman MJ, et al. Ethnic differences in arterial wave reflections and normative equations for augmentation index. Hypertension. 2011;57(6):1108-16.
16. Sell DR, Monnier VM. Molecular basis of arterial stiffening: role of glycation: a mini-review. Gerontology. 2012;58(3):227-37.
17. Baynes JW, Thorpe SR. Role of oxidative stress in diabetic complications: a new perspective on an old paradigm. Diabetes. 1999;48(1):1-9.
18. Powell JT, Vine N, Crossman M. On the accumulation of D-aspartate in elastin and other proteins of the ageing aorta. Atherosclerosis. 1992;97(2-3):201-8.
19. Schnider SL, Kohn RR. Effects of age and diabetes mellitus on the solubility and nonenzymatic glucosylation of human skin collagen. J Clin Invest. 1981;67(6):1630-5.
20. Kawashima S, The two faces of endothelial nitric oxide synthase in the pathophysiology of atherosclerosis. Endothelium. 2004;11(2):99-107.
21. Brillante DG, O'Sullivan AJ, Howes LG. Arterial stiffness in insulin resistance: the role of nitric oxide and angiotensin II receptors. Vasc Health Risk Manag. 2009;5(1):73-8.
22. Semba RD, Najjar SS, Sun K, et al. Serum carboxymethyl-lysine, an advanced glycation end product, is associated with increased aortic pulse wave velocity in adults. Am J Hypertens. 2009;22(1):74-9.
23. O'Rourke MF, Hashimoto J. Mechanical factors in arterial aging: a clinical perspective. J Am Coll Cardiol. 2007;50(1):1-13.
24. Ford ML, Tomlinson LA, Chapman TP, et al. Aortic stiffness is independently associated with rate of renal function decline in chronic kidney disease stages 3 and 4. Hypertension. 2010;55(5):1110-5.
25. Sharman JE, Marwick TH, Gilroy D, et al. Randomized trial of guiding hypertension management using central aortic blood pressure compared with best-practice care: principal findings of the BP GUIDE study. Hypertension. 2013;62(6):1138-45.
26. Vlachopoulos C, Aznaouridis K, O'Rourke MF, et al. Prediction of cardiovascular events and all-cause mortality with central haemodynamics: a systematic review and meta-analysis. Eur Heart J. 2010;31(15):1865-71.
27. Briasoulis A, Oliva R, Kalaitzidis R, et al. Effects of nebivolol on aortic compliance in patients with diabetes and maximal renin angiotensin system blockade: the EFFORT study. J Clin Hypertens (Greenwich). 2013;15(7):473-9.
28. Webb DR, Davies MJ, Gray LJ, et al. Searching for the right outcome? A systematic review and meta-analysis of controlled trials using carotid intima-media thickness or pulse wave velocity to infer antiatherogenic properties of thiazolidinediones. Diabetes Obes Metab. 2010;12(2):124-32.

CHAPTER 50

Telemedicine in Diabetes Management

Krishnam Raju P, Prasad SG

INTRODUCTION

The significant objectives of telemedicine today are to create cutting edge telehealth tools and technologies, thereby enhancing healthcare delivery to medically underserved populations using telecommunication technology, to provide affordable and accessible medical specialty services, and to provide training of healthcare providers, clinical trainees, and students in health-related fields.[1] The advances in the field of Information and Communication Technology (ICT) over the last decade have helped in balancing the supply and demand in the healthcare services in quite an effective way. Telemedicine in particular has become a more viable and feasible model for healthcare delivery with the advent of ICT platform. The emergence of Internet of Things (IoT) has further ensured that a continuum in care can be maintained, with patients having the opportunity to have wearable devices at their homes and using the telemedicine platform for transmission of medical data from these devices for consultations. The impact of social networking platforms and mobile technologies in the healthcare domain needs further work especially in their utility to serving the underserved and remote populations.[1]

The number of people with diabetes is increasing due to population growth, aging, urbanization, and increasing prevalence of obesity and physical inactivity.[2,3] Diabetes is associated with huge human and economic costs. Predictions show that the number of people with diabetes worldwide will double in the next generation. The design and implementation of ICT systems for a longtime now has aimed at supporting the management of diabetes mellitus (DM), mainly in the areas of electronic patient records, decision support systems, and telemedicine.[4-6] During the recent decade, rapid advancements in healthcare services and low-cost wireless communication have greatly assisted in coping with the problem of fewer medical facilities. The integration of mobile communications with wearable sensors has facilitated the shift of healthcare services from clinic-centric to patient-centric and is termed as "Telemedicine" in the literature.[7] In the larger perspective, telemedicine can be of two types: (1) live communication type, where the presence of the doctor and patient is necessary with additional requirements of high bandwidth and good data speed, and (2) store and forward type, which requires acquisition of medical parameters such as vital signs, images, videos, and transmission of patients data to concerned specialist in hospital.[8,9]

The rising prevalence of chronic illnesses in an aging population puts pressure on the supply side of healthcare. Clinicians are not being prepared sufficiently quickly to keep pace with the rate of administration request. What is more, given the increasing expense of care, new models for repaying health centers, and different suppliers have started to underscore quality and proficiency as opposed to units of conveyed administrations. This has led to a competition wherein consumers look out for attractive health insurance policies that require significant deductibles and out-of-pocket expenses. Consequently, a flexible and transparent model for the delivery of healthcare is the need of the hour.

The chronic nature of DM and the need to empower patients make it a "natural" context to test ICT in terms of having continuity of the care being given and the flexibility of supporting home care. DM has taken epidemic proportions throughout the world and is considered among the most challenging health problems in the 21st century.[10] The disease is associated with a number of health-related complications, high morbidity and mortality rates and thus imposes substantial social and economic burdens worldwide.[11] The management of diabetic patients involves lot of challenges and one would require innovative management strategies to improve glycemic and pressure control, as these are frequently above the desired goals.[12] The optimal management requires an organized, systematic, and coordinated approach. Strong evidence demonstrates beneficial effects of patient monitoring and education, focused on a prominent role of the individual self-care with the support of healthcare professionals.[13] This brings into focus the great advances in telecommunication technology and information technology, which can be exploited to improve diabetes management.[14,15] Telemedicine can be a strategy for closer monitoring and intervention to achieve not only better metabolic control, but also to help in the global care of individuals with multiple chronic illnesses.[12,16-18]

IMPACT FACTORS OF TELEMEDICINE IN PATIENT CARE

With the advances made in the field of ICT, telemedicine is now being a good healthcare delivery model for people living remotely. One of the noticeable advantages of this technology is that it has ensured a reduction in the number of clinical visits thereby increasing the convenience factor for the patient. The waiting time in clinics is no longer an issue as the patient can continue with other routine work or rest at home until the specialist is available. The advancement of faster computers and more efficient bandwidth usage has allowed more types of services to be extended to more users. For example, a few decades ago a simple request for medical advice could be obtained by finding a fixed line telephone and dialing in to the clinic where a physician was stationed. With the availability of mobile Voice over Internet Protocol (VoIP) technology, one can now simply pick up a mobile phone and place a video-enabled call to a physician; thereby providing the flexibility to the physician of not being restricted to stay at one clinic to provide medical advice.

Telemedicine helps in bringing up an impact in patient care in the following way (Fig. 1):

- *Informational:* The application of ICT helps in digitizing data thereby facilitating maintaining an electronic medical record (EMR) for remote transmission and enabling a continuity of care.
- *Clinical:* The presence of an EMR tracking all the patient information and test details facilitates frequent communication of information and instructions, which can lead to improved outcomes with lower glycated hemoglobin (HbA1c) levels or fewer adverse sequelae.
- *Behavioral:* The behavioral impact is more frequent therapy adjustments and reminders, leading to greater patient education and empowerment.
- *Structural:* The structural impact is usually time-saving for patients who might need to come into the physician's office for fewer visits; however, the physician workload of reviewing messages and updated data on a regular basis may actually increase.

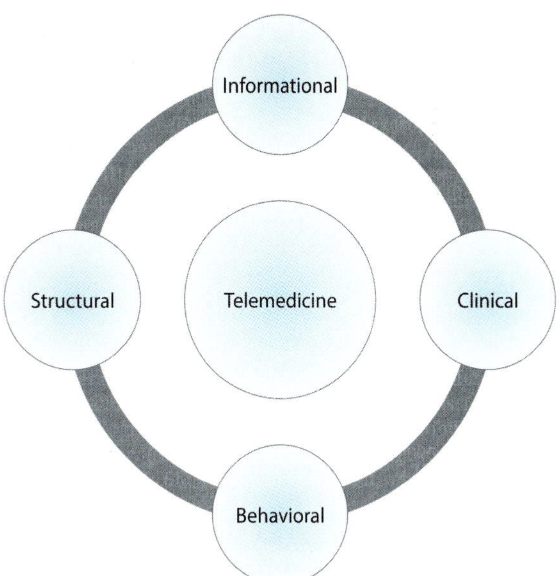

Fig. 1: Importance of telemedicine in patient care

The success for evaluating the effectiveness of telemedicine in the management of diabetes can be categorized in the following way:

- Validated and robust enough technology, which facilitates accurate collection of data, accuracy in terms of input, and verification process along with time stamping for the data collected to help track outcomes.
- Cost-effectiveness in terms of the cost of IoT based medical-assisted devices and application software coupled with transmission of data to specialist for review
- Sustainable and practical working model.

An effective technology allows for the determination of process outcome measures, clinical outcome measures, and patient satisfaction. First, the effectiveness of automated telemedicine systems can be measured to assess the adoption of process outcomes, such as timely foot screenings, retinal evaluations, vaccine administrations, and measurement of laboratory tests. These tests include HbA1c, glucose, and lipids for all patients with diabetes, and other laboratory analytes for selected diabetes patients, including serum creatinine levels in users of metformin, liver tests in users of statins, serum potassium in hypertensive patients on selected blood pressure medications, and serum fructosamine in some patients with hemoglobinopathies. Second, the effectiveness of telemedicine programs can be assessed on the basis of improvements in objective clinical outcomes, such as HbA1c levels, number of hypoglycemic events, glycemic variability according to a predefined formula, or emergency room visits for diabetes-related events. Finally, patient satisfaction can also be used to measure the effectiveness of a telemedicine program. User experience can be quantified by using surveys to measure patient satisfaction, classifying patient feedback in response to provider instructions, and determining the amount of system use by patients.[18] Patients suffering from prolonged diabetes have the potential risk of developing glaucoma, which may result in blindness. So it is important for eye screening of diabetic patients periodically and these retinal images can also be transmitted through telemedicine for identification of glaucoma and retinopathy facilitating further action.

Most telemedicine systems have achieved fair bit of success in dealing with management of diabetes with the advent of IoT based devices. However, a point to be considered and factored is that integration of the data from such systems to become part of the EMR of the patient to enable continuity and management in the care being given.

CLINICAL STUDIES

There is limited data available on the clinical outcomes through telemedicine. A few of them have been listed in Table 1 which had a reasonable success in the management of diabetes through telemedicine.

ROLE OF INTERNET OF THINGS IN DIABETES

The transformation of the healthcare industry has begun. While it may take some time to understand and appreciate the actual impact, the shake-up in patient, provider and payer processes, and analytics systems will leave the industry profoundly different. On the horizon is a much more cost-efficient healthcare industry that offers truly personalized healthcare. Providers and patients will be able to leverage the ever-increasing medical knowledge base and combine that with patient-specific historical and real-time data, including genetics, lifestyle behavior, and environmental data. The adoption of IoT networks, the data collected and the analytics of that data are accelerating the transformation of the healthcare industry.

Some Important Facts to Consider

The development and deployment of remote monitoring sensors for chronic disease management is still a young marketplace, but it is one that is ripe for explosive growth. As healthcare technology vendors begin to craft the industry's own particular IoT, passive big data collection from implantable or wearable medical devices may have a major impact on population health.

- The global IoT healthcare market is expected to grow from $32.47 billion in 2015 to $163.24 billion by 2020[27]
- IoT-enabled connectivity within hospital laboratories will increase total global laboratory test throughput by more than 3.02 billion diagnostic tests over the next 5 year

TABLE 1: Clinical outcomes through telemedicine

Study	*Sample*	*Intervention*	*Effects*
Ahring[19]	42 patients	Home blood sugar monitoring (RCT)	Computer group had HbA1c drop from 10.6% to 9.2% (–13.2%); control group from 11.2% to 10.2% (–8.9%)
Shultz[20]	20 patients	Home blood sugar monitoring (RCT)	Reduced HbA1c levels in computer group but details not given
Billiard[21]	22 patients	Home blood sugar monitoring (RCT)	Computer group had HbA1c drop from 6.7% to 6.0%; control group from 6.8% to 6.7%
DiBiase[22]	20 patients	Home blood sugar monitoring in gestational diabetes (RCT)	Computer group had HbA1c drop from 6.4% to 5.0%; control group from 7.1% to 5.7%
Frost[23]	21 patients	Home blood sugar monitoring in gestational diabetes	Computer group had HbA1c drop from 6.1% to 5.4%; control group from 6.2% to 5.7%
Marrero[24]	106 patients	Home blood sugar monitoring (RCT)	Computer group had HbA1c rise from 9.4% to 10.0%; control group from 9.9% to 10.3%; no difference in ER visits, psychological status, or family functioning
Mease[25]	28 patients	Home blood sugar monitoring (RCT)	Computer group had HbA1c fall from 9.5% to 8.2% vs 9.5% to 8.6% for control group
Biermann[26]	46 patients	Home blood sugar monitoring (RCT)	Computer group had HbA1c fall from 8.3% to 7.3% vs 8.0% to 6.8% for control group

Abbreviations: RCT, randomized controlled trial; HbA1c, glycated hemoglobin; ER, emergency room

- The value of improved health of chronic disease patients through remote monitoring could be as much as $1.1 trillion per year in 2025[27]
- Four million patients globally will remotely monitor their health conditions by 2020
- Consumers utilizing home health technologies will increase from 14.3 million worldwide in 2014 to 78.5 million by 2020. [27]

Over the next few years, patient monitoring devices will improve, and providers will increasingly implement IoT and big data analytics solutions. As a result, the global IoT healthcare market will grow at a significant rate.

Managing diabetes is a difficult ask as "glucose levels change frequently with normal activity like exercising or eating or even sweating. Sudden spikes or precipitous drops are dangerous and not uncommon, requiring round-the-clock monitoring. As a result, many people with diabetes check their blood glucose less often than they should."

The management of diabetes in ambient assisted living (AAL) environments, such as old people and diabetes patients homes, is a very difficult task since many factors affect a patient's blood sugar levels. Several factors such as illness, treatments, physical and psychological stress, physical activity, drugs, intravenous fluids and change in the meal plan cause unpredictable, and potentially dangerous fluctuations in blood sugar levels.

With a number of medical devices now available for measurement of glucose, the IoT platform has enabled monitoring of these patients in a more systematic and comprehensive manner (Fig. 2).

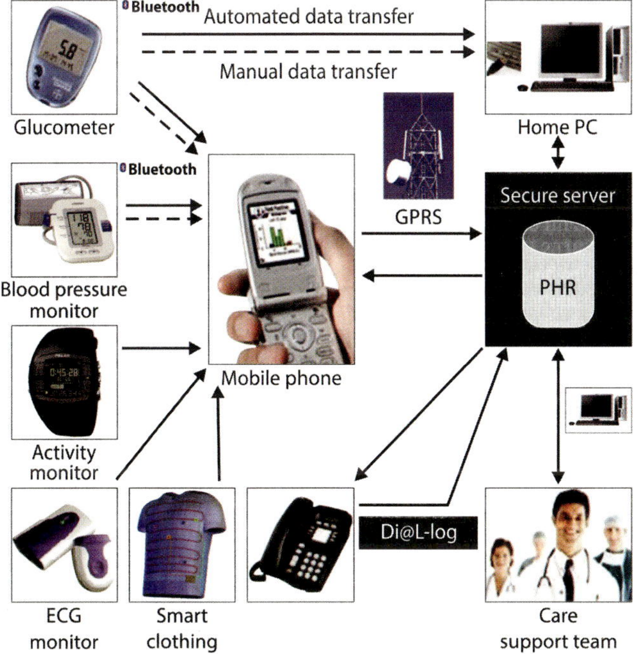

Fig. 2: Internet of Things (IoT) platform for the monitoring of patients in a more systematic and comprehensive manner

There are solutions that offer a diabetic patient with a handheld electronic personal device that could store blood glucose readings and give the patient advice about the next meal and insulin injection. The IoT platform, which provides a global connectivity and management architecture of sensors, devices, users and information, and can be one of the key advances in the areas of mobile diabetes management system. Therefore, this architecture can help us achieve a global connectivity and in the management of diabetes by creating an index for various conditions like hypoglycemia or hyperglycemia with the patient sensors and everything around it to accelerate and enhance the management process. This architecture includes several advanced communication technologies for security, identification, control, and connectivity with internet; among them are Internet Protocol (IPv6) and Low-power Wireless Personal Area Networks (6LoWPAN) and Radio Frequency Identification (RFID) technologies that form the basis of the new generation of personal services based on IoT.

The emergence of IoT-based devices have made telemedicine a more effective tool in the management of diabetes, especially at home in the following ways:

- Uploading food logs to track your food intake, information of medications to be taken, prescribed dosage and blood sugar levels for review by a nurse or doctor who responds electronically
- Providing information on carbohydrate counting app in your mobile to help keep your blood sugar levels in the target range. It also provides an estimate of the amount of insulin you require based on your diet and exercise level
- Enabling you to send queries to the nurse or your doctor through an email or text message
- Ordering diabetes kits, testing supplies, and medications online
- Exploring new treatment options in diabetes management
- Receiving reminders on health check-ups through email and text messages.[28,29]

Smart sensors, which combine a sensor and a micro-controller, make it possible to harness the power of the IoT for healthcare by accurately measuring, monitoring, and analyzing a variety of health status indicators. These can include basic vital signs such as heart rate and blood pressure, as well as levels of glucose or oxygen saturation in the blood. Smart sensors can even be incorporated into pill bottles and connected to the network to indicate, whether a patient has taken a scheduled dose of medication. For smart sensors to work effectively, the microcontroller components must incorporate several essential capabilities:

- *Low-power operation* is essential to keeping device footprint small and extending battery life, characteristics that help make IoT devices as usable as possible

- *Integrated precision-analog capabilities* make it possible for sensors to achieve high accuracy at a low cost
- *Graphical user interfaces (GUIs)* improve usability by enabling display devices to deliver a great deal of information in vivid detail and by making it easy to access that information.

The primary challenge in chronic care diseases is linking the devices so they can communicate reliably and securely. While blood-glucose and heart-rate sensors are widely available, they are rarely setup to export their data to a system that aggregates and shares information with all involved parties. Similarly, a number of companies have sold remote monitoring products for years and it has been observed that the utility to all parties has thus far been limited. To realize the real value, both patients and providers need these sensors to move beyond mere fall detection and be able to measure a wide array of BioSigns and, then, communicate those data to an integrated IoT system. Solving these communication issues can ease the shift to greater home care and increased patient involvement in care, driving better outcomes for patients, and reduced cost for all. With increasing numbers of smartphone users, it is possible to apply mobile app technology to empower patients to better manage their diabetes. Diabetes self-management education (DSME) thereby becomes a possibility with the availability of such technologies. While these IoT based devices help the patient monitor their glucose levels and also provide them with alerts and reminders regarding their medication, telemedicine in turn provides the platform for providing on line consultations too with the specialists, thereby ensuring a continuity in care without the patient having the need to travel.

New era of 5G will bring together improved connectivity, cloud-based storage, and an array of connected devices and services. Extensive computing capability combined with virtual system architecture will open up a mobile IoT. Rather than having computing equipment that is disparate and separate, the 5G world will allow us to enter an era where real-time health services will become the norm rather than the exception. 5G is not simply an extension of 3G and 4G. Instead, it is a transformative ecosystem that includes a heterogeneous network that integrates 4G, Wi-Fi, millimeter wave, and other wireless access technologies. It combines cloud infrastructure, a virtualized network core, intelligent edge services, and a distributed computing model that derives insights from the data generated by billions of devices. By 2020, the 5G network is expected to support 50 billion connected devices and 212 billion connected sensors as well as enable access to 44 zettabytes (ZB) of data.[30]

ROLE OF ARTIFICIAL INTELLIGENCE IN DIABETES MANAGEMENT

One of the core aspects involved in the management of diabetes is pattern recognition. Generally, physicians have a look at the blood glucose readings of the patient over a period of time and make treatment recommendations based on their findings. Some of the key factors that affect these recommendations are desired level of diabetes control, weight of the patient, food habits, other medical problems, current medications, and affordability. But we know that genetic variations can influence how one responds to drugs. It is humanly impossible to understand and keep in mind all those genetic variations and prescribe medications accordingly. So if we have decision support systems and feed the needed data for artificial intelligence (AI), it will become possible to make better judgment calls on diabetes management.

The use of current advances of information technologies and decision-support systems may improve cost-effectiveness of intensive insulin therapy (IIT), by reducing the number of periodical control visits, while increasing the patient or physician communication rate. The use of appropriate AI techniques, such as knowledge-based systems, intelligent data analysis and case-based reasoning, may enhance the design of the overall service. This integrated approach of healthcare devices and systems powered by the AI can analyze the glucose values, dietary patterns, and other factors to come up with treatment recommendations, which can be endorsed by the treating physician before being communicated to the patient. Today, technology companies are open sourcing their machine learning or AI platforms in the healthcare field, which can lead to revolutionizing treatment delivery models especially for patients with chronic diseases.

CONCLUSION

The widespread adoption of ICT in everyday life, including, in particular, the internet and mobile phones, is providing a great opportunity to improve the organization of DM care delivery by improving and optimizing communication among patients, healthcare providers, and healthcare systems. Telemedicine is a good alternative as it helps to avoid unnecessary visits to the specialist or clinic for management and treating diabetes, as compared to other diseases, because diabetes requires interpretation and predetermined responses to many types of data that can be measured in the home by the patient. As technology for communication improves, and better data management and decision support software is available, managing diabetic patients becomes lot easier. There is always a continuity in the care being given and probability of inducing diabetic related complications can reduce significantly through this method. Of course, it is important to note that while telemedicine can support changes and foster communication, and better treatments, it does not cure the disease by itself. Telemedicine interventions will likely improve in their effectiveness as EMRs and decision support software become more ubiquitous and both clinicians and patients develop familiarity with their benefits and drawbacks.

ACKNOWLEDGMENTS

We like to thank the management of CARE Hospital for the support provided for the execution of the telemedicine project. The contribution of the doctors of CARE Hospital by providing valuable insights about the impact of telemedicine in the management of diabetes is duly appreciated and acknowledged.

REFERENCES

1. Ackerman MJ, Filart R, Burgess LP, et al. Developing Next-Generation Telehealth Tools and Technologies: Patients, Systems, and Data Perspectives. Telemed JE Health. 2010;16(1):93-5.
2. Anjana RM, Pradeepa R, Deepa M, et al. Prevalence of diabetes and prediabetes (impaired fasting glucose and/or impaired glucose tolerance) in urban and rural India: Phase I results of the Indian Council of Medical Research-India Diabetes (ICMR-INDIAB) study. Diabetologia. 2011;54(12):3022-7.
3. Wild S, Roglic G, Green A, et al. Global prevalence of diabetes: estimates for the year 2000 and projections for 2030. Diabetes Care,2004;27(5):1047-53.
4. Cavan DA, Hejlesen OK, Hovorka R, et al. Preliminary experience of the DIAS computer model in providing insulin dose advice to patients with insulin dependent diabetes. Comput Methods Programs Biomed. 1998;56(2):157-64.
5. Hetlevik I, Holmen J, Kruger O, et al. Implementing clinical guidelines in the treatment of us in general practice. Evaluation of effort, process, and patient outcome related to implementation of a computer-based decision support system. Int J Technol Assess Health Care. 2000;16(1):210-27.
6. Montani S, Bellazzi R, Portinale L, et al. Diabetic patients management exploiting case-based reasoning techniques. Comput Methods Programs Biomed. 2000;62(3):205-18.
7. Ping W, Jin-Gang W, Xiao-Bo S, et al. The research of telemedicine system based on embedded computer. Proceedings of the 27th Annual International Conference of the Engineering in Medicine and Biology Society (IEEE-EMBS '05). Shanghai, China: IEEE; 2006. pp. 114-7.
8. Johansson AM, Lindberg I, Söderberg S. Patients' experiences with specialist care via video consultation in primary healthcare in rural areas. Int J Telemed Appl. 2014;2014:143824.
9. Gani A, Gribok AV, Lu Y, et al. Universal glucose models for predicting subcutaneous glucose concentration in humans. IEEE Trans Inf Technol Biomed. 2010;14(1):157-65.
10. Guariguata L, Whiting D, Weil C, et al. The International Diabetes Federation diabetes atlas methodology for estimating global and national prevalence of diabetes in adults. Diabetes Res Clin Pract 2011;94(3): 322-32.
11. American Diabetes Association. Standards of medical care in diabetes-2012. Diabetes Care. 2012;35(Suppl 1):S11-S63.
12. Wakefield BJ, Holman JE, Ray A, et al. Effectiveness of home telehealth in comorbid diabetes and hypertension: a randomized, controlled trial. Telemed JE Health. 2011;17(4):254-61.
13. Bujnowska-Fedak MM, Puchała E, Steciwko A. The impact of telehome care on health status and quality of life among patients with diabetes in a primary care setting in Poland. Telemed JE Health. 2011;17(3):153-63.
14. Ajay VS, Prabhakaran D. The scope of cell phones in diabetes management in developing country health care settings. J Diabetes Sci Technol. 2011;5(3):778-83.
15. Costa BM, Fitzgerald KJ, Jones KM, et al. Effectiveness of IT-based diabetes management interventions: a review of the literature. BMC Fam Pract. 2009;10:72.
16. European's Information Society. Thematic Portal: Glossary of Terms. Brussels: European Commission; 2012.
17. van den Berg N, Schumann M, Kraft K, et al. Telemedicine and telecare for older patients: A systematic review. Maturitas. 2012;73(2):94-114.
18. Dalton JE. Web-based care for adults with type 2 diabetes. Can J Diet Pract Res. 2008;69(4):185-91.
19. Ahring KK, Ahring JP, Joyce C, et al. Telephone modem access improves diabetes control in those with insulin-requiring diabetes. Diabetes Care. 1992;15(8):971-5.
20. Shultz EK, Bauman A, Hayward M, et al. Improved care of patients with diabetes through telecommunications. Ann N Y Acad Sci. 1992;670:141-5.
21. Billiard A, Rohmer V, Roques M, et al. Telematic transmission of computerized blood glucose profiles for IDDM patients. Diabetes Care. 1991;14(2):130-4.
22. di Biase N, Napoli A, Sabbatini A, et al. Telemedicine in the treatment of diabetic pregnancy. Annali dell Istituto Superiore di Sanita. 1997;33(3):347-51.
23. Frost D, Beischer W. Telemedicine in the management of pregnancy in type 1 diabetic women. Diabetes Care. 2000;23(6):863-4.
24. Marrero DG, Vandagriff JL, Kronz K, et al. Using telecommunication technology to manage children with diabetes: the Computer-Linked Outpatient Clinic (CLOC) Study. Diabetes Educator. 1995;21(4):313-9.
25. Mease A, Whitlock WL, Brown A, et al. Telemedicine improved diabetic management. Mil Med. 2000;165(8):579-84.
26. Biermann E, Dietrich W, Standl E. Telecare of diabetic patients with intensified insulin therapy: a randomized clinical trial. Stud Health Technol Inform. 2000;77:327-32.
27. Chamberlin B. Healthcare Internet of Things: 18 trends to watch in 2016.
28. Kesavadev J, Saboo B, Shankar A, et al. Telemedicine for diabetes care: an Indian perspective—feasibility and efficacy. Indian J Endocrinol Metab. 2015;19(6):764-9.
29. Mayo Clinic (2014). Telehealth: when technology meets health care. [online]. Available from http://www.mayoclinic.org/healthy-lifestyle/consumer-health/in-depth/telehealth/art-20044878. [Accessed September, 2017].
30. Numbers cited in Carrie MacGillivray, "The Internet of Things Is Poised to Change Everything, Says IDC," Business Wire, October 3, 2013 and Charles McLellan, "The Internet of Things and Big Data," ZDNet, March 2, 2015.

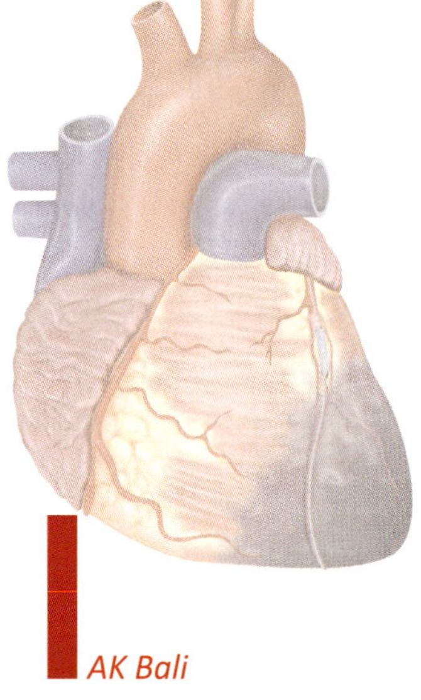

HbA1c: Clinical Relevance in Cardiodiabetes

AK Bali

INTRODUCTION

Diabetes mellitus (DM) is a major public health problem with rapidly increasing prevalence in both developing and developed world. Glycated hemoglobin (HbA1c) is an important marker of long-term glycemic control which reflects the average blood glucose concentration over the course of red blood cell (RBC) lifespan roughly 120 days in normal individual.[1] HbA1c correlates well with risk of long-term diabetes complication. Elevated HbA1c has also found to be independent risk factor for coronary artery disease and stroke in patient with or without diabetes.

Glycated hemoglobin is specific fraction of HbA found in healthy person as well as person with DM. It is formed when "N" terminal valine of beta chain in HbA is modified by addition of sugar moiety, which is nonenzymatic process. The formation of HbA1c is a normal part of physiologic function cycle. However, as the average plasma glucose rises so does the amount of HbA1c. Using the HbA1c as the biomarker for monitoring the level of glucose in diabetic patient was first proposed by Koenig et al. in 1976.[2]

Diabetes is a silent killer. Globally, an estimated 422 million adult were living with diabetes in 2014 compared to 180 million in 1980. The global prevalence (age standardized) of diabetes has nearly doubled since 1980 rising from 4.7% to 8.5% in adult population. Over the past decade diabetes prevalence has risen faster in low-and middle-income countries than in high-income countries. India has approximately 67 million cases of DM (about 8.6%) of total adult population (20–79 years) and continues to grow at alarming rate (2010 estimate 50.8 million).[3]

The American Diabetes Association (ADA) has recommended HbA1c with cut point of more than 6.5% for diagnosing diabetes as an alternative to fasting plasma glucose [fasting blood glucose (FBG) >126 mg/dL] based criteria.[4] Levels of HbA1c are strongly correlated with fasting blood glucose.[5] FBG, 2 hours post-glucose load plasma glucose—oral glucose tolerance test (OGTT) is recommended for diagnosis of diabetes only if HbA1c is not possible due nonavailability of assay, patient factor that precludes its interpretation, and during pregnancy.[5]

POTENTIALS OF GLYCATED HEMOGLOBIN

Glycated hemoglobin is not only useful biomarker of long-term glycemic control but also good predictor of lipid profile, which means that monitoring of glycemic control using HbA1c could have additional benefit of identifying diabetes patient who are at greater risk of cardiovascular complication.[6] In a series of 1,011 type 2 diabetes mellitus (T2DM) patient, there was direct correlation with cholesterol, triglycerides, and low-density lipoprotein and inverse correlation with high-density lipoprotein cholesterol. There was a linear relationship between HbA1c and dyslipidemia, as the level of serum cholesterol and triglycerides was significantly higher and that of high-density lipoprotein cholesterol was significantly lower in patient with worse glycemic control as compared to patient with good glycemic control.[6]

ELEVATED LEVEL OF GLYCATED HEMOGLOBIN: DIAGNOSTIC AND PROGNOSTIC IMPLICATIONS

Elevated level of HbA1c has been identified as a significant risk factor for cardiovascular disease and stroke in subjects who may have diabetes.[7] A community-based population study on 11,092 nondiabetic patients found that elevated HbA1c level was strongly associated with risk of cardiovascular disease and mortality.[8] High levels of HbA1c were associated with an increased risk of recurrence of atrial tachycardia in patients with T2DM and paroxysmal atrial fibrillation undergoing catheter ablation.[9] Even an increase in 1% in HbA1c concentration was associated with about 30% increase in all cause motility and 40% increase in cardiovascular or ischemic heart disease mortality among patients with diabetes. Whereas, lowering HbA1c levels by 0.2% could lower the mortality by 10%.[10] Vagg has suggested that improving glycemic control in patient with T2DM may be more important than treating dyslipidemia for prevention of both microvascular and macrovascular complication.[11] Cick et al.[12] determined the effect of HbA1c on the outcomes of primary percutaneous coronary intervention (PCI) for ST-segment elevation myocardial infarction (STEMI). They observed that in-hospital mortality and major adverse cardiac events were significantly higher in patients with HbA1c more than 6.5% (11%) compared with the group of patients with HbA1c between 5.7% and 6.4% (2.8%) or HbA1c less than 5.6% (0.9%). Out of the total 374 patients, 196 (63.6%) patients without a history of DM had elevated HbA1c more than 5.7%, with 31 (10.1%) of them having HbA1c more than 6.5%.[12] On the basis of 12-month follow-up of 1,433 patients with stable angina who underwent coronary angiography, it was concluded that high level of baseline HbA1c appeared to be an independent predictor for the severity of coronary artery disease and poor outcome in patients with stable coronary artery disease.[13] As the levels of HbA1c increased, patients were more likely to have prior cardiovascular disease and more unfavorable baseline cardiovascular risk profile in a cohort of acute myocardial infarction (AMI) patients.[13] Although the admission glucose levels may represent a marker for increased risk in the acute and subacute setting after AMI, HbA1c being a surrogate for more chronic dysglycemia, is clearly a more useful marker of patients with greater long-term risk of death.[14]

However, in an observational multicenter study of 608 patients with STEMI who underwent primary PCI, the admission level of HbA1c was not found to be an independent prognostic marker for short-term outcome in STEMI patients treated with primary PCI.[15] A prospective cohort of 2,519 nondiabetic patients undergoing elective coronary angiography for suspected stable angina pectoris did not show any association between HbA1c levels and prognosis, questioning an independent role of glycemia in the pathogenesis of atherosclerotic complications in nondiabetic patients.[16] Recently, Wang et al. have shown that HbA1c level is not a significant and independent marker for the severity of angiography (stenosis) in acute coronary syndrome (ACS) patients.[17]

Nondiabetes HbA1c usually falls within the 4.0–5.6% range. The prediabetes usually has the HbA1c levels as 5.7–6.4%, while those with 6.4% or higher HbA1c levels have diabetes.[18,19] Since diabetes is associated with several comorbidities, the recommendations for individuals with diabetes include a healthy lifestyle (diet and exercise) and maintaining the HbA1c levels below 7.0%. Diabetes-related complications are directly proportional to the levels of HbA1c—increase in the HbA1c levels also increase the risk of such complications.

CAVEATS OF GLYCATED HEMOGLOBIN

Using HbA1c as marker for diagnosing and prognosticating in diabetes has some caveats also. For example in anemic patients or those with shorter RBC lifespan [glucose-6-phosphate dehydrogenase (G6PD) deficiency, sickle cell disease, etc.], HbA1c levels may be low indicating false good results.[20] The excessive use of vitamin supplements and increase level of cholesterol, liver, and kidney disease can also present abnormally high levels of HbA1c.[21,22]

CONCLUSION

Glycated hemoglobin evaluation in cardiodiabetes has tremendous diagnostic and prognostic implications and it helps in optimizing therapeutic intervention to reduce cardiodiabetes inflicted morbidity and mortality.

REFERENCES

1. Khan MI, Weinstock RS. Carbohydrates. In: McPherson RA, Pincus MR (Eds). Henry's Clinical Diagnosis and Management by Laboratory Methods, 22nd edition. Philadelphia: Saunders Elsevier; 2011. pp. 210-25.
2. Koenig RJ, Peterson CM, Jones KL, et al. Correlation of glucose regulation and hemoglobin A1c in diabetes mellitus. N Engl J Med. 1976;295(8):417-20.
3. International Diabetes Federation. (2015). IDF 2015 Guidelines. [online] Available from: www.idf.org. [Accessed September, 2015].
4. International Expert Committee. International Expert Committee report on the role of the HbA1c assay in the diagnosis of diabetes. Diabetes care. 2019;32(7):1327-34.
5. Herman WH, Fajans SS. Hemoglobin A1c for diagnosis of diabetes: practical considerations. Pol Arch Med Wewn. 2010;120(1-2):37-40.
6. Khan HA, Sobki SH, Khan SA. Association between glycaemic control and serum lipids profile in type 2 diabetic patients: HbA1c predicts dyslipidemia. Clin Exp Med. 2007;7(1):24-9.

7. Martin-Timon I, Sevillano-Collantes C, segura-Galindo A, et al. Type 2 diabetes and cardiovascular disease: Have all risk factors the same strength? World J diabetes. 2014;5(4):444-70.
8. Selvin E, Steffes MW, Zhu H, et al. Glycated hemoglobin, diabetes, and cardiovascular risk in nondiabetic adults. N Engl J Med. 2010;362(9):800-11.
9. Lu ZH, Liu N, Bai R, et al. HbA1c levels as predictors of ablation outcome in type 2 diabetes mellitus and paroxysmal atrial fibrillation. Herz. 2015;40(Suppl 2):130-6.
10. Khaw KT, Wareham N, Luben R, et al. Glycated haemoglobin, diabetes, and mortality in men in Norfolk cohort of European Prospective Investigation of Cancer and Nutrition (EPIC-Norfolk). BMJ. 2001;322(7277):15-8.
11. Vagg AA. Glycemic control and prevention of microvascular and macrovascular disease in the Steno 2 study. Endocr Pract. 2006;12(Suppl 1):89-92.
12. Cicek G, Uyarel H, Ergelen M, et al. Hemoglobin A1c as a prognostic marker in patients undergoing primary angioplasty for acute myocardial infarction. Coron Artery Dis. 2011;22(3):131-7.
13. Hong LF, Li XL, Guo YL, et al. Glycosylated hemoglobin A1C as a marker predicting the severity of coronary artery disease and early outcome in patients with stable angina. Lipids Health Dis. 2014;13:89.
14. Timmer JR, Hoekstra M, Nijsten MW, et al. Prognostic value of admission glycosylated hemoglobin and glucose in nondiabetic patients with ST-segment elevation myocardial infarction treated with percutaneous coronary intervention. Circulation. 2011;124(6):704-11.
15. Tian L, Zhu J, Liu L, et al. Hemoglobin A1C and short-term outcomes in patients with acute myocardial infarction undergoing primary angioplasty: an observational multicenter study. Coron Artery Dis. 2013;24(1):16-22.
16. Rebnord EW, Pedersen ER, Strand E, et al. Glycated hemoglobin and long term prognosis in patients with suspected stable angina pectoris without diabetes mellitus: a prospective cohort study. Atherosclerosis. 2015;240(1):115-20.
17. Wang X, Han Z, Hao G, et al. Hemoglobin A1c level is not related to the severity of atherosclerosis in patients with acute coronary syndrome. Dis markers. 2015;2015:192108.
18. American Diabetes Association. Standards of medical care in diabetes-2014. Diabetes Care. 2014;37(Suppl 1):S14-80.
19. American Diabetes Association. Diagnosis and classification of diabetes mellitus. Diabetes Care. 2011;34:S62-9.
20. Forbes JM, Soldatos G, Thomas MC. Below the radar: advanced glycation end products that detour "around the side". Is HbA1C not an accurate enough predictor of long term progression and glycaemic control in diabetes? Clin Biochem Rev. 2005;26(4):123-34.
21. Luk AO, Ma RC, Lau ES, et al. Risk association of HbA1c variability with chronic kidney disease and cardiovascular disease in type 2 diabetes: prospective analysis of the Hong Kong Diabetes Registry. Diabetes Metab Res Rev. 2013;29(5):384-90.
22. Xu R, Zhang S, Tao A, et al. Influence of vitamin E supplementation on glycaemic control: a meta-analysis of randomized controlled trials. PLoS One. 2014;9(4):e95008.

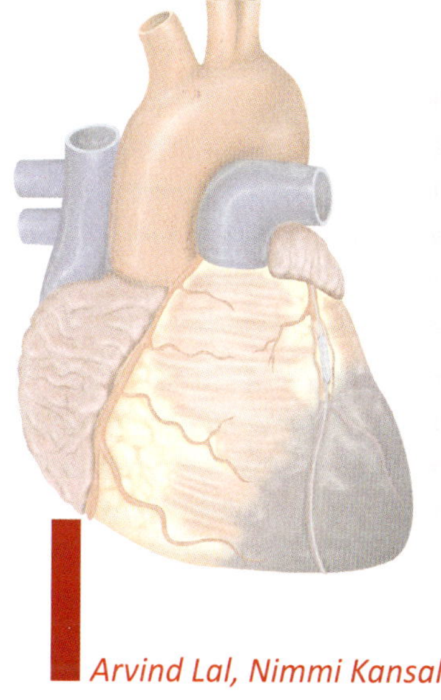

Emerging Role of Cardiac Troponin in Cardiodiabetes

Arvind Lal, Nimmi Kansal

INTRODUCTION

Atherosclerotic cardiovascular disease (ASCVD), including acute coronary syndrome (ACS), myocardial infarction (MI),[1] angina, arterial revascularization, stroke, transient ischemic attack, or peripheral arterial disease, is the leading cause of mortality for individuals with type 2 diabetes (T2D) and is the largest contributor to the economic costs of diabetes. Main ASCVD risk factors include hypertension, dyslipidemia, smoking, a family history of premature coronary disease, and albuminuria. Numerous studies have confirmed the benefits of controlling ASCVD risk factors in patients of T2D. Furthermore, biomarkers have substantial utility in modern cardiovascular (CV) diagnosis, prognosis, and therapy. Cardiac troponin (cTn) concentration is the preferred marker of myocardial necrosis. Elevated concentrations of cTn have a strong association with an adverse prognosis in patients with ACS and are used to identify patients who are likely to benefit from an early invasive management strategy.[2] High-sensitivity troponin (hsTn) assays that allow the measurement of very low cTn levels in patients with stable heart disease are now available for clinical and research use. These low, previously undetectable troponin concentrations have shown strong associations with MI, stroke, and death in a variety of primary and secondary prevention populations, including in patients with stable ischemic heart disease. Although, troponins I and T respond similarly for ACS and acute decompensated heart failure (HF), elevated shTn assays in the setting of T2D without acute cardiac disease have prognostic significance and may justify more intensive risk reduction. Many clinical studies have demonstrated that troponin elevation in patients with T2D and stable ischemic heart disease can be useful in identifying a higher risk cohort.

HIGH-SENSITIVITY TROPONIN IN SCREENING ASCVD RISK IN TYPE 2 DIABETES

Persons with prediabetes and diabetes are at high risk for CV events. However, the relationships of prediabetes and diabetes to development of subclinical myocardial damage are unclear. In the general population, as shown in the Dallas Heart Study, elevated levels of cardiac troponin T (cTnT) were associated with greater rates of structural heart disease, including left ventricular hypertrophy and systolic dysfunction, as well as all-cause mortality within a median follow-up of 6.4 years.[3-9] The Women's Health Study[7] investigated whether high-sensitivity cardiac troponin T (hs-cTnT) levels are associated with adverse CV outcomes in individuals without CVD. In the study, hs-cTnT was detectable (≥0.003 μg/L) in 45.5% of diabetic women and 30.3% of nondiabetic women ($P < 0.0001$). In models adjusted for traditional risk factors and hemoglobin A1c, detectable hs-cTnT was associated with subsequent CVD (MI, stroke, and CV death) in diabetic women [adjusted hazard ratio, 1.79; 95% confidence interval (CI), 1.04–3.07, $P = 0.036$] but not nondiabetic women (adjusted hazard ratio, 1.13; 95% CI, 0.82–1.55; $P = 0.46$). Elevated troponin appears predictive of coronary artery disease (CAD) events, specifically for persons with diabetes. Atherosclerosis Risk in Communities (ARIC) study[10] measured hs-cTnT at two time points, 6 years apart, in 9,331 participants with no diabetes, prediabetes, or diabetes but without CVD. Cumulative probabilities of elevated hs-cTnT at 6 years among persons with no diabetes, prediabetes, and diabetes were 3.7%, 6.4%, and 10.8%, respectively. Compared to normoglycemic persons, the adjusted relative risks for incident elevated hs-cTnT were 1.38 (95% CI 1.07–1.77) for prediabetes and 2.46 (95% CI 1.77–3.42) for diabetes. Persons with diabetes and incident elevations in hs-cTnT were at a substantially higher risk of HF (HR 6.37, 95% CI 4.27–9.51), death (HR 4.36, 95% CI 3.14–6.07), and coronary heart disease (HR 3.84, 95% CI 2.52–5.84) compared to persons without diabetes and no incident elevation in hs-cTnT. Prediabetes and diabetes were independently associated with development of subclinical myocardial damage, as assessed by hs-cTnT, and those persons with evidence of subclinical damage were at highest risk for clinical events.

Thus, hsTn might play a role in screening for structural and coronary heart disease, potentially prompting further evaluation and more aggressive primary prevention measures. However, there are several obstacles to overcome before such a clinical strategy could be used. Biological variability will have to be further explored and quantified to establish reasonable threshold change values.

PROGNOSTIC INFORMATION IN STABLE ISCHEMIC HEART DISEASE

The Bypass Angioplasty Revascularization Investigation 2 Diabetes (BARI 2D) trial demonstrated that hs-cTnT level in 2,285 patients with T2D and stable ischemic disease was predictive of higher CV morbidity and mortality.[11] Of the 2,285 patients, 2,277 (99.6%) had detectable (≥3 ng/L) hs-cTnT concentrations and 897 (39.3%) had abnormal hs-cTnT concentrations at baseline. The 5-year rate of the composite end point was 27.1% among the patients who had abnormal hs-cTnT concentrations at baseline, as compared with 12.9% among those who had normal baseline hs-cTnT concentrations.

The Examination of Cardiovascular Outcomes with Alogliptin versus Standard of Care (EXAMINE) trial described the relationship between changes in high-sensitivity cardiac troponin I (hs-cTnI) and CV outcomes. In this analysis of the EXAMINE trial found that nearly all patients had a measurable concentration of hs-cTnI and that 1 out of 6 patients with T2DM with established ischemic heart disease (1–3 months after ACS) had hs-cTnI levels that were above the 99th percentile upper reference limit (URL). Evaluating serial concentrations of hs-cTnI overtime in this cohort with T2DM and established atherosclerosis, we also found that almost 1 in 4 stable patients had at least a 25% increase in hs-cTnI over a 6-month period. In addition, the majority of patients had stable, rather than declining values, including among those patients with a markedly elevated baseline concentration, pointing to the importance of chronic underlying structural heart disease rather than acute myocardial injury as a determinant of circulating hsTn in this population. Notably, the small cohort of patients with undetectable hs-cTnI was at extremely low risk of future CV events despite their history of T2DM and ischemic heart disease. In contrast, patients with hs-cTnI above the 99th percentile URL either at baseline or 6 months were at considerably higher risk of major established CV events. Moreover, those with intermediate increases in hs-cTnI concentration (2–6 ng/L) were at moderately higher risk of adverse CV events. These findings add to evidence supporting a potential role for hs-cTnI in the risk stratification of patients with T2DM, including those with established atherosclerosis. Serial assessments of hs-cTnI provided additional insight regarding the relationship of changes in hs-cTnI overtime with prognosis.

HIGH-SENSITIVITY TROPONIN IN TYPE 2 DIABETES AND THERAPEUTIC IMPLICATION

Unfortunately, it is common clinical practice to regard low levels of elevated troponin as inconsequential when observed outside of the context of an ACS event. This so called "troponin leak" minimizes mildly elevated troponin values that may be found incidentally in patients with left ventricular hypertrophy, hypertensive emergency, uncontrolled atrial fibrillation, severe sepsis, or acute decompensated HF. Similarly, in the outpatient setting, clinicians may consider mildly elevated circulating troponin as not being reflective of acute plaque rupture and therefore less clinically significant. On the contrary, the recent EXAMINE analysis and the preponderance of data implicate hsTn as a prognostic marker for ASCVD outcomes in an already high-risk population, specifically those with T2D.[12] Thus, clinicians should not succumb to the common practice of discounting mild troponin elevations as merely incidental, as these patients continue to be a population that deserves special attention in terms of implementing intensive medical therapy. Along with hyperglycemia and other conventional risk factors, elevated troponin levels may significantly elevate patient risk to the level of CAD equivalent. Therefore, the use of hs-cTnI assays may greatly assist CV specialists and other clinicians with unveiling patients with T2D who are at "extreme risk" for cardiac events, a new category identified in 2017 by the Association of Clinical Endocrinologists and American College of Endocrinology (AACE) on the comprehensive T2D management algorithm.[13]

ADDITIONAL CLINICAL IMPLICATIONS

The most recent universal definition of MI emphasizes that providers must consider the clinical context of patients in whom biomarkers are measured and found to be elevated. These findings highlight the need to consider the clinical context and to determine whether there is an acutely rising or falling pattern of cTn concentration when ruling in or ruling out the diagnosis of a MI. The measurement of these biomarkers in patients who have diabetes or stable ischemic heart disease and who lack clinical evidence of acute myocardial ischemia increases the possibility of identifying patients with chronic myocardial injury without acute infarction.

CONCLUSION

The ability of hsTn to identify patients at higher risk for a variety of CV events, including CV death, has important prognostic and potential treatment implications. The majority of prevention strategies utilized in clinical practice identify patients at increased risk using only the demographics, lipid levels, and past medical history. Serial assessment of hsTn may enhance risk stratification and reveal a substantial proportion of patients at high risk of recurrent major CV events. Presence of elevated hsTn in diabetes may warrant more aggressive or additional secondary prevention strategies. It is possible that further intensification of secondary prevention strategies may improve outcomes in patients with elevated hsTn.

REFERENCES

1. Thygesen K, Alpert JS, Jaffe AS, et al. Third universal definition of myocardial infarction. J Am Coll Cardiol. 2012;60(16):1581-98.
2. Morrow DA, Cannon CP, Rifai N, et al. Ability of minor elevations of troponins I and T to predict benefit from an early invasive strategy in patients with unstable angina and non-ST elevation myocardial infarction: results from a randomized trial. JAMA. 2001;286(19):2405-12.
3. Amsterdam EA, Wenger NK, Brindis RG, et al. 2014 AHA/ACC guideline for the management of patients with non-ST elevation acute coronary syndromes: a report of the American College of Cardiology/American Heart Association Task Force on Practice Guidelines. J Am Coll Cardiol. 2014;64(24):e139-228.
4. Bhatt DL, Roe MT, Peterson ED, et al. Utilization of early invasive management strategies for high-risk patients with non-ST segment elevation acute coronary syndromes: results from the CRUSADE Quality Improvement Initiative. JAMA. 2004;292(17):2096-104.
5. Omland T, de Lemos JA, Sabatine MS, et al. A sensitive cardiac troponin T assay in stable coronary artery disease. N Engl J Med. 2009;361(26):2538-47.
6. Omland T, Pfeffer MA, Solomon SD, et al. Prognostic value of cardiac troponin I measured with a highly sensitive assay in patients with stable coronary artery disease. J Am Coll Cardiol. 2013;61(12):1240-9.
7. Everett BM, Cook NR, Magnone MC, et al. Sensitive cardiac troponin T assay and the risk of incident cardiovascular disease in women with and without diabetes mellitus: the Women's Health Study. Circulation. 2011;123(24):2811-8.
8. Ferdinand KC, Igari M. Defining cardiovascular risk in diabetes: the emerging role of troponin assays. J Lab Precis Med. 2017;2:37.
9. Wallace TW, Abdullah SM, Drazner MH, et al. Prevalence and determinants of troponin T elevation in the general population. Circulation. 2006;113(16):1958-65.
10. Elizabeth S, Mariana L, Yuan C, et al. Pre-diabetes and incidence of subclinical myocardial damage. Circulation. 2014;130(16):1374-82.
11. Everett BM, Brooks MM, Vlachos HE, et al. Troponin and Cardiac Events in Stable Ischemic Heart Disease and Diabetes. N Engl J Med. 2015;373(7):610-20.
12. Cavender MA, White WB, Jarolim P, et al. Serial Measurement of High Sensitivity Troponin I and Cardiovascular Outcomes in Patients with Type 2 Diabetes Mellitus in the EXAMINE Trial (Examination of Cardiovascular Outcomes With Alogliptin Versus Standard of Care). Circulation. 2017;135(20):1911-21.
13. Garber AJ, Abrahamson MJ, Barzilay JI, et al. Consensus Statement by the American Association of Clinical Endocrinologists and American College of Endocrinology on the Comprehensive Type 2 Diabetes Management Algorithm-2017 Executive Summary. Endocr Pract. 2017;23(2):207-38.

SECTION 3

Management Strategies

CHAPTER 53

Role of Yoga in Cardiodiabetes

SC Manchanda, Kushal Madan

INTRODUCTION

Type 2 diabetes mellitus (T2DM) has become a global health problem and its incidence is rapidly increasing, especially in developing countries.[1,2] T2DM is the major risk factor for cardiovascular diseases (CVDs) increasing the risk by 2–3 folds. Heart disease has always been an immediate cause of mortality and morbidity in patients with T2DM.[3] The health, social, and economic consequences of T2DM are substantial. The current global T2DM epidemic is considered to be fueled largely by lifestyle factors like physical inactivity, overnutrition, obesity, chronic stress, and smoking. There has been tremendous progress in understanding the causes, prevention, and therapeutic options available for its treatment. However, these advances are not without limitations and the implementation of these programs remains challenging, especially in the developing countries. Moreover, lifestyle modification is a complex phenomenon in which lifestyle choices including mind-body interaction and control of stress seems to be important. Stress may contribute significantly to the causation of T2DM and heart disease through the involvement of hypothalamic pituitary axis and sympathetic nervous system (Flow chart 1).[4] Hence, there is a need for newer strategies involving mind-body techniques to control this epidemic. Yoga appears to be one such cost-effective strategy to prevent T2DM.

WHAT IS YOGA?

Yoga is an ancient Indian mind-body technique which is becoming popular all over the globe because of its health benefits. Even the United Nations has also recently realized its importance and declared *21st June as International Day of Yoga*. The word *yoga* comes from a Sanskrit word "Yug" meaning to join the lower human nature to the higher.[5] Ancient texts have described several types of yoga which include:

1. *Bhakti Yoga* emphasizes devotion and spirituality
2. *Gnana Yoga* emphasizes wisdom
3. *Karma Yoga* emphasizes selfless services and offerings
4. *Raj Yoga* emphasizes mastery of mind by focused concentration
5. *Dhyana Yoga* emphasizes meditation
6. *Mantra Yoga* emphasizes repetition of sacred recitation like transcendental meditation
7. *Hatha Yoga* emphasizes psychosocial energies of body.

Yoga is an integrated holistic lifestyle which aims at harmonious development of body, mind, and covers all aspects of human life, which lead to physical, mental, emotional wellbeing culminating into positive thinking, happiness, and peace. Yoga is a universal practical discipline irrespective of caste, creed, sex, nationality, culture, or race. *Hatha yoga* is most commonly practiced and its core components include stretching exercises and physical postures *(Asanas)*, breath control *(Pranayama)*, and concentration and thinking techniques *(Meditation)*. Yoga has been shown to detoxify the body, improve chronic fatigue, and enhance endurance and immune functions.[6] Yoga has also been reported to be beneficial in many chronic lifestyle-related diseases like anxiety, depression, stress, back pain, asthma, acid peptic disease, irritable bowel syndrome, ulcerative colitis, migraine, CVDs, and

Flow chart 1: Possible mechanism of stress causing cardiodiabetes

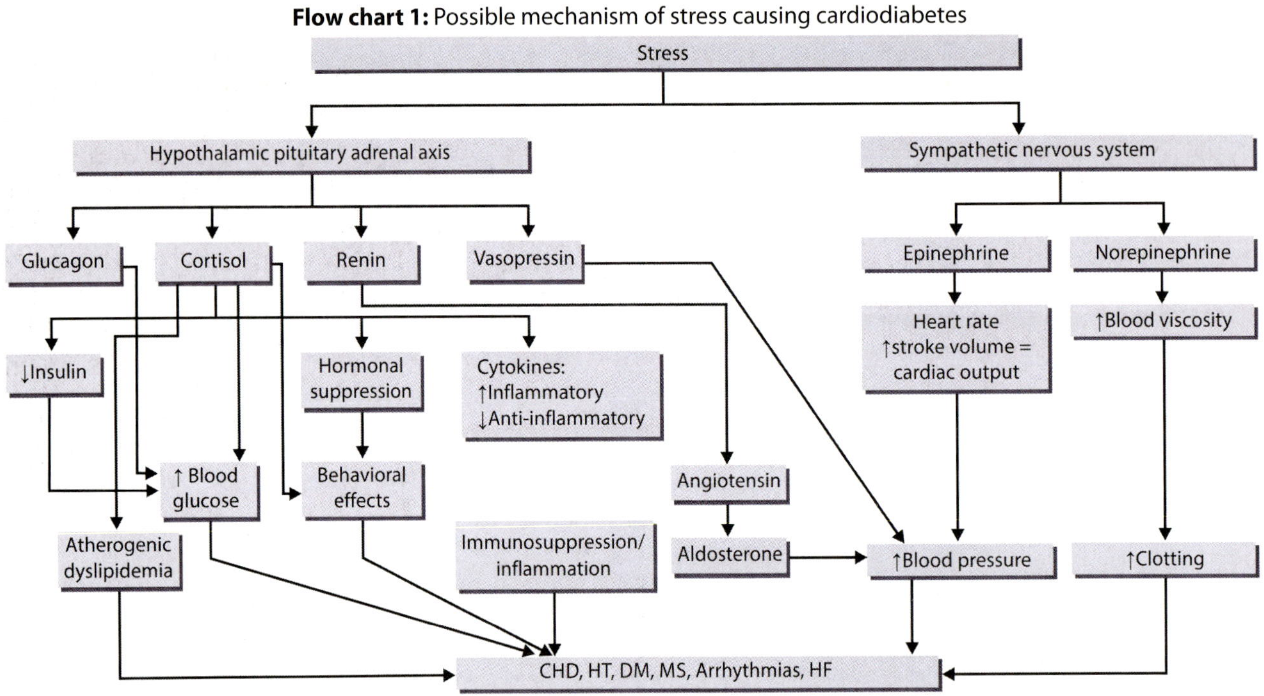

Abbreviations: CHD, coronary heart disease; HT, hypertension; DM, diabetes mellitus; MS, multiple sclerosis; HF, heart failure

diabetes mellitus.[6-13] This chapter will briefly review the scientific evidence regarding the role of yoga in cardiodiabetes.

ROLE OF YOGA

Role of Yoga in Diabetes Mellitus

Several randomized and nonrandomized trials have been reported regarding the role of yoga in T2DM. Table 1 summarizes the results of 14 randomized control trials (RCTs) of yoga in T2DM.[14-27] The number of patients in these studies has varied from 21 to 277 and the yoga intervention duration has varied from 45 days to 9 months. The type and frequency of yoga practices also varied in these studies. Apart from measurement of measures of glucose tolerance and insulin resistance, some studies also evaluated lipid profile, blood pressure, and body weight and composition. It is apparent that majority of these studies have reported beneficial changes in subjects following yogic practices. Therefore, it appears that yoga may have significant beneficial effects on multiple parameters in T2DM including glycemic control, insulin resistance, lipid profiles, body weight and composition, and probable blood pressure.

However, there are several limitations of the reported studies like methodological problems, small numbers, short follow-up, and lack of proper randomization. The compliance of yoga practices have also not been addressed properly. Hence, long-term multicentral well-randomized studies utilizing uniform yoga methodology are needed.

Role of Yoga in Metabolic Syndrome

Metabolic syndrome is a combination of several risk factors like increased waist circumference, increased triglycerides, increased low-density lipoprotein (LDL), decreased high-density lipoprotein (HDL), increased blood pressure, and increased fasting glucose. Metabolic syndrome is widely prevalent throughout the world, especially in the developing countries. It is an important risk factor for T2DM and CVD. Several RCTs have shown that yoga intervention could be useful in controlling metabolic syndrome as well as obesity (Tables 2 and 3).[28-39] Sample size of these studies has varied from 26 to 180 and different types of yoga techniques have been utilized and the follow-up has varied from 8 weeks to 60 weeks (Table 2). These studies demonstrate that systolic blood pressure was significantly improved, as compared to control group. Fasting glucose, triglycerides, and HDL have also been demonstrated to be significantly improved. The waist circumference and body mass index (BMI) have been shown to be decreased in some studies. One study demonstrated a decrease in the early atherosclerosis as assessed by carotid intima media thickness (cIMT) after

TABLE 1: Effect of yoga on diabetes mellitus: Summary of randomized control trials

Author and Year	No. of subjects enrolled	Intervention	Duration	Results
Monro et al., 1992	21	Yoga	12 weeks	Significant decrease in FBG and HbA1c
Khare et al., 1999	80	Yoga	3 months	Significant decrease in blood sugar, TC, and weight
Agrawal et al., 2003	200	Yoga	3 months	Significant decrease in FBG and HbA1c, BMI, TC, LDL,VLDL, SBP, and DBP
Agte et al., 2004	87	Sudarshan kriya, meditation, and lifestyle	4 months	Significant decrease in FBG, PPG, TC, and MDA
Singh et al., 2008	60	Yoga	45 days	Significant decrease in FBG, PPG, insulin, weight, and lipids
Skoro Kondza et al., 2009	59	Yoga	12 weeks	No significant change
Amita et al., 2009	41	Yoga Nidra	90 days	Significant decrease in FBG and PPBG
Pardasany et al., 2010	45	Hatha Yoga and yang-style Tai chi	12 weeks	Significant decrease in FBG, PPBG, HbA1c, TC, and LDL
Hegde et al., 2011	123	Yoga	3 months	Significant decrease in FBG, PPBG, HbA1c, BMI, and MDA
Balalji et al., 2011	44	Yoga	3 months	Significant decrease in FBG, HbA1C, TG, LDL, weight, and BMI
Nagarathna et al., 2012	277	Yoga	9 months	Significant decrease in medicines, FBG, PPBG, HbA1c, TG, TC, LDL, and VLDL
Vaishali et al., 2012	60	Yoga	12 weeks	Significant decrease in FBG, HbA1c, TC, TG, and LDL
Shantakumari et al., 2013	100	Yoga	3 months	Significant decrease in FBG, TG, TC, LDL, SBP, DBP, and weight
Jyotsna et al., 2014	120	Sudarshan kriya	6 months	Significant decrease in PPBG

Abbreviations: FBG, fasting blood glucose; HbA1c, glycated hemoglobin; TC, total cholesterol; BMI, body mass index; LDL, low-density lipoprotein; VLDL, very low-density lipoprotein; SBP, systolic blood pressure; DBP, diastolic blood pressure; PPG, postprandial plasma glucose; MDA, malondialdehyde; PPBG, postprandial blood glucose; TG, triglyceride.

TABLE 2: Effect of yoga on metabolic syndrome: Summary of randomized control trials

Author and Year	No. of subjects enrolled	Intervention	Duration	Results
Cohen et al., 2008	N = 26	Yoga	10 weeks	↓ systolic BP
Corey et al., 2014	N = 171	Restorative yoga + handouts	60 weeks	↓ salivary cortisol
Kanaya et al., 2014	N =180	Yoga	48 weeks	↓ FBG
Kim et al., 2013	N = 41	*Hatha yoga*	12 weeks	↓ SBP
Manchanda et al., 2013	N =100	Yoga	12 months	↓ early athero-sclerosis, BP, lipids, and blood sugar

Abbreviations: BP, blood pressure; FBG, fasting blood glucose; SBP, systolic blood pressure

TABLE 3: Effect of yoga in obesity: Summary of randomized control trials

Author and Year	No. of subjects enrolled	Inter-vention	Duration	Results
Yang et al., 2011	N = 23	Yoga	3 months	↓ weight
Telles et al., 2014	N = 68	Yoga	15 days	↓ BMI ↓ Body fat ↓ Waist circumference
Schmidt et al., 1997	N = 106	Yoga	3 months	↓ weight ↓ BMI
Murugesan et al., 2000	N = 33	Yoga	11 weeks	↓ weight
McCaffrey et al., 2005	N = 61	Yoga	8 weeks	↓ BMI
Manchanda et al., 2000	N = 42	Yoga	1 year	↓ weight
Mahajan et al., 1999	N = 93	Yoga	14 weeks	↓ weight

Abbreviation: BMI, body mass index

TABLE 4: Effect of yoga on hypertension recent review and meta-analysis

Author and year	*Type of study*	*No. of subjects enrolled*	*Intervention*	*Duration*	*Results*
Posadzki et al., 2014	Review of 17 RCT		Yoga		11 RCT—reduction in SBP
					8 RCT—reduction in DBP
					5 RCT—no effect on SBP
					8 RCT—no effect on DBP
Cramer et al., 2014	Review and meta-analysis of 7 RCT	452	Yoga		Low-quality evidence that yoga may be an adjunct in management of HTN
Tyagi et al., 2014	Review of 39 cohort, 30 non RCT, 48 RCT, 3 case report	6,693	Yoga	1 week to 4 years	BP reduced in both normotensive and hypertensive subjects
Wang et al., 2013	Review of 6 RCT	386	Yoga	Variable	Lower DBP and SBP
Hagins et al., 2013	Review of 17 studies		Yoga		Significant fall in SBP and DBP
Okonta et al., 2012	Review of 10 trials		Yoga		Significant fall in BP and glucose
Anderson et al., 2008	Meta-analysis of 7 trials		Transcendental meditation		Significant decrease in SBP and DBP

Abbreviations: RCT, randomized control trial; SBP, systolic blood pressure; DBP, diastolic blood pressure; HTN, hypertension.

1 year practice of yoga.[32] Insulin resistance has also been shown to be decreased in some studies. However, these studies also have methodological problems and short follow-up.

Role of Yoga in Heart Disease

Several studies have demonstrated beneficial effects of yoga in primary and secondary prevention of CVD.[6-13] The risk factors for coronary heart disease like hypertension, diabetes mellitus, obesity, dyslipidemia, mental stress, and smoking have been shown to be benefitted by regular practice of yoga. A large number of control randomized trials and meta-analysis are available regarding the role of yoga in hypertension (Table 4).[40-47] These show a modest decrease of both systolic and diastolic blood pressure. Recently, a scientific statement of American Heart Association has concluded that meditation shows a modest effect in reducing blood pressure [Class IIb, level of evidence B (LOE B)], and hence suggested that it is reasonable for all individuals with blood pressure levels more than 120/80 mm Hg to consider alternative approaches like mediation as adjunct methods to lower the blood pressure when clinically appropriate. Yoga has also been demonstrated to have an anti-inflammatory and antioxidative effect.[48-54] Yoga has also been shown to regress early and advanced atherosclerosis.[32,38,55-58] One study has demonstrated a significant decrease in mortality and morbidity at 5 years by regular practice of meditation as compared to control.[59] Yoga has also been found to be useful in cardiac rehabilitation.[60,61] A few studies also show an improvement in cardiac arrhythmias and heart failure.[62-67] However, several limitations remain in these studies like small sample size, inconsistencies in baseline, nonrandomization and nonuniform methodologies. Hence, large multicenter trials are needed to confirm these findings. However, as yoga is a cost-effective simple technique without any side effects and hence could be recommended for primary and secondary prevention of CVD.

POSSIBLE MECHANISM

Precise mechanism linking yoga and cardiodiabetes is not entirely clear. However, as mental stress has been implicated in the causation of insulin resistance, hypertension, coronary heart diseases, and mortality; yoga by reducing stress may be helpful. There is strong evidence that yoga reduces allostatic load and stress response system so that there is optimal homeostasis.[68] It has been demonstrated that yoga affects the autonomic nervous system with increase in parasympathetic and decrease in sympathetic and under activity of the gamma-aminobutyric acid (GABA) system which is the primary inhibitor of neurotransmitter system. Increased parasympathetic activation results in positive changes and cardiovagal function and associated neuroendocrine, hemodynamic and inflammatory profiles and in related downstream metabolic parameters.

Flow chart 2: Psychophysiology of yoga in cardiodiabetes: Possible mechanisms

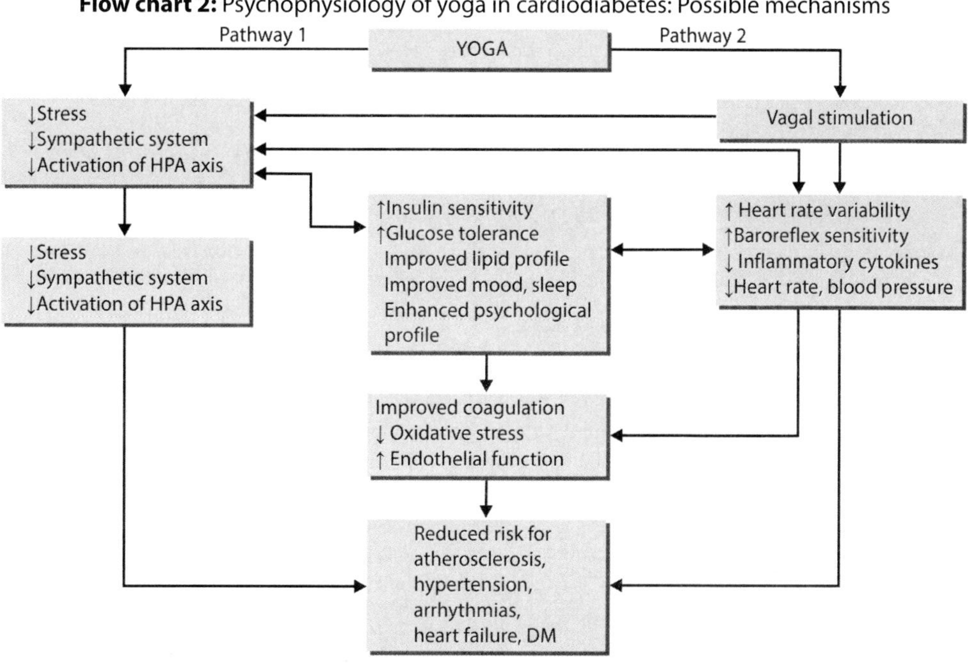

Abbreviations: HPA, hypothalamic pituitary adrenal axis; DM, diabetes mellitus.

(***Source:*** Adapted from Innes KE, Bourguignon C, Taylor AG. Risk indices associated with the insulin resistance syndrome, cardiovascular disease, and possible protection with yoga: a systematic review. J Am Board Fam Pract. 2005;18(6):491-519.

Another mechanism has been postulated which suggests that yoga may reduce the risk of cardiodiabetes through two interconnected pathways—decrease in activity of sympathoadrenal system and hypothalamus pituitary adrenal axis (Flow chart 2).[4] This results in significant reduction in heart and respiratory rate, catecholamines, cortisol and rennin angiotensin levels as well as significant reduction in heart rate variability and baroreflex sensitivity. The alterations in neurohumoral activity also have protective effect against diabetes, metabolic syndrome, coronary heart disease, hypertension, and cardiac arrhythmias. Yoga has also been demonstrated to improve depression, anxiety, and mood, which increase the risk of ischemic heart disease and diabetes. Behavior changes like physical inactivity, alcohol, smoking, and poor diet are also present in many depressed patients. Correction of these behavioral changes by yoga may also play a protective role.[69-72]

CONCLUSION

To conclude yoga, a mind-body technique appears to be promising in the management of cardiodiabetes either alone or in combination with drugs. Several randomized controlled trials suggest that yoga practices significantly reduce blood sugar, lipids, and insulin resistance in diabetic patients. A few studies also have demonstrated an improvement in subjects with metabolic syndrome like decrease in obesity, blood pressure, insulin resistance, and blood sugar. There is extensive literature to show that yoga is extremely beneficial for primary and secondary prevention of coronary heart disease and may even regress atherosclerosis. However, there are several limitations of the reported studies like small sample size, inconsistencies in baseline, nonuniform methodologies, and short follow-up. Therefore, large randomized multicenter trials with long-term follow-up are needed to define the exact role of yoga in cardiodiabetes. However, as yoga is a cost-effective simple technique without any side effects and hence could be recommended for management of cardiodiabetes where it can play a primary or complementary role in this regard.

REFERENCES

1. Danaei G, Finucane MM, Lu Y, et al. National, regional, and global trends in fasting plasma glucose and diabetes prevalence since 1980: systematic analysis of health examination surveys and epidemiological studies with 370 country-years and 2·7 million participants. Lancet. 2011;378(9785):31-40.
2. Chen L, Magliano DJ, Zimmet PZ. The worldwide epidemiology of type 2 diabetes mellitus--present and future perspectives. Nat Rev Endocrinol. 2011;8(4):228-36.
3. Joseph JJ, Golden SH. Type 2 diabetes and cardiovascular disease: what next? Curr Opin Endocrinol Diabetes Obes. 2014;21(2):109-20.
4. Innes KE, Bourguignon C, Taylor AG. Risk indices associated with the insulin resistance syndrome, cardiovascular disease, and possible protection with yoga: a systematic review. J Am Board Fam Pract. 2005;18(6):491-519.

5. Ananda S. The complete book of yoga: harmony of body and mind, 1st edition. New Delhi: Orient Longman; 2001.
6. Raub JA. Psychophysiologic effects of hatha yoga on musculoskeletal and cardiopulmonary function: a literature review. J Altern Complement Med. 2002;8(6):797-812.
7. Ospina MB, Bond K, Karkhaneh M, et al. Meditation practices for health: state of the research. Evid Rep Technol Assess (Full Rep). 2007;155:1-263.
8. Büssing A, Michalsen A, Khalsa SB, et al. Effects of yoga on mental and physical health: a short summary of reviews. Evid Based Complement Alternat Med. 2012;2012:165410.
9. Taneja DK. Yoga and health. Indian J Community Med. 2014;39(2):68-72.
10. Manchanda SC, Madan K. Yoga and meditation in cardiovascular disease. Clin Res Cardiol. 2014;103(9):675-80.
11. Jayasinghe SR. Yoga in cardiac health (a review). Eur J Cardiovasc Prev Rehabil. 2004;11(5):369-75.
12. Manchanda SC. Yoga--a promising technique to control cardiovascular disease. Indian Heart J. 2014;66(5):487-9.
13. Chu P, Gotink RA, Yeh GY, et al. The effectiveness of yoga in modifying risk factors for cardiovascular disease and metabolic syndrome: a systematic review and meta-analysis of randomized controlled trials. Eur J Prev Cardiol. 2016;23(3):291-307.
14. Monro R, Power J, Coumar A, et al. Yoga therapy for NIDDM: a controlled trial. Complemnt Med Res. 1992;6(2):66-8.
15. Khare K, Jain D. Effect of yoga on plasma glucose and serum fructosamine level in NIDDM. Yoga Mimamsa. 1999;33:1-9.
16. Agrawal R, Aradhana R, Hussain S, et al. Influence of yogic treatment on quality of life outcomes, glycemic control and risk factors in diabetes mellitus. Int J Diab Develop Count. 2003;23:130-4.
17. Agte VV, Tarwadi K. Sudarshan Kriya yoga for treating type 2 diabetes: a preliminary study. Alter Complement Thera. 2004;10(4):220-2.
18. Singh S, Kyizom T, Singh KP, et al. Influence of pranayamas and yoga-asanas on serum insulin, blood glucose and lipid profile in type 2 diabetes. Indian J Clin Biochem. 2008;23(4):365-8.
19. Skoro-Kondza L, Tai SS, Gadelrab R, et al. Community-based yoga classes for type 2 diabetes: an exploratory randomised controlled trial. BMC Health Serv Res. 2009;9:33.
20. Amita S, Prabhakar S, Manoj I, et al. Effect of yoga-nidra on blood glucose level in diabetic patients. Indian J Physiol Pharmacol. 2009;53(1):97-101.
21. Pardasany A, Shenoy S, Sandhu JS. Comparing the efficacy of tai chi chuan and hatha yoga in type 2 diabetes mellitus patients on parameters of blood glucose control and lipid metabolism. Indian J Physiother Occup Ther. 2010;4(3):11-6.
22. Hegde SV, Adhikari P, Kotian S, et al. Effect of 3-month yoga on oxidative stress in type 2 diabetes with or without complications: a controlled clinical trial. Diabetes Care. 2011;34(10):2208-10.
23. Balaji PA, Varne SR, Ali SS. Effects of yoga-pranayama practices on metabolic parameters and anthropometry in type 2 diabetes. Int Multidiscip Res J. 2011;1(10):1-4.
24. Nagarathna R, Usharani M, Rao A, et al. Efficacy of yoga-based lifestyle modification program on medication score and lipid profile in type 2 diabetes–a randomized control study. Int J Diabetes Dev Ctries. 2012;32(3):122-30.
25. Vaishali K, Kumar KV, Adhikari P, et al. Effects of yoga-based program on glycosylated hemoglobin level serum lipid profile in community dwelling elderly subjects with chronic type 2 diabetes mellitus: a randomized controlled trial. Phys Occup Ther Geriatr. 2012;30(1):22-30.
26. Shantakumari N, Sequeira S, El deeb R. Effects of a yoga intervention on lipid profiles of diabetes patients with dyslipidemia. Indian Heart J. 2013;65(2):127-31.
27. Jyotsna VP, Dhawan A, Sreenivas V, et al. Completion report: Effect of comprehensive yogic breathing program on type 2 diabetes: a randomized control trial. Indian J Endocrinol Metab. 2014;18(4):582-4.
28. Cohen BE, Chang AA, Grady D, et al. Restorative yoga in adults with metabolic syndrome: a randomized, controlled pilot trial. Metab Syndr Relat Disord. 2008;6(3):223-9.
29. Corey SM, Epel E, Schembri M, et al. Effect of restorative yoga vs. stretching on diurnal cortisol dynamics and psychosocial outcomes in individuals with the metabolic syndrome: the PRYSMS randomized controlled trial. Psychoneuroendocrinology. 2014;49:260-71.
30. Kanaya AM, Araneta MR, Pawlowsky SB, et al. Restorative yoga and metabolic risk factors: the Practicing Restorative Yoga vs. Stretching for the Metabolic Syndrome (PRYSMS) randomized trial. J Diab Complications. 2014;28(3):406-12.
31. Kim HN, Ryu J, Kim KS, et al. Effects of yoga on sexual function in women with metabolic syndrome: A randomized controlled trial. J Sex Med. 2013;10(11):2741-51.
32. Manchanda SC, Mehrotra UC, Makhija A, et al. Reversal of early atherosclerosis in metabolic syndrome by yoga: a randomized controlled trial. J Yoga Phys Ther. 2013;3:132.
33. Yang K, Bernardo LM, Sereika SM, et al. Utilization of 3-month yoga program for adults at high risk for type 2 diabetes: a pilot study. Evid Based Complement Alternat Med. 2011;2011:257891.
34. Telles S, Sharma SK, Yadav A, et al. A comparative controlled trial comparing the effects of yoga and walking for overweight and obese adults. Med Sci Monit. 2014;20:894-904.
35. Schmidt T, Wijga A, Von Zur Mühlen A. Changes in cardiovascular risk factors and hormones during a comprehensive residential three-month kriya yoga training and vegetarian nutrition. Acta Physiol Scand Suppl. 1997;640:158-62.
36. Murugesan R, Govindarajulu N, Bera TK. Effect of selected yogic practices on the management of hypertension. Indian J Physiol Pharmacol. 2000;44(2):207-10.
37. McCaffrey R, Ruknui P, Hatthakit U, et al. The effects of yoga on hypertensive persons in Thailand. Holist Nurs Pract. 2005;19(4):173-80.
38. Manchanda SC, Narang R, Reddy KS, et al. Retardation of coronary atherosclerosis with yoga lifestyle intervention. J Assoc Physicians India. 2001;48(7):687-94.
39. Mahajan AS, Reddy KS, Sachdeva U. Lipid profile of coronary risk subjects following yogic lifestyle intervention. Indian Heart J. 1999;51(1):37-40.
40. Posadzki P, Cramer H, Kuzdzal A, et al. Yoga for hypertension: a systematic review of randomized clinical trials. Complement Ther Med. 2014;22(3):511-22.
41. Cramer H, Haller H, Lauche R, et al. A systematic review and meta-analysis of yoga for hypertension. Am J Hypertens. 2014;27(9):1146-51.
42. Tyagi A, Cohen M. Yoga and hypertension: a systematic review. Altern Ther Health Med. 2014;20(2):32-59.
43. Wang J, Xiong X, Liu W. Yoga for essential hypertension: a systematic review. PLoS One. 2013;8(10):e76357.
44. Hagins M, States R, Selfe T, et al. Effectiveness of yoga for hypertension: systematic review and meta-analysis. Evid Based Complement Alternat Med. 2013;2013:649836.
45. Okonta NR. Does yoga therapy reduce blood pressure in patients with hypertension?: an integrative review. Holist Nurs Pract. 2012;26(3):137-41.
46. Anderson JW, Liu C, Kryscio RJ. Blood pressure response to transcendental meditation: a meta-analysis. Am J Hypertens. 2008;21(3):310-6.
47. Brook RD, Appel LJ, Rubenfire M, et al. Beyond medications and diet: alternative approaches to lowering blood pressure: a scientific statement from the American Heart Association. Hypertension. 2013;61(6):1360-83.
48. Sarvottam K, Magan D, Yadav RK, et al. Adiponectin, interleukin-6, and cardiovascular disease risk factors are modified by a short-term

yoga-based lifestyle intervention in overweight and obese men. J Altern Complement Med. 2013;19(5):397-402.
49. Chohan IS, Nayar HS, Thomas P, et al. Influence of yoga on blood coagulation. Thromb Haemost. 1984;51(2):196-7.
50. Ceriello A, Motz E. Is oxidative stress the pathogenic mechanism underlying insulin resistance, diabetes, and cardiovascular disease? The common soil hypothesis revisited. Arterioscler Thromb Vasc Biol. 2004;24(5):816-23.
51. Bhattacharya S, Pandey US, Verma NS. Improvement in oxidative status with yogic breathing in young healthy males. Indian J Physiol Pharmacol. 2002;46(3):349-54.
52. Singh S, Malhotra V, Singh KP, et al. A preliminary report on the role of yoga asanas on oxidative stress in non-insulin dependent diabetes mellitus. Indian J Clin Biochem. 2001;16(2):216-20.
53. Jatuporn S, Sangwatanaroj S, Saengsiri AO, et al. Short-term effects of an intensive lifestyle modification program on lipid peroxidation and antioxidant systems in patients with coronary artery disease. Clin Hemorheol Microcirc. 2003;29(3-4):429-36.
54. Yadav RK, Ray RB, Vempati R, et al. Effect of a comprehensive yoga-based lifestyle modification program on lipid peroxidation. Indian J Physiol Pharmacol. 2005;49(3):358-62.
55. Ornish D, Brown SE, Scherwitz LW, et al. Can lifestyle changes reverse coronary heart disease? The Lifestyle Heart Trial. Lancet. 1990;336(8708):129-33.
56. Fields JZ, Walton KG, Schneider RH, et al. Effect of a multimodality natural medicine program on carotid atherosclerosis in older subjects: a pilot trial of Maharishi Vedic Medicine. Am J Cardiol. 2002;89:952-8.
57. Yogendra, J, Yogendra HJ, Ambardekar S, et al. Beneficial effects of yoga lifestyle on reversibility of ischaemic heart disease: caring heart project of International Board of Yoga. J Assoc Physicians India. 2004;52:283-9.
58. Gupta SK, Sawhney RC, Rai L, et al. Regression of coronary atherosclerosis through healthy lifestyle in coronary artery disease patients–Mount Abu open heart trial. Indian Heart J. 2001;63:461-9.
59. Schneider RH, Grim CE, Rainforth MV, et al. Stress reduction in the secondary prevention of cardiovascular disease: randomized, controlled trial of transcendental meditation and health education in Blacks. Circ Cardiovasc Qual Outcomes. 2012;5:750-8.
60. Tulpule TH, Tulpule AT. Yoga. A method of relaxation for rehabilitation after myocardial infarction. Indian Heart J. 1980;32(1):1-7.
61. Silberman A, Banthia R, Estay IS, et al. The effectiveness and efficacy of an intensive cardiac rehabilitation program in 24 sites. Am J Health Promot. 2010;24:260-6.
62. Ravindra PN, Madanmohan, Pavithran P. Effect of pranayam (yoga breathing) and shavasan (relaxation training) on the frequency of benign ventricular ectopics in two patients with palpitations. Int J Cardiol. 2006;108(1):124-5.
63. Prakash ES, Ravindra PN, Madanmohan, et al. Effect of deep breathing at six breaths per minute on the frequency of premature ventricular complexes. Int J Cardiol. 2006;111(3):450-2.
64. Lakkireddy D, Atkins D, Pillarisetti J, et al. Effect of yoga on arrhythmia burden, anxiety, depression, and quality of life in paroxysmal atrial fibrillation: the YOGA My Heart Study. J Am Coll Cardiol. 2013;61(11):1177-82.
65. Krishna BH, Pal P, Pal G, et al. A Randomized Controlled Trial to Study the Effect of Yoga Therapy on Cardiac Function and N Terminal Pro BNP in Heart Failure. Integr Med Insights. 2014;9:1-6.
66. Pullen PR, Nagamia SH, Mehta PK, et al. Effects of yoga on inflammation and exercise capacity in patients with chronic heart failure. J Card Fail. 2008;14(5):407-13.
67. Gomes-Neto M, Rodrigues-Jr ES, Silva-Jr WM, et al. Effects of Yoga in Patients with Chronic Heart Failure: A Meta-Analysis. Arq Bras Cardiol. 2014;103(5):433-9.
68. Streeter CC, Gerbarg PL, Saper RB, et al. Effects of yoga on the autonomic nervous system, gamma-aminobutyric-acid, and allostasis in epilepsy, depression, and post-traumatic stress disorder. Med Hypotheses. 2012;78(5):571-9.
69. Kirkwood G, Rampes H, Tuffrey V, et al. Yoga for anxiety: a systemic review of the research evidence. Br J Sports Med. 2005;39(12):884-91.
70. Pilkington K, Kirkwood G, Rampes H, et al. Yoga for depression: the research evidence. J Affect Disord. 2005;89(1-3):13-24.
71. Shapiro D, Cook IA, Davydov DM, et al. Yoga as a complementary treatment of depression: Effects of traits and moods on treatment outcome. Evid-based Complement Alternat Med. 2007;4(4):493-502.
72. Sears SF Jr, Conti JB. Quality of life and psychological functioning of ICD patients. Heart. 2002;87(5):488-93.

CHAPTER

Metabolic Effects of Antihypertensive Drugs

Mohsin Wali, C Venkata S Ram

INTRODUCTION

Cardiovascular (CV) disorders represent a complex pathobiological process precipitated by known and unknown risk factors. Typically, the onset and progression of cardiovascular disease (CVD) occur due to traditional risk factors such as hypertension, diabetes, obesity, tobacco consumption, dyslipidemia, and genetic predisposition. The interaction between risk factors and CVD is well-known and accepted. However, it is not fully established whether certain antihypertensive drugs can have an unfavorable influence on cardiometabolic parameters. In this review, we will cover certain aspects of reactions between antihypertensive drugs and metabolic syndrome. It has become apparent that biomarkers may play a role in the diagnosis and management of CVD. Biomarkers are a reflection of abnormal vascular biology and permit disease and therapeutic monitoring in clinical practice. Biophysical markers of CVD include (but not limited to) central aortic blood pressure (CABP), high-sensitivity C-reactive protein (hs-CRP), adiponectin, cystatin, tumor necrosis factor-alpha (TNF-α), interleukin 6 (IL-6), procollagen, and homeostatic model assessment-insulin resistance (HOMA-IR) (Box 1).

BOX 1: Biomarkers of cardiovascular disease

- Adiponectin
- Procollagen
- HOMA-IR
- C-reactive protein
- TNF-α
- IL-6

Abbreviations: HOMA-IR, homeostatic model assessment-insulin resistance; TNF-α, tumor necrosis factor-alpha; IL-6, interleukin 6.

EFFECTS OF ANTIHYPERTENSIVE DRUGS ON BIOPHYSICAL MARKERS OF CARDIOVASCULAR DISEASE

Adiponectin

Adiponectin is a humoral substance, derived from adipocytes, which exerts anti-inflammatory and antiatherogenic actions. In addition, it also has a modulating effect on glucose and cholesterol metabolism. Reduced adiponectin levels have been reported in patients with CVD or risk factors for CVD. Low levels of adiponectin have been shown to predict vascular disease. Experimental studies have shown an inverse correlation between atherosclerosis and adiponectin levels.[1] Blockers of the renin-angiotensin-aldosterone-system (RAAS) and calcium channel blockers (CCBs) have been shown to increase serum adiponectin levels.[1] In obese patients, low levels of adiponectin have been linked to atherosclerosis and vascular stiffness. Adiponectin increases nitric oxide (NO) levels and inhibits monocyte adherence to the blood vessel site.[2] Angiotensin receptor blockers (ARBs) exert a variable effect on adiponectin levels. For example, telmisartan (but not irbesartan) has been shown to increase the adiponectin levels in hypertension.[3,4] The combination of ARBs with CCBs produces an increase in the adiponectin levels compared to a combination of ARB plus hydrochlorothiazide.[5] ARBs in general produce a greater increase in adiponectin levels compared to CCBs.[6] Compared to angiotensin-converting enzyme inhibitors (ACEIs), ARBs produce a greater increase in adiponectin levels.[7] In contrast to ARBs and CCBs, diuretics and β-blockers do not increase the adiponectin levels.[8]

Procollagen

Collagen and its fractions are linked to atherosclerosis via intricate mechanical and physiological interactions. Altered dynamics of collagen have been observed in hypertension[9] and collagen products correlate with left ventricular mass and vascular stiffness.[10] Therefore, serum levels of procollagen fractions may have some role in the assessment of CV risk.[11]

Small (inconclusive) studies have shown that RAAS blockers but not CCBs lower procollagen levels.[12] ARBs (via procollagen) may protect against CV and renal fibrosis. Procollagen markers are reduced more with ARBs compared to β-blockers.[13]

Homeostatic Model Assessment-Insulin Resistance

Homeostatic model assessment-insulin resistance is a computational mathematical analysis of insulin resistance and diabetes.[14] HOMA-IR predicts cardiometabolic risk.[15] Antihypertensive drugs have an effect on HOMA-IR. RAAS blockers tend to have a favorable effect on HOMA-IR.[15] It is not clear whether the benefits of RAAS blockers on HOMA-IR are a direct consequence or mediated via an intermediary step. Nevertheless, RAAS blockers in general may improve glucose metabolism.

Angiotensin receptor blockers, particularly in combination with ACEIs and CCBs, show a significant reduction in HOMA-IR. Among the CCBs, manidipine appears to exert a significant effect on HOMA-IR.[16] Telmisartan in comparison to losartan, improves HOMA-IR. Several studies have consistently shown that telmisartan improves HOMA-IR.[17,18] In patients with obstructive sleep apnea and insulin resistance, ARBs improve HOMA-IR. The combination of ARBs and CCBs produces a greater improvement in HOMA-IR than combination of ARBs and diuretics. While ARBs and CCBs improve HOMA-IR only the former drugs improve endothelial function.[19] ARBs in addition to improving HOMA-IR also increase adiponectin levels which provide additional CV protection.

High-sensitivity C-reactive Protein

C-reactive protein, an acute-phase reactant, is an important marker of vascular inflammation which is an important pathological step in the development of vascular disease. The precise relationship between hs-CRP and CVD is not conclusive, but it provides a reliable index of CV derangement. Some studies have linked CRP levels to hypertension.[20] A high CRP level in normotensive individuals predicts future risk of hypertension.[21] In a "healthy" population, elevated CRP has been found as a predictor of future CV dysfunction.[22] Whether hs-CRP is a better marker of CVD than low-density lipoprotein cholesterol (LDL-C) is controversial.[23,24] Inhibitors of the RAAS may protect the CV system through decreasing vascular inflammation and hs-CRP levels.[25] In a small study, olmesartan, an ARB has been shown to reduce CRP levels and improve the myocardial function.[26,27] Olmesartan in combination with amlodipine has been shown to reduce indices of vascular inflammation. Various CCB have been shown to decrease hs-CRP levels.[28,29] Newer CCBs like manidipine and azelnidipine appear to have a more pronounced effect on hs-CRP compared to older CCBs. The combination of RAAS blockers plus CCBs produces a significant reduction in hs-CRP levels. Thus, RAAS blockers and certain CCBs have been shown to reduce hs-CRP levels.

Tumor Necrosis Factor-alpha and Interleukin 6

Tumor necrosis factor-alpha, a marker of inflammation may be linked to hypertension and diabetes.[30] TNF-α may promote atherosclerosis by stimulating the cell receptors for advanced glycation end (AGE) products and by causing endothelial damage.[31] TNF-α may contribute to vascular and cardiac dysfunction. IL-6, an inflammatory cytokine has been shown to correlate with CV risk. For example, IL-6 levels have been shown to correlate with CVD, stroke, and congestive heart failure (CHF). IL-C levels have been shown to predict CVD.[32] ARBs have been shown to exert conflicting results on TNF-α levels.[33] Olmesartan has been shown to reduce TNF-α concentrations. In patients with CHF, adding RAAS blockers has been shown to reduce TNF-α levels. Newer CCBs have been shown to decrease TNF-α levels.[16,34] IL-6 levels follow the direction of TNF-α levels. ARBs-olmesartan and losartan reduce IL-6 levels.[35,36] Newer CCBs like azelnidipine appear to have a positive effect on IL-6 levels. The combination of ARBs with CCBs produces additive reductions in IL-6 levels. Although the cytokines described earlier are not specific in terms of CV risk, they do reflect vascular inflammation—an important parameter of vascular dysfunction and markers CV risk, and thus are best utilized in the context of established CVD risk factors.

Altered Potassium Homeostasis

Hyperkalemia can occur in patients with hypertension due to renal insufficiency or it can be drug induced. Hence, hyperkalemia is a marker of an adverse therapeutic effect or due to renal dysfunction. In patients with type 2 diabetes, hyperkalemia can occur even with normal renal function, due to hyporeninemic hypoaldosteronism [type IV renal tubular acidosis (RTA)]. Aldosterone antagonists such as spironolactone or epleronone can cause hyperkalemia. In studies utilizing aldosterone antagonists for the treatment of CHF, hyperkalemia was noted in a small percentage of patients.

CONCLUSION

In addition to the established risk factors in the causation of CVD, certain biomarkers of considerable importance in the early signaling of CV risk. Thus, certain biomarkers are of emerging significance in the diagnosis, prognosis, and management of CVD in the community. However, with the explosion of science and technology in this field, any biomarker measured should be accurate and relevant to the clinical context. Biomarkers have been recognized in the entire spectrum of CVD, hypertension, diabetes, coronary artery disease, diabetes, CHF, obesity, metabolic syndrome, and obstructive sleep apnea. The effect of antihypertensive drugs on biomarkers may be independent of their blood pressure lowering actions, which poses important considerations in the therapy choices. The effects of antihypertensive drugs on HOMA-IR, hs-CRP, and adiponectin may indicate additional vascular protection over and beyond blood pressure reduction. Further research is necessary to shed light on the influence of antihypertensive drugs on biomarkers as a factor for positive outcomes from sustained blood pressure reduction.

REFERENCES

1. Karthikeyan VJ, Lip GY. Antihypertensive treatment, adiponectin and cardiovascular risk. J Hum Hypertens. 2007;21:8-11.
2. Shargorodsky M, Boaz M, Goldberg Y, et al. Adiponectin and vascular properties in obese patients: is it a novel biomarker of early atherosclerosis? Int J Obes (Lond). 2009;33(5):553-8.
3. Negro R, Formoso G, Hassan H. The effects of irbesartan and telmisartan on metabolic parameters and blood pressure in obese, insulin resistant, hypertensive patients. J Endocrinol Invest. 2006;29(11):957-61.
4. Kintscher U, Bramlage P, Paar WD, et al. Irbesartan for the treatment of hypertension in patients with the metabolic syndrome: a sub analysis of the Treat to Target post authorization survey. Prospective observational, two armed study in 14,200 patients. Cardiovasc Diabetol. 2007;6:12.
5. Martinez-Martin FJ, Rodriguez-Rosas H, Peiro-Martinez I, et-al. Olmesartan/amlodipine vs olmesartan/hydrochlorothiazide in hypertensive patients with metabolic syndrome: the OLAS study. J Hum Hypertens. 2011;25(6):346-53.
6. Negro R, Hassan H. The effects of telmisartan and amlodipine on metabolic parameters and blood pressure in type 2 diabetic, hypertensive patients. J Renin Angiotensin Aldosterone Syst. 2006;7(4):243-6.
7. Derosa G, Maffioli P, Ferrari I, et al. Different actions of losartan and ramipril on adipose tissue activity and vascular remodeling biomarkers in hypertensive patients. Hypertens Res. 2011;34(1):145-51.
8. Koh KK, Quon MJ, Han SH, et al. Distinct vascular and metabolic effects of different classes of anti-hypertensive drugs. Int J Cardiol. 2010;140(1):73-81.
9. Szmigielski C, Raczkowska M, Styczynski G, et al. Metabolism of collagen is altered in hypertensives with increased intima media thickness. Blood Press. 2006;15(3):157-63.
10. Ishikawa J, Kario K, Matsui Y, et al. Collagen metabolism in extracellular matrix may be involved in arterial stiffness in older hypertensive patients with left ventricular hypertrophy. Hypertens Res. 2005;28(12):995-1001.
11. Lopez B, González A, Querejeta R, et al. The use of collagen-derived serum peptides for the clinical assessment of hypertensive heart disease. J Hypertens. 2005;23(8):1445-51.
12. Fogari R, Derosa G, Ferrari I, et al. Effect of valsartan and ramipril on atrial fibrillation recurrence and P-wave dispersion in hypertensive patients with recurrent symptomatic lone atrial fibrillation. Am J Hypertens. 2008;21(9):1034-9.
13. Diez J, Querejeta R, López B, et al. Losartan-dependent regression of myocardial fibrosis is associated with reduction of left ventricular chamber stiffness in hypertensive patients. Circulation. 2002;105(21):2512-7.
14. Matthews DR, Hosker JP, Rudenski AS, et al. Homeostasis model assessment: insulin resistance and beta-cell function from fasting plasma glucose and insulin concentrations in man. Diabetologia. 1985;28(7):412-9.
15. Cooper-DeHoff RM, Pacanowski MA, Pepine CJ, et al. Cardiovascular therapies and associated glucose homeostasis: implications across the dysglycemia continuum. J Am Coll Cardiol. 2009;53(5 suppl):S28-34.
16. Martinez-Martin FJ, Macias-Batista A, Comi-Diaz C, et al. Effects of manidipine and its combination with an ACE inhibitor on insulin sensitivity and metabolic, inflammatory and prothrombotic markers in hypertensive patients with metabolic syndrome: the MARCADOR study. Clin Drug Investig. 2011;31(3):201-12.
17. Huang YY, Xu AP, Zhou SS, et al. Effect of losartan on renal expression of monocyte chemoattractant protein-1 and transforming growth factor-β(1) in rats after unilateral ureteral obstruction. Nan Fang Yi Ke Da Xue Xue Bao. 2011;31(8):1405-10.
18. Lan J, Chen X, Wang S, et al. The relationship between visfatin and HOMA-IR in hypertensive patients, and the effect of anti-hypertensive drugs on visfatin and HOMA-IR in hypertensive patients with insulin resistance. Diabetes Res Clin Pract. 2011;94(1):71-6.
19. Nishimura H, Sanaka T, Tanihata Y, et al. Losartan elevates the serum high-molecular weight-adiponectin isoform and concurrently improves insulin sensitivity in patients with impaired glucose metabolism. Hypertens Res. 2008;31(8):1611-8.
20. Bautista LE, Atwood JE, O'Malley PG, et al. Association between C-reactive protein and hypertension in healthy middle-aged men and women. Coron Artery Dis. 2004;15(6):331-6.
21. Dauphinot V, Roche F, Kossovsky MP, et al. C-reactive protein implications in new-onset hypertension in a healthy population initially aged 65 years: the Proof study. J Hypertens. 2009;27(4):736-43.
22. Abramson JL, Weintraub WS, Vaccarino V. Association between pulse pressure and C-reactive protein among apparently healthy US adults. Hypertension. 2002;39(2):197-202.
23. Packard RR, Libby P. Inflammation in atherosclerosis: from vascular biology to biomarker discovery and risk prediction. Clin Chem. 2008;54(1):24-38.

24. Genest J, Preventive cardiology: move over low density lipoprotein cholesterol, hello C-reactive protein? Can J Cardiol. 2004;20(Suppl B):89B-92B.
25. Savoia C, Schiffrin EL. Reduction of C-reactive protein and the use of anti-hypertensives. Vasc Health Risk Manag. 2007;3(6):975-83.
26. Futai R, Ito T, Kawanishi Y, et al. Olmesartan ameliorates myocardial function independent of blood pressure control in patients with mild-to-moderate hypertension. Heart Vessels. 2009;24(4): 294-300.
27. Miyoshi T, Doi M, Hirohata S, et al. Olmesartan reduces arterial stiffness and serum adipocyte fatty acid-binding protein in hypertensive patients. Heart Vessels. 2011;26(4):408-13.
28. Ishimitsu T, Numabe A, Masuda T, et al. Angiotensin-II receptor antagonist combined with calcium channel blocker or diuretic for essential hypertension. Hypertens Res. 2009;32(11):962-8.
29. Fukao K, Shimada K, Hiki M, et al. Effects of calcium channel blockers on glucose tolerance, inflammatory state, and circulating progenitor cells in non-diabetic patients with essential hypertension: a comparative study between Azelnidipine and amlodipine on glucose tolerance and endothelial function–a crossover trial (AGENT). Cardiovasc Diabetol. 2011;10:79.
30. Fogari R, Preti P, Zoppi A, et al. Effects of amlodipine-atorvastatin combination on inflammation markers and insulin sensitivity in normocholesterolemic obese hypertensive patients. Eur J Clin Pharmacol. 2006;62(10):817-22.
31. Fujita M, Okuda H, Tsukamoto O, et al. Blockade of angiotensin-II receptors reduces the expression of receptors for advanced glycation end products in human endothelial cells. Arterioscler Thromb Vasc Biol. 2006;26(10):e138-42.
32. Luc G, Bard JM, Juhan-Vague I, et al. C-reactive protein, interleukin-6, and fibrinogen as predictors of coronary heart disease: the PRIME Study. Arterioscler Thromb Vasc Biol. 2003;23(7):1255-61.
33. Watanabe S, Okura T, Kurata M, et al. The effect of losartan and amlodipine on serum adiponectin in Japanese adults with essential hypertension. Clin Ther. 2006;28(10):1677-85.
34. Nakamura M, Yamashita T, Yajima J, et al. Brachial-ankle pulse wave velocity as a risk stratification index for the short-term prognosis of type-2 diabetic patients with coronary artery disease. Hypertens Res. 2010;33(10):1018-24.
35. Sardo MA, Mandraffino G, Riggio S, et al. Effects of the angiotensin-II receptor blocker losartan on the monocyte expression of biglycan in hypertensive patients. Clin Exp Pharmacol Physiol. 2010;37(9):933-8.
36. Lorenzen JM, Neunhöffer H, David S, et al. Angiotensin-II receptor blocker and statins lower elevated levels of osteopontin in essential hypertension—results from the EUTOPIA trial. Atherosclerosis. 2010;209(1):184-8.

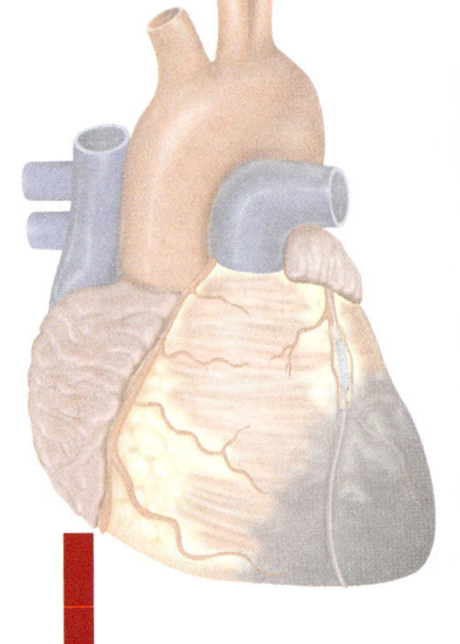

Potential Role of Rosuvastatin in Cardiodiabetes

Saumitra Ray, Sumanta Chatterjee

INTRODUCTION

Diabetes mellitus (DM) is a very commonly occurring metabolic disorder affecting approximately 285 million individuals aged between 20 years and 79 years worldwide. This accounts for 6.4% of the global population and is projected to increase to 438 million by 2030, which should be 7.7% of the global population. A 69% increase in number of adults with diabetes in developing countries and a 20% increase in developed countries, is projected for 2030.[1] In developed countries such as USA, current estimates indicate that 21 million US adults, roughly 10% of the adult population, have diabetes. Owing-in-part to the growing, epidemic of obesity in the United States, the prevalence of diabetes is expected to be more than double to 48 million people by 2050.[2-4] In developing country such as India, current prevalence of diabetes is 50.8 million and it is expected high up to 87 million in 2030.[1] Diabetes is associated with increased oxidative stress due to hyperglycemia. The oxidative damage plays a role in development of micro- and macrovascular complications, including cardiovascular diseases (CVDs). Study established that individuals with diabetes have 2–3 times higher risk of cardiovascular (CV) events than nondiabetic people. Heart disease mortality, however, is two to four times higher in patients with diabetes compared with those without diabetes. During the past three decades, prevalence of diabetes mellitus, hypertension, and dyslipidemia has been increased markedly in India. Diabetic patients tend to have a higher concentration of low-density lipoprotein cholesterol (LDL-C), which is a major risk factor for CVD. Approximately, 80% of deaths in diabetic patients are attributable to CVD and Asian Indians have higher risk of heart attacks than Whites, which, in turn, is highly correlated with diabetic dyslipidemia. Lowering LDL level is the first priority in treating diabetic dyslipidemia.[5]

LOW-DENSITY LIPOPROTEIN CHOLESTEROL LOWERING IN DIABETES MELLITUS

The United Kingdom Prospective Diabetes Study (UKPDS) established the importance of tight glycemic control in patients with diabetes. But, along with glycemic control, control of dyslipidemia is also important to reduce CV events. Efforts to reduce CV morbidity and mortality in people with diabetes have, therefore, focused on overall or global risk factor management, including weight loss and increased physical activity, tight control of blood pressure and blood glucose, and intensive management of diabetic dyslipidemia. In diabetic dyslipidemia, there is high chance of increased level of LDL, small dense LDL, triglycerides (TG), non-high-density lipoprotein (HDL), and low level of HDL.[6]

National Health and Nutrition Examination Survey (NHNES) has suggested target hemoglobin A1c (HbA1c) goal should be less than 7%, while a blood pressure goal should be less than 130/80 mm Hg, and total cholesterol goal of less than 200 mg/dL. Optimal LDL level should be less than 70 mg/dL.[7] Studies have confirmed that aggressive LDL reductions in patients with diabetes contribute to the

TABLE 1: Recommendations for statin and combination treatment in people with diabetes

Age	Risk factors	Recommended statin intensity*
<40 years	None ASCVD risk factor(s)** ASCVD	None Moderate or high High
40–75 years	None ASCVD risk factors ASCVD ACS and LDL cholesterol >50 mg/dL (1.3 mmol/L) in patients who cannot tolerate high-dose statins	Moderate High High Moderate plus ezetimibe
>75 years	None ASCVD risk factors ASCVD ACS and LDL cholesterol >50 mg/dL (1.3 mmol/L) in patients who cannot tolerate high-dose statins	Moderate Moderate or high High Moderate plus ezetimibe

* In addition to lifestyle therapy.
** ASCVD risk factors include LDL cholesterol ≥100 mg/dL (2.6 mmol/L), high blood pressure, smoking, overweight and obesity, and family history of premature ASCVD.

Abbreviations: ASCVD, atherosclerotic cardiovascular disease; ACS, acute coronary syndrome; LDL, low-density lipoprotein

achievement of LDL-C goals. Significant reductions in other highly atherogenic lipids and lipoproteins, such as apolipoprotein B, non-HDL cholesterol, and triglyceride-rich lipoproteins are also possible with intensive statin therapy. Non-HDL cholesterol, which is composed of LDL-C and very low-density lipoprotein (VLDL) cholesterol, is also a viable treatment target in patients with type 2 diabetes and "normal" LDL-C levels. The National Cholesterol Education Program-Adult Treatment Panel III (NCEP ATP III) guidelines consider non-HDL cholesterol a secondary treatment target (after LDL-C) in patients with elevated triglyceride levels (≥200 mg/dL), which includes many diabetic people, because it is a better measure of atherogenic cholesterol than LDL-C alone. The goal level for non-HDL cholesterol is 30 mg/dL higher than that for LDL-C, or less than 130 mg/dL in diabetic patients.[6,8]

American Diabetic Association (ADA), 2016, has recommended statins as a prime drug for dyslipidemia management in DM patients (Table 1).

In clinical practice, providers may need to adjust intensity of statin therapy based on individual patient response to medication (e.g. side effects, tolerability, and LDL-C levels). Combination therapy (statin/fibrate) has not been shown to improve atherosclerotic CVD outcomes and is generally not recommended. However, therapy with statin and fenofibrate may be considered for men with both triglyceride level more than or equal to 204 mg/dL and HDL cholesterol level less than or equal to 34 mg/dL.

TABLE 2: High-intensity and moderate-intensity statin therapy*

High-intensity statin therapy	Moderate-intensity statin therapy
Lowers LDL cholesterol by ≥50%	Lowers LDL cholesterol by 30% to <50%
Atorvastatin 40–80 mg	Atorvastatin 10–20 mg
Rosuvastatin 20–40 mg	Rosuvastatin 5–10 mg Simvastatin 20–40 mg Pravastatin 40–80 mg Lovastatin 40 mg Fluvastatin XL 80 mg Pitavastatin 2–4 mg

* Once-daily dosing.

Abbreviation: LDL, low-density lipoprotein

Dose of statin in diabetic patients is based on need of LDL reduction, and accordingly dose of statin is classified as high, moderate, and low intensity statin (Table 2).[9]

PLEIOTROPIC EFFECTS OF STATINS

Pleiotropic effects of statins include improvement of endothelial dysfunction, increased nitric oxide bioavailability, antioxidant properties, inhibition of inflammatory responses, and stabilization of atherosclerotic plaques. These and several other emergent properties could act in concert with the potent LDL-C lowering effects of statins to exert early as well as lasting CV protective effects. Understanding the pleiotropic effects of statins is important to optimize their use in treatment and prevention of CVD (Fig. 1).[10]

ROLE OF STATIN IN DIABETES MELLITUS PATIENTS

Statins are used for primary and secondary prevention of CVD in DM patients. Several meta-analyses have clearly shown the benefits of statin therapy for either short-term (<5 years) or long-term (>10 years) CV outcomes in primary prevention. These benefits apply to both people at higher risk (>10%) and the lower risk as well. This argument is especially valid in people with diabetes.[11] In 2008, the Cholesterol Treatment Trialists' (CTT) group analyzed 14 trials to ascertain the effects of statins on patients with diabetes. Four primary prevention trials (HPS, ASCOT-LLA, CARDS, and ALLHAT-LLT) accounted for 14,996 (83%) of the 18,686 patients with diabetes. During a mean follow-up of 4.3 years, per 39 mg/dL lowering of LDL-C, the proportional reduction in all-cause mortality was 9% [rate ratio 0.91, 99% confidence interval (CI) 0.82–1.01]. This outcome was primarily driven by a significant 21% reduction in vascular

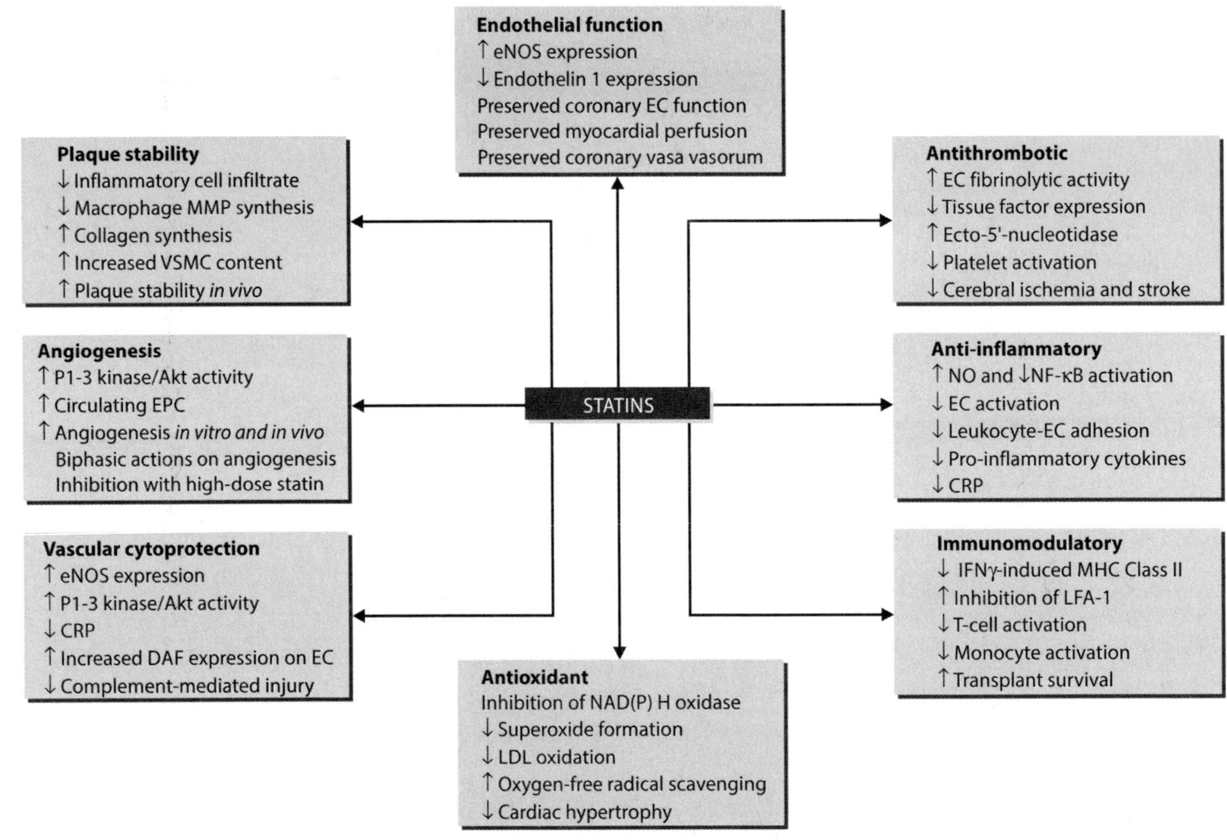

Fig. 1: Pleiotropic effects of statins

Abbreviations: eNOS, endothelial nitric oxide synthase; EC, endothelial cell; MMP, metalloproteinases; VSMC, vascular smooth muscle cell; EPC, endothelial progenitor cell; CRP, C-reactive protein; DAF, decay-accelerating factor; LDL, low-density lipoprotein; IFNγ, interferon-gamma; MHC, major histocompatibility complex; LFA, leukocyte function antigen-1; NO, nitrous oxide; NF-κB, nuclear factor-κB

mortality (rate ratio 0.87, 99% CI 0.76–1.00) with no effect on nonvascular mortality (rate ratio 0.97, 99% CI 0.82–1.16). However, this study did not include major adverse events from microvascular complications (neuropathy or retinopathy) or metabolic disturbances (incidence of diabetic ketoacidosis or nonketotic hyperglycemia). The proportional effects of statins in people with diabetes with vascular disease (secondary prevention) or without vascular disease (primary prevention) were similar. After 5 years, 42 (95% CI 30–55), fewer people had major vascular events (MVEs) per 1,000 among those considered to be at high risk (>10%).[12]

ROLE OF ROSUVASTATIN IN DIABETIC DYSLIPIDEMIA

Rosuvastatin, which is a new generation 3-hydroxy-3-methylglutaryl coenzyme A (HMG-CoA) reductase inhibitor, exhibits some unique pharmacologic and pharmacokinetics properties. It has low extrahepatic tissue penetration, low potential for CYP3A4 interactions, and substantial LDL-C lowering capacity and may, therefore, have some advantages. Its potential impact in primary and secondary prevention of CVD in different groups including heart failure, elderly, renal failure, and diabetes, and also in combination with other lipid lowering drugs, is the subject of ongoing clinical studies.

Although the characteristic statin pharmacophore remains similar to other statins, the addition of a stable polar methane-sulfonamide group provides low lipophilicity and enhanced ionic interaction with HMG-CoA reductase enzyme, thus improving its binding affinity to this enzyme.

Rosuvastatin is one of the synthetic statins which is indicated for primary prevention of CVD. In JUPITER trial 17,802 healthy men and women, rosuvastatin reduces LDL level by 50% and C-reactive protein level by 37%. Consistent effects were observed in all subgroups evaluated. The rosuvastatin group did not have a significant increase in myopathy or cancer, but did have a higher incidence of physician-reported diabetes.[13] It also lowers LDL level very significantly and because of that rosuvastatin is indicated in reduction of CV events.

In one Indian study of 5,000 patients, with LDL levels of more than 140 mg/dL, HDL levels of less than 40 mg/dL and total cholesterol levels of more than 200 mg/dL at the time of enrolment. The study was an open label, nonrandomized, noninterventional, and observational study in India involving type 2 diabetes mellitus (T2DM) patients who require statin therapy to control dyslipidemia. Data were collected at baseline, interim (8 weeks) and subsequently at 16 weeks of rosuvastatin (10 and 20 mg) therapy. Efficacy of the treatment was assessed by evaluating whether subjects reached target LDL and total cholesterol levels. In analysis, it was observed that out of the 5,005 recruited, 4,369 patients, 2,976 males (68.12%) and 1,393 females, (31.88%), completed the study.

Out of 4,369, 1,115 (25.52%) have achieved a target LDL level of less than 100 mg/dL and 1,559 (35.68%) were in the 'near-optimal range' of 100–129 mg/dL of LDL (Table 3).[5]

Out of 4,369 patient population, 2,930 (67.06%) patients achieved HDL levels in the range of 40–60 mg/dL. The mean change in HDL levels was 5.56 (±4.81) mg/dL in females and 4.59 (±4.95) mg/dL in males (Table 4).

In cholesterol less than 200 mg/dL category, 2,794 (63.95%) of patients had achieved the target. The mean change was 51.20 (±46.26) mg/dL in females and 56.10 (±71.35) mg/dL in males (Table 5).

In present study, overall, trial treatment was well tolerated. The percentages of patients who reported adverse events (AEs) during randomized treatment were similar to the previous trials. There were no deaths or serious adverse events (SAEs) reported during the treatment with rosuvastatin. These higher potency statins appear to be safe, even when used at higher dose.[5]

Similarly, the "Use of Rosuvastatin versus Atorvastatin iN type 2 diabetes mellitus" (URANUS) study compared rosuvastatin with atorvastatin for the reduction of LDL-C in patients with T2DM. At the starting dose and following dose titration, rosuvastatin was significantly more effective than atorvastatin at reducing LDL-C and achieving European LDL-C goals in patients with T2DM.[14]

In one Japanese study, low dose of rosuvastatin (2.5 mg or 5 mg) was used in diabetic dyslipidemia patients with low level of HDL (<40 mg/dL) and TG less than 400 mg/dL. Out of 49 patients, all lipid parameters other than TG were significantly improved at 3 and 6 months. At 3 months, 83.3% of patients had achieved the target LDL-C level. Among nonlipid parameters, no changes were observed except for estimated glomerular filtration rate, which was improved by +5.2% and +9.6% at 3 and 6 months, respectively.[15]

Based on CORALL study, high dose of atorvastatin (80 mg) and rosuvastatin (40 mg), both drugs are effective in terms of LDL reduction but both are increasing HbA1c and blood glucose level significantly more at end of study. Future controlled studies are needed to verify these findings and, if confirmed, determine whether such changes represent a true decline in glycemic control or not.[16]

In VOYAGER study,[17-18] an individual patient data pooled analysis of 32,258 patients in studies comparing the efficacy of rosuvastatin with that of atorvastatin or simvastatin, the impact of increasing dose on lowering LDL-C, TG, non-HDL cholesterol, and apolipoprotein B was investigated. Doubling statin dose was associated with greater lowering of LDL-C by 4–6% and non-HDL cholesterol by 3–6%. In another VOYAGER substudy, a meta-analysis of 8,859 patients with DM showed favorable effects on lipids with the three statins studied, in line with results for the overall VOYAGER population.

In MERCURY[19] trial, subgroup of patients with type 2 diabetes, rosuvastatin 10 mg significantly reduced LDL-C levels compared with atorvastatin 10 mg, simvastatin 20 mg, and pravastatin 40 mg (all $p < 0.0001$). In ECLIPSE study, retrospective analysis of 4,754 diabetics in a real world setting, rosuvastatin was more effective in lowering LDL-C and achieving LDL-C treatment goals in the DM population as compared to other statins.[20]

The STELLAR study (comparison of the efficacy and safety of rosuvastatin versus atorvastatin, simvastatin, and pravastatin across doses) showed that at different doses, rosuvastatin reduced total cholesterol better than other statins, and TG better than simvastatin and pravastatin.

At 6 weeks, across-dose analyses showed that rosuvastatin 10–80 mg reduced LDL-C by a mean of 8.2% more than atorvastatin 10–80 mg, 26% more than pravastatin 10–40 mg, and 12–18% more than simvastatin 10–80 mg (all $p < 0.001$).

PULSAR (Prospective Study to Evaluate Low Doses of Atorvastatin and Rosuvastatin) showed that in hypercholesterolemic patients with vascular occlusive disease, rosuvastatin 10 mg reduced LDL-C levels significantly more than atorvastatin 20 mg at week 6 (44.6% vs 42.7%, $p < 0.05$). Significantly more patients achieved NCEP ATP III and 2003 European LDL-C goals with rosuvastatin 10 mg compared with atorvastatin 20 mg (68.8% vs 62.5%, $p < 0.05$; 68.0% vs 63.3%, $p < 0.05$, respectively). HDL cholesterol was increased significantly with rosuvastatin 10 mg versus atorvastatin 20 mg (6.4% vs 3.1%, $p < 0.001$). These results suggest that in high-risk patients with hypercholesterolemia, rosuvastatin 10 mg was more efficacious than atorvastatin 20 mg at reducing LDL-C, enabling LDL-C goal achievement and improving other lipid parameters.

ASTEROID (A Study to Evaluate the Effect of Rosuvastatin on Intravascular Ultrasound-derived Coronary Atheroma Burden) which investigated the impact of high-dose rosuvastatin on regression of atherosclerosis showed that

TABLE 3: Mean change in low-density lipoprotein cholesterol level after treatment for 16 weeks

*Frequency of LDL-C levels**		*Gender (Mean and SD values)*			
		Female		*Male*	
	Frequency (%)	*LDL levels mg/dL (at 16 weeks)*	*% change in LDL levels*	*LDL levels in mg/dL (at 16 weeks)*	*% change in LDL levels*
<100	1115 (25.52%)	–45.94 (38.19)	–36.1%	–44.17 (38.58)	–35.6%
100–129	1559 (35.68%)	–38.53 (35.36)	–25.0%	–57.15 (554.02)	–33.2%
130–159	1144 (26.18%)	–27.54 (56.30)	–16.3%	–25.22 (25.29)	–15.1%
160–189	433 (9.91%)	–14.47 (27.59)	–7.94%	–17.39 (27.22)	–9.28%
≥190	118 (2.70%)	114.89 (282.06)	56.13%	–7.43 (97.53)	–3.2%
		Target achievement			
		Female		Male	Total
Achieved		851 (19.48%)		1823 (41.73%)	2674 (61.20%)
Not achieved		542 (12.41%)		1153 (26.39%)	1695 (38.80%)

Abbreviation: LDL-C, low-density lipoprotein cholesterol

*NCEP ATP III Guidelines

TABLE 4: Mean change in high–density lipoprotein cholesterol level after treatment for 16 weeks

*Frequency of HDL levels**		*Gender (Mean and SD values)*			
		Female		*Male*	
	Frequency (%)	*HDL levels in mg/dL (at 16 weeks)*	*% change in HDL levels*	*HDL levels in mg/dL (at 16 weeks)*	*% change in HDL levels*
<40	935 (21.40%)	–0.92 (10.96)	–2.58%	–1.06 (11.57)	–2.98%
40–60	2930 (67.06%)	5.56 (9.81)	13.42%	4.59 (14.95)	10.8%
>60	504 (11.54%)	20.27 (47.69)	37.37%	16.38 (37.74)	27.77%
		Target achievement			
		Female		Male	Total
Achieved		964 (22.06%)		2056 (47.06%)	3020 (69.12%)
Not achieved		429 (9.82%)		920 (21.06%)	1349 (30.88%)

Abbrevation: HDL, high–density lipoprotein

*NCEP ATP III guidelines

TABLE 5: Mean change in total cholesterol level after treatment for 16 weeks

Frequency of total cholesterol levels*		*Gender (Mean and SD values)*			
		Female		*Male*	
	Frequency (%)	*TC levels in mg/dL (at 16 weeks)*	*% change in TC levels*	*TC levels in mg/dL (at 16 weeks)*	*% change in TC levels*
<200	2794 (63.95%)	–51.20 (46.26)	–23.2%	–56.10 (71.35)	–24.9%
200–239	1097 (25.11%)	–36.31 (41.50)	–14.6%	–37.03 (35.32)	–14.8%
≥240	478 (10.94%)	–43.89 (95.21)	–13.5%	–30.85 (54.64)	–10.3%
		Target achievement			
		Female		Male	Total
Achieved		910 (20.83%)		1884 (43.12%)	2794 (63.95%)
Not achieved		483 (11.06%)		1092 (24.99%)	1575 (36.05%)

Abbreviation: TC, Total cholesterol

*NCEP ATP III Guidelines

rosuvastatin 40 mg produced 53% reduction in LDL-C, 14.7% increase in HDL-C and regression of atheroma volume in the most diseased coronary arteries in 78% of participants. The ORION (Outcome of Rosuvastatin Treatment on Carotid Artery Atheroma: a Magnetic Resonance Imaging Observation) and METEOR (Measuring Effects on Intima Media Thickness: an Evaluation of Rosuvastatin) demonstrated that rosuvastatin 40 mg achieved a 49% LDL-C reduction and slowed progression of atherosclerosis as assessed by carotid intima-media thickness (CIMT), while the COSMOS (Coronary Atherosclerosis Study Measuring Effects of Rosuvastatin Using Intravascular Ultrasound in Japanese Subjects) study found that rosuvastatin achieved significant reduction of coronary plaque volume with good safety in stable Japanese coronary heart disease (CHD) patients. The Archimedes Model was used to simulate head-to-head clinical trials in nine patient populations found that rosuvastatin 20 mg and 40 mg lowers the risk of major adverse cardiovascular event (MACE) more than atorvastatin 40 mg and atorvastatin 80 mg.

ROLE OF ROSUVASTATIN IN DIABETIC HEMODIALYSIS PATIENTS

In AURORA study, among the 731 participants with diabetes who were on hemodialysis were assigned to rosuvastatin. In treatment arm, it was nonsignificant 16.2% reduction in risk for composite primary endpoint of cardiac death, nonfatal myocardial infarction (MI), or fatal or nonfatal stroke (HR 0.84; 95% CI 0.65–1.07). Rosuvastatin treatment significantly reduced the rates of cardiac events by 32% among patients with diabetes (HR 0.68; 95% CI 0.51–0.90). In conclusion, among hemodialysis patients with diabetes mellitus, rosuvastatin might reduce the risk of fatal and nonfatal cardiac events.[21]

ROLE OF ROSUVASTATIN ON INSULIN RESISTANCE IN DIABETIC PATIENTS

In JUPITER trial subanalysis, rosuvastatin was investigated for association of lipoprotein subclasses and size and a novel lipoprotein insulin resistance (LPIR) score (a composite of 6 lipoprotein measures) with incident T2DM among individuals randomized to a high-intensity statin or placebo. Among the 11,918 patients, rosuvastatin lowered the levels of LDL particles (–39.6%; 95% CI, -49.4% to -24.6%), VLDL particles (–19.6%; 95% CI, –40.6% to 10.3%), and VLDL TG (–15.2%; 95% CI, –35.9% to 11.3%) and shifted the lipoprotein subclass distribution toward smaller LDL size, larger VLDL size (2.8%; 95% CI, –5.8% to 12.7%), and lower LPIR score (–3.2%; 95% CI, –20.6% to 16.9%). Rosuvastatin was associated with positive LPIR score in healthy people.[22]

ROLE OF STATIN IN RENOPROTECTION

Cardiovascular disease continues to be the leading cause of morbidity and mortality among people with chronic kidney disease (CKD) worldwide, especially in dialysis patients who have mortality rates up to 40-fold higher than the general population, with CVD being responsible for up to 50% of these deaths. Kidney Disease Outcome Quality Initiative (KDOQI) also recommends statin therapy in CKD patients with high LDL level. A meta-analysis of 31 trials has shown that statin therapy has a 23% relative risk reduction (RRR) for major CV events ($p < 0.001$), with beneficial effect in reduction of coronary event and all-cause mortality as well, but had no significantly effect on stroke (21%, -12 to 44) or no clear effect on kidney failure events (5%, –1 to 10).[23]

ROLE OF STATIN IN CONTRAST-INDUCED NEPHROPATHY

Patients with CKD, congestive heart failure, decreased renal perfusion, advanced age, and DM are at increased risk for developing contrast-induced nephropathy (CIN). Patients with acute coronary syndrome (ACS) are three times more likely to develop CIN and 31% of these cases then developed persistent deterioration of kidney function. In CVD, especially ACS, patients who are going for percutaneous coronary intervention (PCI), statin is much needed to avoid CIN. Pleiotropic effects of statins improve endothelial function and have anti-inflammatory properties and antiapoptotic effects, which make them promising candidates for CIN prevention. Rosuvastatin is least lipophilic but generates more nitrous oxide (NO) and improves endothelial function. In addition, rosuvastatin exhibits strong HMG-CoA reductase inhibition including reduced tubular protein reabsorption. A recent head-to-head trial compared rosuvastatin (10 mg) to atorvastatin (20 mg) for prevention of CIN in statin-naïve patients with CKD undergoing PCI. Both groups had a similar incidence of CIN (5.9 vs. 5.2 %, $p = 0.684$) and in-hospital mortality (0.4 vs 1.5 %, $p = 0.141$) for rosuvastatin and atorvastatin, respectively.[24]

ROLE OF STATIN IN STROKE PREVENTION

Epidemiologic and observational studies have not shown a clear association between cholesterol levels and all causes of stroke. Nonetheless, large, long-term statin trials in patients with established or who are at high risk of CHD have demonstrated that statins decrease stroke incidence. In the Stroke Prevention by Aggressive Reduction in Cholesterol Levels (SPARCL) trial, compared with placebo, the patients with a recent stroke or transient ischemic attack without CHD randomized to atorvastatin 80 mg/day had a significant 16% RRR of stroke, and a 35% reduction in the risk of major coronary events. In trial of 316 stroke patients, where rosuvastatin was compared with placebo and it was found that frequency of new ischemic lesions on diffusion weighted imaging (DWI) was not different between groups (rosuvastatin: 27/137, 19.7% vs placebo: 36/152, 23.6%) (RR-0.83). However, hemorrhagic infarction or parenchymal/subarachnoid hemorrhage occurred less frequently in the rosuvastatin group (6/137, 4.4%) than the placebo group (22/152, 14.5%, p = 0.007). Among 314 patients with at least one dose of study medication, progression or clinical recurrence of stroke tended to occur less frequently in the rosuvastatin group (1/155, 0.6% vs 7/159, 4.4%, p = 0.067).[25]

ROLE OF STATIN IN METABOLIC SYNDROME

Statins are recommended to reach the LDL-C goal in metabolic syndrome with a 10-year CHD risk more than 20% and to correct the other associated lipid and nonlipid abnormalities. Statins also have lowering effect on VLDL and TGs which are responsible for CVD in DM patients. Atorvastatin and rosuvastatin show the stronger triglyceride lowering effect. Their efficacy may reach, at the highest dosages, almost 50% of reduction, but is already present and relevant at lower dosages.[26]

SAFETY OF ROSUVASTATIN

In the pooled safety data of controlled phase II/II trials, the incidence of adverse events during rosuvastatin therapy was comparable to those of other statins. Subsequent meta-analysis of clinical trials and postmarketing experience have consistently shown that rosuvastatin has a comparable safety profile to other available statins when used at 10 mg to 40 mg daily dose. In JUPITER, hepatic injury, myopathy, and cancer did not occur more frequently with rosuvastatin than with placebo, despite the fact that LDL-C less than 55 mg/dL (1.4 mmol/L) were achieved in half of the rosuvastatin group. The overwhelming benefit of statins in the reduction of CV events outweighs the small risk of developing diabetes, therefore, statin therapy should be used in patients with high CV risk. All statins can cause myopathy and rhabdomyolysis, especially at higher doses. Combination of statins with other medications may lead to increased risk if these medications increase plasma concentrations of the statins. One unique effect of rosuvastatin is the dose-dependent transient proximal isolated low-molecular-weight proteinuria which appears to have no effect on glomerular function.

CONCLUSION

Rosuvastatin is one of the promising statins for primary prevention of CV events in diabetes dyslipidemia patients. In various phase-III landmark trials, it has shown increased new onset of diabetes. But in routine practice and clinical study, it reduces LDL level significantly in diabetes dyslipidemia patients without safety concern. It also improves level of low HDL and improves statin resistance with keeping LPIR level positive.

REFERENCES

1. Shaw JE, Sicree RA, Zimmet PZ. Global estimates of the prevalence of diabetes for 2010 and 2030. Diabetes Res Clin Pract. 2010;87(1):4-14.
2. Centers for Disease Control and Prevention. (2005). National diabetes fact sheet. [online] Available from *http://www.cdc.gov/diabetes/pubs/pdf_2005* [Accessed October, 2017].
3. Mokdad AH, Bowman BA, Ford ES, et al. The continuing epidemics of obesity and diabetes in the United States. JAMA. 2001;286(10):1195-200.
4. Beller GA. Noninvasive screening for coronary atherosclerosis and silent ischemia in asymptomatic type 2 diabetic patients: is it appropriate and cost-effective? J Am Coll Cardiol. 2007;49(19):1918-23.
5. Shah NS, Arneja J. Efficacy of rosuvastatin in achieving target HDL, LDL, triglycerides and total cholesterol levels in type 2 diabetes mellitus (T2DM) with newly diagnosed dyslipidaemia: an open label, nonrandomised, non-interventional and observational study in India. J Assoc Physicians India. 2013;61(10):721-6.
6. Nesto RW. LDL cholesterol lowering in type 2 diabetes: what is the optimum approach? Clinical Diabetes. 2008;26(1):1-9.
7. Saydah SH, Fradkin J, Cowie CC. Poor control of risk factors for vascular disease among adults with previously diagnosed diabetes. JAMA. 2004;291(3):335-42.
8. National Cholesterol Education Program (NCEP) Expert Panel on Detection, Evaluation, and Treatment of High Blood Cholesterol in Adults (Adult Treatment Panel III). Third Report of the National Cholesterol Education Program (NCEP) Expert Panel on Detection, Evaluation, and Treatment of High Blood Cholesterol in Adults (Adult Treatment Panel III) final report. Circulation. 2002;106(25):3143-421.
9. Cefalu E, William T. Standards of medical care in diabetes—2016. Diabetes Care. 2016;39(Suppl 1):2-47.
10. Joshi PH, Chaudhari S, Blaha MJ, et al. A point-by-point response to recent arguments against the use of statins in primary prevention. Clin Cardiol. 2012;35(7):404-9.
11. Cholesterol Treatment Trialists' (CTT) Collaborators, Kearney PM, Blackwell L, et al. Efficacy of cholesterol-lowering therapy in 18,686 people with diabetes in 14 randomised trials of statins: a meta-analysis. Lancet. 2008;371(9607):117-25.

12. Ridekr PM, Danielson E, Fonseca FA, et al. Rosuvastatin to prevent vascular events in men and women with elevated C-reactive protein. N Engl J Med. 2008;359(21):2195-207.
13. Berne C, Siewert-Delle A; URANUS study investigators. .Comparison of rosuvastatin and atorvastatin for lipid lowering in patients with type 2 diabetes mellitus: results from the URANUS study. Cardiovasc Diabetol. 2005;4:7.
14. Simsek S, Schalkwijk CG, Wolffenbuttel BH. Effects of rosuvastatin and atorvastatin on glycaemic control in Type 2 diabetes—the CORALL study. Diabet Med. 2012;29(5):628-31.
15. Holdass H, Holme I, Schmieder RE, et al. Rosuvastatin in diabetic hemodialysis patients. J Am Soc Nephrol. 2011;22(7):1335-41.
16. Katabami T, Murakami M, Kobayashi S, et al. Efficacy of low-dose rosuvastatin in patients with type 2 diabetes and hypo high-density lipoprotein cholesterolaemia. J Int Med Res. 2014;42(2):457-67.
17. Dugani SB, Akinkuolie AO, Paynter N, et al. Association of Lipoproteins, Insulin Resistance, and Rosuvastatin With Incident Type 2 Diabetes Mellitus: Secondary Analysis of a Randomized Clinical Trial. JAMA Cardiol. 2016;1(2):136-45.
18. Hou W, Lv J, Perkovic V, et al. Effect of statin therapy on cardiovascular and renal outcomes in patients with chronic kidney disease: a systematic review and meta-analysis. Eur Heart J. 2013;34(24):1807-17.
19. Chyoyu AC, Thodge A, Feldman DN, et al. Statins in the prevention of contrast-induced nephropathy. Curr Treat Options Cardio Med. 2015;17(4):375.
20. Ameracano P, Lavallëe PC, Mazighi M, et al. Statins in Stroke Prevention. Future Lipidol. 2008;3(3):319-25.
21. Averna M, Lo Verde A. Statin and Metabolic syndrome. Int Congr Ser. 2003;1253:243-6.
22. Davignon J. Beneficial cardiovascular pleiotropic effects of statins. Circulation. 2004;109(23 Suppl 1):III39-43.
23. Nicholls SJ, Brandrup-Wognsen G, Palmer M, et al. Meta-analysis of comparative efficacy of increasing dose of Atorvastatin versus Rosuvastatin versus Simvastatin on lowering levels of atherogenic lipids (from VOYAGER). Am J Cardiol. 2010;105(1):69-76.
24. Karlson BW, Barter PJ, Palmer MK, et al. Comparison of the effects of different statins and doses on lipid levels in patients with diabetes: results from VOYAGER. Nutr Metab Cardiovasc Dis. 2012;22(9):697-703.
25. Schuster H, Watkins C, Ditmarsch M. Long-term safety and efficacy analysis from rosuvastatin-treated diabetic patients: results from the MERCURY I Study (Measuring Effective Reductions in Cholesterol Using Rosuvastatin therapY). Diabetologia. 2005;48(A391):1084.
26. Fox KM, Gandhi SK, Ohsfeldt RL, et al. Effectiveness of rosuvastatin in low-density lipoprotein cholesterol lowering and National Cholesterol Education Program Adult Treatment Panel guideline III LDL-C goal attainment compared to other statins among diabetes mellitus patients: a retrospective study using an electronic medical records dataset in the United States. Curr Med Res Opin. 2007;23(9):2125-33.

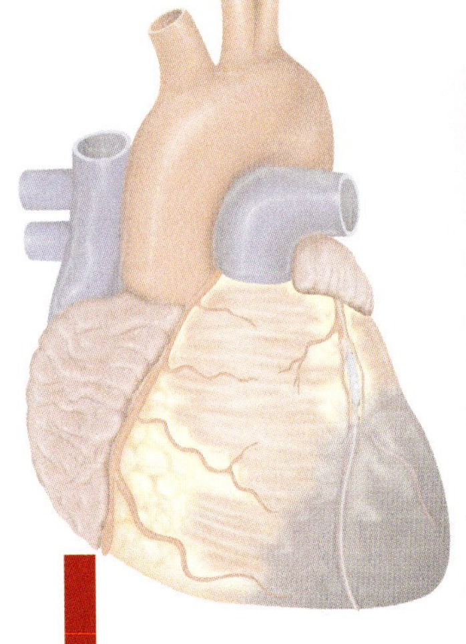

Diabetic Hypertriglyceridemia: Management Strategies

HK Chopra, Ashok Jaiswal, Harmeet Singh

INTRODUCTION

Diabetes mellitus (DM) is a metabolic syndrome that is linked with considerable risk of premature atherosclerosis, mainly coronary heart disease (CHD) and peripheral arterial disease (PAD).[1,2] In the past decade, DM has come up, to be one of the most important cardiovascular disease (CVD) risk factors and even has been considered as an equivalent to myocardial infarction (MI).[3] It is estimated that patients with diabetes have a two-fold to four-fold higher risk of ischemic disease, including CHD, stroke, and PAD, than nondiabetic people[4] and in people without diabetes, elevated fasting blood glucose concentration and glycated hemoglobin (HbA1c) has also been associated with the risk of vascular disease.[5,6] Being a highly populated country, India has a substantial population suffering from DM. The Indian Council of Medical Research-INdia DIABetes (ICMR-INDIAB) study had extrapolated its phase I results in 2011, which estimated 62.4 million individuals with diabetes and 77.2 million with prediabetes in India.[7] In type 2 DM (T2DM), an increased risk for CVD often exists for many years before the actual onset of biochemical hyperglycemia. During this phase, obesity and insulin resistance are usually present, in association with hypertension and dyslipidemia, and is often referred to as metabolic syndrome.[8] These risk factors generally lead to an early development of CHD and an increased incidence of diabetes, subsequent to the diagnosis of the CVD.[9] Dyslipidemia has been found to be a common risk factor and powerful predictor of CVD in high-risk patients, including those with T2DM.[10,11] Presence of T2DM and dyslipidemia have both shown an increase in cardiovascular (CV) risk by 3–4 times as compared to nondiabetic patients with dyslipidemia.[12] Dyslipidemia is one of the main risk factors for macrovascular complications in patients with T2DM.[13] In patients with diabetes, a change in the distribution of lipids increases the risk of atherosclerosis. Specifically, insulin resistance and insulin deficiency have been identified as causes of dyslipidemia in patients with diabetes mellitus.[14] Low-density lipoprotein C (LDL-C) is necessary for the assessment of risk due to lipoproteins. Elevated LDL-C levels have been an established risk factor for CVD and play an important role in diabetes. Current guidelines also suggest that the level of LDL-C is the primary target of cardiovascular (CV) risk in people with diabetes.[15] However, LDL-C levels alone do not reflect the typical characteristics of diabetic dyslipidemia that are hypertriglyceridemia and low high density lipoprotein cholesterol (HDL-C). Although LDL-C is the main target for treatment,[3,16] clinical trials have consistently demonstrated high residual CV risk in statin-treated patients. This may be as statins do not completely correct the vascular risk that is attributed to atherogenic dyslipidemia.[11] The most common pattern of dyslipidemia in T2DM patients is atherogenic dyslipidemia which is reflected by elevated triglycerides (TGs), increased levels of small dense LDL-C (sdLDL-C) particles and decreased HDL cholesterol levels.[17] But multiple evidences from the past two decades, from genetic studies[18-21] and multiple HDL-C increasing trials, which have failed to show CV risk reduction benefit,[22-25] portray low HDL-C to be a simple bystander, rather than a long-term marker of high levels of TGs.[26,27] In the last decade, after tackling LDL-C, the focus has shifted to addressing TGs, rather than HDL-C, supported by multiple insights from emerging evidences in the recent years on the role of hypertriglyceridemia in CVD, especially with diabetes. In this chapter, we will be looking briefly at diabetic hypertriglyceridemia and its management.

DIABETIC HYPERTRIGLYCERIDEMIA AND ATHEROSCLEROSIS

In 1990, Austin et al. were the first to describe a risk-conferring lipid/lipoprotein profile, that was termed "atherogenic dyslipidemia" or the "atherogenic lipoprotein phenotype" that comprised a higher proportion of sdLDL-C particles, reduced HDL-C, and increased TGs.[28] These abnormalities are also reflected by an increase in plasma concentrations of nonHDL-C cholesterol and apolipoprotein B-100 (apoB-100).[29] Atherogenic dyslipidemia is typically seen in patients with obesity, the metabolic syndrome, insulin resistance, and T2DM[30,31] and has emerged as an important marker for atherosclerosis and the increased CVD risk observed in these populations. In diabetes, hypertriglyceridemia is rarely observed alone, rather, it is a combination of hypertriglyceridemia, low HDL-C and high levels of sdLDL-C levels that are generally observed and termed as "atherogenic dyslipidemia" or "atherogenic diabetic dyslipidemia (ADD)". ADD is commonly seen in Asian Indians, though the precise reason for such dyslipidemia is unknown. Genetic predisposition and characteristic body composition (excess intra-abdominal fat) may play a vital role and the common outcome of such a body composition and dyslipidemia in Asian Indians is the tendency to develop insulin resistance.[32] In diabetes, there are multiple factors that influence the changes in lipid metabolism, like hyperglycemia, adipocytokines, and insulin deficiency or resistance.[33] There are multiple facets to the pathophysiology and consequences of diabetic dyslipidemia, that are still not clear, but the process by which hypertriglyceridemia arises and affects, is well understood.[34] Insulin resistance or deficiency seen in DM, activates the hormone sensitive lipase intracellularly, causing an increase in the release of nonesterified free fatty acids (FFA) from TGs that are generally stored in the centrally distributed adipose tissues.[35] The increased levels of FFAs in the circulation lead to an increase in the hepatic production of TGs and increased secretin of apolipoprotein B (apoB) from the liver (Fig. 1).[36] Additionally, the normal effect of insulin of inhibition on the production of apoB from the liver and TG secretion from very-low-density lipoprotein (VLDL) is lost, therefore a larger and more TG rich VLDL is secreted.[37-39] Further, decreased VLDL catabolism also results in increased levels of TGs.[33] In the blood, lipoprotein lipase is the key enzyme which determines the rate of removal of TGs from the circulation, and is normally located on the vascular endothelium. In conditions of insulin resistance or deficiency, there is a downregulation of lipoprotein lipase, which is also known to contribute in the occurrence of postprandial lipemia.[33,40]

Though triglyceride-rich lipoproteins (TGRLs) like chylomicrons and VLDL are not considered to be directly responsible for atherogenesis, they play an important role in the mechanism by which small dense LDL-C particles are generated and HDL cholesterol levels are reduced in diabetes.[1] In type 1 and type 2 diabetes, under the action of cholesteryl ester transfer protein (CETP), the rate of exchange of cholesteryl esters from other lipoproteins into the expanding pool of TGRLs, is greatly increased.[41,42] The TGs are transferred in the opposite direction in such a way that the cholesteryl ester depleted HDL and LDL become rich in TGs. Subsequently, under the action of hepatic lipase, this TG is removed, resulting in smaller denser LDL particles and dysfunctional HDL particles. This increase in the number of sdLDL particles, at relatively normal and unchanged LDL-C and apoB levels in many patients with diabetes, may hide major atherogenic changes.[43,44] These sdLDL-C particles are highly atherogenic and serve as a better predictor of CV risk as compared to LDL-C in diabetics.[45,46] They tend to penetrate the arterial intima more easily and have an enhanced susceptibility of being retained in the extracellular matrix by adhering to arterial proteoglycans and also have decreased antioxidant properties.[47-49] It is necessary to correct a common misunderstanding that TG concentration is a poor marker of CV risk. In fact, in both type 1 and type 2 diabetes, there is a strong connection between TGs and CHD. Increased levels of TGs often portend the development of T2DM, particularly when observed in conjunction with other features of metabolic syndrome or CHD, and continue to predict the risk of CHD even after the development of diabetes, independent of other risk factors.[50]

Extensive recent evidences also point to the fact that both elevated TGs are predictive for CVD. A recent study which analyzed data from 75,725 participants with a median follow-up of 34 years, found that those participants who had a nonfasting TG of less than 90 mg/dL had a 60% lesser risk of ischemic heart disease as compared to participants who had a nonfasting TG of more than 350 mg/dL. The same study also found that heterozygosity for loss-of-function mutations in APOC3 in 260 individuals (which predisposed these individuals to lifelong low levels of TG) were associated with a mean reduction in nonfasting

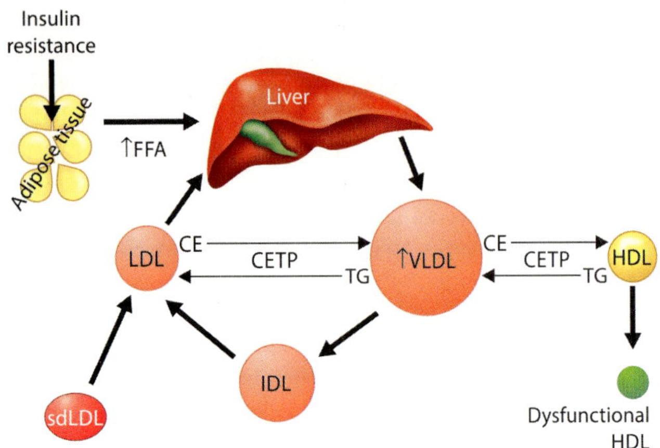

Fig. 1: Consequences of increased triglycerides and triglyceride rich lipoproteins in diabetes

Abbreviations: FFA, free fatty acids; VLDL, very-low density lipoprotein; IDL, intermediate density lipoprotein; LDL, low-density lipoprotein; sdLDL, small dense low density lipoprotein; TG, triglyceride; CE, cholesteryl ester; CETP, cholesteryl ester transfer protein; HDL, high density lipoprotein

TG levels of 44% and a corresponding 41% decrease in the incidence of ischemic vascular disease as compared to the general noncarrier population.[51] In a recent publication in 2016, higher TG levels were found to be independently associated with an increased 22 years, all-cause mortality in more than 15000 patients. The 22-year risk of death in patients with TG levels greater than or equal to 500 mg/dL was significantly increased by 68% as compared to patients who had low normal TG levels (p <0.001), and in the patients who had moderate hypertriglyceridemia (200–499 mg/dL), there was a significant 29% higher risk of death as compared to those patients with a low-to-normal TGs level (p <0.001).[52] The Strong Heart Study, published in 2017, was a prospective cohort of 3216 American Indians who were free from CVD at baseline and were followed up for a period of 17.7 years. It was observed in this study that those participants who had high TG (≥150 mg/dL) and low HDL levels (≤40 mg/dL for men, ≤50 for women) had a 32% higher risk for CHD as compared to those with normal TG and normal HDL levels, and in those participants who had diabetes, high TG levels and low HDL levels were associated with a significant 54% greater risk for CHD (p = 0.003) and 2.13-fold greater risk for stroke (p = 0.060).[53] Another recent analysis of two large randomized controlled trials (RCTs) demonstrated, in patients who had suffered an acute coronary syndrome (ACS) and treated effectively with statins, elevated fasting TG levels predicted recurring CV risk at long term and short term. For long-term evaluation, the authors considered the dal-OUTCOMES trial, which was a randomized, double-blind comparison of dalcetrapib with placebo in 15,871 patients who had ACS. The CV risk up till 31 months was found to increase across quintiles of TG levels, and the HR in the highest/lowest quintile (>175/≤80 mg/dL) was 1.50 (95% CI: 1.05–2.15), and in the MIRACL (Myocardial Ischemia Reduction with Aggressive Cholesterol Lowering) trial, which was a randomized, double-blind comparison of atorvastatin 80 mg daily with placebo in 2086 patients with ACS, the CV risk observed up till 16 weeks increased across tertiles of baseline TGs, with an HR of 1.51 (95% CI: 1.05–2.15) in highest/lowest tertiles (>195/≤135 mg/dL), and more importantly what was observed in this analysis was that this relationship between TGs and cardiovascular risk was independent of LDL cholesterol.[54]

Various guidelines and expert consensus have also recognized the importance of atherogenic dyslipidemia (along with TGs) as one of the key factors of CV risk in insulin-resistant states, even in spite of controlled LDL cholesterol levels.[16,55-58] Thus, targeting TGs in diabetes, secondary to LDL cholesterol reduction has a potential for reducing the residual risk a diabetic might face.

MANAGEMENT OF DIABETIC HYPERTRIGLYCERIDEMIA

For mild-to-moderately raised TGs, other secondary causes of raised TGs such as alcohol intake, hypothyroidism, pregnancy, hepatosteatosis,[59,60] weight regain after substantial weight loss, nephrotic syndrome,[61] and use of some medicines (such as highly active antiretroviral therapy, particularly protease inhibitors; second-generation antipsychotics; glucocorticoids and old types of oral estrogens)[62,63] should be ruled out and treated accordingly.

Lifestyle Management

Lifestyle management is the first and foremost intervention in the management of diabetic dyslipidemia, with the main aim of losing weight through dietary modification and exercising more.[36] Obesity is known to increase insulin resistance and is also linked with elevated levels of TGs and other dyslipidemias.[1] With weight loss, there are improvements seen in lipids and reduction of incidence of T2DM and other CV risk factors has also been observed, and, therefore should be advocated in all diabetics.[64,65] To attain prolonged loss of weight, restriction of calories is paramount and even small degrees of weight loss were linked with betterment of the lipid profile, glycemic and HbA1c control.[66] On the other hand, physical exercise provides additional effect along with dietary restrictions, but is unlikely to be efficacious on its own.[67] The American Diabetes Association (ADA) recommends a diet low in trans fat, saturated fat, and cholesterol.[68] Though dietary interventions are considered the first-line of option for all patients with diabetes, they have yet to be successful in demonstrating a mortality benefit, in spite of prolonged follow-up.[69]

Effect of Hypoglycemic Agents on Hypertriglyceridemia

Diabetic hypertriglyceridemia can be partially rectified by insulin therapy and better blood glucose control. Insulin therapy tends to elevate HDL cholesterol and decrease the circulating TG levels, particularly in patients with poor glycemic control.[70] Metformin in addition to being the first-line hypoglycemic agent, also reduces TGs and improves insulin resistance, but is generally overlooked as a lipid-lowering agent.[71] There are other antidiabetic agents, like gliclazide, pioglitazone and glucagon-like peptide-1 (GLP-1) agonists (exenatide and liraglutide) which also have a moderate effect on TG levels by reducing it.[72-74]

Lipid-lowering Drugs

Statins

Statins are without doubt, the first-line lipid lowering agents used. A linear relationship is clearly distinguishable between the degree of LDL-C lowering achieved with statins and their benefits, with a 10% and 21% reduction seen in all-cause mortality and major vascular events, respectively per 39 mg/dL reduction in LDL-C levels. This is supported further by data showing superiority of intensive LDL-C lowering. Benefits have also been seen in people with CHD, stroke, or diabetes and those who are healthy.[75] Apart from the above effects, statins also decrease TGs in the range of 7% to 37% depending on the TG levels, the statin used and its dose.[3] Statins are generally well-tolerated apart from myalgia, although its frequency is more in clinical settings than in RCTs and as per a recent observational data in more than two million individuals, has shown that acute renal failure might also be a dose-related side effect of statins, although with very low incidence.[76] Another meta-analysis of statin RCTs has shown that one incident case of new type 2 diabetes may occur for every 225 individuals that are treated for 4 years with statins,[77] and, in spite of achieving the LDL-C target with the recommended statin therapy, there is still a high "residual risk" which requires a more aggressive therapy, especially in conditions like diabetes.[11]

Fibrates

Fibrates [peroxisome proliferator-activated receptor-α (PPAR-α) agonists] are one of the major options for treating hypertriglyceridemia, especially in the context of high-risk individuals with insulin resistance.[78] In a subgroup analyses of the FIELD (fenofibrate intervention and event lowering in diabetes) study, T2DM patients with marked atherogenic dyslipidemia, defined as TGs greater than or equal to 204 mg/dL and low HDL cholesterol, obtained greater benefit from fenofibrate treatment than those without this dyslipidemia. About 19% of the total study population fell into this group and a 27% relative reduction in CV risk was seen as compared to the 11% relative risk reduction in the total population.[79] Subsequently, in the ACCORD trial (n = 5,518), a prespecified subgroup analysis demonstrated a substantial benefit associated on adding fenofibrate with background simvastatin in T2DM patients with marked atherogenic dyslipidemia defined by baseline TGs of greater than or equal to 204 mg/dL and baseline HDL cholesterol levels of less than or equal to 34 mg/dL. About 17% of the overall study population was part of this dyslipidemia group. Nearly 30% relative reduction in CV events were observed as compared to the lack of benefit that was observed in the remaining 83% of the study population.[80] Additionally, a meta-analysis of subgroups with similar lipid criteria for atherogenic dyslipidemia in the major fibrate trials confirmed this benefit on residual CV risk.[81] Fibrate therapy was found to be associated with a 35% relative reduction in CV risk in individuals with atherogenic dyslipidemia as compared to 6% in individuals without this dyslipidemia. A subsequent meta-analysis of fibrate trials (n = 45,058) indicated that the reduction in CV risk related with this therapy class is mainly due to prevention of cardiac events.[82] The advantages of TG lowering on residual CV risk may be associated with the effects of endogenous pathways for PPAR-α *activation on atherosclerosis. Lipolysis in certain situations can generate PPAR ligands and also limit some* of the known inflammatory responses.[83] A subsequent study of the ACCORD (Action to Control Cardiovascular Risk in Diabetes) Lipid trial, which evaluated effects on postprandial lipemia, provides a probable reason as to why the benefit of fibrates is specific to patients with atherogenic dyslipidemia.[84] Compared with the simvastatin monotherapy group, treatment with the combination of fenofibrate plus simvastatin led to significant reductions in postprandial exposure to TGs and apoB-48, indicating a decrease in the accumulation of atherogenic, intestinally derived TGRL remnants. This effect of fenofibrate was selective to patients with elevated fasting TGs at baseline. Added to this, there is also evidence of benefit with fenofibrate on diabetes-related microvascular complications, including diabetic retinopathy and nephropathy.[85-89] Despite this favorable profile of macro- and microvascular benefits, the efficacy of the current fibrates may be limited by the increased risk of muscle-related symptoms with the combination of a statin and certain fibrates, specifically gemfibrozil. Other commonly reported adverse effects include increases in homocysteine, creatinine and liver enzymes, markers of CVD, renal disease and hepatic dysfunction, respectively.[80,87]

Omega-3 Fatty Acids

Purified omega-3 fatty acids can lower TGs as much as fibrates, but they have little effect on HDL or LDL-C.[90] There were positive findings from JELIS (Japan Eicosapentaenoic acid Lipid Intervention Study) (n=18,645) with the combination of omega-3 fatty acids [1.8 g/day of eicosapentaenoic acid (EPA)] plus statin versus statin alone, both overall and in patients with the metabolic syndrome.[91] A post-hoc analysis of JELIS evaluated the effect of EPA treatment in individuals with atherogenic dyslipidemia as defined by TGs greater than or equal to 150 mg/dL and HDL cholesterol less than 40 mg/dL, representing 5% of the total study population. In this group, EPA treatment reduced the risk of coronary artery disease by 53% ($p = 0.043$), compared with those individuals without this dyslipidemia.[92] More recently, the ORIGIN (Outcome Reduction with an Initial Glargine Intervention) trial with omega-3 fatty acids did not show any significant effect on the primary outcome (CV death) or any of the secondary or additional outcomes.[11,93] Additionally, a recent meta-analysis of trials of omega-3 supplementation (n = 68,680 subjects in 20 trials, mean dose 1.51 g/day) failed to show any significant association with all-cause mortality, cardiac death, sudden death, MI, or stroke.[94]

Dual PPAR Agonists

A particular area of interest is the next generation of PPAR agonists. PPAR-α *plays a key role in lipid metabolism, whereas PPAR-γ is critical* in regulating energy metabolism in adipose tissue and muscle, as well as being targets for the treatment of insulin resistance.[95] Dual PPAR-α/γ *agonist agents are developed for their dual actions on dyslipidemia and dysglycemia in patients with ADD.* Saroglitazar is currently the only agent of this class approved for clinical usage in India (India, June 2013). Saroglitazar is a nonfibric acid and nonthiazolidinedione derivative. It is a dual PPAR-α and PPAR-γ agonist that has been approved in India for the treatment of diabetic dyslipidemia and hypertriglyceridemia in T2DM, not controlled with statin therapy. Saroglitazar has predominant PPAR-α *action with moderate PPAR-γ action.* Saroglitazar provides a comprehensive management of diabetic dyslipidemia by reducing TGs (46.7%) and non-HDL-C (32%) and also provides moderate glycemic control by reducing glycated hemoglobin levels and fasting blood glucose. It is a safer option for the management of atherogenic dyslipidemia in diabetes.[96,97] Saroglitazar is not associated with weight gain or edema and it does not increase serum creatinine. Currently saroglitazar is being evaluated in Phase III, placebo-controlled, double-blind, randomized clinical trial for its safety and efficacy in patients with nonalcoholic fatty liver disease (NAFLD) and nonalcoholic steatohepatitis (NASH).

RECENT GUIDELINES AND RECOMMENDATIONS

Recent international guidelines recommend addressing diabetic hypertriglyceridemia. With the recent 2016 European Society of Cardiology (ESC) and European Atherosclerosis Society (EAS) guidelines on the management of dyslipidemia recommending that drug treatment should be considered in high-risk patients with TG greater than 2.3 mmol/L (200 mg/dL), wherein a person having diabetes would come under the high-risk category. And in these high-risk patients with TG greater than 2.3 mmol/L (200 mg/dL) despite statin treatment, TG-lowering therapy may be considered in combination with statins.[98] Whereas, the American Diabetes Association suggests that statin and TG lowering may be considered in male patients with both TG level greater than or equal to 204 mg/dL (2.3 mmol/L) and HDL cholesterol level less than or equal to 34 mg/dL (0.9 mmol/L).[68] While, the AACE 2017 guidelines recommended that TG levels should be a part of the routine lipid screening wherein moderate elevations (≥150 mg/dL) may identify individuals at a risk for the insulin resistance and levels greater than or equal to 200 mg/dL may identify individuals at substantially increased atherosclerotic cardiovascular disease (ASCVD) risk and also recommend a TG goal of less than 150 mg/dL. If the TGs levels are severely elevated (>500 mg/dL), begin treatment with a very low-fat diet and reduced intake of simple carbohydrates and initiate combinations of a fibrate, omega-3-fatty acid, and/or niacin to reduce TG levels and to prevent pancreatitis.[99]

CONCLUSION

Diabetic dyslipidemia is a widespread condition, in which insulin resistance is suggested to be the driving force behind the characteristic lipid abnormalities. The frequency of hypertriglyceridemia in T2DM has been found to be reasonably high. Effectively managing diabetic dyslipidemia (high TGs and low HDL-C) has been shown to be significant in reducing the risk of CVD. Evidence from multiple sources strongly support the treatment of diabetic dyslipidemia and with the focus shifting on treating its major components, i.e. hypertriglyceridemia and high small dense LDL levels. Lifestyle and pharmacological interventions are the most important treatment strategies. Treatment with statins is so far the most effective approach to decrease cardiovascular risk in diabetic patients. However, significant residual risk in statin-treated patients and statin intolerance in some patients still remains an unsolved problem. In patients with severe hypertriglyceridemia, triglyceride-lowering therapy should be used to lower triglyceride levels to less than 500 mg/dL and to avert the risk of pancreatitis. In patients with mild-to-moderate hypertriglyceridemia (200–499 mg/dL), consideration should be given to achieve adequate glycemic control and, if required, followed by TG-lowering therapy, to address the residual risk of ASCVD, remaining after statin therapy.

REFERENCES

1. Durrington P. Hyperlipidaemia. Diagnosis and Management, 3rd edition, 2007.
2. Laing SP, Swerdlow AJ, Slater SD, et al. Mortality from heart disease in a cohort of 23,000 patients with insulin-treated diabetes. Diabetologia. 2003;46(6):760-5.
3. National Cholesterol Education Program (NCEP) Expert panel on detection, evaluation, and treatment of high blood cholesterol in adults (adult treatment panel III). Third report of the National Cholesterol Education Program (NCEP) Expert panel on detection, evaluation, and treatment of high blood cholesterol in adults (adult treatment panel III) final report. Circulation. 2002;106(25):3143-421.
4. Solano MP, Goldberg RB. Management of dyslipidemia in diabetes. Cardiol Rev. 2006;14(3):125-35.
5. Emerging Risk Factors Collaboration, Sarwar N, Gao P, et al. Diabetes mellitus, fasting blood glucose concentration, and risk of vascular disease: a collaborative meta-analysis of 102 prospective studies. Lancet. 2010;375:2215-22.
6. Selvin E, Steffes MW, Zhu H, et al. Glycated hemoglobin, diabetes, and cardiovascular risk in nondiabetic adults. N Engl J Med. 2010;362:800-11.
7. Anjana RM, Pradeepa R, Deepa M, et al. Prevalence of diabetes and prediabetes (impaired fasting glucose and/or impaired glucose tolerance) in urban and rural India: phase I results of the Indian Council of Medical Research-INdia DIABetes (ICMR-INDIAB) study. Diabetologia. 2011;54:3022-7.
8. Haffner SM, Stern MP, Hazuda HP, et al. Cardiovascular risk factors in confirmed prediabetic individuals. Does the clock for coronary heart disease start ticking before the onset of clinical diabetes? JAMA. 1990;263:2893-8.
9. Farrer M, Fulcher G, Albers CJ, et al. Patients undergoing coronary artery bypass graft surgery are at high risk of impaired glucose tolerance and diabetes mellitus during the first postoperative year. Metabolism. 1995;44:1016-27.
10. Turner RC, Millns H, Neil AW, et al. Risk factors for coronary artery disease in non-insulin dependent diabetes mellitus: United Kingdom prospective diabetes study (UKPDS:23). Br Med J. 1998; 316(7134):823-8.
11. Fruchart JC, Sacks F, Hermans MP, et al. The Residual Risk Reduction Initiative: A Call to Action to Reduce Residual Vascular Risk in Patients with Dyslipidemia. Am J Cardiol. 2008. 102(10 Supplement 1):1K-34K.
12. Stamler J, Vaccaro O, Neaton JD, et al. Multiple Risk Factor Intervention Trial Research Group. Diabetes, other risk factors, and 12-yr cardiovascular mortality for men screened in the Multiple Risk Factor Intervention Trial. Diabetes Care. 1993;16(2):434-44.
13. Farmer JA. Diabetic dyslipidemia and atherosclerosis: evidence from clinical trials. Curr Diab Rep.2008;8(1):71-7.
14. Chahil TJ, Ginsberg HN. Diabetic dyslipidemia. Endocrinol Metab Clin North Am. 2006;35(3):491-510.
15. Buse JB, Ginsberg HN, Bakris GL, et al. Primary prevention of cardiovascular diseases in people with diabetes mellitus: a scientific statement from the American Heart Association and the American Diabetes Association. Circulation. 2007;115(1):114-26.
16. Brunzell JD, Davidson M, Furberg CD, et al. Lipoprotein management in patients with cardiometabolic risk: consensus statement from the American Diabetes Association and the American College of Cardiology Foundation. J Am Coll Cardiol. 2008;31:811-22.
17. American Diabetes Association. Management of dyslipidemia in adults with diabetes. Diabetes Care. 2003;26(Suppl 1):s83-es86.
18. Andersen RV, Wittrup HH, Tybjaerg-Hansen A, et al. Hepatic lipase mutations, elevated high-density lipoprotein cholesterol, and increased risk of ischemic heart disease: the Copenhagen City Heart Study. J Am Coll Cardiol. 2003;41:1972-82.
19. Frikke-Schmidt R, Nordestgaard BG, Stene MC, et al. Association of loss-of-function mutations in the ABCA1 gene with high-density lipoprotein cholesterol levels and risk of ischemic heart disease. JAMA. 2008;299:2524-32.
20. Haase CL, Tybjærg-Hansen A, Qayyum AA, et al. LCAT, HDL cholesterol and ischemic cardiovascular disease: a Mendelian randomization study of HDL cholesterol in 54,500 individuals. J Clin Endocrinol Metab. 2012;97:E248-E256.
21. Voight BF, Peloso GM, Orho-Melander M, et al. Plasma HDL cholesterol and risk of myocardial infarction: a Mendelian randomisation study. Lancet. 2012;380:572-80.
22. Barter PJ, Caulfield M, Eriksson M, et al, ILLUMINATE Investigators. Effects of torcetrapib in patients at high risk for coronary events. N Engl J Med. 2007;357:2109-22.
23. Schwartz GG, Olsson AG, Abt M, et al, dal-OUTCOMES Investigators. Effects of dalcetrapib in patients with a recent acute coronary syndrome. N Engl J Med. 2012;367:2089-99.
24. Boden WE, Probstfield JL, Anderson T, et al. Niacin in patients with low HDL cholesterol levels receiving intensive statin therapy. N Engl J Med. 2011;365:2255-67.
25. Landray MJ, Haynes R, Hopewell JC, et al. Effects of extended-release niacin with laropiprant in high-risk patients. N Engl J Med. 2014;371:203-12.
26. Nordestgaard BG, Langsted A, Freiberg JJ. Nonfasting hyperlipidemia and cardiovascular disease. Curr Drug Targets. 2009;10:328-35.
27. Nordestgaard BG, Varbo A. Triglycerides and cardiovascular disease. Lancet. 2014;384:626-35.
28. Austin MA, King MC, Vranizan KM, et al. Atherogenic lipoprotein phenotype. A proposed genetic marker for coronary heart disease risk. Circulation. 1990;82:495-506.
29. Watts GF, Karpe F. Triglycerides and atherogenic dyslipidaemia: extending treatment beyond statins in the high-risk cardiovascular patient. Heart. 2011;97(5):350-6.
30. Reaven GM, Chen YD, Jeppesen J, et al. Insulin resistance and hyperinsulinemia in individuals with small, dense low-density lipoprotein particles. J Clin Invest. 1993;92:141-6.
31. Kathiresan S, Otvos JD, Sullivan LM, et al. Increased small low-density lipoprotein particle number: a prominent feature of the metabolic syndrome in the Framingham Heart Study. Circulation. 2006;113:20-9.
32. Misra A, Luthra K, Vikram NK. Dyslipidemia in Asian Indians: determinants and significance. J Assoc Physicians India. 2004;52:137-42.
33. Taskinen MR. Diabetic dyslipidaemia: from basic research to clinical practice. Diabetologia. 2003;46:733-49.

34. Verges B. Pathophysiology of diabetic dyslipidaemia: where are we? Diabetologia. 2015;58:886-99.
35. Nikkila EA, Kekki M. Plasma triglyceride transport kinetics in diabetes mellitus. Metabolism. 1973;22:1-22.
36. Warraich HJ, Wong ND, Rana JS. Role for combination therapy in diabetic dyslipidemia. Curr Cardiol Rep. 2015;17:32.
37. McEneny J, O'Kane MJ, Moles KW, et al. Very low density lipoprotein subfractions in type II diabetes mellitus: alterations in composition and susceptibility to oxidation. Diabetologia. 2000;43:485-93.
38. Malmstrom R, Packard CJ, Caslake M, et al. Defective regulation of triglyceride metabolism by insulin in the liver in NIDDM. Diabetologia. 1997;40:454-62.
39. Cummings MH, Watts GF, Umpleby AM, et al. Acute hyperinsulinemia decreases the hepatic secretion of very-low-density lipoprotein apolipoprotein B-100 in NIDDM. Diabetes. 1995;44:1059-65.
40. Chen YD, Swami S, Skowronski R, et al. Differences in postprandial lipemia between patients with normal glucose tolerance and noninsulin-dependent diabetes mellitus. J Clin Endocrinol Metab. 1993;76:172-7.
41. Bagdade JD, Ritter MC, Subbaiah PV. Accelerated cholesteryl ester transfer in patients with insulin-dependent diabetes mellitus. Eur J Clin Invest. 1991;21:161-7.
42. Bhatnagar D, Durrington PN, Kumar S, et al. Plasma lipoprotein composition and cholesteryl ester transfer from high-density lipoproteins to very low-density and low-density lipoproteins in patients with non-insulin-dependent diabetes mellitus. Diabet Med. 1996;13:139-44.
43. Krauss RM. Lipids and lipoproteins in patients with type 2 diabetes. Diabetes Care. 2004;27:1496-504.
44. Schonfeld G, Birge C, Miller JP, et al. Apolipoprotein B levels and altered lipoprotein composition in diabetes. Diabetes. 1974;23:827-34.
45. Musunuru K. Atherogenic dyslipidemia: cardiovascular risk and dietary intervention. Lipids. 2010;45(10):907-14.
46. Adiels M, Olofsson SO, Taskinen MR, et al. Overproduction of very low-density lipoproteins is the hallmark of the dyslipidemia in the metabolic syndrome. Arterioscler Thromb Vascular Biology. 2008;28(7):1225-36.
47. Vinik AI. The metabolic basis of atherogenic dyslipidemia. Clin Cornerston. 2005;7:27-35.
48. Grundy SM. Hypertriglyceridemia, atherogenic dyslipidemia and the metabolic syndrome. Am J Cardiol. 1998;81:18B-25.
49. Griffin BA, Minihane AM, Furlonger N, et al. Inter-relationships between small, dense low-density lipoprotein (LDL), plasma triacylglycerol and LDL apoprotein B in an atherogenic lipoprotein phenotype in free-living subjects. Clin Sci (Lond). 1999;97:269-76.
50. West KM, Ahuja MM, Bennett PH, et al. The role of circulating glucose and triglyceride concentrations and their interactions with other "risk factors" as determinants of arterial disease in nine diabetic population samples from the WHO multinational study. Diabetes Care. 1983;6(4):361-9.
51. Jørgensen AB, Frikke-Schmidt R, Nordestgaard BG, et al. Loss-of-function mutations in APOC3 and risk of ischemic vascular disease. N Eng J Medicine. 2014;371(1):32-41.
52. Klempfner R, Erez A, Sagit BZ, et al. Elevated Triglyceride Level Is Independently Associated With Increased All-cause Mortality in Patients With Established Coronary Heart Disease. Circ Cardiovasc Qual Outcomes. 2016;9(2):100-8.
53. Lee JS, Chang PY, Zhang Y, et al. Triglyceride and HDL-C dyslipidemia and risks of coronary heart disease and ischemic stroke by glycemic dysregulation status: the Strong Heart Study. Diabetes Care. 2017;40(4):529-37.
54. Schwartz GG, Abt M, Bao W, et al. Fasting triglycerides predict recurrent ischemic events in patients with acute coronary syndrome treated with statins. J Am Coll Cardiol. 2015;65(21):2267-75.
55. Reiner Z, Catapano AL, De Backer G, et al. ESC Committee for Practice Guidelines (CPG) 2008-2010 and 2010-2012 Committees. ESC/EAS guidelines for the management of dyslipidaemias: the Task Force for the management of dyslipidaemias of the European Society of Cardiology (ESC) and the European Atherosclerosis Society (EAS). Eur Heart J. 2011;32:1769-818.
56. Chapman MJ, Ginsberg HN, Amarenco P, et al. European Atherosclerosis Society Consensus Panel: Triglyceride-rich lipoproteins and high-density lipoprotein cholesterol in patients at high risk of cardiovascular disease: evidence and guidance for management. Eur Heart J. 2011;32:1345-61.
57. Perk J, De Backer G, Gohlke H, et al. European Association for Cardiovascular Prevention & Rehabilitation (EACPR); ESC Committee for Practice Guidelines (CPG): European guidelines on cardiovascular disease prevention in clinical practice (version 2012). The Fifth Joint Task Force of the European Society of Cardiology and Other Societies on Cardiovascular Disease Prevention in Clinical Practice (constituted by representatives of nine societies and by invited experts). Eur Heart J. 2012;33:1635-701.
58. Reiner Z. Managing the residual cardiovascular disease risk associated with HDL-cholesterol and triglycerides in statin-treated patients: a clinical update. Nutr Metab Cardiovasc Dis. 2013;23:799-807.
59. Clark JM. The epidemiology of nonalcoholic fatty liver disease in adults. Journal of Clinical Gastroenterology. 2006;40:S5-10.
60. Farrell GC, Larter CZ. Nonalcoholic fatty liver disease: from steatosis to cirrhosis. Hepatology. 2006;43(S1).
61. Kaysen GA. New insights into lipid metabolism in the nephrotic syndrome. Kidney International. 1999;56:S18-21.
62. Calza L, Manfredi R, Chiodo F. Dyslipidaemia associated with antiretroviral therapy in HIV-infected patients. Journal of Antimicrobial Chemotherapy. 2004;53(1):10-4.
63. American Diabetes Association. Consensus development conference on antipsychotic drugs and obesity and diabetes. Diabetes Care. 2004;27(2):596-601.
64. Sjostrom L, Lindroos AK, Peltonen M, et al. Lifestyle, diabetes, and cardiovascular risk factors 10 years after bariatric surgery. N Engl J Med. 2004;351:2683-93.
65. Wood PD, Stefanick ML, Dreon DM, et al. Changes in plasma lipids and lipoproteins in overweight men during weight loss through dieting as compared with exercise. N Engl J Med. 1988;319:1173-9.
66. Rock CL, Flatt SW, Pakiz B, et al. Weight loss, glycemic control, and cardiovascular disease risk factors in response to differential diet composition in a weight loss program in type 2 diabetes: a randomized controlled trial. Diabetes Care. 2014;37:1573-80.
67. Grundy SM. Dietary therapy of hyperlipidaemia. Baillieres Clin Endocrinol Metab. 1987;1:667-98.
68. Marathe PH, Gao HX, Close KL. American Diabetes Association standards of medical care in diabetes 2017. J Diabetes. 2017;9(4):320-4.
69. Look ARG, Wing RR, Bolin P, et al. Cardiovascular effects of intensive lifestyle intervention in type 2 diabetes. N Engl J Med. 2013;369:145-54.
70. Mihailescu DV, Vora A, Mazzone T. Lipid effects of endocrine medications. Curr Atheroscler Rep. 2011;13:88-94.
71. Stumvoll M, Nurjhan N, Perriello G, et al. Metabolic effects of metformin in non-insulin-dependent diabetes mellitus. N Engl J Med. 1995;333:550-4.
72. Monami M, Vitale V, Ambrosio ML, et al. Effects on lipid profile of dipeptidyl peptidase-4 inhibitors, pioglitazone, acarbose, and sulfonylureas: meta-analysis of placebo-controlled trials. Adv Ther. 2012;29:736-46.
73. Schwartz EA, Koska J, Mullin MP, et al. Exenatide suppresses postprandial elevations in lipids and lipoproteins in individuals with impaired glucose tolerance and recent onset type 2 diabetes mellitus. Atherosclerosis. 2010;212:217-22.

74. Hermansen K, Baekdal TA, During M, et al. Liraglutide suppresses postprandial triglyceride and apolipoprotein B48 elevations after a fat-rich meal in patients with type 2 diabetes: a randomized, double-blind, placebo-controlled, cross-over trial. Diabetes Obes Metab. 2013;15:1040-8.
75. Baigent C, Blackwell L, Emberson J, et al. Efficacy and safety of more intensive lowering of LDL cholesterol: a meta-analysis of data from 170,000 participants in 26 randomised trials. Lancet. 2010;376: 1670-81.
76. Dormuth CR, Hemmelgarn BR, Paterson JM, et al. Use of high potency statins and rates of admission for acute kidney injury: multicenter, retrospective observational analysis of administrative databases. BMJ. 2013;346:f880.
77. Sattar N, Preiss D, Murray HM, et al. Statins and risk of incident diabetes: a collaborative meta-analysis of randomised statin trials. Lancet. 2010;375:735-42.
78. Tenenbaum A, Fisman EZ. Fibrates are an essential part of modern anti-dyslipidemic arsenal: spotlight on atherogenic dyslipidemia and residual risk reduction. Cardiovasc Diabetol. 2012;11:125.
79. Scott R, O'Brien R, Fulcher G, et al. Fenofibrate intervention and event lowering in diabetes (FIELD) study investigators: Effects of fenofibrate treatment on cardiovascular disease risk in 9,795 individuals with type 2 diabetes and various components of the metabolic syndrome: the Fenofibrate Intervention and Event Lowering in Diabetes (FIELD) study. Diabetes Care. 2009;32:493-8.
80. ACCORD Study Group, Ginsberg HN, Elam MB, et al. Effects of combination lipid therapy in type 2 diabetes mellitus. N Eng J Med. 2010;362:1563-74.
81. Sacks FM, Carey VJ, Fruchart JC. Combination lipid therapy in type 2 diabetes. N Engl J Med. 2010;363:692-84.
82. Jun M, Foote C, Lv J, et al. Effects of fibrates on cardiovascular outcomes: a systematic review and meta-analysis. Lancet. 2010;375:1875-84.
83. Ziouzenkova O, Plutzky J: Lipolytic PPAR activation: new insights into the intersection of triglycerides and inflammation? Curr Opin Clin Nutr Metab Care. 2004;7:369-75.
84. Reyes-Soffer G, Ngai CI, Lovato L, et al. Effect of combination therapy with fenofibrate and simvastatin on postprandial lipemia in the ACCORD lipid trial. Diabetes Care. 2013;36:422-8.
85. Keech AC, Mitchell P, Summanen PA, et al. Effect of fenofibrate on the need for laser treatment for diabetic retinopathy (FIELD study): a randomised controlled trial. Lancet 2007;370:1687-97.
86. ACCORD Study Group, ACCORD Eye Study Group, et al. Effects of medical therapies on retinopathy progression in type 2 diabetes. N Engl J Med. 2010;363:233-44.
87. Keech A, Simes RJ, Barter P, et al. Effects of long-term fenofibrate therapy on cardiovascular events in 9795 people with type 2 diabetes mellitus (the FIELD study): randomized controlled trial. Lancet. 2005;366:1849-61.
88. Rajamani K, Colman PG, Li LP, et al. Effect of fenofibrate on amputation events in people with type 2 diabetes mellitus (FIELD study): a prespecified analysis of a randomised controlled trial. Lancet. 2009;373:1780-88.
89. Davidson MH, Armani A, McKenney JM, et al. Safety considerations with fibrate therapy. Am J Cardiol. 2007;99(6A):3C-18C.
90. Marchioli R, Barzi F, Bomba E, et al. Early protection against sudden death by n-3 polyunsaturated fatty acids after myocardial infarction: time-course analysis of the results of the Gruppo Italiano per lo Studio della Sopravvivenza nell'Infarto Miocardico (GISSI)-Prevenzione. Circulation. 2002;105:1897-903.
91. Yokoyama M, Origasa H, Matsuzaki M, et al. Japan EPA lipid intervention study (JELIS) Investigators: Effects of eicosapentaenoic acid on major coronary events in hypercholesterolaemic patients (JELIS): a randomized open-label, blinded endpoint analysis. Lancet. 2007;369:1090-8.
92. Saito Y, Yokoyama M, Origasa H, et al. Effects of EPA on coronary artery disease in hypercholesterolemic patients with multiple risk factors: sub-analysis of primary prevention cases from the Japan EPA Lipid Intervention Study (JELIS). Atherosclerosis. 2008;200(1):135-40.
93. ORIGIN Trial Investigators, Bosch J, Gerstein HC, et al. N-3 fatty acids and cardiovascular outcomes in patients with dysglycemia. N Engl J Med. 2012;367:309-18.
94. Rizos EC, Ntzani EE, Bika E, et al. Association between omega-3 fatty acid supplementation and risk of major cardiovascular disease events: a systematic review and meta-analysis. JAMA. 2012;308:1024-33.
95. Fruchart JC. Selective peroxisome proliferator-activated receptor α modulators (SPPARMα): The next generation of peroxisome proliferator-activated receptor α-agonists. Cardiovascular diabetology. 2013;12(1):82.
96. Pai V, Paneerselvam A, Mukhopadhyay S, et al. A Multicenter, Prospective, Randomized, Double-blind Study to Evaluate the Safety and Efficacy of Saroglitazar 2 and 4 mg Compared to Pioglitazone 45 mg in Diabetic Dyslipidemia (PRESS V). J Diabetes Sci Technol. 2014;8(1):132-41.
97. Jani RH, Pai V, Jha P, et al. A Multicenter, Prospective, Randomized, Double-Blind Study to Evaluate the Safety and Efficacy of Saroglitazar 2 and 4 mg Compared with Placebo in Type 2 Diabetes Mellitus Patients Having Hypertriglyceridemia Not Controlled with Atorvastatin Therapy (PRESS VI). Diabetes Technol Ther. 2014;16(2):63-71.
98. Catapano AL, Graham I, De Backer G, et al. 2016 ESC/EAS Guidelines for the Management of Dyslipidaemias. Eur Heart J. 2016;37(39):2999-3058.
99. Jellinger PS, Handelsman Y, Rosenblit PD, et al. American association of clinical endocrinologists and American College of Endocrinology guidelines for management of dyslipidemia and prevention of cardiovascular disease. Endocrine Practice. 2017;23(s2):1-87.

CHAPTER

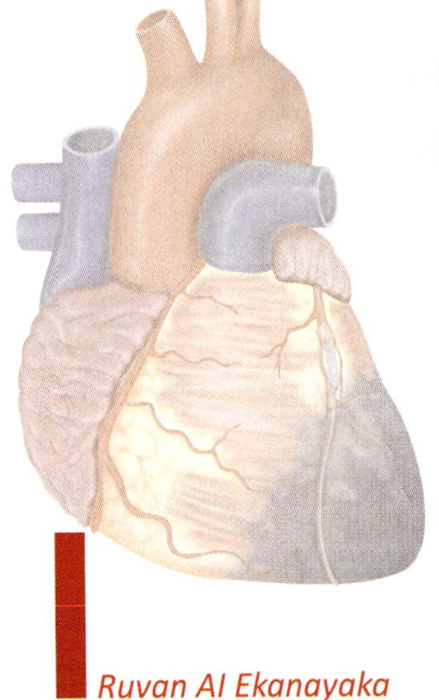

High-density Lipoprotein in Cardiodiabetes

Ruvan AI Ekanayaka

INTRODUCTION

In 2014, the global prevalence of diabetes was 422 million. The most rapid rise was seen in middle- and low-income countries, which makes diabetes mellitus (DM) a very relevant disease in most Asian countries. Diabetes leads to several cardiac complications which are covered by the umbrella term "cardio diabetes". The important cardiodiabetic conditions are coronary atherosclerosis, i.e. ischemic heart disease (IHD), diabetic cardiomyopathy, diabetic cardiac autonomic neuropathy (DCAN), and diabetes related arrhythmias. Of these, coronary atherosclerosis is the most important and will be treated in detail with special reference to high-density lipoprotein cholesterol (HDL-C) levels.

ISCHEMIC HEART DISEASE

Adults with DM have 2 to 3-fold increase of heart attacks and hence it is a major causative factor for IHD, especially in developing countries. Coronary arterial disease is more aggressive, wide spread, and prevalent in diabetics. Young adults with type 1 diabetes mellitus (T1DM have a 10-fold increase in IHD.[1] This aggressive nature of diabetic atherosclerosis is seen also in women.[2]

HDL AND INSULIN RESISTANCE IN THE PATHOGENESIS OF DIABETIC ATHEROSCLEROSIS

In the diabetic scenario, there appears to be a cardiovascular (CV) continuum. The pathophysiological basis of this phenomenon has an important correlation with the patients' lipid status. Type 2 diabetes mellitus (T2DM) usually commences with (1) long standing insulin resistance (IR), (2) subsequent compensatory hyperinsulinemia, and finally (3) raised levels of plasma glucose. These biochemical features can lead to atherosclerosis by different mechanisms. In obese T2DM, adipose tissue releases free fatty acid (FFA), in addition to enhanced de novo synthesis of FFA and increased flux of FFA from systemic pools, which lead to oxidative stress, vascular inflammation, and endothelial dysfunction, all of which are proatherogenic. IR also results in more FFA being released to the liver due to lipolysis. Hence very low-density lipoprotein (VLDL) particles are elevated along with apolipoprotein B (apoB) levels.[3,4] The diabetic lipid profile is characterized by high triglycerides (TG), low HDL-C, increased remnant lipoproteins, elevated apoB, and elevated dense LDL. Recent evidence suggests that the HDL particles in diabetics may be dysfunctional, in that instead of being protective, the HDL particles are pro-oxidative, proinflammatory, and prothrombotic.[5]

Insulin Resistance and Atherosclerosis

The European Society of Cardiology (ESC) guidelines on diabetes, prediabetes, and CV disease [along with the European Association for the Study of Diabetes (EASD); 2013] observes that there is a lack of evidence that early detection and treatment of DM can prevent CV complications.[6] Hence, routine blood sugar checks of the general population is not recommended for reduction of CV disease. This fact raises the question as to whether nonglycemic and nonlipidemic risk factors exist for the cardiodiabetes continuum, although early detection and treatment of diabetes can possibly reduce microvascular complications. In order to answer this justifiable query the hypothesis that hyper insulinemia might contribute to the atherosclerotic process was put forward in the mid-1960s.

However, more recently it is postulated that IR may be the culprit for atherosclerosis seen in T2DM.[7] An angiographic study to investigate the relationship between IR and the atherosclerotic burden in the real world was performed by Karrowni et al. Nondiabetic patients who had suffered an acute myocardial infarction (AMI) had coronary angiography (CA) performed and those with multivessel disease were selected for analysis regarding their IR status. These patients were divided into quartiles depending on their IR. The prevalence of multivessel disease in the quartiles were 37.8%, 42.3%, 47.2%, and 48.0%. Compared with quartile 1, both quartiles 3 and 4 were independently associated with multivessel coronary disease. Low-density lipoprotein cholesterol (LDL-C), HDL-C, TG, hemoglobin A1c (HbA1c), and high-sensitivity C-reactive protein (HS-CRP) were covariates in the analysis model.[8]

Thus, this study demonstrated the association between IR and extensive coronary atherosclerosis in nondiabetic post-myocardial infarction (MI) patients. The IR appears to be a risk factor with greater impact than any lipid parameter including HDL-C, in the genesis of atherosclerosis. The Insulin Resistance Atherosclerosis Study (IRAS) published in 2013, highlighted the fact that the CV risk seems to be higher in the impaired glucose tolerance (IGT) group compared with the group with impaired fasting glucose (IFG). Lipoprotein abnormalities seen even in the prediabetic status, may account for this disparity.[9] In the IFG group, apoB and total LDL particles are increased. However, in the IGT group increases are seen in the TG, VLDL along with structural remodeling of the LDL particles. These latter changes seem to be more atherogenic. IR appears to be a major determinant of acute coronary syndromes too, due to rupture of unstable plaques. The mechanism may be that vascular smooth muscle survival and migration are reduced and apoptosis of smooth muscle cells is increased in IR, which contribute towards an unstable plaque.

It is shown experimentally that insulin receptor substrate 2 (IRS2) silencing leads to (1) expression of inflammatory chemokine fractalkine (CX3CL1) and its receptor and (2) decreased survival of vascular smooth muscles cells.[10] It is important to recall that acute coronary syndromes are the disease entities which lead to death. Hence, cardiodiabetic mortality rates are directly related to acute complications. The evidence available so far indicates that IR and the atherogenic pattern of dyslipidemia seen in diabetics are the main drivers of atherosclerosis in hyperglycemic metabolic disease. The place of HDL in this process is difficult to assess with accuracy as dysfunctional HDL could constitute a major part of the so called protective lipid fraction. However, HDL-C certainly plays a role in diabetic atherosclerosis as a low HDL is taken as a feature of atherogenic dyslipidemia.

OUTLINE OF CLINICAL PHARMACOLOGY OF ORAL ANTIDIABETIC DRUGS WITH SPECIAL REFERENCE TO CARDIOVASCULAR AND HDL-C EFFECTS

There are 12 classes of antidiabetic drugs used in current therapeutics:

1.	Biguanides	Metformin
2.	Glinides (Meglitinides)	Repaglinide
3.	Sulfonylureas	Tolbutamide, Gliclazide
4.	Alpha-glucosidase inhibitors	Acarbose
5.	Thiazolidinediones (Glitazones)	Pioglitazone
6.	Incretin mimetics [glucagon-like peptide 1(GLP-1) mimetics]	Exenatide
7.	Dipeptidyl peptidase 4 inhibitors	Sitagliptin
8.	Dual proliferator-activated receptor (PPAR) α and γ agonists	Saroglitazar
9.	Sodium glucose cotransporter 2 inhibitors	Canagliflozin
10.	Amylin analogs	Pramlintide
11.	Bile acid sequestrants	Colesevelam
12.	Insulin	

Bromocriptine is not widely used in current diabetic therapeutics and hence not included in this listing. As mentioned before, in diabetic patients the risk of IHD, cerebrovascular accidents (CVAs) and ischemic deaths are twice that of nondiabetic patients. Intense glycemic control reduces microvascular complications and this benefit is well established. However, therapeutic effects on macrovascular disease have been inconsistent, trials giving negative, positive or neutral results.[11-17]

Metformin

The United Kingdom Prospective Diabetes Study (UKPDS), in which subpopulation of overweight patients were studied, found that when metformin was initiated early, there was a 32% risk reduction of sudden death, fatal and nonfatal MI, angina, stroke, and amputations. There was also a 36% risk reduction for all-cause mortality. Metformin was significantly better for reduction of diabetes related endpoints than either insulin or sulfonylureas. Additional lower quality data too generally confirms the beneficial effects of metformin in reducing cardiodiabetic complications. The main lipid effects of metformin are on TG (38% decrease) and VLDL. Some studies also show a rise in HDL. The quantification of the contribution that the increased HDL plays in the cardioprotective action of metformin is difficult, but it is probably small as the HDL rise is not universally seen in all studies.

Sulfonylureas

The University Group Diabetes Program (UGDP) study revealed that tolbutamide treated patients had excess cardiac deaths.[18] However, the UKPDS did not substantiate this finding. Also, the Diabetes Mellitus Insulin-Glucose Infusion in Acute Myocardial Infarction (DIGAMI) study demonstrated that patients with AMI did best with insulin glucose infusions, whereas those receiving sulfonylureas had poorer outcomes. The evidence for second generation sulfonylureas seems to be more positive (or, at least neutral). The ADVANCE study used gliclazide and no adverse CV effects were noted. Some data also suggest that gliclazide alone of all the sulfonylureas have a beneficial effect similar to metformin, regarding cardiodiabetic complications.[19,20] Some of data suggest that pancreatic cell specific sulfonylureas such as gliclazide have a beneficial effect in CV outcomes, but additional data is required for confirmation. The majority of trials reveal that both first and second generation sulfonylureas have neutral effects on HDL-C levels.

Thiazolidinediones

These act by an agonist effect at one or more peroxisome—PPARs that regulate gene expression leading to improved glucose utilization and reduced glucose production (primarily at PPAR-γ receptor). The lipid effects of pioglitazone are important. This drug increases HDL, lowers TG, apoB, dense HDL, and increases large fluffy LDL.[21] Rosiglitazone however increases LDL levels.

The PROactive trial with pioglitazone found that in a group of patients with highest propensity for CV disease, pioglitazone reduced all cause mortality, nonfatal MI and CVA. Post-hoc analysis of the PROactive data suggests that the effect on HDL predicts this beneficial effect on CV outcomes.

Glucagon-like Peptide-1 Agonists

Incretins are enteroendocrine peptides which have diverse effects on the stomach, satiety center, glucagon secretion, and augmentation of insulin response to glucose. Glucagon-like peptide 1 (GLP-1) is one such incretin which improves the HbA1c.

The drugs in this group are exenatide, liraglutide, albiglutide, taspoglutide, and lixisenatide. Some GLP-1 agonists can improve CV outcomes as they delay the development of atherosclerosis and reduce plaque burden.[22]

In the DURATION study which utilized exenatide, significant reductions in total cholesterol (TC), LDL, TG, and blood pressure (BP) were seen. These drugs also have a diuretic action. This class of drugs also leads to significant weight loss. A retrospective review of exenatide showed a 20% reduction of CV disease which was statistically significant.[23] This was associated with a rise in the HDL-C levels which phenomenon is seen with the use of exenatide and liraglutide.

Dipeptidyl Peptidase-4 Inhibitors

The dipeptidyl peptidase (DPP) enzyme is widely distributed in tissues. It degrades GLP-1 and other target molecules. The drugs in this class which are in clinical use are sitagliptin, vildagliptin, saxagliptin, linagliptin, and alogliptin. There are numerous associated pleiotropic effects attributed to DPP-4 inhibitors, which are cardioprotective.[24] A few of these pleiotropic effects are restoring endothelial progenitor cell (EPC) activity, activating cardioprotective molecular pathways, and antiarrhythmic effects.

A meta-analysis for DPP-4 inhibitors found a significant reduction in CV events even when compared to metformin. However, metformin and DPP-4 inhibitors have no additive effect with respect to CV risk reduction. The EXAMINE trial showed that the use of alogliptin in the scenario of acute coronary syndromes does not lead to an adverse outcome. The SAVOR-TIMI 53 trial with saxagliptin, CAROLINA trial with linagliptin and TECOS trial with sitagliptin provide evidence for the safety of this class of drugs in the post-MI cohort of patients.

As a class, the gliptins have neutral effects on HDL-C levels. Therefore, the CV benefits must be attributable to their pleiotropic effects or reduction of dysfunctional HDL.

Meglitinides

These secretagogues are similar to sulfonylureas, but act on a different receptor site. However, the effects are like those of sulfonylureas. Repaglinide and nateglinide are currently available.

These drugs have no effects on lipids. CV outcomes are largely unknown. The NAVIGATOR trial did not report improved CV outcomes. The NAVIGATOR trial[24,25] included 9,306 patients with IGT. The subjects also had either CV disease or CV risk factors. Nateglinide for 5 years did not reduce incidence of DM or CV outcomes [death due to CV causes, nonfatal MI, CVA, and heart failure (HF)].

Alpha Glucosidase Inhibitors

These act on the proximal small bowel so that postprandial hypoglycemia is reduced. Acarbose is widely used. The other agent in this class is miglitol. Postprandial hypoglycemia is proatherogenic because of its enhancement of oxidative stress. Acarbose may stimulate GLP-1 secretion which would be cardioprotective. However, data to date do not warrant the conclusion that acarbose is superior to metformin in providing CV protection. Acarbose is largely neutral regarding its HDL effects. However, a minority of trials suggest an increase in HDL with the use of acarbose.

Pramlintide

This is an analogue of amylin. Amylin is a pancreatic hormone that is secreted along with insulin. The secretion is from the beta cells of the pancreas. Pramlintide is used alongside insulin. It has neutral effects on LDL-C and HDL-C levels. There is no data regarding CV outcomes with this drug.

Colesevelam

This molecule is a bile acid sequestrant. It is usually combined with other oral hypoglycemic agents. The HDL-C rises slightly with this drug. It improves CV outcomes probably due to its lipid effects.

Dopamine (D2) Receptor Agonists

Post hoc analysis of the Cycloset safety trial showed a 52% reduction in major CV endpoints (MI, CVA, and deaths), with bromocriptine. Its HDL effects are neutral whereas TGs are reduced.

Saroglitazar

This is a dual PPAR-α/γ agonist. Its main advantage is the significant improvement in the diabetic dyslipidemia, i.e. TG, VLDL, apoB, and non-HDL-C are all reduced, whereas HDL-C levels are elevated.

At present, data is not available regarding macrovascular protection afforded by saroglitazar.

Empagliflozin

The EMPA-REG study was performed enrolling patients with T2DM with high CV risk, in that all participants had established CV disease at baseline.[26] A total of 7,020 patients were followed up for a mean of 3 years. There was no advantage with empagliflozin with respect to MI and CVA.

However, in the empagliflozin group there were significantly lower rates of

- Deaths from CV cause
- Hospitalization for HF
- Deaths from any cause.

There was no reduction in unstable angina.

Summary

Considering the above data, the diabetic drugs having some evidence for reducing CV complications are metformin, gliclazide (a second generation sulfonylureas), pioglitazone, and exenatide. These may be acting at least in part by their HDL raising effect. The DPP-4 inhibitors probably provide CV benefit due to their pleiotropic effects.

EFFECTS OF ORAL ANTIDIABETIC DRUGS ON THE LIPID PROFILE

A meta-analysis done by Monami et al. utilizing trial data up to 2011, yielded importing information.[27] The TC is significantly reduced by pioglitazone, sulfonylureas, and DPP-4 inhibitors but not a by acarbose.

The TGs are significantly reduced by pioglitazone, DPP-4 inhibitors and acarbose but not by sulfonylureas. The HDL-C is increased by metformin, acarbose and pioglitazone but decreased by sulfonylureas. Hence, the worst lipid effects are seen with sulfonylureas. Pioglitazone and DPP-4 inhibitors give the best lipid modifications. Metformin was not assessed in this meta-analysis as it included patients who had other drugs added when metformin failed.

Rosenblit has summarized the HDL effects induced by hypoglycemic agents as follows: metformin-slight ↑, pioglitazone ↑, rosiglitazone ↑, glibenclamide ↔, gliclazide ↔, glimepiride ↔, sitagliptin ↔, vildagliptin ↔, saxagliptin ↔, alogliptin ↔, exenatide ↑, liraglutide ↑, canagliflozin ↑, dapagliflozin ↑, empagliflozin-slight ↑, acarbose ↔/↑, miglitol ↔, bromocriptine ↔, colesevelam-slight ↑, and insulin ↑.[28]

Lipid Effect of Metformin in Patients with Impaired Glucose Tolerance

It is seen from the above summary that although metformin has greatest benefit regarding cardiac disease, its effect on the lipid profile need to be clarified further. In the prediabetics, the TG levels fall by 0.08 mmol/L and the HDL-C is significantly increased (+ 0.008 mmol/L). The LDL phenotype is improved for the better, with the prevalence of phenotype B levels (dense LDL) reducing.[29] However, the lipid profile improved better with lifestyle modification than with metformin.

Lipoproteins and Beta-cell Function

There are pieces of experimental data which suggest that various lipoproteins may directly affect the beta-cell secretion. Natali et al. demonstrated that in nondiabetic individuals, LDL seemed to have no independent association with insulin secretion or clearance (either fasting or stimulated).[30] HDL levels however had a negative association and triglyceride levels demonstrated a positive association with insulin secretion. Neither had an effect on insulin clearance. A low HDL level with a high level of TG is associated with an increase in glucose dependent insulin secretion, but a decrease in non-glucose-dependent insulin secretion. A low HDL and raised triglyceride are associated with increased fasting insulin secretion. Thus, a low HDL and high TG might be contributing to sustain the abnormal prediabetic insulin secretion pattern which is proatherogenic. It is clear that trial evidence of reduction of mortality, CV events, and HF do not strictly follow the patterns set by changes in the lipid profile. Hence, HDL-C cannot be counted as the major determinant of CV morbidity and mortality seen with various oral hypoglycemic drugs and insulin.

Recommended Lipid Targets for Patients with Diabetes Mellitus

The cardiodiabetic forum in 2008 reviewed the literature and made certain observations:

1. Low HDL-C levels are common in the diabetic group.
2. The National Institute for Health and Care Excellence (NICE) and joint British Society (JBS 2) guidelines do not recommend a specific HDL target for diabetics.
3. Most statins raise HDL-C by approximately 0.05–0.1mmol/L, but the group believed that it had only a small impact on outcomes.
4. Lifestyle modification (smoking cessation, exercise, and weight loss) increased HDL by 5–10%. Fibrates did so by 5–15%.

The ESC-EASD guidelines give the following targets for lipid control in diabetics.[31] HDL-C: more than 1.0 mmol/L males and more than 1.2 mmol/L females.

DIABETIC CARDIOMYOPATHY

This refers to a syndrome seen in diabetics which leads to left ventricular dysfunction in the absence of coronary atheroma. In the initial stages of DM, the myocardial cells are preserved but the interstitium is altered so that contractility is impaired. Later on fibrosis of the interstitium and perivascular regions occur. These changes are thought to be mediated by advanced glycation end products (AGEs).

Later in the timeline, hyaline degeneration of the arterioles occurs with capillary microaneurysm formation. Left ventricular mass too increases alongside the inflammatory process.[32-34] Hyperglycemia affects the Na^+–Ca^{2+} channels leading to increased intracellular ironic calcium. In diabetics, the Na^+–K^+ channels too are dysfunctional and this leads to a higher concentration of intra-cellular Na^+ as well.[35]

Genetically determined factors such as insulin like growth factor 1 (IGF-1), which has many effects on the myocardium, can be altered due to dyslipidemia which leads to secondary malfunction of genetic transcription factors.[36] Whether HDL particles are specifically involved in this aspect is as yet unanswered. An additional factor influencing left ventricular function in the diabetic would be cardiac autonomic neuropathy.

Diabetic cardiomyopathy as manifested by diastolic dysfunction seems to be associated with the metabolic syndrome and a higher degree of systemic inflammation.[37] The role played by HDL in this scenario is difficult to evaluate but low HDL is a feature of the metabolic syndrome. In view of the fact that HDL has anti-inflammatory properties, a low HDL may reasonably be implicated as a player in the genesis of diabetic cardiomyopathy. It is experimentally demonstrated that atorvastatin leads to an improvement in myocardial fibrosis and inflammation in diabetic rats. These effects however occurred with no change in the lipid profile and hence it is postulated that the pleiotropic effects of statins are responsible for the benefits seen.[38]

Many epidemiological studies however indicate that HDL-C can be correlated to the incidence of HF. In the specific context of diabetic cardiomyopathy, HDL-C levels are important for a variety of reasons. Firstly, HDLs have an antidiabetic action. They decrease beta-cell apoptosis and this results in better control of blood glucose.[39,40] They have an action of improving insulin sensitivity. A human *apo A-1* gene transfer study (in an experimental rat model) proved that development of diabetic cardiomyopathy could be mitigated.[41] This type of research also confirms that oxidative stress and cardiac fibrosis could be reduced by HDL. All these mechanisms would help in reducing the incidence of diabetic cardiomyopathy and open up avenues for its treatment.

Diabetic Cardiac Autonomic Neuropathy

Diabetic cardiac autonomic neuropathy is important because it predicts the occurrence of diabetic IHD. The data regarding DCAN and HDL-C seems to be very sparse in the literature. In a cohort of Chinese patients, Song et al. found that DCAN was associated with the TG level. The authors say that another key finding was that the severity of lipid profile was independently and significantly associated with DCAN.[42] Some investigators, such as Witte, found that TG and DCAN were not associated but a weak negative relationship existed with HDL.[43] It is postulated that oxidative stress induced by dyslipidemia is a causative mechanism of DCAN, in which case a low HDL could possibly be involved in the pathogenesis of DCAN.

Prince et al. conducted a study to identity any relationship between DCAN and arterial stiffness (as measured by pulse wave analysis) in T1DM. Arterial stiffness is in part regulated by autonomic function.[44] Low levels of HDL-C predicted a higher augmented index (Aix), augmentation pressure (AP), and subendocardial viability ratio (SEVR), all of which indicate an increase in arterial stiffness. This study provides some credibility to the hypothesis that HDL-C influences the occurrence of DCAN as arterial tone is modulated in part by autonomic function.

Arrhythmias in Diabetes

Many investigators report a higher incidence of certain arrhythmias in the diabetic context. The data regarding the role of HDL-C in the genesis and maintenance of these arrhythmias is sparse.

SOME ASPECTS OF THE PATHOBIOLOGY OF HDL IN DIABETICS AND PREDIABETICS

The pathobiology of HDL as pertaining to diabetics is extremely complex. Research abounds in this sphere but in the present synopsis only certain human studies will be selected to be highlighted. Studies at times contradict each other and consensus on certain matters becomes difficult. Only the clinically relevant studies will be summarized in this section.

Diabetic/Atherogenic Dyslipidemia

The dyslipidemia of DM can be described as both ominous and cryptic as LDL levels can be deceptively low due to the B phenotype. The atherogenic dyslipidemia of diabetics is an important clinical parameter which needs aggressive treatment to reduce CV complications. The main constituent of the atherogenic dyslipidemia is an increased triglyceride and reduced HDL-C. The formula log (TG)/HDL-C has been proposed as a measure of atherogenic dyslipidemia.[45] In a study by Herman et al. it was found that atherogenic dyslipidemia (as calculated by the above ratio) correlated with lower beta-cell function and high prevalence of coronary artery disease. The ratio also correlated with macroangiopathy, the risk of which was not captured by LDL estimation.

Silent Coronary Disease and HDL-C

The atherogenic lipid profile seen in T2DM is also predictive of silent myocardial ischemia and clinically silent, but angiographically proven coronary arterial disease. Valensi at al. demonstrated that even in the patient cohort with LDL-C less than 2.6 mmol/L (100 mg %), the atherogenic dyslipidemia (i.e. elevated triglyceride and depressed HDL-C levels) was associated with coronary arterial disease.[46] Silent ischemia is important in diabetic patients. Hence the value of this study. The study also highlights the importance of TG and HDL levels even when LDL levels are within the recommended goals.

High-density Lipoprotein and Endothelial Progenitor Cells[47]

Circulating EPCs seem to be influenced by plasma HDL levels. This is important as EPCs play a role in endothelial function and repair. In an experimental study by Van Oostrum et al. it was demonstrated that one week after an infusion of reconstituted HDL (rHDL) the EPC numbers increased significantly. It is possible that rHDL increases circulating EPCs by prolonging their life span or helping their release from the bone marrow mediated by nitrous oxide.

Extent of Coronary Disease and HDL Activity[48]

The severity of coronary artery disease in T2DM is governed by many factors. Shen at al. conducted a study to determine whether assays of apo A-1 glycation and HDL associated paraoxonase 1 (PON1) and PON3 could predict the severity of coronary artery disease in T2DM. In the presence of increased apo A-1 glycation and decreased PON1 and PON3 activity, there was enhanced coronary artery disease as determined by the extent index (number of coronary artery effected) and the cumulative coronary stenosis score (CCSS). Thus, the angiographic severity of coronary artery disease in T2DM could be assessed by the given parameters which indicate HDL particle activity.

Significance of HDL in Elderly Diabetics[49]

The Japan Cholesterol and DM study was designed to assess the correlation that LDL-C, HDL-C, and glucose levels had with atherosclerotic disease mainly IHD and cerebrovascular disease, in the elderly age group (approximately 70–75 years of age). In the very elderly group (^{3} 75 years), HDL-C was able to predict IHD and CVA. In the nonelderly, LDL-C, HbA1c, systolic BP, and non-HDL-C are risk factors which predict IHD. Thus, in the very elderly diabetics, HDL-C level is an important predictor of atherosclerotic disease.

Genetic Influence on HDL-C in Diabetics[50]

Genetic factors may play a role in the causation of low-HDL levels in T2DM. Diabetic coronary arterial disease is associated with an intergenic locus on chromosome 1 (lead SNP rs10911021). When assaying HDL subclasses, the rs10911021 was associated with the large HDL particle in T2DM. Beaney et al. also found that the minor "protective" allele related to dysfunctional HDL. Hence, the genetic aspects of the HDL story are far from satisfactorily complete at the present time.

Insulin Sensitivity and HDL Levels[51]

High-density lipoprotein cholesterol has many factors that control it. The recognized biochemical factors involved include Lecithin-cholesterol acyltransferase (LCAT), phospholipid transfer protein (PLTP), cholesterol ester transfer protein (CETP), and post-heparin lipoprotein lipases, which are regulated by insulin. The study by Leance et al. suggests that HDL levels are related to increased degree of insulin sensitivity. Even in prediabetics a low-HDL level is associated with higher plasma insulin levels.

Composition of High-density Lipoprotein Particles[52]

The phenotype transformation of LDL particles into the "B" subtype is well documented in diabetics. Along with this phenotype of LDL, several other changes also occur which include higher levels of oxidized LDL, glycated LDL, and lipoprotein phospholipase A2 activity. Along with these changes, alterations in the characteristics of HDL too occur. If the HDL particle contains increased TG content and decreased cholesterol content, such a change is associated with impaired efflux of lipids from adipose tissue. In diabetics with LDL-phenotype B, the cholesterol/TG ratio in HDL is 2.5-fold lower than in normal subjects.

Microvascular Disease and HDL-C Levels[53]

Toth et al. conducted a study in order to correlate lipid fractions with the occurrence of microvascular complications in T2DM. The study found that a 1% decrease of microvascular complications occurred with a 1 mg/dL increase in HDL-C. Patients who achieved the HDL-C goal of the American Diabetes Association (ADA), i.e. more than 40 mg% for males, more than 50 mg% for females, had an 11% lower risk of microvascular complications. Achieving the TG goal (i.e. <150 mg%) also reduced microvascular complications.

Lipoprotein Regulation and HDL in Diabetics[54]

Angiopoietin-like protein 3 (ANGPTL3) is one of the important lipoprotein regulators which has a positive association with HDL-C. Zhao et al. studied the plasma levels of ANGPTL3 in diabetics and nondiabetics subjects. In female diabetic patients, levels of ANGPTL3 levels were decreased which effects the apo A-1 and HDL-C levels.

Racial Disparity in HDL Response to Metformin[55]

The HDL-C levels are improved by using metformin in prediabetics, but there appears to be some degree of racial diversity. In a study by Zhang et al. a significant rise in HDL-C occurred when using metformin 850 mg/BD in American whites and African Americans but not in Hispanics. Hence racial identity is possibly important to consider in assessing the lipid changes induced by metformin.

Treating the Atherogenic Dyslipidemia of Diabetics[56]

Toth et al. studied 529,236 patients in the US, using the database of commercial health plan members. They found that 41.1% patients with two suboptimal lipid levels and 45.1% with three abnormal lipid levels did not receive any lipid modifying treatment. Statin monotherapy was the most common lipid modifying therapy used and less than 30% received a combination of antilipemic therapy. This finding suggests that DM patients are for the most part not treated to ADA recommended lipid goals.

CONCLUSION

Lipid regulation, especially HDL levels, besides TGs and cholesterol are important predictors of appropriate lipid control to reduce cardiodiabetes inflicted morbidity and mortality.

REFERENCES

1. Laing SP, Swerdlow AJ, Slater SD, et al. Mortality from heart disease in a cohort of 23,000 patients with insulin-treated diabetes. Diabetologia. 2003;46:760-5.

2. Nathan DM. Long-term complications of diabetes mellitus. N Engl J Med. 1993;328:1676-85.
3. Saltiel AR, Kahn CR. Insulin signalling and the regulation of glucose and lipid metabolism. Nature. 2001;414(6865):799-806.
4. Kim JA, Montagnani M, Koh KK, et al. Reciprocal relationships between insulin resistance and endothelial dysfunction: molecular and pathophysiological mechanisms. Circulation. 2006;113:1888-904.
5. Sorrentino SA, Besler C, Rohrer L, et al. Endothelial-vasoprotective effects of high-density lipoprotein are impaired in patients with type 2 diabetes mellitus but are improved after extended-release niacin therapy. Circulation. 2010;121:110-22.
6. Ryden L, Grant PJ, Anker SD, et al. ESC Guidelines on diabetes, pre-diabetes, and cardiovascular diseases developed in collaboration with the EASD: the Task Force on diabetes, pre-diabetes, and cardiovascular diseases of the European Society of Cardiology (ESC) and developed in collaboration with the European Association for the Study of Diabetes (EASD). Eur Heart J. 2013;34(39):3035-87.
7. Reaven GM. The insulin resistance syndrome. Curr Atheroscler Rep. 2003;5:364-71.
8. Karrowni W, Li Y, Jones PG, et al. Insulin resistance is associated with significant clinical atherosclerosis in non-diabetic patients with acute myocardial infarction. Arterioscler Thromb Vasc Biol. 2013;33(9):2245-51.
9. Lorenzo C, Hartnett S, Hanley AJ, et al. Impaired fasting glucose and impaired glucose tolerance have distinct lipoprotein and apolipoprotein changes: the insulin resistance atherosclerosis study. J Clini Endocrinol Metab. 2013;98(4):1622-30.
10. Martinez-Herva S, Vinue A, Nunez L, et al. Insulin resistance aggravates atherosclerosis by reducing vascular smooth muscle cell survival and increasing CX3CL1/CX3CR1 axis. Cardiovasc Res. 2014;103(2):324-36.
11. Nathan DM, Cleary PA, Backlund JY, et al. Intensive diabetes treatment and cardiovascular disease in patients with type 1 diabetes. N Engl J Med. 2005;353(25):2643-53.
12. UK Prospective Diabetes Study (UKPDS) Group. Intensive blood-glucose control with sulphonylureas or insulin compared with conventional treatment and risk of complications in patients with type 2 diabetes (UKPDS 33). UK Prospective Diabetes Study (UKPDS) Group. Lancet. 1998;352(9131):837-53.
13. Duckworth W, Abraira C, Moritz T, et al. Glucose control and vascular complications in veterans with type 2 diabetes. N Engl J Med. 2009;360(2):129-39.
14. ADVANCE Collaborative Group, Patel A, MacMahon S, et al. Intensive blood glucose control and vascular outcomes in patients with type 2 diabetes. N Engl J Med. 2008;358(24):2560-72.
15. Holman RR, Paul SK, Bethel MA, et al. 10-year follow-up of intensive glucose control in type 2 diabetes. N Engl J Med. 2008;359(15):1577-89.
16. NICE-SUGAR Study Investigators, Finfer S, Chittock DR, et al. Intensive versus conventional glucose control in critically ill patients. N Engl J Med. 2009;360(13):1283-97.
17. Action to Control Cardiovascular Risk in Diabetes Study Group, Gerstein HC, Miller ME, et al. Effects of intensive glucose lowering in type 2 diabetes. N Engl J Med. 2008;358(24):2545-59.
18. The University Group Diabetes Program. A study of the effects of hypoglycemic agents on vascular complications in patients with adult-onset diabetes. V. Evaluation of pheniformin therapy. Diabetes. 1975;24(Suppl 1):65-184.
19. Zeller M, Danchin N, Simon D, et al. Impact of type of preadmission sulfonylureas on mortality and cardiovascular outcomes in patients with diabetes with acute myocardial infarction. J Clin Endocrinol Metab. 2010;95(11):4993-5002.
20. Schramm TK, Gislason GH, Vaag A, et al. Mortality and cardiovascular risk associated with different insulin secretagogues compared with metformin in type 2 diabetes, with or without a previous myocardial infarction: a nationwide study. Eur Heart J. 2011;32(15):1900-8.
21. Chiquette E, Ramirez G, Defronzo R. A meta-analysis comparing the effect of thiazolidinediones on cardiovascular risk factors. Arch Intern Med. 2004;164(19):2097-104.
22. Nagashima M, Watanabe T, Terasaki M, et al. Native incretins prevent the development of atherosclerotic lesions in apolipoprotein E knockout mice. Diabetologia. 2011;54(10):2649-59.
23. Best JH, Hoogwerf BJ, Herman WH, et al. Risk of cardiovascular disease events in patients with type 2 diabetes prescribed the glucagon-like peptide 1 (GLP-1) receptor agonist exenatide twice daily or other glucose-lowering therapies: a retrospective analysis of the Life Link database. Diabetes Care. 2011;34(1):90-5.
24. NAVIGATOR Study Group, Holman RR, Haffner SM. Effect of nateglinide on the incidence of diabetes and cardiovascular events. N Engl J Med. 2010;362(16):1463-76.
25. Chrysant SG, Chrysant GS. Clinical implications of cardiovascular preventing pleiotropic effects of dipeptidyl peptidase-4 inhibitors. Am J Cardiol. 2012;109(11):1681-5.
26. Zinman B, Wanner C, Lachin JM, et al. Empagliflozin, Cardiovascular Outcomes, and Mortality in Type 2 Diabetes. N Engl J Med. 2015;373(22):2117-28.
27. Monami M, Vitale V, Ambrosio ML, et al. Effects on lipid profile of dipeptidyl peptidase 4 inhibitors, pioglitazone, acarbose, and sulfonylureas: meta-analysis of placebo-controlled trials. Adv Ther. 2012:29(9):736-46.
28. Rosenblit PD. Common medications used by patients with type 2 diabetes mellitus: what are their effects on the lipid profile. Cardiovasc Diabetol. 2016;15:95.
29. Ratner R, Goldberg R, Haffner S, et al. Impact of intensive lifestyle and metformin therapy on cardiovascular disease risk factors in the diabetes prevention program. Diabetes Care. 2005;28(4):888-94.
30. Natali A, Baldi S, Bonnet F, et al. Plasma HDL-cholesterol and triglycerides, but not LDL-cholesterol, are associated with insulin secretion in non-diabetic subjects. Metabolism. 2017;69:33-42.
31. Rydén L, Standl E, Bartnik M, et al. Guidelines on diabetes, pre-diabetes, and cardiovascular diseases: executive summary. The task force on diabetes and cardiovascular disease of the European Society of Cardiology (ESC) and of the Erupean Association for the Study of Diabetes (EASD). Eur Heart J. 2007;28(1):88-136.
32. Vigorita VJ, Morre GW, Hutchens SM. Absence of correlation between coronary arterial atherosclerosis and severity or duration of diabetes mellitus of adult onset. Am J Cardiol. 1980;46(40):535-42.
33. Factor SM, Minase T, Sonnenblick EH. Clinical and morphological features of human hypertensive-diabetic cardiomyopathy. Am Heart J. 1980;99(4):446-58.
34. Palmieri V, Bella JN, Tracy RP, et al. Relationship of left ventricular hypertrophy to inflammation and albuminuria in adults with type 2 diabetes: the strong heart study. Diabetes Care. 2003;26(10):2764-9.
35. Rodrigues B, Cam MC, McNeill JH. Metabolic disturbances in diabetic cardiomyopathy. Mol Cell Biochem. 1998;180(1-2):53-7.
36. Ren J, Sampson WK, Sowers JR. Insulin-like growth factor 1 as a cardiac hormone: physiological and pathophysiological implications in heart disease. J Mol Cell Cardiol. 1999;31(11):2049-61.
37. Diamant M, Lamb HJ, Smit JW, et al. Diabetic cardiomyopathy in uncomplicated type 2 diabetes is associated with the metabolic syndrome and systemic inflammation. Diabetologia. 2005;48(8):1669-70.
38. Van Linthout S, Riad A, Dhayat N, et al. Anti-inflammatory effects of atorvastatin improve left ventricular function in experimental diabetic cardiomyopathy. Diabetologia. 2007;50:1977-86.
39. Abderrahmani A, Niederhauser G, Favre D, et al. Human high-density lipoprotein particles prevent activation of the JNK pathway induced by human oxidised low-density lipoprotein particles in pancreatic beta cells. Diabetologia. 2007;50(6):1304-14.

40. Berg AH, Combs TP, Du X, et al. The adipocyte-secreted protein Acrp30 enhances hepatic insulin action. Nat Med. 2001;7(8):947-53.
41. Van Linthout S, Spillmann F, Graiani G, et al. Down-regulation of endothelial TLR4 signalling after apo A-I gene transfer contributes to improved survival in an experimental model of lipopolysaccharide-induced inflammation. J Mol Med (Beri). 2011;89(2):151-60.
42. Song L, Zhou L, Tang Z. An association analysis of lipid profile and diabetic cardiovascular autonomic neuropathy in a Chinese sample. Lipids Health Dis. 2016;15:122.
43. Witte DR, Tesfaye S, Chaturvedi N, et al. Risk factors for cardiac autonomic neuropathy in type 1 diabetes mellitus. Diabetologia. 2005;48:164-171.
44. Prince CT, Secrest AM, Mackey RH, et al. Cardiovascular autonomic neuropathy HDL-cholesterol and smoking correlate with arterial stiffness markers determined 18 years later in type 1 diabetes. Diabetes Care. 2010;33(3):652-7.
45. Hermans MP, Ahn SA, Rousseau MF. Log(TG)/HDL-C is related to both residual cardiometabolic risk and β-cell function loss in type 2 diabetes males. Cardiovasc Diabetol. 2010;9:88.
46. Valensi P, Avignon A, Sultan A, et al. Atherogenic dyslipidemia and risk of silent coronary artery disease in asymptomatic patients with type 2 diabetes: a cross-sectional study. Cardiovasc Diabetol. 2016;15(1):104.
47. van Oostrom O, Nieuwdorp M, Westerweel PE, et al. Reconstituted HDL increases circulating endothelial progenitor cells in patients with type 2 diabetes. Arterioscler Thromb Vasc Biol. 2007;27(8):1864-5.
48. Shen Y, Ding FH, Sun JT, et al. Association of elevated apoA-I glycation and reduced HDL-associated paraoxonase1, 3 activity, and their interaction with angiographic severity of coronary artery disease in patients with type 2 diabetes mellitus. Cardiovasc Diabetol. 2015;14:52.
49. Hayashi T, Araki A, Kawashima S, et al. Metabolic predictors of ischemic heart disease and cerebrovascular attack in elderly diabetic individuals: difference in risk by age. Cardiovasc Diabetol. 2013;12:10.
50. Beaney KE, Cooper JA, McLachlan S, et al. Variant rs10911021 that associates with coronary heart disease in type 2 diabetes, is associated with lower concentrations of circulating HDL cholesterol and large HDL particles but not with amino acids. Cardiovasc Diabetol. 2016;15(1):115.
51. Leança CC, Nunes VS, Panzoldo NB, et al. Metabolism of plasma cholesterol and lipoprotein parameters are related to a higher degree of insulin sensitivity in high HDL-C healthy normal weight subjects. Cardiovasc Diabetol. 2013;12:173.
52. Sánchez-Quesada JL, Vinagre I, De Juan-Franco E, et al. Impact of the LDL subfraction phenotype on Lp-PLA2 distribution, LDL modification and HDL composition in type 2 diabetes. Cardiovasc Diabetol. 2013;12:112.
53. Toth PP, Simko RJ, Palli SR, et al. The impact of serum lipids on risk for microangiopathy in patients with type 2 diabetes mellitus. Cardiovasc Diabetol. 2012;11:109.
54. Zhao D, Yang LY, Wang XH, et al. Different relationship between ANGPTL3 and HDL components in female non-diabetic subjects and type-2 diabetic patients. Cardiovasc Diabetol. 2016;15:132.
55. Zhang C, Gao F, Luo H, et al. Differential response in levels of high-density lipoprotein cholesterol to one-year metformin treatment in prediabetic patients by race/ethnicity. Cardiovasc Diabetol. 2015;14:79.
56. Toth PP, Zarotsky V, Sullivan JM, et al. Dyslipidemia treatment of patients with diabetes mellitus in a US managed care plan: a retrospective database analysis. Cardiovasc Diabetol. 2009;8:26.

CHAPTER 58

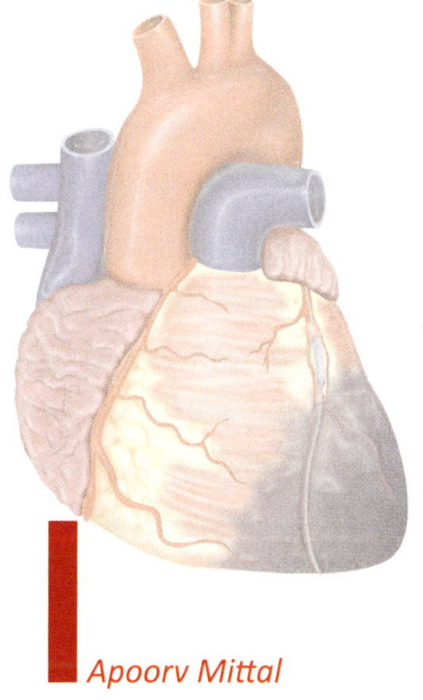

Glucose-lowering Strategies and Cardiovascular Outcomes

Apoorv Mittal

INTRODUCTION

Type 2 diabetes mellitus (T2DM) is a metabolic disease that is diagnosed on the basis of sustained hyperglycemia. People with T2DM are at elevated risk for a number of serious health problems, including cardiovascular (CV) disease, premature death, blindness, kidney failure, amputations, fractures, frailty, depression, and cognitive decline.[1] In prospective epidemiologic studies, the incidence of many of these outcomes is directly associated with the degree of hyperglycemia, as measured by the plasma glucose or the glycated hemoglobin level (HbA1c), a measure of the mean blood glucose level during the previous 2–3 months (Fig. 1).[2] Thus, after adjustment for other risk factors, an increase of 1% in the HbA1c is associated with an increase of 18% in the risk of CV events,[2] an increase of 12–14% in the risk of death,[3,4] and an increase of 37% in the risk of retinopathy or renal failure.[4] People with T2DM have a roughly doubled risk of CV disease, compared with people without T2DM, even after adjustment for established CV risk factors.[5] After diagnosis, patients have a lifetime of attempted strict lifestyle, escalating drug therapy to offset glycemic progression, and management of several risk factors to minimize the risk of DM-related complications. Life expectancy of a person diagnosed with T2DM at age 40 years is estimated to be shortened by about 6–7 years, compared with people without T2DM.[5] A major need exists for evidence-based T2DM treatment strategies that better manage this complex condition by reducing disease progression, improving quality of life, and extending longevity, without causing unwanted or harmful side effects.

Epidemiologic studies have outlined a strong association between T2DM and CV disease.[6,7] It is well-established that patients with T2DM are exposed to a significantly higher risk to develop myocardial infarction (MI) and stroke than matched subjects without T2DM.[7] Diabetic patients hospitalized for unstable angina or non-Q-wave MI display a significantly higher 2-year morbidity and mortality as compared with nondiabetic subjects.[8] In the seminal study by Haffner et al.,[9] the 7-year risk of MI was as high in diabetic patients without prior MI as it was in nondiabetic patients with prior MI, thus establishing diabetes as a "CV disease risk equivalent." The increased prevalence of cardiovascular disease (CVD) in the setting of T2DM can be largely attributed to the heavy atherosclerotic burden and adverse plaque phenotype, as well as the inability to compensate for these alterations.[10] T2DM is characterized by multiple pathophysiologic abnormalities. With time, multiple glucose-lowering medications are commonly required to reduce and maintain plasma glucose concentrations within the normal range. T2DM individuals also are at a very high risk for microvascular complications and the incidence of heart attack and stroke is increased two- to three-fold compared with nondiabetic individuals.[11] Therefore, when selecting medications to normalize glucose levels in T2DM patients, it is important that the agent not aggravate, and ideally even improve cardiovascular risk factors (CVRFs) and reduce CV morbidity and mortality.[11]

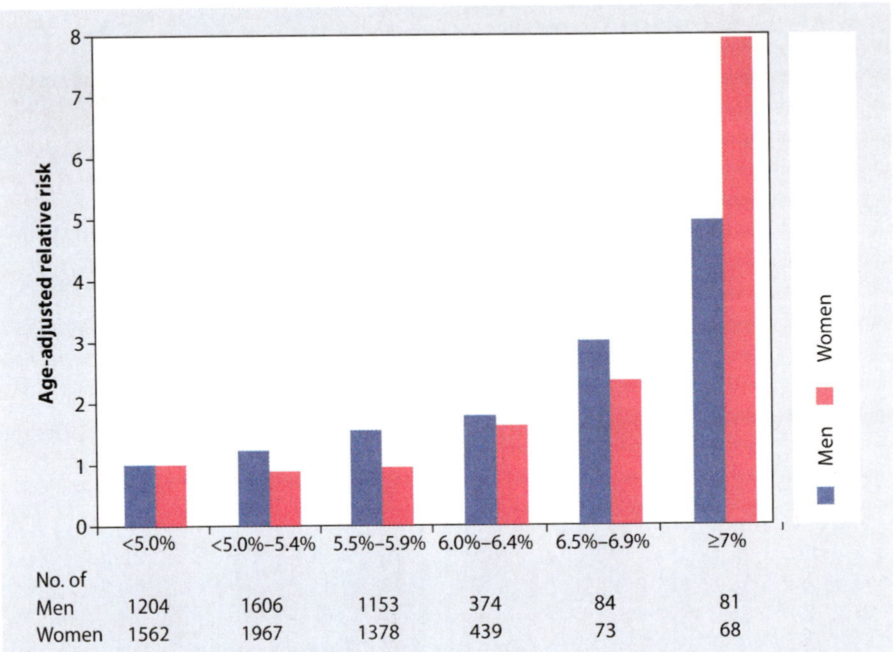

Fig. 1: Age-adjusted relative risks for cardiovascular events by HbA1c category from the European Prospective Investigation

IS LOWER BETTER?

The United Kingdom Prospective Diabetes Study (UKPDS) randomized 3867 patients newly diagnosed as having DM to either intensive therapy (with either a sulfonylurea or insulin) or conventional therapy (predominantly diet alone).[12] The median achieved HbA1c value during the study was 7.0% for the intensive therapy group compared with 7.9% for the conventional group.[13] The intensive therapy group had a 25% lower risk of developing microvascular complications, which was primarily driven by a lower frequency of retinal photocoagulation. A trend toward reduction of MI was noted in the intensive therapy group during 10 years of follow-up; however, it was not statistically significant.[12] Although metformin was less effective at lowering HbA1c values than intensive therapy regimens with a sulfonylurea or insulin, it was associated with a lower risk of death and stroke (although not MI) and, importantly, a much lower risk of hypoglycemia (Fig. 2).[14] In contrast to UKPDS, three recent large randomized trials have shown no reduction in CV events with aggressive versus more conservative glucose control in patients with T2DM, possibly because of a longer mean duration of T2DM and a shorter duration of follow-up than in the UKPDS trial.[13,15,16] Indeed, after 3.5 years, the ACCORD (Action to Control Cardiovascular Risk in Diabetes) trial showed significantly reduced all-cause mortality in T2DM patients randomized to intensive glycemic control as compared with conventional control; as a result, the glycemic control portion of ACCORD was stopped prematurely.[13] Yet, on detailed scrutiny of the data, higher HbA1c values predicted increased risk of death in the intensive arm of the ACCORD trial, in which most of the deaths occurred in the subgroup of patients whose HbA1c values remained high despite attempted intensive glycemic control.[17] Moreover, in the subgroup of patients without documented CV disease at baseline, a subanalysis suggested that intensive glycemic control was associated with a reduced risk of CV death and nonfatal CV events.[13]

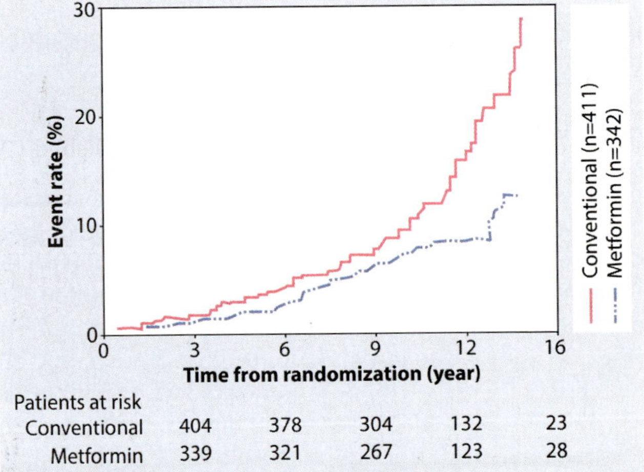

Fig. 2: Kaplan–Meier plot for any type 2 diabetes-related death with metformin and conventional therapy in the UK Prospective Diabetes Study[14]

The Veterans Affairs Diabetes Trial (VADT), which compared intensive and standard treatment strategies in patients with T2DM, did not show a statistically significant difference in the incidence of major CV events after a median follow-up of 5.6 years.[15] In this study, the intensive control group achieved an HbA1c of 6.9% compared with 8.4% in the standard control group.[15] Not surprisingly, 8.5% of the patients in the intensive therapy group were reported to have had at least 1 episode of hypoglycemia versus 3.1% in the standard therapy group.[15] In a substudy of VADT, patients without significant coronary atherosclerosis (as documented by a coronary artery calcium score of less than 100) experienced a decrease in CV events with intensive versus conservative therapy.[18] Although certainly not definitive, these findings from VADT and ACCORD suggest that intensive glucose control may reduce CV events in patients with a shorter duration of DM and in those who do not have significant pre-existing CAD.[14,19] After a median follow-up of 5 years, the ADVANCE (Action in Diabetes and Vascular Disease: Preterax and Diamicron Modified Release Controlled Evaluation) trial showed no difference between intensive control and standard control groups in macrovascular outcomes.[18-20] Mean HbA1c values achieved in the ADVANCE study were 6.5% in the intensive control group and 7.3% in the standard control group.[16] Similar to ACCORD and VADT, the rate of combined primary end point (composite of microvascular and macrovascular events) was significantly lower with intensive versus conservative glucose control among patients who did not have established CV disease at baseline. A recent meta-analysis by Mannucci et al.[21] examined the effects of intensive glycemic control on CV outcomes in pooled data from UKPDS, ACCORD, ADVANCE, and VADT, in addition to the PROACTIVE (Prospective Pioglitazone Clinical Trial in Macrovascular Events) study. This meta-analysis showed that an overall decrease in HbA1c values of 0.9% resulted in modest reduction in the risk of CV events and MI in the intensive therapy groups but no significant reductions in all-cause or CV mortality or stroke. The cumulative data from these studies suggest that the potential for benefit or harm from intensive therapy may be determined by the presence or absence of significant atherosclerosis at the time of therapy initiation[12,13,15,16] and that a less aggressive approach, with an HbA1c target of 7.0–7.5%, appears to be the preferred strategy for patients with limited life expectancy and/or those with established CV disease or long-standing T2DM.

THE CARDIOVASCULAR TOXICITY OF HYPOGLYCEMIA

Hypoglycemia is a common problem in patients with T2DM who need to be treated with insulin or sulfonylureas, and hypoglycemia occurred more frequently in the intensive therapy arms of the ACCORD, ADVANCE, VADT, and UKPDS trials.[12,13,15,16] Hypoglycemia, especially when severe, is a powerful stimulant of the sympathetic nervous system, which in turn may trigger adverse CV events, such as cardiac arrhythmias, sudden cardiac arrest, and acute MI.[22,23] Prolongation of the QT interval, ventricular arrhythmias, and impaired autonomic function are also associated with hypoglycemic episodes.[22-25] Hypoglycemia is also proinflammatory and can increase the risk of plaque inflammation, rupture, and CV events.[26,27]

In their meta-analysis of glycemic control and CV events, Mannucci et al.[21] suggested an association between CV death in the intensive therapy arms and severe hypoglycemia. Although speculative, the CV toxicity caused by recurrent or severe hypoglycemia induced by an aggressive glycemic control strategy (particularly with insulin or sulfonylureas) may supersede the CV benefits of improved glycemic control. This may be particularly true for those who have a predisposition to adverse CV events, such as persons with significant atherosclerosis and/or structural heart disease, such as left ventricular (LV) hypertrophy or systolic and/or diastolic dysfunction. Thus, it is not surprising that patient with long-standing T2DM (with its associations with atherosclerosis and myocardial structural and functional abnormalities) and/or existing CV disease may be more susceptible to the cardiotoxicity induced by hypoglycemia.

THE CARDIOVASCULAR TOXICITY OF POSTPRANDIAL HYPERGLYCEMIA

Another possible reason for the failure of glucose-lowering strategies to improve CV prognosis is the use of glucose lowering therapies that are directed more to the lowering of fasting and preprandial glucose levels than to the lowering of postprandial glucose levels. Postprandial hyperglycemia has been shown to be associated with an increased risk of CV events in patients with and without T2DM.[28] Postprandial glucose excursions, especially when accompanied by increased postprandial triglyceride levels, are pathophysiologically linked to increased oxidative stress, systemic inflammation, and endothelial dysfunction, all of which are related to increases in atherosclerosis and CV events.[29,30] Importantly, even in the setting of controlled fasting glucose levels, postprandial spikes in glucose powerfully increase both atherogenesis and CV events.[28]

A study of postmenopausal women without DM but with coronary artery disease (CAD) showed that the change in the minimal vessel diameter on quantitative coronary angiography during 3 years of follow-up was inversely proportional to the 2-hour postchallenge, but not fasting, glucose levels (Fig. 3).[31] In fact, a 2-hour postprandial glucose level of less than 87 mg/dL (to convert to mmol/L, multiply by 0.0555) was associated with regression of atheroma.[31] Pharmacological lowering of postprandial glucose generally has been shown to decrease CV events.[31] The STOP-NIDDM (STOP-Noninsulin-Dependent Diabetes Mellitus) trial was a large randomized placebo-controlled trial assessing the effects of acarbose in the prevention of T2DM in patients with impaired glucose tolerance.[32] Acarbose, an α-glucosidase inhibitor that slows the digestive breakdown of starch and sucrose to glucose and, therefore almost exclusively affects postprandial glucose, was associated with not only a 25% reduction in progression to T2DM but also a 49% reduction in CV events during the 3.3 years of this randomized trial (Fig. 4).[32] To further investigate the favorable effects of acarbose on CV events, a meta-analysis of seven studies of acarbose in patients with T2DM was performed. Compared with other medications used in the treatment of patients with T2DM, acarbose was associated with a 35% relative risk reduction for any CV event. This statistically significant finding was driven primarily by a markedly decreased risk of MI.[33]

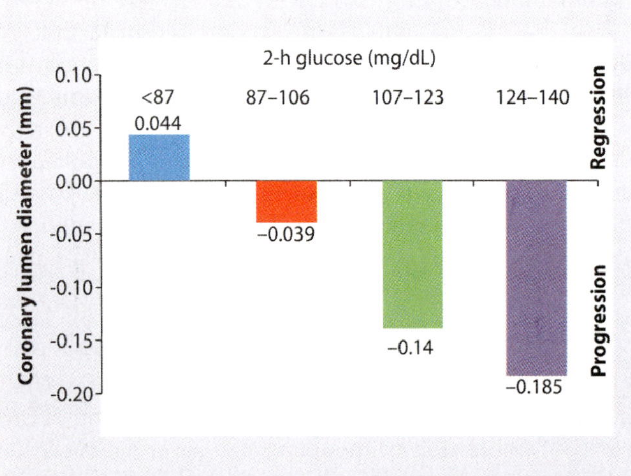

Fig. 3: Postchallenge glucose and coronary atherosclerosis progression. Only women with postchallenge glucose values of less than 87 mg/dL had regression in coronary atherosclerosis[31]

THE CARDIOVASCULAR TOXICITY OF INSULIN RESISTANCE

Insulin resistance is associated with increases in a plethora of CAD risk factors, including hypertension, 38 low-levels of high-density lipoprotein cholesterol (HDL-C),[34] high triglyceride levels,[34] an increased number and decreased size of low-density lipoprotein cholesterol (LDL-C) particles, higher C-reactive protein levels, decreased fibrinolysis, and endothelial dysfunction.[35] Epidemiologically, insulin resistance has also been shown to be associated with increased atherosclerosis and increased CV events.[36] Lowering insulin resistance may also result in less atherosclerosis and decreased CV events.

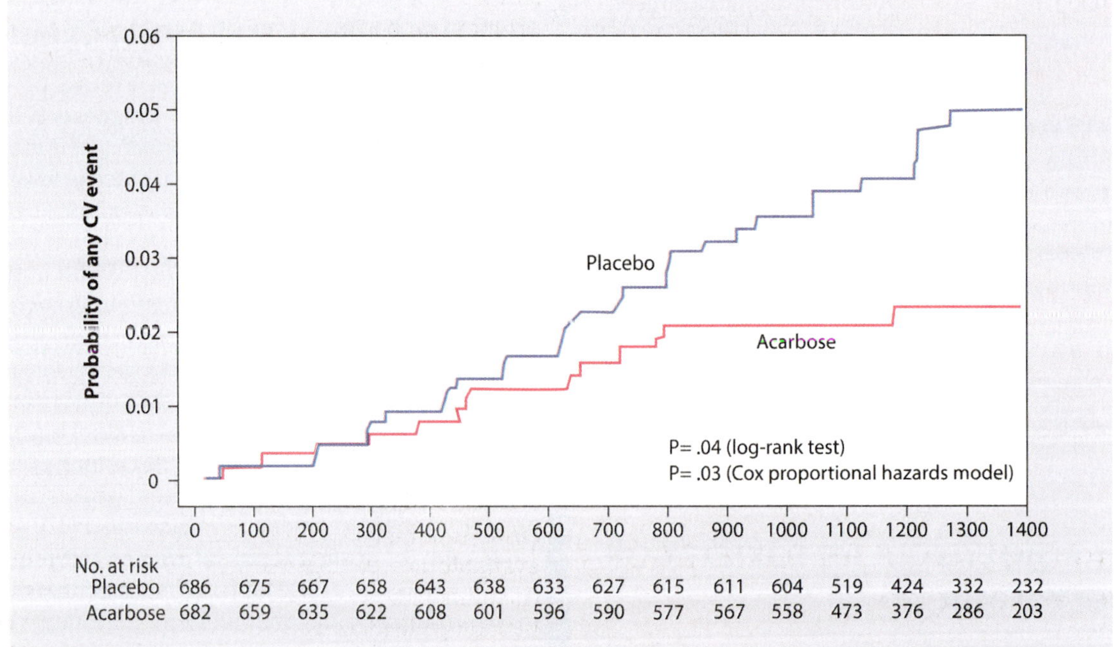

Fig. 4: Cardiovascular (CV) events in STOP-NIDDM. Probability of remaining free of CV disease from STOP-NIDDM[32]

PROMISING APPROACHES TO IMPROVING CARDIOVASCULAR PROGNOSIS IN TYPE 2 DIABETES MELLITUS

Taken together, these data suggest that a logical and promising approach to improving the CV prognosis for the patient with T2DM would be to use therapies that (1) improve glycemic control without leading to hypoglycemia, (2) effectively lower postprandial glucose excursions (or lower both fasting and postprandial glucose), and (3) lower insulin resistance. In fact, therapeutic strategies using agents that have these three features have shown promise for reducing CV events in prospective trials. These therapies include metformin, acarbose, bile acid sequestrants, incretin mimetics, and dipeptidyl peptidase 4 (DPP-4) inhibitors. Bariatric surgery in the treatment of patients with morbid obesity has been shown to confer glucose-lowering and insulin-sensitizing effects. The relative effects of glucose-lowering drugs on the triad of postprandial glucose, insulin resistance, and hypoglycemia are shown in the Table 1.[37] Although insulin use requires injections and can cause hypoglycemia, many patients with T2DM, especially those who have had the disease for a decade or more, will require insulin therapy to maintain reasonable glycemic control. In such patients, as in patients with type 1 DM, modern insulin agents, when used in conjunction with frequent glucose monitoring and close follow-up with a health care professional, have been shown to improve prognosis.[17]

Metformin

The hypoglycemic effect of metformin is due to decreased resistance to the action of insulin on the liver and kidneys, which reduces the hepatic and renal production of glucose. In addition, probably as a result of its anorectic effect and/or the weight loss it induces, metformin lowers peripheral insulin resistance and is associated with a low risk of hypoglycemia. Using the UK General Practice Research Database, a recent retrospective study by Tzoulaki et al.[38] showed that, compared with sulfonylureas, metformin was associated with a lower risk of all-cause mortality and was nonsignificantly associated with a lower risk of a first MI.[38] The differences between metformin and sulfonylureas could simply be due to the low risk of hypoglycemia that occurs with metformin.[14] However, another contributing factor may be that sulfonylureas inhibit myocardial ischemic preconditioning by blocking the adenosine triphosphate-sensitive potassium channels, thereby worsening myocardial ischemia and potentially resulting in larger infarcts, more arrhythmias, and heart failure (HF).[39]

TABLE 1: Effects of antidiabetic drugs on the triad of postprandial glucose, insulin resistance, and hypoglycemia[37]

Drug class	*Lower(s) postprandial glucose*	*Lower(s) insulin resistance*	*Avoid(s) hypoglycemia*
Sulfonylureas	+	-	-
Metformin	-	+	+
Thiazolidinediones	+	+	+
Incretin-based therapies	+	-	+
Bile acid sequestrants	+	-	+
α-glucosidase inhibitors	+	-	+

Thiazolidinediones

Thiazolidinediones (TZDs) lower insulin resistance[40] and increase adiponectin levels,[40] thereby improving CV risk factors. Both rosiglitazone and pioglitazone have been shown to decrease carotid intima-media thickening. However, pioglitazone, but not rosiglitazone, has been shown to decelerate the formation of coronary artery atheroma as assessed by intravascular ultrasonography. The PROACTIVE study randomized 5238 patients with CV disease and suboptimally controlled T2DM to the addition of pioglitazone or placebo to their existing T2DM therapy.[41] After 3 years, a nonsignificant favorable trend in the primary composite end point of adverse CV and peripheral artery disease events was found in the pioglitazone arm. As expected, the frequency of reported HF and hospital admissions for HF in the pioglitazone arm was increased compared with placebo.[42] Rosiglitazone was the TZD used in the RECORD (Rosiglitazone Evaluated for Outcomes and Regulation of Glycaemia in Diabetes), ACCORD, VADT, and BARI-2D (Bypass Angioplasty Revascularization Investigation 2 Diabetes)[43] randomized controlled trials without any significant adverse effect on CV events.[44] However, a possible association between rosiglitazone and an increased risk of MI was reported in a widely publicized meta-analysis by Nissen and Wolski[45] and in some large retrospective database studies.[46] Recently, the European Medicines Agency ruled that rosiglitazone could no longer be marketed or available in Europe, and the US Food and Drug Administration mandated that rosiglitazone remain available only under very restricted access conditions (inability to achieve glycemic control using other agents, including pioglitazone).

In summary, pioglitazone, but not rosiglitazone, appears to be helpful in slowing the progression of atherosclerosis in the carotid and coronary arteries and may decrease CV events. However, the TZDs definitely increase the risk of HF and may also increase the risk of bone fractures.[37] Pioglitazone, which is slated to be available generically in 2012, may be beneficial in selected patients with T2DM, especially when used in combination with metformin. Patients with HF should not be treated with a TZD. Rosiglitazone should not be used because of concerns about CV safety.

α-glucosidase Inhibitors

By blocking the activity of α-glucosidase, α-glucosidase inhibitors slow the digestion of starches and disaccharides into glucose, decreasing both postprandial hyperglycemia and hypertriglyceridemia. Acarbose therapy decreases the progression of thickening of the intima and media of carotid arteries and decreases the incidence of MI and other CV events.[32,33] The improvement in CV events that has been shown with α-glucosidase inhibitors likely results from the lowering of postprandial glucose and triglyceride levels. In addition, α-glucosidase inhibitors do not cause hypoglycemia.[33]

Incretin Mimetics and DPP-4 Inhibitors

Agents that modulate the incretin system, such as incretin mimetics (exenatide and liraglutide), slow gastric emptying, suppress glucagon production, and increase glucose stimulated insulin release, thereby effectively reducing postprandial glucose levels and posing a low risk of hypoglycemia. Dipeptidyl peptidase 4 inhibitors (sitagliptin and saxagliptin) also increase glucose-stimulated insulin release and suppress glucagon production but do not decrease gastric emptying[47] and are, therefore effective in reducing postprandial glucose levels without inducing hypoglycemia.[47] Drugs modulating the incretin system are promising agents for improving the adverse CV prognosis associated with T2DM. By either increasing the levels of glucagon-like peptide 1 (GLP-1) or mimicking its effects, these drugs appear to improve LV function and some CV risk factors.[47] Continuous intravenous infusion of GLP-1 for 5 weeks was shown to improve LV ejection fraction (LVEF) and functional status in patients with class III/IV HF.[48] Additionally, a 72-hour intravenous infusion of GLP-1 after successful primary angioplasty resulted in improved LVEF in patients who had an acute MI and severe LV dysfunction (LVEF <40%).[49] A recent meta-analysis of 41 randomized controlled trials examining CV events with the use of DPP-4 inhibitors suggested that these agents did not increase CV risk or all-cause mortality and were associated with a favorable trend toward lower CV events.[50] By improving postprandial hyperglycemia, CV risk factors, and LV function without causing hypoglycemia, incretin mimetics, and DDP-4 inhibitors may prove to be effective in reducing CV events. The major adverse effect of incretin mimetics is nausea; pancreatitis has been seen rarely in association with both incretin mimetics and DPP-4 inhibitors.[50]

Sodium Glucose Cotransporter 2 Inhibitors

Inhibitors of sodium-glucose cotransporter 2 reduce rates of hyperglycemia in patients with type 2 diabetes by decreasing renal glucose reabsorption, thereby increasing urinary glucose excretion.[51] Empagliflozin is a selective inhibitor of sodium glucose cotransporter 2 that has been approved for type 2 diabetes.[51] Given as either monotherapy or as an add-on therapy, the drug is reported to reduce glycated hemoglobin levels in patients with type 2 diabetes, including those with stage 2 or 3a chronic kidney disease.[51] Furthermore, empagliflozin is associated with weight loss and reductions in blood pressure without increases in heart rate. Empagliflozin also has favorable effects on markers of arterial stiffness and vascular resistance, visceral adiposity, albuminuria, and plasma urate. The most common side effects of empagliflozin are urinary tract infection and genital infection.[51]

In the EMPA-REG OUTCOME trial,[51] a total of 7020 patients were treated (median observation time, 3.1 years) in the empagliflozin group there were significantly lower rates of death from CV causes (3.7% vs 5.9% in the placebo group; 38% relative risk reduction), hospitalization for HF (2.7 and 4.1%, respectively; 35% relative risk reduction), and death from any cause (5.7 and 8.3%, respectively; 32% relative risk reduction) (Table 2). The study concluded that patients with type 2 diabetes at high risk for CV events who received empagliflozin, as compared with placebo, had a lower rate of the primary composite CV outcome and of death from any cause when the study drug was added to standard care.

Bariatric Surgery

Excess abdominal adipose tissue increases insulin resistance and inflammation and markedly increases the likelihood of T2DM and adverse CV events.[37] Bariatric surgery, which increases GLP-1 levels likely as a result of rapid dumping of chyme into the small intestine, is an option for morbidly obese patients with T2DM. The "cure" of T2DM after a Roux-en-Y gastric bypass procedure usually happens early, often before significant weight loss

TABLE 2: Primary and secondary cardiovascular outcomes in EMPA-REG OUTCOME trial[51]

Outcome	*Placebo (N = 2,333)*		*Empagliflozin (N = 4,687)*		*Hazard ratio (95% CI)*	*P-value*
	No. (%)	*Rate/1,000 patient-year*	*No. (%)*	*Rate/1,000 patient-year*		
Death from cardiovascular causes, nonfatal myocardial infarction, or nonfatal stroke: primary outcome	282 (12.1)	43.9	490 (10.5)	37.4	0.86 (0.74–0.99)	
Noninferiority						<0.001
Superiority						0.04
Death from cardiovascular causes, nonfatal myocardial infarction, nonfatal stroke, or hospitalization for unstable angina: key secondary outcome	333 (14.3)	52.5	599 (12.8)	46.4	0.89 (0.78–1.01)	
Noninferiority						<0.001
Superiority						0.08
Death						
From any cause	194 (8.3)	28.6	269 (5.7)	19.4	0.68 (0.57–0.82)	<0.001
From cardiovascular causes	137 (5.9)	20.2	172 (3.7)	12.4	0.62 (0.49–0.77)	<0.001
Fatal or nonfatal myocardial infarction excluding silent myocardial infarction	126 (5.4)	19.3	223 (4.8)	16.8	0.87 (0.70–1.09)	0.23
Nonfatal myocardial infarction excluding silent myocardial infarction	121 (5.2)	18.5	213 (4.5)	16.0	0.87 (0.70–1.09)	0.22
Silent myocardial infarction	15 (1.2)	5.4	38 (1.6)	7.0	1.28 (0.70–2.33)	0.42
Hospitalization for unstable angina	66 (2.8)	10.0	133 (2.8)	10.0	0.99 (0.74–1.34)	0.97
Coronary revascularization procedure	186 (8.0)	29.1	329 (7.0)	25.1	0.86 (0.72–1.04)	0.11
Fatal or nonfatal stroke	69 (3.0)	10.5	164 (3.5)	12.3	1.18 (0.89–1.56)	0.26
Nonfatal stroke	60 (2.6)	9.1	150 (3.2)	11.2	1.24 (0.92–1.67)	0.16
Transient ischemic attack	23 (1.0)	3.5	39 (0.8)	2.9	0.85 (0.51–1.42)	0.54
Hospitalization for heart failure	95 (4.1)	14.5	126 (2.7)	9.4	0.65 (0.50–0.85)	0.002
Hospitalization for heart failure or death from cardiovascular causes excluding fatal stroke	198 (8.5)	30.1	265 (5.7)	19.7	0.66 (0.55–0.79)	<0.001

has occurred.[52] This suggests that a role in the resolution of T2DM is played by an alternative mechanism, such as increased GLP-1 levels that in turn improve β-cell function and insulin production. In a large, prospective, controlled, nonrandomized trial, bariatric surgery was associated with resolution of T2DM in 72% of patients after 2 years and 36% after 10 years. During 7.1 years of follow-up, a large retrospective cohort study showed a 40% reduction in all-cause mortality in morbidly obese patients who underwent gastric bypass surgery compared with age-, sex-, and body mass index-matched controls.[53] Because of the increased insulin production associated with Roux-en-Y gastric bypass, hypoglycemia can be a problem.[52] Other complications of bariatric surgery include dumping syndrome and malabsorption of essential nutrients, such as vitamin B_{12}, iron, and fat-soluble vitamins.[52]

CONCLUSION

Type 2 diabetes mellitus is a major risk factor for CAD. The main target for prevention of CAD remains the strict control of the major associated CV risk factors that tend to cluster with T2DM—primarily hypertension and dyslipidemia. Glycemic control is important for preventing microvascular complications, such as retinopathy, nephropathy, and neuropathy. Improved glycemic control may also confer macrovascular CV benefits, especially in those with a more recent onset of T2DM and without established CAD, and when therapies that lower postprandial hyperglycemia and do not cause hypoglycemia are used. Therapies that lower insulin resistance may also independently reduce CV events. According to the American Diabetes Association, the American College of Cardiology, and the American Heart Association, the current HbA1c target for patients with T2DM is less than 7%.[54] Available data suggest that aggressive control below this goal does not provide benefit and may be harmful, particularly in patients of advanced age, those with a longer duration of T2DM, and those with established CAD. In contrast, younger patients with relatively recently diagnosed T2DM and no known CAD are more likely to benefit from a more aggressive approach to glycemic control.

The major factor in improving CV events with glycemic control may well be the therapies that are used to achieve this control. Preferred treatments rely on drugs that do not cause hypoglycemia (metformin, pioglitazone, α-glucosidase inhibitors, incretin mimetics, and empagliflozin) rather than on insulin or sulfonylureas, which are associated with a higher risk of hypoglycemia. If possible, sulfonylureas should be the last oral agents to be used in patients with T2DM and may be bypassed by using insulin. When insulin therapy is required, insulin analogs, which may be associated with a lower risk of hypoglycemia, are preferred. Furthermore, drugs that have shown favorable effects on insulin resistance, postprandial glucose levels, atherosclerosis, and CV events should be favored. The CV prognosis for patients with T2DM may depend less on the HbA1c level achieved than on the way in which it was attained.

REFERENCES

1. Goff DC Jr, Gerstein HC, Ginsberg HN, et al. Prevention of cardiovascular disease in persons with type 2 diabetes mellitus: current knowledge and rationale for the Action to Control Cardiovascular Risk in Diabetes (ACCORD) trial. Am J Cardiol. 2007;99(12A):4i-20i.
2. Selvin E, Marinopoulos S, Berkenblit G, et al. Meta-analysis: glycosylated hemoglobin and cardiovascular disease in diabetes mellitus. Ann Intern Med. 2004;141(6):421-31.
3. Gerstein HC, Pogue J, Mann JF, et al. The relationship between dysglycaemia and cardiovascular and renal risk in diabetic and non-diabetic participants in the HOPE study: a prospective epidemiological analysis. Diabetologia. 2005;48(9):1749-55.
4. Stratton IM, Adler AI, Neil HA, et al. Association of glycaemia with macrovascular and microvascular complications of type 2 diabetes (UKPDS 35): prospective observational study. BMJ. 2000;321(7258):405-12.
5. Seshasai SR, Kaptoge S, Thompson A, et al. Diabetes mellitus, fasting glucose, and risk of cause-specific death. N Engl J Med. 2011;364(9):829-41.
6. Beckman JA, Paneni F, Cosentino F, et al. Diabetes and vascular disease: pathophysiology, clinical consequences, and medical therapy: part II. Eur Heart J. 2013;34(31):2444-52.
7. Ryden L, Grant PJ, Anker SD, et al. ESC Guidelines on diabetes, pre-diabetes, and cardiovascular diseases developed in collaboration with the EASD: the Task Force on diabetes, pre-diabetes, and cardiovascular diseases of the European Society of Cardiology (ESC) and developed in collaboration with the European Association for the Study of Diabetes (EASD). Eur Heart J. 2013;34(39):3035-87.
8. Malmberg K, Yusuf S, Gerstein HC, et al. Impact of diabetes on long-term prognosis in patients with unstable angina and non-Q-wave myocardial infarction: results of the OASIS (Organization to Assess Strategies for Ischemic Syndromes) Registry. Circulation. 2000;102(9):1014-9.
9. Haffner SM, Lehto S, Ronnemaa T, et al. Mortality from coronary heart disease in subjects with type 2 diabetes and in nondiabetic subjects with and without prior myocardial infarction. N Engl J Med. 1998;339(4):229-34.
10. Yahagi K, Kolodgie FD, Lutter C, et al. Pathology of human coronary and carotid artery atherosclerosis and vascular calcification in diabetes mellitus. Arterioscler Thromb Vasc Biol. 2017;37(2): 191-204.
11. Ferrannini E and DeFronzo RA. Impact of glucose-lowering drugs on cardiovascular disease in type 2 diabetes. Eur Heart J. 2015;36(34):2288-96.
12. UK Prospective Diabetes Study (UKPDS) Group. Intensive blood-glucose control with sulphonylureas or insulin compared with conventional treatment and risk of complications in patients with type 2 diabetes (UKPDS 33). Lancet. 1998;352(9131):837-53.
13. Gerstein HC, Miller ME, Byington RP, et al. Effects of intensive glucose lowering in type 2 diabetes. N Engl J Med. 2008;358(24):2545-59.
14. UK Prospective Diabetes Study (UKPDS) Group. Effect of intensive blood-glucose control with metformin on complications in overweight patients with type 2 diabetes (UKPDS 34). Lancet. 1998;352(9131):854-65.
15. Duckworth W, Abraira C, Moritz T, et al. Glucose control and vascular complications in veterans with type 2 diabetes. N Engl J Med. 2009;360(2):129-39.
16. Patel A, MacMahon S, Chalmers J, et al. Intensive blood glucose control and vascular outcomes in patients with type 2 diabetes. N Engl J Med. 2008;358(24):2560-72.
17. Riddle MC, Ambrosius WT, Brillon DJ, et al. Epidemiologic relationships between A1C and all-cause mortality during a median 3.4-year follow-up of glycemic treatment in the ACCORD trial. Diabetes Care. 2010;33(5):983-90.
18. Piarulli F, Sartore G, Ceriello A, et al. Relationship between glyco-oxidation, antioxidant status and microalbuminuria in type 2 diabetic patients. Diabetologia. 2009;52(7):1419-25.
19. Reaven PD, Moritz TE, Schwenke DC, et al. Intensive glucose-lowering therapy reduces cardiovascular disease events in veterans affairs diabetes trial participants with lower calcified coronary atherosclerosis. Diabetes. 2009;58(11):2642-8.
20. Gerstein HC, Mann JF, Yi Q, et al. Albuminuria and risk of cardiovascular events, death, and heart failure in diabetic and nondiabetic individuals. JAMA. 2001;286(4):421-6.
21. Mannucci E, Monami M, Lamanna C, et al. Prevention of cardiovascular disease through glycemic control in type 2 diabetes: a meta-analysis of randomized clinical trials. Nutr Metab Cardiovasc Dis. 2009;19(9):604-12.
22. Curtis BM, O'Keefe JH Jr. Autonomic tone as a cardiovascular risk factor: the dangers of chronic fight or flight. Mayo Clin Proc. 2002;77(1):45-54
23. DeRosa MA, Cryer PE. Hypoglycemia and the sympathoadrenal system: neurogenic symptoms are largely the result of sympathetic neural, rather than adrenomedullary, activation. Am J Physiol Endocrinol Metab. 2004;287(1):E32-41.
24. Marques JL, George E, Peacey SR, et al. Altered ventricular repolarization during hypoglycaemia in patients with diabetes. Diabet Med. 1997;14(8):648-54.
25. Adler GK, Bonyhay I, Failing H, et al. Antecedent hypoglycemia impairs autonomic cardiovascular function: implications for rigorous glycemic control. Diabetes. 2009;58(2):360-6.
26. Dotson S, Freeman R, Failing HJ, et al. Hypoglycemia increases serum interleukin-6 levels in healthy men and women. Diabetes Care. 2008;31(6):1222-3.

27. Packard RR, Libby P. Inflammation in atherosclerosis: from vascular biology to biomarker discovery and risk prediction. Clin Chem. 2008;54(1):24-38.
28. Cavalot F, Petrelli A, Traversa M, et al. Postprandial blood glucose is a stronger predictor of cardiovascular events than fasting blood glucose in type 2 diabetes mellitus, particularly in women: lessons from the San Luigi Gonzaga Diabetes Study. J Clin Endocrinol Metab. 2006;91(3):813-9.
29. Monnier L, Mas E, Ginet C, et al. Activation of oxidative stress by acute glucose fluctuations compared with sustained chronic hyperglycemia in patients with type 2 diabetes. JAMA. 2006;295(14):1681-7.
30. Ceriello A, Quagliaro L, Piconi L, et al. Effect of postprandial hypertriglyceridemia and hyperglycemia on circulating adhesion molecules and oxidative stress generation and the possible role of simvastatin treatment. Diabetes. 2004;53(3):701-10.
31. Mellen PB, Bittner V, Herrington DM. Post-challenge glucose predicts coronary atherosclerotic progression in non-diabetic, post-menopausal women. Diabet Med. 2007;24(10):1156-9.
32. Chiasson JL, Josse RG, Gomis R, et al. Acarbose treatment and the risk of cardiovascular disease and hypertension in patients with impaired glucose tolerance: the STOP-NIDDM trial. JAMA. 2003;290(4):486-94.
33. Hanefeld M, Cagatay M, Petrowitsch T, et al. Acarbose reduces the risk for myocardial infarction in type 2 diabetic patients: meta-analysis of seven long-term studies. Eur Heart J. 2004;25(1):10-16.
34. Zavaroni I, Bonora E, Pagliara M, et al. Risk factors for coronary artery disease in healthy persons with hyperinsulinemia and normal glucose tolerance. New Engl J Med. 1989;320(11):702-6.
35. Haffner SM, D'Agostino R Jr, Mykkanen L, et al. Insulin sensitivity in subjects with type 2 diabetes: relationship to cardiovascular risk factors: the Insulin Resistance Atherosclerosis Study. Diabetes Care. 1999;22(4):562-8.
36. Despres JP, Lamarche B, Mauriege P, et al. Hyperinsulinemia as an independent risk factor for ischemic heart disease. New Engl J Med. 1996;334(15):952-7.
37. Keefe J, Abuannadi M, Lavie C, et al. Strategies for optimizing glycemic control and cardiovascular prognosis in patients with type 2 diabetes mellitus. Mayo Clin Proc. 2011;86(2):128-38.
38. Tzoulaki I, Molokhia M, Curcin V, et al. Risk of cardiovascular disease and all cause mortality among patients with type 2 diabetes prescribed oral antidiabetes drugs: retrospective cohort study using UK general practice research database. BMJ. 2009;339:b4731.
39. Bell DS. Do sulfonylurea drugs increase the risk of cardiac events? CMAJ. 2006;174(2):185-6.
40. Aso Y, Hara K, Ozeki N, et al. Low-dose pioglitazone increases serum high molecular weight adiponectin and improves glycemic control in Japanese patients with poorly controlled type 2 diabetes. Diabetes Res Clin Pract. 2009;85(2):147-52.
41. Dormandy JA, Charbonnel B, Eckland DJ, et al. Secondary prevention of macrovascular events in patients with type 2 diabetes in the PROactive Study (PROspective pioglitAzone Clinical Trial In macroVascular Events): a randomized controlled trial. Lancet. 2005;366(9493):1279-89.
42. Erdmann E, Charbonnel B, Wilcox RG, et al. Pioglitazone use and heart failure in patients with type 2 diabetes and preexisting cardiovascular disease: data from the PROactive study (PROactive 08). Diabetes Care. 2007;30(11):2773-8.
43. Frye RL, August P, Brooks MM, et al. A randomized trial of therapies for type 2 diabetes and coronary artery disease. New Engl J Med. 2009;360(24):2503-15.
44. Meier M, Hummel M. Cardiovascular disease and intensive glucose control in type 2 diabetes mellitus: moving practice toward evidence-based strategies. Vasc Health Risk Manag. 2009;5:859-71.
45. Nissen SE, Wolski K. Effect of rosiglitazone on the risk of myocardial infarction and death from cardiovascular causes. New Engl J Med. 2007;356(24):2457-71.
46. Lipscombe LL, Gomes T, Levesque LE, et al. Thiazolidinediones and cardiovascular outcomes in older patients with diabetes. JAMA. 2007;298(22):2634-43.
47. Verspohl EJ. Novel therapeutics for type 2 diabetes: incretin hormone mimetics (glucagon-like peptide-1 receptor agonists) and dipeptidyl peptidase-4 inhibitors. Pharmacol Ther. 2009;124(1):113-38.
48. Sokos GG, Nikolaidis LA, Mankad S, et al. Glucagon-like peptide-1 infusion improves left ventricular ejection fraction and functional status in patients with chronic heart failure. J Card Fail. 2006;12(9):694-9.
49. Nikolaidis LA, Mankad S, Sokos GG, et al. Effects of glucagon-like peptide-1 in patients with acute myocardial infarction and left ventricular dysfunction after successful reperfusion. Circulation. 2004;109(8):962-5.
50. Monami M, Iacomelli I, Marchionni N, et al. Dipeptydil peptidase-4 inhibitors in type 2 diabetes: a meta-analysis of randomized clinical trials. Nutr Metab Cardiovasc Dis. 2010;20(4):224-35.
51. Zinman B, Wanner C, Lachin MJ, et al. Empagliflozin, cardiovascular outcomes, and mortality in type 2 diabetes. N Engl J Med. 2015;373(22):2117-8.
52. Thaler JP, Cummings DE. Minireview: Hormonal and metabolic mechanisms of diabetes remission after gastrointestinal surgery. Endocrinology. 2009;150(6):2518-25.
53. Adams TD, Gress RE, Smith SC, et al. Long-term mortality after gastric bypass surgery. New Engl J Med. 2007;357(8):753-61.
54. Skyler JS, Bergenstal R, Bonow RO, et al. Intensive glycemic control and the prevention of cardiovascular events: implications of the ACCORD, ADVANCE, and VA Diabetes Trials: a position statement of the American Diabetes Association and a Scientific Statement of the American College of Cardiology Foundation and the American Heart Association. J Am Coll Cardiol. 2009;53(3):298-304.

CHAPTER

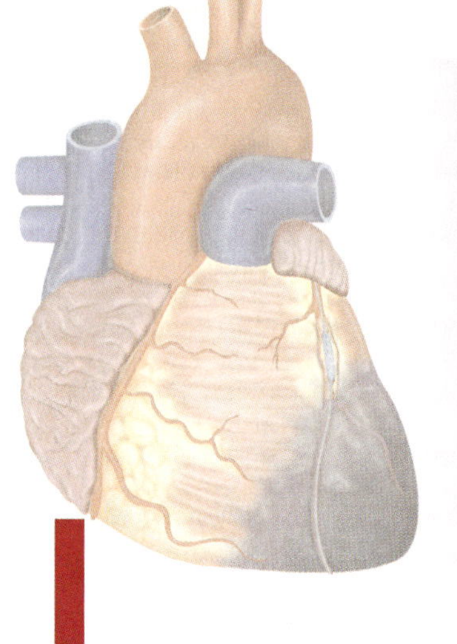

Improving CV Outcomes in Diabetes with New Antidiabetic Medications: A New Era has Begun

PC Manoria, Pankaj Manoria

INTRODUCTION

With better control of infective and metabolic complications, diabetes has emerged as a cardiovascular disease (CVD). About 70% diabetics die because CVD particularly acute myocardial infarction (MI). For close to 100 years, to be precise up to 93 years since the introduction of insulin for clinical use in 1922, no medication designed to treat hyperglycemia associated with type 2 diabetes mellitus (T2DM) had demonstrated benefit for CV risk in randomized CV clinical outcomes trials (CVOTs). The Rosiglitazone controversy created a flutter and the US Food Drug Administration (USFDA) in the year 2008 mandated that all new antidia-betic agents must undergo an adequately powered, glycemic-equipoise CVOTs in high-risk type 2 diabetic patients, during postmarketing phase to demonstrate its safety by showing noninferiority against placebo. The noninferiority was defined as hazard ratio (HR) of less than 1.3 for the upper bound of 95% confidence interval (CI), superiority can also be claimed if upper boundary of 95% CI is found to be less than 1.0 in a subsequent statistical analysis.[1] In 2012, The European Medicines Agency (EMA) also issued similar guidelines.[2] As a consequence of this, since post 2008, all newer antidiabetic agents approved by USFDA and EMA have underwent or currently undergoing CVOT. 2015 came with a breaking news, when three new antidiabetic medications, empagliflozin in the EMPA-REG OUTCOME, liraglutide in Liraglutide Effect and Action in Diabetes—Evaluation of Cardiovascular Outcome Results (LEADER), and semaglutide in Trial to Evaluate Cardiovascular and Other Long-term Outcomes with Semaglutide in Subjects with Type 2 Diabetes (SUSTAIN-6) trial showed CV benefits for the first-time in the history of diabetes. This represents a sea change in the treatment paradigm for type 2 diabetes with CVD. In addition to CV benefits, these medications also improve upon other limitations of older antihyperglycemic medications such as avoidance of weight gain and sodium retention and that too with minimal risk for hypoglycemia. In fact the new medications like sodium-glucose cotransporter 2 inhibitor (SGLT2i) and glucagon-like peptide-1 receptor agonists (GLP-1RA) also decrease weight and blood pressure. In 2017, the Canagliflozin Cardiovascular Assessment Study (CANVAS) trial with canagliflozin also showed improved CV outcomes in diabetics with CVD.

CARDIOVASCULAR OUTCOME TRIALS WITH NEWER AGENTS

Several CVOTs had been initiated to assess the effect of newer antidiabetic medications on CV outcomes. Eight trials have been completed and published, while others are ongoing (Table 1). Indeed four CV outcome trials with newer agents, i.e. EMPA-REG OUTCOME, LEADER and SUSTAIN-6 and CANVAS has shown improved outcomes.

The ongoing CVOT trials are outlined in Table 2.

TABLE 1: Large noninsulin completed CV outcome trials in T2DM.

Trials	*Drug*	*Comparator*	*Status*	*Number*	*Established CVD (%)*	*Results*
DPP-4 inhibitors						
SAVOR[3]	Saxagliptin	Placebo	Declared 2013	16,492	78%	CV neutral, ↑ hospitalization for HF
EXAMINE[4]	Alogliptin	Placebo	Declared 2013	5,380	100%	CV neutral, numerical ↑ HF
TECOS[5]	Sitagliptin	Placebo	Declared 2015	14,735	100%	CV neutral, no increase in hospitalization for HF
SGLT2 inhibitors						
EMPA-REG[6]	Empagliflozin	Placebo	Declared 2015	7,020	99%	Positive CV outcome
CANVAS[6]	Canagliflozin	Placebo	Declared 2017	4,330	67%	Positive CV outcome
GLP-1RA						
LEADER[7]	Liraglutide	Placebo	Declared 2015	9,340	81%	Positive CV outcome
ELIXA[8]	Lixisenatide	Placebo	Declared 2015	6,068	100%	CV neutral
SUSTAIN 6[9]	Semaglutide	Placebo	Declared 2016	3,297	58.8%	Positive CV outcome

Abbreviations: CV, cardiovascular; T2DM, type 2 diabetes mellitus; DPP, dipeptidyl peptidase; SAVOR, the saxagliptin assessment of vascular outcomes recorded in patients with diabetes mellitus; EXAMINE, examination of cardiovascular outcomes with alogliptin versus standard of care; TECOS, the trial evaluating cardiovascular outcomes with sitagliptin; HF, heart failure; CVD, cardiovascular disease; CANVAS, canagliflozin cardiovascular assessment study; LEADER, liraglutide effect and action in diabetes—evaluation of cardiovascular outcome results; ELIXA, evaluation of lixisenatide in acute coronary syndrome; SUSTAIN, trial to evaluate cardiovascular and other long-term outcomes with semaglutide in subjects with type 2 diabetes; GLP-1RA, glucagon-like peptide-1 receptor agonist; EMPA-REG, empagliflozin cardiovascular outcome event trial in type-2 diabetes mellitus patients–Removing excess glucose

TABLE 2: Large noninsulin ongoing CV outcomes trials in T2DM.

Trials	*Drug*	*Comparator*	*Status*	*Number*
DPP-4 Inhibitors				
CAROLINA[10]	Linagliptin	Sulfonylurea	Ongoing	6,000
CARMELINA[11]	Linagliptin	Placebo	Ongoing	8,300
SGLT2 Inhibitors				
DECLARETIMI[12]	Dapagliflozin	Placebo	Ongoing	17,276
VERTIS CV[13]	Ertugliflozin	Placebo	Ongoing	12,600
GLP-1 RA				
EXSCEL[14]	Exenatide	Placebo	Ongoing	14,000
REWIND[15]	Dulaglutide	Placebo	Ongoing	9,622
HARMONY[16]	Albiglutide	Placebo	Ongoing	7,500

Abbreviations: CV, cardiovascular; T2DM, type 2 diabetes mellitus; DPP, dipeptidyl peptidase; CARMELINA, Cardiovascular and Renal Microvascular Outcome Study With Linagliptin in Patients With Type 2 Diabetes Mellitus; CAROLINA, CARdiovascular Outcome Trial of LINAgliptin Versus Glimepiride in Type 2 Diabetes; SGLT2, sodium–glucose cotransporter 2; DECLARE-TIMI, dapagliflozin in Dapagliflozin effect on CardiovascuLAR Events-Thrombolysis in Myocardial Infarction; VERTIS CV; Cardiovascular Outcomes Following Ertugliflozin Treatment in Diabetes Mellitus Participants With Vascular Disease; GLP-1RA, glucagon-like peptide-1 receptor agonist; EXSCEL, Evaluation of Lixisenatide in Acute Coronary Syndrome; REWIND, Researching Cardiovascular Events With a Weekly Incretin in Diabetes

MAJOR ADVERSE CARDIAC EVENTS IN CARDIOVASCULAR CLINICAL OUTCOMES TRIALS

Dipeptidyl Peptidase-4 Inhibitors Trials

All the three dipeptidyl peptidase-4 inhibitors (DPP-4Is) trials, The Saxagliptin Assessment of Vascular Outcomes Recorded in Patients with Diabetes Mellitus (SAVOR), Examination of Cardiovascular Outcomes With Alogliptin versus Standard of Care (EXAMINE) and Trial Evaluating Cardiovascular Outcomes with Sitagliptin (TECOS) achieved the noninferiority margin on major adverse cardiac event (MACE) endpoints as laid down by the FDA in 2008, thereby suggesting that saxagliptin, alogliptin, and sitagliptin all are CV neutral drugs. However, no superiority on MACE was observed with any of the three DPP-4Is.[3-5]

Sodium–Glucose Cotransporter 2 Inhibitors

Surprisingly, empagliflozin in EMPA-REG OUTCOME[6] trial not only achieved by the noninferiority but also demonstrated a substantial superiority against placebo.

EMPA-REG found a significant relative risk reduction in the primary outcome of 3P-MACE (composite of CV death, nonfatal MI, and nonfatal stroke) by 14% (HR = 0.86, 95% CI = 0.74–0.99, *P* = 0.04 for superiority) compared to the placebo.[6]

The CANVAS[6] trial with canagliflozin also showed improved CV outcomes with exactly the same relative risk reduction of 14% in the primary outcome of similar 3P-MACE (HR=,0.86; 95% CI, 0.75–0.97; P< 0.001 for noninferiority; P = 0.02 for superiority) like the EMPA-REG OUTCOME trial. However, in CANVAS, while all three components of MACE moved in the right direction (i.e. HR< 1.0), none actually achieved statistical significance, perhaps reflecting the fact that the study involved a sizable subgroup about one-third of patients who had no prior history of CVD, unlike EMPA which did not included any such patients. Interestingly, in the CANVAS primary prevention subgroup, the HR for the primary outcome was 0.98, suggesting that those without CVD do not experience the CV benefit as those with CVD.

It should also be noted that while 3P-MACE reduction in EMPA-REG was mainly attributed to reduction in the CV death which was majorly due to the reduction in death from HHF; 3P-MACE reduction in LEADER[7] was derived from summation of all CV endpoints, although here also reduction in the CV death contributed majorly. In contrast, the 3P-MACE reduction in SUSTAIN-6[9] was primarily attributed to a significant reduction in the nonfatal stroke. So, in summary, at the present state of time the SGLT2 is, both empagliflozin and canagliflozin show a clear and definite CV advantage in high-risk patients with T2DM and established macrovascular complications. The 'thumbprint,' however, of individual members of the class may be different with regard to not only individual components of MACE but also with regard to adverse effect profiles. The mechanistic underpinnings of the CV effects of SGLT2 is still remain to be fully elucidated. They potentially pertain to the drug's glucoretic-natriuretic properties.[17] Another school of thought points to the tendency for these agents to shift fuel metabolism in favor of the consumption of ketones (instead of glucose and free fatty acids).[18] Such a change, it has been proposed may provide an energy advantage for cardiomyocytes. Clearly, more mechanistic studies are needed to better understand these concepts, which might have implications for the management of CVD.

The results of two ongoing CV outcome trials with other SGLT2 is in T2DM [dapagliflozin in Dapagliflozin Effect on CardiovascuLAR Events (DECLARE)][12] and ertugliflozin in Cardiovascular Outcomes Following Ertugliflozin Treatment in Diabetes Mellitus Participants With Vascular Disease (VERTIS CV)[13] are anticipated over the next several years. We will hopefully then have a better understanding of these issues at that time.

Glucagon-like Peptide-1 Receptor Agonists Trials

From the three GLP-1RAs trials, Evaluation of Lixisenatide in Acute Coronary Syndrome (ELIXA)[8] found lixisenatide to be noninferior (4P-MACE, HR = 1.02; 95% CI = 0.89–1.17; *P* < 0.001 for noninferiority) to placebo while liraglutide in LEADER and semaglutide in SUSTAIN-6 trials showed superiority on similar 3P-MACE compared to placebo.

Liraglutide Effect and Action in Diabetes—Evaluation of Cardiovascular Outcome Results [7] found 13% relative risk reduction (HR = 0.87; 95% CI = 0.78–0.97; P = 0.01) and SUSTAIN-6 demonstrated even a larger 26% relative risk reduction (HR = 0.74; 95% CI = 0.58–0.95; P = 0.02) in 3P-MACE.[6-8]

Interestingly, both LEADER and SUSTAIN-6[9] also demonstrated a significant reduction on the expanded composite outcome [death from CV causes, nonfatal MI, nonfatal stroke, revascularization or hospitalization for unstable angina, or heart failure (HF)] by 12% (HR = 0.88; 95% CI = 0.81–0.96; *P* = 0.005) and 26% (HR = 0.74; 95% CI = 0.62–0.89, *P* = 0.002) respectively, whereas EMP-REG could not demonstrate a significant reduction (HR = 0.89; 95% CI = 0.78–1.01; *P* = 0.08) on expanded 4P-MACE (3P-MACE plus unstable angina). Figure 1 depicts the reduction in MACE in all eight CVOTs.

Cardiovascular Death in Cardiovascular Clinical Outcomes Trials

No benefit was observed in reducing CV death in any CVOTs with DPP-4Is against placebo. Similarly, two GLP-1RAs, lixisenatide, and semaglutide could not show any significant reduction in the CV death in ELIXA and SUSTAIN-6, respectively. However, both empagliflozin in EMPA-REG and liraglutide in LEADER, significantly reduced CV death by 38% (HR = 0.62; 95% CI = 0.49–0.77; *P*< 0.0001) and 22% (HR = 0.78; 95% CI = 0.66–0.93; *P* = 0.007), respectively. This suggests that EMPA-REG showed much larger reduction in CV death compared to LEADER (38% vs. 22%) with more persuasive *P* value (< 0.0001 vs. 0.007). The CANVAS trial published recently showed a trend towards reduction in CVD. Figure 2 depicts the outcome of CV death in all eight CVOTs.

Nonfatal Myocardial Infarction in Cardiovascular Clinical Outcomes Trials

There was a nonstatistical trend in reduction of nonfatal MI in almost all CVOTs except EXAMINE and ELIXA. Figure 3 depicts this outcome. Silent MI was assessed in all patients in LEADER, and SUSTAIN-6, but only in 50% patient in

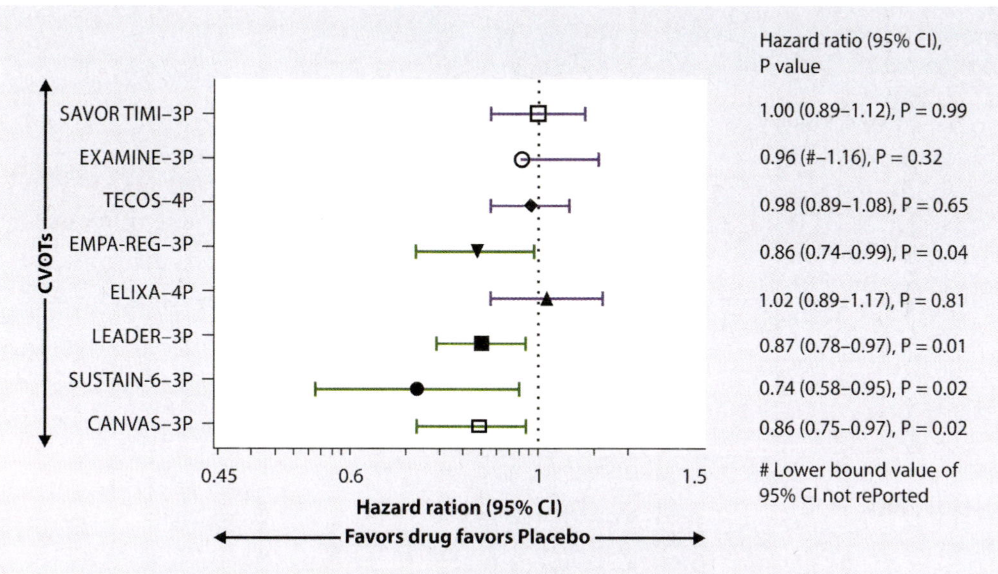

Fig. 1: Primary major adverse cardiac event in cardiovascular outcome trials

Abbreviations: SAVOR; the saxagliptin assessment of vascular outcomes recorded in patients with diabetes mellitus; TIMI, thrombolysis in myocardial infarction; ELIXA: evaluation of lixisenatide in acute coronary syndrome; EXAMINE: examination of cardiovascular outcomes with alogliptin versus standard of care; TECOS, trial evaluating cardiovascular outcomes with sitagliptin; LEADER, liraglutide effect and action in diabetes—evaluation of cardiovascular outcome results; SUSTAIN-6, trial to evaluate cardiovascular and other long-term outcomes with semaglutide in subjects with type 2 diabetes; CANVAS, canagliflozin cardiovascular assessment study; EMPA-REG, empagliflozin cardiovascular outcome event trial in type-2 diabetes mellitus patients–Removing excess glucose

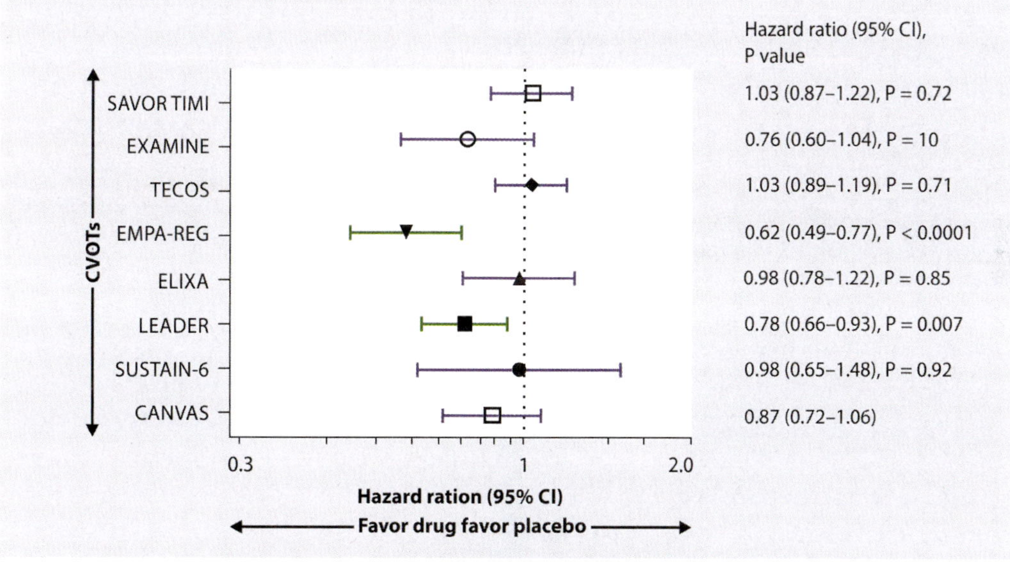

Fig. 2: Cardiovascular death in cardiovascular outcome trials

EMPA-REG. Intriguingly, there was 28% increased trend of silent MI in EMPA-REG although statistically insignificant.

Nonfatal Strokes in Cardiovascular Clinical Outcomes Trials

The Trial Evaluating Cardiovascular Outcomes with Sitagliptin had neutral outcome on nonfatal stroke. SAVOR- Thrombolysis in Myocardial Infarction (TIMI), ELIXA, and EMPA-REG showed a nonsignificant trend of increase in stroke. Stroke increased by 24% in empagliflozin arm (HR = 1.24; 95% CI = 0.92–1.67; $P = 0.16$), although it was statistically not significant. EXAMINE, LEADER, and CANVAS all showed a nonsignificant trend of decrease in stroke. Interestingly, SUSTAIN-6 showed a significant 39% relative risk reduction in nonfatal stroke (HR = 0.61; 95% CI = 0.38–0.99; $P = 0.04$). But its P value just reached statistical significance ($P = 0.04$). Figure 4 depicts the nonfatal stroke

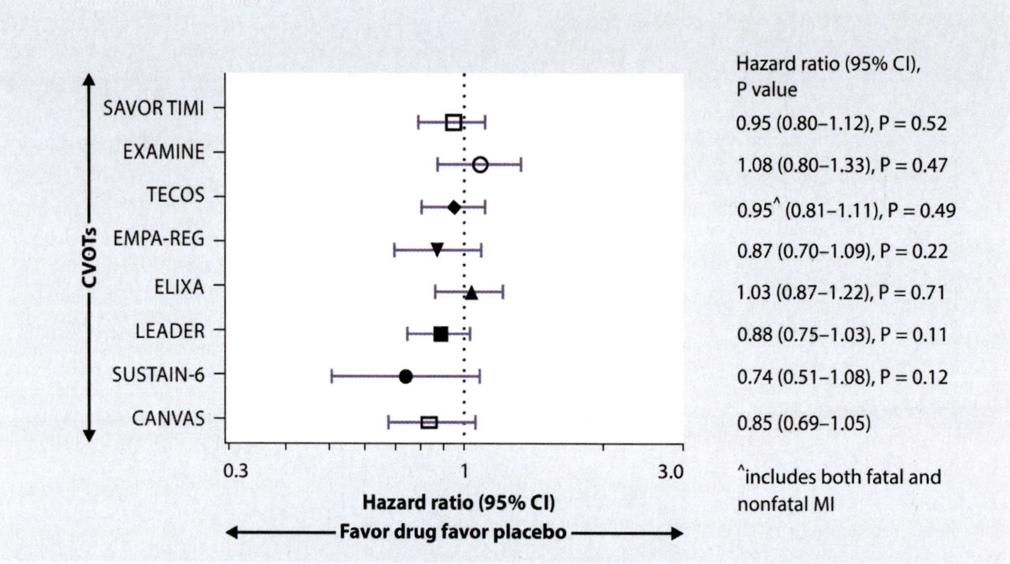

Fig. 3: Nonfatal myocardial infarction in cardiovascular outcome trials

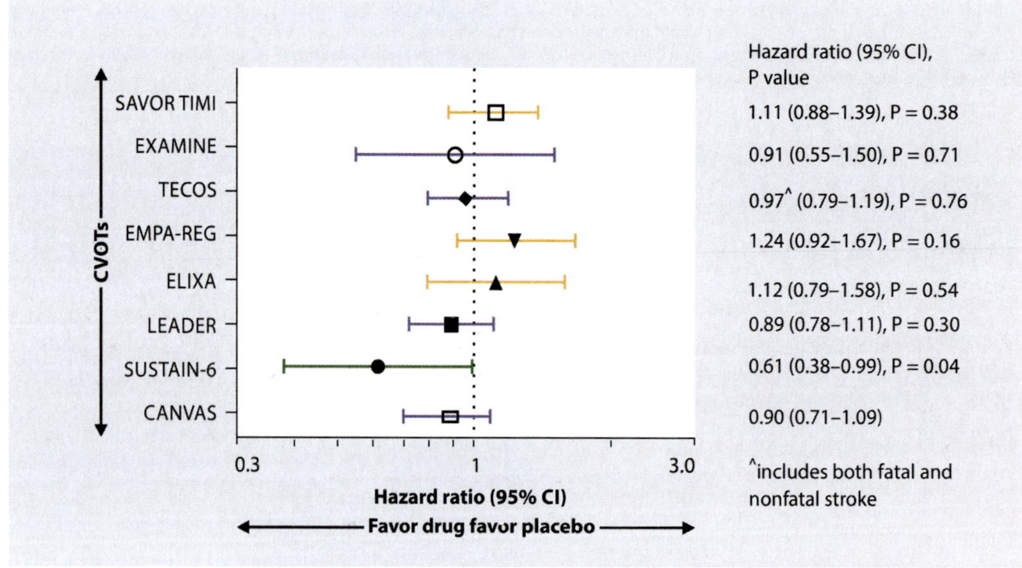

Fig. 4: Nonfatal stroke in cardiovascular outcome trials

outcome of all eight CVOTs. Four subgroups of patients that had significantly higher stroke in EMPA-REG in an independent analysis of FDA are:

1. Patients with age less than 65 years of age (HR = 1.6, 95% CI = 1.03–2.49)
2. Patients from Europe (HR = 2.04, 95% CI = 1.26–3.29)
3. Patients with baseline glycated hemoglobin (HbA1c) more than equal to 8.5% (HR = 2.13, 95% CI = 1.21–3.74)
4. Patients treated with insulin (HR = 1.57, 95% CI = 1.03–2.41).

Hospitalization Due to Unstable Angina in Cardiovascular Clinical Outcomes Trials

No statistically significant difference in hospitalization due to unstable angina was observed in all eight CVOTs as shown in Figure 5.

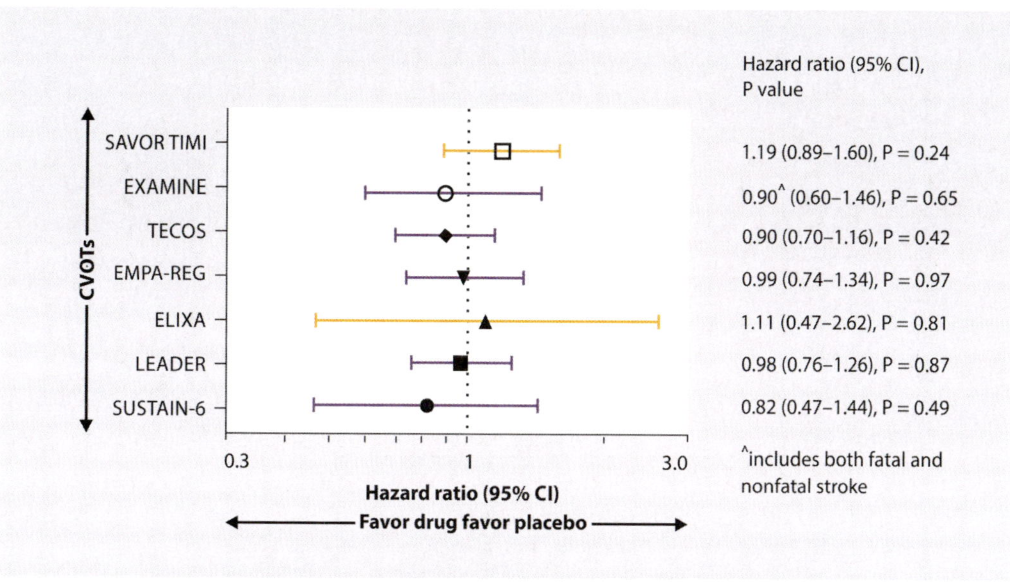

Fig. 5: Unstable angina hospitalization in cardiovascular outcome trials

All-cause Mortality in Cardiovascular Clinical Outcomes Trials

Empagliflozin reduced all-cause mortality by 32% (HR = 0.68; 95% CI = 0.57–0.82; *P*< 0.0001), while LEADER reduced it by 15% (HR = 0.85; 95% CI = 0.74–0.97; *P* = 0.02). This suggests that EMPA-REG had larger and robust reduction in all-cause mortality compared to LEADER (32% vs.15%, respectively) with persuasive *P* value (< 0.0001 vs. 0.02, respectively). The TECOS was neutral in all-cause mortality, while SAVOR-TIMI and SUSTAIN-6 showed a nonsignificant increase in it. The EXAMINE, ELIXA, and CANVAS showed a nonsignificant decrease in all-cause mortality. Figure 6 depicts the all-cause mortality across all eight CVOTs.

Heart Failure Hospitalizations in Cardiovascular Clinical Outcomes Trials

Hospitalization due to HF (HHF) was an exploratory endpoint in all the trials. Saxagliptin in SAVOR-TIMI showed a statistically significant 27% increase in the relative risk of HHF (HR = 1.27; 95% CI = 1.07–1.51, *P* = 0.007). This HHF in SAVOR-TIMI was more pronounced within its first year of randomization. Similar trend of increase (19%) was also observed with alogliptin in EXAMINE (HR = 1.19; 95% CI = 0.89–1.58; *P* = 0.24), although it was statistically insignificant. Intriguingly, the post-hoc analyses from both SAVOR-TIMI and EXAMINE found that certain subgroups had a significant increase in HHF that included, patients with a history of HF and renal disease.[19-21] Curiously, a post hoc analysis of EXAMINE also suggested a significant increase in HHF in patients without any history of HF (HR = 1.76, 95% CI = 1.07–2.90; *P* = 0.026).[22] On the contrary, sitagliptin in TECOS found no signal of HHF. Further extensive analysis of TECOS also could not find any signal of the HF, regardless of time, subgroups and method of statistical analysis applied.[23,24] Meanwhile, FDA put a warning on April 5, 2016 which states that 'safety review' has found that type 2 diabetes medicine containing saxagliptin and alogliptin may increase the risk of HF particularly in the patients who already have heart or kidney disease.[25] It should, however, be noted that HHF was neither a primary or secondary objective of these studies and thus any subanalysis could be subject to statistical error or may be a play of chance.

However, empagliflozin showed a robust reduction in HHF by 35% (HR = 0.65, 95% CI = 0.50–0.85; *P* = 0.002) in EMPA-REG. Interestingly the CANVAS showed identical trend in reduction in HHF (HR=.67; 95% CI 0.52- 0.67). LEADER had a nonsignificant reduction in HHF, which definitely sounds encouraging for liraglutide as earlier two trials conducted in patients with exclusive HF subjects, had disappointing results. While functional impact of GLP-1 for HF treatment (*n* = 300) conducted in patient with advanced HF (median left ventricular ejection fraction of 25%) with liraglutide (FIGHT) had a nonsignificant trend of increase in HHF (HR = 1.30; 95% CI = 0.89–1.88; *P* = 0.17) and death (HR = 1.10; 95% CI = 0.57–2.14; *P* = 0.78), the effect of liraglutide on left ventricular function in chronic HF patients with and without T2DM (LIVE) also had a

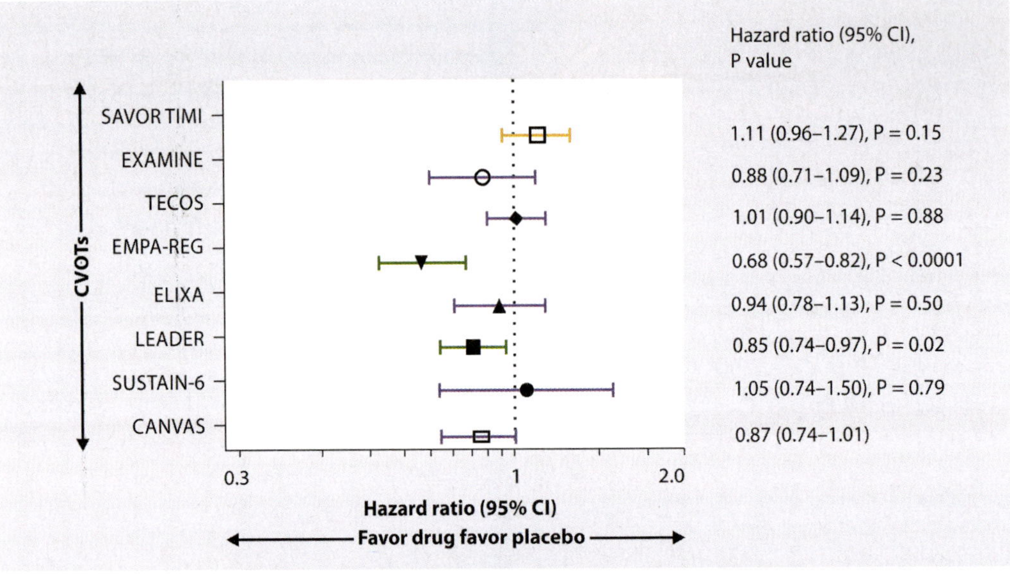

Fig. 6: All-cause mortality in cardiovascular outcome trials

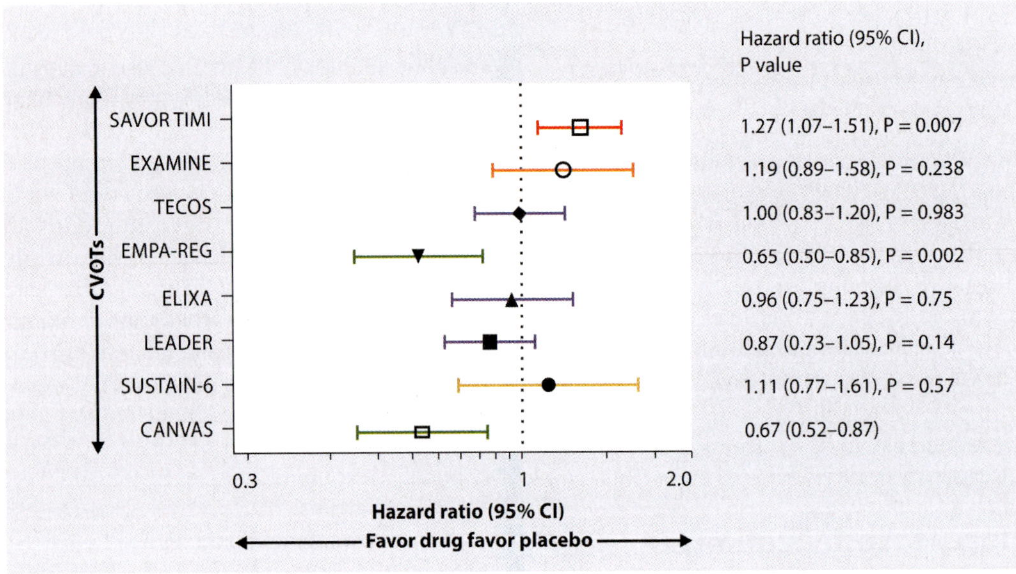

Fig. 7: Heart failure hospitalization in cardiovascular outcome trials

significant increase in serious adverse cardiac events when compared to placebo (12 vs. 3, respectively, $P = 0.04$).[26,27] Intriguingly, SUSTAIN-6 had a nonsignificant increase in trend of HHF. Figure 7 depicts the HHF in all CVOTs.

SAFETY ANALYSIS OF CARDIOVASCULAR CLINICAL OUTCOMES TRIALS

All six CVOTs conducted with incretin-based therapy almost ruled out any real increase in pancreatitis or pancreatic cancer as was perceived earlier. However, there was a slight trend of increase in pancreatitis in DPP-4Is arm compared to the placebo. The only adverse effect observed in the trial was a tripling of genital infections, predominately due to candida, a well-recognized complication of glucosuria. However, CANVAS showed two new side effects not seen in the EMPA, i.e. an increase in lower limb amputations and bone fractures in the canagliflozin group. While LEADER showed a significant increase in acute gallstone disease ($P < 0.001$) and acute cholecystitis ($P = 0.046$), SUSTAIN-6 showed a significant increase (HR = 1.76; 95% CI = 1.11–2.78, $P = 0.02$) in retinopathy complication (includes vitreous hemorrhage, onset of diabetes-related blindness, and the need for treatment with an intravitreal agent or retinal photocoagulation). It should also be noted that liraglutide in LEADER also reported an increased trend in retinopathy complication (HR = 1.15; 95% CI = 0.87–1.52; *P* = 0.33), although it was nonsignificant. From the existing data, it is clear that all the three DPP-4Is saxagliptin, alogliptin, and sitagliptin are CV neutral drugs. Saxagliptin had undoubted increase in HHF in certain subgroups of patients. Alogliptin showed numerical increase in HHF. Sitagliptin in TECOS trial showed no signal of HHF. Among the GLP-1RAs trials, lixisenatide was found to be CV neutral without any obvious safety signals. LEADER had a concordant reduction in all the CV endpoints, some statistically significant and some nonsignificant. SUSTAIN-6 had the largest reduction in 3P-MACE but no reduction in the CV death, all-cause death, and HHF. EMPA-REG had the largest and the most robust reduction in the CV death, all-cause death, and HHF, but a discordant nonsignificant increase in silent MI (assessed in half patients only) and nonfatal stroke.

The progression of kidney disease decreased by 39% ($P< 0.001$) in the EMPA trial and interestingly, the progression of CKD in the CANVAS trial was almost identical to it.

Several CVOT trials are ongoing with linagliptin [Cardiovascular and Renal Microvascular Outcome Study With Linagliptin in Patients With Type 2 Diabetes Mellitus (CARMELINA), CARdiovascular Outcome Trial of LINAgliptin Versus Glimepiride in Type 2 Diabetes (CAROLINA)], canagliflozin (CANVAS-R), dapagliflozin (DECLARE-TIMI), ertugliflozin (VERTIS-CV), exenatide once weekly (EXCEL), dulaglutide [Researching Cardiovascular Events With a Weekly Incretin in Diabetes (REWIND)], and albiglutide (HARMONY), which will further enlighten us in future.

CONCLUSION

Thus the new agents SGLT2i and GLA-1RA have paved the way for a new therapeutic path for diabetes of optimizing glycemic control, minimizing comorbidities and improving CV outcomes coupled with minimal or no hypoglycemia. Indeed this is the beginning of a new revolution which we have desired for many many years.

REFERENCES

1. Center for Drug Evaluation and Research (2008). Guidance for Industry Diabetes Mellitus: Evaluating Cardiovascular Risk in New Antidiabetic Therapies to Treat Type 2 Diabetes. [online] Available from http://www.fda.gov/downloads/Drugs/Guidance Compliance Regulatory Information /Guidances /ucm071627. [Accessed October, 2017].
2. European Medicines Agency (2012). Guideline on Clinical Investigation of Medicinal Products in the Treatment or Prevention of Diabetes Mellitus. [online] Available from http://www.ema.europa.eu/docs/ en_GB/document_library/Scientific_guideline/2012/06/ WC500129256. [Accessed October, 2017].
3. Scirica BM, Bhatt DL, Braunwald E, et al. Saxagliptin and cardiovascular outcomes in patients with type 2 diabetes mellitus. N Engl J Med. 2013;369(14):1317-26.
4. White WB, Cannon CP, Heller SR, et al. Alogliptin after acute coronary syndrome in patients with type 2 diabetes. N Engl J Med. 2013;369(14):1327-35.
5. Green JB, Bethel MA, Armstrong PW, et al. Effect of sitagliptin on cardiovascular outcomes in type 2 diabetes. N Engl J Med. 2015;373(3):232-42.
6. Zinman B, Wanner C, Lachin JM, et al. Empagliflozin, cardiovascular outcomes, and mortality in type 2 diabetes. N Engl J Med. 2015;373(22):2117-28.
7. Marso SP, Daniels GH, Brown-Frandsen K, et al. Liraglutide and cardiovascular outcomes in type 2 diabetes. N Engl J Med. 2016;375(4):311-22.
8. Pfeffer MA, Claggett B, Diaz R, et al. Lixisenatide in patients with type 2 diabetes and acute coronary syndrome. N Engl J Med.2015;373(23):2247-57.
9. Marso SP, Bain SC, Consoli A, et al. Semaglutide and cardiovascular outcomes in patients with type 2 diabetes. N Engl J Med. 2016;375(19):1834-44.
10. Marx N, Rosenstock J, Kahn SE, et al. Design and baseline characteristics of the CARdiovascular Outcome Trial of LINAgliptin Versus Glimepiride in Type 2 Diabetes (CAROLINA®). Diab Vasc Dis Res. 2015;12(3):164-74.
11. CARMELINA. (2017) Cardiovascular and Renal Microvascular Outcome Study With Linagliptin in Patients with Type 2 Diabetes Mellitus. [online] Available from https://www.clinicaltrials.gov/ct2/ show/ NCT01897532. [Accessed October, 2017].
12. Clinical Trials (2017). DECLARE-TIMI58: Dapagliflozin Effects on Cardiovascular Events. [online] Available from https://www. clinicaltrials.gov/ct2/show/ NCT01730534. [Accessed October, 2017].
13. Clinical Trials (2017). VERTIS-CV: Cardiovascular Outcomes Following Ertugliflozin Treatment in Type 2 Diabetes Mellitus Participants with Vascular Disease. Available from https://www. clinicaltrials.gov/ct2/ show/NCT01986881. [Accessed October, 2017].
14. Clinical Trials (2017). EXSCEL: Exenatide Study of Cardiovascular Event Lowering Trial. [online] Available from https://www. clinicaltrials.gov/ct2/show/NCT01144338. [Accessed October, 2017].
15. Clinical Trials (2016). REWIND: Researching Cardiovascular Events with a Weekly Incretin in Diabetes. [online] Available from https:// www.clinicaltrials.gov/ct2/show/. [Accessed October, 2017].
16. Clinical Trials (2017). HARMONY: Effect of Albiglutide, when Added to Standard Blood Glucose Lowering Therapies, on Major Cardiovascular Events in Subjects with Type 2 Diabetes Mellitus. [online] Available from https://www.clinicaltrials.gov/ct2/show/ NCT02465515. [Accessed October, 2017].
17. Sattar N, McLaren J, Kristensen SL, et al. Erratum to: SGLT2 inhibition and cardiovascular events: why did EMPA-REG outcomes surprise and what were the likely mechanisms? Diabetologia. 2016;59(7):1573-74.
18. Ferrannini E, Baldi S, Frascerra S, et al. Shift to fatty substrate utilization in response to sodium-glucose cotransporter 2 inhibition in subjects without diabetes and patients with type 2 diabetes. Diabetes. 2016;65(5):1190-5.
19. Scirica BM, Braunwald E, Raz I, et al. Heart failure, saxagliptin, and diabetes mellitus: Observations from the SAVOR-TIMI 53 randomized trial. Circulation. 2014;130(18):1579-88.
20. US Food and Drug Administration (2015). Briefing Material, NDA 22350: Saxagliptin (Onglyza). NDA 200678: Saxagliptin/Metformin

(Kombiglyze XR). [online] Available from http://www.fda.gov/downloads/AdvisoryCommittees/Committees Meeting Materials/Drugs/Endocrinologic and Metabolic-Drugs Advisory Committee/UCM442060. [Accessed October, 2017].
21. US Food and Drug Administration (2015). EMDAC Briefing Document Cardiovascular Outcomes Trial EXAMINE/NDAs 022271, 022426, & 203414 Nesina (Alogliptin), Oseni (Alogliptin/Pioglitazone), & Kazano (Alogliptin/ MetforminHCl); 2015. [online] Available from http://www.fda.gov/downloads/Advisory Committees/Committees Meeting Materials/Drugs/Endocrinologic and Metabolic Drugs Advisory Committee/UCM442062. [Accessed October, 2017].
22. Zannad F, Cannon CP, Cushman WC, et al. Heart failure and mortality outcomes in patients with type 2 diabetes taking alogliptin versus placebo in EXAMINE: a multicentre, randomised, double-blind trial. Lancet. 2015;385(9982):2067-76.
23. McGuire DK, Van de Werf F, Armstrong PW, et al. Association between sitagliptin use and heart failure hospitalization and related outcomes in type 2 diabetes mellitus: Secondary analysis of a randomized clinical trial. JAMA Cardiol. 2016;1(2):126-35.
24. Scirica BM. The safety of dipeptidyl peptidase 4 inhibitors and the risk for heart failure. JAMA Cardiol. 2016;1(2):123-5.
25. US Food and Drug Administration (2015). FDA Drug Safety Communication: FDA adds warnings about heart failure risk to labels of type 2 diabetes medicines containing saxagliptin and alogliptin. [online] Available from http://www.fda.gov/downloads/Drugs/DrugSafety/UCM493965. [Accessed October, 2017].
26. Margulies KB, Hernandez AF, Redfield MM, et al. Effects of liraglutide on clinical stability among patients with advanced heart failure and reduced ejection fraction: A randomized clinical trial. JAMA. 2016;316(5):500-8.
27. Jorsal A, Kistorp C, Holmager P. Effect of liraglutide, a glucagon-like peptide-i analogue, on left ventricular function in stable chronic heart failure patients with and without diabetes (LIVE)-a multicentre, double-blind, randomised, placebo-controlled trial. Eur J Heart Fail. 2017;19(1):69-77.

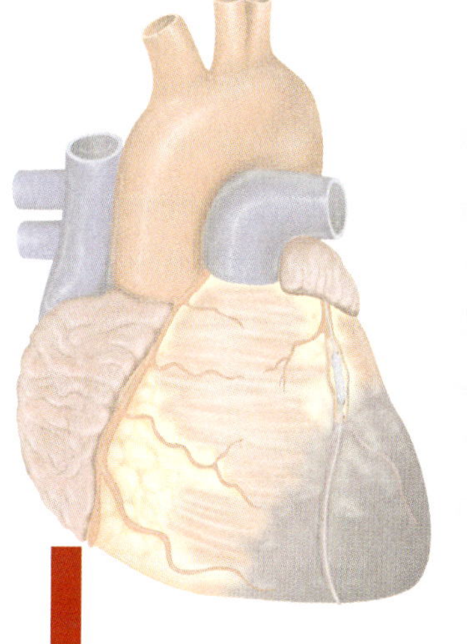

Positioning of Once Weekly GLP–1-based Therapies for Whom and When?

Brij Mohan Makkar, Jugal Kishore Sharma

INTRODUCTION

The incretin concept: Glucagon-like peptide 1 (GLP-1) is an important incretin hormone secreted by L-cells of intestine that plays an important role in glucose and bodyweight homeostasis. The concept of incretin based therapies appeared on the horizon of diabetes management only over last two decades, especially after the approval of exenatide by Food and Drug Administration (FDA) in 2004. However, the incretin concept is at least a century old. The concept of "incretin" was proposed by Bayliss and Starling, who suggested that a chemical which stimulated the pancreas to produce secretions was produced by intestinal mucosa.[1] In 1932 it was called "incretin" by La Barre[2] and later different groups demonstrated independently that orally given glucose showed a better incretin response than intravenous glucose injections.[3,4] Glucose-dependent insulinotropic peptide was first isolated incretin and its insulinotropic properties were identified. It was initially called gastric inhibitory polypeptide (GIP). In following years (1985), a GLP-1 was characterized and shown to have insulinotropic properties. It was further reported that incretin effect was reduced in patients with type 2 diabetes.[5] In 1993, Nauck et al. demonstrated that in poorly controlled diabetic patients a single exogenous infusion of GLP-1 increases insulin levels normalized hyperglycemia in a glucose dependent manner.[6] It was further recognized that GLP-1 is degraded by the ubiquitous protease dipeptidyl peptidase-4 (DPP-4), and that GLP-1 not only stimulates glucose-mediated insulin secretion but also has inhibitory effects on glucagon secretion, gastric emptying, and enhanced satiety. Hence, current therapeutic approaches have utilized either DPP-4 resistant mimetics of GLP-1 or inhibitors of the DPP-4 enzyme to enhance the activity of the endogenously secreted GLP-1 hormone. GLP-1-based therapies can be broadly classified into two categories—GLP-1 receptor agonists (GLP-1RA) and DPP-4 inhibitors (DPP-4i).

GLUCAGON-LIKE PEPTIDE 1 ACTIONS

Glucagon-like peptide 1 is a unique gut peptide with multifaceted actions and plays an important role in regulation of glucose metabolism and bodyweight homeostasis. It stimulates pancreatic beta cells to increase insulin secretion and suppresses alpha cells to decrease glucagon secretion, thereby maintaining the blood glucose levels in normal range. By its action on adipose tissues it increases lipolysis and glucose uptake. At the muscular level, GLP-1 increases glycogen synthesis and increased glucose oxidation. It also decreases gastric emptying and acid secretion in the gastrointestinal tract, playing an important role in reducing postprandial glycemic excursions and decreased gluconeogenesis in liver. By action on the brain, there is decreased appetite, increased satiety, and increased energy expenditure. The myocardial contractility and heart rate are increased with decrease in blood pressure, and it has a natriuretic effect on kidneys.

Glucagon-like peptide 1 has been shown to potentially enhance β-cell proliferation and have antiapoptotic effects on these cells, inducing insulin biosynthesis.[7,8]

Glucagon-like Peptide 1 Receptor Agonists and their Classes

Glucagon-like peptide 1 receptor agonists are injectable anti-hyperglycemic agents which reduce both fasting and postprandial blood glucose levels by acting in a glucose dependent manner. There is no increased risk of hypoglycemia and weight gain typically seen with other antihyperglycemic agents like sulfonylureas and insulins, in fact they are associated with a modest weight loss in most patients. The most frequently reported adverse events associated with this class are nausea, vomiting, and diarrhea, the causes of which are thought to be the effects of GLP-1RAs on gastric emptying or involving the central nervous system.[8] GLP-1RAs have been classified according to their basic structure and pharmacokinetic properties. Structurally, one group exploits the native GLP-1 with some amino acid alterations, which make it resistant to degradation by the DPP-4 enzyme. The other group was synthetically developed by replicating the structure of a naturally occurring protein, exendin-4 (Ex-4), (originally isolated from the saliva of the lizard Heloderma suspectum or Gila monster), with substantial homology to native GLP-1. Like native GLP-1, this protein has GLP-1R-activating properties, and is naturally resistant to degradation by the DPP-4 enzyme.[9] Apart from structural classification, these drugs can also be classified based on the duration of their action,[8-10] i.e. short-acting and long-acting GLP-1RAs (Table 1).[8-10] Although, even short-acting GLP-1RAs are DPP-4 resistant due to structural modifications at their second and third N-terminal amino acids, they are eliminated via the renal tract, thus requiring either a once-daily (QD) or twice-daily (BID) dosing (e.g. exenatide and lixisenatide). Longer acting molecules have undergone some structural modifications to enhance their duration of action, while retaining their ability to act on the GLP-1 receptors [exenatide once-weekly (EQW), dulaglutide, albiglutide, and liraglutide]. Short-acting compounds lead to fluctuations in plasma peptide levels for some time after administration. On the other hand, long-acting compounds tend to have a more consistent supra physiological level of exogenous GLP-1 in the body. Some of the strategies used to prolong the life of these compounds include:

- Albumin binding to prevent renal filtration, e.g. liraglutide, albiglutide, and semaglutide
- Conjugation to a modified immunoglobulin G4 Fc (IgG4 Fc) fragment, e.g. dulaglutide
- Coupling of the molecule to microspheres to delay absorption from the subcutaneous site, e.g. EQW.[8]

TABLE 1: Glucagon-like peptide 1 receptor agonists

	Short-acting GLP-1RAs	*Long-acting GLP-1RAs*
Exendin-4 backbone	Exanetide BID Lixisenatide QD	Exenatide LARQW ITCA 650
Human GLP-1 backbone		Liraglutide QD Dulaglutide QW Albiglutide QW Semaglutide QW

Abbreviation: GLP-1RAs, glucagon-like Peptide 1 receptor agonists

Approved GLP-1RAs:

- Exenatide (Byetta/Bydureon), approved in 2005/2012
- Liraglutide (Victoza and Saxenda), approved in 2010
- Albiglutide (Tanzeum), approved in 2014
- Dulaglutide (Trulicity), approved in 2014
- Lixisenatide (Lyxumia), approved in 2016

Under investigation:

- Semaglutide
- ITCA 650.

Review of Glucagon-like Peptide 1 Receptor Agonists

Exenatide Twice Daily

Exenatide, the first GLP-1RA, was introduced to the Indian market in 2007. Launched in the USA in 2005 and in Europe in 2006, it was discovered in a search for biologically active peptides in the venom of the Gila monster.[11] Exenatide is a synthetic version of Ex-4, and bears 53% homology to the native GLP-1 molecule.[11] It is available in a prefilled pen device and is administered subcutaneously BID within 60 minutes before two major meals. The starting dose is 5 μg BID which, if well tolerated by the patient, may be titrated to 10 μg BID after a month. The mean terminal half-life after administration is 2.4 hours and it remains detectable in plasma for approximately 10 hours after a single dose.[12]

The efficacy and safety of exenatide BID (ExBID) has been studied and established in patients treated with metformin alone, patients treated with a sulfonylurea alone, and patients treated with both metformin and a sulfonylurea.[13-15] Reduction in glycated hemoglobin (Hb) in various trials with 10 μg of ExBID ranged from approximately 0.8 to 0.9% and decrease in weight from baseline observed was up to about 2.8 kg.[12-15] The durability of glycemic effect was noted for up to 3 years.[16] In other comparator studies, glycosylated HbA1c reduction with adjunctive ExBID was generally similar to that of basal insulin,[17] sulfonylureas,[18,19] and lixisenatide;[20] less than that of liraglutide,[21] and EQW.[22,23] The most common adverse effect was mild to moderate nausea and vomiting which decreased with time.[12] The incidence of hypoglycemia was low when not given alongside concomitant sulfonylurea or insulin therap.[12] ExBID is not recommended for use in patients with end-stage renal disease (ESRD) or severe renal impairment.[12] In patients with moderate renal impairment, dose escalation from 5 µg to 10 µg should proceed conservatively.[12] Formation of anti-exenatide antibodies has been reported relatively frequently, which may be a result of only 53% homology to the native GLP-1 molecule and its nonhuman origin.

Liraglutide

Liraglutide is an analog of human GLP-1 produced by recombinant deoxyribonucleic acid (DNA) technology. It was approved for clinical use in Europe in 2009 and in the USA in 2010[9] and has been available in India since 2010.

This engineered peptide shares 97% homology to native human GLP-1.[24] There is no structural modification to render it resistant to DPP-4, but the slow absorption from the site after subcutaneous administration can be attributed to self-association leading to the formation of heptamers at the injection site.[24] Once in plasma, 99% remains bound to plasma albumin, with the bound molecule having a half-life of 13 hours, making it suitable for QD administration. Liraglutide should be initiated with a dose of 0.6 mg QD for 1 week.[24,25] This low starting dose helps in reducing gastrointestinal symptoms during initial titration, but is not effective for glycemic control. After 1 week, the dose should be increased to 1.2 mg QD. If the 1.2 mg dose does not result in acceptable glycemic control, the dose can be further increased to 1.8 mg QD. Liraglutide is available in disposable, prefilled, and multi-dose pens.[9,25]

Liraglutide has been investigated in a clinical development program called Liraglutide effect and Action in Diabetes (LEAD™),[21,26-30] which compared the two licensed doses, 1.2 mg and 1.8 mg of liraglutide, with glimepiride, rosiglitazone, and insulin glargine, as well as a direct comparison (LEAD™ 6) between liraglutide 1.8 mg and ExBID.[24] Liraglutide alone or in combination with oral antihyperglycemic agents was shown to be superior to placebo and active comparators in all LEAD trials except LEAD 2 where both doses were noninferior to glimepiride for HbA1c lowering.[24] Liraglutide had a modest effect on the reduction of gastric emptying, thus the reduction in postprandial plasma glucose (PPG) excursions can be mainly attributed to a reduction in preprandial glucose levels.[9] In a head-to-head trial with ExBID, there was a greater reduction in fasting plasma glucose (FPG) with liraglutide, while better PPG reduction was seen with ExBID after breakfast and dinner.[24]

The most common adverse events were gastrointestinal in nature and tended to decrease over a period of time. Overall, the rate of hypoglycemia was low, except when liraglutide was used in combination with sulfonylureas when there was an increased risk of hypoglycemia. Antiliraglutide antibodies were detected in 8.6% of liraglutide-treated patients, relatively lower than that seen with exenatide owing to high sequence identity with native GLP-1. In general, the presence of antibodies did not impact the clinical efficacy. No dose adjustment is recommended for patients with mild renal impairment. Liraglutide is not recommended in patients with severe renal impairment including those with ESRD.[25]

Lixisenatide

Lixisenatide has been approved for the treatment of adults with type 2 diabetes in various countries.

Lixisenatide is a QD GLP-1RA which, like exenatide, has an Ex-4 backbone, but with some alterations, leading to a half-life of 2–3 hours. Although the short half-life suggested a need for multiple daily dosing, initial dose-finding studies did not show much difference in efficacy between QD dosing and BID dosing. Hence, QD dosing was selected for further evaluation.[9]

Lixisenatide 20 µg QD has been clinically evaluated in the GetGoal program which included monotherapy, add-on therapy to metformin, sulfonylurea or pioglitazone, and in combination with basal insulin. Apart from GetGoal-X, which had an active comparator (ExBID), all these trials compared lixisenatide to placebo.[20,31-37] Lixisenatide showed a significant decrease in HbA1c from baseline in these trials, ranging from 0.7% to 0.94% with an accompanying weight loss of 0.2–2.8 kg.[38] Lixisenatide has a moderate effect on FPG and a predominant effect on PPG, attributed to a reduction in gastric emptying.[9]

The main adverse effects are gastrointestinal in nature. Potentially, immunogenic like other protein/peptide-based products, and 69.8% of patients had a positive-antibody status at the end of the 24-week placebo-controlled studies. The change in HbA1c from baseline was similar, irrespective of antibody status (positive or negative). Lixisenatide is mainly eliminated through the kidneys and should be used with caution in patients with moderate renal impairment. Use is not recommended in patients with severe renal impairment or ESRD.[38]

Exenatide Once Weekly

Exenatide once weekly was approved in Europe in 2011 and the USA in 2012.[9] In this once-weekly formulation, the exenatide molecule is embedded within poly (lactic-co-glycolic acid) microspheres, which once injected subcutaneously, allows a steady and constant release of exenatide through diffusion and erosion of these microspheres, leading to a gradual rise in plasma concentrations. EQW is supplied in a single use, single dose pen.[39]

Exenatide once weekly has been examined in the clinical trial program Diabetes therapy Utilization: Researching changes in HbA1c weight And other factors Through Intervention with exenatide ONce weekly (DURATION) using metformin, sitagliptin, pioglitazone, insulin glargine, liraglutide, and ExBID as active comparators.[22,23,40-44] The HbA1c reduction seen in the DURATION trials ranged from 1.3% to 1.9%. The reduction in weight ranged from 2 kg to 3.7 kg. EQW demonstrated superior FPG reductions compared to ExBID in the two head-to-head studies, whereas ExBID showed greater reductions in the PPG excursions. In the DURATION program, EQW showed superiority or noninferiority to active comparators, except liraglutide, and pioglitazone.[22,23,40-44] It failed to demonstrate noninferiority to liraglutide for HbA1c lowering. Weight loss was also better for liraglutide.[44]

Gastrointestinal side effects were common with rates ranging from 11% to 26.4% across all studies,[22,23,40-44] although less than that seen with the BID regimen. In the head-to-head study against liraglutide 1.8 mg, EQW demonstrated a better tolerability profile in terms of nausea and vomiting.[44] EQW is not recommended for use in patients with ESRD and should be used with caution in moderate renal impairment.

Dulaglutide

Dulaglutide received USFDA approval in September 2014 and European agency approval in November 2014.[45,46] It was approved for use in India in December 2014.[47]

Dulaglutide is a long-acting GLP-1 analog covalently linked to human IgG Fc fragment, modified to increase the duration of pharmacodynamic activity, reduce DPP-4 inactivation, increase solubility, and reduce immunogenicity. The increased duration of pharmacodynamic activity can be attributed to reduced renal clearance; resulting in a plasma half-life of approximately 5 days, allowing for once-weekly dosing.[48-50]

The regulatory approvals of dulaglutide were based on the Assessment of Weekly Administration of LY2189265 in Diabetes (AWARD) 1-6 trials.[48,50-56] In these trials, two doses of dulaglutide once weekly, 0.75 mg and 1.5 mg, were compared to placebo, ExBID, insulin glargine, metformin, and sitagliptin; and dulaglutide 1.5 mg was compared to liraglutide 1.8 mg.[50-56] The duration of these trials ranged from 26 weeks to 104 weeks.[50-56] Dulaglutide met its primary end-point in all six AWARD studies. The 1.5 mg dose further demonstrated superiority to its active comparators in all five registration trials and noninferiority to liraglutide 1.8 mg in the AWARD-6 trial. In various AWARD studies, HbA1c reduction with the 1.5 mg dose ranged from 0.8% to 1.6%. Similarly, weight loss of up to 3.2 kg was seen.[50-56]

Recent studies have demonstrated that dulaglutide is more effective than other antidiabetic agents by reducing the HbA1c by close to or greater than 1%. It is also the only GLP-1 agonist that has had a successful head-to-head trial showing noninferiority to liraglutide. Tolerability profile was similar.

Similar to other agents in the class, dulaglutide has demonstrated weight loss of approximately 6 pounds, which has been sustained over at least 26 weeks. However, one of the substantial benefits dulaglutide provides, and one that patients may place quite a bit of value on, is the convenience of once-weekly dosing compared with other agents' once-daily dosing.

The most common adverse events were gastrointestinal in nature. Dulaglutide exhibited a relatively low immunogenicity with 1.6% of treated patients in the clinical trials developing anti-drug antibodies.[48]

As with any other drug, dulaglutide use is also not without risks, and the adverse effects and contraindications must be considered. It is important to take into careful consideration its long-term safety profile by staying abreast of the current research taking place in regard to major cardiovascular (CV) events and the risk of pancreatitis or pancreatic cancer. Therefore, while dulaglutide has both risks and advantages, it is currently proven to be an adequate choice of treatment for patients with type-2 diabetes in the outpatient setting.[57]

Albiglutide

Albiglutide is a long-acting GLP-1RA approved in the USA as well as Europe, but not yet available on the Indian market.[58,59]

Semaglutide

Semaglutide is a long-acting GLP-1RA developed for once-weekly dosing. Semaglutide has some structural similarities to liraglutide with modifications to increase albumin binding and DPP-4 stability.

COMPARISON OF THE GLUCAGON-LIKE PEPTIDE 1 RECEPTOR AGONISTS

Overall Efficacy

All the GLP-1RAs that were developed after ExBID have been compared in head-to-head comparison trials with previously existing members in this class. In a study that compared two short-acting GLP-1RAs, lixisenatide and ExBID, the glycemic efficacy was similar, with slightly better weight reduction seen with ExBID.[20] Studies comparing long-and short-acting GLP-1RAs typically showed superior HbA1c reduction with long-acting members.[21,22,40,51] In the AWARD-1 study, both doses of once-weekly dulaglutide demonstrated superior glycemic control in terms of HbA1c and fasting glucose versus ExBID.[51]

Differential Effect of Fasting and Postprandial Glucose

Differences in molecular structure of these molecules results in different pharmacokinetic/pharmacodynamics profiles which reflect in their efficacy, safety, and tolerability. While one important benefit of long-acting over short-acting molecules is that they have more stable plasma levels over 24 hours, with a predominant effect on FPG, the effect on delay of gastric emptying is lost in a few hours via modulation of vagal activity. While this may mean less gastrointestinal side effects, it also reflects in the better PPG efficacy of short-acting molecules.[8,9,60] However, this may not always hold true. For example, dulaglutide, however, exhibited clinically relevant postprandial glycemic benefits when compared with ExBID, as described above, somewhat limiting the duration of action-based classification.[51]

Immunogenicity

Consistent with the immunogenic properties of protein and peptide pharmaceuticals, individuals exposed to GLP-1RAs may develop an immune response, including anti-drug antibodies. The molecular structure and homology to the native GLP-1 molecule may also impact the immunogenicity. Exenatide, which has 53% homology to the native GLP-1 molecule,[61] frequently results in formation of anti-exenatide antibodies (up to 43%).[24] The clinical relevance of these antibodies is not certain, but in the majority of patients their presence does not seem to impair the efficacy. In patients with high antibody titers, however, the exenatide-induced reduction in HbA1c level was significantly smaller than in patients with low titers of antibodies.[12] The proportion of patients developing antibodies against liraglutide is lower at 8.6%.[25] In clinical studies, treatment with dulaglutide was associated with a 1.6% incidence of treatment emergent dulaglutide anti-drug antibodies, suggesting that the structural modifications in the GLP-1 and modified IgG4 parts of the dulaglutide molecule, together with high homology with native GLP-1 and native IgG4, minimize the risk of immune response against dulaglutide.[62]

Effect on Weight

Improved glycemic benefit does not always correlate with improved weight loss results. Despite EQW demonstrating superior glycemic control to ExBID in the DURATION 1 and 5 trials, weight loss was similar for both molecules in both trials. Similar results were seen in AWARD-1, with dulaglutide demonstrating superior efficacy but similar weight loss to ExBID. This variability in clinical trial results shows that we are unable to determine the pharmacodynamic action of these drugs from their duration of action. While we may classify drugs according to whether they are long-or short-acting, this does not fully determine their clinical characteristics or mode of action.

Gastrointestinal Effects

Mild to moderate nausea, vomiting, and diarrhea which decline over time, are the most frequent side effects with this class of drugs. While longer-acting molecules may be given independent of meal timing, shorter-acting molecules, like ExBID, should be administered at least an hour before meals to reduce gastrointestinal symptoms. To avoid discontinuation due to these events, appropriate counseling and expectation setting around gastrointestinal symptoms, weight loss, and decreased appetite is critical at the time of prescription. These agents should be avoided in cases of severe gastrointestinal disease, such as gastroparesis.[12,25,38,39,48,63]

CHOOSING THE APPROPRIATE GLUCAGON-LIKE PEPTIDE 1 RECEPTOR AGONIST

It has been shown in the various randomized controlled trials (RCTs) that all GLP-1RAs improve glycemic control, reduce bodyweight, and increase the risk of adverse gastrointestinal symptoms compared with placebo. Although there were no differences when short-acting agents were compared with each other or when long-acting agents were compared with each other, dulaglutide, liraglutide, and once-weekly exenatide were superior to twice-daily exenatide and lixisenatide at lowering HbA1c and FPG levels. There were no differences in hypoglycemia between these three agents, whilst once-weekly exenatide had the lowest risk of vomiting. These results, along with patient's preferences and individualized targets, should be considered when selecting a GLP-1RA.[64]

Once Weekly GLP-1 Receptor Agonists versus Once-a-day GLP-1RAs

In several trials, researchers have compared once weekly GLP-1RAs with daily GLP-1RAs or other glucose-lowering drugs, but no head-to-head comparisons of once-weekly GLP-1RAs have been reported. To assess the comparative efficacy of once-weekly GLP-1RAs, researchers conducted a network meta-analysis of 34 randomized, controlled, phase III trials (≥24 weeks of follow-up) of albiglutide (Tanzuem), dulaglutide (Trulicity), and exenatide (Bydureon) in more than 21,000 adults with type 2 diabetes; analysis also covered taspoglutide, which is no longer being developed.[65]

Network meta-analysis is a statistical method for comparing interventions that have been examined in clinical trials but have not been compared directly with each other.

For the three currently available agents, network meta-analysis revealed mean decreases in HbA1c of –1.4% and –1.2% for dulaglutide (at doses of 1.5 mg and 0.75 mg), –1.3% for exenatide, and –1.0% for albiglutide, relative to placebo. Weight loss was less than 1 kg for all the drugs. Either marginal or no differences among agents were noted for changes in blood pressure and lipids. To varying degrees, all agents were associated with nausea.

Cardiovascular Safety

Three CV outcome studies addressing the CV safety of GLP-1RAs have been published so far—ELIXA, LEADER, and SUSTAIN.[66,67] ELIXA trial showed that lixisenatide added to standard of care vs. placebo was noninferior to placebo and did not increase CV risk in patients with type 2 diabetes with established CV disease. SUSTAIN and LEADER documented the CV safety of semaglutide and CV risk reduction with liraglutide respectively when added to standard of care in patients with type 2 diabetes and established CV disease.

GLP-1-based Therapies—For Whom and When?

The foregoing discussion clearly shows that GLP-1 based therapies have potential to correct more that one underlying pathophysiological mechanisms. In addition, they offer the advantages of low risk of hypoglycemia and clinically meaningful weight loss in addition to significant A1c reduction. GLP-based therapies are currently recommended by all major clinical practice recommendations/guidelines for all type 2 diabetes patients who are not achieving A1c targets with lifestyle interventions and metformin, especially for obese type 2 diabetes patients. They can be also added to two or more oral agents and/or insulin patients with type 2 diabetes patients with inadequately controlled blood sugar levels.

CONCLUSION

Our understanding of diabetes is constantly evolving and GLP-1-RAs represent an important facet of this understanding. The GLP-1RA class improves glycemic control through multiple mechanisms with a low risk of hypoglycemia and facilitates clinically relevant weight loss. Globally, this class is being recognized as an important therapy in the management of type 2 diabetes. Any initial resistance for adopting these therapies could be attributed to fear of daily injections; however, the emerging once-weekly alternatives have the potential for more convenience and greater acceptance by patients, with better efficacy and tolerability. These once-weekly therapies may provide another therapeutic alternative when oral antihyperglycemic medications are unable to provide adequate glycemic control. Nevertheless, the enormous progress in this field has paved the way for other therapeutic options for tailored management of patients with type 2 diabetes.

REFERENCES

1. Bayliss WM, Starling EH. The mechanism of pancreatic secretion. J Physiol. 1902;28:325-53.
2. Kim W, Egan JM. The role of incretins in glucose homeostasis and diabetes treatment. Pharmacol Rev. 2008;60:470-512.
3. Elrick H, Stimmler L, Hlad CJ Jr, et al. Plasma insulin response to oral and intravenous glucose administration. J Clin Endocrinol Metab. 1964;24:1076-82.
4. Perley MJ, Kipnis DM. Plasma insulin responses to oral and intravenous glucose: studies in normal and diabetic subjects. J Clin Invest. 1967;46:1954-62.
5. Nauck M, Stöckmann F, Ebert R, et al. Reduced incretin effect in type 2 (non-insulin-dependent) diabetes. Diabetologia. 1986;29(1):46-52.
6. Nauck MA, Kleine N, Orskov C, et al. Nor-malization of fasting hyperglycaemia by exogenous glucagonlike peptide 1 (7-36 amide) in type 2 (noninsulin dependent) diabetic patients. Diabetologia. 1993;36(8):741-4.
7. Nauck MA, Vilsbøll T, Gallwitz B, et al. Incretin-based therapies: viewpoints on the way to consensus. Diabetes Care. 2009;32 Suppl 2:S223-31.
8. Meier JJ. GLP-1 receptor agonists for individualized treatment of type 2 diabetes mellitus. Nat Rev Endocrinol. 2012;8:728-42.
9. Lund A, Knop FK, Vilsbøll T. Glucagon-like peptide-1 receptor agonists for the treatment of type 2 diabetes: differences and similarities. Eur J Intern Med. 2014;25:407-14.
10. Madsbad S, Kielgast U, Asmar M, et al. An overview of once-weekly glucagon-like peptide-1 receptor agonists—available efficacy and safety data and perspectives for the future. Diabetes Obes Metab. 2011;13(5):394-407.
11. McCormack PL. Exenatide twice daily: a review of its use in the management of patients with type 2 diabetes mellitus. Drugs. 2014;74(3):325-51.
12. Byetta. US Prescribing Information. Princeton, NJ: Bristol-Myers Squibb Company; 2014.
13. Buse JB, Henry RR, Han J, et al. Effects of exenatide (exendin 4) on glycemic control over 30 weeks in sulfonylureatreated patients with type 2 diabetes. Diabetes Care. 2004;27(11):2628-35.
14. DeFronzo RA, Ratner RE, Han J, et al. Effects of exenatide (exendin 4) on glycemic control and weight over 30 weeks in metformin treated patients with type 2 diabetes. Diabetes Care. 2005;28:1092-100.
15. Kendall DM, Riddle MC, Rosenstock J, et al. Effects of exenatide (exendin 4) on glycemic control over 30 weeks in patients with type 2 diabetes treated with metformin and a sulfonylurea. Diabetes Care. 2005;28:1083-91.
16. Klonoff DC, Buse JB, Nielsen LL, et al. Exenatide effects on diabetes, obesity, cardiovascular risk factors and hepatic biomarkers in patients with type 2 diabetes treated for at least 3 years. Curr Med Res Opin. 2008;24:275-86.
17. Heine RJ, Van Gaal LF, Johns D, et al. Exenatide versus insulin glargine in patients with suboptimally controlled type 2 diabetes: a randomized trial. Ann Intern Med. 2005;143(8):559-69.

18. Derosa G, Maffioli P, Salvadeo SA, et al. Exenatide versus glibenclamide in patients with diabetes. Diabetes Technol Ther. 2010;12:233-40.
19. Derosa G, Putignano P, Bossi AC, et al. Exenatide or glimepiride added to metformin on metabolic control and on insulin resistance in type 2 diabetic patients. Eur J Pharmacol. 2011;666:251-6.
20. Rosenstock J, Raccah D, Korányi L, et al. Efficacy and safety of lixisenatide once daily versus exenatide twice daily in type 2 diabetes inadequately controlled on metformin: a 24-week, randomized, open-label, active-controlled study (GetGoal-X). Diabetes Care. 2013;36:2945-51.
21. Buse JB, Rosenstock J, Sesti G, et al. Liraglutide once a day versus exenatide twice a day for type 2 diabetes: A 26-week randomised, parallel-group, multinational, open-label trial (LEAD-6). Lancet. 2009;374:39-47.
22. Blevins T, Pullman J, Malloy J, et al. DURATION-5: exenatide once weekly resulted in greater improvements in glycemic control compared with exenatide twice daily in patients with type 2 diabetes. J Clin Endocrinol Metab. 2011;96(5):1301-10.
23. Drucker DJ, Buse JB, Taylor K, et al. Exenatide once weekly versus twice daily for the treatment of type 2 diabetes: a randomised, open-label, non-inferiority study. Lancet. 2008;372:1240-50.
24. Rigato M, Fadini GP. Comparative effectiveness of liraglutide in the treatment of type 2 diabetes. Diabetes Metab Syndr Obes. 2014;7:107-20.
25. Victoza. US Prescribing Information. Bagsvaerd, Denmark: Novo Nordisk A/S; 2013.
26. Marre M, Shaw J, Brändle M, et al. Liraglutide, a once-daily human GLP-1 analogue, added to a sulphonylurea over 26 weeks produces greater improvements in glycaemic and weight control compared with adding rosiglitazone or placebo in subjects with type 2 diabetes (LEAD1 SU). Diabet Med. 2009;26:268-78.
27. Nauck M, Frid A, Hermansen K, et al. Efficacy and safety comparison of liraglutide, glimepiride, and placebo, all in combination with metformin, in type 2 diabetes: the LEAD (liraglutide effect and action in diabetes)-2 study. Diabetes Care. 2009;32(1):84-90.
28. Garber A, Henry R, Ratner R, et al. Liraglutide versus glimepiride monotherapy for type 2 diabetes (LEAD-3 Mono): a randomised, 52-week, phase III, double-blind, parallel-treatment trial. Lancet. 2009;373:473-81.
29. Zinman B, Gerich J, Buse JB, et al. Efficacy and safety of the human glucagon-like peptide-1 analog liraglutide in combination with metformin and thiazolidinedione in patients with type 2 diabetes (LEAD-4 Met+TZD). Diabetes Care. 2009;32(7):1224-30.
30. Russell-Jones D, Vaag A, Schmitz O, et al. Liraglutide vs insulin glargine and placebo in combination with metformin and sulfonylurea therapy in type 2 diabetes mellitus (LEAD5 met+SU): a randomised controlled trial. Diabetologia. 2009;52(10):2046-55.
31. Fonseca VA, Alvarado-Ruiz R, Raccah D, et al. Efficacy and safety of the once-daily GLP-1 receptor agonist lixisenatide in monotherapy: a randomized, double-blind, placebo-controlled trial in patients with type 2 diabetes (GetGoal-Mono). Diabetes Care. 2012;35(6):1225-31.
32. Ahrén B, Leguizamo Dimas A, Miossec P, et al. Efficacy and safety of lixisenatide once-daily morning or evening injections in type 2 diabetes inadequately controlled on metformin (GetGoalM). Diabetes Care. 2013;36:2543-50.
33. Bolli GB, Munteanu M, Dotsenko S, et al. Efficacy and safety of lixisenatide once daily vs. placebo in people with type 2 diabetes insufficiently controlled on metformin (GetGoal-F1). Diabet Med. 2014;31:176-84.
34. Rosenstock J, Hanefeld M, Shamanna P, et al. Beneficial effects of once-daily lixisenatide on overall and postprandial glycemic levels without significant excess of hypoglycemia in type 2 diabetes inadequately controlled on a sulfonylurea with or without metformin (GetGoal-S). J Diabetes Complications. 2014;28(3):386-92.
35. Pinget M, Goldenberg R, Niemoeller E, et al. Efficacy and safety of lixisenatide once daily versus placebo in type 2 diabetes insufficiently controlled on pioglitazone (GetGoal-P). Diabetes Obes Metab. 2013;15:1000-7.
36. Riddle MC, Aronson R, Home P, et al. Adding once-daily lixisenatide for type 2 diabetes inadequately controlled by established basal insulin: a 24-week, randomized, placebo-controlled comparison (GetGoal-L). Diabetes Care. 2013;36:2489-96.
37. Riddle MC, Forst T, Aronson R, et al. Adding once-daily lixisenatide for type 2 diabetes inadequately controlled with newly initiated and continuously titrated basal insulin glargine: a 24-week, randomized, placebo-controlled study (GetGoal-Duo 1). Diabetes Care. 2013;36:2497-503.
38. Lyxumia. Paris, France: Sanofi-Aventis; 2013.
39. Bydureon. US Prescribing Information. Wilmington, DE: AstraZeneca Pharmaceuticals LP; 2014.
40. Buse JB, Drucker DJ, Taylor KL, et al. DURATION-1: exenatide once weekly produces sustained glycemic control and weight loss over 52 weeks. Diabetes Care. 2010;33:1255-61.
41. Bergenstal RM, Wysham C, Macconell L, et al. Efficacy and safety of exenatide once weekly versus sitagliptin or pioglitazone as an adjunct to metformin for treatment of type 2 diabetes (DURATION-2): a randomised trial. Lancet. 2010;376:431-9.
42. Diamant M, Van Gaal L, Stranks S, et al. Once weekly exenatide compared with insulin glargine titrated to target in patients with type 2 diabetes (DURATION-3): an open-label randomised trial. Lancet. 2010;375:2234-43.
43. Russell-Jones D, Cuddihy RM, Hanefeld M, et al. Efficacy and safety of exenatide once weekly versus metformin, pioglitazone, and sitagliptin used as monotherapy in drug-naive patients with type 2 diabetes (DURATION-4): a 26-week double-blind study. Diabetes Care. 2012;35:252-8.
44. Buse JB, Nauck M, Forst T, et al. Exenatide once weekly versus liraglutide once daily in patients with type 2 diabetes (DURATION-6): a randomised, open-label study. Lancet. 2013;381:117-24.
45. US Food and Drug Administration. Dulaglutide. [online] Available from: http://www.fda.gov/NewsEvents/Newsroom/PressAnnouncements/ucm415180. htm. [Accessed October, 2017].
46. Eli Lilly. (2014). Dulaglutide. [online] Available from: https://investor.lilly.com/releasedetail. cfm?releaseid=871658. [Accessed October, 2017].
47. Central Drugs Standard Control Organization, Government of India. Dulaglutide Approval Letter; 2014.
48. Trulicity US Prescribing Information. Indianapolis, IN: Eli Lilly and Company; 2014.
49. Barrington P, Chien JY, Showalter HD, et al. A 5-week study of the pharmacokinetics and pharmacodynamics of LY2189265, a novel, long-acting glucagon-like peptide-1 analogue, in patients with type 2 diabetes. Diabetes Obes Metab. 2011;13:426-33.
50. Nauck M, Weinstock RS, Umpierrez GE, et al. Efficacy and safety of dulaglutide versus sitagliptin after 52 weeks in type 2 diabetes in a randomized controlled trial (AWARD-5). Diabetes Care. 2014;37:2149-58.
51. Wysham C, Blevins T, Arakaki R, et al. Efficacy and safety of dulaglutide added onto pioglitazone and metformin versus exenatide in type 2 diabetes in a randomized controlled trial (AWARD-1). Diabetes Care. 2014;37:2159-67.
52. Georgino F, Benroubi M, Sun JH, et al. Efficacy and Safety of Once-Weekly Dulaglutide Versus Insulin Glargine in Patients With Type 2 Diabetes on Metformin and Glimepiride (AWARD-2). Diabetes Care;2015;38(12):2241-9.
53. Umpierrez G, Tofé Povedano S, Pérez Manghi F, et al. Efficacy and safety of dulaglutide monotherapy versus metformin in type 2 diabetes in a randomized controlled trial (AWARD-3). Diabetes Care. 2014;37:2168-76.

54. Blonde L, Jendle J, Gross J, et al. Once-weekly dulaglutide versus bedtime insulin glargine, both in combination with prandial insulin lispro, in patients with type 2 diabetes (AWARD-4): a randomised, open-label, phase 3, non-inferiority study. Lancet. 2015;385:2057-66.
55. Weinstock RS, Guerci B, Umpierrez G, et al. Safety and efficacy of once-weekly dulaglutide versus sitagliptin after 2 years in metformin-treated patients with type 2 diabetes (AWARD-5): a randomized, phase III study. Diabetes Obes Metab. 2015;17:849-58.
56. Dungan KM, Povedano ST, Forst T, et al. Once-weekly dulaglutide versus once-daily liraglutide in metformin-treated patients with type 2 diabetes (AWARD-6): a randomised, open-label, phase 3, non-inferiority trial. Lancet. 2014;384:1349-57.
57. Marso SP, Bain SC, Consoli A, et al. Semaglutide and Cardiovascular Outcomes in Patients with Type 2 Diabetes. N Engl J Med. 2016;375(19):1834-44.
58. US Food and Drug Administration. (2014). Albiglutide. [online] Available from: http://www.fda.gov/NewsEvents/Newsroom/PressAnnouncements/ucm393289.htm. [Accessed October, 2017].
59. European Medicines Agency. (2014). Albiglutide. [online] Available from: http://www.ema.europa.eu/ema/index.jsp?curl=pages/medicines/human/medicines/002735/smops/Positive/human_smop_000634.jsp and mid=WC0b01ac058001d127. [Accessed October, 2017].
60. Nauck MA, Kemmeries G, Holst JJ, et al. Rapid tachyphylaxis of the glucagon-like peptide 1-induced deceleration of gastric emptying in humans. Diabetes. 2011;60:1561-5.
61. Dungan K, Buse JB. Glucagon-like peptide 1-based therapies for type 2 diabetes: a focus on exenatide. Clin Diabetes. 2005;23:56-62.
62. Eli Lilly. (2014). Trulicity European Summary of Product Characteristics. [online] Available from: http://ec.europa.eu/health/documents/community-register/2014/20141121130063/anx_130063_en.pdf. [Accessed October, 2017].
63. Tanzeum (albiglutide). Wilmington, DE: GlaxoSmithKline LLC; 2014.
64. Htike ZZ, Zaccardi F, Papamargaritis D, et al. Efficacy and safety of glucagon-like peptide-1 receptor agonists in type 2 diabetes: a systematic review and mixed-treatment comparison analysis. Diabetes Obes Metab. 2017;19(4):524-36.
65. Jamaluddin M. Glucagon-like peptide-1 receptor agonists differed minimally in most respects. Ann Intern Med. 2015.
66. Pfeffer MA, Claggett B, Diaz R, et al. Lixisenatide in Patients with Type 2 Diabetes and Acute Coronary Syndrome. N Engl J Med. 2015;373(23):2247-57.
67. Marso SP, Daniels GH, Brown-Frandsen K, et al. Liraglutide and Cardiovascular Outcomes in Type 2 Diaebtes Patients. N Engl J Med. 2016;375(4):311-22.

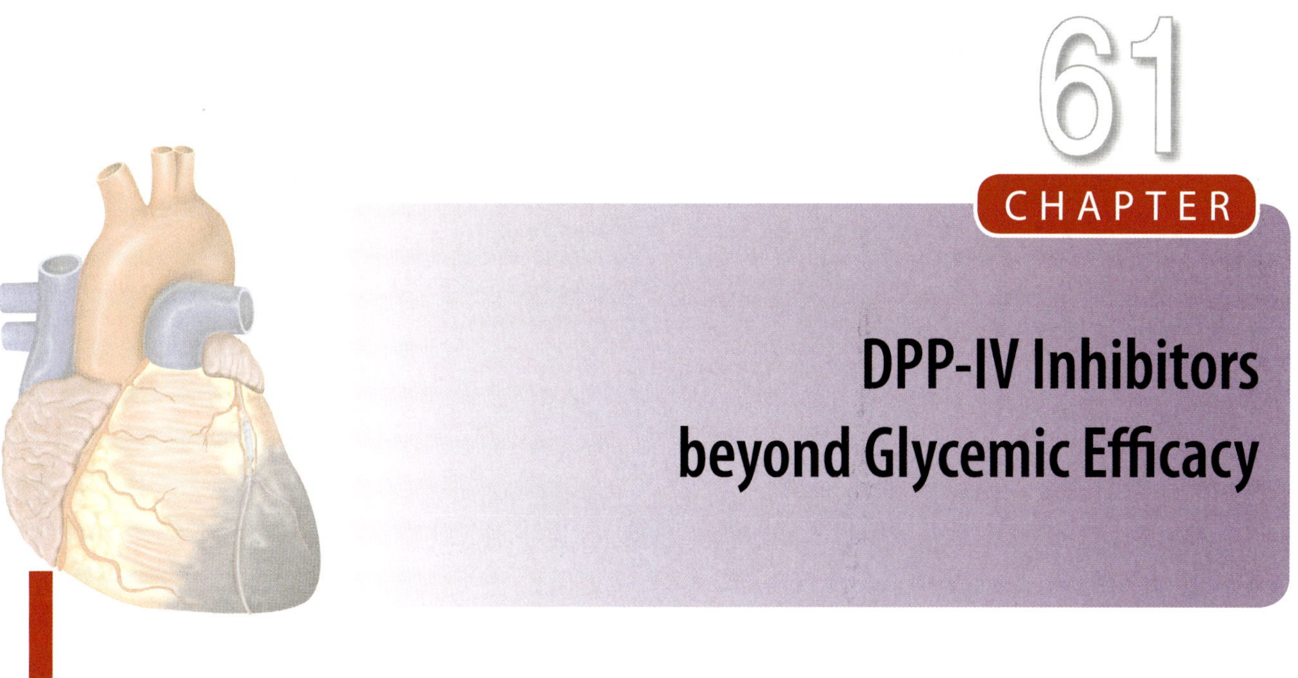

DPP-IV Inhibitors beyond Glycemic Efficacy

Geetha Subramanian, Balaji Lohiya, Vikas Agrawal, Aviraj Chaudhary

INTRODUCTION

Diabetes mellitus is a chronic, progressive, and noncommunicable disease characterized by elevated levels of blood glucose levels due to deficiency of insulin secreted by pancreas or resistance to insulin or both. The worldwide prevalence of diabetes has doubled over last two decades reaching 8.5% in adults currently and is the 8th most common cause of death in both sexes.[1] Cardiovascular diseases are also 2–3 times more prevalent in patients with diabetes mellitus as compared to nondiabetics, and are cause of premature mortality and morbidity in patients with diabetes mellitus. With obesity adversely related to higher blood glucose levels and existing drugs used to treat diabetes like insulin and sulfonylurea class of drugs themselves causing weight gain and significant hypoglycemia there was need for newer molecules as monotherapy or in combination to treat type 2 diabetes. Discovery of incretin effect lead to development of dipeptidyl peptidase-IV (DPP-IV) inhibitors. Glucagon-like peptide-1 (GLP-1) and gastric inhibitory peptide (GIP) are the chief incretins released from gut mucosa in response to oral nutrients, mainly glucose and fat, and they mediate their biological effects through insulin release, glucagon suppression, control of post prandial hyperglycemia as well reduction of gastric emptying and decreased apetite.[2] DPP-IV a cell surface membrane-bound peptidase causes proteolytic degradation of GLP-1 resulting in a half-life of GLP-1 to 1–2 minutes.[3] Thus, DPP-IV inhibitor effects in diabetes mellitus type 2 occurs indirectly by increasing levels of peptides like GLP-1 and GIP. In animal studies it was shown that DPP-IV-deficient mice had improved glucose tolerance after oral glucose. Absence of inhibition leads to higher levels of GLP-1 and GIP peptides resulting in higher insulin levels and better glucose disposal. DPP-IV-deficient mice were resistant to diet-induced obesity.[4] Sitagliptin was the first DPP-IV inhibitor approved in 2006 by Food and Drug Administration (FDA) followed by saxagliptin in 2009 and alogliptin in 2013. Currently available DPP-IV inhibitors are sitagliptin, saxagliptin, vildagliptin, linagliptin, teneligliptin (TEN), and alogliptin. They are recommended as add on therapy if blood glucose is not controlled even after measures like dietary modification, weight reduction, regular exercise, and metformin usage in optimum dosage. DPP-IV inhibitors may be used as monotherapy when metformin use is contraindicated, patients with chronic renal failure and patients at high risk of or prone to hypoglycemia. They reduce hemoglobin 1Ac (Hb1Ac) by 0.7%.

DIPEPTIDYL PEPTIDASE-IV[5-8]

Dipeptidyl peptidase-IV is an exopeptidase enzyme widely distributed in numerous tissues like intestine, pancreas, kidney, liver, spleen, placenta, and adrenal glands. It is also present in lymphocytes and is highly expressed in endothelial cells. Receptor for GLP-1, a substrate for DPP-IV, is also highly expressed in cardiomyocytes, coronary smooth muscle cells, and endothelial cells. DPP-IV is composed of 766 amino acids, is membrane bound, serine-type protease enzyme causing proteolytic degradation.[9] Membrane spanning protein of DPP-IV binds adenosine deaminase and leads to intracellular signals via dimerization and activation of intracellular signaling pathways leading its biological effects with enzymatic activity exhibited by both the membrane-spanning and soluble forms of the molecule.[10] The incretins mainly GLP-1 and GIP are well studied in animal studies and validated in humans for their blood glucose lowering effect. However, the DDP-IV enzyme affects not only GLP-1 and GIP levels but a number of other peptides are also potential substrates for DPP-IV action, e.g. neuropeptide Y, peptide YY, gastrin-releasing polypeptide, insulin-like growth factor-1, substance P, and many more substrates including various chemokines (Table 1).[11,12] Therefore, DPP-IV enzyme may be having a role in processes other than glucose metabolism like blood pressure (BP) regulation, atherosclerosis, angiogenesis, immunomodulatory action, metabolism, and tissue growth.

Wound Healing

Diabetic patients are prone for infection and wound healing is often impaired. Linagliptin has shown better wound healing and re-epithelialization in studies on ob/ob mice after 10 days of linagliptin use as compared to placebo probably explained by tight binding of the linagliptin to DPP-IV in skin and its inhibitory effect on T-cell proliferation and cytokine expression resulting in the improved wound healing and immunomodulatory effect.[13]

Tumor Cells and Dipeptidyl Peptidase-IV Inhibitors[14-17]

Increased expression of DPP-IV enzyme was seen in malignancies of exocrine pancreas, mesothelioma, lung papillary adenocarcinoma, and hepatocellular cancer, whereas decreased expression of DPP-IV was observed in endometrial adenocarcinoma, melanoma, spinocellular lung carcinoma, thyroid papillary carcinoma, follicular cancer, and astrocytic brain tumors suggesting complex relationship of DPP-IV expression and biological properties of tumor cells resulting in pro-oncogenic or antioncogenic effect. According to the FDA report there was increase in neoplasias after sitagliptin (0.8% vs 0.4%) mostly colorectal, skin, and prostate tumors; however the increase was not significant. Low levels of DPP-IV in malignancy are associated with dissemination or metastasis.

Inflammatory Diseases[9,18]

Dipeptidyl Peptidase-IV may have a role as immunomodulator function in conditions like multiple sclerosis, arthritis, and inflammatory bowel disease through its effect on various cytokines. Stromal-cell-derived factor-1, tumor necrosis factor-alpha, and many other inflammatory cytokines may be substrate for DPP-IV. DPP-IV inhibitors had a beneficial effect in rheumatoid arthritis in experimental studies with inhibitory effect on migration of T lymphocyte, T cell deoxyribonucleic acid DNA synthesis, fibroblast activation, production of tumor necrosis factor alpha (TNF-α), and interleukin-11 (IL-11) at the site of inflammation. However, the precise role of DPP-IV in the etiopathogenesis of inflammatory disorders is not clear and human studies and long-term data on clinical effect of DPV-IV inhibitors in inflammatory disorders is lacking.

TABLE 1: Probable substrates for dipeptidyl peptidase-IV enzyme explaining its pleotropic effects[8]

Biological process/ system	*Probable DPP-IV substrate*	*Effect*
Metabolism	GLP-1, GIP, and GLP-2	↑ insulin secretion, ↓ glucagon, ↓ appetite, ↑ acid secretion
	IGF-1	Anabolism and growth, insulin counter-regulatory
Digestion	Aprotinin	Trypsin inhibitor
	PYY	↓ appetite, delayed gastric emptying, and increases water and electrolyte absorption
Inflammation	Bradykinin, Eotaxin, GCP-2, MCP-1,2 and 3, RANTES, Substance P, and IP-10	Vasodilatation and proinflammatory
CNS	β-Casomorphin and endomorphin-2	Opioid like effects
	Chromogranin	Neuroendocrine function
	GHRH	GH production and release by binding to the GRP
	Prolactin	Essential for lactation and regulate fertility
Miscellaneous	SDF-1α, -1β	Chemotaxis, stem/ progenitor cell mobilization, and homing
	IL-2	Specific immunity
	IL-1β	Regulation of cell proliferation, differentiation, and apoptosis
	NPY	Energy balance, memory, and learning

Abbreviations: CNS, central nervous system; DPP-IV, dipeptidyl peptidase-IV; GLP-1, glucagon-like peptide-1; GIP, gastric inhibitory peptide; IGF-1, insulin-like growth factor 1; PYY, peptide YY; GCP-2, granulocyte chemotactic protein-2; IL, interleukin; NPY, neuropeptide Y; GH, growth hormone; GRP, gastrin releasing peptide

Neurological Disorders[10-12]

The pathological abnormalities seen in Alzheimer's disease are abnormal molecules such as p amyloid-β (A β) peptide, hyperphosphorylation, and insulin abnormality. Long-term sitagliptin treatment has shown reduction in brain Aβ peptide and amyloid precursor protein (APP) levels in vivo. There are few reports citing beneficial role of DPP-IV inhibitors in various psychiatric and neurological disorders such as schizophrenia, depression, and Alzheimer disease.

Hypertension and Cardiac Remodeling[19]

Angiotensin II (Ang II) causes retention of sodium through stimulates release of antidiuretic hormones, is involved in prohypertrophic signaling and has proven role in fibrosis, adverse myocardial remodeling, hypertension, and heart failure. TEN in the animal studies has shown to decrease central BP, reduced both systolic blood pressure (SBP) and diastolic blood pressure (DBP) by attenuating a rise in circulating levels of Ang II. In rat models TEN suppressed cardiac sodium-proton pump exchanger-1 (NHE-1) and ameliorated cardiac hypertrophy by inhibiting prohypertrophic signaling responsible for vasoconstriction, fibrosis, and cardiac hypertrophy.

Myocardial Infacrtion[20]

Smaller infarct size was observed in hearts of obese, prediabetic rats with decreased plasma insulin levels after the treatment with the DPP-IV inhibitor.

Antiarrhythmic Effect[21-28]

Dipeptidyl Peptidase-IV inhibitors, GLP-1 and its related molecules may have antiarrhythmic effects during myocardial ischemia by maintaining cardiomyocyte membrane electrical stability apart from its positive effect on reduction of infarct size, reduced inflammation, improved response to oxidative stress, and reduction in myocardial fibrosis. Yamamoto and colleagues reported effect of alogliptin on shortening the duration of atrial fibrillation (AF) in rabbits and suggested probable enhancement of atrial angiogenesis in fibrotic atria of rabbits and increased endothelial nitric oxide. Inhibition of DPP-IV activity may reduce activation of T cells and macrophages with decrease in the plasma markers of inflammation like IL-2, IL-10, IL-12, and interferon-γ (IFN-γ) seen in experimental models. A 6 weeks sitagliptin use reduced serum markers of inflammation while treating type 2 diabetes mellitus patients. Linagliptin monotherapy prostaglandin E2 (PGE2) and IL-6 decreased significantly following 6-month treatment in diabetic hemodialysis patients. DPP-IV deficient isolated cardiomyocytes in rats had lower reactive oxygen species and reduced proapoptotic signaling resistance to oxidative stress. Sitagliptin was shown to reduce expression of transforming growth factor-β1 (TGF-β1) and development of myocardial fibrosis.

Atherosclerosis and Dipeptidyl Peptidase-IV Inhibitors[29-31]

Glucagon-like peptide-1 analog exendin-4 administration reduced atherosclerotic lesion size and recruitment of monocytes to the vascular wall reducing inflammation in plaque independent of effect on lipid levels or glucose tolerance in experimental studies. TEN inhibited atherogenesis with attenuation of the inflammatory phenotype of perivascular adipose tissue and suppression of proinflammatory activation of macrophages and adipocytes. Linagliptin improved endothelial dysfunction, reduced oxidative stress, and inhibited atherogenesis in nondiabetic apolipoprotein E ($ApoE^{-/-}$) mice.

Myocardial Contractility[32]

It was observed that continuous intravenous infusion of GLP-1 improves left ventricular (LV) ejection fraction in patients with myocardial infarction and LV dysfunction. In a pilot study by Read and colleagues sitagliptin improved the myocardial response to dobutamine stress in patients with coronary artery disease and improved myocardial contractility of ischemic segments.

ADVERSE EFFECTS

Available data shows a possible but small risk of nasopharyngitis and urinary tract infection, acute pancreatitis (insufficient data), skin rashes, myalgia, headache, and elevation in liver enzymes. Risk of hypoglycemia is very less and they do not cause weight gain. As cardiovascular disorders are most common cause of death in diabetes mellitus and data showing possible published adverse cardiovascular effects of hypoglycemic drug rosiglitazone in last decade; it became more important to be vigilant regarding cardiovascular safety profile of any new antidiabetic drug.

Heart Failure Risk with Dipeptidyl Peptidase-IV Inhibitors[3,33-37]

In humans studies GLP-1 administration had many beneficial effects like increased LV ejection fraction, improved exercise tolerance in patients with LV dysfunction, reduce SBP and heart rate, and reduced arrhythmia in patients with coronary artery bypass grafting. Levels of GLP-1 are increased by DPP-IV inhibitors and various randomized trial in different phases of studies have shown reduction of major adverse cardiovascular events (MACEs) with DPP-IV inhibitors. Meta-analysis of 53 phase randomized controlled trials (RCTs) involving over 30,000 patients with at least 6 months follow-up showed that the DPP-IV inhibitors use was associated with a 31% relative reduction of MACE. Possible mechanisms responsible for beneficial effects on cardiovascular system postulated were decreased oxidative stress, decreased mitochondrial dysfunction, decreased proapoptotic proteins and decreased ischemia reperfusion injury. However, cardiovascular safety of DPP-IV inhibitors was questioned after publication of results of the Saxagliptin Assessment of Vascular Outcomes Recorded in Patients With Diabetes Mellitus-Thrombolysis in Myocardial Infarction 53 trial (SAVOR-TIMI 53 trial) in 2013 reporting adverse impact on myocardial function with saxagliptin treatment arm having a 27% increase in hospitalization for heart failure as compared to placebo but without an increase in mortality. The findings were seen as a surprise as preclinical studies with GLP-1 infusion had shown a cardioprotective effect like improvement in ejection fraction, decrease in heart rate, and plaque regression. Since then, there has been controversy related to use of DPP-IV inhibitors and risk of heart failure. The Examination of Cardiovascular Outcomes with Alogliptin versus Standard of Care (EXAMINE) trial had no significant rise in the risk of heart failure associated with use of alogliptin. In the Vildagliptin in Ventricular Dysfunction Diabetes (VIVIDD) trial, use of vildagliptin was associated with statistically significant increase in LV end-diastolic volume. Soon after the savor TIMI 53 data published meta-analysis was carried out by M Monami and colleagues in which they found that DPP-IV inhibitors could be associated with an increased risk of heart failure; however, SAVOR-TIMI 53 trial alone contributed for two-third of heart failure events. Thereafter, a large multicenter randomized TEKOS (Trial Evaluating Cardiovascular Outcomes with Sitagliptin) did not show increased heart failure risk or admissions due to heart failure with sitagliptin use. J Kongwatcharapong and colleagues tried to clarify the controversy in their meta analysis of randomized clinical trials involving DPP-IV inhibitors and heart failure. A total of 54 comparative RCTs studies with 74,737 participants with minimum follow-up of 12 weeks were included for analysis with heart failure as primary outcome. They found that use of DPP-IV inhibitors was not associated with an increased risk of heart failure with p value 0.062. However, individually among various DPP-IV inhibitors, saxagliptin was associated with the 21% increased risk of heart failure with p 0.022. They also noted that other factors associated with increased probability of heart failure were age more than and equal to 65 years, duration of diabetes mellitus more than 10 years and obesity (body mass index ≥30 kg/m^2) in patients using saxagliptin. In another study carried out in Taiwan, the authors found no increased risk of hospitalization for heart failure for patients treated with DPP-IV inhibitors including sitagliptin, saxagliptin, and vildagliptin. Thus, the worsened heart failure may not be a class effect and may be related differences in the chemical structure of saxagliptin and should be used with caution in susceptible patients like elderly, obese, uncontrolled diabetics of long duration, and patients with history of previous heart failure with avoidance of use as monotherapy till long-term data becomes available.

CONCLUSION

Dipeptidyl peptidase-IV inhibitors may have a myriad effects on various biological systems considering widespread presence in various tissues and pleotropic effects of DPP-IV enzyme. Animal and preclinical studies have convincingly shown cardioprotective effects of incretin molecule GLP-1 infusion like improvement in myocardial contractility, favorable effect on heart rate and DBP, and atherosclerotic plaque regression which can be extrapolated to DPP-IV inhibitor use as they increase levels of GLP-1. Heart failure may be associated with saxagliptin use; however no data or study has shown any significant linkage of increased heart failure events with other DPP-IV inhibitors. It is important to have large long duration randomized trials sufficiently powered to detect beneficial effects as well as to alleviate safety concerns and strict post marketing surveillance for longer duration to detect harmful effects keeping in mind all potential substrates of DPP-IV enzyme effects. Till the long-term safety data becomes available and relative risk benefit ratio becomes established, DPP-IV inhibitors should not be started as initial monotherapy and warrants a caution before using them in patients with prior heart failure with preferable avoidance of saxagliptin and have close postmarketing vigilance for all physicians while using any new drug and prompt reporting of any adverse outcome.

REFERENCES

1. World Health Organization. Global Report on Diabetes. Geneva: WHO; 2016.
2. Nauck MA. Incretin-based therapies for type 2 diabetes mellitus: properties, functions, and clinical implications. Am J Med. 2011;124:S3-18.
3. Duez H, Cariou B, Staels B. DPP-4 inhibitors in the treatment of type 2 diabetes. Biochem Pharmacol. 2012;83(7):823-32.
4. Conarello SL, Li Z, Ronan J, et al. Mice lacking dipeptidyl peptidase IV are protected against obesity and insulin resistance. Proc Natl Acad Sci USA. 2003;100(11):6825-30.
5. Abbott CA, Baker E, Sutherland GR, et al. Genomic organization, exact localization, and tissue expression of the human CD26 (dipeptidyl peptidase IV) gene. Immunogenetics. 1994;40(5):331-8.

6. Lambeir AM, Durinx C, Scharpe S, et al. Dipeptidyl-peptidase IV from bench to bedside: an update on structural properties, functions, and clinical aspects of the enzyme DPP IV. Crit Rev Clin Lab Sci. 2003;40:209-94.
7. Mentlein R. Dipeptidyl-peptidase IV (CD26)—role in the inactivation of regulatory peptides. Regul Pept. 1999;85:9-24.
8. Drucker DJ. Dipeptidyl peptidase-4 inhibition and the treatment of type 2 diabetes: preclinical biology and mechanisms of action. Diabetes Care. 2007;30(6):1335-43.
9. Ospelt C, Mertens JC, Jungel A, et al. Inhibition of fibroblast activation protein and dipeptidyl peptidase 4 increases cartilage invasion by rheumatoid arthritissynovial fibroblasts. Arthritis Rheum. 2010;62(5):1224-35.
10. Li L, Holscher C. Common pathological processes in Alzheimer disease and type 2 diabetes: a review. Brain Res Rev. 2007;56(2):384-402.
11. Thomas EH. DPP-4 inhibitors for treating neurodegeneration and cognitive disorders. Virginia: US Patent Office; 2009.
12. Hans-Ulrich D, Ants K, Nguyen T, et al. DPP-4 inhibitors for the treatment of schizophrenia and depression. Virginia: US Patent Office; 2012.
13. Linke A, Frank S, Mark M, et al. The DPP IV inhibitor linagliptin (BI 1356) improves wound healing in ob/ob mice. Diabetes. 2009;58(Suppl 1):A161.
14. Stulc T, Sedo A. Inhibition of multifunctional dipeptidyl peptidase-IV: is there a risk of oncological and immunological adverse effects? Diabetes Res Clin Pract. 2010;88(2):125-31.
15. Ghersi G, Zhao Q, Salamone M, et al. The protease complex consisting of dipeptidyl peptidase IV and seprase plays a role in the migration and invasion of human endothelial cells in collagenous matrices. Cancer Res. 2006;66 (9):4652-61.
16. Arscott WT, LaBauve AE, May V, et al. Suppression of neuroblastoma growth by dipeptidyl peptidase IV: relevance of chemokine regulation and caspase activation. Oncogene. 2009;28 (4):479-91.
17. Pro B, Dang NH. CD26/dipeptidyl peptidase IV and its role in cancer, Histol Histopathol. 2004;19(4):1345-51.
18. Detel D, Kehler T, Buljevic S, et al. Is dipeptidyl peptidase IV (DPP IV) associated with inflammation present in human spondylo-arthritides and rheumatoid arthritis. Croat Chem Acta. 2012;85(2): 231-8.
19. Kawase H, Bando YK, Nishimura K, et al. A dipeptidyl peptidase-4 inhibitor ameliorates hypertensive cardiac remodeling via angiotensin-II/sodium-proton pump exchanger-1 axis. J Mol Cell Cardiol. 2016;98:37-47.
20. Zaruba MM, Theiss HD, Vallaster M, et al. Synergy between CD26/DPP IV inhibition and G-CSF improves cardiac function after acute myocardial infarction. Cell Stem Cell. 2009;4(4):313-23.
21. Chinda K, Palee S, Surinkaew S, et al. Cardioprotective effect of dipeptidyl peptidase-4 inhibitor during ischemia-reperfusion injury. Int J Cardiol. 2013;167:451-7.
22. Hu X, Yang X, Jiang H. Glucagon-like peptide-1 and related agents: novel antiarrhythmic agents during myocardial ischemia and reperfusion. Int J Cardiol. 2013;168(3):3119-20.
23. Yamamoto T, Shimano M, Inden Y, et al. Alogliptin, a dipeptidyl peptidase-4 inhibitor, regulates the atrial arrhythmogenic substrate in rabbits. Heart Rhythm. 2015;12(6):1362-9.
24. Tremblay AJ, Lamarche B, Deacon CF, et al. Effects of sitagliptin therapy on markers of low-grade inflammation and cell adhesion molecules in patients with type 2 diabetes. Metabolism. 2014;63(9):1141-8.
25. Nakamura Y, Tsuji M, Hasegawa H, et al. Anti-inflammatory effects of linagliptin in hemodialysis patients with diabetes. Hemodial Int. 2014;18(2):433-42.
26. Bostick B, Habibi J, Ma L, et al. Dipeptidyl peptidase inhibition prevents diastolic dysfunction and reduces myocardial fibrosis in a mouse model of western diet induced obesity. Metabolism. 2014;63:1000-11.
27. Polovina MM, Ostojic MC, Potpara TS. Relation of biomarkers of inflammation and oxidative stress with hypertension occurrence in lone atrial fibrillation. Mediat Inflamm. 2015;2015:653026.
28. Ravassa S, Beaumont J, Huerta A, et al. Association of low GLP-1 with oxidative stress is related to cardiac disease and outcome in patients with type 2 diabetes mellitus: a pilot study. Free Radic Biol Med. 2015;81:1-12.
29. Arakawa M, Mita T, Azuma K, et al. Inhibition of monocyte adhesion to endothelial cells and attenuation of atherosclerotic lesion by a glucagon-like peptide-1 receptor agonist, exendin-4. Diabetes. 2010;59:1030-7.
30. Salim HM, Fukuda D, Higashikuni Y, et al. Teneligliptin, a dipeptidyl peptidase-4 inhibitor, attenuated proinflammatory phenotype of perivascular adipose tissue and inhibited atherogenesis in normoglycemic apolipoprotein-E-deficient mice. Vascul Pharmacol. 2017;96-98:19-25.
31. Salim HM, Fukuda D, Higashikuni Y, et al. Dipeptidyl peptidase-4 inhibitor, linagliptin, ameliorates endothelial dysfunction and atherogenesis in normoglycemic apolipoprotein-E deficient mice. Vascul Pharmacol. 2016;79:16-23.
32. Nikolaidis LA, Mankad S, Sokos GG, et al. Effects of glucagon-like peptide-1 in patients with acute myocardial infarction and left ventricular dysfunction after successful reperfusion. Circulation. 2004;109:962-5.
33. Bonora E, Cigolini M. DPP-4 inhibitors and cardiovascular disease in type 2 diabetes mellitus. Expectations, observations and perspectives. Nutr Metab Cardiovasc Dis. 2016;26(4):273-84.
34. Monami M, Dicembrini I, Mannucci E. Dipeptidyl peptidase-4 inhibitors and heart failure: A meta-analysis of randomized clinical trials. Nutr Metabol Cardiovasc Dis. 2014;24(7):689-97.
35. Green JB, Bethel MA, Armstrong PW, et al. Effect of sitagliptin on cardiovascular outcomes in type 2 diabetes. N Engl J Med. 2015;373(3):232-42.
36. Kongwatcharapong J, Dilokthornsakul P, Nathisuwana S, et al. Effect of dipeptidyl peptidase-4 inhibitors on heart failure: a meta-analysis of randomized clinical trials. Int J Cardiol. 2016;211:88-95.
37. Chang CH, Chang YC, Lin JW, et al. No increased risk of hospitalization for heart failure for patients treated with dipeptidyl peptidase-4 inhibitors in Taiwan. Int J Cardiol. 2016;220:14-20.

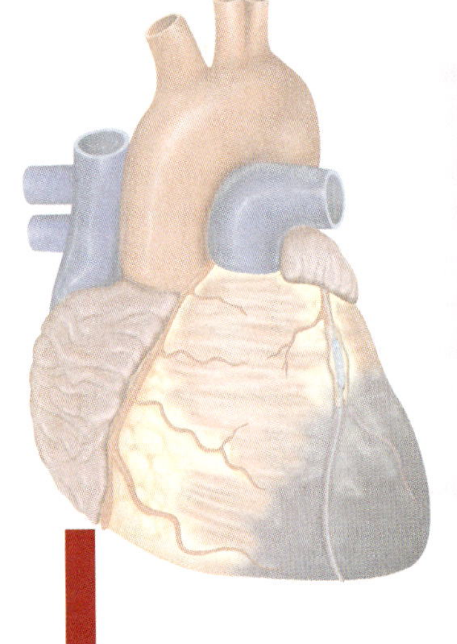

Insulin Therapy and Cardiodiabetes in Critical Care

Surabhi Awasthi, Nikhil Bhat

INTRODUCTION

Hyperglycemia occurs frequently in critically ill patients, including patients with previously known or unrecognized type 1 or type 2 diabetes mellitus (DM), or in those with previous normoglycemia (stress hyperglycemia).[1] Stress hyperglycemia refers to a transient increase in blood glucose (BG) concentration during acute illness in patients with no previous history of diabetes.[2] Several studies in critically ill patients have demonstrated a positive correlation between stress hyperglycemia and poor clinical outcomes, such as longer hospital stay[2,3] and increased morbidity and mortality.[4-6] Complications, such as severe infections and organ failure, are reduced. Several potential mechanisms may explain these benefits—prevention of immune dysfunction, reduction of systemic inflammation, prevention of cellular hypoxia, and protection of the endothelium and of mitochondrial ultrastructure and function. There is no universally accepted definition for stress hyperglycemia. American Diabetes Association (ADA) defined stress hyperglycemia as an elevation of fasting glucose more than and equal to 126 mg/dL or 2-hour postprandial glucose more than or equal to 200 mg/dL in a patient without evidence of previous diabetes.[7,8] Glycosylated hemoglobin (HbA1c) value has been recommended to distinguish between patients with stress hyperglycemia and those with previously undiagnosed diabetes.[7] An HbA1c value more than and equal to 6.5% indicates pre-existing unrecognized diabetes, whereas HbA1c value less than 6.5% indicates stress-induced hyperglycemia (SIH). SIH is a common finding among critically ill patients, particularly among cardiovascular patients, neurocritical patients, and patients undergoing surgical procedures, even in the absence of pre-existing DM.[9] The prevalence of hyperglycemia occurring during a serious illness is especially apparent among patients with cardiovascular disease (CVD). Patients with higher admission glucose levels were more likely to experience subsequent reinfarction, rehospitalization for congestive heart failure, a major cardiovascular event, or death.

PATHOPHYSIOLOGY OF STRESS HYPERGLYCEMIA

Pathophysiology is not well understood. Several conditions, such as surgery, trauma, and acute illness increase the circulatory level of counter-regulatory hormones and proinflammatory cytokines, which alter the effect of insulin on hepatic glucose production and skeletal muscle. Increased counter-regulatory hormones (glucagon, cortisol, catecholamines, and growth hormone)[4,10] contribute to alterations in glucose metabolism, including raised hepatic glucose production and impaired peripheral glucose utilization. Catecholamines inhibit insulin release by pancreatic beta cells and promote glucagon secretion, and cortisol increases hepatic glucose production and stimulates protein catabolism.

Pathogenesis of Stress-induced Hyperglycemia[1]

The pathogenesis of stress-induced hyperglycemia is shown in Flow chart 1.

Flow chart 1: Pathogenesis of stress-induced hyperglycemia

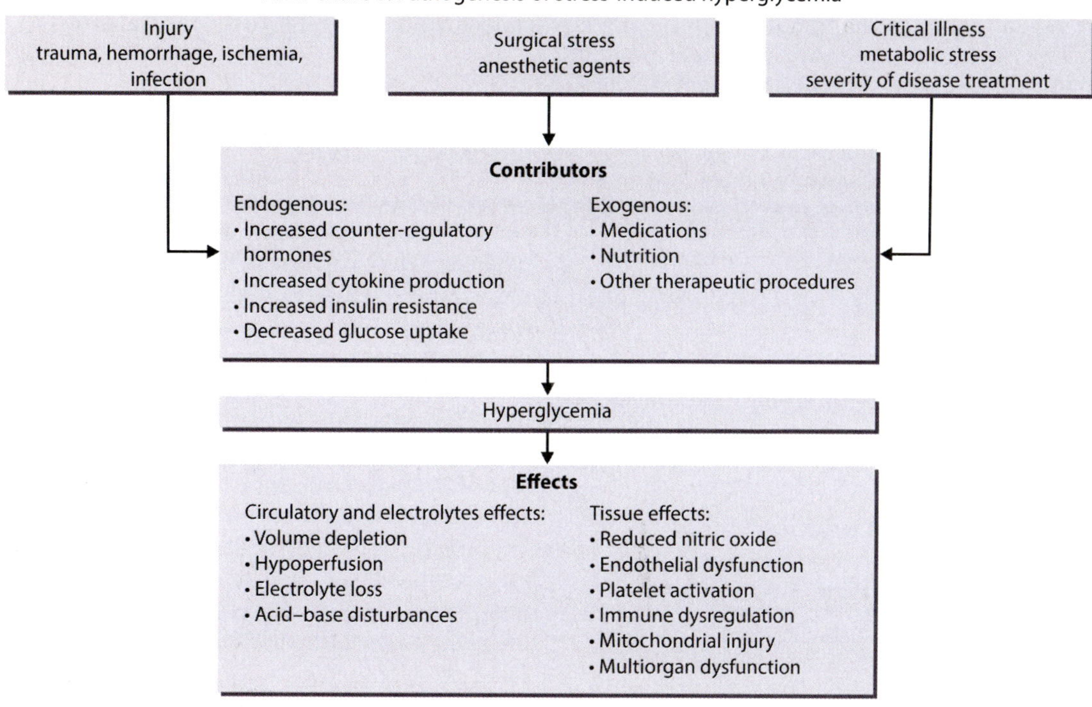

Source: Mukherjee JJ, Chatterjee PS, Saikia M, et al. Consensus recommendations for the management of hyperglycaemia in critically ill patients in the Indian setting. J Assoc Physicians India. 2014;62(7 Suppl):16-25.

Medical therapies may induce hyperglycemia by the administration of exogenous catecholamines and corticosteroids, dextrose infusion, and parenteral nutrition. Acute hyperglycemia may induce a poor outcome in critically ill patients by complications common in chronic diabetic patients, such as increased risk of infections, worse wound healing, and polyneuropathy. Furthermore, acute hyperglycemia may cause injury to endothelial cells, hepatocytes, and renal tubular cells.

HYPERGLYCEMIA AND CARDIOVASCULAR DISEASE IN CRITICAL ILLNESS

Both type 1 diabetes and type 2 diabetes are independent risk factors for chronic heart disease (CHD). One reason for the poor prognosis in patients with both diabetes and ischemic heart disease seems to be an enhanced myocardial dysfunction leading to accelerated heart failure (diabetic cardiomyopathy). Thus, patients with diabetes are unusually prone to congestive heart failure. Several factors probably underlie diabetic cardiomyopathy: severe coronary atherosclerosis, prolonged hypertension, chronic hyperglycemia, microvascular disease, glycosylation of myocardial proteins, and autonomic neuropathy. Most patients with type 2 diabetes have insulin resistance. Indeed, insulin resistance seems to predispose to both CVD and diabetes. Metabolic risk factors that occur commonly in patients with insulin resistance are atherogenic dyslipidemia, hypertension, glucose intolerance, and a prothrombotic state.

Cardioprotective Effect of Insulin[11]

Hyperglycemia leads to glucose toxicity by increasing oxidative stress, flux via the hexosamine pathway, and levels of advanced glycation end products, which are detrimental to the heart.[12] Hyperglycemia may have a prothrombotic effect that augments inflammation.[13,14] It has also long been known that hyperglycemia promotes free radical generation and oxidative stress in DM. In turn, reactive oxygen species may induce insulin resistance and hence perpetuate the hyperglycemia. Oxidative stress damages mitochondrial deoxyribonucleic acid (DNA) and vital cellular proteins, which leads to mitochondrial dysfunction in CVD and the metabolic syndrome. Oxidative stress is also closely associated with inflammation, apoptosis, and vascular dysfunction.

Positive Inotropic Effect[11]

Visscher et al.[15] demonstrated that insulin increased cardiac contractility in isolated heart-lung preparations and increased arterial blood pressure in live animals. Others have later shown that in animal models and in isolated human myocardia, insulin possesses a direct positive inotropic effect that is independent of its modulation of glucose metabolism, although the effect may be species specific. In addition, insulin induces the phosphorylation of heat shock protein.[16] Phosphorylated heat shock protein[16] is associated with improved myocardial contractility after ischemia-reperfusion injury.[17]

Antioxidant Effect[11,14]

Impaired insulin signaling has been implicated in elevated oxidative stress and mitochondrial dysfunction in the murine heart. Insulin can prevent oxidative damage by reducing the formation of peroxynitrite (ONOO) free radicals via the phosphatidylinositol 3-kinase-Akt (PI3K-Akt) pathway after myocardial ischemia.

Antiapoptotic Effect[11,18]

One of the most studied modes of cardioprotection by insulin is the aversion of apoptotic cell death in the context of ischemia-reperfusion. Insulin not only reduces the infarct size, plasma creatine kinase and lactate dehydrogenase (both markers of myocardial injury), and apoptosis (measured by the proportion of apoptotic cells and caspase-3 activity) hours after ischemia, but it better preserves the structure and function of cardiac tissues 4 weeks afterward.[18]

Anti-inflammatory Effect[11]

Hyperglycemia is proinflammatory, whereas insulin is anti-inflammatory. The anti-inflammatory effects of insulin are intimately linked to its antioxidant effects.

Vascular Effects[11]

In humans, insulin increased coronary sinus and myocardial blood flow and reduced coronary resistance.[19,20] Insulin-induced coronary vasodilation is related to nitrous oxide (NO) production.

Other Protective Effects[21]

A recent meta-analysis has concluded that tight glycemic control (TGC) during or after cardiac surgery reduced the incidence of atrial fibrillation (AF) and the use of epicardial pacing. Meanwhile, DM is associated with an increased risk of AF. In addition, insulin may modulate AF by facilitating K^+ uptake in the myocardium, which may help to restore sinus rhythm and stabilize the myocardium.[22]

GUIDELINES OF INSULIN THERAPY IN CRITICAL CARE

The ADA recommends starting insulin in patients with persistent hyperglycemia above 180 mg/dL in critically ill patients,[23] and to maintain the glycemic range between 140 mg/dL and 180 mg/dL. It also states that stricter glycemic control (110–140 mg/dL) can be appropriate for certain patients, such as patients with acute cardiac ischemia or patients with acute neurological event, as long as significant hypoglycemia can be avoided. They also recommend active prevention of hypoglycemia by having a treatment plan if hypoglycemia were to develop and to change the current therapy if serum glucose levels fall below 70 mg/dL. The American College of Physicians recommends serum glucose levels between 140 mg/dL and 200 mg/dL independent of diabetic status, and recommends avoiding blood sugar levels below 140 mg/dL due to the associated risks of hypoglycemia and glycemic variability. The Society of Critical Care Medicine (SCCM) recommends maintaining the serum glucose level between 150 mg/dL and 180 mg/dL. However, it has been shown that patients with uncontrolled diabetes (HbA1c above 7%) had different mortality when hyperglycemia was present when compared to nondiabetic patients or patients with better controlled diabetes (HbA1c <7%).

RECOMMENDATIONS

Blood glucose more than and equal to 150 mg/dL should trigger initiation of insulin therapy, titrated to keep BG less than 150 mg/dL for most adult intensive care unit (ICU) patients and to maintain BG values absolutely less than 180 mg/dL using a protocol that achieves a low rate of hypoglycemia (BG ≤70 mg/dL) despite limited impact on patient mortality. Implementation of moderate glycemic control (GC) (BG <150 mg/dL) in the postoperative period following cardiac surgery is advisable to achieve a reduced risk of deep sternal wound infection and mortality (Table 1). Morbidity benefits for this group of patients included a reduced need for renal replacement therapy, less chance of hyperbilirubinemia, earlier cumulative likelihood of weaning from mechanical ventilation, and ICU and hospital discharge. In critically ill injured (trauma) ICU patients, a BG more than and equal to 150 mg/dL should trigger initiation of insulin therapy, titrated to keep BG less than 150 mg/dL for most adult trauma patients and to

TABLE 1: Glycemic control recommendations based on patient condition[5]

Condition	*Glucose control recommendation*	*Reference*
Nondiabetic ICU patients	140–180 mg/dL	Wiener et al. (2008)[24] Griesdale et al. (2009)[25]
Diabetic ICU patients	If HbA1c < 7%: 140–180 mg/dL If HbA1c > 7%: >200 mg/dL	Egi et al. (2011)[6]
Surgical ICU	If ICU stay is for more than 3 days, ventilator dependent, on dialysis, or with cardiac comorbidities: <150 mg/dL	Furnary et al. (2004)[26]
Neurocritical ICU patients	If not: <180 mg/dL If hypoglycemia can be prevented: 110–140 mg/dL If not: 140–180 mg/dL	Kramer et al. (2012)[27]
STEMI ICU patients	<200 mg/dL	Nice Guidelines (2011)[28]
Sepsis ICU patients	<180 mg/dL	Based of NICE-SUGAR study[29]
Pregnant ICU patients	No consensus	Van de Velde et al. (2013)[16]

Abbreviations: ICU, intensive care unit; HbA1c, glycated hemoglobin; STEMI, ST-elevation myocardial infarction

maintain BG values absolutely less than 180 mg/dL, using a protocol that achieves a low rate of hypoglycemia (BG ≤70 mg/dL) to achieve lower rates of infection and shorter ICU stays in trauma patients. Arterial blood gas (ABG) more than and equal to 150 mg/dL triggers initiation of insulin therapy for most patients admitted to an ICU with the diagnoses of ischemic stroke, intraparenchymal hemorrhage, aneurysmal subarachnoid hemorrhage, or traumatic brain injury (TBI), titrated to achieve BG values absolutely less than 180 mg/dL with minimal BG excursions less than100 mg/dL to minimize the adverse effects of hyperglycemia. BG less than and equal to 70 mg/dL are associated with an increase in mortality, and that even brief episodes of severe hypoglycemia (BG ≤40 mg/dL) is independently associated with a greater risk of mortality and that the risk increases with prolonged or frequent episodes. ABG less than 70 mg/dL (<100 mg/dL in neurologic injury patients) should be treated immediately by stopping the insulin infusion and administering 10–20 g of hypertonic (50%) dextrose, titrated based on the initial hypoglycemic value to avoid overcorrection. The BG should be repeated in 15 minutes with further dextrose administration as needed to achieve BG more than 70 mg/dL with a goal to avoid iatrogenic hyperglycemia. BG should be monitored every 1–2 hours for most patients receiving an insulin infusion. Most point-of-care (POC) glucose meters are acceptable, but not optimal for routine BG testing during insulin infusion therapy. Clinicians must be aware of potential limitations in accuracy of glucose meters for patients with concurrent anemia, hypoxia, and interfering drugs. We should use arterial or venous whole blood sampling instead of finger-stick capillary BG testing for patients in shock, on vasopressor therapy, or with severe peripheral edema, and for any patient on a prolonged insulin infusion. A continuous insulin infusion (1 unit/mL) therapy should be initiated after priming new tubing with a 20 mL waste volume. Insulin may be mixed with 0.9% sodium chloride, lactated Ringer's injection, Ringer's injection, or 5% dextrose. Insulin may be prepared in glass or plastic containers [polyvinyl chloride (PVC), ethylene vinyl acetate, polyethylene, and other polyolefin plastics], although loss will occur through adsorption to containers and to intravenous (IV) tubing and filters. The pump must be able to deliver insulin dose increments of less than 1 unit/h for insulin-sensitive patients. IV insulin infusion is preferred for patients with type 1 DM, hemodynamically unstable patients with hyperglycemia, and also patients in whom long-acting basal insulin should not be initiated due to changing clinical status (hypothermia, edema, frequent interruption of dextrose intake, etc.). Stable ICU patients should be transitioned to a protocol-driven basal/bolus insulin regimen before the insulin infusion is stopped to avoid a significant loss of GC. Calculation of basal and bolus insulin dosing requirements should be based on the patient's IV insulin infusion history and carbohydrate intake. This includes a three-component approach to insulin replacement: (1) basal insulin, (2) nutritional insulin, and (3) correction insulin. Basal insulin is provided as an injection of long-acting insulin given every 24 hours (e.g. glargine) or intermediate-acting insulin given every 6–12 hours (e.g. NPH). Basal insulin will be needed in many diabetic patients on enteral feedings to achieve the desired BG goal. The initial basal insulin dose is recommended at least 2–4 hours before stopping the insulin infusion when possible to prevent rebound hyperglycemia. For nutritional considerations with IV insulin therapy in adult ICU patients, the amount and timing of carbohydrate intake should be evaluated when calculating insulin requirements. We also suggest that GC protocols should include instructions to address unplanned discontinuance of any form of carbohydrate infusion. Consistent intake of nutrition appears to simplify glycemic management during an insulin infusion. Overfeeding may produce hyperglycemia that necessitates insulin infusion therapy, and should be avoided.

TABLE 2: Comparison of the current consensus guideline with existing guidelines for management of hyperglycemia in critically ill patients.

Criteria	*Consensus guideline*	*AACE-ADA*	*API*	*ACP*	*CDA*	*ADS*	*SSC*	*AHA*
Glycemic target	110 mg/dL is not recommended; 110-140 mg/dL in post-CABG, uncomplicated	140–180 mg/dL, <110 mg/dL is not recommended	140–180 mg/dL is in patients with medical morbidity and 110–140 mg/dL for patients	140–200 mg/dL, (MICU/SICU patients on insulin therapy)	144–180 mg/dL (MICU/SICU patients), intraoperative: 99–180 mg/dL (patients with diabetes undergoing CABG) and perioperative 90–180 mg/dL	<180 mg/dL in patients with hyperglycemia along with AMI or acute thrombotic stroke	<180 mg/dL in ICU patients with severe sepsis	90–140 mg/dL in ICU patients with ACS
Initiating insulin therapy	Initiate IIT (continuous IV insulin infusion when BG level >180 mg/dL; short-acting regular insulin preferably with infusion pump; recheck BG before starting IIT in patients without diabetes, start insulin infusion at: BG/100 U/hr)	initiate IIT (continuous IV insulin infusion) when BG Level > 180 mg/dL	Initiate IIT (continuous IV insulin infusion) when BG Level > 180 mg/dL	Do not use IIT to strictly control or normalise BG in MICU/SICU patients with or without diabetes	Initiate IIT (continuous IV insulin infusion) when BG Level > 180 mg/dL. Rest same as consensus		Initiate IIT (continuous IV insulin infusion) when BG Level > 180 mg/dL	Initiate IIT (continuous IV insulin infusion) when BG Level > 180 mg/dL
Monitoring of blood glucose	Monitor capillary BG every 1 hour; every 20-30 minutes till hypoglycemia resolves, restart IIT in modified doses as necessary once	Frequent glucose monitoring in patients with IV insulin therapy, to minimize the risk of hypoglycemia	Initial monitoring should be done on an hourly basis			Frequent monitoring is required in patients on IIT	Monitor BG values every 1–2 hours until BG values and insulin infusion rates are stable, every 4 hours thereafter	Close monitoring of blood glucose in ICU patients with ACS
Transition from IV to SC insulin	Once patient is stable and taking enteral/oral feeds, start transition wherever needed; start SC insuline therapy at least 1 hour prior		Start SC insulin at least 1–2 hours before discontinuing IV insulting or 15–30 min if rapid-acting analogues are used					

Abbreviations: AACE-ADA, American Association of Clinical Endocrinologists and American Diabetes Association; API, Association of Physicians of India; ACP, American College of Physicians; CDA: Canadian Diabetes Association; ADS, Australian Diabetes Society; SSC, surviving sepsis campaign; AHA, American Heart Association, CABG, coronary artery bypass grafting; MICU, medical intensive care unit; SICU, surgical intensive care unit, AMI, acute myocardial infarction; ACS, acute coronary syndrome; IIT, intensive insulin therapy; IV, intravenous; BG, blood glucose; SC, subcutaneous

Source: Mukherjee JJ, Chatterjee PS, Saikia M, et al. Consensus recommendations for the management of hyperglycaemia in critically ill patients in the Indian setting. J Assoc Physicians India. 2014;62(7 Suppl):16-25.

Current Guideline versus Existing Guideline

Comparison of the current consensus guideline with existing guidelines for management of hyperglycemia in critically ill patients has been presented in Table 2.

INSULIN INFUSION PROTOCOLS[30]

The insulin infusion protocols (IIP) have to balance efficacy with safety (avoid hypoglycemia and glycemic variability) and attainability (nursing workload). The Yale protocol has been shown to provide better average glycemia, more time spent in normoglycemia, less time in hypoglycemia, and less glycemic variability.[31]

Yales Protocol

The modified Yales protocol[30] is mentioned below:
Target for ICU patients: 140–180 mg/dL

Indications of IIP

- Diabetic ketoacidosis (DKA)
- Hyperosmolar hyperglycemic state (HHS)
- Very poorly controlled diabetes despite subcutaneous insulin (i.e. BG >350 mg/dL for more than 12 hours)
- Total parenteral nutrition (TPN)
- Type 1 diabetes patients who are NPO, perioperative, or in labor and delivery
- Consider in any ICU patient with hyperglycemia (>180 mg/dL)
- Suspected poor subcutaneous absorption of insulin (rare).

Infusion Preparation

- Mix 100 units of human regular insulin in 100 cc of 0.9% NaCl (or 0.45% NaCl) (1 U = 1 cc).
- Run at least 20 cc through tubing before initiating infusion.

Infusion Initiation

- Start infusion at rate of 1–5 units per hour, depending on degree of hyperglycemia (rate may be higher in highly insulin-resistant individuals, the obese, patients on steroids, and severely hyperglycemic patients).
- Alternatively, when transferring a patient from subcutaneous to IV insulin, divide 50% of the total daily insulin dose by 24 hours for an hourly rate (depending on patient status/condition).
- When patient is NPO, some carbohydrate calories should be provided to prevent catabolism with a D5W solution at rate of 75–125 cc/hr (unless patient is still very hyperglycemic—i.e. >200 mg/dL).
- A reasonable blood sugar target is 140–180 mg/dL in the ICU; higher (e.g. 350–400 mg/dL), insulin infusion should lower the BG by approximately 75 mg/dL/hr.
- If BG is decreased by more than 100 mg/dL/hr, reduce drip rate by 25–50%.
- If greater BG decreases occur, hold the drip for 1 hour and restart at a rate reduced by at least 50%.
- In severely hyperglycemic patients, if BG is increasing or unchanged after 1–2 hours, increase drip rate by 50–100%.
- In patients who are hyperglycemic, but not severely so (i.e. 180–300 mg/dL), and if the BG is increasing or unchanged, more modest insulin drip increases (i.e. 20–50%) are recommended to achieve target.[32]
- If BG falls to 140 mg/dL, hold drip for 1 hour; recheck BG q30 minutes. When BG more than 140 mg/dL, restart drip at 75% of original rate.
- If BG less than 80 mg/dL, treat with oral or IV carbohydrates (depending on level of consciousness); recheck BG q30 minutes. When BG reaches 140 mg/dL, wait 1 hour and then restart drip at 50% of original rate.
- When transferring a patient back to subcutaneous insulin, give short/rapid-acting insulins 1–2 hours or intermediate/long-acting insulins 2–3 hours prior to terminating the drip.

SPECIAL INTENSIVE CARE UNIT POPULATION WITH CARDIODIABETES

Thoracic Surgery

The Society of Thoracic Surgeons created guidelines in 2009 for glucose management in adult cardiac surgery patients, including diabetics.[11] For preoperative care, maintenance with insulin therapy with a serum glucose goal below 180 mg/dL was recommended along with Preoperative HbA1c level. Intraoperatively, insulin therapy was also recommended for glycemic values above 180 mg/dL, and intravenous insulin infusion was recommended for persistent glycemic levels above 180 mg/dL intraoperatively or postoperatively in the ICU.[11,31,33] The recommendation was to keep a goal of 180 mg/dL throughout their stay in the ICU unless they are expected to remain in the critical care unit more than 3 days, or if the patient is ventilator-dependent, or requires therapy with inotropes, intra-aortic balloon pump, left ventricular assist device, antidysrhythmic medications, dialysis, or hemofiltration. In aforementioned cases, it is recommended to have the BG levels below 150 mg/dL.[32,34]

Patients with Acute Myocardial Infarction

Hyperglycemia has been found to be associated with poor clinical outcome in acute myocardial infarction (AMI) patients.[35] TGC may not contribute toward any increased mortality but it definitely reduces the risk of complications associated with MI, such as congestive cardiac failure and reinfarction.[36] It has been seen that even a moderately elevated HbA1c concentration, although within the normal range, indicated an increased risk of CVD and mortality. Critically ill patients with new-onset hyperglycemia, in addition, appear to have significantly higher inhospital mortality and worse functional outcomes than those with previously diagnosed diabetes or normoglycemia.[37] In 2008, the American Heart Association released a statement on glucose management in acute coronary syndrome, which recommended a glucose levels between 90 mg/dL and 140 mg/dL in ICU patients with acute coronary syndrome.[32] The recommendations were later updated in 2009, suggesting an upper limit of serum glucose to 180 mg/dL.[37]

Patients with Neurological Events[27]

Loose glycemic control (>200 mg/dL) was shown to increased mortality when compared to a moderate glycemic control (140–180 mg/dL).[27] The ADA states that BG level of 110–140 mg/dL may be appropriate if significant hypoglycemia can be avoided.[38]

Patients with Sepsis

In patients with sepsis/septic shock, the surviving sepsis campaign had earlier recommended a stricter range of glycemic control, with an upper goal of 110 mg/dL of serum glucose.[29] With the advent of the Normoglycemia in Intensive Care Evaluation and Surviving Using Glucose Algorithm Regulation (NICE-SUGAR) trial in 2009, which also included septic patients, the 2013 update of the Surviving Sepsis Campaign modified its recommendation to a looser goal of 180 mg/dL.[39] Due to increased risk of hypoglycemia and hypoglycemia-related mortality, the Surviving Sepsis Campaign deemed that there was no apparent benefit from strict glucose control. Intensive insulin therapy during intensive care prevents morbidity, but does not significantly reduce the risk of death among all patients in the medical ICU. However, among those who stay in the ICU for three or more days, IIP reduces morbidity and mortality.[29] The reduced morbidity results from the prevention of acquired kidney injury, earlier weaning from mechanical ventilation, and earlier discharge from the medical ICU and the hospital. While conventional glucose-lowering interventions that aim to maintain BG levels between 140 mg/dL and 180 mg/dL are recommended for critically ill patients, intensive glucose-lowering protocols having target glucose levels set at less than 110 mg/dL remain controversial. Benefits with such protocols, in terms of increased survival and shorter ICU stays, have been shown in surgical ICU patients[25] and those who remained in the ICU for 3 days or longer.[29] An alternative and more likely explanation for the difference in the effect of intensive insulin therapy in patients staying in the ICU for at least 3 days is that the benefit from intensive insulin therapy requires time to be realized. Indeed, the intervention is aimed not at curing disease, but at preventing complications that occur during and perhaps in part as a result of intensive care. Prevention probably does not occur when the patient has a high risk of death from the disease causing admission to the ICU and when the intervention is administered for a relatively short time. However, among patients in whom complications resulting from intensive care contribute to an adverse outcome, such a preventive strategy, if continued long enough, is likely to be effective.[40] Hyperglycemia and insulin resistance are common in severe illness and are associated with adverse outcomes. Glycemic control in critically ill patients is a unique challenge for both intensivist and endocrinologist, as these patients invariably have multiorgan dysfunction.[41-53]

CONCLUSION

Insulin therapy is the mainstay of diabetes control in setting of cardiodiabetes with other comorbidities. It helps us in appropriate glycemic control, thereby improves fast recovery.

REFERENCES

1. Mukherjee JJ, Chatterjee PS, Saikia M, et al. Consensus recommendations for the management of hyperglycaemia in critically ill patients in the Indian setting. J Assoc Physicians India. 2014;62(7 Suppl):16-25.
2. Jacobi J, Bircher N, Krinsley J, et al. Guidelines for the use of an insulin infusion for the management of hyperglycemia in critically ill patients. Crit Care Med. 2012;40(12):3251-76.
3. Kovalaske MA, Gandhi GY. Glycemic control in the medical intensive care unit. J Diabetes Sci Technol. 2009;3(6):1330-41.
4. McDonnell ME, Umpierrez GE. Insulin therapy for the management of hyperglycemia in hospitalized patients. Endocrinol Metab Clin North Am. 2012;41(1):175-201.
5. Silva-Perez LJ, Benitez-Lopez MA, Varon J, et al. Management of critically ill patients with diabetes. World J Diabetes. 2017;8(3): 89-96.
6. Egi M, Bellomo R, Stachowski E, et al. The interaction of chronic and acute glycemia with mortality in critically ill patients with diabetes. Crit Care Med. 2011;39:105-11.
7. Reider J, Lin H, DiNardo M, et al. Efficacy of a guideline for treatment of corticosteroid related hyperglycemia in the hospital. Diabetes. 2008;57:A574.

8. Clore JN, Thurby-Hay L. Glucocorticoid-induced hyperglycemia. Endocr Pract. 2009;15:469-74.
9. Viana MV, Moraes RB, Fabbrin AR, et al Assessment and treatment of hyperglycemia in critically ill patients. Rev Bras Ter Intensiva. 2014;26:71-6.
10. Gearhart M, Parbhoo SK. Hyperglycemia in the critically ill patient. AACN Clin Issues.2006;17(1):50-5.
11. Wooi Ng K, Allen ML, Desai A, et al. Cardioprotective effects of insulin: how intensive insulin therapy may benefit cardiac surgery patients. Circulation. 2012;125:721-8.
12. Muniyappa R, Montagnani M, Koh KK, et al. Cardiovascular actions of insulin. Endocr Rev. 2007;28:463-91.
13. Lemkes BA, Hermanides J, Devries JH, et al. Hyperglycemia: a prothrombotic factor? J Thromb Haemost. 2010;8:1663-9.
14. Maritim AC, Sanders RA, Watkins JB 3rd. Diabetes, oxidative stress, and antioxidants: a review. J Biochem Mol Toxicol. 2003;17(1):24-38.
15. Visscher MB, Muller EA. The influence of insulin upon the mammalian heart. J Physiol. 1927;62:341-8.
16. Van de Velde MSH, Plante L. Maternal Critical Care. United Kingdom: Cambridge University Press; 2013.
17. Li G, Ali IS, Currie RW. Insulin-induced myocardial protection in isolated ischemic rat hearts requires p38 MAPK phosphorylation of Hsp27. Am J Physiol Heart Circ Physiol. 2008;294:H74-H87.
18. Xing W, Yan W, Fu F, et al. Insulin inhibits myocardial ischemia-induced apoptosis and alleviates chronic adverse changes in post-ischemic cardiac structure and function. Apoptosis. 2009;14:1050-60.
19. Rogers WJ, Russell RO Jr, McDaniel HG, et al. Acute effects of glucose-insulin-potassium infusion on myocardial substrates, coronary blood flow and oxygen consumption in man. Am J Cardiol. 1977;40:421-8.
20. Lautamaki R, Airaksinen KE, Seppanen M, et al. Insulin improves myocardial blood flow in patients with type 2 diabetes and coronary artery disease. Diabetes. 2006;55:511-6.
21. Pancorbo-Hidalgo PL, García-Fernandez FP, Ramírez-Pérez C. Complications associated with enteral nutrition by nasogastric tube in an internal medicine unit. J Clin Nurs. 2001;10(4):482-90.
22. Haga KK, McClymont KL, Clarke S, et al. The effect of tight glycaemic control, during and after cardiac surgery, on patient mortality and morbidity: a systematic review and meta-analysis. J Cardiothorac Surg. 2011;6:3.
23. American Diabetes Association. Standards of medical care in diabetes—2010. Diabetes Care. 2010;33 (Suppl 1):S11-S61.
24. Wiener RS, Wiener DC, Larson RJ. Benefits and risks of tight glucose control in critically ill adults: a meta-analysis. JAMA. 2008;300:933-44.
25. Griesdale DE, de Souza RJ, van Dam RM, et al. Intensive insulin therapy and mortality among critically ill patients: a meta-analysis including NICE-SUGAR study data. CMAJ. 2009;180(8):821-7.
26. Okabayashi T, Shima Y, Sumiyoshi T, et al. Intensive versus intermediate glucose control in surgical intensive care unit patients. Diabetes Care. 2014;37(6):1516-24.
27. Kramer AH, Roberts DJ, Zygun DA. Optimal glycemic control in neurocritical care patients: a systematic review and meta-analysis. Crit Care. 2012;16(5):R203.
28. Centre for Clinical Practice at NICE (UK). Hyperglycaemia in acute coronary syndromes: management of hyperglycaemia in people with acute coronary syndromes. London: National Institute for Health and Clinical Excellence (UK); 2011.
29. Van den Berghe G, Wilmer A, Hermans G, et al. Intensive insulin therapy in the medical ICU. N Engl J Med. 2006;354:449-61.
30. Inzucchi SE. Diabetes Facts and Guidelines. New Haven Yale Diabetes Centre and Yale School of Learning; 2008.
31. De Block CEM, Rogiers P, Jorens PG, et al. A comparison of two insulin infusion protocols in the medical intensive care unit by continuous glucose monitoring. Ann Intensive Care. 2016;6(1):115.
32. Furnary AP, Wu Y, Bookin SO. Effect of hyperglycemia and continuous intravenous insulin infusions on outcomes of cardiac surgical procedures: the Portland Diabetic Project. Endocr Pract. 2004;10(suppl 2):21-33.
33. Kushner FG, Hand M, Smith SC, et al. 2009 focused updates: ACC/AHA guidelines for the management of patients with ST-elevation myocardial infarction (updating the 2004 guideline and 2007 focused update) and ACC/AHA/SCAI guidelines on percutaneous coronary intervention (updating the 2005 guideline and 2007 focused update) a report of the American College of Cardiology Foundation/American Heart Association Task Force on Practice Guidelines. J Am Coll Cardiol. 2009;120:2271-306.
34. Lazar HL, McDonnell M, Chipkin SR, et al. The Society of Thoracic Surgeons practice guideline series: blood glucose management during adult cardiac surgery. Ann Thorac Surg. 2009;87:663-9.
35. Pinto DS, Skolnick AH, Kirtane AJ, et al. U-shaped relationship of blood glucose with adverse outcomes among patients with ST-segment elevation myocardial infarction. J Am Coll Cardiol. 2005;46:178-80.
36. Malmberg K, Rydén L, Wedel H, et al. Intense metabolic control by means of insulin in patients with diabetes mellitus and acute myocardial infarction (DIGAMI 2): effects on mortality and morbidity. Eur Heart J. 2005;26(7):650-61.
37. Umpierrez GE, Isaacs SD, Bazargan N, et al. An independent marker of in-hospital mortality in patients with undiagnosed diabetes. J Clin Endocrinol Metab. 2002;87(3):978-82.
38. Professional Practice Committee for the Standards of Medical Care in Diabetes-2016. Diabetes Care. 2016;39(Suppl 1):S107-8.
39. Dellinger RP, Levy MM, Rhodes A, et al. Surviving Sepsis Campaign: international guidelines for management of severe sepsis and septic shock, 2012. Intensive Care Med. 2013;39(2):165-228.
40. Van den Berghe G, Wouters P, Weekers F, et al. Intensive insulin therapy in critically ill patients. N Engl J Med. 2001;345:1359-67.
41. Bajwa SS, Baruah MP, Kalra S. et al. (2013). Guidelines on Inpatient Management of Hyperglycemia. [online] available from http://www.apiindia.org/medicine_update_2013/chap35.pdf. [Accessed October, 2017]
42. Svensson AM, McGuire DK, Abrahamsson P, et al. Association between hyper-and hypoglycaemia and 2 year all-cause mortality risk in diabetic patients with acute coronary events. Eur Heart J. 2005;26:1255-61.
43. Mehta SR, Yusuf S, Diaz R, et al. Effect of glucose-insulin-potassium infusion on mortality in patients with acute ST-segment elevation myocardial infarction: the CREATE-ECLA randomized controlled trial. JAMA. 2005;293(4):437-46.
44. Sodi-Pallares D, Testelli MR, Fishleder BL, et al. Effects of an intravenous infusion of a potassium-glucose-insulin solution on the electrocardiographic signs of myocardial infarction: a preliminary clinical report. Am J Cardiol. 1962;9:166-81.
45. Yates AR, Dyke PC, Taeed R, et al. Hyperglycemia is a marker for poor outcome in the postoperative pediatric cardiac patient. Pediatr Crit Care Med. 2006;7:351-5.
46. Lecomte P, Foubert L, Coddens J, et al. Management of tight intraoperative glycemic control during off-pump coronary artery bypass surgery in diabetic and nondiabetic patients. J Cardiothorac Vasc Anesth. 2011;25 (6):937-42.
47. Yuan J, Liu T, Zhang X, et al. Intensive versus conventional glycemic control in patients with diabetes during enteral nutrition after gastrectomy. J Gastrointest Surg. 2015;19:1553-8.
48. Umpierrez G, Cardona S, Pasquel F, et al. Randomized controlled trial of intensive versus conservative glucose control in patients

undergoing coronary artery bypass graft surgery: GLUCO-CABG trial. Diabetes Care. 2015;38:1665-72.

49. Kar P, Plummer MP, Bellomo R, et al. Liberal glycemic control in critically ill patients with type 2 diabetes: an exploratory study. Crit Care Med. 2016;44:1695-703.
50. Bellodi G, Manicardi V, Malavasi V, et al. Hyperglycemia and prognosis of acute myocardial infarction in patients without diabetes mellitus. Am J Cardiol. 1989;64:885-8.
51. Ingels C, Debaveye Y, Milants I, et al. Strict blood glucose control with insulin during intensive care after cardiac surgery: impact on 4-years survival, dependency on medical care, and quality-of-life. Eur Heart J. 2006;27(22):2716-24.
52. Moghissi ES, Korytkowski MT, DiNardo M, et al. American Association of Clinical Endocrinologists and American Diabetes Association consensus statement on inpatient glycemic control. Endocr Pract. 2009;15(4):353-69.
53. Khaw KT, Wareham N, Bingham S, et al. Association of hemoglobin A1c with cardiovascular disease and mortality in adults: the European Prospective Investigation into Cancer in Norfolk. Ann Intern Med. 2004;141(6):413-20.

CHAPTER

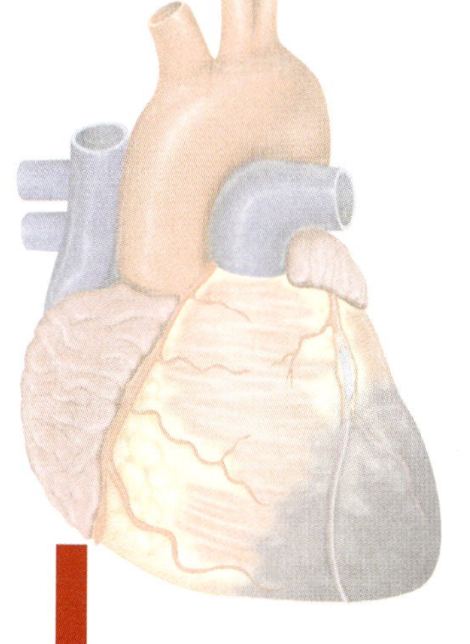

Lixisenatide: A Cardiodiabetes Perspective

Vijay Panikar, Jimit Vadgama, Tejas Kamat

INTRODUCTION

In recent years, glucagon-like peptide-1 receptor agonists (GLP-1RAs) have shown promise as an important therapeutic option in the management of type 2 diabetes mellitus (T2DM). They have multiple and complex glucose and weight-regulating actions, which are due to the combination of enhanced insulin secretion and suppression of glucagon secretion, delayed gastric emptying, and promotion of satiety. Unlike other secretagogues, GLP-1RAs enhance insulin secretion in a glucose dependent manner, hence have low propensity to cause hypoglycemia. Most global guidelines like the American Diabetes Association/European Association for the Study of Diabetes (ADA/EASD) 2017 and American Association of Clinical Endocrinologists (AACE) 2017 for management of T2D recommend GLP-1RAs as an effective at initiation, intensification of oral therapy and in patients failing on basal insulin regimes for intensification.

CLASSIFICATION ON GLUCAGON-LIKE PEPTIDE 1 RECEPTOR AGONISTS[1]

Glucagon-like peptide-1 receptor agonists based on their duration of action are categorized as short-acting and long-acting compounds.

Short-acting compounds, which provide short-lived receptor activation such as exenatide and lixisenatide, primarily lower postprandial blood glucose levels by activating the GLP-1 receptor and also through inhibition of gastric emptying, hence referred to as prandial GLP-1RAs.

Long-acting compounds for example, albiglutide, dulaglutide, exenatide long-acting release, and liraglutide activate the GLP-1 receptor continuously at their recommended dose. They have a stronger effect on fasting glucose levels, which is mediated predominantly through their insulinotropic and glucagonostatic actions, hence referred as nonprandial GLP-1RAs.

However, these two types of GLP-1RAs appear to have similar effects on food intake and body weight.

The availability of these two different types allows for individualized care within the GLP-1RA class. In most patients with poor control who need a second or third antihyperglycemic drug, where the main abnormality is basal hyperglycemia will benefit from long-acting or nonprandial GLP-1RAs.

Patients receiving basal insulin may specially benefit with prandial GLP-1RAs. While basal insulin primarily affects fasting plasma glucose (FPG), a prandial GLP-1RA primarily affects postprandial glucose (PPG). In addition, while basal insulin is associated with modest weight gain, prandial GLP-1RA therapy is associated with weight loss and low risk of hypoglycemia.

LIXISENATIDE: A ONCE DAILY PRANDIAL GLUCAGON-LIKE PEPTIDE 1 RECEPTOR AGONIST ANALOG

Lixisenatide is a synthetic GLP-1RA with a plasma half-life of 1.5–4.5 hours. It is a potent and selective GLP-1RA action and is more resistant to proteolysis by dipeptidyl peptidase-4 (DPP4) than native GLP-1 with a binding affinity that is approximately 4 times greater than human GLP-1 hormone. These factors collectively enable once-a-day dosing of lixisenatide.[2,3]

Global clinical development program included series of randomized and placebo-controlled trials; lixisenatide was evaluated across the spectrum of T2D care as monotherapy, as add-on therapy to metformin, sulfonylureas, or thiazolidinediones, and in combination with basal insulin. Three studies investigated the combined effects of lixisenatide and basal insulin with the rationale that targeting both PPG (with lixisenatide) and FPG and preprandial plasma glucose (with basal insulin) may provide additive effects, leading to enhanced glycemic control. In all of the completed studies, the efficacy of lixisenatide once daily in reducing blood glucose levels with a pronounced effect on PPG has been demonstrated.

Lixisenatide and Markers of Cardiovascular Safety: Weight Change and Glycemic Variability

When combined with basal insulin and metformin or sulfonylurea, lixisenatide 20 µg once daily had a beneficial effect on body weight.

In the GetGoal-L study, patients with T2D with uncontrolled glucose values despite use of a stable dose of basal insulin (with or without a stable dose of metformin more than and equal to 1,500 mg per day) were randomized to receive lixisenatide 20 µg daily or placebo for 24 weeks. There was a mean weight reduction of 1.8 kg, which was significantly more compared to a 0.5 kg weight reduction with placebo ($P < 0.0001$).[4]

In GetGoal-L Asia, there was a mean decrease of 0.38 kg weight with lixisenatide, which was statistically nonsignificant compared with a 0.06 kg weight gain with placebo ($P = 0.09$). In GetGoal-Duo1, patients on lixisenatide experienced a mean increase of 0.28 kg, which was statistically less than the 1.16 kg mean weight gain observed in placebo patients (P 0.0012).[5]

Studies suggest that glycemic variability, particularly with excursions into the hyperglycemic range, rather than chronic sustained hyperglycemia, could have a greater causative role in promoting cardiovascular (CV) complications.

A pooled analysis of patient-level data of 1,198 patients from three 24-week, randomized, phase 3 clinical trials showed that when added to insulin with or without oral agents, lixisenatide significantly reduced glycemic variability and PPG excursions versus placebo, without increased risk of hypoglycemia. This reduction in glycemic variability was primarily associated with a significant reduction in high blood glucose index (HBGI) in the lixisenatide group; glycemic variability fell from an HBGI of 10.63 (representing a high-risk for hyperglycemia) to 6.99 (representing a moderate risk for hyperglycemia). Low blood glucose index (LBGI) was unchanged from baseline to week 24 in both groups (0.41 and 0.44 at baseline and week 24, respectively, in the lixisenatide group; 0.38 and 0.38 at baseline and week 24, respectively, in the placebo group), representing an overall low risk for hypoglycemia. This may have relevance in patients with advanced T2DM where glycemic variability is increased.[6]

Lixisenatide in Elderly Patients[7]

In GetGoal-O study, 350 elderly patients (age more than 70 years, duration of diabetes 13–14 years) with high-risk of hypoglycemia, comorbidities and polypharmacy, lixisenatide has proven to be an effective glycatyed hemoglobin (HbA1c) reduction and in targeting postprandial hyperglycemia, with no unexpected safety findings. The relative contribution of PPG is higher than FPG in older patients; thus, agents such as lixisenatide that preferentially lower postprandial hypoglycemia may be more effective in achieving glycemic goals without increasing the risk of hypoglycemia in these patients.

The First GLP-1RA Cardiovascular Outcomes Study: Evaluation of Lixisenatide in Acute Coronary Syndrome[8]

Evaluation of Lixisenatide in Acute Coronary Syndrome (ELIXA) was a randomized, double-blind, placebo-controlled, parallel-group, and multicenter phase III event-driven trial that assessed the effects of lixisenatide added to standard T2DM therapy on CV morbidity and mortality in patients with a recent acute coronary syndrome (ACS).

The study was designed to demonstrate the CV safety of lixisenatide in accordance with the 2008 US Food and Drug Administration (FDA) guidance for the evaluation of new antidiabetic therapies.

This study included 6,068 patients (317 from India) with T2D who had a myocardial infarction or who had been hospitalized for unstable angina within the previous 180 days to receive lixisenatide or placebo in addition to locally determined standards of care. The trial was designed with 96% and 90% statistical power to assess whether lixisenatide was noninferior as well as superior to placebo respectively, as defined by an upper boundary of the 95% confidence interval for the hazard ratio of less than 1.3 and

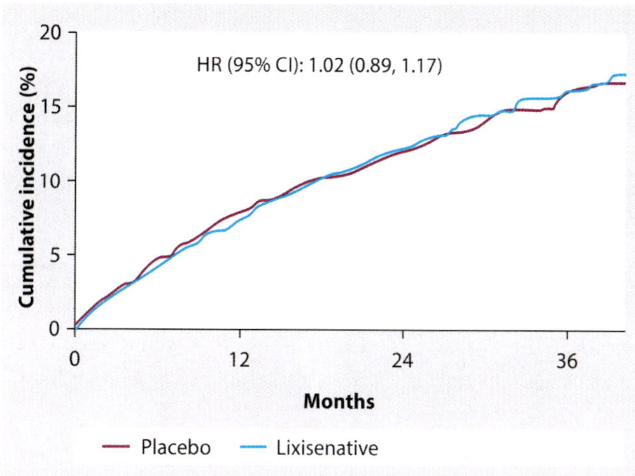

Fig. 1: Primary endpoint-4 point MACE (cardiovascular death, nonfatal myocardial infarction, nonfatal stroke, and hospitalization for unstable angina)

Abbreviations: HR, hazard ratio; CI, confidence interval; MACE, major adverse cardiac events

1.0, respectively, for the primary composite endpoint of CV death, myocardial infarction, stroke, or hospitalization for unstable angina.

The 6,068 patients who underwent randomization were followed for a median of 25 months. A primary endpoint event occurred in 406 patients (13.4%) in the lixisenatide group and in 399 (13.2%) in the placebo group [hazard ratio, 1.02; 95% confidence interval (CI), 0.89–1.17], which showed the noninferiority of lixisenatide to placebo ($P < 0.001$) but did not show superiority ($P = 0.81$) (Fig. 1). There were no significant between group differences in the rate of hospitalization for heart failure (hazard ratio in the lixisenatide group, 0.96; 95% CI, 0.75–1.23) or the rate of death (hazard ratio, 0.94; 95% CI, 0.78–1.13). Lixisenatide was not associated with a higher rate of serious adverse events or severe hypoglycemia, pancreatitis, pancreatic neoplasms, or allergic reactions than was placebo.

In patients with T2D and a recent acute coronary syndrome, the addition of lixisenatide to usual care did not significantly alter the rate of major CV events or other serious adverse events.

CONCLUSION

Lixisenatide is a prandial GLP-1RA that complements basal insulin to provide an ideal basal-prandial approach to glycemic control. ELIXA demonstrated the long-term CV safety of lixisenatide. Over a period of 3.1 years, lixisenatide as compared to placebo decreased the worsening of albuminuria, lowered HbA1c, lowered body weight and did not increase the risk of severe hypoglycemia, pancreatitis, or pancreatic cancer.

REFERENCES

1. Fineman MS, Cirincione BB, Maggs D, et al. GLP-1 based therapies: differential effects on fasting and postprandial glucose. Diabetes Obes Metab. 2012;14(8):675-88.
2. Barnett AH. Lixisenatide: evidence for its potential use in the treatment of type 2 diabetes. Core Evid. 2011;6:67-79.
3. Christensen M, Knop FK, Holst JJ, et al. Lixisenatide, a novel GLP-1 receptor agonist for the treatment of type 2 diabetes mellitus. IDrugs. 2009;12(8):503-13.
4. Clinical Trials.gov. (2016). GLP-1 receptor agonist lixisenatide in patients with type 2 diabetes for glycemic control and safety evaluation, on top of basal insulin (GETGOAL-L). [online] available from http://www.clinicaltrials.gov/ct2/show/NCT00715624?term=lixisenatide&rank=17 [Accessed October, 2017].
5. Seino Y, Min KW, Niemoeller E, et al. Randomized, double-blind, placebo-controlled trial of the once-daily GLP-1 receptor agonist lixisenatide in Asian patients with type 2 diabetes insufficiently controlled on basal insulin with or without a sulfonylurea (GetGoal-L-Asia). Diab Obesity Metab. 2012;14(10):910-7.
6. Umpieacrrez GE, O'Neal D, DiGenio A, et al. Lixisenatide reduces glycemic variability in insulin-treated patients with type 2diabetes. Diabetes Obes Metab. 2017;19(9):1317-21.
7. Meneilly GS, Roy-Duval C, Alawi H, et al. Lixisenatide Therapy in older patients with type 2 diabetes inadequately controlled on their current antidiabetic treatment: The GetGoal-O randomized Trial. Diabetes Care. 2017;40(4):485-93.
8. Pfeffer MA et al. Lixisenatide in patients with type 2 diabetes and acute coronary syndrome. NEJM. 2015;373:2247-57.

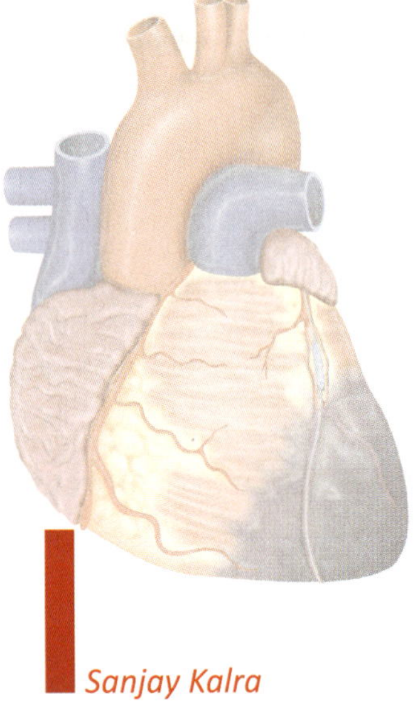

SGLT2-i Agents and Cardiovascular Diabetology

Sanjay Kalra

INTRODUCTION

The burden of cardiovascular disease (CVD), in the background of type-2 diabetes mellitus (T2DM), is well recognized. Subclinical CVD is evident in atleast two out of every three patients of diabetes.[1] CVD manifests as rapidly developing atherosclerosis and heart failure in patients of T2DM, accounting for majority of the deaths in these patients.[2] However, contrary to logical understanding, a good control of glycemia has failed to demonstrate consistent improvement in macrovascular outcomes of T2DM.[3,4] In fact, the pathogenesis of T2DM is closely associated with CVD; hence, any therapeutic target for T2DM, may possibly influence the vascular pathology as well. In the past, antidiabetic drugs like tolbutamide and rosiglitazone have demonstrated worsening of the cardiovascular (CV) outcomes. Hence, it is compulsory for any new glucose-lowering agent to conclusively prove a safe CV profile for clinical use.[5] The CV safety of an antidiabetic preparation is generally assessed through a dedicated cardiovascular outcome trial (CVOT). With the well-designed CVOTs, it may be possible to also identify if CV protection is afforded by the medicine under evaluation. In September 2015, the CVOT 'Empa-Reg outcome' demonstrated a clear evidence of CV protection with the antidiabetic medicine empagliflozin.[6] This was the first time when any therapy for T2DM had conclusively demonstrated CV protection, over and above the existing cardioprotective therapies. With this landmark result demonstrated by the selective sodium–glucose cotransporter type-2 (SGLT2) inhibitor empagliflozin, our understanding of the pathological nexus between CVD and T2DM, and the clinical implications for such therapeutic approach, have tremendously progressed.

SODIUM-GLUCOSE COTRANSPORTER TYPE-2 INHIBITORS

The SGLT2 inhibitors represent a class of antidiabetic agents that facilitates elimination of glucose through the urine. These agents selectively inhibit the SGLT2. The SGLT2 transporter is located specifically in the proximal convoluted tubules of the kidneys and facilitates the reabsorption of glucose from the ultrafiltrate. In T2DM, the activity of SGLT2 transporter is upregulated, resulting in increased tubular reabsorption of glucose. An inhibitor of the SGLT2 transporter by preventing the reabsorption of glucose results in lowering of the blood glucose levels. The specific role of the different SGLT transporters is described in Table 1.[7-9]

Clinically, the SGLT2 transporter plays a more important role in the renal reabsorption of glucose. Sodium–glucose cotransporter type-1 (SGLT1) transporter is present more ubiquitously in the body, having a predominant role in the gut, skeletal, and cardiac muscle cells. SGLT1 transporter also has a minor role in the kidneys, accounting for a small fraction of glucose reabsorption. The first SGLT-inhibitor "phlorizin", was derived from the bark of apple tree in the year 1835. Phlorizin had a nonselective blocking action on the SGLT1 and SGLT2 transporters. The potential antidiabetic effects of phlorizin, in reducing the blood glucose levels and improving insulin sensitivity, were

TABLE 1: Sodium-glucose cotransporter (SGLT) transporters

SGLT-1 transporter	*SGLT-2 transporter*
Main uptake mechanism for glucose and galactose in the intestine	Maximally expressed in the brush-border membrane of proximal renal tubular cells
S2 and S3 segments of the proximal renal tubule are responsible for ≈10% of the total renal glucose reabsorption	S1 and S2 segments of proximal renal tubule are responsible for ≈90% of the total renal glucose reabsorption
High-affinity, low-capacity transporter that transfers Na^+ and glucose in a ratio of 2:1	Low-affinity, high-capacity transporter that transfers Na^+ and glucose in a ratio of 1:1

TABLE 2: Currently available sodium-glucose cotransporter 2 inhibitors

	Empagliflozin	*Dapagliflozin*	*Canagliflozin*
SGLT2: SGLT1 selectivity[@]	>2,500[14]	>1,200[14]	>250[14]
Nonspecific* tissue distribution	Lowest[15]	Intermediate[15]	Highest[15]
Risk of hyperkalemia	No imbalance[$16]	No imbalance[$17]	↑ in moderate renal impairment[$18]
Risk of bone fractures	No imbalance[11,16]	No imbalance[12,17]	Increased risk[13,18]
Risk of malignancy	No imbalance[11,16]	Imbalance for bladder cancer[#12,17]	No imbalance[13,18]
Cardiovascular outcome trial	CV Protection (Empa-Reg outcome)[6]	Study ongoing (declare-TIMI 58)[19]	Study ongoing (CANVAS program)[20]
Risk of leg and foot amputations	No imbalance[11,16]	No imbalance[12,17]	≈2-fold ↑ in risk with canagliflozin[21] (both doses)

Abbreviations: SGLT2: sodium-glucose cotransporter type-2; SGLT1, sodium-glucose cotransporter type 1; CV, cardiovascular; DECLARE, dapagliflozin effect on cardiovascular event; TIMI, thrombolysis in myocardial infarction; CANVAS, canagliflozin cardiovascular assessment study

@The clinical relevance of SGLT transporter selectivity is incompletely understood at present.

*Nonspecific: organs other than target organ (kidney), or the organs of absorption and elimination (gut and liver). This is an extrapolation from the observed preclinical data, based on the respective maximum concentration (C_{max}) and area under the curve (AUC) values observed at clinically used doses of the 3 agents.

$In case of conditions that may lead to fluid loss, careful monitoring of volume status, and electrolytes is recommended.

#An imbalance in bladder cancers was observed in clinical trials. Dapagliflozin should not be used in patients with active bladder cancer and should be used with caution in patients with a prior history of bladder cancer.

characterized in the late 1980s. However, phlorizin could not be developed as a clinically viable medicine because of various reasons, including its nonselectivity for the SGLT transporters. The blockade of SGLT1 transporter in the gut resulted in multiple gastrointestinal adverse reactions, including diarrhea, malabsorption, and dehydration. As the SGLT2 transporter has a more specific action on the kidneys, the selective inhibition of SGLT2 has a clinical relevance in T2DM.[10]

At present, three such selective SGLT2-i agents are available in the Indian market including canagliflozin, dapagliflozin, and empagliflozin. These agents facilitate elimination of nearly 60–80 g of glucose per day, in patients of T2DM. The extent of glucose elimination is proportionate to the blood-glucose levels. All these agents are approved for the management of T2DM, whereas empagliflozin is additionally approved by the US Food and Drug Administration (USFDA) and European Medicines Agency (EMA), for the prevention of CV death in patients of T2DM with CVD.[11-13] The characteristics of the available SGLT2 inhibitors are summarized in Table 2.

SODIUM-GLUCOSE COTRANSPORTER TYPE 2 INHIBITION AND CARDIOVASCULAR MECHANISMS

The glycosuria is mediated by a selective SGLT2 inhibitor, results in multiple hemodynamic and metabolic effects in the body (Fig. 1). As an acute outcome, a transient natriuresis is evident for a few days, along with glucose-mediated osmotic diuresis. This effect results in 1–2 extra voids (350 mL urine) per day, for a few initial days. However, unlike diuretics, the SGLT2-i agents result in a modest amount of hemoconcentration, which persists throughout the course of SGLT2-i therapy.[22] These agents have generally not demonstrated significant increases in plasma renin activity or serum aldosterone levels, except in conditions of dehydration or concomitant diuretic use.[23,24] These agents also do not increase the sympathetic activity. The resting heart rate does not get altered over long-term empagliflozin therapy, in the Empa-Reg outcome study.[6] As a result of clearance of glucotoxicity, the vascular oxidative stress is decreased; this may be a key contributor to the improvement in arterial stiffness[25] within the kidneys, an improved sodium delivery to the distal tubule results in normalization of the tubulo-glomerular feedback (TGF) mechanism. This effect reduces the intraglomerular pressure, thus preserving the renal function in long-term.[26]

A modest reduction in systolic and diastolic blood pressure is consistently evident with the SGLT2-i agents. In fact, some difficult cases of hypertension in T2DM, maybe clinically benefited with an SGLT2-i based therapy.[27] Resistant hypertension often results from ineffective diuresis. In patients of T2DM, multiple mechanisms like hyperinsulinemia, and hyperactivity of the SGLT2 transporter could facilitate ineffective diuresis.

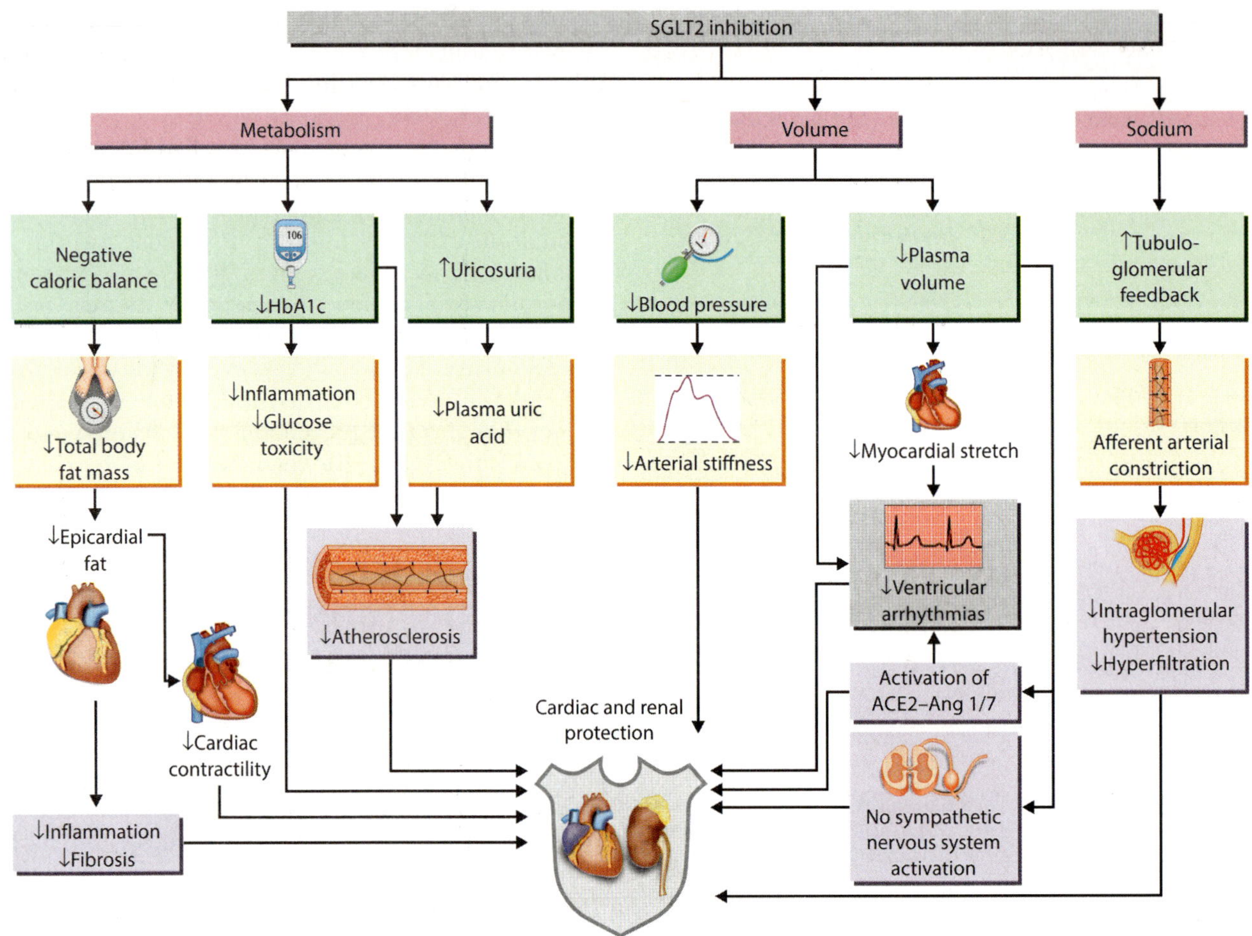

Fig. 1: SGLT2 inhibition and resultant cardiovascular effects

Abbreviations: SGLT2, sodium-glucose cotransporter type-2; HbA1C, glycated hemoglobin; ACE2, angiotensin-converting enzyme 2

Patients of T2DM classically have hyperinsulinemia, secondary to insulin resistance. Insulin possesses a strong fluid and sodium-retaining property. SGLT2-i therapy lowers the plasma insulin concentration as a consequence of reduction in blood glucose level, and improvement in peripheral insulin sensitivity. This partial reversal of hyperinsulinemia in T2DM could benefit the complex pathologies of hypertension in these patients.

Apart from this mechanism, the patients of T2DM also demonstrate an increased activity of SGLT2 transporters in proximal tubule, resulting in increased sodium reabsorption. This could be a contributory mechanism to ineffective diuresis. The kidneys adapt through a TGF mechanism, resulting in the dilatation of afferent glomerular arterioles. This leads to increased inflow within the glomeruli, raising the intraglomerular pressure, and resulting in hyperfiltration. Chronically raised intraglomerular pressure contributes to the progression of diabetic kidney disease. The SGLT2-i agents directly counter this mechanism in the proximal tubules, leading to normalization of the TGF, and facilitation of a more effective diuresis process.

The metabolic adaptive changes following glucose elimination result in weight loss, consequent to persistent calorie deficit. The weight loss plateaus over 4–6 months of therapy, as a new metabolic equilibrium is gradually achieved. The free fatty acids released from the adipose tissue are metabolized to ketone bodies within the liver, in a glucagon-dominated milieu. This effect results in mild ketosis. These metabolic changes may be beneficial for diabetic cardiomyopathy, a condition characterized by cardiac lipotoxicity and inefficient myocardial metabolism which manifests as an accelerated pump failure. Ketone bodies are efficient substrates which may be utilized by the myocardium, resulting in improved myocardial metabolism. This 'thrifty-substrate' hypothesis suggests an improved metabolic efficiency in various organ-systems, as a result of SGLT2-i therapy (Fig. 2).[28,29]

The combination of all these hemodynamic and metabolic effects, leads to reductions in preload, in

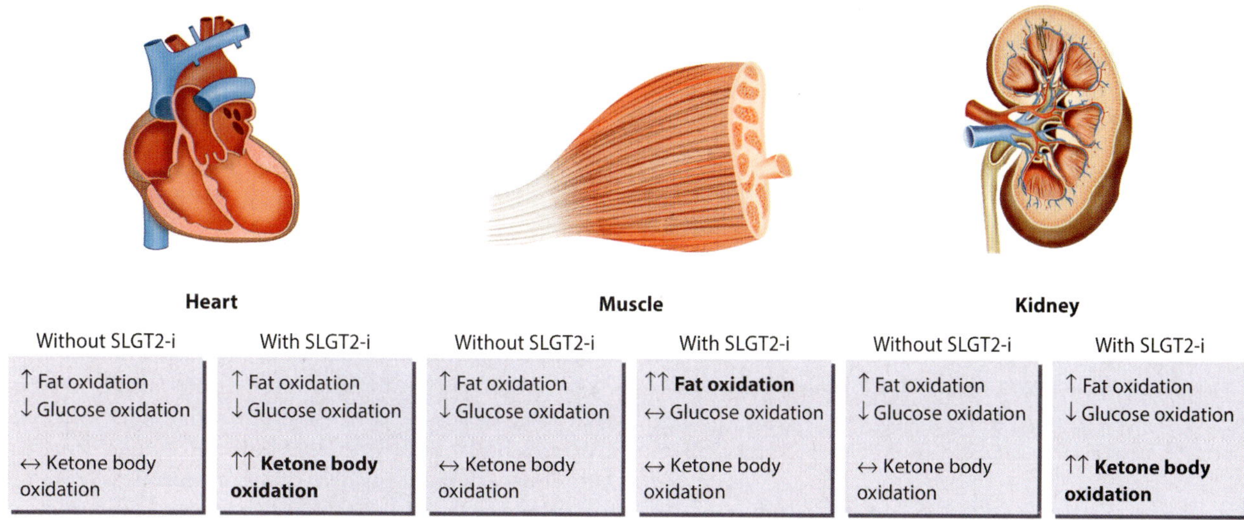

Fig. 2: SGLT2-inhibitors and fuel energetics: thrifty-substrate hypothesis[28,29]

Abbreviation: SGLT2, sodium-glucose cotransporter type-2

afterload, and a possible improvement in myocardial metabolism. Consequent to the reduction in hemodynamic workload on the heart, in a milieu supporting improved metabolic efficiency, the pathophysiology of diabetic cardiomyopathy may be favorably influenced. Apart from these effects, SGLT2-i based therapy results in clinically relevant reductions in serum uric acid levels. Empagliflozin has also demonstrated a direct effect on the myocardium in preclinical studies, resulting in improvement in the mitochondrial calcium homeostasis.[30]

EMPAGLIFLOZIN AND CV OUTCOMES: EVIDENCE AND CLINICAL INFERENCE

In the patients of T2DM with CVD, empagliflozin therapy demonstrated a 14% reduction in major adverse CV events, as compared to placebo.[6] This incremental CV benefit with empagliflozin, was evident on the top of optimum cardioprotective therapies in the background (including the blockers of renin-angiotensin system, antiplatelet agents, statins, antihypertensive, and antidiabetic medications). The overall CV benefit was driven by a 38% reduction in CV mortality with empagliflozin, as compared to placebo. In patients who received empagliflozin, the hospitalizations for heart failure reduced by 35%, and the incidence or worsening of nephropathy reduced by 39%, as compared to placebo.[31] These effects resulted in an overall mortality benefit of 32%, as compared to placebo. All these CV outcomes were statistically significant, and suggestive of a much desirable clinical benefit of empagliflozin in patients with T2DM and CVD.

The clinical inferences of these study results are highly promising. In patients of CVD who have T2DM, the currently available cardioprotective therapies are insufficient to address the residual CV risk. In such patients, prevention of one additional death is possible by treating 39 such patients with empagliflozin over 3.1 years. More importantly, treating only 21 patients having heart failure burden, with empagliflozin over 3.1 years, will prevent one additional CV death.[32] To draw an analogy, in the PARADIGM-HF trial, 32 patients had to be treated with sacubitril-valsartan over 2.2 years to prevent one additional CV death.[33] These trials are different in their principle context, and their outcomes cannot be compared directly. However, the analogy reflects the clinical relevance of empagliflozin in patients with CVD and T2DM, beyond the existing armamentarium of cardioprotective therapies. Based on the available evidence, the European Society of Cardiology guidelines for the management heart failure (2016), recommend the use of empagliflozin in patients with T2DM, for preventing or delaying the onset of heart failure, or prolonging life (Class IIa, Level B recommendation).[34]

Practical inferences of study-evidence are also reasonably drawn from Bayesian statistical analysis. Bayesian analysis marry the new study results, with the historical evidence supporting such outcomes, to derive a clinical interpretation of the data. This analysis of Empa-Reg outcome study suggested a high likelihood of atleast 15% reduction in CV mortality, if empagliflozin is added to the existing therapies, in patients of CVD and T2DM.[35]

SAFETY CONSIDERATIONS

The SGLT2 inhibitors are associated with pertinent safety aspects, necessitating clinical consideration. Many of these aspects are pertinent to the patient's

BOX 1: Considerations associated with sodium-glucose cotransporter 2 inhibitors (SGLT2-i) agents

Prohibit use of SGLT2-i therapy, in:
- Moderate to severe CKD (eGFR <45mL/min/1.73 m^2
- Pregnant and breastfeeding women: Risk not known
- Acute stressful states (severe medical/surgical considerations)

Observe caution in:
- Risk of volume depletion (frail elderly, concomitant loop diuretics, and predisposition to dehydration/renal impairment)
- Complicated UTIs: Temporary discontinuation recommended
- History of recurrent UTIs: Risk of UTIs
- Conditions of fasting: Risk of starvation and precipitation of eu-DKA
- Existing elevation in hematocrit
- Predisposition to amputations of lower limb (specifically canagliflozin)

Abbreviation: SGLT2, sodium-glucose cotransporter type-2; CKD, chronic kidney disease; eGFR, estimated glomerular filtration rate; UTI, urinary tract infection; eu-DKA, euglycemic diabetic ketoacidosis.

phenotype, necessitating appropriate patient selection for these medicines. The aspects are briefly summarized in Box 1.[36,37]

These medicines may increase the risk of genital fungal infections (observed in around 5–10% of the patients). Urinary tract infections (UTIs) are not specifically increased, unless the patient has a history of recurrent UTIs. Volume-depletion related adverse events may be possible, in patients who cannot tolerate lowering of blood volume (hypotensive patients, frail elderly patients, concomitant use of loop diuretics, or states of dehydration). In acute stressful conditions (severe medical or surgical stress, excessive alcoholism, fasting, or dehydration), these agents may facilitate development of diabetic ketoacidosis. Hence, these agents should be avoided during such conditions. The use of SGLT2-i agents should be discontinued about 2–3 days prior to any planned events like surgical procedures, or radiocontrast studies. In patients having an elevated hematocrit due to any background comorbidity, the use of SGLT2-i agents may be avoided. Some adverse reactions, including an increased risk of bone fractures and lower-limb amputations, have been specifically evident with canagliflozin.

The use of SGLT2-i agents may result in an initial rise in the serum creatinine levels (similar to the renin-angiotensin inhibitors), due to a hemodynamic adaptation in the nephrons. This is a protective mechanism, secondary to the lowering of intraglomerular pressure. However, the risk of acute renal impairment should be considered, if these agents are concomitantly used with other nephrotoxic agents, or in a state of dehydration. A modest increase in the serum levels of low-density lipoprotein-cholesterol (LDL-C) and high-density lipoprotein-cholesterol (HDL-C) are also observed with SGLT2-i agents, which are partly explained by hemoconcentration. The ratio of LDL-C to HDL-C does not get altered, and the clinical significance of this effect is not known.

These agents do have an insulin-sparing effect; however, the SGLT2-i agents should not be used as substitutes for insulin. In a patient receiving insulin, the addition of an SGLT2-i agent should prompt a gradual down-titration of insulin, rather than a drastic reduction or stopping of insulin.

CONCLUSION

Sodium-glucose cotransporter type 2 inhibitors are an important class of drugs, which help to reduce glucose as well as CV risk. Use of these drugs in persons with type 2 diabetes helps improve CV health and reduce mortality. One must ensure, however, that contraindications to use are ruled out, and that proper monitoring is ensured.

REFERENCES

1. Ingelsson E, Sullivan LM, Murabito JM, et al. Prevalence and prognostic impact of subclinical cardiovascular disease in individuals with the metabolic syndrome and diabetes. Diabetes. 2007;56(6):1718-26.
2. Low Wang CC, Hess CN, Hiatt WR, et al. Clinical Update: Cardiovascular Disease in Diabetes Mellitus: Atherosclerotic Cardiovascular Disease and Heart Failure in Type 2 Diabetes Mellitus-Mechanisms, Management, and Clinical Considerations. Circulation. 2016;133(24):2459-502.
3. Control G, Turnbull FM, Abraira C, et al. Intensive glucose control and macrovascular outcomes in type 2 diabetes. Diabetologia. 2009;52(11):2288-98.
4. Bergenstal RM, Bailey CJ, Kendall DM. Type 2 diabetes: assessing the relative risks and benefits of glucose-lowering medications. Am J Med. 2010;123(4):374.e9-18.
5. CDER. (2008). Diabetes Mellitus-Evaluating Cardiovascular Risk in New Antidiabetic Therapies to Treat Type 2 Diabetes (Guidance for Industry). [online]. Available from: http://www.fda.gov/Downloads/Drugs/Guidancecomplianceregulatoryinformation/Guidances/Ucm071627.pdf. [Accessed September, 2017].
6. Zinman B, Wanner C, Lachin JM, et al. Empagliflozin, Cardiovascular Outcomes, and Mortality in Type 2 Diabetes. N Engl J Med. 2015;373(22):2117-28.
7. Chao EC, Henry RR. SGLT2 inhibition--a novel strategy for diabetes treatment. Nat Rev Drug Discov. 2010;9(7):551-9.
8. Mather A, Pollock C. Glucose handling by the kidney. Kidney Int Suppl. 2011;120:S1-6.
9. Wright EM, Hirayama BA, Loo DF. Active sugar transport in health and disease. J Intern Med. 2007;261(1):32-43.
10. Rosenwasser RF, Sultan S, Sutton D, et al. SGLT-2 inhibitors and their potential in the treatment of diabetes. Diabetes Metab Syndr Obes. 2013;6:453-67.
11. USFDA. (2014). Jardiance: Prescribing information (Ingelheim B). [online] Available from: https://www.accessdata.fda.gov/drugsatfda_docs/label/2016/204629s008lbl.pdf. [Accessed September, 2017].
12. USFDA. (2014). Farxiga: prescribing information (AstraZeneca). [online] Available from: https://www.accessdata.fda.gov/drugsatfda_docs/label/2014/202293s003lbl.pdf. [Accessed September, 2017].

13. USFDA (2013). Invokana: prescribing information (Janssen). [online] Available from: http://www.accessdata.fda.gov/drugsatfda_docs/label/2013/204042s000lbl.pdf. [Accessed September, 2017].
14. Grempler R, Thomas L, Eckhardt M, et al. Empagliflozin, a novel selective sodium glucose cotransporter-2 (SGLT-2) inhibitor: characterisation and comparison with other SGLT-2 inhibitors. Diabetes Obes Metab. 2012;14(1):83-90.
15. Liebig S, Martin HJ, Mark M, et al. 52nd annual conference of EASD, Sep 2016. Munich, Germany. 2016.
16. EMA. Jardiance: Summary of Product Characteristics (Ingelheim B). [online] Available from: http://www.ema.europa.eu/docs/en_GB/document_library/EPAR-Product_Information/human/002677/WC500168592.pdf. [Accessed September, 2017].
17. EMA. Forxiga: summary of Product Characteristics (AstraZeneca). [online] Available from: http://www.ema.europa.eu/docs/en_GB/document_library/Referrals_document/SGLT2_inhibitors__20/European_Commission_final_decision/WC500206510.pdf. [Accessed September, 2017].
18. EMA. Invokana: summary of Product Characteristics (Janssen). [online] Available from: http://www.ema.europa.eu/docs/en_GB/document_library/EPAR_-_Product_Information/human/002649/WC500156456.pdf. [Accessed September, 2017].
19. ClinicalTrials. Multicenter Trial to Evaluate the Effect of Dapagliflozin on the Incidence of Cardiovascular Events (DECLARE-TIMI58). [online] Available from: https://clinicaltrials.gov/ct2/show/NCT01730534?term=DECLARE+TIMI&rank=1. [Accessed September, 2017].
20. Clinicaltrials. CANVAS-CANagliflozin cardioVascular Assessment Study (CANVAS). [online] Available from: https://clinicaltrials.gov/ct2/show/NCT01032629?term=CANVAS&rank=1. [Accessed September, 2017].
21. USFDA-Drug Safety Communication (2016). FDA confirms increased risk of leg and foot amputations with the diabetes medicine canagliflozin (Invokana, Invokamet, and Invokamet XR). [online] Available from: https://www.fda.gov/downloads/Drugs/DrugSafety/UCM558427.pdf. [Accessed September, 2017].
22. Inzucchi S (2016). SGLT2 inhibition and cardiovascular outcomes. Oral Presentation #S33.1. Presented at 52nd annual meeting of EASD. Munich. [online] Available from: http://www.easdvirtualmeeting.org/resources/sglt2-inhibition-and-cardiovascular-outcomes. [Accessed September, 2017].
23. Heise T, Jordan J, Wanner C et al. Pharmacodynamic Effects of Single and Multiple Doses of Empagliflozin in Patients with Type 2 Diabetes. Clin Ther. 2016;38(10):2265-76.
24. Lambers Heerspink HJ, de Zeeuw D, Wie L, et al. Dapagliflozin a glucose-regulating drug with diuretic properties in subjects with type 2 diabetes. Diabetes Obes Metab. 2013;15(9):853-62.
25. Chilton R, Tikkanen I, Cannon CP, et al. Effects of empagliflozin on blood pressure and markers of arterial stiffness and vascular resistance in patients with type 2 diabetes. Diabetes Obes Metab. 2015;17(12):1180-93.
26. van Bommel EJ, Muskiet MH, Tonneijck L, et al. SGLT2 Inhibition in the diabetic kidney-from mechanisms to clinical outcome. Clin J Am Soc Nephrol. 2017;12(4):700-10.
27. Obeid A, Pucci M, Martin U, et al. Sodium glucose co-transporter 2 inhibitors in patients with resistant hypertension: a case study. JRSM Open. 2016;7(9):2054270416649285.
28. Ferrannini E, Mark M, Mayoux E. CV Protection in the EMPA-REG OUTCOME Trial: A "Thrifty Substrate" Hypothesis. Diabetes Care. 2016;39(7):1108-14.
29. Mudaliar S, Alloju S, Henry RR. Can a shift in fuel energetics explain the beneficial cardiorenal outcomes in the EMPA-REG OUTCOME study? A unifying hypothesis. Diabetes Care. 2016;39(7):1115-22.
30. Vettor R, Inzucchi SE, Fioretto P. The cardiovascular benefits of empagliflozin: SGLT2-dependent and -independent effects. Diabetologia. 2017;60(3):395-8.
31. Wanner C, Inzucchi SE, Lachin JM, et al. Empagliflozin and progression of kidney disease in type 2 diabetes. N Engl J Med. 2016;375(4):323-34.
32. Fitchett D, Zinman B, Lachin JM, et al. Effects of empagliflozin on cardiovascular mortality by prevalent or incident heart failure in the Empa-Reg Outcome trial. Can J Cardiol. 2016;32(Suppl 1):s90-1.
33. McMurray JJ, Packer M, Desai AS, et al. Angiotensin-neprilysin inhibition versus enalapril in heart failure. N Engl J Med. 2014;371(11):993-1004.
34. Ponikowski P, Voors AA, Anker SD, et al. 2016 ESC Guidelines for the diagnosis and treatment of acute and chronic heart failure: The Task Force for the diagnosis and treatment of acute and chronic heart failure of the European Society of Cardiology (ESC). Developed with the special contribution of the Heart Failure Association (HFA) of the ESC. Eur J Heart Fail. 2016;18(8):891-975.
35. Kaul S. Is the mortality benefit with empagliflozin in type 2 diabetes mellitus too good to be true. Circulation 2016;134(2):94-6.
36. Rajput R, Ved J. SGLT2-inhibitors in type-2 diabetes: the remaining questions! Diabetes Metab Syndr. 2017;pii:S1871-4021(17)30016-4.
37. Kalra S, Ghosh S, Aamir AH, et al. Safe and pragmatic use of sodium-glucose co-transporter 2 inhibitors in type 2 diabetes mellitus: South Asian Federation of Endocrine Societies consensus statement. Indian J Endocrinol Metab. 2017;21(1):210-30.

CHAPTER

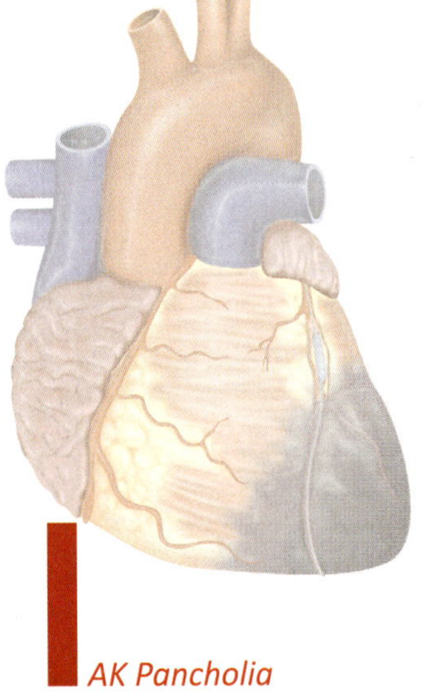

SGLT2-i for the Reduction of Cardiovascular Events in High-risk Patients with Diabetes Mellitus

AK Pancholia

INTRODUCTION

Type 2 diabetes mellitus (T2DM) is associated with a substantially increased cardiovascular (CV) risk,[1,2] and several international guidelines statements addressing the management of T2DM[3,4] underscore the need to prevent and reduce CV complications. Although, it is conceivable that glycemic control plays an important role in this process, as suggested by epidemiological studies, there remains great controversy concerning the impact of glucose lowering on CV outcomes from intensive glycemic control trials.[5] Thus, and in light of the multiple CV risk factors beyond hyperglycemia that exist in most patients with T2DM, a multifactorial approach to addressing CV risk has been emphasized. This includes, in addition to glucose lowering, the control of blood pressure (BP) and lipids, weight management, smoking cessation and, when indicated, antiplatelet therapy.[3,4] Despite these recommendations, it is known to be difficult for most patients in clinical practice to reach their therapeutic goals. Explanations include prevailing patient factors and clinician factors superimposed upon the progressive nature of the disease, as well as the inherent limitations of our current pharmaceutical armamentarium. In light of the multifaceted pathogenesis of CV disease in diabetes, it would be viewed as an advantage if a specific intervention could attenuate atherosclerosis risk in a multidimensional fashion, and beyond glycemic control alone.

The CV safety of antidiabetic medications has become an acute area of concern. Rosiglitazone, sulfonylureas, and insulin are three traditional antidiabetic medications that have been associated with increased risk of CV events in patients with T2DM.[6] In 2008, the US Food and Drug Administration (FDA) mandated all new antidiabetic medications to provide evidence that they do not increase risk of CV diseases.[7,8]

However, to date, the potential effects of specific glucose-lowering agents, that is, sulfonylurea (SU), glinides, metformin, thiazolidinediones, insulin, and glucagon-like peptide-1 receptor analogues or dipeptidyl-peptidase-4 (DPP-4) inhibitors, on CV events in patients with T2DM remain uncertain.[9] This was recently illustrated with the neutral effect for the composite CV death, myocardial infarction (MI) or stroke from the first-two placebo-controlled trials involving the DPP-4 inhibitors saxagliptin (i.e. saxagliptin assessment of vascular outcomes recorded in patients with diabetes mellitus–thrombolysis in myocardial infarction 53 [SAVOR-TIMI53])[10] and alogliptin (i.e. examination of cardiovascular outcomes with alogliptin versus standard of care [EXAMINE]),[11] a class associated with beneficial effects on several factors and biological processes linked to atherogenesis in mechanistic and preclinical studies.[12] It should be noted that both SAVOR-TIMI 53 and EXAMINE were relatively short in duration (median follow-up 2.2 and 1.5 years, respectively) and included patients predominantly, or exclusively, with overt CV disease. A sufficient duration of treatment might be important since macrovascular (as well as microvascular) disease may be a relatively late complication of a complex and progressive pathogenic process that spans years.[13] In addition, in T2DM patients with established CV complications, who are often targeted by these studies, it may be more difficult to further reduce the residual CV risk beyond that which standard of care can offer.[14] However, the CV safety profile of sodium-glucose cotransporter type-2 (SGLT2) inhibitors and information related to CV outcomes [e.g. MI, stroke, cardiac death, heart failure (HF), and arrhythmia] is currently under investigation. In addition, study quality and risks of bias were rarely considered in previous papers that have assessed the CV risks associated with SGLT2 inhibitors. Therefore, the objective of this review was to provide a comprehensive summary and critical analysis of the available literature pertaining to CV safety (MI, stroke, angina, and CV-related death) of SGLT2 inhibitors in patients with T2DM.

ROLE OF THE KIDNEY IN GLUCOSE METABOLISM

Through its contribution to gluconeogenesis and its capacity to reabsorb glucose from the urine, the kidney plays an important role in glucose homeostasis. In humans without diabetes, ~160–180 g of glucose are filtered by the kidneys per day[15] and in healthy individuals without diabetes, virtually all filtered glucose is reabsorbed in the proximal tubule. As long as the filtered glucose does not exceed the maximum renal glucose reabsorption capacity, filtered glucose is reabsorbed thus allowing energy conservation.[16] About 90% of glucose filtered in the glomeruli is reabsorbed in the first segment of the proximal tubule by SGLT2, which is a low-affinity, high-capacity transporter.[17] The remaining 10% is reabsorbed in the more distal part of the tubule by sodium-glucose cotransporter type-1 (SGLT1), a high-affinity, low-capacity transporter (Fig. 1).[18,19] Sodium glucose cotransporter proteins are proteins localized in the apical membrane capable of actively transporting glucose along with sodium against a concentration gradient into the cell. This process is driven by the active transport of sodium out of the cell by the adenosine triphosphate-dependent sodium-potassium pump. Once in the intracellular space, glucose then passively diffuses from the basolateral membrane of the tubule cell into the blood via glucose transporter 2 (GLUT2), a member of the GLUT family of proteins[20] (Fig. 2). However, if the blood glucose load exceeds the renal tubular glucose excretion threshold of ~180 mg/dL, glucosuria occurs. In patients with diabetes and chronic hyperglycemia, the threshold paradoxically increases to ~220 mg/dL due to an enhanced maximum renal glucose reabsorption capacity mediated by up-regulation of SGLT2 in the proximal tubule. This maladaptive mechanism seems to be explained by increased SGLT2 transcription and translation resulting in increased SGLT2 density on the apical membrane in the proximal tubule.[17,19]

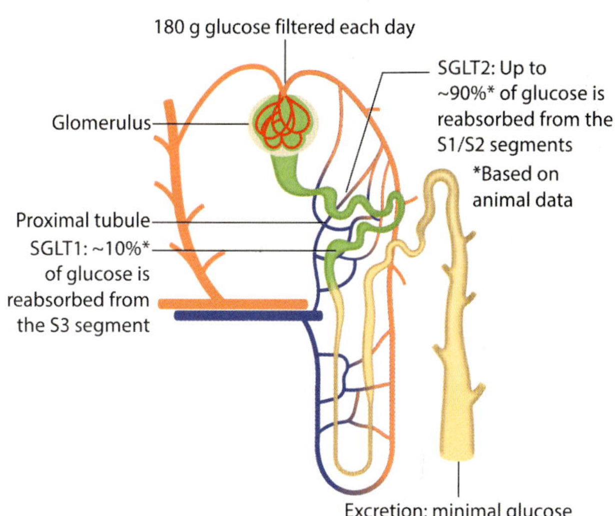

Fig. 1: Renal glucose handling

Abbreviation: SGLT, sodium-glucose cotransporter type

SODIUM-GLUCOSE COTRANSPORTER-2 INHIBITORS MODE OF ACTION AND GLUCOSE-LOWERING PROPERTIES (EHJ)

Sodium-glucose cotransporter-2 inhibitors are a novel class of glucose-lowering drugs that act in the kidney by inhibiting SGLT2-mediated glucose reabsorption in the proximal tubule. The resulting increase in urinary glucose excretion leads to a reduction in plasma glucose levels (Fig. 2).[21-23] The concept of SGLT2 inhibition is different from other glucose-lowering strategies since glucose is removed from the 'system', thus reducing total-body and cellular glucose toxicity, a mechanism that is completely independent of insulin. Overall, 24-hour urinary glucose excretion in patients treated with SGLT2 inhibitors lies between 60 and 100 g/day, corresponding to a loss of 240–400 kcal/day upon chronic administration.[24] In addition to their glucosuric effects, SGLT2 inhibitors lead—at least temporarily—to an increase in sodium excretion,[25] as well as a reduction in plasma volume due to glucose osmotic diuretic effects and natriuresis.[26] Currently, three SGLT2 inhibitors are approved in Europe and the USA: dapagliflozin, canagliflozin, and empagliflozin.[27] Meta-analyses for these SGLT2 inhibitors suggest that they lower glycated hemoglobin (HbA1c) levels between 0.7 and 0.8% relative to placebo.[28] SGLT2 inhibitor effects are glucose-dependent, thus leading to a very low-risk of hypoglycemia. In addition, SGLT2 inhibitors can be combined with any other antihyperglycemic medication since the mechanism of action is different from all other agents presently available and is completely independent of insulin.[29] Interestingly,

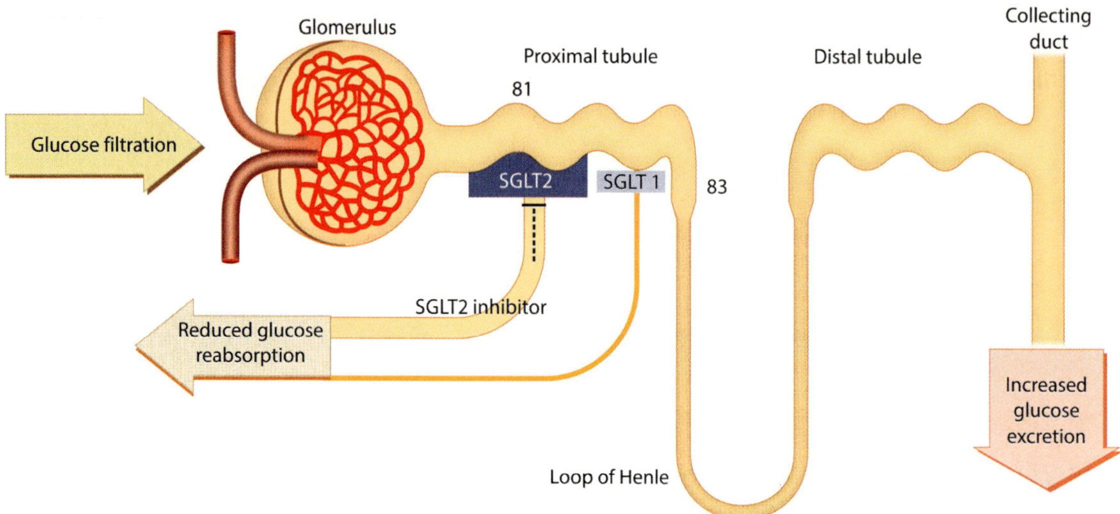

Fig. 2: Reduction of renal glucose reabsorption by SGLT2 inhibition

Abbreviation: SGLT, sodium-glucose cotransporter type

various studies suggest that SGLT2 inhibitors may improve insulin sensitivity potentially through an increase in insulin-mediated glucose tissue disposal,[30,31] and overtime, due to the net caloric loss and enhanced insulin-sensitivity mediated by weight loss. Moreover, recent data have shown that SGLT2 inhibitors increase glucagon secretion from alpha-cells in the pancreatic islet, a mechanism that may contribute to enhanced endogenous glucose production in treated patients.[32] In addition to these effects on glucose homeostasis, SGLT2 inhibitors exhibit potential beneficial effects on CV risk factors, as has been previously published with selected observations summarized below.[33,34]

EFFECTS OF SODIUM-GLUCOSE COTRANSPORTER-2 INHIBITORS BEYOND GLUCOSE CONTROL (FIG. 3)

- *Anthropometrics:* The glucosuric effect of SGLT2 inhibitors causing a negative energy balance results in an average weight reduction of 2–3 kg that occurs gradually over the first few months on treatment, a consistent observation across the class of medications in studies over 1–2 years.[35] Interestingly, the weight loss appears to reach a nadir and thereafter stabilizes after 3–6 months, most likely through a compensatory increased energy intake.[36] These medications seem to have no effect on energy expenditure.[37-39]
- *Blood pressure and diuresis:* A reduction in BP in patients treated with SGLT2 inhibitors is another effect beyond glucose control consistently observed across the class of medications. Several trials have shown that SGLT2 inhibitors lead to a reduction in systolic BP in a range of 3–5 mm Hg and 2–3 mm Hg in diastolic BP. In addition, SGLT2 inhibitors reduce pulse pressure, mean arterial pressure, and the product of heart rate-X-systolic BP (aka 'double product', or rate-pressure product) versus placebo suggesting an effect on different markers and mediators of arterial stiffness.[40] Interestingly, these BP effects occurred without a compensatory increase in heart rate, suggesting a lack of compensatory sympathetic activation. In addition, clamp studies in patients with uncomplicated type 1 diabetes suggest that empagliflozin reduces carotid-radial pulse wave velocity also without inducing a reflex sympathomimetic activity.[41]
- *Renal hemodynamic effects:* Sodium-glucose cotransporter-2 inhibition has been suggested to directly affect the tubuloglomerular feedback mechanism in the kidney. The increased delivery of solute (sodium and chloride) to the macula densa in the setting of SGLT2 inhibition may reduce hyperglycemia-induced glomerular hyperfiltration via tubuloglomerular feedback invoking adenosine-dependent pathways, with direct effects on afferent glomerular arteriolar tone that may diminish hyperfiltration acutely and consistently during treatment.[42]
- *Effects on mediators and markers of cardiovascular risk:* With respect to lipids, SGLT2 inhibitors mildly increase both low-density lipoprotein cholesterol (LDL-C) as well as high-density lipoprotein cholesterol (HDL-C) through as of yet unexplained mechanism.[43,44] These observations may reflect direct effects on lipoprotein particle metabolism, but could also simply reflect

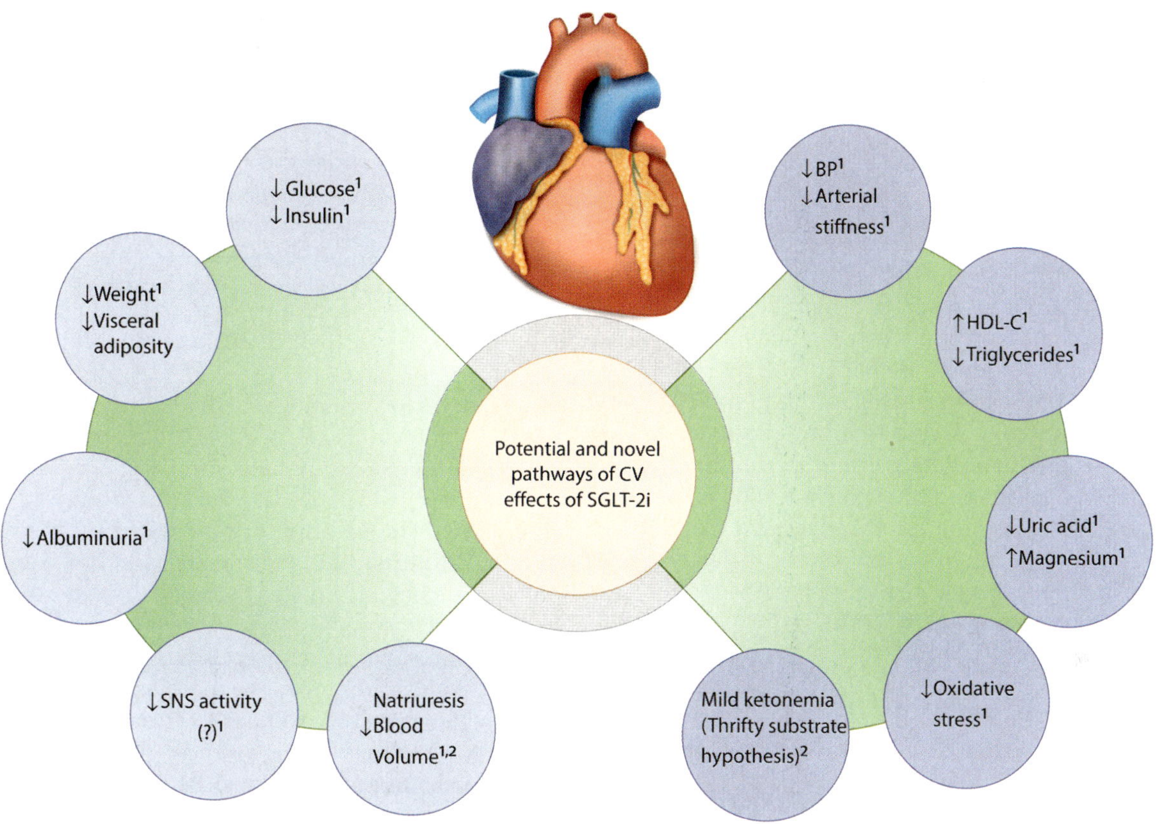

Fig. 3: Pleotropic effects of SGLT 2 inhibitor

Abbreviations: SGLT, sodium-glucose cotransporter type; BP, blood pressure; HDL-C, high-density lipoprotein cholesterol; SNS, sympathetic nervous system.

hemoconcentration resulting from the diuretic effects of SGLT2 inhibition, thereby having no net effect on circulating lipid particle numbers.

- *Cardiac effects:* Experimental data in obese and diabetic mice demonstrated that the SGLT2 inhibitor empagliflozin significantly ameliorates cardiac fibrosis, coronary arterial thickening, as well as cardiac macrophage infiltration suggesting a direct cardiac effect along with an attenuation of oxidative stress on the myocardium.[45] Other potential direct or indirect cardiac effects might include alterations of myocardial energetics and potential antiarrhythmic effects, postulated mechanisms that have arisen in attempts to understand the EMPA-REG OUTCOME trial results, but with little data to date to evaluate. From a myocardial energetics perspective, SGLT1 but not SGLT2 is expressed in cardiac myocytes.[46] In the kidney, SGLT2 inhibition results in increased SGLT1-mediated glucose reabsorption,[47] and if this is a humoral-mediated response, the possibility remains for upregulation of cardiac SGLT1. This could directly affect myocardial substrate metabolism and energetics with enhanced glucose and decreased fatty acid (FA) metabolism that could favorably affect myocardial function. In addition, shifting from β-oxidation of free FA to glycolysis in the myocardium might reduce the potential proarrhythmia effects of free FA metabolites.[48]
- *Reduction in levels of uric acid:* Uric acid is the end product of purine metabolism in humans, and hyperuricemia is a diagnostic marker for gout. Increased uric acid levels have, however, also been associated with chronic kidney disease,[49] CV complications[50] and congestive HF,[51] although a cause and effect relationship of uric acid, and CV outcomes is far from proven.[52] Reduction in levels of uric acid has been consistently seen with SGLT-2 inhibitors,[18,53,54] presumably mediated by the actions of solute carrier family 2, facilitated glucose transporter member 9 (SLC2A9), also called GLUT9, an urate transporter which secretes urate back into the urine in exchange for glucose. It is entirely unclear whether these uric acid effects might translate into long-term beneficial outcomes on either renal function or macrovascular complications.
- *Effect on lipid parameters:* SGLT-2 inhibitors are associated with a small increase in HDL-C as well as an increase in LDL-C with concomitant reductions

in triglyceride levels.[43,55,56] Whether these small lipid changes are clinically relevant and whether they could potentially offset any potential CV benefit with SGLT-2 inhibitors will need further clarification.

- *Effects on other cardiovascular risk pathways:* In animal and mechanistic models, SGLT-2 inhibitors have been shown to reduce leukocytosis induced by hyperglycemia[57] and to reduce inflammation and oxidative stress,[58-60] which are processes involved in the pathophysiology of atherosclerosis. Since inhibition of SGLT-2 leads to glucosuria with an accompanying diuresis, weight and BP reductions, all of which are theoretically beneficial in patients with HF, it is also conceivable that impaired ventricular function and remodeling could be improved with such an intervention. Although clinical data are yet to be reported, an animal study suggested that SGLT-2 inhibition could attenuate the increase in left ventricle mass and left ventricle end diastolic diameter in a rat model of progressive HF.[61]

CLINICAL LANDMARK TRIALS OF SODIUM–GLUCOSE COTRANSPORTER TYPE-2 INHIBITORS AND CARDIOVASCULAR RISK

Dapagliflozin Effect on Cardiovascular Event Thrombolysis in Myocardial Infarction 58 Trial with Dapagliflozin[62]

It has been done in patients with type 2 diabetes (T2D), both overall and with different levels of CV risk, including CV disease (CVD) history, age, and other CV risk factors, were analyzed. Analyses were based on time to first event using a Cox proportional hazards model stratified by study comparing dapagliflozin versus control. Results: in total, 9,339 patients were included in this meta-analysis; 5,936 patients received dapagliflozin 2.5–10 mg (6,668 patient-years) and 3,403 received control (3,882 patient-years). Dapagliflozin is not associated with increased CV risk and results further suggest the potential for a beneficial effect both in the overall population [hazard ratio (HR) 0.77; 95% confidence interval (CI) (0.54 and 1.10) for major adverse cardiac event (MACE)] and in those with a history of CVD [HR 0.80 (0.53 and 1.22)]. These findings were consistent in patients with varying degrees of CV risk, including age, number and type of CVD events in medical history, and number of CV risk factors present. Furthermore, there was no increased risk of MACE in patients who experienced a hypoglycemic event compared with those who did not (Fig. 4).

EMPA-REG OUTCOME TRIAL WITH EMPAGLIFLOZIN

The EMPA-REG OUTCOME study[63] is the first study to provide evidence that an antidiabetes agent decreases CV events. In 7,020 T2DM patients with established CVD, empagliflozin significantly reduced [HR 0.86 (95% CI 0.74–0.99), $P = 0.04$] the primary MACE outcome (CV death, nonfatal MI, and nonfatal stroke). However, several outcomes were surprising. First, the primary outcome was driven by decreased CV mortality and a striking disconnect between the three MACE components was observed: (1) for nonfatal MI, HR (0.87) decreased slightly but not significantly ($P = 0.22$); (2) for stroke, HR (1.24) increased slightly but not significantly ($P = 0.22$) and (3) for CV death, HR (0.62) decreased significantly by 38% ($P = 0.001$). Unlike other interventions that reduce CV risk, e.g. lowering LDL cholesterol[64] and BP[65], separation between empagliflozin and placebo curves occurred very early, and reduction in the primary outcome was evident 3 months after starting empagliflozin. The beneficial effect of empagliflozin on mortality and hospitalization for HF widened progressively over the 3.1 years of treatment. Both empagliflozin doses (10 mg and 25 mg) had a similar effect on outcome measures with no dose-response relationship. (Figs 5A and B).

Potential Mechanisms Explaining the Results in EMPA-REG OUTCOME

The surprising and unexpected results of EMPA-REG OUTCOME on mortality and HF cannot be explained by glucose control per se nor by a reduction of atherosclerotic events since the effect of empagliflozin on nonfatal MI and hospitalization for unstable angina was not statistically significant. More likely, the favorable outcomes are related to effects of empagliflozin on HF and CV mortality, direct or indirect, that are independent of effects on hyperglycemia or on atherosclerotic CVD. In the trial, 10% of the patients enrolled had a history of HF, but no data on left ventricular function or surrogate parameters like N-terminal pro b-type natriuretic peptide (NT-proBNP) were collected. Empagliflozin led to a highly significant reduction in hospitalization for HF with an effect that became evident very early in the trial in the overall study population. Subgroup analyzes stratified by presence or absence of HF at baseline suggest a consistent benefit observed in patients with and without baseline HF with no evident heterogeneity of efficacy by HF status.[66] It is important to note that the outcomes analyzed in the study only evaluated first events, and no conclusion on the effects of empagliflozin therapy on total HF events (i.e. first + recurrent) can yet be made. Various factors may contribute to the observed

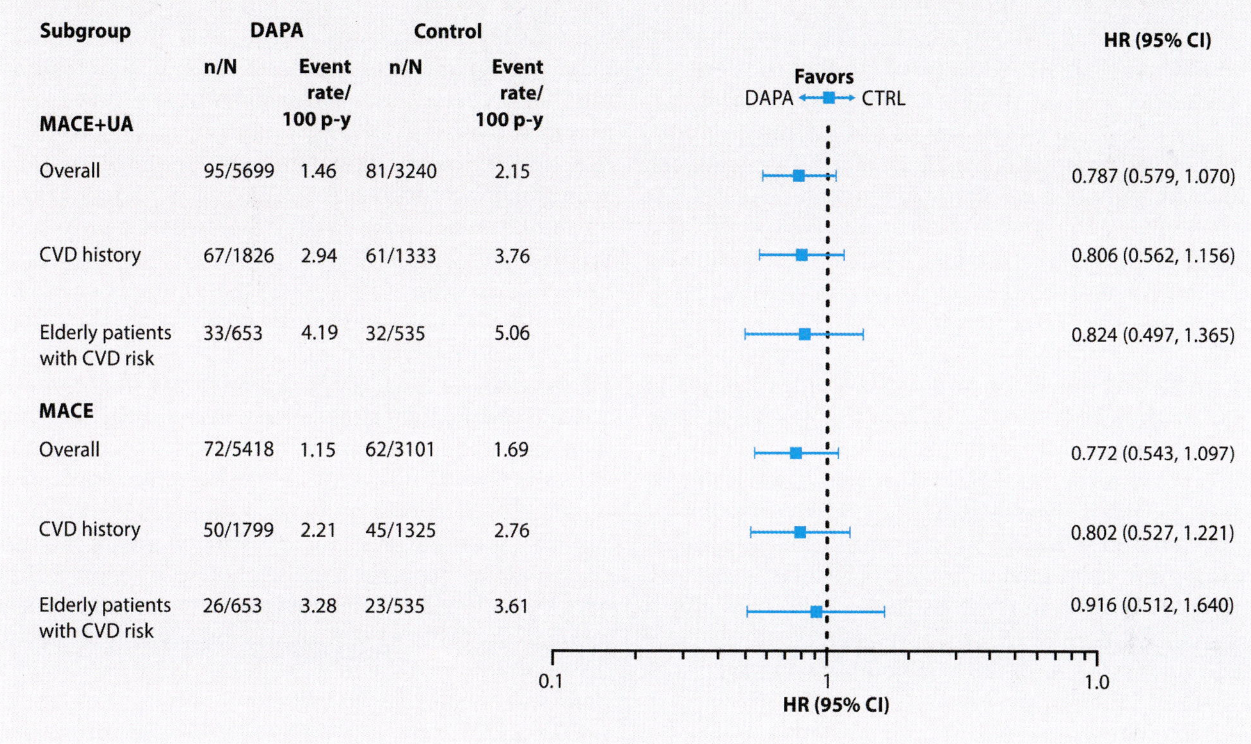

Fig. 4: DECLARE TIMI 58 trial.

Abbreviations: DECLARE, dapagliflozin effect on cardiovascular event; TIMI, thrombolysis in myocardial infarction; DAPA, dapagliflozin; MACE, major adverse cardiac event; CVD, cardiovascular disease; HR, hazard ratio; CI, confidence interval; UA, unstable angina.

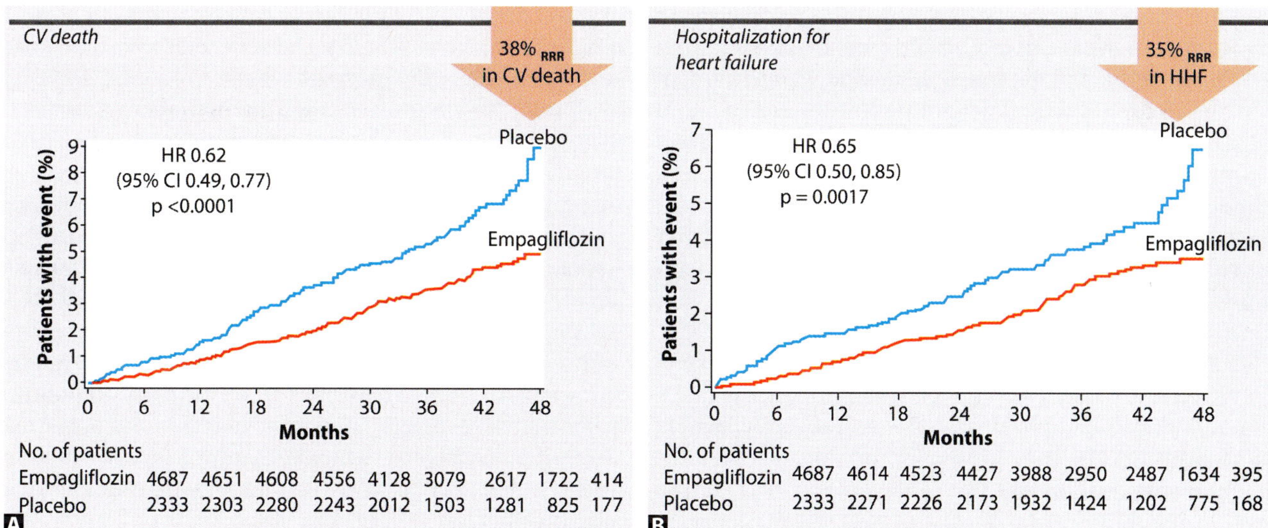

Figs 5A and B: EPMA-REG OUTCOME results with empagliflozin

reduction in CV death and HF hospitalization. As with the atherosclerotic event endpoints discussed above, blood glucose reduction itself is very unlikely to account for the results observed given the minor difference in HbA1c levels between groups as well as the fact that previous studies showed that intensified glucose control does not influence the incidence of these events in similar populations. The significant reductions in BP and body weight seen in EMPA-REG OUTCOME have been proposed as potential contributors to the beneficial results. However, BP lowering only translates into CV risk reduction after 6–12 months or even longer, making the early beneficial effects seen unlikely to be attributable to BP reduction per se. Still, the decrease in markers of arterial stiffness found in SGLT2 inhibitor-treated patients, all closely linked to BP reduction, may have a direct, potentially beneficial effect on myocardial oxygen consumption via afterload reduction. Weight loss seems to play a minor role in this context given the data from the Look Action for Health in Diabetes study, showing that intensive lifestyle intervention, focused on weight loss, did not improve CV risk in patients with T2D.[67]

The diuretic effect of empagliflozin has been discussed as a potential contributor to the observed reduction of hospitalization for HF through at least temporary reduction in plasma volume as shown for SGLT2-inhibitors.[25] However, similar or greater decreases in intravascular volume and net sodium balance is affected by most commonly used diuretic medications but—in contrast to empagliflozin—treatment with loop diuretics or thiazides has not been demonstrated to reduce CV death in previous studies, and their effects on hospitalization for HF risk, when demonstrated, have been much more modest in magnitude compared with the large reduction observed with empagliflozin. Yet, SGLT2 inhibitors are different from the loop and thiazide diuretics in several important ways. First, they do not lead to a reflex activation of the sympathetic nervous system. In addition, thiazides work in the distal tubule while SGLT2 inhibitors act proximal of the macula densa, thus leading to an increased urinary sodium and chloride delivery to the juxtaglomerular apparatus. This has been suggested to restore the tubuloglomerular feedback mechanism in diabetes with afferent arteriolar vasoconstriction and subsequent reduction of hyperfiltration, and normalization of transglomerular perfusion pressures. Similarly, the increased sodium and chloride delivery to the macular densa upon SGLT2 inhibitor treatment may affect other neurohormonal factors such as local renin-angiotensin-aldosterone system (RAAS) inhibition,[68-70] which may have contributed to preglomerular vasoconstriction in diabetes. It is tempting to speculate that these effects possibly result in aldosterone withdrawal and reduced sympathetic nerve activity—either or both of which could directly benefit CV death and HF risk. Moreover, other yet unknown mechanisms influencing the renal-cardiac interaction may be of important in this context. Still, the depletion of sodium and potential reduction in body sodium content by SGLT2 inhibition may play a crucial in HF in diabetes. It has been hypothesized that patients with diabetes exhibit an excess of total-body sodium, mainly because of increased sodium retention in the kidney as a consequence of hyperglycemia and hyperinsulinemia.[71-73] Sodium-loading studies in animals and humans suggest that excess sodium is not only distributed in the extracellular space but possibly also intracellularly as well as in osmotically inactive compartments, e.g. matrix components of skin and muscle. Increased intracellular sodium in the myocardium may increase the risk of arrhythmias and impair myocardial function,[74,75] most likely through an impairment of mitochondrial function. Interestingly, experimental data in an animal model of HF showed an increase in myocardial intracellular sodium and in this model, blockade of the mitochondrial Na^+/Ca^{2+} exchange prolonged survival of these animals, and significantly decreased arrhythmias.[76] SGLT2 inhibition leads to an early and transient increase in urinary sodium excretion that normalizes after 2 weeks.[77] This increase in sodium depletion is not reflected by changes in plasma sodium concentration, but since plasma sodium does not directly mirror whole body sodium content, the increase in urinary sodium excretion is likely to rapidly reduce total-body sodium. This mechanism may thus contribute to the early beneficial effect of empagliflozin on CV death and HF hospitalization not only through a reduction of volume load but also through direct effects in the myocardium. Still, to date, little is known about these potential effects of empagliflozin and future research is warranted to further explore this issue. Other mechanisms that may explain the profound effects of empagliflozin on CV events include antioxidative, anti-inflammatory, or antiapoptotic properties of SGLT2 inhibitors as shown in experimental models, as well as counterbalancing effects of these drugs on cellular senescence.[58,78] Still, hitherto, it remains speculative whether such effects seen in preclinical studies translate into humans.

Finally, the increase in glucagon secretion induced by SGLT2 inhibition[32] may be interesting in light of the EMPA-REG OUTCOME results. Work in the 1970s suggested that glucagon exhibits inotropic effects with an increased myocardial contractility and cardiac output in glucagon-treated patients with MI.[79,80] In the myocardium, glucagon generates cyclic adenosine monophosphate (cAMP), thus exhibiting positive inotropic and chronotropic action without the need for beta-1 adrenoreceptor stimulation.[70] In addition, glucagon has been shown to exhibit antiarrhythmic effects. Clinically, glucagon has previously been employed as an adjunctive therapy in shock situations and HF, but given that catecholamines are much more effective in these conditions, glucagon is no longer used for this indication. Still, a continuous increase in glucagon levels in SGLT2 inhibitor-treated patients could contribute to a cardioprotective effect.

Empagliflozin has been included in European Society of Cardiology (ESC) 2016 Guidelines for diagnosis and treatment of acute and chronic HF as class 2A, level b recommendation (Fig. 6).

Recommendations	Class[a]	Level[b]
Treatment of hypertension is recommended to prevent or delay the onset of HF and prolong life.	I	A
Treatment with statins is recommended in patients with or at high-risk of CAD whether or they have LV systolic dysfunction, in order to prevent or delay the onset of HF and prolong life.	I	A
Counseling and treatment for smoking cessation and alcohol intake reduction is recommended for people who smoke or who consume excess alcohol in order to prevent or delay the onset of HF.	I	C
Treating other risk factors of HF (e.g. obesity, dysglycemia) should be considered in order to prevent or delay the onset of HF.	IIa	C
Empagliflozin should be considered in patients with type 2 diabetes in order to prevent or delay the onset of HF and prolong life.	IIa	B
ACE-I is recommended in patients with asymptomatic LV systolic dysfunction and a history of myocardial infraction in order to prevent or delay the onset of HF and prolong life.	I	A
ACE-I is recommended in patients with asymptomatic LV systolic dysfunction without a history of myocardial infraction, in order to prevent or delay the onset of HF.	I	B

Fig. 6: European Society of Cardiology 2016 Guidelines for diagnosis and treatment of acute and chronic HF as class 2A, level B recommendation

Abbreviations: HF, heart failure; CAD, coronary artery disease; ACE, angiotensin-converting enzyme; LV, left ventricle.

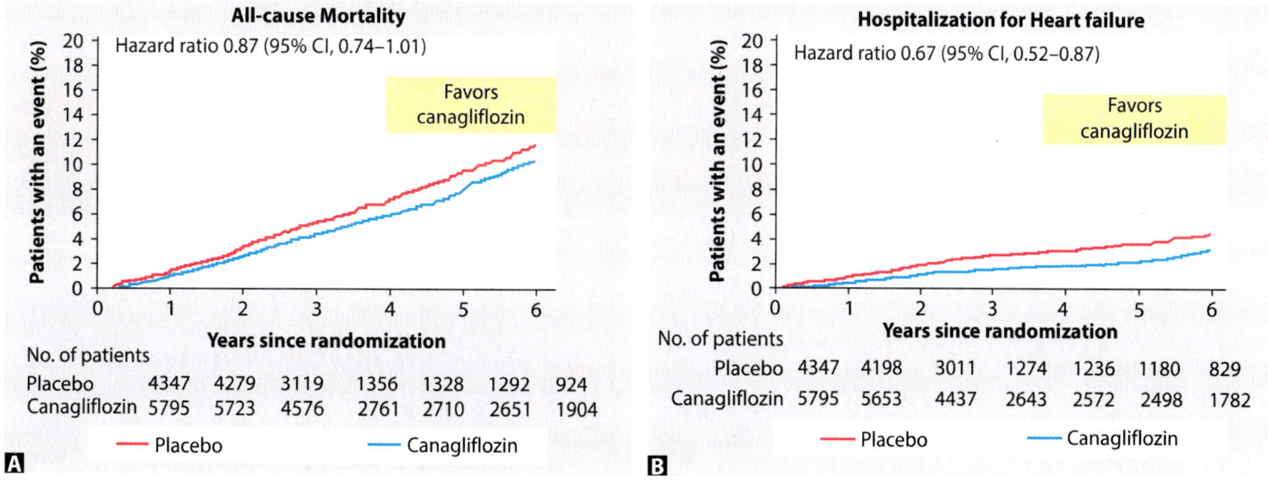

Figs 7A and B: CANVAS trial result

Abbreviations: CANVAS, canagliflozin cardiovascular assessment study; CI, confidence interval

CANAGLIFLOZIN CARDIOVASCULAR ASSESSMENT STUDY TRIAL WITH CANAGLIFLOZIN

Canagliflozin cardiovascular assessment study (CANVAS) trial was presented recently in American Diabetes Association (ADA), June 2017,[81] canagliflozin reduces CV events by 14%, all cause and CV deaths by 13%, HF by 33%,cuts renal decline by 40% but doubles the risk of lower limb amputations (Figs 7A and 7B).

CONCLUSION

Given the increasing prevalence of T2DM in populations worldwide and suboptimal control of glycemia and other CV risk factors achieved with currently available agents, the need for therapies with novel modes of action remains an important clinical priority. Of the large number of antihyperglycemic drug classes now available for patients with T2DM, none is recognized unequivocally to reduce CV events over and above any modest effects of glucose lowering itself. Metformin, which is widely viewed as having CV benefits, has actually never been studied in a large properly designed randomized clinical trial powered to answer this specific question. SGLT-2 inhibitors are novel oral glucose-lowering agents that offer the potential to improve glycemic control, independent of insulin secretion, offering a modest reduction in BP and body weight. Their mode of action, which is independent of endogenous insulin secretion, enables their use in any stage of T2DM. Pleotropic effects of SGLT-2 inhibitors showed the potential for its CV benefits. Results of EPMA REG OUTCOME with empagliflozin and CANVAS trial with canagliflozin are encouraging. Empagliflozin because of its proven benefit in HF, has found its place in ESC 2016 HF guidelines.

REFERENCES

1. Huxley R, Barzi F, Woodward M. Excess risk of fatal coronary heart disease associated with diabetes in men and women: meta-analysis of 37 prospective cohort studies. BMJ. 2006;332(7533):73-8.
2. Sloan FA, Bethel MA, Ruiz D Jr, et al. The growing burden of diabetes mellitus in the US elderly population. Arch Intern Med. 2008;168(2):192-9.
3. Inzucchi SE, Bergenstal RM, Buse JB, et al. Management of hyperglycemia in type 2 diabetes: a patient-centered approach: position statement of the American Diabetes Association (ADA) and the European Association for the Study of Diabetes (EASD). Diabetes Care. 2012;35(6):1364-79.
4. Ryden L, Grant PJ, Anker SD, et al. ESC Guidelines on diabetes, pre-diabetes, and cardiovascular diseases developed in collaboration with the EASD: the Task Force on diabetes, pre-diabetes, and cardiovascular diseases of the European Society of Cardiology (ESC) and developed in collaboration with the European Association for the Study of Diabetes (EASD). Eur Heart J. 2013;34(39): 3035-87.
5. Skyler JS, Bergenstal R, Bonow RO, et al. Intensive glycaemic control and the prevention of cardiovascular events: implications of the ACCORD, ADVANCE, and VA diabetes trial; A position statement of American Diabetes Association and a Scientific Statement of the American College of Cardiology Foundation and the American Heart Association. Diabetes Care. 2009;32(1):187-92.
6. Singh S, Bhat J, Wang PH. Cardiovascular effects of anti-diabetic medications in type 2 diabetes mellitus. Curr Cardiol Rep. 2013;15(1):327.
7. Nam M. Clinical trial for antidiabetic drugs: FDA guidance for diabetes mellitus-evaluation of cardiovascular risk in new antidiabetic therapies. J Korean Diabetes. 2011;12:129.
8. Division of Metabolism and Endocrinology Products in the Center for Drug Evaluation and Research (CDER) at Food and Drug Administration. (2008). Guidance for Industry Diabetes Mellitus-Evaluating Cardiovascular Risk in New Antidiabetic Therapies to Treat Type 2 Diabetes 2008. [online] Available from https://www.fda.gov/. [Accessed September, 2017].
9. Bennett WL, Maruthur NM, Singh S, et al. Comparative effectiveness and safety of medications for type 2 diabetes: an update including new drugs and 2-drug combinations. Ann Intern Med. 2011;154(9):602-13.
10. Scirica BM, Bhatt DL, Braunwald E, et al. Saxagliptin and cardiovascular outcomes in patients with type 2 diabetes mellitus. N Engl J Med. 2013;369(14):1317-26.
11. White WB, Cannon CP, Heller SR, et al. Alogliptin after acute coronary syndrome in patients with type 2 diabetes. N Engl J Med. 2013;369(14):1327-35.
12. Fadini GP and Avogaro A. Cardiovascular effects of DPP-4 inhibition: beyond GLP-1. Vascul Pharmacol. 2011;55(1-3): 10-6.
13. Dzau V, Braunwald E. Resolved and unresolved issues in the prevention and treatment of coronary artery disease: a workshop consensus statement. Am Heart J. 1991;121(4 Pt 1):1244-63.
14. Lee SJ, Leipzig RM, Walter LC. Incorporating lag time to benefit into prevention decisions for older adults. JAMA. 2013;310(24):2609-10.
15. Gerich JE. Role of the kidney in normal glucose homeostasis and in the hyperglycaemia of diabetes mellitus: therapeutic implications. Diabet Med. 2010;27(2):136-42.
16. Marsenic O. Glucose control by the kidney: an emerging target in diabetes. Am J Kidney Dis. 2009;53(5):875-83.
17. Rahmoune H, Thompson PW, Ward JM, et al. Glucose transporters in human renal proximal tubular cells isolated from the urine of patients with non-insulin-dependent diabetes. Diabetes 2005;54(12):3427-34.
18. Bailey CJ, Gross JL, Pieters A, et al. Effect of dapagliflozin in patients with type 2 diabetes who have inadequate glycaemic control with metformin: a randomised, double-blind, placebo-controlled trial. Lancet. 2010;375(9733):2223-33.
19. Chao EC, Henry RR. SGLT2 inhibition–a novel strategy for diabetes treatment. Nat Rev Drug Discov. 2010;9(7):551-9.
20. Saeed MA, Narendran P. Dapagliflozin for the treatment of type 2 diabetes: a review of the literature. Drug Des Devel Ther. 2014;8:2493-505.
21. Abdul-Ghani MA, Norton L, Defronzo RA. Role of sodium-glucose cotransporter 2 (SGLT 2) inhibitors in the treatment of type 2 diabetes. Endocr Rev. 2011;32(4):515-31.
22. Whalen K, Miller S, Onge ES. The role of sodium-glucose co-transporter 2 inhibitors in the treatment of type 2 diabetes. Clin Ther. 2015;37(6):1150-66.
23. Wright EM, Loo DD, Hirayama BA. Biology of human sodium glucose transporters. Physiol Rev. 2011;91(2):733-94.
24. Nauck MA. Update on developments with SGLT2 inhibitors in the management of type 2 diabetes. Drug Des Devel Ther. 2014;8:1335-80.
25. DeFronzo RA, Hompesch M, Kasichayanula S, et al. Characterization of renal glucose reabsorption in response to dapagliflozin in healthy subjects and subjects with type 2 diabetes. Diabetes Care. 2013;36(10):3169-76.
26. Sha S, Polidori D, Heise T, et al. Effect of the sodium glucose co-transporter 2 inhibitor canagliflozin on plasma volume in patients with type 2 diabetes mellitus. Diabetes Obes Metab. 2014;16(11):1087-95.
27. Ferrannini E, DeFronzo RA. Impact of glucose-lowering drugs on cardiovascular disease in type 2 diabetes. Eur Heart J. 2015;36(34):2288-96.
28. Ferrannini E, Solini A. SGLT2 inhibition in diabetes mellitus: rationale and clinical prospects. Nat Rev Endocrinol. 2012;8(8):495-502.
29. Clar C, Gill JA, Court R, et al. Systematic review of SGLT2 receptor inhibitors in dual or triple therapy in type 2 diabetes. BMJ Open. 2012;2(5):pii:e001007.
30. Ferrannini E, Muscelli E, Frascerra S, et al. Metabolic response to sodium-glucose cotransporter 2 inhibition in type 2 diabetic patients. J Clin Invest 2014;124(2):499-508.
31. Merovci A, Solis-Herrera C, Daniele G, et al. Dapagliflozin improves muscle insulin sensitivity but enhances endogenous glucose production. J Clin Invest 2014;124(2):509-14.
32. Bonner C, Kerr-Conte J, Gmyr V, et al. Inhibition of the glucose transporter SGLT2 with dapagliflozin in pancreatic alpha cells triggers glucagon secretion. Nat Med. 2015;21(5):512-7.
33. Inzucchi SE, Zinman B, Wanner C, et al. SGLT-2 inhibitors and cardiovascular risk: proposed pathways and review of ongoing outcome trials. Diab Vasc Dis Res. 2015;12(2):90-100.

34. Ptaszynska A, Hardy E, Johnsson E, et al. Effects of dapagliflozinon cardiovascular risk factors. Postgrad Med. 2013;125(3):181-9.
35. Vasilakou D, Karagiannis T, Athanasiadou E, et al. Sodium-glucose cotransporter 2 inhibitors for type 2 diabetes: a systematic review and meta-analysis. Ann Intern Med. 2013;159(4):262-74.
36. Ferrannini G, Hach T, Crowe S, et al. Energy balance after sodium-glucose cotransporter 2 inhibition. Diabetes Care. 2015;38(9): 1730-5.
37. Ridderstrale M, Andersen KR, Zeller C, et al. Comparison of empagliflozin and glimepiride as add-on to metformin in patients with type 2 diabetes: a 104-week randomised, active-controlled, double-blind, phase 3 trial. Lancet Diabetes Endocrinol. 2014;2(9):691-700.
38. Bolinder J, Ljunggren Ö, Johansson L et al. Dapagliflozin maintains glycaemic control while reducing weight and body fat mass over 2 years in patients with type 2 diabetes mellitus inadequately controlled on metformin. Diabetes Obes Metab. 2014;16(2):159-69.
39. Cefalu WT, Leiter LA, YoonKH, et al. Efficacy and safety of canagliflozin versus glimepiride in patients with type 2 diabetes inadequately controlled with metformin (CANTATA-SU): 52 week results from a randomised, double-blind, phase 3 non-inferiority trial. Lancet. 2013;382(9896):941-50.
40. Chilton R, Tikkanen I, Cannon CP, et al. Effects of empagliflozin on blood pressure and markers of arterial stiffness and vascular resistance in patients with type 2 diabetes. Diabetes Obes Metab. 2015;17(12):1180-93.
41. Cherney DZ, Perkins BA, Soleymanlou N, et al. The effect of empagliflozin on arterial stiffness and heart rate variability in subjects with uncomplicated type 1 diabetes mellitus. Cardiovasc Diabetol. 2014;13:28.
42. Cherney DZ, Perkins BA, Soleymanlou N, et al. Renal hemodynamic effect of sodium-glucose cotransporter 2 inhibition in patients with type 1 diabetes mellitus. Circulation. 2014;129(5):587-97.
43. Monami M, Dicembrini I, Nardini C, et al. Effects of glucagon-like peptide-1 receptor agonists on cardiovascular risk: a meta-analysis of randomized clinical trials. Diabetes Obes Metab. 2014;16(1):38-47.
44. Sinclair A, Bode B, Harris S, et al. Efficacy and safety of canagliflozin compared with placebo in older patients with type 2 diabetes mellitus: a pooled analysis of clinical studies. BMC Endocr Disord. 2014;14:37.
45. Lin B, Koibuchi N, Hasegawa Y, et al. Glycemic control with empagliflozin, a novel selective SGLT 2 inhibitor, ameliorates cardiovascular injury and cognitive dysfunction in obese and type 2 diabetic mice. Cardiovasc Diabetol. 2014;13:148.
46. Banerjee SK, McGaffin KR, Pastor Soler NM, et al. SGLT1 is a novel cardiac glucose transporter that is perturbed in disease states. Cardiovasc Res 2009;84(1):111-8.
47. Rieg T, Masuda T, Gerasimova M, et al. Increase in SGLT1-mediated transport explains renal glucose reabsorption during genetic and pharmacological SGLT2 inhibition in euglycemia. Am J Physiol Renal Physiol. 2014;306(2):F188-93.
48. Taegtmeyer H, McNulty P, Young ME. Adaptation and maladaptation of the heart in diabetes: Part I: general concepts. Circulation. 2002;105(14):1727-33.
49. Madero M, Sarnak MJ, Wang X, et al. Uric acid and long-term outcomes in CKD. Am J Kidney Dis. 2009;53(5):796-803.
50. Ndrepepa G, Braun S, King L, et al. Association of uric acid with mortality in patients with stable coronary artery disease. Metabolism. 2012;61(12):1780-6.
51. Huang H, Huang B, Li Y, et al. Uric acid and risk of heart failure: a systematic review and meta-analysis. Eur J Heart Fail. 2014;16(1): 15-24.
52. Zand S, Shafiee A, Boroumand M, et al. Serum uric acid is not an independent risk factor for premature coronary artery disease. Cardiorenal Med. 2013;3(4):246-53.
53. Hach T, Gerich J, Salsali A, et al. Empagliflozin improves glycaemic parameters and cardiovascular risk factors in patients with type 2 diabetes: pooled data from four pivotal phase III trials. Diabetes. 2013;62(Suppl. 1):LB19 [69-LB].
54. Rosenstock J, Aggarwal N, Polidori D, et al. Dose-ranging effects of canagliflozin, a sodium-glucose cotransporter 2 inhibitor, as add-on to metformin in subjects with type 2 diabetes. Diabetes Care. 2012;35(6):1232-8.
55. Monami M, Nardini C, Mannucci E. Efficacy and safety of sodium glucose co-transport-2 inhibitors in type 2 diabetes: a meta-analysis of randomized clinical trials. Diabetes Obes Metab. 2014;16(5): 457-66.
56. Hardy E, Ptanszynska A, de Bruin TW, et al. Changes in lipid profiles of patients with type 2 diabetes mellitus on dapagliflozin therapy. Diabetologia. 2013;(Suppl 947):61.
57. Nagareddy PR, Murphy AJ, Stirzaker RA, et al. Hyperglycaemia promotes myelopoiesis and impairs the resolution of atherosclerosis. Cell Metabolism. 2013;17(5):695-708.
58. Tahara A, Kurosaki E, Yokono M, et al. Effects of SGLT2 selective inhibitor ipragliflozin on hyperglycemia, hyperlipidemia, hepatic steatosis, oxidative stress, inflammation, and obesity in type 2 diabetic mice. Eur J Pharmacol. 2013;715(1-3):246-55.
59. Panchapakesan U, Pegg K, Gross S, et al. Effects of SGLT2 inhibition in human kidney proximal tubular cells–renoprotection in diabetic nephropathy? PLoS ONE. 2013;8(2):e54442.
60. Osorio H, Coronel I, Arellano A, et al. Sodium-glucose cotransporter inhibition prevents oxidative stress in the kidney of diabetic rats. Oxid Med Cell Longev. 2012;2012:542042.
61. Younis FM, Hollander K, Mayoux EW, et al. Effect of prophylactic treatment with empagliflozin on cardiac function and diabetes in CRDH rats. Diabetes. 2014;63(Suppl 1):A273 (1056-P).
62. Sonesson C, Johansson PA, Johnsson E, et al. Cardiovascular effects of dapagliflozin in patients with type 2 diabetes and different risk categories: a meta-analysis. Cardiovasc Diabetol. 2016;15:37.
63. Zinman B, Wanner C, Lachin JM, et al. EMPA-REG OUTCOME Investigators. Empagliflozin, cardiovascular outcomes, and mortality in type 2 diabetes. N Engl J Med. 2015;373(22):2117-28.
64. The Long-Term Intervention with Pravastatin in Ischaemic Disease (LIPID) Study Group. Prevention of cardiovascular events and death with pravastatinin patientswithcoronaryheart disease and a broad range of initial cholesterol levels. N Engl J Med. 1998;339(19): 1349-57.
65. Patel A, MacMahon S, Chalmers J, et al. ADVANCE Collaborative Group. Effects of a fixed combination of perindopril and indapamide on macrovascular and microvascular outcomes in patients with type 2 diabetes mellitus (the ADVANCE trial): a randomised controlled trial. Lancet. 2007;370(9590):829-40.
66. Fitchett D, Zinman B, Wanner C, et al. Heart failure outcomes with empagliflozin in patients with type 2 diabetes at high cardiovascular risk: results of the EMPA-REG OUTCOME(R) trial. Eur Heart J. 2016;37(39):1526-34.
67. Wing RR, Reboussin D, Lewis CE, et al. Intensive life style intervention in type 2 diabetes. N Engl J Med. 2013;369(24):2358-9.
68. Cherney DZ, Perkins BA, Soleymanlou N, et al. Sodium glucose cotransport-2 inhibition and intrarenal RAS activity in people with type 1 diabetes. Kidney Int. 2014;86(5):1057-8.
69. Baker WL, Smyth LR, Riche DM, et al. Effects of sodium-glucose co-transporter 2 inhibitors on blood pressure: a systematic review and meta-analysis. J Am Soc Hypertens. 2014;8(4):262-75.
70. Lambers Heerspink HJ, de Zeeuw D, Wie L, et al. Dapagliflozin a glucose-regulating drug with diuretic properties in subjects with type 2 diabetes. Diabetes Obes Metab. 2013;15(9):853-62.
71. DeFronzo RA, Cooke CR, Andres R, et al. The effect of insulin on renal handling of sodium, potassium, calcium, and phosphate in man. J Clin Invest. 1975;55(4):845-55.

72. Weder AB. Sodium metabolism, hypertension, and diabetes. Am J Med Sci. 1994;307(Suppl 1):S53-9.
73. Weidmann P, Ferrari P. Central role of sodium in hypertension in diabetic subjects. Diabetes Care 1991;14(3):220-32.
74. Remme CA, Wilde AA. Late sodium current inhibition in acquired and inherited ventricular (dys)function and arrhythmias. Cardiovasc Drugs Ther 2013;27(1):91-101.
75. van Emous JG, Nederhoff MG, Ruigrok TJ, et al. The role of the Na+ channel in the accumulation of intracellular Na+during myocardial ischemia: consequences for post-ischemic recovery. J Mol Cell Cardiol 1997;29(1):85-96.
76. Liu T, Takimoto E, Dimaano VL, et al. Inhibiting mitochondrial Na^+/Ca^{2+} exchange prevents sudden death in a Guinea pig model of heart failure. Circ Res. 2014;115(1):44-54.
77. Komoroski B, Vachharajani N, Feng Y, et al. Dapagliflozin, a novel, selective SGLT2 inhibitor, improved glycemic control over 2 weeks in patients with type 2 diabetes mellitus. Clin Pharmacol Ther. 2009;85(5):513-9.
78. Kitada K, Nakano D, Ohsaki H, et al. Hyperglycemia causes cellular senescence via a SGLT2- and p21-dependent pathway in proximal tubules in the early stage of diabetic nephropathy. J Diab Complications 2014;28(5):604-11.
79. Diamond G, Forrester J, Danzig R, et al. Haemodynamic effects of glucagon during acute myocardial infarction with left ventricular failure in man. Br Heart J. 1971;33(2):290-5.
80. Murtagh JG, Binnion PF, Lal S, et al. Haemodynamic effects of glucagon. Br Heart J. 1970;32(3):307-15.
81. Neal B, Perkovic V, Mahaffey KW, et al. Optimizing the analysis strategy for the CANVAS Program: a prespecified plan for the integrated analyses of the CANVAS and CANVAS-R trials. Diabetes Obes Metab. 2017;19(7):926-35.

CHAPTER

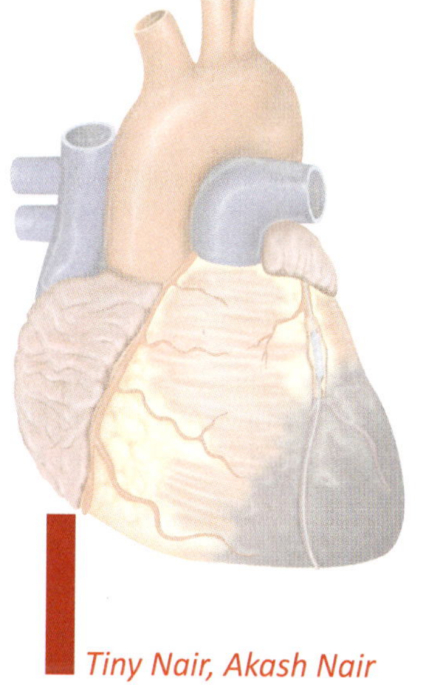

Diabetes and Heart Failure: New Data on the Role of SGLT 2 Inhibitors—A Change of Concept?

Tiny Nair, Akash Nair

INTRODUCTION

Around 40% of patients hospitalized for heart failure (HF) have diabetes mellitus (DM), while 30% of all diabetic patients would eventually develop HF. Diabetes increases propensity for atherosclerosis, resulting in higher incidence of obstructive coronary artery disease (CAD) and myocardial infarction, which in turn, increases the chances of LV dysfunction.[1] The spectrum of left ventricular (LV) dysfunction in diabetes may range from silent and asymptomatic to severely symptomatic. Treatment of HF has changed with introduction of newer drugs [mineralocorticoid receptor antagonists (MRA), ivabradine, angiotensin neprilysin inhibitors (ARNI)], while indication and scope for device therapy has broadened. But, despite all these advances, HF still carries a high-rate of morbidity, mortality, and hospitalization. These overall outcome indices of HF in diabetic subset continue to be worse than the nondiabetic counterpart.

ORAL ANTIDIABETIC DRUGS AND CARDIOVASCULAR EVENTS

All antidiabetic drugs reduce glycemic parameters like fasting plasma glucose (FPG), postprandial plasma glucose (PPG), and glycated hemoglobin (HbA1c) in different proportions; but its effects on cardiovascular (CV) events are variable. Many antidiabetic drugs increase CV events, while some tend to worsen HF by fluid retention. Most sulfonylureas tend to increase CV events and carry a black-box warning in the US.[2] Glitazones retain fluid, worsen pedal edema, and HF.[3] The dipeptidyl peptidase-4 (DPP4) inhibitors (gliptins) are generally tend to be safe despite some signals of an increased HF hospitalization in some trials.[4-6] Sodium–glucose cotransporter type-2 (SGLT2) receptors are involved in reabsorption of glucose from the kidneys. The new group of drugs SGLT2 inhibitors tend to reduce diabetes by reduction of glucose absorption, increased glucose excretion, and reluctant lowering of blood sugar. Being a cotransporter, it also results in increased urinary excretion of sodium and resultant loss of volume.[7,8] These drugs have shown to improve CV outcomes and has a propensity to reduce incidence of HF as well as HF hospitalization. Empagliflozin, canagliflozin, and dapagliflozin are marketed in India. The EMPA-REG OUTCOME trial has shown positive outcome on most CV events including HF hospitalization.[9] The new canagliflozin cardiovascular assessment study (CANVAS) program with canagliflozin also shows improvement of triple primary endpoint of death, myocardial infarction (MI), and stroke.[10]

Cardiovascular Safety of Antidiabetic Drugs

The Food and Drug Administration (FDA) mandates that if the hazard ratio (HR) 95% and confidence interval (CI) crosses 1.8, the result is considered inferior while below that it is noninferior. If the HR 95%, CI is below 1.3, the study drug can be considered as noninferior and accepted, while values between 1.3 and 1.8 needs a postmarketing surveillance to prove CV safety. A HR below 1 with a significant p value would make the drug superior to standard therapy, though that is not a mandatory primary endpoint for CV safety trials.

EMPA-REG OUTCOME

The EMPA-REG OUTCOME trial randomized 7,020 patients of diabetes (4,687 empagliflozin; 2,333 placebos) for a period of 3 years. The primary triple end point of death, MI and stroke was reduced by 14% (HR 0.86 95% and CI 0.74–0.99). CV death was reduced by 38% while HF hospitalization was reduced by 33%.[9] This study showed that SGLT2 inhibitors reduce CV events (superior) compared to the present gold standard therapy for diabetes. Thus, SGLT2 inhibitors joined select band of antidiabetic drugs (metformin) to offer CV protection and not mere CV safety. The transition of SGLT2 inhibitors from CV safe drugs to CV protecting agents has been truly remarkable. FDA approved empagliflozin on basis of EMPA-REG OUTCOME trial.

CANVAS

The CANVAS was a huge and ambitious program, involving 30 countries and 667 sites [North America 2, Latin America 4, Europe 17, and Asia pacific 7. The original program (CANVAS) was initiated in 2009, while CANVAS-R started rolling in 2013]. While CANVAS randomized 4,330 patients and CANVAS-R randomized 5,813 patients. In total 4,347 patients were on placebo while 5,795 on canagliflozin. The mean follow-up was 188 weeks. Both the groups were well matched. The average duration of diabetes was roughly 14 years. Interesting aspects from the CV standpoint was that 90% had hypertension, 15% HF and 65% CV disease. The majority (78%) were whites, and 15% Asian population. Roughly, 75% were on metformin and 50% insulin. Both were well treated, renin-angiotensin aldosterone system (RAAS) inhibitors in 80%, statins 75%, and more than 70% received antithrombotic therapy. The average HbA1c was 8.2%, average blood pressure (BP) 136/78, and average LDL 90 mg%.

On follow-up the HbA1c was consistently lower by 0.6%, systolic BP (SBP) lower by 4 mm Hg, and a weight reduction of 1.6 Kg in the canagliflozin group compared to placebo. In CANVS the primary major adverse cardiac event (MACE) outcome consisting of CV death, nonfatal MI, or nonfatal stroke had a HR of 0.86, (CI 0.75–0.97), thus proving clear superiority which puts this drug in par with empagliflozin (EMPA-REG). Individual endpoints like CV death (HR 0.87), MI (HR 0.85), stroke (HR 0.90), all-cause mortality (HR 0.87), HF hospitalization (HR 0.67), CV death, or hospitalization for HF (HR 0.78).[10]

LEADER

Liraglutide Effect and Action in Diabetes: Evaluation of Cardiovascular Outcome Results (LEADER) trial withy liraglutide [once a day glucagon-like peptide-1 (GLP-1) agonist] showed triple postexposure prophylaxis (PEP) reduction by 13%, CV death 22%, MI 12%, and HF hospitalization by 13%.[11]

SUSTAIN-6

SUSTAIN-6 used semaglutide (once a week GPL-1 agonist) and showed triple PEP reduction by 26%, CV death reduced by 2%, and MI by 26% with little effect on HF hospitalization.[12]

DISCUSSION

The benefit of canagliflozin in CANVAS is impressive and clearly shows that it follows the same line and direction of empagliflozin. SGLT2 inhibitors work primarily by inhibiting absorption of glucose in the kidneys. This in consequence results in loss of sugar and sodium in urine resulting in volume contraction. Calorie loss results in loss of weight and BP goes down. Though primarily reduction of BP and body weight has been ascribed to calorie and volume loss, there seems to be effects beyond simple loss of sodium and sugar. Decreased nephron hyperfiltration imparts nephroprotection. The cardiac benefits include decreased cardiac preload and afterload, decreased systolic and diastolic dysfunction, decreased HF hospitalization, and possible reduction of major (fatal) arrhythmias.

A new hypothesis suggests that perhaps GLP-1 agonists slow atherothrombosis, while SGLT2 inhibitors improve cardiac function. Liver produces increased betahydroxy butyrate because of the relative ketotoc state. In HF the mitochondria uses it to increase myocardial energetics. It reduces progressive myocardial fibrosis.

Coronary Artery Disease and Sodium–glucose Cotransporter Type-2 Inhibitors

Sodium–glucose cotransporter type-2 inhibitors cause loss of sugar in urine resulting in loss of calorie and thus reduction of body weight. Loss of sodium results in volume loss and reduction of BP. Combination of a better glycemic control, improved BP control, and a lower body weight result in better CV outcome. But the timeframe of CV event reduction and the degree of benefit is more than could be explained by simple control of these risk factors. Hence, a pleotropic effect of SGLT2 inhibitors might also play a role.

Heart Failure and Sodium–glucose Cotransporter Type-2 inhibitors

The benefit of SGLT2 inhibitors in HF is more than could be explained by simple volume depletion and BP control. So several new 'out-of-the-box' hypothesis are being proposed.

Fuel Shift

Sodium–glucose cotransporter type-2 inhibitors result in a shift of metabolism from glucose to fat. This result in increased production of acetyl coenzyme A (coA), which again preferentially tend to go to produce ketone rather than the tricarboxylic acid cycle (TCA cycle) in view of higher glucagon levels produced by the drug. The resultant low-level ketosis acts as a new energy substrate for the mitochondria of the failing myocardium. This may be an explanation for improvement of myocardial energetics.[13]

Uric Acid

Sodium–glucose cotransporter type-2 inhibitors tend to lower serum uric acid levels, which might be beneficial for a better CV outcome since uric acid tertiles have been clearly linked to the prognosis of CV disease.[14]

Increased glucagon, decreased sodium, and reduced central aortic pressure may be responsible for reduced myocardial fibrosis, improved diastolic function, and better outcome. [15]

CONCLUSION

A failing heart in diabetes is a bad combination; the thrust lies in SGLT2 inhibitors bring about a new promise in the prevention and treatment of HF in diabetes.

REFERENCES

1. Dei Cas A, Khan SS, Butler J, et al. Impact of diabetes on epidemiology, treatment outcome of patients with heart failure. JACC Heart failure. 2015;3(2):136-45.
2. Bain S, Druyts E, Balijepalli C, et al. Cardiovascular events and all-cause mortality associated with sulphonylureas compared with other antihyperglycemic drugs: a Bayesian meta-analysis of survival data. Diabetes Obes Metab. 2017;19(3):329-35.
3. Nissen SE, Wolski K. Effect of rosiglitazone on the risk of myocardial infarction and death from cardiovascular causes. N Eng J Med. 2007;356(24):2457-71.
4. Scirica BM, Bhatt DL, Braunwald E. SAVOR-TIMI 53 steering committee and investigators. Saxagliptin and cardiovascular outcomes in patients with type 2 diabetes mellitus. N Eng J Med. 2013;369(14):1317-26.
5. White WP, Canon CP, Heller SR, et al. EXAMINE investigators. Alogliptin after acute coronary syndrome in patients with type 2 diabetes. N Eng J Med. 2013;369(14):1327-35.
6. Green JB, Bethel MA, Armstrong PW, et al. TECOS study group. Effect of sitagliptin on cardiovascular outcomes in type 2 diabetes. N Eng J Med. 2015;373(3):232-42.
7. List JF, Woo V, Morales E, et al. Sodium-glucose cotransport inhibition with dapagliflozin in type 2 diabetes. Diabetes Care. 2009;32(4):650-7.
8. Baker WL, Smyth LR, Riche DM, et al. Effects of sodium- glucose co-transporter 2 inhibitors on blood pressure: a systematic review and meta-analysis. J Am Soc Hypertens. 2014;8(4):262-75.
9. Zinman B, Wanner C, Lachin JM, et al. EMPA-REG OUTCOME investigators. Empagliflozin cardiovascular outcome and mortality in type 2 diabetes. N Eng J Med. 2015;373(22):2117-28.
10. Neal B, Perkovic V, Mahaffey KW, et al. CANVAS colloborators group. Canagliflozin and cardiovascular and renal events in type 2 diabetes. N Engl J Med. 2017;377(7):644-57.
11. Marso SP, Daniels GH, brown-Frandsen K, et al. LEADER steering committee on behalf of the LEADER investigators. Liraglutide and cardiovascular outcomes in type 2 diabetes. N Eng J Med. 2016;375(4):311-25.
12. Marso SP, Bain SC, Consoli A, et al. SUSTAIN-6 investigators. Semaglutide and cardiovascular outcomes in type 2 diabetes. N Eng J Med. 2016;375(19):1834-44.
13. Ferannini E, Muscelli E, Frascerra S, et al. Metabolic response to sodium glucose cotransporter 2 inhibition in type 2 diabetes patients. J Clin Invest. 2014;124(2):499-508.
14. Odden MC, Amadu AR, Smit E, et al. Uric acid levels, kidney function, and cardiovascular mortality in US adults: national health and Nutrition Examination Survey (NHANES) 1988-1994 and 1999-2002. Am J Kidney Ds. 2014;64(4):550-7.
15. Bonner C, Kerr-Conte J, Gymr V, et al. Inhibition of glucose transporter SGLT2 with dapagliflozin in pancreatic alpha cells triggers glucagon secretion. Nat Med. 2015;21(5):512-7.

CHAPTER

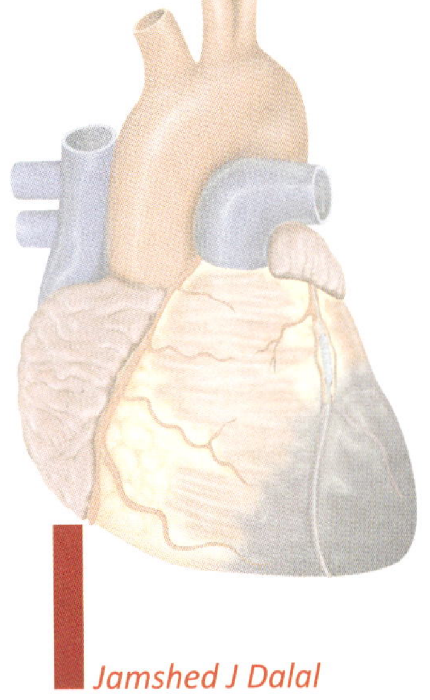

Bisoprolol: Is It Superior in Cardiodiabetes?

Jamshed J Dalal

INTRODUCTION

Abundant evidence is present that patients with type 1 diabetes or type 2 diabetes are at a high-risk for several cardiovascular disorders (CVDs): coronary heart disease, stroke, peripheral arterial disease, cardiomyopathy, and congestive heart failure (HF), and diabetes have long been recognized to be an independent risk factors for CVD. Prospective studies, such as the Framingham, Honolulu, and San Antonio Heart Studies, as well as numerous more recent population studies in the United States and other countries, have documented the excess CVD risk in patients with diabetes from multiple racial and ethnic groups. Several explanations are behind this increase. First, the incidence of diabetes rises with advancing age, and the number of older people in the world is growing rapidly. Second, insulin and other modern treatment for patients with type 1 diabetes has prolonged their lives significantly, and with each year of additional life comes an increased risk for CVD complications. Third, type 2 diabetes occurs at an earlier age in obese and overweight persons, and the prevalence of obesity is rising in the United States.[1] Patients with diabetes mellitus type 2 (DM-2) with hypertension have an increased sympathetic activity and cardiovascular risk profile[2] and in association with metabolic syndrome, is associated with poor outcomes after acute coronary syndromes (ACS), including an increased in-hospital death rate and progression to more severe HF.[3,4] Blood pressure-lowering trials, such as the Systolic Hypertension in the Elderly Program (SHEP) and the United Kingdom Prospective Diabetes Study (UKPDS), likewise have shown a reduction in cardiovascular events in patients with diabetes comparable to benefits found in those without diabetes. The Diabetes Control and Complication Trial (DCCT) showed that improved glycemic control could prevent or reduce microvascular disease and may reduce macrovascular disease in patients with type 1 diabetes.[1]

BETA-BLOCKERS IN CARDIOVASCULAR DISEASE

Beta-blockers (BBs) are a multiform group of drugs with multiple applications in the treatment of patients with cardiovascular disease. They are used in a variety of cardiac diseases (arterial hypertension, coronary artery disease, HF, cardiomyopathies, and arrhythmias) and it is worth emphasizing that their use has improved the survival of the patients with cardiovascular diseases.[5]According to the current literature review and guidelines, BBs are not the first line agents for the treatment of hypertension. As per the Joint National Committee (JNC 8) report, they are the reserve drugs for the management of hypertension postmyocardial infarction (MI) and congestive HF.[6] Despite controversy, BBs still have an important place in the management of hypertension[7] for certain patient populations, especially those with comorbid conditions such as coronary heart disease, recent history of MI, arrhythmia, atrial fibrillation, chronic stable HF, resistant hypertension, thyrotoxicosis, migraine, and essential tremors.[8-10] BBs may be a valuable option for treatment of hypertension in patients with these comorbidities.

A large study in treatment of naïve hypertensive patients without hypertension-related complication treated with BB monotherapy showed better treatment persistence in nonatenolol group compared to atenolol. The patients treated with atenolol had earlier treatment discontinuation whereas new BBs had lower risk of treatment discontinuation as compared with atenolol. Betaxolol, which is no longer used, performed poorer compared to atenolol in terms of risk of discontinuation.[11] BBs can reduce cardiovascular mortality in patients with renal disease. Moreover, they also have renal benefits; which could be important in patients with chronic renal disease. Recently, it has been shown that BBs may reduce or prevent progression of renal impairment in people having hypertension, diabetes, and renovascular disease possibly because of reduced renal oxygen consumption.[12] BBs are the first-line of treatment in secondary prevention after an acute MI (AMI).[13] The use of BBs in patients with ST-segment elevation MI (STEMI) is recommended in all the major guidelines. The use of BBs for secondary prevention post-STEMI is recommended as class IIa by the European Society of Cardiology (ESC) guidelines, and as class Ib by the American College of Cardiology Foundation/American Heart Association (ACCF/AHA) guidelines regardless of the method of reperfusion. In patients with HF or left ventricular (LV) dysfunction, the recommendation to use BBs is listed in class Ia. Oral BB therapy should be initiated in the first 24 hours for patients as recommended by these guidelines. Further, BBs should be continued during and after hospitalization for all patients with STEMI and with no contraindications to their use (level of evidence: B). During the past two decades, based on impressive RCT data, BBs have become one of the most important pharmacological treatments for improving the CV prognosis for patients with systolic HF.[1]

Recently, completed retrospective analyses of subgroups of patients from several large landmark HF trials, such as Metoprolol CR/XL Randomized Intervention Trial in Congestive HF (MERIT-HF), Cardiac Insufficiency Bisoprolol Study II (CIBIS-II), and the Carvedilol Prospective Randomized Cumulative Survival (COPERNICUS) trial,[14] have established the beneficial effects of BBs in diabetic patients with HF. BBs are as beneficial and well-tolerated in patients with HF and diabetes as they are in those without diabetes. These observations strongly support a role for the use of BBs in patients with both HF and diabetes.

Concern of Beta-blockers in Cardiovascular Disease in Diabetes Patients

The risk of development of new-onset DM with BBs was assessed in a systematic review.[15] This review included 12 studies with a total of 94,492 participants and found that there was a 22% increase in the risk of development of new-onset DM with BB therapy as compared with nondiuretic antihypertensive (anti-HTN) therapy [relative risk (RR) = 1.22, 95% confidence interval (CI) 1.12–1.33]. There was also an increased risk of DM with BB therapy as compared with placebo (fixed-effects model: 33% increase, RR = 1.33, 95% CI 1.00–1.76, p = 0.05; random-effects model: 44% increase, RR = 1.44, 95% CI 0.69–3.00, p = 0.33; heterogeneity χ^2-6.18, p = 0.013). The risk of DM, death, and stroke is, therefore, increased by BB therapy as compared with other nondiuretic anti-HTN drugs and this effect was more pronounced with atenolol therapy.[16] One of the anxieties associated with the primary use of BBs is the concern about adverse metabolic effects, such as unfavorable effects on lipids or insulin sensitivity and a propensity to cause weight gain in some patients.[17-19] However, studies have shed a light on these issues and also described the common reasons for withholding BBs from diabetic patients. Hypoglycemia, which is thought to be obscured by BBs, is touted as the common reason. However, cardioselective BBs have neither been found to prolong hypoglycemia nor interfere with glucagon and adrenaline-mediated recovery.[20,21] Other studies also did not find an association between use of BB therapy in diabetic patients and an increased risk of hospitalization or serious hypoglycemia.[22,23] Thus, it is important to note that not only the efficacy, but β-1 selectivity also affects the safety profile. Using a highly selective β-1 agent leads to avoidance of metabolic disturbance involving blood sugar, glycated hemoglobin (HbA1C), insulin sensitivity, free fatty acids, plasma triglycerides, very low-density lipoproteins, and high-density lipoproteins.[24]

BISOPROLOL

Benefits of β-1 Selectivity

An important point to consider is that β-1 selectivity varies with different drugs and the higher the β-1 selectivity, better the blood pressure control. Considering propranolol (which blocks β-1 and β-2 receptors equally) and taking it as a reference, the β-1 selectivity is highest for bisoprolol followed by atenolol and metoprolol.[25] In other words, highly β-1 selective bisoprolol even if given at the relatively low dosage would effectively block majority of β-1 receptors.[26] Bisoprolol does not possess intrinsic sympathomimetic activity (ISA) and membrane-stabilizing effects. It was noted to have minimal effects on glucose tolerance and plasma lipid profiles.[27] Using a highly selective β-1 agent may lead to avoidance of metabolic disturbance involving blood sugar, HbA1C, insulin sensitivity, free fatty acids, plasma triglycerides, very low-density lipoproteins, and high-density lipoproteins.[24] In some earlier studies done to investigate the common adverse event of sexual dysfunction associated with BB therapy, newly diagnosed men with hypertension as well as those already taking hypertensives were administered bisoprolol and extensively studied for sexual parameters like firmness of erection during coitus, centeredness with sexual functioning and satisfaction with sexuality. It was observed that bisoprolol did not have any detrimental effect on these sexual parameters, and in the group of patients shifted to bisoprolol from other antihypertensive medication.[24] A long elimination half-life of 10–14 hours makes bisoprolol an ideal choice for once-a-day administration.[28] Bisoprolol does not occupy β-2-adrenoreceptors, even at peak plasma levels, 2–3 hours after its administration within a dose range of 5–10 mg and once a day dosage regimen. [26]

Role of Bisoprolol in Cardiovascular Disease

Hypertension

Wang B et al. study showed that bisoprolol when compared with captopril appears to be a beta-1 selective blocker possessing a satisfactory antihypertensive effect without any adverse effects on glucose metabolism and is, therefore, a choice for treating hypertensive patients with type 2 diabetes mellitus (T2DM).[29] In a randomized controlled trial (RCT), that compared bisoprolol and atenolol, it was found that bisoprolol at lower doses was significantly effective at lowering diastolic blood pressure throughout the day (–11.6 vs –8.7 mm Hg).[30] Channaraya et al. conducted an open label, multicenter observational study on 2,418 patients to evaluate the efficacy and tolerability of a bisoprolol as a first-line antihypertensive in Indian patients diagnosed with essential hypertension (BRIGHT). They found bisoprolol as an effective and safe option for controlling blood pressure up to a dose of 10 mg/day.[31] The CREATIVE study concluded that bisoprolol provided superior dynamic heart rate (HR) reduction in the last 4 hours of the treatment period and noninferior dynamic blood pressure reduction versus metoprolol CR/ZOK in patients with mild-to-moderate hypertension.[32]

Heart Failure

The CIBIS-II trial was conducted to assess the effect of BBs on the survival of patients with HF. This study randomized 2,647 patients with congestive heart failure New York Heart Association (CHF NYHA) class III or IV and LV ejection fraction (LVEF) of less than 35% to receive either bisoprolol or placebo in addition to diuretics and angiotensin-converting enzyme (ACE) inhibitors. This study was stopped early because bisoprolol showed a significant reduction in the incidence of all-cause mortality. As compared with the placebo group, the group receiving bisoprolol had significantly lower mortality rates (11.8% versus 17.3%, HR = 0.66, 95% CI 0.54 to 0.81, p <0.0001) and the incidence of SCD was also lower in the bisoprolol group (3.6% versus 6.3%, HR = 0.56, 95% CI 0.39 to 0.80, p = 0.0011). Similarly, CV deaths (p = 0.0049), hospitalizations for any cause (p = 0.0006) and the combined end point of CV death and hospitalization for CV event (p = 0.0004) were also seen more infrequently in the group treated with bisoprolol. Hospitalizations due to ventricular tachycardia (VT) and fibrillation (p = 0.006), and hypotension (p = 0.03) were also less common in the bisoprolol group.[16] Bisoprolol and carvedilol did not worsen glycemic control, lipid profile or albuminuria status in subjects with systolic heart failure (SHF), and T2DM. There was not significant difference between the glycemic control between carvedilol and bisoprolol in subjects with SHF and T2DM. Therefore, BBs should not be withheld from patients with T2DM and SHF.[33] Not only is bisoprolol an effective BB, it has fewer adverse events (AEs) as well when compared with other BBs. In a study of 22 HF patients suffering from dizziness and hypotension, initially on carvedilol therapy; switching to bisoprolol significantly reduced these AEs after 6 months.[34]Marazzi G and colleagues[35] showed that bisoprolol is more effective than carvedilol in reducing atrial fibrillation (AF) after coronary bypass surgery in such patients. In a prospective trial, both drugs were initiated after 4–5 days postsurgery. Bisoprolol was started at the dose of 1.25 mg/day while carvedilol was given as 3.125 mg BD. Bisoprolol group was associated with significantly less incidence of postoperative AF compared to carvedilol (RR 0.6, CI 0.4–0.9, p = 0.032). After 4 weeks, the patients receiving bisoprolol had significantly less HR (p = 0.021) compared to carvedilol, without significant difference in the blood pressure.

Coronary Artery Disease

Total Ischemic Burden Bisoprolol Study (TIBBS) that involved 330 patients with stable angina with ST-segment depression, bisoprolol was observed to be highly effective in suppressing the ischemic episodes over 24-hour period as compared with nifedipine. Bisoprolol significantly reduced the HR at onset of episodes by 13.7 +/– 1.4 beats/min from baseline (99.5 +/– 1.2 beats/min; *p* <0.001). It was further observed that bisoprolol had a distinctive advantage in reducing the ischemic episodes in the vulnerable period between 6:00 am and noon.[36] Highly cardioselective bisoprolol not only alleviates the symptoms but also reduces silent ischemia. When compared with atenolol (100 mg) or verapamil, bisoprolol demonstrated equipotent effect in reducing anginal attack rate and nitroglycerin consumption as well as the rate-pressure product in previous studies.[37-39] In yet another study of patients with chronic obstructive bronchitis, it was found that bisoprolol could be an effective option in treatment of angina pectoris and it did not lead to a clinically significant deterioration of already existing chronic obstructive bronchitis in these patients. Further, there was no significant change observed in parameters like total cholesterol and triglycerides.[40]

CONCLUSION

Diabetes has long been recognized to be an independent risk factor for CVD. BBs have a role in a variety of cardiac diseases such as arterial hypertension, coronary artery disease, HF, cardiomyopathies and arrhythmias, and their use has improved the survival of the patients with cardiovascular diseases. Selection of the right type of BB is important and can have an impact on the overall efficacy and safety. Bisoprolol is β-1 selective BB with no ISA and membrane-stabilizing effects. Bisoprolol also has minimal effects on glucose tolerance and plasma lipid profiles. Efficacy of bisoprolol is proved in various clinical trials for indications such as HF, hypertension, and coronary artery disease. Overall, bisoprolol is very well tolerated without significant serious AEs and may be considered as a preferred BB in patients having cardiovascular disease with diabetes mellitus.

REFERENCES

1. Diabetes mellitus: a major risk factor for cardiovascular disease. A joint editorial statement by the American Diabetes Association; The National Heart, Lung, and Blood Institute; The Juvenile Diabetes Foundation International; The National Institute of Diabetes and Digestive and Kidney Diseases; and The American Heart Association. Circulation. 1999; 100(10):1132-33.
2. Perin PC, Maule S, Quadri R. Sympathetic nervous system, diabetes, and hypertension. Clin Exp Hypertens. 2001;23(1-2):45-55.
3. Zeller M, Steg PG, Ravisy J, et al. Prevalence and impact of metabolic syndrome on hospital outcomes in acute myocardial infarction. Arch Intern Med. 2005;165(10):1192-8.
4. Lee MG, Jeong MH, Ahn Y, et al. Impact of the metabolic syndrome on the clinical outcome of patients with acute ST-elevation myocardial infarction. J Korean Med Sci. 2010;25(10):1456-61.
5. Boudonas GE. β-blockers in coronary artery disease management. Hippokratia. 2010;14(4):231-5.
6. James PA, Oparil S, Carter BL, et al. 2014 evidence-based guideline for the management of high blood pressure in adults: report from the panel members appointed to the Eighth Joint National Committee (JNC 8). JAMA. 2014;311(5):507-20.
7. Mancia G. Prevention of risk factors: beta-blockade and hypertension. Eur Heart J Suppl. 2009;11(Suppl A):A3-A8.
8. Hwang AY, Dave C, Smith SM. Trends in Antihypertensive Medication Use among US Patients with Resistant Hypertension, 2008 to 2014. Hypertension. 2016;68(6):1349-54.
9. Cruickshank JM. Beta-blockers continue to surprise us. Eur Heart J. 2000;21(5):354-64.
10. Larochelle P, Tobe SW, Lacourcière Y. β-blockers in hypertension: studies and meta-analyses over the years. Can J Cardiol. 2014; 30(5 Suppl):S16-22.
11. Choi YJ, Ah YM, Kong J, et al. Implication of different initial beta blockers on treatment persistence: atenolol vs new-generation beta blocker, a population-based study. Cardiovasc Ther. 2016;34(4):268-75.
12. Hall ME, Rocco MV, Morgan TM, et al. Beta-blocker use is associated with higher renal tissue oxygenation in hypertensive patients suspected of renal artery stenosis. Cardiorenal Med. 2016; 6(4):261-8.
13. Freemantle N, Cleland J, Young P, et al. β blockade after myocardial infarction: systematic review and meta regression analysis. BMJ. 1999; 318(7200):1730-7.
14. Parker M, Fowler MB, Roecker EB, et al. Effect of carvedilol on morbidity in patients with severe heart failure: results of the carvedilol prospective randomized cumulative survival (COPERNICUS STUDY). Circulation. 2002;106(17):2194-9.
15. Bangalore S, Parkar S, Grossman E, et al. A meta-analysis of 94,492 patients with hypertension treated with beta blockers to determine the risk of new-onset diabetes mellitus. Am J Cardiol. 2007;100(8):1254-62.
16. DiNicolantonio JJ, Farres H, Niazi AK, et al. β-blockers in hypertension, diabetes, heart failure and acute myocardial infarction: a review of the literature. Open Heart 2015;2(1):e000230.
17. Black HR. Metabolic considerations in the choice of therapy for the patient with hypertension. Am Heart J. 1991;121(2 Pt 2):707-15.
18. Kaplan NM. Effects of antihypertensive therapy on insulin resistance. Hypertension. 1992;19(1 Suppl):I116-8.
19. Rössner S, Taylor CL, Byington RP, et al. Long-term propranolol treatment and changes in body weight after myocardial infarction. BMJ. 1990;300(6729):902-3.
20. Giugliano D, Acampora R, Marfella, R et al. Metabolic and cardiovascular effects of carvedilol and atenolol in non-insulin-dependent diabetes mellitus and hypertension. A randomized, controlled trial. Ann Intern Med. 1997;126(12):955-9.
21. Lager I, Blohme G, Smith U. Effect of cardioselective and non-selective beta-blockade on the hypoglycaemic response in insulin-dependent diabetics. Lancet. 1979;1(8114):458-62.
22. Herings RM, de Boer A, Stricker BH, et al. Hypoglycaemia associated with use of inhibitors of angiotensin-converting enzyme. Lancet. 1995;345(8959):1195-8.
23. Shorr RI, Ray WA, Daugherty JR. Antihypertensives and the risk of serious hypoglycemia in older persons using insulin or sulfonylureas. JAMA. 1997;278(1):40-3.
24. Cruickshank JM. Are we misunderstanding beta-blockers. Int J Cardiol. 2007;120(1):10-27.
25. Wellstein A, Palm D, Belz GG. Affinity and selectivity of beta-adrenoceptor antagonists in vitro. J Cardiovasc Pharmacol. 1986;8 Suppl 11:S36-40.
26. Wellstein A, Palm D, Belz GG et al. Reduction of exercise tachycardia in man after propranolol, atenolol and bisoprolol in comparison to beta-adrenoceptor occupancy. Eur Heart J. 1987;8 Suppl M:3-8.
27. Johns TE, Lopez LM. Bisoprolol: is this just another beta-blocker for hypertension or angina? Ann Pharmacother. 1995;29(4):403-14.
28. Leopold G, Ungethum W, Pabst J, et al. Pharmacodynamic profile of bisoprolol, a new beta. 1 selective adrenoceptor antagonist. British Journal of Clinical Pharmacology. 1986;22(3):293-300.
29. Wang B, Song WH, Liu GZ. Multi-center Cooperation Group of Bisoprolol. The effect long-term administration of a selective beta. 1 blocker bisoprolol on glucose metabolism in patients with essential hypertensive and type 2 diabetes mellitus. Zhonghua Nei Ke Za Zhi. 2005; 44(7):503-5.
30. Neutel JM, Smith DH, Ram CV, et al. Application of ambulatory blood pressure monitoring in differentiating between antihypertensive agents. Am J Med. 1993;94(2):181-7.

31. Channaraya V, Marya RK, Somasundaram M, et al. Efficacy and tolerability of a beta-1 selective beta blocker, bisoprolol, as a first-line antihypertensive in Indian patients diagnosed with essential hypertension (BRIGHT): an open-label, multicentric observational study. BMJ Open. 2012;2(3).
32. Yang T, Jiang Y, Hao Y, et al. Comparison of bisoprolol to a metoprolol CR/ZOK tablet for control of heart rate and blood pressure in mild-to-moderate hypertensive patients: the CREATIVE study. Hypertens Res. 2017;40(1):79-86.
33. Wai B, Kearney LG, Hare DL, et al. Beta blocker use in subjects with type 2 diabetes mellitus and systolic heart failure does not worsen glycaemic control. Cardiovasc Diabetol. 2012;11:14.
34. Taniguchi T, Ohtani T, Mizote I, et al. Switching from carvedilol to bisoprolol ameliorates adverse effects in heart failure patients with dizziness or hypotension. J Cardiol. 2013;61(6):417-22.
35. Marazzi G, Iellamo F, Volterrani M, et al. Comparison of effectiveness of carvedilol versus bisoprolol for prevention of postdischarge atrial fibrillationafter coronary artery bypass grafting in patients with heart failure. Am J Cardiol. 2011;107(2):215-9.
36. von Arnim T. Medical treatment to reduce total ischemic burden: total ischemic burden bisoprolol study (TIBBS), a multicenter trial comparing bisoprolol and nifedipine. The TIBBS Investigators. J Am Coll Cardiol. 1995;25(1):231-8.
37. Kohli RS, Khurmi NS, Kardash MM, et al. Efficacy of once daily bisoprolol in stable angina pectoris: an objective comparison with atenolol and long-term follow-up. Eur Heart J. 1985;6(10):845-50.
38. Maltz MB, Dymond DS, Nathan AW, et al. A comparison of once daily bisoprolol, 5 and 10 mg, and atenolol 100 mg in the treatment of angina pectoris. Eur Heart J. 1987;8 Suppl M:37-42.
39. De Divitiis O, Liguori V, Di Somma S, et al. Bisoprolol in the treatment of angina pectoris: a double blind comparison with verapamil. Eur Heart J. 1987;8 Suppl M:43-54.
40. Dorow P, Thalhofer S, Bethge H, et al. Long-term treatment of angina pectoris with bisoprolol or atenolol in patients with chronic obstructive bronchitis: a randomized, double-blind crossover study. J Cardiovasc Pharmacol. 1990;16 Suppl 5:S36-44.

CHAPTER

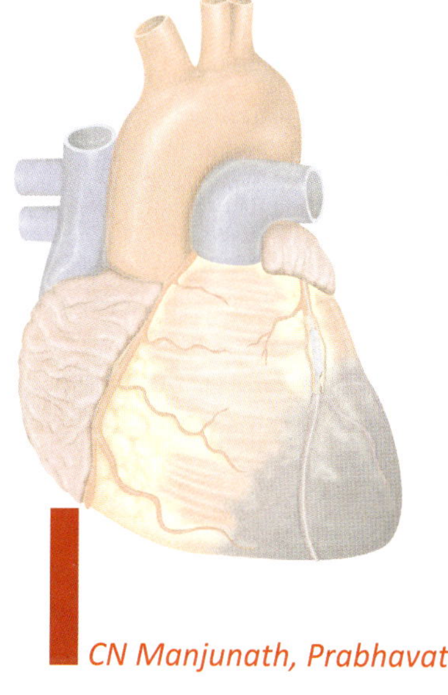

Bisoprolol: A Choice of Beta Blocker in Hypertension and ACS in Cardiodiabetes

CN Manjunath, Prabhavathi

INTRODUCTION

Beta blocker therapy is recommended as part of the emergency treatment of suspected acute coronary syndrome (ACS), especially if the patient has tachycardia or hypertension.[1] The benefit is even more in patients with left ventricular (LV) dysfunction. Hypertension guidelines recommend use of beta blockers in hypertension with compelling indications, such as heart failure, postmyocardial infarction (MI), high-risk for coronary disease, and diabetes.[2] However, their usage has been limited in patients with diabetes. The patients with diabetes have been largely excluded from trials where beta blockers demonstrated efficacy and safety.[2,3]

REASONS FOR UNDERUTILIZATION OF BETA BLOCKERS IN DIABETES

- *Adverse metabolic effects:* One of the myths associated with the use of beta blockers is the concern about its unfavorable effects on lipids, insulin sensitivity, and propensity to cause weight gain.[4-6] All these are largely overcome by highly beta-1 selective beta blocker bisoprolol.
- *Hypoglycemia* was thought to be obscured and prolonged by beta blockers. However, cardioselective beta blockers have neither been found to prolong hypoglycemia nor to interfere with glucagon and adrenaline-mediated recovery.[7,8]
- *Increased insulin resistance* remains a questionable clinical issue. But the United Kingdom Prospective Diabetes Study (UKPDS) found no difference in glycated hemoglobin (HbA1c) levels with atenolol and captopril after 9 years. However, atenolol group required an additional hypoglycemic medication.[9]

A review article, which discussed all these issues, concluded that β-blockers are not contraindicated in patients with diabetes.[10] In fact, one of the largest studies, Systolic Hypertension in the Elderly Program (SHEP) study with a follow-up of 14 years observed that beta blocker therapy did not harm patients as compared to naturally occurring diabetes. Study further suggested that, a beta blocker without intrinsic sympathomimetic activity (ISA) or alpha blocking activity like low-dose bisoprolol should be used.[11] Beta blockers, particularly atenolol, is not considered as the first-line agent for treatment of hypertension in the absence of compelling indications. This is based on the fact that stroke reduction is lesser in patients on atenolol. An explanation is the absence of reduction of central aortic pressure with atenolol. A registry looking at the differential effect of atenolol in different age groups showed that this effect was more important in the elderly but not in the younger patients. Since most of the studies were done with atenolol, we do not have much data on beta blockers like bisoprolol, which is highly cardioselective and does have an effect on reducing central aortic pressure.[12]

BISOPROLOL

Bisoprolol is a highly selective beta-1 adrenoceptor antagonist. It has no partial agonist (intrinsic sympathomimetic) activity or membrane stabilizing (local anesthetic) activity. Oral bioavailability of bisoprolol is high (90%) and the drug has a long elimination half-life of 10–12 hours, which allows once daily administration. In addition, it is hepatically and renally cleared in equal proportions. In noncomparative studies and comparative trials, bisoprolol proved effective and as efficacious as atenolol, low doses of metoprolol, diuretics, and nifedipine SR in hypertension. Bisoprolol is well tolerated in most patients.[13] It is approved by the US Food and Drug Administration (FDA) in 1992.[14] It is also listed as an essential cardiovascular medicine in the World Health Organization (WHO) model list of essential medicines.[15]

Absence of ISA and the potent inhibition of chronic beta-1 stimulation induced myocardial apoptosis or necrosis or inflammation are the invaluable features of bisoprolol. It can be safely used in young and elderly patients with heart failure as it does not cause the harmful effects of beta-2 blockade and alpha-1 blockade.[16] Highly selective beta-1 blockade of bisoprolol also renders it a powerful antisupraventricular and ventricular arrhythmic agent. Bisoprolol does not occupy beta-2 receptors even at peak plasma levels at 2–3 hours within a dose range of 5–10 mg.[17] Bisoprolol has been shown to be effective and safe in a wide spectrum of cardiovascular disorders.[18]

Bisoprolol: A Beta Blocker of Choice

Bisoprolol has shown to have several advantages over other beta blockers (Box 1). Highly beta-1 selective bisoprolol has shown to reduce blood pressure with a single dose. It was noted to have minimal effects on glucose tolerance and plasma lipid profiles.[19] Studies have shown bisoprolol to be 5–10 times more potent than propranolol, atenolol, and metoprolol, in reducing exercise-induced tachycardia. In a randomized control trial that compared bisoprolol and atenolol, it was found that bisoprolol at lower doses was significantly effective at lowering diastolic blood pressure throughout the day.[20]

In an open-label, multicenter observational study on 2,418 patients to evaluate the efficacy and tolerability of bisoprolol as first-line antihypertensive in Indian patients diagnosed with essential hypertension (BRIGHT), bisoprolol was found to be effective and safe up to a dose of 10 mg/day.[21] In another study, use of bisoprolol was shown to avoid any metabolic disturbances involving blood sugar, insulin sensitivity, free fatty acids, plasma triglycerides (TGL), and high-density lipoproteins (HDL).[21] A study that compared five different beta blockers showed that bisoprolol had no significant effect on TGL and HDL-cholesterol (HDL-C).[21] Unlike other beta blockers, bisoprolol does not cause sexual dysfunction.[22]

BOX 1: Advantages of bisoprolol

- Highest β-1 selectivity
- No ISA and membrane stabilizing activity
- Highly effective in reducing exercise-induced tachycardia
- Minimal effect on plasma lipid profile
- No significant effect on parameters of glucose metabolism
- No bronchoconstriction in 5–10 mg/day dosage
- No sexual dysfunction

Abbreviation: ISA, intrinsic sympathomimetic activity.

Bisoprolol has been found to be beneficial in treatment of angina pectoris in patients with chronic obstructive bronchitis without an increased risk of clinically significant deterioration. Bisoprolol also causes lesser bronchospasm in ischemic patients with obstructive airway disease as compared to atenolol.[23] Bisoprolol has fewer adverse effects. In a study of 22 heart failure patients suffering from dizziness and hypotension initially on carvedilol, switching to bisoprolol significantly reduced these side effects after 6 months.[24] The usual oral dose of bisoprolol in mild to moderate essential hypertension or stable angina pectoris is 10 mg once daily with a maximum recommended dose of 20 mg/day. In some patients, 5 mg/day may be adequate. However, in end-stage renal or hepatic insufficiency, dosage should not exceed 10 mg once daily.

Bisoprolol in Postmyocardial Infarction Patients

In post-MI patients, bisoprolol is the preferred beta blocker with high efficacy and safety profile. A comparative study between bisoprolol and metoprolol succinate in 6,349 patients with heart failure showed no significant differences in all-cause mortality and/or cardiovascular mortality.[25] In another study, bisoprolol was compared with atenolol in patients with acute MI. Bisoprolol was found to be safe, effective and well tolerated.[26] In a retrospective survival analysis of patients from the database of the Lower Austrian MI Network that recommended use of bisoprolol in patients with MI, it was found that after a follow-up duration of 31 months, the probability of a fatal event was higher (19.2%) in the patients who were given bisoprolol late in the course of treatment as compared with those who were given bisoprolol immediately (10.7%). This was maintained at 30 days and 1 year.[27] In a prospective nonrandomized observational study in patients with ST-segment elevation MI (STEMI) undergoing emergent percutaneous coronary intervention (PCI), 343 patients received immediate (within 30 minutes) oral bisoprolol 2.5 mg and 321 patients received delayed (> 24 hours) bisoprolol. Immediate bisoprolol group had a significant reduction in all-cause mortality at 30 days and in 1 year. In the multivariate analysis, immediate bisoprolol administration was independently associated with reduction in all-cause mortality.[27]

BETA BLOCKERS AND DIABETICS WITH OVERT CORONARY ARTERY DISEASE

Beta blockers have powerful anti-ischemic properties, which are significantly superior to those of dihydropyridine, calcium antagonists, and resulting in an improved prognosis.[28] In the Bezafibrate Infarction Prevention Study,[29] 19% of the 14,417 recruits had type 2 diabetes of which one-third received beta blockers. Over 3 years, the diabetics who received beta blockers experienced a 42% increase in survival compared to the nonbeta blocker group. A meta-analysis of randomized, controlled post-MI studies[30] revealed that chronic beta-blockade was associated with an impressive 48% reduction in mortality in diabetics compared to 33% in nondiabetics (Fig. 1).

Beta Blockers and Diabetics with Hypertension

Unlike diuretics, calcium antagonists, and angiotensin-converting enzyme (ACE) inhibitors, there are no prospective, randomized, placebo-controlled mortality trials in hypertensives involving diabetics who received beta blockers. A study which came close to this was the Standardized Treatment of Pulmonary Exacerbations II (STOP2) study[31] in the elderly wherein 719 hypertensive diabetics, so called conventional therapy (an unspecified mix of diuretics and beta blockers given as first-line therapy), did not differ from ACE inhibitors or calcium antagonists in preventing cardiovascular event.

There are, however, two classic prospective, randomized, comparative studies involving atenolol, namely the UKPDS study[9,32] comparing atenolol and the ACE inhibitor captopril, and the Losartan Intervention For Endpoint reduction (LIFE) study[33,34] comparing atenolol and the angiotensin-II type 1-receptor antagonist losartan.

In UKPDS study, 1,148 mild-to-moderate hypertensive patients with type 2 diabetes, mean age 56 years, were randomly allocated to either 'less tight' or 'tight', control of blood pressure. The tight control group was further randomly allocated to receive either captopril or atenolol as first-line therapy. After a mean of 8.4 years follow-up the blood pressure was 10/5 mm Hg lower in the tight control group. All seven primary clinical endpoints were less frequent in the tight control group, achieving significance for any diabetes-related endpoint, deaths related to diabetes, stroke, and microvascular disease. The major surprise, however, was that the ACE inhibitor was not superior to the beta-blocker in reducing either primary or secondary clinical endpoints. The blood pressure at baseline and after 9 years of follow-up was the same in both drug groups. Although, no significant differences existed between the two drugs the trends of all 7 primary endpoints (i.e. any diabetes endpoint, deaths related to diabetes, all-cause mortality, MI, stroke, peripheral vascular disease and microvascular disease) favored the beta blocker (Fig. 2).

Also a large majority of the secondary endpoints showed trends favoring the beta blocker. Beta-1 blockade was atleast as 'renoprotective' as ACE inhibition in the UKPDS study. At baseline, 20% of patients assigned to atenolol and 16% of those assigned to captopril had albuminuria (>50 mg/L). After 9 years, the proportions were 26% and 31% respectively, and there was no difference

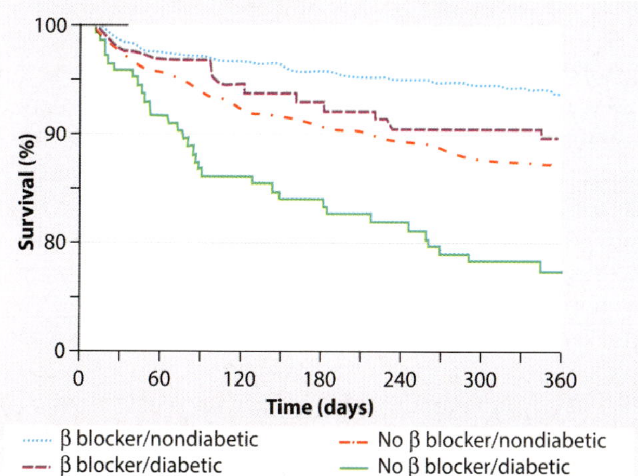

Fig. 1: Beta blockers markedly improve one-year survival of postmyocardial infarction patients with diabetes.[29]

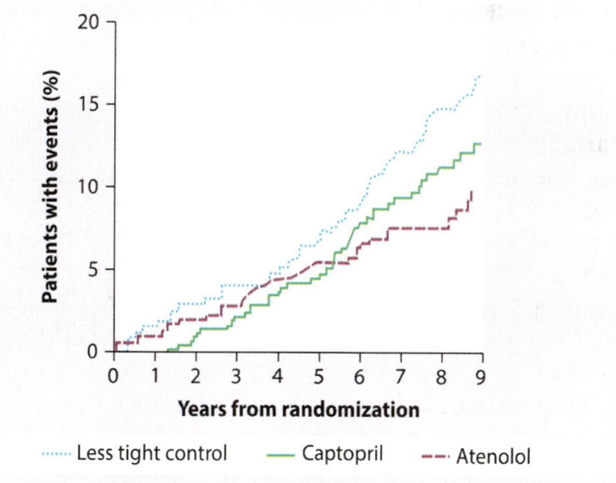

Fig. 2: UKPDS 39—over a 9-year period atenolol was atleast as effective as captopril in preventing deaths due to diabetes (with permission[59]). Kaplan–Meier plots of patients who died of disease related to diabetes (myocardial infarction, sudden death, stroke, peripheral vascular disease, and renal failure).

Abbreviation: UKPDS, United Kingdom Prospective Diabetes Study.

in the plasma creatinine concentration (or in those who had more than a two-fold increase in plasma creatinine concentration between the atenolol and captopril groups). Noncompliance was slightly worse on atenolol due to cold feet (4%) and bronchospasm (6%).

Why Type 2 Diabetes is Associated with Higher Cardiovascular Risk?

High insulin levels (as occur in type 2 diabetes) result in increased sympathetic nervous activity via mainly central (brain) stimulation. Sustained increased sympathetic nervous activity, including at night, has been linked to poor cardiovascular outcome. Noradrenaline has been shown to (1) lower the threshold to lethal ventricular arrhythmias thus increasing the risk of sudden death, (2) cause myocardial myocyte necrosis, apoptosis, arterial wall damage which predisposes to atheroma and local hemodynamic changes which could increase the likelihood of atheromatous plaque rupture, (3) cause high blood pressure, particularly at night (nondipping), and (4) to stimulate renin release from the kidney leading on to angiotensin II formation; angiotensin II not only increases intraglomerular pressure and predisposes to nephropathy but also stimulates centrally noradrenaline release from peripheral nerve endings, particularly within the heart—thus a vicious cycle between high noradrenaline and angiotensin II activity is setup.[35]

How Beta-1 Blockade Reduces This Risk?

Beta-1 blockade might be expected to inhibit the above harmful actions of sustained high noradrenaline activity. Certainly, beta-1 selective blockade inhibits lethal ventricular arrhythmias and normalizes low heart rate variability (reflecting high sympathetic tone), which predisposes to ventricular arrhythmias and sudden death. Beta-1 selective blockade also effectively (compared to a calcium antagonist) reduces circumferential coronary artery wall stress and thus diminishes the risk of plaque rupture. Beta blockade inhibits catecholamine-induced vascular necrosis and slows the progression of atheroma in a man. Beta-1 selective blockade inhibits catecholamine-induced cardiac myocyte necrosis in a man and apoptosis in animals. Even angiotensin II-induced myocardial and vascular damage is largely inhibited by beta blockade.[35]

Is the Choice of Beta blocker Important?

The answer is yes, in terms of both safety and efficacy in lowering blood pressure. For optimal efficacy and safety, selective blocking of the beta-1 receptor appears to be the crucial factor, avoiding blocking of the beta-2 receptor. Beta blockers that also possess alpha blocking activity, e.g. nonselective labetalol and carvedilol, can cause, in some patients. Symptomatic postural hypotension, particularly after exercise.

Degree of Beta-1 Selectivity

Beta-1 selectivity is not an absolute property and some agents are more selective than others. In relation to propranolol (which blocks beta-1 and -2 receptors equally), the hierarchy of beta-1 selectivity of some commonly used agents, in ascending order, is metoprolol, atenolol, and bisoprolol.[35] A recent direct comparison, involving human tissue, between bisoprolol and nebivolol,[35] revealed that bisoprolol was 4–5 times more beta-1 selective than nebivolol. It is worth remembering that beta-1 selectivity is dose-dependent, so that low doses should be given to patients susceptible to beta-2 blockade. Thus, highly beta-1 selective bisoprolol given at the relatively low dosage of 5–10 mg occupies 30–80% of beta-1 receptors with zero occupancy of beta-2 receptors.[36,37]

A large randomized study comparing moderately beta-1 selective atenolol 50–100 mg/day with highly beta-1 selective bisoprolol 10–20 mg/day revealed that in 203 patients who underwent 24-hour blood pressure recording, bisoprolol was significantly more effective in lowering diastolic blood pressure throughout the whole day (–11.6 versus –8.7 mm Hg) and both systolic and diastolic blood pressure (–14.2/–11.5 versus –9.9/–7.7 mm Hg) during the 'vulnerable' period from 6.00 am to noon (Figs 3A and B).[20]

CONCLUSION

Prevalence of type 2 diabetes is increasing steeply, due to lifestyle factors, like obesity and physical inactivity. Type 2 diabetes is associated with a clustering of coronary risk factors and 60–80% of patients have hypertension so that the risk of a premature cardiovascular event or death is increased 4–5 fold. Oral beta blockers are cornerstone in the treatment of patients with ACS. ACS is frequent in patients with type 2 diabetes. Beta blocker use is even more important in this group of patients. They have additional benefit of reducing morbidity and mortality in patients with reduced LV function or heart failure. Beta blockade is atleast as effective as 'favored' ACE inhibition in the prevention of both macrovascular and microvascular events in young and middle-aged hypertensive diabetics. Selection of the right type of beta blocker is important. Drugs with high beta-1 selectivity like bisoprolol will ensure optimal lowering of blood pressure, including central blood pressure. It will also reduce the risk of potentially dangerous adverse events arising from blockade of the

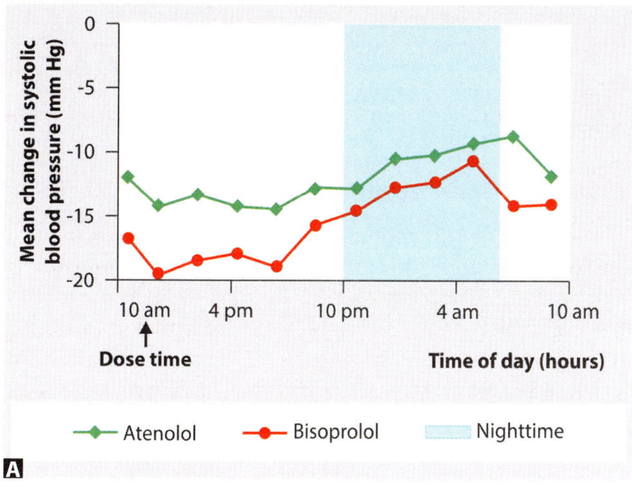

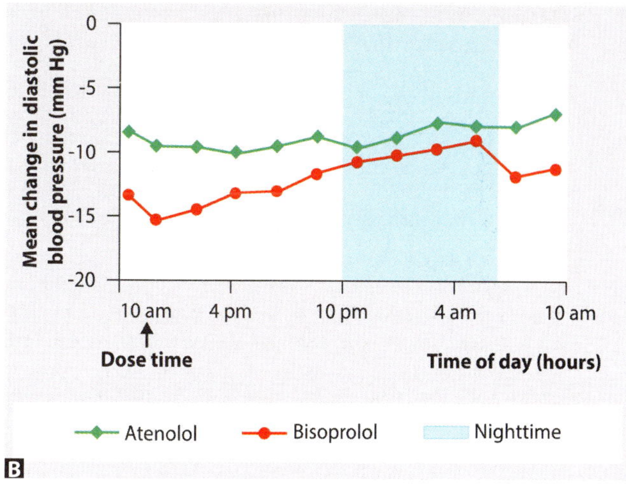

Figs 3A and B: Control of 24-hour blood pressure by atenolol and bisoprolol, randomized study in 203 hypertensives. (A) Systolic blood pressure. (B) Diastolic blood pressure. Atenolol dose = 50–100 mg/day and bisoprolol dose = 10–20 mg/day; * $p < 0.05$; ** $p < 0.01$.

beta-2 receptor like bronchospasm and metabolic effects on lipids and sugar. Recent importance of heart rate control in reducing mortality further emphasizes the need for use of bisoprolol. Beta blockers are class effect. All cardioselective beta blockers are beneficial. Bisoprolol being highly beta-1 selective is preferred. Beta blockers are still significantly underprescribed to post-MI diabetics and hypertensive diabetics. Comprehensive education programs are required to change these practices.

REFERENCES

1. Roffi M, Patrono C, Collet JP, et al. 2015 ESC Guidelines for the management of acute coronary syndromes in patients presenting without persistent ST-segment elevation: Task Force for the Management of Acute Coronary Syndromes in Patients Presenting without Persistent ST-segment Elevation of the European Society of Cardiology (ESC). Eur Heart J. 2016;37(3): 267-315.
2. Statement on hypertension in diabetes mellitus. Final report. The Working Group on Hypertension in Diabetes. Archives of Internal Medicine. 1987:147(5):830-42.
3. Psaty BM, Smith NL, Siscovick DS, et al. Health outcomes associated with antihypertensive therapies used as first-line agent. A systemic review and meta-analysis. JAMA. 1997:227(9):739-45.
4. Black HR. Metabolic consideration in the choice of therapy for the patient with hypertension. Am Heart J. 1991;121(2Pt2):707-15.
5. Kaplan NM. Effects of antihypertensive therapy on insulin resistance. Hypertension. 1992;19(1 Suppl):1116-8.
6. Rossner S, Taylor CL, Byington RP, et al. Long-term propronol treatment and changes in body weight after myocardial infarction. BMJ.1990;300(6729):902-3.
7. Guigliano D, Acampora R, Marfella Ra, et al. Metabolic and cardiovascular effects of carvedilol and atenolol in noninsulin-dependent diabetes mellitus and hypertension. A randomized, controlled trial. Ann Intern Med. 1997;126(12):955-9.
8. Lager I, Blohme G, Smith U. Effect of cardioselective and nonselective beta-blockade on the hypoglycaemic response in insulin-dependent diabetics. Lancet. 1979;1(8114);458-62.
9. Tight blood pressure control and risk of macrovscular and microvascular complication in type 2 diabetes: UKPDS 38. UK prospective Diabetes study group. BMJ. 1998;317(7160):703-13.
10. Majumdar SR. Beta blockers for the treatment of hypertension in patients with diabetes: exploring the contraindication myth. Cardiovasc Drugs Ther. 1999;13(5):435-9.
11. Kostis JB, Wilson AC, Freudenberger RS, et al. Long-term effect of diuretic-based therapy on fatal outcomes in subjects with isolated systolic hypertension with and without diabetes. Am J Cardiol. 2005;95(1):29-35.
12. Dalal JJ. Bisoprolol: A beta blocker of choice in hypertension with metabolic syndrome during an ACS. STEMI—A Cardiology update 2016.
13. Simon G. Lancaster, Eugene M. Bisoprolol: A Preliminary Review of its Pharmacodynamic and Pharmacokinetic Properties, and Therapeutic Efficacy in Hypertension and Angina Pectoris. Drugs.1988;36:256-85.
14. Official FDA information. Bisoprolol side effects and uses. [online] Available from: http://www.drugs.com/pro/bisoprolol.html [Accessed September 2017].
15. WHO. 19th WHO Model List of Essential Medicines (April 2015). [online] Available from: http://www.who.int/medicines/publications/essentialmedicnies/ EML 2015_8-May-15.pdf.2015 [Accessed September, 2017].
16. Fogari R, Zoppi A. The clinical benefits of beta-1 sensitivity. Rev Contemp Pharmacolther. 1997;8:45-54.
17. Wellstein A, Palm D, Belz GG, et al. Reduction of exercise tachycardia in man after propranolol, atenolol and bisoprolol in comparison to beta-adrenoceptor occupancy. Eur Heart J. 1987;8(Suppl M):3-8.
18. Manjunath CN. Bisoprolol is a preferred beta blocker in STEMI protocol. STEMI—A Cardiology update 2016.
19. Johns TE, Lopez LM. Bisoprolol: is this just another beta-blocker for hypertension or angina? Ann Pharmacother. 1995;29(4):403-14.
20. Neutel JM, Smith DH, Ram CV, et al. Application of ambulatory blood pressure monitoring in differentiating between antihypertensive agents. Am J Med. 1993;94(2):181-7.

21. Channaraya V, Marya RK, Somasundaram M, et al. Efficacy and tolerability of a β-1 selective β-blocker, bisoprolol, as a first-line antihypertensive in Indian patients diagnosed with essential hypertension (BRIGHT): an open-label, multicentric observational study. BMJ Open. 2012;2(3).
22. Brokman CP, Haensel SM, Van de Ven LL, et al. Bisoprolol and hypertension: effects on sexual functioning in men. J Sex Marital Ther. 1992;18(4):325-31.
23. Dorow P, Bethge H, Tonnesmann U. Effects of single oral doses of bisoprolol and atenolol on airway function in nonasthmatic chronic obstructive lung disease and angina perctoris. Eur J Clin Pharmacol. 1986;31(2):143-7.
24. Taniguchi T, Ohtani T, Mizote I, et al. Switching from carvedilol to bisoprolol ameliorates adverse effects in heart failure patients with dizziness or hypotension. J Cardiol. 2013;61(6):417-22.
25. Pasternak B, Mattsson A, Svanstrom H, et al. Comparative effectiveness of bisoprolol and metoprolol succinate in patients with heart failure. Int J Cardiol. 2015;190:4-6.
26. Van den Ven LLM, Spanjaard JN, De Jongste MJL, et al. Safety of beta-blocker therapy with and without thrombolysis: a comparison of bisoprolol and atenolol in acute myocardial infarction. Current Therapeutics Research. 1996;57(5):313-26.
27. Hirschi MM, Wollmann CG, Erhart F, et al. Benefit of immediate beta-blocker therapy on mortality in patients with ST-segment elevation myocardial infarction. Crit Care Med. 2013;41(6):1396-404.
28. Von Armin T. Prognostic significance of transient ischaemic episodes: Response to treatment shows improved prognosis. Results of the Total Ischemic Burden Bisoprolol Study (TIBBs) follow-up. J Am Coll Cardiol. 1996;28:20-4.
29. Jonas M, Reicher-Reiss H, BoykoV, et al. Usefulness of beta-blocker therapy in patients with non-insulin dependent diabetes mellitus and coronary artery disease. Bezafibrate Infarction Prevention (BIP) Study Group. Am J Cardiol. 1996;77(15):1273-7.
30. Kjekshus J, Gelpin E, Cali G, et al. Diabetic patients and beta blockers after acute myocardial infarction. Europ Heart J. 1990;11(1):43-50.
31. Lindholm LH, Hansson L, Ekbom T, et al. Comparison of antihypertensive treatments in preventing cardiovascular events in elderly diabetic patients: Results from Swedish Trial in Old Patients with Hypertension-2. STOP Hypertension-2 Study Group. J Hypertens. 2000;18(11):1671-5.
32. UK Prospective Diabetes Study Group. Efficacy of atenolol and captopril in reducing risk of macrovascular and microvascular complications of type 2 diabetes: UKPDS 39. BMJ. 1998;317(7):713-20.
33. Gress TW, Nieto FJ, Shahar E, et al. Hypertension and antihypertensive therapy as risk factors for type 2 diabetes mellitus. Atherosclerosis Risk in Communities Study. N Engl J Med. 2000;342(13):905-12.
34. Erkens JA, Klungel OH, Stolk RP, et al. Cardiovascular drug use and hospitalizations attributable to type 2 diabetes. Diabeties Care. 2001;24(8):1428-32.
35. Cruickshank JM. Beta blockers and diabetes: The Bad Guys Come Good. Cardiovascular drugs and therapy. 2002;16(5):457-70.
36. Wellstein A, Palm D, Belz GG. Affinity and selectivity of beta receptor antagonists in vitro. J Cardiovasc Pharmacol. 1986;8(Suppl 11):536-40.
37. Maack C, Tyroller S, Schnabel P, et al. Characterisation of beta-1 selectivity, adrenoceptor-Gs-protein interaction and inverse agonism of nebivolol in human myocardium. Br J Pharmacol. 2001;132(8):1817-26.

CHAPTER

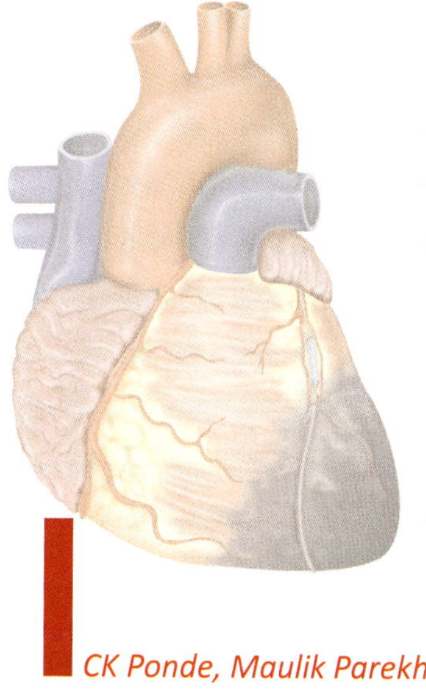

Bisoprolol in Heart Failure in Cardiodiabetes

CK Ponde, Maulik Parekh

INTRODUCTION

Heart failure (HF) is a global health hazard. It has assumed a mammoth proportion in recent times. Around sixty-two million adults are estimated to be living with HF and this number is expected to rise due to mainly three reasons, namely aging population, increasing prevalence of risk factors, and improved post-infarct survival.[1,2] About 1% of total population or estimated 10 million people are living with HF in India. Annual mortality of HF in our country is estimated to be 0.1–0.15 million.[3] HF is a bigger challenge in India since our HF patients are relatively younger and in-hospital as well as 6 months mortality rates are significantly higher in our country compared to western world.[4] Despite the newer advances in treatment and its better availability, the 5-year post-diagnosis mortality in chronic HF patients is nearly 50%.[5] Diabetes mellitus (DM) is a risk factor for HF independent of coronary artery disease (CAD) and hypertension. Diabetic cardiomyopathy is defined as ventricular dysfunction in diabetics independent of a recognizable cause.[6] The Framingham study has demonstrated that diabetes increased the risk of HF 2.4 folds in men and five-fold in women. A number of other studies have reported similar findings. Based on various studies, the important risk factors for development HF in diabetics include age, duration of DM, insulin use, CAD, poor glycemic control, and microalbuminuria among others. Glycemic control and risk of HF are closely related. A report from Kaiser et al. of more than 48,000 patients with DM showed that each 1% rise in glycated hemoglobin (HbA1c) was associated with 8% increase in relative risk of HF.[7] Another study of 31,546 adults with DM also revealed that each 1 mmol/L (18 mg/dL) increase in fasting glucose was associated with significant rise in the risk of HF hospitalization.[8] However, current data does not suggest a causal relationship, i.e. tight glycemic control has not been shown to reduce the incident of HF in patients with type 2 DM.[9]

CHARACTERISTICS OF HEART FAILURE IN CARDIODIABETES

Diabetes mellitus patients have both systolic and diastolic left ventricular (LV) dysfunction. The Strong Heart Study also showed that DM patients had higher LV mass, wall thickness, and arterial stiffness compared with nondiabetics. Patients with DM also are known to have higher E/e' values and impaired global longitudinal strain values, even in asymptomatic individuals. On pathological studies, DM patients have been reported to have higher diastolic LV stiffness irrespective of LV ejection fraction (LVEF). Other microstructural abnormalities like myocardial fibrosis and advanced glycation end-product deposition have also been noted.[10]

Beta-blockers in Therapy of Heart Failure

Earlier, HF was considered as a hemodynamic disorder and sympathetic activation was thought to be beneficial in terms of increased contractility and cardiac output. As the understanding of the pathophysiology of HF evolved, the role of neurohormonal mechanism was established. Increased cardiac sympathetic tone was shown to be associated with higher energy expenditure and possible ischemia in the failing heart muscle. Beta-1 adrenergic receptors (ARs) activation has been shown to accelerate the cell death and abnormal intracellular calcium handling by sarcoplasmic reticulum. Beta-blockade helps in HF by counteracting these deleterious effects. It slows the heart rate (HR), which-in-turn reduces the myocardial oxygen (O_2) demand. It also improved coronary perfusion because of longer diastolic periods (Fig. 1).

Clinical trials have proven this beyond doubt that LV remodeling and mitral regurgitation are reduced by long-term administration of beta-blocker with significant improvement in the LVEF.[11-14] The mortality benefit and magnitude of these changes are greater than that described with angiotensin-converting enzyme (ACE) inhibitors. Over a period of time, the indications of beta-blockers in HF have expanded. Various trials have proved its beneficial effect on mortality and HF hospitalizations.[15-17] Bisoprolol has been studied widely in patients with HF. Here we discuss the salient pharmacodynamics, pharmacokinetics, efficacy, and safety of bisoprolol in cardiodiabetes and HF.

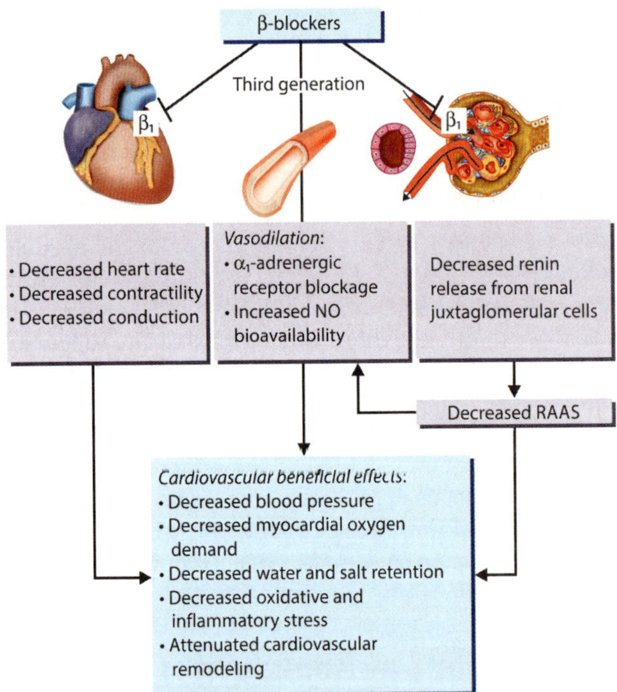

Fig. 1: Beta adrenergic blockade effect

Abbreviation: RAAS, renin–angiotensin–aldosterone system

TABLE 1: Pharmacological properties of various beta-blockers

β-blocker	*β-1/β-2 selectivity*	*Oral absorption*	*Oral bioavailability*
Metoprolol	45	90%	50%
Bisoprolol	119	80%	90%
Carvedilol	7.3	>90%	30%
Nebivolol	293	Variable	Variable (12–96%)

Beta-receptor Selectivity

Bisoprolol has high selectivity for β-1 ARs amongst all available cardioselective beta-blockers. The ratio of β-1–β-2 antagonist activity of bisoprolol is 119, compared with a ratio of 45 for metoprolol. This selectivity leads to better tolerability of the drug in patients with concomitant lung problems and peripheral vascular disease (Table 1).

Bisoprolol is very well absorbed in the gastrointestinal (GI) tract (90%) and has a very low first-pass metabolism (10%). It has low plasma protein binding (30%) with a 1:1 ratio between hepatic metabolism and renal excretion. In normal subjects, its half-life is long (10–11 hours) and is further prolonged in patients with HF (17 ± 5 hours) and/or with severe renal failure allowing once daily administrations (Leopold et al. 1997). Bisoprolol does not interfere with the metabolism of other drugs. Bisoprolol should be initiated at very low doses with gradual uptitration. Recommended starting dose is 1.25 mg once daily and target dose is up to 10 mg daily, if tolerated. In Cardiac Insufficiency Bisoprolol Study (CIBIS) trial, bisoprolol 5 mg did not reduce the mortality. However, in CIBIS II trial, 10 mg dose showed significant mortality reduction. The dose of beta-blockers may have to be decreased during hemodynamic compromise (hypotension and bradycardia) in HF. The only absolute contraindication for use of beta-blockers in HF is patients with active asthma. However, patients with bronchial asthma show better tolerance to bisoprolol because of high β-1 selectivity. Bisoprolol, like all other beta-blockers, should not be stopped suddenly. It may result in tachycardia, tachyarrhythmias, angina, and worsening HF.

BISOPROLOL EFFECTS IN PATIENTS WITH HEART FAILURE

Heart Rate

Bisoprolol administration causes a reduction in HR, which is consistently shown in all the trials, CIBIS (–16.3 ± 15.3 versus –1.6 ± 13.4 bpm with placebo and bisoprolol, respectively; p <0.001), as well as in CIBIS II (–9.8 ± 14.7

versus –0.2 ± 13.7 bpm with placebo).[18,19] In both these trials, it was established that changes in HR were predictable of better survival. However, the analysis also showed that *beneficial effects of bisoprolol was independent of HR changes*, i.e. patients on bisoprolol, who did not have much change in HR, were also shown to have survival benefit with the therapy.

Blood Pressure

The antihypertensive effect of bisoprolol is comparable to that of metoprolol, with slightly better tolerability. In CIBIS-II, bisoprolol reduced blood pressure (BP) from baseline (–4.1 ± 16.4 versus –2.3 ± 16.4 mmHg with placebo for systolic BP, and –2.6 ± 10.7 versus –0.9 ± 10.9 mm Hg with placebo, $p < 0.0001$ in both cases).[18,19] However, lower BP has not been shown to have any impact on mortality benefit in HF. Interestingly, too lower BP has been associated with increased mortality in HF (Metra et al. 2005).

Left Ventricular Function

The hemodynamic effect of bisoprolol was examined in various studies. In the study by Dubach et al. (2002),[20] the effects of bisoprolol on LV function were studied by nuclear magnetic resonance myocardial tagging in 28 patients with chronic HF randomized to bisoprolol or placebo. One-year treatment with bisoprolol was associated with an increase in LVEF (from 25 ± 7 to 36 ± 9%; $p < 0.05$) and a nonsignificant decline in LV end-diastolic and end-systolic volumes (–54 and –62 mL, respectively). No change occurred with placebo. In a retrospective analysis of CIBIS, the changes in LV fractional shortening were related to subsequent prognosis both in the bisoprolol and the placebo groups. Patients who had a fractional shortening change >0.014 (median value) had a better survival than the others. The change in LV fractional shortening, the changes in HR, and bisoprolol administration were independent predictors of survival.[18] These results were consistent with other studies showing the changes in LVEF after beta-blocker therapy predict subsequent outcome.[21]

EFFECT ON NEUROHORMONAL PARAMETERS AND INFLAMMATORY MARKERS

Cardiac Insufficiency Bisoprolol Study trial subgroup was analyzed by Pousset et al. (1996) for HR variability and R-R interval scatter plots. They established that there was a significantly increase in parameters related to parasympathetic activity and decrease in parameters of sympathetic activity.[22] Belenkov et al. also established that bisoprolol treatment can also decrease other neurohormonal parameters such as plasma rennin activity, plasma level of norepinephrine, angiotensin II, and aldosterone. Bisoprolol has also been associated with favorable effects on markers of inflammatory activity [tumor necrosis factor (TNF) alpha, interleukin (IL)].[23,24]

OVERALL OUTCOMES

The CIBIS was a placebo-controlled, randomized, double-blind multicenter trial assessing the effect of bisoprolol on outcome and its tolerability in 641 patients with symptomatic HF. [New York Heart Association (NYHA) III or IV, LVEF <40%]. Bisoprolol did not significantly reduce the mortality. HF hospitalization rate was lower in patients on bisoprolol, compared with placebo. The NYHA functional class also improved significantly in bisoprolol group. CIBIS was underpowered to detect the effect on mortality. CIBIS-II provided answer to the questions left unanswered by the previous trial, by having a sample size large enough to detect mortality differences inhibitors. This trial was prematurely stopped, after a mean follow-up of 1.3 years, for the significant reduction in mortality in the patients randomized to bisoprolol, compared with those on placebo. Mortality reduction was mainly caused by a reduction in sudden cardiac death (SCD). Pump failure deaths were reduced but this result did not reach statistical significance because of the lower number of events. All cause hospitalizations were also significantly lower in bisoprolol group. Subgroup analyses of CIBIS-II showed that the beneficial effects of bisoprolol on mortality and hospitalizations were independent from cause of HF, HF severity, and bisoprolol dose. Patients assuming higher doses of the study drug had less severe HF at baseline and showed a reduction in mortality of greater magnitude with bisoprolol, compared with the patients who could tolerate only low doses (Simon et al. 2003). CIBIS-II showed excellent tolerability of bisoprolol. A meta-analysis of CIBIS and CIBIS-II trials combined confirmed that bisoprolol is associated with a highly significant reduction in overall death, HF death and hospitalization ($p = 0.0001$) (Leizorovicz et al. 2002).

The Cardiac Insufficiency Bisoprolol Study–III Trial: Which Drug to Start First in Heart Failure?

Starting a patient of HF on beta-blockers before ACE inhibitor may be beneficial because of following reasons. First, sympathetic activation may precede the activation of renin-angiotensin system in HF. Second, beta-blockers may reduce the activation of renin-angiotensin system to a great extent. Third, SCD is the most important cause of death HF, and beta-blockers have greater protection from SCD compared with that from ACE inhibitors. The hypothesis of the CIBIS-III trial was that initiation of treatment of HF with the beta-1 selective beta-blocker bisoprolol (to which enalapril is subsequently added) is as effective and safe as a treatment regimen based on the initiation with the ACE inhibitor enalapril (to which bisoprolol is subsequently added). Thus, the primary endpoint of the study was showing that initiation of therapy with bisoprolol, followed by combination therapy with enalapril after 6 months, was comparable (noninferior) to initiation of therapy with enalapril, followed by combination therapy with bisoprolol, after 6 months, with respect to the prevention of all-cause death and all-cause hospitalizations.[25]

Another analysis regarded the effects of treatment on SCD rate. During the first 6 months of monotherapy, 8 of 23 deaths in the bisoprolol-first group were sudden, compared with 16 of 32 in the enalapril-first group (HR 0.50, p = 0.107). During the first year, 16 of 42 deaths in the bisoprolol-first group were sudden versus 29 of 60 deaths in the enalapril-first group, representing a significant 46% reduction (HR, 0.54, p = 0.049). The incidence of other causes of death was, in contrast similar between the two treatment groups.

Bisoprolol Compared to Other Beta-blockers

Bisoprolol is found to be more tolerable in elderly and coexisting chronic obstructive pulmonary disease (COPD) patients. In a study by Su VT et al. it was shown that in patients with coexisting HF and COPD, use of bisoprolol demonstrated a dose-response survival benefit of bisoprolol use, but not of carvedilol or metoprolol use.[26] Another study in 63 patients with COPD and HF, bisoprolol induced demonstrable improvement in pulmonary function and caused less adverse event compared to carvedilol.[27] A study done by Taniguchi et al. found that switching from carvedilol to bisoprolol may help with continuation of β-blocker treatment as well as dosage increase in HF patients with adverse symptoms or signs, allowing them to reach the target dose (Table 2).[28]

TABLE 2: Equi-effective dose of bisoprolol for switching to and from metoprolol

β-blocker	Dose	Equi-effective bisoprolol dose
Metoprolol tartrate IR	50 mg	2.5 mg
	100 mg	5 mg
	200 mg	10 mg
Metoprolol succinate CR/XL	50 mg	2.5 mg
	100 mg	5 mg
	200 mg	10 mg

Tolerability

Various controlled trials have shown that bisoprolol is well tolerated. In CIBIS trial, withdrawal rates for lack of tolerance were similar to placebo. The contraindications to bisoprolol use are asthma, advanced atrioventricular block, and sinus bradycardia. Recent episode of HF is also relative contraindications to use of beta-blockers. There is a lot of concern about hyperglycemia and poor glycemic control in diabetic HF patients with bisoprolol. However, various small and large studies have shown that glycemic control is not affected by bisoprolol. In their study on 125 patients, Bryan Wai et al. observed that beta-blockers did not worsen glycemic control, lipid profile or albuminuria in subjects with HF, and type 2 DM.[29]

CONCLUSION

Independent of CAD and hypertension, diabetes is a cause or systolic and/or diastolic HF. Despite the relationship of glycemia to the risk of developing HF, there is no evidence that tight glycemic control affects the natural history of HF. Beta-blockers, which were once considered a contraindication in HF, today form the cornerstone of HF therapy. This shift is due to better understanding of HF pathophysiology and evidence. Bisoprolol is highly β_{-1} selective agent, which has proven mortality and morbidity (hospitalization) benefits, well tolerated, and does not affect the glycemic control in cardiodiabetes. Beta-blocker therapy in all eligible HF patients, in right doses, is the need of the hour.

REFERENCES

1. Mozaffarian D, Benjamin EJ, Go AS, et al. Heart disease and stroke statistics--2015 update: a report from the American Heart Association. Circulation. 2015;131(4):e29-e322
2. GBD 2013 DALYs and HALE Collaborators, Murray CJ, Barber RM, et al. Global, regional, and national disability-adjusted life years (DALYs) for 306 diseases and injuries and healthy life expectancy (HALE) for 188 countries, 1990-2013: quantifying the epidemiological transition. Lancet. 2015;386(10009):2145-91
3. Chaturvedi V, Parekh N, Seth S, et al. Heart failure in India: The INDUS (INDia Ukieri Study) study. J Pract Cardiovasc Sci. 2016;2(1):28-35.
4. Seth S, Khanal S, Sivasubramanian R, et al. Epidemiology of acute decompensated heart failure in India: The AFAR study (Acute failure registry study). J Pract Cardiovasc Sci. 2015;1(1):35-8.
5. Owan TE, Hodge DO, Herges RM, et al. Trends in Prevalence and Outcome of Heart Failure with Preserved Ejection Fraction. N Engl J Med. 2006;355(3):251-9.
6. Boudina S, Abel ED. Diabetic cardiomyopathy revisited. Circulation. 2007;115(25):3213-23.

7. Iribarren C, Karter AJ, Go AS, et al. Glycemic control and heart failure among adult patients with diabetes. Circulation. 2001; 103(22): 2668-73.
8. Held C, Gerstein HC, Yusuf S, et al. Glucose levels predict hospitalization for congestive heart failure in patients at high cardiovascular risk. Circulation. 2007; 115(11):1371-5.
9. Lind M, Bounias I, Olsson M, et al. Glycaemic control and incidence of heart failure in 20,985 patients with type 1 diabetes: an observational study. Lancet. 2011;378(9786):140-6.
10. van Heerebeek L, Hamdani N, Handoko ML, et al. Diastolic stiffness of the failing diabetic heart: importance of fibrosis, advanced glycation end products, and myocyte resting tension. Circulation. 2008;117(1):43-51.
11. Lechat P, Packer M, Chalon S, et al. Clinical effects of β-adrenergic blockade in chronic heart failure: a meta-analysis of double-blind, placebo-controlled, randomized trials. Circulation. 1998;98: 1184-91.
12. Bristow MR. Beta-adrenergic receptor blockade in chronic heart failure. Circulation. 2000;101(5):558-69.
13. Metra M, Nardi M, Giubbini R, et al. Effects of short- and long-term carvedilol administration on rest and exercise hemodynamic variables, exercise capacity and clinical conditions in patients with idiopathic dilated cardiomyopathy. J Am Coll Cardiol. 1994;24(7):1678-87.
14. Metra M, Giubbini R, Nodari S, et al. Differential effects of beta-blockers in patients with heart failure. A prospective, double-blind comparison of the long-term effects of metoprolol versus carvedilol. Circulation. 2000;102(5):546-51.
15. CIBIS-II Investigators and Committees. The Cardiac Insufficiency Bisoprolol Study: a randomised trial. Lancet. 1999;353(9146):9-13.
16. MERIT-HF Study Group. Effect of metoprolol CR/XL in chronic heart failure: Metoprolol CR/XL Randomised Intervention Trial in Congestive heart failure (MERIT-HF). Lancet. 1999;353(9169):2001-7.
17. Packer M, Coats A, Fowler M, et al. Effect of carvedilol on survival in severe chronic heart failure. N Engl J Med. 2001;344(22):1651-8.
18. Lechat P, Escolano S, Golmard JL, et al. Prognostic value of bisoprolol-induced hemodynamic effects in heart failure during the Cardiac Insufficiency Bisoprolol Study (CIBIS). Circulation.1997;96(7):2197-205.
19. Lechat P, Hulot JS, Escolano S, et al. Heart rate and cardiac rhythm relationships with bisoprolol benefit in chronic heart failure in CIBIS II trial. Circulation. 2001;103(10):1428-33.
20. Dubach P, Myers J, Bonetti P, et al. Effects of bisoprolol fumarate on left ventricular size, function, and exercise capacity in patients with heart failure: analysis with magnetic resonance myocardial tagging. Am Heart J. 2002;143(4):676-83.
21. Metra M, Nodari S, Parrinello G, et al. Marked improvement in left ventricular ejection fraction during long-term beta-blockade in patients with chronic heart failure: clinical correlates and prognostic significance. Am Heart J. 2003;145(2):292-9.
22. Pousset F, Copie X, Lechat P, et al. Effects of bisoprolol on heart variability in heart failure. Am J Cardiol. 2003;77(8):612-7.
23. Ohtsuka T, Hamada M, Hiasa G, et al. Effect of beta-blockers on circulating levels of inflammatory and anti-inflammatory cytokines in patients with dilated cardiomyopathy. J Am Coll Cardiol. 2001;37(2):412-7.
24. Ichihara S, Yamada Y, Ichihara G, et al. Attenuation of oxidative stress and cardiac dysfunction by bisoprolol in an animal model of dilated cardiomyopathy. Biochem Biophys Res Commun. 2006;350(1):105-13.
25. Willenheimer R, Van Veldhuisen DJ, Silke B, et al. Effect on survival and hospitalization of initiating treatment for chronic heart failure with bisoprolol followed by enalapril, as compared with the opposite sequence. Results of the Randomized Cardiac Insufficiency Bisoprolol Study (CIBIS) III. Circulation. 2005;112(16):2426-35.
26. Su VY, Chang YS, Hu YW, et al. Carvedilol, bisoprolol, and metoprolol use in patients with coexistent heart failure and chronic obstructive pulmonary disease. Medicine (Baltimore). 2016;95(5):e2427.
27. Lainscak M, Podbregar M, Kovacic D, et al. Differences between bisoprolol and carvedilol in patients with chronic heart failure and chronic obstructive pulmonary disease: a randomized trial. Respir Med. 2011;105(Suppl 1):S44-9.
28. Taniguchi T, Ohtani T, Mizote I, et al. Switching from carvedilol to bisoprolol ameliorates adverse effects in heart failure patients with dizziness or hypotension. J Cardiol. 2013;61(6):417-22.
29. Wai B, Kearney LG, Hare DL, et al. Beta-blocker use in subjects with type 2 diabetes mellitus and systolic heart failure does not worsen glycaemic control. Cardiovasc Diabetol. 2012;11:14.

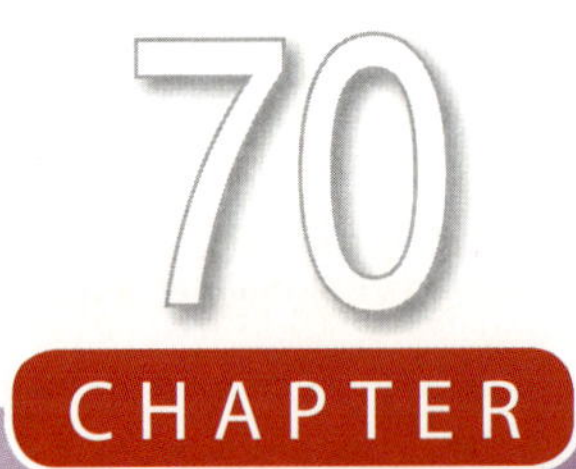

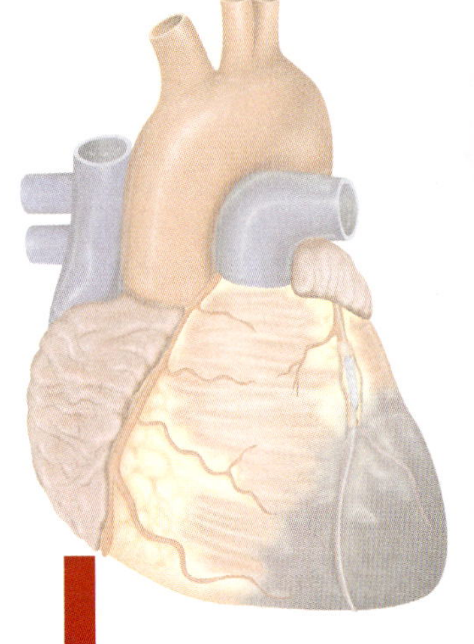

Nebivolol for Hypertension in Cardiodiabetes

Abhirup Chatterjee, Soumitra Kumar

INTRODUCTION

The global problem of hypertension (HTN) is now well known, so is its association with diabetes mellitus (DM). Almost 66% of hypertensives have been found to be prediabetic or diabetic,[1] an evil association which synergistically increase all-cause and cardiovascular (CV) mortality. A review article by R Gupta states that statistics indicate 111% increase in CV mortality by 2020 in India. Approximately, 47% of ischemic heart disease (IHD) and 54% of stroke worldwide are caused due to high blood pressure (BP). In 2010, about 9.4 million people died of HTN globally. By 2015, more than 1.5 billion people are estimated to suffer from HTN. In South-East Asia and Pacific region prevalence of HTN ranges from 5–47% and 7–38% in males and females, respectively. According to World Health Organization (WHO), 2015 data 69.2 million people (8.7% of total population) in India have diabetes. With an increasing trend to adapt Western lifestyle and population aging, the problem is on the rise.[4] In an Indian study, the prevalence of HTN varied between 28.1–31.5% in urban and 19.8–26.2% in rural areas. The journey of beta-blockers (BBs) to treat HTN was never smooth. In 1962, Sir James Black first introduced BBs in clinical medicine and pharmacology with the rationale of reduction in chest pain in IHD with myocardial beta-adrenoreceptor antagonism.[4] Later, BB became one of the first choice-drugs in antihypertensive armamentarium. Modern times have seen BBs evolving from first generation ones like propranolol and pindolol, through more selective second generation ones like atenolol to third generation ones like carvedilol and nebivolol having additional vasodilatory property.[2-4]

BETA-BLOCKERS IN HYPERTENSION: AN EQUIPOISE

Primarily BBs exert antihypertensive effects through their negative chronotropic and inotropic actions, resulting in reduction in cardiac output.[2-4] In earlier guidelines for HTN, BBs were included in first-line treatment, but as newer outcome data came in, BBs went through a set-back from being used as first-line antihypertensive [refer to Joint National Committee 8 (JNC8) and National Institute for Health and Clinical Excellence (NICE) 2011 guidelines]. Earlier studies conducted in 1992 by Medical Research Council on British, elderly patients found that atenolol is of no benefit against coronary events and provide minor protection against stroke. In a systematic review of trials in the elderly conducted by Messerli et al. reveals worse outcome with BBs than diuretics when used as monotherapy for HTN. More recently Lindholm et al. in a meta-analysis of 13 randomized control trials compared BBs to other antihypertensive drugs and have shown about 19% reduction in stroke risk as compared to placebo or no treatment but this risk reduction was not comparable with the reduction reported in other trials using angiotensin receptor blockers (ARBs) or angiotensin converting enzyme (ACE) inhibitors or calcium channel blocker (CCBs). Multiple other studies [Carlberg et al 2004; Bangalore et al 2008; LIFE (2002) etc.] have proven the

TABLE 1: Comparison of pharmacological properties of newer beta-blockers (BBs)

Newer BBs	Receptor selectivity	Additional α-1 blocking	ISA	Vasodilatory property	Remarks
Nebivolol	β_1 selective	No	No	Yes	Release of NO
Carvedilol	Nonselective	Yes	No	Yes	-
Labetalol	Nonselective	Yes	Minimal	Yes	Rapid ↓ BP

Abbreviations: ISA, intrinsic sympathomimetic activity; NO, nitric oxide; BP, blood pressure.

inferiority of BBs in CV-protection as compared to others in this category. Traditional BBs like atenolol, metoprolol, and propranolol have suboptimal antihypertensive effects; they create a state of unfavorable hemodynamics by increasing systemic vascular resistance (SVR) (secondary to reduced cardiac output), and causing end-organ hypoperfusion (like skeletal muscle); they also cause unwanted metabolic effects (reducing insulin-mediated glucose uptake by reducing insulin sensitivity). A substudy of the ASCOT (2012) trial has shown more reduction in central aortic pressure (an independent variable associated directly with increased risk of vascular events including stroke) with amlodipine compared to atenolol, whereas reduction in brachial systolic BP (SBP) was comparable.

The important point in this perspective is that in these studies only older BBs, particularly atenolol was compared to other antihypertensive drugs like ARB or CCB or diuretics, and few of these studies are limited because of the significant heterogeneity of the study population. The unfavorable outcome results of certain BBs used in trials, especially of first and second generation ones, has led to an apparent 'BB phobia'. In contrast to JNC8 and NICE guidelines, European Society of Cardiology/European Society of Hypertension (ESC/ESH) 2013 guideline recommend that ACE inhibitors, ARBs, CCBs, BBs, and diuretics are all suitable for initiation and maintenance therapy of HTN as mono or combination therapy. Several Asian countries like China, Korea, India, Singapore, and Indonesia, in their HTN guideline have considered BBs as one of the first-line drugs. The 2009 reappraisal of ESC/ESH guideline also highlighted that beta-1 selective blockers or those with additional vasodilatory action may be preferred as first-line antihypertensives.

NEWER BBS: BETTER OR OLD WINE IN A NEW BOTTLE?

Newer BBs differ from their contemporary counterparts in having a more favorable physiological effect through various actions like receptor selectivity, vasodilatory property, intrinsic sympathomimetic action, additional alpha-1 blocking action, and few novel actions like nitric oxide (NO) mediated effect on vascular endothelium. The physiological benefits are: (1) reduction in SVR while maintaining cardiac output, (2) reduction in afterload and preload, and (3) possible reversal of arterial remodeling leading to lowering of central aortic pressure (Table 1).

Pharmacological Properties of Nebivolol[4,6]

Nebivolol is one of the third generation BBs with highest beta-1 selectivity, devoid of any alpha-1 blocking action (Van Bortel et al. 1997). It is a racemic mixture of its 'd'- and 'l'-isomers in equal amount. The d-isomer contributes to its beta-1 adrenoreceptor selective antagonism and the both l- and d-isomers (primarily l-isomer) to its vasodilatory property. Naturally, racemic nebivolol is pharmacologically most effective.

In contrast to carvedilol, nebivolol exerts its vasodilatory activity not by alpha-1 blockade rather by stimulating endothelial L-arginine/nitric oxide (NO) pathway. This novel mechanism leads to increased availability of NO, a property first demonstrated in isolated canine coronary arteries. Nebivolol is rapidly absorbed when used orally and reaches its peak plasma concentration within 30–120 minutes. It undergo extensive first pass metabolism by CYP450 system in liver and excreted through feces and urine. Age does not alter its pharmacokinetics, but as applicable to other class of antihypertensive agents, a reduced dose should be advocated in elderly.

Nebivolol Above other BBs: The Physiological and Clinical Superiority

The main reasons of superiority of nebivolol above other BBs are (1) highest beta-1 selectivity (321-fold higher than that for beta-2 in human myocardium;[4] (2) dual mechanism (beta-1 antagonism plus NO-mediated vasodilatation) of antihypertensive action; and (3) its effect on endothelium through beta-3 receptor mediated activation of endothelial nitric oxide synthases (eNOS) and thereby NO production. These effects summate to exert antihypertensive effect as well as improve endothelial dysfunction, which on its own is a predecessor of vascular microinflammation,[5] atherosclerosis, neurodegeneration, and vascular events.

Activation of eNOS leads to increased production of NO which activates NO or cyclic GMP signal cascade. Nebivolol also stimulates NO production indirectly by lowering an endogenous inhibitor of eNOS known as asymmetrical dimethylarginine (ADMA), which is related to CV-mortality and morbidity due to endothelial dysfunction in a concentration dependent manner. Moreover interacting with free radicals, NO mediates scavenging reactive oxygen species (ROS) in a receptor independent manner. Few studies have also proven that NO reduces production of proatherogenic free radicals like O_2^- by inhibiting eNOS uncoupling and probably by upregulating eNOS level in glomerulus.[7-9]

Multiple studies have shown that nebivolol and other BBs reduce plasma renin activity (PRA), which is presumably due to sympatholytic effect on juxtaglomerular apparatus (JGA) as a consequence of inhibition of renin release by beta-1 blocking property.[7] Reduction in plasma aldosterone level, in some studies, has been shown with nebivolol. But few studies show statistically insignificant result.[8]

Recent studies demonstrated that nebivolol-mediated vasodilatation is dose-dependent and independent of beta-1 receptor antagonism. Inhibitory effect of nebivolol has been shown on nicotinamide adenine dinucleotide phosphate (NADPH) oxidase. This enzyme is critical in increasing the production of ROS. It reduces oxidative stress in end-organs like skeletal muscle through this mechanism. A small study by Katie Ayers et al. in 2012 show an insignificant increase of plasma F_2-isoprostanes unlike that with metoprolol. Impaired fibrinolysis as a result of increased level of plasminogen activator inhibitor (PAI-1) (a physiological inhibitor of fibrinolysis) raises the risk of thrombotic CV events. NO decreases the expression of PAI-1.[8]

In rat models, the vasodilatory effect has been found beneficial in reducing pulmonary arterial pressure and also correct the endothelial dysfunction and proinflammatory phenotype of endothelium in pulmonary arterial HTN patients.[7] More recently a study revealed benefit of nebivolol in pulmonary arterial hypertension (PAH), improving pulmonary vascular remodeling, and right heart failure.[13] Effect of BBs on insulin-glucose homeostasis has been extensively studied. Traditional BBs have been shown to precipitate insulin resistance and worsening of glycemic status of the patient, an add-on to the increased risk of CV-mortality. The exact mechanism behind, this is unknown. It is hypothesized that it is because of unopposed alpha-adrenoreceptor mediated vasoconstriction, which results in decreased blood flow. Studies have shown that nebivolol has no or insignificant effect in decreasing insulin sensitivity or altering acute insulin response to glucose. These findings are in contrast with BBs like metoprolol which has been shown to increase insulin resistance (IR) as measured by homeostatic model assessment-IR (HOMA-IR) index.[8] The inhibitory effect of nebivolol on NADPH oxidase also contributes to its beneficial effect in preventing decrement in insulin metabolic signaling, thereby engaging insulin receptor substrate (IRS-1) to the regulatory element of phosphoinositide-3-kinase (PI3K) and protein kinase-B. This causes better insulin dependent glucose transport as well as glucose metabolism in insulin sensitive tissue like skeletal muscle.[10]

Nebivolol as Antihypertensive

The efficacy of nebivolol as antihypertensive has been studied in much detail in both animal and human subjects. In late 20th century, two double-blind placebo-controlled trial were conducted by van Bortel and van Baak in 1992 and by van Nueten et al. in 1997 using nebivolol 5 mg for HTN both of which show significant reduction in BP. This study also show lower exercise capacity and higher rate of fatigue with atenolol compared with nebivolol. In 2001, a study enrolling 3,741 patients by Cleophas et al. found nebivolol to be well-tolerated in long-term and its efficacy as antihypertensive increasing at first 6 months of monotherapy. About 73% of patients reported to feel better after 6 months of nebivolol therapy, whereas 67% reported to have tolerated the drug better than their previous monotherapy with any drug. In another observational study by Fallois and Faulhaber (2001), nebivolol has been found to reduce both systolic BP (SBP) and diastolic BP (DBP) without significant adverse effects seen with first generation BBs, including adverse metabolic effects on lipid profile and blood glucose level. Other studies have shown nebivolol to be equally effective in blacks (with notable absence of side effects), highly effective in isolated systolic hypertension (ISH) whether used as monotherapy or as add-on. Nebivolol also reduced total peripheral resistance during exercise significantly than placebo.

Data on Diabetes and Glucose Metabolism

Role of endothelial dysfunction, decreased availability and activity of NO have been proven to have definite role in atherogenesis and development of metabolic syndrome. A study by Palatini et al. (1999) has shown that tight control of BP is more important than tight glycemic control in prevention of CV events in known diabetic patients. A number of studies show proven benefit of nebivolol in diabetic patients because of its neutral effect on insulin sensitivity and glucose tolerance, in contrast with other BBs.[6] In a recent study, Prakash Deedwania et al. (2013) nebivolol used as add-on with ACE-i/ARB resulted in significant additional reduction in DBP in hypertensive patients with prediabetes, compared with placebo, without having little or no effect on metabolic parameters when compared with hydrochlorothiazide (HCTZ) treatment.[3] In one recent study, nebivolol has been shown to improve insulin sensitivity in transgenic rat models with a side-by-side decrease in oxidative stress[10] (Camila Manrique et al. 2011).

Data on Lipid Metabolism

Available data claims nebivolol to be at least lipid neutral if not beneficial. Patients when treated with 10 mg/day dose of nebivolol, no change in serum triglyceride, cholesterol, lipoproteins, and apolipoproteins were observed even at 3 months of continuous treatment. In 2006, a study conducted by P Peter et al. show no significant change in serum cholesterol and triglyceride level but a significant increase in high-density lipoprotein (HDL) level over 6 months of treatment, suggesting cardioprotection. Interestingly this study has also shown a significant reduction in anti-oxidant capacity and increased low-density lipoprotein (LDL) score with a minimal change in baseline lipid hydroperoxides, implying a more atherogenic state.[11,12] More robust evidences are awaited in this respect.

Arterial Stiffness and Cardiovascular Risk Data

Many studied reveal arterial wall stiffness to be a risk factor for CV-related events, an important predictor of all-cause mortality, and an independent predictor of diastolic dysfunction in hypertensive patients. There is a correlation between arterial wall stiffness and endothelial dysfunction and less NO bioavailability (Wilkinson et al. 2004), both of which contribute to atheroma formation as detailed earlier. Thus drugs like Nebivolol which upregulate NO production and bioavailability can potentially reduce stiffness of large arterial wall, as measured by aortic pulse wave velocity (PWV), irrespective of its effect on BP (McEniery et al. 2004). This is again in contrast with other traditional BBs like atenolol, which actually increase pulse wave deflection and central aortic pressure, aggravating the atherogenic process. However, larger long-term intervention trials are needed to have concrete evidence. A large randomized, double-blind, placebo-controlled trial in elderly population with a mean age of 76 years show comparable benefit to those of other BBs that were previously studied in heart failure (SENIORS study 2004).[6] Additional vasodilatory property may attribute to better tolerability of nebivolol in elderly.

SAFETY AND TOLERABILITY DATA

Meta-analysis shows that adverse effects of nebivolol are no different with placebo. It is well-tolerated at doses up to 30 mg/day. Reportedly, it does not interfere with quality of life too. Thus, it shows positive safety and tolerability in hypertensive patients. In elderly population, also nebivolol show adverse effect similar to typically used BBs and tolerability similar to placebo (SENIORS study).

CONCLUSION

While treating HTN in a background of cardiodiabetes clinicians must keep in mind that (1) there are few strong benefit of BBs, (2) there is a wide spectrum of BBs intrinsically varying in their therapeutic benefit and pharmacological profile, (3) BBs with vasodilatory action, especially nebivolol has few proven benefit in cardiodiabetes and few potential, benefits which should change the dictum regarding unfavorable metabolic effects as seen with traditional BBs like metoprolol or atenolol, and (4) an overall neutral effect on healthcare cost has been found when patients switched to nebivolol from metoprolol.[13,14] Advantage of nebivolol lies in (1) its efficacy as antihypertensive both as monotherapy as well as add-on (recent studies on nebivolol valsartan combination has been found to outweigh the benefit of component therapy and is well-tolerated), (2) single dosing which improves compliance, (3) no harmful effect on pulmonary airways [well-tolerated in hypertensive patients with chronic obstructive pulmonary disease (COPD)], (3) novel mechanism involving NO pathway, which attenuate atherogenesis and endothelial dysfunction, reduce SVR, and (4) potential beneficial role in erectile dysfunction, thus being an ideal BB for male hypertensives. These benefits of nebivolol should make it a suitable first-line drug for hypertensive patients especially in a background of metabolic syndrome and diabetes.[15,16] However, these recommendations are based on clinical data and more large scale comparative studies and outcome trials on nebivolol are required to establish its benefit unquestionably.

REFERENCES

1. Kim CH, Abelardo N, Buranakitjaroen P, et al. Hypertension treatment in the Asia-Pacific: the role of and treatment strategies with Nebivolol. Heart Asia. 2016;8(1):22-26.
2. R Gupta. Trends in hypertension epidemiology in India. J Hum Hypertens. 2004;18:73-8.
3. Deewania P, Shea J, Chen W, et al. Effects of add-on nebivolol on blood pressure and glucose parameters in hypertensive patients with prediabetes. J Clin Hypertens (Greenwich). 2013;15(4):270-8.
4. Bhansali A, Dhandania VK, Deepa M, et al. Prevalence of and risk factors for hypertension in urban and rural India: the ICMR-INDIAB study. J Hum Hypertens. 2014;29(3):204-9.

5. Ram CV. Beta-blockers in hypertension. Am J Cardiol. 2010;106(12):1819-25.
6. Fogari R, Zoppi A, Lazzari P, et al. Comparative effects of nebivolol and atenolol on blood pressure and insulin sensitivity in hypertensive subjects with type II diabetes. J Hum Hypertens. 1997;11(11):753-7.
7. Cockcroft J. A Review of the safety and efficacy of nebivolol in the mildly hypertensive patient. Vasc Health Risk Manag. 2007:3(6): 909-17.
8. Fici F, Celik T, Balta S, et al. Comparative effects of nebivolol and metoprolol on red cell distribution width and neutrophil/lymphocyte ratio in patients with newly diagnosed essential hypertension. J Cardiovasc Pharmacol. 2013;62(4):388-93.
9. Giles Td, Cockcroft JR, Pitt B, et al. Rationale for nebivolol/valsartan combination for hypertension: review of preclinical and clinical data. J Hypertens. 2017;35(9):1758-67.
10. Ayres K, Byrne LM, deMatteo A, et al. Differential effects of nebivololand metoprolol on insulin sensitivity and plasminogen activator inhibitior in the metabolic syndrome. Hypertension. 2012;59(4):893-8.
11. Fongemie J, Felix-Getzik E. A Review of Nebivolol Pharmacology and Clinical Evidence. Drugs. 2015;75:1349-71.
12. Perros F, Ranchoux B, Izikki M, et al. Nebivolol for improving endothelial dysfunction, pulmonary vascular remodeling, and right heart function in pulmonary hypertension. J Am Coll Cardiol. 2015;65(7):668-80.
13. van Bortel LM. Efficacy, tolerability and safety of nebivolol in patients with hypertension and diabetes: a post-marketing surveillance study. Eur Rev Med Pharmacol Sci. 2010;14: 749-58.
14. Manrique C, Lastra G, Habibi J, et al. Nebivolol Improves Insulin Sensitivity in the TGR(Ren2)27 Rat. Metabolism. 2011;60(12): 1757-66.
15. Sindaco DD, Tinti MD, Monzo L, et al. Clinical and economic aspects of the use of nebivolol in the treatment of elderly patients with heart failure. Clin Interv Aging. 2010:5:381-93.
16. Peter P, Martin U, Sharma A, et al. Effect of treatment with nebivolol on parameters of oxidative stress in type 2 diabetics with mild to moderate hypertension. J Clin Pharm Ther. 2006;31(2):153-9.

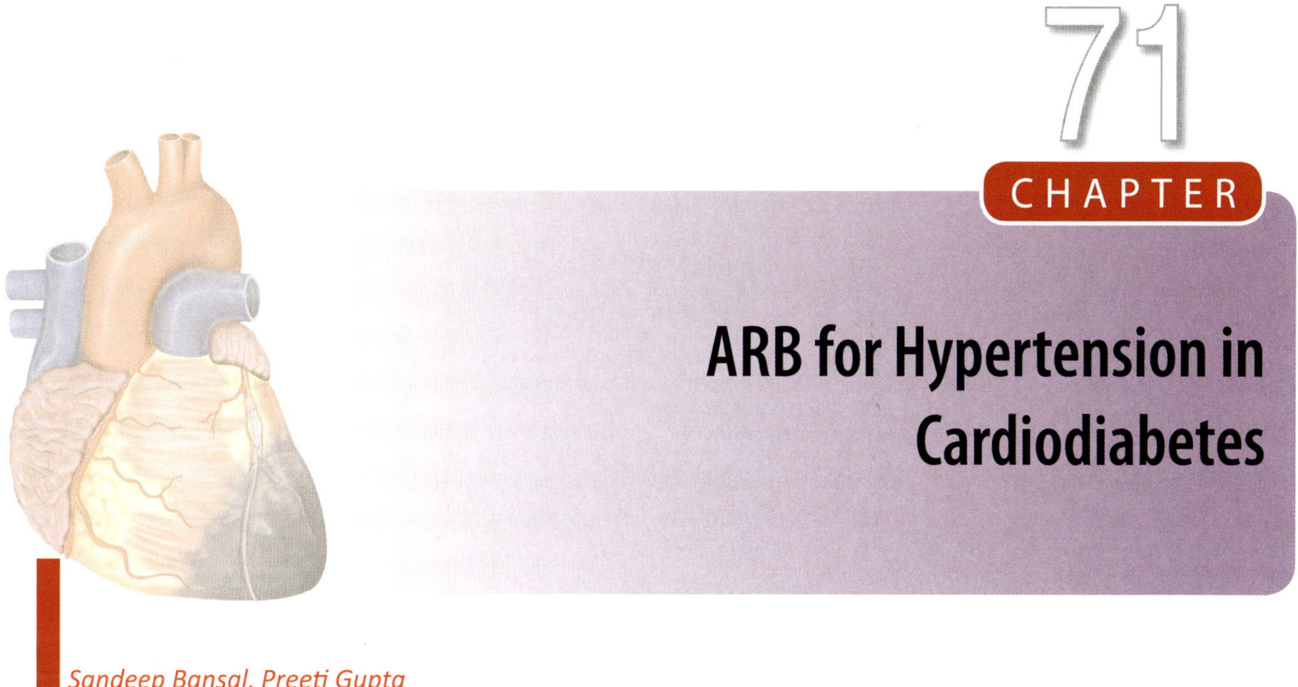

71

CHAPTER

ARB for Hypertension in Cardiodiabetes

Sandeep Bansal, Preeti Gupta

INTRODUCTION

Angiotensin receptor blockers (ARBs) are the most recommended antihypertensive agents by various guidelines, globally as an initial therapy or as an add-on to the existing antihypertensive regimen. ARBs also demonstrated incremental lowering of blood pressure (BP) when combined with other antihypertensive class of drugs like thiazide diuretics or dihydropyridine calcium channel blockers (CCBs). ARBs are considered as the mainstay in the management of stage 1 and 2 of hypertension (HTN). The ARBs are in vogue for more than two decades demonstrating excellent tolerability profile as monotherapy and in combination with other antihypertensive class of drugs. This characteristic feature of tolerability over other drugs has increased therapy adherence, thus it has become the mainstay of therapeutic class. In addition to above features, series of trials have demonstrated expanded therapeutic spectrum of ARBs that is beyond their antihypertensive effects. ARBs have proven effects on mortality and morbidity in heart failure (HF) and chronic renal disease, specifically in patients with type 2 diabetes. The fundamental reason behind increased mortality and morbidity in type 2 diabetes patients is due to complications caused by macrovascular derangements. Angiotensin II (ANG II), through its multiple mechanisms contributes to this increased risk of macrovascular derangements in diabetes. Many therapeutic agents or regimens have their goal in reducing these disease-attributable vascular events in these comorbid patients.[1]Although, the underlying mechanism for angiotensin converting enzyme inhibitors (ACEIs) and ARBs are similar through block renin-angiotensin-aldosterone system (RAAS) blockade, ARBs have been the most opted strategy to block RAAS. ARBs tolerability profile is a distinctive feature over ACEI. Among all available ARBs, telmisartan seems to be the only ARB with a broad indication for cardiovascular (CV) risk reduction in patients with atherothrombotic disease or diabetes with end-organ damage as the evidence from other ARBs remains largely restricted to patients with HF, diabetic nephropathy or specific subsets of hypertensive patients. All sartans (ARBs) are approved for the management of HTN. Based on the results of Ongoing Telmisartan Alone and in Combination with Ramipril Global Endpoint Trial (ONTARGET), telmisartan is the first ARB to be granted additional approval by US Food and Drug Administration (FDA) for CV risk reduction in patients intolerant to ACEIs.

Hypertension seems to be related to insulin resistance, which contributes to the pathogenesis of the cardiometabolic syndrome (CMS).[2,3] Hypertensive patients might have higher fasting as well as the postprandial insulin level which would not relate with body mass index or body fat distribution.[4] Insulin resistance plays a pivotal role in the pathophysiology of chronic kidney disease (CKD) and CV disease (CVD). Human studies have shown insulin, sensitizers have positive effect on the BP by managing the insulin resistance. Incorrect activation of RAAS is one of the important pathophysiologic factors involved in CMS and HTN. In the management of CVD, RAAS plays an important role. ACEIs and ANG II type 1 (AT_1) receptor antagonism are main agents, which blocks RAAS system. Previous studies revealed the systemic effects of RAAS on BP regulation, glucose metabolism, and inflammation. Latest studies showed influence of RAAS in the skeletal muscle, heart, vasculature, adipocytes, and pancreas and its activation impacts the insulin resistance, and diabetes in humans.[5] The ANG II contributes to insulin resistance.

BRIEF HISTORY OF DEVELOPMENT OF RENIN–ANGIOTENSIN–ALDOSTERONE SYSTEM BLOCKERS

The RAAS has always been the key targeted pathway in the development of various antihypertensive agents. There are four major classes of medications that block at different levels in this pathway, viz. ARBs, ACEIs, aldosterone antagonists, and direct renin inhibitors (DRIs). As stated earlier, ANG II has multiple effects of on the vascular system, renal sodium and water handling, and cellular proliferation.[6]

In 1981, first oral active ACEI drug that was discovered and available commercially was captopril. Subsequent to the discovery of captopril, other early members of the class (enalapril and lisinopril) were released in the market by mid-1980s. Within a span of few months, four drugs (fosinopril, quinapril, benazepril, and ramipril) were released commercially in 1991. Between 1993 and 1996, the other three ACEIs (perindopril, moexipril, and trandolapril) were available in the market.[7]

The discovery of ARBs has been important breakthrough in the treatment of CVDs as well as in the management history of HTN. It gave the opportunity to personalize the therapy to ACEI intolerant patients.[8] The key attributable features of ARBs such as excellent efficacy and tolerability allowed these to be an acceptable therapy of choice for many physicians. Particularly, these ARBs have no negative metabolic effect and no accumulation of bradykinin, which scored over the existing agents (ACEI). Like ACEI, ARBs also cause vasodilation of small vessels by activation of AT_2 receptors. This feature of ARBs leads to additional cardiac and renal protection. Commercially approved and available ARBs in USA and Europe are candesartan, olmesartan, irbesartan, losartan, valsartan, telmisartan, eprosartan, and azilsartan.[8]

Mineralocorticoid receptor antagonists (MRAs) competitively inhibit mineralocorticoid receptor present in the distal renal tubule causing a reduction in the number of available epithelial sodium channels.[9]

Conventional RAAS blocking induce rebound concentrations in renin, which may lead to RAAS 'escape'. DRIs inhibit the RAAS cascade at the initial step, which is specific, and rate-limiting step.[10] Aliskiren is the first in class and only available DRI, which is approved for the use in HTN (Table 1).

The table provide clinical summary of its evidence-based use beyond hypertension.

TABLE 1: Landmark clinical trials featuring ARBs

Indication	*Therapy group*	*Therapy*	*Trial*	*Brief summary*
Coronary heart disease	ACE inhibitors and ARBs	Ramipril and telmisartan	ONTARGET	Telmisartan noninferior to Ramipril. No benefit from both agents
	Angiotensin receptor blockers	Telmisartan	ONTARGET	Telmisartan noninferior to Ramipril. No benefit from both agents
		Valsartan	VALUE	Valsartan inferior BP control versus amlodipine; similar CV event rate
Heart failure	ARBs	Candesartan	CHARM	ARBs reduced death in CCF; may add to ACEI benefit (N.B. Val-HF); no benefit in preserved LV dysfunction
		Diastolic dysfunction	CHARM, I-PRESERVE	Irbesartan no benefit in NYHA-II or diastolic dysfunction
		Valsartan	ValHeFT	Valsartan improved symptoms and mortality in NYHA2 +; no benefit added to ACEI
Hypertension	ARB	Losartan	LIFE	Losartan reduced mortality above atenolol for same BP reduction
		Valsartan	VALUE	Valsartan inferior BP control versus amlodipine; similar CV event rate

Abbreviations: ACE, angiotensin converting enzyme; ARB, angiotensin receptor blocker; BP, blood pressure; CV, cardiovascular; LV, left ventricular; NYHA, New York Heart Association; ONTARGET, ongoing telmisartan alone and in combination with ramipril global endpoint trial; VALUE, valsartan antihypertensive long-term use evaluation; CHARM, candesartan in heart failure assessment of reduction in mortality and morbidity; I-PRESERVE, irbesartan in heart failure with preserved systolic function; Val-HeFT, valsartan heart failure trial; LIFE, losartan intervention for endpoint reduction

CLINICAL COMPARISON OF ANGIOTENSIN RECEPTOR BLOCKERS

Antihypertensive efficacy of ARBs was evaluated in a meta-analysis, which comprised of 43 randomized clinical trials involving a total of 11,281 patients. In these trials, ARBs were compared with placebo, other antihypertensive class, and other ARBs. The results showed comparable BP reductions with a response rates ranging from 48% to 55%. The results of these studies suggest that candesartan, irbesartan, and telmisartan may be slightly more effective than losartan.[11]

There is accumulating evidence on the comparative safety and efficacy of azilsartan. There are two trials with olmesartan and valsartan, and one trial with candesartan. The results showed that it is effective in office and ambulatory BP reduction (Table 2).[12]

The efficacy of ACEIs and ARBs from the available evidence shows similar effects on BP control. However,

TABLE 2: Comparative clinical trials involving angiotensin II receptor blockers[11]

Study design (ref)	*Drug, dosage, and number of patients*	*Results*
8-week double-blind, randomized, multicenter (CLAIM II)	Candesartan 16 mg × 2 weeks, then 32 mg × 6 weeks (307 patients) Losartan 50 mg × 2 weeks, then 100 mg × 6 weeks (304 patients)	At 8 weeks, candesartan lowered sitting blood pressure (BP) more than losartan (P < 0.05). Response rates were 58.8% for candesartan and 52.1% for losartan* ; difference has statistical significance but questionable clinical significance
8-week double-blind, randomized, parallel, forced titration	Candesartan 8 mg × 4 weeks, then 16 mg × 4 weeks (115 patients) Losartan 50 mg × 4 weeks, then 100 mg × 4 weeks (115 patients), Placebo (38 patients)	Both candesartan and losartan reduced systolic and diastolic BP when compared with placebo. Differences between candesartan 8 mg and losartan 50 mg were not significant. Candesartan 16 mg lowered systolic BP more effectively than either losartan dose (P < 0.05)
8-week double-blind, randomized, parallel	Irbesartan 300 mg (142 patients) Irbesartan 150 mg (142 patients) Losartan 100 mg (141 patients) Placebo (142 patients)	Irbesartan 300 mg was superior to both irbesartan 150 mg and losartan 100 mg in lowering sitting diastolic BP (P = 0.05) Irbesartan 150 mg and losartan 100 mg did not differ in response. Irbesartan was better tolerated than losartan
6-week double-blind, randomized	Telmisartan 40 mg (57 patients) Telmisartan 80 mg (54 patients) Losartan 50 mg (57 patients)	Telmisartan 40 mg and 80 mg had significantly greater reductions of ambulatory BP assessment (from baseline) than losartan (P <0.05).† Telmisartan 80 mg had greater reductions in diastolic and systolic BP from baseline than losartan at all evaluation periods
4-way, double-blind, placebo-controlled crossover; patients received each drug for 4 weeks followed by a 2-week washout	Losartan 50 mg (30 patients) Telmisartan 40 mg (30 patients) Valsartan 80 mg (30 patients)	Mean 24-hour diastolic BP was significantly lower with valsartan than with losartan or telmisartan (P < 0.001). Heart rate was not affected by any agent
Randomized open-label crossover; patients received drug for 4 weeks followed by a 2-week washout	Valsartan 80 mg (40 patients) Losartan 50 mg (40 patients)	Mean 24-hour BP, daytime and nighttime systolic and diastolic BP were lower with valsartan (P < 0.01). Trough or peak ratio of BP was significantly greater with valsartan (P < 0.05) (Both agents main-tained antihypertensive effects throughout the 24 hours)
8-week randomized, double-blind, placebo-controlled	Valsartan 80 mg × 4 weeks, then 160 mg × 4 weeks (551 patients) Losartan 50 mg × 4 weeks, then 100 mg × 4 weeks (273 patients)	There was no significant difference between the 2 drug treatments. Valsartan showed a slightly greater response rate at the end of 8 weeks (P < 0.021)
8-week double-blind, randomized, parallel	Olmesartan 20 mg (147 patients) Losartan 50 mg (150 patients) Valsartan 80 mg (145 patients) Irbesartan 150 mg (146 patients)	Reduction of sitting diastolic BP with olmesartan was greater than with losartan (P = 0.0002), valsartan (P < 0.0001), or irbesartan (P = 0.0412). Reductions of systolic BP were not significantly different. Reduction in mean 24-hour diastolic and systolic BP with olmesartan was significantly greater than with losartan and valsartan (P = 0.05)
Comparative trial‡	Eprosartan 600 mg (60 patients) Losartan 50 mg (60 patients)	Mean change in BP was greater for eprosartan but did not reach statistical significance

*Response defined as a decrease in diastolic BP to <90 mm Hg or at least a decrease of 10 mm Hg.
†Ambulatory blood pressure assessed continuously throughout the 18- to 24-hour period after dosing.
‡Personal communication, Maryann T. Travaglini, PharmD, SmithKline Beecham Pharmaceuticals, April 2, 1998.
BP indicates blood pressure.
Source: Adapted from Barreras A, Gurk-Turner C. Angiotensin II receptor blockers. Proc (Bayl Univ Med Cent) . 2003;16(1):123-6.

ARBs scores over ACEIs in tolerability profile. The patients reported higher rates of cough in ACEIs group than ARBs. Data regarding other outcomes are limited.[13]

Comparison of Sartans among Themselves and with Angiotensin Converting Enzyme Inhibitors in Cardiodiabetes

Based on World Health Organization (WHO) report, an estimated 422 million adults were living with diabetes in 2014 globally.[14] This number is projected to increase to 642 million by 2040.[15] ANG II contributes to increased risk of macrovascular derangements in diabetes and ARBs have been the most opted strategy over ACEI to address in diabetes patients as they block through RAAS cascade.[16]

Latest studies demonstrated that RAAS blockade has favorable effect on glucose metabolism and even diabetes incidence and CVD.[17] It is known that ARBs have effect on biomarkers level such as urinary albumin and plasma brain natriuretic peptide (BNP).

The results of a trial of telmisartan prevention of CVD (ATTEMPT-CVD) trial provided first evidence that use of ARB (telmisartan) treatment caused a greater decrease in urinary albumin creatinine ratio (UACR) and small increase in plasma BNP levels, which are predictors of CKD and CVD, respectively.[18]

Ongoing Telmisartan Alone and in Combination with Ramipril Global Endpoint Trial has shown that telmisratan is an equally effective alternative to ACEI (ramipril) in patients with vascular disease or high-risk diabetes. A subgroup analysis of ONTARGET trial also has shown progressive decrease in systolic BP resulted in reduced risk of primary outcomes like CV death or myocardial infarction (MI).[19]

The meta-analysis of four trials on the metabolic effects of new sartan, azilsartan has shown potent antihypertensive effect over olmesartan and valsartan; however there were no significant difference observed in metabolic parameters like blood glucose, insulin levels, and adiponectin levels. Long-term trials might be required to assess potential benefits.[12]

Different Angiotensin Receptor Blockers with Different Benefits

Angiotensin receptor blockers have common structural features but pharmacologic properties differ (Table 3).

There are no set guidelines on, which ARBs should be used in which conditions. Lack of comparative trial between different ARBs to show additional benefit beyond BP lowering control.[8] However, from few studies and comparative trials, telmisartan has shown the pleiotropic properties which stands apart from other ARBs. Telmisartan is unique in terms of interacting and activating structurally with ligand-activated transcription factor that called peroxisome proliferator-activated receptor gamma (PPARγ), which regulates the lipid metabolism and insulin sensitivity.[16]

Telmisartan has shown the highest agonist activity toward PPARγ followed by other ARBs such as candesartan and irbesartan. Whereas losartan, valsartan and olmesartan seem to have little PPARγ agonist activity. Also telmisartan is partial PPARγ agonist, which is related to improve the surrogate markers of CV health in type 2 diabetes patients. However, telmisartan is not associated with adverse effects like sodium and water retention, edema, and HF as it is not show full agonistic activity.

PPARγ activity of telmisartan was compared with other ARB that does not show or known to have this property in terms of reducing the risk of macrovascular events in 50,000 older adult diabetic patients. The results of the study are showed telmisartan and valsartan were associated with a reduced risk of hospital admission for stroke, acute MI, or HF in comparison with irbesartan.[16]

The evidence from this study denotes the statistically important differences exist in the effectiveness of ARBs when used for the prevention of diabetes related macrovascular disease and telmisartan, and valsartan are most preferred ARBs in this indication.[16] This study reinforces the small trial results with diabetes patients where telmisartan in comparison to other ARBs showed significantly greater reductions in serum lipid levels, plasma glucose concentration, glycated hemoglobin (HbA1c) levels, and markers of insulin resistance.

There are few preclinical studies that support azilsartan to be as potential agent with beneficial in diabetic patients beyond its antihypertensive efficacy.[12]

Table 4 shows a summary of available evidence on the advantage of ARBs beyond BP lowering effects, done by Casaba Andra De´zsi. This table also highlights the preferred ARBs in various comorbid conditions.[8]

A summary of conclusions is mentioned in the Table 4.

Telmisartan proved to be superior over other ARBs in reduction of fasting plasma glucose levels and increasing adiponectin levels based on the meta-analysis of eight trials. Telmisartan at higher doses of 80 mg may also show reduction in fasting plasma insulin levels as well as homeostasis model assessment of insulin resistance (HOMA-IR).[17]

Studies have also shown decreased incidence of new onset diabetes using ARB therapy as compared to placebo in patients with high CV risk and/or HTN. ARBs like losartan, candesartan, and valsartan also showed decrease

TABLE 3: Summary of pharmacologic properties of ARBs

When?	*Which one to give?*		*Which one to avoid?*
Clinical condition of concern	First ARBs of choice	ARBs with potentially beneficial effects	ARBs with potentially negative effect
Cardiovascular prevention	Telmisartan	Losartan	
Heart failure	Valsartan		
	Candesartan		
	Losartan		
Myocardial infarction	Valsartan	Telmisartan	
Stroke	Losartan	Telmisartan	
		Candesartan	
		Eprosartan	
Atrial fibrillation	Telmisartan	Losartan	
		Candesartan	
		Valsartan	
Diabetes mellitus	Telmisartan	Losartan	Olmesartan
	Valsartan	Irbesartan	
		Candesartan	
Diabetic nephropathy	Losartan	Telmisartan	Olmesartan
	Irbesartan	Valsartan	
		Candesartan	
Metabolic syndrome	Telmisartan	Valsartan	
Hyperuricemia	Losartan	Irbesartan	Candesartan
Erectile dysfunction	Valsartan		
	Losartan		
	Irbesartan		
Cognitive decline		Candesartan	
		Irbesartan	
		Losartan	
		Valsartan	
		Eprosartan	
		Telmisartan	

Abbreviation: ARB, angiotensin receptor blocker.

Source: D Csaba, The Different Therapeutic Choices with ARBs. Which One to Give? When? Why? Am J Cardiovasc Drugs. 2016;16:255-266

TABLE 4: Summary of available evidence on the advantage of ARBs

Drug	*Biological half-life [h]*	*Protein binding [%]*	*Bioavailability [%]*	*Renal or hepatic clearence*	*Food effect*
Losartan	2	98.7	33	90/10	Minimal
Candesartan	9	>99	15	40/60	No
Valsatan	6	95	25	30/70	40–50% decreased
Irbesartan	15	90–95	70	20/80	No
Telmisartan	24	>99	42–58	NS/~100	No
Eprosartan	5	98	13	30/70	No
Olmesartan	14–16	>99	29	40/60	No
Azilsartan	11	>99%	60%	55%/42%	No

Abbreviation: ARB, angiotensin receptor blocker

in the incidence of new onset diabetes in landmark trials like Losartan Intervention for Endpoint reduction (LIFE), Study on Cognition and Prognosis in the Elderly (SCOPE), and Valsartan Antihypertensive Long-term Use Evaluation (VALUE) trials, respectively. The combined estimated relative risk (RR) of 0.80 was observed for all the three agents. 16% reduction in the risk of new onset diabetes as compared to placebo was observed in the meta-analysis of two landmark trials [Telmisartan Randomized Assessment Study in ACE Intolerant Subjects with Cardiovascular Disease (TRANSCEND) and Prevention Regimen For Effectively Avoiding Second Strokes (PRoFESS)] of telmisartan.

The effect of telmisartan in diabetic patients in prevention and progression of proteinuria was evaluated in a meta-analysis of 20 randomized controlled trials. This meta-analysis included all landmark trials of telmisartan like A comparison of telMisartan versus losArtan in hypertensive type 2 DiabEtic patients with Overt nephropathy (AMADEO), ONTARGET, TRANSCEND, The INcipieNt to OVert: Angiotensin II receptor blocker, Telmisartan, Investigation On type 2 diabetic Nephropathy (INNOVATION), Diabetes Exposed to Telmisartan And enalaprIL (DETAIL) and study to inVestIgate the efficacy of telmIsartan versus VALsartan in hypertensive type 2 DIabetic patients with overt nephropathy (VIVALDI), which concluded telmisartan shows statistically significant reduction in percent changes of albuminuria or proteinuria. In comparison to other ARBs, ACEIs, and other therapies UACR ratio was also reduced by 20%, 14%, and 40% respectively.

Another meta-analysis showed telmisartan when used in patients with metabolic syndrome significantly improved metabolic parameters such as insulin, fasting glucose, hemoglobin A1c: HbA1c levels and HOMA index.

Telmisartan resulted in significant improvement in hyperinsulin response to glucose loading in obese patients with HTN and insulin resistance [ARB trial of hypertension in obese patients with hyperinsulinemia assessed by oral glucose tolerance test (ATHLETE) study]. Number of telmisartan studies has also shown that telmisartan to reduce visceral fat and TNF-α levels improvement in vascular inflammation, and increase in serum adiponectin levels. Other ARBs like valsartan, losartan, and eprosartan were also studied in obese hypertensive subjects, however were unable to show the above effects in obese hypertensive patients.

The results of Saga Telmisartan Aggressive Research (STAR) study showed the cholesterol (total cholesterol and triglycerides) lowering effects of telmisartan. Considering the above study, hypertensive patients with dyslipidemic profile, telmisartan can be preferred choice.[20]

COMBINATION THERAPIES WITH ANGIOTENSIN RECEPTOR BLOCKERS AND THEIR ROLE IN HYPERTENSION MANAGEMENT

The recommended goal BP in hypertensive diabetic patients is 140/90 mm Hg, which is difficult to attain in most of the patients.[2] Studies have shown for greater reduction of clinical CV endpoints tight BP control is required.[3,4] Single treatment is effective; however HTN being progressive disease, nearly 50% require more than one drug for adequate control of their BP. Hence, combination therapy brings adequate BP control in patients where BP is poorly managed on a single agent.[20]

Angiotensin Receptor Blockers with Calcium Channel Blockers

There are adequate evidences available to support a combination of agents that block RAAS and CCB or diuretic to reach goal BP.

Fogari et al. has studied the combination effect of other drugs using telmisartan 40 mg and amlodipine 2.5 mg. The results showed comparable BP reduction with high dose of telmisartan or amlodipine. However, additional effects were observed in the reduction of UACR in patients with increased telmisartan dose. This combination offers an effective and tolerable option to comorbid patients who consider combination therapy with high dose telmisartan therapy.

In a study, amlodipine or an ARB administered as a separate agents or as a combination in once daily dosage for the duration of 8–16 weeks. The results showed combination therapy was effective in moderate-to-severe HTN along with maintenance of BP for approximately for one year in follow-up study.[21]

The results of the two randomized trials have shown significant BP reduction in combination of azilsartan plus amlodipine as compared to monotherapy.

Angiotensin Receptor Blockers with Diuretics

Diuretics induces increase in renin activity, addition of RAAS inhibitor with diuretic therapy nullifies this effect of diuretic. RAAS blockers effect which leads to loss of salt in the body attributed to its antihypertensive activity. Moreover, an ARB will also nullify the metabolic effects of thiazide diuretics like hypokalemia and hyperglycemia. This combination at low doses has demonstrated greater BP reductions and higher response rates in several studies in comparison with monotherapy (single agent).[20]

In moderate-to-severe HTN cases, it was observed that combination therapy [irbesartan with hydrochlorothiazide (HCTZ)] was found to be safe and effective irrespective of baseline BP level, age, obesity, race, diabetic status, and metabolic syndrome.[20] Patients whose BP is uncontrolled using an ARB (candesartan 8 mg/day or valsartan 80 mg/day) were selected for a trial. These patients were administered a combination therapy of telmisartan 40 mg/day and HCTZ 12.5 mg/day. In 12 weeks, there was significant reduction in office and home BP along with reduction in early morning BP. Reduction in early morning BP signifies the duration of activity of the combination.

Switching from amlodipine to telmisartan + HCTZ at low-doses was evaluated by ONgoing Evaluation of depressor effect And Safety of combination therapy with Telmisartan and low-dose hydrochlorothiazide (ONEAST) study group. The results showed significant BP reduction in combination therapy (telmisartan + low-dose HCTZ) group than monotherapy (amlodipine) group alone. All the above evidences points toward the combination of a RAAS blocker and a low-dose thiazide is effective in hypertensive patients where BP cannot be controlled with CCB alone.[20]

A combination of azilsartan and chlorthalidone was compared with olmesartan plus hydrochlorothiazide. The azilsartan combination was found to be efficient in reduction of BP.[12]

Angiotensin Receptor Blocker with Angiotensin Converting Enzyme Inhibitor

Theoretically, combination of ACEI + ARB offer complete blockade of the RAAS. Treatment with ACEI alone causes increase ANG II levels, despite continuous treatment with ACEI. This ACEI escape phenomenon gets reduces by the addition of ARB. Additionally, the ACEI itself inhibits bradykinin degradation.

The therapeutic efficacy of combination of ACEI and ARB were assessed in two major landmark trials. Candesartan and Lisinopril Microalbuminuria (CALM) trial investigators showed the combination was more effective in reducing BP levels than monotherapy. Statistically significant decrease in albuminuria was observed when combination therapy was compared to monotherapy (candesartan alone).

The efficacy of the combination of ARB and ACEI were evaluated in ONTARGET trial, which evaluated the efficacy of two individual agents as monotherapy vis-à-vis combination therapy. Telmisartan (ARB) and ramipril (ACEI) demonstrated as equally effective in CV even prevention in high-risk patients. However, the combination did not provide any additional benefit. On the contrary, the combination showed increased adverse effects than either monotherapy in this patient population. ONTARGET does not rule out use of the ACEI plus ARB combination in severe HF, where angiotensin escape mechanisms are expressed and dual blockade may be needed.

Nevertheless, the potential danger of ARB plus ACEI combinations needs to be taken into consideration. This kind of combination usually produces worsening of hyperkalemia, and may be associated with a decline in the hematocrit in chronic renal failure (CRF) patients with renal anemia. Therefore, combination treatment to be used with caution and monitored carefully and closely, especially in patients with renal artery stenosis, those receiving concomitant cyclooxygenase inhibitors, or in the elderly, salt depleted, or anemic patients.

Though various agents are available that can be used in combination with ARB for the management of HTN, the choice of agent to combine with ARB depends upon the associated risk factors, presence of comorbidities like diabetes, renal dysfunction and the adverse effects. The combination regimen needs to be tailored according to individual patient.

Currently, there are ARB combination options are available for managing HTN. But this combination use depends upon risk factors, comorbidities such as diabetes, renal dysfunction, and the adverse effects. Therefore treatment should be individualized as per the patient need.

CURRENT AND FUTURE ROLE OF ANGIOTENSIN RECEPTOR BLOCKERS IN CARDIOVASCULAR RISK REDUCTION AND HEART FAILURE

Cardiovascular Risk Reduction

Globally, an estimated 17.7 million (31%) deaths from CVDs in 2015.[22] CVDs; ischemic heart disease and stroke form the majority reasons for these deaths. Atherosclerosis is underlying pathophysiology in 75% of death cases.[4] ARBs block systemic effects of RAAS through selective inhibition of ANG II on AT_1 receptors. RAAS inhibition prevents vascular inflammation, which may prevent the development of atherosclerosis, consequently reducing the risk of major CV events. Selective blockade of AT_1 receptors can contribute to additional CV protection by ARBs.

Based on the ONTARGET study results, telmisartan is the only ARB indicated for the reduction of CV morbidity in patients who manifest atherothrombotic CVD. Telmisartan also demonstrated similar reduction to that of ramipril in the composite endpoint of CV death, MI, stroke, or hospitalization due to HF. The TRANSCEND study failed to reach the composite primary endpoint; however, telmisartan did reduce hospitalizations for CV reasons and left ventricular hypertrophy. Both macrovascular and microvascular events plus microalbuminuria were also observed in fewer patients. A combined analysis of PRoFESS data showed telmisartan to contribute significant benefit in CV death as well as MI and stroke. Another ARB, losartan in a landmark trial (LIFE) demonstrated 13% RR reduction when compared to atenolol; also showed 39% mortality reduction in diabetic patients.

Heart Failure

Valsartan in Valsartan Heart Failure Trial (Val-HeFT) trial showed 33% reduction in all-cause mortality and 44% in composite mortality and morbidity in HF patients who were not on ACEIs. Valsartan has shown significant improvements in New York Heart Association (NYHA) class, ejection fraction, and HF signs and symptoms and reduced the rate of hospitalization in overall study population.

In another landmark study [Randomized Evaluation of Strategies for Left Ventricular Dysfunction (RESOLVD)] where candesartan was used showed similar benefits to that of enalapril on left ventricular function and NYHA functional classification (NYHA-FC). Candesartan in Heart Failure: Assessment of Reduction in Mortality and Morbidity (CHARM) trial also demonstrated that candesartan when compared with placebo reduced significantly the risk of CV deaths and hospitalizations due to HF.

Study involving elderly HF patients [Evaluation of Losartan in the Elderly I and II (ELITE I and ELITE II)] where losartan was compared with captopril showed NYHA class improvement in terms of all-cause mortality, sudden death, or resuscitated arrests. Also, this study showed that there was reduction in sudden cardiac death due to losartan therefore less mortality. The 150 mg dose of losartan as compared with 50 mg dose has additional benefit of reducing death rate or hospitalizations due to HF and left ventricular ejection fraction.

CONCLUSION

The aim of therapeutic strategy for the management of CVD is to control and minimize the risk factors and thereby CV events, which in turn impact morbidity and mortality rates. In prospective randomized trials, ARBs have shown the ability to reduce the risk of stroke and HF as well as the risk of major CV events. They can play a significant role in the near future. With an aim to prevent CV events, primarily telmisartan and eventually losartan are the ARBs of choice in patients with high CV risk and a general need for CV risk reduction.

REFERENCES

1. Akhrass P, McFarlane S. Telmisartan and cardioprotection. Vasc Health Risk Manag. 2011;7:677-83.
2. Ferrannini E, Buzzigoli G, Bonadonna R, et al. Insulin resistance in essential hypertension. N Engl J Med. 1987;317(6):350-7.
3. Bonora E, Capaldo B, Perin PC, et al. Hyperinsulinemia and insulin resistance are independently associated with plasma lipids, uric acid and blood pressure in nondiabetic subjects. The GISIR database. Nutr Metab Cardiovasc Dis. 2008;18(9):624-31.
4. Manrique C, Lastra G, Whaley-Connell A, et al. Hypertension and the cardiometabolic syndrome. J Clin Hypertens (Greenwich). 2005;7(8):471-6.
5. Underwood P, Adler G. The Renin Angiotensin Aldosterone System and Insulin Resistance in Humans. Curr Hypertens Rep. 2013;15(1):59-70.
6. Brown NJ, Vaughn DE. Angiotensin-converting enzyme inhibitors. Circulation. 1998;97(14):1411-20.
7. Sica D. The evolution of renin-angiotensin blockade:angiotensin-converting enzyme inhibitors as the starting point. Curr Hypertens Rep. 2010;12(2):67-73.
8. Dézsi CA. The Different Therapeutic Choices with ARBs. Which One to Give? When? Why? Am J Cardiovasc Drugs. 2016;16:255-66.
9. de Gasparo M, Joss U, Ramjoue HP, et al. Three new epoxy-spirolactone derivatives: characterization in vivo and in vitro. J Pharmacol Exp Ther. 1987;240(2):650-6.
10. Gradman AH, Kad R. Renin inhibition in hypertension. J Am Coll Cardiol. 2008;51(5):519-28.
11. Barreras A, Gurk-Turner C. Angiotensin II receptor blockers. Proc (Bayl Univ Med Cent). 2003;16(1):123-6.
12. Georgiopoulos G, Katsi V, Oikonomou D, et al. Azilsartan as a Potent Antihypertensive Drug with Possible Pleiotropic Cardiometabolic Effects: A Review Study. Front Pharmacol. 2016;7:235.
13. Matchar DB, McCrory DC, Orlando LA, et al. Systematic review: comparative effectiveness of angiotensin-converting enzyme inhibitors and angiotensin II receptor blockers for treating essential hypertension. Ann Intern Med. 2008;148(1):16-29.
14. World Health Organization. Global Report on Diabetes. Geneva: World Health Organization; 2016.
15. International Diabetes Federation. IDF Diabetes Atlas, 7th edition. Brussels: International Diabetes Federation; 2015.
16. Antoniou T, Camacho X, Yao Z, et al. Comparative effectiveness of angiotensin-receptor blockers for preventing macrovascular disease in patients with diabetes: a population-based cohort study. CMAJ. 2013;185(12):1035-41.
17. Suksomboon N, Poolsup N, Prasit T. Systematic review of the effect of telmisartan on insulin sensitivity in hypertensive patients with insulin resistance or diabetes. J Clin Pharm Ther. 2012;37(3):319-27.
18. Ogawa H, Soejima H, Matsui K, et al. A trial of telmisartan prevention of cardiovascular diseases (ATTEMPT-CVD): Biomarker study. Eur J Prev Cardiol. 2016;23(9):913-21.
19. Liebson PR, Amsterdam EA. Ongoing Telmisartan Alone and in Combination with Ramipril Global Endpoint Trial (ONTARGET): implications for reduced cardiovascular risk. Prev Cardiol. 2009;12(1):43-50.
20. Kalra S, Kalra B, Agrawal N. Combination therapy in hypertension: An update. Diabetol Metab Syndr. 2010;2:44.
21. Sabbah Z, Mansoor A, Kaul U. Angiotensin Receptor Blockers-Advantages of the New Sartans. J Assoc Physicians India. 2013;61(7):464-70.
22. WHO. (2017). Cardiovascular diseases (CVDs). [online] Available from *www.who.int/mediacentre/factsheets/fs317/en/*. [Accessed September, 2017].

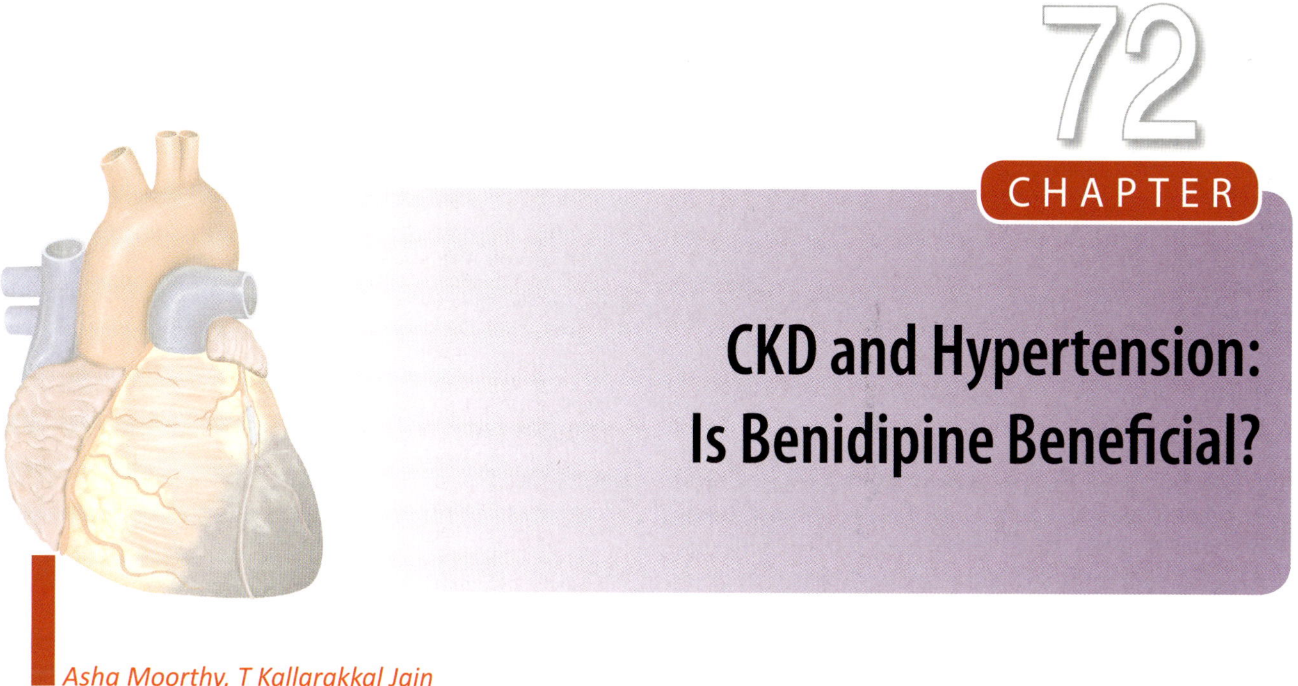

CKD and Hypertension: Is Benidipine Beneficial?

Asha Moorthy, T Kallarakkal Jain

INTRODUCTION

Calcium (Ca) channels have been classified into five subtypes, namely, L, T, N, P/Q, and R, according to their location and function.[1] Three types of Ca channel blockers (CCBs), the L-, T-, and N-type CCBs, are in clinical use. Both L-type and T-type Ca channels are present in the afferent arterioles, whereas only T-type Ca channels are present in the efferent arterioles. Benidipine has been shown to block both L-type and T-type Ca channels and causes dilatation of both efferent and afferent arterioles.

BENIDIPINE

Benidipine is the only CCB of all the CCBs that has the triple Ca^{2+} channel blocking property. It not only has an inhibitory effect on muscular (L-type) Ca^{2+} channel, but also has an inhibitory effect on N- and T-type Ca^{2+} channels. It is an orally active drug approved for the treatment of hypertension and angina pectoris. Adverse reactions of this drug include palpitations, facial flushing, hot flushes, headache, dizziness, sleepiness, constipation, nausea, abdominal discomfort, edema, malaise, redness and warm feeling in the fingers, shoulder stiffness, and increased frequency of micturition. Elevations in serum glutamic-oxaloacetic transaminase (SGOT), serum glutamic pyruvic transaminase (SGPT), alkaline phosphatase, total bilirubin, creatinine, and uric acid are also reported.

Usual CCBs combine directly with the dihydropyridine (DHP) binding site in the cell membrane, thereby inhibiting the intracellular influx of Ca ions. Benidipine enters the lipid layer of the cell membrane and then diffuses extremely rapidly to the Ca channels. This action of benidipine binding to the Ca channels is called the 'membrane approach' (approach to the cell membrane followed by long retention in the DHP binding site). This 'membrane approach' of benidipine results in its slow binding and dissociation.

Antihypertensive Features

Benidipine has a durable and consistent BP reduction over 24 hours. A 4-mg dose of benidipine once daily in the morning for 2 weeks adequately decreased the 24-hour blood pressure (BP). The mean systolic BP (SBP) decreased after drug administration by 18 mm Hg (from 172 ± 18 mmHg to 154 ± 18 mm Hg) at 90% level and mean diastolic BP (DBP) decreased by 10 mm Hg (from 99 ± 12 mm Hg to 89 ± 13 mm Hg) at 90% level. Benidipine may also prevent left ventricular hypertrophy (LVH) by improving collagen type I degradation abnormalities in essential hypertensive patients. In a comparison study with amlodipine, benidipine resulted in a 12/9 mm Hg greater reduction of SBP/DBP than amlodipine.

Renoprotection

Proteinuria is detrimental to the kidney because ultrafiltration of proteins across the glomerular basement membrane brings about mesangial and tubular protein overload, which provokes inflammation and ultimately results in glomerulosclerosis and tubulointerstitial interstitial fibrosis.[2] It is known that proteinuria is associated with the risk of cardiovascular disease. Therefore, because of the antiproteinuric effect, benidipine would seem to be more advantageous than an L-type CCB, not only by slowing the progression of renal tissue injuries but also by reducing the incidence of cardiovascular events in patients with chronic kidney disease (CKD).

Furukawa et al.[3] surveyed the blocking activity of various CCBs on L-/T-/N-type Ca current in Xenopus oocytes. Although both benidipine and amlodipine exhibited blocking function on both L- and T-type Ca channels, benidipine predominantly blocked the T-type Ca channel, whereas amlodipine predominantly blocked the L-type Ca channel. Furthermore, the concentration required for benidipine to exert the inhibitory effect on T-type Ca channels can be achieved at clinically relevant doses of benidipine used for the treatment of hypertension.[4] Therefore, benidipine, which is an L-/T-type CCB, should offer additive benefits over CCB-inhibiting L-type Ca channels, but not T-type Ca channels.

It has been demonstrated that aldosterone can directly damage various organs, including the heart and blood vessels, via mineralocorticoid receptors, independent of changes in BP. Benidipine decreased plasma aldosterone levels without any effect on serum Na and K levels when administered to patients with mild-to-moderate stage CKD. Thus, in addition to lowering BP, benidipine would be expected to provide renoprotection by inhibiting aldosterone production. Long-term treatment with angiotensin-converting enzyme (ACE) inhibitors or angiotensin-receptor blockers (ARBs) can cause escape or rebound of plasma aldosterone levels. In such a situation, addition of a mineralocorticoid receptor blocker has been shown to reduce proteinuria in patients taking inhibitors of the renin–angiotensin–aldosterone system (RAAS) for the treatment of hypertension and kidney disease; a T-type CCB might be a suitable addition for the purpose of inhibiting aldosterone production and managing aldosterone escape.

Role in Cardiovascular System

In cardiac muscle, two types of Ca^{+2} channels, the low-threshold (L-type) and T-type (transient-type), contributes to the upstroke of the action potential. Basic research has shown that benidipine increases nitrogenoxide in the coronary circulation and stimulates endothelial cell-type nitric oxide synthesis (eNOS) independently of its antihypertensive action. LVH is particularly common in elderly hypertensive patients and is an independent risk factor for heart failure, coronary heart disease, stroke, arrhythmias, sudden cardiac death, and cardiovascular morbidity and mortality in elderly patients. Benidipine has been reported to reduce left ventricular mass index (LVMI) in essential hypertensive patients with severe LVH. Benidipine also improved arterial compliance significantly and thus potentially improved arterial function and perhaps arterial properties.

Benidipine in Diabetics

Benidipine has shown a significant reduction in urinary protein excretion in diabetic patients. It also causes a significant change of platelet activation markers, microparticles, chemokines, and soluble adhesion markers in hypertensive patients with type 2 diabetes. It is also found that benidipine improve insulin sensitivity after 12 weeks of treatment as compared to placebo group in subject with essential hypertension.

CONCLUSION

Benidipine is the only CCB of all the CCBs that has the triple Ca^{2+} channel blocking property. It has a durable and consistent BP reduction over 24 hours. Treatment with benidipine results in a greater reduction of albuminuria and plasma aldosterone than other CCBs, in patients with CKD. These effects of benidipine would seem to make the drug more advantageous in terms of the progression of renal dysfunction and preventing cardiovascular tissue and organ injuries in patients with hypertension, diabetes, and CKD.

REFERENCES

1. Perez-Reyes E. Molecular physiology of low-voltage-activated t-type calcium channels. Physiol Rev. 2003;83(1):117-61.
2. Abbate M, Benigni A, Bertani T, et al. Nephrotoxicity of increased glomerular protein traffic. Nephrol Dial Transplant. 1999;14(2):304-12.
3. Furukawa T, Nukada T, Miura R, et al. Differential blocking action of dihydropyridine Ca2+ antagonists on T-type Ca2+ channel (a1G) expressed in xenopus oocytes. J Cardiovasc Pharmacol. 2005;45(3):241-6.
4. Akizuki O, Inayoshi A, Kitayama T, et al. Blockade of T-type voltage-dependent Ca2+ channels by benidipine, a dihydropyridine calcium channel blocker, inhibits aldosterone production in human adrenocortical cell line NCI-H295R. Eur J Pharmacol. 2008;584(2-3):424-34.

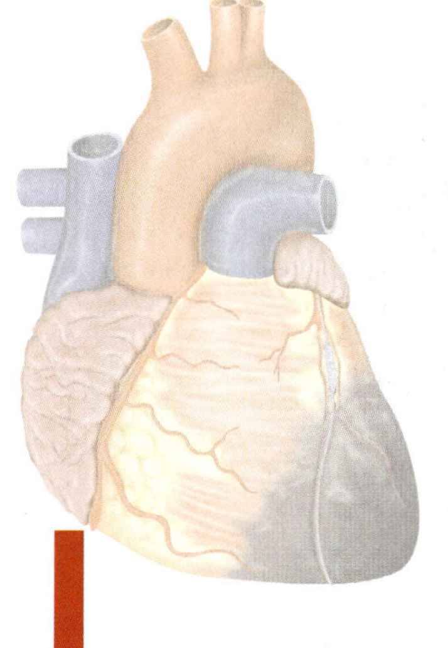

73

CHAPTER

Azilsartan: Promise and Power for Hypertension in Cardiodiabetes

Lal C Daga, Suman Bhandari

INTRODUCTION

Blood Pressure (BP) demonstrates tolerability profiles similar to placebo.[1,2] The clinical outcome trials have shown that the angiotensin II receptor blockers (ARBs) reduces the proportion of hypertensive patients who develop type 2 diabetes mellitus and improve cardiovascular outcomes in such conditions as high-risk hypertension,[3,4] heart failure,[5] and diabetic kidney disease.[6,7] Improved control of BP in patients with hypertension is required to produce the maximum reduction in clinical cardiovascular events,[8,9] and expert consensus guidelines advocate BP levels 140/90 mm Hg in patients lacking target organ involvement and 130/80 mm Hg in patients with diabetes mellitus, heart disease, or kidney disease.[10,11]

AZILSARTAN MEDOXOMIL

Azilsartan medoxomil (AZL-M) is a prodrug quickly hydrolyzing to the active moiety azilsartan, a potent and highly selective ARB with estimated bioavailability of 60% and half-life of 12 hours.[12] The other major metabolite M-II is formed via CYP2C9 and has low affinity for the angiotensin II type 1 receptor. On the basis of dose-ranging studies and supporting pharmacokinetic data, the expected plateau of BP reduction for AZL-M in the large majority of patients with hypertension is 40 mg or 80 mg once daily (Flow chart 1).[12]

It has superior ambulatory and clinical BP-lowering effects compared with Olmesartan and Valsartan at their highest clinically used doses and are well tolerated in patients with hypertension. BP control and response rates by this drug at its highest dose are greater than other drugs in the same class by absolute rates of 8–10%. On the basis of these data, we would expect that AZL-M could lead to enhanced BP control in patients with stages 1 to 2 hypertension.[13] The latest evaluation of the National Health and Nutrition Examination Survey in the United States (NHANES)[14] estimates that 50.1% of patients with hypertension, with some variance according to age and ethnicity, are controlled. AZL-M was found to be more effective in terms of reducing indices of blood pressure over alternative ARBs or angiotensin-converting enzyme (ACE) inhibitors with minimal side effects. Preclinical studies have established pleiotropic effects (Flow chart 1) for AZL-M beyond its primary antihypertensive role through differential gene expression, upregulation of membrane receptors and favorable effect on selective intracellular biochemical and pro-atherosclerotic pathways. Indirect but accumulating evidence from recent literature supports the efficacy and safety of AZL-M among diabetic patients. However, no clinical data exist to date that convinces a beneficial role of AZL-M in patients with metabolic disorders on top of its antihypertensive effect.[15]

Many preclinical studies (Table 1) have proven it as a pleiotropic drug that may exert beneficial cardiometabolic effects beyond its antihypertensive properties (Flow chart 1).[16-21] These favorable effects are probably due to higher affinity, tighter binding, and slower dissociation from angiotensin I receptor (AT1) receptors and its superiority was observed even when AZL-M was used in therapeutic doses in comparison to other ARBs that were administered

TABLE 1: Clinical trials comparing azilsartan medoxomil as a monotherapy or in specific drug combinations to established antihypertensive medication[15]

				Azilsartan medoxomil as monotherapy		
Bakris et al. 2011	Double-blind RCT	1,275	6 weeks	AZL-M $20, 40, 80 mg or OLM 40 mg or placebo	Change from baseline in 24-hr mean SBP	AZL-M 80 mg (−14.6 mm Hg) vs OLM (−12.6 mm Hg) ($p = 0.038$) AZL-M 40 mg (−13.4 mm Hg) was non-inferior to OLM 40 mg
White et al. 2011	Double-blind RCT	1,291	6 weeks	AZL-M 40, 80 mg or VAL 320 mg or OLM 40 mg or placebo	Change from baseline in 24-h mean SBP	AZL-M 80 mg (−14.5 mm Hg) vs OLM (−12.0 mm Hg) ($p = 0.009$) and VAL (−10.2 mm Hg) ($p < 0.001$) AZL-M 40 mg (−13.4 mm Hg) was non-inferior to OLM 40 mg
Sica et al. 2011	Double-blind RCT	984	24 weeks	AZL-M 40, 80 mg or VAL 320 mg	Change from baseline in 24-hr mean SBP	AZL-M 40 mg (−14.9 mm Hg) and 80 mg (−15.3 mm Hg) vs VAL (−11.3 mm Hg) ($p < 0.001$ for both)
Rakugi et al. 2012	Double-blind RCT	622	16 weeks	AZL-M 20–40 mg or CAND 8–12 mg	Change from baseline in the sitting trough DBP	AZL-M (−12.4 mm Hg) vs CAND (−9.8 mm Hg) ($p = 0.0003$)
Bönner et al. 2013	Double-blind RCT	884	24 weeks	AZL-M 20–80 mg or RAM 2.5–10 mg	Change from baseline in the sitting trough SBP	AZL-M 40 mg (−20.6 mm Hg) and AZL-M 80 mg (−21.2 mm Hg) vs RAM (−12.2 mm Hg) ($p < 0.001$)
Kario and Hoshide, 2015	Open-label RCT	718	8 weeks	AZL-M 20 mg or AML 5 mg	Differences between sleep SBP	AZL-M 20 mg (−12.6 mm Hg) vs AML 5 mg (−17.5 mmHg) ($p < 0.001$)
EARLY Gitt et al. 2016	Observational, prospective	3,849	12 months	AZL-M or any ACE-i	• Documentation of the achievement of target BP values set according to recent guidelines • Description of the safety profile of AZL-M	Target BP level achieved in AZL-M group (61.1% of patients) vs. ACE-I group (56.4% of patients) ($p < 0.05$) Equivalent safety profile ($p = 0.73$)
Bakris et al., 2012	Double-blind RCT	609	10 weeks	AZL-M/CLD 40/12.5 – 40/25 mg or AZL-M/HCTZ 40/12.5 – 40/25 mg	Change from baseline in clinic SBP	AZL-M/CLD 40/12.5 mg (−35.1 mm Hg) vs AZL-M/HCTZ 40/12.5 (−29.5 mm Hg) ($p < 0.001$)
Sica et al., 2012	Double-blind RCT	1,714	8 weeks	AZL-M 0, 20, 40, 80 mg and/or CLD 0, 12.5, 25 mg	Change from baseline in trough SBP by ABPM	AZL-M/CLD 40/25 and 80/25 mg (−28.9 mm Hg) vs AZL-M 80 mg (−15.1 mm Hg) and CLD 25 mg (−15.9 mm Hg) ($p < 0.001$ for both)
Cushman et al., 2012	Double-blind RCT	1,071	12 weeks	AZL-M/CLD 40/25 mg or AZL-M/CLD 80/25 mg or OLM/HTCZ 40/25 mg	Changes from baseline in trough, seated, clinic SBP	AZL-M/CLD 40/25 mg (−42.5 mm Hg) and AZL-M/CLD 80/25 mg (−44.0 mm Hg) vs OLM/HTCZ 40/25 mg (−37.1 mm Hg) ($p < 0.001$)
Weber et al., 2014b	Double-blind RCT	566	6 weeks	AZL-M/AML 40/5, 80/5 mg or AML 5 mg + placebo	Change from baseline in 24-h SBP	AZL-M/AML 40/5 mg (−24.8 mm Hg) and AZL-M/AML 80/5 mg (−24.5 mm Hg) vs AML 5 mg + placebo (13.6 mm Hg) ($p < 0.001$)
Rakugi et al., 2014	Double-blind RCT	603	8 weeks	AZL-M/AML 20/5 mg or AZL-M/AML 20/2.5 mg or AZL 20 mg or AML 5 mg or AML 2.5 mg	Change from baseline in the seated trough DBP	AZL-M/AML 20/5 mg (−35.3 mm Hg) and AZL-M/AML 20/2.5 mg (−31.4 mm Hg) vs. AZL-M 20 mg (−21.5 mm Hg), AML 5 mg (−26.4 mm Hg), AML 2.5 mg (−19.3 mm Hg) ($p < 0.001$)
Kipnes et al., 2015	Double-blind RCT	299	6 weeks	AZL-M ± CLD ± other antihypertensive or Placebo±CLD ± other antihypertensive (*depending on the open-label phase*)	Change in trough clinic sitting DBP	Mean difference between AZL-M and placebo (−7.8 mm Hg) ($p < 0.001$)

Abbreviations: RCT, randomized controlled trial; OLM, olmesartan; VAL, valsartan; AZL-M, azilsartan medoxomil; SBP, systolic blood pressure; AML, amlodipine; CAND, candesartan; ACE-i, acetylcholine inhibitors; ACE-1, acetylcholine inhibitor 1; CLD, chlorthalidone; HTCZ, hydrochlorothiazide; DBP, diastolic blood pressure

Flow chart 1: Azilsartan: Pleiotropic effects and positive mechanisms

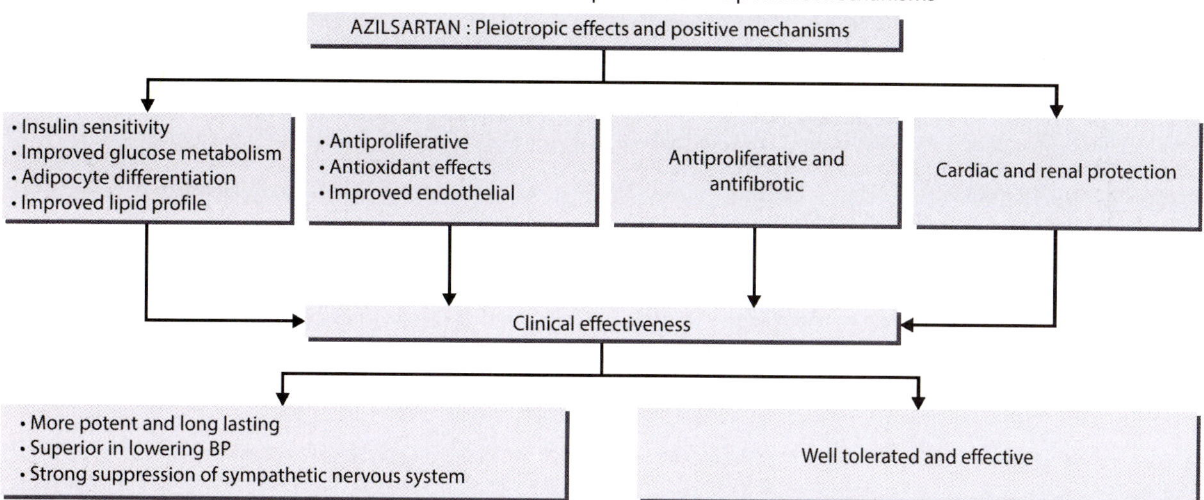

above recommended clinical doses.[16,18] The proposed mechanisms of pleiotropic effects are mostly related to AT1 receptor but at cellular level there is evidence of actions beyond AT1 receptor as well.[22] Experimental studies mentioned that the activation of peroxisome proliferator-activated receptors (PPARγ) pathway from AZL-M as a possible favorable pathophysiological mechanism on top of the AT1 receptor blockage but the data is limited at clinical level.[23] In general, preclinical trials support AZL-M as a possible beneficial treatment strategy for diabetic patients, beyond its antihypertensive effect. AZL-M is a potent and well-tolerated antihypertensive drug and, furthermore, there is indirect evidence of its efficacy and safety among diabetic patients.[15] Moreover, it is more potent and efficient when combined with other antihypertensive drugs.

CONCLUSION

Azilsartan is possibly a promising molecule for control of hypertension especially in setting of cardio-diabetes because of its multiplicity of actions. However more data is required to reveal its superiority as compared to other ARBs. At present, there are no large clinical trials assessing the effect of AZL-M on metabolic profile and on cardiovascular morbidity and mortality.

REFERENCES

1. Ruddy MC, Kostis JB. Angiotensin II receptor antagonists. In: Oparil S, Weber MA (Eds.) Hypertension. Philadelphia: WB Saunders Co.; 2000. pp. 621-37.
2. McGill JB, Reilly PA. Telmisartan plus hydrochlorothiazide versus telmisartan or hydrochlorothiazide monotherapy in patients with mild to moderate hypertension: a multicenter, randomized, double-blind, placebo-controlled parallel-group trial. Clin Ther. 2001;23:833-50.
3. Dahlof B, Devereux RB, Kjeldsen SE, et al. Cardiovascular morbidity and mortality in the Losartan Intervention for Endpoint Reduction in Hypertension Study (LIFE): a randomized trial against atenelol. Lancet. 2002;359:995-1003.
4. Weber MA, Julius S, Kjeldsen SE, et al. Blood pressure dependent and independent effects of antihypertensive treatment on clinical events in the VALUE trial. Lancet. 2004;363:2049-51.
5. Cohn JN, Tognoni G. Valsartan Heart Failure Trial Investigators. A randomized trial of the angiotensin-receptor blocker valsartan in chronic heart failure. N Engl J Med. 2001;345:1667-75.
6. Brenner BM, Cooper ME, deZeeuw D, et al. Effects of losartan on renal and cardiovascular outcomes in patients with type 2 diabetes and nephropathy. N Engl J Med. 2001;345:861-69.
7. Lewis EJ, Hunsicker LG, Clarke WR, et al. Renoprotective effect of the angiotensin-receptor antagonist irbesartan in patients with nephropathy due to type 2 diabetes. N Engl J Med. 2001;345:851-60.
8. Staessen JA, Wang JG, Thijs L. Cardiovascular protection and blood pressure reduction: a meta-analysis. Lancet. 2001;358:1305-15.
9. Turnbull F. Blood Pressure Lowering Treatment Trialists' Collaboration. Effects of different blood-pressure-lowering regimens on major cardiovascular events: results of prospectively-designed overviews of randomized trials. Lancet. 2003;362:1527-35.
10. Chobanian AV, Bakris GL, Black HR, et al. Joint National Committee on Prevention, Detection, Evaluation, and Treatment of High Blood Pressure. National Heart, Lung, and Blood Institute; National High Blood Pressure Education Program Coordinating Committee. Seventh report of the Joint National Committee on Prevention, Detection, Evaluation and Treatment of High BP. Hypertension. 2003;42:1206-52.
11. European Society of Hypertension-European Society of Cardiology Guidelines Committee. 2003 European Society of Hypertension-European Society of Cardiology guidelines for the management of arterial hypertension. J Hypertens. 2003;21:2203-4.
12. Deerfield IL. (TAK 491) Azilsartan Medoxomil Global Investigator's Brochure, 6th edition. Deerfield: Takeda Global Research & Development Center, Inc.; 2007.
13. White WB, Weber MA, Sica D, et al. Effects of the Angiotensin-Receptor Blocker Azilsartan Medoxomil versus Olmesartan and Valsartan on Ambulatory and Clinic Blood Pressure in Patients With Stages 1 and 2 Hypertension. Hypertension. 2011;57:413-20.

14. Egan BM, ZhaoY, Axon RN. US trends in prevalence, awareness, treatment and control of hypertension, 1988-2008. JAMA. 2010;303:2043-50.
15. Georgios G, Vasiliki K, Dimitrios O, et al. Azilsartan as a potent antihypertensive drug with possible pleiotropic cardiometabolic effects: a review study. Front Pharmacol. 2016;7:235.
16. Iwai M, Chen R, Imura Y, et al. TAK-536, a new AT1 receptor blocker, improves glucose intolerance and adipocyte differentiation. Am J Hypertens. 2007;20:579-86.
17. Kusumoto K, Igata H, Ojima M, et al. Antihypertensive, insulin-sensitising and renoprotective effects of a novel, potent and long-acting angiotensin II type 1 receptor blocker, azilsartan medoxomil, in rat and dog models. Eur J Pharmacol. 2011;669:84-93.
18. Zhao M, Li Y, Wang J, et al. Azilsartan treatment improves insulin sensitivity in obese spontaneously hypertensive Koletsky rats. Diabetes Obes Metab. 2011;13:1123-9.
19. Lastra G, Santos FR, Hooshmand P, et al. The novel angiotensin II receptor blocker azilsartan medoxomil ameliorates insulin resistance induced by chronic angiotensin II treatment in rat skeletal muscle. Cardiorenal Med. 2013;3:154-64.
20. Tarikuz Zaman AK, McLean DL, Sobel BE. The efficacy and tolerability of azilsartan in obese insulin-resistant mice with left ventricular pressure overload. J Cardiovasc Pharmacol. 2013;62:381-7.
21. Kajiya T, Ho C, Wang J, et al. Molecular and cellular effects of azilsartan: a new generation angiotensin II receptor blocker. J Hypertens. 2011;29:2476-83.
22. Kurtz TW, Klein U. Next generation multifunctional angiotensin receptor blockers. Hypertens Res. 2009;32:826-34.
23. Kusuyama T, Ogata H, Takeshita H, et al. Effects of azilsartan compared to other angiotensin receptor blockers on left ventricular hypertrophy and the sympathetic nervous system in hemodialysis patients. Ther Apher Dial. 2014;18:398-403.

CHAPTER

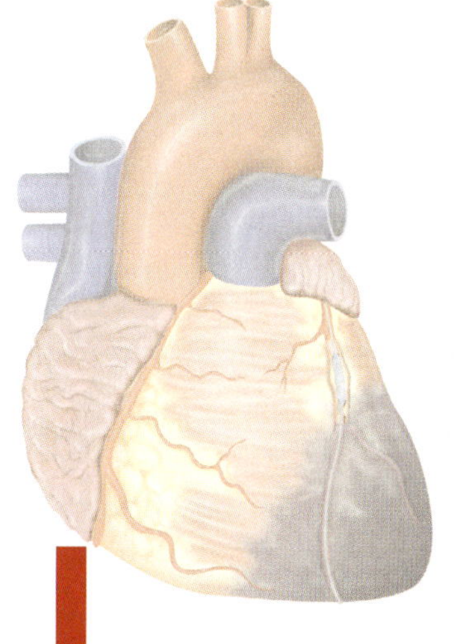

Benidipine for Hypertension in Cardiodiabetes

HK Chopra, Ravi R Kasliwal, Manish Bansal

INTRODUCTION

It is a well-known fact that hypertension is often complicated by diabetes and vice-versa. Both these conditions are the major risk factors for arteriosclerosis, which significantly and synergistically increase the risk of cardiovascular events.[1] Additionally, hypertension is also regarded as a large contributing factor to the progress of renal disorders associated with diabetes. Hence, normalization of hypertension is a key treatment goal for renal protection and possibly cardio protection in type 2 diabetes patients.

Various guidelines have proposed that strict blood pressure (BP) control is necessary in the treatment of diabetes. Efficacy of angiotensin converting enzyme (ACE) inhibitors and angiotensin II receptor blockers (ARB) for preventing cardiovascular events in diabetic hypertensives is well-established. On the other hand, the use of calcium channel blockers (CCBs) with potent antihypertensive effect to treat diabetes has also been recommended.[1] Benidipine is a dihydropyridine (DHP)-derived CCB developed in Japan in 1991. It exhibits unique mechanisms of action which make this molecule different from the other molecules from the same class apart from being a potent antihypertensive.

Unique Mechanisms of Benidipine[1,2]

- A membrane approach
- High vascular selectivity
- Vascular endothelial cells protective effect
- Enhancement of nitric oxide (NO) production
- Antioxidative action and antiatherosclerotic effect
- Triple calcium channels (L, N, and T) blocking action
- Renal protective effects
- Beneficial effect on insulin resistance.

Hence, benidipine not only shows potent antihypertensive effects in diabetic hypertensives but also has beneficial effects on glucose metabolism and renal functions, and consequently seemed to be useful to treat hypertension with diabetes.[1] Importantly, the cardioprotection with benidipine is independent of its potent antihypertensive effect.

Unique Membrane Approach[2]

Benidipine shows genuine 24 hours BP control with least chances of nocturnal BP changes in cardiodiabetic patients. The T/P ratio, an indicator of the duration of antihypertensive activity, has also been studied for benidipine and calculated as from systolic BP (SBP) and diastolic BP (DBP) were 82 and 64, respectively, thus satisfying the World Health Organization (WHO)-recommended T/P ratio (over 50). These results are comparable or superior to the results for other long-lasting CCBs. The strong and long-lasting activity of benidipine can be explained by the concept called as 'membrane approach'. Benidipine has a high affinity for the DHP binding site and cell membranes. Exhibits slow binding to and slow dissociation from the DHP binding site and hence the concept of the (approach to the cell membrane followed by long retention in the DHP binding site) is applicable to benidipine (Figs 1A and B).

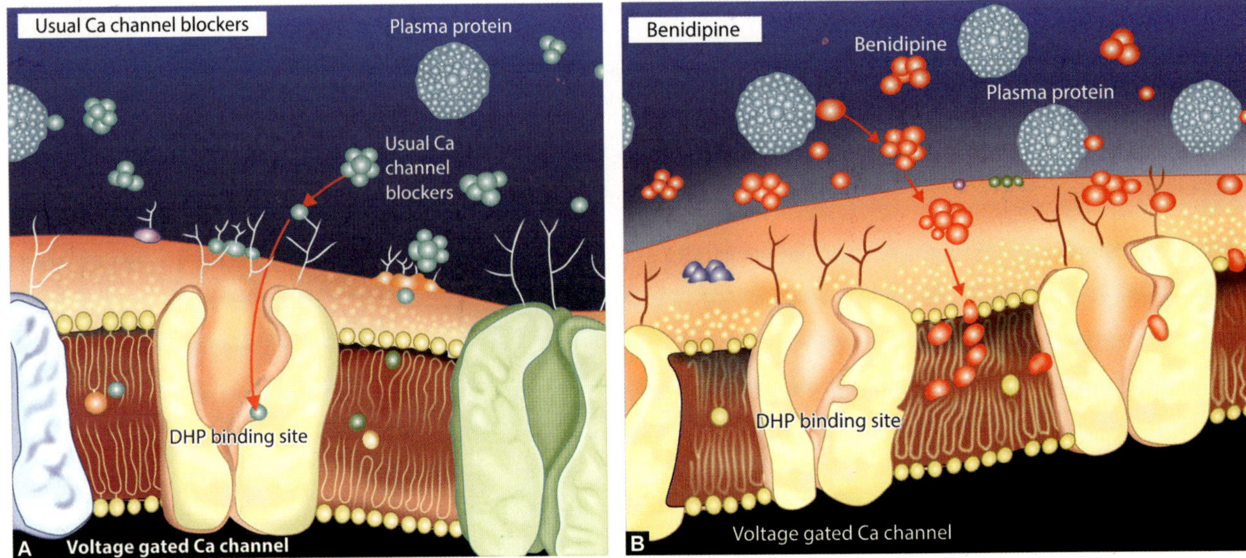

Figs 1A and B: (A) Usual Ca channel blockers; (B) Benidipine

High Vascular Selectivity[2]

In the preclinical studies, coronary artery selectivity of benidipine was 14.4 times higher than that of nifedipine and 19 times higher than that of amlodipine. In addition, the ratio of binding to peripheral blood vessels to binding to the heart was higher with benidipine than with nifedipine or amlodipine. This high vascular selectivity seems to be associated with the pharmacological actions of this drug such as its vasodilative and vasoprotective effects, which are the very useful for the management of hypertension and related complications especially in diabetic patients.

Vascular endothelial cells protective effect[3]: Benidipine improves oxidized low-density lipoprotein (oxLDL) dependent monocyte and endothelial dysfunction in hypertensive patients with type 2 diabetes mellitus. Activation of platelets and/or monocytes is very important for the development of vascular disorder in hypertensive patients with type 2 diabetes. Levels of platelet, monocyte, and endothelial cell activation markers, microparticles, chemokines, and soluble adhesion molecules are higher in hypertensive diabetic patients with than in those without type 2 diabetes. Administration of benidipine decreases the concentrations of all these markers along with the significant reduction in SBP and DBP. The effect of this drug is significant in diabetes patients with high levels of anti-oxLDL antibody. Hence, benidipine is effective for the treatment of oxLDL-dependent vascular disorders in hypertensive patients with type 2 diabetes.

Anti-Oxidative Effect:[4] Hypertension along with diabetes is associated with increased oxidative stress. Oxidative stress reduction may have similar advantages with antihypertensive treatment for prevention of cardiovascular disease. Plasma thiobarbituric acid reactive substances (TBARS), one of the markers of oxidative stress, reflect plasma malondialdehyde concentrations resulting from lipid or cell thiobarbituric acid peroxidation. They are known to be increased in patients of hypertension and diabetes is associated with a further increased TBARS level. Benidipine alone decreased plasma TBARS levels not only in the patients demonstrating strong decrease (< 140 mm Hg) in BP, but also in those with only a slight decrease (< 150 mm Hg). Hence, benidipine exerts effects on oxidative stress independent of its antihypertensive action. As per Suzuki et al. of 85 patient's data where 23 patients were diabetic, benidipine treatment resulted in a significant decrease in BP (SBP/DBP) from 154 ± 22/87 ± 11 mm Hg to 133 ± 18/76 ± 9 mm Hg ($p < 0.001$) and a significant reduction in plasma TBARS levels from 3.3 ± 0.9 to 2.7 ± 0.7 nmol/mL ($p < 0.001$). When patients were stratified according to patient characteristics (sex, age, smoking, hypertension, diabetes, dyslipidemia, ischemic heart disease, and old myocardial infarction), benidipine was found to have significantly reduced plasma TBARS levels in all subsets (Figs 2 and 3).

Probable mechanisms of antioxidative effects of benidipine include lipophilic nature of benidipine, benidipine has the highest partition coefficient among calcium antagonists. A high concentration of a lipophilic calcium antagonist in the membrane can prevent oxidative injury, independent of antihypertensive actions. Benidipine was found to be associated with a lower incidence of total cardiovascular events in diabetic patients.[4]

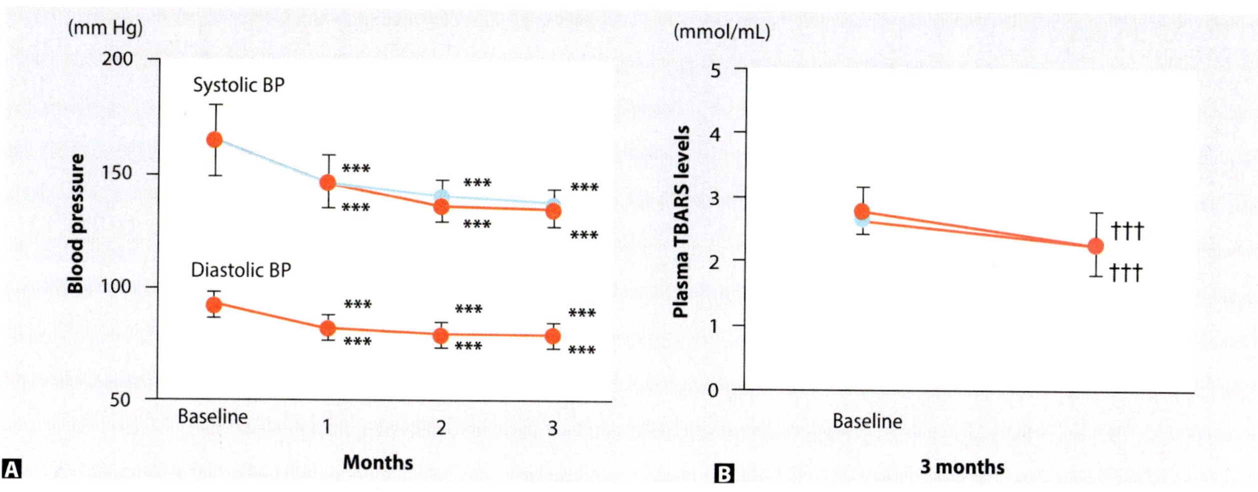

Figs 2A and B: Changes in (A) blood pressure and (B) plasma TBARS levels in high-risk, essential hypertensive patients treated with benidipine

- or amlodipine
- Values are means ± SD.

***p<0.001, versus before drug treatment by the Dunnett's multiple comparison

†††p<0.001 versus before drug treatment by the paired t-test.

Abbreviations: TBARS, thiobarbituric acid reactive substance; BP, blood pressure

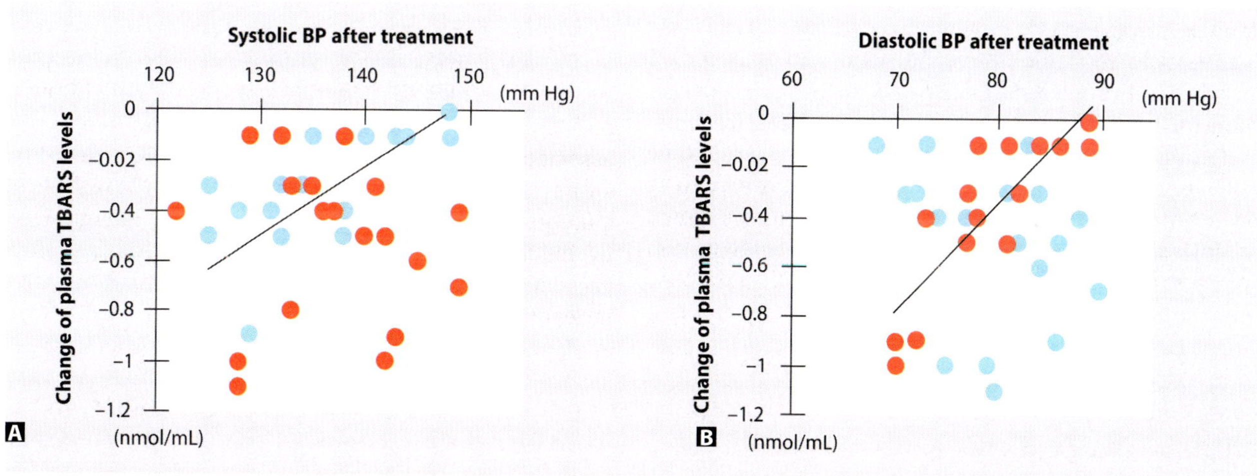

Figs 3A and B: Correlation between blood pressure and reduction in plasma TBARS levels in essential hypertensive patients treated with amlodipine

Abbreviations: BP, blood pressure; TBARS, thiobarbituric acid reactive substances; r, Pearson's correlation coefficient. A significant positive correlation was found for the amlodipine group (solid line: systolic BP, P<0.01; diastolic BP, p<0.001).

These antioxidative and vascular endothelium-protective activities of benidipine seem to appear at dose levels lower than those required by other CCBs due to the 'membrane approach'. In anesthetized dogs, benidipine (100 ng/kg/min) elevated coronary blood flow through the ischemic myocardium, alleviated the reduction in myocardial contractility, and reduced metabolic disorders such as diabetes.[2]

Antiatherosclerosis effect: Shown effects on reduction of P and S selectin and reduces the chances of atherosclerosis (Fig. 4).[5]

Benidipine is expected to suppress the progression of atherosclerosis also by stimulating the formation of NO by its direct action on vascular endothelial cells in addition to exerting antioxidative effects.[2]

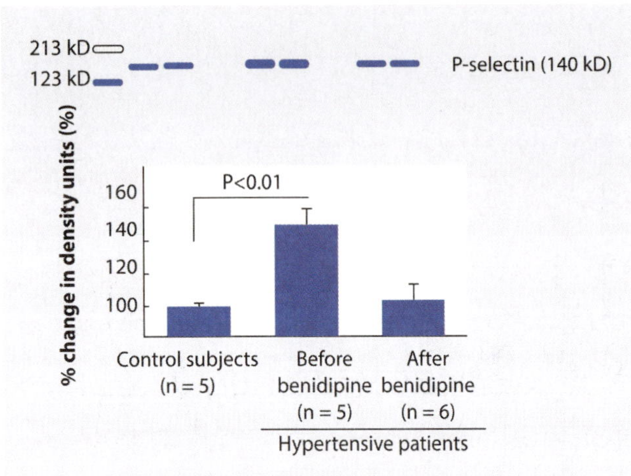

Fig. 4: Western blot analysis of P-selectin in human platelets before and after benidipine treatment

Prognostic Effects of Benidipine in Patients with Vasospastic Angina

Fukumoto et al. performed a prospective study involving 527 patients with vasospastic angina who were treated with one of the three CCBs (amlodipine, diltiazem, and benidipine) and were followedup for a mean period of 5.2 years. For risk factors including smoking, hypertension, diabetes mellitus, and reduced left ventricular ejection fraction, were found to be significant risk factors for cardiovascular events in this cohort. Compared with amlodipine and diltiazem, benidipine was associated with a lower incidence of total events, cardiovascular events, and cerebral infarction. Moreover, benidipine significantly reduced the incidence of vascular infarction events, suggesting the possible role of atherosclerosis in causation of vasospastic angina. These findings suggested that benidipine might be useful for the treatment of vasospastic angina in patients with diabetes.[6]

The nitric oxide-increasing effect: The increase in NO seems to be one of the mechanisms responsible for increased in the coronary blood flow observed with benidipine. Benidipine increases NO formation associated with endothelial NO synthase (eNOS) but does not increase NO formation associated with inflammatory inducible NOS (iNOS). Treatment with benidipine resulted in a reduction in cardiac hypertrophy and an increase in left ventricular NO formation and eNOS messenger ribonucleic acid (mRNA) levels. Benidipine is known to increase the renal NO levels as well.[2]

Effect on sympathetic nervous system: Activation of the sympathetic nervous system seems to be responsible for aggravation of diabetes and hypertension. Benidipine does not cause heart rate increase, tachycardia or facial flush, indicating the maintenance of N-type calcium channel blocking activity. Benidipine is reported to block the N-type calcium channel and inhibit the sympathetic nervous system.[1]

Lipid lowering effect: 17 hypertensive patients with noninsulin dependent diabetes mellitus were treated with benidipine for 6 months. The time courses of blood neutral fat, high-density lipoprotein (HDL) cholesterol, LDL-cholesterol levels were followed. A significant decrease in blood triglyceride level accompanied by significant reduction in apo C-II, C-III, and E. Furthermore, serum oxygen radical scavenger activity (like superoxide dismutase activity) was significantly increased, whereas serum lipid peroxide levels was significantly decreased.[2]

Renal Protective Effect of Benidipine

It is known that renal disorders are a major factor in the prognosis of diabetic patients. Benidipine was shown in this study to be effective in controlling BP and lowering up.[1]

- *Triple calcium channel blocking effect of benidipine:* Glomerular hypertension is an important factor in the mechanism for the onset of hypertensive glomerular injury in diabetic patients. T-type calcium channel is involved in the constriction and dilation of renal efferent arterioles.[1] Benidipine dilates both the afferent and efferent arterioles and reduces the glomerular pressure.
- *Reduction in urinary protein excretion:*[7] It was suggested that benidipine has the potential to be more effective at reducing proteinuria in the case of diabetic patients.[7] Benidipine also suppresses the progression of albuminuria and sclerotic changes in the glomeruli with significant reduction in SBP and DBP.
- *Beneficial effect on renal tissue:* Benidipine exerts natriuretic effects by acting on both the upper segment of tubules and the distal tubules. Suppresses both the necrosis and apoptosis of tubules.[2]
- *Effect on Aldosterone:*[9] It has been demonstrated that aldosterone can directly damage various organs including the heart and blood vessels, via mineralocorticoid receptors, independent of changes in BP. It has been suggested that hypertensive incidents and organ damage in humans may occur even at plasma aldosterone levels within the normal physiological range. Therefore, targeting aldosterone synthesis and release may be clinically important in preventing cardiovascular disease. Ca^{2+} ions are conveyed through the T-type Ca channel to the mitochondria where they activate aldosterone synthesis which in turn

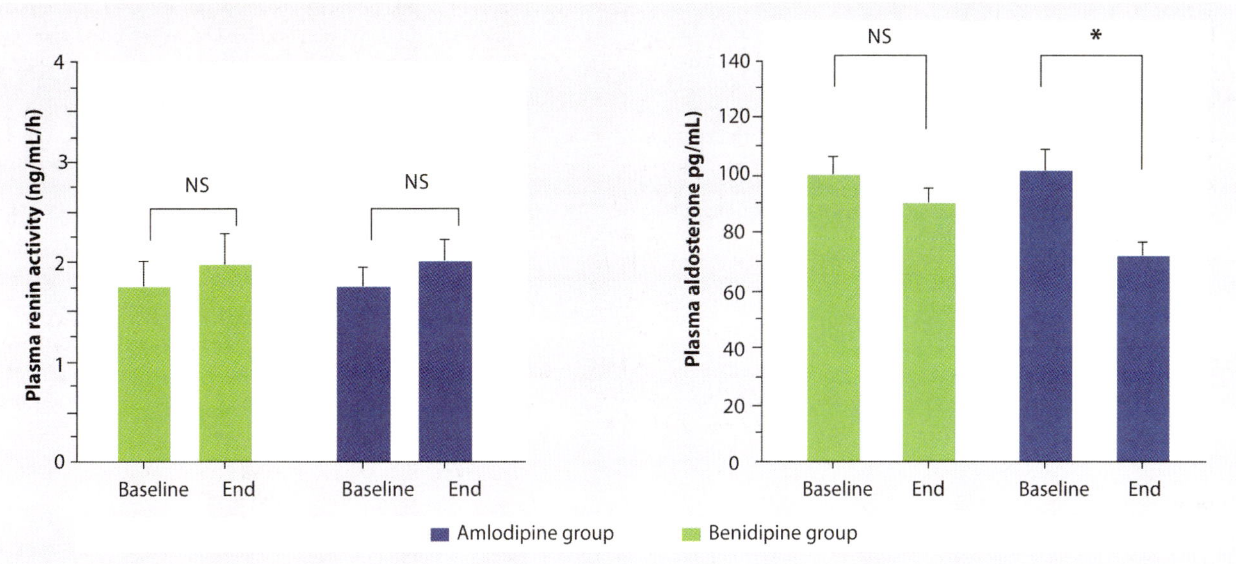

Fig. 5: Changes in plasma renin activity and plasma aldosterone levels in the two groups

Abbreviation: NS, not significant;
*P<0.01 vs. baseline; †P<0.05

stimulates T-type Ca channel expression, creating a positive feedback loop of aldosterone biosynthesis in adrenal cells. As per the data published in Hypertension Research (2011) plasma aldosterone level were significantly decreased in the benidipine treatment group-type CCBs[8] inhibit renin secretion and renin gene expression *in vivo*, whereas L-type CCBs function as stimulators of the renin system-type CCBs have a dual effect on plasma renin activity and renin mRNA expression *in vivo*, with low concentrations stimulating and high concentrations inhibiting the renin system. Benidipine decreases plasma aldosterone levels without any effect on serum Na and K levels when administered to patients with mild-to-moderate stage chronic kidney disease (CKD) (Fig. 5).

Thus, in addition to lowering BP benidipine would be expected to provide renoprotection by inhibiting aldosterone production. Long-term treatment with ACE inhibitors or ARBs can cause escape or rebound of plasma aldosterone levels. In such a situation, addition of a mineralocorticoid receptor blocker has been shown to reduce proteinuria in patients taking inhibitors of the renin-angiotensin-aldosterone system for the treatment of hypertension and kidney disease; a T-type CCB benidipine might be a suitable addition for the purpose of inhibiting aldosterone production and managing aldosterone escape in diabetic and nondiabetic patients.[9]

- *Effects on insulin resistance*: In view of trial findings on the effects of benidipine in reducing insulin resistance and protecting organs from injury due to diabetes mellitus, it seems likely that benidipine is also useful in the treatment of hypertension complicated by diabetes mellitus.[2]

CONCLUSION

Being a unique triple CCB, Benidipine with reno- and cardioprotective actions and other inimitable antihypertensive effects compared to other CCBs in hypertensive diabetics patients is indeed a way forward to manage hypertension in cardiodiabetic patients, thereby help reducing morbidity.

REFERENCES

1. Seino G, Miyaguchi S, Yamazaki T, et al. Benidipine hydrochloride effect of benidipine hydrochloride, a long-acting T-type calcium channel blocker, on blood pressure and renal function in hypertensive patients with diabetes mellitus. Analysis after switching from cilnidipine to benidipine. Arzneimittelforschung. 2007;57(8):526-31.
2. K Yao, Nagashima K, Miki H. Pharmacological, pharmacokinetic, and clinical properties of benidipine hydrochloride, a novel, long-acting calcium channel blocker. J Pharmacol Sci.2006;100(4):243-61.
3. Nomura S, Shouzu A, Omoto S, et al. Benidipine improves oxidized LDL-dependent monocyte and endothelial dysfunction in hypertensive patients with type 2 diabetes mellitus. J Hum Hypertens. 2005;19(7):551-7.
4. Suzuki O, Yoshida T, Tani S, et al. Antioxidative effects of benidipine hydrochloride in patients with hypertension independent of antihypertensive effects. Relationship between blood pressure and oxidative stress. Arzneimittelforschung. 2004;54(9):505-12.

5. Sanada H, Midorikawa S, Yatabe J, et al. Elevation of Serum Soluble E- and P-Selectin in patients with hypertension is reversed by Benidipine, a long-acting calcium channel blocker. Hypertens Res. 2005;28(11):871-8.
6. Fukumoto Y, Yasuda S, Ito A, et al. Prognostic Effects of Benidipine in Patients With Vasospastic Angina: Comparison With Diltiazem and Amlodipine. J Cardiovasc Pharmacol. 2008;51(3):253-7.
7. Abe M, Okada K, Maruyama N, et al. Comparison between the antiproteinuric effects of the calcium channel blockers benidipine and cilnidipine in combination with angiotensin receptor blockers in hypertensive patients with chronic kidney disease. Expert Opin Investig Drugs. 2010;19(9):1027-37.
8. Yousef WM, Omar AH, Morsy MD, et al. The mechanism of action of calcium channel blockers in the treatment of diabetic nephropathy. Int J Diabetes & Metabolism. 2005;13:76-82.
9. Abe M, Okada K, Maruyama N, et al. Benidipine reduces albuminuria and plasma aldosterone in mild-to-moderate stage chronic kidney disease with albuminuria. Hypertension Research. 2011;34(2):268-73.

CHAPTER 75

Azilsartan: A Molecule of First Choice for Hypertension in Cardiodiabetes

HK Chopra, Viveka Kumar, AK Pancholia

INTRODUCTION

Hypertension (HTN) is ranked as third most important risk factor for attributable burden of cardiovascular (CV) disease in South Asia.[1] It has been reported that at ages around 40–69 years, an increase of 20 mm Hg in systolic blood pressure (SBP) or 10 mm Hg in diastolic BP (DBP) is associated with more than two-fold increase in risk of death from stroke or ischemic heart disease (IHD).[2] Antihypertensive medications significantly reduce adverse CV outcomes by decreasing BP. Among different antihypertensive therapies, Renin-angiotensin-aldosterone system (RAAS) blockers like, angiotensin converting enzyme inhibitors (ACEIs) and angiotensin (ANG) receptor blockers (ARBs) are recommended among first-choice therapy in treatment of HTN.[3-6]

Azilsartan medoxomil (AZM) is a new ARB recently approved for treatment of HTN. Azilsartan differs to candesartan by modification of the tetrazole ring (Fig. 1).[7]

PHARMACOLOGY

Mechanism of Action

Azilsartan is a selective ANG II type 1 (AT1) subtype ANG II receptor blocker (ARB). AZM selectively blocks the binding of ANG II to the AT1 receptor and thereby diminishes the vasoconstrictor and aldosterone-secreting effects of ANG II.

Pharmacodynamics

In vitro and *in vivo* studies demonstrated that AZM is a potent selective AT1 subtype ANG II receptor antagonist. It has a strong potency and causes long-lasting AT1 receptor blockade due to its slow dissociation from AT1 receptor. Azilsartan has more than a 10,000-fold greater affinity for the AT1 receptor than for the ANG II type 2 (AT2) receptor. AZM binds to the AT1 receptor in a concentration dependent manner with high affinity. Azilsartan was found to be approximately twice as potent as olmesartan (OLM) or telmisartan and 5–20 times more potent than irbesartan and valsartan (VAL).[8]

Role of Angiotensin Converting Enzyme-2 and Angiotensin 1–7 and Pleiotropic Benefits

Experimental evidence suggests that ANG-(1–7), generated by ACE-2, has vasoprotective and atheroprotective effects. Studies have shown that plasma ANG-(1–7) levels (pg/mL) were increased with azilsartan treatment. Increase in ANG-(1–7) level during AT1 receptor blockade by azilsartan could result in mas receptor activation and the induction of cardioprotective and renoprotective effects. ACE-2/ANG-(1–7)/mas pathway activation can lead to increased afferent arteriolar dilatation, increase renal flow, and reduction in protein loss in kidneys; results in release of prostaglandins and nitric oxide (NO) which probably results in reduced matrix protein deposition and reduced glomerulosclerosis.[9] Amplification of ACE-2/ANG (1–7)/mas signaling opposes the effects of classical RAAS,

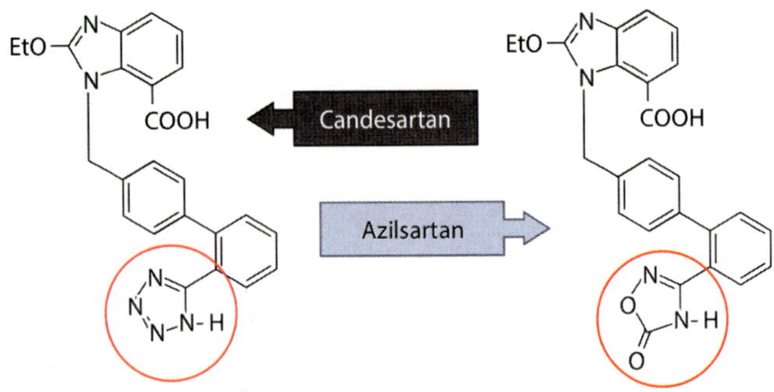

Fig. 1: Difference between azlisartan and candesartan by tetrazole ring modification

additionally lowers BP and prevents or reverses related target organ damage.

Pharmacokinetics

Azilsartan medoxomil is a prodrug, which is metabolized by CYP2C9 to bioactive molecule, azilsartan. Time required to reach peak plasma concentration is 1.5–3 hours. Azilsartan is metabolized to the inactive major M-II metabolite by O-dealkylation, and the minor M-I metabolite via decarboxylation. M-I and M-II metabolites do not contribute to the pharmacologic activity of azilsartan. Terminal half-life ($t_{1/2}$) of azilsartan is nearly 11 hours. Estimated renal clearance of azilsartan is 2.3 mL/min. Accumulation in body does not occur with continuous once-daily dosing.[10] Steady state concentration is achieved in 5 days.

ANIMAL STUDIES

Fractional Sodium Excretion (Fig. 2)

Effect of azilsartan on sodium handling in renal tubules was examined in an animal model study in subtotal nephrectomized C57BL/6 mice. Mice received azilsartan (1.0 mg/kg/day), candesartan (0.3 mg/kg/day), or vehicle via the oral route in conjunction with a normal (0.3%) or high-salt (8.0%) diet. Two weeks later, the azilsartan group showed significantly lower BP during the light period than the candesartan and vehicle groups (azilsartan: 103.1 ± 1.0; candesartan: 111.7 ± 2.7; vehicle: 125.5 ± 2.5 mm Hg; $P < 0.05$; azilsartan or candesartan vs. vehicle). The azilsartan

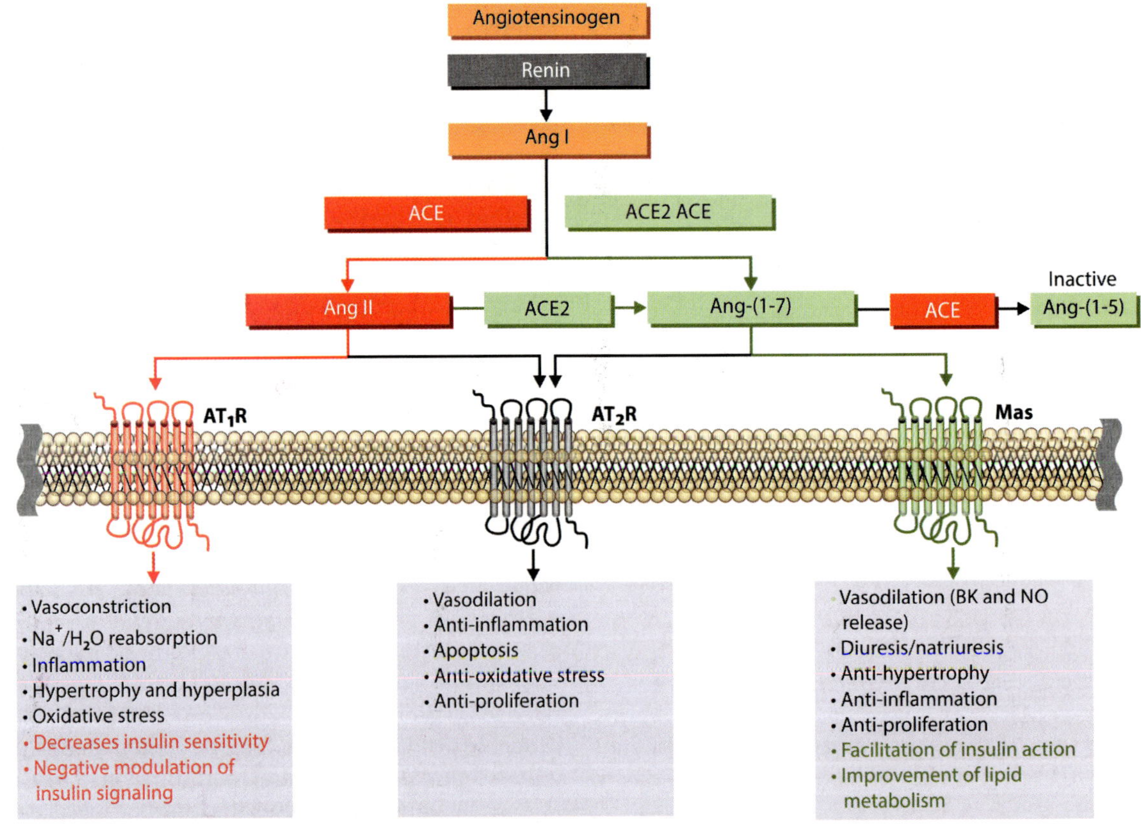

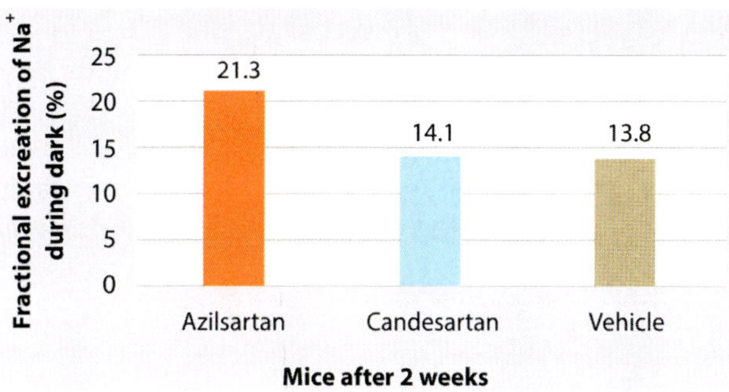

Fig. 2: Fractional excretion of Na+ in high salt fed mice after 2 weeks

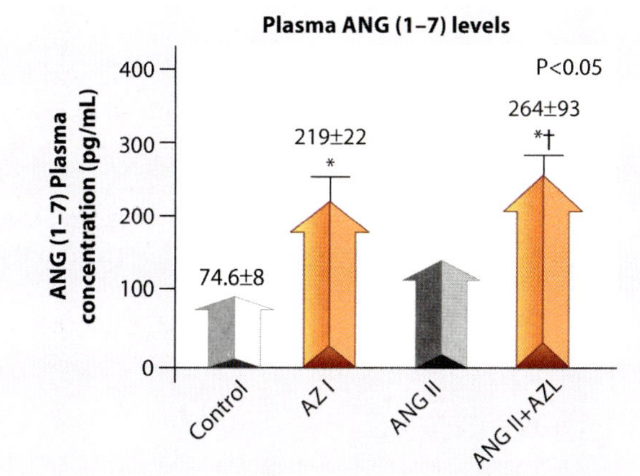

Fig. 3: Plasma ANG (1–7) level after 10 days of ANG II infusion and azlisartan treatment

group also showed higher urinary fractional excretion of sodium during the dark period than the candesartan and vehicle groups (azilsartan: 21.37 ± 3.69%; candesartan: 14.17 ± 1.42%; vehicle: 13.85 ± 5.30%; *P*< 0.05 azilsartan vs. candesartan or vehicle).[11]

Effect on Angiotensin 1–7

To understand the ability of azilsartan to modulate levels of plasma ANG-(1–7) and renal epoxyeicosatrienoic acids (EETs) and 20-hydroxyeicosatetraenoic acid (20-HETE) an animal model study was conducted on Sprague-Dawley rats infused with ANG-II (125 ng/min) or vehicle. Azilsartan (3 mg/kg/day) or vehicle was administered starting 1 day prior to ANG-II or vehicle infusion. On day 10, plasma was obtained for measurement of ANG-(1–7) and kidneys for isolation of microvessels for histological evaluation. The BP elevation with ANG-II infusion (121 ± 5 mm Hg) was completely normalized with azilsartan cotreatment (86 ± 3 mm Hg). Plasma ANG-(1–7) levels (pg/mL) were increased with azilsartan treatment (219 ± 22) and azilsartan + ANG-II infusion (264 ± 93) compared to vehicle controls (74.62 ± 8) (Fig. 3).

Study concluded that treatment with azilsartan completely antagonized the elevation of BP induced by ANG II, prevented cardiac hypertrophy, attenuated renal damage, and increased ANG-(1–7) levels.[12]

CLINICAL EVIDENCES

Hypertension and Ambulatory Blood Pressure Monitoring

Azilsartan versus Valsartan

Azilsartan was compared with VAL in a randomized, double-blind, multicenter study using ambulatory and clinic BP measurements (24-week duration). In total, 984 patients were randomized to AZM 40 mg (n = 327), AZM 80 mg (n = 329), and VAL 320 mg (n = 328). Changes in both 24-hour and clinic DBP were significantly greater for AZM 40 mg and 80 mg than with VAL 320 mg. The proportion of patients who achieved a reduction in clinic SBP to less than140 mm Hg and/or a reduction of more than equal to 20 mm Hg was significantly greater with AZM 40 mg (56%) and AZM 80 mg (59%) than with VAL 320 mg (47%; *P* = 0.016 and *P* = 0.002, respectively).

Treatment-emergent adverse events (AEs) were mostly mild-to-moderate in severity. Rates of AEs were similar in azilsartan 40 mg (65.4%) and 80 mg (65.3%) groups but were numerically lower in VAL 320 mg (59.2%) group.[13]

Azilsartan versus Olmesartan

In a randomized, double-blind, placebo controlled, multicenter study, Bakris et al.[14] assessed change in 24-hour mean SBP at week 6 as assessed by ambulatory BP monitoring (ABPM). Change in trough sitting clinic SBP at week 6 was key secondary endpoint.

Patients with primary HTN (n = 1,275) and baseline 24-hour mean ambulatory systolic pressure more than equal to 130 mm Hg and less than equal to 170 mm Hg were enrolled. Reduction in 24-hour mean SBP and clinic SBP were significantly greater with azilsartan 80 mg than OLM 40 mg by 2.1 mm Hg (95% confidence interval (CI), -4.0 -0.1; *P* = 0.038) and by 2.7 mm Hg (95% CI, -5.3–0.1; *P* = 0.043), respectively.

Reduction was significantly greater in 80 mg dose compared to highest strength of OLM (40 mg). Azilsartan 40 mg was also noninferior to OLM 40 mg.

Azilsartan versus Ramipril

Bonner et al.[15] in a randomized, double blind, placebo-controlled trial compared azilsartan 40 mg (n = 295) and 80 mg (n = 294) with ramipril 10 mg once daily (n = 295) in patients who had clinic SBP between 150–180 mm Hg. The primary endpoint was change in trough, seated, and clinic SBP at 24 weeks.

Responder rate was significantly higher for both doses of azilsartan than ramipril. AEs leading to discontinuation were less frequent with AZM 40 mg and 80 mg (2.4% and 3.1%, respectively) than with ramipril (4.8%).

Study Group	BP	Change in clinic BP (mm Hg) (SD)	Change in 24-hour mean BP (mm Hg) (SD)
AZM 40	SBP	−20.6 (0.9)	−12.7 (1.0)
	DBP	−10.2 (0.6)	−8.0 (0.7)
AZM 80	SBP	−21.2 (0.9)	−12.3 (1.0)
	DBP	−10.5 (0.6)	−8.3 (0.6)
RAM 10	SBP	−12.2 (0.9)	−7.8 (1.0)
	DBP	−4.9 (0.6)	−5.3 (0.7)

Abbreviations: BP, blood pressure; SD, standard deviation; AZM, azilsartan medoxomil; SBP, systolic blood pressure, DBP, diastolic blood pressure; RAM, ramipril.

Hypertension with Diabetes

- White et al.[16] compared efficacy, safety, and metabolic effects of azilsartan with OLM and VAL in prediabetic and diabetic patients. In pooled analysis of 3,821 patients from 3 randomized controlled trials (RCTs), reduction in 24-hour mean SBP and clinic SBP are shown in Figure 4.
  Azilsartan can be considered in prediabetes and diabetes to provide additional 3–7 mm Hg SBP reduction over existing ARBs.
- Rakugi et al.[17] in a 16-week randomized double-blind clinical trial found that AZL-M (40–80 mg; n = 313) compared to candesartan (8–12 mg; n = 309) was associated with significantly greater reduction in sitting systolic (mean difference -4.4 mm Hg, p< 0.0001) and diastolic (mean difference: -2.6 mm Hg, p = 0.0003) BP. On ambulatory BP monitoring, AZL-M significantly reduced 24-hour, day-time, night-time, and early morning BP.

Diabetes mellitus	Changes at week 16 in sitting trough DBP (mm Hg)		Changes at week 16 in sitting trough SBP (mm Hg)	
	Azilsartan	Candesartan	Azilsartan	Candesartan
Presence	−11.5 (10.19) (n = 61)	−9.7 (8.96) (n = 73)	−20.9 (16.27) (n = 61)	−16.4 (12.95) (n = 73)
Absence	−12.7 (9.80) (n = 250)	−9.8 (8.37) (n = 236)	−22.1 (15.08) (n = 250)	−17.8 (12.62) (n = 236)

Azilsartan versus angiotensin converting enzyme inhibitors: 1-year outcomes of the EARLY registry:

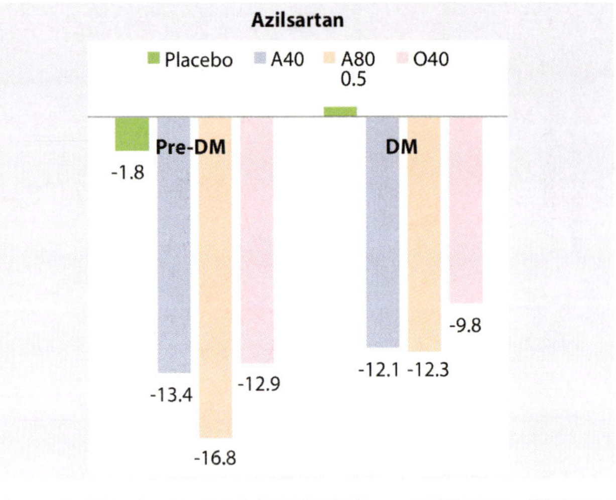

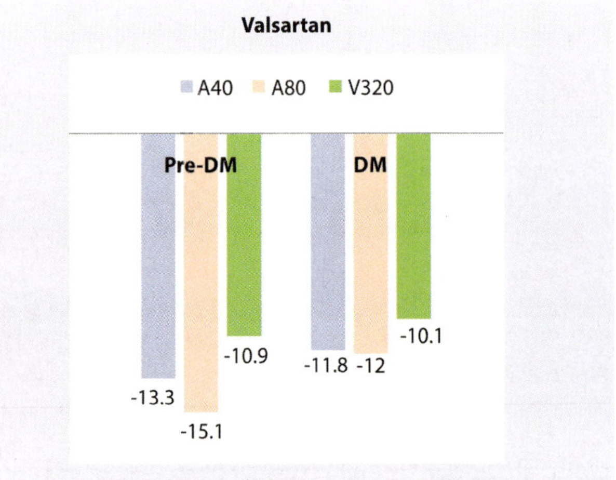

Fig. 4: 24-hour SBP: Azilsartan versus valsartan

Abbreviations: SBP, systolic blood pressure; DM, diabetes mellitus.

Gitt et al.[18] assessed efficacy and safety of AZL-M (n = 2,809) in comparison to ACEIs (n = 1,040) from their prospective, observational EARLY registry with a follow-up of 12-months.

Results in diabetic subgroup: Distribution of patients who had diabetes was similar in AZL-M and ACEIs groups (19.4% vs. 19.3%, $p = 0.96$). AZL-M was associated with significant reductions BP with achievement of target BP of less than 140/90 mm Hg at end of 12-months.

- *In patients with diabetes:* Odds ratio (OR) 1.05 (95% CI 0.74–1.49).
- *In patients without diabetes*: OR 12.6 (95% CI 1.05–1.51) Thus, findings from this observational study suggest that when BP reduction is taken alone as efficacy measure, azilsartan is more effective than ACEIs.
- *Azilsartan versus valsartan and olmesartan: Achievement of SBP goals among hypertensive patients with diabetes.* Sussman et al.[19] created a Monte Carlo

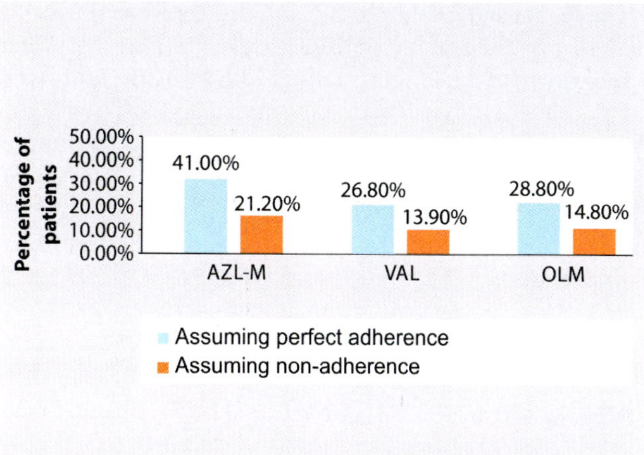

Fig. 5: Percentage of patient achieving BP goal of less than 140/90 assuming adherence and nonadherence in three groups

Abbreviations: AZL-M, azilsartan medoxomil; VAL, valsartan; OLM, olmesartan.

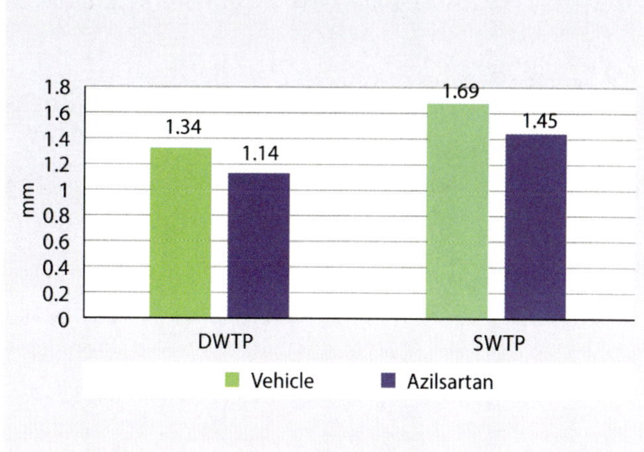

Fig. 6: Effect of azilsartan on left ventricular wall thickness in obese mice

Abbreviations: DWTP, diastolic wall thickness; SWTP, systolic wall thickness.

simulation model to determine the number of patients with HTN and diabetes who can achieve SBP goal of less than 130 mm Hg with AZL-M, OLM and VAL after 12 months of treatment. They created hypothetical cohort of patients with diabetes and uncontrolled HTN from National Health and Nutrition Examination Survey (NHANES) 1999–2006 cohort and assigned them a baseline SBP. Diabetes subpopulation data from azilsartan clinical trial program was used to generate follow-up SBPs by randomly sampling mean and standard deviation (SD) of percentage change from baseline. With a baseline SBP of 151 ± 19 mm Hg SBP goals would be achieved in better in AZL-M than other treatments as shown in Figure 5.

OTHER STUDIES

Azilsartan versus Angiotensin Receptor Blockers: Effect on Left Ventricular Hypertrophy and the Sympathetic Nervous System in Hemodialysis Patients

- Kusuyama et al. (2014)[20] assessed 17 patients on hemodialysis (HD) being treated with ARBs like losartan, VAL, telmisartan, or OLM for more than 6 months before enrolment. Once enrolled, their ARB was switched to azilsartan. During the study period, patients' records of major adverse cardiovascular and cerebrovascular AEs were obtained (all-cause death, myocardial infarction, coronary revascularization, or cerebrovascular disease). Echocardiographic assessment was done at baseline and at the 6-month follow-up. Holter monitoring was done top record ambulatory BP monitoring.
  In 16 patients analyzed (one excluded), mean age was 66.8 years, all had HTN. Noradrenaline level reduced significantly (p = 0.002) from baseline (550.1 ± 282.9 ng/mL) to 6 months (351.7 ± 152.3 ng/mL). Significant reduction in left ventricular (LV) mass and LV mass index (LVMI) were evident after switching to azilsartan (Fig. 6). The ABPM data showed that azilsartan significantly reduced 24-hr SBP (from 150.9 ± 16.2 mm Hg to 131.3 ± 21.7 mm Hg; p = 0.008), awakening time SBP (from 152.1 ± 16.9 mm Hg to 131.7 ± 23.2 mm Hg, p = 0.01), and sleep-time SBP (from 148.1 ± 19.7 mm Hg to 130.0 ± 20.1 mm Hg, p = 0.005).
- *Azilsartan in obese insulin-resistant mice with left ventricular pressure overload:* Zaman et al. (2013)[21] studied effect of azilsartan on LV wall thickness and cardiac function in obese and insulin resistant mice with LV pressure overload. LV pressure overload was created. Azilsartan was administered as 10 mg/kg body weight/day from 4 weeks before surgery to 14 weeks after surgery. Echocardiographic assessment of LV wall thickness and cardiac function was done. Compared to vehicular control, azilsartan treatment was associated with significant reduction in left ventricle anterior diastolic wall thickness (DWTA) and left ventricle posterior systolic wall thickness (SWTP) (Fig. 6).
  Further, a significant increment in cardiac output was seen with azilsartan compared to control.
- *Azilsartan in mice with left ventricular pressure overload or acute myocardial infarction:* Bauman et al. (2013)[22] studied effect of azilsartan on LV wall thickness, LV mass

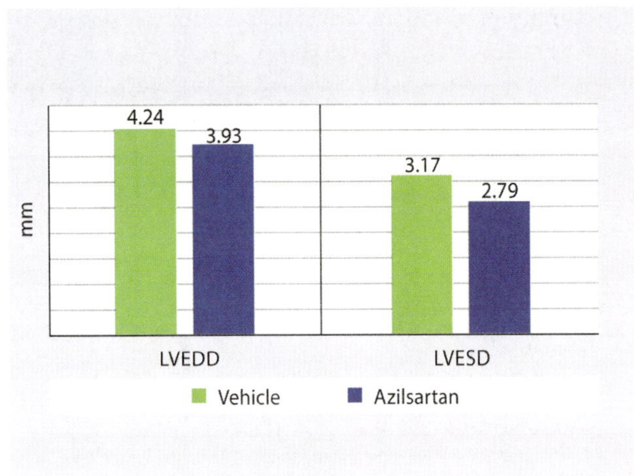

Fig. 7: LVEDD and LVESD in azilsartan and vehicle treatment

Abbreviations: LVEDD, left ventricular end diastolic internal diameter; LVESD, left ventricular end systolic internal diameter.

and cardiac function in mice with surgically induced LV pressure overload or acute infarction. LV pressure overload was created by surgical aortic banding in each mice. Azilsartan was administered as 10 mg/kg body weight/day from 4 week before surgery to 14 weeks after surgery and peanut butter was used as vehicle. For discussion purpose, results in aortic banding mice are described here. BP measure 1 week after surgery was reduced significantly in azilsartan treatment than vehicle (80 ± 7 mm Hg vs. 109 ± 9, $p = 0.007$). Azilsartan was associated with significantly less LV hypertrophy (LVH) than vehicle treatment as described by LV weight: body weight ratio (0.0035 vs. 0.0041, $p < 0.05$). Further, azilsartan resulted in significantly lower LV dilatation as suggested by LV end-diastolic internal diameter (LVEDD) and LV end-systolic internal diameter (LVESD) in Figure 7.

Changes in cardiac output and stroke volume were nearly similar in two treatment groups but fractional shortening (FS) was significantly higher in the azilsartan than vehicle treatment (30.36 ± 8.6 vs. 25.26 ± 3.6, $p = 0.03$).

RENAL SAFETY WITH AZILSARTAN

Early registry was designed to document BP control and its impact on cardiovascular and renal events during a 12-month follow-up period in patients administered either AZL-M or an ACEI at baseline. A total of 3, 849 patients with essential arterial HTN were recruited from primary care offices in Germany. Patients who initiated monotherapy at baseline comprising either AZL-M or an ACEI were included at a ratio of 7:3.

In terms of the safety of AZL-M, there was no difference in the proportion of patients experiencing an AE in comparison to those being treated with an ACEI. There were no significant differences in laboratory values between the groups, creatinine, potassium, and estimated glomerular filtration rate (eGFR).[18]

A 52-week, randomized, open-label, titrate-to-target BP study evaluated the safety and tolerability of the fixed-dose combinations AZM /chlorthalidone (AZL-M/CLD) versus OLM medoxomil/hydrochlorothiazide (OLM/HCTZ) in hypertensive subjects (clinic SBP 135–160 mm Hg on stable doses of 2–3 antihypertensive medications) with stage three chronic kidney disease (CKD) (eGFR 30–<60 mL/min/1.73 m^2). Serious AEs were reported in 10.4% on AZL-M/CLD versus 11.8% on OLM/HCTZ. One death (pulmonary artery thrombosis) occurred in the OLM/HCTZ arm. Common AEs (AZL-M/CLD vs OLM/HCTZ) were blood creatinine increased (44.2% vs. 38.2%), dizziness (7.8% vs. 6.6%), and headache (10.4% vs.2.6%). Subjects with consecutive SCr elevations more than 50% from baseline and more than upper limit of normal (ULN) or eGFR less than 20 mL/min/1.73 m^2 were similar between groups (5.3% in AZL-M/CLD vs. 5.4% in OLM/HCTZ).

The safety and tolerability of long-term treatment with AZL-M/CLD and OLM/HCTZ in a titrate-to-target BP study were comparable in hypertensive subjects with stage three CKD.[23]

In a 56-week phase three, open-label, treat-to-target study, involving two consecutive, nonrandomized cohorts, evaluated the safety and tolerability of AZM (AZL-M) in essential HTN. All subjects (n = 669) initiated AZL-M 40 mg QD, force-titrated to 80 mg QD at week 4, if tolerated. From week 8, subjects could receive additional medications, starting with CLD 25 mg QD (Cohort 1) or HCTZ 12.5–25 mg QD (Cohort 2), if required, to reach BP targets.

In safety analysis, consecutive creatinine elevations more than equal to 50% of baseline and more than ULN were reported in 21 (3.2%) subjects overall, mostly in those who received add-on CLD [n = 18 (8.3%)]. For all subjects with an elevated creatinine value at the final visit, the follow-up serum creatinine returned to within normal levels of the reference range, to baseline or screening values or to near baseline values [≤0.2 mg/dL (18 µmol/L) above baseline value].

In general, subjects with serum creatinine elevations tended to have greater SBP reductions. Mean changes in serum fasting glucose, lipids, and urinalysis parameters were small. Shifts from normal to high uric acid and from normal to low potassium were more common in subjects who received AZL-M + CLD than in those who received AZL-M alone.[24]

PLACE IN THERAPY

Azilsartan is an ANG-II AT1 receptor blocker indicated for the treatment of HTN, either as monotherapy or in combination with other antihypertensive agents. Dose adjustment is not necessary with azilsartan in patients with mild-to-severe renal impairment, or end-stage renal disease, mild-to-moderate hepatic impairment, or in geriatric patients. The mean reduction in 24-hour SBP and clinic SBP with azilsartan 80 mg is 15.3 mm Hg and 17.6 mm Hg, respectively, which is much higher than maximum approved doses of most of the ARBs. The responder rate is around 58–59%, which is much higher than other ARBs. Thus, azilsartan can be considered as initial choice of antihypertensive for intensive BP lowering in all patients with HTN including both young and elderly, irrespective of gender, and with any degree of renal dysfunction.

SYSTOLIC BLOOD PRESSURE INTERVENTION TRIAL: BENEFITS OF INTENSIVE BLOOD PRESSURE LOWERING ON CV OUTCOMES

This was a randomized, controlled, open-label, multicenter trial in hypertensive patients with SBP of 130–180 mm Hg and who were at an increased risk of CV events. Patients with diabetes mellitus or prior stroke were excluded. Patients were randomized to SBP target of either less than 140 mm Hg (the standard-treatment group) or less than 120 mm Hg (the intensive-treatment group). The primary outcome was the composite outcome of myocardial infarction, acute coronary syndrome not resulting in myocardial infarction, stroke, acute decompensated heart failure, or death from CV causes. Trial was prematurely stopped after a median follow-up of 3.26 years owing to a significantly lower rate of the primary composite outcome in the intensive-treatment group than in the standard-treatment group ($P < 0.001$).

Supplementary appendix published by Systolic Blood Pressure Intervention Trial (SPRINT) authors, highlighted that 39.7% patients in the intensive-treatment group were on ARBs of which azilsartan was one of the ARB used at the dose of 40–80 mg once daily. Azilsartan was found to potentially reduce SBP, DBP and 24-hour mean ambulatory BP greater than currently available ARBs like OLM, VAL, and candesartan as well as than ramipril.[25]

CONCLUSION

Azilsartan is a promising ANG-II AT1 receptor blocker indicated for the treatment of HTN, either as monotherapy or in combination with other antihypertensive agents such as CLD, especially in cardiodiabetes. It is cardioprotective, renoprotective, vesoprotective and brain protective and has cardiovascular inflicted morbidity and mortality benefits.

REFERENCES

1. Lim SS, Vos T, Flaxman AD, et al. A comparative risk assessment of burden of disease and injury attributable to 67 risk factors and risk factor clusters in 21 regions, 1990-2010: a systematic analysis for the Global Burden of Disease Study 2010. Lancet. 2012;380(9859): 2224-60.
2. Lewington Clarke R, Qizilbash N, Peto R, et al. Prospective Studies Collaboration. Age-specific relevance of usual blood pressure to vascular mortality: a meta-analysis of individual data for one million adults in 61 prospective studies. Lancet. 2002;360(9349):1903-13.
3. Mancia G, Fagard R, Narkiewicz K, et al. 2013 ESH/ESC Guidelines for the management of arterial hypertension The Task Force for the management of arterial hypertension of the European Society of Hypertension (ESH) and of the European Society of Cardiology (ESC). J Hypertens. 2013;31(7):1281-357.
4. James PA, Oparil S, Carter BL, et al. 2014 Evidence-Based Guideline for the Management of High Blood Pressure in Adults: Report from the Panel Members Appointed to the Eighth Joint National Committee (JNC 8). JAMA. 2014;311(5):507-20.
5. Weber MA, Schiffrin EL, White WB, et al. Clinical Practice Guidelines for the Management of Hypertension in the Community: A Statement by the American Society of Hypertension and the International Society of Hypertension. J Clin Hypertens (Greenwich). 2014;16(1):14-26.
6. Association of Physicians of India. Indian guidelines on hypertension (I.G.H.) - III. 2013. J Assoc Physicians India. 2013;61:6-36.
7. Dargad RR, Parekh JD, Dargad RR, et al. Azilsartan: Novel Angiotensin Receptor Blocker. J Assoc Physicians India. 2016;64(3):96-8.
8. Kurtz TW, Kajiya T. Differential pharmacology and benefit/risk of azilsartan compared to other sartans. Vasc Health Risk Manag. 2012;8:133-43.
9. Simões e Silva AC, Silveira KD, Ferreira AJ, et al. ACE2, angiotensin-(1-7) and Mas receptor axis in inflammation and fibrosis. Br J Pharmacol. 2013;169(3):477-92.
10. Baker WL, White WB. Azilsartan Medoxomil: A New Angiotensin II Receptor Antagonist for Treatment of Hypertension. Ann Pharmacother. 2011;45(12):1506-15.
11. Hatanaka M, Kaimori JY, Yamamoto S, et al. Azilsartan Improves Salt Sensitivity by Modulating the Proximal Tubular Na^+-H^+ Exchanger-3 in Mice." PloS one. 2016;11(1):e0147786.
12. Kautzky-Willer A, Handisurya A. Metabolic diseases and associated complications: sex and gender matter!. Eur J Clin Invest. 2009; 39(8):631-48.
13. Sica D, White WB, Weber MA, et al. Comparison of the novel angiotensin II receptor blocker azilsartan medoxomil vs valsartan by ambulatory blood pressure monitoring. J Clin Hypertens (Greenwich). 2011.; 3(7):467-72.
14. Bakris GL, Sica D, Weber M, et al. The comparative effects of azilsartan medoxomil and olmesartan on ambulatory and clinic blood pressure. J Clin Hypertens (Greenwich). 2011;13(2):81-8.
15. Bönner G, Bakris GL, Sica D, Weber MA, White WB, Perez A, et al. Antihypertensive efficacy of the angiotensin receptor blocker azilsartan medoxomil compared with the angiotensin-converting enzyme inhibitor ramipril. J Hum Hypertens. 2013;27(8):479-86.
16. White WB, Weber MA, Sica D, et al. Effects of the angiotensin receptor blocker azilsartan medoxomil versus olmesartan and valsartan on ambulatory and clinic blood pressure in patients with stages 1 and 2 hypertension. Hypertension. 2011;57(3):413-20.

17. Rakugi H, Enya K, Sugiura K, et al. Comparison of the efficacy and safety of azilsartan with that of candesartan cilexetil in Japanese patients with grade I–II essential hypertension: a randomized, double-blind clinical study. Hypertens Res. 2012;35(5):552-8.
18. Gitt AK, Baumgart P, Bramlage P, et al. EARLY treatment with azilsartan compared to ACE-inhibitors in anti-hypertensive therapy–rationale and design of the EARLY hypertension registry. BMC Cardiovasc Disord. 2013;13(1):46.
19. Sussman M, Leahy M, Friedman M, et al. PCV21 effects of azilsartan medoxomil versus valsartan and olmesartan medoxomil on the achievement of systolic blood pressure goals among hypertensive patients with diabetes. Value in Health. 2011;14(3):A36.
20. Kusuyama T, Ogata H, Takeshita H, et al. Effects of azilsartan compared to other angiotensin receptor blockers on left ventricular hypertrophy and the sympathetic nervous system in hemodialysis patients. Ther Apher Dial. 2014;18(5):398-403.
21. Tarikuz Zaman AK, McLean DL, Sobel BE. The efficacy and tolerability of azilsartan in obese insulin-resistant mice with left ventricular pressure overload. J Cardiovasc Pharmacol. 2013;62(4):381-7.
22. Baumann PQ, Zaman AK, McElroy-Yaggy K, et al. The efficacy and tolerability of azilsartan in mice with left ventricular pressure overload or acute myocardial infarction. J Cardiovasc Pharmacol. 2013;61(5):437-43.
23. Sica D, Zhao L, Oparil S, et al. Long-term safety of fixed-dose combinations: azilsartan medoxomil/chlorthalidone (AZL-M/CLD) vs olmesartan medoxomil/hydrochlorothiazide (OLM/HCTZ) in hypertensive subjects with stage 3 chronic kidney disease. Journal of the American Society of Hypertension. 2014;8(4):e32.
24. Handley A, Lloyd E, Roberts A, et al. Safety and tolerability of azilsartan medoxomil in subjects with essential hypertension: a one-year, phase 3, open-label study. Clin Exp Hypertens. 2016;38(2):180-8.
25. Cushman WC, Whelton PK, Fine LJ, et al. SPRINT Trial Results. Latest News in Hypertension Management. Hypertension. 2016;67(2):263-5.

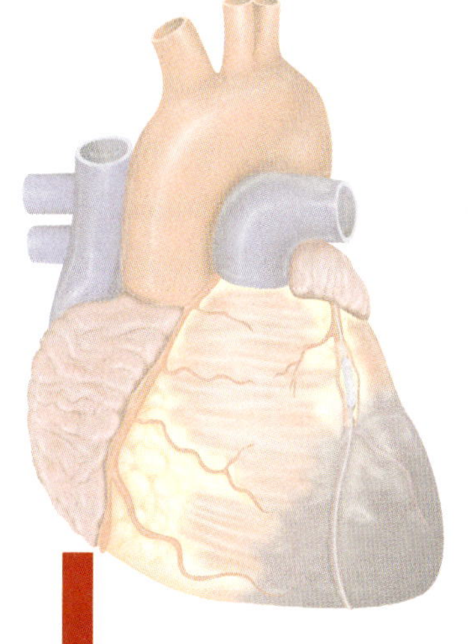

Superiority of Telmisartan: ARB, the First Choice in Cardiodiabetes

Kajal Ganguly, Santanu De, Auriom Kar, Biswadev Basu

INTRODUCTION

All antihypertensive drugs lower blood pressure (BP) (by definition), and the main benefit based on a large number of randomized trials is due to lowering of BP *per se* and is largely independent of the drugs employed. However, differences between drugs exist with respect to target-organ damage and prevention of cardiovascular events. Treatment should be individualized according to concomitant risk factors and diseases, and depend on age, biochemical, and hemodynamic measurements of the patients.

OVERALL APPROACH FOR SELECTING A THERAPY

The choice of antihypertensive agents in diabetic patients is based upon their ability to do the following: prevent mortality; prevent adverse cardiovascular events, such as myocardial infarction (MI), stroke, and heart failure; prevent the progression of renal disease, if present. The choice is not based upon retinopathy endpoints since comparative trials have not demonstrated superiority of one agent over another for retinopathy. Meta-analyses published in 2008 and 2009, the 2007 American Heart Association statement on the treatment of blood pressure, and the 2013 European Society of Hypertension/European Society of Cardiology (ESH/ESC) guidelines on the management of hypertension, all concluded that the degree of blood pressure reduction is the major determinant of reduction in cardiovascular risk in both younger and older patients with hypertension (including diabetic patients), not the choice of antihypertensive drug; this is also true in diabetic patients.[1] There are also known differences in diabetogenic effect between the different drug regimens. A network meta-analysis has calculated the odds ratio for new-onset diabetes to be 0.62 (0.51–0.77) for angiotensin II receptor blockers (ARBs), 0.67 (0.57–0.79) for angiotensin-converting enzyme inhibitors (ACEIs), 0.75 (0.63–0.89) for placebo, 0.79 (0.67–0.92) for calcium channel blockers (CCBs), and 0.93 (0.78–1.11) for β-blockers compared with treatment with diuretics (reference drug = 1). There is no doubt that β-blockers and diuretics, especially when combined, have adverse metabolic effects and increase the risk of new-onset diabetes in predisposed patients. The ESH guidelines therefore argue against the combination of diuretics and β-blockers in primary prevention among people with a high risk of developing diabetes.[2] However, in patients with diabetic nephropathy, angiotensin inhibitors ACEIs and ARBs may slow kidney disease progression more effectively than other antihypertensive drugs.

Thus, our overall approach in diabetic patients who require antihypertensive therapy is as follows: In patients with severely increased albuminuria ('macroalbuminuria'), we treat with an ACE inhibitor or an ARB. We also use these drugs in patients with moderately increased albuminuria ('microalbuminuria'), even though the benefits of angiotensin inhibition on kidney disease progression in such patients are unproven. In patients without increased albuminuria, initial monotherapy can consist of an ACE inhibitor, ARB, thiazide diuretic, or calcium channel blocker. However, because angiotensin inhibitors can prevent albuminuria, and because thiazide diuretics have the disadvantage of an adverse effect on glucose metabolism, many experts will choose an ACE inhibitor or ARB even in patients without albuminuria. In patients who require more than one drug to control their blood pressure, we treat with a combination of an ACE inhibitor (or ARB if unable to take an ACE inhibitor) and a dihydropyridine calcium channel blocker (e.g. amlodipine).[3]

ACE INHIBITORS VERSUS ARB IN DIABETES

Angiotensin converting enzyme inhibitors block the conversion of angiotensin I into angiotensin II by inhibition of ACE. The reduced levels of angiotensin II lead not only to vasodilatation and a fall in BP but also to a reduction of potential harmful effects of angiotensin II on the cardiorenovascular system, such as structural damage to the heart, blood vessels, and kidneys ACEIs also increase bradykinin levels through inhibition of degradation with potential effects and side effects (cough). The ARBs block angiotensin II Type I receptors leading to vasodilatation, but owing to their angiotensin II type I receptor selectivity, they lack the effect of potentiation of bradykinin and possibly other vasoactive peptides. In diabetic patients, combination treatment is commonly needed to effectively lower BP, so the discussion of which medication to be used first is not always important. However, a blocker of the renin-angiotensin system (RAS) should almost invariably be included because of the evidence of its superior protective effects. Especially, in proteinuric-diabetic nephropathy, RAS blockade is clearly indicated. Large hypertension and heart failure trials have also reported an impact on diabetes development in favor of RAS blockade. So for persons with cardiovascular or kidney disease, including microalbuminuria, or with cardiovascular risk factors in addition to diabetes and hypertension, an ACEI or ARB should be started.

ALLHAT TRIAL

The ALLHAT trial is by far the largest prospective study of the treatment of mild hypertension and assessed the efficacy of different medications (Fig. 1). Over 33,000 patients (36% had type 2 diabetes) with hypertension (mean 146/84 mm Hg) and at least one other coronary risk factor were randomly assigned to chlorthalidone (12.5–25 mg/day), amlodipine, or lisinopril, a fourth arm of doxazosin therapy was prematurely terminated because of an increased incidence of heart failure.[4]

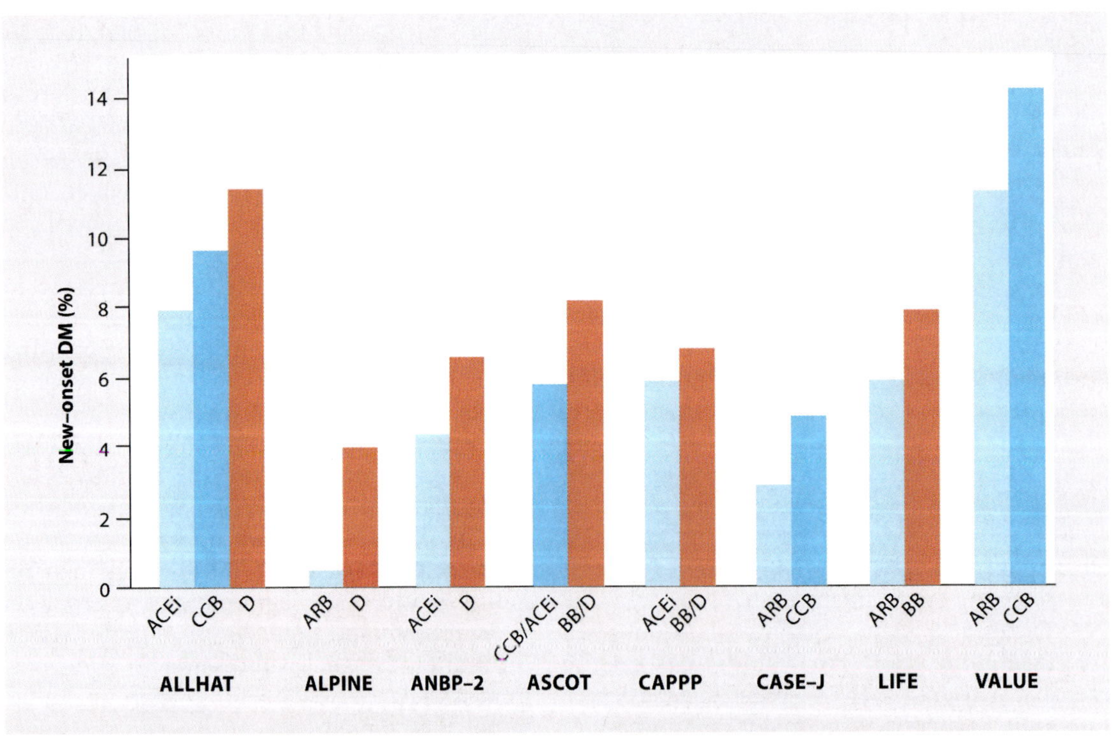

Fig. 1: Percentage development of new cases of diabetes mellitus (DM) in various studies

Which ARB is Preferred in Diabetes?

'In clinical practice, most of us assume that the effect of ARBs as a class is similar', said Bangalore. 'However, intergroup differences have long been debated. We have shown that of all the ARBs the antihypertensive efficacy of losartan is the lowest. It is therefore interesting to see these data from a large observational study showing probable superiority of telmisartan and valsartan.'

More Than 54,000 Patients Analyzed

The population-based retrospective study included an analysis of 54,186 Canadian patients with diabetes who started taking an ARB between 2001 and 2011. All patients were 66 years of age or older, the average age being 73 years, and the average duration of diabetes was approximately 6 years. Overall 20.2% of patients were treated with candesartan, 23.4% with irbesartan, 15.5% with losartan, 15.1% with telmisartan, and 25.8% with valsartan.[5] The primary end point, a composite of admission to the hospital for MI, heart failure, or stroke, occurred in 2,712 patients taking an ARB. In an adjusted risk model, telmisartan was associated with a 15% lower risk of the primary end point, while valsartan was associated with a 14% lower risk when compared with irbesartan. In a dose-response analysis, the group found no difference in the risk of the primary outcome with moderate or high doses of ARBs, although the effectiveness of valsartan was 'somewhat attenuated' when adjusted for dose.

Risk of the Composite Outcome of Hospitalization for MI, Stroke, or Heart Failure (Table 1)

The reduction in the primary end point, however, was driven primarily by a reduction in the risk of heart failure hospitalizations. Analyzed separately, telmisartan was associated with a 20% lower risk of heart failure hospitalizations, while valsartan was associated with a borderline 13% nonsignificant reduction [hazard ratio 0.87; 95% confidence interval (CI) 0.75–1.00].[5]

TABLE 1: Risk of the composite outcome of hospitalization for MI, stroke, or heart failure

Drug	*Adjusted hazard ratio (95% CI)*
Irbesartan	1.00 (reference)
Telmisartan	0.85 (0.74–0.97)
Candesartan	0.99 (0.89–1.11)
Losartan	0.93 (0.83–1.05)
Valsartan	0.86 (0.77–0.96)

Abbreviation: CI, confidence interval.

WHY TELMISARTAN IS PREFERRED

PPAR-γ Agonist Effect of Telmisartan (Fig 2)

- Telmisartan is the only ARB which acts as a partial agonist of PPAR-γ.
- PPAR-γ is a ligand activated transcription factor that regulates cell growth, inflammation, lipid metabolism, and insulin sensitivity.
- It has been successfully shown that PPAR-γ agonists limit high glucose-induced inflammation in proximal tubular cells (PTC). PPAR-γ agonists also exert anti-fibrotic effects in human proximal tubular cells under high glucose conditions by attenuating the increase in AP-1, TGF-β1, and downstream production of the extracellular matrix protein, fibronectin.
- PPAR-γ agonists can improve insulin sensitivity, reduce triglyceride levels and decrease the risk of atherosclerosis.

A study examined the ability of different ARBs to activate PPAR-γin a cell-based transient transfection assay. This assay was designed to eliminate interference from endogenous nuclear receptors. In the results shown here, each ARB was used at a concentration of 10 mmol/L. *Telmisartan was the only ARB to show strong (27-fold) activation*, although irbesartan also showed a slight activation (two-fold to three-fold). By comparison, full PPAR-γ agonists show approximately 140-fold activation in this assay. Importantly, telmisartan was also the only ARB that activated PPAR-γ when tested at lower concentrations that can be achieved physiologically (1–5 mmol/L). Telmisartan therefore acts as a partial agonist of PPAR-γ(Fig. 2).[6]

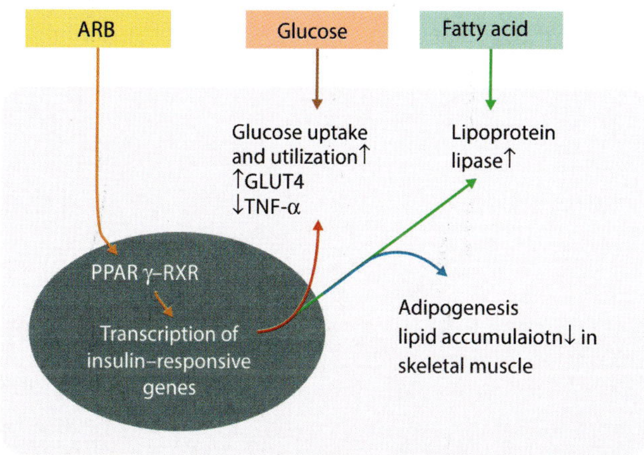

Fig. 2: Mechanism of how ARBs improve insulin sensitivity

The ONTARGET Study

The ONgoing Telmisartan Alone and in combination with Ramipril Global Endpoint Trial (ONTARGET®) was the largest ever study of an angiotensin II receptor blocker (ARB). It compared telmisartan with ramipril and the combination with treatment duration of upto 5.5 years. ONTARGET® was notable not only for the size of the patient population (over 25,000), but also for the broad inclusion criteria (patients could have coronary artery disease, peripheral arterial occlusive disease, cerebrovascular event or diabetes mellitus with end-organ damage). Patients were screened for tolerance to angiotensin-converting enzyme (ACE) inhibitors before trial entry.[7] ONTARGET® showed that telmisartan was as effective as ramipril, the ACE inhibitor whose efficacy in reducing cardiovascular events was established in the Heart Outcomes Prevention Evaluation (HOPE) study and that has since become a widely used intervention for cardiovascular protection.[7] Telmisartan was better tolerated than ramipril, despite intolerance of an ACE inhibitor being screened for in the study run-in period. The parallel trial, Telmisartan Randomized AssessmeNt Study in aCE iNtolerant subjects with cardiovascular Disease (TRANSCEND®), in nearly 6,000 patients intolerant of ACE inhibitors, showed that telmisartan significantly reduced the cardiovascular composite of cardiovascular death, myocardial infarction and stroke (although not heart failure) compared with placebo, when administered on a background of otherwise optimal standard of care.[7] The ONTARGET® trial established telmisartan as a proven option for the prevention of cardiovascular events in patients at high risk. Both ARBs and ACE inhibitors are currently used to slow the onset and progression of diabetic nephropathy. Recent analyses of the ONTARGET® trial have provided evidence for slowing the progression of renal disease demonstrated by level of microalbuminuria in at-risk patients, including those with diabetes, being treated with telmisartan or ramipril. These data are of particular interest given the link between renal and cardiovascular disease.

Telmisartan in Diabetic Nephropathy

The efficacy of telmisartan in diabetic patients with varying degrees of renal dysfunction, ranging from initial endothelial dysfunction to overt nephropathy, has been investigated in a total of five studies comprising the Programme of Research to show Telmisartan End-organ protection (PROTECTION®)[8] The Telmisartan versus Ramipril in renal ENdothelium DYsfunction (TRENDY®) study showed that treatment with telmisartan or ramipril for 9 weeks significantly improved ($p < 0.001$) the response of the renal vasculature to nitric oxide, an indicator of basal nitric oxide activity and thereby of endothelial function of the renal vasculature . The magnitude of the effect of telmisartan appeared somewhat greater than that of ramipril; this may explain why only temisartan improved resting renal plasma flow.[9] The INcipieNt to OVert: Angiotensin II receptor blocker, Telmisartan, Investigation On type 2 diabetic Nephropathy (INNOVATION®) study, which was conducted exclusively in Japanese patients with microalbuminuria, assessed the transition to overt nephropathy when treated with telmisartan 40 or 80 mg or with placebo for upto 2 years. Rates of transition were 16.7% with telmisartan 80 mg, 22.6% with telmisartan 40 mg, and 49.9% with placebo. The renoprotective effect of telmisartan was similar in the normotensive patient population and was again dose-dependent.[10] The Diabetics Exposed to Telmisartan And enalaprIL (DETAIL®) study compared the effects of the two drugs on the decline in glomerular filtration rate (GFR) over 5 years in patients with type 2 diabetes and early nephropathy. The DETAIL® study used a direct, iohexol-based, measure of GFR rather than an indirect estimation from serum creatinine levels. Both drugs provided similar renal protection. Comparison between the shorter-term ARB studies, showed that the annual decline in GFR was lowest with telmisartan , but the cumulative benefit due to the longer duration of the DETAIL® study cannot be discounted, but it may be that the full renal protective effect of other ARBs is not achieved within the short-term follow-up.[11] A prospective 1-year trial to compare Micardis® versus losArtan in hypertensive type 2 DiabEtic patients with Overt nephropathy (AMADEO™) suggests that renoprotection provided by different ARBs is not the same when given at doses licensed for the treatment of hypertension (Fig. 3). The patients who were studied, all had urinary albumin levels >900 mg/24 hours and elevated serum creatinine (97–265 μmol/L) in women and

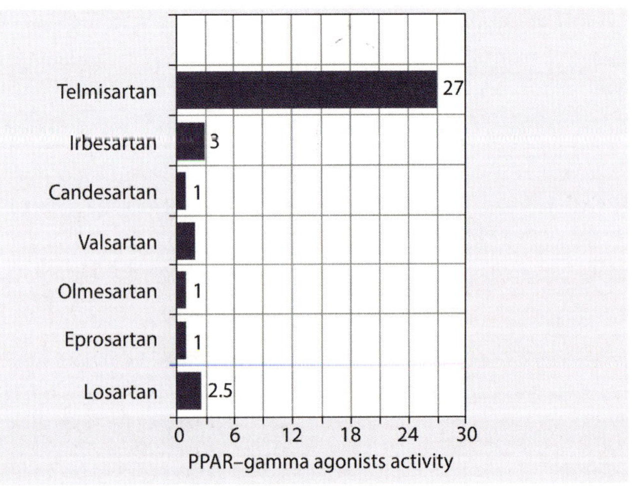

Fig. 3: PPAR-gamma agonist activity

115–285 μmol/L in men). When given for 1 year, telmisartan produced a 29.8% reduction in urine albumin-to-creatinine ratio (UACR), whereas that with losartan was only 21.4% (p = 0.027). This represents an approximately 30% difference in reduction of proteinuria with telmisartan 80 mg versus losartan 100 mg in favor of telmisartan. The sister trial, a trial to inVestigate the efficacy of telmIsartan versus VALsartan in hypertensive type 2 DIabetic patients with overt nephropathy (VIVALDI®) showed that telmisartan and valsartan provided equivalent reductions in proteinuria.[12]

Renoprotection in the ONTARGET® Trial Program

Results from TRANSCEND® assessed the changes in albuminuria from baseline to after 2 years of treatment and at the end of the study. The changes in albuminuria were significantly smaller with telmisartan than in the placebo plus best standard of care group. It should be noted that these data are based on observations in the overall patient population of 5,926, approximately 36% of whom had diabetes. ONTARGET®, the larger of the two studies demonstrated that telmisartan was more effective than ramipril in slowing down the change in albuminuria in a population of 25,620 high-risk patients and that the effect was similar to the one observed for the combination of ramipril and telmisartan. The difference between treatments was apparent after 2 years, and differences between telmisartan and ramipril, and between telmisartan plus ramipril and ramipril alone, were significant at the end of the 5-year study (both p <0.001)(Fig. 4).

Although the combination of telmisartan plus ramipril provided superior control of albuminuria, the incidence of the primary renal endpoint for ONTARGET®, a composite of dialysis (either acute or chronic), doubling of serum creatinine, and death, which is the same as used in IDNT, was significantly higher for telmisartan plus ramipril versus ramipril alone [HR 1.08 (95% CI 1.00, 1.16)]. The most frequent endpoint within the composite was all-cause mortality. If one differentiates between patients who underwent acute dialysis (i.e. <2-months duration) and chronic dialysis (an indicator of end-stage renal disease), the incidence of chronic dialysis was no different in the telmisartan and the telmisartan plus ramipril groups.[14] The decline in estimated GFR in ONTARGET® has been critically examined. Over 5 years, the loss in estimated GFR was 5.94, 3.96, and 2.66 mL/min in the telmisartan plus ramipril, telmisartan and ramipril groups, respectively (Fig. 5). The greatest loss in estimated GFR was observed in the first 6 weeks of therapy and was greatest in the patients treated with telmisartan plus ramipril. High-risk patients with cardiovascular disease are also likely to have intraglomerular vascular disease, and GFR is maintained in these patients because of the effect of angiotensin II. Hence, blockade of the RAS is expected to generate a short-term loss of GFR. The more effective the blockade, the greater the loss in GFR which can precipitate acute renal failure and the need for short-term dialysis, which may in turn explain the high need for acute dialysis in the combination treatment arm. This decline is likely to be exacerbated if there are challenges to renal autoregulation by virtue of vascular pathology, as was likely in the ONTARGET®

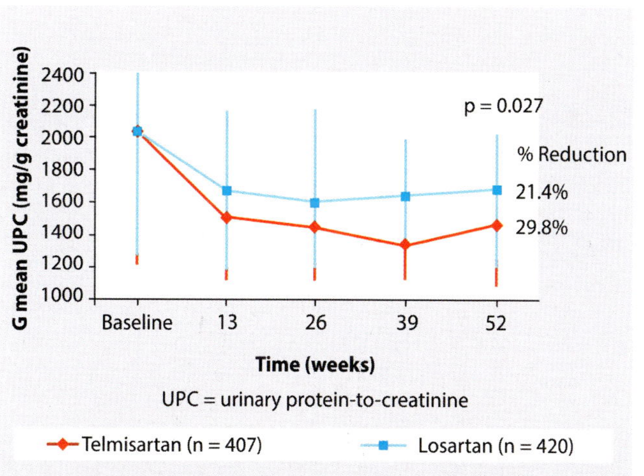

Fig. 4: Effects of treatment with telmisartan 80 mg or losartan 100 mg on urinary protein/creatinine ratio (UPCR) in patients with type 2 diabetes and overt nephropathy (morning spot UPCR ≥ 700 mg/g creatinine)[12]

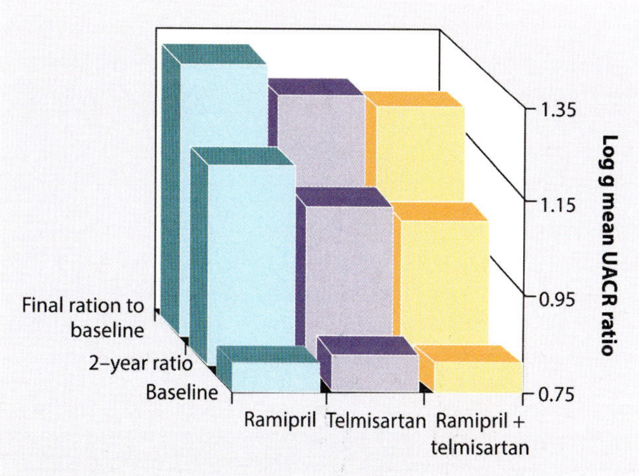

Fig. 5: Ratio of change in log geometric (g) mean urinary albumin/creatinine ratio (UACR) after 2-years' treatment and final ratio in patients in ONTARGET® treated with ramipril, telmisartan or telmisartan plus ramipril[13]

patient population. If the annual loss of estimated GFR recorded in ONTARGET® is compared with those observed in IDNT , IRbesartan in patients with type 2 diabetes and MicroAlbuminuria (IRMA-2) and RENAAL, the decline in estimated GFR over 5 years was actually quite acceptable with all three treatments, comparing favorably with that observed in a general population aged between 65 and 85 years.[15] Of important note is the increase in adverse events in the combined telmisartan and ramipril arm of the study with no added benefit. This increased adverse event rate with ARB plus ACE inhibitor with no efficacy benefit was also seen in the VALsartan In Acute myocardial iNfarcTion (VALIANT) trial with valsartan and captopril. For this reason, the combination of ARB and ACE inhibitor is not advised.[15]

CONCLUSION

An essential component of the management of the diabetic patient, especially those with other risk factors such as nephropathy, is the control of blood pressure to prevent cardiovascular events and premature death. Blood pressure targets are in most cases not being met. A multifactorial approach is needed for the management of risk factors (i.e. total cholesterol, hyperglycemia, and anemia, as well as blood pressure) in patients with diabetes. However, management of risk is lamentably poor, even by diabetologists and nephrologists. Albuminuria provides a simple means of identifying the onset of kidney and vascular disease and charts the progression of chronic disease in patients with type 2 diabetes. As well as being a risk factor for end stage renal disease, albuminuria is a prognostic factor for cardiovascular morbidity and mortality. Clinical studies in patients with type 2 diabetes show that the use of ARBs effectively protects the renal function, the effect being not exclusively attributed to blood pressure control. Post-hoc analysis of studies evaluating ARBs suggests that this approach to treatment also provides cardiovascular benefit. Telmisartan provides superior reductions of proteinuria, compared with losartan, and is effective in reducing renal endpoints. Coupled with evidence of cardiovascular protection in ONTARGET®, this reinforces the potential for telmisartan as an alternative to ramipril to reduce the progression of diabetic nephropathy and to reduce cardiovascular risk in a high-risk population.[15]

REFERENCES

1. Epstein M, Sowers JR. Diabetes mellitus and hypertension. Hypertension. 1992;19(5):403-18.
2. KDIGO. Definition and classification of CKD. Kidney Int Suppl. 2013;3(1):19-62.
3. Parving HH, Hommel E, Mathiesen E, et al. Prevalence of microalbuminuria, arterial hypertension, retinopathy and neuropathy in patients with insulin dependent diabetes. Br Med J (Clin Res Ed). 1988;296 (6616):156-60.
4. Mogensen CE, Hansen KW, Pedersen MM, et al. Renal factors influencing blood pressure threshold and choice of treatment for hypertension in IDDM. Diabetes Care. 1991;14(Suppl 4):13-26.
5. Hypertension in Diabetes Study (HDS): I. Prevalence of hypertension in newly presenting type 2 diabetic patients and the association with risk factors for cardiovascular and diabetic complications. J Hypertens. 1993;11(3):309-17.
6. Nosadini R, Sambataro M, Thomaseth K, et al. Role of hyperglycemia and insulin resistance in determining sodium retention in non-insulin-dependent diabetes. Kidney Int. 1993;449(1):139-46.
7. Cruickshank K, Riste L, Anderson SG, et al. Aortic pulse-wave velocity and its relationship to mortality in diabetes and glucose intolerance: an integrated index of vascular function? Circulation. 2002;106(16):2085-90.
8. Gaede P, Vedel P, Parving HH, et al. Intensified multifactorial intervention in patients with type 2 diabetes mellitus and microalbuminuria: the Steno type 2 randomised study. Lancet. 1999;353(9153):617-22.
9. American Diabetes Association. Cardiovascular disease and risk management. Diabetes Care. 2015;38(Suppl):S49-S57.
10. Buse JB, Ginsberg HN, Bakris GL, et al. Primary prevention of cardiovascular diseases in people with diabetes mellitus: a scientific statement from the American Heart Association and the American Diabetes Association. Circulation. 2007;115(1):114-26.
11. Yusuf S, Teo K, Anderson C, et al. Telmisartan Randomised AssessmeNt Study in ACE iNtolerant subjects with cardiovascular Disease (TRANSCEND®) Investigators: effects of the angiotensin-receptor blocker telmisartan on cardiovascular events in high-risk patients intolerant to angiotensin-converting enzyme inhibitors: a randomised controlled trial. Lancet. 2008;372(9644): 1174-83.
12. Mann JF, Schmieder RE, Dyal L, et al. TRANSCEND® (Telmisartan Randomised Assessment Study in ACE Intolerant Subjects with Cardiovascular Disease) Investigators: effect of telmisartan on renal outcomes: a randomized trial. Ann Intern Med. 2009;7(1):1-10.
13. Levey AS, Bosch JP, Lewis JB, et al. Modification of Diet in Renal Disease Study Group: A more accurate method to estimate glomerular filtration rate from serum creatinine: a new prediction equation. Ann Intern Med. 1999;130(6):461-70.
14. Stevens LA, Coresh J, Greene T, et al. Assessing kidney function-measured and estimated glomerular filtration rate. N Engl J Med. 2006;354(23):2473-83.
15. Levey AS, Stevens LA, Schmid CH, et al. CKD-EPI (Chronic Kidney Disease Epidemiology Collaboration): a new equation to estimate glomerular filtration rate. Ann Intern Med. 2009;150(9): 604-12.

CHAPTER

ARNI in Heart Failure with Cardiodiabetes: The Way Forward

Srikant Sharma, Surabhi Chhabra

INTRODUCTION

With the improvement in healthcare system, heart failure (HF) and diabetes remain one of the major concerns across the Globe. Coexistence of the two has been repeatedly confirmed by many clinical researches and trials. The prevalence of diabetes is as high as 35–40% in patients with HF,[1] which is independent of degree of impaired ejection fraction. Also, two- to four-fold increase of incidence of HF is noticed in diabetes mellitus, as it affects in the form of diabetic cardiomyopathy, asymptomatic abnormalities of ventricle, derangement of systolic and diastolic functions, systemic hypertension, elevated hemoglobin A1C (HbA1C) level, microalbuminuria [are also solely independent risk factors of congestive heart failure (CHF)].

The American College of Cardiology Foundation/ American Heart Association guideline defines HF as "a complex clinical syndrome that results from any structural or functional impairment of ventricular filling or ejection of blood".[2] HF prevalence and the number of HF-related hospitalizations are increasing, and the prognosis remains poor, with a 5-year mortality worse than many cancers.[3,4] There has been significant progress in HF therapy, but mostly in HF with reduced ejection fraction (HFrEF), refers to impaired systolic function with left ventricular ejection fraction (LVEF) less than 40%,[5] while for patients with preserved ejection fraction (HFpEF), no therapy has improved clinical outcomes.[6,7] Despite such advances, however, morbidity and mortality of HFrEF still remain high and HF continues to progress. Hence, the time demands for remodeling ventricular structure in improvement of HF. The angiotensin receptor neprilysin inhibitor (ARNI) was designed with the aim of inhibiting neprilysin while blocking the adverse effects of renin angiotensin aldosterone system (RAAS) and thereby was remodeling the heart structure.

EVOLUTION OF THERAPEUTIC INTERVENTION IN HEART FAILURE

For the past 25 years, an add-on therapy approach to chronic HF has been used, beginning with diuretics, then adding angiotensin-converting enzyme (ACE) inhibitors [or angiotensin-receptor blockers (ARBs)] and beta-blockers, followed by mineralocorticoid receptor antagonists.[7,8] Ivabradine, which reduces heart rate, is also approved as an add-on therapy in HF.[9] Intravenous (IV) iron therapy (if serum ferritin < 100 μg/L and transferrin saturation is less than 20%), sodium-glucose co-transporter-2 (SGLT2) inhibitors were also approved to improve mortality in HF. Nevertheless, morbidity and mortality remain still high and there is, therefore, a need for new therapeutic targets in HF.

The modern history of therapy for HF with HFrEF began with the introduction of vasodilatation as a treatment for HF. The Vasodilator Heart Failure Trial (V-HeFT I) study (1986; see Heart-Failure Therapy Articles in the *New England Journal of Medicine* for cited *Journal* articles) demonstrated that treatment with hydralazine plus isosorbide dinitrate, as compared with either placebo or prazosin, reduced mortality. Soon thereafter, the Consensus (1987) and SOLVD-Treatment (1991a) Trials established that ACE inhibition with enalapril reduced overall mortality by 16–40%. V-HeFT II (1991b) showed that enalapril was superior to the combination of hydralazine and isosorbide dinitrate. The SOLVD-Prevention Trial (1992) showed that enalapril benefit in reducing the rate of hospitalizations for HF extended to asymptomatic patients with HFrEF. These landmark trials ushered in the era of ACE inhibition, which has been the centerpiece of heart-failure therapy for 25 years.

Angiotensin-receptor blockers interfere with the action of angiotensin II at its type 1 receptor, resulting in vasodilatation. These agents interrupt the angiotensin pathway by a different mechanism than ACE inhibitors, which block the conversion of angiotensin I to angiotensin II and also interfere with the breakdown of kinins. The V-HeFT trial (2001c) introduced the concept of ARB therapy for HF, but because treatment with ARBs is not superior to treatment with ACE inhibitors, ARBs have generally been reserved for patients who cannot take ACE inhibitors because of cough or angioedema.

The use of beta-blocker therapy, now a cornerstone of heart-failure treatment, was once considered counterintuitive, because of concern that patients with HFrEF either would not benefit or would have unacceptable side effects from adrenergic blockade. However, evidence of a mortality benefit emerged for three beta-blockers—(1) bisoprolol, (2) carvedilol, (3) and sustained-release metoprolol. In the timeline, we include two studies on the alpha- and beta-adrenergic blocker carvedilol (the US Carvedilol Heart Failure Study, 1996, and Copernicus, 2001a). Both studies demonstrated that carvedilol led to a substantial reduction in mortality and contributed to our understanding of the role of adrenergic activation in the pathophysiology of HF.

Another paradigm shift in HF therapy occurred with the RALES trial (1999) of spironolactone, a mineralocorticoid receptor antagonist (MRA). The investigators reported a 30% reduction in mortality among patients already receiving an ACE inhibitor and a loop diuretic. The EMPHASIS-HF trial (2011a), in which investigators studied the MRA eplerenone in patients with systolic HF and mild symptoms, confirmed and extended this finding. Together, these trials added another important drug class to the heart-failure armamentarium.

Not all therapies listed on the timeline proved successful. Drugs with positive inotropic effects, such as the phosphodiesterase inhibitor milrinone, provide a striking example. In a large clinical trial (PROMISE, 1991c)—oral milrinone, as compared with placebo, increased mortality among patients with HF by 28%. Being novel inotropic agents proved disappointing.

An older class of inotropic agents, the cardiac glycosides, also met with disappointment. Since, the classic observations of William Withering recorded 230 years ago in his extraordinary document, *An Account of the Foxglove, and Some of Its Medical Uses: With Practical Remarks on Dropsy, and Other Diseases,* digitalis glycosides were a mainstay of therapy for HF. However, a trial published in the *Journal* (Digitalis Investigation Group, DIG, 1997) showed unequivocally that digoxin had no beneficial effect on mortality in HF, though it did reduce overall hospitalizations and specifically reduced hospitalizations for HF by 28%. Despite their long history, cardiac glycosides are no longer first-line therapy for HF, though they may be used to mitigate symptoms and prevent hospitalizations for HF.

The story of nesiritide, a recombinant B-type natriuretic peptide with vasodilator properties, reinforces the fundamental importance of evidence-based practice. Nesiritide was approved for use in acute HF in 2001 to improve dyspnea. Given by infusion, the drug was administered at many outpatient centers established specifically for this purpose. However, the ASCEND-HF trial (2011b) demonstrated no benefit of nesiritide on the co-primary endpoint of death or rehospitalization for HF and no significant improvement in dyspnea. Thus, an interesting and widely used biological agent proved to be ineffective when subjected to a rigorous clinical trial.

The introduction of cardiac devices represents perhaps the most fundamental paradigm shift exhibited on the timeline. Not appearing on the timeline until 2001, device trials nevertheless appear more frequently than trials of any single class of medical therapy. The timeline includes three types of cardiac devices—(1) the left ventricular assist device (LVAD) in REMATCH (2001b), (2) the implantable cardioverter-defibrillator (ICD) in SCD-HeFT (2005a), and (3) cardiac resynchronization therapy (biventricular pacemakers, CRT) in COMPANION (2004), CARE-HF (2005b), MADIT-CRT (2009), and RAFT (2010). All three types of devices have been shown to reduce mortality in HF. LVADs may be used as a bridge to cardiac transplantation or, in some patients, as destination therapy. ICDs may be used alone or together with CRT (CRT-D). A recent follow-up study of the MADIT-CRT trial (2014a) demonstrated that as compared with ICD alone, CRT-D reduced mortality among patients with HF and mild symptoms, but only when the QRS complex was greater than 130 ms with a left bundle-branch block pattern.

The final entry in the timeline is the PARADIGM-HF trial (2014b), (prospective comparison of ARNI with ACEI to determine impact on global mortality and morbidity in HF trial) now published in the *Journal.* The study showed that a novel approach to HF therapy, angiotensin-receptor and neprilysin inhibition with LCZ696, a combination of sacubitril and valsartan, reduced cardiovascular mortality by 20% and overall mortality by 16%, as compared with enalapril. Neprilysin is a neutral endopeptidase involved in the metabolism of a number of vasoactive peptides. The inhibitor blocks the action of neprilysin, resulting in higher levels of peptides such as natriuretic peptides, which have vasodilator properties, facilitate sodium excretion, and most likely have effects on remodeling. The timeline reveals steady progress, punctuated by paradigm shifts, in the treatment of HF. ACA/AHA guidelines 2016, recommended as category Class 1, in patients with chronic symptomatic HFrEF NYHI Class 2 or 3 who tolerated ACEI/ARB, replacement by an ARNI is believed to further reduce morbidity and mortality.[10]

Sacubitril/valsartan is recommended as 1B category as a replacement for ACEI to further reduce the rise of HF, hospitalization, and death in ambulatory patients with HFrEF who remains symptomatic despite optimal treatment with an ACEI, a beta-blocker and an MRA.[11]

Mechanism of Action

The novel mechanism of action of an ARNI is by two steps involving sacubitril and valsartan, simultaneously.

Sacubitril is a neprilysin inhibitor. Neprilysin, an enzyme expressed in a wide variety of tissues (endothelial, epithelial, and smooth muscle cells, cardiac myocytes and adipocytes),[12,13] degrades endogenous vasoactive peptides including natriuretic peptide, bradykinin, adrenomedullin, and glucagon-like peptide 1 (GLP1).[14] Inhibition of neprilysin results in increase of concentration of these proteins and their activities leading to consequences (vasodilatation, natriuresis, and diuresis). Inhibition of neprilysin (neutral endopeptidase—NEP) occurs via LBQ657, the active metabolite of the prodrug sacubitril. NPs (natriuretic peptides) exert their effects by activating membrane-bound guanylyl cyclase-coupled receptors, resulting in increased concentrations of the second messenger cyclic guanosine monophosphate (cGMP), thereby promoting vasodilation, natriuresis and diuresis, increased glomerular filtration rate, and renal blood flow (Fig. 1). Second action is by blocking the angiotensin II type-1 (AT1) receptor via valsartan. It causes inhibition of renin and aldosterone release, reduction of sympathetic activity, and antihypertrophic and antifibrotic effects.

Sustained activation of the renin-angiotensin-aldosterone system results in vasoconstriction, renal

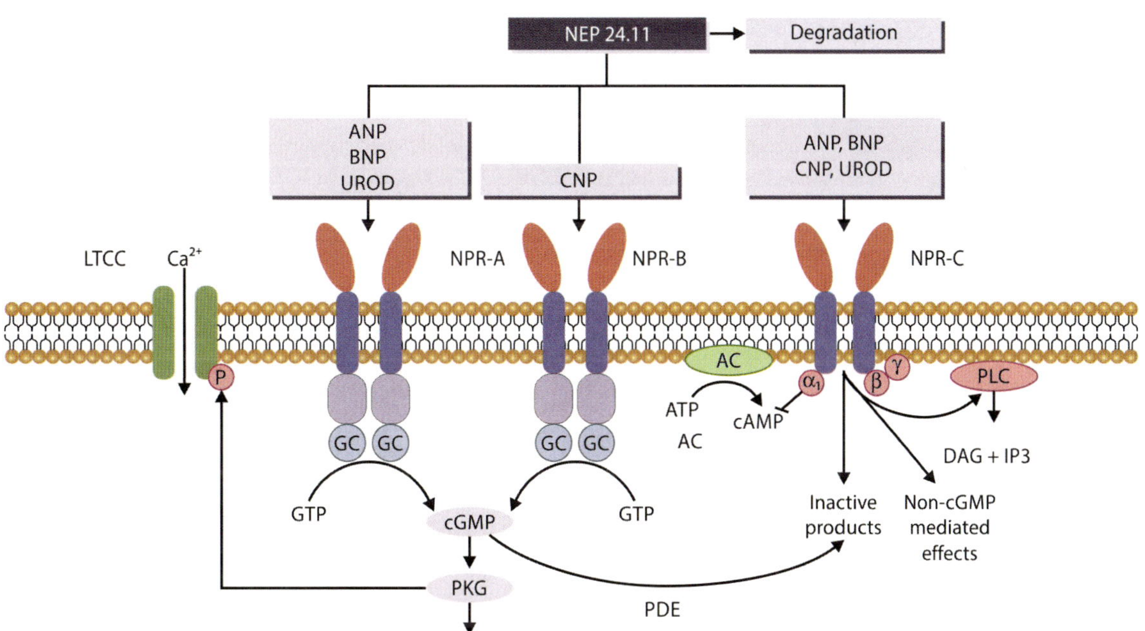

Fig. 1: Mechanisms of action of LCZ696 on natriuretic peptide

Abbreviations: ANP, atrial natriuretic peptide; BNP, B-type natriuretic peptide; CNP, C-type natriuretic peptide; cGMP, cyclic guanosine monophosphate; DAG, diacilglicerol; GC, guanylyl cyclase-A; GMP, guanosine monophosphate; GTP, guanosine triphosphate; IP3, inositol 1,4,5-trifosfato; LTCC, L-type calcium channel; NEP, neprilysin (neutral endopeptidase); NPR, natriuretic peptide receptor, PDE, phosphodiesterase; PKG, protein kinase G; PLC, phospholypase C; RAAS, renin-angiotensin-aldosterone system; UROD, urodilatin

sodium and fluid retention, activation of cellular growth and proliferation, and subsequent maladaptive cardiovascular remodeling.

Valsartan inhibits detrimental cardiovascular and renal effects of angiotensin II by selectively blocking the AT1 receptor, and also inhibits angiotensin II-dependent aldosterone release.

Hence, the complementary cardiovascular benefits and renal effects in HF patients are attributed to the enhancement of peptides and the simultaneous inhibition of the deleterious effects of angiotensin II by valsartan.

While the activation of the RAAS and sympathetic nervous system is detrimental in HF, other counter-regulatory pathways are activated in HF, including the natriuretic peptide (NP) system (see Fig. 2). The NP system consists of atrial (ANP),[15] B-type (BNP),[16] and C-type (CNP) NPs; these hormones regulate BP and fluid homeostasis.[17-19] ANP is synthesized and secreted in atria, BNP is secreted from the ventricles in response to mechanical stretch and increased intracardiac volume/pressure and CNP mostly originates from endothelial and renal cells and is secreted in response to endothelium-dependent agonists and proinflammatory cytokines.[17,18,20] NPs activate three transmembrane receptors—(1) natriuretic peptide receptor (NPR)-A, (2) NPR-B, (3) and NPR-C.[19] The binding of NPs to type A (NPR-A) and type B (NPR-B) receptors activates guanylate cyclase, increasing levels of the second messenger cyclic guanosine monophosphate (cGMP) and its effector molecule protein kinase G. This induces natriuresis, diuresis, vasodilation, and inhibition of the RAAS system and the sympathetic nervous system, as well as antifibrotic, antiproliferative, and antithrombotic effects (see Fig. 2).[17,18,20]

A growing body of evidence suggests that hypertension and HF may be consequences of a dysregulated NP system and that patients with HF and hypertension may have a deficiency of biologically active NPs.[20,21] NPR-C clears NP from the circulation through receptor-mediated internalization and degradation. Urodilatin, a renally synthesized isoform of ANP, stimulates NPR-A located in the glomeruli and collecting ducts and promote Na^+ excretion.[22]

Another key component of the NP system is neprilysin (neutral endopeptidase), which catalyzes the degradation of ANP, BNP, and CNP as well as the degradation of bradykinin, adrenomedullin, endothelin-1, substance P, and angiotensin II.[23] Neprilysin is a potentially useful therapeutic target in HF.[24,20] Inhibition of neprilysin

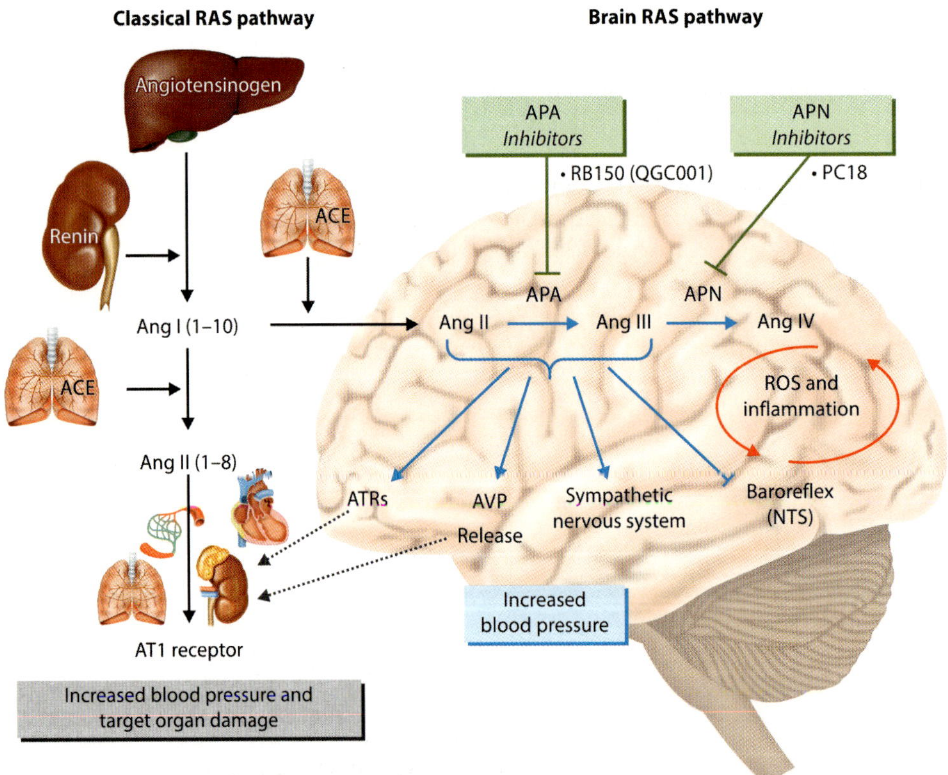

Fig. 2: Reticular-activating system (RAS) pathway

Abbreviations: ACE, angiotensin-converting enzyme; AT1, angiotensin II receptor type 1; APA, aminopeptidase A; APN, aminopeptidase N.

increases the levels of NP, causing vasodilation and a reduction in extracellular fluid volume.

ARNI IN HEART FAILURE WITH DIABETES

There are several potential mechanisms, which have been studied suggesting this drug might lead to the improvement in glycemic control by inhibition of neprilysin. Promotion of mobilization of lipids from adipose tissue,[24] postprandial lipid oxidation,[25] promotion of adiponectin release,[26] and muscular oxidative capacity[27] has also been studied in this regard.

Atrial natriuretic peptide system regulates postprandial lipid oxidation by attenuation of postprandial decline in lipid mobilization leading to increase in free fatty acids.

Infusion of BNP leads to decrease glucose concentration in blood.[28] Bradykinin (a neprilysin substrate) has been studied to improve sensitivity of insulin and attenuation of breakdown of lipids.[29] Role of kinins in adipocytes have systemic contributions to metabolic homeostasis, since exclusive expression of these receptors in fat cells is able to control whole body insulin sensitivity and predisposition to obesity.

Cyclic guanosine monophosphate, which is also increased by neprilysin inhibition, has known vasodilatory effects in skeletal muscles.[14] GLP-1 (neuropeptide of incretin family), which is a potent antiglycemic hormone and has a very short-circulating half-life is partially degraded by neprilysin.

Inhibition of RAAS has also been studied to improve glycemic control,[30,31] where angiotensin-2 promotes resistance of insulin while angiotensin-1 receptor blockade modestly improves insulin sensitivity.[2]

Sacubitril/valsartan was shown in PARADIGM-HF to reduce the risk of cardiovascular death, all-cause mortality, and hospital readmission rates in comparison to enalapril in HFrEF. The rates of these outcomes increased with increasing HBA1C at baseline.[32] ARNI improved peripheral insulin sensitivity in obese hypertensive patients.[33]

ABOUT ANGIOTENSIN RECEPTOR BLOCKER NEPRILYSIN INHIBITOR (FIG. 3)

Active Substances

Sacubitril/Valsartan

It contains a salt complex of the anionic forms of sacubitril and valsartan, sodium cations, and water molecules in the molar ratio of 1:1:3:2.5, respectively. Following oral administration, it dissociates into sacubitril (which is further metabolized to LBQ657) and valsartan.

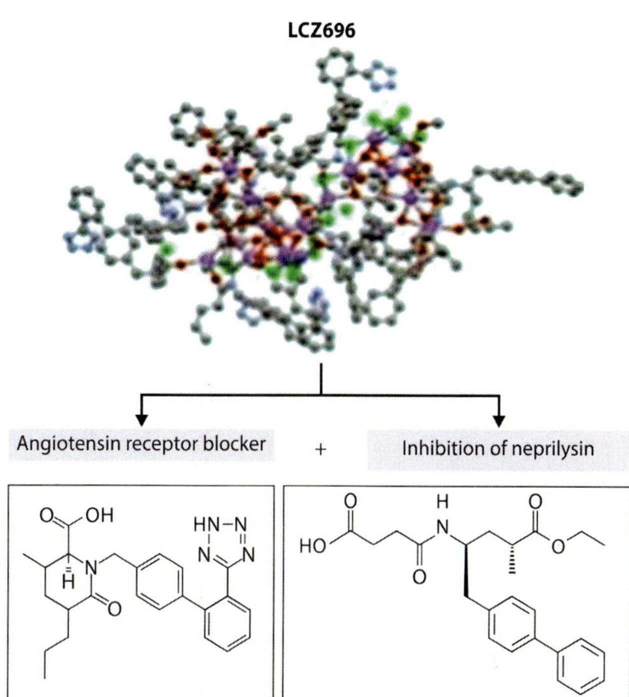

Fig. 3: Angiotensin receptor neprilysin inhibition

Pharmacodynamics

The pharmacodynamic effects of sacubitril/valsartan were evaluated after single and multiple dose administrations in healthy subjects and in patients with HF, and are consistent with simultaneous neprilysin inhibition and RAAS blockade. In a 7-day valsartan-controlled study in patients with HFrEF, administration resulted in a significant nonsustained increase in natriuresis, increased urine cGMP, and decreased plasma MR-proANP and N-terminal prohormone of brain NP (NT-proBNP) compared to valsartan. In a 21-day study in HFrEF patients, it significantly increased urine ANP and cGMP and plasma cGMP, and decreased plasma NT-proBNP, aldosterone, and endothelin-1 compared to baseline. It blocked the AT1-receptor as evidenced by increased plasma renin activity and plasma renin concentrations. In PARADIGM-HF, sacubitril/valsartan decreased plasma NT-proBNP and increased plasma BNP and urine cGMP compared with enalapril.

Neprilysin is one of multiple enzymes involved in the clearance of amyloid-β (A-β) from the brain and cerebrospinal fluid (CSF). Administration of sacubitril/valsartan 400 mg once daily for 2 weeks to healthy subjects was associated with an increase in CSF A-β 1-38 compared to placebo; there were no changes in concentrations of CSF A-β 1-40 and 1-42. The clinical relevance of this finding is unknown.

Neprilysin has been implicated in the catabolism of amyloid beta peptides in the brain and as such has received considerable attention, particularly as a therapeutic target for Alzheimer's disease. An inverse relationship between neprilysin levels and A-β peptide levels and between neprilysin levels and amyloid plaque formation has been observed in human brain. Neprilysin levels decline with aging in the temporal and frontal cortex possibly contributing to higher A-β peptide levels. A number of studies have shown that increasing neprilysin levels in the brain leads to a decrease in brain A-β peptide levels. Most recently, a potential relationship between A-β peptide synthesis from the amyloid precursor protein and neprilysin activity has been proposed.

Dementia- and cognition-related adverse effects were not increased by LCZ696 in PARADIGM-HF (or omapatrilat in OVERTURE), and the beneficial cardiovascular actions of angiotensin receptor neprilysin inhibition might prevent cognitive decline in other ways.[34,35] However, as a precaution, serial cognitive function testing is planned in the recently initiated efficacy and safety of LCZ696 compared to valsartan, on morbidity and mortality in HF patients with preserved ejection fraction (PARAGON-HF).

Pharmacokinetics

Absorption

Following oral administration, sacubitril/valsartan dissociates into sacubitril, which is further metabolized to LBQ657, and valsartan, which reaches peak plasma concentrations in 0.5 hours, 2 hours, and 1.5 hours, respectively. The oral absolute bioavailability of sacubitril and valsartan is estimated to be more than or equal to 60% and 23%, respectively. Following twice daily dosing of sacubitril/valsartan, steady state levels of sacubitril, LBQ657, and valsartan are reached in 3 days. At steady state, sacubitril and valsartan do not accumulate significantly, while LBQ657 accumulates by 1.6-fold. Sacubitril/valsartan administration with food has no clinically significant impact on the systemic exposures of sacubitril, LBQ657, and valsartan.

Distribution: Sacubitril/valsartan is highly bound to plasma proteins (94–97%). Based on the comparison of plasma and CSF exposures, LBQ657 does cross the blood-brain barrier to a limited extent (0.28%).

Biotransformation/Metabolism

Sacubitril is readily converted to LBQ657 by esterases; LBQ657 is not further metabolized to a significant extent. Valsartan is minimally metabolized, as only about 20% of the dose is recovered as metabolites. A hydroxyl metabolite has been identified in plasma at low concentrations (<10%). Since CYP450 enzyme-mediated metabolism of sacubitril and valsartan is minimal, coadministration with drugs that impacts CYP450 enzymes is not expected to impact the pharmacokinetics.

Elimination

Following oral administration, 52–68% of sacubitril (primarily as LBQ657) and ~13% of valsartan and its metabolites are excreted in urine; 37–48% of sacubitril (primarily as LBQ657), and 86% of valsartan and its metabolites are excreted in feces.

Sacubitril, LBQ657, and valsartan are eliminated from plasma with a mean elimination half-life (T1/2) of approximately 1.43 hours, 11.48 hours, and 9.90 hours, respectively.

Linearity/Nonlinearity

The pharmacokinetics of sacubitril, LBQ657, and valsartan are linear in the dose range tested (50–400 mg of sacubitril/valsartan).

Impaired Renal Function

A correlation was observed between renal function and systemic exposure to LBQ657, but not to valsartan. In patients with mild-to-moderate renal impairment [30 mL/min/1.73 m^2 ≤ estimated glomerular filtration rate (eGFR) < 60 mL/min/1.73 m^2] the AUC for LBQ657 was up to two-fold higher. No dosage adjustment is required in patients with mild or moderate renal impairment. A 2.7-fold higher AUC for LBQ657 was observed in patients with severe renal impairment (eGFR < 30 mL/min/1.73 m^2).

Caution should be exercised when administering sacubitril/valsartan in patients with severe renal impairment.

Impaired Hepatic Function

In patients with mild-to-moderate hepatic impairment, the exposures of sacubitril increased by 1.5- and 3.4-fold, LBQ657 increased by 1.5- and 1.9-fold, and valsartan increased by 1.2-fold and 2.1-fold, respectively, compared to matching healthy subjects. No dosage adjustment is recommended when administering sacubitril/valsartan to patients with mild-hepatic impairment (Child-Pugh A classification) including patients with biliary obstructive disorders. A low starting dose is recommended in patients with moderate hepatic impairment (Child-Pugh B classification).

In severe hepatic impairment (Child-Pugh C classification), its use is not recommended.

Adverse Effects (Table 1)

Hypotension

Cases of symptomatic hypotension have been reported in patients treated with this drug during clinical trials. Symptomatic hypotension is more likely to occur, if the patient has been volume-depleted, e.g. by diuretic therapy, dietary salt restriction, diarrhea, or vomiting. Sodium and/or volume depletion should be corrected before starting treatment.

Hyperkalemia

As for any drug that acts on the RAAS, use of sacubitril/valsartan may be associated with an increased risk of hyperkalemia. In PARADIGM-HF, the incidence of clinically relevant hyperkalemia was low, resulting in treatment discontinuation in 0.26% of sacubitril/valsartan-treated patients compared to 0.35% of enalapril-treated patients. Medications known to raise potassium levels (e.g. potassium-sparing diuretics and potassium supplements) should be used with caution when coadministered with sacubitril/valsartan. Monitoring of serum potassium is recommended especially in patients with risk factors such as severe renal impairment, diabetes mellitus, hypoaldosteronism, or receiving a high-potassium diet.

Angioedema

Angioedema has been reported in patients treated with sacubitril/valsartan. If angioedema occurs, it should be immediately discontinued and appropriate therapy and monitoring should be provided until complete and sustained resolution of signs and symptoms has occurred. Sacubitril/valsartan must not be readministered.

In cases of confirmed angioedema where swelling has been confined to the face and lips, the condition has generally resolved without treatment, although antihistamines have been useful in relieving symptoms.

Angioedema associated with laryngeal edema may be fatal. Where there is involvement of the tongue, glottis, or larynx, likely to cause airway obstruction, appropriate therapy, e.g. subcutaneous epinephrine/adrenaline solution 1:1,000 (0.3 mL to 0.5 mL) and/or measures necessary to ensure a patent airway, should be promptly administered. Sacubitril/valsartan must not be used in patients with a known history of angioedema related to previous ACE inhibitor or ARB therapy. Due to potential risk of angioedema when used along with an ACE inhibitor, it must not be started until 36 hours after discontinuing ACE inhibitor therapy. If treatment with ARNI (sacubitril/valsartan) is stopped, ACE inhibitor therapy must not be initiated until 36 hours of last dose of ARNI.

TABLE 1: Adverse effect of vymada and enalapril

Adverse drug reactions	*Vymada 200 mg twice daily (%)**	*Enalapril 10 mg twice daily (%)**	*Frequency category*
Metabolism and nutrition disorders			
Hyperkalemia	11.61	14.00	Very common
Hypokalemia	3.31	2.53	Common
Nervous system disorders			
Dizziness	6.33	4.87	Common
Dizziness postural	0.57	0.28	Uncommon
Headache	2.45	2.51	Common
Ear and labyrinth disorders			
Vertigo	1.45	1.40	Common
Vascular disorders			
Hypotension	17.61	11.97	Very common
Syncope	2.24	2.70	Common
Orthostatic hypotension	1.52	0.80	Common
Respiratory, thoracic and mediastinal disorders			
Cough	8.78	12.60	Common
Gastrointestinal disorders			
Diarrhea	4.62	4.47	Common
Nausea	2.09	2.36	Common
Skin and subcutaneous tissue disorders			
Angioedema	0.45	0.24	Uncommon
Renal and urinary disorders			
Renal impairment	10.14	11.52	Very common
Renal failure (renal failure, acute renal failure)	4.76	5.30	Common
General disorders and administration site conditions			
Fatigue	2.97	3.05	Common
Asthenia	2.09	1.84	Common

** Safety analysis set*

VYMADA/ENTRESTO/SACUBITRIL + VALSARTAN

Special Considerations

Females of Childbearing Potential (and Contraceptive Measures, if Applicable)

Female patients of childbearing potential should be advised about the consequences of exposure to sacubitril/valsartan during pregnancy and to use contraception during treatment with sacubitril/valsartan and for 1 week after their last dose.

Pregnancy

As for other drugs that also act directly on the RAAS, sacubitril/valsartan must not be used during pregnancy. Sacubitril/valsartan exerts its effects via angiotensin II antagonism. As a result, a risk to the fetus cannot be excluded. There have been reports of injury to the developing fetus (e.g. spontaneous abortion, oligohydramnios, and newborn renal dysfunction), when pregnant women have taken valsartan. Patients should be advised to discontinue sacubitril/valsartan as soon as pregnancies occur and to inform their physicians.

Breastfeeding

It is not known whether sacubitril/valsartan is excreted in human milk. The components of sacubitril/valsartan, sacubitril and valsartan, were excreted in the milk of lactating rats because of the potential risk for adverse drug reactions in breastfed newborns/infants, sacubitril/valsartan is not recommended during breastfeeding. A decision should be made whether to abstain from breastfeeding or to discontinue sacubitril/valsartan while breastfeeding, taking into account the importance of sacubitril/valsartan to the mother.

Fertility

There are no available data on the effect of sacubitril/valsartan on human fertility. No impairment of fertility was demonstrated in studies with sacubitril/valsartan in male and female rats.

Elderly patients (aged over 65 years):

- No dosage adjustment is necessary.

Pediatric patients (aged below 18 years):

- Sacubitril/valsartan has not been studied in pediatric patients.

How to start LCZ696, if patient on ACEI—stop it for 36 hours. Starting dose 50 mg twice a day. Maintenance dose is 100 mg twice, as tolerability by the patient. Reduce starting dose 25 mg twice daily for patients not on ACEI/ARBs with renal impairment or with moderate hepatic impairment.

Toxicity

Overdosage: In healthy volunteers, a single dose of sacubitril/valsartan 1,200 mg and 900 mg multiple doses (14 days) have been studied and were well tolerated. Hypotension is the most likely symptom of overdosage due to the blood pressure-lowering effects of sacubitril/valsartan.

Symptomatic treatment should be provided. This drug is highly bound to plasma protein and, therefore unlikely to be removed by dialysis.

HOW TO CHECK FOR HEART FAILURE IN ARNI PATIENTS?

Neprilysin does not hydrolyze NT-proBNP, therefore the latter is a useful cardiac biomarker to assess therapeutic effect and prognosis in patients treated with neprilysin inhibitors.[36,37]

CONCLUSION

First-line treatment for symptomatic class I, class II HF (NYHA).[5] If patient has good BP with ACEI tolerability and is recently hospitalized with slightly increased BNP, ARNI is the treatment of choice.[12] In patient with HFrEF taking ACEI/ARB with beta blocker, if symptoms are not resolved then ACEI is replaced by ARNI.[13] In patients with DM and HFrEF, ARNI decreases HbA1C more than enalapril (PARADIGM-HF study), hence is recommended. ARNI improves peripheral insulin sensitivity also in high-HbA1C, obese, and hypertensive patients (ESC 2016 ARNI and ACEI for HFrEF). ARNI is a novel drug for HFrEF therapy, which reduces cardiovascular mortality (20%), total mortality (16%), and hospital readmission, as compared with enalapril. Patient's volume status, diuretic therapy, salt status, and dehydration status are supposed to be checked before starting the drug. After starting, BP and serum potassium levels to be monitored especially in patients with diabetes, hypoaldosteronism, renal impairment, etc. If patient is using ACEI, then sacubitril/valsartan is to be used only after stopping it for 36 hours. Not to be used in children less than 18 years, pregnancy and breastfeeding females. Potential female of childbearing age should use contraception, if ARNI is to be used. Patient not on ACEI/ARB with renal or moderate hepatic impairment should start with low-dose ARNI followed by gradual increase of dose may be done as per the tolerability of patient. The ARNI's efficacy in HF can be monitored by periodical NT-ProBNP evaluation. Timely administration of ARNI in HF patient with diabetes has tremendous potential of reducing the cardiac morbidity and mortality.

REFERENCES

1. McMurray JJ, Gerstein HC, Holman RR, et al. Heart failure: a cardiovascular outcome in diabetes that can no longer be ignored. Lancet Diab Endocrinol. 2014;2:843-51.
2. van der Zijl NJ, Moors CC, Goossens GH, et al. Valsartan improves {beta}-cell function and insulin sensitivity in subjects with impaired glucose metabolism. Diabetes Care. 2011;34:845-51.
3. Lindenfeld J, Albert NM, Boehmer JP, et al. HFSA 2010 Comprehensive heart failure practice guideline. J Card Fail. 2010;16:e1-e194.
4. McMurray JJ, Packer M, Desai AS, et al. Angiotensin neprilysin inhibition versus enalapril in heart failure. N Engl J Med. 2014;371:993-1004.
5. Yancy CW, Jessup M, Bozkurt B, et al. 2013 ACCF/AHA guideline for the management of heart failure: a report of the American College of Cardiology Foundation/American Heart Association Task Force on practice guidelines. Circulation. 2013;128:e240-e327.
6. Mann DL, Bristow MR. Mechanisms and models in heart failure: the biomechanical model and beyond. Circulation. 2005;111:2837-49.
7. Sliwa K, Norton GR, Kone N, et al. Impact of initiating carvedilol before angiotensin-converting enzyme inhibitor therapy on cardiac function in newly diagnosed heart failure. J Am Coll Cardiol. 2004;44:1825-30.
8. McMurray JJ, Ostergren J, Swedberg K, et al. Effects of candesartan in patients with chronic heart failure and reduced left-ventricular systolic function taking angiotensin-converting-enzyme inhibitors: the CHARM-Added trial. Lancet. 2003;362:767-71.
9. Swedberg K, Komajda M, Böhm M, et al. Ivabradine and outcomes in chronic heart failure (SHIFT): a randomised placebo-controlled study. Lancet. 2010;376:875-85.
10. Ponikowski P, Voors AA, Anker SD, et al. 2016 ESC Guidelines for the diagnosis and treatment of acute and chronic heart failure: The Task Force for the diagnosis and treatment of acute and chronic heart failure of the European Society of Cardiology (ESC) Developed with the special contribution of the Heart Failure Association (HFA) of the ESC. Eur Heart J. 2016;37:2129-200.
11. Yancy CW, Jessup M, Bozkurt B, et al. 2016 ACC/AHA/HFSA Focused Update on New Pharmacological Therapy for Heart Failure: An Update of the 2013 ACCF/AHA Guideline for the Management of Heart Failure: A Report of the American College of Cardiology/American Heart Association Task Force on Clinical Practice Guidelines and the Heart Failure Society of America. J Am Coll Cardiol. 2016;68:1476-88.
12. Turner AJ, Isaac RE, Coates D. The neprilysin (NEP) family of zinc metalloendopeptidases: genomics and function. Bioessays. 2001;23:261-9.
13. Turner AJ. Neprilysin. In: Barret AJ, Rawlings ND, Woessner JF (Eds). Handbook of Proteolytic Enzymes. Amsterdam: Elsevier; 2004. pp. 419-26.
14. Messerli FH, Weber MA, Brunner HR. Angiotensin II receptor inhibition: a new therapeutic principle. Arch Intern Med. 1996;156:1957-2019.
15. de Bold AJ, Borenstein HB, Veress AT, et al. A rapid and potent natriuretic response to intravenous injection of atrial myocardial extract in rats. Life Sci. 1981;28:89-94.
16. Sudoh T, Kangawa K, Minamino N, et al. A new natriuretic peptide in porcine brain. Nature. 1988;332:78-81.
17. Potter LR, Abbey-Hosch S, Dickey DM. Natriuretic peptides, their receptors, and cyclic guanosine monophosphate-dependent signaling functions. Endocr Rev. 2006;27:47-72.
18. Boerrigter G, Burnett JC Jr. Recent advances in natriuretic peptides in congestive heart failure. Expert Opin Investig Drugs. 2004;13:643-52.
19. Zois NE, Bartels ED, Hunter I, et al. Natriuretic peptides in cardiometabolic regulation and disease. Nat Rev Cardiol. 2014;11:403-12.
20. Mangiafico S, Costello-Boerrigter LC, Andersen IA, et al. Neutral endopeptidase inhibition and the natriuretic peptide system: an evolving strategy in cardiovascular therapeutics. Eur Heart J. 2013;34:886-93c.
21. Macheret F, Heublein D, Costello-Boerrigter LC, et al. Human hypertension is characterized by a lack of activation of the antihypertensive cardiac hormones ANP and BNP. J Am Coll Cardiol. 2012;60:1558-65.
22. Forssmann W, Meyer M, Forssmann K. The renal urodilatin system: clinical implications. Cardiovasc Res. 2001;51:450-62.
23. Ferro CJ, Spratt JC, Haynes WG, et al. Inhibition of neutral endopeptidase causes vasoconstriction of human resistance vessels in vivo. Circulation. 1998;97:2323-30.
24. Birkenfeld AL, Boschmann M, Moro C, et al. Lipid mobilization with physiological atrial natriuretic peptide concentrations in humans. J Clin Endocrinol Metab. 2005;90:3622-8.
25. Birkenfeld AL, Budziarek P, Boschmann M, et al. Atrial natriuretic peptide induces postprandial lipid oxidation in humans. Diabetes. 2008;57:3199-204.
26. Coué M, Badin PM, Vila IK, et al. Defective natriuretic peptide receptor signaling in skeletal muscle links obesity to type 2 diabetes. Diabetes. 2015;64:4033-45.
27. Engeli S, Birkenfeld AL, Badin PM, et al. Natriuretic peptides enhance the oxidative capacity of human skeletal muscle. J Clin Invest. 2012;122:4675-9.
28. Heinisch BB, Vila G, Resl M, et al. B-type natriuretic peptide (BNP) affects the initial response to intravenous glucose: a randomised placebo-controlled cross-over study in healthy men. Diabetologia. 2012;55:1400-05.
29. Mori MA, Sales VM, Motta FL, et al. Kinin B1 receptor in adipocytes regulates glucose tolerance and predisposition to obesity. PLoS One. 2012;7:e44782.
30. Jing F, Mogi M, Horiuchi M. Role of renin-angiotensin-aldosterone system in adipose tissue dysfunction. Molecular Cell Endocrinol. 2013;378:23-8.
31. Messerli FH, Weber MA, Brunner HR. Angiotensin II receptor inhibition: a new therapeutic principle. Arch Intern Med. 1996;156:1957-2019.
32. Kristensen SL, Preiss D, Jhund PS, et al. PARADIGM-HF Investigators and Committees. Risk Related to Pre-Diabetes Mellitus and Diabetes Mellitus in Heart Failure With Reduced Ejection Fraction: Insights From Prospective Comparison of ARNI With ACEI to Determine Impact on Global Mortality and Morbidity in Heart Failure Trial. Circ Heart Fail. 2016;9:pii: e002560.
33. Jordan J, Stinken R, Jox T, et al. Improved insulin sensitivity with Angiotensin Receptor Neprilysin inhibition in individuals with obesity and hypertension. Clin Pharmacol Ther. 2017;101:254-63.
34. Saido T, Leissring MA. Proteolytic degradation of amyloid β-protein. Cold Spring Harb Perspect Med. 2012;2:a006379.
35. Howell S, Nalbantoglu J, Crine P. Neutral endopeptidase can hydrolyze β-amyloid (1–40) but shows no effect on β-amyloid precursor protein metabolism. Peptides. 1995;16:647-52.
36. Martinez-Rumayor A, Richards AM, Burnett JC, et al. Biology of the natriuretic peptides. Am J Cardiol. 2008;101:3-8.
37. Plamboeck A, Holst JJ, Carr RD, et al. Neutral endopeptidase 24.11 and dipeptidyl peptidase IV are both mediators of the degradation of glucagon-like peptide 1 in the anaesthetised pig. Diabetologia. 2005;48:1882-90.

78

CHAPTER

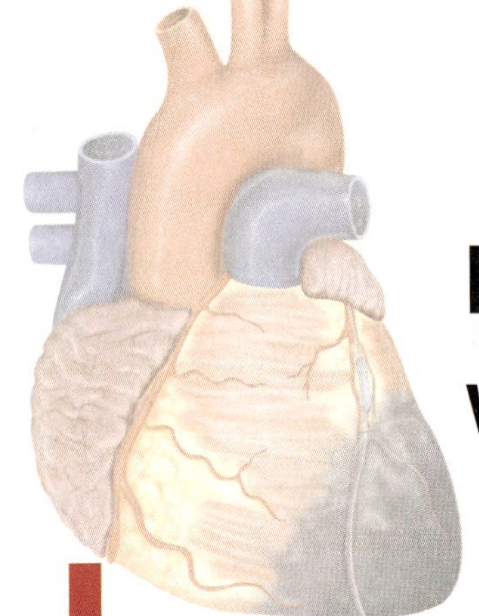

Indapamide versus Hydrochlorothiazide versus Chlorthalidone in Cardiodiabetes

Debabrata Roy, Md Saiyed Rana

INTRODUCTION

Until middle of the 20th centuries, before era of antihypertensive agents started, hypertension was considered as a compensatory mechanism of human physiology to maintain vital organ perfusion and it was widely believed that it should not be controlled even if somebody has a way to do it, earning it the so called name of 'essential hypertension'.[1] A series of randomized controlled trial (RCT) around 1960 broke this myth and proved that controlling blood pressure (BP) is actually beneficial measured by so-called hard outcomes such as stroke, myocardial infarction and mortality.[2] Thiazide diuretics did better compare to other antihypertensive medications as proved in recent RCTs such as ALLHAT, HYVET, PROGRESS, MRFIT, SHEP, INSIGHT, etc. allowing it to enjoy the status of first line of drugs from the very beginning till in most recent guidelines on hypertension (Table 1).[3] Not surprisingly thiazide diuretics are the second most common prescribed drugs worldwide, the first being angiotensin converting enzyme inhibitors (ACEI). Thiazides obviously come with side effects specific to them at recommended therapeutic doses used in those trials. These are proarrhythmic dyselectrolemia, hyperuricemia, altered lipid and glucose metabolism and new onset diabetes (NOD) in patients who are prone to develop so. In a post-hoc analysis of the Valsartan Antihypertensive Long-Term Use Evaluation (VALUE) study, the hypertensive subjects who developed NOD showed a 43% higher risk of cardiac morbidity when compared with individuals who did not develop diabetes and NOD was associated with a marginally higher risk of myocardial infarction (P = 0.057) and a significantly higher risk of congestive HF (P = 0.017).[4] These findings are consistent with a report from the Ongoing Telmisartan Alone and In Combination with Ramipril Global End Point Trial (ONTARGET), in which NOD was associated with a 74% excess risk of congestive HF requiring hospitalization.[5] The situation is worrisome if we consider the fact that global prevalence (age-standardized) of diabetes has nearly doubled since 1980, rising from 4.7% to 8.5% in the adult population mainly because of rise of metabolic syndrome and diabetes related complications will be one of the leading killer by 2030.[6] There is substantial overlap between diabetes and hypertension in etiology and disease mechanisms with obesity, inflammation, oxidative stress, and insulin resistance are thought to be the common pathways.[7] In reality, diabetes and hypertension are found in the same individual more often than would occur by chance, whereas the overlap between insulin resistance and raised blood pressure is even more substantial than that between diabetes and hypertension.[8] So, if we want to treat a patient with hypertension for long-term, the least we want him/her to become diabetic or his/her glycemic and lipid profile to be deranged. Our discussion here will be limited to the pros and cons of three thiazide group of diuretics namely hydrochlorothiazide (HCTZ), chlorthalidone (CTDN) and indapamide (INDAP) in patients with diabetes mellitus.

TABLE 1: Most recent international guidelines on Hypertension and their recommendation

	UK, NICE	*CHEF*	*ESH/ESC*	*ACA/AHA*	*JNC – 8*	*ISH/ASH*
Year	2011	2012	2013	2013	2014	2014
HTN Diagnosis	≥ 140/90	≥ 140/90	≥ 140/90	≥ 140/90	≥ 140/90	≥ 140/90
Target BP Uncomplicated	< 140/90	< 140/90	<140/90	<140/90	<140/90	<140/90
Elderly	<150/90 80+ year	<140/90	<140/90	<150/90 60+ year	< 140/90	< 150/90 80+ year
Diabetes	-	<130/80	<140/85	<140/90	<140/90	<140/90
1st line drugs	CCB, ACEI, ARB	CCB, ACEI, ARB	CCB, ACEI, ARB	CCB, ACEI, ARB	CCB, ACEI, ARB	CCB, ACEI, ARB
Diuretics as 1st line	CTDN, INDAP	THZ	CTDN, IDAP, HCTZ	THZ	CTDN, IDAP, HCTZ	CTDN, IDAP, HCTZ

Abbreviations: THZ, thiazides; CTDN, chlorthalidone; HCTZ, hydrochlorothiazide; INDAP, indapamide

PHARMACOLOGY OF THIAZIDE DIURETICS AS A WHOLE (TABLE 1)

Mechanism of Action

Thiazides blocks the Na-Cl cotransporter in distal convoluted tubule (DCT), thereby causing natriuresis, diuresis, reduced preload causing reduced stroke volume and cardiac output which ultimately leads to decrease of BP. With chronic administration, plasma volume returns to normal, but peripheral vascular resistance is decreased and this is probably the reason for sustained antihypertensive effect. Chlorothiazide (CTZ) was the prototype molecule in this group and HCTZ, CTDN, and INDAP were developed one by one with chemical modification. INDAP has additional vasorelaxant property which may explain its capacity to reduce BP in CKD patients.

Pharmacokinetics and Metabolism

Hydrochlorothiazide is well absorbed (65–75%) following oral administration. Peak plasma concentrations are observed within 1-5 hours of dosing. Binding to serum proteins has been reported to be approximately 40–68%. HCTZ is eliminated primarily by renal pathways. Following oral doses of 12.5–100 mg, 55–77% of the administered dose appears in urine and greater than 95% of the absorbed dose is excreted in urine as unchanged drug. In patients with renal disease, plasma concentrations of HCTZ are increased and the elimination half-life is prolonged. CTDN has bioavailability of 100% even when taken with food. CTDN and INDAP have a longer half-life and duration of action as compared with HCTZ. Indeed, CTDN is twice as potent in reducing 24-hour ambulatory BP compared with HCTZ.

Pharmacodynamics

Onset of action occurs within 2 hours of dosing, peak effect is observed at about 4 hours, and activity persists for less than 24 hours in case of HCTZ. HCTZ is less potent than INDAP, CTDN, ACEI, ARB, beta blockers, and CCB by 4.2–6.2 mm Hg SBP.[9] The recommended dose used in clinical trials is 50–100 mg daily with two divided doses to compensate for short-duration of action.

SIDE EFFECT PROFILE OF THIAZIDES (TABLE 2)

Hyponatremia

Symptomatic hyponatremia can occur up to 7–21% of patients treated with thiazides and is more common in elderly, females and patients with low body weight. Compared to HCTZ, hyponatremia is more common in CTDN at doses more than 25 mg daily. Hyponatremia is rare with INDAP sustained release preparation.

Hypokalemia

Hypokalemia is a serious complication of thiazide diuretics, which is associated with an increased risk of ventricular arrhythmias and cardiac arrest at doses used in RCT (50–100 mg daily). It is equally found in CTDN, HCTZ and may be the reason behind hyperglycemia. However incidence of hypokalemia was significantly lower in patients receiving INDAP at therapeutic doses, more so when they are on sustained release (SR) formulation. Hypomagnesemia and hypercalcemia are seen more commonly during therapy with HCTZ and CTDN and rarely happens during therapy with INDAP.

Hyperuricemia

In a retrospective cohort analysis, CTDN was shown to result in significantly higher uric acid level compared with HCTZ ($p < 0.0001$). In SHEP study, it was demonstrated that patients with coexisting elevated serum uric acid (>1 mg/dL) had lost cardiovascular (CV) benefit of CTDN therapy [hazard ratio: 0.95 (95% CI: 0.67–1.39) and 0.56 (95% CI: 0.37–0.85) for patients with and without serum uric acid >1

TABLE 2: Pharmacological property and metabolic side effects of INDAP, CTDN and HCTZ

Variable	*HCTZ*	*CTDN*	*INDAP*	*Remarks*
Bioavailability after oral dose	60%	100%	90%	CTDN, INDAP can be taken with food
Half life (hr)	3–10	24–72	6–15	
Duration of action (hr)	12–18	24–72	24–36	CTDN, INDAP can be used as single daily dose
Daily dose	12.5–50	12.5–25	1.25–2.5	INDAP dose is 1/10th of HCTZ for similar BP reduction
Single dose	No	Yes	Yes	
Antihypertensive effects	Weak	Strong	Intermediate	INDAP, CTDN converts non-dippers to dippers when used as add on
Pleotropic effects	No	Yes	Yes	HCTZ has negligible pleotropic effects compared to INDAP and CTDN
New onset diabetes	Yes	Yes	No	NOD is dose dependent side effects. Earlier trials used 50–100 mg CTDN daily, much higher than now
Hyperuricemia	Yes	Yes	No	Hyperuricemia counterbalance the beneficial effects of CTDN
Deranged lipid profile	Yes	Yes	No	
Use in low GFR	No	Yes	Yes	INDAP still can reduce BP in compromised renal function
Dyselectrolemia	Yes	Yes	Uncommon	Dyselectrolemia is rare in INDAP sustained release preparation
Nephron independent action	No	No	Yes	INDAP has role mediated through L type Ca Channel, can lower BP in CKD patients

mg/dL, respectively]. However, INDAP has been shown to cause only modest increases in uric acid levels as compared with HCTZ.

Dyslipidemia and New Onset Diabetes Mellitus

Thiazide diuretics notoriously disturbs glycemic control in diabetics, precipitate NOD in susceptible population, increase total cholesterol, low-density lipoprotein cholesterol (LDL-C) and triglycerides, and decrease HDL in a dose dependent manner. In the Multiple Risk Factor Intervention Trial (MRFIT), CTDN has been shown to cause less increases in total cholesterol (overall $p < 0.0001$) and LDL-C (overall $p = 0.0009$) as compared with HCTZ. ALLHAT trial showed a significantly higher incidence of diabetes mellitus (DM) with CTDN versus lisinopril in patients with existing metabolic syndrome, and a significantly higher incidence of DM compared with lisinopril and amlodipine in those without metabolic syndrome. Natrilix SR versus Enalapril Study in hypertensive Type 2 diabetics with Microalbuminuria (NESTOR) trial also demonstrated that INDAP has a neutral effect on lipids and glucose levels in patients with type 2 DM. Thus, INDAP may be considered a metabolically neutral diuretic, both during short- and long-term administration.

THE CLINICAL EVIDENCE

HCTZ versus CTDN

There are very few prospective RCTs which did the head-to-head comparison between HCTZ versus CTDN. So we have to rely mainly on retrospective data and drug adjusted and office BP adjusted network meta-analysis. Compared to other antihypertensive agents HCTZ was found to be less effective in preventing cardiovascular events (CVE). It was found to be inferior to enalapril in the ANBP2 trial, to amlodipine in the ACCOMPLISH trial, and to CTDN and HCTZ—amiloride combination in network analyses of several trials. On the other hand in ALLHAT trial CTDN was found to be superior to the α-blocker doxazosin mesylate in the prevention of stroke and was superior to the ACE inhibitor lisinopril in the prevention of stroke in black individuals. In office BP adjusted network meta-analysis of trials, it was found that for a comparable decrease in blood pressure, the risk of developing cardiovascular event was found to be higher with HCTZ than with CTDN. In head-to-head comparison between HCTZ and CTDN in MRFIT trial CTDN arm was associated with significantly fewer CVD events; lower SBP, more hypokalemia, lower total and LDL-C levels; and significantly higher uric acid levels compared with HCTZ arm. CHD mortality rates in clinics that switched from HCTZ to CTDN decreased by 28%, suggesting that CTDN may be the preferred thiazide diuretic for hypertension in patients at high risk of CVD events like in DM.[10] In 1992, the Systolic Hypertension in the Elderly Program (SHEP) concluded that 12.5-25 mg. CTDN daily causes a 36% risk reduction in stroke (primary end point, $p = 0.0003$) versus placebo. In another network analysis by Roush et al.[11] to assess the efficacy of CTDN compared to HCTZ, in reducing CVE it was found that though the percentage of risk reduction in CCF for CTDN versus HCTZ was 23 (95% CI, 2–39; P-0.032); but in composite CVE it was 21 (95% CI, 12–28; $P < 0.0001$) proving again the superiority of CTDN over HCTZ.[11]

INDAP versus HCTZ

INDAP SR 1.5 mg is equally efficacious as HCTZ 25 mg or amlodipine 5 mg in reducing BP, more efficacious than enalapril 20 mg in reducing LVH, and equal to enalapril in reducing microalbuminuria in hypertension patients with type 2 DM.[12] In a recent systemic meta-analysis, by Roush GC et al. it was found that like CTDN, INDAP is more potent than HCTZ at commonly prescribed doses without evidence for greater adverse metabolic effects. There were no detectable differences between HCTZ and INDAP in metabolic adverse effects including effects on serum potassium.[9] INDAP has reduced left ventricular mass index by 17% ($P < 0.001$), while HCTZ or CTDN has no effect in this end organ process.[13] INDAP was found to be comparable with captopril and enalapril in reducing albuminuria in diabetes mellitus whereas in another study, HCTZ had no effect on urinary microalbuminuria.[14] INDAP is more effective in scavenging oxygen radicals and in inhibiting platelet aggregation and unlike HCTZ, INDAP has no effect on serum lipids.[15] That is why INDAP is considered the most metabolically neutral diuretics so far. INDAP can still reduce BP in end-stage renal disease, mediated via L type Ca^{++} channel blocking property[16] whereas CTDN, HCTZ is dependent on GFR for optimum action. A single trial demonstrated an increase in creatinine clearance by 28.5% with INDAP, but a 17.4% decrease with HCTZ ($p < 0.01$, for the difference) despite a similar BP control.[17] In a meta-analysis, it was found that type 2 DM with mild-to-moderate hypertension when prescribed INDAP (1.5 mg SR) therapy, showed no alteration in serum sodium, potassium, chloride, uric acid, liver enzymes, BUN, creatinine, lipid profiles, FBS, HbA1C levels.[18] Another recent RCT compared effects of INDAP versus HCTZ on CV outcome when added to ACEI in patients with type 2 DM and hypertension and it was found that INDAP plus ACEI combination significantly improved mean longitudinal systolic velocity and longitudinal strain by 7 and 14% respectively (from 5.6 ± 1.8 to 6.0 ± 1.1 cm/s and from 16.2% ± 1.8% to 18.5% ± 1.1%, both $p < 0.05$)[19] proving superiority of INDAP over HCTZ.

CONCLUSION

When we compare HCTZ versus CTDN, there is no doubt that CTDN is better drug, reducing CV outcome comparable to ACEI, CCB whereas HCTZ failed to do so. On the other hand INDAP is also a better drug than HCTZ as proved in trials. Both INDAP and CTDN can be used as a monotherapy or as add-on therapy. Both has long duration of action providing sustained BP reduction and can convert nondippers to dippers. HCTZ and CTDN come with their metabolic side effects specially if used at doses, which has been found to provide beneficial outcome in therapeutic trials, i.e. 50–100 mg daily for HCTZ and 25–50 mg daily for CTDN. INDAP is considered the metabolically neutral thiazides with some favorable pleiotropic effects not shown by other two. Despite this, among three, 80% prescription are for HCTZ mostly in combination with other class of antihypertensives. The dose of HCTZ used is also less (<50 mg) than what has been recommended in clinical trials. So in our opinion we should stop using HCTZ in not only in diabetic patients but also in all patients. Whether to use INDAP or CTDN in hypertension in diabetics is very difficult to answer. CTDN at recommended doses (12.5–50 mg daily) has definitely some adverse metabolic side effects which in long run can increase MACE as shown in some study and INDAP at recommended dose (1.25–2.5 mg daily) is metabolically neutral with some favorable pleiotropic effects as good as ACEI. In our opinion INDAP should be the winner among three but we need RCT with head-to-head comparison between INDAP and CTDN.

REFERENCES

1. White PD. Heart Disease, 3rd edition. New York: Macmillan; 1944. pp21-23.
2. Zanchetti A. Interventional trials in hypertension: what have we learned and what remains to be learned? In: Manual of Hypertension of the European Society of Hypertension, 2nd edition. Boca Raton: CRC Press; 2014.
3. Chobanian AV, Bakris GL, Black HR, et al. The Seventh Report of the Joint National Committee on Prevention, Detection, Evaluation, and Treatment of High Blood Pressure: the JNC 7 report. JAMA. 2003;289:2560-72.
4. Aksnes TA, Kjeldsen SE, Rostrup M, et al. Impact of new-onset diabetes mellitus on cardiac outcomes in the Valsartan Antihypertensive Long-term Use Evaluation (VALUE) trial population. Hypertension. 2007;50:467-73.
5. Held C, Gerstein HC, Yusuf S, et al. Glucose levels predict hospitalization for congestive heart failure in patients at high cardiovascular risk. Circulation. 2007;115:1371-5.
6. Forouzanfar MH, Alexender L, Anderson HR, et al. GBD 2013 Risk Factors Collaborators. Global, regional, and national comparative risk assessment of 79 behavioural, environmental and occupational, and metabolic risks or clusters of risks in 188 countries, 1990–2013: a systematic analysis for the Global Burden of Disease Study 2013. Lancet. 2015;386(1010):2287-323.
7. Cheung BMY, Wat NMS, Tso AWX, et al. Association between raised blood pressure and dysglycemia in Hong Kong Chinese. Diabetes Care. 2008;31:1889-91.
8. Gress TW, Nieto FJ, Shahar E, et al. Hypertension and antihypertensive therapy as risk factors for type 2 diabetes mellitus. Atherosclerosis Risk in Communities Study. N Engl J Med. 2000;342(13):905-12.
9. Roush GC, Ernst ME, Kostis JB, et al. Head-to-head comparisons of hydrochlorothiazide with indapamide and chlorthalidone: antihypertensive and metabolic effects. Hypertension. 2015;65(5):1041-6.
10. Dorsch MP, Gillespie BW, Erickson SR, et al. Chlorthalidone reduces cardiovascular events compared with hydrochlorothiazide:

a retrospective cohort analysis. Hypertension. 2011;57(4): 689-94.
11. Roush GC, Holford TR, Guddati AK, et al. Chlorthalidone compared with hydrochlorothiazide in reducing cardiovascular events systematic review and network meta-analyses. Hypertension. 2012;59:1110-7.
12. Puig JG, Marre M, Kokot F, et al. Efficacy of indapamide SR compared with enalapril in elderly hypertensive patients with type 2 diabetes. Am J Hypertens. 2007;20(1):90-7.
13. Gosse P, Sheridan DJ, Zannad F, et al. Regression of left ventricular hypertrophy in hypertensive patients treated with indapamide SR 1.5 mg versus enalapril 20 mg: the LIVE study. J Hypertens. 2000;18:1465-75.
14. Hallab M, Gallois Y, Chatellier G, et al. Comparison of reduction in microalbuminuria by enalapril and hydrochlorothiazide in normotensive patients with insulin dependent diabetes. BMJ. 1993;306(6871):175-82.
15. Rendu F, Bachelot C, Molle D, et al. Indapamide inhibits human platelet aggregation in vitro: comparison with hydrochlorothiazide. J Cardiovasc Pharmacol. 1993;22(Suppl 6):557-63.
16. Acchiardo SR, Skoutakis VA. Clinical efficacy, safety, and pharmacokinetics of indapamide in renal impairment. Am Heart J. 1983;106(1 Pt 2):237-44.
17. Madkour H, Gadallah M, Riveline B, et al. Indapamide is superior to thiazide in preservation of renal function, in patients with renal insufficiency and systemic hypertension. Am J Cardiol. 1996;77(6):23B-25B.
18. Carey PA, Sheridan DJ, de Cordoue, A, et al. Effect of indapamide on left ventricular hypertrophy in hypertension: a meta-analysis. Am J Cardiol. 1996;77:17B-19B.
19. Vinereanu D, Dulgheru R, Magda S, et al. The effect of indapamide versus hydrochlorothiazide on ventricular and arterial function in patients with hypertension and diabetes: results of a randomized trial. Am Heart J. 2014;168(4):446-56.

CHAPTER 79

Polypill for Cardiovascular Protection in Diabetes

Jugal Bihari Gupta, Rajeev Gupta

INTRODUCTION

Polypill is a drug product in pill form (i.e. tablet or capsule) that combines multiple active pharmaceutical ingredients. The prefix 'poly' means 'multiple,' referring to the multiplicity of distinct drugs in a given 'pill.' It is commonly manufactured as a Fixed-Dose Combination (FDC) drug product targeting treatment or prevention of chronic disease.[1] It can reduce the number of tablets or capsules that need to be taken which in turn may facilitate handling and administration of pharmaceuticals as well as alleviate the pill-burden.[2] Sometimes these multiple drugs in a given polypill might all be aimed at a single underlying condition or group of related conditions. The term polypill was first coined in the context of cardiovascular disease (CVD) prevention.[3] Combinatorial drug products were proposed for treating diagnosed conditions long before they were proposed for preventative medicine including for those diagnosed with CVD.[4] Fixed-dose combination products today are also common for treating other diseases, such as diabetes tuberculosis, and human immunodeficiency virus/acquired immunodeficiency syndrome (HIV/AIDS).

Diabetes particularly type 2 diabetes is a major cause of morbidity and mortality worldwide including India. Diabetes also contributes substantially to cardiovascular risk and more than 60–70% of mortality in diabetics is due to CVD.[5] The initial polypill proposed by Wald and Law contained six ingredients, an angiotensin-converting enzyme (ACE) inhibitor enalapril, a β-blocker atenolol, hydrochlorothiazide, aspirin, a statin simvastatin, and folic acid.[3] A polypill for diabetes could include a statin [to reduce low-density lipoprotein (LDL) cholesterol and for their anti-inflammatory properties], an ACE inhibitor [for blood pressure (BP) control and to protect the kidneys], aspirin (for antiplatelet and anti-inflammatory properties), and metformin (a medication for diabetes that is also associated with weight loss). Thiazide and β-blocker may not be indicated and included because of side effects. Relatedly people who have high cholesterol, high BP, and/or are overweight can have metabolic syndrome, and may be a candidate for an appropriate polypill due to the quantity of different medications potentially involved. However, in this case also the polypill as proposed by Wald and Law falls short because of potential of drug-induced diabetes because of thiazides, statins, and β-blockers.[6]

WHAT IS POLYPILL

For CVD prevention, primary or secondary, polypill is currently defined as any drug combination containing BP-lowering drugs along with a statin.[4] On the basis of a series of meta-analyses, Wald and Law proposed a polypill for use in both primary and secondary prevention containing low-dose aspirin (50–125 mg/day), folic acid 0.8 mg/day, a potent statin (atorvastatin 10 mg or simvastatin 40 mg/day), and three BP-lowering drugs at half the standard dose (thiazide diuretics, β-blocker, and ACE inhibitors).[3]

However, some of the assumptions of Wald and Law are refuted by recent evidence. Folic acid has not prevented CVD in large randomized trials.[4] Low-dose aspirin is beneficial in secondary prevention, but its value in primary prevention remains unproven as the modest reduction in CVD events is counterbalanced by increased major bleeds.[4] On the other hand, statins and BP-lowering drugs are proven in both primary and secondary prevention.[4] Wald and Law estimated that a low to moderate dose of a potent statin is safe, lowers LDL cholesterol by about 37% or 70 mg/dL from an average pretreatment level of 180 mg/dL, and would reduce ischemic heart disease (IHD) by about 60% and stroke by 17% after 2 years of treatment.[3] However, in contemporary settings, average pretreatment LDL cholesterol levels are substantially lower than 180 mg/dL, and in long-term statin trials 70 mg/dL reduction in LDL was not achieved (in most trials it was closer to 35–40 mg/dL). The Cholesterol Treatment Trialists' collaboration found that for each 1 mmol/L (38 mg/dL) reduction in LDL cholesterol over 5 years, there was a 11% relative risk reduction in total mortality, 26% in major IHD events, and 16% in strokes, lower than estimated by Law and Wald but nevertheless very important, and treatment was very safe.[7] The only serious adverse effects of statins, myopathy (rates of about 11 per 100,000 person-years), rhabdomyolysis (rates of 3–4 per 100,000 person-years), and persistent elevation in transaminases (<0.1% of patients) are rare, although myalgia may be more common and affect adherence.[8] In recent meta-analysis, statins slightly increased the risk of developing diabetes mellitus but the risk was low in absolute terms and very low when compared with the reduction in coronary events.[9]

Wald and Law further suggested that the combination of three different antihypertensive agents used at half standard doses safely reduces BP from all pretreatment levels with greater reductions for higher pretreatment levels and with lowering of systolic and diastolic BP by about 20 mm Hg and 11 mm Hg respectively in people with a pretreatment BP of 150/90 mm Hg (the average BP in people aged 50–69 years who experience a stroke or a coronary event).[3] They estimated that this BP-lowering would reduce stroke by 63% and IHD by 46%. Combining several drugs at low doses was proposed to minimize side effects which are more common at high doses, while maintaining efficacy because most of the BP-lowering effect occurs at low doses. Furthermore, side effects of some drugs could be counterbalanced by simultaneous use of other drugs (e.g., hypokalemia and hyperglycemia from diuretics could be avoided by the simultaneous use of ACE inhibitors). An independent meta-analysis of individual patient data from 29 trials of hypertensive individuals (mostly with BP ≥160/100 mm Hg) or those with preexisting CVD confirmed that lowering systolic BP by 5 mm Hg over 4–5 years reduced the risk of IHD by 20%, stroke by 28%, and major CVD events by 22%, with additional reductions in heart failure.[10] Larger reductions in BP led to greater benefits, and treatment was generally safe. However, till date there are no data on the effects of long-term therapy with three BP-lowering drugs at half doses in individuals selected by risk level rather than established hypertension. In a recent small study form Australia, however, the short-term efficacy of a quadruple dose polypill has been established. In addition, the hypothesis that BP-lowering drugs may benefit a wide range of individuals without CVD, including those with 'normal' entry BP levels remains largely untested.[11] In fact, critical appraisals of available data including the HOPE-3 trial suggest that even for patients with mild hypertension (systolic BP of 140–160 mm Hg), the evidence for treatment benefit remains scant, and new trials in high-risk patients with established CVD and/or diabetes mellitus challenge the notion of a consistent relationship between BP-lowering and reduction of vascular events.[12] There have been no trials for efficacy or effectiveness of a polypill in diabetes but we could learn from general cardiovascular prevention trials.[13]

POLYPILL FOR PRIMARY PREVENTION

Primary prevention should include multiple strategies: Health policy and environmental changes, individual behavioral changes, and use of proven and safe drugs.[14] In theory, lifestyle interventions are attractive because of their inherent appeal, perceived low cost, and simplicity and safety. However, behavioral interventions to modify individual lifestyles are costly have generally only modest and unsustainable impact, and have failed to reduce CVD events when tested in large, long-term trials. Changes in health policy, the environment, and cultural attitudes are likely to have a greater impact. For example, antismoking legislation reduces CVD outcomes and has been adopted by a large number of countries.[15] Similarly, health policy changes directed at dietary modifications and smoking cessation in combination with community interventions have reduced CVD mortality in some regions, most notably in Finland and other Scandinavian countries.[16] However, such interventions have not been successfully adapted to other regions and are not implemented in most developed and developing countries, and evidence for their success is required from a wide range of settings.

A complementary approach which can be implemented immediately is the use of drugs to lower risk factor levels.[4] Long-term use of multiple drugs given separately in healthy asymptomatic individuals to lower multiple risk factor levels is impractical and likely to succeed only in unusually motivated individuals. A FDC drug administered once daily (i.e. a polypill) could intervene simultaneously on several common risk factors and theoretically reduce CVD to a large extent.[3] Among people without existing CVD, the most discriminatory screening factor is age because it is greater than 90% of CVD, deaths occur in people aged which is greater than or equal to 55 years. Therefore, using a polypill in people aged greater than or equal to 55 years, especially those with at least one additional risk factor (i.e. at moderate risk) could prevent the majority of CVD events in both high- and low-income countries.

Several trials are currently evaluating the effects of a polypill on risk factor levels.[4] TIPS-1 conducted in India is a prime example. In this trial, 2,053 individuals aged 45–80 years without CVD and with at least one risk factor were randomized to a Polycap consisting of thiazide (12.5 mg), atenolol (50 mg), ramipril (5 mg), simvastatin (20 mg), and aspirin (100 mg), or eight other groups (aspirin alone, simvastatin alone, hydrochlorothiazide alone, three combinations of two BP-lowering drugs, three BP-lowering drugs alone, three BP-lowering drugs plus aspirin) administered for 12 weeks. At baseline, mean BP was 134/85 mm Hg, and LDL cholesterol was 3.0 mmol/L.[17] All study participants received lifestyle advice. Compared with groups not receiving BP-lowering drugs, the Polycap reduced systolic and diastolic BP by 7.4 mm Hg and 5.6 mm Hg, respectively which was similar to the groups with three individual BP-lowering drugs with or without aspirin, LDL cholesterol lowering in the Polycap group was 0.73 mmol/L which was less than with simvastatin alone at 0.83 mmol/L, heart rate was reduced by 7.0 bpm, similar to atenolol; and urinary 11-dehydrothromboxane B2 (a measure of platelet activation) was reduced to a degree similar to that with aspirin. There was a 5% absolute reduction in rates of smoking in all groups.

Although the rates of drug discontinuation were relatively high (≈15% over 3 months), these were similar in all treatment groups and occurred largely for 'social' reasons and not because of side effects (3.8%). On the basis of the magnitude of risk factor lowering observed and utilizing calculations similar to those used by Wald and Law, the authors estimated that the Polycap could reduce IHD by 62% and stroke by 42%.[17] The study proved the feasibility of formulating a polypill (or capsule) that can effectively and safely lower risk factor levels in asymptomatic individuals at moderate risk. It also emphasized the need to test every polypill preparation in the population intended for treatment without assuming effects equal to the combined effects of its components (LDL cholesterol lowering with the Polycap was slightly lower than with simvastatin alone) or effects equal to those derived from theoretical models (the effects on BP and cholesterol were lower than those projected by Law and Wald even after nonadherence was taken into consideration). Several other feasibility trials have been conducted and show a cardiovascular risk reduction from 30 to 70% in all patients with high-risk, including those with diabetes (Fig. 1).

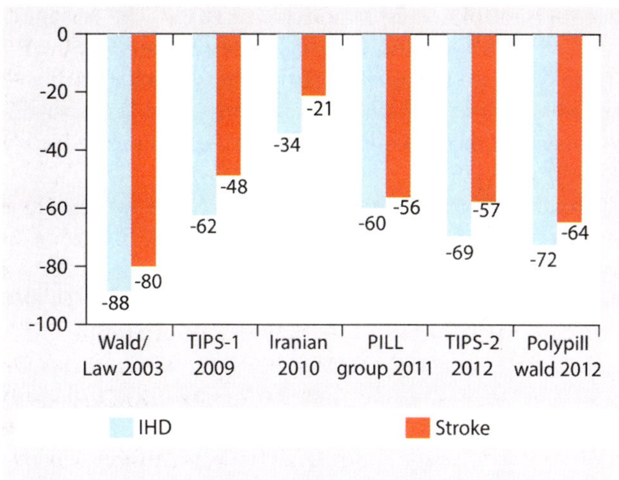

Fig. 1: Hypothesized cardiovascular risk reduction in various polypill trials

Abbreviation: IHD, ischemic heart disease

POLYPILL FOR SECONDARY PREVENTION

Aspirin, statins, β-blockers, and blockers of the renin-angiotensin system (ACE inhibitors and angiotensin receptor blockers [ARBs]) are proven to reduce CVD in secondary prevention.[18] Approximately half of the decline in cardiovascular mortality observed in developed countries during the last two decades is attributable to medical therapy.[19] However, despite clear evidence of effectiveness, a large treatment gap exists. Multiple barriers to better implementation of secondary prevention exist—First, proven therapies are not prescribed to all who may benefit; for example, the third European Action on Secondary Prevention Through Intervention to Reduce Events (EUROASPIRE IV) survey in 9 European countries found that the prevalence of smoking (17%), obesity (35%), uncontrolled BP (56%), and elevated cholesterol (25%) among patients with IHD in the community remains high, and the use of statins and ACE inhibitors/ARBs, although improved compared with previous surveys, remains suboptimal at 71% and 78% respectively.[20] Similar results have emerged from other registries in developed countries. Use of proven therapies is lower in developing countries. The World Health Organization study on Prevention of Recurrence of Myocardial Infarction and Stroke (WHO-PREMISE) survey conducted in 10 low- and middle-income countries found that 81.2% of patients with IHD and 70.6% of patients with cerebrovascular disease were prescribed aspirin, 48.1% and 22.8% β-blockers, 39.8% and 37.8% ACE inhibitors, and 29.8% and 14.1% statins.[21] A recent community-based study conducted in 53 villages in India found that among patients with IHD or cerebrovascular disease only 14% were taking aspirin, 41% a BP-lowering drug, and 5% a cholesterol-lowering medication.[22] These findings are further supported by data from 600 communities from 17 high-, medium-, and low-income countries in the Prospective Urban Rural Epidemiology (PURE) study.[23,24]

Second, long-term adherence with prescribed medications is poor, often less than 50% because of social, cultural, psychological, economic, and clinical factors related to patients, health care providers, health care systems, and their interactions. Nonadherence has major consequences because medication discontinuation is associated with higher rates of recurrent events and mortality in patients with established CVD. Third, cost and affordability are major additional barriers. Although drugs used in secondary prevention are cost-effective, these drugs are still not affordable to the majority of individuals in middle- and low-income countries, where the cost of 1-month supply of standard generic secondary prevention drugs ranges from 1.5 to 18.4 days' wages of government workers.[23,24]

Fixed-dose combination drugs, polypills especially those based largely on generic preparations could overcome some but not all of these barriers.[18] Furthermore, when combined with new models of health care delivery (e.g. by nonphysician health care workers and with little or no monitoring), the use of the polypill may lead to more widespread and cost-effective secondary prevention.

ADVANTAGES AND DISADVANTAGES OF POLYPILL

The polypill concept is an important concept in providing ease in CVD prevention and care of patients with diabetes. It has several advantages and shortcomings. The advantages include improved delivery of care, better adherence and reduced costs while shortcomings could be lack of evidence of effectiveness (improved patient outcomes), pharmacological and biocompatibility issues and need to better define an ideal combination pharmacotherapy.[4,18,24] The advantages and disadvantages are discussed here.

Improved Delivery of Care

By avoiding complex algorithms to identify individuals for therapy, increasing the ease of prescribing, and avoiding multiple steps for dose titration of each drug more at risk individuals could be treated. Although such advantages are as yet unproven, a study in high-risk patients with IHD with diabetes mellitus in the United States showed that use of a cardioprotective bundle, a simplified regimen involving fixed doses of generic statin and ACE inhibitor/ARB, delivered with minimal physician visits, laboratory tests, and dose titration was feasible and scalable and led to reduced the risk of hospitalizations for IHD or stroke within 1 year. Moreover, FDC drugs are already widely used in diabetes and also in hypertension and in other conditions such as AIDS and tuberculosis.

Improved Adherence

Individuals would need to take only one versus several pills per day which may enhance adherence. However, this is not proven, and improving adherence is complex and requires further study.

Reduced Cost

Costs of a polypill using generic components are likely to be much lower than the costs of individual drugs. Savings may be realized from reduced packaging, distribution, and marketing costs, fewer physician visits, and laboratory tests. An example of potential cost savings is provided by the pricing of the Polycap used in The Indian Polycap Study (TIPS) trial in India where it is currently approved for use and marketed at a substantially lower cost than its component drugs.

Polypill as a Platform for Novel Approaches to Widespread CVD Prevention

Current CVD prevention approaches (detailed selection of individuals who require therapy, prescribing one drug at a time, frequent dose titration, monitoring of tests, and physician visits) cannot be scalable to tackle a global epidemic. Novel approaches that use trained nonphysician health care workers to deliver the polypill plus lifestyle advice in those at moderate risk in primary prevention and in patients with CVD with physician referral for side effects, new symptoms, or when alternative drugs or a dose escalation appears warranted (e.g. if BP remains above critical levels), will reach a much wider number of at-risk individuals and thus will have a larger impact.

Lack of Evidence for Risk Reduction and Primary Prevention

Although the efficacy of a polypill in secondary prevention can be inferred from the independent effects of each of its components in patients with established CVD, no data on the benefits and long-term safety of a polypill in primary prevention in individuals with average levels of risk factors are available. Such information is critical before a polypill is used in primary prevention. Multiple trials are under way to address this issue (TIPS-3, etc.).

Pharmaceutical Formulation Issues

Formulation of a polypill involving four or five active components is complex. (Therefore, for each formulation of the bioavailability, pharmacokinetics, possible interactions, and effects on risk factors need to be). Although the combined effects of the components of the polypill are assumed to be additive, studies examining these assumptions are required for each proposed polypill preparation. For example, in the TIPS-1 study, there was attenuation of efficacy of simvastatin when this was combined with aspirin.

Ideal Polypill Uncertain

In the TIPS-1 trial, the BP and cholesterol lowering were of lesser magnitude than projected. This finding raises many questions, such as the potential need for full doses of some BP-lowering drugs or the addition of a fourth BP-lowering drug (e.g. calcium channel blocker at half dose) and the use of simvastatin 40 mg or a more potent statin. Side effects of a more potent polypill will require evaluation. In primary prevention, the benefits of aspirin are small, and there is an increased risk of gastrointestinal bleeding and some risk of allergy. Cough with ACE inhibitors may reduce adherence, and an ARB may be considered instead. The need for a few different polypill preparations requires consideration, such as a polypill without a β-blocker for people with asthma and different strength polypills especially in secondary prevention in which very low LDL cholesterol levels are desirable. If, indeed, polypills with more potent components become available, there may be a need for dose titration in some patients. However, even if this were the case, treatment could still be considerably simplified compared with current practice with only a few 'upfront' decisions and one single-dose titration needed in some high-risk patients. Wald and Law estimated the rates of adverse effects of the polypill to be about 8–15% resulting in permanent discontinuation in only 1–2%. However, the actual rates of adverse effects of long-term treatment with a polypill are not known.

Regulatory Issues

Given that any polypill will comprise drugs already approved for clinical use and widely available, it was suggested that for registration purposes demonstration of efficacy with the use of surrogate markers (risk factor levels) and acceptable safety will suffice. This strategy may be acceptable in secondary prevention but is not adequate in primary prevention in which large and long-term randomized trials will be required.

Adherence

Adherence is dependent on side effects as well as additional factors such as self-motivation, cost, ease of use (e.g. a very large tablet or capsule may be difficult to swallow), and availability. Wald and Law estimated a low rate of treatment discontinuations partly on the basis of data from short-term trials. Longer-term treatment may result in higher rates of adverse effects and poorer adherence. Moreover, in primary prevention subjects feel healthy and may not be motivated to use medications in long-term. Even minor side effects to one component of the polypill may lead to its discontinuation and hence loss of benefit from all component drugs.

Cost-effectiveness

The cost-effectiveness of each individual component of the polypill was demonstrated in various populations. Although no health economic analysis exists for a polypill such an analysis was conducted for a multidrug regimen containing aspirin, a calcium channel blocker or a β-blocker, an ACE inhibitor, and a statin found this to be cost-effective in secondary and high-risk primary prevention. It is expected that a polypill may be cheaper than such a multidrug regimen and therefore even more cost-effective. However, the real cost of a polypill is not known and will depend not only on the costs of the 'raw ingredients' and packaging but also costs of formulating the product, research and development, registration, marketing and distribution as well as 'profit' margins for manufacturers.

Interference with Adoption of Healthy Lifestyle

There are concerns that a single 'magic bullet' for CVD prevention may lead people to abandon healthy lifestyles. Educational initiatives to address this concern are needed. Moreover, use of a polypill would allow physicians to spend less time prescribing and monitoring multiple drugs and to allocate more time and resources to lifestyle counseling.

Acceptability

Acceptance of the polypill concept will require both more evidence and more time. Emphasis on education about prevention, low cost, and tolerability is essential for the acceptance of the polypill by individuals targeted for therapy. Among physicians who used to prescribing drugs sequentially and used to dose titration based on measured risk factor levels, acceptance of the polypill requires a change in conventional thinking. The polypill may also be perceived as a threat to the traditional role of physicians in many countries and to the perceived superiority of the individualized, titrated, target-driven approach to CVD prevention, but new data may alleviate such concerns.

Ultimately, as with any therapy the polypill may not be suitable for all. Patients at extremely high-risk (e.g. those with very aggressive manifestations of atherothrombotic disease) or those with side effects to multiple medications may still require individualized therapy, and therefore the polypill should be considered as a complementary strategy.[25]

CONCLUSION

In patients with type 2 diabetes, the major cause of mortality and morbidity is CVDs including coronary heart disease, stroke and peripheral arterial disease. Although diabetes contributes substantially to cardiovascular risk, yet some ingredients appropriate for a cardiovascular polypill may not be advisable for patients with diabetes. These include β-blockers and thiazide diuretics. Theoretically, a polypill for diabetes would include a statin (to reduce LDL cholesterol and for their anti-inflammatory properties), an ACE inhibitor (for BP control and to protect the kidneys), aspirin (for antiplatelet and anti-inflammatory properties), and metformin (a medication for diabetes that is also associated with weight loss). Relatedly, people who have high cholesterol, high BP, and/or are overweight can have metabolic syndrome, and may be a candidate for an appropriate polypill due to the quantity of different medications involved as mentioned earlier. However, there are no large randomized outcome based trials that have focused on polypill in diabetes. Such trials are urgently required given the huge global burden of diabetes related CVDs.

REFERENCES

1. World Health Organization. Secondary prevention of non-communicable disease in low- and middle-income countries through community-based and health service interventions. WHO-Wellcome Trust Meeting Report. 2002.
2. Xavier D, Pais P, Sigamani A, et al. The need to test the theories behind the polypill: rationale behind the Indian Polycap study. Nat Clin Pract Cardiovasc Med. 2009;6(2):96-7.
3. Wald NJ, Law MR. A strategy to reduce cardiovascular disease by more than 80%. BMJ. 2003;326(7404):1419.
4. Huffman MD, Xavier D, Perel P. Uses of polypills for cardiovascular disease and evidence to date. Lancet. 2017;389(10073):1055-65.
5. Unnikrishnan R, Anjana RM, Mohan V. Diabetes mellitus and its complications in India. Nat Rev Endocrinol. 2016;(6):357-70.
6. DBarzilay JI, Davis BR, Whelton PK. The glycemua effects of antihypertensive medications. Curr Hypertens Rep. 2014;16:410.
7. Baigent C, Blackwell L, Emberoon J, et al. Cholesterol Treatment Trialists' Collaboration. Efficacy and safety of more intensive lowering of LDL cholesterol: a meta-analysis of data from 170,000 participants in 26 randomised trials. Lancet. 2010;376(9753):1670-81.
8. Armitage J. The safety of statins in clinical practice. Lancet. 2007;370(9601):1781-90.
9. Beckett RD, Schepers SM, Gordon SK. Risk of new-onset diabetes associated with statin use. SAGE Open Med. 2015;3:2050312115605518.
10. Bundy JD, Li C, Stuchlik P, et al. Systolic blood pressure reduction and risk of cardiovascular disease and mortality: a systematic review and network meta-analysis. JAMA Cardiol. 2017;2(7):775-81.
11. Bennett A, Chow CK, Chou M, et al. Efficacy and safety of quarter-dose blood pressure-lowering agents: A systematic review and meta-analysis of randomized trials. Hypertension. 2017;70(3):85-93.
12. Lonn EM, Bosch J, Lopez-Jaramillo P, et al. Blood pressure lowering in intermediate risk persons without cardiovascular disease. N Engl J Med. 2016;374(21):2009-20.
13. Volpe M, Chin D, Paneni F. The challenge of polypharmacy in cardiovascular medicine. Fundam Clin Pharmacol. 2010;24(1):9-17.
14. Gupta R, Deedwania PC. Interventions for cardiovascular disease prevention. Cardiol Clin. 2011;29(1):15-34.
15. Tan CE, Glantz SA. Association between smoke-free legislation and hospitalizations for cardiac, cerebrovascular and respiratory diseases: a meta-analysis. Circulation. 2012;126(18):2177-83.
16. Puska P, Vartiainen E, Nissinen A, et al. Background, principles, implementation and general experiences of the North Karelia Project. Glob Heart. 2016;11(2):173-8.
17. Yusuf S, Pais P, Afzal R, et al. The Indian Polycap Study (TIPS). Effects of a polypill (Polycap) on risk factors in middle aged individuals without cardiovascular disease (TIPS): a phase II, double-blind, randomized trial. Lancet. 2009;373(9672):1341-51.
18. Webster R, Castalleno JM, Onuma OK. Putting polypills into practice: challenges and lessons learned. Lancet. 2017;389(10073):1066-74.
19. Huffman MD, Lloyd-Jones DM, Ning H, et al. Quantifying options for reducing coronary heart disease mortality by 2020. Circulation. 2013;127(25):2477-84.
20. Kotseva K, Wood D, Backer G, et al. EUROASPIRE IV: A European Society of Cardiology survey on the lifestyle, risk factor and therapeutic management of coronary patients from 24 European countries. Eur J Prev Cardiol. 2016;23(6):636-8.
21. Mendis S, Abegunde D, Yusuf S, et al. WHO study on prevention of recurrences of myocardial infarction and stroke (WHO-PREMISE). Bull WHO. 2005;83(11):820-9.
22. Joshi R, Chow CK, Raju PK, et al. Fatal and nonfatal cardiovascular disease and the use of therapies for secondary prevention in a rural region of India. Circulation. 2009;119(14):1950-55.
23. Yusuf S, Islam S, Chow CK, et al. Low use of secondary prevention medications for cardiovascular disease in the community in 17 high, middle and low income countries (The PURE Study). Lancet. 2011;378(9798):1231-43.
24. Gupta R, Mony P, Shankar Factors K, et al. Socioeconomic status and use of secondary preventive therapies for cardiovascular diseases in South Asia: The PURE study. Eur J Prev Cardiol. 2015;22(10):1261-71.
25. Vierra AJ. Whatever happened to the polypill? BMJ. 2017;356:j1474.

CHAPTER 80

Clopidogrel in Patients of Diabetes with Acute Coronary Syndrome

A Gupta, MP Girish, Mohit D Gupta

INTRODUCTION

Diabetes mellitus (DM) represents a major public health concern because of its prevalence and the poorer cardiovascular prognosis of patients with this disease; thus, strategies aimed at improving cardiovascular outcomes in patients with DM may have relevant epidemiological, economic, and clinical effects.[1] Acute coronary syndromes (ACS) are a spectrum of cardiovascular conditions characterized by the presence of an unstable atherosclerotic plaque with overlying thrombus. ACS is precipitated by the ischemic effect of an occlusive intracoronary thrombus that develops over a ruptured atheromatous plaque as a result of platelet adhesion and aggregation.[2]

PLATELETS IN DIABETES: ANGRY DIABETIC PLATELETS

Patients with DM have increased atherothrombotic risk and elevated rates of recurrent cardiac events, which may be in part attributable to abnormalities of platelet function resulting in increased platelet reactivity (Fig. 1). Among diabetic individuals, increased platelet aggregation and adhesion are due to the following:[3]

- Reduced platelet membrane fluidity due to changes in the lipid composition of the membrane or glycation of membrane proteins.
- Increased production of thromboxane A2 (TXA2) from arachidonic acid metabolism, which increases platelet sensitivity.
- Increased expression of platelet adhesion molecules such as CD31, CD36, CD49b, CD62P, and CD63 (when assessed by flow cytometry).
- Upregulation of platelet adenosine diphosphate (ADP) P2Y12 receptor signaling, which suppresses cyclic adenosine monophosphate (cAMP) levels and lowers insulin responsiveness, thereby leading to increased adhesion, aggregation, and procoagulant activity.
- Increased expression of platelet surface receptors such as P-selectin, glycoprotein (GP) Ib, and GPIIb/IIIa. GPIb mediates platelet binding to von Willebrand factor (vWF), an important step in platelet dependent thrombosis, and GPIIb/IIIa binds to fibrinogen resulting in platelet cross-linking as a part of the aggregation process.
- Increased generation of platelet dependent thrombin.
- Platelets are less sensitive to the effects of prostaglandin 12 (PGI2) and nitric oxide (NO).
- Platelets in type 2 diabetes mellitus (T2DM) show disordered calcium and magnesium hemostasis. Intraplatelet calcium regulates a variety of activities including platelet shape change, secretion, aggregation, and TXA2 formation. Increased intracellular calcium and decreased intracellular magnesium has been linked to platelet hyperaggregability and adhesiveness.
- Active platelets in DM patients are also rich in cytokines and chemokines such as platelet factor-4, interleukin-1β, and CD40L and hence contribute to inflammation and atherogenesis alongside a procoagulant milieu.

Clopidogrel is a well-established antiplatelet therapy for patients with ACS and those undergoing percutaneous

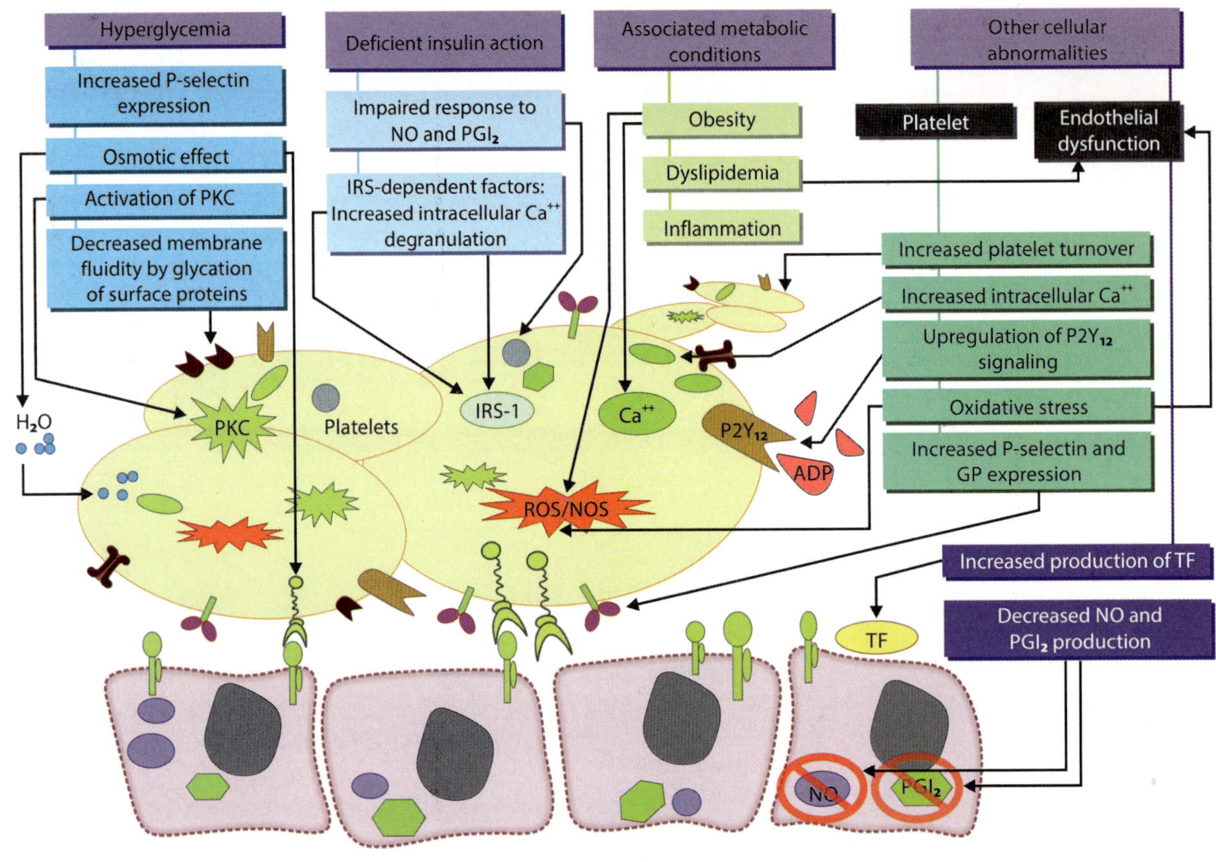

Fig. 1: Mechanisms involved in platelet dysfunction in patients with diabetes mellitus

coronary intervention (PCI), and has been part of the standard of care in the treatment of ACS for several years.[4] Patients with diabetes are more likely to be resistant to aspirin, and in addition, have increased P2Y12 receptor signaling. Outcomes of patients with diabetes with ACS on clopidogrel monotherapy are superior to those on aspirin. It is, therefore, not surprising that when clopidogrel is combined with aspirin, the outcomes are favorable in reduction of ischemic events, versus placebo with aspirin.[5]

CLOPIDOGREL PHARMACOLOGY

Clopidogrel is the most widely used thienopyridine and has a faster onset of action through the administration of a loading dose. When administered orally, clopidogrel is normally, rapidly, and extensively absorbed. Its absorption is limited by the drug efflux transporter P-glycoprotein (encoded by the *ABCB1* gene). Polymorphisms of the *ABCB1* gene contribute to the wide interpatient variability of clopidogrel bioavailability. Upon absorption, a majority of clopidogrel is metabolized into inactive metabolites by de-esterification. The remaining 15% of clopidogrel is converted to its active metabolite by two CYP-dependent steps. CYP1A2, CYP3A4/CYP3A5, CYP2C9, and CYP2C19 are considered the main contributors to active metabolite formation (Fig. 2).[6]

Active metabolite generation and the degree to which clopidogrel inhibits platelet function vary widely from patient to patient, ranging from near-complete platelet inhibition to almost no inhibition with a roughly normal distribution. Significant pharmacokinetic and pharmacodynamic benefits have been observed with a higher than standard clopidogrel dose. However, not all clopidogrel hyporesponsiveness can be overcome with high doses, and significant interpatient variability remains. Clinical studies investigating the clinical benefit of higher than standard clopidogrel doses have yielded mixed results, with some showing higher clopidogrel doses to be associated with a significant clinical benefit, whereas others have not.[7]

CAPRIE: The Rise of New Star

The clopidogrel versus aspirin in patients at risk of ischemic events (CAPRIE) trial compared the efficacy of clopidogrel (75 mg/day) and aspirin (325 mg/day) in reducing the risk

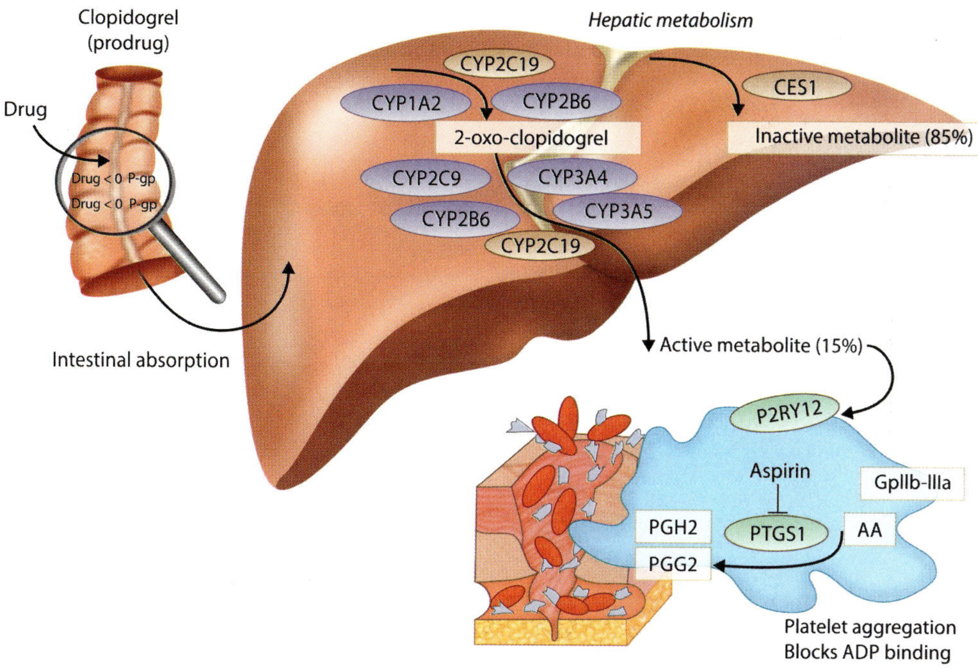

Fig. 2: Absorption, metabolism and target of clopidogrel

Source: EUR Heart JE 2009. Oxford University Press.

of ischemic outcomes in patients (n = 19,185) with recent myocardial infarction (MI), recent ischemic stroke, or established peripheral arterial disease. The results showed a significantly low annual rate of ischemic events (ischemic stroke, MI, or vascular death) in patients who received clopidogrel (5.32% vs 5.83%; p = 0.043). DM subgroup had a significantly higher benefit (15.6% vs 17.7%; p = 0.042). For every 1,000 DM patients treated with clopidogrel, vascular events were prevented. Several large scale trials have shown clear benefit of clopidogrel in addition to aspirin in preventing recurrent ischemic events, including stent thrombosis in the setting of ACS [including unstable angina/non-ST segment elevation myocardial infarction (UA/NSTEMI), ST-segment elevation myocardial infarction (STEMI), PCI, compared to aspirin alone (Table 1).[8]

Among patients with documented prior MI, ischemic stroke, or symptomatic peripheral artery disease in the CHARISMA trial (n = 9,478, ~30% were diabetics), the rate of cardiovascular death, MI, or stroke was significantly lower in the clopidogrel group than in the placebo group: 7.3% versus 8.8% [hazard ratio (HR), 0.83; 95% CI, 0.72–0.96; p = 0.01]; this benefit was more prominent in patients with prior MI or ischemic stroke than symptomatic peripheral artery disease (HR, 0.774 vs 0.780 vs 0.869). There was no significant difference in the rate of severe bleeding (1.7% vs 1.5%; HR, 1.12; 95% CI, 0.81–1.53; p = 0.50). Therefore, the antiplatelet effect of dual antiplatelet therapy (DAPT) may reduce the risk of ischemic event occurrence in selected patients with overt cardiovascular disease (CVD) outside ACS.[9]

The clopidogrel for high atherothrombotic risk and ischemic stabilization, management, and avoidance (CHARISMA) trial found no benefit of dual aspirin and clopidogrel therapy in the long term in a wide range of non-ACS patients (n = 15,603) with risk factors for, and established atherothrombotic disease, including DM patients (n = 6,555; 42% of the study population). Hence, DAPT is not recommended even in DM patients outside ACS/PCI setting.[9]

High-dose versus Low-dose Clopidogrel Therapy

CURRENT-OASIS 7 trial evaluated the 30-day clinical benefit of high-dose (600 mg loading followed by 150 mg daily for 1 week) versus standard-dose clopidogrel (300 mg loading followed by 75 mg daily) in ACS patients; the subgroup undergoing PCI suggested a clinical benefit in the high-dose group, with a significant reduction in the ischemic event rate (3.9% vs 4.5%, p = 0.039) and stent thrombosis (0.7% vs 1.3%, p = 0.0001) at the expense of major bleeding (1.6% vs 1.1%, p = 0.009). Reduction in ischemic events by high-dose clopidogrel was similar in patients with versus without DM.[10]

Current guidelines recommend DAPT with aspirin and clopidogrel for patients of diabetes with ACS, including UA/NSTEMI, STEMI, and patients undergoing PCI. The recommended clopidogrel dose is 300 mg loading dose (up to 600 mg in PCI setting) followed by a maintenance dose of 75 mg daily.[10]

TABLE 1: Outcomes from large-scale randomized placebo-controlled trials evaluating the efficacy of dual antiplatelet therapy with aspirin and clopidogrel versus aspirin alone in ACS/PCI patients in the overall study population and in DM patients.

Study	Scenario	Primary endpoint	n (overall)	% of events and association measure (overall)	n (DM)	% of events and association measure (DM)
CURE RR (95% CI)	UA/NSTEMI	Cardiovascular death, nonfatal MI, or stroke at 1 year	12,562	9.3 versus 11.4 0.80 (0.72–0.90)	2,840	14.2 versus 16.7 0.84 (0.70–1.02)
PC1-CURE RR (95% CI)	CURE patients undergoing PCI	Cardiovascular death, MI, or urgent TVR at 30 days	2,658	4.5 versus 6.4 0.70 (0.50–0.97)	504	12.9 versus 16.5 0.77 (0.48–1.22)
CREDO RRR (95% CI), %	Elective PCI	Death, MI or stroke at 1 year	2,116	8.5 versus 11.5 26.9 (3.9–44.4)	560	NR 11.2 (-46.8–46.2)
COMMIT OR (95% CI)	Acute MI (93% STEMI)	Death, reinfarction or stroke at discharge or 28 days	45,852	9.2 versus 10.1 0.91 (0.86–0.97)	NR	NR
CLARITY OR (95% CI)	STEMI with fibrinolysis	Occluded infarct-related artery on angiography or death or recurrent MI before angiography	3,491	15.0 versus 21.7 0.64 (0.53–0.76)	575	NR
PCI-CLARITY OR (95% CI)	CLARITY patients undergoing PCI	Cardiovascular death, recurrent MI or stroke at 30 days	1,863	3.6 versus 6.2 0.54 (0.35–0.85)	282	6.0 versus 10.1 0.61 (0.24–1.53)

Abbreviations: CURE, clopidogrel in unstable angina to prevent recurrent events; CREDO, clopidogrel for reduction of events during observation; COMMIT, clopidogrel and metoprolol in myocardial infarction trial; CLARITY, clopidogrel as adjunctive reperfusion therapy; RR, relative risk; RRR, relative risk reduction; OR, odds ratio; NR, not reported; DM, diabetes mellitus; MI, myocardial infarction; TVR, target vessel revascularization; UA/NSTEMI, unstable angina/non-ST-segment elevation myocardial infarction; ACS, acute coronary syndromes; PCI, percutaneous coronary intervention.

CLOPIDOGREL RESISTANCE

Clopidogrel resistance is a phenomenon encountered in daily medical practice. The prevalence of clopidogrel resistance is 5–44% in various studies. Increasing the loading dose of clopidogrel to 600 mg is helpful in reducing resistance. If the pre- and post-treatment ADP induced platelet aggregation was less than 10%, these patients were in its broadest sense defined as having clopidogrel resistance. It refers to the continued chance of ischemic events despite adequate clopidogrel therapy and compliance.[11]

Several mechanisms of clopidogrel resistance are possible and can be classified into two categories: (1) extrinsic, and (2) intrinsic. Extrinsic mechanisms that reflect a reduced bioavailability of clopidogrel may include noncompliance to clopidogrel therapy, underdosing, or inappropriate dosing of clopidogrel, and drug-drug interactions affecting the biotransformation of clopidogrel into its active metabolite. Possible intrinsic mechanisms may include polymorphisms of the P2Y12 receptor gene leading to an increased number of P2Y12 receptors, and polymorphisms of the CYP3As. There are also possibilities of increased release of ADP and upregulation of other platelet activation pathways (such as thrombin, ADP, collagen, TXA2, and epinephrine).[12]

Diabetes is a major risk factor for diminished clopidogrel response, independent of the CYP2C19 genotype. To date, the etiology of this phenomenon has largely been attributed to systemic inflammation and insulin resistance, the latter leading to platelet P2Y12 receptor signaling abnormalities.

Role of Phenotypic Testing in Overcoming Clopidogrel Resistance

A standardized method to evaluate in-vivo platelet response is still lacking. Clopidogrel inhibits one of the two ADP receptors; ex-vivo measurement of ADP-nduced platelet aggregation by light transmittance aggregometry is the most commonly used "gold standard" method to evaluate clopidogrel responsiveness.

Lately, it was suggested that since clopidogrel-induced platelet disaggregation was better demonstrated by measuring late platelet aggregation at 6 minutes after stimulation with ADP rather than maximum aggregation. Flow cytometric measurements of expression of GpIIb/IIIa receptor and p-selectin expression after ADP stimulation can also identify clopidogrel nonresponsiveness. In addition, measurements of ADP-induced fibrin clot strength is measured by whole blood thromboelastography and the *VerifyNow P2Y12* receptor assay using ADP as agonist.[13]

The PFA-100 method using collagen ADP-based cartridges and whole blood aggregometry are associated with inconsistent estimates of platelet reactivity to ADP. The phosphorylation state of vasodilator stimulated phosphoprotein is a specific intracellular marker for residual P2Y12 receptor reactivity in patients treated with clopidogrel, but the method is difficult.[14]

There are accumulating evidence that have shown that patients with laboratory-defined resistance have an increased risk of atherothrombosis. Thrombotic events, stent thrombosis, in particular, occurs more frequently in patients who have high on-treatment platelet reactivity while taking clopidogrel, suggesting that a poor response to clopidogrel is a major factor in thrombosis development.[6]

Role of Genotypic Testing in Overcoming Clopidogrel Resistance

For reliable genotyping of genetic variants (especially CYP2C19*2) in clopidogrel-treated patients, conventional use of laboratory-based methods such as DNA sequencing or TaqMan genotyping will be best suited primarily for research purposes.

At present, only two point-of-care assays are available for CYP2C19*2 genotyping: (1) the Verigene CYP2C19 XP system (Nanosphere, Northbrook, IL, United States), and (2) the Spartan RX CYP2C19 system (Spartan Bioscience Inc., Ottawa, ON, Canada). The Verigene system uses whole blood, with a detection technology based on gold nanoparticles. It allows the genotyping of different CYP2C19 allelic variants in parallel, but the time from probe sampling to results takes about 3 hours. The Spartan system uses a buccal swab with a detection technology based on end-point PCR. In its present form, this system allows for genotyping of CYP2C19*2 only, but results are available with 1 hour after probe sampling.[15]

Individuals with CYP2C19 variant alleles designated *2 and *3 have nonfunctional enzyme activity compared to *1 (wild-type) individuals, leading to absent or markedly decreased metabolite that may require increased maintenance doses of clopidogrel. Individuals with CYP2C19 variant alleles designated *17 have increased enzyme activity compared to *1 (wild-type) individuals, leading to increased levels of active metabolite and may require lower maintenance doses of clopidogrel.

At present, the best available evidence for individualizing P2Y12 inhibitor treatment and a possible role of genotyping in this setting comes from TRITON-TIMI 38. In fact, for the primary end point of the trial (death from cardiovascular causes, nonfatal MI, nonfatal stroke) the overall risk was comparable in prasugrel treated patients from the entire cohort.

Flow chart 1: Planned treatment with more potent agent for high-risk patients

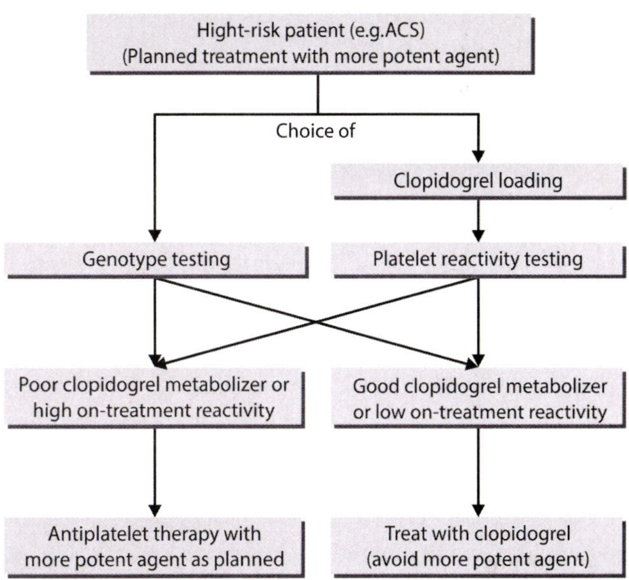

One should "consider alternative treatment or treatment strategies in patients identified as CYP2C19 poor metabolizers." The term "poor metabolizer status" was defined by the US FDA as a subject being homozygous for the CYP2C19*2 allele. Defining only the homozygous *2 allele carriers as poor metabolizer.

Recently updated "ACCF/AHA Guidelines for the Management of Patients with Unstable Angina/Non-ST-elevation Myocardial Infarction" now include new class IIb recommendations for both approaches (level of evidence: B for platelet function testing, level of evidence: C for CYP2C19*2 genotyping). With randomized studies including genotyping-directed treatment options still lacking, these guideline recommendations offer the treating physician some reassurance in case one opts to change treatment, based on testing results (Flow chart 1).[15]

STATUS OF CLOPIDOGREL AS ANTIPLATELET AT THE TIME OF ACUTE CORONARY SYNDROMES PRESENTATION

The main goal of optimal antiplatelet therapy for patients with ACS is to minimize the risk of early and long-term thrombotic adverse events, as well as to reduce risk of bleeding complications. The combination of aspirin and clopidogrel has been the mainstay of ACS and PCI antiplatelet therapy for the past decade. The use of this combination is supported by several large-scale studies and practitioners have a large amount of real-world experience with this combination. Yet, serious CV events recur in approximately 11% of patients with ACS, most of which occur early after the index event.[16]

Perhaps the most advantageous way to use clopidogrel in preparation for PCI is to tailor the loading dose of clopidogrel using platelet function monitoring. In this approach, patients have their platelet reactivity measured following the administration of a clopidogrel loading dose. If a patient meets the criteria for clopidogrel resistance, before undergoing PCI, he or she receives additional clopidogrel loading doses in 600-mg increments until a target clopidogrel response is achieved or up to a maximum of 2,400 mg. At that point, the patient will undergo PCI.[16]

This approach has been examined using vasodilator-stimulated phosphoprotein (VASP) index to measure the clopidogrel response. Clopidogrel resistance was defined as a VASP index is greater than 50%, and additional clopidogrel loading doses were administered to achieve a VASP index is less than 50% before PCI was performed. The rate of stent thrombosis 1 month after undergoing PCI was significantly lower in patients who received VASP index-guided care than in control subjects who did not (0.5% vs 4.2%; $p = 0.01$), even though approximately 8% of patients who received 2,400 mg clopidogrel under VASP index-guided care continued to have a low response. VASP index-guided care was also associated with a significantly reduced risk of major adverse CV events, including CV death, MI, or urgent revascularization (0.5% vs 8.9%; $p = 0.001$), without significantly increasing the risk of major or minor bleeding (3.7% vs 2.8%; $p = 0.08$).[17]

In the CLEAR PLATELETS (clopidogrel loading with eptifibatide to arrest the reactivity of platelets) study; 600 mg loading dose was associated with a superior pharmacodynamic antiplatelet profile compared to a 300 mg clopidogrel loading dose, in the absence of a GPIIb/IIIa inhibitor.[18]

However, in the recent ISAR-CHOICE (intracoronary stenting and antithrombotic regimen: choice between high oral doses for immediate clopidogrel effect) study, there was a ceiling effect in unchanged clopidogrel and clopidogrel metabolite levels and platelet inhibition with the 600 mg loading dose, and no significant additional effect was seen with the 900 mg loading dose.[19]

Recently, ACC/AHA guidelines recommended a class IIb recommendation that "in patients in whom subacute thrombosis may be catastrophic or lethal, platelet aggregation studies may be considered and the dose of clopidogrel needs to be increased to 150 mg per day if less than 50% inhibition of platelet aggregation is demonstrated." Tailored approach to dosing clopidogrel in patients before PCI has been shown to be effective at reducing early rates of recurrent CV events and stent thrombosis.[20]

STATUS OF CLOPIDOGREL AS MAINTENANCE ANTIPLATELET THERAPY

Nonadherence to antiplatelet therapy is an important risk factor for recurrent CV events the introduction of lower cost generic clopidogrel may significantly increase patient compliance, improve outcomes, and make the drug a more viable therapeutic option.

The question remains as to whether a strategy of tailoring dose of clopidogrel using platelet function monitoring can be applied to maintenance therapy. Thus far, platelet reactivity testing-guided antiplatelet management has not been shown to improve clinical outcomes. The gauging responsiveness with a 'verify now' assay-impact on thrombosis and safety (GRAVITAS) trial demonstrated no improvement in clinical outcomes with high-dose clopidogrel (150 mg/d) when compared with standard-dose clopidogrel (75 mg/d) despite an improvement in hyporesponsiveness.[21]

The responsiveness to clopidogrel and stent-related events in acute coronary syndromes (RECLOSE2-ACS) trial showed a poor pharmacodynamic response to clopidogrel to be associated with increased event rates in patients with ACS undergoing PCI; however, increasing the clopidogrel dose in patients with a poor response was not associated with clinical benefits in these patients.

Routine platelet monitoring to guide antiplatelet therapy should not be encouraged in low-risk patients. Higher-risk populations are likely more dependent on adequate inhibition of platelet reactivity. The prognostic utility of serial platelet function testing may become more evident in such a patient population. Prospective clinical trials using on-treatment platelet reactivity to guide clinical decision making are needed to demonstrate the clinical benefits of this strategy.

Another method of overcoming clopidogrel nonresponsiveness is to switch treatment from clopidogrel to either prasugrel or ticagrelor. This concept was studied in the testing platelet reactivity in patients undergoing elective stent placement on clopidogrel to guide alternative therapy with prasugrel (TRIGGER-PCI) trial, in which nonresponders who had undergone stenting were either treated with prasugrel or continued on the standard clopidogrel dose. Prasugrel improved platelet reactivity in nonresponders to clopidogrel compared with clopidogrel continuation.[22]

An OPTIMUS-2 study of randomized crossover platelet function study in patients with type 2 DM and coronary

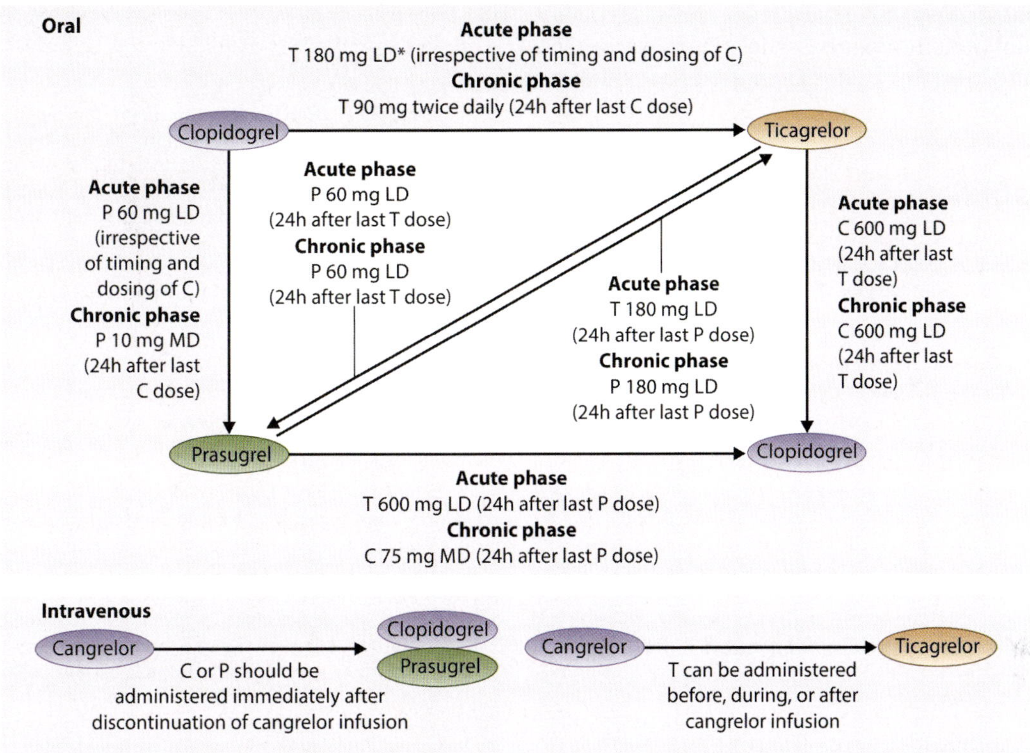

Fig. 3: Practical recommendations for switching between oral and intravenous antiplatelet agents.

artery disease following DAPT revealed that the reduced platelet inhibition of P2Y12 signaling can be enhanced by adjunctive treatment with cilostazol when compared with DAPT. Thus, cilostazol led to significantly increased P2Y12 platelet inhibition, as measured by flow cytometry and light transmission aggregometry. These findings were similar to the results of a study conducted by Yang et al. Several clinical studies have shown that triple antiplatelet therapy has better clinical outcomes than DAPT in patients undergoing PCI and coronary stenting.[23]

CLOPIDOGREL VERSUS NEWER ANTIPLATELETS

Prasugrel and ticagrelor accomplished a reduction in ischemic events as compared with clopidogrel in TRITON-TIMI 38 and PLATO. In diabetic patients, prasugrel use led to an even greater reduction in ischemic endpoints than clopidogrel with a comparable bleeding risk whereas ticagrelor led to a comparable reduction in ischemic events and a reduction in coronary artery bypass surgery-related bleeding. The latter effect is likely the result of reversible drug-binding to the P2Y12 receptor.

How should we translate the given evidence into our clinical pathways? Is there still a place for clopidogrel? Should ticagrelor or prasugrel be used preferentially? First, limitations of the TRITON-TIMI 38 and the PLATO diabetes sub-studies should not be forgotten. Even though prespecified groups were analyzed, randomization was not performed. Importantly, most outcome differences in relation to the randomized treatment did not reach statistical significance.[24,25]

SWITCHING OF ANTIPLATELETS

Data on switching antiplatelet therapies are primarily based on pharmacodynamic studies (Fig. 3). These studies were not powered to assess the clinical impact of switching. Specifically designed studies evaluating the efficacy and safety with respect to clinical outcomes from switching are currently not available. Therefore, the recommendations should be used as a guide only.[26,27]

CONCLUSION

The role of clopidogrel in patients of diabetes with ACS is supported by many several large scale studies and years of real world experience. There are some cons such as response variability, susceptibility to genetic variation and drug-to-drug interaction though inexpensiveness, long history of use, once daily dose makes it easy-to-use drug. At present, individualization of treatment seems appropriate, but necessitates a deep understanding of clinical evidence and individual patient characteristics. Furthermore, we need to try hard to improve guideline adherence in diabetic patients.

REFERENCES

1. Malmberg K, Yusuf S, Gerstein HC, et al. Impact of diabetes on long-term prognosis in patients with unstable angina and non-Q-wave myocardial infarction: Results of the OASIS Registry. Circulation. 2000;102(9):1014-9.
2. Ferreiro JL, Angiolillo DJ. Diabetes and antiplatelet therapy in acute coronary syndrome. Circulation. 2011;123(7):798-813.
3. Li Y, WooV, Bose R. Platelet hyperactivity and abnormal Ca^{2+} homeostasis in diabetes mellitus. Am J Physiol. 2001;280(4): H1480-9.
4. Yusuf S, Zhao F, Mehta SR, et al. Effects of clopidogrel in addition to aspirin in patients with acute coronary syndromes without ST-segment elevation. N Engl J Med. 2001;345(7):494-502.
5. Yusuf S, Mehta SR, Zhao F, et al. Early and late effects of clopidogrel in patients with acute coronary syndromes. Circulation. 2003;107(7):966-72.
6. Savi P, Pereillo JM, Uzabiaga MF, et al. Identification and biological activity of the active metabolite of clopidogrel. Thromb Haemost. 2000;84(5):891-6.
7. Angiolillo DJ, Fernández-Ortiz A, Bernardo E, et al. High clopidogrel loading dose during coronary stenting: effects on drug response and interindividual variability. Eur Heart J. 2004;25(21):1903-10.
8. CAPRIE Steering Committee. A randomised, blinded, trial of clopidogrel versus aspirin in patients at risk of ischaemic events (CAPRIE). Lancet. 1996;348(9038):1329-39.
9. Bhatt DL, Fox KA, Hacke W, et al. Clopidogrel and aspirin versus aspirin alone for the prevention of atherothrombotic events. N Engl J Med. 2006;354(16):1706-17.
10. Mehta SR, Tanguay JF, Eikelboom JW, et al. Double-dose versus standard-dose clopidogrel and high-dose versus low-dose aspirin in individuals undergoing percutaneous coronary intervention for acute coronary syndromes (CURRENT-OASIS 7): a randomised factorial trial. Lancet. 2010;376(9748):1233-43.
11. Gurbel PA, Bliden KP, Hiatt BL, et al. Clopidogrel for coronary stenting: response variability, drug resistance, and the effect of pretreatment platelet reactivity. Circulation. 2003;107(23):2908-13.
12. Wiviott SD, Antman EM. Clopidogrel resistance: a new chapter in a fast-moving story. Circulation. 2004;109(25):3064-7.
13. Nicholson NS, Panzer-Knodle SG, Haas NF, et al. Assessment of platelet function assays. Am Heart J. 1998;135(5):S170-8.
14. Michelson AD. Platelet function testing in cardiovascular diseases. Circulation. 2004;110(19):e489-93.
15. Lau WC, Gurbel PA, Watkins PB, et al. Contribution of hepatic cytochrome P450 3A4 metabolic activity to the phenomenon of clopidogrel resistance. Circulation. 2004;109(2):166-71.
16. Bonello L, Camoin-Jau L, Armero S, et al. Tailored clopidogrel loading dose according to platelet reactivity monitoring to prevent acute and subacute stent thrombosis. Am J Cardiol. 2009;103(1):5-10.
17. Barragan P, Bouvier JL, Roquebert PO, et al. Resistance to thienopyridines: clinical detection of coronary stent thrombosis by monitoring of vasodilator-stimulated phosphoprotein phosphorylation. Catheter Cardiovasc Interv. 2003;59(3):295-302.
18. Gurbel PA, Bliden KP, Zaman KA, et al. Clopidogrel loading with eptifibatide to arrest there activity of platelets: results of the clopidogrel loading with eptifibatide to arrest the reactivity of platelets (CLEARPLATELETS) study. Circulation. 2005;111(9):1153-9.
19. von Beckerath N, Taubert D, Pogatsa-Murray G, et al. Absorption, metabolization, and antiplatelet effects of 300-, 600-, and 900-mg loading doses of clopidogrel. Results of the ISAR-CHOICE (Intracoronary stenting and antithrombotic regimen: choose between 3 high oral doses for immediate clopidogrel effect). Trial Circ. 2005;112(19):2946-50.
20. Parodi G, Marcucci R, Valenti R, et al. High residual platelet reactivity after clopidogrel loading and long-term cardiovascular events among patients with acute coronary syndromes undergoing PCI. JAMA. 2011;306(11):1215-23.
21. Price MJ, Angiolillo DJ, Teirstein PS, et al. Platelet reactivity and cardiovascular outcomes after percutaneous coronary intervention: a time-dependent analysis of the Gauging Responsiveness with a VerifyNow P2Y12 assay: Impact on Thrombosis and Safety (GRAVITAS) trial. Circulation. 2011;124(10):1132-7.
22. Trenk D, Stone GW, Gawaz M, et al. A randomized trial of prasugrel versus clopidogrel in patients with high platelet reactivity on clopidogrel after elective percutaneous coronary intervention with implantation of drug-eluting stents: results of the TRIGGER-PCI (Testing Platelet Reactivity in Patients Undergoing Elective Stent Placement on Clopidogrel to Guide Alternative Therapy With Prasugrel) study. J Am Coll Cardiol. 2012;59(24):2159-64.
23. Angiolillo DJ, Capranzano P, Goto S, et al. A randomized study assessing the impact of cilostazol on platelet function profiles in patients with diabetes mellitus and coronary artery disease on dual anti-platelet therapy: results of the OPTS-2 study. Eur Heart J.2008;29(18):2202-11.
24. Wiviott SD, Braunwald E, McCabe CH, et al. Prasugrel versus clopidogrel in patients with acute coronary syndromes. N Engl J Med. 2007;357(20):2001-15.
25. Wallentin L, Becker RC, Budaj A, et al. Ticagrel or versus clopidogrel in patients with acute coronary syndromes. N Engl J Med. 2009;361(11):1045-57.
26. AngiolilloDJ, SaucedoJF, DeraadR, et al. Increased platelet inhibition after switching from maintenance clopidogrel to prasugrel in patients with acute coronary syndromes: results of the SWAP (SWitching Anti Platelet) study. J Am Coll Cardiol. 2010;56(13):1017-23.
27. Gurbel PA, Bliden KP, Butler K, et al. Response to ticagrelor in clopidogrel nonresponders and responders and effect of switching therapies: the RESPOND study. Circulation. 2010;121(10):1188-99.

Acute Coronary Syndrome in Cardiodiabetes: Is It Different?

Gaurav Mohan, Ravina Sharma, GS Wander

INTRODUCTION

Diabetes mellitus (DM) is a rapidly growing pandemic disease affecting more than 350 million[1] patients all over the world. There appears a strong association between type 2 diabetes mellitus (T2DM) and cardiovascular disease (CVD) as suggested by one of the meta-analysis conducted by the Emerging Risk Factors Collaboration,[2] that included over 700,000 subjects with no history of myocardial infarction (MI), angina or stroke at baseline [diabetes confers an approximately two-fold excess risk for coronary heart disease (CHD), major stroke and deaths attributed to other vascular causes]. The negative impact of DM on the outcomes is maintained across the acute coronary syndrome (ACS) spectrum, including unstable angina and non-ST elevation myocardial infarction (NSTEMI),[3] ST elevation myocardial infarction (STEMI)[4] treated medically, and acute coronary syndrome (ACS) undergoing percutaneous coronary intervention (PCI).[5] DM patients have more progressive, diffuse, and multivessel coronary disease compared to nondiabetic patients and have poorer outcomes after both PCI and coronary artery bypass graft surgery (CABG), compared to nondiabetic patients. The advent of drug eluting stents (DES)[5] has improved PCI outcomes but the problem of atherothrombotic complications, including stent thrombosis, persists in diabetic patients.

PATHOPHYSIOLOGY OF ATHEROSCLEROSIS IN PATIENTS WITH TYPE 2 DIABETES MELLITUS POST-ACUTE CORONARY SYNDROME

Diabetes mellitus generates a state of prothrombosis in the body which is responsible for increased cardiovascular events (Fig. 1).

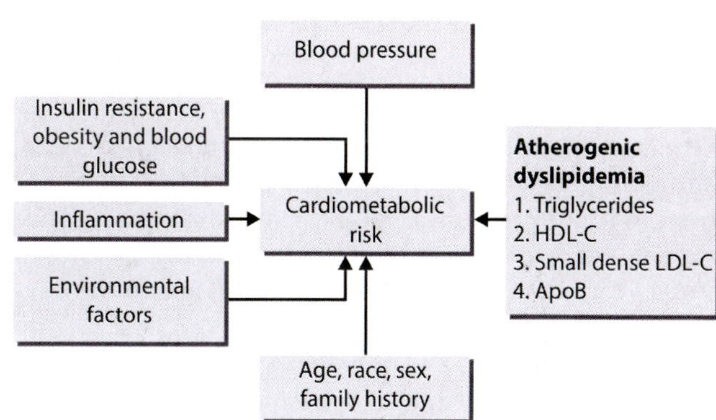

Fig. 1: Cardiovascular disease risk markers contributing to cardiometabolic risk

Abbreviations: HDL-C, high-density lipoprotein cholesterol; LDL-C, low-density lipoprotein cholesterol; ApoB, apolipoprotein B.

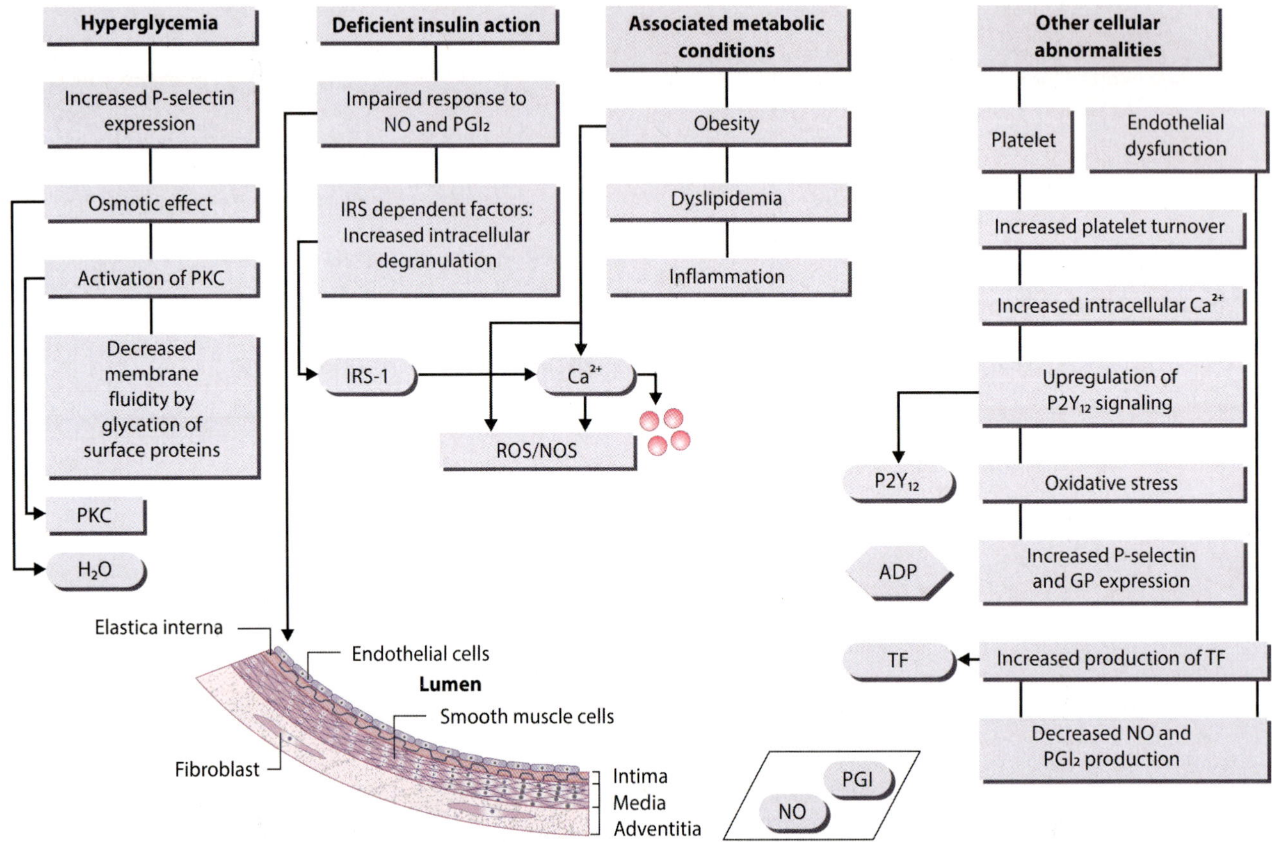

Fig. 2: Mechanisms involved in platelet dysfunction in patients with diabetes mellitus

Abbreviations: PKC, protein kinase C; NO, nitric oxide; PGI_2, prostaglandin I_2; ADP, adenosine diphosphate; TF, tissue factor; GP, glycoprotein

Detrimental Effects of Hyperglycemia and Insulin Resistance

Chronic hyperglycemia can lead to prothrombotic milieu inside the body thereby increasing the cardiovascular events.[6] DM leads to formation of advanced glycation end-products (AGEs)[7] that alter tissue function and mechanical properties. Hyperglycemia-induced reactive oxygen species (ROS) along with AGEs binds to cell-surface receptors (RAGEs)[7] and induce signaling pathways promoting inflammation and vasoconstriction. In the vulnerable plaque, AGE/RAGE expression correlates with the expression of matrix metalloproteinase-9,[8] an enzyme responsible for plaque destabilization and rupture accounting for increased incidence of ACS in diabetics.

Platelet Hyperactivity

Ruptured atheromatous plaque, hallmark of ACS, results in platelet adhesion and aggregation causing occlusive intracoronary thrombus (Fig. 2). Hyperglycemia results in increased production of thromboxane A2 (TXA2)[9] and expression of platelet adhesion molecules (CD31, CD36, CD49b, CD62P, and CD63) along with upregulation of platelet ADP P2Y12[10,11] receptor signaling, leading to increased adhesion, aggregation and procoagulant activity of platelets. Further platelets of diabetic patients are shown to be less sensitive to the effects of prostaglandin I2 (PGI2) and nitric oxide (NO).

These characteristics may be responsible for frequent occurrence of ACS with poorer outcomes observed in DM and also may account for the poorer response of usual antiplatelet strategy for secondary prevention.

Diabetic Dyslipidemia and Systemic Inflammation

Dyslipidemia in diabetes [increased triglycerides and low high-density lipoprotein (HDL)] is often associated with normal low-density lipoprotein cholesterol (LDL-C) levels.[6] These high levels of TGs and low levels of high-density lipoprotein cholesterol (HDL-C), contribute to chronic inflammation and oxidative stress. In addition there is shift of the LDL-C pool towards small, dense LDL-C particles which are prone to oxidation by nitric oxide synthase (NOS) and contribute to atherosclerotic process through internalization by macrophages and foam cell formation and also increased plaque destabilization.[11]

IS MANAGEMENT OF ACUTE CORONARY SYNDROME IN DIABETES DIFFERENT?

Blood glucose control is imperative not only in the treatment of ACS but also prevention of reinfarction. Contrary to the earlier belief that strict control of blood sugar level improves outcomes, recent studies have rather shown increased adverse events related to more frequent hypoglycemic episodes in patients allocated to tight glucose control.[12]Modern consensus now favor rather modest approach in controlling blood sugar particularly for those with more advanced CV disease, older age and longer diabetes duration. Treatment target should be to avoid severe hyperglycemia (glucose concentration >180–200 mg/dL) as well as hypoglycemia (<90 mg/dL). Baring few studies (immediate trial)[13] suggesting small benefit of glucose–insulin–potassium infusion, largely the data is unsupportive.[14]

Antithrombotics

Most of the available data is suggestive of similar drugs and dosages of antiplatelets in both diabetic and nondiabetic patients presenting with ACS. However, more potent P2Y12 inhibitors prasugrel and ticagrelor proved superior compared to clopidogrel in diabetic patients in the TRITON-TIMI 38[15] and PLATO[16] studies. In diabetics patients, prasugrel reduced the composite endpoint of CV death or MI or stroke without excess major bleeding (12.2% vs 17.0%; HR = 0.70; $P < 0.001$) proving superiority compared to clopidogrel. Risk of stent thrombosis in the DM subgroup was significantly reduced.[15] Similarly in the PLATO study, ticagrelor compared to clopidogrel, reduced rate of ischemic events in ACS without increased major bleeding irrespective of diabetic status and glycemic control.[16] Earlier studies showed beneficial effects glycoprotein IIb/IIIa (GPIIb/IIIa) receptor inhibitors in diabetic population, but mostly without concomitant use of thienopyridines.[17] This led to popular practice of routine upstream use of these agents along with dual antiplatelet. This rather produced excess bleeding[18] as seen in most of the recent studies (EARLY-ACS trial).[19] Currently with availability of prasugrel or ticagrelor, routine upstream use of these agents should be avoided it appears reasonable to use them for bailout of thrombotic complications following PCI.

Revascularization Procedures

Diabetic patients are often older with atypical symptoms and have frequent comorbidities like hypertension and renal failure and are more likely to develop complications,[20] such as heart failure, stroke, reinfarction, renal failure, and bleeding. Therefore, in diabetic patients with ongoing ischemia or hemodynamic instability, immediate coronary angiography is indicated and the best revascularization should be chosen.

Timing of Revascularization: Early versus Delayed

Multiple observational studies and meta-analyses of randomized trials demonstrate the benefit of an early invasive strategy in management of diabetic NSTE-ACS patients, mainly through reduction of composite clinical event rates and MI.[21]Multiple trials have been done comparing an early invasive strategy to an initial conservative strategy, such as (TACTICS-TIMI 18; 4–48 hours),[22] (ICTUS; 24–48 hours),[23]and (FRISC II; 24–48 hours)[24] trials, with mixed results.

Fragmin and fast revascularization during instability in coronary artery disease II (FRISC II) with over 2,000 subjects demonstrated a benefit in terms of 1-year death or MI, particularly with diabetes patients causing relative risk reduction of 39% and absolute risk reduction of 9.3%.[24] Somewhat similar data emerged from the TACTICS-TIMI 18 trial (n = 2,220) where compared to initial conservative approach, an early invasive strategy resulted in significant reduction in death, MI, or rehospitalization for ACS at 6 months.[22] Similar to other studies with early invasive approach diabetic patients inferred a larger benefit (RRR of 27% and 13%, respectively and ARR 7.6% and 1.8%, respectively). Based on existing data current international guidelines, endorse a routine invasive strategy (within 72 hours of hospitalization) for diabetics presenting with NSTE-ACS.[25]

Percutaneous Coronary Intervention versus Coronary Artery Bypass Graft Surgery

The revascularization strategy in diabetic patients presenting with ACS remains uncertain because no randomized clinical trial (RCT) has compared different strategies in this setting. These patients frequently have extensive disease and multiple comorbidities making the best choice of revascularization modality difficult. Under such circumstances individualized approach seems to be the best bet with due consideration given to clinical presentation, ischemic burden, suitability of the coronary lesions for PCI or bypass grafting, left ventricle (LV) function and comorbidities. In a meta-analysis of 10 randomized trials mostly involving over 7,000 patients,[26] CABG was associated with significantly lower mortality at 5.9-year follow-up than with PCI in diabetic patients (23% vs 29%; HR = 0.70). BARI-2D trial[27] showed that at end of 5-years all-cause mortality or MI were significantly lower in the CABG group compared to intensive medical therapy alone (21.1% vs 29.2%; $P < 0.010$). Recent data with studies using DES in PCI have also provided similar results. The Coronary Artery Risk Development in Young Adults (CARDIA) study (small and underpowered), and subgroup analysis of SYNTAX[28] study showed an increased rate of major adverse cardiac and cerebrovascular event (MACCE) at 12 months for patients with multivessel disease who underwent PCI with DES, as compared with CABG. MACCE rate was doubled primarily because of repeat revascularization with no significant difference in rates of death or MI. In SYNTAX trial 3-year follow-up, similar trends were noted. Over 1,900 patients studied in FREEDOM trial,[29] which provided further evidence of superior effectiveness of CABG versus PCI. 947 patients in CABG arm after 5 years had significantly lower mortality (10.9% vs 16.3%) and fewer MI (6.0% vs 13.9%), but significantly more strokes (5.2% vs 2.4%). However, it has to be pointed out that these trials incorporated mostly—if not only—chronic stable patients, and it is unclear whether these data can be extrapolated to patients with ACS.

Relevance of Drug-eluting Stents and Conduits

Repeat target vessel revascularization was considerably less frequent with a DES than a bare metal stents (BMS) [or 0.29 for sirolimus (SES) eluting; 0.38 for paclitaxel (PES) eluting].[30] In the diabetic subgroup of HORIZONS-AMI study, PES compared to BMS resulted in a 70% reduction in target lesion revascularization (TLR), 46% reduction in major adverse cardiovascular events (MACE) at 3 year.[31] Based on overwhelming data, current guidelines recommend DES to reduce rates of repeat revascularization. Several observational studies support arterial grafts over saphenous vein grafts in terms of outcome, however, no data confined to ACS patients alone are available.

CONCLUSION

Diabetes mellitus not only increases the mortality but also the subsequent complication rates of patients presenting with ACS. Based on available data these patients require aggressive therapy with a nearly invasive strategy with both SES and PES having comparable outcome. In diabetic patients, Prasugrel leads to better and ticagrelor leads to a comparable reduction in ischemic events. Trials of chronic stable angina favor CABG as a better revascularization strategy compared to PCI in these patients but, individualization based on comorbidities, extent of plaque burden and age should be taken into account particularly in ACS patients as none of the studies have specifically studied this subgroup.

REFERENCES

1. Van Dieren S, Beulens JW, van der Schouw YT, et al. The global burden of diabetes and its complications: an emerging pandemic. Eur J Cardiovasc Prev Rehabil. 2010;17(Suppl 1):S3-8.
2. Sarwar N, Gao P, Seshasai SR, et al. Emerging Risk Factors Collaboration. Diabetes mellitus, fasting blood glucose concentration, and risk of vascular disease: a collaborative meta-analysis of 102 prospective studies. Lancet. 2010;375(9733):2215-22.
3. O'Donoghue ML, Vaidya A, Afsal R, et al. An invasive or conservative strategy in patients with diabetes mellitus and non- ST-segment elevation acute coronary syndromes: a collaborative meta-analysis of randomized trials. J Am Coll Cardiol. 2012;60(2):106-11.
4. Woodfield SL, Lundergan CF, Reiner JS, et al. Angiographic findings and outcome in diabetic patients treated with thrombolytic therapy for acute myocardial infarction: the GUSTO-I experience. J Am Coll Cardiol. 1996;28(7):1661-9.
5. West NE, RuyGrok PN, Disco CM, et al. Clinical and angiographic predictors of restenosis after stent deployment in diabetic patients. Circulation. 2004;109(7):867-73.
6. Ginsberg HN, MacCallum PR. The obesity, metabolic syndrome, and type 2 diabetes mellitus pandemic: part I. Increased cardiovascular disease risk and the importance of atherogenic dyslipidemia in persons with the metabolic syndrome and type 2 diabetes mellitus. J Cardiometab Syndr. 2009;4(2):113-9.
7. Cipollone F, Iezzi A, Fazia M, et al. The receptor RAGE as a progression factor amplifying arachidonate-dependent inflammatory and proteolytic response in human atherosclerotic plaques: role of glycemic control. Circulation. 2003;108(9):1070-77.
8. Ishibashi T, Kawaguchi M, Sugimoto K, et al. Advanced glycation end product-mediated matrix metallo-proteinase-9 and apoptosis via renin-angiotensin system in type 2 diabetes. J Atheroscler Thromb. 2010;17(6):578-89.
9. Ferreiro JL, Gomez-Hospital JA, Angiolillo DJ. Platelet abnormalities in diabetes mellitus. DiabVasc Dis Res. 2010;7(4):251-9.
10. Blankenberg S, Barbaux S, Tiret L. Adhesion molecules and atherosclerosis. Atherosclerosis. 2003;170(2):191-203.
11. Eibl N, KruglugerW, Streit G, et al. Improved metabolic control decreases platelet activation markers in patients with type-diabetes. Eur J Clin Invest. 2004;34(3):205-9.
12. Finfer S, Chittock DR, Su SY, et al. Intensive versus conventional glucose control in critically ill patients. N Engl J Med. 2009;360(13):1283-97.
13. Selker HP, Beshansky JR, Sheehan PR, et al. Out-of-hospital administration of intravenous glucose-insulin-potassium in patients with suspected acute coronary syndromes: the IMMEDIATE randomized controlled trial. JAMA. 2012;307(18):1925-33.
14. Jin PY, Zhang HS, Guo XY, et al. Glucose-insulin-potassium therapy in patients with acute coronary syndrome: a meta-analysis of randomized controlled trials. BMC Cardiovasc Disord. 2014;14:169.

15. Wiviott SD, Braunwald E, Angiolillo DJ, et al. Greater clinical benefit of more intensive oral antiplatelet therapy with prasugrel in patients with diabetes mellitus in the trial to assess improvement in therapeutic outcomes by optimizing platelet inhibition with prasugrel-thrombolysis in myocardial infarction 38. Circulation. 2008;118(16):1626-36.
16. James S, Angiolillo DJ, Cornel JH, et al. Ticagrelor vs. clopidogrel in patients with acute coronary syndromes and diabetes: a substudy from the PLATelet inhibition and patient Outcomes (PLATO) trial. Eur Heart J. 2010;31(24):3006-16.
17. Roffi M, Chew DP, Mukherjee D, et al. Platelet glycoprotein IIb/IIIa inhibitors reduce mortality in diabetic patients with non-ST-segment-elevation acute coronary syndromes. Circulation. 2001;104(23):2767-71.
18. Eikelboom JW, Mehta SR, Anand SS, et al. Adverse impact of bleeding on prognosis in patients with acute coronary syndromes. Circulation. 2006;114(8):774-82.
19. Giugliano RP, White JA, Bode C, et al. Early versus delayed, provisional eptifibatide in acute coronary syndromes. N Engl J Med. 2009;360(21):2176-90.
20. Norhammar A, Lagerqvist B, Saleh N. Long-term mortality after PCI in patients with diabetes mellitus: results from the Swedish Coronary Angiography and Angioplasty Registry. Euro Intervention. 2010;5(8):891-7.
21. Milosevic A, Vasiljevic-Pokrajcic Z, Milasinovic D, et al. Immediate invasive strategy for patients with both new ischemic electrocardiographic changes and troponin elevation. JACC: Cardiovasc Interven. 2016;9(7):541-9.
22. Cannon CP, Weintraub WS, Demopoulos LA, et al. Comparison of early invasive and conservative strategies in patients with unstable coronary syndromes treated with the glycoprotein IIb/IIIa inhibitor tirofiban. N Engl J Med. 2001;344(25):1879-87.
23. deWinter RJ, Windhausen F, Cornel JH, et al. Early invasive versus selectively invasive management for acute coronary syndromes. N Engl J Med. 2005;353(11):1095-104.
24. Wallentin L, Lagerqvist B, Husted S, et al. Outcome at 1 year after an invasive compared with a non-invasive strategy in unstable coronary-artery disease: the FRISC II invasive randomised trial. FRISC II Investigators. Fast Revascularisation during Instability in Coronary artery disease. Lancet. 2000;356(9223):9-16.
25. Roffi M, Patrono C, Collet J-P, et al. 2015 ESC Guidelines for the management of acute coronary syndromes in patients presenting without persistent ST-segment elevation: task force for the management of acute coronary syndromes in patients presenting without persistent ST-segment elevation of the European Society of Cardiology (ESC). Eur Heart J. 2016;37(3):267-315.
26. Hlatky MA, Boothroyd DB, Bravata DM, et al. Coronary artery bypass surgery compared with percutaneous coronary interventions for multivessel disease: a collaborative analysis of individual patient data from ten randomised trials. Lancet. 2009;373(9670):1190-7.
27. Chaitman BR, Hardison RM, Adler D, et al. The Bypass Angioplasty Revascularization Investigation 2 Diabetes randomized trial of different treatment strategies in type 2 diabetes mellitus with stable ischemic heart disease: impact of treatment strategy on cardiac mortality and myocardial infarction. Circulation. 2009;120(25):2529-40.
28. Banning AP, Westaby S, Morice MC, et al. Diabetic and nondiabetic patients with left main and/or 3-vessel coronary artery disease: comparison of outcomes with cardiac surgery and paclitaxel-eluting stents. J Am Coll Cardiol. 2010;55(11):1067-75.
29. Farkouh ME, Domanski M, Sleeper LA, et al. Strategies for multivessel revascularization in patients with diabetes. N Engl J Med. 2012;367(25):2375-84.
30. Stettler C, Allemann S, Wandel S, et al. Drug eluting and bare metal stents in people with and without diabetes: collaborative network meta-analysis. BMJ. 2008;337:a1331.
31. Witzenbichler B, Guagliumi G, Peruga JZ, et al. Impact of Paclitaxel-Eluting Stents in diabetic and non-diabetic patients with Acute Myocardial Infarction undergoing primary angioplasty: 3-year results from the HORIZONS AMI Trial. J Am Coll Cardiol. 2011;57:E1650.

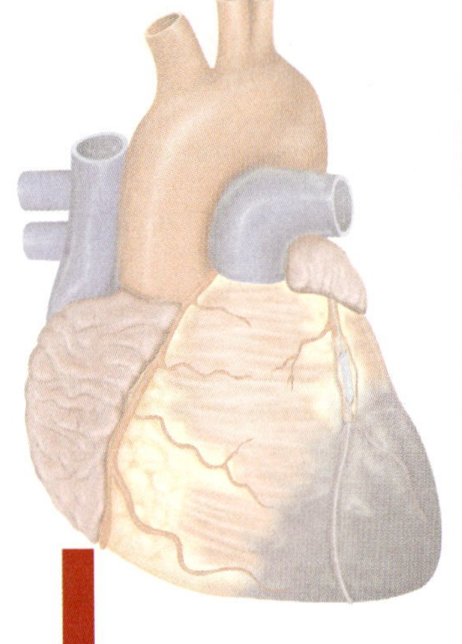

Newer Drugs in Heart Failure and Changes in Our Clinical Approach

Vatchsala Sree Varadharajan

INTRODUCTION

Heart failure (HF) is a major public health concern affecting as many as 23 million people worldwide. The goals of treatment in patients with HF include improving their clinical status, functional capacity and quality of life, prevent hospitalization, and to reduce mortality. HF still carries significant morbidity and mortality with 5-year mortality that rival those of many cancers. Substantial progress has been made in the management of HF with drugs. Despite the advancement, one ongoing challenge is to ensure that proven HF therapies are used at tolerated target doses. A number of risk factors including ischemic heart disease, hypertension, smoking, obesity, and diabetes have been identified that both predict the incidence of HF as well as its severity. Because of high morbidity and mortality, there is a compelling need for new therapies that are safe in improving outcomes in HF patients.[1]

DEFINITION OF HEART FAILURE

Heart failure due to left ventricular (LV) dysfunction is categorized according to LV ejection fraction (LVEF) into HF with reduced ejection fraction (HFrEF) (with LVEF≤ 40%; known as HFrEF: also referred to as systolic HF) and HF with preserved ejection fraction (HFpEF) (with LVEF ≥50%; known as HFpEF; also referred to as diastolic HF). HFpEF is further classified into HFpEF borderline (EF 41–49%) and HFpEF improved (EF >40%). Predominantly all randomized controlled trials (RCTs) have been conducted only in patients with HFrEF and only in those patients that efficacious therapies are available to date. Diagnosing HFpEF is challenging and different, criteria are applied to make a diagnosis and no efficacious therapy have been identified to date. Considering HFpEF borderline, their characteristics, treatment pattern, and outcomes appear similar to those of patients with HFpEF. However, HFpEF improved are those patients who had a reduced EF previously and have made an improvement in their EF. More research is needed in this subset of population. [2]

ETIOLOGY OF HEART FAILURE

The causes for HF or more precisely the risk factors for developing HF are multifactorial. The list is vast. In a broader sense, it can be grouped into causes in a structurally abnormal heart and the causes in a structurally normal heart. Coronary artery disease (CAD), previous myocardial infarction (MI), stenotic, and regurgitant valvular lesions including infective endocarditis, different cardiomyopathies (dilated and hypertrophic), congenital heart disease, severe lung disease, diabetes, obesity, and sleep apnea are major causes for HF in a structurally abnormal heart. Anemia, hyperthyroidism, and dysrhythmia are major causes for HF in a structurally normal heart. All cardiomyopathies predisposes to HF. A detailed discussion of it is beyond the scope of this article. However, the MOGE(S) classification of cardiomyopathy is an useful tool to simplify the etiology of cardiomyopathy.[3]

HEART FAILURE CLASSIFICATION

The American College of Cardiology/American Heart Association (ACC/AHA) stages of HF and the New York Heart Association (NYHA) functional classification provide useful and complementary information about the presence and severity of HF. The NYHA classes that focus on exercise capacity grades, the symptoms from class I to IV where class I has no limitation to physical activity and class IV is unable to carry on any physical activity without symptoms of HF or symptoms of HF at rest. The ACC/AHA classification categorizes the stages of HF into four viz. A, B, C, and D. Stage A is at high-risk for HF but without structural heart disease or symptoms of HF. Stage B is structural heart disease but without signs or symptoms of HF. Stage C is structural heart disease with prior or current symptoms of HF and stage D is refractory HF requiring specialized interventions.[2]

MANAGEMENT OF HEART FAILURE WITH REDUCED EJECTION FRACTION

A holistic approach in the management of HF includes treating associated conditions, lifestyle modifications, drug therapy, device therapy, cardiac rehabilitation, and preventive care. Adequate treatment of associated conditions such as hypertension, ischemic heart disease, valvular heart disease, diabetes, thyroid dysfunction, and infection is imperative in the overall treatment of HF. Pharmacological treatment with drugs includes established drugs like angiotensin converting enzymes inhibitor (ACEI), beta-blockers and mineralocorticoid or aldosterone receptor blockers (MRA), and newer agents like angiotensin receptor neprilysin inhibitor (ARNI) and I_f-channel inhibitor.

Angiotensin converting enzymes inhibitors have been shown to reduce mortality and morbidity in patients with HFrEF[4] and are recommended unless contraindicated or not tolerated in all symptomatic patients. ACEIs should be uptitrated to the maximum tolerated dose in order to achieve adequate inhibition of the renin-angiotensin-aldosterone system (RAAS). ACEIs are also recommended in patients with asymptomatic LV systolic dysfunction to reduce the risk of HF development, HF hospitalization, and death.

Beta-blockers should be initiated in clinically stable patients at a low dose and gradually uptitrated to the maximum tolerated dose. Beta-blockers reduce mortality and morbidity in symptomatic patients with HFrEF, despite treatment with an ACEI. However, they are not tested in congested or decompensated patients. In patients admitted due to acute HF (AHF), beta-blockers should be cautiously initiated in hospital, once the patient is stabilized. Beta-blockers should be considered for rate control in patients with HFrEF and atrial fibrillation (AF), especially in those with a high heart rate (HR). Beta-blockers are recommended in patients with a history of MI and asymptomatic LV systolic dysfunction to reduce the risk of death.[5]

MRA (spironolactone and eplerenone) block receptors bind aldosterone and with different degrees of affinity. Spironolactone or eplerenone is recommended in all symptomatic patients (despite treatment with an ACEI and a beta-blocker) with HFrEF and LVEF less than equal to 35%, to reduce mortality and HF hospitalization .Caution should be exercised when MRA are used in patients with impaired renal function and in those with serum potassium levels more than 5.0 mmol/L. Regular checks of serum potassium levels and renal function should be performed according to clinical status.[6]

Angiotensin II type I receptor blockers (ARBs) are recommended only as an alternative in patients intolerant of an ACEI because of serious side effects. The combination of ACEI or ARB should be restricted to symptomatic HFrEF patients receiving a beta-blocker who are unable to tolerate an MRA, and must be used under strict supervision.

ANGIOTENSIN RECEPTOR NEPRILYSIN INHIBITOR

Background

Currently, blockade of the RAAS is the cornerstone of the treatment of HF. However, the combination of RAAS blockade with inhibition of neprilysin, an enzyme that degrades natriuretic peptides (NPs), has recently emerged as a potentially superior treatment strategy. In July 2015, the Food and Drug Administration (FDA) approved sacubitril/valsartan (previously known as LCZ696) for use in patients who have chronic and stable but symptomatic HF and who have an LVEF of less than 40%. The drug should be used in conjunction with other HF therapies but in place of ACE inhibitors or ARBs, and is contraindicated in patients with a history of ACE inhibitor or ARB-induced angioedema.

Mechanism of Action

The first in class is LCZ696 which is a molecule that combines a neprilysin inhibitor (sacubitril) and an ARB (valsartan) in a single substance. Neprilysin is a zinc-dependent neutral endopeptidase. It is responsible for the degradation of several vasoactive peptides such as NPs, bradykinin, and adrenomedullin and contributes to the breakdown of angiotensin II.[7] High circulating A-type NP (ANP) and B-type NP (BNP) exert physiologic effects through binding to NP receptors and the augmented generation of current good manufacturing practice (cGMP), thereby enhancing diuresis, natriuresis and myocardial relaxation, and antiremodeling. ANP and BNP also inhibit renin and aldosterone secretion. Selective AT1-receptor blockade reduces vasoconstriction, sodium and water retention, and myocardial hypertrophy. Neprilysin inhibition is thought to be the therapeutic target for counteracting the neurohormonal activation and complementarily inhibiting the RAAS. [8]

PARADIGM TRIAL

The Prospective comparison of ARNI with ACEI to Determine Impact on Global Mortality and morbidity in Heart Failure (PARADIGM-HF) trial was conducted in 8,399 patients with NYHA class II–IV HF and LVEF of less than equal to 35%. They were randomly assigned to LCZ696 or enalapril. LCZ696 was associated with significant reductions in all-cause mortality, cardiovascular mortality, and hospitalization for worsening HF. The differences were apparent within 4 weeks of treatment and were maintained when patients were assessed again 8 months later. This trial provided strong evidence for superiority of the ARNI in patients with HFrEF. Important safety issues remain when initiating therapy with this drug in clinical practice. Symptomatic hypotension was more often present in the LCZ696 group compared to the enalapril group. The risk of angioedema in the trial was reduced by recruiting only those who tolerated therapy with enalapril 10 mg bid and LCZ696 during an active run-in phase of 5–9 weeks to minimize the risk of angioedema caused by overlapping ACE and neprilysin inhibition, the ACEI should be withheld for at least 36 hours before initiating LCZ696. Combined treatment with an ACEI (or ARB) and LCZ696 is contraindicated.[7]

IF-CHANNEL INHIBITOR

Background

Heart rate (HR) control is a novel potential therapeutic option for HF. An elevated HR is associated with worse cardiovascular outcomes. Although beta-blockers are used mainly for reducing HR in HF treatment, uptitration of beta-blockers can be associated with an increased risk of adverse reactions.[9] Ivabradine which acts by directly and selectively inhibiting the IF current in the sinoatrial node and therefore should only be used for patients in sinus rhythm, has potential benefits of pharmacologic modification of HR in HF. Ivabradine lowers HR by inhibiting a specific sinus node pacemaker, if current without affecting the myocardial contractility or relaxation, ventricular repolarization, or intracardiac conduction. This is rather different from the mechanism induced by beta-blockers which acts wherever beta-adrenergic receptors are present, causing negative inotropism, and vasoconstriction in the bronchi; and calcium channel blockers act on the calcium channels of the heart and smooth muscle causing negative inotropism, hypotension, and constipation.

BEAUTIFUL Trail

The Morbidity-Mortality Evaluation of the I_f Inhibitor Ivabradine in Patients with Coronary Disease and Left Ventricular Dysfunction (BEAUTIFUL) trial was an RCT to test the efficacy of ivabradine in 10,917 patients with stable coronary disease and an LVEF of less than 40% and an HR of more than 60 bpm. In this trial, ivabradine reduced HR but had no effect on the primary endpoint of cardiovascular death or admission to a hospital for new-onset or worsening HF. However, in a subgroup of patients with an HR of at least 70 bpm, ivabradine revealed a clear benefit with respect to the secondary endpoints of admission to a hospital for a fatal or nonfatal MI and coronary revascularization.[10]

SHIFT Trial

The Systolic Heart Failure Treatment with the If Inhibitor Ivabradine Trial (SHIFT) enrolled 6,558 patients with stable symptomatic HF and an LVEF of less than 35% in sinus rhythm with an HR of at least 70 bpm. In this trial, ivabradine significantly reduced the primary endpoint of cardiovascular death or hospitalization for worsening HF and deaths due to HF. The effect was consistent across all prespecified subgroups including the elderly. Further analyses proved that high HR is a risk factor in HF and lowering HR improve outcomes. One problem with interpreting the results of the SHIFT trial is that many patients were not on target doses of beta-blockers. If indeed these patients were intolerant of higher doses of beta-blockers, then these results are quite important for clinical care. Given its promising therapeutic value, ivabradine is clearly desirable in patients with symptomatic LV systolic dysfunction, elevated HR, and intolerance to beta-blockers.[11]

INCORPORATION OF THE NEWER AGENTS INTO CURRENT CLINICAL PRACTICE

The ACC, the AHA, and the HF Society of America (HFSA) recognize that the introduction of effective new therapies that potentially affect a large number of patients presents both opportunities and challenges. The introduction of ARNI (valsartan/sacubitril) and ivabradine, when applied judiciously, complements established pharmacological and device-based therapies and represents a milestone in the evolution of care for patients with HF. Accordingly, the writing committees of the '2016 ACC/AHA/HFSA Focused Update on New Pharmacological Therapy for HF' and the '2016 ESC Guideline on the Diagnosis and Treatment of Acute and Chronic HF' concurrently developed recommendations for the incorporation of these therapies into clinical practice. Working independently, each writing committee surveyed the evidence, arrived at similar conclusions, and constructed similar, but not identical recommendations. Given the concordance, the respective organizations simultaneously issued aligned recommendations on the use of these new treatments to minimize confusion and improve the care of patients with HF. The ACC/AHA recommendation includes:[12]

- Sacubitril/valsartan is recommended as a replacement for an ACEI to reduce further the risk of HF hospitalization and death in ambulatory patients with HFrEF who remain symptomatic despite optimal treatment with an ACEI, a beta-blocker and an MRA[a] [class I level of evidence B (LOE B)]
- Ivabradine should be considered to reduce the risk of HF hospitalization and cardiovascular death in symptomatic patients with LVEF less than equal to 35%, in sinus rhythm and a resting HR more than equal to 70 bpm despite treatment with an evidence-based dose of beta-blocker (or maximum tolerated dose below that), ACEI (or ARB), and an MRA (or ARB)-or have contraindications for a beta-blocker. Patients should also receive an ACEI (or ARB) and an MRA (or ARB) (Class IIa LOE C).

NEWER AGENTS TO PREVENT HYPERKALEMIA DURING RAAS INHIBITION:

Hyperkalemia is a common electrolytic abnormality in HF patients treated with RAAS inhibitors and MRA particularly with they have concomitant chronic kidney disease (CKD). This warrants treatment with agents that control plasma concentration of potassium while maintaining the use of RAAS inhibitors. Now, there are two novel potassium absorbents, patiromer calcium and zirconium silicate (ZS-9), that are designed to increase potassium loss via the gastrointestinal tract. Although they have not yet been approved by the FDA, both have demonstrated efficacy and safety in recent trials. Patiromer is a nonabsorbable polymer that binds potassium in exchange for calcium throughout the gastrointestinal tract. This agent which is an orally administered drug, increases fecal excretion of potassium and consequently decreases plasma potassium levels.[13] ZS-9 is a high-specificity inorganic crystal that entraps potassium in the intestinal tract. Instead of exchanging calcium, ZS-9 exchanges sodium and hydrogen ions for potassium. Dose-dependent excretion of potassium occurs in the feces, whereas urinary excretion decreases with dose. Initial results from the Hyperkalemia Randomized Intervention Multidose ZS-9 Maintenance (HARMONIZE) study is promising that tested the ZS-9 efficacy in achieving normokalemia. Further studies assessing the long-term efficacy and safety profile of this novel drug are ongoing.[14]

Relaxin

Serelaxin is a recombinant form of the human hormone relaxin, which is a naturally occurring hormone that is produced by the corpus luteum and placenta in pregnancy. Recent studies have shown that relaxin is also produced by the vasculature and failing myocardium. Relaxin is a potent nitric oxide generator that interacts with G-protein-coupled receptor resulting in an increase in cyclic adenosine monophosphate (cAMP). Activation of the endothelin-B receptor is probably involved in the relaxin-mediated increases in renal blood. Thus, relaxin increases cardiac output, arterial compliance, and renal blood flow, supporting important physiological changes during pregnancy. Given its potent vasodilator properties as well as its ability to increase renal perfusion, relaxin became of interest as a potential therapy for AHF.[15]

URODILATIN

Decongestion is an important part of managing both acute and chronic HF, and retention of fluid and sodium metabolism play a fundamental role in this. NPs are activated in HF and exert compensatory effects by inhibiting the RAAS and inducing vasodilation and natriuresis. Therefore, NPs have received much interest as a potential therapy in acute decompensated HF (ADHF). NPs consist of ANP, BNP, C-type NP (CNP), D-type NP (DNP), and urodilatin. Urodilatin was first isolated from human urine in 1988 as a modified version of pro-ANP. It is produced mainly by distal renal tubule cells and is secreted into urine and is involved in renal sodium handling. Ularitide is a synthetic form of urodilatin. Synthetic NPs such as carperitide (a recombinant form of ANP) and nesiritide (a recombinant form of BNP) are currently used to treat congestive HF (carperitide is available only in Japan). When it is administered to patients with ADHF, a rapid reduction of pulmonary capillary pressure and consequent relief of dyspnea often result because of natriuresis, diuresis, and venous and arterial dilation. In contrast to ANP and BNP, urodilatin is effective in more distal parts of the renal tubular system because of its slower elimination rate.[16]

CONCLUSION

The treatment of HF has evolved rapidly over the past few years and many aspects of this are considered in this article. Patients are often complex, with multiple comorbidities, and being under specialist care has been shown to be associated with greater use of evidence-based therapies and improved survival. Future clinical trials with adequately powered, more appropriate study designs, optimal clinical endpoints, and proper patient selection are mandatory to assess the true efficacy of these treatments.

REFERENCES

1. Bui AL, Horwich TB, Fonarow GC. Epidemiology and risk profile of heart failure. Nat Rev Cardiol. 2011;8(1):30-41.
2. Yancy CW, Jessup M, Bozkurt B, et al. 2013 ACCF/AHA guideline for the management of heart failure: executive summary: a report of the American College of Cardiology Foundation/American Heart Association Task Force on practice guidelines. Circulation. 2013;128(16):1810-52.
3. Arbustini E, Narula N, Tavazzi L, et al. The MOGE(S) Classification of Cardiomyopathy for Clinicians. J Am Coll Cardiol. 2014;64(3): 304-18.
4. SOLVD Investigators, Yusuf S, Pitt B, et al. Effect of Enalapril on Survival in Patients with Reduced Left Ventricular Ejection Fractions and Congestive Heart Failure. N Engl J Med. 1991;325(5):293-302.
5. Willenheimer R, van Veldhuisen DJ, Silke B, et al. Effect on Survival and Hospitalization of Initiating Treatment for Chronic Heart Failure With Bisoprolol Followed by Enalapril, as Compared With the Opposite Sequence. Results of the Randomized Cardiac Insufficiency Bisoprolol Study (CIBIS) III. Circulation. 2005;112(16):2426-35.
6. Pitt B, Zannad F, Remme WJ, et al. The Effect of Spironolactone on Morbidity and Mortality in Patients with Severe Heart Failure. N Engl J Med. 1999;341(10):709-17.
7. Packer M, McMurray JJV, Desai AS, et al. Angiotensin Receptor Neprilysin Inhibition Compared With Enalapril on the Risk of Clinical Progression in Surviving Patients With Heart Failure. Circulation. 2015;131(1):54-61.
8. Mangiafico S, Costello-Boerrigter LC, Andersen IA, et al. Neutral endopeptidase inhibition and the natriuretic peptide system: an evolving strategy in cardiovascular therapeutics. Eur Heart J. 2013;34(12):886-93.
9. Böhm M, Borer J, Ford I, et al. Heart rate at baseline influences the effect of ivabradine on cardiovascular outcomes in chronic heart failure: analysis from the SHIFT study. Clin Res Cardiol. 2013;102(1):11-22.
10. Fox K, Ford I, Steg PG, et al. Ivabradine for patients with stable coronary arterydisease and left-ventricular systolic dysfunction (BEAUTIFUL): a randomised, double-blind, placebo-controlled trial. Lancet. 2008;372(9641):807-16.
11. Böhm M, Swedberg K, Komajda M, et al. Heart rate as a risk factor in chronic heart failure (SHIFT): the association between heart rate and outcomes in a randomised placebo-controlled trial. Lancet. 2010;376(9744):886-94.
12. Yancy CW, Jessup M, Bozkurt B, et al. 2016 ACC/AHA/HFSA Focused Update on New Pharmacological Therapy for Heart Failure: An Update of the 2013 ACCF/AHA Guideline for the Management of Heart Failure. A Report of the American College of Cardiology/ American Heart Association Task Force on Clinical Practice Guidelines and the Heart Failure Society of America. Circulation. 2016 Sep 27;134(13):e282-93.
13. Weir MR, Bakris GL, Bushinsky DA, et al. Patiromer in Patients with Kidney Disease and Hyperkalemia Receiving RAAS Inhibitors. N Engl J Med. 2015;372(3):211-21.
14. Anker SD, Kosiborod M, Zannad F, et al. Maintenance of serum potassium with sodium zirconium cyclosilicate (ZS-9) in heart failure patients: results from a phase 3 randomized, double-blind, placebo-controlled trial. Eur J Heart Fail. 2015;17(10):1050-6.
15. Jeyabalan A, Novak J, Danielson LA, et al. Essential Role for Vascular Gelatinase Activity in Relaxin-Induced Renal Vasodilation, Hyperfiltration, and Reduced Myogenic Reactivity of Small Arteries. Circ Res. 2003;93(12):1249-57.
16. Mitrovic V, Seferovic PM, Simeunovic D, et al. Haemodynamic and clinical effects of ularitide in decompensated heart failure. Eur Heart J. 2006;27(23):2823-32.

CHAPTER 83

Role of Oral Anticoagulants in Atrial Fibrillation with Cardiodiabetes

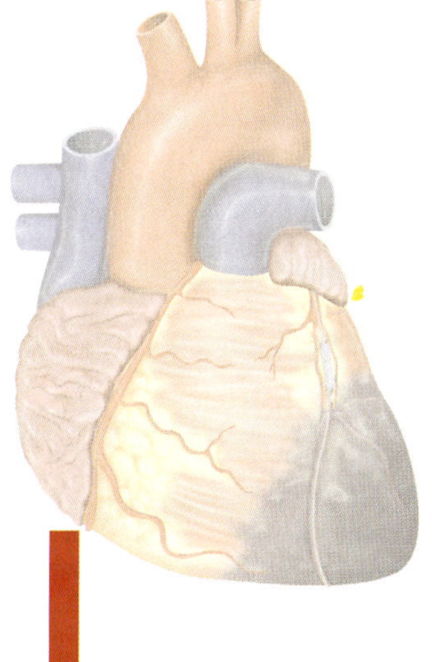

Chetan P Shah, Priyank Mody

INTRODUCTION

Diabetes and heart are hand in glove and together have emerged as the deadliest global epidemic of the 21st century. Diabetic patients have a high risk of developing arterial disease due to endothelial dysfunction, smooth muscle cell migration, and platelet hyperreactivity.[1] Atrial fibrillation (AF) is now the most common arrhythmia encountered in daily practice. The risk of AF is 2.1 times higher in a patient with diabetes.[2] Management of AF can be divided under two paradigms—the first involving control of ventricular rate and/or restoring sinus rhythm in select subgroup population for effective treatment of disabling symptoms and the second, but equally important is protecting from thromboembolism, which remains the most important cause of morbidity and mortality in a patient with AF. With the advent of non-vitamin K oral anticoagulants (NOACs), warfarin and its analogues, which has practically been the only option for prevention of stroke in AF for more than 50 years, will face a tough competition for survival particularly with recently published superiority trials published in favor of newer NOACs.

EPIDEMIOLOGY

Atrial fibrillation is one of the main cardiovascular complications associated with diabetic disease. Data from the Framingham Heart Study showed that in addition to intrinsic cardiac causes such as valve disease and congestive heart failure, risk factors for cardiovascular disease like hypertension, obesity, and diabetes also predispose to AF. Between these, diabetes mellitus (DM) conferred an odds ratio of 1.4 for men and 1.6 for women, after multivariable adjustment, for developing AF.[3] The incidence of AF in patients with DM is reported to be 14.9%, and in the same study atrial flutter occurred in 4% of DM patients versus 2.5% of the control group (P-value less than 0.003).[4] Furthermore, DM is cohesive to metabolic syndrome, including obesity which is an established risk factor for AF.[5]

RISK STRATIFICATION

For limiting ourselves to the need of anticoagulation in a patient who comes with AF, the first important step would be to risk stratify the patient according to his risk of thromboembolic event vis-a-vis his/her risk of bleeding. 2010 European Society of Cardiology (ESC) guidelines has established CHA_2DS_2-VASc score[6] as the most widely used score to assess the thromboembolic risk and of all the available risk scores for bleeding, i.e. HAS-BLED, ATRIA, and $HEMORR_2HAGES$, HAS-BLED is the most validated scoring system (Table 1).[7-9]

CHA_2DS_2-VASc includes DM as a risk factor, contributing to improve the accuracy of such score in predicting stroke risk.[6] On the other hand, DM is not included among well-established risk factors employed to assess bleeding risk in AF recipients on oral anticoagulation therapy (HAS-BLED, ATRIA, $HEMORR_2HAGES$).[7-9] Evidence accumulated so far strongly suggests that oral

TABLE 1: Stroke and bleeding risk stratification with the CHA_2DS_2-VASc and HAS-BLED schemas

CHA_2DS_2-VASc	Score	HAS-BLED	Score
Congestive heart failure/ LV dysfunction	1	Hypertension, i.e. uncontrolled BP	1
Hypertension	1	Abnormal renal/liver function	1 or 2
Aged ≥75 years	2	Stroke	1
Diabetes mellitus	1	Bleeding tendency or predisposition	1
Stroke/TIA/TE	2	Labile INR	1
Vascular disease (prior MI, PAD, or aortic plaque)	1	Age (e.g. >65)	1
Aged 65–74 years	1	Drugs (e.g. concomitant aspirin or NSAIDs) or alcohol	1
Sex category (i.e. female gender)	1		
Maximum score	9		9

Abbreviations: NSAIDs, nonsteroidal anti-inflammatory drugs; MI, myocardial infarction; PAD, peripheral artery disease; INR, international normalized ratio.

anticoagulation is mandatory when diabetes coexists in AF patients. Both the North American and European guidelines agree on systemic anticoagulation with an OAC when the CHA_2DS_2-VASc score is 2 or greater, but the guidelines differ on recommendations for systemic anticoagulation for a score of 1 (optional in North America, recommended in European). However, not all risk factors in the CHA_2DS_2-VASc score carry the same weight in estimating stroke risk. In a recent retrospective study of 186,570 patients with AF,[10] in men with a CHA_2DS_2-VASc score of 1, the highest risk for stroke was associated with age older than 65 years and diabetes. These findings were also consistent in women with a CHA_2DS_2-VASc score of 2. The presence of vascular disease alone accounted for 1.68-fold and 2.15-fold increased risks for ischemic stroke in men and women, respectively. In patients with both AF and type 2 diabetes, anticoagulation management is more complex and recommendations vary based on the presence of additional risk factors and which guidelines are followed. For example, the 2016 ESC guidelines for management of atrial fibrillation recommends anticoagulation for all patients with a CHA_2DS_2-VASc score of 1 or higher.[11] This implies that all patients with diabetes and AF should be treated with an OAC to prevent stroke and systemic embolism, provided no absolute contraindication exists. In contrast, according to the 2014 American College of Cardiology Foundation (ACCF)/ American Heart Association (AHA)/Heart Rhythm Society (HRS) guidelines,[12] younger men with diabetes as the only risk factor (CHA_2DS_2-VASc score, 1) may be treated

TABLE 2: Scores and risk factors of the patients with atrial fibrillation and type 2 diabetes

CHA_2DS_2-VASc risk score and factors	2014 AHA/ACC/ HRS recommendations	2016 ESC guidelines	Expert opinion
0	No antithrombotic	No antithrombotic	No antithrombotic
1	No antithrombotic or aspirin or OAC (NOAC or VKA)	Antithrombotic in male patients (IIa recommendation)	NOAC>OAC
≥2	NOAC or VKA	NOAC preferred over VKA if no contraindication to NOACs*	NOAC>OAC
≥2 and CKD with CrCl is less than 15 mL/ min/1.73 m^2 or requiring HD	VKA	VKA	VKA preferred; may consider apixaban in patients with stable HD
≥2 and moderate–severe CKD	Reduced dose of NOAC or VKA	Reduced dose of NOAC or VKA	Reduced dose of factor Xa inhibitor is greater than VKA or dabigatran

****Moderate to severe mitral stenosis and mechanical heart valve.***

Abbreviations: AHA, American Heart Association; HRS, Heart Rhythm Society; ACC, American College of Cardiology; ESC, European Society of Cardiology; NOAC, non-vitamin K oral anticoagulants; VKA, vitamin K antagonist; CKD, chronic kidney disease

with no antithrombotic, aspirin, or an OAC. However, the ACCF/AHA/HRS guidelines recommend that all women with diabetes, and all patients age 65 years or older with diabetes, in the setting of AF, be treated with an OAC (Table 2).

ORAL ANTICOAGULANTS FOR PREVENTION OF THROMBOEMBOLISM IN PATIENTS WITH ATRIAL FIBRILLATION

Warfarin

The superiority of warfarin in preventing stroke has been well established by large clinical trials as compared to aspirin. Target international normalized ratio (INR) maintained between 2 and 3 provides the best balance between stroke prevention (64% relative risk reduction in all cause stroke)[13] and hemorrhagic complications (1–2% per year based on the risk factors previously discussed).[14] It is this narrow therapeutic index, need for continuous monitoring of INR and the wide variety of drug–drug and food–drug interactions of warfarin, which creates a large unmet need for safer yet equally efficacious drugs. Even in controlled environment of clinical trials, patients spend only a mean 55% (95% CI = 51–58%) of their time in the therapeutic INR range [time in therapeutic range, (TTR)] 10.[15] Moreover, DM has emerged as one of the clinical factors affecting quality of anticoagulation control during warfarin treatment, as assessed by SAMe-TT2R2 score.[16] These data imply that warfarin may not be the best option in diabetic patients with AF.

To overcome the inherent limitations of warfarin, along with INR monitoring, the evolution of specialized clinics and genomics is appreciable.

- *Specialized INR monitoring* clinics comprising of the primary physician, treating cardiologist, and trained nursing staff have been able to optimize TTR to more than two-thirds of total time, hence, achieving optimum benefit from thromboembolic episode.
- *Genomics*: The testing of CYP2C9 (isoform of cytochrome P-450 enzyme) and VKORC1 (a vitamin K epoxide reductase complex subunit) may help in determining the possibility of pharmacokinetic and pharmacodynamic resistance, respectively. The same has not been validated in randomized trials.
- *Management of warfarin resistance*: Some patients need higher-than-expected doses of warfarin (Coumadin) to get their INR into the therapeutic range. The cause of warfarin resistance can be either acquired (e.g., poor compliance, drug interactions, dietary interactions) or hereditary. The simple Flow chart 1 would help in evaluating and managing patients of warfarin resistance. 2016 ESC guidelines gives class 1 recommendation for preference of NOACs over warfarin in nonvalvular AF.[17]

NEWER ANTICOAGULANTS: NON-VITAMIN K ORAL ANTICOAGULANTS

The benefit of non-vitamin K oral anticoagulants (NOACs) in reducing arterial thromboembolism in patients with AF when compared with warfarin has been demonstrated in four warfarin-controlled phase 3 trials.[18-21] In a pooled analysis of these four trials, the combined rates of stroke/systemic embolism across the four trials in patients with diabetes were 3.16% (in the 9,096 patients treated with NOACs) vs. 3.96% (in the 8990 patients treated with warfarin) (relative risk, 0.80; 95% CI, 0.69–0.93). The

Flow chart 1: Algorithm for evaluating suspected warfarin resistance[17]

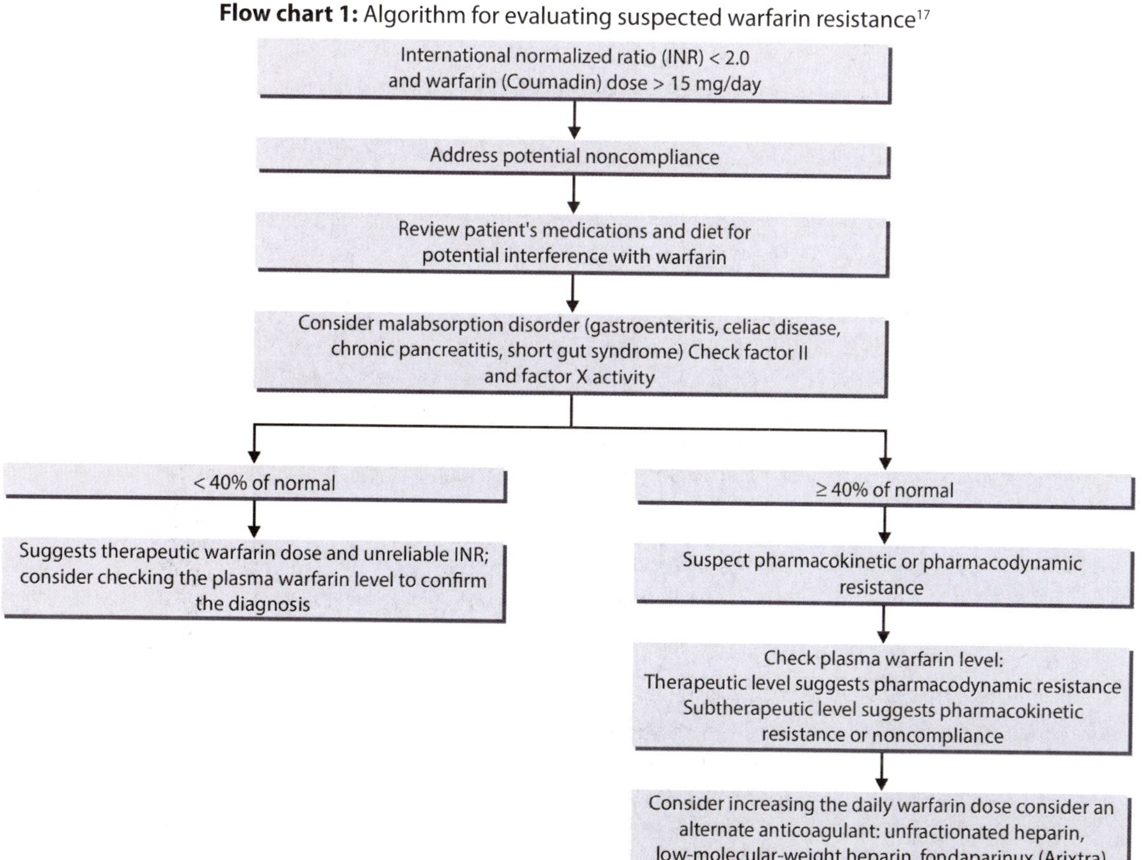

corresponding event rates in the 20,216 NOAC-treated and 20,238 warfarin treated patients without diabetes were lower at 3.08% vs. 3.73%, respectively. However, the relative treatment benefit of NOACs as compared with warfarin in patients without diabetes was not different (HR, 0.83; 95% CI, 0.74–0.93; *P*-value for interaction = 0.73) (Fig. 1).[22] Likewise, there was no heterogeneity of effect by diabetes status on the comparative rates of major bleeding in patients treated with NOACs vs. warfarin (Fig. 2). However, as patients with diabetes were at increased absolute risk for stroke/systemic embolism compared with those without diabetes, the similar relative risk reduction across the diabetes strata translates into greater absolute benefits and smaller numbers needed to treat with NOACs among patients with diabetes.

- *Dabigatran*: Dabigatran is a direct thrombin inhibitor which competitively and reversibly binds to the active site of free and clot bound thrombin, thereby blocking its procoagulant activity. RE-LY trial[18] which *compared Dabigatran to Warfarin in 18,113 Patients with Atrial Fibrillation at Risk of Stroke* concluded that dabigatran 150 mg significantly reduced stoke compared to warfarin with similar risk of major bleeding while dabigatran 110 mg had a similar rate of stroke as warfarin with significantly reduced major bleeding. Both doses markedly reduced intracerebral, life-threatening, and total bleeding. Dabigatran had no major toxicity, but did increase dyspepsia and gastrointestinal (GI) bleeding.
- *Apixaban*: In the ARISTOTLE (Apixaban for Reduction in Stroke and Other Thromboembolic Events in AF) trial,[21] apixaban 5 mg twice daily reduced stroke or systemic embolism by 21% compared with warfarin, combined with a 31% reduction in major bleeding and an 11% reduction in all-cause mortality (all statistically significant). Rates of hemorrhagic stroke and intracranial hemorrhage, but not of ischemic stroke, were lower on apixaban. Rates of GI bleeding were similar between the two treatment arms.[23] Apixaban is the only NOAC that has been compared with aspirin in AF patients; apixaban significantly reduced stroke or systemic embolism by 55% compared with aspirin, with only a small difference in rate of major bleeding or intracranial hemorrhage.[24,25]
- *Edoxaban*: In the ENGAGE AF-TIMI 48 (Effective Anticoagulation with Factor Xa Next Generation in Atrial Fibrillation-Thrombolysis in Myocardial Infarction 48) trial,[20] edoxaban 60 mg once daily and edoxaban 30 mg once daily (with dose reductions in certain patients, were compared with adjusted-dose warfarin.[26] Edoxaban 60 mg once daily was noninferior to warfarin.

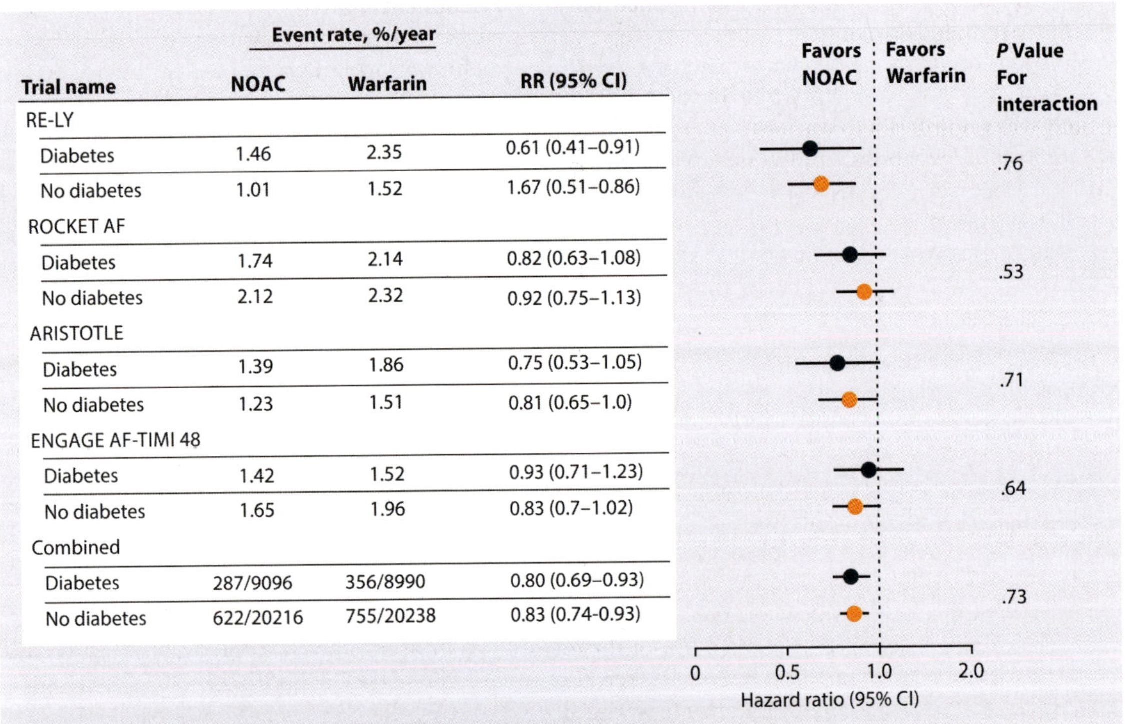

Trial name	NOAC (Event rate, %/year)	Warfarin (Event rate, %/year)	RR (95% CI)	P Value For interaction
RE-LY				
Diabetes	1.46	2.35	0.61 (0.41–0.91)	.76
No diabetes	1.01	1.52	1.67 (0.51–0.86)	
ROCKET AF				
Diabetes	1.74	2.14	0.82 (0.63–1.08)	.53
No diabetes	2.12	2.32	0.92 (0.75–1.13)	
ARISTOTLE				
Diabetes	1.39	1.86	0.75 (0.53–1.05)	.71
No diabetes	1.23	1.51	0.81 (0.65–1.0)	
ENGAGE AF-TIMI 48				
Diabetes	1.42	1.52	0.93 (0.71–1.23)	.64
No diabetes	1.65	1.96	0.83 (0.7–1.02)	
Combined				
Diabetes	287/9096	356/8990	0.80 (0.69–0.93)	.73
No diabetes	622/20216	755/20238	0.83 (0.74-0.93)	

Fig. 1: Efficacy of non-vitamin K oral anticoagulants (NOACs) versus warfarin in patients with atrial fibrillation stratified by diabetes status

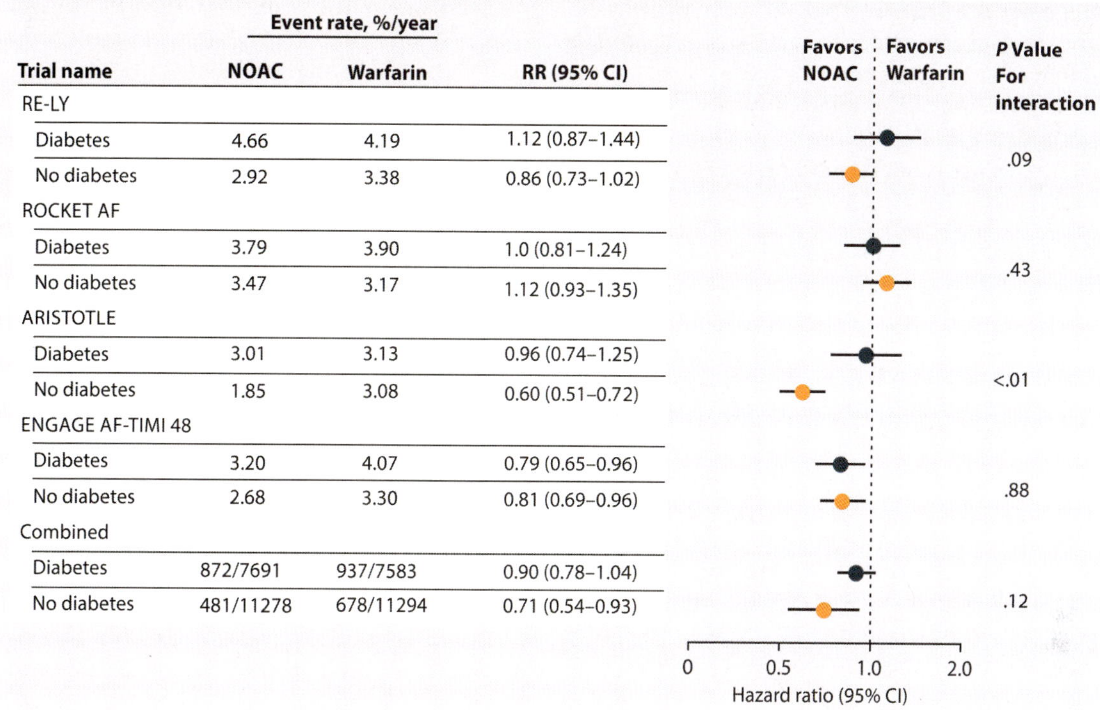

Fig. 2: Safety of non-vitamin K oral anticoagulants (NOACs) versus warfarin in patients with atrial fibrillation stratified by diabetes status

In an on-treatment analysis, edoxaban 60 mg once daily significantly reduced stroke or systemic embolism by 21% and significantly reduced major bleeding events by 20% compared with warfarin, while edoxaban 30 mg once daily was noninferior to warfarin for prevention of stroke and systemic embolism but significantly reduced major bleeding events by 53%. Cardiovascular death was reduced in patients randomized to edoxaban 60 mg once daily or edoxaban 30 mg once daily compared with warfarin. Only the higher dose regimen has been approved for stroke prevention in AF.

- *Rivaroxaban*: Oral direct coagulation factor Xa inhibitor. It reversibly binds to the active site of coagulation. Factor Xa without ant thrombin mediation affecting free and platelet-bound factor Xa. In the ROCKET-AF (Rivaroxaban Once Daily Oral Direct Factor Xa Inhibition Compared with Vitamin K Antagonism for Prevention of Stroke and Embolism Trial in Atrial Fibrillation) trial,[19] 320 patients were randomized to rivaroxaban 20 mg once daily or vitamin K antagonist (VKA), with a dose adjustment to 15 mg daily for those with estimated CrCl 30–49 mL/min by the Cockcroft-Gault formula. Rivaroxaban was noninferior to warfarin for the prevention of stroke and systemic embolism in the intent-to-treat analysis, while the per-protocol on-treatment analysis achieved statistical superiority with a 21% reduction in stroke or systemic embolism compared with warfarin. Rivaroxaban did not reduce the rates of mortality, ischemic stroke, or major bleeding events compared to VKA. There was an increase in GI bleeding events, but a significant reduction in hemorrhagic stroke and intracranial hemorrhage with rivaroxaban compared with warfarin. Comparable event rates have been reported in post authorization analyses, which are part of the postapproval risk management process.[27]

LIMITATIONS OF NON-VITAMIN K ORAL ANTICOAGULANTS

- No established laboratory test to monitor the efficacy of anticoagulation
- Cost
- Lack of long-term safety data
- *Antidote*:
    - *Idarucizumab* (*Praxbind*): Antidote for direct thrombin inhibitor, FDA approved October 2015 based on REVERSE AD[28] study and is now available in India, however, the present cost (₹ 1.5 lakhs) may be a limiting factor in most of our patients
    - *Andexanet alfa*: Reversal of factor Xa

- *Pregnancy and breastfeeding*: Not recommended
- *Renal dysfunction*: It is not recommended for those with CrCl less than 30 mL/min per 1.73 m^2.
- *Hepatic dysfunction*: In moderate to severe hepatic dysfunction (Child–Pugh class B or C) or impaired coagulation, its use is not recommended.

LABORATORY TESTING WITH NON-VITAMIN K ORAL ANTICOAGULANTS

Non-vitamin K oral anticoagulants do not require monitoring owing to rapid onset of action, stable pharmacokinetic properties and no significant drug interactions, however, in clinical situations like overdoses, emergency preoperative settings, or bleeding laboratory test to monitor activity and plan reversal is of utmost importance.

For dabigatran: Ecarin clotting time (ECT) and ecarin chromogenic assay (ECA) may be helpful (limited to research labs) while *rivaroxaban and apixaban* can be monitored using modified chromogenic anti-Xa assays that use specific rivaroxaban and apixaban standards, respectively.

SOME SPECIAL CLINICAL CIRCUMSTANCES

Acute Stroke

Thrombolysis is a relative contraindication, if the patient is on OAC. If on warfarin and INR is less than 1.7, one can safely thrombolyse the patient. Safety of thrombolysis in patients receiving NOA is not established and poses a very high risk of bleeding, few case reports of dabigatran when the last dose was given before 24 hours and activated partial thromboplastin time (aPTT) being normal, thrombolysis was safe. However, similar reports with rivaroxaban and apixaban are lacking.

MANAGEMENT OF BLEEDING/ OVERDOSE DUE TO NON-VITAMIN K ORAL ANTICOAGULANTS

Given the relatively short half-lives of the NOAs in patients with normal renal function, most of the anticoagulant effect should dissipate within 48 hours.

However, when the need arises.

- Use of antidote, if available
- Activated charcoal
- *Hemodialysis*: Might be useful only for dabigatran (as only 35% of drug is protein bound). In case of rivaroxaban and apixaban, dialysis is unlikely to be effective as more than 80–90% of drug is protein bound
- Prothrombin complex concentrates (PCCs)
- A randomized controlled study using a nonactivated 4-factor PCC showed normalization of the prothrombin time (PT) alone in patients taking rivaroxaban but not dabigatran. No studies have evaluated PCCs in patients receiving the NOAs with clinical bleeding; however, its use seems reasonable in the setting of serious bleeding.

Cardioversion: Anticoagulation is recommended at least 3 weeks prior and 4 weeks after electrical or pharmacological cardioversion. Data on the safety of warfarin and dabigatran (RE-LY) trial is well-established. Similar data on other molecules is awaited.

Switching between Anticoagulants

- *From VKA to NOACs*: Discontinue VKA and start dabigatran, when INR is less than 2 (same for apixaban) and rivaroxaban, when INR is less than 3.
- *From IV anticoagulants to oral anticoagulants*: Warfarin to be started before 5 days and bridging IV or subcutaneous (SC) anticoagulants used till INR more than 2 is achieved NOACs initiate NOA 2 hours before the next regularly scheduled dose of the discontinued SC anticoagulant and for continuous IV unfractionated heparin (UFH), initiate NOA at the time of discontinuation of the continuous infusion.

CONCLUSION

Diabetes puts the patient of AF at extra risk of thromboembolism. The present recommendation is to anticoagulate all patients with AF and diabetes (2016 ESC Recommendation). Warfarin remains the standard of care for patients with valvular AF or mechanical heart valves until further safety and efficacy data regarding the use of NOAs in these situations is available. The NOAs are not all superior in terms of efficacy compared with warfarin, if TTR is maintained more than 70% of time patients with hepatic dysfunction or associated coagulopathies or impaired renal function (CrCl <30 mL/min per 1.73 m^2) are not good candidates for NOAs owing to their hepatic metabolism and renal excretion. Choice amongst NOACs—no head to head trails to prove superiority of any single molecule. In patients with a recent history of GI bleeding, apixaban may be a better choice as it has a lower incidence of GI bleeding than dabigatran and rivaroxaban. Given the association of dabigatran with a trend toward an increase in the incidence of myocardial infarction, rivaroxaban or apixaban should possibly be considered when selecting an NOA in this subset of patients. In patients with a history of ischemic strokes while taking warfarin, dabigatran, and apixaban may be suitable alternatives as they are the only NOAs with a lower rate of ischemic stroke than warfarin. When compliance is an issue once daily rivaroxaban may be the drug of choice.

REFERENCES

1. Martin-Timon I, Sevillano-Collantes C, Segura-Galindo A, et al. Type 2 diabetes and cardiovascular disease: have all risk factors the same strength? World J Diabetes. 2014;5(4):444-70.
2. Movahed MR, Hashemzadeh M, Jamal MM. Diabetes mellitus is a strong, independent risk for atrial fibrillation and flutter in addition to other cardiovascular disease. Int J Cardiol. 2005;105(3):315-8.
3. Benjamin EJ, Levy D, Vaziri SM, et al. Independent risk factors for atrial fibrillation in a population-based cohort. The Framingham Heart Study. JAMA. 1994;271(11):840-4.
4. Movahed MR, Hashemzadeh M, Jamal MM. Diabetes mellitus is a strong, independent risk for atrial fibrillation and flutter in addition to other cardiovascular disease. Int J Cardiol. 2005;105(3):315-8.
5. Pathak RK, Mahajan R, Lau DH, et al. The implications of obesity for cardiac arrhythmia mechanisms and management. Can J Cardiol. 2015;31(2):203-10.
6. European Heart Rhythm Association, European Association for Cardio-Thoracic Surgery, Camm AJ, et al. Guidelines for the management of atrial fibrillation: the Task Force for the Management of Atrial Fibrillation of the European Society of Cardiology (ESC). Eur Heart J. 2010;31(19):2369-429.
7. Olesen JB, Lip GY, Hansen PR, et al. Bleeding risk in 'real world' patients with atrial fibrillation: comparison of two established bleeding prediction schemes in a nationwide cohort. J Thromb Haemost. 2011;9(8):1460-7.
8. Gage BF, Yan Y, Milligan PE, et al. Clinical classification schemes for predicting hemorrhage: results from the National Registry of Atrial Fibrillation (NRAF). Am Heart J. 2006;151(3):713-9.
9. Fang MC, Go AS, Chang Y, et al. A new risk scheme to predict warfarin-associated hemorrhage: The ATRIA (Anticoagulation and Risk Factors in Atrial Fibrillation) Study. J Am Coll Cardiol. 2011;58(4):395-401.
10. Chao TF, Liu CJ, Wang KL, et al. Should atrial fibrillation patients with 1 additional risk factor of the CHA2DS2-VASc score (beyond sex) receive oral anticoagulation? J Am Coll Cardiol. 2015;65(7):635-42.
11. Kirchhof P, Benussi S, Kotecha D, et al. 2016 ESC guidelines for the management of atrial fibrillation developed in collaboration with EACTS. Revista espanola de cardiologia. 2017;70(1):50.
12. January CT, Wann LS, Alpert JS, et al. American College of Cardiology/ American Heart Association Task Force on Practice Guidelines. 2014 AHA/ACC/HRS guideline for the management of patients with atrial fibrillation: a report of the American College of Cardiology/ American Heart Association Task Force on Practice Guidelines and the Heart Rhythm Society. J Am Coll Cardiol. 2014;64(21): e1-e76.
13. Hart RG, Pearce LA, Aguilar MI. Meta-analysis: antithrombotic therapy to prevent stroke in patients who have nonvalvular atrial fibrillation. Ann Intern Med. 2007;146(12):857-67.
14. Cairns JA, Connolly S, McMurtry S, et al. Canadian Cardiovascular Society atrial fibrillation guidelines 2010: prevention of stroke and systemic thromboembolism in atrial fibrillation and flutter. Can J Cardiol. 2011;27(1):74-90.
15. Baker WL, Cios DA, Sander SD, et al. Meta-analysis to assess the quality of warfarin control in atrial fibrillation patients in the United States. J Manage Care Pharm. 2009;15(3):244-52.
16. Apostolakis S, Sullivan RM, Olshansky B, et al. Factors affecting quality of anticoagulation control among patients with atrial fibrillation on warfarin: the SAMe-TT2R2 score. Chest. 2013;144(5):1555-63.
17. Osinbowale O, Al Malki M, Schade A, et al. An algorithm for managing warfarin resistance. Cleve Clin J Med. 2009;76(12):724-30.
18. Connolly SJ, Ezekowitz MD, Yusuf S, et al. RE-LY Steering Committee and Investigators. Dabigatran versus warfarin in patients with atrial fibrillation. N Engl J Med. 2009;361(12):1139-51.
19. Patel MR, Mahaffey KW, Garg J, et al. ROCKET AF Investigators. Rivaroxaban versus warfarin in nonvalvular atrial fibrillation. N Engl J Med. 2011;365(10):883-91.
20. Giugliano RP, Ruff CT, Braunwald E, et al. ENGAGE AF-TIMI 48 Investigators. Edoxaban versus warfarin in patients with atrial fibrillation. N Engl J Med. 2013;369(22):2093-104.
21. Granger CB, Alexander JH, McMurray JJ, et al. ARISTOTLE Committees and Investigators. Apixaban versus warfarin in patients with atrial fibrillation. N Engl J Med. 2011;365(11):981-92.
22. Ruff CT, Giugliano RP, Braunwald E, et al. Comparison of the efficacy and safety of new oral anticoagulants with warfarin in patients with atrial fibrillation: a meta-analysis of randomised trials. Lancet. 2014;383(9921):955-62.
23. Hylek EM, Held C, Alexander JH, et al. Major bleeding in patients with atrial fibrillation receiving apixaban or warfarin: The ARISTOTLE Trial (Apixaban for Reduction in Stroke and Other Thromboembolic Events in Atrial Fibrillation): Predictors, Characteristics, and Clinical Outcomes. J Am Coll Cardiol. 2014;63(20):2141-7.
24. Flaker GC, Eikelboom JW, Shestakovska O, et al. Bleeding during treatment with aspirin versus apixaban in patients with atrial fibrillation unsuitable for warfarin: the apixaban versus acetylsalicylic acid to prevent stroke in atrial fibrillation patients who have failed or are unsuitable for vitamin K antagonist treatment (AVERROES) trial. Stroke. 2012;43(12):3291-7.
25. Connolly SJ, Eikelboom J, Joyner C, et al. Apixaban in patients with atrial fibrillation. N Engl J Med. 2011;364(9):806-17.
26. Ruff CT, Giugliano RP, Braunwald E, et al. Association between edoxaban dose, concentration, anti-Factor Xa activity, and outcomes: an analysis of data from the randomised, double-blind ENGAGE AF-TIMI 48 trial. Lancet. 2015;385(9984):2288-95.
27. Camm AJ, Amarenco P, Haas S, et al. XANTUS: a real-world, prospective, observational study of patients treated with rivaroxaban for stroke prevention in atrial fibrillation. Eur Heart J. 2016;37(4):1145-53.
28. Pollack CV Jr, Reilly PA, van Ryn J, et al. Idarucizumab for Dabigatran Reversal - Full Cohort Analysis. N Engl J Med. 2017;377(5):431-41.

CHAPTER

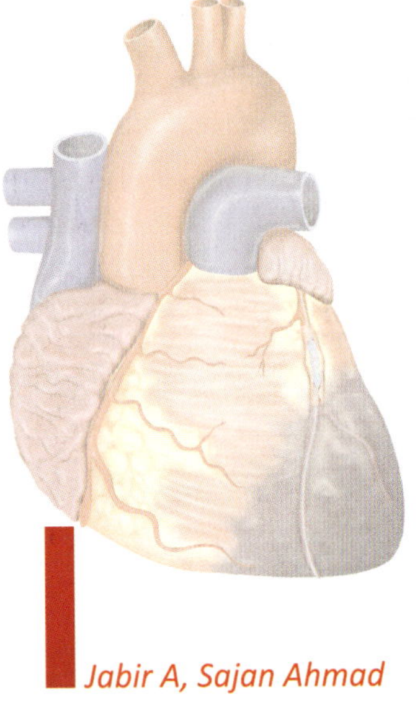

Low-molecular-weight Heparin in Acute Coronary Syndrome in Cardiodiabetes

Jabir A, Sajan Ahmad

INTRODUCTION

Diabetes mellitus is an established risk factor for cardiovascular disease (CVD). With the incidence of diabetes increasing in both urban and rural populations in India, the cardiologist is already facing the challenge of managing the "diabetic subset" of coronary artery disease (CAD) patients.

Coronary artery disease accounts for 75% of all deaths in patients with diabetes mellitus and approximately 20–25% of all patients with acute coronary syndromes (ACS)-UA/NSTEMI (unstable angina/non-ST-elevation myocardial infarction) have diabetes. Patients with UA/NSTEMI and diabetes have more severe CAD, and diabetes is an important independent predictor for adverse outcomes [death, myocardial infarction (MI), or readmission with UA at 1 year; RR 4.9]. Diabetic ACS patients, hence, are more likely to derive greater clinical benefit from optimal guideline directed medical therapy.[1]

DIABETES AND ACUTE CORONARY SYNDROME: THE INTERFACE

Patient-related factors and pathophysiologic factors interact to produce the clinical impact (Fig. 1).

Patient-related Factors

- *Age*: Diabetic patients with ACS may fall into the extremes of age, young patients with premature atherosclerosis, and older patients with diffuse or multivessel disease.
- *Gender*: Women with diabetes lose the so called "female advantage" in CAD. They tend to be older and are likely to have more severe forms of CAD.
- *Comorbidities*: Diabetic patients with ACS often have coexistent medical disorders that might require alteration in evaluation and management of CAD. Diabetic nephropathy is of course the most important among these. Dose modifications in pharmacotherapy may need to be done in this setting. Diabetic patients tend to have more noncoronary vascular comorbidities,

Diabetes – ACS interface

Patient	Pathophysiology
☐ Age	☐ Platelet
☐ Gender	☐ Coagulation
☐ Comoribidity	☐ Inflammation
☐ Risk category	☐ Vascular

Fig. 1: Interface between diabetes and acute coronary syndrome—patient-related factors and pathophysiologic factors influence the clinical outcome.

Abbreviations: ACS, acute coronary syndrome.

hypertension, left ventricular hypertrophy, cardiomyopathy, and heart failure.[2] Diabetic autonomic neuropathy can have adverse effects on heart rate and blood pressure regulation, and may also raise the threshold for perception of angina. Anemia is often seen in patients with chronic kidney disease (CKD).

- *Risk category*: Diabetes has a ubiquitous presence in all the risk-stratification scores in ACS. In the thrombolysis in myocardial infarction (TIMI) risk score for unstable angina/NSTEMI, diabetes is one among the major CAD risk factors. Diabetic patients undoubtedly belong to a high-risk group, and have more adverse events. On angiography, diabetic patients are more likely to have unstable, ulcerated plaques and more of intracoronary thrombi.[2]

Pathophysiologic Factors

- *Platelet activation*: The platelets in diabetes are more "active," with adhesion and aggregation occurring more robustly when compared to nondiabetic patients. Both insulin deficiency and insulin resistance increase platelet reactivity.[3]
- *Coagulation system*: Diabetes can promote a prothrombotic milieu, with higher concentrations of procoagulant factors and less active fibrinolytic systems. Diabetic patients have higher levels of circulating tissue factor (TF), fibrinogen, as well as elevated levels of factor VII.[4] Hyperglycemia is a stimulant for thrombin production.[5,6]
- *Inflammation*: Diabetes produces a state of chronic low grade inflammation, with elevated levels of IL-6.[7]
- *Vascular pathology*: Diabetic patients have abnormal macrovascular and microvascular systems. Endothelial response to vasodilatory stimuli is less.

ANTICOAGULATION IN ACUTE CORONARY SYNDROMES

The factors considered while choosing an anticoagulant in ACS are the established efficacy, safety (particularly bleeding risk), cost, ease of administration, comfort with dosage regimens, especially when intervention or surgical management is likely, and the desire to reverse the effect, should the need arise.

Unfractionated Heparin

It exerts its anticoagulant effect by accelerating the action of circulating antithrombin, a proteolytic enzyme that inactivates factor IIa (thrombin), factor IXa, and factor Xa. It prevents thrombus propagation but does not lyse existing thrombi. Unfractionated heparin (UFH) has got poorer bioavailability and marked variability in action that is probably related to its pharmacokinetic limitation of binding to plasma proteins and cells.[2] Target activated partial thromboplastin time (aPTT) should be 1.5- to 2.5-fold.[8] No dose adjustment is needed in CKD.

Low-molecular-weight Heparins

These are obtained through chemical or enzymatic depolymerization of the polysaccharide chains of heparin to provide chains with different molecular weight distributions. Low-molecular-weight heparin (LMWH) chains that are fewer than 18 saccharide units retain their ability to inactivate factor Xa but not thrombin. Therefore, LMWHs are relatively more potent in facilitating inhibition of factor Xa than in the inactivation of thrombin.[2]

Low-molecular-weight Heparin versus Unfractionated Heparin

The well-accepted benefits of LMWH over UFH include: Equivalent or superior efficacy, longer duration and more predictable action, lesser frequency of administration, less bleeding, less risk of heparin-induced thrombocytopenia–thrombosis, and no requirement for laboratory based monitoring of action. On the flip side, the cost is higher, LMWH requires dose reduction in diabetic nephropathy, and there is no effective antidote (unlike UFH which is cheap, does not require dose adjustment in renal dysfunction and has an effective antidote in the form of protamine).

Enoxaparin: Enoxaparin is the most commonly used LMWH. It is also the most studied LMWH in clinical trials. The dose is 1 mg/kg administered subcutaneously twice daily, but the dose is reduced to 1 mg/kg once daily, if estimated glomerular filtration rate (eGFR) is less than 30 mL/min/1.73 m^2. LMWH should not be administered, if eGFR is less than 15 mL/min/1.73 m^2.[9]

Fondaparinux: Fondaparinux is a synthetic pentasaccharide and has an established role in the management of ACS, except in patients undergoing an interventional procedure (due to a higher risk of catheter-related thrombosis when fondaparinux is used as the sole agent for anticoagulation). Ease of administration (subcutaneous, once daily) and less bleeding risk, especially in the elderly diabetic confer special advantages. However, it must not be used in patients with advanced diabetic nephropathy with a creatinine clearance (CrCl) of less than 30 mL/min.

DATA FROM MAJOR TRIALS

- *ExTRACT TIMI 25 Trial* (effect of enoxaparin versus UFH in diabetic patients with STEMI in the enoxaparin and thrombolysis in myocardial infarction study 25):[10] Among 20,479 patients with STEMI treated with fibrinolysis and randomized to enoxaparin or UFH, 3,060 patients (15%) had diabetes. Patients with diabetes were older, more likely to be women and presented more often with heart failure. Superior net clinical benefit was found with enoxaparin, with less mortality (9.5% vs 11.8%) and death/MI/urgent revascularization (16% vs 19.7%). However, there was a trend toward higher major bleeding (2.6% vs 1.6%).
- *ENTIRE TIMI 23 Trial* (enoxaparin as adjunctive antithrombin therapy for ST-elevation myocardial infarction):[11]

  In patients with STEMI who were thrombolysed with tenecteplase, enoxaparin was associated with similar TIMI 3 flow rates as UFH, with better reduction in ischemic events at similar risk of major hemorrhage. The 14% of patients in this study had diabetes.
- *INTERACT Trial* (randomized evaluation of the safety and efficacy of enoxaparin versus UFH in high-risk patients with non-ST-segment elevation ACS receiving glycoprotein IIb/IIIa inhibitor eptifibatide):[12]

  About 22.1% of the patients randomized to enoxaparin in this study were diabetic. Enoxaparin produced less ischemia (14.3% vs 25.4%), and death or MI (5% vs 9%) compared to UFH. Major noncoronary artery bypass grafting (non-CABG) related bleeding was lower in the enoxaparin group (1.8% vs 4.6%); however, minor bleeding was more in the enoxaparin group.
- *OASIS 5 Trial (fifth organization to assess strategies in ischemic syndromes)*:[13]

  About 25% of patients in this study were diabetic. Fondaparinux reduced major bleeding (5.2% vs 8.3%) and had similar ischemic events, thereby demonstrating an improved net clinical outcome compared to enoxaparin.

SPECIAL CONSIDERATIONS FOR ENOXAPARIN USE

- *Diabetic nephropathy on hemodialysis*: Enoxaparin at therapeutic doses may be as safe and effective as intravenous UFH. However, in patients not on dialysis, the dose clearly depends on the renal function and should be reduced to approximately 64% of the usual dose in patients with CrCl less than 30 mL/min.[14,15]
- *Elderly diabetic*: No specific dose modification is recommended with enoxaparin, although consideration of bleeding risk is essential.
- *Hepatic impairment*: No specific dose modification is required.
- *Pregnancy*: Enoxaparin does not cross the placenta, and is safe for the fetus.[16]

CONCLUSION

Low-molecular-weight heparin has a pivotal role in the management of diabetic patients with ACS. The efficacy and safety has been well-established in randomized clinical trials with a sizeable diabetic population. Since diabetic patients are a high-risk subset, the expected benefit of treatment is also likely to be more robust. A patient-centric and balanced approach to anticoagulation, considering the benefits, risks and the effect of comorbidities in diabetes is of paramount importance.

REFERENCES

1. Amin AP, Marso SP. Acute coronary syndrome in the patient with diabetes: is the management different? Curr Cardiol Rep. 2010;12(4):321-9.
2. Anderson JL, Adams CD, Antman EM, et al. 2012 ACCF/AHA focused update incorporated into the ACCF/AHA 2007 guidelines for the management of patients with unstable angina/non-ST-elevation myocardial infarction. Circulation. 2013;127(23):e663-e828.
3. Schneider DJ. Factors contributing to increased platelet reactivity in people with diabetes. Diabetes Care. 2009;32(4):525-7.
4. Boden G, Vaidyula VR, Homko C, et al. Circulating tissue factor procoagulant activity and thrombin generation in patients with type 2 diabetes: effects of insulin and glucose. J Clin Endocrinol Metab. 2007;92(11):4352-8.
5. Undas A, Wiek I, Stepien E, et al. Hyperglycemia is associated with enhanced thrombin formation, platelet activation, and fibrin clot resistance to lysis in patients with acute coronary syndrome. Diabetes Care. 2008;31(8):1590-5.
6. Klein RL, Hunter SJ, Jenkins AJ, et al. Fibrinogen is a marker for nephropathy and peripheral vascular disease in type 1 diabetes: studies of plasma fibrinogen and fibrinogen gene polymorphism in the DCCT/EDIC cohort. Diabetes Care. 2003;26(5):1439-48.
7. Ajjan R, Grant PJ. Coagulation and atherothrombotic disease. Atherosclerosis. 2006;186(2):240-59.
8. Harenberg J. Past, present and future perspectives of heparins in clinical settings and the role of impaired renal function. Int J Card. 2016;212(Suppl 1):S10-13.
9. Roffi M, Patrono C, Collet JP, et al. 2015 ESC guidelines for the management of acute coronary syndromes in patients presenting without persistent ST-segment elevation: task force for the Management of Acute Coronary Syndromes in Patients Presenting

without Persistent ST-Segment Elevation of the European Society of Cardiology (ESC). Eur Heart J. 2016;37(3):267-315.
10. Morrow DA, Antman EM, Murphy MA, et al. Effect of enoxaparin versus unfractionated heparin in diabetic patients with ST-elevation myocardial infarction in the ExTRACT TIMI 25 trial. Am Heart J. 2007;154(6):1078-84.
11. Antman EM, Louwerenburg HW, Baars HF, et al. Enoxaparin as adjunctive antithrombin therapy for ST-elevation myocardial infarction: results of the ENTIRE TIMI 23 Trial. Circulation. 2002;105(14):1642-9.
12. Fitchett D, Goodman SG, Armstrong PW, et al. Randomized evaluation of the safety and efficacy of enoxaparin versus unfractionated heparin in high-risk patients with non-ST-segment elevation acute coronary syndromes receiving the glycoprotein IIb/IIIa inhibitor eptifibatide. Circulation. 2003;107(2):238-44.
13. Jolly SS, Faxon DP, Fox KA, et al. Efficacy and safety of fondaparinux versus enoxaparin in patients with acute coronary syndromes treated with glycoprotein IIb/IIIa inhibitors or thienopyridines. J Am Coll Cardiol. 2009;54(5):468-76.
14. Pon TK, Dager WE, Roberts AJ, et al. Subcutaneous enoxaparin for therapeutic anticoagulation in hemodialysis patients. Thromb Res. 2014;133(6):1023-8.
15. Collet J, Montalescot G, Choussat R, et al. Enoxaparin in unstable angina patients with renal failure. Int J Card. 2001;80(1):81-2.
16. Brenner B. Enoxaparin use in pregnancy: state of the art. Women's Health. 2007;3(1):9-14.

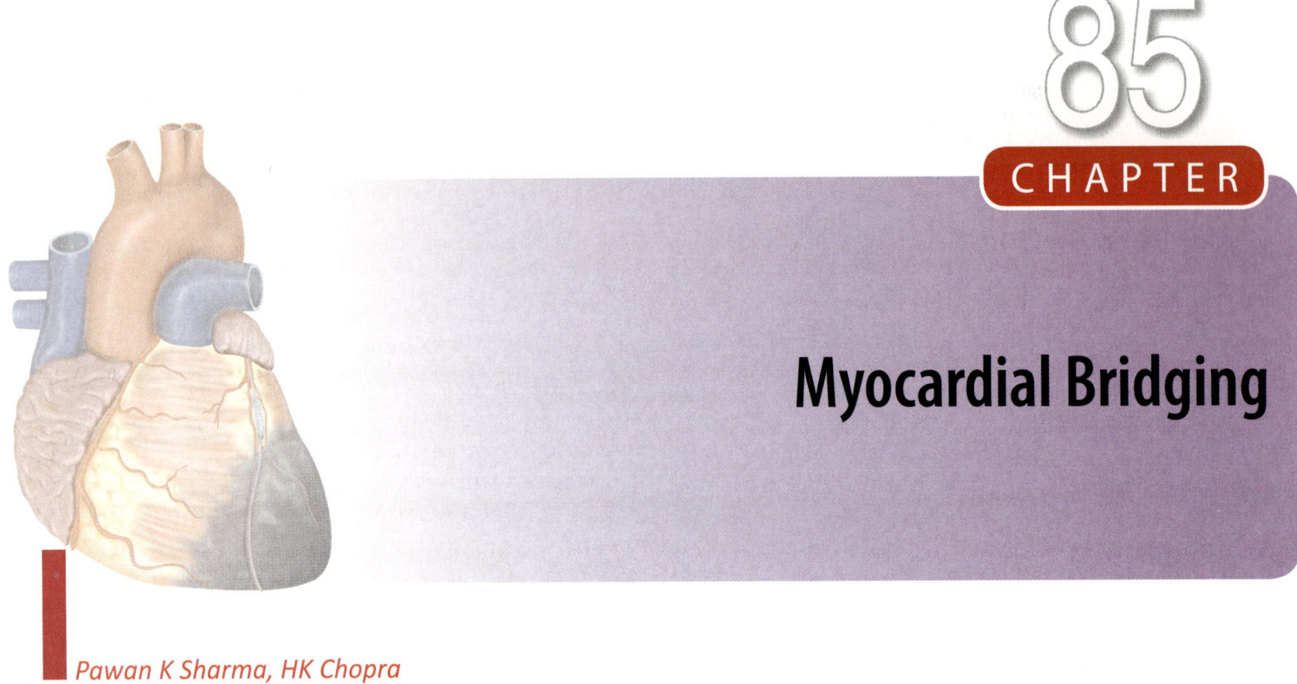

85

CHAPTER

Myocardial Bridging

Pawan K Sharma, HK Chopra

INTRODUCTION

Usually, the coronary arteries are epicardial but in myocardial bridging a segment of the coronary artery takes a "tunneled" intramuscular course under a "bridge" of overlying myocardium.[1] Myocardial bridge affects left anterior descending (LAD) artery most commonly and occurs in 67–98% cases.[2,3] The middle segment of LAD is most frequently affected.[1] Other arteries such as diagonal (18%) and marginal (40%) branches may also be involved.[4] One of the initial angiographic imaging of myocardial bridge was described by Portsmann in 1960.[5] Other diagnostic modalities such as coronary computed tomographic angiography (CCTA),[6] intravascular ultrasound (IVUS),[7] intracoronary Doppler,[8] and fractional flow reserve (FFR)[9] provide better analysis of the anatomic and hemodynamic consequences of the systolic compression, including effects on coronary flow.[10] Despite these advancements, treatment options remain limited.

PREVALENCE

Prevalence rates of myocardial bridging differ based on the mode of evaluation. Angiographically reported rates of bridging vary from 0.5% to 12%.[11] Higher rates varying from 5% to 86%, with a mean of 25% have been reported in autopsy series compared to angiographically reported bridging.[4] The autopsy series and CCTA studies[6,12] find myocardial bridges at similar rates. Patients with hypertrophic cardiomyopathy[13,14] and heart transplant[15] have higher rates of myocardial bridging than the general population.

MORPHOLOGY

Ferreira et al.[16] described two subtypes of myocardial bridges:

1. *Superficial bridging less than 2 mm* occurs in approximately 75% of cases. It involves LAD situated in the intraventricular groove and crossed by a muscle bundle perpendicularly or at an acute angle. Systolic compression of the superficial subtype occurs only infrequently.
2. In the *deep bridging greater than 2 mm*, LAD deviates toward the right ventricle and dips into the intraventricular septum. The overlying longitudinal muscle bundle arises from the right ventricular apex and crosses the tunneled segment transversely, obliquely or helically before terminating in the intraventricular segment.[16] This orientation and degree of overlying bridging in the deep variant results in twisting of the tunneled segment over the course of the cardiac cycle, resulting in hemodynamic compromise during coronary flow.

Another subset of myocardial bridging is known as the *myocardial loop*, in which an epicardial vessel (artery or vein) runs through a segment of atrial myocardium.[17] Myocardial loops are usually 10–15 mm long and 0.1–0.3 mm thick, typically involving the distal left circumflex (LCX) and distal right coronary artery (RCA).[18] Because of the shorter and thinner size compared to ventricular tunnels and the minimal compression exerted by atrial muscle, these loops are without much clinical consequence.

Myocardial bridges may range from 0.3 mm to 28 mm in depth.[2,19] Typical myocardial bridge depth is 1–10 mm, with length of 10–30 mm.[7] There does not appear to be a difference in prevalence of bridging by gender or age. Bridges greater than 5 mm deep are less amenable to surgical myotomy.[20]

PATHOPHYSIOLOGY OF ISCHEMIA

As majority of coronary filling occurs in diastole, systolic compression of the artery should have only a minimal impact on total effective myocardial perfusion.[21] Studies using quantitative coronary angiography (QCA) along with IVUS, have shown that vessel compression of bridged arteries extend into mid to late diastole and thus affect the predominant phase of coronary perfusion.[22-24] In symptomatic bridging, combined angiography with intracoronary Doppler flow and pressure measurements show hemodynamic abnormalities characterized by a persistent decrease in diastolic vessel diameter, increase in blood flow velocities and retrograde flow, and a reduced flow reserve.[25] The diameter of the intramuscular segment is smaller compared to the adjacent proximal segment overall, and during diastole there is a persistent reduction of 34–51% in the bridged segment.[8] In addition, the greater the systolic narrowing, the greater the reduction in diastolic diameter, associated with a corresponding decrease in flow and flow reserve. A scoring system has been proposed to quantify the degree of systolic narrowing (Table 1).[26] A usual score varies from 2 to 5, with a score of 5 being the most severe.

In 90% cases, the vessel segment proximal to the bridge develops atherosclerosis.[7] Expression of vasoactive agents endothelial nitric oxide synthase, endothelin-1, and angiotensin-converting enzyme are all increased in the proximal segment.[27] The intramural and distal segments of bridged vessels remain free from atherosclerotic disease.[7,28]

TABLE 1: Scoring system to quantify degree of systolic narrowing

	Score
Systolic narrowing	
<50%	1
50–75%	2
>75%	3
Length of compressed segment	
<1 cm	1
>1 cm	2

Biomechanical forces may explain these observations. Low and oscillatory wall shear stress (WSS) are associated with increased expression of vascular cell adhesion molecule 1[29,30] and reactive oxygen species production[31] as well as development of a proatherogenic endothelial cell phenotype.[32] Another proposed mechanism of plaque formation proximal to a myocardial bridge involves solid mechanical forces that result from the motion and deformity of the coronary tree and myocardial material properties. Specifically, compression within the bridge and severe vessel angulation at the junction of the bridge result in a heterogeneous stress field in the proximal segment. The induced stresses are hypothesized to be conducive to plaque development and possible fissuring in the proximal segment.[33] It is still not well-understood that despite the presence of low WSS, why the segment distal to myocardial bridge is spared from atherosclerosis.

Histology shows that the intima of the tunneled segment is significantly thinner than the proximal segment, and contains a predominance of the "contractile" subtype of smooth muscle cells thought to be negatively associated with the development of atherosclerotic lesions.[34] Foam cells, an important component of atherosclerosis, also appeared to be missing in the tunneled segments.[35] In addition, the expression of known vasoactive agents endothelial nitric oxide synthase, endothelin-1, and angiotensin-converting enzyme is reduced in the bridged vessel wall.[27] These agents have been implicated in the proliferation of smooth cells resulting in increased size of atherosclerotic lesions. Systolic kinking of the bridged segments, coupled with the afore mentioned endothelial dysfunction, may also predispose to coronary vasospasm and thrombus formation.[36]

CLINICAL PRESENTATION

Myocardial bridging can be an incidental finding on angiography or autopsy. Symptomatic patients with myocardial bridging can present with myocardial ischemia,[37] acute coronary syndrome,[38-40] coronary spasm,[37,41] exercise-induced dysrhythmias such as supraventricular tachycardia,[40] ventricular tachycardia[42,43] or atrioventricular conduction block,[44] myocardial stunning,[45] transient ventricular dysfunction,[46] syncope[40,43] or even sudden death.[47,48]

Following pathophysiological changes can induce symptoms of myocardial ischemia in previously asymptomatic patients (Figs 1A and B).

- Aging, hypertension, and coronary atherosclerosis by increasing left ventricular diastolic dysfunction can exacerbate the supply-demand mismatch imposed by the bridge.

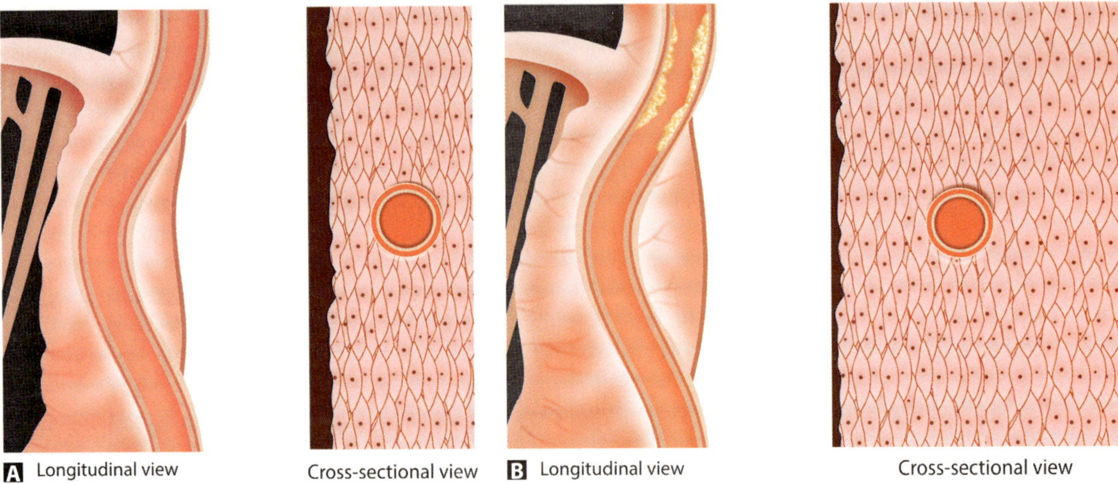

Figs 1A and B: Effects of aging on the myocardial bridging: (A) Early stage, (B) Late stage

Source: Adapted from Corban MT, Hung OY, Eshtehardi P, et al. Myocardial bridging: contemporary understanding of pathophysiology with implications for diagnostic and therapeutic strategies. J Am Coll Cardiol. 2014;63:2346-55.

- Development of left ventricular hypertrophy can increase compression and reduce the coronary microvascular reserve.
- Coronary vasospasm, microvascular dysfunction, or endothelial dysfunction.
- Plaque development proximal to the bridge can augment coronary obstruction by the bridge.
- The negative remodeling within the bridge can reduce myocardial flow.

DIAGNOSTIC TESTING

Noninvasive Diagnostic Techniques

Multiple-slice computed tomography (MSCT), stress single-photon emission computed tomography and stress echocardiography have been used in the diagnosis of myocardial bridging. Physiological assessment by MSCT may enhance its diagnostic utility for identifying hemodynamically significant bridges. In patients with myocardial bridging, the severity of reversible myocardial perfusion defects on stress single-photon emission computed tomography is proportional to the degree of systolic luminal narrowing.[49,50] However, myocardial perfusion imaging does not appear to have the sensitivity required to adequately identify myocardial bridging.[49,51] Stress echo has been proposed as a noninvasive functional test for myocardial bridging. Lin et al., identified septal wall motion abnormalities on two-dimensional imaging in 14 patients with IVUS and FFR proven bridging.[52] Contrast stress echocardiography has been used for detection of myocardial bridging but is not as well validated.[53] Further studies will be necessary to improve and validate these techniques before they can be accepted as a method for the diagnosis of bridging.

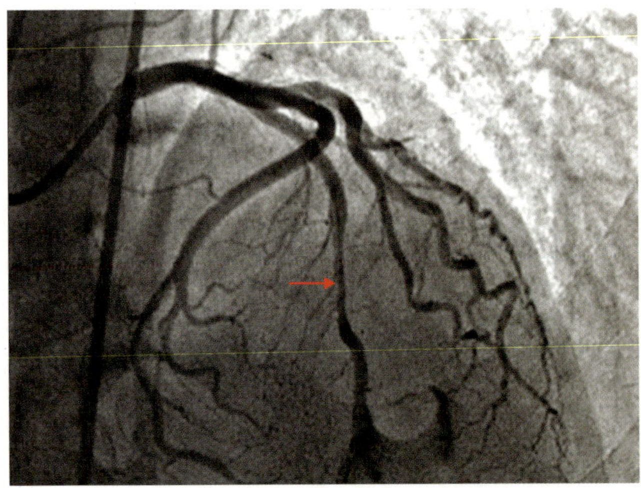

Fig. 2: Systolic compression of the myocardial bridge (red arrow)

Invasive Diagnostic Techniques

Coronary Angiography

Coronary angiography remains the most common technique for diagnosing myocardial bridging (Fig. 2). Bridging involves a systolic narrowing, or "milking" of an epicardial artery, with a "step-down" and "step-up" demarcating the impacted area. For significant "milking effect" to be present there is greater than or equal to 70%

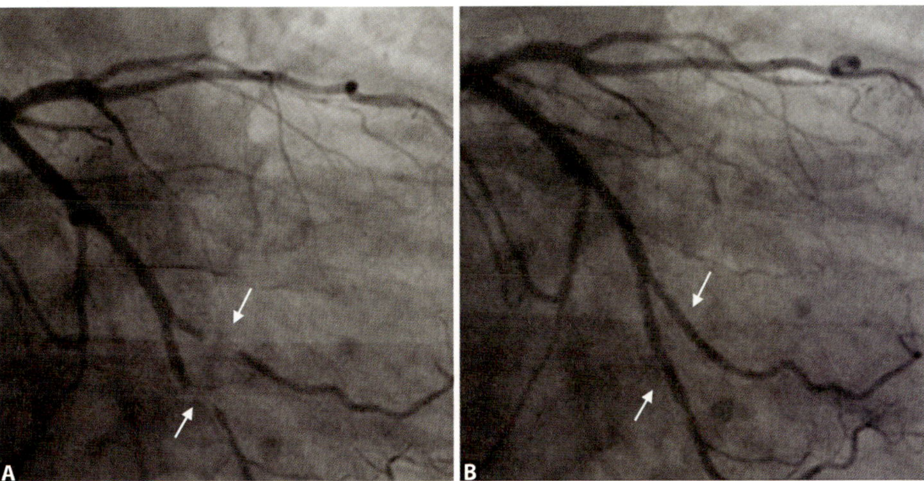

Figs 3A and B: Milking effect on coronary angiography: white arrows indicate areas of myocardial bridging. (A) Systolic compression "the milking effect", (B) Increase in vessel lumen diameter during diastole

Source: Adapted from Corban MT, Hung OY, Eshtehardi P, et al. Myocardial bridging: contemporary understanding of pathophysiology with implications for diagnostic and therapeutic strategies. J Am Coll Cardiol. 2014;63:2346-55.

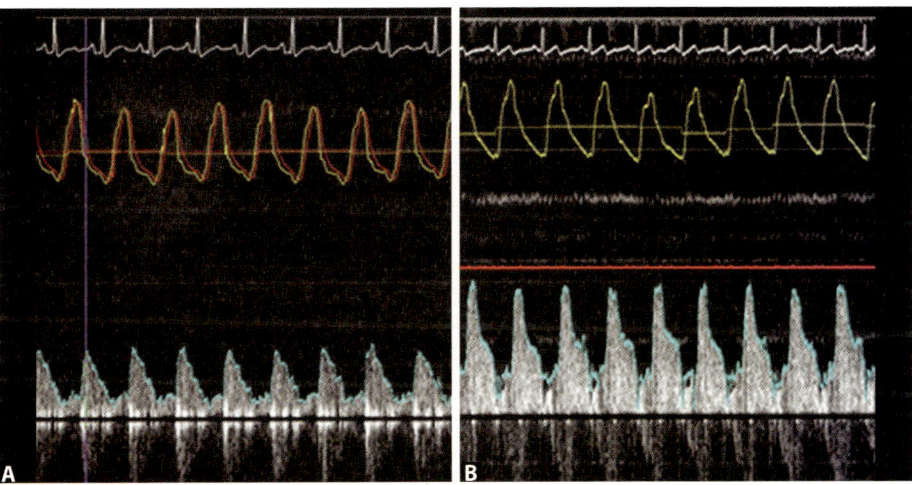

Figs 4A and B: Fingertip phenomenon during intracoronary Doppler measurements. (A) Normal flow pattern. (B) Fingertip phenomenon showing abrupt early diastolic acceleration, rapid mid-diastolic deceleration and mid-to-late diastolic plateau

Source: Adapted from Corban MT, Hung OY, Eshtehardi P, et al. Myocardial bridging: contemporary understanding of pathophysiology with implications for diagnostic and therapeutic strategies. J Am Coll Cardiol. 2014;63:2346-55.

reduction in minimal luminal diameter during systole and persistent greater than or equal to 35% reduction in minimal luminal diameter during mid-to-late diastole (Figs 3A and B).[48]

Intracoronary Doppler

Doppler-tipped guidewires allow accurate measurement of intracoronary flow velocity.[47] Myocardial bridges reveal a characteristic "spike-and-dome" pattern or "fingertip" phenomenon, with abrupt early diastolic flow acceleration, rapid mid-diastolic flow deceleration, and a mid-to-late diastolic plateau.[25] Retrograde flow during the systolic period can be detected immediately proximal to the bridged segment, exacerbated by nitroglycerin provocation, especially in deep bridges (Figs 4A and B).[54]

Intravascular Ultrasound

On IVUS, the tunneled segment of artery demonstrates systolic compression that persists into diastole. There is also a highly specific echolucent "half-moon" appearance

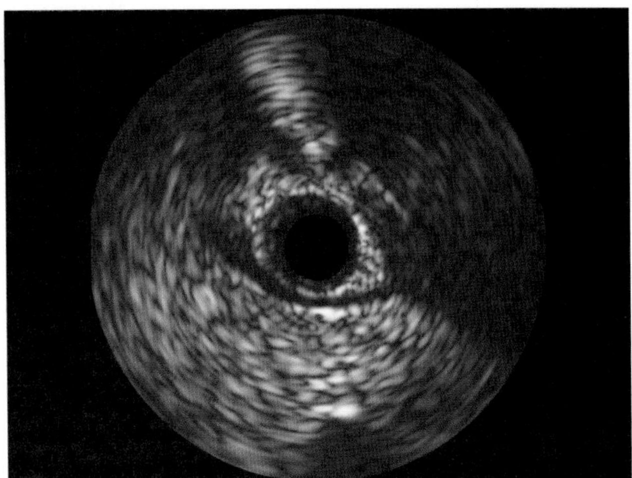

Fig. 5: Intravascular ultrasound "half-moon sign"

Source: Adapted from Corban MT, Hung OY, Eshtehardi P, et al. Myocardial bridging: contemporary understanding of pathophysiology with implications for diagnostic and therapeutic strategies. J Am Coll Cardiol. 2014;63:2346-55.

throughout the cardiac cycle, the etiology of which is not well understood (Fig. 5).[7] IVUS can detect vessel compression with coronary provocation testing even in the absence of angiographically significant "milking".[24] In patients with de novo LAD artery lesions, IVUS-detected bridging in 23% of patients, while angiographic bridging was noted only in 3% of patients.[55]

Fractional Flow Reserve

In 12 patients with LAD artery bridging on angiography, Escaned et al. measured FFR both at baseline and with dobutamine provocation.[9] The mean FFR decreased to a lesser extent (0.90 down to 0.84) and there was significant decrease in diastolic FFR (0.88 down to 0.77). It is thought that mean FFR measurement are artifactually elevated by overshooting of systolic pressures, and thus diastolic FFR evaluation should be the technique of choice. Dobutamine provocation appears to be more accurate when compared with adenosine for FFR evaluation of bridging, highlighting the importance of inotropic state in the development of vessel compression.[56]

Cardiac Computed Tomography Angiography

Computed tomography (CT) angiography detects anatomical myocardial bridging at much higher rates than by angiography.[6,12,57,58] Since CT provides structural information rather than functional information, further correlation is required to determine clinical relevance. CT based noninvasive FFR may provide useful information for combined anatomical/hemodynamic study of myocardial bridge, but such application has not yet been reported.[59]

SPECIAL PATIENT POPULATIONS

Patients with hypertrophic cardiomyopathy have high prevalence of myocardial bridging, with rates up to 80% on angiography.[60] Multiple studies in children with hypertrophic obstructive cardiomyopathy (HOCM) and myocardial bridging have greater rates of chest pain, ventricular tachycardia, history of resuscitated cardiac arrest, and positive changes on exercise testing.[61] Interestingly, this relationship does not hold in the adult population. In a series of 425 adult patients with hypertrophic cardiomyopathy with (15%) and without (85%) myocardial bridging, there was no difference in all-cause mortality and cardiac death at 6.8 year follow-up.[14] An autopsy study of 255 patients with sudden cardiac death, did not find an independent contribution of myocardial bridging to mortality in patients with hypertrophic cardiomyopathy, despite occurring at a higher prevalence.[62] Orthotopic heart transplantation patients also have higher prevalence of myocardial bridging. In a series of 64 heart transplant recipients, 33% were found to have angiographically significant bridging.[15] This was thought to be related to the increased stiffness and hypertrophy of the myocardium post-transplant, resulting in increased rates of systolic vessel compression. While the presence of bridging was previously thought to be a risk factor for early death after cardiac transplantation,[63] more recent experience[64,65] suggests that this may not be the case.

PROGNOSIS

Generally, myocardial bridging is considered a benign condition, but it has also been proposed as a cause of angina-like chest pain, coronary spasm, myocardial ischemia, acute coronary syndromes, left ventricular dysfunction/stunning, arrhythmias (including supraventricular tachycardia and ventricular tachycardia), and even sudden cardiac death. Schwartz has proposed a classification scheme for myocardial bridging based on symptoms as well as noninvasive and invasive measurement of hemodynamic and anatomical parameters in order to guide therapy (Table 2).[66] While some data exist on the long-term follow up of patients with myocardial bridging,[67] there is lack of studies that establish the natural history of the condition in response to intervention to validate such a classification scheme.

TABLE 2: Schwartz's classification scheme and therapeutic strategy for myocardial bridging[66]

	Clinical symptoms	*Signs of ischemia*	*Initial treatment strategy*	*Secondary treatment, if no improvement*
Type A	Yes	No (incidental finding on angiography)	Reassurance	–
Type B	Yes	Yes, by noninvasive stress test	Beta-blockers[b]	Intracoronary hemodynamic evaluation[a] → surgery or stenting, if abnormal
Type C	Yes	Yes, by altered intracoronary hemo-dynamics[a]	Beta-blockers[b]	Surgery or stenting

[a]By quantitative coronary arteriography, fractional flow reserve (FFR) or intracoronary Doppler.
[b]If beta-blockers are contraindicated, non-dihydropyridine calcium-channel blockers can be used.

TREATMENT

Medical Therapy

For patients experiencing symptoms due to myocardial bridging, first-line therapy consists of beta-blockers[68,69] and non-dihydropyridine calcium-channel blockers.[70] There is limited evidence to support their use, and rationale is based on theoretical improvement in coronary hemodynamics with decreased chronotropy and inotropy. It is thought that the prolongation of diastole with reduction in heart rate and reduced chronotropy with exercise is a major contributor to reduction in symptoms. But while beta-blockade has been shown to decrease vessel compression and improve angina symptoms, no studies have ever evaluated clinical endpoints of morbidity and mortality.[68] Nitrates are contraindicated in patients with myocardial bridging. Nitroglycerin has shown to accentuate systolic compression of bridged segments and vasodilating segments proximal to the bridge and thereby, reducing the myocardial ischemia.[7,54] It is used as an agent for provocation of these lesions.[71] This effect likely relates to an increase in vessel wall compliance, as well as a reflex sympathetic increase in contractility.[54]

Surgery

Surgical options for myocardial bridging include surgical myotomy and coronary artery bypass graft surgery. Surgical myotomy involving resection of the overlying muscle fibers should be limited to patients with refractory symptoms despite medical therapy, especially in those with demonstrated inducible ischemia and those who are at high risk for myocardial infarction, ventricular tachycardia, or resuscitated cardiac arrest. Surgical myotomy has been shown to eliminate symptoms[72,73] and increase coronary flow.[74] However, risks include dissection into the right ventricle in patients with myocardial bridges that take a deep subendocardial course.[75] Coronary artery bypass graft surgery has been reported as a treatment for bridging, and typically involves anastomosis of the left internal mammary artery to the LAD artery.[20,76] Both techniques, surgical myotomy and coronary artery bypass graft surgery for myocardial bridging show excellent symptom relief, with no surgical complications reported.[19,77,78] Despite the risk of graft occlusion in the presence of competitive flow, there were no graft failures when followed up to 35 months. Coronary artery bypass grafting can be considered a treatment option for myocardial bridging, especially in extensive and deep bridges.

Percutaneous Coronary Intervention

The first case of coronary stenting for severe myocardial bridging refractory to medical therapy was reported in 1995 by Stables et al.[79] Stenting can resolve hemodynamic abnormalities and symptoms[34] but some studies have shown high rates of target lesion revascularization. In a study of 70 patients with myocardial bridging who received stents [primarily drug-eluting stents (DES)], for a LAD artery lesion proximal to the bridge, rate of target vessel revascularization at 1 year were much higher (24% vs 3%) in patients whose stent extended into the bridged segment.[80] Another study reported target lesion revascularization rate of 36% (4 out of 11) in a group of patients receiving bare-metal stents specifically for symptomatic myocardial bridging, despite significant improvements in the minimal luminal area (from 0.6 mm^2 to 1.9 mm^2) and cross-sectional area (from 3.3 mm^2 to 6.8 mm^2) at the time of stenting.[87] Complications like coronary perforation[81-84] and stent fracture[85,86] in a stented myocardial bridge could be related to stent oversizing. As with surgical intervention, percutaneous coronary intervention should only be considered as a therapeutic option in patients with bridging refractory to medical therapy, with the expectation that revascularization rates will be high even with drug-eluting stents.

CONCLUSION

Myocardial bridging is a congenital anomaly in which an epicardial coronary artery takes an intramyocardial course. It is detectable angiographically in less than 10% of patients whereas anatomically it is noted in approximately 25% of patients based on autopsy and CT. Flow alterations can cause accelerated atherosclerosis in the coronary segment immediately proximal to the bridged segment. The bridged portion itself is "spared" from atherosclerosis, likely through favorable shear forces resulting in increased expression of vasoactive agents as well as morphological changes in endothelial and smooth muscle cells in the area. Hemodynamic effects of bridging include systolic flow reversal proximal to the bridge, as well as a decrease in coronary flow reserve. Clinical consequences range from angina to acute coronary syndrome to sudden cardiac death. First-line therapy involves medical treatment with beta-blockers and non-dihydropyridine calcium channel blockers, while nitrates are contraindicated due to secondary tachycardia and hypercontractility from reflex sympathetic activation. For refractory symptom, multiple interventional strategies have been attempted such as surgical myotomy, coronary artery bypass surgery, and stenting. A prospective randomized trial is required to identify the best treatment strategy for patients with myocardial bridging.

REFERENCES

1. Angelni P, Velasco JA, Flamm S. Coronary anomalies: incidence, pathophysiology, and clinical relevance. Circulation. 2002;105(20):2449-54.
2. Loukas M, Curry B, Bowers M, et al. The relationship of myocardial bridges to coronary artery dominance in the adult human heart. J Anat. 2006;209(1):43-50.
3. Qian JY, Zhang F, Dong M, et al. Prevalence and characteristics of myocardial bridging in coronary angiogram: data from consecutive 5525 patients. Chin Med J (Engl). 2009;122(6):632-35.
4. Mohlenkamp S, Hart W, Ge J, et al. Update on myocardial bridging. Circulation. 2002;106:2616-22.
5. Portsmann W, Iwig J. Die intramurale koronarie im angiogramm. Fortschr Geb Rontgenstr Nuklearmed. 1960;92:129-32.
6. Konen E, Goitein O, Sternik L, et al. The prevalence and anatomical patterns of intramuscular coronary arteries: a coronary computed tomography angiographic study. J Am Coll Cardiol. 2007;49(5):587-93.
7. Ge J, Jeremias A, Rupp A, et al. New signs characteristic of myocardial bridging demonstrated by intracoronary ultrasound and Doppler. Eur Heart J. 1999;20(23):1701-16.
8. Schwarz ER, Klues HG, vom Dahl J, et al. Functional characteristics of myocardial bridging: a combined angiographic and intracoronary Doppler flow study. Eur Heart J. 1997;18(3):434-42.
9. Escaned J, Cortes J, Flores A, et al. Importance of diastolic fractional flow reserve and dobutamine challenge in physiologic assessment of myocardial bridging. J Am Coll Cardiol. 2003;42:226-33.
10. Alegria JR, Herrmann J, Holmes DR Jr, et al. Myocardial bridging. Eur Heart J. 2005;26(12):1159-68.
11. Soran O, Pamir G, Erol C, et al. The incidence and significance of myocardial bridge in a prospectively defined population of patients undergoing coronary angiography for chest pain. Tokai J Exp Clin Med. 2000;25(2):57-60.
12. La Grutta L, Runza G, Lo Re G, et al. Prevalence of myocardial bridging and correlation with coronary atherosclerosis studies with 64-slice CT coronary angiography. Radiol Med. 2009;114(7):1024-36.
13. Mohiddin SA, Begley D, Shin J, et al. Myocardial bridging does not predict sudden death in children with hypertrophic cardiomyopathy but is associated with more severe cardiac disease. J Am Coll Cardiol. 2000;36:2270-8.
14. Sorajja P, Ommen SR, Nishimura RA, et al. Myocardial bridging in adult patients with hypertrophic cardiomyopathy. J Am Coll Cardiol. 2003;42(5): 889-94.
15. Wymore P, Yedlicka JW, Garcia-Medina V, et al. The incidence of myocardial bridges in heart transplants. Cardiovasc Intervent Radiol. 1989;12(4):202-6.
16. Ferreira AG, Trotter SE, Konig B, et al. Myocardial bridges: morphological and functional aspects. Br Heart J. 1991;66(5):364-7.
17. Polacek P, Kralove H. Relation of myocardial bridges and loops on the coronary arteries to coronary occlusions. Am Heart J. 1961;61(1):44-52.
18. Giampalmo A, Bronzini E, Bandini T. Sulla minor compromissione aterosclerotica delle arterie coronarie quando siano (per variante anatomica) in situazione intramiocardica. Giornale Ital Arterioscl. 1964;2:1-14.
19. Wu QY, Xu ZH. Surgical treatment of myocardial bridging: report of 31 cases. Chin Med J. 2007;120(19):1689-93.
20. Attaran S, Moscarelli M, Athanasiou T, et al. Is coronary artery bypass grafting an acceptable alternative to myotomy for the treatment of myocardial bridging? Interact Cardiovasc Thorac Surg. 2013;16(3):347-49.
21. Marcus JT, Smeenk HG, Juijer JP, et al. Flow profiles in the left anterior descending and the right coronary artery assessed by MR velocity quantification: effects of through-plane and in-plane motion of the heart. J. Comput Assist Tomogr. 1999;23(4):567-76.
22. Erbel R, Rupprecht HJ, Ge J, et al. Coronary artery shape and flow changes induced by myocardial bridging. Assessment by intravascular ultrasound. Echocardiography. 1993;10(1): 71-7.
23. Bourassa MG, Butnaru A, Lesperance J, et al. Symptomatic myocardial bridges: overview of ischemic mechanisms and current diagnostic and treatment strategies. J Am Coll Cardiol. 2003;41(3):351-9.
24. Ge J, Erbel R, Rupprecht HJ, et al. Comparison of intravascular ultrasound and angiography in the assessment of myocardial bridging. Circulation. 1994;89(4):1725-32.
25. Klues HG, Schwarz ER, vom Dahl, et al. Disturbed intracoronary hemodynamics in myocardial bridging. Early normalization by intracoronary stent placement. Circulation. 1997;96(9):2905-13.
26. Angelini P, Tivellato M, Donis J, et al. Myocardial bridges: a review. Prog Cardiovasc Dis. 1983;26(1):75-88.
27. Masuda T, Ishikawa Y, Akasaka Y, et al. The effect of myocardial bridging of the coronary artery on vasoactive agents and atherosclerosis localization. J Pathol. 2001;193(3):408-14.
28. Ishikawa Y, Akasaka Y, Suzuki K, et al. Anatomic properties of myocardial bridge predisposing to myocardial infarction. Circulation. 2009;120(5):376-83.
29. Cheng C, Tempel D, van Haperen R, et al. Atherosclerotic lesion size and vulnerability are determined by patterns of fluid shear stress. Circulation. 2006;113(23):2744-53.
30. Walpola PL, Gotlieb AI, Cybulsky MI, et al. Expression of ICAM-1 and VCAM-1 and monocyte adherence in arteries exposed to altered shear stress. Arterioscler Thromb Vasc Biol. 1995;15(1):2-10.
31. McNally JS, Davis ME, Giddens DP, et al. Role of xanthine oxidoreductase and NAD(P)H oxidase in endothelial superoxide production in response to oscillatory shear stress. Am J Physiol Heart Circ Physiol. 2003;285(6):H2290-7.
32. Malek AM, Alper SL, Izumo S. Hemodynamic shear stress and its role in atherosclerosis. JAMA. 1999;282:2035-42.
33. Ge J, Erbel R, Gorge G, et al. High wall shear stress proximal to myocardial bridging and atherosclerosis: intracoronary ultrasound and pressure measurements. Br Heart J. 1995;73(5):462-5.

34. Risse M, Weiler G. Die koronare Muskelbrucke und ihre Beziehung zu lokaler Koronarsklerose, regionaler Myokardischamie und Koronarspasmus. Eine morphometrische Studie. Z Kardiol. 1985;74:700-5.
35. Ishil T, Asuwa N, Masuda S, et al. The effects of a myocardial bridge on coronary atherosclerosis and ischaemia. J Pathol. 1998;185(1):4-9.
36. Ciampricotti R, el Gamal M. Vasospastic coronary occlusion associated with a myocardial bridge. Cathet Cardiovasc Diagn. 1988;14(2):118-20.
37. Berry JF, von Mering GO, Schmalfuss C, et al. Systolic compression of the left anterior descending coronary artery: a case series, review of literature, and therapeutic options including stenting. Catheter Cardiovasc Interv. 2002;56(1):58-63.
38. Gowda RM, Khan IA, Ansari AW, et al. Acute ST segment elevation myocardial infarction from myocardial bridging of left anterior descending coronary artery. Int J Cardiol. 2003;90(1):117-8.
39. Tio RA, Ebels T. Ventricular septal rupture caused by myocardial bridging. Ann Thorac Surg. 2001;72(4):1369-70.
40. Ural E, Bildirici U, Celikyurt U, et al. Long-term prognosis of non-interventionally followed patients with isolated myocardial bridge and severe systolic compression of the left anterior descending coronary artery. Clin Cardiol. 2009;32(8):454-7.
41. Kodama K, Morioka N, Hara Y, et al. Coronary vasospasm at the site of myocardial bridge: report of two cases. Angiology. 1998;49(8):659-63.
42. Feld H, Guadanino V, Hollander G, et al. Exercise-induced ventricular tachycardia in association with a myocardial bridge. Chest. 1991;99(5):1295-6.
43. Kracoff OH, Ovsyshcher I, Gueron M. Malignant course of a benign anomaly: myocardial bridging. Chest. 1987;92(6):1113-5.
44. Den Dulk K, Brugada P, Braat S, et al. Myocardial bridging as a cause of paroxysmal atrioventricular block. J Am Coll Cardiol. 1983;1(3): 965-9.
45. Marchionni N, Chechi T, Falai M, et al. Myocardial stunning associated with a myocardial bridge. Int J Cardiol. 2002;82(1):65-7.
46. Roul G, Sens P, Germain P, et al. Myocardial bridging as a cause of acute transient left heart dysfunction. Chest 1999;116(2):574-80.
47. Tio RA, Van Gelder IC, Boonstra PW, et al. Myocardial bridging in a survivor of sudden cardiac near-death: role of intracoronary Doppler flow measurements and angiography during dobutamine stress in the clinical evaluation. Heart. 1997;77(3):280-2.
48. Morales AR, Romanelli R, Boucek RJ. The mural left anterior descending coronary artery, strenuous exercise and sudden death. Circulation. 1980;62(2):230-7.
49. Gawor R, Kusmierek J, Plachcinska A, et al. Myocardial perfusion GSPECT imaging in patients with myocardial bridging. J Nucl Cardiol. 2011;18(6):1059-65.
50. Galbraith EM, Eshtehardi P, Samady H. SPECT perfusion imaging and myocardial bridges: bridging the gap of diagnostic uncertainty. J Nucl Cardiol. 2011;18(6):1000-2.
51. Tang K, Wang L, Shi R, et al. The role of myocardial perfusion imaging in evaluating patients with myocardial bridging. J Nucl Cardiol. 2011;18(1):117-22.
52. Lin S, Tremmel JA, Yamada R, et al. A novel stress echocardiography pattern for myocardial bridge with invasive structural and hemodynamic correlation. J Am Heart Assoc. 2013;2(2):1-11.
53. Gaibazzi N, Rigo F, Reverberi C. Severe coronary tortuosity or myocardial bridging in patients with chest pain, normal coronary arteries, and reversible myocardial perfusion defects. Am J Cardiol. 2011;108(7):973-8.
54. Hongo T, Tada H, Ito K, et al. Augmentation of vessel squeezing at coronary-myocardial bridge by nitroglycerin: study by quantitative coronary angiography and intravascular ultrasound. Am Heart J. 1999;138(2):345-50.
55. Tsujita K, Maehara A, Mintz GS, et al. Comparison of angiographic and intravascular ultrasonic detection of myocardial bridging of the left anterior descending coronary artery. Am J Cardiol. 2008;102(12):1608-13.
56. Hakeem A, Cilingiroglu M, Leesar MA. Hemodynamic and intravascular ultrasound assessment of myocardial bridging: fractional flow reserve paradox with dobutamine versus adenosine. Catheter Cardiovasc Interv. 2010;75(2): 229-36.
57. Kim PJ, Hur G, Kim SY, et al. Frequency of myocardial bridges and dynamic compression of epicardial coronary arteries: a comparison between computed tomography and invasive coronary angiography. Circulation. 2009;119(10):1408-16.
58. Wang MH, Sun AJ, Qian JY, et al. Myocardial bridging detection by non-invasive multi-slice spiral computed tomography: comparison with intravascular ultrasound. Chin Med J (Engl). 2008;121(1):17-21.
59. Taylor CA, Fonte TA, Min JK. Computational fluid dynamics applied to cardiac computed tomography for noninvasive quantification of fractional flow reserve: scientific basis. J Am Coll Cardiol. 2013;61(22):2233-41.
60. Navarro-Lopez F, Soler J, Magrina J, et al. Systolic compression of coronary artery in hypertrophic cardiomyopathy. Int J Cardiol. 1986;12:309-20.
61. Yetman AT, McCrindle BW, MacDonald C, et al. Myocardial bridging in children with hypertrophic cardiomyopathy: a risk factor for sudden death. N Engl J Med. 1998;339(17): 1201-9.
62. Basso C, Thiene G, Mackey-Bojack S, et al. Myocardial bridging, a frequent component of the hypertrophic cardiomyopathy phenotype, lacks systematic association with sudden cardiac death. Eur Heart J. 2009;30(13):1627-34.
63. Pittaluga J, de Marchena E, Posoda JD, et al. Left anterior descending coronary artery bridge: a cause of early death after cardiac transplantation. Chest. 1997;111(2):511-3.
64. Singhal AK, McClurken JB, Fisher CA, et al. Successful transplantation of an older donor heart with documented myocardial bridging: a case report. J Heart Lung Transplant. 2005;24(3):340-2.
65. D'Ancona G, Baglini R, Clemenza F, et al. Left anterior descending coronary artery bridge: contraindication to cardiac transplantation? J Heart Lung Transplant. 2007;26(6):637-8.
66. Schwarz ER, Gupta R, Haager PK, et al. Myocardial bridging in absence of coronary artery disease: proposal of a new classification based on clinical-angiographic data and long-term follow-up. Cardiology. 2009;112(1):13-21.
67. Haager PK, Schwarz ER, vom Dahl J, et al. Long term angiographic and clinical follow-up in patients with stent implantation for symptomatic myocardial bridging. Heart. 2000;84(4):403-8.
68. Schwarz ER, Klues HG, vom Dahl J, et al. Functional, angiographic and intracoronary Doppler flow characteristics in symptomatic patients with myocardial bridging: effect of short-term intravenous beta-blocker medication. J Am Coll Cardiol. 1996;27(7):1637-45.
69. Nair CK, Dang B, Heintz MH, et al. Myocardial bridges: effect of propranolol on systolic compression. Can J Cardiol. 1986;2(4): 218-21.
70. Alessandri N, Dei Giudici A, De Angelis S, et al. Efficacy of calcium channel blockers in the treatment of the myocardial bridging: a pilot study. Eur Rev Med Pharmacol Sci. 2012;16(6):829-34.
71. Ishimori T, Raizner AE, Chahine RA, et al. Myocardial bridges in man: clinical correlations and angiographic accentuation with nitroglycerin. Cathet Cardiovasc Diagn. 1977;3(1):59-65.
72. Betriu A, Tabau J, Sanz G, et al. Relief of angina by periarterial muscle resection of myocardial bridges. Am Heart J. 1980;100(2):223-6.
73. Katznelson Y, Petchenko P, Knobel B, et al. Myocardial bridging: surgical technique and operative results. Mil Med. 1996;161(4):248-50.

74. Hill RC, Chitwood WR Jr, Bashore TM, et al. Coronary flow and regional function before and after supra-arterial myotomy for myocardial bridging. Ann Thorac Surg. 1981;31(2):176-81.
75. Iversen S, Hake U, Mayer E, et al. Surgical treatment of myocardial bridging causing coronary artery obstruction. Scand J Thorac Cardiovasc Surg. 1992;26(2):107-11.
76. Pratt JW, Michler RE, Pala J, et al. Minimally invasive coronary artery bypass grafting for myocardial muscle bridging. Heart Surg Forum. 1999;2(3):250-3.
77. Wan L, Wu Q. Myocardial bridge, surgery or stenting? Interact Cardiovasc Thorac Surg. 2005;4(6):517-20.
78. Huang XH, Wang SY, Xu JP, et al. Surgical outcome and clinical follow-up in patients with symptomatic myocardial bridging. Chin Med J. 2007;120(18):1563-6.
79. Stables RH, Knight CJ, McNeill JG, et al. Coronary stenting in the management of myocardial ischaemia caused by muscle bridging. Br Heart J. 1995;74(1):90-2.
80. Tsujita K, Maehara A, Mintz GS, et al. Impact of myocardial bridge on clinical outcome after coronary stent placement. Am J Cardiol. 2009;103(10):1344-8.
81. Broderick TM, Kereiakes DJ, Whang DD, et al. Myocardial bridging may predispose to coronary perforation during rotational atherectomy. J Invasive Cardiol. 1996;8(3):161-3.
82. Hering D, Horstkotte D, Schwimmbeck P, et al. Acute myocardial infarct caused by a muscle bridge of the anterior interventricular ramus: complicated course with vascular perforation after stent implantation. Z Kardiol. 1997;86(8):630-8.
83. Li W, Li Y, Sheng L, et al. Myocardial bridge: is the risk of perforation increased? Can J Cardiol. 2008;24(11):e80-81.
84. Zhang M, Kang WC, Moon CI, et al. Coronary artery perforation following implantation of a drug-eluting stent rescued by deployment of a covered stent in symptomatic myocardial bridging. Korean Circ J. 2010;40(3):148-51.
85. Tandar A, Whisenant BK, Michaels AD. Stent fracture following stenting of a myocardial bridge: report of two cases. Catheter Cardiovasc Interv. 2008;71(2):191-6.
86. Srinivasan M, Prasad A. Metal fatigue in myocardial bridges: stent fracture limits the efficacy of drug-eluting stents. J Invasive Cardiol. 2011;23(6):E150-52.
87. Corban MT, Hung OY, Eshtehardi P, et al. Myocardial bridging: contemporary understanding of pathophysiology with implications for diagnostic and therapeutic strategies. J Am Coll Cardiol. 2014;63(22):2346-55.

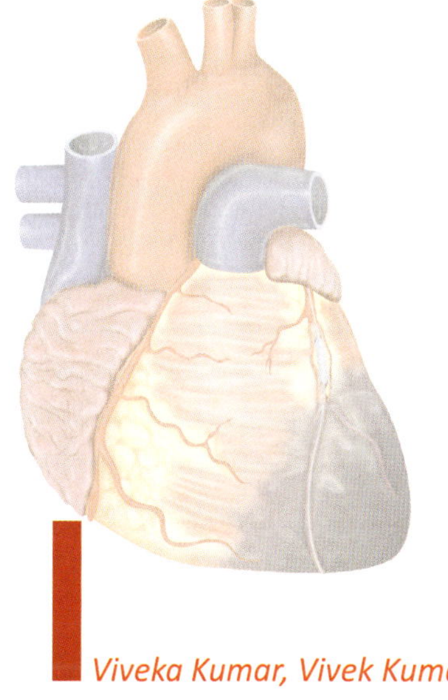

Benidipine for Hypertension in STEMI with Cardiodiabetes

Viveka Kumar, Vivek Kumar

INTRODUCTION

Calcium (Ca^{2+}) channel blockers are used for the treatment of ischemic heart disease and systemic hypertension because of their ability to effectively dilate coronary and systemic arteries..[1,2] Since Ca^{2+} overload is deleterious for the maintenance of cellular homeostasis, Ca^{2+} channel blockers are believed to be effective in attenuating Ca^{2+} overload. However, Ca^{2+} overload in ischemic and hypoxic cardiomyocytes is reportedly mediated by Na^+/H^+ and Na^+/Ca^{2+}exchangers, not by Ca^{2+} channels. Thus, Ca^{2+} channel blockers may not attenuate Ca^{2+}overload during myocardial ischemia and reperfusion. Also endothelial cell function is important for the preservation of organ functions during ischemic or hypertensive stress.[3-5] Indeed, endothelial-dependent coronary vasodilation is impaired in patients with either coronary artery disease or systemic hypertension, both of which reduce the levels of nitric oxide (NO) more so in the setting of diabetes. Benidipine reportedly has a cardioprotective effect during myocardial ischemia and reperfusion injury as well.[6] Since myocardial ischemia impairs endothelial cell function by the activation of platelets and leukocytes,[7,8] benidipine may attenuate endothelial cell dysfunction and increase the production of NO in ischemic hearts. We review here the clinical, pharmacological, and cardiovascular properties of benidipine and the role of NO in benidipine-induced cardioprotection in context of cardiodiabetes.

CHEMISTRY AND MECHANISMS OF ACTION

Benidipine hydrochloride is a racemic mixture of two isomers, having high lipid solubility and it was developed as a long-acting, L-type Ca^{2+} channel blocker.[9] The racemate nature of benidipine seems to play a role in its slow-onset antihypertensive effect, which results in minimal tachycardia or palpitation. In the clinical setting, this property is very important in the treatment of heart disease, because it is undesirable to induce acute systemic hemodynamic changes in patients with ischemic or failing hearts.

CARDIOHEMODYNAMIC EFFECTS

Although benidipine is a dihydropyridine Ca^{2+} channel blocker, the cardiohemodynamic effects of this drug are quite different from other Ca^{2+} channel blockers.[10] First, pharmacological activity appears gradually and persists for a long time following oral administration. Because of this, the activation of the sympathetic and renin-angiotensin systems, both of which are deleterious to the diseased heart, are avoided. Indeed in contrast to short-acting Ca^{2+} channel blockers, amlodipine, the other long-acting Ca^{2+} channel blocker and a long-acting formulation of nifedipine have also been reported to attenuate mortality of patients with non-ischemic chronic heart failure[11] and mortality due to cardiovascular and cerebral diseases in elderly patients with essential hypertension,[12] respectively. Second, benidipine selectively dilates the vasculature with minimal effect on cardiac contractility.[13,14] Both in vitro and in vivo experiments have shown that vascular selectivity of benidipine is quite high[13-15] and that benidipine is more selective than nifedipine or amlodipine. This property of benidipine may be especially advantageous in patients who exhibit cardiac dysfunction after ST-elevation myocardial infarction (STEMI).

Third, benidipine has potent antihypertensive effects[16-18] with minimal daily variability.[19] Via a reflex mechanism, most Ca^{2+} channel blockers induce tachycardia and a marked elevation of plasma catecholamines (i.e. neurohumoral activation) that increase the risk of adverse cardiac events.[20] In contrast, benidipine elevates plasma catecholamine levels only slightly (unpublished observation of Karasawa A. et al., Pharmaceutical Research Institute, Kyowa Hakko Kogyo Co., Ltd., Sunto, Shizuoka, Japan). And that too, it is reversed within 2 weeks following chronic treatment of hypertensive patients with benidipine.[21]

PROTECTIVE EFFECTS ON THE ENDOTHELIUM

One of the distinguishing characteristics of benidipine is its protective effect on the endothelium. In several experimental models of endothelial cell damage, benidipine was shown to protect the endothelium from injury following ischemia and from reperfusion injury.[22-24] These protective effects may be due to either an inhibitory effect against Ca^{2+} overload, selective vasodilation, or a protective effect on the endothelium. It is reported that benidipine attenuates the extent of ischemia through NO-dependent mechanisms,[25] which is independent of adenosine-induced coronary vasodilation as reported with other Ca^{2+} channel blockers. Benidipine increases coronary blood flow (CBF) dose-dependently, by its action on the enzyme NO synthase directly or indirectly. Though adenosine-induced, and/or to some extent, NO-induced coronary vasodilation have been reported with amlodipine and nifedipine, this action may be blunted in ischemic myocardium because of decreased probability of open Ca^{2+} channels in ischemic cells. Additionally, benidipine can increase production of endothelium-derived relaxing factors (EDRF) in addition to increased NO, and activated Ca^{2+}-activated K^{+} channels,[26-28] which may contribute to the cardioprotective effects.[27] Since benidipine has a high affinity for cell membranes, where endothelial cell NO synthase is located, benidipine may be more potent in its action. Further, clinical studies are required to ascertain its clinical value.

ROLE OF BENEDIPINE IN ISCHEMIC AND DIABETIC HEARTS

Endothelial dysfunction and high inflammatory burden is a hallmark of diabetic heart and it has been reported that in the presence of hypertension, NO levels in systemic blood are also decreased.[5] Evidence is accumulating in support of the hypothesis that the effects of benidipine on the cardiovascular system are at least partly attributable to NO. Nitric oxide is believed to attenuate the severity of myocardial ischemia since it increases CBF, attenuates myocardial anaerobic metabolism inhibits platelet aggregation and leukocyte activation, and attenuates the activation of sympathetic activity in ischemic hearts. NO also reportedly mediates cardioprotection during the late phase of ischemic preconditioning resulting in limiting infarct size[29,30] or the attenuation of myocardial stunning.[31] Taken together, the data supported the idea that benidipine mediates or enhances NO-dependent cardioprotection in diseased hearts which may be more rewarding in the setting of endothelial dysfunction as seen in diabetic heart. The effect of potentiation of endogenous NO can inhibit both cardiac hypertrophy and coronary vascular remodeling. Obesity, which may cause or be associated with hyperinsulinemia, as seen in diabetic patients, has a deleterious effect on the cardiovascular system. Interestingly, benidipine may have an antiobesity effect. Animal studies have shown that benidipine activated brown adipose tissue, presumably by increasing the blood flow to this tissue.[32] Chronic treatment with benidipine induced a decrease in visceral fat and body weight without affecting food intake, and it did not adversely influence the plasma lipid profile.[33] Another closely associated aspect of cardiodiabetes is diabetic nephropathy. Benidipine has been found to have greater renal-protective effect than amlodipine, it has greater efficacy than amlodipine in reducing blood pressure and proteinuria/albuminuria. Not only this, it has also been found to decrease plasma aldosterone level suggesting its action on renin-angiotensin system.[34,35] Also it is reported that benidipine decreases in oxidative stress.[36]

CONCLUSION

Compared with other Ca^{2+} channel blockers, benidipine, a new dihydropyridine Ca^{2+} channel blocker, has been recently reported to have several unique properties. It has a slow onset of action and long-acting effects in vivo, resulting in minimal sympathetic activation. Its high lipid solubility confers to its high specificity and access to interact from within the membrane with Ca^{2+} channels in the cell membrane of target cells even in ischemic cells. The vascular selectivity of benidipine is very high compared with the other Ca^{2+} channel blockers, which may be especially advantageous in treating patients with cardiac dysfunction. Most remarkably benidipine attenuates endothelial cell injury, decreases oxidative stress and also has effect on renin-angiotensin system. Taken together, these data suggest that benidipine may be a potent primary drug for the treatment of cardiovascular diseases in the setting of cardiodiabetes that exerts its effect, at least in part, by enhancing NO-dependent mechanisms.

REFERENCES

1. Maseri A, Chierchia S. Coronary artery spasm: demonstration, definition, diagnosis, and consequences. Prog Cardiovasc Dis. 1982;25(3):169-92.
2. Opie LH. Should calcium antagonists be used after myocardial infarction? Ischemia selectivity versus vascular selectivity. Cardiovasc Drugs Ther. 1993;6(1):19-24.
3. Bassenge E, Heusch G. Endothelial and neuro-humoral control of coronary blood flow in health and disease. Rev Physiol Biochem Pharmacol. 1990;116:77-165.
4. Moncada S, Palmer RMJ, Higgs EA. Nitric oxide: physiology, pathophysiology, and pharmacology. Pharmacol Toxicol. 1990;30:535-60.
5. Node K, Kitakaze M, Yoshikawa H, et al. Decreased plasma levels of nitric oxide in patients with essential hypertension. Hypertension. 1997;30(1):405-8.
6. Fujimura Y, Tsuboi H, Esato K. Efficacy of benidipine hydrochloride on myocardial ischemia and reperfusion. J Surg Res. 1995;59:321-5.
7. Engler RL, Dahlgren MD, Morris DD, et al. Role of leukocytes in response to acute myocardial ischemia and reflow in dogs. Am J Physiol. 1986;251(2 Pt 2):H314-22.
8. Willerson JT. Serotonin and thrombotic complications. J Cardiovasc Pharmacol. 1991;17(Suppl 5):S13-20.
9. Suzuki H, Ono E, Ueno H, et al. Physico-chemical properties and stabilities of the highly potent calcium antagonist benidipine hydrochloride. Arzneim-Forsch/Drug Res. 1988;38:1671-80.
10. Suzuki H, Saruta T. Benidipine. Cardiovasc Drug Rev. 1989;7:22-38.
11. Packer M, O'Connor CM, Ghali JK, et al. Effects of amlodipine on morbidity and mortality in severe chronic heart failure. New Engl J Med. 1996;335(15):1107-14.
12. Gong L, Zhang W, Zhu Y, et al. Shanghai trial of nifedipine in the elderly (STONE). J Hypertens. 1996;14(10):1237-45.
13. Karasawa A, Kubo K. Calcium antagonistic effects and the in vitro duration of actions of KW-3049, a new 1,4-dihydropyridine derivative, in isolated canine coronary arteries. Jpn J Pharmacol. 1988;47(1):35-44.
14. Karasawa A, Kubo K, Oka T, et al. Effects of the new calcium antagonist benidipine hydrochloride on cardiohemodynamics in anesthetized dogs. Arzneim-Forsch/Drug Res. 1988;38(II):1713-6.
15. Moriyama T, Karasawa A. Cardiovascular effects of benidipine and amlodipine in isolated tissues and anesthetized dogs. Biol Pharm Bull. 1994;17(11):1468-71.
16. Dohi Y, Kojima M, Sato K. Benidipine improves endothelial function in renal resistance arteries of hypertensive rats. Hypertension. 1996;28(1):58-63.
17. Kobayashi N, Kobayashi K, Kouno K, et al. Effect of benidipine on microvascular remodeling and coronary flow reserve in two kidneys, one-clip Goldblatt hypertension. J Hypertens. 1997;15(11): 1285-94.
18. Nito M, Sato H, Hara T, et al. Suppressive effects of benidipine on the development of hypertension and renal lesions in salt-loaded stroke-prone hypertensive rats. Clin Exp Pharmacol Physiol. 1995;(Suppl 1):S337-38.
19. Nakanishi T, Nishimura M, Takahashi H, et al. Beneficial effect of benidipine hydrochloride from the analysis of 24-h blood pressure monitoring. Rinsho to Kenkyu. 1992;69:4067-70.
20. Grossman E, Messerli FH. Effect of calcium antagonists on plasma norepinephrine levels, heart rate, and blood pressure. Am J Cardiol. 1997;80(11):1453-8.
21. Fuji Y, Suzuki H, Katsumata H, Nakajima S, Saruta T. Hormonal and renal responses to oral once-daily calcium entry blocker in normotensive and hypertensive persons. J Cardiovasc Pharmacol. 1988;11(4):438-43.
22. Kitakaze M, Minamino T, Node K, et al. Beneficial effects of inhibition of angiotensin-converting enzyme on ischemic myocardium during coronary hypoperfusion in dogs. Circulation. 1995;92(4):950-61.
23. Tanaka H, Deguchi T. The protective effect of benidipine hydrochloride against hypoxic myocardial injury of cultured mouse fetal heart cells. Folia Pharmacol Jpn. 1995;105(3):161-9.
24. Yao K, Karasawa A. Protective effect of benidipine against myocardial damage following ischemia and reperfusion in the isolated perfused rat heart. Biol Pharm Bull. 1994;17(4):517-21.
25. Kitakaze M, Node K, Minamino T, et al. A Novel Ca Channel Blocker, Benidipine, Increases Coronary Blood Flow and Attenuates the Severity of Myocardial Ischemia via NO-dependent Mechanisms in the Dogs. J Am Coll Cardiol (in press).
26. Node K, Kitakaze M, Kosaka H, et al. Bradykinin mediation of Ca^{2+}-activated K^+ channels regulates coronary blood flow in ischemic myocardium. Circulation.1997;95:1560-67.
27. Node K, Kitakaze M, Kosaka H, et al. Role of Ca^{2+}-activated K^+ channels in the protective effect of ACE inhibition against ischemic myocardial injury. Hypertension. 1998;31:1290-8.
28. Sauve R, Parent L, Simoneau C, et al. External ATP triggers a biphasic activation process of a calcium-dependent K^+ channel in cultured bovine aortic endothelial cells. Pflugers Arch. 1988;412(5):469-81.
29. Bolli R, Bhatti ZA, Tang XL, et al. Evidence that late preconditioning against myocardial stunning in conscious rabbits is triggered by the generation of nitric oxide. Circ Res. 1997;81(1):42-52.
30. Li WJ, Kitakaze M, Minamino T, et al. Nitric oxide opens the second window of cardioprotection of ischemic preconditioning: role of induction of heat shock protein (HSP72). J Am Coll Cardiol. 1997;29:12A.
31. Qui Y, Tang XL, Manchikalapudi S, et al. Nitric oxide triggers late preconditioning against myocardial infarction in conscious rabbits. Am J Physiol. 1997;273(6 Pt 2):H2931-6.
32. Kajita J, Kobayashi S, Yoshida T. Effect of benidipine hydrochloride on regional blood flow of the adipose tissue in anesthetized rats. Arzneim-Forsch/Drug Res. 1994;44(I):297-300.
33. Sakamoto T, Murakado M, Utusmi E, et al. Long-term effects of oral benidipine hydrochloride on plasma lipids and visceral fat accumulation in rats. Jpn Pharmacol Ther. 1996;24:1257-61.
34. Ohishi M, Takagi T, Ito N, et al. Renal-protective effect of T-and L-type calcium channel blockers in hypertensive patients: an amlodipine-to-benidipine changeover (ABC) study. Hypertens Res. 2007;30(9):797-806.
35. Abe M, Okada K, Maruyama N, et al. Benidipine reduces albuminuria and plasma aldosterone in mild-to-moderate stage chronic kidney disease with albuminuria. Hypertens Res. 2011;34(2):268-73.
36. Yasunari K, Maeda K, Nakamura M, et al. Benidipine, a long-acting calcium channel blocker, inhibits oxidative stress in polymorphonuclear cells in patients with essential hypertension. Hypertens Res. 2005;28:107-12.

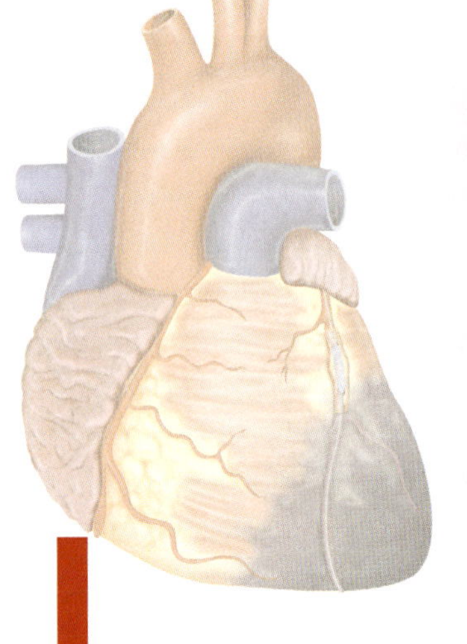

Thrombolytic Therapy of Choice in STEMI with Cardiodiabetes

KN Srinivasan, I Sathyamurthy

INTRODUCTION

ST-segment elevation myocardial infarction (STEMI) is caused by complete occlusion of a major epicardial coronary artery and is usually trigged by rupture of vulnerable plaque, with formation of fibrin-rich occlusive thrombus. Fast restoration of myocardial blood flow is the main stay in the treatment of STEMI, in order to restrict the infarct size and improve the outcome. This can be achieved either by mechanical reperfusion by primary percutaneous intervention (PPCI) or by pharmacological reperfusion by thrombolysis. Wherever, PPCI facility is not available, thrombolysis is the main stay in the treatment of STEMI patients. Diabetic patients presenting with STEMI (cardiodiabetics) were older, more likely to be female, more often present with anterior wall myocardial infarction. They are likely to receive thrombolysis later and majority of them have multivessel disease by coronary angiogram. Because of associated autonomic neuropathy, silent myocardial infarction and atypical presentations are more common in cardiodiabetics. They often present late to the hospital and receive the thrombolysis less often than the nondiabetic STEMI patients. Fear of thrombolysis-related bleeding among physicians also accounts for the failure to institute lysis in cardiodiabetics. Despite early use of potent thrombolytic agents, cardiodiabetics have more morbidity and mortality, due to reduced ventricular function at the noninfarct area (distant ischemia) secondary to multivessel disease and metabolic derangements during the acute phase of STEMI. Hence, choosing the right thrombolytic agent utmost important in the treatment of STEMI in cardiodiabetics. Thrombolytic agents are classified as fibrin-specific and nonfibrin-specific agents (Table 1). Efficacy assessment of a thrombolytic agent is done by vessel patency by coronary angiogram, TIMI flow grading, preservation of myocardial function and reduction in the mortality. Safety assessment of a thrombolytic agent is primarily driven by the bleeding risk. Ideal thrombolytic agent should be more efficacious and safe in clinical use. Among the available thrombolytic agents, tenecteplase is the most ideal fibrin-specific agent in clinical use (Tables 2 to 4 and Box 1).

STREPTOKINASE

Streptokinase (SK) is the poor man thrombolytic agent and was available for clinical use since 1958. It is produced by beta-hemolytic Streptococci and is antigenic. It is not a

TABLE 1: Thrombolytic agents

Fibrin specific	*Nonfibrin specific*
Alteplase (r-tPA)	Streptokinase (SK)
Tenecteplase (TNK-tPA)	Anistreplase
Reteplase (r-PA)	Urokinase
Staphylokinase	
Lanoteplase	
Monteplase	
Pametiplase	
Amediplase	

TABLE 2: Dosing regimens of thrombolytic agents

- *Streptokinase (SK)*
  - 1.5 million IU/hour
- *Alteplase:* Accelerated (total dose should not exceed 100 mg)
  - 15 mg IV bolus
  - 0.75 mg/kg over 30 min (max 50 mg)
  - 0.5 mg/kg over 60 min (max 35 mg)
- *Reteplase*
  - Initial 10 IU bolus, ½ hour later second 10 IU bolus
- *Tenecteplase*
  - Weight adjusted single bolus

Patient weight (kg)	TNK-tPA (elaxim) dose (mg)	Volume of TNK-tPA to be administered (mL)
<60	30	6
≥60 to <70	35	7
≥70 to <80	40	8
≥80 to <90	45	9
≥90	50	10

Note: Half-dose, if age >75 years: TNK-tPA is not mentioned in the label.

TABLE 3: Comparison of thrombolytic agents

	STK	*Alteplase*	*Reteplase*	*TNK-tPA*
Bolus administration	No	No	Yes	Yes
Antigenic	Yes	No	No	No
Allergic reaction (hypotension common)	Yes	No	No	No
Systemic fibrinogen depletion	Marked	Mild	Moderate	Minimal
90-min patency rate %	~50	~75	~75	~75
TIMI grade 3 flow%	32	54	60	63
Cost/dose ₹	3,500	80,000	30,000	30,000
Fibrin specificity	_	↑	↓	↑↑
Half-life (min)	18–23	3–4	15–18	20–24
PAI-I resistance	_	_	_	+

TABLE 4: International tissue plasminogen activator/streptokinase mortality trial

ISG	*NonDM*	*DM*	
		Insulin	*Noninsulin*
Hospital mortality	7.5%	16.9%	11.8%
Six-month mortality	10.7%	23.1%	17.8%
p-value	<0.0001	<0.0001	<0.0001

Abbreviations: DM, diabetes mellitus.

fibrin-specific agent. TIMI-1 trial[1] has shown 31% coronary artery patency at 90 minutes after lysis with SK. Intravenous streptokinase in acute myocardial infarction (ISAM) study[2] has shown preservation of left ventricular function with SK. Gruppo Italiano per lo Studio della Sopravvivenza nell'Infarto Miocardico (GISSI) trial[3] has shown reduction in mortality in SK arm compared to control arm (10.7% vs 13.1%) in less than 6 hours postlysis, 20% at 3-week postlysis, and 13% at 1 year.

BOX 1: Advantages of TNK-tPA (tenecteplase)

1. *Ease of administration:* Anytime, anywhere
2. *Rapid action:* Saves myocardium
3. More potent than alteplase
4. *Weight adjusted dosing:* Prevents over under dosing
5. No allergic reactions/hypotension
6. *Fibrin specificity:* Reduces bleeding
7. *Reduced plasma clearance:* Long half-life, single dose
8. *High PAI-1 resistance:* Stays longer in blood
9. Efficacy comparable with alteplase
10. More effective than alteplase in late treated patients
11. Less incidence of bleeding than alteplase
12. Best suited for pre-hospital thrombolysis

ALTEPLASE

Alteplase (r-tPA) is the first recombinant tissue plasminogen activator and is a fibrin-specific agent. It is not antigenic and can be safety re-administered, whenever needed. TIMI-I trial has shown 62% coronary patency at 90 minutes after lysis with r-tPA ($p < 0.0001$). Mortality reduction with r-tPA was found to be similar to SK arm in Anglo-Scandinavian study of early thrombosis (ASSET),[4] GISSI-2[5] and Third International Study of Infarct Survival (ISIS-3)[6] trials. Subgroup analysis in cardio-diabetics who received SK versus r-tPA was done in International Study Group (ISG),[7] Thrombolysis and Angioplasty in Myocardial Infarction (TAMI),[8] GISSI-2,[9] Fibrinolytic Therapy Trialists (FTT)[10] and Global Use of Strategies to Open Occluded Coronary Arteries 1 (GUSTO-1) trials. In international tissue plasminogen activator/SK mortality trial (ISG), thrombolysis with SK versus r-tPA was compared in cardio-diabetics. Among diabetic patients, in-hospital mortality was lowest with SK with heparin-treated arm (9.8%) and was highest with SK without heparin (16.1%). Patients treated with SK and heparin had a nonsignificant lower mortality rate than that of patients treated with r-tPA and heparin (9.87 vs 12.5%, $p = 0.50$). Hospital mortality was significantly higher in patients with a diabetes duration of greater than 10 years (odds rate 1.99). There was no difference in incidence of reinfarction in all four diabetic arms and was 7.0% in nondiabetic arm.

Global use of strategies to open occluded coronary arteries-1 trial[11] was the first landmark trial that has shown superiority of r-tPA over SK, when it was administered in accelerated infusion fashion over 1.5 hours instead of regular 3 hours infusion. There was significantly higher 30-day mortality for cardiodiabetics (10.5%) than that for nondiabetic patients (6.2%) and was highest among diabetic patients on insulin (12.5%) compared to non-insulin treated diabetics (9.7%) and was lowest among those who received accelerated r-tPA as thrombolytic agent. Although stroke occurred more frequently among diabetics (1.9%) than nondiabetic patients, there was no significant difference in the intracranial hemorrhage (ICH). Diabetes remained an independent predictor for mortality at 1-year follow-up (14.5% vs. 8.9%) ($p = 0.0001$) (Tables 5 to 7; Figs 1 and 2). GUSTO-1 angiographic substudy[12] showed a coronary patency of 54% with r-tPA as against 32% with SK arm in the overall study population. But there was no major difference in the infarct-related artery (IRA) patency rates between diabetics and nondiabetics (41% vs 38%) following thrombolysis. Similarly, in TAMI study,[8] there was no difference in 90-minute patency rates between cardio-diabetics and nondiabetics (71% vs 70%). With r-tPA, there is actual benefit of 10 additional lives saved for every 1,000 patients treated and 9 deaths and disabling stroke prevented per every 1,000 patients treated.

RETEPLASE

Reteplase (r-PA) is a second-generation lytic agent and is a mutant of alteplase. It has longer half-life than r-tPA, making its administration as bolus injection. But it is less fibrin specific than r-tPA. Coronary patency was higher with r-PA (two boluses at half an hour interval) as against r-tPA (both 90 minutes and 3 hours regimen) in RAP1DI-II trials. But these early patency rates did not translate into better outcomes. International Joint Efficacy Comparison of Thrombolytics (INJECT) trial[13] did not find any difference in 35-day mortality between double-bolus r-PA and SK. In GUSTO III trial,[14] 30-day and 1-year mortality were similar

TABLE 5: 30-day outcome according to thrombolytic strategy (GUSTO-1)[11]

	Nondiabetic	*Diabetic patients*	
		Noninsulin treated	*Insulin treated*
t-PA	*n* = 8,865	*n* = 1,079	*n* = 412
Mortality*	504 (5.7)	86 (8.0)	51 (21.4)
Reinfarction$	347 (3.9)	49 (4.5)	25 (6.1)
Stroke*	132 (1.5)	18 (1.7)	12 (2.9)
Streptokinase+	*n* = 17,143	*n* = 2,181	*n* = 824
Mortality*	1,100 (6.4)	222 (10.2)	114 (13.9)
Reinfarction	658 (3.9)	87 (4.5)	33 (4.0)
Stroke+	21 (1.2)	31 (1.4)	23 (2.8)
t-PA plus streptokinase	*n* = 1,041	*n* = 1,041	*n* = 407
Mortality*	559 (6.3)	111 (10.7)	41 (10.1)
Reinfarction	361 (4.1)	45 (4.3)	17 (4.2)
Stroke	138 (1.6)	22 (2.1)	10 (2.5)

*p < 0.001, +p = 0.017, patients with versus without diabetes. $p = 0.053, insulin-treated diabetic versus nondiabetic patients. Pooled streptokinase study arms. Data presented are number (%) of patients.

Abbreviations: t-PA, tissue-type plasminogen activator; GUSTO-I, global utilization of streptokinase and tissue plasminogen activator for occluded coronary arteries

TABLE 6: Early mortality and diabetic status in randomized trials[11]

	30-day mortality rate (%)			
Study	*No. of patients*	*NonDM*	*DM*	*OR (95% CI)**
TAMI[8]	1,071	5.7	11.5	2.04 (1.10–3.74)
ISG[7]	8,055	7.5	12.7	1.79 (1.43–2.24)
GISSI-2[9]	11,667	7.3	12.3	1.82 (1.55–2.14)
FTT[10]	21,659	8.7	13.6	1.64 (1.43–1.87)
GUSTO-I[11]	40,832	6.2	10.5	1.77 (1.61–1.95)
Pooled	83,284	7.1	11.6	1.71 (1.60–1.83)

*Patients with versus without diabetes. Insulin-treated versus noninsulin treated diabetic patients. In-hospital mortality. 35-day mortality. 30-day mortality.

Abbreviations: CI, confidence interval; FTT, fibrinolytic therapy trialists study; GISSI-2, Gruppo Italiano per lo Studio della Sopravvivenza nell'Infarto Miocardico; GUSTO-I, global utilization of streptokinase and tissue plasminogen activator for occluded coronary arteries; ISG, international tissue plasminogen activator/streptokinase mortality trial; DM, diabetes mellitus; OR, odds ratio; TAMI, thrombolysis and angioplasty in myocardial infarction trial.

TABLE 7: Early mortality and diabetic status in randomized trials for insulin-treated versus noninsulin treated diabetic patient[11]

	30-day mortality rate (%)			
Study	*No. of patients*	*Noninsulin Rx*	*Insulin Rx*	*OR (95% CI)**
TAMI[8]	1,071	10.7	15.0	148 (0.44–4.77)
ISG[7]	8,055	11.8	16.9	1.52 (0.92–2.50)
GISSI-2[9]	11,667	11.7	16.4	1.49 (1.04–2.12)
FTT[10]	21,659	NA	NA	NA
GUSTO-I[11]	40,832	9.7	12.5	1.34 (1.11–1.60)
Pooled	83,284	10.4	13.5	1.34 (1.15–1.56)

*Patients *with* versus *without* diabetes. Insulin-treated versus noninsulin treated diabetic patients. In-hospital mortality. 35-day mortality. 30-day mortality.

Abbreviations: CI, confidence interval; FTT, fibrinolytic therapy trialists study; GISSI-2, Gruppo Italiano per lo Studio della Sopravvivenza nell'Infarto Miocardico; GUSTO-I, global utilization of streptokinase and tissue plasminogen activator for occluded coronary arteries; ISG, international tissue plasminogen activator/streptokinase mortality trial; NA, not available; OR: odds ratio; TAMI, thrombolysis and angioplasty in myocardial infarction trial.

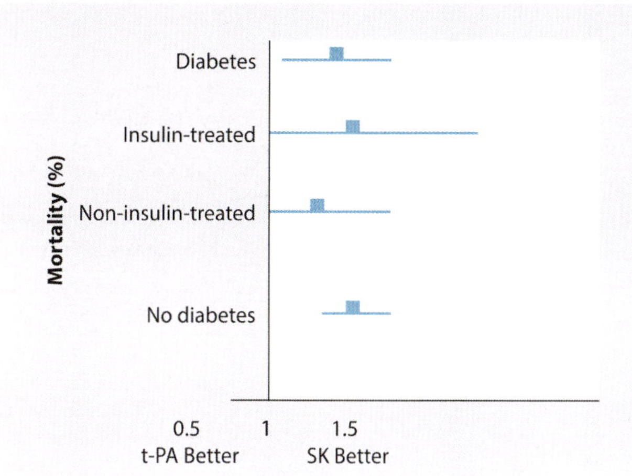

Fig. 1: Odds ratio and 95% confidence intervals for 30-day mortality in patients with and without diabetes. GUSTO I trial data.[11]

Abbreviations: SK, streptokinase; t-PA, alteplase

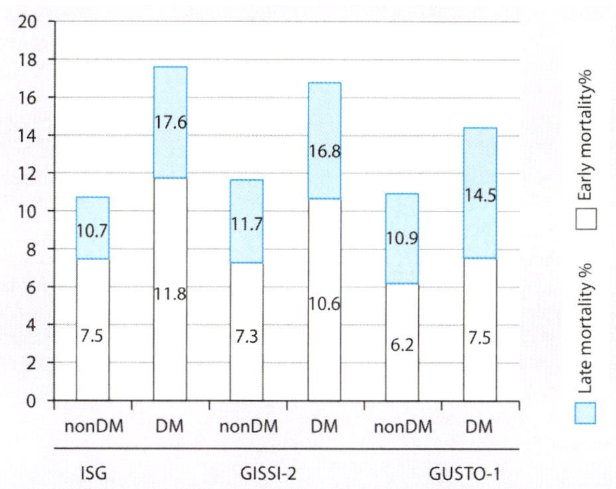

Fig. 2: Early (30–35 days) and late (6–12 months) mortality among nondiabetics and diabetics.[11]

Abbreviations: DM, patients with diabetes; nonDM, patients without diabetes. ISG, international tissue plasminogen activator/streptokinase mortality trial

between r-PA and r-tPA (7.47 vs 7.24). Hemorrhagic stroke was higher with r-PA as against r-tPA (0.91% vs 0.93%). Alteplase is better than r-PA in late treated patients because of better fibrin specificity with former than later.

TENECTEPLASE

Tenecteplase (TNK-tPA) is produced by recombinant DNA technology using Chinese hamster ovary cells. There are three modifications in the structure of r-tPA which makes this molecule to have a longer half-life, greater fibrin specificity and resistant to plasminogen

TABLE 8: Assessment of the safety and efficacy of a new thrombolytic (ASSENT-2) trial[16]

ASSENT-2 trial	*30-day mortality*	
	TNK-tPA	*r-tPA*
Primary analysis	6.17%	6.15%
Diabetes: Yes	8.8%	8.7%
Diabetes: No	5.6%	5.7%

Abbreviations: TNK-tPA, tenecteplase; r-tPA, alteplase

activator inhibitor-1 (PAI-I). Long half-life makes it to be administered as single bolus and greater fibrin specificity makes it safer with less bleeding risk. Nitrates do not appear to affect TNK-tPA levels unlike r-tPA. In TIMI 10A, 10 B[15] trials, 40 mg of TNK-tPA was compared with accelerated tPA and showed similar patency rates (63% vs 63%). The 50 mg of TNK-tPA was discontinued in the trial due to excess bleeding. In ASSENT-2 trial,[16] 30-day mortality was similar between TNK-tPA and r-tPA arms (6.18% vs 6.21%) in primary analysis and (8.8% vs 8.7%) in diabetic subgroup analysis (Table 8) and severe bleeding including ICH was also similar (0.93 vs 0.94). There was decreased rate in noncerebral bleeds (26.43 vs 28.95, $p = 0.0003$), in major bleeds (4.68% vs 5.94%, $p = 0.0002$) and in need for blood transfusion (4.25% vs 5.49%, $p = 0.0002$) with TNK-tPA as against r-tPA, showing TNK-tPA is also safer than r-tPA. These general results were comparable in all major subgroups including the diabetes status. These positive results were found persisting even after 1 year. TNK-tPA scores over other molecules in both efficacy and safety in two special groups namely late presenters (>4 hours after symptom onset) and in high risk MI group (women aged >75 years, weighing <67 kg) because of high fibrin specificity. Late presenters responded significantly better with TNK-tPA with absolute 2% difference in 30-day mortality. STREAM trial[17] has shown half-dose TNK-tPA is safe and efficacious in patients who are greater than 75 years of age with no excess ICH.

In our Indian registry data,[18] on cardiodiabetics treated with tenecteplase, the mortality was 3.9% in diabetics and 2.63% in nondiabetics with no significant difference between the groups and the overall mortality of 3.2%, was much lower than earlier reported incidence of 6.18% in the ASSENT-2 and up to 6.5% in TIMI-10B study. The incidence of bleeding, myocardial reinfarction and heart failure was similar to that reported in TIMI 10B and ASSENT-2 trials. The overall stroke was 0.41% only as against 1.4% reported in GUSTO-1 trial and there was no difference in the incidence of stroke between diabetic and nondiabetic patients unlike GUSTO-1 trial data.

Low molecular weight heparin (LMWH) is an attractive alternative to unfractionated heparin (UFH) when given in combination with TNK-tPA (ASSENT-3[19] and ENTIRE-

TIMI-23[20] trials). 30-day mortality and in-hospital reinfarction and refractory ischemia were less with LMWH arm as against UFH arm (11.4% vs 15.4%, $p = 0.0002$) and there was similar reduction noted in in-hospital ICH or major bleeds. The concept of prehospital thrombolysis came to light because late presentation to the hospital, and delayed institution of reperfusion therapy was associated with poor outcomes. Late presentation to the hospital is mostly driven by the transport delay. It is feasible today to institute thrombolysis with single bolus fibrinolytic agent (e.g. weight adjusted tenecteplase) with bolus enoxaparin in the ambulance itself. In ASSENT-3 plus trial,[21] the fraction of patients received reperfusion therapy within 2 hours of symptom onset has increased from 29% to 52% with institution of TNK-tPA in the ambulance which was associated with lower mortality. 5-year follow-up data from CAPTIM[22] (Comparison of Angioplasty and Pre-hospital Thrombolysis in Acute Myocardial Infarction) and FAST-MI[23] (French Registry on Acute ST-elevation Myocardial Infarction) trials did not show any superiority of PPCI over prehospital fibrinolysis.

CONCLUSION

Diabetes mellitus is an independent predictor of adverse outcomes including mortality in patients presenting with STEMI and with the use of thrombolytic treatment, this has significantly come down. Patients with fasting hyperglycemia have worse outcomes than known diabetics on admission with STEMI. Although TIMI flow by coronary angiogram following thrombolysis was similar in diabetics with STEMI in various randomized studies, myocardial perfusion grading was not so. Postlysis complete ST-segment resolution (a marker of successful myocardial reperfusion) was found less frequently in diabetic STEMI patients because of microvascular dysfunction. No-reflow phenomenon on cardio-diabetics could be secondary to diminished flow reserve, endothelial dysfunction, and microvascular structural abnormalities and found to be key predictor of mortality at 2 years. Hence, it becomes mandatory to choose the right thrombolytic agent and administer it at the earliest to get the desired results.

REFERENCES

1. The TIMI Study Group. The Thrombolysis in Myocardial Infarction (TIMI) Trial: phase I findings. N Engl J Med. 1985;312(4):932-6.
2. The ISAM Study Group. Prospective trial of intravenous streptokinase in acute myocardial infarction (ISAM). N Engl J Med. 1986;314(23):1465-71.
3. GISSI. Effectiveness of intravenous thrombolytic treatment in acute myocardial infarction. Lancet. 1986;1(8478):397-402.
4. Wilcox RG, von der Lippe G, Olsson CG, et al. Trial of tissue plasminogen activator for mortality reduction in acute myocardial infarction: Anglo-Scandinavian Study of Early Thrombosis (ASSET). Lancet. 1988;2(8610):525-30.
5. The International Study Group. In-hospital mortality and clinical course of 20,891 patients with suspected acute myocardial infarction randomized between alteplase and streptokinase with or without heparin. Lancet. 1990;336(8707):71-5.
6. ISIS-3 (Third International Study of Infarct Survival) Collaborative Group. ISIS-3: a randomised comparison of streptokinase vs tissue plasminogen activator vs anistreplase and of aspirin plus heparin vs aspirin alone among 41,299 cases of suspected acute myocardial infarction. Lancet. 1992;339(8796):753-70.
7. Barbash GI, White HD, Modan M, et al. Significance of diabetes mellitus in patients with acute myocardial infarction receiving thrombolytic therapy. Investigators of the International Tissue Plasminogen Activator/Streptokinase Mortality Trial. J Am Coll Cardiol. 1993;22(3):707-13.
8. Granger CB, Califf RM, Young S, et al. Outcome of patients with diabetes mellitus and acute myocardial infarction treated with thrombolytic agents. The Thrombolysis and Angioplasty in Myocardial Infarction (TAMI) study group. J Am Coll Cardiol. 1993;21(4):920-5.
9. Zuanatte G, Latini R, Maggioni AP, et al. Influence of diabetes on mortality in acute myocardial infarction: data from the GISSI-2 study. J Am Coll Cardiol. 1993;22(7):1788-94.
10. Fibrinolytic Therapy Trialists (FTT) Collaborative Group. Indications for fibrinolytic therapy in suspected acute myocardial infarction. Collaborative overview of early mortality and major morbidity results from all randomised trials of more than 1000 patients. Lancet. 1994;343(8893):311-22.
11. Mak KH, Moliterno DJ, Granger CB, et al. Influence of diabetes mellitus on clinical outcome in the thrombolytic era of acute myocardial infarction. GUSTO-1 Investigators. Global Utilization of Streptokinase and Tissue Plasminogen Activator for Occluded Coronary Arteries. J Am Coll Cardiol. 1997;30(1):171-9.
12. Simes RJ, Topol EJ, Holmes DR Jr, et al. Link between the angiographic substudy and mortality outcomes in a large randomized trial of myocardial reperfusion. Importance of early and complete infarct artery. GUSTO-1 Investigators. Circulation. 1995;91(7):1923-8.
13. Schröder R, Wegscheider K, Schröder K, et al. Extent of early ST segment elevation resolution: a strong predictor of outcome in patients with acute myocardial infarction and a sensitive measure to compare thrombolytic regimens. A substudy of the International Joint Efficacy Comparison of Thrombolytics (INJECT) trial. J Am Coll Cardiol. 1995;26(7):1657-64.
14. The Global Use of Strategies to Open Occluded Coronary Arteries (GUSTO III) Investigators. A comparison of reteplase with alteplase for acute myocardial infarction. N Engl J Med. 1997;337(16):1118-23.
15. Cannon CP, Gibson CM, McCabe CH, et al. TNK-tissue plasminogen activator compared with front-loaded alteplase in acute myocardial Infarction: results of the TIMI 10B trial. Thrombolysis in Myocardial Infarction (TIMI) 10B Investigators. Circulation. 1998;98(25):2805-14.
16. Fu Y, Goodman S, Chang W, et al. Time to treatment influences the impact of ST-segment resolution on one-year prognosis: Insights from the assessment of the safety and efficacy of a new thrombolytic (ASSENT-2) trial. Circulation. 2001;104(22):2653-9.
17. Larson DM, Duval S, Sharkey SW, et al. Safety and efficacy of a pharmaco-invasive reperfusion strategy in rural ST-elevation myocardial infarction patients with expected delays due to long-distance transfers. Eur Heart J. 2012;33(10):1232-40.
18. Sathyamurthy I, Jayanthi K, Iyengar SS, et al. Efficacy and Safety of Tenecteplase in Diabetic and Non-diabetic Patients of STEMI-Indian Registry Data. JAPI. 2010;58:229-30.
19. Assessment of the Safety and Efficacy of a New Thrombolytic Regimen (ASSENT)-3 Investigators. Efficacy and safety of

tenecteplase in combination with enoxaparin, abciximab, or unfractionated heparin: the ASSENT-3 randomised trial in acute myocardial infarction. Lancet. 2001;358(9282):605-13.
20. Antman EM, Louwerenburg HW, Baars HF, et al. Enoxaparin as adjunctive antithrombin therapy for ST-elevation myocardial infarction: results of the ENTIRE-Thrombolysis in Myocardial Infarction (TIMI) 23 trial. Circulation. 2002;105(14):1642-9.
21. Wallentin L, Goldstein P, Armstrong P W, et al. Efficacy and safety of tenecteplase in combination with the low-molecular-weight heparin enoxaparin or unfractionated heparin in the prehospital setting: The Assessment of the Safety and Efficacy of a New Thrombolytic Regimen (ASSENT)-3 PLUS Randomized Trial in Acute Myocardial Infarction. Circulation. 2003;108(2):135-42.
22. Bouneloy E, Lapostolle F, Leizorovicz A, et al. Primary angioplasty versus pre-hospital thrombolysis in acute myocardial infarction: a randomized study. Lancet. 2002;360(9336):825-9.
23. Danchin N, Puymirat E, Steg PG, et al. Five-year survival in patients with ST-segment-elevation myocardial infarction according to modalities of reperfusion therapy: the French Registry on Acute ST-elevation and Non-ST-elevation Myocardial Infarction (FAST-MI) 2005 Cohort. Circulation. 2014;129(16):1629-36.

CHAPTER

Tenecteplase and ST-elevation Myocardial Infarction with Cardiodiabetes

SS Iyengar

INTRODUCTION

Diabetes is a growing and major global as well as national problem amongst the challenges posed by the noncommunicable diseases. It is a major risk factor for atherosclerotic vascular disease (ASCVD) and is often conceived as a coronary artery disease (CAD) equivalent. Moreover, cardiovascular disease is the main cause of mortality and morbidity amongst diabetics. Diabetes plays an important role in accelerated atherogenesis and atherothrombosis. Atherothrombotic process involves a sequence of an unstable atheromatous plaque in the coronary artery developing an erosion or a rupture, activation of clotting cascade and formation of an occlusive thrombus, leading to ST-elevation myocardial infarction (STEMI). Diabetic patients with STEMI respond well to reperfusion therapy, be it primary percutaneous coronary intervention (PCI) or fibrinolytic therapy followed by a strategy of pharmacoinvasive therapy.

DIABETES AND ATHEROSCLEROSIS: PREVALENCE AND PATHOPHYSIOLOGY

The National Urban Survey conducted across the metropolitan cities of India reported prevalence of diabetes as follows:[1,2]

- 11.7% in Kolkata (Eastern India)
- 6.1% in Kashmir Valley (Northern India)
- 11.6% in New Delhi (Northern India)
- 9.3% in West India (Mumbai)
- 13.5% in Chennai (South India)
- 16.6% in Hyderabad (South India) and
- 12.4% Bengaluru (South India).

It is predicted that by 2030, diabetes mellitus may afflict up to 79.4 million individuals in India.[3] Thus, diabetes is a major problem and is a causative risk factor in a substantial number of patients with CAD and MI. Diabetes increases the risk of MI, and continues to contribute to a high risk of adverse events in these patients, though there has been a decline in the risk in recent years.[4-6] In a study from Sweden (1998–2014), mortality and the incidence of cardiovascular outcomes showed a substantial decline in diabetic patients, but fatal outcomes declined less in diabetics than in controls.[7] Diabetes accelerates atherosclerotic process, and might well initiate the process, lead to progression and contribute to the instability of the atheromatous plaque. Its usual association with other ASCVD risk factors like hypertension, dyslipidemia and obesity partly accounts for the risk of developing atherosclerosis. But diabetes with its complex underlying pathophysiology has direct implications in the development of atherosclerosis. The factors involved are endothelial dysfunction, circulating fatty acids and inflammatory milieu.[8] Diabetes also creates a prothrombotic state. It has an unfavorable effect on the coagulation pathways and platelet function. There is an increased level of tissue factor, factor VII, von Wille brand factor and plasminogen activator inhibitor, while activity of antithrombin III and protein C is decreased.[9]

DIABETES AND STEMI: STUDIES

Studies have clearly demonstrated that reperfusion therapies are effective and there is a decline in the rate of adverse outcome events in diabetic patients with STEMI. In fact, there was a time in the past when the presence of hemorrhagic diabetic retinopathy was an absolute contraindication for thrombolytic therapy because of the risk for retinal hemorrhage. However, in the GUSTO-I trial, 6,011 patients were diabetics and about 2,000 had nonproliferative retinopathy and 300 had proliferative retinopathy.[10] There were no signals of increased risk of retinal bleed with thrombolytic treatment. A large number of studies have included diabetic patients with STEMI and intraocular bleed was not an issue of concern.[11] Diabetic retinopathy should *not* be considered as a contraindication to fibrinolytic therapy in STEMI. In the ISIS-2 trial, amongst 17,187 participants, diabetic patients receiving streptokinase had a greater improvement compared to placebo than nondiabetics (31% vs 23%).[12]

GISSI-2 trial studied 11,667 patients and all of them received thrombolytic therapy; 32% of women and 16% of men were diabetics. The adverse events were more in diabetics. The in-hospital mortality was 10.1% for type 2 diabetics versus 5.8% for nondiabetics.[13] In GUSTO-I trial,[14] over 40,000 patients received thrombolysis, 15% being diabetics. Diabetic patients were older, and had more often hypertension and heart failure, prior infarctions and coronary artery bypass graft (CABG) procedures. Between diabetics and nondiabetics, there was no difference in the infarct-related arterial patency rates (TIMI flow grade III) at 90 minutes (40% vs 38%), in reocclusion rates (9.2% vs 5.3%), or LV systolic function at 90 minutes or 5–7 days. Despite this, the diabetic patients had a significantly higher mortality rate at 30 days (11.3% vs 5.9%) and 1 year (14.5% vs 8.9%). Diabetes is an independent risk factor for short- and long-term mortality. In an Indian prospective registry study of 15,222 STEMI patients, 41.33% were diabetics with a mean age of 57.59 years, a mean body weight of 70.24 kg and a male to female ratio of 4.64. All of them received tenecteplase as a fibrinolytic agent. Thrombolysis was equally successful in diabetics as compared to the overall population (95.14% vs 95.43%). Bleeding (other than intracranial) was seen in 2.18% in diabetics versus 1.89% in nondiabetics. Diabetics had a mortality of 2.19% versus 1.28% in nondiabetics. The study showed that diabetics respond equally well to reperfusion therapy with tenecteplase, and are at a higher risk of adverse events.[15] Severity and extent of ASCVD, multivessel CAD, intrinsic myocardial abnormality, microvascular disease, pre-existing CAD, and associated comorbidities have an adverse impact on the outcome in diabetics patients.

BOX 1: Factors favoring tenecteplase as a preferred fibrinolytic agent in patients with ST-elevation myocardial infarction (STEMI) and diabetes

- Ease of administration—IV single bolus over 5 seconds
- Rapid action—induces 50% lysis three times faster than tPA
- Potency—13.5-fold more potent in lysing platelet rich clots in vivo than tPA
- Weight adjusted dosing—0.53 mg/kg
- Fibrin specificity—14-fold greater than tPA
- Reduced plasma clearance—50% remained in circulation after 15 minutes of injection (1% tPA)
- High PAI-1 resistance—80-fold more than tPA
- Noncerebral bleed less than tPA
- Clinical efficacy comparable with tPA
- Pharmacoinvasive strategy—best suited
- Supported by clinical data

Abbreviations: IV: intravenous; tPA: tissue plasminogen activator

Source: Modified from Saran RK, Sethi R, Nagori M. Tenecteplase: the best among the equals. Indian Heart J. 2009;61:4454-8

In Strategic Reperfusion Early After Myocardial Infarction (STREAM) study, 1,892 patients with STEMI were studied and were randomized to undergo either primary PCI or fibrinolytic therapy with bolus tenecteplase (which was amended later to half dose in patients ≥75 years of age) 12–13% were diabetics. The incidence of the primary end point (a composite of death, shock, congestive heart failure, or reinfarction up to 30 days) in the prespecified subgroups that included diabetics versus nondiabetics, was no different and there was no significant treatment interactions.[16]

In the management of patients with STEMI, fibrinolytic therapy has a role as an initial reperfusion method even in this era of intervention.[17] Where time and transport barriers cannot be overcome to institute primary PCI, pharmaco-invasive strategy of thrombolysis with tenecteplase[18] followed by coronary angiogram and PCI, if required within 3 to 24 hours of thrombolysis saves the situation and achieves equally good results in diabetic patients with STEMI (Box 1).

CONCLUSION

Diabetes and CAD are reaching epidemic proportions in our country. A substantial number of patients with STEMI would be harboring diabetes. There are effective means of reperfusion therapies—primary PCI or pharmacoinvasive strategy (along with adjunctive measures) to face this challenge and achieve better outcomes. Tenecteplase fits well into the scheme of management of diabetic patients with STEMI and is well-supported by various national and international studies.

REFERENCES

1. Zargar AH, Khan AK, Masoodi SR, et al. Prevalence of type 2 diabetes mellitus and impaired glucose tolerance in the Kashmir Valley of the Indian subcontinent. Diabetes Res Clin Pract. 2000;47(2):135-46.
2. Ramachandran A, Snehalatha C, Kapur A, et al. Diabetes Epidemiology Study Group in India (DESI). High prevalence of diabetes and impaired glucose tolerance in India: National Urban Diabetes Survey. Diabetologia. 2001;44(9):1094-101.
3. Whiting DR, Guariguata L, Weil C, et al. IDF Diabetes atlas: global estimates of the prevalence of diabetes for 2011 and 2030. Diabetes Res Clin Pract. 2011;94:311-21.
4. Fang J, Alderman MH. Impact of the increasing burden of diabetes on acute myocardial infarction in New York City: 1990-2000. Diabetes. 2006;55:768.
5. Gore MO, Patel MJ, Kosiborod M, et al. Diabetes mellitus and trends in hospital survival after myocardial infarction, 1994 to 2006: data from the National Registry of Myocardial Infarction. Circ Cardiovasc Qual Outcomes. 2012;5:791.
6. Wiviott SD, Braunwald E, Angiolillo DJ, et al. Greater clinical benefit of more intensive oral antiplatelet therapy with prasugrel in patients with diabetes mellitus in the trial to assess improvement in therapeutic outcomes by optimizing platelet inhibition with prasugrel-thrombolysis in myocardial infarction 38. Circulation. 2008;118:1626.
7. Aidin R, Araz R, Stefan F, et al. Mortality and cardiovascular disease in type 1 and type 2 diabetes. N Engl J Med. 2017;376:1407-18.
8. Orasanu G, Plutzky J. The pathologic continuum of diabetic vascular disease. J Am Coll Cardiol. 2009;53:S35.
9. Mathewkutty S, McGuire DK. Platelet perturbations in diabetes: implications for cardiovascular disease risk and treatment. Expert Rev Cardiovasc Ther. 2009;7:541.
10. Mahaffey KW, Granger CB, Toth CA, et al. Diabetic retinopathy should not be a contraindication to thrombolytic therapy for acute myocardial infarction: review of ocular hemorrhage incidence and location in the GUSTO-I trial. Global Utilization of Streptokinase and t-PA for Occluded Coronary Arteries. J Am Coll Cardiol. 1997;30(7):1606.
11. Ward H, Yudkin JS. Thrombolysis in patients with diabetes. BMJ. 1995;310(6971):3.
12. Randomised trial of intravenous streptokinase, oral aspirin, both, or neither among 17,187 cases of suspected acute myocardial infarction: ISIS-2. ISIS-2 (Second International Study of Infarct Survival) Collaborative Group. Lancet. 1988;2(8607):349.
13. Zuanetti G, Latini R, Maggioni AP, et al. Influence of diabetes on mortality in acute myocardial infarction: data from the GISSI-2 study. J Am Coll Cardiol. 1993;22(7):1788.
14. Mak KH, Moliterno DJ, Granger CB, et al. Influence of diabetes mellitus on clinical outcome in the thrombolytic era of acute myocardial infarction. GUSTO-I Investigators. Global Utilization of Streptokinase and Tissue Plasminogen Activator for Occluded Coronary Arteries. J Am Coll Cardiol. 1997;30(1):171.
15. Iyengar SS, Nair T, Hiremath JS, et al. Pharmacologic reperfusion therapy with indigenous tenecteplase in 15,222 patients with ST Elevation Myocardial Infarction: The Indian Registry. Indian Heart J. 2013;65:436-41.
16. Armstrong PW, Gershlick AH, Goldstein P, et al. Fibrinolysis or primary PCI in ST-Segment Elevation Myocardial Infarction. N Engl J Med. 2013;368:1379-87.
17. Iyengar SS, Girish SG. Thrombolysis in the era of intervention. JAPI. 2011;59:26-30.
18. Saran RK, Sethi R, Nagori M. Tenecteplase: the best among the equals. Indian Heart J. 2009;61:4454-8.

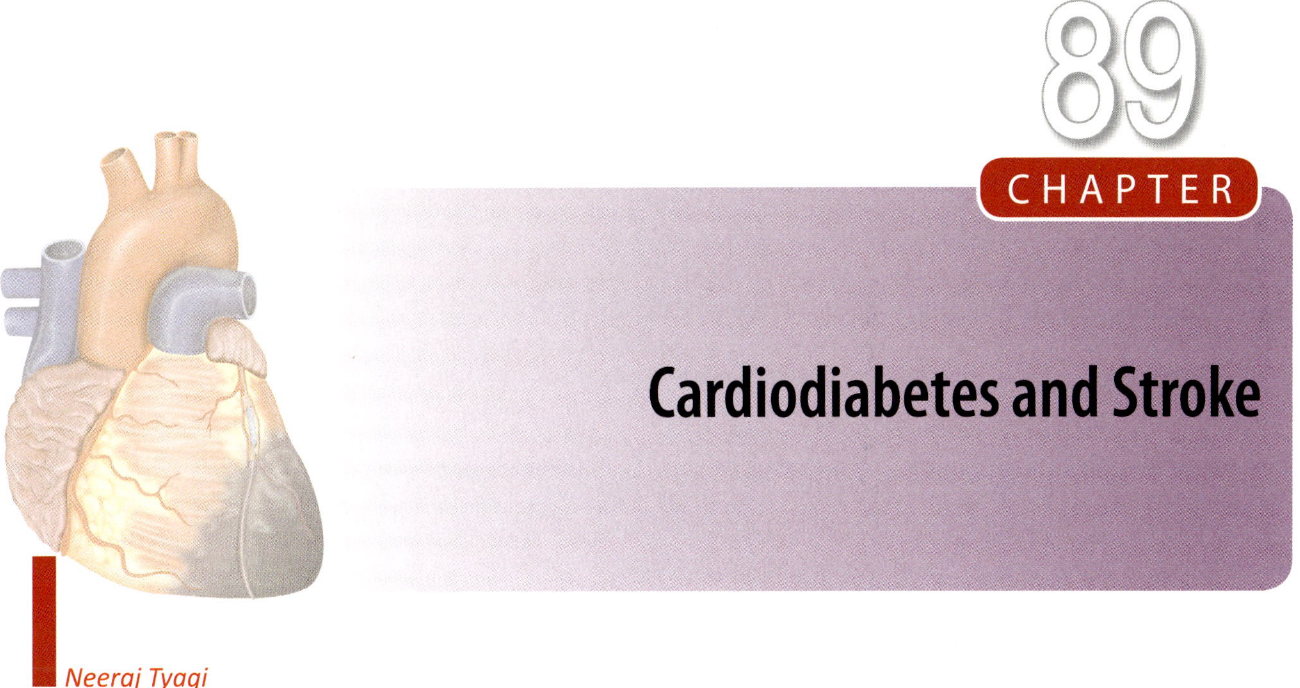

Cardiodiabetes and Stroke

Neeraj Tyagi

INTRODUCTION

Stroke is being considered the second most common cause of death and the third most common cause of disability worldwide.[1] For each patient of ischemic stroke, the prognosis, treatment strategy, and further risk of recurrence depend on the presumed etiology. Cardioembolic causes of stroke are responsible for up to 20% of ischemic strokes with a high rate of recurrence.[2] Atrial fibrillation (AF) is the most common risk factor for cardioembolic stroke. This chapter will address the aspects of cardioembolic stroke except AF due to vastness of the topic. AF reader is advised to read a comprehensive update on AF.[3] Diabetes mellitus is a major risk factor for cardiovascular disease including stroke. Cardiometabolic risk factors, including obesity, hypertension, and dyslipidemia often coexist with diabetes mellitus and can contribute to the higher reported relative stroke risks when compared to patients with similar risk profile without diabetes.[4] This chapter will briefly touch the complex aspect of cardiodiabetes and stroke as the name suggests.

CLINICAL FEATURES OF CARDIOEMBOLIC STROKE

Clinical features that support the diagnosis of cardioembolic stroke include sudden onset to maximal deficit (<5 minutes) and decreased level of consciousness compared to thrombotic. Another important feature is onset of symptoms after a valsalva-provoking activity. Lacunar infarction is only rarely caused by cardiac embolism (2.65% of cases).[5] Hemorrhagic transformation of an ischemic infarct occurs in up to 71% of cardioembolic strokes. As many as 95% of hemorrhagic infarcts are caused by cardioembolism.[6] Box 1 enumerates the causes of cardioembolic stroke.[7]

ACUTE MYOCARDIAL INFARCTION AND STROKE

The risk factor for myocardial infarction (MI) and ischemic stroke is common, both often coexist. Acute MI is a risk factor for ischemic stroke and vice-versa, particularly in the initial 30 days. Approximately, 12.2 patients per 1,000 develop ischemic stroke after MI, while 3% of ischemic stroke patients develop MI within 1 year.[8] Various factors associated with acute MI can cause ischemic stroke, most important are—ventricular hypokinesis, arrhythmia, and increased sympathetic activity, and less commonly—hypoperfusion because of pump failure. Unfortunately, the prognosis after ischemic stroke and acute MI is poor.[9] Patients with acute MI and left ventricular (LV) thrombus are especially at high risk of ischemic stroke. Treatment with warfarin was associated with a decreased risk of ischemic stroke after MI, but a greater risk of significant bleeding. Current American Heart Association (AHA) guideline recommendations are that anticoagulation is reasonable in patients with LV thrombus as well as in patients with anterior apical akinesis or dyskinesis. Patients with an anterior MI should be evaluated with echocardiography to assess for LV thrombus. The use of novel oral anticoagulants in the context of LV thrombus is not clear (Box 1).[10]

BOX 1: Cardiac causes of ischemic stroke based on TOAST (trial of ORG 10172 in acute stroke treatment) classification

High-risk sources:
1. Atrial fibrillation (AF)
2. Left ventricular dysfunction:
   - Recent myocardial infarction
   - Left ventricular aneurysm
   - Cardiomyopathies
3. Valvular pathology:
   - Mitral stenosis
   - Endocarditis
   - Mechanical valve prosthesis
4. Cardiac masses:
   - Tumors
   - Proximal aortic atheroma

Low-risk or undetermined risk sources:
1. Valvular pathology:
   - Mitral valve prolapse
   - Calcific aortic stenosis
   - Mitral annular calcification
   - Giant Lambl's excrescences
2. Paradoxical embolism:
   - Patent foramen ovale
   - Atrial septum aneurysm

VALVULAR HEART DISEASE AND STROKE

The patients of valvular heart disease are also at risk of ischemic stroke. Rheumatic heart disease and mechanical prosthetic heart valves are well-recognized risk factors for ischemic stroke. Risk of ischemic stroke is higher in patients of mitral stenosis, particularly with prior history of stroke, atrial thrombus, or enlarged LA (>55 mm in diameter) and needs anticoagulation.[11] Mitral regurgitation with sinus rhythm has lower risk and risk in mitral valve, prolapse is less clear.[12,13] Diseases of the aortic valve including aortic regurgitation, stenosis, sclerosis, and annular calcification do not appear to independently increase the risk of ischemic stroke.[14] Valve replacement increases the risk of ischemic stroke via thromboembolism and this risk is greater with mechanical than bioprosthetic valves. Most patients with mechanical valves should be treated with warfarin with a target INR of 2.0–3.0 for low-risk aortic valve patients, or of 2.5–3.5 for patients with additional risk factors or mitral valves.[15] Mitral annular calcification is a chronic degenerative process characterized by calcium and lipid deposition in the fibrous support of the mitral valve. Mitral annular calcification has been cited as a possible source of cerebral embolism with a relative risk of stroke of 2.1 in the Framingham study but anticoagulation with warfarin is not warranted.[16]

CARDIOMYOPATHY AND STROKE

Cardiomyopathy increases the risk of embolic ischemic stroke, even in patients in sinus rhythm with estimated risk of 1–2% annually.[17] Despite extensive research, the optimal antithrombotic management for stroke prevention is yet not clear. A meta-analysis of the major randomized trials comparing warfarin with aspirin supported the conclusion that treatment of non-AF cardiomyopathy patients with warfarin resulted in fewer strokes. However, there were significantly more major hemorrhages. Mortality was not significantly different between the aspirin and warfarin groups.[18] Presently, the treatment choice of antithrombotic drugs should be individualized with respect to the perceived risks of ischemic stroke and hemorrhage.

HEART FAILURE AND STROKE

The risk of ischemic stroke is 2–3 times higher for patients with congestive heart failure (CHF) than it is for patients without CHF.[19] The stroke risk is highest within 1 month after the diagnosis of heart failure but returns to normal within 6 months.[20] Advancing age, diabetes, and prior stroke are additional risk factor for recurrent stroke in CHF. Various pathophysiological mechanisms have been proposed like activation of the sympathetic nervous system and of the renin-angiotensin-aldosterone system leading to hypercoagulable state, increased aggregation of thrombocytes, endothelial dysfunction, and reduced fibrinolysis in patients with CHF.[21-23] There is no evidence of a clinical benefit of anticoagulation compared with antiplatelet therapy with regard to stroke prevention in CHF patients with persisting sinus rhythm.[24] Within the Sudden Cardiac Death in Heart Failure Trial (SCD-HeFT) study, the use of an implantable cardioverter-defibrillator [odds ratio (OR) 0.57; 95% confidence interval (CI), 0.3–0.99] and the intake of amiodarone (OR 0.44; 95% CI, 0.2–0.8) reduced the rate of thromboembolic complications (predominantly ischemic strokes) in patients with CHF and persisting sinus rhythm.[25]

PATENT FORAMEN OVALE AND STROKE

A stroke is considered cryptogenic when a cause has not been identified. Cryptogenic strokes account for almost 30% of cases and are more common in younger patients.[26] Multiple studies have demonstrated an association between patent foramen ovale (PFO) and cryptogenic stroke.[27] The foramen ovale is an important fetal structure that closes after birth in most individuals and remains open as PFO in approximately 25% of the healthy population.

In these individuals, bypass of the pulmonary circulation via shunting from the right-sided venous circulation to the left-sided arterial circulation is possible.[28] The search for possibility of PFO should be sought in any young patient of ischemic stroke in which there are radiographic evidence of cortical infarct and absence of traditional risk factors like hypertension, diabetes, smoking, prior transient ischemic attack (TIA) or stroke. The more likely the stroke caused by PFO, the lower the risk of recurrence.[29] PFOs have a wide variability in size as detected on transesophageal echocardiography (TEE). However, the relationship of PFO size, physiologic shunt size and presence of shunting of rest, and the development of cryptogenic stroke are conflicting, with early studies suggesting that larger PFOs are associated with cryptogenic stroke,[30] but observations from the risk of paradoxical embolism (RoPE) database showing no relationship.[31] Contrast TEE allows for direct anatomic visualization of shunting across a PFO and is considered the gold standard for diagnosis.[32]

Currently, it is recommended that patients with cryptogenic stroke and PFO should be treated with antiplatelet therapy. There is currently no evidence to suggest a benefit of warfarin over aspirin.[33] Advances in catheter-based techniques have made PFO closure an attractive treatment option. Percutaneous closure is highly effective, with more than 90% success rate and a low rate of adverse events (<5%).[34] Three randomized clinical trials comparing percutaneous PFO closure versus medical therapy have been performed. Based on the three randomized clinical trials, the 2014 American Heart Association and American Stroke Association guidelines recommend against closure of PFO in cryptogenic stroke.[33] Myxomas account for more than half of primary cardiac tumors and thromboembolism is the most common presenting symptom in patients with myxomas. Other primary cardiac tumors include papillary fibroelastoma. The atheromatous aortic arch with plaque thickness of 4 mm and mobile components are other causes.

DIABETES AND STROKE

The number of people suffering from diabetes is projected to increase to 439 million worldwide by 2030.[35] It has been proved beyond doubt that diabetes is an independent and modifiable risk factor for stroke. The adjusted hazard ratio with diabetes for ischemic stroke has been calculated to be 2.27.[36] Even prediabetes (defined as impaired glucose tolerance or a combination of impaired fasting glucose plus impaired glucose tolerance) has been linked to a greater risk of stroke.[36] The incidence of ischemic stroke is higher compared to hemorrhagic stroke in diabetic patients.[37] Among ischemic stroke subtypes, the lacunar infarcts is the most common. This may be due to the higher prevalence of microvascular disease and the coexistence of hypertension seen in this patient group.[36]

Pathophysiology of Stroke in Diabetes

Hyperglycemia induces oxidative stress that leads to microvascular complications by various mechanisms. Hyperglycemia-induced overproduction of reactive oxygen species (ROS) inhibits the action of glyceraldehyde-3-phosphate dehydrogenase (GADPH), a key enzyme in glycolysis. This results in the accumulation of glycolytic intermediates upstream of GAPDH, which leads to activation of various pathogenic pathways contributing to endothelial dysfunction and diabetes complications.[38] Nitric oxide (NO) mediates vasodilation, and in diabetes, there is increased inactivation of NO. This can cause endothelial dysfunction and increased atherosclerosis. Individuals with type II diabetes have stiffer arteries and decreased elasticity compared with subjects having normal glucose level. More recent evidence indicates hyperglycemia-induced ROS production triggers persistent epigenetic changes leading to changes in gene expression.[39]

GLYCEMIC CONTROL AND STROKE

Hyperglycemia is frequently seen in acute stress condition like stroke patients, even without preexisting diabetes diagnosis. It has been shown that even moderately elevated admission glucose level was a significant predictor of larger infarct volumes, mortality, or poor functional recovery after stroke independent of other prognostic factors.[40] In many patients, the first diagnosis of diabetes is often made in the event of an acute stroke and, especially in the elderly. As hyperglycemia is associated with poor outcomes, proper management of post-stroke hyperglycemia is critical for improving outcomes. The American Heart Association (AHA)/American Stroke Association guidelines for the early management of patients with acute ischemic stroke recommends to achieve serum glucose concentrations in the range of 140–180 mg/dL (7.8–10 mmol/L) during the first 24 hours after acute ischemic stroke in all hospitalized patients.[41] There is still debate on how to manage hyperglycemia in acute stroke. The largest efficacy trial to date, the United Kingdom Glucose Insulin in Stroke Trial, showed no difference in mortality or functional outcomes in patients with mild-to-moderate blood glucose elevations. Episodes of hypoglycemia were also observed in 41% of subjects in the treatment arm. Therefore, the use of insulin infusion regimens with mild-to-moderate hyperglycemia is not advisable.[42] Typically, hyperglycemia in the acute setting is treated with subcutaneous insulin.

The evidence of glycemic management after the patient recovers enough to resume oral feeding is also controversial. Although there are chances that there will be diurnal fluctuations and postprandial glucose excursions, but there are no evidences that tight glycemic control by insulin administration can lead to better outcome in randomized, prospective interventional studies.[43] The most appropriate target for hemoglobin A1c (HbA1c) should remain less than 7.

Heart failure is common in subjects with diabetes that is associated with higher risk for stroke. A recent study demonstrated heart failure patients with diabetes and no AF was associated with a 27% increased relative risk of ischemic stroke.[44] The relationship to the duration of diabetes was not established. With the emergence of newer oral and injectable antidiabetic agents in the management of type 2 diabetes mellitus (T2DM), the use of older agents with hypoglycemia risk such as insulin and sulfonylureas as well as glinides is less favored by physicians recently. While metformin and pioglitazone have demonstrated cerebrovascular benefit in the insulin-resistant population, the glucagon-like peptide-1 (GLP-1) analogs have proved their efficacy in cardiovascular outcomes along with weight and blood pressure reduction. The EMPA-REG Trial showed significant cardiovascular benefit with weight and blood pressure reduction though there was a marginal signal of higher stroke rates.[45]

CONCLUSION

Cardiovascular abnormalities and diabetes mellitus are important risk factors for stroke and their presence should be sought in every case. Individualized care plan for stroke patients depending on the clinical scenario should be tailored with considerations of disease comorbidities, including diabetes.

REFERENCES

1. Lozano R, Naghavi M, Foreman K, et al. Global and regional mortality from 235 causes of death for 20 age groups in 1990 and 2010: a systematic analysis for the Global Burden of Disease Study 2010. Lancet. 2012;380:2095-128.
2. Arboix A, Alio J. Acute cardioembolic cerebral infarction: answers to clinical questions. Curr Cardiol Rev. 2012;8:54-67.
3. Chopra HK, Wander GS, Chandra P, et al. Atrial Fibrillation Update "A Textbook of Cardiology", 1st edition. New Delhi: Jaypee Brothers Medical Publishers (P) Ltd. 2017.
4. Shou J, Zhou L, Zhu S, et al. Diabetes is an Independent Risk Factor for Stroke Recurrence in Stroke Patients: A Meta-analysis. J Stroke Cerebrovasc Dis. 2015;24:1961-8.
5. Bogousslavsky J, Cachin C, Regli F, et al. Cardiac sources of embolism and cerebral infarction-clinical consequences and vascular concomitants: The Lausanne Stroke Registry. Neurology. 1991;41:855-9.
6. Bogousslavsky J, Regli J, Uské A, et al. Early spontaneous hematoma in cerebral infarct: is primary cerebral hemorrhage overdiagnosed? Neurology. 1991;41:837-40.
7. Adams HP Jr, Bendixen BH, Kappelle LJ, et al. Classification of subtype of acute ischemic stroke. Definitions for use in a multicenter clinical trial. TOAST. Trial of Org 10172 in Acute Stroke Treatment. Stroke J Cereb Circ. 1993;24:35-41.
8. Gunnoo T, Hasan N, Khan MS, et al. Quantifying the risk of heart disease following acute ischaemic stroke: a meta-analysis of over 50000 participants. BMJ Open. 2016;6:e009535.
9. Wienbergen H, Schiele R, Gitt AK, et al. for the MIR and MITRA Study Groups. Incidence, risk factors, and clinical outcome of stroke after acute myocardial infarction in clinical practice. Am J Cardiol. 2001;87:782-5, A8.
10. O'Gara PT, Kushner FG, Ascheim DD, et al. American College of Cardiology Foundation/American Heart Association Task Force on Practice Guidelines. 2013 ACCF/AHA guideline for the management of ST-elevation myocardial infarction: A report of the American College of Cardiology Foundation/American Heart Association Task Force on Practice Guidelines. Circulation. 2013;127:e362-e425.
11. Whitlock RP, Sun JC, Fremes SE, et al; American College of Chest Physicians. Antithrombotic and thrombolytic therapy for valvular disease: Antithrombotic Therapy and Prevention of Thrombosis, 9th edition: American College of Chest Physicians Evidence Based Clinical Practice Guidelines. Chest. 2012;141:e576S-e600S.
12. Avierinos JF, Brown RD, Foley DA, et al. Cerebral ischemic events after diagnosis of mitral valve prolapse: A community-based study of incidence and predictive factors. Stroke. 2003;34:1339-44.
13. Enriquez-Sarano M, Akins CW, Vahanian A. Mitral regurgitation. Lancet. 2009;373:1382-94.
14. Rodriguez CJ, Bartz TM, Longstreth, et al. Association of annular calcification and aortic valve sclerosis with brain findings on magnetic resonance imaging in community dwelling older adults: The Cardiovascular Health Study. J Am Coll Cardiol. 2011;57: 2172-80.
15. Bonow RO, Carabello BA, Chatterjee K, et al. 2008 Focused update incorporated into the ACC/AHA 2006 guidelines for the management of patients with valvular heart disease: A report of the American College of Cardiology/American Heart Association Task Force on Practice Guidelines (Writing Committee to Revise the 1998 Guidelines for the Management of Patients With Valvular Heart Disease). Circulation. 2008;118:e523-e661.
16. Benjamin EJ, Plehn JF, D'Agostino RB, et al. Mitral annular calcification and the risk of stroke in an elderly cohort. N Engl J Med. 1992;327:374-9.
17. Stöllberger C, Blazek G, Dobias C, et al. Frequency of stroke and embolism in left ventricular hypertrabeculation/noncompaction. Am J Cardiol. 2011;108:1021-3.
18. Kumar G, Goyal MK. Warfarin versus aspirin for prevention of stroke in heart failure: A meta-analysis of randomized controlled clinical trials. J Stroke Cerebrovasc Dis. 2013;22:1279-87.
19. Witt BJ, Brown RD Jr, Jacobsen SJ, et al. Ischemic stroke after heart failure: a community-based study. Am Heart J. 2006;152:102-9.
20. Alberts VP, Bos MJ, Koudstaal PJ, et al. Heart failure and the risk of stroke: the Rotterdam Study. Eur J Epidemiol. 2010;25:807-12.
21. Pullicino P, Homma S. Stroke in heart failure: atrial fibrillation revisited? J Stroke Cerebrovasc Dis. 2010;19:1-2.
22. Georgiadis D, Sievert M, Cencetti S, et al. Cerebrovascular reactivity is impaired in patients with cardiac failure. Eur Heart J. 2000;21: 407-13.

23. Hunt SA, Abraham WT, Chin MH, et al. ACC/AHA 2005 guideline update for the diagnosis and management of chronic heart failure in the adult. Circulation. 2005;112:e154-235.
24. Freudenberger RS, Hellkamp AS, Halperin JL, et al. Risk factors for thromboembolism in the SCD-Heft Study. Circulation. 2007;115:2637-41.
25. Putaala J, Metso AJ, Metso TM, et al. Analysis of 1008 consecutive patients aged 15 to 49 with first-ever ischemic stroke: The Helsinki young stroke registry. Stroke. 2009;40:1195-203.
26. Di Tullio M, Sacco RL, Gopal A, et al. Patent foramen ovale as a risk factor for cryptogenic stroke. Ann Intern Med. 1992;117:461-5.
27. Hagen PT, Scholz DG, Edwards WD. Incidence and size of patent foramen ovale during the first 10 decades of life: An autopsy study of 965 normal hearts. Mayo Clin Proc. 1984;59:17-20.
28. Kent DM, Ruthazer R, Weimar C, et al. An index to identify stroke-related vs incidental patent foramen ovale in cryptogenic stroke. Neurology. 2013;81:619-25.
29. Goel SS, Tuzcu EM, Shishehbor MH, et al. Morphology of the patent foramen ovale in asymptomatic versus symptomatic (stroke or transient ischemic attack) patients. Am J Cardiol. 2009;103:124-9.
30. Wessle BS, Thaler DE, Ruthazer R, et al. Transesophageal echocardiography in cryptogenic stroke and patent foramen ovale: Analysis of putative high-risk features from the risk of paradoxical embolism database. Circ Cardiovasc Imaging. 2014;7:125-31.
31. Schneider B, Zienkiewicz T, Jansen V, et al. Diagnosis of patent foramen ovale by transesophageal echocardiography and correlation with autopsy findings. Am J Cardiol. 1996;77:1202-9.
32. Kernan WN, Ovbiagele B, Black H, et al. Guidelines for the prevention of stroke in patients with stroke and transient ischemic attack: A guideline for healthcare professionals from the American Heart Association/American Stroke Association. Stroke. 2014;45:2160-236.
33. Carroll JD, Saver JL, Thaler DE, et al. Closure of patent foramen ovale versus medical therapy after cryptogenic stroke. N Engl J Med. 2013;368:1092-100.
34. Heidenreich PA, Trogdon JG, Khavjou OA, et al. Forecasting the future of cardiovascular disease in the United States: a policy statement from the American Heart Association. Circulation. 2011;123:933-44.
35. Collaboration TERF. Diabetes mellitus, fasting blood glucose concentration, and risk of vascular disease: a collaborative meta-analysis of 102 prospective studies. Lancet. 2010;375:2215-22.
36. Lee M, Saver JL, Hong KS, et al. Effect of pre-diabetes on future risk of stroke: meta-analysis. Br Med J. 2012;344:e3564.
37. Tuttolomondo A, Pinto A, Salemi G, et al. Diabetic and non-diabetic subjects with ischemic stroke: differences, subtype distribution and outcome. Nutr Metab Cardiovasc Dis. 2008;18:152-7.
38. Brownlee M. The pathobiology of diabetic complications: a unifying mechanism. Diabetes. 2005;54:1615-25.
39. El-Osta A, Brasacchio D, Yao D, et al. Transient high glucose causes persistent epigenetic changes and altered gene expression during subsequent normoglycemia. J Exp Med. 2008;205:2409-17.
40. Hankey GJ, Anderson NE, Ting RD, et al. Rates and predictors of risk of stroke and its subtypes in diabetes: a prospective observational study. J Neurol Neurosurg Psychiatry. 2013;84:281-7.
41. Jauch EC, Saver JL, Adams HP, et al. Guidelines for the early management of patients with acute ischemic stroke a guideline for healthcare professionals from the American Heart Association/American Stroke Association. Stroke. 2013;44:870-947.
42. Gray CS, Hildreth AJ, Sandercock PA, et al. Glucose potassium-insulin infusions in the management of post-stroke hyperglycaemia: the UK Glucose Insulin in Stroke Trial (GIST-UK). Lancet Neurol. 2007;6:397-406.
43. Raz I, Wilson PW, Strojek K, et al. Effects of prandial versus fasting glycemia on cardiovascular outcomes in type 2 diabetes: the HEART2D trial. Diabetes Care. 2009;32:381-6.
44. Melgaard L, Gorst-Rasmussen A, Søgaard P, et al. Diabetes mellitus and risk of ischemic stroke in patients with heart failure and no atrial fibrillation. Int J Cardiol 2016;209:1-6.
45. Zinman B, Wanner C, Lachin JM, et al. Empagliflozin, Cardiovascular Outcomes, and Mortality in Type 2 Diabetes. N Engl J Med. 2015;373:2117-28.

CHAPTER

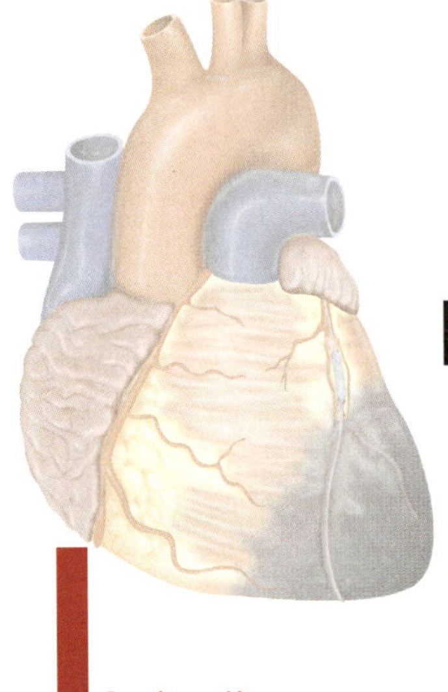

Hemorrhagic Stroke and Cardiodiabetes

Sanjeev Kumar

INTRODUCTION

The hemorrhagic stroke, which accounts for 15% of all cases of stroke, represents the most devastating form of neurological disorder with the mortality approaching 70% at the end of one year. Amongst the survivors, it is the leading cause of severe disability. The sudden development of persistent focal neurological deficit secondary to a vascular event is classical of stroke. The hemorrhagic stroke is caused by bleeding directly into or around the brain. Depending upon the location, it can take the form of intracerebral hemorrhage (ICH) when the bleeding occurs in the brain substance, subarachnoid hemorrhage (SAH) when the bleed occurs in subarachnoid space or intraventricular bleed (IVH) where the ventricles are involved. It causes the neurological symptoms by producing a mass effect on neural structures, from toxic effects of blood itself or by increasing the intracranial pressure (ICP) (Fig. 1). In contrast to ischemic stroke which typically has significant sensory or motor deficit with little or no impairment of consciousness (except massive or brain stem stroke), intracerebral bleed is associated with smooth onset of symptoms over minutes or hours, presence of severe headache, frequent vomiting with depression of consciousness at the outset.

Heart disease is an important risk factor for the stroke. *This in part reflects the common underlying precursor's for stroke and heart disease—hypertension and atherosclerosis.* The risk of stroke is doubled in individuals with coronary artery disease, which accounts for the majority of deaths amongst the stroke survivors. *Of the modifiable risk factors, hypertension is most important for the stroke.* The degree of risk increases with higher levels of blood pressure and becomes particularly strong with levels higher than 160/95 mm Hg. The successful long-term treatment of hypertension results in substantial risk reduction. The early diagnosis and effective management of hypertension limits the secondary changes of hypertensive vascular disease. The treatment of hypertension after a patient has had a stroke is much less effective in reducing the future risk of vascular events.

Atrial fibrillation (AF) and valvular heart disease increases the risk of cerebral infarctions secondary to cerebral emboli and their prevention needs long-term anticoagulation which carries the danger of ICH especially in elderly with impaired balance who are likely to fall. Diabetes is an independent risk factor and doubles the risk of stroke. However, good sugar control alone does not seem to significantly slow down the progression of CVA. Stroke and diabetes accounts for third and fifth leading cause of death in the United States of America. Patients with diabetes mellitus who have heart disease or stroke usually fare worse than their nondiabetic counterparts.

Hyperglycemia is common in acute stroke settings. There is approximate 30% risk of poor outcome of patients with immediate poststroke hyperglycemia as compared to euglycemic patients. Further research is needed to define the degree of glucose control that is optimal for better neurological outcome. SAH accounts for 7% of all cases of stroke. The most common cause of SAH is rupture of arterial aneurysm at the base of brain. The aneurysm develops from small defects in the wall of arteries and slowly increase in the size with eventual hemorrhage. The aneurysm often forms at the site of hemodynamic stress and hypertension

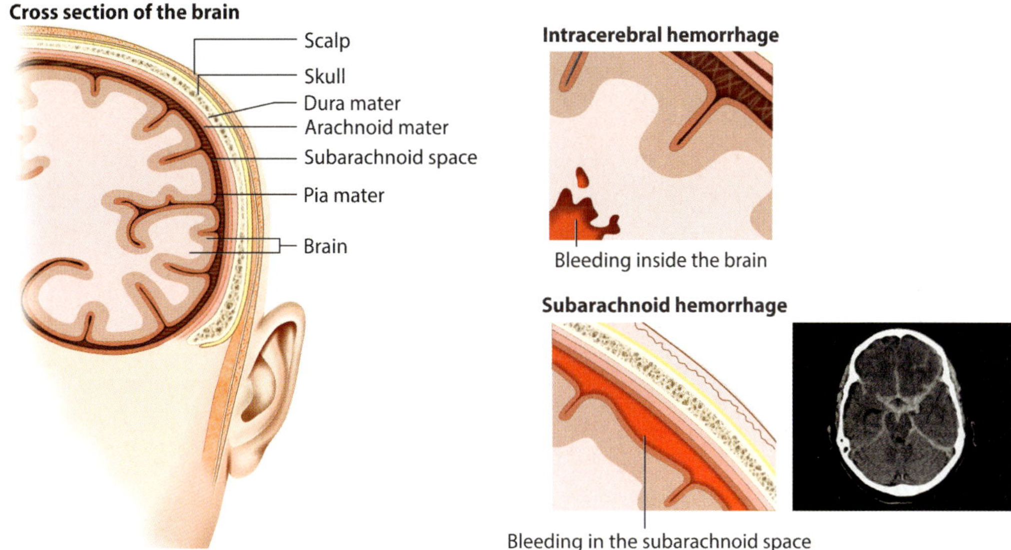

Fig. 1: Major types of intracranial bleed

may play a role. More than half of the patients with ruptured aneurysm have pre-existing evidence of hypertension.

Neural tissues are very sensitive and once insulted, they cannot regenerate. Therefore, in spite of advancements in neurological surgery, neurocritical care and diagnostic modalities, each year hemorrhagic stroke adds significantly to the pool of severe disabilities with its huge emotional, social and financial implications. The importance of stress on preventive measures for hemorrhagic stroke cannot be overemphasized (Fig. 2). This chapter attempts further to explore the crucial link of the "heart-brain connect" in the genesis of stroke and keeps a stress on collaborative approach amongst cardiac and neuroscientists in pursuit to optimize our efforts in the larger interest of humanity (Fig. 3).

Fig. 2: Human brain: a mystery

REVIEW OF LITERATURE

Hypertension and Hemorrhagic Stroke

In Framingham heart study, a sevenfold increased risk of cerebral infarction was observed in patients who were hypertensive. Hypertension increases the risk of several stroke types including thrombotic, lacunar, hemorrhagic and SAH. Successful long-term treatment of hypertension results in substantial risk reduction. Early diagnosis and effective management of hypertension limits the secondary changes of hypertensive vascular disease. Treatment of hypertension after a patient has had a stroke is much less effective in reducing the risk of future vascular event.[1] The International Society of Hypertension labels hypertension as the most important modifiable risk factor for stroke. The Seventh Report of Joint National Commission (JNC7)

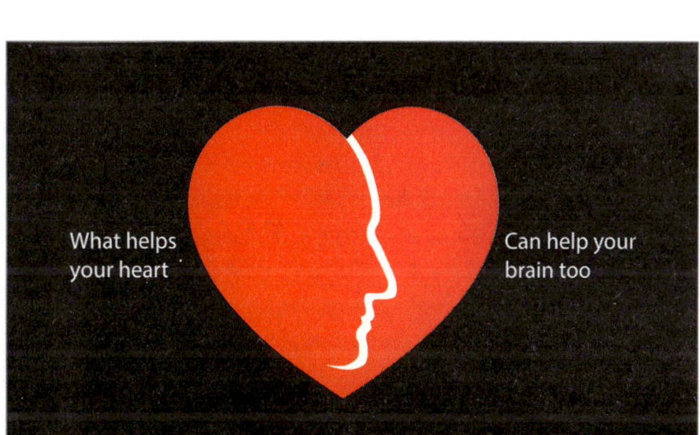

Fig. 3: Heart-brain connect

Target organ damage with hypertension

- Brain
  - Stroke or transient ischemic attack

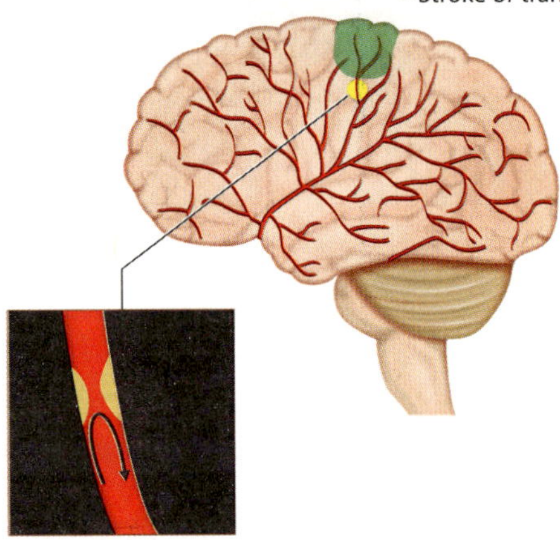

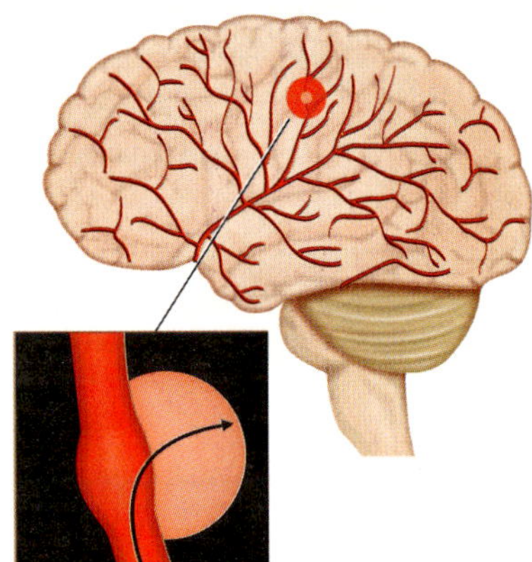

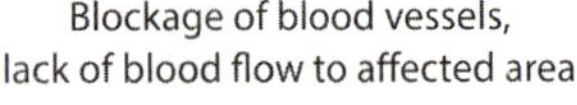

Ischemic stroke

Rupture of blood vessels,
leakage of blood in affected area

Hemorrhage stroke

Fig. 4: Hypertension: a modifiable giant killer

defines hypertension as systolic pressure higher than 140 mm Hg and diastolic pressure higher than 90 mm Hg. The association of hypertension is stronger with hemorrhagic stroke than ischemic and it rises with an increase in blood pressure (Fig. 4).[2,3]

Ambulatory blood pressure monitoring is indicated when the person suspects episodic hypertension, "white coat" hypertension and autonomic hypertension. Aspirin therapy should not be started in uncontrolled hypertension as it can increase the risk of hemorrhagic stroke. If a patient has diabetes or chronic kidney disease, the goal of blood pressure should be less than 130/80 mm Hg. The higher-pressure category determines the goal, i.e. systolic or diastolic. Increased systolic blood pressure (SBP) is an important risk factor and requires treatment, especially in elderly. When treating isolated systolic hypertension in older patients more than 65 years, increased risk of stroke was noted at diastolic blood pressure (DBP) less than 65 mm Hg. Blood pressure should be treated cautiously in these patients. Special consideration must be given to patients with significant cerebral atherosclerosis. Overly tight blood pressure control in some cases with severe stenosis can lead to hypoperfusion and stroke. The degree and location of stenosis should be considered when prescribing and managing hypertension in poststroke patients.

Hypertension together with age is the leading risk factor for silent or symptomatic cerebrovascular disease. High blood pressure multiplies the risk for stroke as much as four-fold. Both factors are also related to the probability of suffering some degree of cognitive impairment. The risk of cerebral hemorrhage in hypertensive patients is 3.9 times higher than in non-hypertensive individuals. In aneurysmal SAH , the relative risk is 2.8 higher.

The diagnosis and control of hypertension is one of the main strategies for primary and secondary prevention of stroke. The effect of chronic hypertension on cerebral vessels and tissue (microhemorrhages, silent infarctions, white matter lesions and atrophy) also supports a physiopathological mechanism for the association between hypertension and cognitive impairment.[4,5]

To better define the etiologic importance of hypertension for spontaneous ICH, hospital records were studied for all patients sustaining ICH during 1982 in the Cincinnati metropolitan area. Hypertension predating the hemorrhage was present in 45% (69 of 154), as determined by history. A more inclusive definition of hypertension, combining those with a positive history with those found to have left ventricular hypertrophy by electrocardiogram or cardiomegaly by chest radiography, applied in 56% (87 of 154). The cases were compared to controls with and without hypertension derived from the National Health and Nutrition Examination Survey (NHANES) II study of blood pressure (n = 16,204) to determine the relative risk. For the presence of hypertension by history, the relative risk of ICH was 3.9 (95% confidence interval, 2.7–5.7). For the inclusive definition of hypertension, the relative risk was 5.4 (3.7–7.9). Relative risk was also determined for hypertension in blacks (= 4.4), age greater than 70 (= 7), prior cerebral infarction (= 22), and diabetes (= 3). The study concluded that the term "hypertensive hemorrhage" should be used very selectively and proposed that hypertension be viewed as one of several important risk factors for spontaneous ICH.[6] Elevated blood pressure is seen in 46–56% of patients with ICH.[7] It remains unclear if elevated blood pressure directly causes hematoma expansion but studies have shown elevated systolic, diastolic, and mean arterial pressure are associated with a poor outcome in ICH.[8] However, physicians have been reluctant to treat hypertension in ICH patients because of the fear of overaggressive treatment of blood pressure which may decrease cerebral perfusion pressure (CPP) and theoretically worsen brain injury, particularly in the setting of increased ICP. In 1999, a special group consisting of healthcare professionals from the American Heart Association Stroke Council addressed these two rational theoretical concerns while attempting to write guidelines for the management of ICH. The task force recommended maintaining a mean arterial pressure below 130 mm Hg in patients with a history of hypertension (level of evidence V, grade C recommendation). In patients with elevated ICP who have an ICP monitor, cerebral perfusion pressure [Mean arterial pressure (MAP)–ICP] should be kept more than 70 mm Hg (level of evidence V, grade C recommendation).[9]

In summary, hypertension, smoking, and regular heavy alcohol use are important, modifiable risk factors for ICH in the young and middle-aged present an opportunity for prevention of this devastating type of stroke. The association of ICH with menopause and caffeine consumption deserves further investigation.[10]

Diabetes Mellitus and Hemorrhagic Stroke

According to the World Health Organization (WHO) statistics, there are 150,000,000 diabetic patients worldwide and this rate is estimated to reach more than 300,000,000 patients by 2025. Furthermore, given the gigantic costs, diabetes can be considered as the most significant challenge of the 21st century in developing countries (Fig. 5).[11]

Diabetes is the major risk factor that contributes significantly to the incidence of stroke. Patients with diabetes who develop heart disease or stroke fare worse than their nondiabetic counterparts. Although tight control of serum glucose level is desirable for the microvascular complication of diabetes, its role in stroke prevention seems minor. Rigid control of blood pressure appears to be crucial for stroke prevention in diabetic patients. Angiotensin-converting enzyme (ACE) inhibitors should be considered as first line treatment for diabetic patients with hypertension.

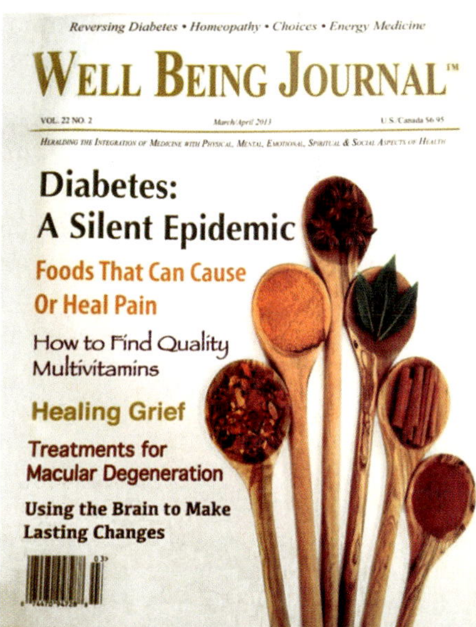

Fig. 5: Diabetes: a global silent killer

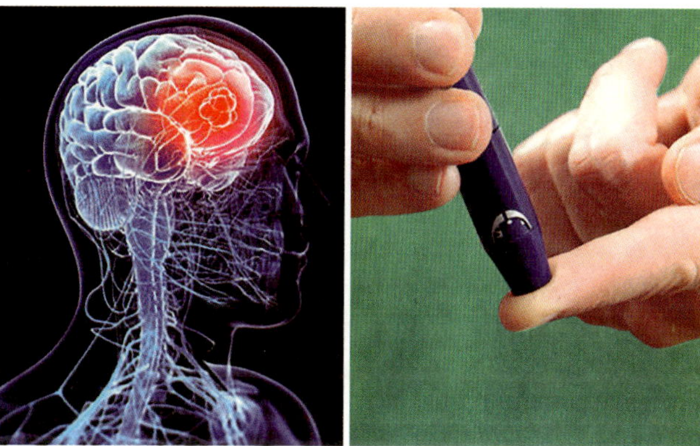

Fig. 6: Diabetes and brain attack: an intricate association

In a study by Hitt et al., it confirmed the correlation between diabetes mellitus and ICH in individuals less than 55 years of age. In older age groups, though, no such direct correlation was found, but there was a compounding risk along with other risk factors. However, the etiology of this correlation is not clear and must be investigated in future studies (Fig. 6).[12]

Another important issue, which should be taken into consideration, is the role of high blood glucose or diabetes mellitus in prognosis of patients with ICH. It has been shown that high plasma glucose at the admission time is an independent predictor of death after ICH. High blood sugar also has a high impact on mortality from hemorrhagic stroke. The present study also could not find a significant relationship between diabetes mellitus and ICH (except in patients younger than 60 years). Further prospective studies with a larger sample size are required to evaluate the relationship of diabetes mellitus and ICH separately in the elderly and young individuals.[13]

The brain is a site of both macrovascular and microvascular complications of diabetes. Microvessel structural and functional changes due to acute and chronic hyperglycemia lead to increased incidence and worsened outcomes from stroke in diabetic patients. Acute hyperglycemia also reduces both the safety and efficacy of reperfusion therapy in acute ischemic stroke patients. Lessons learned from experimental models of acute, chronic, mild and severe diabetes help explain some, but not all, of these clinical observations. More investigations need to be performed to identify novel targets for therapeutic intervention so that the consequences of cerebrovascular complications can be mitigated in patients with diabetes.

The importance of serum glucose in the complications of reperfusion therapy for acute ischemic stroke was first reported by Demchuk et al. when 138 consecutive patients that received recombinant tissue plasminogen activator (rtPA) within 3 hours of the onset of stroke were studied. Symptomatic intracerebral hemorrhage (sICH), the dreaded complication of reperfusion therapy, occurred in 9% of patients and admission serum glucose was the only independent predictor of sICH in multivariate analysis. In patients with admission glucose more than 11.2 mmol/L, the rate was more than 25%. This was replicated in the Prolyse in Acute Cerebral Thromboembolism (PROACT) II study, where acute ischemic stroke patients were treated with intra-arterial prourokinase within 6 hours of onset of symptoms. In this study, patients with blood glucose more than 200 mg/dL (11 mmol/L) experienced sICH at a rate of 36%.

Diabetic patients are at 2- to 6-fold increased risk of stroke, compared to their age-matched counterparts, and the highest relative risks occur in young type 1 diabetics. In addition, hyperglycemia at the time of acute ischemic stroke is associated with increased death and dependency. Acute hyperglycemia, especially more than 200 mg/dL, increases the risk of severe ICH after treatment with reperfusion therapy and decreases the likelihood of neurologic recovery. Although trials are ongoing to test the efficacy of glucose control in the acute stroke period, the risk of hypoglycemia is an ever-present threat. Understanding the mechanisms and consequences of cerebrovascular damage due to diabetes, using experimental models, may assist in the design of therapeutic strategies that are vascular protective.[14]

Dyslipidemia, hypertension and obesity are atherogenic risk factors frequently found in type 2 diabetes patients. Also, diabetes is an independent risk factor of ischemic stroke of atherothrombotic cause. The influence of diabetes upon increasing the stroke risk is higher in women than in men. Diabetes is the main risk factor following hypertension of cerebral small vessel disease and has been identified as a significant independent variable of symptomatic recurrence in patients with first-ever cerebral infarction of the lacunar type. The combination of hypercholesterolemia and hypertension increases the frequency of vascular complications in patients with diabetes.[15,16]

Cardiac Diseases and Hemorrhagic Stroke

Heart diseases are the second cause of acute cerebrovascular events and are diagnosed in one-third of patients with stroke. AF and atrial flutter are the most important and modifiable risk factor frequently associated with cardioembolic stroke. Cardioembolic infarction is the most severe stroke subtype due to the very low percentage of symptom-free patients at hospital discharge, the non-negligible risk of early recurrent embolic events and the high mortality in the acute stroke phase (27% in the Sagrat Cor of Barcelona Stroke Registry).

The prevalence of AF increases with age. It has been shown that 5% of subjects older than 70 years have AF (the mean age of patients with AF is 75 years), and about one-fourth of acute strokes in very old patients (> 80 years) are caused by AF. Future embolism is also more frequent in patients with underlying comorbid heart diseases, such as AF and stenosis of the mitral valve. The risk of stroke is 3–4 times higher in the absence of organic heart disease or risk factors (lone atrial fibrillation). On the other hand, AF associated to hypertensive heart disease is the most common cardiogenic source of cerebral embolization in industrialized countries. Similar rates of cardioembolism for paroxysmal and chronic AF have been reported, so that preventive therapy should not be different for patients with paroxysmal AF and those with chronic AF. In patients without history of transient ischemic attack (TIA) or stroke, AF carries a risk of stroke of 2–4% per year. Cardiac emboli arising from cardiac chambers are often large and hence especially likely to cause severe stroke, disability and death.

A number of cardiac conditions are potential sources of embolism, such as dilated cardiomyopathy, heart valve disease (mechanical prosthetic valve, mitral rheumatic stenosis, infectious endocarditis, marantic endocarditis), left ventricular hypertrophy, atrial myxoma and congenital heart diseases (such as patent foramen ovale, atrial septal aneurysm and ventricular septal defects). Acute coronary syndromes are minor causes of cardioembolism. There is an inverse correlation between ejection fraction of the left ventricle and the incidence of ischemic stroke.[15,16]

For prevention of cardioembolic events, anticoagulants and antiplatelets are used which increases the chances of hemorrhagic stroke, making this association very intricate.

INTRACEREBRAL HEMORRHAGE

Definition

Intracerebral hemorrhage is a type of intracranial bleed that occurs within the brain tissue or ventricles.

Epidemiology

Intracerebral hemorrhage affects about 2.5 per 10,000 people each year. It occurs more often in males and older people. About 44% of those affected die within a month. A good outcome occurs in about 20% of those affected.[17] It accounts for 10% of all cases of stroke with 50% case fatality rate.

Etiology

Brain trauma, aneurysms, arteriovenous malformations (AVMs), brain tumors and idiopathic varieties are the main causes. The largest risk factors for spontaneous bleeding are high blood pressure and amyloidosis. Other risk factors include alcoholism, dyslipidemia, anticoagulants and antiplatelet treatment, diabetes mellitus, menopause, cigarette smoking, excessive alcohol consumption, and coagulation disorder.[18,19]

Symptoms

It can include headache, one-sided weakness, vomiting, seizures, decreased level of consciousness, and neck stiffness. Often symptoms get worse over time. Fever is also common. In many cases, bleeding is present in both the brain tissue and the ventricles.

Location

When due to high blood pressure, they typically occur in the putamen or thalamus (60%), cerebrum (20%), cerebellum[13] or pons (7%).[20]

Pathological Effects

Space occupying effects and increasing mass effects inside the brain. Most hypertensive hemorrhages develop over 30–90 minutes whereas those associated with anticoagulant therapy develop over 24–48 hours. Edema is a prominent feature. Hematoma resolution occurs in 1–6 months leaving a cystic cavity.

Investigation

CT Scan

The investigation of choice for acute focal hemorrhage in supratentorial space. MRI of the brain is generally not recommended unless CT scan is inconclusive.

Angiography

Magnetic resonance angiography or CT angiography or digital subtraction angiography (DSA) may be needed to rule out AVM or underlying aneurysm if there is atypical presentation like temporal hematoma in a young non-hypertensive patient may be due to middle cerebral artery aneurysm.

For diagnosing hemorrhagic stroke in the emergency setting:

- CT scans (*without* contrast enhancements)
  - Sensitivity = 89%
  - Specificity = 100%
- MRI scan
  - Sensitivity = 81%
  - Specificity = 100%[21]

Clinical Effects

The clinical effects depend upon the location of the hematoma. It generally presents as abrupt onset of focal neurological deficit. This focal deficit typically worsens steadily over 30–90 minutes and is associated with diminishing level of consciousness and signs of raised ICP like headache or vomiting.

Management

Basic Principles

Treatment should ideally be carried out in an intensive care unit. Antihypertensive therapy started to bring down the blood pressure in acute phases appears to improve outcome. The American Heart Association and American Stroke Association guidelines in 2015 recommended decreasing the blood pressure to a SBP of 140 mm Hg.[18]

Systemic reviews have shown that increased risk of death, deterioration, dependency with increased blood pressure after ICH. Extremes of blood pressure should be corrected immediately to minimize the potential for hematoma expansion and to maintain adequate CPP, which is MAP–ICP. Treatment of hypertension should be aggressive but one has to be very careful to avoid excessive reduction of CPP, which might precipitate ischemia in peri-hematoma zone (Fig. 7).

HEMATOMA GROWTH

- In a meta-analysis of 218 patients with spontaneous ICH who had a head CT scan within 3 hours of onset and follow-up head CT within 24 hours, each 10% increase in ICH growth was associated with increased mortality (hazard ratio 1.05, 95% CI 1.03–1.08) and worse outcome as measured by the modified Rankin scale (odds ratio 0.84, 95% CI 0.75–0.92).[1]
- That is, for each 10% increase in hematoma volume, patients were 5% more likely to die and 16% more likely to increase one point on the modified Rankin scale.

1. Davis SM, Broderick J, Hennerici M, et al. Hematoma growth is a determinant of mortality and poor outcome after intracerebral hemorrhage. Neurology 2006; 66:1175.

Fig. 7: Risk of hematoma growth with hypertension

American Stroke Association recommends MAP be maintained less than 130 mm Hg for ICH patients with history of hypertension. In patients who have undergone craniotomy, MAP should be less than 100. In all cases, systolic blood pressure should be maintained more than 90 mm Hg. In patients with ICP monitor, CPP should be maintained more than 70 mm Hg. Hypertension should be controlled with repeated IV dose of labetalol every 10 minutes with doses escalating from 20 mg to 80 mg.

In ICU settings, blood pressure is best controlled with continuous infusion of labetalol/esmolol/nicardipine. Sodium nitroprusside should be avoided because of the tendency of this agent to cause cerebral vasodilation and elevated ICP. NIH trial gives highest priority to a trial of aggressive blood pressure control (MAP 100–120 mm Hg) within first three hours of ICH onset.

Antiplatelets should be reversed if possible and blood sugar kept in the normal range.

In general, supratentorial hematoma with volume less than 30 mL has favorable prognosis. 30–60 mL has intermediate prognosis and more than 60 mL has poor prognosis. Extension into ventricular system, advancing age, location in posterior fossa, poor GCS at the time of presentation are associated with poor outcomes. Though Surgical Treatment for Ischemic Heart Failure (STICH) trial did not support routine surgical evacuation of ICH, it does have a definite role in patient with deteriorating sensorium and worsening neurological deficit. The cerebellar hematoma more than 3 cm requires surgery and less than 1 cm surgical removal is unnecessary. If hematoma is between 1–3 cm, it needs careful observation and surgical intervention if clinical worsening or rise in ICP. Pontine or brain stem bleed has poorer prognosis. Intraventricular bleed has poor outcome. External ventricular drain (EVD) may be considered to relieve the ICP.

TYPES OF SURGERY

- *Intracranial pressure monitoring*: For close monitoring of patients being managed conservatively. May be coupled with external ventricular drainage.
- *External ventricular drain or reservoir*: EVD may be considered to relieve the ICP. It allows the therapeutic advantage of cerebrospinal fluid drainage but has the disadvantage of infection.
- *Craniotomy and evacuation of hematoma*: The standard surgical intervention for ICH. The drain may be placed in situ in view of high risk of recollection (Figs 8A to D).
- Decompressive craniectomy: To relieve the intracranial pressure.
- Endoscopic or stereotactic removal of hematoma aspiration by stereotactic surgery or endoscopic drainage may be used in basal ganglia hemorrhages, although successful reports are limited.[22]

PROGNOSIS

Extension into ventricular system, advancing age, location in posterior fossa, poor Glasgow Coma Scale (GCS) at presentation are associated with poor outcomes. For spontaneous ICH seen on CT scan, the death rate (mortality) is 34–50% by 30 days after the insult and half of the deaths occur in the first 2 days. Even though the majority of deaths occur in the first days after ICH, survivors have a long-term excess mortality of 27% compared to the general population.[23]

SUBARACHNOID HEMORRHAGE (FIG. 9)

Definition

The intracranial vessels lie in subarachnoid space (the area between arachnoid membrane and pia mater that surrounds the brain) and give off small perforating branches to brain tissue. Bleeding from these vessels or from an associated aneurysm occurs primarily into this space and therefore known as subarachnoid hemorrhage or SAH. It occurs in 10–15 per 100,000 persons per year.

Causes

The most common cause of SAH is aneurysm formation (75%) in whose formation of hypertension can play an important role. Hypertension can also precipitate SAH. Other risk factors for spontaneous cases include smoking, family history, alcoholism, oral contraceptive pills, and cocaine use.[24]

Symptoms and Signs

A severe headache of rapid onset (classical description is "sudden onset of the worst headache of my life", which is present in 97% of cases), vomiting, decreased level

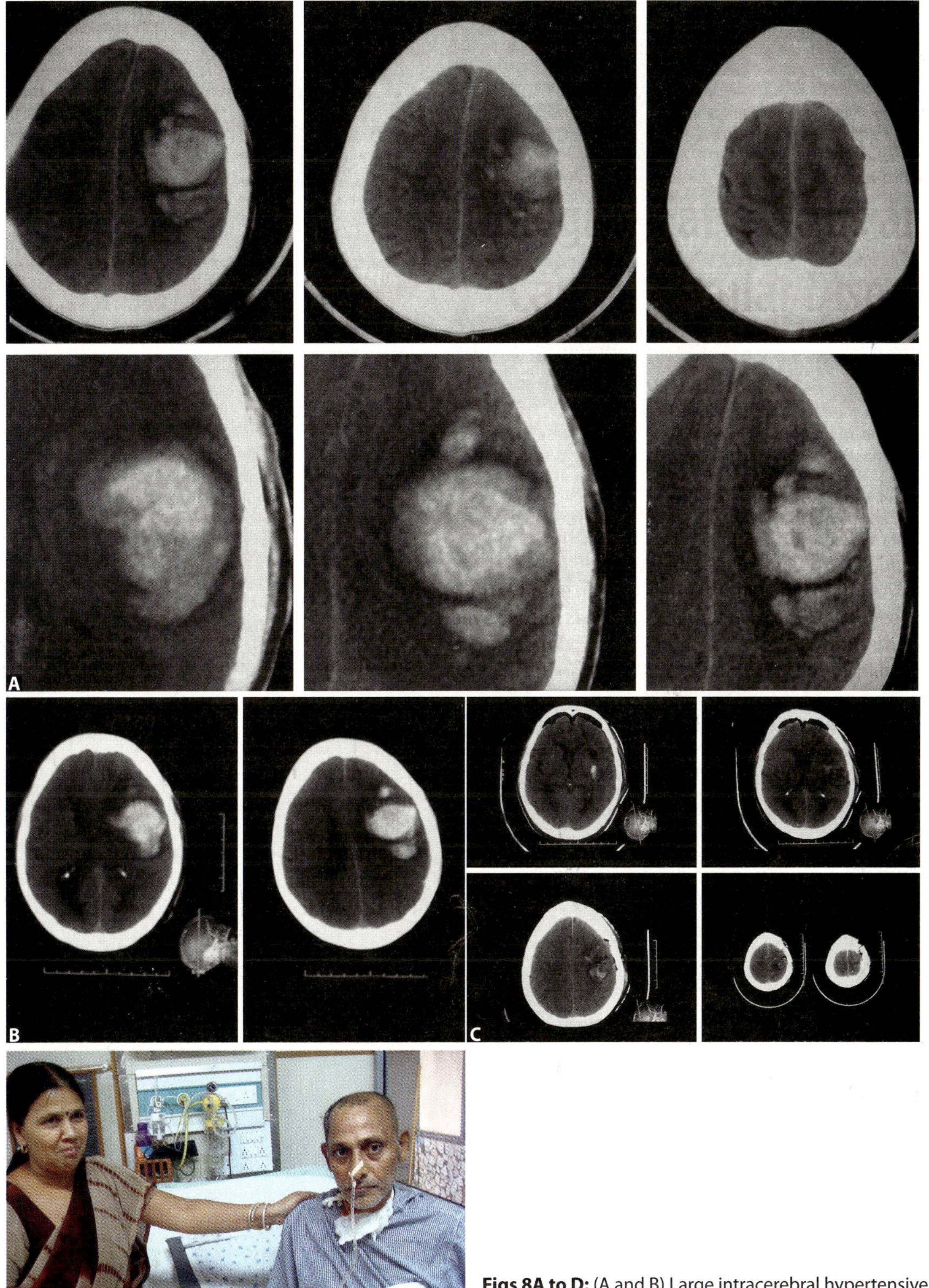

Figs 8A to D: (A and B) Large intracerebral hypertensive bleed with mass effect with poor Glasgow Coma Score; (C) Postoperative CT scan day 1—significant decrease of mass effect following craniotomy; (D) The patient in postoperative state

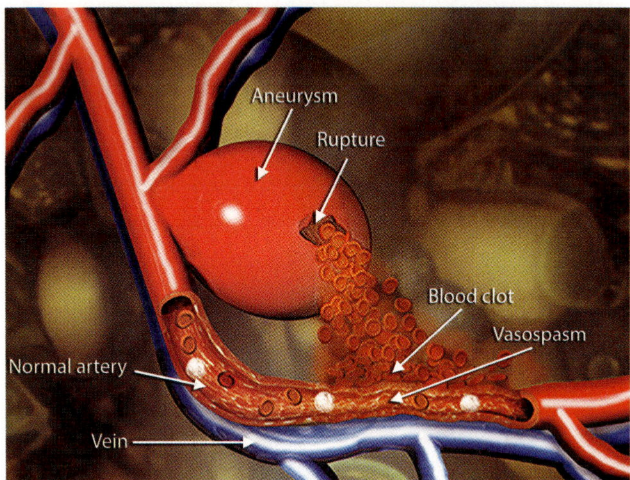

Fig. 9: The intracranial aneurysm

of consciousness, fever, and sometimes seizures. Neck stiffness or neck pain is also relatively common. In about a quarter of people, a small bleed with resolving symptoms occurs within a month of a larger bleed which is known as "sentinel bleed". The focal neurological deficit (diplopia, ptosis from third nerve palsy), hemiparesis, etc. may occur. Sign of meningism (neck stiffness) develops 3–12 hours later. Fundus examination may reveal papilledema or subhyaloid hemorrhage. There may be reactive hypertension with no pre-existing history.

Investigations

- CT head: The best modality for the initial assessment. Confirms the diagnosis in 95%.
- Lumbar puncture: If CT does not reveal SAH and index of suspicion is very high, lumbar puncture may be done.
- Digital subtraction angiography: A dedicated 4-vessel angiogram is the gold standard in all the cases of SAH.
- CT angiography: With sensitivity of 95% and specificity of 83% in detecting aneurysm more than 2.2 mm, it is considered superior to DSA in showing the three-dimensional image of aneurysm and its relation to bony structures.
- Magnetic resonance angiography: It has sensitivity of 86–95% in detecting aneurysm more than 3 mm. It is accepted as screening test in patient who is at high risk of harboring intracranial aneurysm.[25-27]

Pathogenesis of Aneurysm Formation

Aneurysms were once thought to have congenital origin. It however appears that they appear because of defects of internal elastic lamina and are probably related to arteriosclerotic changes.

Severity Grading of Subarachnoid Hemorrhage[28]

- Hunt and Hess Grading.
- World Federation of Neurological Surgeons (WFNS) Grading.

Management of Subarachnoid Hemorrhage

- Bed rest
- Prevention of rebleed
  - *Clipping of aneurysm:* The historical gold standard to secure the neck of aneurysm by applying clips after craniotomy and dissection of aneurysm (Fig. 10).
  - *Endovascular treatment:* A landmark multicenter prospective randomized trial (The International Subarachnoid Aneurysm trial [(ISAT)] compared clipping and endovascular treatment of ruptured aneurysm and demonstrated that the endovascular coil embolization had superior outcomes compared with craniotomy for clip ligation in certain patients (Fig. 11):[29]
    - *Coil embolization*: Stent assisted coiling for wide neck aneurysm (Fig. 12).
    - *Balloon embolization*: A balloon is placed inside the lumen using endovascular technique and coils placed.
  - *Trapping*: In giant or intracavernous aneurysm, trapping may be considered in which proximal and distal arterial occlusion is done surgically or by balloon followed by extracranial-intracranial bypass to continue flow distally (Fig. 13).

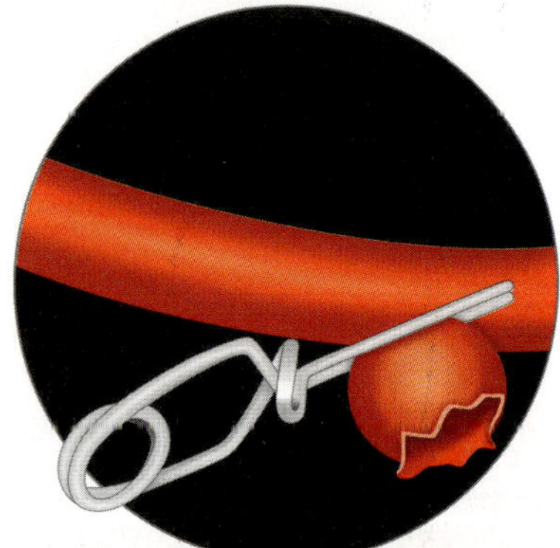

Fig. 10: Clipping of the neck of aneurysm: a thrill for neurosurgeons

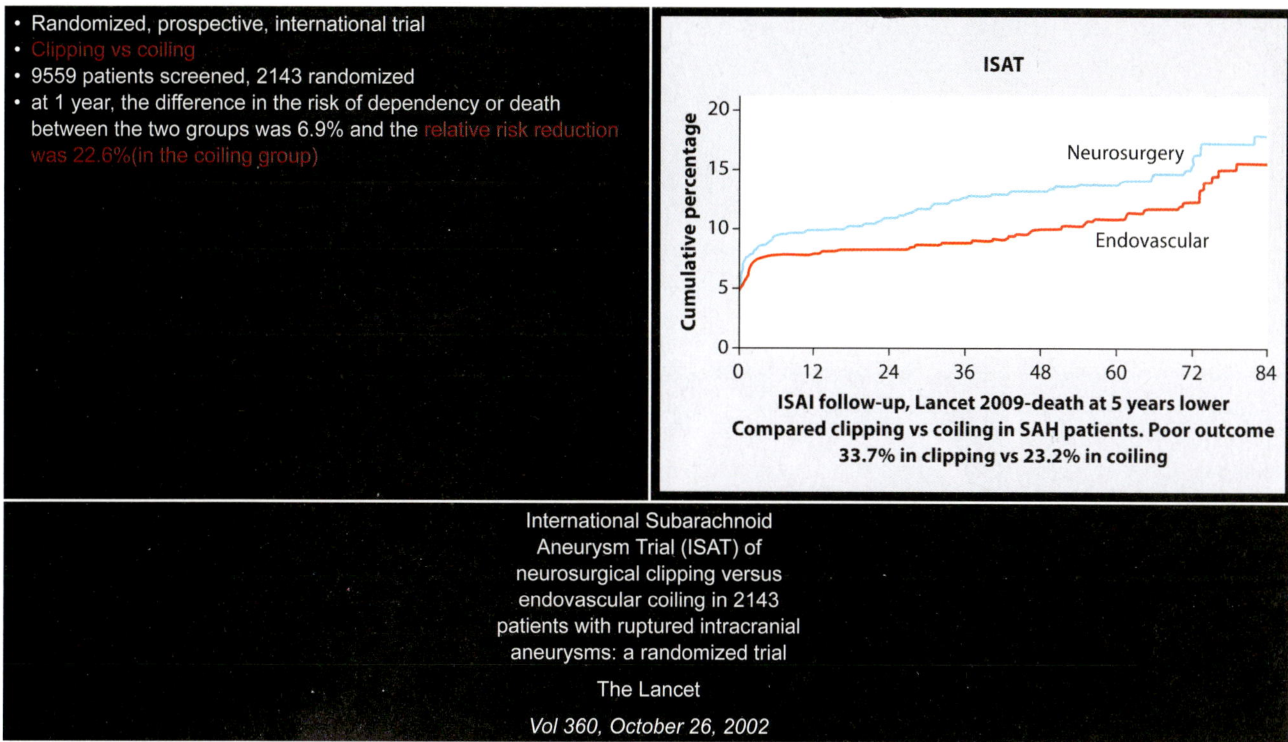

Fig. 11: The International Subarachnoid Aneurysm trial (ISAT)—a landmark trial published in Lancet changed the way aneurysmal subarachnoid hemorrhage is treated

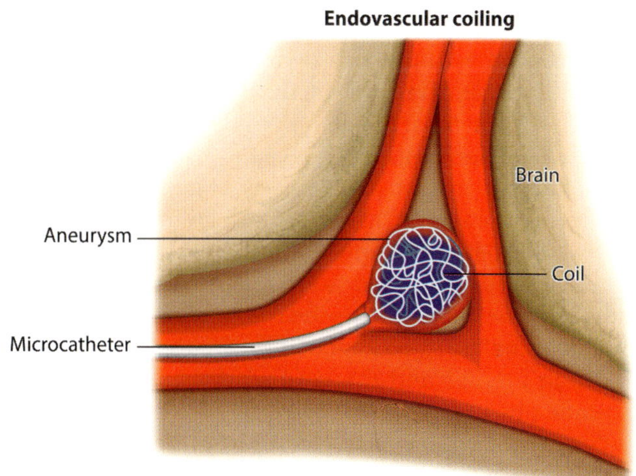

Fig. 12: Endovascular coiling of aneurysm—schematic

- Prevention of cerebral ischemia
  - *Calcium antagonists*: Nimodipine oral or intravenous is the most commonly used agent.
  - *3H therapy*: It is often used as a measure to treat vasospasm when it causes symptoms. This is the use of intravenous fluids to achieve a state of hypertension, hypervolemia and hemodilution (mild dilution of the blood).[30]

    Systolic blood pressure should be maintained at 120–150 mm Hg by cuff for unsecured aneurysm to avoid re-rupture. Once aneurysm is secured, blood pressure needs to be elevated. Standard treatment of patient in vasospasm includes hyperdynamic therapy or 3H therapy which is believed to result in indirect arterial dilation and enhanced perfusion of ischemic areas of brain by alteration of rheological properties of blood. Iatrogenic hypertension by expansion of blood volume has been shown to be beneficial in this population.

    It is important to note that hypertension in a patient with an unsecured ruptured aneurysm can provoke devastating re-hemorrhage. Hyperdynamic therapy may be dangerous in patient with massive cerebral edema or large ischemic infarcts as edema may be exacerbated or hemorrhagic conversion of infarct may ensue, respectively.
  - Neuroprotective agents.

Prognosis

Subarachnoid hemorrhage is often associated with a poor outcome.[31] Aneurysmal SAH carries a very high initial mortality risk which gradually declines with time. Of those

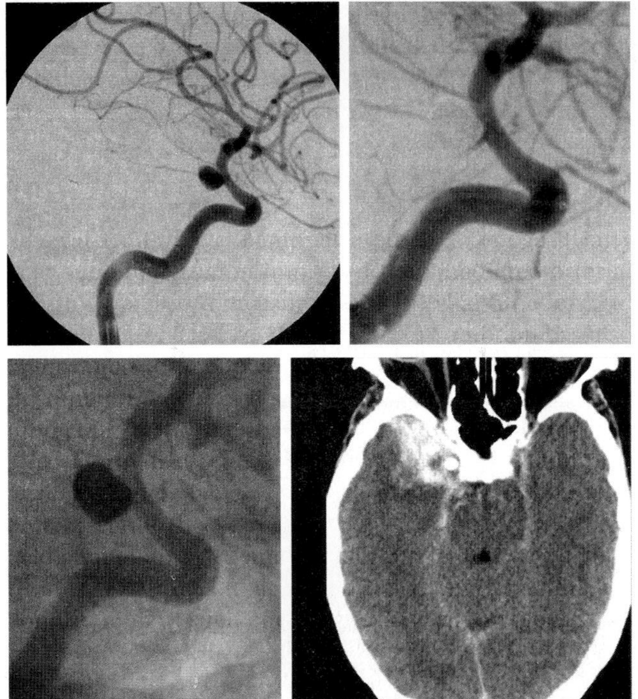

Fig. 13: Pre- and postcoiling angiographic images of an intracranial aneurysm

who survive the initial bleed, re-bleeding and cerebral infarctions are the major causes of death.

In an analysis in 1960s when just conservative management of SAH was done, out of 100 patients with aneurysm:

- 15 die before reaching hospital
- 15 die in first 24 hours
- 15 die between 24 hours and 2 weeks
- 15 die between 2 weeks and 2 months
- 15 die between 2 months to 2 years.

With advances in techniques to treat the aneurysm and management of vasospasm current death rate for SAH is between 40% and 50%, but trends for survival are improving. Factors found on admission that are associated with poorer outcome include delay in diagnosis, poorer neurological grade, systolic hypertension; a previous diagnosis of heart attack or SAH; liver disease, more blood and larger aneurysm on the initial CT scan; location of an aneurysm in the posterior circulation and higher age. Factors that carry a worse prognosis during the hospital stay include occurrence of delayed ischemia resulting from vasospasm, development of intracerebral hematoma or intraventricular hemorrhage and other complications of SAH including hydrocephalus.[32]

CONCLUSION

In spite of tremendous amount of progress medical sciences has made in the recent times, hemorrhagic stroke continues to be the most devastating neurological disorder with very high mortality. Probably, in no other sphere in medicine the needs of preventive measures are felt more desperately than hemorrhagic stroke because of its huge emotional, social and financial impact on its victims being the leading cause of severe disability worldwide. Hypertension is the most important modifiable cause of intracranial hemorrhage. Popularization of ambulatory blood pressure monitoring and optimal treatment of blood pressure at the right time can go a long way in saving countless lives worldwide and prevent disasters from happening in view of direct relation between hypertension and ICH, its role in genesis of aneurysm formation and its rupture amongst other issues described in the text. A direct relation between diabetes mellitus and ICH in young population and the fact that outcome of stroke is worse in diabetics as compared to nondiabetic counterparts makes this silent killer in global pandemic, a very important consideration. The management of spontaneous intracranial hemorrhage on "time is brain" model requires greater awareness in society and simultaneously, the integration of various levels of healthcare along with development and execution of better protocols by the multitasked stroke team. The management of aneurysmal SAH has undergone phenomenal change following landmark publication of ISAT trial in Lancet 2002. However, age old neurosurgical clipping of aneurysm practiced by generations of neurosurgeons is still a precious art that must get adequate attention and must be considered whenever it is believed to be a better option for the patient. It seems the journey to human brain and attempts to unravel its mysteries must go through human heart. "Heart–brain connect" symbolizing the need for value-based collaborative association between cardiac and neuroscientists world over is the best way to move forward if we are to make a significant headway in the management of "brain attack" and the cardiac diseases in view of common precursors of hypertension, DM, atherosclerosis and metabolic syndromes.

REFERENCES

1. Kannel WB, Dawber TR, Sorlie P, et al. components of blood pressure and risk of atherothrombotic brain infarction: the Framingham study. Stroke. 1976;7:327-31.
2. Chalmers J, Todd A, Chapman N, et al. International Society of Hypertension (ISH): Statement on blood pressure lowering and stroke prevention. J Hypertension. 2003;21(4):651-63.

3. Chobanian AV, Bakris GL, Black HR et al. The Seventh Report of Joint National Committee on Prevention, Detection, Evaluation and Treatment of blood pressure. The JNC 7 report. JAMA. 2003;289(19):2560-72.
4. Shimbo D, Newman JD, Aragaki AK, et al. Association between annual visit-to-visit blood pressure variability and stroke in postmenopausal women: data from the Women's Health Initiative. Hypertension. 2012;60:625-30.
5. Kang J, Ko Y, Park JH, et al. Effect of blood pressure on 3-month functional outcome in the subacute stage of ischemic stroke. Neurology. 2012;79:2018-24.
6. Brott T, Thalinger K, Hertzberg V. Hypertension as a risk factor for spontaneous intracerebral hemorrhage. Stroke. 1986;17:1078-83.
7. Dandapani BK, Suzuki S, Kelley RE, et al. Relation of blood pressure and outcome in intracerebral hemorrhage. Stroke. 1995;26:21-4.
8. Leonardi-Bee J, Bath PM, Phillips SJ, et al. Blood pressure and clinical outcomes in the International Stroke Trial. Stroke. 2002;33:1315-20.
9. Broderick JP, Adams HP, Barsan W, et al. Guidelines for the management of spontaneous intracerebral hemorrhage: a statement for health professionals from a special writing group of the Stroke Council, American Heart Association. Stroke. 1999;30:905-15.
10. Edward F, Broderick JP, Kernan WN, et al. Major risk factors for intracerebral hemorrhage in the young are modifiable. Stroke. 2005;36:1881-5.
11. WHO Expert Consultation. Appropriate body mass index for Asian populations and its implications for policy and intervention strategies. Lancet. 2004;363(9403):157-63.
12. Hitt Emma. (2007). Diabetes mellitus associated with increased intracerebral hemorrhage risk in younger patients. [online]. Medscape. Available from *http://www.medscape.com/viewarticle/559428*. [Accessed Oct. 2017].
13. S Tetri S Juvela, P Saloheimo, et al. Hypertension and diabetes as predictors of early death after spontaneous intracerebral hemorrhage. J Neurosurg. 2009;110(3):411-7.
14. Kase CS, Furlan AJ, Wechsler LR, et al. Cerebral hemorrhage after intra-arterial thrombolysis for ischemic stroke: the PROACT II trial. Neurology. 2001;57(9):1603-10.
15. Arboix A, Oliveres M, Massons J, et al. Early differentiation of cardioembolic from atherothrombotic cerebral infarction: a multivariate analysis. Eur J Neurol. 1999;6:677-83.
16. Kishore A, Vail A, Majid A, et al. Detection of atrial fibrillation after ischemic stroke or transient ischemic attack: a systematic review and meta-analysis. Stroke. 2014;45:520-6.
17. Caceres JA, Goldstein JN. Intracranial hemorrhage. Emerg Med Clin North Am. 2012;30(3):771-94.
18. Hemphill JC 3rd, Greenberg SM, Anderson CS, et al. Guidelines for the Management of Spontaneous Intracerebral Hemorrhage: A Guideline for Healthcare Professionals from the American Heart Association/American Stroke Association. Stroke. 2015;46(7):2032-60.
19. Feldmann E, Broderick JP, Kernan WN, et al. Major Risk factors for intracerebral bleed are modifiable. Stroke. 2005;36:1881.
20. Prayson Richard A. Neuropathology. Los Angeles, CA: Elsevier Health Sciences; 2012. p. 49.
21. Chalela JA, Kidwell CS, Nentwich LM, et al. Magnetic resonance imaging and computed tomography in emergency assessment of patients with suspected acute stroke. Lancet. 2007;369(9558):293-8.
22. David S Liebeskind. Intracranial hemorrhage: treatment and medication: emedicine specialities. Updated: 2006.
23. Hansen BM, Nilsson OG, Anderson H, et al. Long term (13 years) prognosis after primary intracerebral hemorrhage: a prospective population based study of long term mortality, prognostic factors and cause of death. J Neurol Neurosurg Psychiatry. 2013;84(10):1150-5.
24. Abraham MK, Chang WW. Subarachnoid Hemorrhage. Emerg Med Clin North Am. 2016;34(4):901-16.
25. Hunt WE, Hess RM. Surgical risk as related to time of intervention in the repair of intracranial aneurysms. J Neurosurg. 1968;28(1):14-20.
26. Hunt WE, Meagher JN, Hess RM. Intracranial aneurysm. A nine-year study. Ohio State Med J. 1966;62(11):1168-71.
27. Teasdale GM, Drake CG, Hunt W, et al. A universal subarachnoid hemorrhage scale: report of a committee of the World Federation of Neurosurgical Societies. J Neurol Neurosurg Psychiatry. 1988;51(11):1457.
28. Hemphil JC III, Bonowich DC, Besmertis L, et al. The ICH score: a simple, reliable grading scale for ICH. Stroke. 2001;32(4):891-7.
29. Molyneux A, Kerr R, Stratton I, et al. International subarachnoid aneurysm trial (ISAT) of neurosurgical clipping versus endovascular coiling in 2143 patients with ruptured intracranial aneurysms: A randomized trial. Lancet. 2002;360(9342):1267-74.
30. Sen J, Belli A, Albon H, et al. Triple H therapy in the management of aneurysmal subarachnoid hemorrhage. Lancet Neurol. 2003;2(10):614-21.
31. Feigin VL, Rinkel GJ, Lawes CM, et al. Risk factors for subarachnoid hemorrhage: an updated systemic review of epidemiological studies. Stroke. 2005;36(12):2773-80.
32. Lindsay KW, Bone I, Callender R (Eds.). The Textbook of Neurology and Neurosurgery, Illustrated, 5th Edition. London: Churchill Livingstone; 2010. p. 278.

Prognostication of STEMI in Cardiodiabetes

Kewal C Goswami, Deepti Siddharthan

INTRODUCTION

The global burden of diabetes mellitus is substantial with current trends pointing toward a continual rise. According to the estimates by International Diabetes Federation,[1] 415 million adults aged 20–79 years worldwide had diabetes in the year 2015. This figure is projected to rise to 642 million by 2040. This increase in the burden of diabetes is closely mirrored by a substantial rise in the incidence of cardiovascular disease, which is the most prevalent cause of morbidity and mortality in diabetes.[2] The GRACE investigators[3] reported a history of diabetes in 21%, 26%, and 25% of patients presenting with ST-elevation myocardial infarction (STEMI), non-ST elevation myocardial infarction (NSTEMI), and unstable angina, respectively. The CREATE[4] and the Thai ACS[5] registries reported nearly 30% and 40% of patients presenting with STEMI as having diabetes. This chapter reviews the influence of diabetes in determining the prognosis in patients with STEMI.

MORBIDITY AND MORTALITY AFTER STEMI IN DIABETIC PATIENTS

Diabetes is associated with a threefold increase in age-adjusted cardiovascular mortality.[6] In fact, diabetes has now been accorded the status of being a risk equivalent of coronary artery disease for future myocardial infarction (MI) and cardiovascular death.[7] In addition to being an important cardiovascular risk factor, diabetes significantly influences the outcomes after MI. Diabetes is associated with significantly worse morbidity and mortality after STEMI. In hospital case, fatality rates are doubled for diabetic patients compared to those without diabetes.[3] The 30-day mortality among patients with diabetes presenting with STEMI is 8.5%, which is significantly higher compared to 5.4% among non diabetic patients.[8] The odds ratio (OR) for mortality at 30 days after STEMI for diabetic patients is 1.40 [95% confidence interval (CI) 1.24–1.57]. Similarly, diabetes at presentation is associated with significantly higher 1-year mortality after STEMI with a hazard ratio of 1.22 (95% CI 1.08–1.38). The increased risk of mortality persists at a follow up of 20 years.[9] The median survival among diabetic patients after STEMI is 11 years compared to 15 years in those without diabetes. A recent study[10] reported a decrease in in-hospital mortality (5%) in diabetic patients presenting with STEMI compared to that reported in GRACE registry. This decline has been attributed to a decrease in the percentage of active smokers and an increase in the rates of revascularization in this subset of patients. In this study, no differences were noted in terms of mortality between insulin-dependent and noninsulin-dependent diabetes.[10]

In addition to the increase in mortality, higher morbidity has also been observed in diabetic patients with STEMI. Diabetic patients tend to have higher thrombolysis in myocardial infarction (TIMI) risk indices (median TIMI risk index of 22.2 vs 18.8) at presentation with STEMI and are more likely to have heart failure (Killip classes 2–4) (14.7% vs 10.4%) at presentation.[8] The incidence of heart failure during the index hospitalization is nearly twice than that observed in nondiabetic patients.[3] The incidence of cardiogenic shock is likewise increased. Baseline serum creatinine levels were observed to be elevated in diabetic patients in the GRACE registry[3] at presentation. Renal failure was diagnosed nearly twice as often in diabetic patients compared to nondiabetic patients.

The reasons for the increased morbidity and mortality in diabetic patients presenting with STEMI are not completely understood. Diabetic patients presenting with STEMI tend to be older, are more often women, and have higher body mass indices. There is a higher incidence of other risk factors including hypertension and known dyslipidemia. Patients with diabetes tend to have lower initial low-density lipoprotein (LDL) levels because of increased statin use before presentation with STEMI. However, they have lower high-density lipoprotein (HDL) levels and high-serum-triglyceride levels.[10] Diabetic patients are more likely to have a history of angina, prior MI, heart failure, and coronary artery bypass graft (CABG) surgery compared to STEMI patients without diabetes. The prevalence of current smoking is however lower in diabetic patients compared to their nondiabetic counterparts. However, regression analyses controlling for these adverse risk factors have demonstrated that the worse outcomes cannot be explained by the worse risk profile alone.[6] Other putative factors have been proposed to be contributing to the poor prognosis in STEMI patients with diabetes.[11] The worse in hospital outcomes including mortality, heart failure, and renal failure have been linked to pre-existing ventricular dysfunction due to diabetic cardiomyopathy and severe coronary artery disease including multivessel disease and small-vessel disease. There is decreased vasodilatory reserve of epicardial and resistance arteries, and possibly abnormal metabolism of myocardial substrate. Late outcomes have been related to the diffuse nature of the atherosclerotic disease, increased platelet activity, decreased fibrinolysis and autonomic neuropathy leading to ventricular arrhythmias.

MEDICAL MANAGEMENT IN DIABETIC PATIENTS PRESENTING WITH STEMI

Patients with diabetes mellitus are more likely to be on aspirin, statins, beta blockers, angiotensin-converting enzyme inhibitors (ACEI), and angiotensin receptor blockers (ARBs) at the time of presentation with STEMI.[10] However, differences have been noted in the medical therapy received by diabetic patients after STEMI compared to those without diabetes. Even though diabetic patients have been shown to benefit to a greater extent from the use of beta-blockers in the immediate post-infarction period,[12] in the GRACE registry,[3] the rate of use of these agents was found to be lower than those without diabetes. The lower rates of use of beta-blockers were attributed to apprehensions about exacerbation of glucose intolerance and masking of hypoglycemic symptoms. On the other hand, the use of ACEI and ARBs was greater than that in nondiabetic patients. The use of calcium channel antagonists (CCBs) and nitrates was higher in diabetic patients probably because of higher percentage of patients having angina and hypertension prior to MI. Similarly, diabetic patients received diuretics more often due to higher risk profile at baseline including hypertension and heart failure.[9]

THROMBOLYSIS IN DIABETIC PATIENTS PRESENTING WITH STEMI

In the GRACE population,[3] the use of thrombolytic agents was lower in diabetic patients possibly due to delayed presentation and atypical symptoms. However, even after adjusting for the extent of delay in presentation, diabetic patients fared worse. The underuse of thrombolysis in diabetic patients with STEMI is also due to the concern about the increased risk of bleeding complications in diabetic patients. The benefit of thrombolysis has been shown to be similar in both diabetic and nondiabetic patients.[13] There are no significant differences between diabetic and nondiabetic patients in terms of patency of the infarct-related artery at 90 minutes (71% vs 70%) or left ventricular ejection fraction (LVEF) (50% vs 52%).[14] However in spite of these benefits, the in-hospital, 30-day, and 1-year mortality rates are worse in diabetic patients due to severe pre-existing disease with the worst outcomes in women with type 1 diabetes.[15] In the past, hemorrhagic diabetic retinopathy was an absolute contraindication for thrombolytic therapy. Though the risk of ocular hemorrhage has not been systematically evaluated in major thrombolytic trials, major intraocular bleeding has not been reported in trials including a good percentage of diabetic patients. Consequently, diabetic retinopathy is no longer considered a contraindication to thrombolysis.

CORONARY ANGIOGRAPHY AND PRIMARY PERCUTANEOUS CORONARY INTERVENTION IN STEMI IN DIABETIC PATIENTS

According to the coronary angiography data available,[8,14] dia betic patients are more likely to have multivessel disease (OR 1.68, 95% CI 1.56–1.82) and more advanced atherosclerotic lesions. Patients with diabetes are more likely to undergo revascularization in the index hospitalization compared to their nondiabetic counterparts. However, the mode of revascularization in this subset is more likely to be CABG rather than primary percutaneous coronary intervention (PCI), which also accounts for the higher rates of revascularization. The influence of diabetes on outcomes after primary PCI for STEMI has also been described.[16] Subset analysis of diabetic patients in clinical trials comparing primary PCI with thrombolysis has shown a significant reduction in death or MI at 30 days (9.2% vs 19.3%; $P < 0.05$),[17] a higher infarct-related artery patency rate (88% vs 31%; $P < 0.001$), and improved left ventricular function (LVEF 49% vs 36%; $P < 0.05$), and long-term survival.[18]

In diabetic patients, primary PCI is more often associated with distal embolization, impaired perfusion, and higher mortality.[19-21] Final postprocedure TIMI grade 3 flow is observed in fewer diabetic patients (84.7%) compared to those without diabetes (91.7%).[16] The use of glycoprotein (GP) IIb/IIIa inhibitors is less frequent in diabetic patients undergoing primary PCI. The 30-day cardiac mortality after primary PCI has been observed to be higher in diabetic patients (11.7%) compared to nondiabetic patients (4.2%).[16] The 3-year rates of stent thrombosis are similar between diabetic (1.6%) and nondiabetic patients (1.5%). The rates of target lesion revascularization (TLR) and target vessel revascularization (TVR) are higher in diabetic patients, with 3-year follow-up rates of TLR being 12.1% vs 8.7% and TVR being 16.8% vs 11.9% in diabetic versus nondiabetic patients. At 3-year follow-up after primary PCI, diabetic patients have higher rates of MI (12.3% vs 5.6%), cardiac mortality (15.8% vs 6.9%) and all-cause mortality (23.7% vs 12.7%) compared to their nondiabetic counterparts.[16] The risk of a 30-day bleeding event following primary PCI is higher in diabetic STEMI patients than in those without diabetes (6.2% vs 0.9%).[22]

INFLUENCE OF GENDER ON PROGNOSTICATION OF STEMI IN DIABETES

The effect of gender on prognosis after STEMI in diabetes has been studied.[23,24] Women were found to have worse early and 12-month outcomes after MI compared to men. The prevalence of hypertension and obesity increases far more with age in women, though after multivariate analysis, none of the known risk factors except age is a significant predictor of mortality. An additional reason for the poorer prognosis in women is the underuse of modern medical treatments. About 45% of the women in the Polish Registry of Acute Coronary Syndromes (PL-ACS)[24] received conservative treatment and were not offered any reperfusion therapy.

ATRIAL FIBRILLATION IN DIABETIC PATIENTS PRESENTING WITH STEMI

One-fifth of diabetic patients presenting with STEMI have atrial fibrillation (AF) at presentation.[25] The risk of stroke is high in this subset and therefore oral anticoagulation is indicated, which in turn increases the risk of bleeding complications with triple antiplatelet and anticoagulant therapy. In such situations, the selection of stent (bare metal versus drug eluting) should be made individually balancing the risk of stroke and bleeding complications.

DIAGNOSIS OF DIABETES MELLITUS AT PRESENTATION WITH STEMI

The effect of diagnosis of diabetes at presentation with STEMI has also been studied. In the 2014 NCDR report,[10] 14% of patients presenting with STEMI were diagnosed to have diabetes at presentation. These patients were found to have a higher BMI, higher initial LDL levels, slightly lower HDL levels, and higher triglyceride levels. These patients were more likely to be discharged on ACEI and clopidogrel than patients without DM. The in-hospital clinical events rates were similar to nondiabetic patients. The level of hyperglycemia at presentation with STEMI is a significant predictor of mortality and morbidity.[26] The treatment of hyperglycemia remains an open issue. Intensive control of glycemia is associated with risk of increasing mortality.[27] Hypoglycemia during treatment increases cardiovascular events and even mortality. A glycemic target of 180 mg/dL or less is recommended by the guidelines.[28]

CONCLUSION

Diabetes mellitus is an important negative prognostic factor for mortality and morbidity in patients presenting with STEMI. About a quarter of patients presenting with STEMI are diabetic. These patients tend to be older and are more likely to have hypertension, dyslipidemia, higher BMI, pre-existing angina, heart failure, and history of CABG. The atherosclerotic process tends to be diffuse in nature in this subset with increased platelet activity, decreased fibrinolysis, and autonomic neuropathy. They are more likely to receive ACEI, ARBs, CCBs, and nitrates. However, there is continued underuse of beta-blockers and thrombolysis in these patients in spite of proven benefits. The mode of revascularization is more likely to be CABG rather than primary PCI due to higher incidence of multivessel disease. The rates of MI, TLR, TVR, cardiac mortality, all-cause mortality, and bleeding events after primary PCI are higher in diabetic patients. Diabetic women tend to fare worse than their male counterparts after STEMI.

REFERENCES

1. Ogurtsova K, da Rocha Fernandes JD, Huang Y, et al. IDF Diabetes Atlas: Global estimates for the prevalence of diabetes for 2015 and 2040. Diabetes Res Clin Pract. 2017;128:40-50.
2. Matheus AS, Tannus LR, Cobas RA, et al. Impact of diabetes on cardiovascular disease: an update. Int J Hypertens. 2013;2013:653-789.
3. Franklin K, Goldberg RJ, Spencer F, et al. GRACE Investigators. Implications of diabetes in patients with acute coronary syndromes. The Global Registry of Acute Coronary Events. Arch Intern Med. 2004;164:1457-63.
4. Xavier D, Pais P, Devereaux PJ, et al. CREATE registry investigators. Treatment and outcomes of acute coronary syndromes in India (CREATE): a prospective analysis of registry data. Lancet. 2008;371:1435-42.
5. Boonsom W, Ratanasumawong K, Hutayanon P, et al. Implications of diabetes mellitus in patients with STEMI: data from Thai ACS Registry. J Med Assoc Thai. 2007;90:12-20.
6. Garcia MJ, McNamara PM, Gordon T, et al. Morbidity and mortality in diabetics in the Framingham population: sixteen year follow-up study. Diabetes. 1974;23:105-11.
7. Nayor M, Vasan RS. Recent Update to the US Cholesterol Treatment Guidelines. A Comparison with International Guidelines. Circulation. 2016;133:1795-806.
8. Donahoe SM, Stewart GC, McCabe CH, et al. Diabetes and mortality following acute coronary syndromes. JAMA. 2007;298:765-75.
9. Nauta ST, Deckers JW, Akkerhuis KM, et al. Short- and long-term mortality after myocardial infarction in patients with and without diabetes. Changes from 1985 to 2008. Diabetes Care. 2012;35:2043-7.
10. Rousan TA, Pappy RM, Chen AY, et al. Impact of diabetes mellitus on clinical characteristics, management, and in-hospital outcomes in patients with acute myocardial infarction (from the NCDR). Am J Cardiol. 2014;114:1136-44.
11. Aronson D, Rayfield EJ, Chesebro JH. Mechanisms determining course and outcome of diabetic patients who have had acute myocardial infarction. Ann Intern Med. 1997;126:296-306.
12. Lowel H, Koenig W, Engel S, et al. The impact of diabetes mellitus on survival after myocardial infarction: can it be modified by drug treatment? Results of a population-based myocardial infarction register follow-up study. Diabetologia. 2000;43:218-26.
13. Baigent C, Collins R, Appleby P, et al. ISIS-2: 10 year survival among patients with suspected acute myocardial infarction in randomised comparison of intravenous streptokinase, oral aspirin, both, or neither. The ISIS-2 (Second International Study of Infarct Survival) Collaborative Group. BMJ. 1998;316:1337-43.
14. Mak KH, Moliterno DJ, Granger CB, et al. Influence of diabetes mellitus on clinical outcome in the thrombolytic era of acute myocardial infarction. GUSTO-I Investigators. Global Utilization of Streptokinase and Tissue Plasminogen Activator for Occluded Coronary Arteries. J Am Coll Cardiol. 1997;30:171-9.
15. Zuanetti G, Latini R, Maggioni AP, et al. Influence of diabetes on mortality in acute myocardial infarction: data from the GISSI-2 study. J Am Coll Cardiol. 1993;22:1788-94.
16. Jensen LO, Maeng M, Thayssen P, et al. Influence of diabetes mellitus on clinical outcomes following primary percutaneous coronary intervention in patients with ST-segment elevation myocardial infarction. Am J Cardiol. 2012;109:629-35.
17. Grines C, Patel A, Zijlstra F, et al. PCAT Collaborators. Percutaneous transluminal coronary angioplasty. Primary coronary angioplasty compared with intravenous thrombolytic therapy for acute myocardial infarction: six-month follow up and analysis of individual patient data from randomized trials. Am Heart J. 2003;145:47-57.
18. Timmer JR, Ottervanger JP, Thomas K, et al. Myocardial Infarction Study Group. Long-term, cause-specific mortality after myocardial infarction in diabetes. Eur Heart J. 2004;25:926-31.
19. De Luca G, Gibson CM, Bellandi F, et al. Diabetes mellitus is associated with distal embolization, impaired myocardial perfusion, and higher mortality in patients with ST-segment elevation myocardial infarction treated with primary angioplasty and glycoprotein IIb-IIIa inhibitors. Atherosclerosis. 2009;207:181-5.
20. Marso SP, Miller T, Rutherford BD, et al. Comparison of myocardial reperfusion in patients undergoing percutaneous coronary intervention in ST-segment elevation acute myocardial infarction with versus without diabetes mellitus (from the EMERALD Trial). Am J Cardiol. 2007;100:206-10.
21. De LG, Malek LA, Maciejewski P, et al. STEMI 2003 Registry Collaborators. Impact of diabetes on survival in patients with ST-segment elevation myocardial infarction treated by primary angioplasty: insights from the POLISH STEMI registry. Atherosclerosis. 2010;210:516-20.
22. Zhang H, Hu X, Wu Q, et al. Impact of diabetes on bleeding events in ST-elevation myocardial infarction patients after urgent percutaneous coronary intervention: A retrospective cohort study. Medicine (Baltimore). 2016;95:e4470.
23. Dotevall A, Hasdai D, Wallentin L, et al. Data from the Euro Heart Survey ACS. Diabetes mellitus: clinical presentation and outcome in men and women with acute coronary syndromes. Diabet Med. 2005;22:1542-550.
24. Poloński L, Gasior M, Gierlotka M, et al. Polish Registry of Acute Coronary Syndromes (PL-ACS). Characteristics, treatments and outcomes of patients with acute coronary syndromes in Poland. Kardiol Pol. 2007;65:861-72.
25. Dabek J, Bałys M, Majewski M, et al. Diabetic Patients with an Acute Myocardial Infarction in Terms of Risk Factors and Comorbidities Management: Characteristics of the Highest-Risk Individuals. Adv Clin Exp Med. 2016;25:655-63.
26. Deedwania P, Kosiborod M, Barrett E, et al. Hyperglycemia and acute coronary syndrome: a scientific statement from the American Heart Association Diabetes Committee of the Council on Nutrition, Physical Activity, and Metabolism. Anesthesiology. 2008;109:14-24.
27. NICE-SUGAR Study Investigators, Finfer S, Chittock DR, et al. Intensive versus conventional glucose control in critically ill patients. N Engl J Med. 2009;360:1283-97.
28. Steg PG, James SK, Atar D. ESC Guidelines for the management of acute myocardial infarction in patients presenting with ST-segment elevation. Eur Heart J. 2012;33:2569-619.

CHAPTER

Management of Hypertension in Diabetes: Special Consideration

Naveen Mittal, Rohin Vinayak, GS Wander

INTRODUCTION

Hypertension, defined as a sustained blood pressure greater than or equal to 140/90 mm Hg, is a common comorbidity of type 1 and type 2 diabetes. The prevalence of hypertension depends on the type of diabetes, age, sex, body mass index (BMI), and race/ethnicity. Hypertension is a major risk factor for both macrovascular and microvascular complications. In type 1 diabetes, hypertension is often the result of underlying diabetic kidney disease; while in type 2 diabetes, it usually coexists with other cardiometabolic risk factors. Hypertension care is guided by recommendations from professional bodies, which collate evidence and propose rational means of assessing and managing high blood pressure. We analyze three documents[1-3] which guide blood pressure management in persons with diabetes and make an effort to find concordance between them. This chapter utilizes the evidence-based recommendations of the American Diabetes Association's (ADA) Standards of Medical Care in Diabetes 2017,[1] the European Society of Hypertension/European Society of Cardiology (ESH/ESC) 2013,[2] and the panel members of the Eighth Joint National Committee (JNC8).[3] It reinforces the need to interpret and follow their guidance, utilizing "good clinical sense," without losing sight of our aim: To provide optimal health to people with diabetes and hypertension.

REPORT OF PANEL MEMBERS OF EIGHTH JOINT NATIONAL COMMITTEE

The panel members of the JNC8 have defined the target threshold, for various subgroups of people with hypertension. Eighth Joint National Committee, however, does not specify any cutoff above which lifestyle modification should be initiated. In the general population, the blood pressure threshold for initiating pharmacologic treatment is greater than or equal to 140/90 mm Hg in those aged less than 60 years, and greater than or equal to 150/90 mm Hg in those aged 60 or above. Eighth Joint National Committee does not suggest lower targets for persons with diabetes. At the same time, it reiterates that a person who has lower blood pressure should not modify therapy, as long as it is well-tolerated.

The panelists of JNC8 justify their recommendation by explaining that the various trials used to support lower blood pressure targets for persons with diabetes have certain shortcomings. According to them, Action in Diabetes and Vascular Disease: Preterax and Diamicron MR Controlled Evaluation (ADVANCE) included participants irrespective of baseline blood pressure and did not have randomized blood pressure treatment thresholds or goals. ADVANCE studied both macrovascular and microvascular outcomes, rather than focusing only on blood pressure. Blood pressure control, using a perindopril + indapamide-based strategy was used as a method of achieving better outcomes, and not as an end in itself.[4] Therefore, the JNC8 omitted a large study with good outcome data.

The panelists also disregarded the lower incidence of stroke observed with lower blood pressure (systolic blood pressure goal <120 mm Hg, as compared to <140 mm Hg) in Action to Control Cardiovascular Risk in Diabetes (ACCORD)-Blood Pressure,[5] because of the low absolute numbers involved. The Hypertension Optimal Trial (HOT),[6] which showed reduction in a composite cardiovascular disease outcome with a diastolic blood pressure goal of less than or equal to 80 mm Hg as compared to less than or equal to 90 mm Hg, was disregarded, perhaps because of the smaller number of participants with diabetes. Eighth Joint National Committee panelists also disregarded the United Kingdom Prospective Diabetes Study (UKPDS),[7] because it was a "mixed systolic and diastolic goal study and because it did not use a diastolic cutoff of 90 mm Hg in one of its groups." No evidence from recent, large trials has been published in the past few years to support these earlier reports.

Eighth Joint National Committee panelists do recommend ethnicity-based choice of therapy including thiazide-type diuretic or calcium channel blocker (CCB) for the general black population (including those with diabetes), and angiotensin-converting enzyme inhibitor (ACEi) or angiotensin-receptor blocker (ARB) for Blacks with chronic kidney disease (CKD). No specific guidance is provided for South Asians.

Eighth Joint National Committee panelists suggest initiating monotherapy or combination. Some members recommend initiation of combination therapy (2 or more drugs) when blood pressure is greater than 160/100 mm Hg or when it is greater than 20/10 mm Hg above goal and then titrating drug treatment by either maximizing dosage, or adding a second medication, or starting a fixed-dose combination. It reiterates that more than one class of drugs will frequently be necessary and advocates use of thiazide-like diuretics, ACE or ARB and CCB, in varying combination. Only if these three classes prove inadequate, along with lifestyle modification, do they recommend the addition of beta-blockers, aldosterone antagonists, or other classes.

AMERICAN DIABETES ASSOCIATION STANDARD OF CARE-2017

American Diabetes Association[1] reviews the very same evidence, including ACCORD, ADVANCE-Blood Pressure, and HOT trials,[4-6] analyzing their design and results.

It suggests a target of less than 140/90 mm Hg for all people with diabetes, but advocates lower (not specified) targets in specific situations. These include "younger patients" those with albuminuria, and/or those with one or more additional atherosclerotic cardiovascular disease (ASCVD) risk factors (dyslipidemia, obesity, and smoking). Such targets are proposed only if they can be achieved "without undue treatment burden." Lower targets are especially important in persons with a high risk of stroke (systolic blood pressure control) or worsening of albuminuria, and "long life expectancy." At the same time, when palliative care is needed in older adults (>65 years of age), ADA suggests that strict blood pressure control may not be necessary, and therapy may be withdrawn.[8] The threshold for beginning nonpharmacological intervention is also lower, at greater than 120/80 mm Hg.

American Diabetes Association states that high ASCVD risk associated with diabetes, and the high prevalence of undiagnosed ASCVD in these patients, favor the use of renin-angiotensin system (RAS) inhibitors. American Diabetes Association suggests administration of one or more antihypertensive medications at bedtime and reminds us that more often than not, multiple drugs will be needed to achieve control. No attempt is made to prioritize either ACEi or ARBs over each other, but mention is made of outcomes benefits with perindopril + indapamide and benazepril + amlodipine combinations. Angiotensin, converting enzyme inhibitor and ARB may be substituted for each other if one class is not tolerated. Both should never be used together. Serum creatinine/estimated glomerular filtration rate (eGFR) and serum potassium levels should be monitored during long term of RAS blockers.

EUROPEAN SOCIETY OF HYPERTENSION/EUROPEAN SOCIETY OF CARDIOLOGY- 2013 GUIDELINES

The 2013 ESH/ESC guidelines[2] propose a therapeutic approach based on an assessment of overall cardiovascular risk, aiming to reduce it by appropriate diagnosis, management and follow-up of hypertension. The authors describe their literature search methodology, including a description of the Appropriate Blood Pressure Control in Diabetes and Randomized Olmesartan and Diabetes Microalbuminuria Prevention Trials.[9,10]

All persons with diabetes are classified alongside those with organ damage of hypertension or with CKD stage 3. Patients with diabetes and evidence of organ damage, or with other risk factors, as categorized, are being equivalent to those with symptomatic cardiovascular disease or CKD stage 4. Thus, the ESH/ESC taxonomy classifies diabetes into two grades of risk. A color-coded table, using shades of green, yellow, and red is used to emphasize this concept. To paraphrase the ESH/ESC guidance—persons with uncomplicated diabetes have a risk equivalent to that of CKD stage 3 or end-organ damage in those with diabetes + other risk factors, or diabetes + end-organ damage, are equivalent in risk to CKD stage 4.

The role of asymptomatic organ damage is thought to be crucial in risk stratification. Four markers (microalbuminuria, increased pulse wave velocity, left ventricular hypertrophy, and carotid plaques) are considered important risk prognosticators. Among investigations, echocardiography with Doppler is considered to have the highest predictive value, while electrocardiography, eGFR, microalbuminuria, carotid intima-media thickness, arterial stiffness, ankle-brachial index, and fundoscopy are considered useful, available, reproducible, and cost-effective alternatives.

The 2013 ESH/ESC guidelines suggest institution of pharmacotherapy above a threshold of 140/90 mm Hg, in all patients with low-moderate cardiovascular risk, or previous stroke/transient ischemic attack, or coronary heart disease or diabetic/nondiabetic kidney disease. The only exception is made for the elderly (who are offered a higher systolic target) and for diabetes (who are given a lower diastolic target). The recommended diastolic target in diabetes is less than 85 mm Hg, with the reminder that values between 80 mm Hg and 85 mm Hg are safe and well-tolerated. If overt proteinuria is present, systolic blood pressure targets of less than 130 mm Hg may be considered, provided that a change in eGFR is monitored. Lifestyle modification is encouraged in all diabetics at a level of 130/85 mm Hg or more.

The 2013 ESH/ESC authors list metabolic syndrome and glucose intolerance as possible contraindications for thiazide diuretics and beta-blockers but refrain from describing this contraindication as compelling. The choice of class of drugs, or an individual drug, is expected to be based on comorbidities. All classes of antihypertensive drugs can be used in diabetes, but RAS blockers are preferred, especially in the presence of proteinuria or microalbuminuria. Again, no attempt is made to compare ACEi and ARB, though simultaneous administration is strongly discouraged. They also favor the use of fixed-dose combinations, and initiation of combination therapy in persons with marked blood pressure elevation, or those at high/very high cardiovascular risk.

TABLE 1: Comparison of blood pressure targets and interventional thresholds in diabetes

Parameter	*JNC8*	*ADA-2017*	*ESH/ESC-2013*
Target SBP	<140 mm Hg	<140 mm Hg	<140 mm Hg
Target DBP	<90 mm Hg	<90 mm Hg	<85 mm Hg
Threshold for initiating lifestyle changes	Not discussed	>120/80 mm Hg	>130/85 mm Hg
Higher targets suggested for	>60 years (SBP > 150 mm Hg)	Older adults (>65 years) requiring palliative care	Elderly (SBP > 150 mm Hg)
Lower targets suggested for		Younger patients High risk of stroke, albuminuria Additional ASCVD risk factors	Overt proteinuria (SBP < 130 mm Hg)

Abbreviations: JNC8, Eighth Joint National Committee; ADA, American Diabetes Association; ESH, European Society of Hypertension; ESC, European Society of Cardiology; SBP, systolic blood pressure; DBP, diastolic blood pressure; ASCVD, atherosclerotic cardiovascular disease.

TABLE 2: Criteria for stringent and relaxed targets of blood pressure

	Stringent targets	*Relaxed targets*
Age	Young	Elderly
Expected life expectancy	Long	Short
Symptoms	Symptomatic	Asymptomatic
Risk factors	AVSCD risk factors: obesity, dyslipidemia, smoking	Chances of deyhdration (fasting, hot climate), risk of falls
Patient motivation	High	Low

Abbreviation: ASCVD, atherosclerotic cardiovascular disease.

WHAT SHOULD WE DO?

We have compared blood pressure targets and interventional thresholds in diabetes given by panel members of JNC8, ADA 2017, and ESH/ESC 2013 (Table 1). Both ADA and EHC/ESC convey the message of choosing patient-centered targets and goals while managing hypertension in diabetes. While the general target for blood pressure may be made more stringent for younger individuals with longer life expectancy, having additional risk factors (smoking, obesity, and dyslipidemia) or showing progression of albuminuria (Table 2). At the same time, less stringent targets may be in order for the elderly, those with a high risk of postural hypotension, or falls (such as limited fluid intake, frequent fasting, leading to dehydration, especially in hot climate), and inability or unwillingness to cope with prescribed pills.

However, the superiority of ACE inhibitors or ARBs over other antihypertensive agents for prevention of cardiovascular outcomes has not been consistently shown for all patients with diabetes.[11-14] In particular, a recent meta-analysis suggests that thiazide-type diuretics or dihydropyridine CCBs have cardiovascular benefit similar to that of ACE inhibitors or ARBs.[11] Therefore, among patients without albuminuria for whom cardiovascular disease prevention is the primary goal of blood pressure control, a thiazide-like diuretic or dihydropyridine CCB may be considered instead of or in addition to an ACE inhibitor or ARB.

CONCLUSION

So for lowering of blood pressure, a variety of antihypertensive agents, including ACE inhibitors, ARBs, diuretics, and CCBs may be used to reduce cardiovascular events. Consider administering one or more antihypertensive medications at bedtime, as there is an association between absence of nocturnal blood pressure dipping and the incidence of cardiovascular disease in diabetes patients. An important caveat is that most patients with diabetes and hypertension require multiple-drug therapy to reach blood pressure treatment goals. Identifying and addressing barriers to medication adherence (such as cost and side effects) should routinely be done. If blood pressure remains uncontrolled despite confirmed adherence to optimal doses of at least three antihypertensive agents of different classes, one of which should be a diuretic, clinicians should consider an evaluation for secondary causes of hypertension.

REFERENCES

1. American Diabetes Association. Cardiovascular disease and risk management (Section 8). In: Standards of medical care in diabetes 2017. Diabetes Care. 2017;40(Suppl 1):S75-87.
2. Mancia G, Fagard R, Narkiewicz K, et al. 2013 ESH/ESC guidelines for the management of arterial hypertension: the task force for the management of Arterial Hypertension of the European Society of Hypertension (ESH) and of the European Society of Cardiology (ESC). Blood Press. 2013;22:193-278.
3. James PA, Oparil S, Carter BL, et al. 2014 evidence-based guideline for the management of high blood pressure in adults: report from the panel members appointed to the Eighth Joint National Committee (JNC 8). JAMA. 2014;311(5):507-20.
4. Patel A, MacMahon S, Chalmers J, et al. ADVANCE Collaborative Group. Effects of a fixed combination of perindopril and indapamide on macrovascular and microvascular outcomes in patients with type 2 diabetes mellitus (the ADVANCE trial): a randomised controlled trial. Lancet. 2007;370(9590):829-40.
5. Margolis KL, O'Connor PJ, Morgan TM, et al. Outcomes of combined cardiovascular risk factor management strategies in type 2 diabetes: the ACCORD randomized trial. Diabetes Care. 2014;37(6):1721-8.
6. Hansson L, Zanchetti A, Carruthers SG, et al. Effects of intensive blood-pressure lowering and low-dose aspirin in patients with hypertension: principal results of the Hypertension Optimal Treatment (HOT) randomised trial. HOT study group. Lancet. 1998;351(9118):1755-62.
7. American Diabetes Association. Older adults (Section 10). In: Standards of medical care in diabetes, 2016. Diabetes Care. 2016;39(Suppl 1):S81-5.
8. UK Prospective Diabetes Study Group. Tight blood pressure control and risk of macrovascular and microvascular complications in type 2 diabetes: UKPDS 38. BMJ. 1998;317:703-13.
9. Estacio RO, Jeffers BW, Hiatt WR, et al. The effect of nisoldipine as compared with enalapril on cardiovascular outcomes in patients with non-insulin-dependent diabetes and hypertension. N Engl J Med. 1998;338(10):645-52.
10. Haller H, Ito S, Izzo JL Jr, et al. Olmesartan for the delay or prevention of microalbuminuria in type 2 diabetes. N Engl J Med. 2011;364(10):907-17.
11. Bangalore S, Fakheri R, Toklu B, et al. Diabetes mellitus as a compelling indication for use of renin-angiotensin system blockers: systematic review and meta-analysis of randomized trials. BMJ. 2016;352:i438.
12. Palmer SC, Mavridis D, Navarese E, et al. Comparative efficacy and safety of blood pressure-lowering agents in adults with diabetes and kidney disease: a network meta-analysis. Lancet. 2015;385(9982):2047-56.
13. Whelton PK, Barzilay J, Cushman WC, et al. ALLHAT Collaborative Research Group. Clinical outcomes in antihypertensive treatment of type 2 diabetes, impaired fasting glucose concentration, and normoglycemia: Antihypertensive and Lipid-lowering Treatment to Prevent Heart Attack Trial (ALLHAT). Arch Intern Med. 2005;165(12):1401-9.
14. Remonti LR, Dias S, Leitão CB, et al. Classes of antihypertensive agents and mortality in hypertensive patients with type 2 diabetes-Network meta-analysis of randomized trials. J Diabetes Complications. 2016;30(6):1192-200.

Benidipine: A New Calcium Channel Blocker for Management of Hypertension and Angina in Cardiodiabetes

CK Ponde, Maulik Parekh

INTRODUCTION

Forty years after the first report of calcium channel blockers (CCBs) in 1969 by Fleckenstein et al., who demonstrated inhibition of calcium influx into cells can have an antihypertensive effect; CCBs are most frequently used class of drugs for hypertension and angina. Type II diabetes mellitus increases risk of cardiovascular disease and it has been shown in several studies that it leads to premature atherosclerosis and left ventricular hypertrophy with or without hypertension, both of which adversely affect prognosis. Angiotensin-converting enzyme (ACE) inhibitors and angiotensin receptor blockers (ARBs) should always be the first choice in treatment of hypertension and diabetes. However, in almost 40% of patients, these drugs alone are not enough to achieve optimal control of blood pressure. Microalbuminuria occurs in 20% of type II diabetics and is a prognostic marker. Once again, in these subsets, ACE/ARBs, alone or in combination with N-type and N- + T-type CCBs are needed to control proteinuria. Benidipine is a newest dihydropyridine CCB with many unique properties.

CHEMISTRY

Benidipine hydrochloride is a racemic mixture of two isomers (S and R), and odorless to slightly yellowish crystalline powder which is stable under varying light conditions and does not decompose even in high humidity. Unique properties of benidipine include the following:

- *Benidipine has very high affinity for cell membranes* and has slow binding to and slow dissociation from dihydropyridine (DHP) binding site. Benidipine is lipophilic (highly lipid soluble), enters the cell membrane and then diffuses to the calcium channel protein and this concept is called "membrane approach".[1]
- *Benidipine inhibits all the three calcium channels* viz., L-type, N-type, and T-type. The triple calcium channel blocking effect translates into the pharmaco-clinical advantages of this drug such as renoprotective effect, vascular selectivity and inhibition of aldosterone secretion.[1]
- *Vascular selectivity of benidipine.* The coronary selectivity of benidipine is 14 times greater than that of nifedipine and 19 times greater than amlodipine. The ratio of binding to peripheral vessels compared to coronaries is higher with this drug compared to any other CCB.[1]
- *Benidipine stimulates nitric oxide (NO) production from the vascular endothelium.* Endothelial nitric oxide production is reduced in patients with coronary artery disease, systemic hypertension and diabetes. By virtue of this effect it shows cardioprotective effect during myocardial ischemia and reperfusion injury.[2]
- *Benidipine suppresses aldosterone formation.* Aldosterone is known to induce diffuse vascular endothelial injury and interstitial fibrosis in myocardium and renal parenchyma. The inhibition of T-type of calcium channels by benidipine in adrenal glomerulosa results in suppression of aldosterone formation. This results in profound beneficial effects in patients with hypertension.[3]

- *Benidipine has a profound renoprotective effect*[1]
  - Unlike traditional CCBs which preferentially dilate the afferent renal arterioles leading to intraglomerular hypertension, benidipine dilates both afferent and efferent arterioles leading to reduction in intraglomerular pressure
  - Increases renal blood flow
  - Has natriuretic effect
  - The increased NO production by benidipine suppresses progression of nephropathy.
- *Benidipine improves insulin sensitivity* in patients with essential hypertension and diabetes. Insulin resistance leads to hyperinsulinemia which is responsible for accelerated atherosclerosis and acceleration of blood pressure. Benidipine improves insulin sensitivity without affecting insulin secretion per se.[1]

PHARMACOKINETICS OF BENIDIPINE

Benidipine is rapidly absorbed after the oral dose reaching maximum drug concentration in 2 hours.The absorption is more complete when the drug is consumed after the meal. It is highly protein bound (98%) and predominantly metabolized in liver. The antihypertensive effect starts within 1 hour, peaks at 4 hours and is sustained up to 24 hours. This is in contrast with the fact that the plasma levels of the drug at around 8 hours after the oral dose are almost undetectable proving the concept of "membrane approach of this drug."

COMPARISON WITH OTHER CALCIUM CHANNEL BLOCKERS[4]

The comparison of benidipine with other calcium channel blockers is shown in Table 1.

CLINICAL EVIDENCES WITH BENIDIPINE

Benidipine versus Amlodipine

- In a small study of 40 hypertensive patients with chronic kidney disease (CKD) randomly assigned to benidipine 8 mg once daily versus amlodipine 5 mg once daily and followed up for 1 year it was shown that benidipine is more effective than amlodipine in protecting renal function and reducing carotid intima media thickness.[5]
- In a another study of 108 patients with CKD it was shown that benidipine reduces augmentation index (AI) and urinary albumin excretion greater than amlodipine in patients already on renin-angiotensin system (RAS) inhibitors.[6]
- In a study of Fukumoto et al., 527 patients with vasospastic angina treated with benidipine (N = 148), amlodipine (N = 111), and diltiazem (N = 313), benidipine showed beneficial prognostic effect compared to other two CCBs with much lower incidence of total major adverse cardiac events (MACE).[7]
- In a meta-analysis of a total 1997 patients with positive coronary spasm provocation tests who were treated with four different CCBs it was observed that benidipine showed significantly more prognostic benefits in terms of far lower occurrence of MACE as compared to all the other three CCBs namely amlodipine, nifidipine, and diltiazem.[8]
- In a retrospective real world study on renal function in hypertensive patients treated with different CCBs in combination with ARBs it was found that benidipine has stronger renoprotective effect than other CCBs when combined with ARBs.[9]

TABLE 1: The comparison of benidipine with other calcium channel blockers

		Blocking activity			
Drugs		*L-type*	*T-type*	*N-type*	
Nifedipine		+	–	–	
Amlodipine		+	–	?	
Benidipine		+	+	+	
Cilnidipine		+	–	+	
Clinical significance					
Heart	Contractility ↓	Heart rate ↓		Heart rate ↓	
Sympathetic nervous system	Pulse rate ↑	Pulse rate ↓		Pulse rate ↓	
Kidney	Glomerular pressure ↑	Glomerular pressure ↓		Glomerular pressure ↓	
Adrenal		Aldosterone secretion ↓			

Benidipine versus Cilnidipine

In 40 hypertensive patients with diabetes and poor BP control despite Cilnidipine it was observed that after switching over to benidipine the blood pressure control was better alongwith reduction in albumin urea suggesting that benidipine is more potent in reducing blood pressure and albumin excretion in diabetic hypertensive patients.[10]

Hypertensive patients with CKD who were already receiving ARBs for blood pressure and protein urea were randomly assigned to addition of cilnidipine versus benidipine and followed for 12 months. Benidipine exerted greater antiproteinuric effect compared to Cilnidipine and this effect was even more profound in those who has diabetes.[11]

Benidipine and Lipids

Nomura et al. investigated the effects of long-term benidipine treatment on levels of monocyte and endothelial cell activation markers in hypertensive patients with or without diabetes. Benidipine showed significant reduction in oxidized **low-density lipoprotein** (LDL) dependent endothelial dysfunction in hypertensive patients with Type 2 diabetes.[12]

In a recent meta-analysis of data from 24 studies (1,696 patients) assessing the effects of different T-type CCBs on renal function and aldosterone it was seen that the protective effects of T-type CCBs on renal function were far much profound than the L-type CCBs. Moreover, these protective effects from renal function were independent of blood pressure reduction and were associated with significant decline in plasma aldosterone levels.[13]

Benidipine and Cardioprotection

Various studies have elucidated the cardioprotective effect of benidipine and its possible mechanisms. The studies suggest that the cardioprotective effects are likely due to increase in coronary blood flow, suppression of calcium overload and antioxidative and vascular endothelium protecting activities. In the presence of ischemia, benidipine suppressed coronary artery spasm more effectively.[14,15] Benidipine, due to its antioxidant effect, also has been shown to reduce infarct size and reperfusion injury in experimental dog heart.[16] Studies have shown beneficial effects of combination of diltiazem with benidipine for angina. Benidipine increases the coronary blood flow more effectively than diltiazem, while diltiazem reduces myocardial O_2 consumption by negative inotropic and chronotropic effect more.[17]Benidipine also has been shown to suppress cardiac hypertrophy in hypertensive rats.[18]This effect, in addition to antihypertensive effect, may add to cardioprotection.

Other Effects of Benidipine

Benidipine increases the cerebral blood flow with much longer lasting effect than nifedipine.[19] It is also found to decrease the lower limit of the autoregulation of cerebral blood flow. Thus, it is a promising molecule for treatment of hypertension complicated by cerebrovascular disease. Benidipine has also been shown to exert beneficial effect on bone in terms of increased differentiation of osteoblasts.[20] The dose of benidipine required for this action is far more lower than that of amlodipine or nifedipine. In a small study, benidipine decreased serum levels of uric acid, ammonia and hypoxanthine.[21] It is postulated that this effect is independent of calcium channel blocking action, and is due to pleotropic effect of benidipine. It could be due to increase in renal excretion of uric acid and suppression of formation of hypoxanthine in skeletal muscles.

Safety and Tolerability

Benidipine is a relatively well-tolerated drug. In a prospective 3 year post-marketing surveillance study in elderly hypertensive patients, the overall incidence of adverse reactions was only 4.9%. Even once daily dosage of benidipine improves compliance significantly.

CONCLUSION

Benidipine is triple CCB with long duration of action and membrane selective binding. It has vascular protecting qualities namely NO production, prevention of oxidation of LDL and suppression of aldosterone production. It has 19 times more vascular selectivity than amlodipine and is twice as potent as amlodipine for hypertension control. It has profound renoprotective effect compared to other CCBs. It is the only CCB as effective as β-blocker in reduction of MACE post-MI. All these qualities make it an excellent drug for use in cardio diabetes.

REFERENCES

1. Yao K, Nagashima K, Miki H. Pharmacological, pharmacokinetic, and clinical properties of benidipine hydrochloride, a novel, long-acting calcium channel blocker. J Pharmacol Sci. 2006;100(4):243-61.
2. Fujimura Y, Tusboi H, Esato K. Efficacy of benidipine hydrochloride on myocardial ischemia and reperfusion. J Surg Res. 1995;59(3):321-5.
3. Tomino Y. Renoprotective effects of the L-/T-type calcium channel blocker benidipine in patients with hypertension.Curr Hypertens Rev. 2013;9(2):108-14.
4. Furukawa T, Nukada T, Namiki Y, et al. Five different profiles of dihydropyridines in blocking T-type Ca^{2+} channel subtypes ($Ca_v3.1$ (α_{1G}), $Ca_v3.2$ (α_{1H}), and $Ca_v3.3$ (α_{1I})) expressed in *Xenopus* oocytes. Eur J Pharmacol. 2009;613(1-3):100-7.

5. Nakamura T, Sato E, Fujiwara N, et al. Comparative effects of benidipine and amlodipine on proteinuria, urinary 8-OHdG, urinary L-FABP, and inflammatory and atherosclerosis markers in early-stage chronic kidney disease. Am J Med Sci. 2010;339(2):157-63.
6. Takayama T, Yoda S, Yajima Y, et al. Improvements in augmentation index and urinary albumin excretion with benidipine in hypertensive patients with chronic kidney disease. Int Heart J. 2016;57(1):53-60.
7. Fukumoto Y1, Yasuda S, Ito A, et al. Prognostic effects of benidipine in patients with vasospastic angina: comparison with diltiazem and amlodipine. J Cardiovasc Pharmacol. 2008;51(3):253-7.
8. Nishigaki K, Inoue Y, Yamanouchi Y, et al. Prognostic effects of calcium channel blockers in patients with vasospastic angina: a meta-analysis. Circ J. 2010;74(9):1944-9.
9. Yamada, H,Suga1N, Maeda K, et al. Effects of combination therapy with angiotensin II type I receptor blockers and calcium channel blockers on renal function in hypertensive patients A retrospective, "real-world" comparative study. Arzneimittelforschung. 2010;60(2):64-70.
10. Seino H, Miyaguchi S, Yamazaki T, et al. Effect of benidipine hydrochloride, a long-acting T-type calcium channel blocker, on blood pressure and renal function in hypertensive patients with diabetes mellitus. Analysis after switching from cilnidipine to benidipine. Arzneimittelforschung. 2007;57(8):526-31.
11. Abe M, Okada K, Maruyama N, et al. Comparison between the antiproteinuric effects of the calcium channel blockers benidipine and cilnidipine in combination with angiotensin receptor blockers in hypertensive patients with chronic kidney disease. Expert Opin Investig Drugs. 2010;19(9):1027-37.
12. NomuraS, ShouzuA, OmotoS, et al. Benidipine improves oxidized LDL-dependent monocyte and endothelial dysfunction in hypertensive patients with type 2 diabetes mellitus. J Hypertens. 2005;19(7):551-7.
13. LiX, Yang MS. Effects of T-Type calcium channel blockers on renal function and aldosterone in patients with hypertension: a systematic review and meta-analysis. PLoS One. 2014;9(10):e109834.
14. Karasawa A, Kubo K, Shuto K, et al. Antianginal effects of the new calcium antagonist benidipine hydrochloride in anesthetized rats and spontaneously hypertensive rats. Electrocardiographic study. Arzneimittelforschung. 1988;38(11A):1702-7.
15. Karasawa A, Kubo K, Shuto K, et al. Pharmacological actions of benidipine hydrochloride in several isolated smooth muscles and myocardium. Arzneimittelforschung. 1988;38(11A):1722-30.
16. Wang N, Minatoguchi S, Chen XH, et al. Benidipine reduces myocardial infarct size involving reduction of hydroxyl radicals and production of protein kinase C-dependent nitric oxide in rabbits. J Cardiovasc Pharmacol. 2004;43(6):747-57.
17. Yao K, Shirakura S. Combined effects of benidipine and diltiazem in a rat model of experimental angina. J Pharmacol Sci. 2004;95(3): 394-7.
18. Kobayashi N, Kobayashi K, Kouno K, et al. Effect of benidipine on microvascular remodeling and coronary flow reserve in two-kidney, one clip Goldblatt hypertension. J Hypertens. 1997;15(11):1285-94.
19. Karasawa A, Kubo K, Shuto K, et al. Vasodilating effects of the new calcium antagonist benidipine hydrochloride in anesthetized dogs and cats. Arzneimittelforschung. 1988;38(11A):1707-12.
20. Nishiya Y, Sugimoto S. Effects of various antihypertensive drugs on the function of osteoblast. Biol Pharm Bull. 2001;24(6):628-33.
21. Hamada T, Matsubara K, Igawa G, et al. Inhibitory effect of benidipine hydrochloride on myogenic hyperuricemia in essential hypertensive patients. Ther Res. 2003;24:1987-91.

CHAPTER

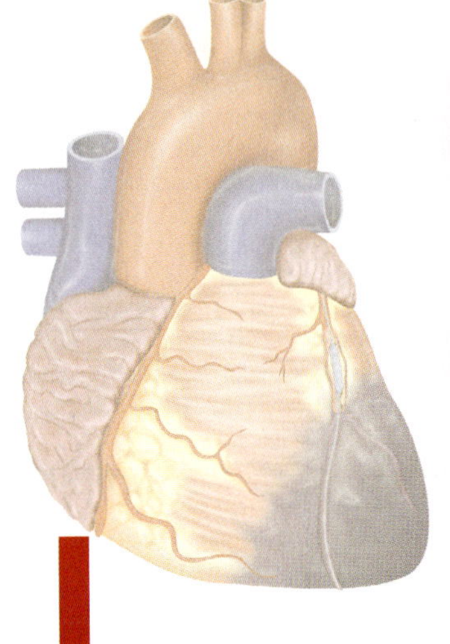

Azilsartan for Hypertension Management in Cardiodiabetes

Harsh Wardhan, Nitin Aggarwal

INTRODUCTION

According to the 2015 AHA statistical report,[1-6] over 75% of the population aged at least 40 years has elevated blood pressure (BP) levels (65.3% among those aged 40–59 years, and 84.3% among those aged above 59 years). Furthermore, only 60% of patients achieve good BP control, and despite the decreasing cardiovascular (CV) morbidity, BP is still a leading cause of death in developing as well as in Western countries, affecting nearly 230 of every 100,000 individuals.[6] In India about 33% urban and 25% rural Indians are hypertensive. Out of these 25% rural and 42% urban Indians are aware of their hypertensive status. Only 25% rural and 38% of urban Indians are being treated for hypertension. One-tenth of rural and one-fifth of urban Indian hypertensive population have their BP under control.[7] The target BP advocated in current treatment guidelines is generally less than 140/90 mm Hg, with a lower target (<130/80 mm Hg) for patients with diabetes mellitus or heart or renal disease.[8] A meta-analysis of 61 prospective, observational studies has shown that a 10 mm Hg lower systolic blood pressure (SBP) would be associated over the long term with a 40% lower risk of stroke death and a 30% lower risk of death from ischemic heart disease (IHD) or other vascular causes. Even a small, 2 mm Hg falls in mean SBP would be associated with large reductions in stroke mortality (10%) and death due to IHD and other vascular diseases (7%) in middle age.[9] Numerous guidelines for the effective management of hypertension have been published. Selection of a suitable antihypertensive drug is dependent on a number of factors, including concurrent diseases, tolerability profile, efficacy of drug, 24 hour blood pressure control, and cost. Several classes of drugs are available in India for the treatment of patients with essential hypertension. These include drugs such as diuretics, beta adrenergic antagonists (blockers), alpha-adrenergic blockers, calcium channel blockers, and drugs that affect the renin-angiotensin system (RAS), such as the direct renin inhibitors, the angiotensin-converting enzyme (ACE) inhibitors and the angiotensin II receptor antagonists (blockers) also known as angiotensin receptor blockers (ARBs). But adequate blood pressure control is still a great challenge in India. In spite of the availability of numbers of drugs for hypertension, it still remains poorly controlled. There is always a search for potent and safer new antihypertensive. Ability of ARBs to protect against target organ damage and improve clinical outcomes is still considered to be largely mediated by their ability to decrease BP. Despite the fact that all approved AT1 receptor blockers can lower BP, many patients treated with currently available ARBs do not achieve BP treatment goals.[10] Azilsartan medoxomil (AZL-M) is a recent addition to the angiotensin II receptor antagonist class of drugs and is the eighth approved drug in this class for the management of hypertension.

PHARMACOLOGY

Azilsartan medoxomil is the newest approved ARB for the management of hypertension. It is a prodrug that is quickly hydrolyzed to the active moiety Azilsartan and reaches its peak plasma concentration between 1.5 hours and 3 hours

TABLE 1: Favorable drug specific pharmacological properties of azilsartan medoxomil in comparison to other angiotensin receptor blockers[11]

Inhibitory effects on the specific binding of radiolabeled AII to human AT1 receptors		
Compound	IC50 (nM)	
	No washout	After washout
Azilsartan	2.6	7.4
Olmesartan	6.7	242.5
Telmisartan	5.1	191.6
Irbesartan	15.8	>10,000
Valsartan	44.9	>10,000
Dissociation rate		
Compound	Reduction (%) of inhibitory effects on the specific binding of radiolabeled AII to human	
	AT1 receptors 240 minutes after washout	
Azilsartan	25	
Olmesartan	44	
Telmisartan	70	
Valsartan	99	

Abbreviations: IC50, half maximal inhibitory concentration; nM, nanomolar concentration (10^{-6} mol/m^3); AII, angiotensin II; AT1, angiotensin II receptor 1.

following oral administration. It is an ARB with estimated bioavailability of 60% and elimination half-life of 11 hours. Metabolism of AZL-M occurs in the liver via cytochrome P450 (CYP) 2C9 and to a lesser extent by CYP2B6 and CYP2C8, resulting in the formation of inactive metabolites. Azilsartan medoxomil is primarily excreted by the kidney, as inactive metabolites, with a clearance of 2.3 mL/min. *Azilsartan medoxomil is a potent and highly selective and insurmountable AT1 receptor antagonist that binds tightly to and dissociates slowly from AT1 receptors compared with other ARBs.*[11] Ojima et al. using indirect kinetic methods showed that AZL-M remained substantially bound to the receptors after washout of the compound compared with other ARBs, such as olmesartan, telmisartan, valsartan, and irbesartan (Table 1).[11] As a consequence, the inhibitory effect of AZL-M on AT1 was reduced only by 25%, 4 hours after washout, while inhibitory effects of olmesartan, telmisartan, and valsartan were reduced by 44%, 70%, and 99%, respectively (Table 1). The high-affinity and tight binding properties of AZL-M are expected to induce potent and long-lasting antihypertensive effects in preclinical and clinical settings while inverse agonism may offer organ protective effects.[11] Interestingly, in a small study of hemodialysis patients with crossover design, AZL-M exerted more prominent suppression of sympathetic nervous system in comparison to other ARBs that resulted in stronger anti-hypertensive effect.[12] Sympathoinhibition is a specific class effect of ARBs, and can be quantified by plasma noradrenaline levels—a sensitive index of the activity of the sympathetic nervous system.[13] Thus, the significant decrease in noradrenaline levels following substitution of losartan, valsartan, telmisartan, or olmesartan with AZL-M, suggests an amplified primary class effect for this member of ARBs.

CARDIOVASCULAR AND OTHER EFFECTS

Azilsartan medoxomil produces antihypertensive effects in adults with essential hypertension and reduce SBP to a clinically relevant extent in clinical trials.[14-16] The BP-lowering efficacy of AZL-M in 3,672 patients with mild, moderate or severe hypertension has been evaluated in seven randomized, double-blind, controlled trials.[14,17] These studies included active treatment arms (n = 1,468) and placebo arms (n = 801). In addition to its effect on BP in adults with hypertension, azilsartan medoxomil has shown beneficial effects on cellular mechanisms of cardiovascular disease and on insulin sensitivity in several animal studies and cellular experiments.[18,19] In blood vessel walls, plasminogen activator inhibitor type-1 (PAI-1) protein expression can be increased by angiotensin II and this may result in the acceleration of atherosclerosis.[18] Furthermore, after myocardial infarction, PAI-1 overexpression in the heart may contribute to negative left ventricular modeling and heart failure. Inhibition of the AT1, receptor may potentially blunt expression of the PAI-1 protein in the wall of the aorta, thereby reducing the risk of atherosclerosis by decreasing atherosclerotic plaque formation and the likelihood of plaque rupture, a significant cause of morbidity and mortality globally.[18] In a preclinical study, azilsartan medoxomil, administered orally for 16 weeks, suppressed vascular wall expression of PAI-1 protein in overexpressing PAI-1 vascular smooth muscle cells in mice. Across three dose regimens (0.1-10 mg/kg), the mice exposed to azilsartan had a decrease in aortic wall PAI-1 as well as increases in both the cellularity and collagen content of atherosclerotic plaques, consistent with the presence of more biologically stable plaques less likely to rupture.[18] Some angiotensin II receptor antagonist drugs are known to be pleiotropic molecules and exhibit pharmacological effects beyond AT1 receptor blockade related effects that may be clinically relevant in terms of cardiovascular protection or in the treatment of conditions concomitant to cardiovascular disease.[10,20] In addition, several angiotensin II receptor antagonist drugs have been shown to have a direct effect at several types of peroxisome proliferator activated receptors (PPARs) that are known to regulate various inflammatory and metabolic responses.[21,22] Although the BP-lowering effects and mechanism of action of azilsartan as an AT1 receptor antagonist are well known and its inhibitory effects on vascular contractility documented,[11] data are currently reasonably limited on its pleiotropic characteristics, such as its effects on vascular cell proliferation, adipogenesis and adipocyte gene expression.[20] In an in vitro study that used cell-based assay systems, adipogenesis in cultured preadipocytes was enhanced by the presence of azilsartan, which also exerted more marked effects than valsartan on the expression of genes that encoded peroxisome proliferator-activated receptor-α (PPAR-α) PPAR-γ, adipsin, adiponectin and leptin.[20] Furthermore, in the absence of exogenously supplemented angiotensin II, azilsartan produced potent inhibition of vascular cell proliferation. At low concentrations (<1 ηmol/L), azilsartan inhibited the proliferation of aortic endothelial cells, whereas antiproliferative effects were not observed or were minimal with valsartan at concentrations greater than 10 ηmol/L. Azilsartan also displayed antiproliferative effects in cells without AT1 receptors and, in vascular smooth muscle cells, blocked the activation of mitogen activated protein kinase induced by angiotensin II; the latter effect was not observed with valsartan.[20]

EVIDENCE FROM CLINICAL TRIALS

Antihypertensive Effects of Azilsartan Medoxomil in Comparison to Other Angiotensin Receptor Blockers

A number of double-blind randomized clinical trials have investigated the antihypertensive efficacy and safety of AZL-M compared to other ARBs (Table 2).[14-16,23] Azilsartan medoxomil was compared with olmesartan in two trials,[14,15] with valsartan in two trials[15,16] and with candesartan in one trial.[23] The trials ranged in duration from 6 weeks to 24 weeks while the recruited population ranged from 622 to 1,291 participants. Azilsartan medoxomil was found to be more effective toward the primary end point of

TABLE 2: Clinical trials comparing azilsartan medoxomil as a monotherapy with other antihypertensives

Study (year)	*Type of study*	*Patients*	*Time*	*Treatment*	*End point*	*Result*
Bakris et al., 2011[14]	Double-blind RCT	1,275	6 weeks	AZL-M $20,40,80 mg or OLM 40 mg or placebo	Change from baseline in 24-h mean SBP	AZL-M 80 mg (–14.6 mm Hg) vs. OLM (–12.5 mm Hg) (p = 0.038) AZL-M 40 mg (–13.4 mm Hg) was noninferior to OLM 40 mg
White et al., 2011[15]	Double-blind RCT	12,791	6 weeks	AZL-M 40,80 mg or VAL 320 mg or OLM 40 mg or placebo	Change from baseline in 24-h mean SBP	AZL-M 80 mg (–14.5 mm Hg) vs. OLM (–12.0 mm Hg) (p = 0.009) and VAL (–10.2 mm Hg) (p< 0.001) AZL-M 40 mg (–13.4 mm Hg) was noninferior to OLM 40 mg
Sica et al., 2011[16]	Double-blind RCT	984	24 weeks	AZL-M 40,80 mg or VAL 320 mg	Change from baseline in 24-h mean SBP	AZL-M 40 mg (–14.9 mm Hg) and 80 mg (–15.3 mm Hg) vs. VAL (–11.3 mm Hg) (p < 0.001 for both)
Rakugi et al., 2012[23]	Double-blind RCT	622	16 weeks	AZL-M 20–40 mg or CAND 8–12 mg	Change from baseline in the sitting trough DBP	AZL-M (–12.4 mm Hg) vs. CAND (–9.8 mm Hg) (p = 0.0003)
Bönner et al., 2013[33]	Double-blind RCT	884	24 weeks	AZL-M 20–80 mg or RAM 2.5–10 mg	Change from baseline in the sitting trough SBP	AZL-M 40 mg (–20.6 mm Hg) and AZL-M 80 mg (–21.2 mm Hg) vs. RAM (–12.2 mm Hg) (p< 0.001)
Kario and Hoshide, 2015[34]	Open-label RCT	718	8 weeks	AZL-M 20 mg or AML 5 mg	Differences between sleep SBP	AZL-M 20 mg (–12.6 mm Hg) vs. AML 5 mg (–17.5 mm Hg) (p < 0.001)
EARLY Gitt et al., 2016[35]	Observational, prospective	3,849	12 months	AZL-M or any ACE-i	Documentation of the achievement of target BP values set according to recent guidelines Description of the safety profile of AZL-M	Target BP level achieved in AZL-M group (61.1% of patients) vs. ACE-I group (56.4% of patients) (p < 0.05) Equivalent safety profile (p= 0.73)

Abbreviations: RCT, randomized controlled trial; AZL-M, Azilsartan Medoxomil; OLM, olmesartan; RAM, ramipril; VAL, valsartan; CAND, candesartan; AML, amlodipine; SBP,: systolic blood pressure; DBP, diastolic blood pressure.

reduction in office or ambulatory systolic BP over each of its comparators. Adverse events were reported similarly in all treatment groups and were mostly mild to moderate in severity, including mainly dizziness, headache, urinary infection, and upper respiratory tract inflammation. The incidence of treatment-associated adverse events ranged from 35.9% to 65.4 % for AZL-M and from 37.9% to 59.2 % for alternative ARBs ($p > 0.05$ for all).[14-16,23] Discontinuations due to adverse events were infrequent in all groups. In detail, discontinuation rates for AZL-M ranged from 1.1% to 8.2 % as compared with 1.3% to 6.1 % for other ARBs ($p > 0.05$ for individual comparisons). It should be emphasized that the clinical trials that established the efficacy of AZL-M, analyzed data from 24 hours ambulatory blood pressure monitoring (ABPM) for comparisons with alternative antihypertensive agents, in addition to other hemodynamic indices. Superiority of AZL-M in lowering BP during a 24-h period could be partially explained by its selective binding and tighter binding properties.[11]

Metabolic Effects of Azilsartan Medoxomil in Comparison to Other Angiotensin Receptor Blockers

Although AZL-M has been approved for hypertension, it remains to be determined whether this new drug can offer clinical benefits beyond its antihypertensive action.[24] In general, accumulating evidence suggests that ARBs could decelerate the progression of diabetic nephropathy, independently of their BP lowering effect.[25,26] In addition, some ARBs may be more effective than others in reducing proteinuria in patients with diabetic nephropathy despite similar induced reductions in BP. Most important, specific ARBs are pleiotropic molecules with additional cellular actions beyond the blockade of AT1 receptors that might confer favorable cardiometabolic effects.[27] Several preclinical studies have shown beneficial effects of AZL-M regarding pro-atherosclerotic pathways, insulin sensitivity, and adipocyte (Flow chart 1).[20,28-32] In specific, Kajiya et al.,[20] investigated pleiotropic features of AZL-M in cell-based assay systems independently of its effects on blood pressure and showed that AZL-M, but not valsartan, blocked AII-induced activation of mitogen-activated protein kinases (MAPK) in vascular smooth muscle cells (VSMCs) after delayed washout of the drug.[20] This phenomenon is consistent with the intrinsic high-affinity and tight binding properties of AZL-M.[11] However, in the same study AZL-M exerted anti-proliferative effects in vascular cells in the absence of AII that could be explained by its inverse agonist properties, but also in cells lacking AT1 receptors, suggesting involvement of mechanisms beyond AT1 receptor blockade.

Results from another animal study suggest that azilsartan restores endothelial function more effectively than does candesartan cilexetil, by normalizing eNOS function and by reducing inflammation and oxidative stress in diabetic mice.[31] The higher affinity for and slower dissociation

Flow chart 1: Possible pleiotropic effects and proposed mechanisms in subjects with unfavorable metabolic profile combined with antihypertensive properties of azilsartan medoximil

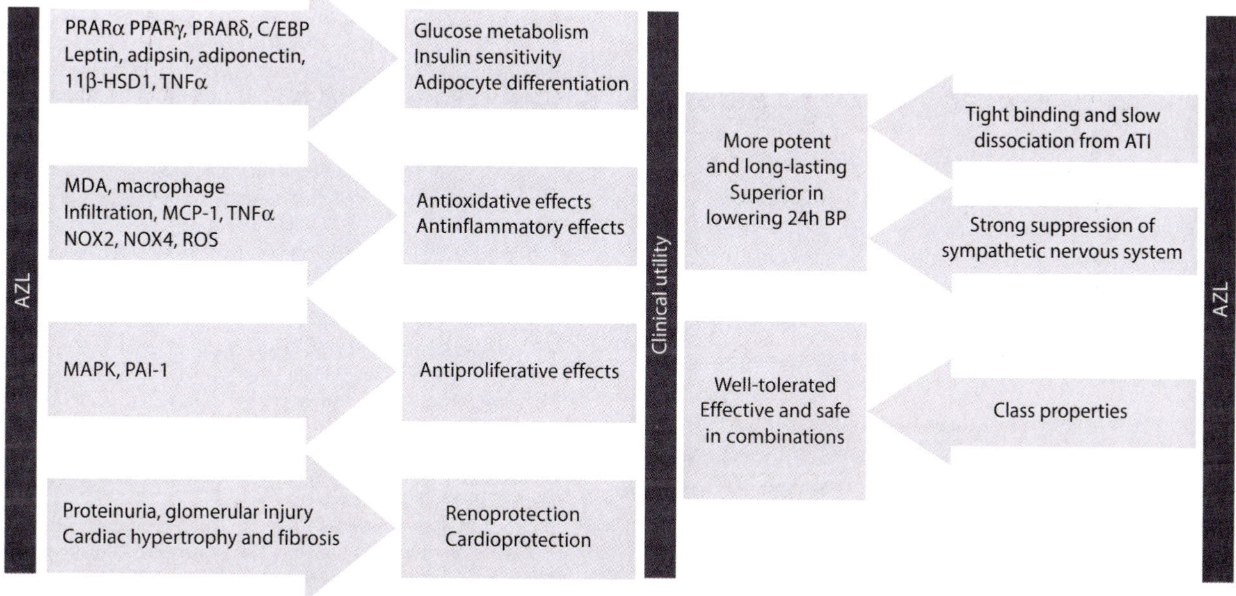

from AT1 receptors may underlie AZL-M efficacy in diabetic vascular dysfunction.[28,31] Iwai et al.[28] reported an upregulated expression of PPAR-γ in adipose tissue, but, Zhao et al.[32] failed to reproduce this effect. In support of the results from Iwai et al.,[28] additional data have linked AZL-M with protection of brain endothelial cells from oxidative stress, through preserved mitochondrial function; eNOS mediated anti-inflammatory activity and activation of the PPAR-γ pathway.[30] However, notable exclusion criteria for most clinical trials assessing AZL-M were previous history of major cardiovascular events or significant cardiac conduction abnormalities, severe renal impairment as well as type I or poorly controlled type II diabetes. As a result, there is limited evidence regarding treatment with AZL-M in diabetic patients. However, three out of the four clinical trials[14-16] reported the recruitment of patients with well-controlled DM II (HbAC1 < 8 mg/dL). Although no prespecified subgroup analysis for the presence of DM II was provided in these studies, we can assume that AZL-M may be effective and well-tolerated in the subgroup of diabetic patients as part of the total population. This assumption is reinforced by the results of the fourth trial by Rakugi et al.[23]. Diabetic patients were included without any limitations and the subgroup analysis based on the presence of DM showed similar effectiveness of AZL-M in the diabetic subgroup compared to the nondiabetic and superiority over candesartan in diabetic subgroup.[23,33-35] In a meta-analysis[15] of three of the four randomized controlled clinical trials mentioned, the efficacy, safety and metabolic effects of AZL-M were compared to alternative ARBs (valsartan and olmesartan), separately in patients with impaired fasting glucose (prediabetes mellitus) and DM. A total of 3,821 patients were randomized to AZL-M, olmesartan, valsartan, or placebo and further stratified by subgroups of normoglycemic, prediabetic, and DM status. Azilsartan medoxomil exhibited more potent antihypertensive efficacy than olmesartan or valsartan in patients with prediabetes mellitus and DM based on both office and ambulatory BP results. As far as metabolic parameters were concerned (including among others blood glucose, insulin levels, and biomarkers, such as adiponectin and lipoproteins), no significant differences were established among treatment subgroups.

CONCLUSION

Azilsartan medoxomil emerges as a pleiotropic drug that may exert beneficial cardiometabolic effects beyond its antihypertensive properties. These favorable effects are more profound in comparison to other ARBs, probably due to higher affinity, tighter binding, and slower dissociation from AT1 receptors. This superiority was observed even when AZL-M was used in therapeutic doses in comparison to other ARBs that were administered above recommended clinical doses. Azilsartan medoxomil is a potent and well-tolerated antihypertensive drug and there is indirect evidence of its efficacy and safety among diabetic patients. In comparison to other ARBs, the superior antihypertensive effect of AZL-M could be attributed to its unique binding properties. In general, preclinical trials support AZL-M as a possible beneficial treatment strategy for diabetic patients, beyond its antihypertensive effect. We anticipate the results from the ongoing trials to fully adjudicate AZL-M as the most promising member of the ARB class toward primary and secondary cardiometabolic prevention.

REFERENCES

1. Turnbull F, Neal B, Algert C, et al. Effects of different blood pressure-lowering regimens on major cardiovascular events in individuals with and without diabetes mellitus: results of prospectively designed overviews of randomized trials. Arch Intern Med. 2005;165(12):1410-19.
2. Mancia G, Fagard R, Narkiewicz K, et al. 2013 ESH/ESC practice guidelines for the management of arterial hypertension. Blood Press. 2014;23(1):3-16.
3. Hao G,Wang Z, Guo R, et al. Effects of ACEI/ARB in hypertensive patients with type 2 diabetes mellitus : a meta-analysis of randomized controlled studies. BMC Cardiovasc Disord. 2014;14:148.
4. Chen G, McAlister FA, Walker RL, et al. Cardiovascular outcomes in Framingham participants with diabetes: the importance of blood pressure. Hypertension. 2011;57:891-7.
5. Olivares-Reyes JA, Arellano-Plancarte A, Castillo-Hernandez JR. Angiotensin II and the development of insulin resistance: implications for diabetes. Mol Cell Endocrinol. 2009;302(2):128-39.
6. Heart Disease and Stroke Statistics–2015 update. A report from the American Heart Association. Circulation. 2015;131(4):e29-e322.
7. Anchala R, Kannuri NK, Pant H, et al. Hypertension in India: a systematic review and meta-analysis of prevalence, awareness, and control of hypertension. J Hypertens. 2014;32(6):1170-7
8. Perry CM. Azilsartan Medoxomil: a review of its use in hypertension. Clin Drug Investig. 2012; 32(9):621-39.
9. Lewington S, Clarke R, Qizilbash N, et al. Age-specific relevance of usual blood pressure to vascular mortality: a meta-analysis of individual data for one million adults in 61 prospective studies. Lancet. 2002;360:1903-13.
10. Kurtz TW, Kajiya T. Differential pharmacology and benefit/risk of Azilsartan compared to other sartans. Vasc Health Risk Manag. 2012;8:133-43.
11. Ojima M, Igata H, Tanaka M, et al. In vitro antagonistic properties of a new angiotensin type1 receptor blocker, azilsartan, in receptor binding and function studies. J Pharmacol Exp Ther. 2011;336(3):801-8.
12. Kusuyama T, Ogata H, Takeshita H, et al. Effects of azilsartan compared to other angiotensin receptor blockers on left ventricular hypertrophy and the sympathetic nervous system in hemodialysis patients. Ther Apher Dial. 2014;18(5):398-403.
13. Bakris GL, Williams M, Dworkin L, et al. Preserving renal function in adults with hypertension and diabetes: a consensus approach. Am J Kidney Dis. 2000;36(3):646-61.
14. Bakris GL, Sica D, Weber M, et al. The comparative effects of azilsartan medoxomil and olmesartan on ambulatory and clinic blood pressure. J Clin Hypertens (Greenwich). 2011;13(2):81-8.

15. White WB, Weber MA, Sica D, et al. Effects of the angiotensin receptor blocker azilsartan medoxomil versus olmesartan and valsartan on ambulatory and clinic blood pressure in patients with stages 1 and 2 hypertension. Hypertension. 2011;57(3):413-20.
16. Sica D, White WB, Weber MA, et al. Comparison of the novel angiotensin II receptor blocker azilsartan medoxomil vs valsartan by ambulatory blood pressure monitoring. J Clin Hypertens (Greenwich). 2011;13(7):467-72.
17. Edarbi azilsartan medoxomil. European public assessment report. [online] Available from https://www.edarbi.com/edarbi. [Accessed August, 2017].
18. French CJ, Zaman AK, Sobel BE. The angiotensin receptor blocker, azilsartan medoxomil (TAK-491), suppresses vascular wall expression of plasminogen activator inhibitor type-I protein potentially facilitating the stabilization of atherosclerotic plaques. J Cardiovasc Pharmacol. 2011;58(2):143-8.
19. Kusumoto K, Igata H, Ojima M, et al. Antihypertensive, insulin-sensitising and renoprotective effects of a novel, potent and long-acting angiotensin II type 1 receptor blocker, azilsartan medoxomil, in rat and dog models. Eur J Pharmacol. 2011;669(1-3):84-93.
20. Kajiya T, Ho C, Wang J, et al. Molecular and cellular effects of azilsartan; a new generation angiotensin II receptor blocker. J Hypertens. 2011;29(12):2476-83.
21. Schupp M, Janke J, Ciasen R, et al. Angiotensin type 1 receptor blockers induce peroxisome proliferator-activated receptor-γ activity. Circulation. 2004;109(17):2054-7.
22. Clemenz M, Frost N, Schupp M, et al. Liver-specific peroxisome proliferator-activated a target gene regulation by the angiotensin type 1 receptor blocker telmisartan. Diabetes. 2008;57(5):1405-13.
23. Rakugi H, Enya K, Sugiura K, et.al. Comparison of the efficacy and safety of azilsartan with that of candesartan cilexetilin Japanese patients with grade I-II essential hypertension: a randomized , double-blind clinical study. Hypertens Res. 2012;35:552-8.
24. Kurtz TW, Kajiya T. Differential pharmacology and benefit/risk of azilsartan compared to other sartans. Vasc Health Risk Manag. 2012;8:133-43.
25. Isaacs AN, Vincent A. Antihypertensive therapy for the prevention of nephropathy in diabetic hypertensive patients. J Clin Pharm Ther. 2016;41:111-5.
26. Weber MA, Schiffrin EL, White WB, et al. Clinical practice guidelines for the management of hypertension in the community: a statement by the American Society of Hypertension and the International Society of Hypertension. J Clin Hypertens. 2014;16(1):14-26.
27. Kurtz TW, Pravenec M. Molecule-specific effects of angiotensin II-receptor blockers independent of the renin-angiotensin system. Am J Hypertens. 2008;21:852-9.
28. Iwai M, Chen R, Imura Y, et al. TAK-536,a new AT1 receptor blocker, improves glucose intolerance and adipocyte differentiation. Am J Hypertens. 2007;20(5):579-86.
29. Lastra G, Santos FR, Hooshmand P, et al. The novel Angiotensin II receptor blocker Azilsartan Medoxomil Ameliorates insulin resistance induced by Chronic Angiotensin II treatment in Rat Skeletal Muscle. Cardiorenal Med. 2013;3:154-64.
30. Liu H, Mao P, Wang J, et al. Azilsartan, an angiotensin II type 1 receptor blocker, attenuates tertbutyl hydroperoxide-induced endothelial cell injury through inhibition of mitochondrial dysfunction and anti-inflammatory activity. Neurochem Int. 2016;94:48-56.
31. Matsumoto S, Shimabukuro M, Fukuda D, et al. Azilsartan, an angiotensin II type 1 receptor blocker, restores endothelial function by reducing vascular inflammation and by increasing the phosphorylation ratio Ser(1177)/Thr(497) of endothelial nitric oxide synthase in diabetic mice. Cardiovasc Diabetol. 2014;13:30.
32. Zhao M, Li Y, Wang J, et al. Azilsartan treatment improves insulin sensitivity in obese spontaneously hypertensive Koletsky rats. Diabetes Obes Metab. 2011;13(12):1123-9.
33. Bönner G, Bakris GL, Sica D, et al. Antihypertensive efficacy of the angiotensin receptor blocker azilsartan medoxomil compared with the angiotensin-converting enzyme inhibitor ramipril. J Hum Hypertens. 2013;27(8):479-86.
34. Kario K, Hoshide S. Age-related difference in the sleep pressure-lowering effect between an angiotensin II receptor blocker and a calcium channel blocker in Asian hypertensives: the ACS1 Study. Hypertension. 2015;65(4):729-35.
35. Gitt AK, Bramlage P, Potthoff SA, et al. Azilsartan compared to ACE inhibitors in anti-hypertensive therapy: one-year outcomes of the observational EARLY registry. BMC Cardiovasc Disord. 2016; 16:56.

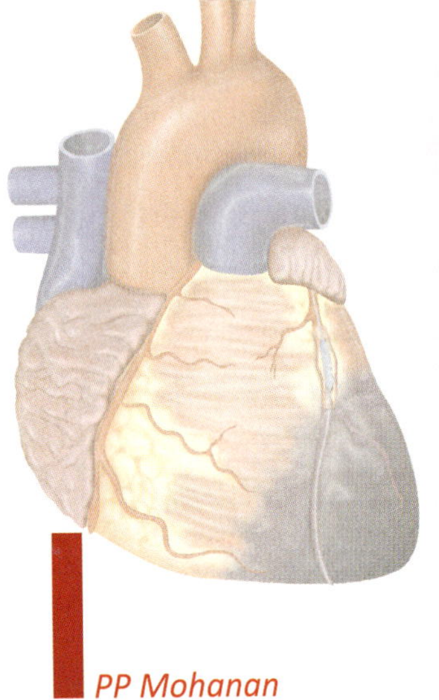

Need for Registry of Cardiodiabetes in India

PP Mohanan

INTRODUCTION

Cardiovascular diseases (CVD), comprising coronary heart (CHD) and cerebrovascular diseases, are currently the leading cause of death globally, accounting for 21.9% of total deaths, and are projected to increase to 26.3% by 2030.[1] The factors that coalesce to increase the risk of developing atherosclerotic CHD were demonstrated in Framingham in the mid-20th century[2] and have subsequently been shown to be pervasive across ethnicities and regions of the world.[3] These are not new risks, but the ubiquity of smoking, dyslipidemia, obesity, diabetes, and hypertension has been gradually escalating,[4] and is thought to be the driving influence behind the epidemic of heart disease faced today.

Of the risk factors, diabetes, and its predominant form, type 2 diabetes mellitus (T2DM), have a distinctive association with CHD. Those with diabetes have two- to four-fold higher risk of developing coronary disease than people without diabetes[5] and CVD accounts for an overwhelming 65–75% of deaths in people with diabetes.[6,7] The prevalence of T2DM is increasing worldwide major contribution from China and India which in the present scenario called as Chindia World Health Organization (WHO) estimates that nearly 347 million people all over the world suffer from diabetes and this number is likely to be doubled by 2030. In the year 2002, 32 million Indians were suffering from diabetes and the International Diabetes Federation (IDF) estimates that the number of diabetics in India can rise up to 109 million by the year 2030. There has been an increase in the prevalence of diabetes among rural population in India. Results of a national study conducted by the ICMR (ICMR-INDIAB) which assessed the prevalence of diabetes and prediabetes (impaired fasting glucose and/or impaired glucose tolerance) in urban and rural India, have been published in 2011.

More significantly however, the age- and sex-adjusted mortality risk in diabetic patients without pre-existing coronary artery disease was found to be equal to that of nondiabetic individuals with prior myocardial infarction.[8] These remarkable findings regarding higher risk of mortality[9-11] have led to suspicion that common precursors predispose to diabetes and CHD,[12,13] with subsequent implications that insulin resistance, visceral adiposity, and excess inflammation[14-16] underlie the pathophysiology of thrombogenesis. In addition, a complex mix of mechanistic processes such as oxidative stress, enhanced atherogenecity of cholesterol particles, abnormal vascular reactivity, augmented hemostatic activation, and renal dysfunction have been proposed as features characteristic of T2DM that may confer excess risk of CHD.[17] People of Indian Asian descent make up over a fifth of the world's population, combining inhabitants of the subcontinent and the Indian diaspora living elsewhere. The so-called "Asian Indian Phenotype" refers to an amalgamation of clinical (larger waist-to-hip and waist-to-height ratios signaling excess visceral adiposity), biochemical (insulin resistance, lower adiponectin, and higher C-reactive protein levels) and metabolic abnormalities [raised triglycerides, low high-density lipoprotein (HDL)] cholesterol that are more prevalent in individuals of South Asian origin and predispose this group to developing diabetes and premature CHD.[18-20] It is expected that individuals of Indian Asian ethnicity will account for between 40% and 60% of global.[21] The astonishingly higher risk in this particular ethnic group has been attributed to underlying genetic susceptibility[22,23] unmasked by environmental factors (permeation of contemporary lifestyle practices)[24] or intrauterine programming which predisposes to asymmetric energy metabolism and rapid, excess accumulation of visceral body fat in adult life.[25]

GLYCEMIC CONTROL IN CARDIOVASCULAR RISK REDUCTION: AN ACTIVELY EVOLVING PARADIGM

In patients with diabetes, where excess CVD risk has already been demonstrated, the relationship between glycemia itself and CVD should not, theoretically, be in doubt. Even studies in nondiabetic subjects[26,27] including a meta-regression analysis combining data from greater than 95,000 participants,[28] have shown an association between fasting blood glucose and CVD. Another meta-analysis of prospective cohort studies[29] examined glycosylated hemoglobin (HbA1C a more stable, accurate, less error-prone measure of long-term glycemic levels) and CVD in persons with diabetes and found 18% (pooled RR 1.18; 95% CI 1.10–1.26) and 15% (pooled RR 1.15; 95% CI 0.92–1.43) greater relative risk per 1% increase in HbA1C in T2DM and T1DM, respectively. However, the converse of this association, whether reducing glucose levels to near-normal targets results in lower CVD events, is still a controversial topic. Despite impressive reduction in microvascular complications and retrospective cohort data showing lower risk of strokes (21%) and MI (23% with lower levels of glycemia, the early prospective trial data evaluating macrovascular outcomes classically provided equivocal results [e.g. 16% ($P = 0.052$) nonsignificant reduction in MI in United Kingdom Prospective Diabetes Study (UKPDS)], citing reasons of inadequate power, follow-up[30] or design deficiencies. More recent multicenter trials sought to conclusively evaluate the influence of achieving lower therapeutic targets for glycemic control on the incidence of CVD endpoints. Since a variety of pharmacological and nonpharmacological treatments are established, cost-effective, and safe interventions for glycemic control,[31] the more contemporary theme of what level of glycemia to achieve holds topical interest, requiring more in-depth discussion. Three large prospective randomized trials attempted to definitively address the glycemia and CVD debate. The Action to Control Cardiovascular Risk in Diabetes (ACCORD) Action in Diabetes and Vascular Disease: Preterax and Diamicron Modified Release Controlled Evaluation (ADVANCE) and Veterans Affairs Diabetes Trial (VADT) studies randomized 10,251, 11,140, and 1,791 T2DM patients, respectively, with coexisting risk factors and/or history of diabetic complications (including previous CVD events) into intensive (aiming for bold "near-normal" glycemic targets) or conventional therapy groups, using different treatment regimens. After a 1.1% relative difference in median HbA1C between the groups (6.4 vs 7.5%) and 3.5 years of follow-up, ACCORD was prematurely discontinued due to 54 excess deaths in the intensive therapy arm. The ADVANCE trial achieved a 0.8% lower median HbA1C (6.5%) in the intensive therapy arm compared to the standard group over a 5 year follow-up period and demonstrated a 10% reduction in composite of major micro- and macrovascular events (HR 0.90, 95% CI 0.82–0.98; $P = 0.01$), which did not remain significant after adjustment for reduction in nephropathy (21% reduction in intensive therapy group; HR 0.79, 95% CI 0.66–0.93; $P = 0.006$). From a baseline median HbA1C level of 9.4%, the VADT achieved A1C levels of 6.9% and 8.4% in the intensive and standard groups, respectively. However, there was no significant between-group difference in the composite primary outcome (HR 0.88; 95% CI, 0.75–1.05; $P = 0.14$), nor in the number of new, or progression of, microvascular complications. Across these three studies,[32] the intensive therapy arms all reported higher incidence of hypoglycemia requiring medical assistance and weight gain among participants. A very convincing point is that glycemia is not the sole consideration in CVD risk, but rather plays a role in the confluence of multifactorial influences.

The case for concerted multiple risk factor modification and drawing well-informed lessons from the literature is therefore compelling. Cardiologists have been very proactive and comfortable in treating most of the cardiometabolic contributors associated with T2DM. Yet data from the PINNACLE Registry reveal persistent gaps in the treatment of lipids in T2DM patients, with nearly 30% not treated with a statin.[33]

To better understand the changing epidemiology of T2DM, prevalent in patients with an array of cardiovascular disorders including hypertension, coronary artery disease, peripheral vascular disease, congestive heart failure, and stroke. To better understand the metabolic syndrome associated with T2DM and its relationship to cardiac and vascular disease beyond measures directed at glycemic control. To set the stage for gauging the impact of recently published randomized clinical trials showing clear cardiovascular protection with the use of specific diabetic therapies. To identify trends in the comprehensive care of patients with T2DM that include treatments of lipids, hypertension, and obesity, and approaches to the treatment of hemodynamically significant coronary and vascular disease and identify treatment gaps.

CONCLUSION

Glycemic and CVD risk factors control can be challenging in any context, not least in the subcontinent. Evidence-based recommendations for diabetes care, mainly based on trials in Anglo-Caucasian populations, are available, but there is no indication of how well these guidelines are implemented in South Asia, nor any randomized trial evidence is available from this particular population group. The Delhi Diabetes Community (DEDICOM) and DiabCare Asia[34] surveys suggest that quality of diabetes care is suboptimal [participants reported low frequency of self-monitoring and poor glycemic control (HbA1c >8%) amongst 42–50% of diabetes patients, only 17.5% were taking aspirin while lipid and BP targets were not met in almost half the subjects surveyed] in a region where dedicated, diligent follow-up of diabetes patients should be a priority, given the amplified risks. Poor clinical practices such as these help explain the remarkable proportion (54%) that reported severe late-stage complications. Focused, context-specific research and careful analyses that integrate medication therapy and preventative lifestyle choices may pave the way for alignment of resources with needs, health systems development, and consequent reductions in morbidity and mortality. The Diabetes Collaborative Registry (DCR) has been designed to track and improve the quality of care of diabetes and metabolic syndrome across the continuum of primary and specialty care. The participation of primary care physicians, endocrinologists, cardiologists, and other healthcare providers managing diabetes is encouraged. The registry is a partnership of the ACC, American Diabetes Association, American College of Physicians, American Association of Clinical Endocrinologists, and Joslin Diabetes Center.[35] The National Diabetes Registry (NDR) was established to keep track of the target achievement and clinical outcomes of patients with diabetes managed at primary healthcare. A similar national registry in India is the need of the hour.

Simply having a chronic disease registry does not guarantee higher quality care. There must be a culture of improvement and quality from within the organization to continually strive to improve diabetes care while tapping on advancing health information technology as an enabler or tool to achieve its mean.

REFERENCES

1. Department of Measurement and Health Information Systems of the Information, Evidence and Research Cluster. Geneva: WHO Press; 2008. pp. 29-31.
2. Kannel WB. Some lessons in cardiovascular epidemiology from Framingham. Am J Cardiol. 1976;37(2):269-82.
3. Yusuf S, Hawken S, Ounpuu S, et al. Effect of potentially modifiable risk factors associated with myocardial infarction in 52 countries (the INTERHEART study): case-control study. Lancet. 2004;364(9438):937-52.
4. Gupta R, Joshi P, Mohan V, et al. Epidemiology and causation of coronary heart disease and stroke in India. Heart. 2008;94(1):16-26.
5. Kannel WB, McGee DL. Diabetes and cardiovascular disease. The Framingham study. JAMA. 1979;241(19):2035-8.
6. Moss SE, Klein R, Klein BE. Cause-specific mortality in a population-based study of diabetes. Am J Public Health. 1991;81(9):1158-62.
7. Geiss LS, Herman WM, Smith PJ. Diabetes in America. In: National Diabetes Data Group (Ed). Mortality in non-insulin-dependent diabetes, 2nd edition. Bethesda, MD: NIH & NIDDK: National Diabetes Information Clearinghouse; 1995. pp. 233-55.
8. Haffner SM, Lehto S, Ronnemaa T, et al. Mortality from coronary heart disease in subjects with type 2 diabetes and in nondiabetic subjects with and without prior myocardial infarction. N Engl J Med. 1998;339(4):229-34.
9. Donahoe SM, Stewart GC, McCabe CH, et al. Diabetes and mortality following acute coronary syndromes. JAMA. 2007;298(7):765-75.
10. Stamler J, Vaccaro O, Neaton JD, et al. Diabetes, other risk factors, and 12-yr cardiovascular mortality for men screened in the Multiple Risk Factor Intervention Trial. Diabetes Care. 1993;16:434-44.
11. Franco OH, Steyerberg EW, Hu FB, et al. Associations of diabetes mellitus with total life expectancy and life expectancy with and without cardiovascular disease. Arch Intern Med. 2007;167(11): 1145-51.
12. Laakso M, Kuusisto J. Epidemiological evidence for the association of hyperglycemia and atherosclerotic vascular disease in non-insulin-dependent diabetes mellitus. Ann Med. 1996;28:415-8.
13. Haffner SM. Epidemiology of insulin resistance and its relation to coronary artery disease. Am J Cardiol. 1999;84:11J-14J.
14. Plutzky J, Viberti G, Haffner S. Atherosclerosis in type 2 diabetes mellitus and insulin resistance: mechanistic links and therapeutic targets. J Diabetes Complications. 2002;16(6):401-15.
15. Haffner SM. Abdominal adiposity and cardiometabolic risk: do we have all the answers? Am J Med. 2007;120(9 Suppl 1):S10-S16.
16. Barnett AH. The importance of treating cardiometabolic risk factors in patients with type 2 diabetes. Diab Vasc Dis Res. 2008;5(1):9-14.
17. Deedwania PC, Fonseca VA. Diabetes, prediabetes, and cardiovascular risk: shifting the paradigm. Am J Med. 2005;118(9):939-47.
18. Mohan V, Sandeep S, Deepa R, et al. Epidemiology of type 2 diabetes: Indian scenario. Indian J Med Res. 2007;125(3):217-30.
19. McKeigue PM, Ferrie JE, Pierpoint T, et al. Association of early-onset coronary heart disease in South Asian men with glucose intolerance and hyperinsulinemia. Circulation. 1993;87(1):152-61.
20. Enas EA, Mehta J. Malignant coronary artery disease in young Asian Indians: thoughts on pathogenesis, prevention, and therapy. Coronary artery disease in Asian Indians (CADI) Study. Clin Cardiol. 1995;18:131-5.
21. Gaziano TA, Reddy KS, Paccaud F, et al. Cardiovascular disease. In: Jamison DT, Breman JG, Measham AR, Alleyne G, Claeson M, Evans DB (Eds). Disease control priorities in developing countries, 2nd edition. New York: Oxford University Press; 2006. pp. 645-62.
22. Radha V, Mohan V. Genetic predisposition to type 2 diabetes among Asian Indians. Indian J Med Res. 2007;125(3):259-74.
23. Chambers JC, Elliott P, Zabaneh D, et al. Common genetic variation near MC4R is associated with waist circumference and insulin resistance. Nat Genet. 2008;40(6):716-8.
24. Gupta M, Brister S. Is South Asian ethnicity an independent cardiovascular risk factor? Can J Cardiol. 2006;22(3):193-7.
25. Yajnik CS. Early life origins of insulin resistance and type 2 diabetes in India and other Asian countries. J Nutr. 2004;134(1):205-10.
26. Ramachandran A. Epidemiology of diabetes in India—three decades of research. J Assoc Physicians India. 2005;53:34-8.
27. Fuller JH, Shipley MJ, Rose G, et al. Mortality from coronary heart disease and stroke in relation to degree of glycaemia: the Whitehall study. Br Med J (Clin Res Ed). 1983;287(6396):867-70.

28. Coutinho M, Gerstein HC, Wang Y, et al. The relationship between glucose and incident cardiovascular events. A metaregression analysis of published data from 20 studies of 95,783 individuals followed for 12.4 years. Diabetes Care. 1999;22:233-40.
29. Selvin E, Marinopoulos S, Berkenblit G, et al. Meta-analysis: glycosylated hemoglobin and cardiovascular disease in diabetes mellitus. Ann Intern Med. 2004;141(6):421-31.
30. The effect of intensive treatment of diabetes on the development and progression of long-term complications in insulin-dependent diabetes mellitus. The Diabetes Control and Complications Trial Research Group. N Engl J Med. 1993;329(14):977-86.
31. Turner R, Cull C, Holman R. United Kingdom prospective diabetes study 17: a 9-year update of a randomized, controlled trial on the effect of improved metabolic control on complications in noninsulin-dependent diabetes mellitus. Ann Intern Med. 1996;124:136-45.
32. Skyler JS, Bergenstal R, Bonow RO, et al. Intensive glycemic control and the prevention of cardiovascular events: implications of the ACCORD, ADVANCE, and VA diabetes trials: a position statement of the American Diabetes Association and a scientific statement of the American College of Cardiology Foundation and the American Heart Association. Diabetes Care. 2009;32(1):187-92.
33. Pokharel Y, Gosch K, Nambi V, et al. Practice-level variation in statin use among patients with diabetes: Insights from the PINNACLE registry. J Am Coll Cardiol. 2016;68:1368-9.
34. Brown JB, Nichols GA, Perry A. The burden of treatment failure in type 2 diabetes. Diabetes Care. 2004;27(7):1535-40.
35. Arnold SV, Inzucchi SE, McGuire DK, et al. Evaluating the quality of comprehensive cardiometabolic care for patients with type 2 diabetes in the U.S.: the diabetes collaborative registry. Diabetes Care. 2016;39:e99-e101.

CHAPTER

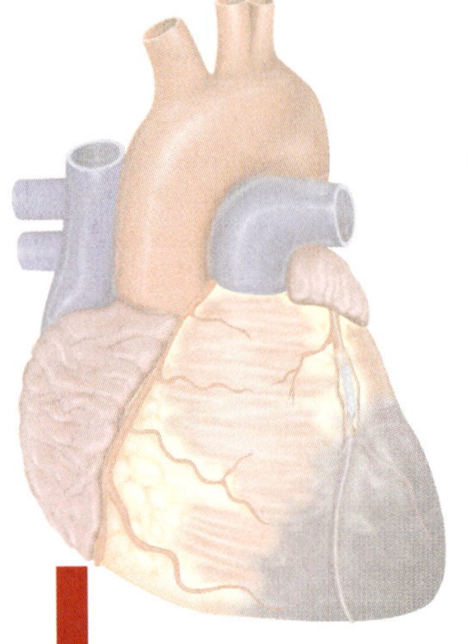

Nonpharmacological Management of Cardiodiabetes

Dharmendra Jain, Geetha Subramanian, Aviraj Chaudhary

INTRODUCTION

Diabetes mellitus is a chronic disease for which self-management is of the utmost importance.[1] Diabetes can be diagnosed on the basis of plasma glucose criteria, either the fasting plasma glucose (FPG) or the 2-h plasma glucose (2-h PG) value after a 75-g oral glucose tolerance test (OGTT) or glycated hemoglobin (HbA1C) criteria (Box 1).[2]

A large body of epidemiological and pathological data suggests that diabetes is an independent risk factor for cardiovascular disease (CVD) in both men and women.[3-5] Women with diabetes seem to lose most of their inherent protection against developing CVD.[3,6] Cardiovascular diseases are listed as the cause of death in around 65% of persons with diabetes.[7] Diabetes acts as an independent risk factor for several forms of CVD. To make matters worse, when patients with diabetes develop clinical CVD, they sustain a worse prognosis for survival than do CVD patients without diabetes.[8-10] These considerations have convinced the Scientific Advisory and Coordinating Committee of the American Heart Association (AHA) that diabetes mellitus deserves to be designated a major risk factor for CVD. This formal designation commits the AHA to a greater emphasis on diabetes as a risk factor in its scientific and educational programs. This statement provides the scientific rationale for the decision to classify diabetes as a major risk factor for CVD.

DIABETES AND SPECIFIC CARDIOVASCULAR DISEASE

Atherosclerotic Coronary Heart Disease

The diabetes is an independent risk factor for cardiovascular heart disease.[3-5] Moreover, in diabetic patients myocardial ischemia due to coronary atherosclerosis commonly occurs without symptoms.[11] As a result, multivessel atherosclerosis often is present before ischemic symptoms occur and before treatment is instituted. A delayed recognition of various forms of coronary heart disease (CHD) worsens the prognosis for survival for many diabetic patients.

Diabetic Cardiomyopathy

One reason for the poor prognosis in patients with both diabetes and ischemic heart disease seems to be an enhanced myocardial dysfunction leading to accelerated heart failure (diabetic cardiomyopathy).[12-19] Thus, patients with diabetes are unusually prone to congestive heart failure. Several factors probably underlie diabetic cardiomyopathy: severe coronary atherosclerosis, prolonged hypertension, chronic hyperglycemia, microvascular disease, glycosylation of myocardial proteins, and autonomic neuropathy. Improved glycemic control, better control of hypertension, and prevention of atherosclerosis with

BOX 1: American diabetes association diagnostic criteria for diabetes mellitus[2]

- Fasting plasma glucose ≥7.0 mmol/L(126 mg/dL) fasting is defined as no calorie intake at least 8 hr
  or
- 2-hour plasma glucose ≥11.1 mmol/L (200 mg/dL) during standardized 75-g oral glucose tolerance test
  or
- Symptoms of hyperglycemia plus nonfasting plasma glucose ≥11.1 mmol/L (200 mg/dL)
  or
- HbA1c ≥6.5% (200 mg/dL)

cholesterol-lowering therapy may prevent or mitigate diabetic cardiomyopathy. An early clinical trial[20] suggested that sulfonylureas used for control of hyperglycemia are cardiotoxic and may exacerbate diabetic cardiomyopathy. This side effect, however, was not confirmed in a recent large clinical trial.[21]

Stroke

Mortality from stroke is almost three times higher in diabetic patients than nondiabetics patients.[22] The most common site of cerebrovascular disease in patients with diabetes is occlusion of small paramedian penetrating arteries.[23] Diabetes also increases the risk of severe carotid atherosclerosis.[24,25] Patients with diabetes, moreover, are likely to suffer irreversible brain damage with carotid emboli that otherwise would produce only transient ischemic attacks in persons without diabetes. Approximately 13% of patients with diabetes greater than 65 years old have had a stroke.[26]

Renal Disease

Chronic renal disease is a common and dreaded complication of diabetes.[27] Approximately 35% of patients with type 1 diabetes of 18 years duration will have signs of diabetic renal involvement.[28] Up to 35% of new patients beginning dialysis therapy have type 2 diabetes.[29] End-stage renal disease (ESRD) appears to be especially common among Hispanics, blacks, and Native Americans with diabetes.[30-34] For patients with diabetes who are on renal dialysis, mortality rates probably exceed 20% per year.[29] When diabetes is present, CVD is the leading cause of death among patients with ESRD.[35-37].

NONPHARMACOLOGICAL MANAGEMENT

This fact is emphasized in the 1998 Clinical Practice Guidelines for the Management of Diabetes in Canada, in which Step 1 of the approach to type 2 diabetes is nonpharmacological therapy consisting of lifestyle modifications such as nutrition therapy, physical activity, avoidance of smoking and diabetic education.[38] If individualized goals for glucose control are not achieved after 2–4 months of such therapy, only then are oral agents and/or insulin usually recommended for most newly-diagnosed patients. For patients with type 2 diabetes, including elderly patients, individualized attention to food portions and weight management, combined with physical activity, may help to improve glycemic control.[39]

Diet, Physical Activity, and Behavioral Therapy[40]

Diet, physical activity, and behavioral therapy designed to achieve greater than 5% weight loss and should be prescribed for overweight and obese patients with type 2 diabetes ready to achieve weight loss. Such interventions should be high intensity (>16 sessions in 6 months) and focus on diet, physical activity, and behavioral strategies to achieve a 500–750 kcal/day energy deficit. Diets should be individualized, as those that provide the same caloric restriction but differ in protein, carbohydrate, and fat content are equally effective in achieving weight loss. For patients who achieve short-term weight loss goals, long-term (>1 year) comprehensive weight maintenance programs should be prescribed. Such programs should provide at least monthly contact and encourage ongoing monitoring of body weight (weekly or more frequently), continued consumption of a reduced calorie diet, and participation in high levels of physical activity (200–300 min/week). To achieve weight loss of greater than 5%, short-term (3-month) interventions that use very low-calorie diets (<800 kcal/day) and total meal replacements may be prescribed for carefully selected patients by trained practitioners in medical care settings with close medical monitoring. To maintain weight loss, such programs must incorporate long-term comprehensive weight maintenance counseling.

Nutrition

For many individuals with diabetes, the most challenging part of the treatment plan is determining what to eat and following a food plan. There is not a one-size-fits-all eating pattern for individuals with diabetes. Nutrition therapy has an integral role in overall diabetes management, and each person with diabetes should be actively engaged in education, self-management, and treatment planning with his or her healthcare team, including the collaborative development of an individualized eating plan.[41,42]

There is a large and ever-growing number of dietary patterns that are marketed to improve weight and cardiovascular health. Unfortunately, however, few of these interventions have been studied rigorously, and most dietary interventions are found to be unsustainable in the long term. In the case of motivated patients, there are some specific dietary patterns with high-quality evidence to recommend them. The simplest intervention is the implementation of a vegetarian or vegan diet. Over 18 months, this has been shown to improve fasting glucose and cholesterol profile, and promote weight loss.[43] In another study, a calorie-restricted vegetarian diet led to a reduction in diabetes medication in 46% of participants (versus 5% with conventional diet).[44] A Mediterranean diet is comprised of large amounts of fruits, vegetables, legumes, nuts, and whole grains. In addition, it includes moderate consumption of olive oil, dairy, fish and poultry, with low consumption of red meat. This dietary pattern has been extensively studied, and in a meta-analysis has been shown to improve glycemic control, blood pressure, and lipid profile.[45] The PREDIMED study evaluated the efficacy of two versions of the Mediterranean diet, one supplemented with olive oil or mixed nuts, for reducing cardiovascular events. This multicenter randomized control trial of 7,447 participants at high cardiovascular risk (48.5% of whom had diabetes) was stopped early due to benefit. Both versions of the diet reduced cardiovascular events by 30% over 5 years of follow-up.[46]

Nutrition, referred to as the "cornerstone of diabetes care", is a complex, controversial and evolving area. Nutritional management of diabetes has the goal of improving or maintaining quality of life, in addition to the physiological health and nutritional status of patients. In general, nutrition recommendations for elderly patients with diabetes follow the principles of Canada's Guidelines for Healthy Eating.[47] These include enjoying a variety of foods from the four food groups, while emphasizing cereals, breads, whole grains, vegetables and fruits. In addition, the choice of lower-fat dairy products, leaner meats and foods prepared without fat are stressed.[47] Achieving and maintaining a healthy body weight and limiting salt, alcohol and caffeine intake are also points of focus. Nutrition therapy seeks to improve glycemic control by balancing a patient's food intake with their endogenous insulin levels.[38] Current recommendations suggest that all patients with diabetes should receive individualized nutrition counseling from a registered dietician who can make specific dietary recommendations according to the patient's preferences, type and severity of disease, medication use, complications, lifestyle, socioeconomic status and degree of obesity.[38,39] In type 2 diabetes, these recommendations are aimed at improving glucose and lipid levels through diet modification and weight loss where appropriate.[38]

Carbohydrates: Sugars and sweeteners carbohydrates from cereals, breads and other grain products, vegetables, fruits, legumes, dairy products as well as any added sugars, should provide 50–60% of the individual's energy requirements.[39,48] Emphasizing carbohydrates with a low glycemic index may be helpful in controlling blood glucose. Glycemic index expresses the rise in blood glucose elicited by a carbohydrate food as a percentage of the rise that would occur if an equal amount of carbohydrate from white bread or glucose was consumed. The website of the Canadian Diabetes Association (www.diabetes.ca) offers a tool that clinicians can use to help educate patients about glycemic index. Examples of foods that have a low glycemic index include 100% stone ground whole wheat bread, oatmeal cereal, yams and legumes such as lentils and chickpeas. Up to 10% of the daily energy requirement can take the form of added sugars, such as table sugar and/or sugar containing products, without impairing diabetes control in most type 2 patients.[39] The moderate use of nutritive (sucrose, fructose, xylitol, mannitol, sorbitol, isomalt, lactitol, maltitol, and aspartame) and non-nutritive sweeteners (sucralose) also can be part of a well-balanced diabetic diet.[39]

Fiber: Traditional Indian diet is rich in fibers. Achieving a total dietary fiber intake of approximately 30 g per day from a variety of sources is recommended. Asoluble fiber intake of 5–10 g per day from oats, barley and legumes can reduce serum cholesterol by up to 10%.[49] The insoluble fiber from cereals may reduce the risk of coronary heart disease by up to 30% for each 10 g increase in intake.[50]

Protein: The recommended protein intake for patients with diabetes is the same as for other healthy adults: 0.86 g/kg per day. Excessive protein intake represents a load on the kidneys and may contribute to diabetic nephropathy. Vegetable protein, low fat milk and milk products should be considered as a favored alternative to animal protein with respect to reducing cholesterol and improving nephropathy.[39]

Fats: The current recommendations for fat intake in patients with diabetes mirrors those for the general population—total fat should be limited to less than or equal to 30% of daily energy requirements. Saturated and polyunsaturated fats each should contribute less than or equal to 10% of daily energy requirements. Monounsaturated fats should be used whenever possible and the use of foods containing saturated or transfatty acids should be avoided. Fish containing omega-3 fatty acids may reduce serum cholesterol and should be consumed at least once per week.[39]

Alcohol: Alcohol intake is best avoided and if used must be in moderation. Moderate use of alcohol (less than or equal to 5% of total daily energy intake or up to two standard drinks per day) can be part of the diet of diabetics with well controlled blood glucose, lipids and blood pressure.[39]

Micronutrients: The daily vitamin and mineral requirements for patients with diabetes should be obtained from a well-balanced diet, as there is no conclusive evidence recommending the routine use of vitamin or mineral supplements.[39]

Physical Activity

There are numerous benefits of physical activity in patients with diabetes, and these extend to the elderly. The benefits include increased insulin sensitivity, improved glycemic control, weight loss or maintenance, lower blood pressure, improved cardiovascular fitness, improved lipid profile and an increased sense of well-being.[38] These benefits may even result in a decreased need for medications. In general, a stepwise increase in physical activity that becomes an extension of the person's lifestyle should be part of the treatment plan for every patient with type 2 diabetes who is able to increase activity. Individualized modifications need to be made for patients with occlusive vascular disease (or even a high risk of subclinical disease), significant sensory neuropathy or microvascular complications. Before an exercise program is initiated, each patient with diabetes should undergo a detailed medical evaluation with appropriate diagnostic studies. Special consideration is given to screening for macro- and microvascular complications that may be exacerbated by exercise. The history and physical examination should focus on the heart and blood vessels, eyes, kidneys, and nervous system.[51] A graded exercise stress test should be considered if the patient is about to start a moderate to high-intensity exercise program, and is at high-risk for CVD based on having one of the criteria presented in Box 2. If nonspecific electrocardiogram (ECG) changes occur in response to exercise or if there are nonspecific ST and T wave changes on the resting ECG, alternative tests such as radionuclide stress testing may be necessary.[51]

Canada's Physical Activity Guide to Healthy Active Living provides exercise recommendations for patients with uncomplicated diabetes and no other related medical conditions.[48,52] The 1998 clinical practice guidelines for the management of diabetes in Canada also provide excellent general advice for physical activity in patients with diabetes, including the use of proper footwear and daily foot assessment, avoiding exercise when metabolic control is poor, ingesting a rapidly absorbed carbohydrate if pre-exercise blood glucose is less than 5 mmol/L, and avoiding exercise in extreme weather conditions.[38] The American Diabetes Association provides some recommendations for exercise prescription in the face of diabetic complications. For instance, patients with known coronary artery disease should undergo a supervised evaluation of ischemic response to exercise, ischemic threshold and the propensity to arrhythmia during exercise.[38] The basic treatment for peripheral arterial disease is smoking cessation and a supervised exercise program. For patients with active, proliferative diabetic retinopathy, strenuous activity may cause vitreous hemorrhage or retinal detachment. As a result, such patients should avoid anaerobic exercise and exercise with straining, jarring or valsalva maneuvers.[44] Strenuous exercise also should likely be curtailed in patients with overt nephropathy. Peripheral neuropathy may result in loss of sensation to the feet, and is an indication to limit weight-bearing exercise.[51]

BOX 2: Criteria indicting patients with diabetes are at high risk of cardiovascular disease[51]

1. Age > 35
2. Type 2 diabetes for >10 years duration
3. Presence of any additional risk factor for coronary artery disease
4. Presence of microvascular disease (proliferative retinopathy or nephropathy, including vascular disease)
5. Peripheral vascular disease
6. Autonomic neuropathy

CONCLUSION

Diabetes mellitus type 2 is a common and important chronic disease affecting the cardiovascular system. The nonpharmacological measures such as nutrition, counseling, and physical activity play an important role in improving disease control and limiting disease-related complications. Specific recommendations regarding these lifestyle measures for the elderly are similar to those made for adults in general.

REFERENCES

1. Wheeler ML. Nutrition management and physical activity as treatments for diabetes. Prim Care. 1999;26:857-68.
2. American Diabetes Association. Diagnosis and classification of diabetes mellitus. Diabetes Care. 2014;37(Suppl 1):S81-S90.
3. Wilson PW, D'Agostino RB, Levy D, et al. Prediction of coronary heart disease using risk factor categories. Circulation. 1998;97(18):1837-47.
4. Wilson PW. Diabetes mellitus and coronary heart disease. Am J Kidney Dis. 1998;32(5 Suppl 3):S89-S100.
5. McGill HC Jr, McMahan CA. Determinants of atherosclerosis in the young: Pathobiological Determinants of Atherosclerosis in Youth (PDAY) research group. Am J Cardiol. 1998;82(10B):30T-36T.
6. Brezinka V, Padmos I. Coronary heart disease risk factors in women. Eur Heart J. 1994;15(11):1571-84.
7. Geiss LS, Herman WH, Smith PJ. National Diabetes Data Group. Diabetes in America. Bethesda, MD: National Institutes of Health, National Institute of Diabetes and Digestive and Kidney Diseases; 1995. pp. 233-57.
8. Stone PH, Muller JE, Hartwell T, et al. The MILIS Study Group. The effect of diabetes mellitus on prognosis and serial left ventricular function after acute myocardial infarction: contribution of both coronary disease and diastolic left ventricular dysfunction to the adverse prognosis. J Am Coll Cardiol. 1989;14(1):49-57.
9. Singer DE, Moulton AW, Nathan DM. Diabetic myocardial infarction: interaction of diabetes with other preinfarction risk factors. Diabetes. 1989;38:350-57.

10. Smith JW, Marcus FI, Serokman R. Prognosis of patients with diabetes mellitus after acute myocardial infarction. Am J Cardiol. 1984;54:718-21.
11. Wingard DL, Barrett-Connor EL, Scheidt-Nave C, et al. Prevalence of cardiovascular and renal complications in older adults with normal or impaired glucose tolerance or NIDDM: a population-based study. Diabetes Care. 1993;16:1022-5.
12. Rubler S, Dlugash J, Yuceoglu YZ, et al. New type of cardiomyopathy associated with diabetic glomerulosclerosis. Am J Cardiol. 1972;30(6):595-602.
13. Regan TJ, Lyons MM, Ahmed SS, et al. Evidence of cardiomyopathy in familial diabetes mellitus. J Clin Invest.1977;60(4):884-99.
14. Regan TJ. Congestive heart failure in the diabetic. Annu Rev Med. 1983;34:161-8.
15. Ettinger PO, Regan TJ. Cardiac disease in diabetes.Postgrad Med.1989;85(6):229-32.
16. van Hoeven KH, Factor SM. A comparison of the pathological spectrum of hypertensive, diabetic, and hypertensive-diabetic heart disease. Circulation. 1990;82:848-55.
17. Gotzsche O, Darwish A, Gotzsche L, et al. Incipient cardiomyopathy in young insulin-dependent diabetic patients: a seven-year prospective Doppler echocardiographic study. Diabet Med. 1996;13:834-40.
18. Spector KS. Diabetic cardiomyopathy. Clin Cardiol. 1998;21(12):885-7.
19. Mahgoub MA, Abd-Elfattah AS. Diabetes mellitus and cardiac function. Mol Cell Biochem. 1998;180(1-2):59-64.
20. Klimt CR, Knatterud GI, Meinert CL, et al. University Group Diabetes Program. A study of the effects of hypoglycemic agents on vascular complications in patients with adult-onset diabetes, II: mortality results. Diabetes. 1970;19(Suppl):789-830.
21. UK Prospective Diabetes Study (UKPDS) Group. Intensive blood-glucose control with sulphonylureas or insulin compared with conventional treatment and risk of complications in patients with type 2 diabetes (UKPDS 33). Lancet. 1998;352(9131):837-53.
22. Stamler J, Vaccaro O, Neaton JD, et al. Diabetes, other risk factors, and 12-year cardiovascular mortality for men screened in the Multiple Risk Factor Intervention Trial (MRFIT). Diabetes Care. 1993;16:434-44.
23. Bell DSH. Stroke in the diabetic patient. Diabetes Care. 1994;17:213-9.
24. Folsom AR, Eckfeldt JH, Weitzman S, et al. Atherosclerosis risk in communities study investigators. Relation of carotid artery wall thickness in diabetes mellitus, fasting glucose and insulin, body size, and physical activity. Stroke. 1994;25:66-73.
25. O'Leary DH, Polak JF, Kronmal RA, et al. Distribution and correlates of sonographically detected carotid artery disease in the cardiovascular health study. Stroke. 1992;23(12):1752-60.
26. Kuller LH. National diabetes data group. Stroke and diabetes. Diabetes in America. Bethesda, MD: National Institutes of Health, National Institute of Diabetes and Digestive and Kidney Diseases; 1995. pp. 449-56.
27. Nelson RG, Knowler WC, Pettitt JD, et al, National Diabetes Data Group. Kidney diseases in diabetes. Diabetes in America. Bethesda, MD: National Institutes of Health, National Institute of Diabetes and Digestive and Kidney Diseases; 1995. pp. 349-400.
28. Mogensen CE, Christensen CK, Vittinghus E. The stages of diabetic renal disease: with emphasis on the stage of incipient diabetic nephropathy.Diabetes.1983;32(Suppl 2):64-78.
29. US Renal Data System. USRDS 1994 Annual data report. In: Bethesda, MD; National Institutes of Health, National Institute of Diabetes and Digestive and Kidney Diseases; 1994.
30. Cowie CC, Port FK, Wolfe RA, et al. Disparities in incidence of diabetic end-stage renal disease according to race and types of diabetes. N Engl J Med. 1989;321(16):1074-9.
31. Rostand SG, Kirk KA, Rutsky EA, et al. Racial differences in the incidence of treatment for end-stage renal disease. N Engl J Med. 1982;306(21):1276-9.
32. Stephens GW, Gillaspy JA, Clyne D, et al. Racial differences in the incidence of end-stage renal disease in types I and II diabetes mellitus. Am J Kidney Dis. 1990;15(6):562-7.
33. Lopes AA, Port FK, James SA, et al. The excess risk of treated end-stage renal disease in blacks in the United States. J Am Soc Nephrol. 1993;3(12):1961-71.
34. Nelson RG, Pettitt DJ, Carraher MJ, et al. Effect of proteinuria on mortality in NIDDM. Diabetes .1988;37(11):1499-504.
35. McMillan MA, Briggs JD, Junor BJ. Outcome of renal replacement treatment in patients with diabetes mellitus. BMJ. 1990;301(6751):540-4.
36. Hirschl MM, Heinz G, Sunder-Plassmann G, et al. Renal replacement therapy in type 2 diabetic patients: 10 years' experience. Am J Kidney Dis. 1992;20:564-8.
37. Rischen-Vos J, van der Woude FJ, Tegzess AM, et al. Increased morbidity and mortality in patients with diabetes mellitus after kidney transplantation as compared with non-diabetic patients. Nephrol Dial Transplant. 1992;7:433-7.
38. Meltzer S, Leiter L, Daneman D, et al. 1998 clinical practice guidelines for the management of diabetes in Canada. CMAJ. 1998;159(8 Suppl):S1-29.
39. Wolever T, Barbeau MC, Charron S, et al. Guidelines for the nutritional management of diabetes mellitus in the new millennium: a position statement by the Canadian Diabetes Association. Can J Dia Care. 1999;23:56-69.
40. American Diabetes Association. Obesity management for the treatment of type 2 diabetes (Section 7). Standards of Medical Care in Diabetes 2017. Diabetes Care 2017;40(Suppl 1):S57-S63.
41. Inzucchi SE, Bergenstal RM, Buse JB, et al. Management of hyperglycemia in type 2 diabetes, 2015: a patient-centered approach: update to a position statement of the American Diabetes Association and the European Association for the Study of Diabetes. Diabetes Care. 2015;38(1):140-9.
42. Evert AB, Boucher JL, Cypress M, et al. Nutrition therapy recommendations for the management of adults with diabetes. Diabetes Care. 2014;37(Suppl 1):S120-S143.
43. Barnard ND, Cohen J, Jenkins DJ, et al. A low-fat vegan diet and a conventional diabetes diet in the treatment of type 2 diabetes: a randomized, controlled, 74-wk clinical trial. Am J Clin Nutr. 2009;89:1588-96.
44. Kahleova H, Matoulek M, Malinska H, et al. Vegetarian diet improves insulin resistance and oxidative stress markers more than conventional diet in subjects with type 2 diabetes. Diabet Med. 2011;28(5):549-59.
45. Esposito K, Maiorino MI, Ceriello A, et al. Prevention and control of type 2 diabetes by Mediterranean diet: a systematic review. Diabetes Res Clin Pract. 2010;89(2):97-102.
46. Estruch R, Ros E, Salas-Salvado J, et al. Primary prevention of cardiovascular disease with a Mediterranean diet. N Engl J Med. 2013;368(14):1279-90.
47. Health and Welfare Canada. Action towards healthy eating Canada's guidelines for healthy eating and recommended strategies for implementation. The report of the communications/ implementation committee. Ottawa: Minister of Supply and services Canada; 1990.
48. Health and Welfare Canada. Nutrition recommendations. The report of the scientific review committee. Ottawa: Canadian Government Publications Centre; 1990 (Cat no H49-42/ 1990E).
49. Jenkins DJA, Wolever TM, Rao AV, et al. Effect on serum lipids of very high fiber intakes in diets low in saturated fats and cholesterol. N Engl J Med. 1993;329(1):21-6.
50. Rimm EB, Ascherio A, Giovannucci E, et al. Vegetable, fruit, and cereal fiber intake and risk of coronary heart disease among men. JAMA. 1996;275(6):447-51.
51. American Diabetes Association. Position statement: diabetes mellitus and exercise. Diabetes Care. 2002;25(1 Suppl): S64-S68.
52. Health Canada. Canada's physical activity guide to healthy active living. [online] Available from http://www.hc-sc.gc.ca/hppb/paguide/. [Accessed August, 2017].

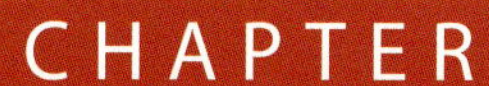

Maternal Diabetes Mellitus and Fetal Cardiac Malformations: Antenatal and Postnatal Management and Outcome

Smita Mishra, Neha Gupta

INTRODUCTION

Diabetes mellitus (DM) complicates 3–10% of pregnancies. These pregnancies are at increased risk of fetal malformations (FMs), especially neural tube and cardiac abnormalities, abortions, stillbirths, and early neonatal complications.[1-4] There is nearly a fivefold (8.5) increase in congenital heart diseases (CHD) in pregnancies complicated by diabetes from the general population.[1] Up to 80% of them may be diagnosed to have hyperglycemia in the latter half of the pregnancy (gestational DM), when organogenesis is already over. Rest of them (20%) have preexisting DM either of type 1 (35%) or type 2 (65%). According to one estimate, 2.7% of all live births are complicated by maternal hyperglycemia.[1-7] Nowadays active surveillance is recommended due to its potential for causing perinatal morbidity and mortality. The pregnancies that are complicated by gestational DM are at increased risk of later developing type 2 DM. In an infant of diabetic mother (IDM)—it may be difficult to identify underlying cardiac problem unless the echocardiography has been done proactively as it may have multiple underlying issues. This review article analyzes the evidence obtained from the literature about the effects of antenatal hyperglycemia in relation to fetal cardiac malformations (CMs), preventive strategies and issues related to the early management of newborn.[1-3]

INCIDENCE

The risk of CMs is about 2.5–12% in women with pregestational diabetes or gestational diabetes.[1-5] Ventricular septal defect (VSD) is the most common congenital cardiac defect seen in the diabetic pregnant population followed by conotruncal defects, more commonly D-transposition of great vessels.[1-4,8,9] Women with gestational diabetes have malformation rates no different from the general nondiabetic obstetric population. The most important cardiac effect seen beyond the age of organogenesis is hypertrophic cardiomyopathy (HCM), with an estimated incidence of 10–12% of IDM who underwent selective echocardiography. However, if echocardiography done routinely, HCM may be found in 30–40% cases.[2-4,8]

In one large study-cohort, 142,509 nondiabetic pregnant women had 2,075 (1.5%) FM; out of which, 206 were CM (0.1%).[3] While those with pregestational diabetes had 25 FM/5CM out of 410 (6.1% FM, 1.2% CM), gestational diabetes (normal fasting sugar) had 24 FM/2CM out of 2,047 (1.2% FM, 0.1% CM), gestational diabetes (elevated fasting sugar) had 11 FM/1 CM out of 230 (4.8% FM, 0.4% CM) pregnant women.[2]

PATHOGENESIS

It is well documented that initially the blood sugar level is low in normal pregnancy but subsequently, with the linear rise in placental steroid and peptide hormones (e.g. estrogen, progesterone, and chorionic somatomammotropin) in second and third trimester, there is increased tissue resistance to insulin.[8,9] Resultant hyperglycemia needs compensatory escalation in the insulin secretion up to 50% higher than the prepregnancy levels.

Maternal inadequate pancreatic response to hyperglycemia reflects as the fetal hyperinsulinemia, a normal response to the fetal hyperglycemic state. Insulin helps in lipogenesis from the excess glucose in fetal blood and hence causes accelerated growth. The typical postprandial hyperglycemic episodes in the mother act as a significant source of the accelerated growth exhibited by the fetus. Many studies have found that high level of glycated hemoglobin (HbA1c) is a red-flag sign. Lisowski et al. (2010) published a meta-analysis—in a study of three different populations of diabetic pregnancies, a rise in HbA1c value to mean 6.4% escalated the risk of CHD from 2.5% to 6.1%.[4] However, fetal hyperglycemia is considered as the primary teratogen for alteration in cardiac development, though its mechanism of action is not fully understood and hence, is a matter of speculation and research. Three major factors resulting from the fetal hyperglycemia are: (1) Modulating insulin levels; (2) altered fat levels; (3) increased reactive oxygen species. Ornoy et al. found, in the rat models, that severe hyperglycemia also can cause hypoxia as was shown by increased level of HIF1α.[9] Both may then lead to oxidative stress as evident by increased lipid peroxidation and increased level of nitrotyrosine as well as low-molecular-weight antioxidants.[9] In the embryo and fetus, antioxidant defense mechanism is immature and hence exposure to any oxidative stress during a vulnerable period leads to the embryotoxicity.[9]

EFFECT OF MATERNAL HYPERGLYCEMIA ON CARDIOVASCULAR SYSTEM

Congenital Heart Disease

Congenital heart disease is defined as a malformation of heart and intrathoracic vessels that is actually or potentially of functional importance, has its onset before the birth, affects 5–15 per 1,000 live births, in general population.[10] Moreover, it has emerged as the major cause of neonatal morbidity and mortality. It is multifactorial etiologically and fetal targeted screening between 18 weeks and 20 weeks in those pregnant women who have *identifiable maternal factors* and termination of pregnancy for severe CM, is the only preventive method.[5] As discussed earlier, fetal hyperglycemia secondary to the maternal hyperglycemia, is *teratogenic* and if happens during the period of organogenesis, predisposes for various kind of CMs. Wren et al. compared cardiovascular malformations reported in six series (Pederson et al.1964, Rowland et al. 1973, Mills et al. 1988, Ferencz et al. 1990, Becerra et al. 1990, and Wren et al. 2003).[6] Total number of CHDs detected in six series was 125. The most common cardiac defects were—VSD (28%) followed by D-transposition of great vessels (14.4%), and coarctation of aorta (8.8%). Tabib et al. in a case-control study [170 pregnant women with DM (case) and 85 nondiabetic pregnant women (control)] classified diabetic pregnant women in two groups: (1) pre-GDM Group (68, 40%), (2) gestational DM (102, 60%). Fetal echocardiography was performed at the mean gestational age (GA) of 24.7 ± 5.4 (range: 17–38 weeks) in DM group and 20.27 ± 3.9 (16–33 weeks) in nondiabetic (control) group. The cardiac disease was detected in 1 (1.17%) fetus in nondiabetic group and 15 (8.8%) fetuses of DM group. The screening recognized two cases of VSD.[7] Besides VSD, study reported: tetralogy of Fallot (ToF) (1), truncus arteriosus (1), dextrocardia (1), severe mitral and aortic stenosis (1), pulmonary atresia severe tricuspid regurgitation (1), transposition of the great arteries (TGA-1); double outlet right ventricle (1). HCM was detected in 6 (3.5%) fetus of DM group.[5]

Diabetic Mellitus as the Maternal Risk Factor for CHD

In a statement from the American Heart Association, DM has been included as the maternal risk factor for group of CHDs.[11] Liu et al. selected five groups of CHDs (heterotaxy, conotruncal malformation, atrioventricular septal defect and left ventricular outflow obstruction) and looked into the contributory maternal factors.[5] They found preexisting maternal DM (types 1 and 2) to be a notable risk factor for CHD in general and for almost every selected group of CHD (Fig. 1).

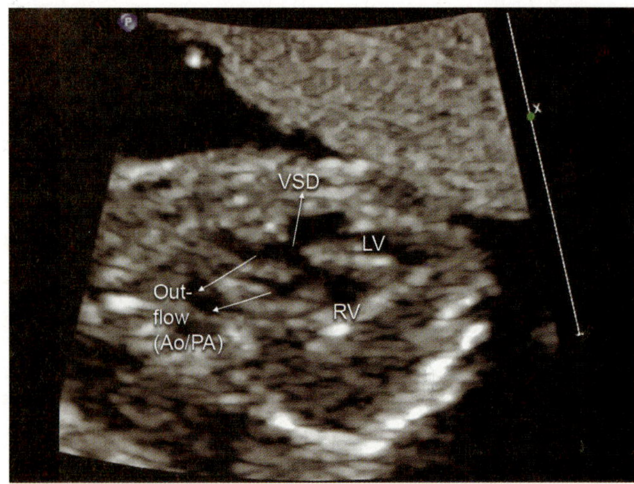

Fig. 1: Ultrasound showing the 18 weeks of gestational age (HbA1c = 11%, DORV, VSD, and PS)

Abbreviations: DORV, double outlet right ventricle; VSD, ventricular septal defect; PS, pulmonic stenosis

Hypertrophic Cardiomyopathy[12-16]

Cardiac hypertrophy of IDM is due to the anabolic effect of fetal hyperinsulinism causing hyperplasia and hypertrophy of myocardium (Fig. 2). In a recent study published in 2015, right ventricular/left ventricular (RV/LV) wall thickness and interventricular septum (IVS) thickness values were increased in 69% of the fetuses of mothers with GDMs.[12] Moreover, 10–15% of theses newborns may become symptomatic. Microscopically, like in HCM, there is also a disarray of the myofibrils. The dominance of IVS hypertrophy is common and has been speculated to be, because of abundance of insulin receptors in the IVS. Fetal insulin levels during exposure to maternal diabetes are often elevated due to the fetal beta-cell response to hyperglycemia. For this reason, it has been difficult to determine whether it is fetal hyperglycemia or fetal hyperinsulinemia, or both, that drive cardiac overgrowth in response to maternal diabetes. Tight control of HbA1c has been proposed as the preventive measure for cardiac hypertrophy, though evidence exists in literature, to suggest that HCM may present despite good control of HbA1c. The fetal hypertrophic response to hyperglycemia can be of two types:

1. Isolated asymmetrical septal hypertrophy.
2. Left ventricular hypertrophy mimicking HCM with increased LV mass, left ventricular outflow tract (LVOT) obstruction, systolic anterior motion of anterior mitral leaflet, and mitral regurgitation.

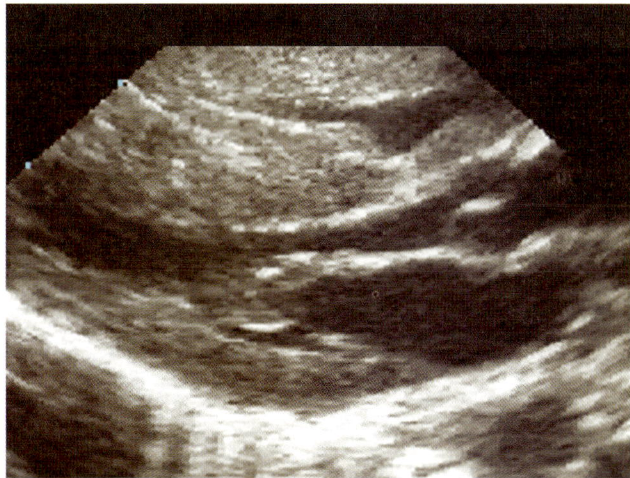

Fig. 2: Gestational diabetes (HbA1c = 10%)

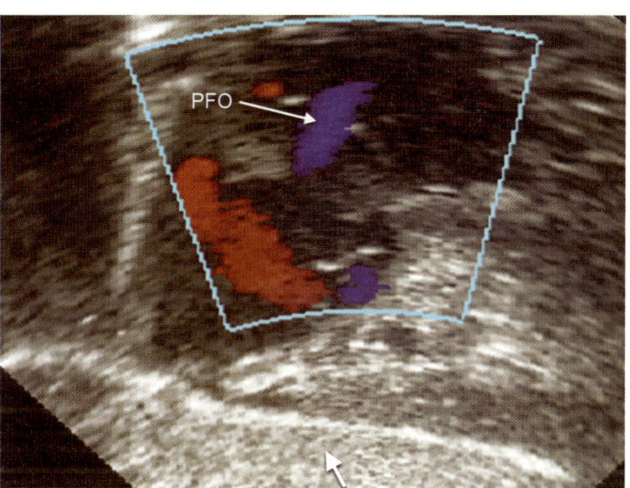

Fig. 3: Newborn with hypertrophic cardiomyopathy (HCM). Patent foramen ovale (PFO) shunting right to left shunt (subcostal coronal view) in a neonate with HCM born to a mother with gestational diabetes

Abbreviation: PFC, persistent fetal circulation

Isolated Right Ventricular Hypertrophy with or without Right to Left Shunting at Atrial Level[17]

Transient isolated RV hypertrophy has been reported in the literature. Hayrullah et al. compared the 27 reported cases with transient isolated RVH in recent English literature. Maternal diabetes was found in only in one case, suggesting that maternal hyperglycemia do not have strong correlation in this subgroup.

Persistent Fetal Circulation[18,19]

Persistent fetal circulation (PFC) has not been correlated directly to the maternal hyperglycemia. But PFC is not uncommon in IDM, probably secondary to the polycythemia, increased viscosity and secondary pulmonary hypertension. Clinically, PFC can be suspected, if difference of PaO_2 between radial artery and descending aorta blood, is greater than 15 mm Hg (Fig. 3).

Functional Fetal Cardiac Evaluation in Pregnancy with DM

Walther et al. reported diminished cardiac output (per kilogram) linearly in infants of mothers with DM, with increasing septal thickness which can be attributed to decrease in stroke volume at comparable heart rate. IDMs had higher LA/Ao ratio, greater RV systolic time interval than the control group.[20] Costa et al. reported relatively higher fetal heart rate in IDM.[21]

Chen et al. compared echocardiographic parameters of fetal cardiac anatomy and function like wall thickness, mitral, tricuspid, aortic and pulmonary valve Doppler velocities, Tei index, ventricular ejection fraction and fractional shortening between 40 GDM [DM with poorly controlled blood sugar (BS) vs. DM with good control of BS] and 70 nondiabetic pregnant women.[22] They succeeded to record all the parameters at different GA (<28, 28–34, >34 weeks of GA) for both the groups. They reported high LV/

RV Tei index, increased LV/RV free wall and IVS thickness, reduced diastolic function but comparable ventricular ejection fraction and fractional shortening, and relatively higher aortic velocities. In our own institutional experience of 2 years, we detected 14 cases of fetal CHD. In one case, who got referred to us in 17th gestational week of pregnancy, had high HbA1c level (11%), she was referred for fetal echo due to abnormal triple vessel view seen on the anomaly scan. On fetal echo, she had double outlet right ventricle with subpulmonary VSD (transposition physiology). Family opted for termination. Another case of double inlet left ventricle, aorta from RV and pulmonary atresia presented to us as the duct-dependent cyanotic neonate. Historically, mother had HbA1c of 9% in first month after detection of pregnancy. She was put on metformin but was never recommended a fetal anomaly scan.

MANAGEMENT

Prevention of Congenital Heart Disease

The milder gestational diabetes (Class A1, normal fasting glucose) is not an incremental risk factor for the FMs. A meticulous plan is essential to keep blood sugar under control with or without pharmacotherapy or insulin, to keep HbA1c levels below 6.5% during the pregnancy. Preconception screening for DM in high-risk pregnancies, and proactive diabetic management may be able to prevent some of these anomalies. High HbA1c levels in first trimester must be treated as the teratogenic factor and fetal anomaly scan must be recommended to rule out any FMs. Now, there is paradigm shift in approach towards the prenatal care and adoption of inverted pyramid[23] model is recommended in which more antenatal visits are planned in first trimester, rather than in the third trimester. First trimester assessment of various fetomaternal parameters allows early diagnosis of fetal complications. If recognized early, medical termination of pregnancy may be recommended. In India, medical termination of pregnancy (MTP) cannot be done beyond the GA of 20th weeks.[24,25]

Care of Newborn

In utero transfer[26]*:* For the fetal critical CM or duct-dependent CHDs, delivery can be planned in a tertiary care multispecialty hospital or near a tertiary care center to accomplish an early transfer of baby to a desired center having facility for cardiac intervention. D-transposition of great vessels is most common critical CHD associated with DM which may be life-threatening, if intervention is delayed. However, a timely arterial switch operation gives the opportunity to a baby to have almost completely normal life.

Postnatal care of an IDM: All of these babies may need intensive care to begin with! Screening for critical CHDs is mandatory. A thorough clinical examination, which includes palpation of pulses including femorals, blood pressure measurement of all four limbs, X-ray chest, electrocardiogram, SpO_2 in right upper and lower limbs and hyperoxia test (10 minutes 100% oxygen then assessment of PO_2), is recommended. These babies may need oxygen, noninvasive or invasive ventilation, intravenous fluid, inotrope and routine care like vitamin K injection. Echocardiography, if available, is the gold standard for the diagnosis.

Role of prostaglandin infusion: In cases, where cyanotic CHD is suspected and SPO_2 is below 90%, a prostaglandin infusion must be kept ready before planning the transport. Whenever prostaglandin infusion is planned, one must be ready to provide invasive or noninvasive ventilation to manage the impending apnea. There may be a need for inotropic support to manage the systemic hypotension.

Management of hypoglycemia: The IDMs are prone to hyperinsulinemic hypoglycemia[27] and need to be kept under observation to avoid low blood sugar and consequent irreversible neuronal damage, as the glucose is the main energy source of brain cells. Therefore, prompt recognition and treatment of these infants with hypoglycemia is paramount for a long-term good prognosis.

Transport: Exact echo-diagnosis is ideal before the transfer of a baby to a tertiary care center, usually situated far away. A long distance transfer by road or train may cause significant morbidity and mortality. Air ambulances are costly and may not be within reach of common public. It is the cost-effective effort to differentiate critical from noncritical CHD and normal heart. In absence of echo-diagnosis, a thorough screening as mentioned earlier, must be done and clinical findings as well reports of the bedside investigations, can be exchanged with a pediatric cardiologist on mobile phone or E-mail. Mostly, the pulse oximeter or hyperoxia test is of great help. However, they may be misleading in cases of PFC. Usually, there is difference of 15 mm Hg of PO_2 in right upper limb and lower limb in PFC.

Routinely, complete blood counts, platelet count, sepsis screen, blood sugar, liver and kidney function tests, and arterial/venous gas analysis (ABG/VBG) must be done before the transport to rule out acidosis, electrolyte imbalance, high lactate levels, and abnormal PCO_2/PO_2 levels. A baby must be assessed for central and peripheral temperature difference. Maintenance fluid and oxygen source, sedation, must be adequately planned. A trained person, ideally a doctor, who can perform intubation and put intravenous lines must accompany the baby. Baby must be stabilized and adequately ventilated, supported with inotropes before starting the journey.

TABLE 1: Pregnancy with hyperglycemia–glycemic targets: American Diabetes Association-2016 Guidelines about diabetes in pregnancy

Glycemic targets for gestational diabetes mellitus	
Fasting	≤95 mg/dL (5.3 mmol/L)
1st hour postprandial	≤140 mg/dL(7.8 mmol/L)
2nd hour postprandial	≤120 mg/dL (6.7 mmol/L)
HBA1C: 6.0–6.5% (42–48 mmol/L) recommended <6.0% may be optimal (avoid hypoglycemia)	
Glycemic targets for pregestational diabetes mellitus	
Fasting	≤90 mg/dL (5.0 mmol/L)
1st hour postprandial	≤130–140 mg/dL (7.2–7.8 mmol/L)
2nd hour postprandial	≤120 mg/dL (6.7 mmol/L)
HBA1c: 6.0–6.5% (42–48 mmol/L) recommended <6.0% may be optimal (avoid hypoglycemia)	

Source: National Diabetes Education Initiative. (2016). American Diabetes Association (ADA) 2016 Guidelines: Diabetes Management Guidelines. [online] http://www.ndei.org/ADA-diabetes-management-guidelines-diabetes-in-pregnancy-GDM.aspx.html. [Accessed August, 2017]

It may be a challenge to maintain the blood sugar of an IDM during the transfer and hence glucometer and concentrated dextrose must be there in resuscitation trolley.

Family must be explained about financial requirement before reaching to the tertiary care center. There may be more than one congenital malformations, hence it is obligatory to assess all of them and discuss with family about the individual outcome for different malformations, need for multiple intervention by a team of specialists, underlying genetic abnormalities and financial implications of this complex situation. Sometimes, nongovernment organizations may come forward for financial assistance but they may need related documents like residential proof and income certificate. Henceforth, family must be advised to carry essential documents.

We must know that central government provides financial assistance to children suffering from CHD through Rashtriya Bal Swasthya Karyakram (RBSK) and Chief Medical Officer of every city is empowered to provide approval letter for the intervention for those centers which are empaneled with different states.

Detailed recommendations have been published by the American Heart Association scientific statements and all caregiver must go through it (Table 1).

CONCLUSION

Congenital heart diseases are common cause of neonatal mortality and morbidity and its primary prevention may be possible by identifying the predisposing genetic, maternal and environmental factors. Uncontrolled DM is now well-documented teratogenic factor for spectrum of FMs in general and CHD in particular. Conotruncal anomalies like D-TGA, truncus arteriosus, TOF, DORV, are most common critical CHDs associated with maternal hyperglycemia happening during the period of organogenesis, usually in women having preconception diagnosed or undiagnosed type 1 or type 2 DM. One of the red-flag signs is maternal HbA1c level. A rise in HbA1c value to mean 6.4% escalated the risk of CHD from 2.5% to 6.1%. Therefore, preconception screening and control of blood sugar with the diet or pharmacotherapy, is very important preventive strategy of FMs. Second most important step is to identify group of women having hyperglycemia in first trimester and put them through anomaly scan and fetal echocardiography within 20 weeks of gestation. Also, a keen watch is needed to avoid late hyperglycemia or gestational diabetes, to avoid fetal macrosomia and HCM. The IDMs need intensive care and blood sugar monitoring just after the birth. Those who fail to maintain SPO_2, need screening to rule out critical CHD. They may need prostaglandin infusion and transport to tertiary cardiac care facility. Overall, fetal outcome for a pregnancy with DM depends on the strict control of maternal blood sugar, fetal monitoring, and care of newborn.

REFERENCES

1. Becerra JE, Khoury MJ, Cordero JF, et al. Diabetes mellitus during pregnancy and the risks for specific birth defects: a population-based case-control study. Pediatrics.1990;85(1):1-9.
2. Sheffield JS, Butler-Koster EL, Casey BM, et al. Maternal diabetes mellitus and infant malformations. Obstet Gynecol. 2002;100(5Pt 1):925-30.
3. Arroyo R, Rodriguez-Pinilla E, Cordero JF. Maternal diabetes: the risk for specific birth defects. Eur J Epidemiol. 1992;8(4):503-8.
4. Lisowski LA, Verheijen PM, Copel JA, et al. Congenital heart disease in pregnancies complicated by maternal diabetes mellitus. Herz. 2010;35(1):19-26.
5. Liu S, Joseph KS, Lisonkova S, et al. Association between maternal chronic conditions and congenital heart defects:a population-based cohort study. Circulation. 2013;128(6):583-9.
6. Wren C, Birrell G, Hawthorne G. Cardiovascular malformations in infants of diabetic mothers. Heart. 2003;89(10):1217-20.
7. Tabib A, Shirzad N, Sheikhbahaei S, et al. Cardiac malformations in fetuses of gestational and pregestational diabetic mothers. Iran J Pediatr. 2013;23(6):664-8.
8. Costrini NV, Kalkhoff RK. Relative effects of pregnancy, estradiol, and progesterone on plasma insulin and pancreatic islet insulin secretion. J Clin Invest. 1971;50(5):992-9.
9. Ornoy A, Rand SB, Bischitz N. Hyperglycemia and hypoxia are interrelated in their teratogenic mechanism: studies on cultured rat embryos. Birth defects Res B. 2010;89(2):106-15
10. Hoffman JI, Kaplan S. The incidence of congenital heart disease. J Am Coll Cardiol. 2002;39(12):1890-900.
11. Donofrio MT, Moon-Grady AJ, Hornberger LK, et al. Diagnosis and treatment of fetal cardiac disease:a scientific statement from the American Heart Association. Circulation. 2014;129(21):2183-242.

12. Han SS, Wang G, Jin Y, et al. Investigating the mechanism of hyperglycemia-induced fetal cardiac hypertrophy. PLoS One. 2015;10(09):e0139141.
13. Palmieri C, Simões MA, Silva JC, et al. Prevalence of hypertrophic cardiomyopathy in fetuses of mothers with gestational diabetes before initiating treatment. Rev Bras Ginecol Obstet. 2017;39(1):9-13.
14. Oberhoffer R, Högel J, Stoz F, et al. Cardiac and extracardiac complications in infants of diabetic mothers and their relation to parameters of carbohydrate metabolism. Eur J Pediatr.1997;156(4):262-5.
15. Gordon EE, Reinking BE, Hu S, et al. Maternal hyperglycemia directly and rapidly induces cardiac septal overgrowth in fetal rats. J Diabet Res. 2015;2015(479565):11
16. Grunberger G, Taylor SI, Dons RF, et al. Insulin receptors in normal and disease states. Clin Endocrinol Metab. 1983;12(1):191-219.
17. Hayrullah A, Zehra K, Tamer B. Transient severe isolated right ventricular hypertrophy in neonates. J Clin Neonatol. 2014;3(3):161-3.
18. D'cunha C, Sankaran K. Persistent fetal circulation. Paediatr Child Health. 2001;6(10):744-50.
19. Goldberg JF, Mery CM, Griffiths PS, et al. Extracorporeal membrane oxygenation support in severe hypertrophic obstructive cardiomyopathy associated with persistent pulmonary hypertension in an infant of a diabetic mother. Circulation. 2014;130(21):1923-5.
20. Walther FJ, Siassi B, King J, et al. Cardiac output in infants of insulin-dependent diabetic mothers. J Pediatr.1985;107(1):109-14.
21. Costa VN, Nomura RM, Reynolds KS, et al. Effects of maternal hyperglycemia on fetal heart rate in pregnancies complicated by pregestational diabetes mellitus. Eur J Obstet Gynecol Reprod Biol. 2009;143(1):14-7.
22. Chu C, Gui YH, Ren YY, et al. The impacts of maternal gestational diabetes mellitus (GDM) on fetal hearts. Biomed Environ Sci. 2012;25(1):15-22.
23. NicolaidesKH. Turning the pyramid of prenatal care. Fetal Diagn Ther. 2011;29(3):183-96.
24. National Diabetes Education Initiative. (2016). American Diabetes Association (ADA) 2016 Guidelines: Diabetes Management Guidelines. [online] http://www.ndei.org/ADA-diabetes-management-guidelines-diabetes-in-pregnancy-GDM.aspx.html. [Accessed August, 2017].
25. Boinpally T, Jovanovic L. Management of type 2 diabetes and gestational diabetes in pregnancy. Mt Sinai J Med. 2009;76(3):269-80.
26. British Association of Perinatal Medicine. (2008). Acute In utero transfer guidelines (Fenton A, Peebles D, Ahluwalia J). [online] Available from http://www.bapm.org/publications/documents/guidelines/IUTs_Jun08_final.pdf. [Accessed August, 2017].
27. Vora S, Chandan S, RajaduraiVS, et al. Hyperinsulinemic hypoglycemia in infancy: current concepts in diagnosis and management. Indian Pediatr. 2015;52(12):1051-9.

CHAPTER 98

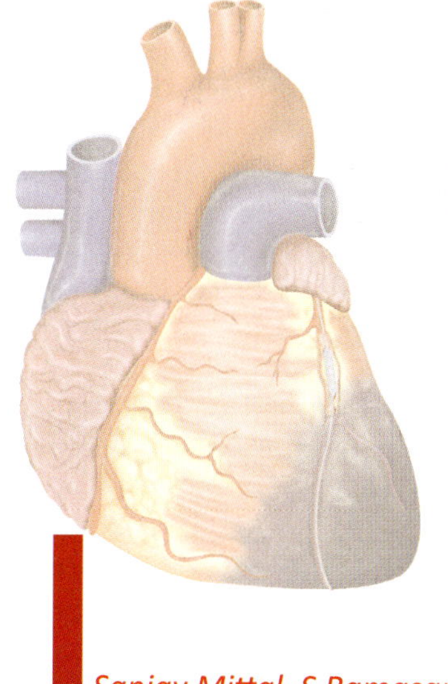

Role of Enhanced External Counterpulsation: Future Perspectives

Sanjay Mittal, S Ramasamy

INTRODUCTION

The treatment for refractory angina and heart failure poses a great challenge to the cardiologists since these patients have recurrent symptoms, demonstrable residual ischemia, repeat emergency visit, repeat hospitalization, and poor quality of life in spite of optimal medical management and exhausted or not amendable for further interventional procedures. The presence of diabetes in these groups is usually associated with worse outcomes with higher rate of restenosis[1,2] graft occlusion[3] and higher complication rate when repeat revascularization procedures are attempted.[4] Currently, the evidence shows clear role of revascularization in patients with unstable coronary syndrome, but still these procedures like coronary artery bypass graft (CABG) and percutaneous transluminal coronary angioplasty (PTCA) role in stable patients beyond improving the quality of life is not clearly understood and still under investigation.[5,6] The recent Clinical Outcomes Utilizing Revascularization and Aggressive Drug Evaluation (COURAGE) and (Bypass Angioplasty Revascularization Investigation 2 Diabetes (BARI 2D) randomized trials have supported the view that patient's benefit derived from optimal medical management is comparable to that of intervention without any difference in rate of death or myocardial infarction (MI). This has recently increased attention on the US Food and Drug Administration (FDA) approved noninvasive treatment options like enhanced external counterpulsation (EECP) to improve the patient's symptoms and decrease the ischemic burden when added above optimal medical therapy. The treatment strategy other than standard interventional procedures like CABG and PTCA were EECP treatment, stem cell-induced neovascularization, gene therapy, intramyocardial angiogenic growth factor delivery, neurostimulation, percutaneous transmyocardial laser revascularization, and extracorporeal shockwave myocardial revascularization. Of all these treatment modalities, EECP is the widely used treatment as its mechanism of action is well established and also supported by two randomized trial showing its benefit in angina and heart failure patients.

HISTORY OF ENHANCED EXTERNAL COUNTERPULSATION

Evolution of counterpulsation from beginning to the current advance form is designed to achieve two important hemodynamic treatment goals, to augment diastolic pressure and to reduce left ventricular afterload. This was expected to have a favorable effect in patients with coronary artery disease by improving coronary perfusion pressure and reducing myocardial oxygen consumption. Augmenting diastolic pressure concept was first tested in 1953 by Kantrowitz and showed in an animal study that coronary blood flow could be increased by 20–40% by elevating the pressure during the diastolic phase.[7] Sarnoff and colleagues described myocardial workload is directly proportionate to the left ventricular contraction time and pressure.[8] Then in 1957, Birtwell combined both the principle of Kantrowitz and Sarnoff and design a counterpulsation device as a circulatory-assist device. In 1963, Denis and coworkers began clinical studies using a G-suite (hydraulic compression of legs), a rigid case enclosing a single pant-like bag filled with water, put around the lower extremities of the patients. Water was pumped in and out of the rigid metallic case in synchronization with patients electrocardiogram (ECG).[9] The initial clinical objective of the device is to support and stabilize the patients with acute myocardial infarction (AMI) and cariogenic shock. Early clinical papers in 1960s to 1970s were on these two acute indications. This leads to development of two parallel research in counterpulsation treatment—one led by Moulopoulos in developing invasive intra-aortic balloon pump (IABP) counterpulsation and other led by Birtwell in developing noninvasive EECP.[10,11] One randomized control trial on AMI by external counterpulsation demonstrated by applying 1–4 hours of counterpulsation within first 24 hours of onset of MI, there is significant reduction in mortality when compared to control group.[12] In 1964, Birtwell device showed by applying external pressure to the arterial system demonstrated similar benefit of increased diastolic pressure and reduce myocardial oxygen consumption, when compared to IABP. Cohen in 1973 showed EECP increases cardiac output by an average of 25% compared with 4% for IABP. This effect is due to increase venous return achieved by the compression of lower extremities.[13] In 1975, the water-driven hydraulic system was replaced by the advanced air-driven pneumatic counterpulsation for humans. In 1983, finally addition of the upper thigh cuffs or buttocks cuff and sequential pattern of inflation was introduced into the EECP system. The system performance significantly improved within increased diastolic augmentation (DA) and afterload reduction with these new additions. The current EECP system is shown in the Figure 1.

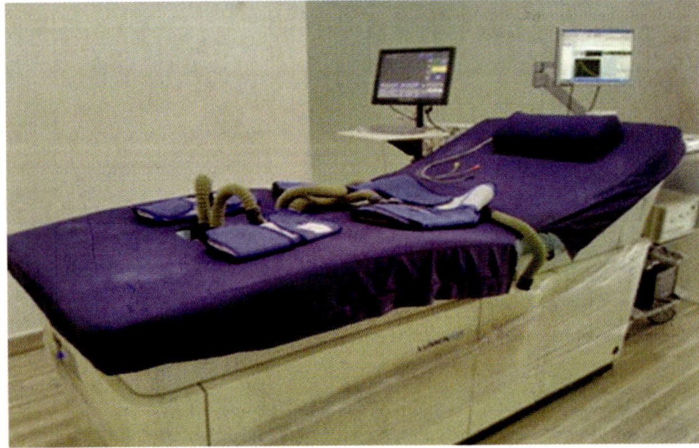

Fig. 1: Enhanced external counterpulsation (EECP) treatment system

ENHANCED EXTERNAL COUNTERPULSATION THERAPY

Enhanced external counterpulsation therapy system is an electromechanical system consisting of a specialized treatment table with integrated valve regulatory system, attached to specialized two sets three cuffs and a treatment console. The console comprises air compressor and touch screen panel to control inflation and deflation of the cuffs in synchronization with the patient's own ECG with microsecond precision. The cuffs inflate sequentially from lower calves proceeding upwards to lower thigh, then to upper thigh with a 50 millisecond delay with each cuff inflation in order to milk the blood flow in early diastolic phase and deflate simultaneously at the end of the diastolic or presystolic phase (Fig. 2). This sequential compression results in increased retrograde blood flow from the femoral artery towards the descending aorta. When the movement of column of blood reaches the root of aorta exactly during the diastole, the aortic valve will be in closed position and thereby significantly increasing blood flow to the coronary arteries at the time when coronary vascular resistance is at its lowest level. This is called DA. The inflation of the cuffs also increases the retrograde venous blood flow to the right side of the heart, providing greater ventricular filling and increase cardiac output. At the end of diastole and when the ventricle is prepared for systole all three cuffs simultaneous deflate, results in significant reduction in total systemic peripheral vascular resistance leaving the heart to empty the stroke volume into relatively lesser resistance peripheral vascular pathway and intern significantly reducing the after-load of the heart and overall myocardial oxygen demand. The cuff pressure can be increased from 80 mm Hg to 300 mm Hg. The central DA can be roughly estimated by using finger plethysmography. The pressure is adjusted in the cuffs to reach the DA ratio of more than one, which has been shown to have a favorable hemodynamic effect. The treatment is given on an outpatient day care basis, 1 hour session per day, 6 days per week over 6 weeks or 2 hours per day, 6 days per week for 3 weeks as tolerated for a total of 35 hours. In some patients a short course of 15, one-hour session is given to prepare the patients for high-risk CABG.

Major Randomized Trial of Enhanced External Counterpulsation

Multicenter study of enhanced external counterpulsation (MUST-EECP) is a multicenter, prospective, randomized, blinded, and control trial of EECP in angina patients with proven coronary artery disease and positive exercise treadmill test.[14] They were treated with either active

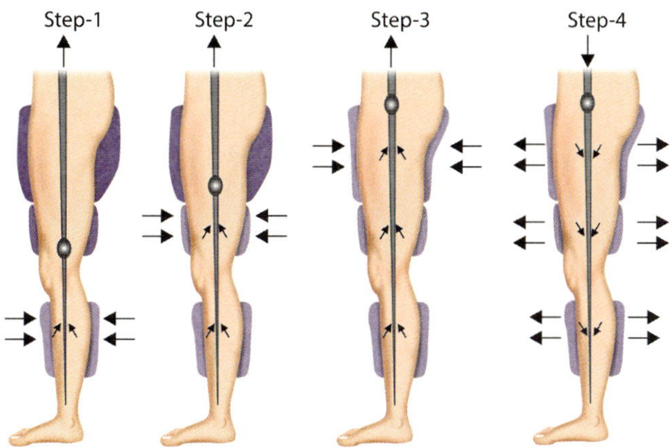

Fig. 2: Technique of enhanced external counterpulsation (EECP) therapy. Three pairs of pneumatic cuffs are applied to the calves, lower thighs, and upper thighs. The cuffs are inflated sequentially during diastole, distal to proximal. The compression of the lower extremity vascular bed increases diastolic pressure and flow and increases venous return. The pressure is then released at the onset of systole. Inflation and deflation are timed according to the R-wave on the patient's cardiac monitor. The pressures applied and the inflation-deflation timing can be altered by using the pressure wave forms and electrocardiogram on the EECP therapy monitor

(Adapted from Manchanda and Soran)

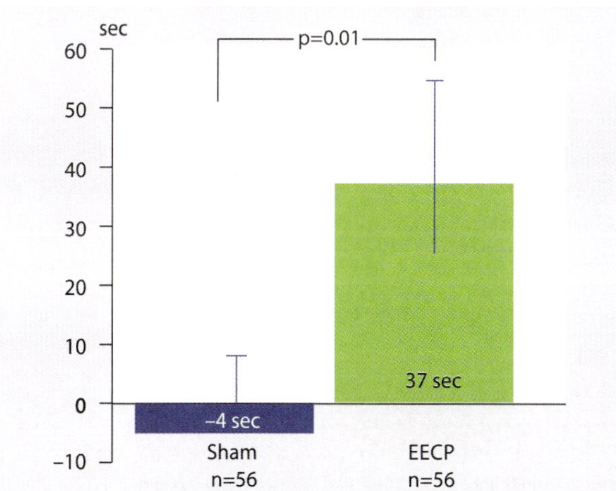

Fig. 3: Change in time to exercise-induced ST-segment depression significant in active treatment group

counterpulsation (applied cuff pressure upto 300 mm Hg) and inactive counterpulsation (<75 mm Hg). Time to 1 mm ST-segment depression increased significantly from baseline in active group compared with inactive group (p = 0.01) (Fig. 3). The treatment also significantly reduces the number of angina episodes and nitroglycerin usage in the active group. A substudy with 12-month follow-up also showed sustained improvement in health-related quality of life in active EECP group when compared to sham group.[15]

PEECH-EECP is a prospective evolution of enhanced external counterpulsation in heart failure patients with mild- to-moderate symptoms.[16] Patients are randomized to either EECP with protocol-defined pharmacologic therapy (PT) or PT alone. About 35% in EECP and 25% in control groups increased their exercise time by at least 60 seconds (p = 0.016) at 6 months (Figs 4A and B). New York Heart Association (NYHA) functional class improved in the active treatment group significantly at 1 week, 3 months, and 6 months. The Minnesota Living with Heart Failure score also improved significantly in the treated group at 1 week ($p < 0.002$) and 3 months (p = 0.01) after treatment, versus no significant changes in the control group. In subgroup analysis of elderly patients 65 years or older in addition to mean changes in exercise duration, peak oxygen consumption from baseline were significantly increased when compared to the control at 1 week, 3 months, and 6 months following completion of treatment.[17]

Acute Hemodynamic Benefit during Enhanced External Counterpulsation

Enhanced external counterpulsation hemodynamic effects are similar to that of IABP counterpulsation. During EECP treatment, the cuff pressure given in the lower extremities results in significant change in central hemodynamic circulation similar to that of what achieved in IABP except the increase in venous return (preload). When the cuffs inflate sequentially, it increases the central aortic and intracoronary diastolic pressure up to 92% and 93%, respectively, and the intracoronary flow velocity increase by 150% and the coronary flow increase by 28%.[18] Similarly, the cuff inflation also causes increase in venous return, which causes increase in right arterial pressure, pulmonary capillary wedge pressure, increase in blood flow into left ventricle, and cardiac output.[19] During EECP, cardiac output has shown to increase up to 25%.[20] When the cuffs deflate simultaneously, it decreases the central aortic and intracoronary systolic pressure by 11% and 15%, respectively. It lowers the left ventricular afterload and thereby reduces myocardial workload.[18]

Enhanced Myocardial Blood Flow

The long-time effect of EECP is presumably achieved through the development of new capillaries from the pre-existing vessels and by enhancing the collateral flow. EECP has been shown to associate with significant increase of

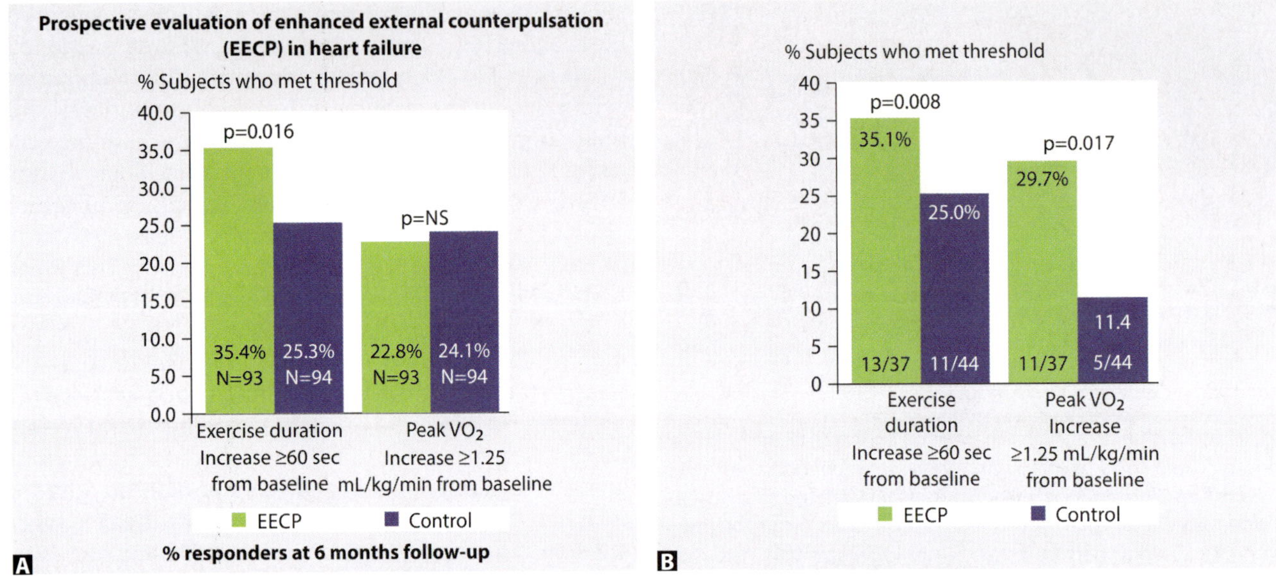

Figs 4A and B: (A) Increase in exercise duration and peak VO_2% responders at 6-month follow-up; (B) Increase in exercise duration and peak VO_2 in older patients ≥65% responders at 6-month follow-up

TABLE 1: Summary of the published radionuclide stress perfusion studies demonstrating EECP treatment improves perfusion to ischemic regions of the myocardium

Author	*Year*	*Method*	*n*	*Perfusion changes*
Lawson et al.	1992	Thallium	18	78% pts (↑Maximal Exercise)
Sjukri et al.	1995	Thallium	35	87% pts (↑Maximal Exercise)
Urano et al.	2000	Thallium	12	46% (↑same workload)
Masuda et al.	2001	PET	11	23% (↑overall) 47% (↑ischemic region)
Stys et al. Ramasamy S	2002	Thallium sestamibi	175	83% pts (↑same workload) 54% pts (↑maximal exercise)
Tartaglia et al. Ramasamy S	2003	Sestamibi	25	64% pts (↑maximal exercise)

angiogenic factor including plasma vascular endothelial growth factor (VEGF), hepatocyte growth factor (HGF), and basis fibroblast growth factors (bFGF).[21] The recruitment of new myocardial collateral arteries has been shown clinically by improved stress radionuclide coronary perfusion and N-ammonia positron emission tomography studies.[22-26] The improvement in myocardial blood flow is further confirmed by 2 randomized control trials by measuring pressure-derived collateral flow index (CFIp) and pressure-derived fractional flow reserve (FFR).[27,28] Both the parameters improved significantly in EECP treated group while there is no change in control group. Table 1 shows all the study done using myocardial perfusion scan.

Improves Endothelial Function

The increase in pressure and velocity in circulation achieved through counterpulsation by compressing the lower extremities not only causes shear stress to the vascular endothelium in coronary vascular bed but also to the entire systemic vascular system. The improvement in endothelial function is achieved by significant increase in plasma nitric oxide and reduction in plasma endothelin levels.[29] This plasma change in nitric oxide and endothelin were sustained even after the completion of EECP treatment up to 3 months. So in addition to improvement in coronary blood flow, endothelial function also has been shown to improve after a course of EECP treatment.[30]

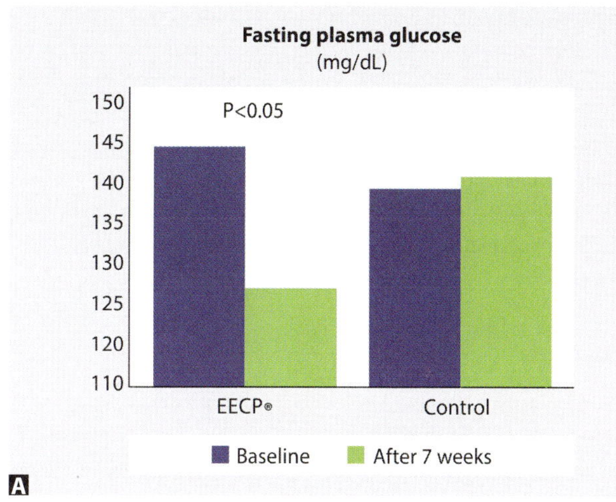

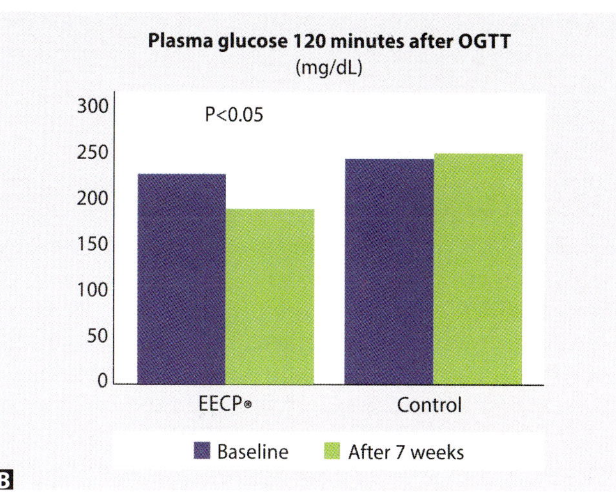

Figs 5A and B: (A) Fasting blood sugar reduce significantly in treatment group 143.9 ± 8.5–127 ± 66 mg/dL ($p < 0.05$) and no change in control group; (B) Two hours after an oral glucose tolerance test (OGTT) with 75 g of glucose, plasma blood sugar reduce significantly in treatment group 224.4 ± 24.6–196.1 ± 24.7 mg/dL ($p < 0.05$) when compared to control group

EECP therapy has also shown to decrease the proinflammatory cytokines like tumor necrosis factor- α (TNF-α), monocyte chemoattractant protein-1 (MCP-1), vascular cell adhesion molecule, and increase of endothelial progenitor cells, which are actually a circulating repair cells in patient with symptomatic coronary artery disease.[31,32]

Enhanced External Counterpulsation in Diabetes

Patients with diabetes are at greater risk of adverse cardiovascular events and they respond poorly to revascularization and aggressive antiplatelet therapy when compared to patients with no diabetes. Patients who are high-risk and diabetic with prior surgical and catheter-based revascularization and currently not an eligible candidate for further intervention who have undergone EECP treatment for their symptom relief, have shown similar reduction in angina symptoms compared to patients without diabetes. In 1-year follow-up study, both the groups maintain their benefit in anginal class and on demand nitrate intake. The incidence of PTCA, CABG, and MI are also similar in both these groups. When these groups of patients with diabetes treated with EECP compared to patient treated with elective PCI in National Heart, Lung, and Blood Institute (NHLBI) dynamic registry of coronary intervention and BARI the cumulative 1 year mortality are comparable with no increase in mortality in EECP-treated diabetic group.[33]

Enhanced external counterpulsation mechanism of action of improving the nitric oxide bioavailability and peripheral arterial function has also shown to manage better glycemic control in patients with abnormal glucose tolerance (AGT), which is a prediabetic status with greater risk of developing diabetes and cardiovascular disease. This was shown in a randomized control trial, where fasting plasma glucose declined 16.9 mg/dL (Fig. 5A) and plasma glucose 120 minutes after initiation of oral glucose tolerance testing decreases 28.3 mg/dL (Fig. 5B) significantly in EECP group while there was no change in the control group. In addition, the homeostasis model assessment of insulin resistance (HOMA-IR), a measure of insulin resistance decreases by 31%, while the whole body composite insulin sensitivity index (CISI) increases by 21% in the EECP-treated group and no change in the control group. There was also 47% increase in glucose transporter 4 (GLUT-4) protein expression only in the EECP group.[34] This provides evidence that EECP sensitizes transport of insulin into skeletal muscle thereby providing help to manage glycemic control in patient with AGT. In another study the patients with left ventricular dysfunction (LVD) are grouped into diabetes and nondiabetes and the effect of EECP was studied. In this study, ejection fraction (EF), cardiac output, and stroke volume increases similarly in both groups. The effect of EECP seems to be independent of the status of diabetes.[35]

ENHANCED EXTERNAL COUNTERPULSATION INDICATIONS

Enhanced External Counterpulsation as Primary Treatment

- Chronic stable angina patients symptomatic with optimal medical management but not willing or not a candidate for PTCA or CABG.

- Coronary angiogram shows diffuse coronary atherosclerosis in distal vessels or challenging coronary anatomy.
- Target lesion is inaccessible for stenting or grafting the vessels.
- Patient symptomatic with evidence of ischemia and lesions are nonflow limiting and less than 70%.
- Patients with multivessel disease without left main involvement and only partial revascularization is possible.
- Patients with comorbid states like uncontrolled diabetes, chronic renal failure stroke or pulmonary disease which create high-risk for any interventional procedures.
- Patients with severe LVD recommended for CABG if the risk is higher than the benefit.
- Patients with cardiac syndrome X (microvascular angina).

Preparation for High-Risk Coronary Artery Bypass Graft

- Severe LVD with hibernating myocardium to improve myocardial blood.
- Flowing to stabilize the cardiac function prior to CABG.
- Waiting for CABG.

Enhanced External Counterpulsation as Secondary Treatment

- Post-CABG/post-PTCA residual ischemia and symptomatic.
- Restenosis after PTCA.
- Graft occlusion after CABG.
- Native vessel disease progression post-CABG and post-PTCA, where further intervention is not planned.

Enhanced External Counterpulsation in Heart Failure

- Symptomatic heart failure patients.
- Recurrent admission due to left ventricular failure/pulmonary edema.
- Ischemic and non-ischemic cardiomyopathy.

ENHANCED EXTERNAL COUNTERPULSATION CONTRAINDICATIONS

Absolute

- Severe aortic insufficiency (reduced coronary perfusion).
- Aortic aneurysm more than 5 cm or dissection (diastolic augmentation can cause rupture).
- Decompensated heart failure with fluid overload.
- Severe peripheral vascular disease/aortoiliac occlusive disease (prevent retrograde blood flow beyond the obstruction).
- Right heart failure with fluid overloads (increase venous return can cause pulmonary edema).
- Severe pulmonary hypertension (pulmonary artery pressure systolic pressure more than 50 mm Hg).
- Pregnancy (safety study not done).

Relative

- International normalized ratio (INR) greater than 2.5 (may cause bleeding).
- Arrhythmias interfering with system triggering (atrial fibrillation/flutter and frequent premature ventricular contraction).
- Uncontrolled severe hypertension more than 180/110 mm Hg (further augmenting diastolic pressure may be deleterious).
- Deep vein thrombosis (may cause pulmonary embolism).
- Thrombophlebitis and cellulitis.

ENHANCED EXTERNAL COUNTERPULSATION IN REFRACTORY ANGINA PATIENTS

Refractory angina poses a great challenge to the treating physician as these patients have already exhausted all treatment options and are in maximal tolerated medical management with objective evidence of ischemia. EECP treatment has shown consistently in many clinical trials improvement in clinical symptom of angina, decreases nitrate use, increases exercise tolerance, enhances quality of life accompanied by favorable psychosocial effects, prolongation of time to exercise induced ST-segment depression, and resolution of myocardial reversible perfusion defects.[36-39] The EECP therapy clinical benefits has been shown in wider range of patients, who include severe triple vessel disease, diabetes, LVD, elderly, patient with systolic, and diastolic dysfunction.[40,41] EECP has not only been demonstrated to be effective in treating these groups of patients with severe coronary artery disease, it has also been reported to be safe during treatment with only minor side effects, such as leg pain, skin abrasion, and temporary paresthesia. The International EECP Patient Registry (IEPR) with follow-up study of 1 year, 2 years, and 3 years has shown EECP benefits are sustained during the follow-up period in 75–85% of the patients.[42-44] In another independent study, 18 refractory angina patients were followed upto 5 years and they have been shown to maintain their clinical benefits.[45] Repeat EECP therapy after completion of first course is necessary in 10% of the patients in 1 year follow-up, 20% in 2 years follow-up, and 22% in 3 years follow-up. Most common reason for the repeat EECP therapy is failure to complete at least 30 sessions, recurrent symptoms, or residual symptoms after completing full course.[46]

ENHANCED EXTERNAL COUNTERPULSATION IN HEART FAILURE PATIENTS

Enhanced external counterpulsation therapy initially was considered to be contraindicated in patient with LVD based on path physiological reasoning that EECP increases preload and therefore may precipitate pulmonary edema. However, it has been reported that in patients with severe LVD (EF <25%), EECP is not only shown to be safe but also effective in significantly reducing systolic and diastolic volume and improving their LV function.[47] In a multicenter feasibility study, Soran and coworkers reported in patients with stable heart failure NYHA class II and III with both ischemic and nonischemic etiology, EECP therapy was associated with significant improvement in peak oxygen uptake (+27%), exercise capacity (16%), and functional status. These benefits were sustained for a period of 6 months even after completion of standard 35 sessions of EECP.[41] In IEPR patients with history of LVD (EF < 35%), who completed EECP treatment, 2 years follow-up have shown 83% survival rate and major cardiovascular event-free survival rate of 70%.[48]

In another prospective cohort study of 450 patients with LVD (EF < 30 ± 8%) a course of EECP therapy has significantly reduced all-cause emergency department visit by 78% and hospitalization rate by 73% at 6-months follow-up period, when compared to 6 months before EECP therapy.[49]

Enhanced external counterpulsation treatment has also shown significantly decrease in the heart failure readmission when started 90 days in post-discharges patients. The rehospitalization for heart failure reduced to 6% compared to predicted rate of 30–34%. These patients also show a significant improvement in 6 minutes walk distance, NHYA class, and Duke Activity Status Index (DASI) score suggesting that improvements in functional status and symptoms were contributing to very low rates of rehospitalization.[50]

Enhanced external counterpulsation therapy as per current evidence is on effective treatment option for patients with heart failure to improve their clinical symptoms, exercise tolerance, heart failure readmission, quality of life, peak oxygen consumption, and also to improve the LV function. The overall benefit of EECP has also been shown to be similar in both diastolic and systolic heart failure patients.[38]

CONCLUSION

Enhanced external counterpulsation treatment has been under focus in recent times due to its application in wide variety of patients' population who are high risk with poor quality of life. Its role in restoring blood supply to the ischemic myocardium by angiogenesis has opened up a lot of opportunity in this subgroup of patients who are not willing or not a candidate for revascularization. Any reduction in ischemic burden or improvement in quality of life with increase in exercise time will immensely benefit these patients. EECP's potential role in improving glycemic control in type II diabetic patients and favorably altering endothelial function by shear stress on vascular wall can protect or possibly can reverse the progression of vascular disease. EECP may play a greater role as cardiovascular protection therapy in patients with refractory angina and heart failure. The American College of Cardiology foundation guidelines for patients with stable ischemic heart disease recommends it as a class IIb (level of evidence B). The European Society of Cardiology guideline on the management of stable coronary artery disease recommends it as a Class IIa (level of evidence B). EECP is a validated, effective, safe, and noninvasive outpatient treatment for patients with angina and heart failure.

REFERENCES

1. Rozenman Y, Sapoznikov D, Gotsman MS. Restenosis and progression of coronary disease after balloon angioplasty in patients with diabetes mellitus. Clic Cardiol. 2000;23:890-4.
2. Przewlocki T, Pieniazek P, Ryniewicz W, et al. Long-term outcome of coronary balloon angioplasty in diabetic patients. Int J cardiol. 2000;76:7-16.
3. Lytle BW, Loop FD, Cosgrove DM, et al. Long-term (5 to 12 years) serial studies of internal mammary artery and saphenous vein coronary bypass grafts. J Thorac Cardiovasc Surg. 1985;89:248-58.
4. Stephan WJ, O'Keefe JH Jr, Piehler JM, et al. Coronary angioplasty versus repeat coronary artery bypass grafting for patients with previous bypass surgery. J Am Coll Cardiol. 1996;28:1140-6.
5. Boden WE, O'Rourke RA, Teo KK, et al. Optimal Medical Therapy with or without PCI for stable coronary disease. N Engl J Med. 2007;356:1503-16.
6. Frye RL, August P, Brooks MM, et al. BARI 2D study Group: a randomized trial of therapies for type 2 diabetes and coronary artery disease. N Engl J Med. 2009;306-2503-15.
7. Kantrowitz A. Experimental augmentation of coronary flow by retardation of arterial pressure pulse. Surgery. 1953;34(4):678-87.
8. Sarnoff SJ, Braunwald E, Welch GH Jr, et al. Hemodynamic determinants of oxygen consumption of heart with special reference to tension-time index. Am J Physiol. 1958;192:148-56.

9. Dennis C, Moreno JR, Hall DP, et al. Studies on external counterpulsation as a potential measure for acute left heart failure. Trans Am Soc Artif Intern Organs. 1963;9:186-91.
10. Moulopoulos SD, Topaz S, Kolff WL. Diastolic balloon pumping (with carbon dioxide in aorta: mechanical assistance to failing circulation. Am Heart J. 1962;63:669-75.
11. Soroff HS, Ruiz U, Birtwell WC, et al. Synchronous external circulatory assist. Trans Am Soc Artif Intern Organs. 1964;10:79-88.
12. Amsterdam EA, Banas J, Criley JM, et al. Clinical assessment of external pressure circulatory assistance in acute myocardial infarction: report of a cooperative clinical trial. Am J Cardiol. 1980;45:349-56.
13. Soroff HS, Hui J, Giron F. Historical Review of the Development of Enhance External Counterpulsation Technology and its physiologic Rationale. Cardiovasc Rev Rep. 1997;18:34-40.
14. Arora RR, Chou TM, Jain D, et al. The Multicenter Study of Enhanced External Counterpulsation (MUST-EECP): effect of EECP on exercise-induced myocardial ischemia and anginal episodes. J Am Coll Cardiol. 1999;33:1833-40.
15. Arora RR, Chou TM, Jain D, et al. Effects of enhanced external counterpulsation on health-related quality of life continue 12 months after treatment: a substudy of the multicenter study of enhanced external counterpulsation. J Investing Med. 2002;50: 25-32.
16. Feldman AM, Siver MA, Francis GS, et al. Enhanced external counterpulsation improves exercise tolerance in patients with chronic heart failure. J Am Coll Cardiol. 2006;48:1198-205.
17. Abbottsmith CW, Chung ES, Varricchione T, et al. Enhanced external counterpulsation improves exercise duration and peak oxygen consumption in older patients with heart failure: a subgroup analysis of the PEECH trail. Congest Heart Fail. 2006;12:307-11.
18. Michaels AD, Accad M, Ports TA, et al. Left ventricular systolic unloading and augmentation of intracoronary pressure and Doppler flow during enhanced external counterpulsation. Circulation. 2002;106(10):1237-42.
19. Taguchi I, Ogawa K, Oida A, et al. Comparison of hemodynamic effects of enhanced external counterpulsation and intra-aortic balloon pumping in patients with acute myocardial infarction. Am J Cardiol. 2000;86(10):1139-41.
20. Barsness GW. Enhanced external counterpulsation in unrevascularizable patients. Curr Intrerv Cardiol Rep. 2001;3(1):37-43.
21. Masuda D, Nohara K, Kataoka K, et al. Enhance External Counterpulsation promotes angiogenesis factors in patients with chronic stable angina. Circulation. 2001;104:II445.
22. Urano H, Ikeda H, Ueno T, et al. Enhanced external counterpulsation improves exercise tolerance, reduces exercise-induced myocardial ischemia and improved left ventricular diastolic filling in patients with coronary artery disease. J Am Coll Cardiol. 2001;37:93-9.
23. Masuda D, Nohara R, Horai T, et al. External counterpulsation improved myocardial perfusion and coronary flow reserve in patients with chronic stable angina. Eur Heart J. 2001;22:1451-8.
24. Stys TP, Lawson WE, Hui JC, et al. Effects of enhanced external counterpulsation on stress radionuclide coronary perfusion and exercise capacity in chronic stable angina pectoris. Am J Cardiol. 2002;89(7):822-4.
25. Tartaglia J, Stenerson J Jr, Charney R, et al. Exercise capability and myocardial perfusion in chronic angina patients treated with enhanced external counterpulsation. Clin Cardiol. 2003;26(6): 287-90.
26. Sjukri K, Setal A. Enhanced external counterpulsation in the treatment and rehabilitation of coronary patients in Indonesia. Asian Cardiovasc Thorac Ann. 1995;3(1):26-28.
27. Buschmann EE, Utz W, Pagonas N, et al. Improvement of fractional flow reserve and collateral flow by treatment with external counterpulsation (Art.Net.-2 Trial). Eur J Clin Invest. 2009;39(10):866-75.
28. Gloekler S, Meier P, de Marchi SF, et al. Coronary collateral growth by external counterpulsation: a randomised controlled trial. Heart. 2010;96(3):202-7.
29. Akhtar M, Wu GF, Du ZM, et al. Effect of enhanced external counterpulsation on plasma nitric oxide and endothelin-1 levels. Am J Cardiol. 2006;98(1):28-30.
30. Bonetti PO, Barsness GW, Keelan PC, et al. Enhanced external counterpulsation improves endothelial function in patients with symptomatic coronary artery disease. J Am Coll Cardiol. 2003;41(10):1761-8.
31. Casey DP, Conti CR, Nichols WW, et al. Effect of enhanced external counterpulsation on inflammatory cytokines and adhesion molecules in patients with angina pectoris and angiographic coronary artery disease. Am J Cardiol. 2008;101(3):300-2.
32. Barsheshet A, Hod H, Shechter M, et al. The effect of external counterpulsation therapy on circulating endothelial progenitor cells in patients with angina pectoris. Cardiology. 2008:110(3):160-6.
33. Linnemeier G, Rutter MK, Barness G, et al. Enhanced external counterpulsation for the relief of angina in patients with diabetes: safety, efficacy and 1 year clinical outcomes. Am Heart J. 2003;146:453-8.
34. Martin JS, Beck DT, Arnanda JM, et al. Enhanced external counterpulsation improves peripheral artery function and glucose tolerance in subject with abnormal glucose tolerance. J Appl Physiol. 2012;112:868-76.
35. Ramasamy S, Sivakadaksham N, Pradeep G, et al. Is the benefits of enhanced external counterpulsation in patient with moderate left ventricular dysfunction independent of diabetes? J Am Coll Cardiol. 2015;66(16):142.
36. Fitzgerald CP, Lawson WE, Hui JC, et al. Enhanced external counterpulsation as initial revascularization treatment for angina refractory to medical therapy. Cardiology. 2003;100(3):129-35.
37. Lawson WE, Hui JC, Lang G. Treatment benefit in the enhanced external counterpulsation consortium. Cardiology. 2000;94(1):31-5.
38. Lawson WE, Silver MA, Kennard L, et al. Angina patients with diastolic or systolic heart failure demonstrate comparable immediate and one year benefit from enhanced external counterpulsation. J Card Fail. 2003;9(5):107.
39. Lawson WE, Hui JCK, Guo T, et al. Prior revascularization increases the effectiveness of enhanced external counterpulsation. Clin Cardiol. 1998;21(11):841-4.
40. Soran O, Kennard ED, Kelsey S, et al. Enhanced External Counterpulsation as treatment for chronic angina in patients with left ventricular dysfunction: a report from international EECP registry (IEPR). Congest Heart Fail. 2002;8(6):297-302.
41. Soran O, Flesishman B, DeMarco T, et al. Enhanced External Counterpulsation in patients with heart failure—a multicenter feasibility study. Congest Heart Fail. 2002;8:204-8.
42. Pettersson T, Bondesson S, Cojocaru D, et al. One-year follow-up of patients with refractory angina pectoris treated with enhanced external counterpulsation. BMC Cardiovasc Disord. 2006;6:28.
43. Michaels AD, Linnemeier G, Soran O, et al. Two-year outcomes after enhanced external counterpulsation for stable angina pectoris (from the International EECP Patient Registry [IEPR]). Am J Cardiol. 2004;93(4):461-4.
44. Loh PH, Cleland JG, Louis AA, et al. Enhanced external counterpulsation in the treatment of chronic refractory angina: a long-term follow-up outcome from the International Enhanced External Counterpulsation Patient Registry. Clin Cardiol. 2008;31:159-64.
45. Lawson WE, Hui JCK, Cohn PF. Long-term prognosis of patients with angina treated with enhanced external counterpulsation: five-year follow-up study. Clin Cardiol. 2000;23:254-8.
46. Lawson EW, Barsness G, Michaels AD, et al. Effectiveness of repeat enhanced external counterpulsation for refractory angina in

patients failing to complete an initial course of therapy. Cardiology. 2007;108:170-5.

47. Gorcscan J III, Crawford L, Soran O, et al. Improvement in left ventricular performance in Enhanced External Counterpulsation in patients with heart failure. J Am Coll Cardiol. 2000;35 Supple:230A.
48. Soran O, Kennard ED, Kfoury AG, et al. IEPR Investigators. Two-year clinical outcomes after enhanced external counterpulsation (EECP) therapy in patients with refractory angina pectoris and left ventricular dysfunction (report from the international EECP patient registry). Congest Heart Fail. 2002;8(6):297-302.
49. Soran O, Kennard ED, Bart BA, et al. Impact of external counterpulsation treatment on emergency department visits and hospitalizations in refractory angina patients with left ventricular dysfunction. Congest Heart Fail. 2007;13(1):36-40.
50. Tecson KM, Silver MA, Brune SD, et al. Impact of enhanced external counterpulsation on heart failure rehospitalization in patients with ischaemic cardiomyopathy. Am J Cardiol. 2016;117:901-5.

SECTION 4

Nutraceutical and Obesity Care

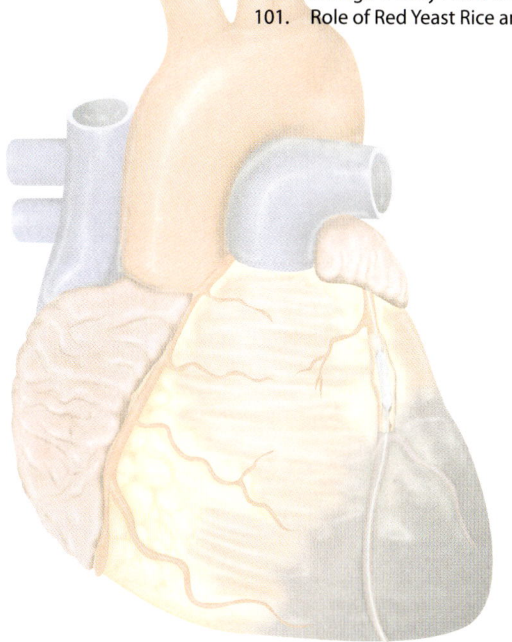

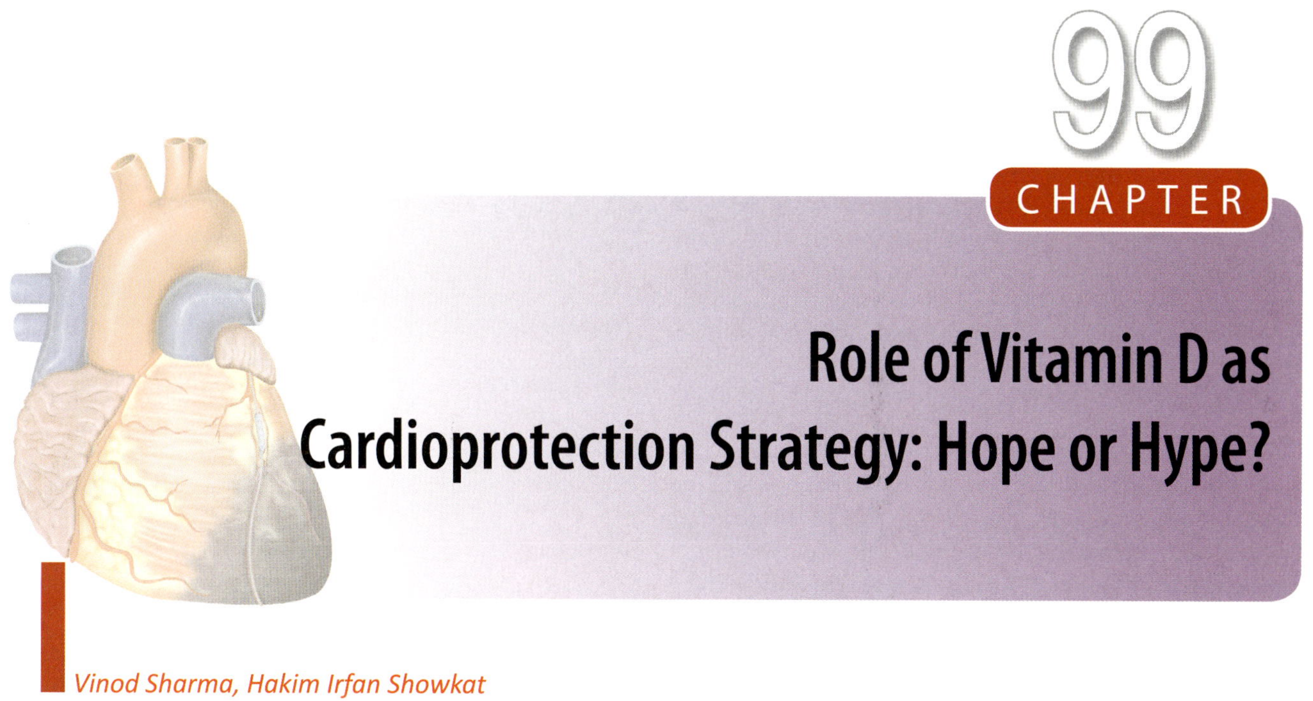

99

CHAPTER

Role of Vitamin D as Cardioprotection Strategy: Hope or Hype?

Vinod Sharma, Hakim Irfan Showkat

INTRODUCTION

A growing body of evidence suggests that people who are deficient in 25-hydroxyvitamin D [25(OH)D] have higher risks for numerous chronic medical conditions. Vitamin D is either produced in the skin via the effects of ultraviolet light or ingested with food and/or supplements. This vitamin D undergoes hydroxylation in the liver to produce 25(OH) D. It is widely believed that the renal enzyme 25(OH)D-1-hydroxylase is primarily responsible for producing the circulating levels of the activated form of vitamin D, the hormone 1,25(OH)D. 25(OH)D-1-hydroxylase is located in the inner mitochondrial membrane and is a cytochrome P-450 monooxygenase. Most of the biologic activities of 1,25(OH)D are mediated by its binding to a high-affinity receptor that acts as a ligand-activated transcription factor. The major steps involved in the control of gene transcription by the vitamin D receptor (VDR) include ligand binding, heterodimerization with retinoid X receptor, binding of the heterodimer to vitamin D response elements, and recruitment of other nuclear proteins into the transcriptional preinitiation complex. 1,25(OH)D may also act through nonVDR or nongenomic VDR-mediated pathways.[1-3]

Vitamin D deficiency is widely prevalent. Low levels of 25(OH)D the principal circulating storage form of vitamin D, are present in one-third to one-half of otherwise healthy middle-aged to elderly adults.[4-7] Although most consequences of vitamin D deficiency involve the musculoskeletal system, there is a growing body of evidence suggesting that low levels of vitamin D may adversely affect the cardiovascular system.[4] A serum 25(OH)D level below 75 nmol/L (30 ng/L) is generally regarded as vitamin D insufficiency in both adults and children, while a level below 50 nmol/L (20 ng/L) is considered deficiency in both populations.[8,9] Vitamin D deficiency which is affected by multiple factors and appears to have an association with diverse cardiac diseases starting with its direct effect on the cardiac cell, its association with coronary artery disease (CAD), and its risk factors such as diabetes and hypertension (HTN); ending at last and probably not least in its relation with congestive heart failure (CHF). Similarly, there is some evidence that links vitamin deficiency to increased-risk of stroke.

CARDIOVASCULAR BIOLOGY AND VITAMIN D[10]

Both VDR and 1-a-hydroxylase that convert vitamin D into the hormonal 1, 25-OH-D2 (calcitriol) form are actively expressed in cardiovascular tissues including cardiomyocytes, endothelial, and vascular smooth muscle cells.

Cardiomyocytes

In ventricular myocytes isolated from neonatal rat hearts, calcitriol regulated the number of cells entering the synthesis phase of the cell cycle, therefore affecting subsequent maturation and differentiation. In addition, murine models lacking VDR exhibit increased ventricular mass, higher levels of atrial natriuretic peptide, in addition to cardiac metalloproteinases and fibroblast dyshomeostasis that precipitate a fibrotic extracellular matrix. These changes eventually lead to ventricular dilation and impaired electromechanical coupling. Moreover, rats fed a vitamin D-deficient diet show higher systolic pressure and serum creatine phosphokinase that parallel decreases in calcium levels. All these effects are readily corrected by vitamin D analogs. Finally, vitamin D analogs attenuated the left ventricular hypertrophy associated with increased sodium load in salt sensitive rats via modulation of several protein kinase pathways.

Vascular Endothelial Cells

Endothelial cells express VDR and its activation affects the development of immature cells, partly by modulating response elements in the vascular endothelial growth factor (VEGF) promoter. While VDR is upregulated under stress in endothelial cells, active vitamin D analogs decrease cytokine induced expression of adhesion molecules and protect against advanced glycation products. Furthermore, vitamin D metabolites reduced endothelium-dependent vascular smooth muscle contractions and vascular tone in hypertensive models, an effect mediated by affecting calcium influx across endothelial cells.

Renin-angiotensin-aldosterone System

Renin expression was shown to be highly deregulated in VDR knockout murine models, despite maintenance of a normal electrolyte balance. Tonic scission of angiotensinogen sharply increased angiotensin II levels and resulted in hypertensive heart disease. Similar abnormalities were observed with defective calcitriol synthesis in a wild-type model, independent of calcium metabolism which were normalized following calcitriol administration. These findings suggest an active role for vitamin D in the pathogenesis of cardiovascular disorders and parallel results from clinical investigations.

ROLE OF VITAMIN D IN MODULATING ADAPTIVE IMMUNITY, VASCULAR INFLAMMATION, AND ENDOTHELIAL FUNCTION[10]

Other potential consequences of vitamin D metabolism on human vasculature derive from several lines of experimental investigation and include exacerbation of atherogenesis and acceleration of arterial calcification. For example, the established anti-lymphoproliferative effects of vitamin D extend to regulation of monocyte/macrophage differentiation and the concomitant response to and secretion of inflammatory cytokines. This in turn may determine monocyte infiltration and cholesterol retention in the vascular wall and may corroborate clinical evidence of increased plaque instability and incident myocardial infarctions in vitamin D-deficient patients in addition to the observed improvements in inflammatory biomarker levels in heart failure patients following vitamin D therapy. Additionally, aberrant vitamin D signaling induced in murine models caused extensive calcification of medium and small sized arteries, resembling human age-related Mönckeberg's disease. In humans, vitamin D deficiency independently predicted prevalence, incidence, and progression of coronary calcification in 374 diabetic patients over 6 years of follow-up. Similar to experimental studies that show endothelial cell function modulation by vitamin D analogs; indices of endothelial function and microvascular reactivity assessed as brachial artery flow-mediated dilation and reactive hyperemia index, respectively were independently correlated with 25(OH)D levels in a study we conducted in asymptomatic individuals (Table 1).

TABLE 1: Vitamin D deficiency and cardiovascular diseases[11]

Pathology	*Proposed Mechanism of Action*
Hypertensive vascular disease	• Increased intracellular calcium leading to decreased renin activity • Calcitriol suppression of renin promoter gene • Alteration of the sensitivity of vascular smooth muscle cells
Peripheral vascular disease and, Diabetes mellitus	• Increased calcification • Immunomodulatory effects by reducing tumor necrosis factor– α; parathyroid hormone, and interleukin-10 • Decreased insulin receptor expression leading to peripheral resistance of insulin • Effect on intracellular calcium levels leading to decreased insulin secretion
Lipid metabolism	• Increase peripheral insulin resistance contributing to high lipid profile • Statins may increase vitamin D levels by increasing 7-dehydrocholesterol • Increased vessel free radicals lead to oxidation of low-density lipoprotein and increased engulfment by macrophages, an early sign of atherosclerosis
Coronary artery disease	• Indirect effect through risk factor modification • Altering endothelial function • Increased coronary artery calcification
Heart failure	• Direct effect on myocardial contractility • Regulation of brain natriuretic peptide secretion • Reduction of left ventricular hypertrophy with effects on extracellular remodeling • Regulation of inflammatory cytokines • Secondary hyperparathyroidism which leads to vasodilatation and positive inotropic stimulation
Arrhythmias	• Direct myocardial substrate modification • Indirectly via calcium levels and metabolism at a cellular level

Vitamin D Deficiency and Hypertension

Vitamin D deficiency and HTN is associated with inappropriate stimulation of the renin-angiotensin-aldosterone system (RAAS). Calcitriol is known to be one of the negative endocrine regulators of RAAS. In VDR receptor knockout mice, HTN was more prevalent, probably secondary to the stimulation of RAAS as it was corrected by angiotensin-converting enzyme inhibitors and angiotensin II receptor antagonists. In several trials, calcitriol supplementation was shown to reduce plasma renin activity, angiotensin II levels, blood pressure, and myocardial hypertrophy. It has been demonstrated that regular exposure to ultraviolet B radiation increases circulating 25(OH)D above a level of 100 nmol/L and significantly reduces blood pressure by approximately 6 mm Hg in hypertensive patients with initial 25(OH)D levels of 26 nmol/L within an intervention period of 6 weeks.

So as per the current evidence, vitamin D is probably one of the mechanisms leading to HTN and its adverse effects and should always be taken into consideration while treating such cases.

Vitamin D Deficiency and Coronary Artery Disease

Many studies show an association of vitamin D deficiency with well-established atherosclerosis risk factors including obesity, glucose intolerance, metabolic syndrome, HTN, and hyperlipidemia. The Third National Health and Nutrition Examination Survey, a cross-sectional representative sample of the United States population, also showed a significant increase in the prevalence of HTN, diabetes mellitus, and hypertriglyceridemia, in patients with vitamin D levels less than 21 ng/mL compared to those with levels higher than 37 ng/mL. That association was further supported by a recent study from the University of Utah that linked vitamin D deficiency to an increased risk of hyperlipidemia, diabetes and HTN in vitamin D deficient individuals. The presumed role of vitamin D in the pathogenesis of CAD is not necessarily linked only to atherosclerosis, but may involve vascular calcification. The basis of this presumption comes from patients with end-stage renal disease. As a consequence of reduced renal calcitriol synthesis, in addition to other factors, secondary hyperparathyroidism emerges in the early stages of chronic kidney disease. In patients with end-stage renal disease, secondary hyperparathyroidism is considered an important risk factor in the pathogenesis of CAD leading to vascular calcification. In hemodialysis patients, the use of active vitamin D and synthetic vitamin D analogs has been shown to reduce the risk of death from cardiovascular disease (CVD). In the general population, the presence of vascular calcification is a predictor of poorer 5-year survival rates. Interestingly, the use of calcitriol was found to be inversely correlated with the extent of vascular calcification, independently from other risk factors for ischemic heart disease. Nonetheless, a recent study showed that vitamin D levels could be independently linked to the risk of CVD. In a cohort of 14,641 men and women living in Norfolk, United Kingdom, aged 42–82, during the period between 1997 and 2000, and who were followed upto 2012, an increase of 20-nmol/L 25(OH)D levels was associated with total mortality and for prevalence of CVD, even after adjustment for multiple variants in both men and women.

There is a growing enormous data of CAD with vitamin D deficiency as well as excess. CAD is definitely showing the importance of vitamin D as per the current data. So deficiency of the vitamin D has shown correlation with the CAD and its treatment in some of the quoted series has shown some improvement and positive influence.

Vitamin D Deficiency and Heart Failure

There is an increasing evidence that vitamin D deficiency may be an important factor in the pathogenesis of heart failure. Vitamin D deficiency seems to be linked to various mechanisms that play a significant role in the pathogenesis of CHF. These mechanisms include the activation of RAAS, the presence of oxidative stress in different tissues including the skin, skeletal muscles, heart, peripheral blood mononuclear cells, and activation of proinflammatory cytokines as interleukin (IL)-8 and tumor necrosis factor (TNF)-alpha. Vitamin D suppresses the proinflammatory state by downregulating nuclear factor-κB activity and decreasing IL-6, IL-12, interferon-c, and TNF-α production. At the same time, it increases anti-inflammatory cytokines. Vitamin D deficiency therefore, leads to a reduction in the downregulation of nuclear factor-κB activity, a decrease in IL-10 production, and an increase in IL-6, IL-12, interferon-c, and TNF-α production, all of which lead to the proinflammatory state of CHF (Flowchart 1).

Vitamin D deficiency seems to be linked to various mechanisms that play a significant role in the pathogenesis of CHF. These mechanisms include the activation of RAAS, the presence of oxidative stress in different tissues including the skin, skeletal muscles, heart, and peripheral blood mononuclear cells, and activation of proinflammatory cytokines as IL-8 and TNF-α. So vitamin D has a definite role in heart failure and its proper management is important in all cases of heart failure and it shows positive role of vitamin D in a subset of patients.

The summary of interventional studies evaluating the effect of vitamin D supplements on CVD risk is given in Table 2.[12]

Flow chart 1: Vitamin D deficiency role in the pathogenesis of congestive heart failure

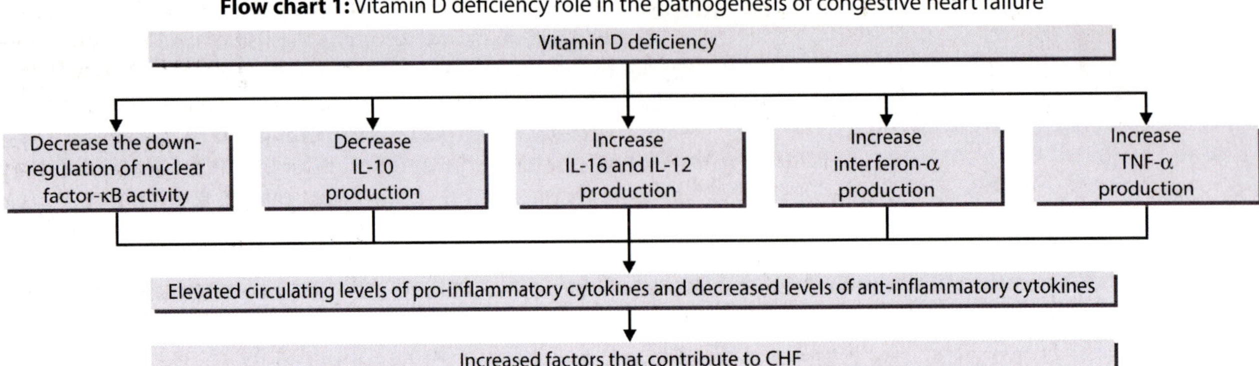

Abbreviations: CHF, congestive heart failure; TNF-α, tumor necrosis factor-alpha; IL, interleukin

TABLE 2: Summary of interventional studies evaluating the effect of vitamin D supplements on cardiovascular disease risk[12]

Source	Study design	Condition	Population (cases)	Main outcome(s)
Harris et al.	Randomized, placebo-controlled trial	Vitamin D (2,000 IU/day) for 16 weeks	57 African American adults	Vitamin D supplements (2,000 IU/day) for 16 weeks were effective at improving vascular endothelial function in African American adults
Zittermann et al.	Randomized, placebo-controlled trial	Vitamin D (83 µg/day) for 1 year	200 overweight subjects (mean 25[OH]D_3 levels = 12 ng/mL)	Vitamin D supplements enhanced the beneficial effects of weight loss on CVD risk including decreasing lipid levels and inflammation
Sun et al.	Cross-sectional (prospective study)	Vitamin D (≥600 IU/day) or vitamin D (<100 IU/day)	2,280,324 person-years of follow-up	Higher intake of vitamin D was associated with a lower risk of CVD in men but not in women
Cauley et al.	Cross-sectional (prospective study)	Calcium plus vitamin D supplementation	29,862 postmenopausal women	There was no difference in CVD morbidity between groups
Ponda et al.	Randomized, placebo-controlled trial	Vitamin D (50,000 IU/week) for 8 weeks	151 vitamin D-deficient (25[OH]D levels <20 ng/mL) patients	Correcting vitamin D deficiency in the short-term did not improve the lipid profile
Yiu et al.	Randomized, placebo-controlled trial	Vitamin D (5,000 IU/day) for 12 weeks	100 type 2 diabetes mellitus patients	12 weeks of oral supplementation with vitamin D did not significantly affect vascular function or serum biomarkers of inflammation and oxidative stress
Stricker et al.	Randomized, placebo-controlled trial	Vitamin D (100,000 IU/single oral dose)	76 patients with peripheral arterial disease	Vitamin D supplementation did not influence endothelial function, arterial stiffness, coagulation, or inflammation parameters
Gepner et al.	Randomized, placebo-controlled trial	Vitamin D (2,500 IU/day) for 4 months	114 subjects	Vitamin D supplementation did not improve endothelial function, arterial stiffness, or inflammation

Abbreviations: 25[OH]D, 25-hydroxyvitamin D; CVD, cardiovascular disease

TREATMENT AND PREVENTION OF VITAMIN D DEFICIENCY AND ROLE IN CARDIOVASCULAR DISEASE[10]

In healthy individuals, prevention of vitamin D deficiency can be readily achieved by a combination of casual sunlight exposure, consumption of fatty fish or fish oils in addition to fortified foods and/or supplements. While the current recommended dietary allowance of vitamin D in the United States ranges between 400 IU/day and 800 IU/day as much as 2,000 IU/day may be needed to maintain sufficient 25(OH)D levels (≥30 ng/mL) in at-risk adults. As most diets generally provide less than the recommended daily allowance of vitamin D, pharmacological supplementation with vitamin D2 or D3 is therefore, often required particularly in locations where few foods are fortified with vitamin D or in individuals with

Flow chart 2: The relationship between vitamin D levels and the clinical and laboratory parameters of congestive heart failure

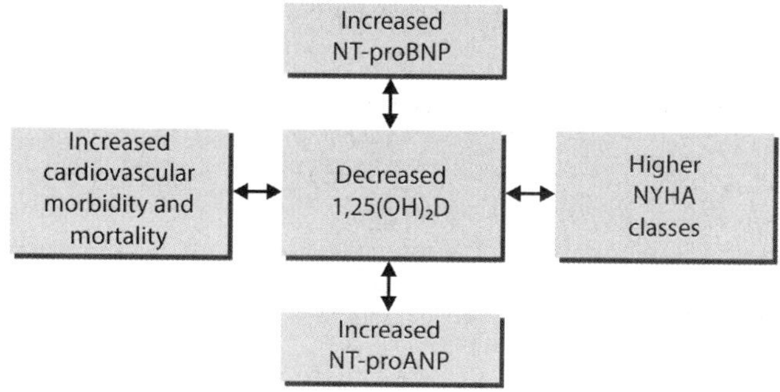

Abbreviations: 25(OH)D, 25-hydroxyvitamin D; NYHA, New York Heart Association; NT-proANP, N-terminal proatrial natriuretic peptide; NT-proBNP, N-terminal B-type natriuretic peptide

increasing risk factors. Importantly while an inverse linear dose-response relationship between 25(OH)D and CVD risk exists at levels between 20 nmol/L and 60 nmol/L (≈8–24 ng/mL), higher serum levels were not associated with a definitive increase or decrease in CVD risk (Flow chart 2). Thus, whereas vitamin D sufficiency confers a protective CVD effect compared with deficiency, further increases in 25(OH)D by means of pharmacological supplementation may have no effects on CVD. For treatment of documented vitamin D deficiency, a recent practice guideline statement by The Endocrine Society recommends oral administration of 50,000 IU/week of either vitamin D2 or D3 for 8 weeks, followed by daily maintenance doses between 1,500 IU and 2,000 IU. Both loading and maintenance doses may be folds higher to in those with increasing risks for the development or recurrence of vitamin D deficiency. Concurrent calcium supplementation is a key component of effective therapy, and a preventative strategy should always address underlying causes, if possible.

ONGOING TRIAL: VITAL TRIAL

Despite continued appreciation of the potential role of vitamin D and omega-3 fatty acids in the prevention of cancer and CVD, there remain no completed large-scale, randomized trials of these agents for the primary prevention of cancer or CVD in a population that has not been selected on the basis of elevated risk. The Vitamin D and omega-3 Trial (VITAL) is a 2 × 2 factorial randomized, double-blind, placebo-controlled trial of the benefits and risks of vitamin D [vitamin D3 (cholecalciferol), 2,000 IU/day] and marine omega-3 fatty acids (Omacor® fish oil, a 1 g/day) in the primary prevention of cancer and CVD among 25,875 men and women, aged greater than or equal to 50 and greater than or equal to 55 years respectively. Randomization began in November 2011 and was completed in March 2014. This report will describe the rationale for the trial and currently available randomized trial data, summarize related ongoing large-scale trials, and provide a brief overview of study design, and an update on randomization milestones, racial/ethnic diversity, biorepository activities, in-depth phenotyping of a subcohort, and ancillary studies. Results are awaited as of now.

Vitamin D deficiency is a highly prevalent condition and is independently associated with most CVD risk factors and to CVD morbidity and mortality. Despite a large body of experimental, cross-sectional, and prospective evidence that implicate vitamin D deficiency in the pathogenesis of CVD, the causality of this relationship remains to be established. Despite the widespread prevalence of vitamin D deficiency, the strong and consistent association with CVD risk factors and mortality, as well as biological plausibility from mechanistic laboratory studies, it is still unclear whether vitamin D is just a marker for increased CVD risk or actually plays a role in the pathogenesis of CVD. Potential confounders to the observational data include obesity, physical activity, sun exposure, and nutritional status.

CONCLUSION

Abundant evidence now points to the numerous cardioprotective functions of vitamin D. Restoring vitamin D to normal levels has been found to help reduce inflammation, normalize blood pressure, and improve insulin sensitivity—all factors that reduce heart disease risk. Vitamin D deficiency has been shown to diminish contractile function of heart muscle cells, contribute to endothelial dysfunction, distort heart muscle structure (triggering hypertrophy or abnormal heart muscle growth), and increase smooth muscle growth in the coronary artery wall—a process that leads to atherosclerotic plaque formation. Low levels of serum 25(OH)D have been linked with CHF, a condition in which the heart is unable to keep up with the body's demands for blood and oxygen. A recent analysis showed that individuals with low serum levels of vitamin D had higher rates of high blood pressure, diabetes, and elevated triglycerides than those with higher vitamin D levels.

REFERENCES

1. Yuan W, Pan W, Kong J, et al. 1,25-Dihydroxyvitamin D3 suppresses renin gene transcription by blocking the activity of the cyclic AMP response element in the renin gene promoter. J Biol Chem. 2007;282(41):29821-30.
2. Revelli A, Massobrio M, Tesarik J. Nongenomic effects of 1 alpha, 25-dihydroxyvitamin D(3). Trends Endocrinol Metab. 1998;9(10):419-22.

3. Zanello LP, Norman A. 1 Alpha, 25(OH)2 vitamin D3 actions on ion channels in osteoblasts. Steroids. 2006;71(4):291-7.
4. Von der Recke P, Hansen MA, Hassager C. The association between low bone mass at the menopause and cardiovascular mortality. Am J Med. 1999;106(3):273-8.
5. Aoyagi K, Ross PD, Orloff J, et al. Low bone density is not associated with aortic calcification. Calcif Tissue Int. 2001;69(1):20-4.
6. Samelson EJ, Kiel DP, Broe KE, et al. Metacarpal cortical area and risk of coronary heart disease: the Framingham Study. Am J Epidemiol. 2004;159(6):589-95.
7. Rajasree S, Rajpal K, Kartha CC, et al. Serum 25-hydroxyvitamin D3 levels are elevated in South Indian patients with ischemic heart disease. Eur J Epidemiol. 2001;17(6):567-71.
8. Holick MF. Vitamin D deficiency. N Engl J Med. 2007;357(3):266-81.
9. Contreras JJ, Hiestand B, O'Neill JC, et al. Vitamin D deficiency in children with fractures. Pediatr Emerg Care. 2014;30(11):777-81.
10. Al Mheid I, Patel RS, Tangpricha V, et al. Vitamin D and cardiovascular disease: is the evidence solid? Eur Heart J. 2013;34(48):3691-8.
11. Fanari Z, Hammami S, Hammami MB, et al. Vitamin D deficiency plays an important role in cardiac disease and affects patient outcome: Still a myth or a fact that needs exploration? J Saudi Heart Assoc. 2015;27(4):264-71.
12. Yin K, Agrawal DK. Vitamin D and inflammatory diseases. J Inflamm Res. 2014;7:69-87.

CHAPTER

Omega-3 Fatty Acids and Cardiovascular Disease

Pawan K Sharma, HK Chopra

INTRODUCTION

Omega-3 fatty acids are a class of polyunsaturated fatty acids and have a double carbon-to-carbon bond in the third position from the omega (or methyl, or *n*) end of the fatty acid chain. There are four main omega-3 fatty acids of clinical importance (Table 1). Most of the cardiovascular research on the omega-3 family has been on eicosapentaenoic acid (EPA), docosahexaenoic acid (DHA), and alpha-linolenic acid (ALA). EPA and DHA are found primarily in fatty fish.

Docosapentaenoic acid (DPA), a long-chain omega-3 fatty acid metabolite of EPA is present in smaller amounts in fish.[1] Circulating DPA levels correlate weakly with fish consumption[2] suggesting that DPA levels in humans are predominantly determined by endogenous metabolism rather than diet. Although DPA may have relevant physiological effects,[1] relatively little is known about its clinical effects. A few studies have observed inverse associations between circulating DPA and risk of coronary events.[2,3] In addition to omega-3 fatty acid, fish provide specific proteins, vitamin D, selenium, and other minerals and elements.[4-6]

Alpha-linolenic acid is the plant-derived omega-3 fatty acid found in flaxseed, walnuts and soybeans. ALA is an essential dietary fatty acid and cannot be synthesized in humans. A small amount of ALA can be converted to EPA and EPA to DHA in humans. About 0.2–8% of ALA is converted to EPA with conversion being higher in women and 0–4% of ALA to DHA.[7-9] Thus, the tissue and circulating levels of EPA and DHA levels primarily depend on the dietary source. Some observational studies suggest that ALA might have cardiovascular benefits, but overall evidence remains inconclusive.[10,11] Currently, it is not known whether ALA is active itself or only via its metabolites. Thus, plant sources of omega-3 fatty acids cannot currently be considered as a replacement for seafood-derived omega-3 fatty acid.[10] Additional studies of ALA's effects are needed because of the lower cost and greater potential global supply of ALA as opposed to EPA plus DHA. In this review, the term omega-3 fatty acid refers to EPA and DHA only.

There are some contaminants in certain fish species which include methylmercury, dioxins, and polychlorinated biphenyls (PCBs) (Table 2).[12-14] In most fish species, mercury levels are quite low; few species contain moderate levels (e.g. albacore tuna approximately 0.36 μg/g) or higher levels of 1 μg/g [e.g. tilefish (golden bass), swordfish, shark, Gulf of Mexico King mackerel[15]]. Mercury exposure from fish consumption has no relations with higher cardiovascular disease (CVD) risk.[16] Most commercially sold fish contain low levels of PCBs and dioxins, and overall fish consumption contributes a minority of dietary exposure compared with other foods.[17] In general population, the health benefits of modest fish consumption significantly outweigh the potential risks due to these contaminants.[10,18]

In general, nursing or pregnant women should limit their consumption of certain fish, as some fish (but not fish oil) contain high levels of mercury. The highest levels of mercury are usually found in the larger, older predatory fish such as swordfish, tilefish and mackerel and the United States Food and Drug Administration (USFDA) advises

TABLE 1: Omega-3 fatty acids

Omega-3 fatty acid	*Source*
Eicosapentaenoic acid (EPA)	Fatty fish
Docosahexaenoic acid (DHA)	Fatty fish
Docosapentaenoic acid (DPA)	Fatty fish
Alpha-linolenic acid (ALA)	*Plant source only*: Flaxseed, walnuts, and soybeans

TABLE 2: Common contaminants in fish

S. No.	*Contaminants*
1.	Methylmercury
2.	Dioxins
3.	Polychlorinated biphenyls (PCBs)

women who are nursing or pregnant to avoid these fish completely. Tuna, red snapper and orange roughy are lower in mercury, but nursing or pregnant women should still limit consumption of these fish to 12 oz per week.[19]

EFFECTS OF OMEGA-3 FATTY ACIDS ON VARIOUS RISK FACTORS (TABLE 3)

Effects on Plasma Triglycerides

Hypertriglyceridemia is believed to increase the risk of coronary heart disease (CHD) by two mechanisms. First, triglyceride-rich lipoproteins such as very low-density lipoprotein (VLDL) and intermediate-density lipoprotein (IDL) are thought to be atherogenic. Secondly, triglyceride-lipoprotein metabolism involves competition with high-density lipoprotein (HDL) leading to a decrease in HDL production and to denser LDL particles.[20] The omega-3 fatty acids lower triglyceride levels and the mechanisms include reduced fatty acid availability for triglyceride synthesis due to decreased de novo lipogenesis (DNL) which is the process of converting carbohydrates into fat, increased fatty acid beta-oxidation, and reduced delivery of nonesterified fatty acids to the liver, reduced hepatic enzyme activity for triglyceride synthesis, and increased hepatic synthesis of phospholipids rather than triglycerides.[21-23] Another proposed mechanism is that EPA and DHA increase the activity of lipoprotein lipase leading to an increase in chylomicron clearance. Khan et al.[24] showed that lipoprotein lipase activity increased in patients who received omega-3 fatty acids 3 g/day for 6 weeks. The degree of triglyceride-lowering is linearly dependent on the dose of omega-3 fatty acid but has variable individual response including greater absolute reductions among individuals with higher baseline levels. Habitual consumption of omega-3 fatty acid over time reduces hepatic DNL, reduces hepatic steatosis and hepatic insulin resistance. This could partly contribute to lower cardiovascular risk.[25,26]

TABLE 3: Possible effects of omega-3 fatty acids

Factor	*Effect*	*Clinical implications*
Triglycerides	Decrease	May reduce atherogenesis
Heart rate	Decrease	May reduce blood pressure
Systolic/diastolic blood pressure	Decrease	Improve diastolic filling and augments vagal tone, arterial compliance improved
Platelet aggregation and thrombosis	Decrease	Inhibit arachidonic acid pathway, may have antithrombotic effect
Inflammation	Decreased	Decreased eicosanoids, leukotriene E4, reduce inflammation
Endothelial/ autonomic function	Improved	Decreased E-selectin, reduces VCAM-1, decreased intercellular adhesion molecules. May promote arterial dilatation and improve endothelial function
Cardiac filling and myocardial efficiency	Improved	Augments early and late diastolic filling. Benefit in congestive heart failure
Insulin resistance and diabetes	Unclear effect	Unclear clinical effect
Plaque	Stabilizes	Thick plaque cap. Stabilize coronary artery plaque
Restenosis	No effect	
Arrhythmias—atrial or ventricular	Reduced	Act via ion channels. May have role in preventing sudden death

Abbreviations: VCAM-1, vascular cellular adhesion molecule 1

Advantage of Fish Oil plus a Statin

Statin therapy is a very effective in lowering LDL-C but has modest effects on triglycerides. Omega-3 fatty acids effectively reduce triglycerides but have been known to increase LDL-C levels. This net LDL-C increase averaged around 10 mg/dL.[27] However, despite the net effect of an increase in LDL-C, it is hypothesized that the larger LDL particles produced by omega-3 fatty acid treatment may be less atherogenic.[28] The effectiveness of combined therapy in reducing triglycerides has been widely studied. In a randomized, placebo controlled trial[29] looking at the effectiveness of atorvastatin and EPA/DHA, 52 obese men were randomized to receive atorvastatin 40 mg/day, EPA/DHA 4 g/day both in combination or placebo. After 6 weeks, triglyceride levels decreased by 26% from baseline in the atorvastatin group, 25% in the EPA/DHA group and 40% in the combination therapy group ($P = 0.002$). LDL-C levels decreased to a similar degree with either atorvastatin monotherapy or combination therapy. Combination therapy may also lower the rate of major coronary events.

The Japan EPA Lipid Intervention Study (*JELIS*)[30] was an open label study which randomized more than 18,000 patients to receive either a statin alone or a statin plus

EPA 1,800 mg daily. It was the largest randomized trial to date comparing statin use alone and in combination with omega-3 fatty acids. The statins used were pravastatin 10 mg daily or simvastatin 5 mg daily; if hypercholesterolemia remained uncontrolled, these doses were doubled. There were 5,859 men and 12,786 postmenopausal women (mean age 61) with or without coronary artery disease who had total cholesterol levels of 251 mg/dL or greater. The mean baseline LDL-C level was 180 mg/dL. People who had an acute myocardial infarction in the past 6 months or unstable angina were excluded. The primary end point was any major coronary events defined as sudden death, fatal or nonfatal myocardial infarction, unstable angina, angioplasty, or coronary artery bypass grafting (CABG). After 5 years, patients with a history of coronary artery disease had a 19% lower rate of major coronary events in the EPA group than in the control group ($P = 0.011$). There was no significant difference between the two groups in the rates of sudden cardiac death (SCD), fatal myocardial infarction, nonfatal myocardial infarction, CABG, or percutaneous coronary interventions. The JELIS trial showed that combination therapy may reduce the risk of coronary events. The limitation of this study was that it was performed in Japan where people already have a high intake of fatty fish and the results may not be applicable to other countries.

Effects on Heart Rate and Blood Pressure

Omega-3 fatty acid consumption reduces resting heart rate (HR) and systolic and diastolic blood pressure.[31] The HR lowering could result from direct effects on cardiac electrophysiological pathways.[32] Omega-3 fatty acids may also lower HR by indirect effects such as by improving left ventricular diastolic filling or augmenting vagal tone.[33] In short-term trials, omega-3 fatty acid consumption increases nitric oxide production, mitigates vasoconstrictive responses to norepinephrine and angiotensin II, enhances vasodilatory responses, and improves arterial compliance.[34-38] Such effects could contribute to lowering of systemic vascular resistance and blood pressure. In a meta-analysis,[39] the reduction in blood pressure was estimated to be 2.1 mm Hg systolic and 1.6 mm Hg diastolic. The median intake of fish oil was 3.7 g/day. The largest reductions were in patients with known hypertension and those over age 45. These findings seem consistent with the hypothesis that omega-3 fatty acids affect the endothelium given that the arterial wall tends to become stiffer with age. Overall, however, the results of a number of studies show that fish oil supplementation is of limited clinical use in lowering blood pressure.

Effect on Platelet Aggregation (may reduce)

Arachidonic acid is an omega-6 fatty acid, i.e. metabolized into prostaglandins, leukotrienes and thromboxanes which are important for cell function. Many of these by-products (e.g. leukotriene B4) have inflammatory effects and others (e.g. prostaglandin I2 E2) promote arrhythmias. EPA and DHA competitively inhibit the arachidonic acid cascade leading to different by-products that promote vasodilation and inhibit platelet aggregation among other effects.[40] The impact of this effect in clinical practice is still unclear.

Effect on Thrombosis

Omega-3 fatty acids are considered to have antithrombotic effects because by inhibiting the arachidonic acid pathway, they increase bleeding times at very high doses (e.g. 15 g/day). Conversely in human trials omega-3 fatty acid consumption has no consistent effects on platelet aggregation or coagulation factors.[41,42] In a trial in 511 patients undergoing CABG who were receiving aspirin or warfarin, the bleeding time, and the number of bleeding episodes were no higher in those who were randomized to receive 4 g/day of omega-3 fatty acids daily than in a control group.[43] Harris[44] reviewed 19 studies of omega-3 fatty acids in patients undergoing CABG, carotid endarterectomy, or femoral artery catheterization, and none of the studies found a significantly increased risk of bleeding.

Effect on Inflammation

Although omega-3 fatty acid could alter several inflammatory pathways, it remains unclear whether such anti-inflammatory effects are clinically meaningful especially at usual dietary doses. It has been shown that omega-3 fatty acid supplementation reduce plasma and urine levels of eicosanoids such as leukotriene E_4.[45,46] Findings for other circulating inflammatory biomarkers such as interleukin-1-beta and tumor necrosis factor-alpha are mixed.[47-49] Fish oil has been proposed as an adjunctive therapy for inflammatory diseases such as rheumatoid arthritis,[50] and meta-analysis of placebo-controlled trials found that high-dose omega-3 fatty acid supplementation (1.7–9.6 g/day) reduced morning stiffness and joint pain in patients with rheumatoid arthritis.[51] EPA and DHA could also have local anti-inflammatory effects that might be difficult to detect with circulating biomarkers. Omega-3 fatty acids are precursors to resolvins, protectins, and other inflammation-resolving mediators that might have potent anti-inflammatory properties and assist in the resolution of inflammation.[52] Further studies are needed to study the influence of dietary fish consumption or usual fish oil supplement doses on levels of these inflammation-resolving mediators and the clinical relevance of such potential effects.

Effect on Endothelial and Autonomic Function

Several trials have demonstrated that omega-3 fatty acid supplementation improved flow-mediated arterial dilation which is a measure of endothelial function and health.[36,37,47,53,54] Omega-3 fatty acid consumption has also been noted to lower circulating markers of endothelial dysfunction such as E-selectin, vascular cell adhesion molecule-1, and intercellular adhesion molecule-1.[55,56] Thus, normalization of endothelial function could play a role in protective effects of omega-3 fatty acid against CVD. Overall these studies suggest that omega-3 fatty acid might improve autonomic function especially related to augmentation of vagal activity or tone, but further confirmation of such effects and their dose–responses is required.

Effect on Cardiac Filling and Myocardial Efficiency

Some animal experiments and human studies suggest that omega-3 fatty acid consumption improves cardiac filling and myocardial efficiency. In observational studies of habitual fish consumption; and in trials of fish oil in healthy adults and in patients with chronic heart failure omega-3 fatty acid consumption augments both early (energy-dependent) and late (compliance-dependent) left ventricular diastolic filling.[57-59] Such effects could lead to long-term improvements in ventricular compliance due to reduced systemic vascular resistance. In animal experiments and in a randomized controlled trial (RCT) in humans, fish oil consumption has shown to improve myocardial efficiency, reducing workload-specific myocardial oxygen demand without reducing peak performance.[60,61] In two placebo-controlled trials, omega-3 fatty acid consumption also improved left ventricular ejection fraction in patients with established heart failure.[58,62]

Effect on Insulin Resistance and Diabetes

In a meta-analysis of 26 RCTs, fish oil supplementation (2–22 g/day) slightly raised fasting glucose in patients with noninsulin-dependent diabetes and lowered fasting glucose in patients with insulin-dependent diabetes; hemoglobin A1c levels were not significantly affected.[63] Meta-analysis of RCTs found no overall effects of fish oil (0.9–18 g/day) on fasting glucose or hemoglobin A1c in patients with noninsulin-dependent diabetes.[64] Omega-3 fatty acid directly regulate hepatic genes, suppressing triglyceride production by means of decreased DNL and other possible effects.[21,25] It may be possible that this decrease in triglyceride synthesis from carbohydrates as a substrate could result in some increased shunting of carbohydrates and/or glycerol to glucose production which could raise fasting plasma glucose levels but reduce hepatic steatosis and insulin resistance and not adversely affect peripheral insulin resistance or systemic metabolic dysfunction.[26,65] Further investigation is needed, but at present it is unclear whether omega-3 fatty acid has clinically relevant effects on insulin resistance or diabetes risk in humans.

Effect on Plaque (may stabilize plaque)

In a study, 188 patients were randomized to receive fish oil supplements before carotid endarterectomy. It was found that the carotid plaque of patients who received the supplements had higher levels of EPA and DHA and had thicker fibrous caps and fewer signs of inflammation (e.g. macrophages) compared with a control group and a group that received sunflower oil. These findings show that omega-3 fatty acids are readily incorporated into atheromatous plaque and can help to stabilize it. An inference from this study is that fish oil could also play a role in stabilizing coronary artery plaque.[66]

Effect on Restenosis (no effect on restenosis)

These agents, however, have no effect on restenosis rates after coronary angioplasty as restenosis is mediated less by plaque formation than by intimal hyperplasia and negative remodeling within the endothelium. Even at high doses of 5 mg/day before angioplasty, omega-3 fatty acids failed to reduce the incidence of restenosis at 6 months.[67]

Effect on Arrhythmias

In vitro and animal experiments suggest that omega-3 fatty acid directly influence atrial and ventricular myocyte electrophysiology, potentially mediated by effects on membrane ion channels or cell-cell connexins.[68,69] Confirmation of such effects in humans has been limited by absence of reliable physiological measures or biomarkers to quantify antiarrhythmic potential. Several smaller trials have attempted to address this hypothesis by studying patients at higher risk for arrhythmias including patients with implantable cardioverter-defibrillators (ICDs) for recurrent tachyarrhythmias, patients with recurrent paroxysmal atrial fibrillation (AF), and patients undergoing cardiac surgery. Findings have been mixed with some trials demonstrating lower risk of arrhythmias and others finding with no significant effects.[70-72] Overall, clinically relevant antiarrhythmic effects of omega-3 fatty acid has remained unclear. It is also unclear whether such benefits if present are due to direct effects on myocyte electrophysiology or more indirect influences such as improvements in myocardial efficiency, autonomic tone, local inflammatory responses. The Gruppo Italiano per lo Studio della Sopravvivenza nell'Infarto Miocardico Prevenzione (GISSI-Prevention) trial[73] was a large randomized trial of fish oil therapy as secondary prevention. In this trial, 11,323 patients who had a myocardial infarction less than 3 months before enrolment were randomized to receive either EPA/DHA 850 mg daily, vitamin E, both or no treatment. The primary end points were death from any cause, nonfatal myocardial infarction and nonfatal stroke. At 3 months, 63 (1.1%) patients in the EPA/DHA group had died, compared with 88 (1.6%) in the no-treatment group, ($P = 0.037$), and the benefit persisted for the duration of the study. However, the difference between the groups in the rates of nonfatal myocardial infarction did not reach statistical significance. Vitamin E seemed to have no effect. EPA/DHA is thought to have prevented deaths in this study, not by reversing atherosclerosis, but rather by suppressing arrhythmias and inflammation. In support of this theory, Getz and Reardon[74] noted that in GISSI the treatment showed its maximal benefit on the incidence of sudden death by 9 months, whereas statin treatment takes 1–2 years to reach its maximal effect. This point suggests that the role of omega-3 fatty acids in secondary prevention will be different from that of statins. Several animal and human studies have shown that omega-3 fatty acid supplements reduce the incidence of sudden death and ventricular fibrillation[75] and prevent arrhythmias by stabilizing the myocardial membrane through interaction with voltage gated sodium and L-type calcium channels. During an ischemic event, the affected heart cells allow potassium ions to escape. Since potassium ions carry a positive charge, the resting membrane potential is increased, lowering the threshold for initiating an action potential through sodium channels and increasing the risk of fatal arrhythmias. It is hypothesized that omega-3 fatty acids inhibit sodium channels by being incorporated into the membrane phospholipid bilayer, increasing its fluidity and thereby affecting the sodium channel. This reduces membrane excitability and arrhythmic potential.[75] Mixed results were observed in large randomized clinical trials specifically looking at ventricular arrhythmias in patients with an ICD.[76,77] Raitt et al.[76] found that patients who recently received an ICD had higher rates of ventricular tachycardia and fibrillation, if they received EPA/DHA than if they received placebo, 65% versus 59% ($P = 0.07$). In contrast, Leaf et al.[77] reported a lower rate of ventricular arrhythmias with EPA/DHA than with placebo, 28% versus 39%. In another study, Calo et al.[78] randomized 160 patients to receive omega-3 fatty acids 2 g/day or placebo starting at least 5 days before elective coronary artery bypass surgery and continuing until discharge. The primary end point measured was the development of AF after surgery. The incidence of AF in the omega-3 fatty acid group was 15.2%, compared with 33% in the control group ($P = 0.013$). The experts generally believe that these agents may reduce arrhythmic events, but they lack clear evidence of their clinical effectiveness, and their use for such purposes is off-label.

TRIALS ON CARDIOVASCULAR OUTCOMES WITH OMEGA-3 FATTY ACID CONSUMPTION

Prevention of Cardiovascular Disease Mortality in Diabetes/Prediabetes

In the ORIGIN trial, the 12,536 patients randomized to omega-3 fatty acid or placebo were at high-risk of CVD with the majority having had a prior CHD event.[79] Supplementation with omega-3 fatty acids did not affect the risk of death resulting from cardiovascular causes or the other secondary cardiovascular outcomes. Available data do not support omega-3 fatty acid supplementation among patients with diabetes mellitus or prediabetes to prevent cardiovascular events. Overall the current evidence from RCTs suggests no benefit of omega-3 fatty acid supplementation among patients with or at risk for diabetes mellitus to prevent CVD (treatment not indicated: Class III—no benefit recommendation).[80]

Randomized Controlled Trials of Omega-3 Fatty Acid: Clinical Cardiovascular Events and Coronary Heart Disease Mortality

Several prospective observational studies and large RCTs indicate that consumption of fish or fish oil significantly reduces CHD mortality including fatal myocardial infarction and SCD, in populations with and without established CVD.[18,81,82] The final common pathway for most cardiac deaths is arrhythmia. *In vitro* and animal models have shown that omega-3 fatty acids stabilize partially depolarized ischemic myocytes reducing susceptibility to triggered ventricular arrhythmias and clinical reductions in cardiac death. Other physiologic benefits of omega-3 fatty acid on blood pressure, triglycerides, or inflammation could over many years or at higher doses alter chronic atherogenesis and/or acute plaque rupture, modestly lowering nonfatal coronary syndromes.[18,83] However, clinical effects on nonfatal coronary events are not yet established. The effects of omega-3 fatty acid on CHD do not differ by sex, age, or race/ethnicity. Prospective cohort studies among both men and women, in those of middle age and older adults, and in different races/ethnicities have demonstrated similar findings.[18] Women convert ALA to EPA in modestly greater amounts,[7] but the clinical significance of this is not established. Not all RCTs have demonstrated reductions in CHD mortality with omega-3 fatty acid consumption.[84-88] Although, the DART 2 trial,[87] an open-label, dietary advice trial among men with stable angina was adequately powered to detect reductions in CHD mortality with omega-3 fatty acid consumption but it had several limitations including lack of participant blinding, inadequate funding that interrupted recruitment over 7 years, little follow-up to reinforce dietary advice or evaluate long-term compliance, and no evaluation of changes in medications or other behaviors. Additionally, the control group and intervention groups were not provided similar dietary advice. These limitations make it difficult to interpret this trial's findings. The JELIS,[85] Alpha-Omega,[89] Omega,[86] and SU.FOL.OM3[88] trials were all underpowered to detect effects on CHD mortality, although the JELIS trial did find modest benefits for nonfatal coronary events. In the JELIS trial,[85] the risk reduction occurred from a reduction in unstable angina, CABG, or percutaneous transluminal coronary angioplasty. There was a little evidence of risk reduction in the hard end points of nonfatal MI and CHD death. Also due to lower than expected event rates, the Alpha–Omega trial compared the effects of low-dose EPA plus DHA (376 mg/day) with a combined control group that received either placebo or active treatment with the plant-derived omega-3 ALA (1.9 g/day). In this study, subjects also consumed relatively with high background dietary EPA plus DHA (median 120–130 mg/day) which could minimize effects of the additional low-dose omega-3 fatty acid supplement on the basis of evidence for a threshold of benefit for CHD mortality at approximately 250 mg/day.[18] Both the Omega and SU.FOL.OM3 trials were markedly underpowered.[85,88] Since there was a lack of consensus, therefore, majority of coauthors from American Heart Association Science Advisory concluded that treatment is not indicated (Class III: no benefit recommendation), a minority of coauthors concluded that treatment of these patients is reasonable (Class IIb recommendation).[80]

Secondary Prevention of CHD and SCD among Patients with Prevalent CHD

Five large RCTs evaluated the effects of omega-3 fatty acid supplementation on clinical cardiovascular events in patients with prior clinical CHD.[73,83,87,89,90] The average dose of omega-3 fatty acid was 1,000 mg/day and the average mean duration of the trial was 2 years. The cumulative findings from RCTs suggest that omega-3 fatty acid supplements may reduce CHD death possibly through a reduction in ischemia-induced SCD among patients with prior CHD, but the treatment does not reduce the incidence of recurrent nonfatal MI. Additionally given that the benefit likely outweighs any risk of treatment, the majority of coauthors from American Heart Association Science Advisory concluded that treatment with omega-3 fatty acid supplements is reasonable for the secondary prevention of CHD death (Class IIa recommendation); a minority of coauthors gave IIb recommendation.[80]

Ischemic Stroke

Meta-analyses of observational studies suggest that fish consumption reduces risk of ischemic stroke,[91] but stroke incidence has not been significantly affected in fish oil trials.[92] Reasons for these differing findings remain unclear, with possibilities including residual confounding (bias) in the observational studies, inadequate statistical power in the trials (which were not designed to evaluate stroke as an endpoint), insufficient duration of treatment in the trials, or benefits for stroke from other nutrients present in fish but not fish oil. Appropriately powered RCTs of fish or fish oil consumption and ischemic stroke are needed.

Primary Prevention of Stroke

Nine studies in a meta-analysis,[93] showed that there was little evidence of a reduction in stroke events in those treated with omega-3 fatty acid supplement. Overall, there is no benefit of omega-3 fatty acid supplementation as a means to reduce the risk of stroke among patients without a history of stroke (Class III: no benefit recommendation).[80]

Secondary Prevention of Stroke

Overall, there is no evidence of benefit of omega-3 fatty acid supplementation as a means to reduce the risk of stroke or other CVDs among patients with a prior stroke (no recommendation).[80]

Atrial Fibrillation

Some in vitro and animal studies suggest that omega-3 fatty acid could reduce onset of AF.[94,95] The possible mechanisms of such effects could be direct antiarrhythmic effects or favorable changes in left ventricular performance, autonomic tone, or inflammation. Estimated fish or dietary omega-3 fatty acid consumption was associated with lower AF incidence in some[96] but not in other[97,98] large observational cohorts. In a prospective evaluation of plasma omega-3 fatty acid biomarkers, DHA levels were inversely associated with incident AF.[99] Another trial demonstrated no effects of omega-3 fatty acid supplements on AF recurrence in 663 patients with pre-existing paroxysmal AF.[100] Due to these mixed results, it is still unclear whether omega-3 fatty acid can prevent AF.

Primary Prevention of Atrial Fibrillation

Since there are no data from large randomized, placebo-controlled RCTs of the effects of omega-3 fatty acid supplementation on the primary prevention of AF. On this basis, no recommendation for treatment with omega-3 fatty acid supplements can be made for primary prevention of AF.[80]

Secondary Prevention of Atrial Fibrillation in Patients with Prior Atrial Fibrillation

Results from multiple RCTs,[99,101,102] do not support omega-3 fatty acid supplementation to prevent recurrent AF (Class III: no benefit recommendation).[80]

Atrial Fibrillation after Cardiac Surgery

Overall results from a large placebo-controlled RCT,[103] do not show a benefit of omega-3 fatty acid supplementation as a means to prevent postoperative AF in patients undergoing cardiac surgery (Class III: no benefit recommendation).[80]

Recurrent Ventricular Tachyarrhythmias

Based partly on antiarrhythmic effects in animal experiments, few placebo-controlled RCTs have evaluated whether omega-3 fatty acids reduce recurrent ventricular tachycardia or fibrillation (VT/VF) in patients with ICDs and pre-existing VT/VF. One of these trials showed 31% reduction in definite or probable recurrent VT/VF (p = 0.03),[104] whereas the other showed no statistically significant effects.[105] Heterogeneity of results could relate to varying patient populations or omega-3 fatty acid dosing (from 0.8 g/day to 2.6 g/day EPA + DHA). Overall, the relatively small sizes (n = 200–546) and brief treatment durations (1–2 years) of these trials limit definitive conclusions for effects of omega-3 fatty acid on recurrent VT/VF in patients with ICDs. Benefits seen in at least one of these trials, when considered with in vitro and animal-experimental evidence, lend further support to antiarrhythmic effects of omega-3 fatty acid. Confirmation of such effects would be clinically important for this patient subset.

Congestive Heart Failure

Primary Prevention of Heart Failure

To date, no published RCTs have assessed the effect of omega-3 fatty acid supplements on the primary prevention of heart failure. On this basis, no recommendation for treatment with omega-3 fatty acid supplements can be made for the primary prevention of heart failure.[80]

Secondary Prevention of Outcomes in Patients with Heart Failure

Fish or dietary omega-3 fatty acid consumption has been associated with lower incidence of heart failure in few prospective observational studies.[106,107] An investigation using EPA as circulating biomarkers found this relationship to be strongest, with 50% lower incidence of congestive heart failure (CHF) in the highest versus lowest quartile.[108] In a double-blind, placebo-controlled clinical RCT among nearly 7,000 patients with established heart failure, omega-3 fatty acid supplementation (1 g/day) reduced total mortality by 8% (p = 0.009),[90] accompanied by significant improvements in left ventricular ejection fraction,[58] when given in addition to maximal modern drug therapies. On the basis of this trial, recommendations for fish consumption or fish oil use should be considered in patients with established heart failure. A large RCT[109] trial showed that the omega-3 fatty acid supplements reduced the risk of total mortality by 9% and the risk of cardiovascular-related hospitalizations or death by 8%. It should be noted that 91% of the patients had heart failure with reduced ejection fraction (LVEF < 40%). Based on this trial, omega-3 fatty acid supplements is reasonable among patients with heart failure with reduced ejection fraction (Class IIa recommendation). RCTs are needed among patients with heart failure and preserved ejection fraction.[80]

DIETARY GUIDELINES

Dietary guidelines for omega-3 fatty acid consumption are not different by sex or race/ethnicity (Table 4). The 2010 US Dietary Guidelines for Americans recommended that individuals at both higher and average CVD risk can consume two servings of seafood per week (4 oz per serving), with types of fish selected to provide an average of at least 250 mg/day EPA plus DHA (1,750 mg/week).[10] People with known coronary artery disease should take in 1 g of EPA/DHA per day, according to the American Heart Association.[110] Generic 1-g fish oil supplements may contain variable amounts of DHA and EPA, and some may have less than 300 mg. Therefore, buyers need to carefully examine the label of over-the-counter fish oil supplements. Data are insufficient on

TABLE 4: Dietary recommendations of omega-3 fatty acids

Subject	Recommendation
Healthy person	250 mg/day EPA + DHA Two servings of oily fish per week
Patients with known CAD	1 g/day EPA + DHA
Sex/race/ethnicity	Same recommendation as above
Pregnancy	Avoid high-mercury fish consumption

Abbreviations: CAD, coronary artery disease; EPA, eicosapentaenoic acid; DHA, docosahexaenoic acid

relative importance of EPA versus DHA or any specific "ratio" of their intakes for CVD benefits, and thus guidelines are based on their combined consumption. For women who are or might become pregnant and nursing mothers and young children, additional specific recommendations are available for avoidance of selected higher-mercury fish species[10] as well as for minimum DHA consumption[111] to optimize brain development in their children.

Fish versus Fish Oil

Most studies of CHD death in generally healthy populations have evaluated fish consumption, not fish oil supplementation. Fish contain several potentially beneficial nutrients not contained in fish oil. Thus, we agree with clinical and policy recommendations that focus on dietary omega-3 fatty acid from fish consumption rather than from supplements. For individuals who cannot consume sufficient amounts of fish or who consume fish but wish to further supplement their dietary omega-3 fatty acid consumption, use of fish oil is reasonable. Many over-the-counter supplements and few prescription formulations are available. Depending on the brand, the combined content of EPA plus DHA per 1 g capsule varies from approximately 300 mg to 850 mg.[112,113] Fish oil supplements contain no mercury (which is tightly protein-bound) and contain low absolute quantities of dioxins/PCBs. Thus, the choice among different brands can be determined by other factors such as price, availability, and taste for flavored brands. If significant triglyceride-lowering is a goal, then concentrated over-the-counter or prescription formulations are preferable to facilitate sufficiently high doses (>3 g/day EPA + DHA) with reasonable daily numbers of capsules. A common symptom from fish oil is "fishy" taste or eructation. Taking the capsule frozen, switching to a different formulation, or taking the capsule with meals or at a different time of day can minimize this symptom in most people.

CLINICAL IMPLICATIONS AND RECOMMENDATIONS

Although some RCTs have questioned the benefits of omega-3 supplementation to prevent clinical CVD events, we make the following recommendations (Table 5):

TABLE 5: Recommendation for clinical use of omega-3 fatty acid supplementation for prevention of cardiovascular events.

Indication	Recommendation/class of recommendation
Primary prevention of CHD	No recommendation
Prevention of CVD mortality in DM/ prediabetes	Treatment not indicated (III)
Prevention of CHD among high CVD risk patients	Treatment not indicated (III)
Secondary prevention of CHD and SCD among patients with prevalent CHD	Treatment is reasonable (IIa)
Primary prevention of stroke	Treatment not indicated (III)
Secondary prevention of stroke	No recommendation
Primary prevention of heart failure	No recommendation
Secondary prevention of outcomes in patients with heart failure	Treatment is reasonable (IIa)
Primary prevention of AF	No recommendation
Secondary prevention of AF in patients with prior AF	Treatment not indicated (III)
AF after cardiac surgery	Treatment not indicated (III)

Abbreviations: AF, atrial fibrillation; CHD, coronary heart disease; CVD, cardiovascular disease; DM, diabetes mellitus; SCD, sudden cardiac death

- Treatment with omega-3 fatty acid supplements is not recommended in the general population who are not at high risk, including those with diabetes and prediabetes.
- Omega-3 fatty acid supplementation is reasonable for secondary prevention of CHD death in patients with a recent CHD event such as a recent MI. Even a 10% reduction in CHD mortality would justify treatment with a relatively safe therapy.
- Treatment with omega-3 fatty acid supplements is not recommended to prevent incident stroke among patients at high CVD risk or recurrent stroke and recurrent AF.
- No recommendations can be made for primary prevention of CHD, heart failure, and AF because there are no RCTs related to primary prevention.
- Omega-3 fatty acid supplementation can be considered for patients with heart failure with reduced ejection fraction.
- Omega-3 fatty acid supplementation is not recommended to prevent postoperative AF in patients undergoing cardiac surgery.

CONCLUSION

Omega-3 fatty acid consumption improves vascular and cardiac hemodynamics, triglycerides, and possibly endothelial function, autonomic control, inflammation, thrombosis, and arrhythmia. Not all trials of omega-3 fatty acid have demonstrated reductions in CVD, but several clinical trials have documented significant benefits. When combined with the evidence from observational studies, the documented effects on risk factors in short-term trials, and the experimental and mechanistic evidence, it is clear that omega-3 fatty acid are bioactive nutrients that play an important role in cardiovascular health, in particular for reducing risk of cardiac mortality. Various omega-3 fatty acid trials demonstrated inconclusive results and had several limitations. These included small number of patients enrolled, underpowered trials, selection bias and lack of patient blinding, inadequate funding to support the trials, inconsistent dietary advice, insufficient duration and follow up of trials. Appropriately designed and powered clinical trials are needed to assess effects of omega-3 fatty acid on cardiovascular endpoints, including nonfatal coronary events, ischemic stroke, recurrent ventricular arrhythmias, AF, and heart failure. Additional studies should also address the role of ALA and DPA in improving CVD risk factors and outcomes. As a part of routine healthier dietary advice which includes fruits, vegetables, whole grains, nuts, vegetable oils, and dairy,[114] the physicians should also recommend fish consumption for their patients. The government and public health agencies should implement strategies to improve attainment of the recommended levels of fish and omega-3 fatty acid consumption to reduce population burdens of CHD mortality and sudden cardiac death.

REFERENCES

1. Kaur G, Cameron-Smith D, Garg M, et al. Docosapentaenoic acid (22:5n-3): a review of its biological effects. Prog Lipid Res. 2011;50(1):28-34.
2. Sun Q, Ma J, Campos H, et al. Blood concentrations of individual long-chain n-3 fatty acids and risk of nonfatal myocardial infarction. Am J Clin Nutr. 2008;88(1):216-23.
3. Oda E, Hatada K, Katoh K, et al. A case-control pilot study on n-3 polyunsaturated fatty acid as a negative risk factor for myocardial infarction. Int Heart J. 2005;46(4):583-91.
4. Roos N, Wahab MA, Chamnan C, et al. The role of fish in food-based strategies to combat vitamin A and mineral deficiencies in developing countries. J Nutr. 2007;137(4):1106-9.
5. Fox TE, Van den Heuvel EG, Atherton CA, et al. Bioavailability of selenium from fish, yeast and selenate: a comparative study in humans using stable isotopes. Eur J Clin Nutr. 2004;58(2):343-9.
6. Holden JM, Lemar LE, Exler J. Vitamin D in foods: development of the US Department of Agriculture database. Am J Clin Nutr. 2008;87(4):1092S-6S.
7. Burdge G. Alpha-linolenic acid metabolism in men and women: nutritional and biological implications. Curr Opin Clin Nutr Metab Care. 2004;7(2):137-44.
8. Burdge GC, Finnegan YE, Minihane AM, et al. Effect of altered dietary n-3 fatty acid intake upon plasma lipid fatty acid composition, conversion of [13C] alpha-linolenic acid to longer-chain fatty acids and partitioning towards beta-oxidation in older men. Br J Nutr. 2003;90(2):311-21.
9. Burdge GC, Jones AE, Wootton SA. Eicosapentaenoic and docosapentaenoic acids are the principal products of alpha-linolenic acid metabolism in young men. Br J Nutr. 2002;88(4): 355-63.
10. U.S. Department of Agriculture, U.S. Department of Health and Human Services. Dietary Guidelines for Americans, 2010, 7th edition. Washington, DC: U.S. Government Printing Office; 2010.
11. Mozaffarian D. Does alpha-linolenic acid intake reduce the risk of coronary heart disease? A review of the evidence. Altern Ther Health Med. 2005;11(3):24-30, quiz 31, 79.
12. U.S. Environmental Protection Agency (2010). Mercury Study Report to Congress. [online] Available from *http://www.epa.gov/mercury/report.htm.* [Accessed August, 2017].
13. National Center for Environmental Assessment, U.S. Environmental Protection Agency (2010). Dioxin and related compounds. [online] Available from *http://cfpub.epa.gov/ncea/CFM/nceaQFind.cfm?keyword=Dioxin.* [Accessed August, 2017].
14. U.S. Environmental Protection Agency. (2010). Polychlorinated biphenyls (PCBs). [online] Available from *http://www.epa.gov/epawaste/hazard/tsd/pcbs/index.htm.* [Accessed August, 2017].
15. Mozaffarian D, Shi P, Morris JS, et al. Mercury exposure and risk of cardiovascular disease in two U.S. cohorts. N Engl J Med. 2011;364(12):1116-25.
16. Schecter A, Cramer P, Boggess K, et al. Intake of dioxins and related compounds from food in the U.S. population. J Toxicol Environ Health A. 2001;63(1):1-18.
17. FAO/WHO. (2010). Joint FAO/WHO expert consultation on the risks and benefits of fish consumption. [online] Available from *http://www.globefish.org/upl/Health/files/risk%20and%20benefits%20of%20fish%20consumption.pdf.* [Accessed August, 2017].
18. Mozaffarian D, Rimm EB. Fish intake, contaminants, and human health: evaluating the risks and the benefits. JAMA. 2006;296(15):1885-99.
19. U.S. Food and Drug Administration (2009). Mercury in fish: cause for concern? [online] Available from *www.fda.gov/fdac/reprints/mercury.html.* [Accessed August, 2017].
20. Jacobson TA. Secondary prevention of coronary artery disease with omega-3 fatty acids. Am J Cardiol. 2006;98(4A):61i-70i.
21. Faeh D, Minehira K, Schwarz JM, et al. Effect of fructose overfeeding and fish oil administration on hepatic de novo lipogenesis and insulin sensitivity in healthy men. Diabetes. 2005;54(7):1907-13.
22. Rivellese AA, Maffettone A, Iovine C, et al. Long-term effects of fish oil on insulin resistance and plasma lipoproteins in NIDDM patients with hypertriglyceridemia. Diabetes Care. 1996;19(11):1207-13.
23. Jump DB. Fatty acid regulation of hepatic lipid metabolism. Curr Opin Clin Nutr Metab Care. 2011;14(2):115-20.
24. Khan S, Minihane AM, Talmud PJ, et al. Dietary long-chain n-3 PUFAs increase LPL gene expression in adipose tissue of subjects with an atherogenic lipoprotein phenotype. J Lipid Res. 2002;43(6):979-85.
25. Tanaka N, Zhang X, Sugiyama E, et al. Eicosapentaenoic acid improves hepatic steatosis independent of PPARalpha activation through inhibition of SREBP-1 maturation in mice. Biochem Pharmacol. 2010;80(10):1601-12.
26. Masterton GS, Plevris JN, Hayes PC. Review article: omega-3 fatty acids- a promising novel therapy for non-alcoholic fatty liver disease. Aliment Pharmacol Ther. 2010;31(7):679-92.
27. Harris WS. N-3 fatty acids and serum lipoproteins: human studies. Am J Clin Nutr. 1997;65(Suppl 5):1645S-1654S.
28. Robinson JG, Stone NJ. Antiatherosclerotic and antithrombotic effects of omega-3 fatty acids. Am J Cardiol. 2006;98(4A):39i-49i.
29. Chan DC, Watts GF, Mori TA, et al. Factorial study of the effects of atorvastatin and fish oil on dyslipidaemia in visceral obesity. Eur J Clin Invest. 2002;32(6):429-36.
30. Yokoyama M, Origasa H, Matsuzaki M, et al. Japan EPA lipid intervention study (JELIS) Investigators. Effects of eicosapentaenoic acid on major coronary events in hypercholesterolaemic patients (JELIS): a randomised open-label, blinded endpoint analysis. Lancet. 2007;369(9567): 1090-8.

31. Mozaffarian D, Geelen A, Brouwer IA, et al. Effect of fish oil on heart rate in humans: a meta-analysis of randomized controlled trials. Circulation. 2005;112(13):1945-52.
32. O'Keefe JH Jr, Abuissa H, Sastre A, et al. Effects of omega-3 fatty acids on resting heart rate, heart rate recovery after exercise, and heart rate variability in men with healed myocardial infarctions and depressed ejection fractions. Am J Cardiol. 2006;97(8):1127-30.
33. Kenny D, Warltier DC, Pleuss JA, et al. Effect of omega-3 fatty acids on the vascular response to angiotensin in normotensive men. Am J Cardiol. 1992;70(15):1347-52.
34. Stirban A, Nandrean S, Gotting C, et al. Effects of n-3 fatty acids on macro- and microvascular function in subjects with type 2 diabetes mellitus. Am J Clin Nutr. 2010;91(3):808-13.
35. Dangardt F, Osika W, Chen Y, et al. Omega-3 fatty acid supplementation improves vascular function and reduces inflammation in obese adolescents. Atherosclerosis. 2010;212(2):580-5.
36. Goodfellow J, Bellamy MF, Ramsey MW, et al. Dietary supplementation with marine omega-3 fatty acids improve systemic large artery endothelial function in subjects with hypercholesterolemia. J Am Coll Cardiol. 2000;35(2):265-70.
37. Mori TA, Watts GF, Burke V, et al. Differential effects of eicosapentaenoic acid and docosahexaenoic acid on vascular reactivity of the forearm microcirculation in hyperlipidemic, overweight men. Circulation. 2000;102(11):1264-9.
38. Nestel P, Shige H, Pomeroy S, et al. The n-3 fatty acids eicosapentaenoic acid and docosahexaenoic acid increase systemic arterial compliance in humans. Am J Clin Nutr. 2002;76(2):326-30.
39. Geleijnse JM, Giltay EJ, Grobbee DE, et al. Blood pressure response to fish oil supplementation: metaregression analysis of randomized trials. J Hypertens. 2002;20(8):1493-9.
40. Harris WS, Assaad B, Poston WC. Tissue omega-6/omega-3 fatty acid ratio and risk for coronary artery disease. Am J Cardiol. 2006;98(4A):19i-26i.
41. Balk E, Chung M, Lichtenstein A, et al. Effects of omega-3 fatty acids on cardiovascular risk factors and intermediate markers of cardiovascular disease. Evid Rep Technol Assess (Summ). 2004; 93:1-6.
42. Kristensen SD, Iversen AM, Schmidt EB. n-3 polyunsaturated fatty acids and coronary thrombosis. Lipids. 2001;36(Suppl):S79-S82.
43. Eritsland J, Arnesen H, Seljeflot I, et al. Long-term effects of n-3 polyunsaturated fatty acids on haemostatic variables and bleeding episodes in patients with coronary artery disease. Blood Coagul Fibrinolysis. 1995;6(1):17-22.
44. Harris WS. Expert opinion: omega-3 fatty acids and bleeding—cause for concern? Am J Cardiol. 2007;99(6A):44C-46C.
45. Nakamura K, Kariyazono H, Komokata T, et al. Influence of preoperative administration of omega-3 fatty acid-enriched supplement on inflammatory and immune responses in patients undergoing major surgery for cancer. Nutrition. 2005;21(6): 639-49.
46. Accinni R, Rosina M, Bamonti F, et al. Effects of combined dietary supplementation on oxidative and inflammatory status in dyslipidemic subjects. Nutr Metab Cardiovasc Dis. 2006;16(2):121-7.
47. Tagawa H, Shimokawa H, Tagawa T, et al. Long-term treatment with eicosapentaenoic acid augments both nitric oxide-mediated and non-nitric oxide-mediated endothelium-dependent forearm vasodilatation in patients with coronary artery disease. J Cardiovasc Pharmacol. 1999;33(4):633-40.
48. Mori TA, Woodman RJ, Burke V, et al. Effect of eicosapentaenoic acid and docosahexaenoic acid on oxidative stress and inflammatory markers in treated-hypertensive type 2 diabetic subjects. Free Radic Biol Med. 2003;35(7):772-81.
49. Yusof HM, Miles EA, Calder P. Influence of very long-chain n-3 fatty acids on plasma markers of inflammation in middle-aged men. Prostaglandins Leukot Essent Fatty Acids. 2008;78(3):219-28.
50. Goldberg RJ, Katz J. A meta-analysis of the analgesic effects of omega-3 polyunsaturated fatty acid supplementation for inflammatory joint pain. Pain. 2007;129(1-2):210-23.
51. Serhan CN. Novel lipid mediators and resolution mechanisms in acute inflammation: to resolve or not? Am J Pathol. 2010;177(4): 1576-91.
52. Dlugosova K, Okruhlicova L, Mitasikova M, et al. Modulation of connexin-43 by omega-3 fatty acids in the aorta of old spontaneously hypertensive rats. J Physiol Pharmacol. 2009;60(3):63-9.
53. Schiano V, Laurenzano E, Brevetti G, et al. Omega-3 polyunsaturated fatty acid in peripheral arterial disease: effect on lipid pattern, disease severity, inflammation profile, and endothelial function. Clin Nutr. 2008;27(2):241-7.
54. Doshi SN, Naka KK, Payne N, et al. Flow-mediated dilatation following wrist and upper arm occlusion in humans: the contribution of nitric oxide. Clin Sci (Lond). 2001;101(6):629-35.
55. Kris-Etherton PM, Harris WS, Appel LJ. Fish consumption, fish oil, omega-3 fatty acids, and cardiovascular disease. Circulation. 2002;106(21):2747-57.
56. de Roos B, Mavrommatis Y, Brouwer IA. Long-chain n-3 polyunsaturated fatty acids: new insights into mechanisms relating to inflammation and coronary heart disease. Br J Pharmacol. 2009;158(2):413-28.
57. Ghio S, Scelsi L, Latini R, et al. Effects of n-3 polyunsaturated fatty acids and of rosuvastatin on left ventricular function in chronic heart failure: a substudy of GISSI-HF trial. Eur J Heart Fail. 2010;12(12):1345-53.
58. Grimsgaard S, Bonaa KH, Hansen JB, et al. Effects of highly purified eicosapentaenoic acid and docosahexaenoic acid on hemodynamics in humans. Am J Clin Nutr. 1998;68(1):52-9.
59. Peoples GE, McLennan PL, Howe PR, et al. Fish oil reduces heart rate and oxygen consumption during exercise. J Cardiovasc Pharmacol. 2008;52(6):540-7.
60. Pepe S, McLennan PL. Cardiac membrane fatty acid composition modulates myocardial oxygen consumption and postischemic recovery of contractile function. Circulation. 2002;105(19):2303-8.
61. Nodari S, Triggiani M, Campia U, et al. Effects of n-3 polyunsaturated fatty acids on left ventricular function and functional capacity in patients with dilated cardiomyopathy. J Am Coll Cardiol. 2011;57(7):870-9.
62. Djousse L, Gaziano JM, Buring JE, et al. Dietary omega-3 fatty acids and fish consumption and risk of type 2 diabetes. Am J Clin Nutr. 2011;93(1):143-50.
63. Hartweg J, Perera R, Montori V, et al. Omega-3 polyunsaturated fatty acids (PUFA) for type 2 diabetes mellitus. Cochrane Database Syst Rev, 2008;1:CD003205.
64. Montori VM, Farmer A, Wollan PC, et al. Fish oil supplementation in type 2 diabetes: a quantitative systematic review. Diabetes Care. 2000;23(9):1407-15.
65. Giacco R, Cuomo V, Vessby B, et al. Fish oil, insulin sensitivity, insulin secretion and glucose tolerance in healthy people: is there any effect of fish oil supplementation in relation to the type of background diet and habitual dietary intake of n-6 and n-3 fatty acids? Nutr Metab Cardiovasc Dis. 2007;17(8):572-80.
66. Thies F, Garry JM, Yaqoob P, et al. Association of n-3 polyunsaturated fatty acids with stability of atherosclerotic plaques: a randomised controlled trial. Lancet. 2003;361(9356):477-85.
67. Johansen O, Brekke M, Seljeflot I, et al. N-3 fatty acids do not prevent restenosis after coronary angioplasty: results from the CART study. Coronary Angioplasty Restenosis Trial. J Am Coll Cardiol. 1999;33(6):1619-26.
68. Fischer R, Dechend R, Qadri F, et al. Dietary n-3 polyunsaturated fatty acids and direct renin inhibition improve electrical remodeling in a model of high human renin hypertension. Hypertension. 2008;51(2):540-6.

69. Radosinska J, Bacova B, Bernatova I, et al. Myocardial NOS activity and connexin-43 expression in untreated and omega-3 fatty acids-treated spontaneously hypertensive and hereditary hypertriglyceridemic rats. Mol Cell Biochem. 2011;347(1-2):163-73.
70. Saravanan P, Bridgewater B, West AL, et al. Omega-3 fatty acid supplementation does not reduce risk of atrial fibrillation after coronary artery bypass surgery: a randomized, double-blind, placebo-controlled clinical trial. Circ Arrhythm Electrophysiol. 2010;3(1):46-53.
71. Heidarsdottir R, Arnar DO, Skuladottir GV, et al. Does treatment with n-3 polyunsaturated fatty acids prevent atrial fibrillation after open heart surgery? Europace. 2010;12(3):356-63.
72. Farquharson AL, Metcalf RG, Sanders P, et al. Effect of dietary fish oil on atrial fibrillation after cardiac surgery. Am J Cardiol. 2011;108(6):851-6.
73. Gruppo Italiano per lo Studio della Sopravvivenza Nell'Infarto Miocardico. Dietary supplementation with n-3 polyunsaturated fatty acids and vitamin E after myocardial infarction: results of the GISSI-Prevenzione trial. Lancet. 1999;354(9177):447-55.
74. Getz GS, Reardon CA. Nutrition and cardiovascular disease. Arterioscler Thromb Vasc Biol. 2007;27(12):2499-506.
75. Reiffel JA, McDonald A. Antiarrhythmic effects of omega-3 fatty acids. Am J Cardiol. 2006;98(4A):50i-60i.
76. Raitt MH, Connor WE, Morris C, et al. Fish oil supplementation and risk of ventricular tachycardia and ventricular fibrillation in patients with implantable defibrillators: a randomized controlled trial. JAMA. 2005;293(23):2884-91.
77. Leaf A, Albert CM, Josephson M, et al. Prevention of fatal arrhythmias in high-risk subjects by fish oil n-3 fatty acid intake. Circulation. 2005;112(18):2762-8.
78. Calo L, Bianconi L, Colivicchi F, et al. N-3 fatty acids for the prevention of atrial fibrillation after coronary artery bypass surgery: a randomized, controlled trial. J Am Coll Cardiol. 2005;45(10):1723-8.
79. Bosch J, Gerstein HC, Dagenais GR, et al. ORIGIN Trial Investigators. n-3 fatty acids and cardiovascular outcomes in patients with dysglycemia. N Engl J Med. 2012;367(4):309-18.
80. Siscovick DS, Barringer TA, Fretts AM, et al. Omega-3 Polyunsaturated Fatty Acid (Fish Oil) Supplementation and the Prevention of Clinical Cardiovascular Disease: a Science Advisory From the American Heart Association. Circulation. 2017;135(15):e867-e884.
81. Marik PE, Varon J. Omega-3 dietary supplements and the risk of cardiovascular events: a systematic review. Clin Cardiol. 2009;32(7):365-72.
82. Feskens EJ, Kromhout D. Epidemiologic studies on Eskimos and fish intake. Ann N Y Acad Sci. 1993;683:9-15.
83. Rauch B, Schiele R, Schneider S, et al. OMEGA, a randomized, placebo-controlled trial to test the effect of highly purified omega-3 fatty acids on top of modern guideline-adjusted therapy after myocardial infarction. Circulation. 2010;122(21):2152-9.
84. Albert CM, Campos H, Stampfer MJ, et al. Blood levels of long-chain n-3 fatty acids and the risk of sudden death. N Engl J Med. 2002;346(15);1113-8.
85. Yokoyama M, Origasa H, Matsuzaki M, et al. Effects of eicosapentaenoic acid on major coronary events in hypercholesterolaemic patients (JELIS): a randomised open-label, blinded endpoint analysis. Lancet. 2007;369(9567):1090-8.
86. Burr ML, Ashfield-Watt PA, Dunstan FD, et al. Lack of benefit of dietary advice to men with angina: results of a controlled trial. Eur J Clin Nutr. 2003;57(2):193-200.
87. Burr ML, Fehily AM, Gilbert JF, et al. Effects of changes in fat, fish, and fibre intakes on death and myocardial reinfarction: diet and reinfarction trial (DART). Lancet. 1989;2(8666):757-61.
88. LaRosa JC, He J, Vupputuri S. Effect of statins on risk of coronary disease: a meta-analysis of randomized controlled trials. JAMA. 1999;282(24):2340-6.
89. Kromhout D, Giltay EJ, Geleijnse JM. n-3 fatty acids and cardiovascular events after myocardial infarction. N Engl J Med. 2010;363(21):2015-26.
90. Galan P, Kesse-Guyot E, Czernichow S, et al. Effects of B vitamins and omega 3 fatty acids on cardiovascular diseases: a randomised placebo controlled trial. BMJ. 2010;341:c6273.
91. He K, Song Y, Daviglus ML, et al. Accumulated evidence on fish consumption and coronary heart disease mortality: a meta-analysis of cohort studies. Circulation. 2004;109(22):2705-11.
92. Hooper L, Thompson RL, Harrison RA, et al. Risks and benefits of omega 3-fats for mortality, cardiovascular disease, and cancer: systematic review. BMJ. 2006;332(7544):752-60.
93. Rizos EC, Ntzani EE, Bika E, et al. Association between omega-3 fatty acid supplementation and risk of major cardiovascular disease events: a systematic review and meta-analysis. JAMA. 2012;308(10):1024-33.
94. Kitamura K, Shibata R, Tsuji Y, et al. Eicosapentaenoic acid prevents atrial fibrillation associated with heart failure in a rabbit model. Am J Physiol Heart Circ Physiol. 2011;300(5):H1814-21.
95. Mozaffarian D, Psaty BM, Rimm EB, et al. Fish intake and risk of incident atrial fibrillation. Circulation. 2004;110(4):368-73.
96. Frost L, Vestergaard P. n-3 Fatty acids consumed from fish and risk of atrial fibrillation or flutter: the Danish Diet, Cancer, and Health Study. Am J Clin Nutr. 2005;81(1):50-4.
97. Brouwer IA, Heeringa J, Geleijnse JM, et al. Intake of very long-chain n-3 fatty acids from fish and incidence of atrial fibrillation: The Rotterdam Study. Am Heart J. 2006;151(4):857-62.
98. Berry JD, Prineas RJ, van Horn L, et al. Dietary fish intake and incident atrial fibrillation (from the Women's Health Initiative). Am J Cardiol. 2010;105(6):844-8.
99. Kowey PR, Reiffel JA, Ellenbogen KA, et al. Efficacy and safety of prescription omega-3 fatty acids for the prevention of recurrent symptomatic atrial fibrillation: a randomized controlled trial. JAMA. 2010;304(21):2363-72.
100. National Institute of Health Clinical Trials Registry (2010). Evaluating the effectiveness of fish oil supplements at reducing the recurrence of atrial fibrillation. [online] Available form *http://clinicaltrials.gov/ct2/show/NCT00552084?term=atrial+fibrillation&intr=fish+oil&rank=1*. [Accessed August, 2017].
101. Macchia A, Grancelli H, Varini S, et al. GESICA Investigators. Omega-3 fatty acids for the prevention of recurrent symptomatic atrial fibrillation: results of the FORWARD (Randomized Trial to Assess Efficacy of PUFA for the Maintenance of Sinus Rhythm in Persistent Atrial Fibrillation) trial. J Am Coll Cardiol. 2013;61(4):463-8.
102. Mariani J, Doval HC, Nul D, et al. N-3 polyunsaturated fatty acids to prevent atrial fibrillation: updated systematic review and meta-analysis of randomized controlled trials. J Am Heart Assoc. 2013;2(1):e005033.
103. Mozaffarian D, Marchioli R, Macchia A, et al. OPERA Investigators. Fish oil and post-operative atrial fibrillation: the Omega-3 Fatty Acids for Prevention of Post-operative Atrial Fibrillation (OPERA) randomized trial. JAMA. 2012;308(19):2001-11.
104. Raitt MH, Connor WE, Morris C, et al. Fish oil supplementation and risk of ventricular tachycardia and ventricular fibrillation in patients with implantable defibrillators: a randomized controlled trial. JAMA. 2005;293(23):2884-91.
105. Brouwer IA, Zock PL, Camm AJ, et al. Effect of fish oil on ventricular tachyarrhythmia and death in patients with implantable cardioverter defibrillators: the Study on Omega-3 Fatty Acids and Ventricular Arrhythmia (SOFA) randomized trial. JAMA. 2006;295(22): 2613-9.
106. Levitan EB, Wolk A, Mittleman MA. Fish consumption, marine omega-3 fatty acids, and incidence of heart failure: a population-based prospective study of middle-aged and elderly men. Eur Heart J. 2009;30(12):1495-500.

107. Mozaffarian D, Bryson CL, Lemaitre RN, et al. Fish intake and risk of incident heart failure. J Am Coll Cardiol. 2005;45(12): 2015-21.
108. Chee KM, Gong JX, Rees DM, et al. Fatty acid content of marine oil capsules. Lipids. 1990;25(9):523-8.
109. Tavazzi L, Maggioni AP, Marchioli R, et al. Gissi-HF Investigators. Effect of n-3 polyunsaturated fatty acids in patients with chronic heart failure (the GISSI-HF trial): a randomised, double-blind, placebo-controlled trial. Lancet. 2008;372(9645):1223-30.
110. American Heart Association (2009). Fish and Omega-3 fatty acids. [online] Available from *www. americanheart.org/presenter. jhtml?identifier=4632.* [Accessed August, 2017].
111. Roger VL, Go AS, Lloyd-Jones DM, et al. Heart disease and stroke statistics—2011 update: a report from the American Heart Association. Circulation. 2011;123(4):e18-e209.
112. Tatarczyk T, Engl J, Ciardi C, et al. Analysis of long-chain omega-3 fatty acid content in fish-oil supplements. Wien Klin Wochenschr. 2007;119(13-14):417-22.
113. Abete P, Testa G, Galizia G, et al. PUFA for human health: diet or supplementation? Curr Pharm Des. 2009;15(36):4186-90.
114. World Health Organization (2010). Joint FAO/WHO expert consultation on fats and fatty acids in human nutrition, 2008. [online] *http://www.who.int/nutrition/topics/FFA_summary_rec_conclusion.pdf.* [Accessed August, 2017].

Role of Red Yeast Rice and Phytosterols in Dyslipidemia

Pawan K Sharma, Paul N Hopkins, HK Chopra

INTRODUCTION

Red yeast rice (RYR) is also known as Red Koji, Hong Qu, Ang-kak, red mold rice, and Beni-Koji. In 1989, Stephen DeFelice used the term "nutraceutical" for a food or part of a food, which can be of plant or animal origin, that has a potential pharmaceutical activity.[1] Red yeast rice is a nutraceutical made by fermenting white rice with the red yeast *Monascus purpureus*. RYR is used as an herbal supplement and in the East Asian countries for flavoring, coloring, and preservation of food.[2] RYR contains many compounds including monacolins, plant sterols (beta-sitosterol, campesterol, stigmasterol, and sapogenin), isoflavones, isoflavone glycosides, zinc, selenium, and monounsaturated fatty acids.[3] Monacolins inhibit HMG-CoA (3-hydroxy-3-methyl-glutaryl-coenzyme A) reductase, the rate limiting step in cholesterol synthesis. At least 13 monacolins have been isolated from RYR, of which monacolin K (also known as mevicolin) is chemically identical to lovastatin.[4] The hydroxy acid form of monacolin K is called monacolin KA, which is the activated form of lovastatin after it passes through the liver.

CLINICAL TRIALS INVOLVING RED YEAST RICE IN DYSLIPIDEMIA

In a trial involving 83 healthy adults with dyslipidemia, patients were randomized to receive either RYR supplementation (2.4 g/day in the form of Cholestin) or placebo for 12 weeks. RYR supplementation significantly reduced low-density lipoprotein (LDL) cholesterol by 22% ($p < 0.05$) as well as total cholesterol and triglycerides in comparison with placebo. High-density lipoprotein (HDL) did not significantly differ from baseline in either group.[5] In a Chinese study involving 79 patients with a mean baseline LDL of 204 mg/dL, patients were randomized to receive either RYR 600 mg twice daily or placebo for 8 weeks. Compared to baseline, LDL was reduced by 27.7%, total cholesterol by 21.5%, triglycerides by 15.8%, and apolipoprotein B by 26% in the RYR supplementation group which were statistically significant. An increase of HDL of 0.9% was not statistically significant.[6]

Liu et al. in a meta-analysis of 93 randomized trials involving 9,265 dyslipidemic participants, compared the lipid-lowering effects of RYR with placebo. Three different preparations of RYR (Cholestin, Xuezhikang, and Zhibituo) were analyzed in the trials. All preparations showed significant reductions in total cholesterol, triglycerides, and LDL compared with placebo ($p < 0.00001$). Only Zhibituo preparation showed a significant improvement of HDL levels ($p < 0.00001$).[7] Becker et al. evaluated simvastatin 40 mg daily versus RYR, fish oil, and life-style changes for a period of 12 weeks. Significant reductions in LDL cholesterol from baseline was found in both groups ($p < 0.001$), but no significant differences were found between the two groups. However, the group receiving RYR, fish oil, and life-style changes had significant reduction in triglycerides ($p = 0.003$) in comparison to the simvastatin group.[8]

A meta-analysis in 2015 examined 20 randomized trials consisting of 6,663 patients and showed a clinically and statistically significant reduction in LDL cholesterol of 1.02 mmol/L when compared with RYR and placebo groups. This has been reported to correspond to a cardiovascular risk reduction of 15–20%. There was no difference in LDL between RYR and statin therapy, with an incidence of kidney injury and liver abnormalities of less than 5% in both the RYR and control group.[9] RYR is also reported to reduce blood pressure, and may possess anti-inflammatory, antidiabetic, anticancer, and osteogenic properties.[10]

A large, randomized controlled trial examined RYR in *secondary cardiovascular prevention* in 4,870 Chinese patients with previous myocardial infarction. Patients were randomized to receive either Xuezhikang 300 mg or placebo and monitored for 4.5 years. Patients treated with Xuezhikang had a significant 20% reduction in LDL cholesterol ($p < 0.01$) and a significant decrease in frequency of major coronary events ($p < 0.001$) from baseline. Overall, this study showed that RYR reduces nonfatal myocardial infarction, coronary disease mortality, coronary revascularization, and total mortality in patients with a history of myocardial infarction and moderate hypercholesterolemia.[11]

Safety and Efficacy of Red Yeast Rice

Safety and efficacy of RYR was evaluated in 62 dyslipidemic patients with prior history of statin-associated myalgias. They were randomized to receive either RYR 1800 mg twice daily or placebo twice daily for 24 weeks. The LDL cholesterol decreased by 23% and total cholesterol decreased by 16% in the RYR group compared with baseline at the end of 24 weeks. In the RYR group, the LDL cholesterol levels at 12 and 24 weeks were significantly lower than that in the placebo group; $p < 0.001$ and $p = 0.011$, respectively. There was no difference in liver transaminase and creatine phosphokinase levels, and the presence of myalgias in either group compared with baseline levels.[12]

Multiple studies evaluating a specific RYR extract, Xuezhikang, on dyslipidemia and coronary events have been conducted in China. Liu et al.[13] randomized 50 patients with coronary heart disease to receive the study medication Xuezhikang at a dose of 1,200 mg daily or placebo for 6 weeks. After 6 weeks, the Xuezhikang group had significantly decreased C-reactive protein concentrations ($p < 0.05$), serum lipoprotein(a) ($p < 0.05$), and triglyceride levels ($p < 0.001$) compared with baseline levels.

Although statins raise glucose slightly but significantly, a 2014 meta-analysis of five trials consisting of 352 patients showed that RYR does not significantly increase glucose compared to placebo.[11] In addition, RYR in combination with antioxidants has been demonstrated to reduce high sensitivity C-reactive protein (hs-CRP) and endothelial dysfunction.[14]

In a subgroup analysis, 591 diabetic patients with cardiovascular disease were randomized to either receive Xuezhikang or placebo and followed for 4 years. In the Xuezhikang group, the risk reduction for cardiovascular heart disease events was 64%, fatal myocardial infarction by 59%, and cardiovascular sudden death by 27% from baseline.[15]

Xuezhikang extract, independent of lipid-lowering effects, is beneficial in improving left-ventricular diastolic function in patients with hypertension as well as efficacious in lowering morbidity and mortality in elderly patients with a history of myocardial infarction.[16,17]

Adverse Effects of Red Yeast Rice

Adverse effects of RYR include gastrointestinal effects, myopathy, hepatotoxicity, rhabdomyolysis, and anaphylaxis similar to the statins.[18,19] The mycotoxin citrinin, found in poorly produced RYR products, can be mutagenic as found in animal models, genotoxic to human lymphocytes, and can cause kidney failure although acute toxicity is quite rare.[20-23]Administration of RYR with cytochrome P450 (CYP) enzyme inhibitors [e.g. ketoconazole, human immunodeficiency virus (HIV) protease inhibitors, erythromycin] can lead to worsening adverse effects such as myopathy.[10,24] But clinical studies which showed effectiveness of RYR in dyslipidemia also showed that it is a relatively safe product.[9,25]

The European Food Safety Authority (EFSA) allows the health claims that consumption of monacolin K in RYR preparations maintains normal blood LDL concentration provided that the daily dietary intake is at least 10 mg of monacolin K from RYR.[26] This value is considered acceptable even though different RYR products may have variable amounts, thus representing a health risk in the absence of appropriate information for the customer.[24]

The US Food and Drug Administration (FDA) consider monacolin K an unapproved drug because it is identical to lovastatin. Therefore, all RYR products that contain a specified amount of monacolin K are prohibited. The RYR supplements in the market are not standardized and contain variable amounts of monacolins including monacolin K, citrinin, and other contaminants. The manufacturers do not report the monacolin content in their RYR products on the packaging for fear it would prompt regulatory action from the FDA.[18,27]

POSSIBLE CLINICAL IMPLICATIONS OF RED YEAST RICE

Besides the coronary disease prevention studies cited earlier, RYR has been studied in diabetes, hypertension, obesity, depression, osteoporosis, cancer, and has antioxidant and anti-inflammatory properties. Studies

TABLE 1: Potential clinical uses of red yeast rice but need human studies.

- *Coronary Heart disease:* Lower total cholesterol, LDL cholesterol and triglyceride
- *Diabetes:* Decrease plasma glucose, delay insulin resistance and increase insulin secretion
- *Hypertension:* May lower BP
- Improve cardiac diastolic function
- *Obesity:* Prevent weight gain
- *Depression:* Monoamine oxidase inhibitory activity may have a use in the treatment of depression
- Promote bone growth and prevent osteoporosis
- Inhibit cancer cell proliferation
- Antioxidant effect
- Anti-inflammatory effect and may prevent Alzheimer's dementia

mainly involve cellular and animal research; however, further investigation could translate these findings to human medicine (Table 1).

Diabetes

A study in rats showed that orally administered RYR can decrease plasma glucose, delay insulin resistance, and increase insulin sensitivity.[28] RYR increases the release of acetylcholine, resulting in increased insulin secretion in rats.[29] These studies suggest that RYR could be useful in prediabetic patients, although further research is needed to confirm this benefit in humans.

Hypertension

Red yeast rice is reported to produce antihypertensive effects by three mechanisms.

The first mechanism is through gamma-aminobutyric acid (GABA) content in *Monascus purpureus* M9011.[30] When RYR was compared with pure GABA in rats with fructose-induced hypertension, the RYR had a more potent antihypertensive effect.[30] The study indicated that other components besides the GABA content contributed to the antihypertensive effect of RYR. The second mechanism is through acetylcholine that was identified in *Monascus pilosus* IFO4520.[31] The third mechanism is through inhibition of angiotensin I—converting enzyme by four active peptides that were found in *Monascus purpureus* IFO = 4489.[32]

Based on these results, RYR could be helpful in reducing blood pressure in diabetic patients and in the general population; however, human studies are needed before it can be recommended for the treatment of hypertension.

Obesity

Potential use of RYR in obesity was seen in Wistar rats on a high fat diet. The rats fed RYR had less weight gain and decreased cholesterol and insulin levels.[33] These effects of RYR have not been studied in humans, although use as an appetite suppressant would be particularly useful.

Depression

Monoamine oxidase inhibitors have therapeutic use in the treatment of depression. Some components of RYR have been found to have monoamine oxidase inhibitory activity.[34] Monankarins A to D had monoamine oxidase, inhibiting activity, with monankarin C showing strong monoamine oxidase-B inhibition in mice brain cells.[34]

Osteoporosis

In a study, RYR was found to increase the proliferation of osteoblasts, thus promoting the synthesis of collagenous proteins and factors essential for bone growth.[35] These bone-promoting qualities of RYR were further tested on parietal bones of white rabbits. RYR was mixed with a collagen matrix and applied to the damaged bones. There was more bone formation in rabbits treated with the RYR mixture than in those treated with just a collagen matrix alone.[36] Based on animal research, RYR may have potential role in bone formation but more research is needed to determine if this effect translates into human studies.

Cancer

Lovastatin and monacolin-rich RYR have similar abilities to stop colon cancer cell proliferation; however, whole RYR and pigment-rich RYR also decreased colon cancer cell proliferation. This suggests that there are components in RYR, other than just monacolins, that inhibit cancer cell proliferation. There is also evidence to suggest that components other than the monacolins in RYR decreased androgen-dependent and -independent prostate cancer growth.[37,38] A study in mice with prostate cancer showed that there was a decrease in tumor size in those receiving RYR in comparison to those mice that received placebo.[39] The use of RYR to prevent cancer or slow tumor progression needs more human studies to delineate its role in cancer.

Antioxidant

A component of RYR, dimerumic acid, has antioxidant properties. In molecular studies, dimerumic acid donates an electron to produce its antioxidant effect, and when dimerumic acid (12 mg/kg) was administered to mice, it was able to reduce drug-induced liver toxicity.[40,41]

Anti-inflammatory Effect

Various constituents of RYR have anti-inflammatory properties of varying potency.[41] The antioxidant and anti-inflammatory properties of RYR could be protective against amyloid beta-peptide induced plaques.[42] Amyloid beta-peptide plaque formation in the brain can contribute to the development of Alzheimer's disease. A cellular study found that RYR protected cells from the effects of the amyloid beta-peptide.[42] When studied in rats, RYR was found to reverse the memory loss caused by amyloid beta peptide.[43]

Discussion

In order to reduce variability of the monacolin content of different RYR preparations and to minimize toxic compounds, such as citrinin, quality control policy should be implemented and enforced by the responsible authorities for food and supplement oversight.

PHYTOSTEROLS

Phytosterols are steroid compounds similar to cholesterol in structure and function. They are present in plants and modestly lower plasma total cholesterol and LDL-cholesterol levels by blocking intestinal cholesterol absorption. Therefore, it is believed that phytosterols may promote health when consumed regularly for a period of time. We, in this review, discuss the bioavailability, biological activities, and possible health benefits of phytosterols.

Types of Phytosterols

There are two types of phytosterols:

1. *Sterols:* These have a double bond in the sterol ring and are *unsaturated* compounds. The most abundant sterols are beta-sitosterols, campesterols, and stigmasterol which account for 65, 30, and 3% of dietary phytosterols contents respectively.[44]
2. *Stanols*: These do not have double bond in the sterol ring and are *saturated* compounds. They form only 10% of total dietary phytosterols. The most common plant stanols in the human diet are sitostanol and campestanol and both of them combined make up to 5% of dietary phytosterols.[45]

Sources of Phytosterols

Humans cannot synthesize phytosterols. Therefore, all phytosterols in human blood and tissue are derived from the diet. The richest naturally occurring sources of phytosterols are vegetable oils. Dietary phytosterols can be present in free form and as esters of fatty acid/cinnamic acid or as glycosides. The bound form is usually hydrolyzed in the small intestine by pancreatic enzymes.[46] Other sources of phytosterols are nuts, cereals, vegetables, fruits, and berries.[47] Seeds, whole grain, and legumes are also dietary sources of phytosterols.[48]

Plant sterols and stanols are often esterified which makes them fat-soluble, so that they can be easily incorporated into fat-containing foods including margarines and salad dressing.

Absorption and Metabolism of Phytosterols

The serum phytosterol concentrations are usually several hundred times lower than serum cholesterol levels in humans.[49] Less than 10% of dietary phytosterols are systemically absorbed, in contrast to 50–60% of dietary cholesterol.[50]

Phytosterols are incorporated into mixed micelles before they are taken up by enterocytes. Once inside the enterocytes their systemic absorption is inhibited by the activity of efflux transporters, consisting of a pair of ATP-binding cassette (ABC) proteins known as ABCG5 and ABCG8.[51] ABCG5 and ABCG8 form two halves of a transporter that secretes phytosterols and unesterified cholesterol from the enterocytes into the intestinal lumen. Phytosterols are secreted back into the intestine by ABCG5/G8 transporters at a much greater rate than cholesterol, resulting in much lower intestinal absorption of dietary phytosterol than cholesterol. Within the enterocytes, phytosterols are not readily esterified, so they are incorporated into chylomicrons at much lower concentrations. The phytosterols that are incorporated into chylomicrons enter blood circulation and are taken up by the liver. Once inside the liver, phytosterols are metabolized into cholesterol and other metabolites, by the action of several enzymes and a key enzyme called cholesterol 7 alpha-hydroxylase into bile acids, and rapidly secreted into bile by hepatic ABCG5/G8 transporters. This enzyme is a regulatory enzyme in bile acid biosynthesis.[52] Therefore, the lower concentrations of phytosterols compared to cholesterol can be explained by decreased intestinal absorption and increased excretion of phytosterols into bile.

Biological Activities of Phytosterols (Table 2)

Effect on Cholesterol Absorption and Lipoprotein Metabolism

It is well-established that phytosterols can lower serum total and LDL cholesterol.[53,54] In the intestinal lumen, phytosterols displace cholesterol from mixed micelles and inhibit cholesterol absorption.[55] Increased phytosterol intake leads to increased endogenous cholesterol synthesis, as well as increased LDL receptor expression. The net result is a reduction in serum LDL cholesterol concentration.

TABLE 2: Possible clinical effects of phytosterols but need human studies

- Reduction of total cholesterol and LDL cholesterol and prevent coronary heart disease
- Anti-inflammatory effect
- Induction of apoptosis in cancer cells and prevent lung, colon, ovarian and breast cancer
- Treatment of BPH

Health Canada reviewed 84 randomized trials published between 1994 and 2007 which showed that phytosterol supplementation results in 8.8% reduction in LDL cholesterol concentration at a mean intake of 2 grams of phytosterols per day.[56] Health Canada concluded that sufficient scientific evidence exists to support a relationship between phytosterol consumption and blood cholesterol lowering. Saturated phytosterols were found to be more effective than unsaturated forms in lowering cholesterol levels.[57]

Anti-inflammatory Effects

Limited data from cell culture and animal studies suggest that phytosterols may attenuate the inflammatory activity of immune cells, including macrophages and neutrophils.[58] Thus, they may have anti-inflammatory activities in living systems.

Induction of Apoptosis in Cancer Cells

Sitosterols have been found to induce apoptosis when added to cultured human prostate,[59] breast,[60] and colon cancer cells.[61] Therefore, they may play significant roles in the management and prevention of human cancers.

Disease Prevention

The cholesterol level can be reduced by 11.3% if a person consumes 1.5–3.0 grams of phytosterols every day. The EFSA concluded that by reducing blood cholesterol and LDL cholesterol levels, the phytosterols may reduce the risk of coronary heart disease.[62] The FDA and Health Canada have also adopted similar positions. The FDA has authorized the claim on food labels that regular consumption of food enriched with plant sterols or stanol esters may reduce the risk of heart disease. It is also reported that phytosterols may inhibit lung, stomach, ovarian, and breast cancers.[63]

Disease Treatment

In a 6 month study of 200 men with symptomatic benign prostatic hyperplasia (BPH) 60 mg/day of a beta-sitosterol preparation improved symptoms, increased peak urinary flow, and decreased postvoid residual urine volume compared to placebo.[64] However, few controlled studies have examined the efficacy of phytosterol supplements in men with symptomatic BPH.

Safety of Phytosterols

In the United States, plant sterols and stanols added to food products are generally recognized as safe (GRAS) by the FDA. The scientific committee on foods of the European Union (EU) also concluded that plant sterols and stanols added to food products are safe for human use.[62] However, the committee also recommended that intakes of plant sterols and stanols from food products should not exceed 3 g/day because there is no evidence of health benefits at higher intakes and there might be undesirable effects when they are consumed in high amounts.

Phytosterols are usually well tolerated, however, nausea, indigestion, diarrhea, and constipation have sometimes been reported.[64] In epidemiological studies, higher levels of serum phytosterols were associated with increased risk of coronary artery disease.[65-67] In a mouse study, food supplementation with plant sterol esters was found to impair endothelial function, aggravate ischemic brain injury, and promote atherogenesis and persons consuming margarine supplemented with plant sterol esters had increased tissue sterol concentrations.[68]

Sitosterolemia (Phytosterolemia)

Sitosterolemia is a very rare hereditary disease that results from homozygous or compound heterozygous absence of normally functioning ABCG5 or ABCG8.[69] Affected individuals have elevated serum phytosterol concentrations due to its increased intestinal absorption and decreased biliary excretion. Though, the serum cholesterol or LDL-cholesterol concentrations may range from normal to severely elevated, individuals with sitosterolemia are at higher risk for premature atherosclerosis. Patients with sitosterolemia are routinely treated with a low phytosterol diet but also greatly benefit from ezetimibe.[53]

Phytosterols in Pregnancy and Lactation

Plant sterols or stanols added to food or supplements are not recommended for pregnant or breastfeeding women because their safety has not been studied.[53]

Phytosterol: Drug Interaction

The LDL cholesterol lowering effects of plant sterols or stanols may be additive to those of HMG-CoA reductase inhibitors (statins).[69] The results of controlled clinical trials suggest that consumption of 2–3 g/day of plant sterols or stanols on statin therapy may result in additional 7–11% reduction in LDL cholesterol, an effect comparable to doubling the statin dose.[70] Another study showed that consumption of 4.5 g/day of stanol esters for 8 weeks did not affect prothrombin time [international normalized ratio (INR)] in patients on warfarin.[71]

Phytosterol: Nutrient Interaction

Fat soluble vitamins (Vitamins A, D, E, and K): The effect of plant sterols and stanols on fat-soluble vitamins status has also been studied in clinical trials because they are known to decrease cholesterol absorption and serum LDL cholesterol concentrations. Plasma vitamin A (retinol) concentrations were not affected by plant stanol or sterol esters consumption for upto 1 year.[72] The majority of studies found no change in plasma vitamin D(25-hydroxyvitamin D3) concentrations. However, one placebo-controlled study in individuals consuming 1.6 g/day of sterol esters for 1 year observed a small (7%) but statistically significant decrease in plasma 25-hydroxyvitamin D3 concentration. There is little evidence that plant sterol or stanol consumption adversely affects vitamin K status.[72]

Carotenoids: Dietary carotenoids are fat-soluble phytochemicals that circulate in lipoproteins. Some studies have shown 10–20% reductions in plasma carotenoids after short-term and long-term consumption of plant sterol- or stanol-enriched foods. It is not clear whether reductions in plasma carotenoids concentrations could cause any health risks but several studies have found that increasing intakes of carotenoid-rich fruits and vegetables can prevent phytosterol-induced decrease in plasma carotenoids.[73]

CONCLUSION

Red yeast rice has been shown to be an efficacious option in decreasing serum lipid levels in patients with dyslipidemia, with the greatest effect being on LDL cholesterol. Preparations containing active monacolins and relatively free of citrinin appear to be a safe, viable option in patients intolerant to statins because of myalgias and/or other statin related side effects. Currently, RYR is the only supplement that has been proven to reduce the occurrence of adverse cardiac events in a comparable degree to statins. Multiple animal studies also suggest potential uses in other diseases. Despite these favorable effects, a major limitation to the use of RYR is the lack of consistency in ingredients between different manufacturers and the inability to determine appropriate dosing. There is scientific evidence to support the fact that phytosterols and their derivatives can lower LDL-cholesterol. However, the net benefit has yet to be demonstrated and significant precautions have been raised with regard the atherogenesis. Reports of anti-inflammatory activities; prevention of colon, breast and prostate cancers, and treatment of BPH will need to be confirmed. Therefore, the potential benefit or harm of supplementation with plant sterols and stanols has yet to be demonstrated clearly. Their consumption in natural foods is generally considered safe and potentially beneficial for persons without phytosterolemia. It is, therefore, recommended that future work should focus on randomized controlled clinical trials in humans, to determine if cholesterol-lowering activity of phytosterols could reduce risk of cardiovascular diseases, and if the apparent adverse effects on endothelial health or decrease in absorption of fat-soluble nutrients such as carotenoids by phytosterols could cause any health risk.

REFERENCES

1. DeFelice SL. The nutraceutical revolution: its impact on food industry R&D. Trends Food Sci Tech. 1995;6(2):59-61.
2. Burke FM. Red yeast rice for the treatment of dyslipidemia. Curr Atheroscler Rep. 2015;17(4):495.
3. Journoud M, Jones PJ. Red yeast rice: a new hypolipidemic drug. Life Sci. 2004;74(22):2675-83.
4. Zhang Z, Ali Z, Khan SI, et al. Cytotoxic monacolins from red yeast rice, a Chinese medicine and food. Food Chem. 2016,202:262-8.
5. Heber D, Yip I, Ashley JM, et al. Cholesterol-lowering effects of proprietary Chinese red-yeast-rice dietary supplement. Am J Clin Nutr. 1999;69(2):231-6.
6. Lin CC, Li TC, Lai MM. Efficacy and safety of *Monascus purpureus* Went rice in subjects with hyperlipidemia. Eur J Endocrinol. 2005;153(5):679-86.
7. Liu J, Zhang J, Shi Y, et al. Chinese red yeast rice (*Monascus purpureus*) for primary hyperlipidemia: a meta-analysis of randomized controlled trials. Chin Med. 2006:1-4.
8. Becker DJ, Gordon RY, Morris PB, et al. Simvastatin vs therapeutic lifestyle changes and supplements: randomized primary prevention trial. Mayo Clin Proc. 2008;83(7):758-64.
9. Gerards MC, Terlou RJ, Yu H, et al. Traditional Chinese lipid-lowering agent red yeast rice results in significant LDL reduction but safety is uncertain–a systematic review and meta-analysis. Atherosclerosis. 2015;240(2):415-23.
10. Patel S. Functional food red yeast rice (RYR) for metabolic syndrome amelioration: a review on pros and cons. World J Microbiol Biotechnol. 2016;32:2035-42.
11. Lu Z, Kou W, Du B, et al. Effect of Xuezhikang, an extract from red yeast Chinese rice, on coronary events in a Chinese population with previous myocardial infarction. Am J Cardiol. 2008;101(12):1689-93.
12. Becker DJ, Gordon RY, Halbert SC, et al. Red yeast rice for dyslipidemia in statin-intolerant patients: a randomized trial. Ann Intern Med. 2009;150(12):830-39.
13. Liu L, Zhao SP, Cheng YC, et al. Xuezhikang decreases serum lipoprotein(a) and C-reactive protein concentrations in patients with coronary heart disease. Clin Chem. 2003;49(8):1347-52.
14. Cicero AF, Morbini M, Parini A, et al. Effect of red yeast rice combined with antioxidants on lipid pattern, hs-CRP level, and endothelial function in moderately hypercholesterolemic subjects. Ther Clin Risk Manag. 2016;12:281-6.
15. Zhao SP, Lu ZL, Du BM, et al. Xuezhikang, an extract of cholestin, reduces cardiovascular events in type 2 diabetes patients with coronary heart disease: subgroup analysis of patients with type 2

diabetes from China coronary secondary prevention study (CCSPS). J Cardiovasc Pharmacol. 2007;49(2):81-4.

16. Ye P, Wu CE, Sheng L, et al. Potential protective effect of long-term therapy with Xuezhikang on left ventricular diastolic function in patients with essential hypertension. J Altern Complement Med. 2009;15(7):719-25.
17. Li JJ, Lu ZL, Kou WR, et al. Beneficial impact of Xuezhikang on cardiovascular events and mortality in elderly hypertensive patients with previous myocardial infarction from the China Coronary Secondary Prevention Study (CCSPS). J Clin Pharmacol. 2009;49(8):947-56.
18. Gordon RY, Cooperman T, Obermeyer W, et al. Marked variability of monacolin levels in commercial red yeast rice products: buyer beware! Arch Intern Med. 2010;170(19): 1722-7.
19. Klimek M, Wang S, Ogunkanmi A. Safety and efficacy of red yeast rice (*Monascus purpureus*) as an alternative therapy for hyperlipidemia. PT. 2009;32:313-27.
20. Endo A, Kuroda M. Citrinin, an inhibitor of cholesterol synthesis. J Antibiot. 1976;29:841-3.
21. Sabater-Vilar M, Maas RF, Fink-Gremmels J. Mutagenicity of commercial Monascus fermentation products and the role of citrinin contamination. Mutat Res. 1999;444(1):7-16.
22. Donmez-Altuntas H, Dumlupinar G, Imamoglu N, et al. Effects of the mycotoxin citrinin on micronucleus formation in a cytokinesis-block genotoxicity assay in cultured human lymphocytes. J Appl Toxicol. 2007;27(4):337-41.
23. Pascual-Ahuir A, Vanacloig-Pedros E, Proft M. Toxicity mechanisms of the food contaminant citrinin: application of a quantitative yeast model. Nutrients. 2014;6:2077-87.
24. Venhuis BJ, van Hunsel F, van de Koppel S, et al. Pharmacologically effective red yeast rice preparations marketed as dietary supplements illustrated by a case report. Drug Test Anal. 2016;8(3-4):315-8.
25. Li Y, Jiang L, Jia Z, et al. A meta-analysis of red yeast rice: An effective and relatively safe alternative approach for dyslipidemia. PLoS One. 2014;9(6):e98611.
26. Agostoni C, Bresson JL, Fairweather-Tait S, et al. Scientific opinion on the substantiation of health claims related to monacolin K from red yeast rice and maintenance of normal blood LDL cholesterol concentrations (ID 1648, 1700) pursuant to Article 13 (1) of Regulation (EC) No 1924/2006. EFSA J. 2011;9(7):2304-20.
27. Childress L, Gay A, Zargar A, et al. Review of red yeast rice content and current Food and Drug Administration oversight. J. Clin Lipidol. 2013;7(2):117-22.
28. Su CF, Liu IM, Cheng JT. Improvement of insulin resistance by Hon-Chi in fructose-rich chow-fed rats. Food Chem. 2007;104(1):45-52.
29. Chen CC, Liu IM. Release of acetylcholine by Hon-Chi to raise insulin secretion in Wistar rats. Neurosci Lett. 2006;404(1-2):117-21.
30. Hsieh PS, Tai YH. Aqueous extract of *Monascus purpureus* M9011 prevents and reverses fructose-induced hypertension in rats. J Agric Food Chem. 2003;51(14):3945-50.
31. Li X-M, ShenXH, Duan ZW, et al. Advances on the pharmacological effects of red yeast rice. Chin J Nat Med. 2011;9(3):161-6.
32. Kuba M, Tanaka K, Sesoko M, et al. Angiotensin I-converting enzyme inhibitory peptides in red-mold rice made by *Monascus purpureus*. Process Biochem. 2009;44(10):1139-43.
33. Chen WP, Ho BY, Lee CL, et al. Red mold rice prevents the development of obesity, dyslipidemia and hyperinsulinemia induced by high-fat diet. Int J Obes (Lond). 2008;32(11):1694-704.
34. Hossain CF, Okuyama E, Yamazaki MA. A new series of coumarin derivatives having monoamine oxidase inhibitory activity from *Monascus anka*. Chem Pharm Bull (Tokyo). 1996;44(8):1535-9.
35. Cho YE, Alcantara E, Kumaran S, et al. Red yeast rice stimulates osteoblast proliferation and increases alkaline phosphatase activity in MC3T3-E1 cells. Nutr Res. 2010;30(7):501-10.
36. Wong RW, Rabie B. Chinese red yeast rice (*Monascus purpureus*-fermented rice) promotes bone formation. Chin Med. 2008;3:4.
37. Poynter JN, Gruber SB, Higgins PD, et al. Statins and the risk of colorectal cancer. N Engl J Med. 2005;352(21):2184-92.
38. Hong MY, Seeram NP, Zhang Y, et al. Chinese red yeast rice versus lovastatin effects on prostate cancer cells with and without androgen receptor overexpression. J Med Food. 2008;11(4):657-66.
39. Hong MY, Henning S, Moro A, et al. Chinese red yeast rice inhibition of prostate tumor growth in SCID mice. Cancer Prev Res (Phila). 2011;4(4):608-15.
40. Taira J, Miyagi C, Aniya Y. Dimerumic acid as an antioxidant from the mold, *Monascus anka*: the inhibition mechanisms against lipid peroxidation and hemeprotein-mediated oxidation. Biochem Pharmacol. 2002;63(5):1019-26.
41. Aniya Y, Ohtani II, Higa T, et al. Dimerumic acid as an antioxidant of the mold, *Monascus anka*. Free RadicBiol Med. 2000;28(6):999-1004.
42. Lee CL, Wang JJ, Pan TM. Red mold rice extract represses amyloid beta peptide-induced neurotoxicity via potent synergism of anti-inflammatory and antioxidative effect. Appl Microbiol Biotechnol. 2008;79(5):829-41.
43. Lee CL, Kuo TF, Wu CL, et al. Red mold rice promotes neuroprotectives APP alpha secretion instead of Alzheimer's risk factors and amyloid beta expression in hyperlipidemic A40-infused rays. J Agric Food Chem. 2010;58(4):2230-8.
44. Weihrauch JL, Gardner JM. Sterol content of foods of plant origin. J Am Dietet Assoc. 1978;73(1):39-47.
45. Andersson SW, Skinner J, Ellegard L, et al. Intake of dietary plant sterols is inversely related to serum cholesterol concentration in men and women in the EPIC Norfolk population: a cross-sectional study. Eur J Clin Nutr. 2004;58(10):1378-85.
46. Moreau RA, Hicks KB. The in vitro hydrolysis of phytosterol conjugates in food matrices by mammalian digestive enzymes. Lipids. 2004;39(8):769-76.
47. Valsta LM, Lemsrom A, Ovaskainen ML, et al. Estimation of plant sterol and cholesterol intake in Finland: quality of new values and their effect on intake. Brit J Nutr. 2007;92(4):671-8.
48. de Jong A, Pat J, Mensink RP. Metabolic effects of plant sterols and stanols (Review). J Nutr Biochem. 2003;14(7):362-9.
49. von Bergmann K, Sudhop T, Lutjohann D. Cholesterol and plant sterol absorption: recent insights. Am J Cardiol. 2005;96(1):S10-14.
50. Ostlund RE Jr, McGill JB, Zeng CM, et al. Gastrointestinal absorption and plasma kinetics of soy Delta(5)-phytosterols and phytostanols in humans. Am J Physiol Endocrinol Metab. 2002;282:E911-6.
51. Sudhop T, Lutjohann D, von Bergmann K. Sterol transporters: targets of natural sterols and new lipid lowering drugs. Pharmacol Ther. 2005;105(3):333-41.
52. Sudhop T, Sahin Y, Lindenthal B, et al. Comparison of the hepatic clearances of campesterol, sitosterol, and cholesterol in healthy subjects suggests that efflux transporters controlling intestinal sterol absorption also regulate biliary secretion. Gut. 2002;51(6):860-3.
53. Berger A, Jones PJ, Abumweiss SS. Plant sterols: factors affecting their efficacy and safety as functional food ingredients. Lipids Health Dis. 2004;3:5.
54. Katan MB, Grundy SM, Jones P, et al. Efficacy and safety of plant stanols and sterols in the management of blood cholesterol levels. Mayo Clin Proc. 2003;78(8):965-78.
55. Nissinen M, Gylling H, Vuoristo M, et al. Micellar distribution of cholesterol and phytosterols after duodenal plant stanol ester infusion. Am J Physiol Gastrointest Liver physiol. 2002;282(6):G1009-15.
56. Health Canada. (2010). Plant Sterols and Blood Cholesterol Lowering. [online] www.hc-sc.gc.ca [Accessed September, 2017].
57. Ling WH, Jones PJ. Dietary phytosterols: a review of metabolism, benefits and side effects. Life Sci. 1995;57(3):195-206.
58. Awad AB, Toczek J, Fink CS. Phytosterols decrease prostaglandin release in cultured P388D1/MAB macrophages. Prostaglandins Leukot Essent Fatty Acids. 2004;70(6): 511-20.

59. von Holtz RL, Fink CS, Awad AB. Beta-sitosterol activates the sphingomyelin cycle and induces apoptosis in LNCaP human prostate cancer cells. Nutr Cancer. 1998;32(1):8-12.
60. Awad AB, Roy R, Fink CS. Beta-sitosterol, a plant sterol, induces apoptosis and activates key caspases in MDA-MB-231 human breast cancer cells. Oncol Rep. 2003;10(2):497-500.
61. Choi YH, Kong KR, Kim YA, et al. Induction of Bax and activation of caspases during beta-sitosterol-mediated apoptosis in human colon cancer cells. Int J Oncol. 2003;23(6):1657-62.
62. European Food Safety Authority: Scientific Opinion. Scientific Opinion on the substantiation of a health claim related to 3 g/day plant sterols/stanols and lowering blood LDL-cholesterol and reduce risk of (coronary) heart disease pursuant to Article 19 of Regulation (EC) No 1924/2006. EFSA Panel on Dietetic Products, Nutrition and Allergies (NDA). EFSA J. 2012;10(5): 2693.
63. Woyengo TA, Ramprasath VR, Jones PL. Anticancer effects of phytosterols. Eur J Clin Nutr. 2009;63(7):813-20.
64. Berges RR, Windeler J, Trampisch HJ, et al. Randomised, placebo-controlled, double-blind clinical trial of beta-sitosterol in patients with benign prostatic hyperplasia. Beta-sitosterol Study Group. Lancet. 1995;345(8964):1529-32.
65. Assman G, Cullen P, Erbey J, et al. Plasma sitosterol elevations are associated with an increased incidence of coronary events in men: results of a nested case-control analysis of the Prospective Cardiovascular Munster (PROCAM) study. Nutr Metab Cardiovasc Dis. 2006;16(1):13-21.
66. Sudhop T, Gottwald BM, von Bergmann K. Serum plant sterols as a potential risk factor for coronary heart disease. Metabolism. 2002;51(12):1519-21.
67. Rajaratnam RA, Gylling H, Miettinen TA. Independent association of serum squalene and noncholesterol sterols with coronary artery disease in postmenopausal women. J. Am Coll Cardiol. 2000;35:1185-91.
68. Weingartner O, Lutjohann D, Ji S, et al. Vascular effects of diet supplementation with plant sterols. J. Am Coll Cardiol. 2008;51(16):1553-61.
69. Normen L, Holmes D, Frohlich J. Plant sterols and their role in combined use with statins for lipid lowering. Curr Opin Investig Drugs. 2005;6(3):307-16.
70. Simons LA. Additive effect of plant sterol-ester margarine and cerivastatin in lowering low-density lipoprotein cholesterol in primary hypercholesterolemia. Am J Cardiol. 2002;90(7):737-40.
71. Nguyen TT, Dale LC. Plant stanol esters and vitamin K (letter). Mayo Clin Proc. 1999;74(6):642-3.
72. Hendriks HF, Brink EJ, Meijer GW, et al. Safety of long-term consumption of plant sterol esters-enriched spread. Eur J Clin Nutr. 2003;57(5):681-92.
73. Ntanios FY, Duchateau GS. A healthy diet rich in carotenoids is effective in maintaining normal blood carotenoid levels during the daily use of plant sterol-enriched spreads. Int J Vitam Nutr Res. 2002;72(1):32-9.

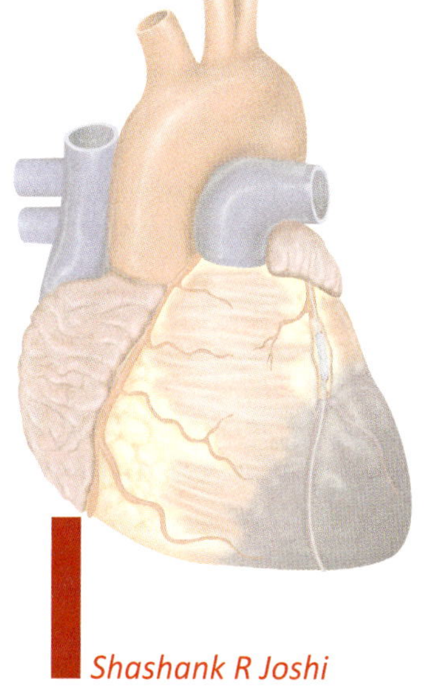

Meal Replacement Therapy for Obesity Care in Cardiodiabetes

Shashank R Joshi

INTRODUCTION

The prevalence of obesity in India is increasing rapidly and recent data show that 13–50% of the urban population and 8–38.2% of the rural population suffer from obesity.[1] The increase in obesity has led to increase in associated comorbidities like type 2 diabetes mellitus (T2DM), hypertension, dyslipidemia, coronary heart disease (CHD), nonalcoholic fatty liver disease (NAFLD), obstructive sleep apnea, and certain cancers.[1] Cardiovascular disease (CVD) and T2DM are strongly associated with obesity and there is very good evidence that weight loss lowers glucose, blood pressure, low-density lipoprotein (LDL) cholesterol, and triglyceride.[2] Being overweight or obese is a major risk factor for developing T2DM, and weight loss is a recommended treatment strategy for the prevention and management of this condition. Excess body fat is recognized to result in key metabolic disturbances in obese subjects with T2DM and excess body fat is a common trait among many patients with T2DM. Weight loss intervention in obese patients with T2DM has been shown to be capable of correcting many of the metabolic abnormalities associated with T2DM, such as hyperinsulinemia, hyperglycemia, and hypertriglyceridemia.[3] A healthful eating pattern, regular physical activity, and often pharmacotherapy are key components of diabetes management. For many individuals with diabetes, the most challenging part of the treatment plan is determining what to eat. It is now well established that there is not a "one-size-fits-all" eating pattern for individuals with diabetes.[4,5]

ADIPOSITY AND DIABETES

A number of factors may be responsible for increasing adiposity in people with diabetes, including a reduction in glycosuria and thus retention of calories otherwise lost as an effect of therapeutic intervention, changes in food intake, or changes in energy expenditure. If adiposity is a concern, medications that are weight neutral or weight reducing [e.g. metformin, incretin-based therapies, and sodium glucose cotransporter 2 (SGLT-2) inhibitors] could be considered. Several intensive diabetes self-management education (DSME) and nutrition intervention studies show that glycemic control can be achieved while maintaining weight or even reducing weight when appropriate lifestyle counseling is provided.[5] More than three out of every four adults with diabetes are at least overweight, and nearly half of individuals with diabetes are obese. Because of the relationship between body weight specifically the adiposity and insulin resistance, weight loss has long been a recommended strategy for overweight or obese adults with diabetes. Prevention of weight gain is also equally important. Long-term reduction of adiposity is difficult for most people to achieve, and even harder for individuals with diabetes to achieve given the impact of some medications used to improve glycemic control like insulin, insulin secretagogues, and thiazolidinediones. Intentional weight loss in people with diabetes is very effective at reducing CV risk. In a systematic review, Aucott et al. (2004) found that people with diabetes who lost weight intentionally significantly reduced their mortality risks by 25% with weight loss of 9–13 kg being most protective. Therefore, development and use of effective weight loss strategies are very important in people with diabetes.[2]

MANAGEMENT

Metabolic control, including weight loss can be considered the cornerstone of diabetes management. Achieving A1c goals decreases the risk for microvascular and macrovascular complications, especially the CVD risk. In addition, achieving blood pressure and lipid goals can help reduce risk for CVD events. An individualized nutrition intervention plan and ongoing support of behavior changes by a team of healthcare professionals can facilitate the achievement of their patients' health goals.[5] A 5–15% weight loss over a period of 6 months is realistic and of proven health benefit. A greater (20% or more) weight loss may be considered for those with greater degrees of obesity [body mass index (BMI) ≥35 kg/m^2).[6] Findings from randomized controlled trials (RCTs) and from systematic and Cochrane reviews demonstrate the effectiveness of nutrition therapy for improving glycemic control and various markers of CV and hypertension risk. In the general population, medical nutrition therapy (MNT) provided to patients with an abnormal lipid profile has been shown to reduce daily fat (5–8%), saturated fat (2–4%), energy intake (232–710 kcal/day), lower triglycerides (11–31%), LDL cholesterol (7–22%), and total cholesterol (7–21%) levels.[5]

MEDICAL NUTRITION THERAPY

The MNT is outcome based. Considering an individualized dietary requirements, the MNT can be planned in a structured way.

Goals of Medical Nutrition Therapy

To promote and support nutritious eating patterns, emphasizing a variety of nutrient dense foods in appropriate portion sizes, in order to improve overall health and specifically to:

- Attain individualized glycemic, blood pressure, and lipid goals.

General recommended goals from the American Dietetic Association (ADA) for these markers are as follows:*

- HbA1c, 7%
- Blood pressure, 140/80 mm Hg
- Low-density lipoprotein cholesterol, 100 mg/dL; triglycerides, 150 mg/dL; high-density lipoprotein (HDL) cholesterol, 40 mg/dL for men; and HDL cholesterol 50 mg/dL for women
- Achieve and maintain body weight goals
- Delay or prevent complications of diabetes.[5]

Research has shown that those with prediabetes can reduce their risk of developing T2DM by nearly 60–80% by weight loss accomplished through participation in a structured lifestyle change program with or without pharmacotherapy. In people with T2DM, modest weight loss of just 2–5% can improve glycemic control, and therapeutic weight loss of more than or equal to 5% can further improve glycemia and produce cardiometabolic benefits. Weight loss of more than or equal to 10% in patients with T2DM has been associated with a reduced rate of CV events and deaths.[7] Results from lifestyle intervention programs like the Diabetes Prevention Program (DPP) have shown considerable outcomes. Those patients who had the goal of a minimum weight loss of 7% body weight through dietary modification (hypocaloric diet) and 150 minutes of moderate intensity physical activity per week were found to have a 58% reduction in the incidence rate of diabetes. Also, in the look Action for Health in Diabetes (AHEAD) study, a 5–10% weight loss over 1 year led to improvement in glycemic control along with improvement in CVD risk factors. Other benefits of weight loss include improvement in NAFLD, osteoarthritis, urinary incontinence, depression, obstructive sleep apnea, mobility, and quality of life.[1]

A 15–30% decrease in energy (calorie) intake from habitual intake in a weight-stable individual is sufficient and appropriate. There is a great variation in energy requirements between the individuals, which is dependent on the individual's gender, age, BMI, and physical activity level. Energy requirements must be calculated by taking into account gender, age, BMI, and physical activity. The recommended weight-reducing dietary regimen tailored to an individual's need usually provides an energy deficit of 500–600 kcal/day. A 600 kcal (2,600 kJ) daily deficit will predict a weight loss of about 0.5 kg weekly. Diets providing 1,200 kcal/day or more are classified as hypocaloric balanced diets (HBD) or balanced deficit diets. Diets providing less than 1,200 kcal/day might yield micronutrient deficiencies, which could exert untoward effects not only on nutritional status but also on the weight management outcome. However, in clinical practice, a further reduction in caloric intake might be required. In this case, the appropriate use of dietary supplements may prevent such nutritional deficits. In clinical practice, low-calorie diets (LCDs) and very-low-calorie diets (VLCDs) are used. LCDs, consisting of normal meals and partial meal replacements (MRs), have an energy content between 800 kcal/day and 1,200 kcal/day. VLCDs usually provide less than 800 kcal/day and may be used only as part of a comprehensive program under the medical supervision. Their administration should be limited for specific patients and for short periods of time. VLCDs are unsuitable as a sole source of nutrition for children and adolescents, pregnant or lactating women, and the elderly. MR diets (substitution of one or two daily meal portions by

VLCD) may contribute to nutritionally well-balanced diet and weight loss maintenance.[6]

Efficacy of weight loss programs has frequently referred to nutritional adequacy of diets in relation to general composition or recommended daily intakes (RDIs) or specific health measures (e.g. bone resorption).[8]

Meal Replacement—An Effective Medical Nutrition Therapy

Commercial MRs have become increasingly popular as a strategy among people trying to lose weight, in both diabetic and nondiabetic population. In a country like US, 15% of women and 13% of men reportedly use MRs as their weight-loss strategy, showing its rising preference in lifestyle intervention plan.[8] Use of MR plans prescribed by trained medical practitioners and registered dietitians, with close patient monitoring, can be beneficial. Within the intensive lifestyle intervention group of the Look AHEAD trial, for example, use of a partial MR plan was associated with improvements in diet quality. Meal replacements was being used in the Look AHEAD Diabetes study in the USA as part of a comprehensive behavioral strategy and at 12 months a weight loss of 8.6% versus 0.8% in the control group had occurred which had reduced to 4.7% and 1.1% in 4 years.[2]

In a systematic review of controlled trials of lifestyle interventions, Brown et al. observed that when MRs were added to a low-fat diet, there was a significant improvement in weight loss of 5.4 kgs. In another study of 57 subjects with T2DM comparing MRs with an exchange diet plan for 12 weeks, Yip et al. (2001) found that weight loss in the two MR groups were greater (6.4% and 6.7%, respectively) compared with weight loss in the diet plan group (4.9%), although this was not significant. In addition, fasting glucose, total cholesterol, and LDL cholesterol levels were reduced in the MR groups and the glucose change was significant compared with the diet plan group ($p = 0.01$), but glycated hemoglobin (HbA1c) was not different (0.2% difference between groups). Similarly, Li et al. (2005) in a longer 12-month study found that percentage weight loss was greater in the MR group (4.6%) than in diet plan group (2.3%) although BMI change was not significant ($p = 0.07$). Fasting glucose was reduced in MRs group at 6 months and HbA1c level improved in MR at 6 months compared to the diet plan group by 0.49% ($p = 0.1$ for comparison), but this difference had disappeared by 12 months (0.15%, $p = 0.6$) and neither group had a significant change in HbA1c compared to baseline. Each participant in both groups received individual consultation with a registered dietitian at baseline, weeks 2, 4, 6, 8 and then monthly for the duration of the 1-year study and 77 out of 104 subjects completed the study. More subjects in MRs group reduced their use of medications. In a study of 119 subjects, Cheskin et al. (2008) found that weight loss on an MR program for 34 weeks with 1-year follow-up was greater than on a standard diet with more subjects 40% versus 12% achieving more than equal to 5% weight loss. HbA1c dropped by 0.28% in the MR group versus an increase of 0.32% in the standard diet ($p = 0.06$). In a report by Ditschuneit (2006), patients with diabetes on a MR program achieved weight loss of 5.2% and 4.4% of their body weight at 6 months and 12 months, respectively. In comparison, patients on a diet plan achieved weight loss of 2.9% and 2.4% at 6 months and 12 months.[2]

Meal replacements have been examined in a small number of long-term studies that suggest weight loss is maintained by using this strategy. For example, in a 116-week follow-up study that used MRs, weight loss was 6 kg overall. After 1 year, 77% of subjects maintained more than 80% of the initial weight loss and 62% maintained more than 80% of the initial weight loss after 2 years, with only 7.4% of subjects above baseline weight. Flechtner-Mors et al. found that after 4 years in a single-arm intervention study using MRs, which had an initial 12-week 2-arm MR and a conventional diet intervention period, the original conventional diet group had a 3.2% weight loss versus 8.4% in the MR group.[8] In a nutshell, the use of MRs for 6 months can increase weight loss by 2.5 kg compared with nonprofessional advice from a diet book, but HbA1c was not significantly different between the groups. In order to achieve a greater reduction in HbA1c, professional advice is probably required, although this is not a guarantee of success as the Li study showed no significant effect on HbA1c at 12 months in either group despite extensive professional advice.[2]

FAT LOSS VERSUS WEIGHT LOSS

It is scientifically proven that the immediate reduction in carbohydrate using the protein-rich MRs was the most important cause of a fall in HbA1c at 3 months in the MR group. Medication dosage reduction clearly had an effect on the results as well, particularly in the MR group. It's important to note that a greater weight loss is required to maintain the early changes in HbA1c.[2] MR simplifies the weight loss regimens by replacing one or two meals a day with a product of defined nutrient and calorie content. An increase in dietary protein content has been proposed to be effective for body weight regulation through effects on satiety, thermogenesis, and substrate partitioning. Protein has specific effects on satiety hormones, including PYY 3–36. When protein replaces carbohydrate within a low-fat diet, reduced insulinemic and glycemic responses have been observed resulting in increased fat oxidation.[9] Retention of lean mass during weight loss is important for long-term weight maintenance and also for maintaining physical function after weight loss. The amount of fat lost on an absolute basis, and as a proportion of the total weight lost, was similar between the two cohorts, suggesting there was not a difference in the way these cohorts utilized adipose tissue to meet the caloric deficit in their diets. This is in contrast to other research which found that individuals with T2DM lost less fat per unit of body weight than those without T2DM. Indeed, the only body composition differences in this study occurred at week 4, where the cohort with D/HBS lost less lean mass compared with controls and had a greater percentage of weight loss from fat. At later time points, the losses in fat mass were similar, with 48% of weight loss due to loss of fat mass in both cohorts. Thus, both cohorts had good retention of lean mass (6% or less absolute loss of lean mass across the study period). Although modest exercise was encouraged during the weight-loss program, there was no formal exercise component. The nutritional composition of these meal plans, which provide a relatively high level of protein (~100–150 g per day), is likely an important contributing factor in the retention of lean mass.[7]

Because individuals with T2DM are at a higher risk for CVD, weight loss-related improvements in cardiometabolic risk factors are an important outcome measure. Clinically relevant and similar improvements in both blood pressure (systolic and diastolic) and pulse were observed in both cohorts. The reduction in both systolic and diastolic blood pressure and pulse occurred early in weight loss, with the majority of the response occurring within the first 4 weeks, corresponding to the time interval when individuals lost an average of 5% of baseline body weight. The magnitude of the blood pressure reductions observed in this study (10–11 mmHg systolic and 4–6 mmHg diastolic) has been associated with a substantial reduction in CVD risk.

MEAL REPLACEMENT THERAPY IN INDIA

In Indian context, the role of MR therapy is essentially to limit food choices. Most of the people who go on weight loss diets find it extremely challenging to adhere to meal plans, especially when they are travelling or at work place. This is so because there are no food options available which will ensure caloric restriction. Also most of foods available like biscuits, etc. although low in calories, are very poor in nutritional composition. They are typically only carbohydrate-containing foods which lack proteins, vitamins, and essential fats. Use of meal replacers in such cases ensures dietary regimen is followed and nutritionally diets are complete. Globally, meal replacers are available in various formats like shakes, bars, soup, etc. while in India, they are typically available as shakes. Among MR therapy, partial MR therapy works the best and has highest compliance. Essentially, snacks are replaced by replacer and individuals are still allowed to eat their main meals.

CONCLUSION

In people with diabetes, MRs are most often used as part of a multidisciplinary weight management program as they are viable and potentially cost-effective solution to weight management in T2DM.[2] Meal replacers provide portion control and can bring structure to weight-loss interventions. Weight-loss success can also be enhanced by providing behavioral support to improve adherence to a reduced calorie diet, using either in-person or telephone counseling. Including both meal replacers and support provides a more comprehensive approach to weight reduction and is associated with weight loss success.[7] The overall impact of weight loss in patients with T2DM is not only the tighter glycemic control, but also the reduction in the CV risk among many others.

REFERENCES

1. Behl S, Misra A. Management of obesity in adult Asian Indians. Ind Heart J. 2017;69(4):539-44.
2. Keogh JB, Clifton PM. Meal Replacements for Weight Loss in Type 2 Diabetes in a Community Setting. J Nutr Metab. 2012;2012:918571.
3. Yip I, Go VLW, DeShields S, et al. Liquid Meal Replacements and Glycemic Control in Obese Type 2 Diabetes Patients. Obes Res. 2001;9(4):341s-7s.
4. American Diabetes Association. Obesity Management for the Treatment of Type 2 Diabetes. Diabetes Care. 2017;40(Suppl 1):S57-63.
5. Evert AB, Boucher JL, Cypress M, et al. Nutrition Therapy Recommendations for the Management of Adults with Diabetes. Diabetes Care. 2014;37(1):s120-43.
6. Yumuk V, Tsigos C, Fried M, et al. European Guidelines for Obesity Management in Adults. Obes Facts. 2015;8(6):402-24.
7. Coleman CD, Kiel JR, Mitola AH, et al. Comparative effectiveness of a portion-controlled meal replacement program for weight loss in adults with and without diabetes/high blood sugar. Nutr Diabetes. 2017;7(7):e284.
8. Noakes M, Foster PR, Keogh JB, et al. Meal replacements are as effective as structured weight-loss diets for treating obesity in adults with features of metabolic syndrome. J Nutr. 2017;134(8):1874-99.
9. Treyzon L, Chen S, Hort K, et al. A controlled trial of protein enrichment of meal replacements for weight reduction with retention of lean body mass. Nutr J. 2008;7:23.

CHAPTER

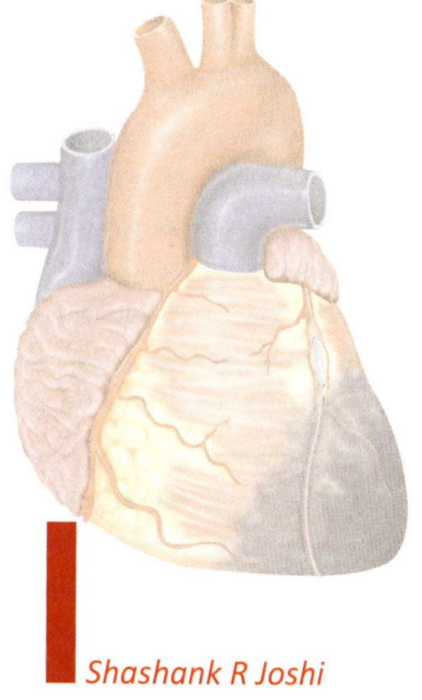

Ideal Edible Oil in Cardiodiabetes

Shashank R Joshi

INTRODUCTION

Dietary fat plays an essential role in our diet. Fats form an important part of our diet. National Institute of Nutrition (NIN), India recommends that diet should consist of 15–30% fats. Nutrition also goes beyond the quantity and quality of food; it also depends on the way food is cooked and the manner in which food is consumed. Edible oils are one of the major contributors of fat in our diet. The way oils are used especially in Indian cooking makes it important to choose them wisely and to select oils that are designed especially for Indian cooking.

FATS AND OILS: BASICS

Fats consist of a group of compounds that is chemically insoluble in water. It has lower density than water and may range from being in liquid state to solid state at room temperature depending on its structure. Even though the words 'fats', 'oils', and 'lipids' are synonymous, 'oils' is usually referred to the fats that are liquids at room temperature, and 'fats' are solids. 'Lipids' is used to refer to both.[1] Triacylglycerols are the predominant components of most food. The nonglyceride or minor components are mono and diacylglycerols, sterols, free fatty acids, phosphatides, fat-soluble vitamins, fatty alcohols, and other substances.[2]

The brief description of different components is given here:

- *Triacylglycerols:* Dietary triacylglycerols are the major lipid components in the human diet and they are carriers of energy as well as important fatty acids. Various factors affect the digestion and absorption of triacylglycerols. Increasing evidence shows that, in addition to the overall fatty acid profile, the triacylglycerol structure and the species composition are of importance when considering the nutritional effects of a fat. There is also enough evidence that in addition to its short-term effects in the intestine on absorption of fatty acids, the triacylglycerol structure also has long-term effects resulting from differences in the profile of absorbed fatty acids. Studies analyzing the different atherogenic potential of dietary fats have given us a clear indication of the importance of the triacylglycerol structure for absorption of saturated fatty acids (SFAs). Hence, contextually one may focus on the effects of the structure of dietary fats as such, or may speculate also on the possibilities of modifying the structure of fats to affect their absorption and the distribution of the fatty acids in the body after digestion and uptake.[3] One hundred g of fat yield approximately 95 g of fatty acids.[4]
- *Minor Components of Oils:*[4]
  - *Mono and Diacylglycerols:* Mono-and diacylglycerols are mono-and diesters of fatty acids and glycerol. They are prepared commercially by the reaction of glycerol and triacylglycerols or by the esterification of glycerol and fatty acids. They also occur naturally in very minor amounts in both animal fats and vegetable oils.
  - *Free Fatty Acids:* Free fatty acids are unattached fatty acids present in a fat. Refining processes reduce the levels of fatty acids.

- *Phosphatides:* Phosphatides consist of alcohols (usually glycerols), combined with fatty acids, phosphoric acid, and a nitrogen-containing compound. Cephalin and lecithin are common phosphatides found in edible fats. Refining removes the phosphatides from fat or oil.
- *Sterols:* Sterols, also referred to as steroid alcohols, are a class of molecules that contain the common steroid nucleus plus an 8–10 carbon side chain and an alcohol group found in both animal fats and vegetable oils. Cholesterol is the major animal fat sterol and is only found in vegetable oils in trace amounts. Vegetable sterols are collectively termed as 'phytosterols'. Sitosterol and stigmasterol are best known vegetable oil sterols.
- *Vitamins:* Tocopherols are important minor constituents of most vegetable fats described as series of organic compounds consisting of methylated phenols. They serve as a sources of vitamin E. Amongst tocopherols, alpha-tocopherol have the highest activity of vitamin E and lowest antioxidant potential. Fat soluble vitamins A and D are sometimes added to foods which contain fat because they serve as good carriers and are widely consumed.

Fats: Classification

Irrespective of the way they have been classified structurally from the nutrition perspective, the fats are classified usually on the basis of their unsaturation (Fig. 1).[5]

- *Saturated fat* is a fat that consists of triglycerides containing only SFAs. SFAs do not have any double bonds between the individual carbon atoms of the fatty acid chain. The chain of carbon atoms is fully 'saturated' with hydrogen atoms. Single bonds between carbon atoms are more stable than double bonds. Thus, compared to unsaturated fats, saturated fats are more stable and are usually solid at room temperature. The dietary sources of these fats include fat in milk, cream, butter, ghee, animal tallow, and among vegetarian sources such as coconut oil, palm oil, etc. Many studies have found that consuming diets which are low in saturated fat reduces total and low-density lipoprotein cholesterol (LDL-C) and also reduces the incidence of heart diseases. There is also a large evidence to show relation between higher SFA intake and prevalence of various kinds of cancer especially breast cancer and colorectal cancer. Also there is enough evidence to prove that higher SFA intakes decreases insulin sensitivity.[6] One of the homologous series, palmitic acid is implicated as atherogenic. SFAs are known to increase high-density lipoprotein (HDL).
- *Partially Hydrogenated or Trans Fatty Acids:* These solid fats are made from mostly unsaturated vegetable oils (liquids) which have been added some hydrogen atoms through the process called hydrogenation, until the desired food characteristics of flavor, texture, and stability are achieved. During the hydrogenation process, some hydrogen atoms change their configuration from being on the same side (cis) of a carbon-carbon double

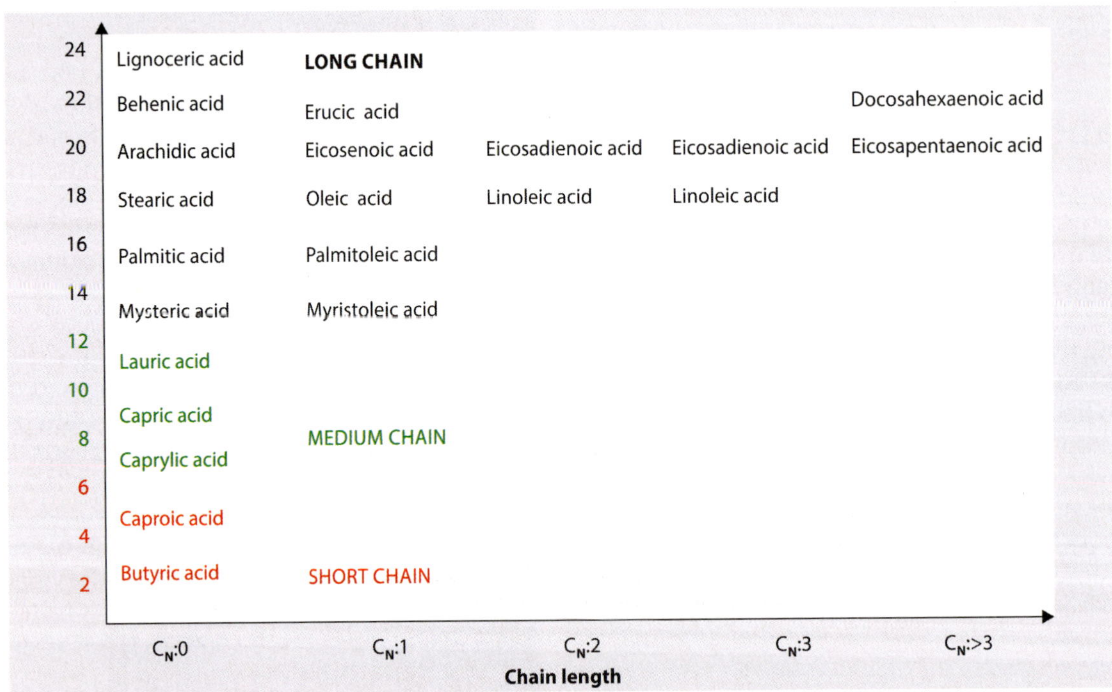

Fig. 1: Graphical depiction of classification of fat

bond to being on opposite sides (trans). If complete hydrogenation is achieved than no trans fats and saturated fats result. If only partial hydrogenation is obtained, some double bonds remain, and trans fats are produced. Trans fats were believed to have more structural stability and provide required texture to foods. Naturally occurring transfatty acids are found in smaller amounts in beef and lamb. In India, transfats are available as *Vanaspati* and baking shortening. They are also present in stick margarines and shortening. Most of the food which is baked like cookies, pastries, puff, khari, and toast, etc. have a large amount of transfatty acid in them. Ready to eat and processed foods tend to have more transfats in them as trans fats are also generated at high temperature cooking. Research has shown that consumption of trans fatty acid have been associated with coronary artery diseases, increase in LDL-C, decreasing in HDL cholesterol (HDL-C) and increase in C-reactive protein (CRP).[7]

- *Unsaturated Fatty Acids:* An unsaturated fat is a fat or fatty acid in which there is atleast one double bond within the fatty acid chain. The fat molecule is monounsaturated if it contains one double bond and polyunsaturated if it contains more than one double bond.
  - *Monounsaturated Fatty Acids:* These have fatty acids containing one double bond. As they have lesser double bonds as compared to polyunsaturated fatty acids (PUFAs), they are less vulnerable to lipid peroxidation. Foods containing higher amount of monounsaturated fatty acid (MUFA) are shown to reduce LDL-C and increase HDL-C. Dietary sources of MUFA are olive oil, groundnut oil, rice bran oil, mustard oil, and canola oil. Lot of nuts like almonds, peanuts, etc. have high proportions MUFA in them. Fruits like olives and avocados are rich sources of monounsaturated fatty acids. Fats such as mustard oil, groundnut oil, olive oil, rice bran oil, and soybean oil are rich in monounsaturated fats as compared to other oils. These oils when used in prescribed amounts lower total cholesterol and LDL-C levels in the blood.[8]
  - *Polyunsaturated Fatty Acids:* Polyunsaturated lipids are triacylglycerols in which the hydrocarbon tails of this ester constitutes PUFA (fatty acids possessing more than a single carbon–carbon double bond). Use of PUFA as fats is shown to reduce LDL-C and improve insulin sensitivity. These are recommended fats for patients with cardiac diseases. Oils such as sunflower oil, safflower oil (SO), and corn oil are polyunsaturated fats. Besides these all invisible fats present in cereals and pulses are majorly polyunsaturated. These fats are known to lower cholesterol. This is so because they are prone to oxidation in cooking.[9] Hence, great precaution should be taken in using these oils. Never recycle these.

EDIBLE OIL INDUSTRY: INDIAN PERSPECTIVE

In India, cooking oil forms an integral part of every household and right choice of edible oil is needed for maintaining a healthy life. In western and southern states mainly there is a strong preference for groundnut oil, and in the north and east, mustard oil is preferred. Palm oil is consumed the most however, the large quantity of palm oil is utilized for the manufacture of *'Vanaspati'* which is mostly used in commercial establishments.[10] Studies have shown that it is not a single fat source, but a combination or a blend of various fats having fatty acid compositions and additional minor components like tocotrienols, oryzanol, and a good balance of saturated and unsaturated fats that will bring about favorable serum lipid profiles which help in guarding against suffering or mortality from coronary heart disease (CHD).

Different oils have unique constituents like oryzanol, tocopherols, tocotrienols and phytosterols. Hence, the NIN India, in their recent recommendations state that a correct combination or blend of two or more oils should be used to achieve all kinds of fatty acids in the diet (Table 1).[11]

Edible Oils: Indian Cooking Conditions

Indian cooking conditions subjects food at very temperatures especially their fat components. Oil is mainly used from the beginning of the process, starting with sautéing ginger and garlic and then adding chilies and onions. The temperature of this form of shallow frying reaches upto 120–130°C. The deep frying process subjects oil upto more than 150°C. However, a series of complex reactions such as oxidation, isomerization, hydrolysis, and polymerization take place during the deep-fat frying course and influence quality attributes of the final product such as sensory parameters like flavor, texture, and functional attributes like shelf life and nutrient composition. The effect of these reactions results from a number of their products including volatile compounds, oxidized triacylglycerol monomers, hydrolysis products, trans configuration compounds, polymers, nitrogen-and sulfur-containing heterocyclic compounds, acrylamide, etc. which are present in both frying oil and the fried food. Additionally, these reactions are interacted and influenced by various impact factors such as frying oil

TABLE 1: Fatty acid profile of different commonly consumed oils in India[11]

Common Edible Oils and Fats	Total SFA (g/100 g)	Total MUFA (g/100 g)	Total PUFA (g/100 g)	Omega 3 (g/100 g)	Omega 6 (g/100 g)	Omega 6: Omega 3 (5:1 to 10:1)	SFA:MUFA:PUFA
Coconut oil	89.5	7.8	2		2	-	1:0.9:0.02
Palm olein	47.7	41.4	10.6	0.3	10.3	34.3: 1	1:0.9:0.2
Olive oil	14.8	74.5	10		10	-	1:5:0.6
Mustard oil	10.7	56	32.6	14.5	18.1	1.2: 1	1:5.2:3
Groundnut oil	20.9	49.3	30.9		30.9	-	1:2.3:1.5
Rice bran oil	22.1	41	35.7	1.4	34.3	24.5: 1	1:1.8:1.6
Safflower oil	10.7	16.7	73.5		73.5	-	1:1.5:6.8
Sunflower oil	9.1	25.1	66.2		66.2	-	1:2.7:7
Corn oil	12.7	29.6	57.6		57.6	-	1:2.3:4.5
Soybean oil	13.1	28.9	57.2	6.5	50.7	7.8: 1	1:2.2:4.3

Abbreviations: SFA, saturated fatty acid; MUFA, monounsaturated fatty acid; PUFA, polyunsaturated fatty acid

type, frying conditions (time, fryer conditions, temperature, etc.), and fried material type.

There is some evidence that highly oxidized and heated lipids may have carcinogenic properties because of potentially toxic substances which are forming as the result of the former reactions throughout frying process. Animal studies have also shown that these compounds increase the levels of cholesterol and phospholipids in plasma and HDL and the levels of Thiobarbituric acid reactive substance (TBARS) in liver and plasma lipoproteins. Malondialdehyde (MDA) is the principal and most studied product of polyunsaturated fatty acid peroxidation. The aldehyde is a toxic molecule and should be considered as more than just a marker of lipid peroxidation. Its interface with deoxyribonucleic acid (DNA) and proteins has often been referred to as potentially mutagenic and atherogenic.

Hence, there is a need to choose oils that are suitable for Indian cooking conditions. Oils with an antioxidant system in built can be seen as a possible solution. Every antioxidant works in a different manner and thus, it is essential to design and develop a system of antioxidants that prevent oil from degrading in cooking conditions.[12-15]

Antioxidants: In Human Health

In living systems, free radicals which often incorporate the highly reactive oxygen in their structure are known to attack healthy cells of the body in oxidation reactions that result in their loss of structure and function.

Reactive oxygen species (ROS) and reactive nitrogen species (RNS) [e.g. nitric oxide (NO)] are well recognized for playing a dual role as both beneficial and deleterious species. ROS and RNS are generated by tightly regulated enzymes, such as NO synthase (NOS) and NAD(P)H oxidase isoforms, respectively. Overproduction of ROS [arising either from mitochondrial electron-transport chain or excessive stimulation of NAD(P)H] results in oxidative stress, a process that can be an important mediator of damage to cell structures including DNA, lipids, and proteins. In contrast, beneficial effects of ROS/RNS (e.g. superoxide radical and NO) occur at low/moderate concentrations and involve physiological roles in cellular responses to noxia, for example in defense against infection, and the induction of a mitogenic response. Ironically, many ROS-mediated actions in fact protect cells against ROS-induced oxidative stress and re-establish or maintain 'redox balance' termed also 'redox homeostasis'. The 'double edged sword' character of ROS is clearly substantiated.

In the development of atherosclerosis, LDL particles accumulate within the arterial subendothelial space. These residents LDL particles then undergo chemical alteration, like oxidized LDL (oxLDL), resulting in the formation of a modified LDL that is capable of inducing local vascular cells to stimulate monocyte recruitment and their differentiation into macrophages. These accumulating cells further oxidize resident LDL particles. As the protein component of LDL (apoprotein B-100) becomes more negatively charged, the LDL particles are recognized by scavenger receptors on macrophages that, in turn, internalize these LDL particles resulting in the formation of foam cells. As additional monocytes are recruited to the subendothelial space, the already present macrophages and foam cells remain trapped within the vasculature, unable to escape due to their internal build-up of oxLDL. Adjacent endothelial cells, respond to the cytotoxic build-up of oxLDL by releasing lipids and lysosomal enzymes that further enhance the progression of atherosclerotic lesions.

Antioxidants in living systems are capable of stabilizing or deactivating free radicals, thus controlling their formation. If the balance is disturbed, however, 'oxidative stress' occurs, leading to deterioration of normal cell functions and even cell death. All antioxidants mainly work by neutralizing the free radical and hence, preventing formation of free radical species.[16-18]. Thus, it is essential to ensure that we get enough of antioxidants in our diet.

Edible Oils: Antioxidants

In Indian cooking conditions, oil is subjected to high cooking temperatures and in these conditions the oxidative degradation of oil is accelerated. Even the shelf life stability of vegetable oils in food uses and their applicability depends on its oxidative stability. The oxidative damage of PUFAs is the highest followed by MUFA and SFA. Hence, it becomes essential to protect the fatty acids from degradation to maximize their benefits in the body. Oxidization of LDL-C (oxLDL-C) *in vivo* is also known to be the first step of atherosclerosis. Antioxidants are known to maintain the integrity of vegetable oils by preventing the oxidation reactions mainly by scavenging free radicals. Different antioxidants work on different levels and hence, no one antioxidant is sufficient to interact at all levels. All oils have minor components present and hence, it becomes a good source of antioxidants. Also different oils have different antioxidants hence, it becomes essential to combine oils or blend oils to get a variety of antioxidants in the diet.

A study conducted in the year 2011, stated that SO which is a rich source of essential, n = 6 PUFA linoleic acid; showed an increase in lean body mass and decrease in fat mass in the trunk region, another observation of the study was the SO improved fasting glucose, hemoglobin A1c, CRP, HDL-C, and adiponectin levels. Human study revealed that when 300 mg/day gamma-oryzanol was administered for a period of 3 months on hyperlipidemic patients there was a significant decrease in plasma total cholesterol (TC) and LDL-C levels, another observation in the study was that there was an increase in HDL-C levels in the hypercholesterolemic group.[19]

Selection of Oil

All vegetables oils are composed of three types of fatty acids mainly, SFA, MUFA, and PUFA (Table 2). Some of the naturally occurring vegetables oils are rich in one of the above components e.g. high SFA oils—coconut oil and palm kernel oil; high PUFA (omega-6) oil—sunflower oil and SO. Vegetable oils are also rich in various nonfat components such as sterols, carotenoids, and vitamin E.[20] While single oils have their own set of unique nonglyceride component, such as rice bran oil has oryzanol and olive oils have polyphenols, etc. there is no single oil that would provide all the required nutritional benefits. NIN, Hyderabad suggests that it is important to obtain right amount of different fatty acids in the diet and avoid excess intake of any one group of fatty acids. Thus, it becomes important to use different single oils such as to get all kinds of fatty acids.

Physically blending two or more commonly available oils is one of the most common methods employed to obtain the desired fatty acids ratio. A combination of two healthy cooking oils keep a balance of three fatty acids is beneficial to the body. Better fatty acid profile that is nutritionally healthy with better balance of SFA, MUFA, and PUFA. The stability of the oil is also maintained. It is much more convenient to have single blended oil for all cooking purposes than having different oils for different cooking purposes. Recent guidelines (2010) by NIN, India suggests that one should use a blend of two or more vegetable

TABLE 2: Minor components in oil and their effect

Minor components	*Oil*	*Biological effect*	*Mechanism of action*
Plant sterols	All vegetable oils	Hypocholesterolemic	Inhibits cholesterol absorption
Tocopherols	All vegetable oils	Vitamin and antioxidant	Scavenge reactive oxygen species (ROS)
Tocotrienols	Palm, rice bran	Vitamin and antioxidant	Scavenge ROS
Carotenes	Red palm	Provitamin A and antioxidant	Scavenge ROS
Oryzanols	Rice bran	Hypocholesterolemic	Inhibits cholesterol biosynthesis
Hydroxytyrosol, phenolic acids	Olive	Antioxidant	---
Sesamin	Sesame	Hypocholesterolemic; increases DGLA and eicosanoids of 1 series; anti-inflammatory	Inhibits cholesterol absorption and biosynthesis; inhibits D5 desaturase activity
Sesamolin, Sesamol	Sesame	Antioxidant	Potentiates antioxidant effects of tocopherols

Abbreviation: DGLA, dihomo-γ-linolenic acid

oils such as to get all the fatty acids in a balance. Thus, by blending different oils, the benefits of individual oils can be combined together. Currently under the Indian Regulatory framework (FDA/PFA) blend can contain maximum two vegetable oil and each oil should be minimum 20% in a blend.

Indian culinary practices involve deep frying which involves heating oil at 180°C and drying of the moisture at high temperature.[21] At this temperature, oil and its components comes in contact with the oxygen and water at very high temperature. These severe conditions lead to generation of free radicals which lead to breakdown of unsaturated fatty acids leading to harmful secondary oxidation products. Also there is a practice in India to recycle once used oils till 4–5 times and refill with fresh oil to maintain the optimal frying levels in pan which increase the content of secondary oxidation products. Thus the Indian deep frying practices are harmful to larger extent on nutritional quality of oils which is generally experienced by user as an off flavor, dark color, and increased viscosity due to polymerization. The by-products generated in due course of frying are many and a few of these are MDA, ketones, 4-hydroxynonenal (HNE), hydroperoxides, and are known to be carcinogenic and detrimental to health.[22] PUFA has always been known to have cardioprotective effect. Hence, there is a need to protect PUFA and the oil from deterioration and the same can be achieved by providing an antioxidant system in the oil in Indian scenario which can protect oil as much as possible against the oxidation.[23-33]

CONCLUSION

Research has constantly showcased the correlation between lifestyle changes and health. Hence, to tackle health problems in India it becomes pivotal to ensure that the lifestyle changes are customized to suit Indian lifestyle. Edible oil forms an integral part of Indian cooking and hence, it is essential to realize the difference of different single oils and acknowledge its uniqueness as well but at the same time, it is essential to understand that no single oil is perfect. Hence, on the basis of scientific research, it is essential to design oil solutions that will be customized to Indian cooking conditions. Also, free radical generation is an important health threat that needs to be looked into. Free radicals are generated during normal metabolic process and their production is accelerated due to environmental factors. They need to be kept in control and hence, attention should be given to antioxidants especially the naturally present antioxidants in the form of nonglyceride components in edible oils. Thus, it can be concluded that lifestyle modifications along with substitution of cooking oil by the blend oil with antioxidant technology results in significant lowering of LDL-C levels and has positive benefits on the inflammatory markers thus having a positive impact in overall health especially cardiac health in hyperlipidemic subjects.

REFERENCES

1. Maton A, Hopkins J, Johnson S, et al. Human biology and health. New Jersey, USA: Prentice Hall, Englewood Cliffs; 1993.
2. Dennis S, Belcher M, Dawson T, et al. Food Fats and oils. New York: Institute of Shortening and Edible Oils; 2006.
3. Mu H, Høy CE. The digestion of dietary triacylglycerols. Prog Lipid Res. 2004;43(2):105-33.
4. Sapna J, Saikia N, Mathur HB, et al. Fatty acids profile of edible oils and fats in India. New Delhi: Centre for Science and Environment; 2009.
5. Baez RV, Baez AV. (2013). Overview about lipid structure. [online] Available from https://www.intechopen.com/books/lipid-metabolism/overview-about-lipid-structure. [Accessed October, 2017].
6. Harvard School of Public Health. (2014). Fats and Cholesterol: Out with the bad in with the good. [online] Available from https://www.hsph.harvard.edu/nutritionsource/fats-full-story/. [Accessed October, 2017].
7. Centers for Disease Control and Prevention. (2014). Trans Fat. [online] Available from https://www.cdc.gov/nutrition/everyone/basics/fat/transfat.html. [Accessed October, 2017].
8. Kris-Etherton PM, Pearson TA, Wan Y, et al. High-monounsaturated fatty acid diets lower both plasma cholesterol and triacylglycerol concentrations. Am J Clin Nutr. 1999;70(6):1009-15.
9. American Heart Association. (2014). The Skinny on Fats. [online] Available from http://www.heart.org/HEARTORG/Conditions/Cholesterol/PreventionTreatmentofHighCholesterol/Know-Your-Fats_UCM_305628_Article.jsp. [Accessed October, 2017].
10. Srinivasan PV. Impact of trade liberalization on India's oilseed and edible oils sector. Report prepared for IGIDR-ERS/USDA Project: Indian Agricultural Markets and Policy. 2005.
11. Indian Council of Medical Research. Nutrient requirements and recommended dietary allowances for Indians. Report of the expert group of the Indian Medical Research. Hyderabad: National Institute of Nutrition; 2010.
12. Zhang Q, Saleh AS, Chen J, et al. Chemical alterations taken place during deep-fat frying based on certain reaction products: a review. Chem Phys Lipids. 2012;165(6):662-81.
13. Ganbi HH. Alteration in Fatty Acid Profiles and Formation of Some Harmful Compounds in Hammour Fish Fillets and Frying Oil Medium Throughout Intermittent Deep-Fat Frying Process. World Appl Sci J. 2011;12(4):536-44.
14. Garrido-Polonio C, García-Linares MC, García-Arias MT, et al. Thermally oxidized sunflower-seed oil increases liver and serum peroxidation and modifies lipoprotein composition in rats. Br J Nutr. 2004;92(2):257-65.
15. Ringseis R, Gutgesell A, Dathe C, et al. Feeding oxidized fat during pregnancy up-regulates expression of PPARα-responsive genes in the liver of rat fetuses. Lipids Health Dis. 2007;6:6.
16. Shahidi F. Bailey's Industrial Oil and Fat Products. Edible Oil and Fat Products: Chemistry, Properties and Health Effects, 6th edition. New York: Wiley; 2005.
17. Valko M, Leibfritz D, Moncol J, et.al. Free radicals and antioxidants in normal physiological functions and human disease. Int J Biochem Cell Biol. 2007;39(1):44-84.

18. Dutta A, Dutta SK. Vitamin E and its role in the prevention of atherosclerosis and carcinogenesis: a review. J Am Coll Nutr. 2003;22(4):258-68.
19. Lynch SM, Gaziano JM, Frei B. Ascorbic acid and atherosclerotic cardiovascular disease. Subcell Biochem. 1996;25:331-67.
20. Simopoulos AP. The importance of the ratio of omega-6/omega-3 essential fatty acids. Biomed Pharmacother. 2002;56(8):365-79.
21. Upadya H, Devaraju CJ, Joshi SR. Anti-inflammatory properties of blended edible oil with synergistic antioxidants. Indian J Endocrinol Metab. 2015;19(4):511-9.
22. Ayala A, Muñoz MF, Argüelles S. Lipid peroxidation: production, metabolism, and signaling mechanisms of malondialdehyde and 4-hydroxy-2-nonenal. Oxid Med Cell Longev. 2014;2014:1-31.
23. Read NW, Welch IM, Austen CJ, et al. Swallowing food without chewing; a simple way to reduce postprandial glycaemia. Br J Nutr. 1986;55(1):43-7.
24. Brand JC, Nicholson PL, Thorburn AW, et al. Food processing and the glycemic index. Am J Clin Nutr. 1985;42(6):1192-6.
25. Rosillo-Calle F, Pelkmans L, Walter A. A global overview of vegetable oils, with reference to biodiesel. A Report for the IEA Bioenergy Task 40. IEA Bioenergy. 2009.
26. Del Rio D, Stewart AJ, Pellegrini N. A review of recent studies on malondialdehyde as toxic molecule and biological marker of oxidative stress. Nutr Metab Cardiovasc Dis. 2005;15(4):316-28.
27. McCord JM. The evolution of free radicals and oxidative stress. Am J Med. 2000;108(8):652-9.
28. Halliwell B. Free radicals, antioxidants, and human disease: curiosity, cause, or consequence? Lancet. 1994;344(8924):721-4.
29. Vollaard NB, Shearman JP, Cooper CE. Exercise-induced oxidative stress: myths, realities and physiological relevance. Sports Med. 2005;35(12):1045-62.
30. Valko M, Rhodes CJ, Moncol J, et al. Free radicals, metals and antioxidants in oxidative stress-induced cancer. Chem Biol Interact. 2006;160(1):1-40.
31. Kalra J, Chaudhary AK, Prasad K. Increased production of oxygen free radicals in cigarette smokers. Int J Exp Pathol. 1991; 72(1):1-7.
32. Pham-Huy LA, He H, Pham-Huy C. Free radicals, antioxidants in disease and health. Int J Biomed Sci. 2008;4(2):89-96.
33. Niki E. Assessment of antioxidant capacity in vitro and in vivo. Free Radic Biol Med. 2010;49(4):503-15.

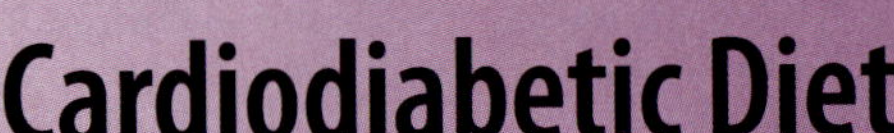

Cardiodiabetic Diet

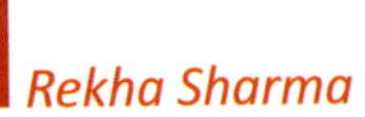

Rekha Sharma

INTRODUCTION

Key factors for the prevention and management of cardio-diabetic diet are maintenance of body weight, healthy eating practices, and regular exercise. It is important to control and maintain body weight. The best way to assess the body weight is by body mass index (BMI),

$$BMI = \frac{\text{Weight in kilogram}}{\text{Height in meter}^2}.$$

Obesity cut-offs for Asian Indians[1] normal weight range is 20 to 23, overweight greater than 23, obese greater than 25. It is advisable to keep BMI in the normal weight range. Healthy eating practices, reduce fat, especially saturated fats and cholesterol. Increase fiber and eat whole grains, vegetables, and fruits. Reduce sodium in the diet.

WORLD HEALTH ORGANIZATION DIETARY GUIDELINES[2] ON "HEALTHY EATING"

Key Facts

- A healthy diet protects against malnutrition and noncommunicable diseases (NCDs), like diabetes, heart disease, stroke, and cancer.
- Physical inactivity and unhealthy diet are the greatest risk factors for diabetes and heart disease.
- Healthy dietary practices start early in life, breastfeeding helps in healthy growth and improves cognitive development, also prevents overweight and obesity, thus preventing the development of NCDs later in life.
- Energy intake (calories) should be in balance with energy expenditure. Evidence suggests that total fat should not exceed 30% of total energy intake, saturated fats should be reduced to less than 10% in favor of unsaturated fats[3]and trans fats should be avoided.
- Intake of free sugars[4] to be limited to less than 10% of total energy intake. A further reduction to less than 5% of total energy intake is suggested for additional health benefits.
- Keep salt intake to[5] less than 5 g per day as it helps in the prevention of hypertension and reduces the risk of heart disease and stroke in the adult population.
- World Health Organization (WHO) Member States have agreed to reduce the global population's intake of salt by 30% and halt the rise in diabetes and obesity in adults, adolescents, and in children by 2025.[6]

The Nutritional Goals

- Provide adequate calories for achieving and maintaining normal body weight, normal growth, and development.
- Improve overall health through healthy food choices.
- Maintain normal or near normal blood glucose levels for diabetics, by integrating physical activity pattern and, if necessary, oral hypoglycemic drugs or insulin therapy into their diet.
- Achieve and maintain optimal blood pressure and lipid levels.

- Address individual nutrition needs, incorporating personal and cultural preferences, willingness to change, and maintaining diets within a family meal.

The relative importance of each nutritional goal will vary based on the patient's complete clinical, biochemical, and nutritional assessment.

Diet Planning

The diet plan[7] has to be individualized based on one's age, sex, lifestyle, physical activity, eating pattern, and food availability, however, the basic principles remain the same that optimally manage the "ABCs" of diabetes controls, i.e. glycated hemoglobin (HbA1c), blood pressure, and low-density lipoprotein (LDL)-cholesterol. The prescription must be individualized for the individual patient, based on the risk of complications if any.

Healthy Diet for Adults[2]

- *Energy:* Sufficient to maintain weight.
- *Carbohydrates* should provide 45–65% of total daily calories. The type and amount of carbohydrate are both important. Patients should monitor their carbohydrate intake either through carbohydrate counting or meal planning exchange lists.[8] Fruits, vegetables, legumes (e.g. lentils and beans), nuts, and whole grains (e.g. unprocessed maize, millet, oats, wheat, and brown rice)[2] are beneficial. Watch for free sugars, most free sugars[4] are added to foods or drinks by the manufacturer, cook or consumer, and also found naturally in honey, syrups, fruit juices, and fruit juice concentrates.
- *Fats* should provide less than 30%[3,9,10] of total energy intake. Unsaturated fats (e.g. found in fish, nuts, sunflower, canola, and olive oils) are preferable to saturated fats (e.g. found in fatty meat, butter, palm and coconut oil, cream, cheese, and ghee)and industrial trans fats (e.g. found in processed food, fast food, snacks, fried food, cookies, margarines, and spreads). Monounsaturated fatty acids (MUFA) should provide (olive, peanut, canola oil; rice bran oil; nuts) greater than 10%, poly unsaturated fatty acids (PUFA) (fish, flaxseed oil, and walnuts) less than 10%, saturated fatty acids (SFA) (red meat and butter) less than 7% when the blood lipids are high and trans fats less than 1% of total calories. For more details, please see "*Take Low Fat Diet and Avoid Cholesterol, Saturated Fats and Trans Fats*" section given later.
- *Protein* should provide 12–20% of total energy intake, although this may vary depending on a patient's individual health requirements. Patients with kidney disease should limit protein intake.
- A diet that is high in fiber (25–30 grams per day) can help control blood sugar levels and HbA1C.
- Less than 5 g of salt (equivalent to approximately 1 teaspoon) per day[5] and use iodized salt.
- Artificial sweeteners may be consumed in moderation. Sugar alcohols (sorbitol, xylitol, lactitol, and mannitol) generally increase the blood sugar levels slightly and should be used with caution, and they can also lead to diarrhea in children.

For Infants and Young Children

For infants and young children, the diet is same as for adults except the following considerations:

- Infants should be breastfed exclusively during the first 6 months of life.
- Infants should be breastfed continuously until 2 years of age and beyond.
- From 6 months of age, breast milk should be complemented with a variety of adequate, safe, and nutrient dense complementary foods. Salt and sugars should not be added to complementary foods.

Take Low-fat Diet and Avoid Cholesterol, Saturated Fats and Trans Fats

Cholesterol is a natural component of animal foods such as mutton, pork, ham, sausages, lamb, chicken, eggs (yellow), whole milk, cheese, ice cream, butter, and *desi ghee*. Increased cholesterol in blood is called hypercholesterolemia, which leads to atherosclerosis.

Saturated fats are solid at room temperature like milk fat, butter, ghee, coconut oil, and palm oil. These saturated fats in the diet also give rise to high LDL in blood, thus leading to atherosclerosis and should be avoided in the diet.

Trans fats are partially hydrogenated fats, *vanaspati*, margarine, reused oil for more than 6 hours. These are known to raise LDL in blood, enhancing atherosclerosis.

Monounsaturated fats are liquid at room temperature, the food sources being olive oil, canola oil, mustard oil, rice bran oil, til oil, and ground nut oil. MUFA is good for heart and diabetes, as it reduces LDL (bad cholesterol) and increases high-density lipoprotein (HDL) (good cholesterol) in the blood, thereby preventing heart diseases and hence should be encouraged in the diet.

Polyunsaturated fats are liquid at room temperature and consist mainly of two components, n-6 linoleic acid (safflower, corn or sunflower oil) and n-3 alpha-linolenic acid (mustard oil or rapeseed oil). To get a healthy ratio, it is important to combine n-6 and n-3 rich oils and achieve ratio of n6/n3 between 5 and 10. Too much of n-6 can reduce HDL.

Sources of fat in our diet: Fat in our diet is of two types—(1) visible fat, and (2) invisible fat. Visible fat (cooking medium) is extracted either from oil seeds (vegetable oils) or milk (butter and ghee). While the sources of invisible fat in our diet are milk and milk products, eggs, meat and meat products, pulses, cereals, and nuts. 15–20 g of visible fat (cooking medium) along with 15–20 g of invisible fat a day is enough to fulfill our daily recommendations.

Salt

Indian population consumes too much sodium through salt and salty foods (corresponding to an average of 9–12 g of salt per day) and not enough potassium. High salt consumption and insufficient potassium intake (less than 3.5 g/day) contribute to high blood pressure, which in turn increases the risk of heart disease and stroke.[5,11]

1.7 million deaths could be prevented each year if people's salt consumption were reduced to the recommended level of less than 5 g per day.[12]

People are often unaware of the amount of salt they consume. The salt comes from processed foods (e.g. pickles, *chutney, papad, ketchup,* processed meats like bacon, ham, and sausages; cheese and salty snacks) or from food consumed frequently in large amounts (e.g. bread). Salt is also added to food during cooking, and table salt on salads, etc.

Reduce salt consumption by:
- Avoid the use of sauces during the preparation of food
- Avoid having salt on the table
- Limit the consumption of salty snacks, pickles, and *chutneys*
- Choose foods with low sodium content.

Fiber

Increase fiber in the diet, soluble fiber helps in bringing down the blood lipids. Common sources of soluble fiber are pulses, especially, soy and Bengal gram, fruits, and vegetables along with Psyllium (isabgol). In addition, they are also sources of antioxidants, vitamins, and minerals which have a great role to play in the prevention and management of hypertension.

Meal Timings

All meal plans have to be individualized based on eating pattern, cultural factors, and meal timings which could vary according to one's daily schedule.

Most persons with type 2 diabetes mellitus (DM) could follow a traditional pattern of 3–4 meals/day. However, it is advisable that diabetics follow a pattern of three small meals along with three snacks, to avoid overload of carbohydrate coming from a large meal. This will also avoid a higher peak in the patient's blood sugar.

Carbohydrate Counting

Based on the research, for most people with diabetes, especially type 1, the first tool for managing blood glucose is some type of carbohydrate counting. Balancing total carbohydrate intake with physical activity and diabetes medication or insulin is a key for managing blood glucose levels.

The type of carbohydrate has an effect on blood glucose, using glycemic index (GI) may be helpful in "fine-tuning" blood glucose management. Carbohydrate counting is a method of calculating grams of carbohydrate consumed at meals and snacks. We count carbohydrates because they have the greatest effect on glucose. Use exchange lists to count carbohydrates. 1 carbohydrate count = 10–15 g of carbohydrate (approximate).

Counting carbohydrates is a good solution to incorporate a wider range of foods into the meal plan.

Food Exchange System and Exchange List

An exchange list is a grouping of foods in which specified amounts of all the foods are approximately equal in carbohydrates, proteins, and fats (Table 1). For example in a cereal list, one *chapati* can be exchanged for rice, potato,

TABLE 1: Exchange list with food value of each exchange.

Exchange	*Amount*	*Energy (kcal)*	*Proteins (g)*	*Carbohydrates(g)*	*Fat (g)*
Milk	240 mL, 3% fat (1 glass)	145	8	12	7
S'Milk	240 mL (1 glass)	60	5	10	0
Meat	40 g (2 pieces)/(1 Egg)	70	7	0	5
Pulse	25 g raw weight/1bowl 125 gm	80	5	15	0
Cereals	20 g raw weight	70	2	15	0
Veg A	100 g/1 bowl	20	1	3	0
Veg B	100 g/1 bowl	32	2	6	0
Fruit	100 g, 1 medium	40	0	10	0
Fat	5 g, 1 teaspoon	45	0	0	5

Source: Sharma R, Ahuja MMS. Diabetes and Its Dietary management, 3rd edition. BI Publications; 2011.

TABLE 2: Food exchanges list

1. *Cereal exchange*: Each exchange contains 15 g carbohydrates and 2 g protein (70 calories)	
Chapati	20 gatta, 1(5" ´ 0.1")
Cooked rice	75 g,3 tablespoons
Idli	1 medium size
Bread	30 g, 1 large slice (4" ´ 3½ ´ 0.4")
Potato	75 g, ½ medium size
Cornflakes	20 g, dry weight 3tablespoons
Porridge	180 g, cooked weight¾ cup
Noodles cooked	75 g, ½ cup
Biscuits medium size	2 nos.
Ragi	20 g raw, 1½ tablespoons
2. *Meat exchange*: Each exchange contains 7 g protein and 5 g fat (75 calories)	
Mutton	40 g
Chicken	25 g
Fish	30 g
Lamb	30 g
Egg 1 medium	50 g
Pork	30 g
Sausage	20 g
Ham, Shredded	20 g
Cheese	40 g, 2 inch cube/2 slice
Cottage cheese	50 g, One 2" × 1½" cube
3. *Milk exchange (240 mL)*: Each exchange contains 12 g carbohydrates, 8 g proteins, and 7 g fats (145 calories)	
Milk	240 mL, 1 glass (3" diameter top) (3% fat)*
Curd	240 g, 2 bowls (3% fat)*
Cottage cheese (*Paneer*)	50 g, 2"× 3"× ½" cube
Buttermilk	750 mL, 3 glasses
Skimmed milk powder	45 g, 3 tablespoons
Khoa	30 g, 2 tablespoons
4. *Pulses and legumes exchange*: Each exchange contains 15 g carbohydrates, 5 g proteins (80 calories)	
Moong	25 g, 1 medium bowl (125 g cooked)
Urad	25 g
Arhar	25 g

Contd...

Contd...

Rajma	25 g
Lobia	25 g
Bengal gram	25 g
Soya nuggets (soy bean)	20 g
5. *Fruit exchange:* Each exchange contains 10 g carbohydrates (40 calories)	
Orange	100 g, 1 medium
Pear	90 g, 1 small
Apple	90 g, 1 small
Banana	40 g, ½ medium
Mango	60 g, ½ medium
Ber	70 g, 5–8 in numbers
Water-melon	300 g, 1 large slice
Papaya	120 g, 1–2" slice
Grapes	55 g, 8–10 in numbers (small)
Guava	100 g, 1 medium
Loquat	100 g,5–6 in numbers
Tomato juice	240 g, 1 glass
Dry fruit (almond, cashew nuts, peanuts, and walnuts)	6 g, 3–4 in numbers
Dates (dry)	12 g, 4–5 in numbers
6. *Fat/Oil exchange*: Each exchange contains 5 g fat (45 calories)	
Oil: Safflower, sunflower, soya, peanut, maize, til, mustard or any refined oil	5 g (1 tsp.)
Ghee, vanaspati	5 g, 1 tsp.
Butter	5 g, 1 tsp.
Cream (heavy)	10 g, 2 tsp.
Mayonnaise	8 g, 2 tsp.
Bacon	7 g, 1 strip
7. *Vegetable exchange*: Vegetables are broken into three groups as follows:	
A group (100 g, 1 bowl) 3 g carbohydrates, 1 g proteins (16 calories) cabbage, spinach, mustard green, cauliflower, brinjal, capsicum, *lauki*, and *tori*. *B group* (100 g, 1 bowl) 6 g carbohydrates, 2 g proteins (32 calories) Peas, green beans, carrots, pumpkin, *bhindi*, onions, and radish. *Roots and tubers* (25 g) 5 g carbohydrates (20 calories) Potatoes, sweet potato, colocasia, beet root, and yam.	

*DMS toned milk/other dairy toned milk.

idli or whole wheat bread in varying amounts. Exchange lists are made according to the different food groups, like cereals, milk and milk products, legumes, meats, vegetables, fruits, fats, and oils.

Regulation of diets on daily basis is one of the important factors in a diabetic's diet. Exchange lists give variety by substituting one food with other one of one's choice (Table 2).

Rules for Food Substitution

1. Substitute within the same meal, e.g. if bread is not eaten at breakfast, some other items from the cereal list can be added at breakfast.
2. Substitute in correct amounts, e.g. one medium-sized *chapati* (20 g wheat flour) is approximately equal to three tablespoons or 75 g of cooked rice.

3. Substitute from the same food group. Since different foods have different functions, therefore, substitution should be made from within the same food group.,

SPECIAL SITUATIONS REQUIRING DIETARY MODIFICATION

Fasting

Can a diabetic fast? This would depend on whether one is a type 1-insulin dependent diabetic on insulin therapy, or type 2 DM-noninsulin dependent diabetic on oral hypoglycemic agents. The absence of insulin and food in type 1 may lead to hypoglycemic coma. Fasting is thus only advised under the guidance of a physician, in the noninsulin dependent type 2 diabetics, as metabolic adjustments in such individuals can be tolerated and this helps in reduction of weight.

Periodic fasting undertaken at regular intervals is well tolerated in type 2 DM (not on oral hypoglycemic and on diet alone) and if the person adjusts to the regime. Unsupervised fasting should be avoided.

Sick Days

In the case of any sickness, a diabetic on insulin or oral drugs must consult a doctor even though the illness might not seem serious. The physician will advise the dose of the antidiabetic agent and modify the diet accordingly. It is, thus advised, one should keep taking fluids or items like thin soup, buttermilk, tea or fresh lime.

In the event of fever or other illness, the diet should be modified by changing the consistency and texture of foods. During sickness, the diabetic has to be very careful that acetone does not appear in the urine, as it can lead to coma.

Take plenty of fluids (fresh lime with salt, clear soups, buttermilk, and an added intake of salt should be encouraged).

If there is no nausea/vomiting, light meals may be taken (half boiled/poached egg, toast, *khichri, curd*, and fruits are acceptable).

Traveling

The timing of meals may have to be adjusted. This would mean adjustment in the schedule of insulin or oral drugs to what is being taken as food. One should carry nutritious snacks while traveling, as they may be of additional help, in planning a major meal. This would also safeguard one from eating wayside foods, the chances of infection, or inaccessibility in case one is unwarily delayed on the way due to the late schedule of the transport one is traveling. Some biscuits, a slice of cheese or some home-made snacks are easy items to carry and can replace a cooked meal. Something sweet (chocolate and candy) should also be carried as it helps in the event of early symptoms of hypoglycemia. It would be beneficial to always carry an identification card which declares that one is a diabetic or a cardiac patient and is on a particular medication for this purpose. This would facilitate diagnosis and timely management in case of an emergency.

At Parties/Eating Out

The most important fact is to have confidence and be discrete in calculating the calories. One should not make oneself or one's host conscious of being a diabetic or a cardiac patient. Self-restraint is a great virtue. Select foods that are plainly cooked without too much of oil and sugar. Avoid refined cereals, rich gravies, and meats with fats. For example, in chicken curry, eat just the chicken pieces and leave the curry aside or in *dahi vada,* eat only the *dahi* and leave *vada* alone. Salads add to the bulk of food and at the same time make the plate look full. Some fresh fruits can be opted for as dessert. At a birthday party, a diabetic child may share the cake, but manage with a smaller helping (50% of what others take), go in for fruit chat or *channa* chat or plain biscuits. Estimate the extra calories and adjust these in the next meal or go for a brisk and long walk to use them up. If one can learn to eat slowly, one can easily avoid second or third helping.

The purpose of a diet for a diabetic/cardiac patient is not to deny food, but rather to enable them to select the right items in appropriate amounts. The care exercised in this direction is well-rewarded.

OTHER DIETARY COMPONENTS

Sweeteners

Nutritive Sweeteners

Nutritive sweeteners include fructose, honey, corn syrup, molasses, fruit juice or fruit juice concentrates, dextrose, maltose, mannitol, sorbitol, xylitol, as well as sucrose. Fructose, which occurs naturally in fruits, vegetables, and honey, provides 4 kcal/g, as do other carbohydrates, but causes a smaller rise in plasma glucose than do sucrose and other starches.

Nonnutritive Sweeteners

Aspartame, acesulfame K, sucralose, saccharin, and stevia are currently approved for use by the US Food and Drug Administration (FDA). All can be used safely by people with diabetes. The average intake of all the nonnutritive sweeteners is much less than the acceptable daily intake (ADI), which is determined by the FDA. The ADI represents the amount of a food additive that even if consumed on a daily basis throughout an individual's lifetime, is still considered safe by a 100-fold safety margin. It is not a toxic threshold, and even if an individual occasionally ingested a substance in amounts greater than the ADI, it would not pose a health risk.

Nonnutritive sweeteners—noncaloric sweeteners (approved by FDA):

- Acesulfame K (Sunnet): Moderate use in pregnancy, lactation, and renal
- Aspartame (Equal, Nutrasweet): Moderate use in pregnancy and lactation
- Saccharin (Sweet N low): Avoid in pregnancy and lactation
- Sucralose (Splenda): Safe in pregnancy and lactation
- Stevia: Avoid in pregnancy and lactation.

Food and Agriculture Organization (FAO)/WHO, approved by European Parliament and council directive.

Cyclamate, not approved by FDA.

Alcohol

If diabetes and body weight is well-controlled, moderate use of alcohol is unlikely to have adverse affect on blood glucose. However, it is important to verify this through blood glucose monitoring. Patients who take insulin should limit their intake to not more than two drinks per day (one drink equals 250 mL beer, 120 mL wine, or 30 mL distilled alcohol). If alcohol is consumed, it should not be counted as part of the meal plan, but in addition to the meal plan. In the fasting state, alcohol may produce hypoglycemia. This is because alcohol cannot be converted to glucose, it inhibits gluconeogenesis, and augments or increases the effect of insulin by interfering with the counter-regulation of insulin-induced hypoglycemia. Alcohol is metabolized in a manner similar to fat. Even though extra calories are consumed, total food intake should not be reduced. When calorie intake is being restricted, as in individuals trying to reduce their body weight, alcohol may be substituted for fat (one drink equals two fat exchanges, or about 100 kcal that would have been consumed as fat).

Women could drink fewer alcoholic beverages a day.

Alcohol is allowed provided there is good glycemic control, IBW, and no dyslipidemia.

Arning: Alcohol masks hypoglycemia.

CONCLUSION

We are what we eat. Optimization of nutrients is the need of the hour to have perfect control of cardiodiabetes. *For insulin users*, limit to two small drinks per day. Drink only with food. Do not cut back on food except fat in case of the obese. *For noninsulin users*, substitute for fat calories. Limit to promote weight loss or maintenance. Limit if triglycerides are elevated. Therefore, nutritional intervention and optimization may help reducing cardiodiabetes inflicted morbidity and mortality.

REFERENCES

1. Singh SP, Sibri G, Garg MK. Obesity cut offs for Asian Indian. Med J Armed Forces. 2008;64(4):350-3.
2. World Health Organization. WHO Healthy Diet Guidelines 2015. Geneva: World Health Organization; 2015.
3. FAO. Fats and fatty acids in human nutrition: report of an expert consultation. In: FAO Food and Nutrition Paper 91. Rome: Food and Agriculture Organization of the United Nations; 2010.
4. World Health Organization. Guideline: Sugars Intake for Adults and Children. Geneva: World Health Organization; 2015.
5. World Health Organization. Guideline: Sodium Intake for Adults and Children. Geneva: World Health Organization; 2012.
6. World Health Organization. Global status report on noncommunicable diseases 2014. Geneva: World Health Organization; 2014.
7. American Diabetes Association. 2011.
8. Kajnuma H. Exchange List. Diet Management, Diabetes and its Dietary Management Guideline. Asian Med J. 2001;44(2):57-63.
9. Hooper L, Abdelhamid A, Moore HJ, et al. Effect of reducing total fat intake on body weight: systematic review and meta-analysis of randomised controlled trials and cohort studies. BMJ. 2012;345:e7666.
10. World Health Organization. Diet, nutrition and the prevention of chronic diseases: report of a Joint WHO/FAO Expert Consultation. In: WHO Technical Report Series, No. 916. Geneva: World Health Organization; 2003.
11. World Health Organization. Potassium intake for adults and children. Geneva: World Health Organization; 2012.
12. Mozaffarian D, Fahimi S, Singh GM, et al. Global sodium consumption and death from cardiovascular causes. N Engl J Med. 2014;371(7):624-34.

SECTION 5

Arrhythmia Management

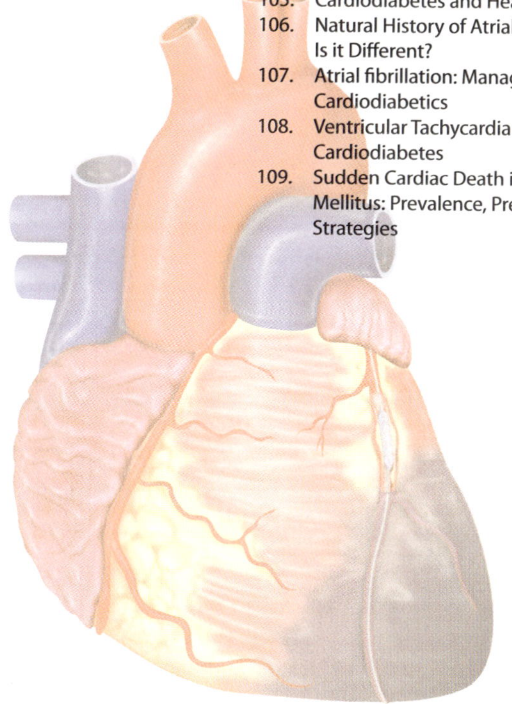

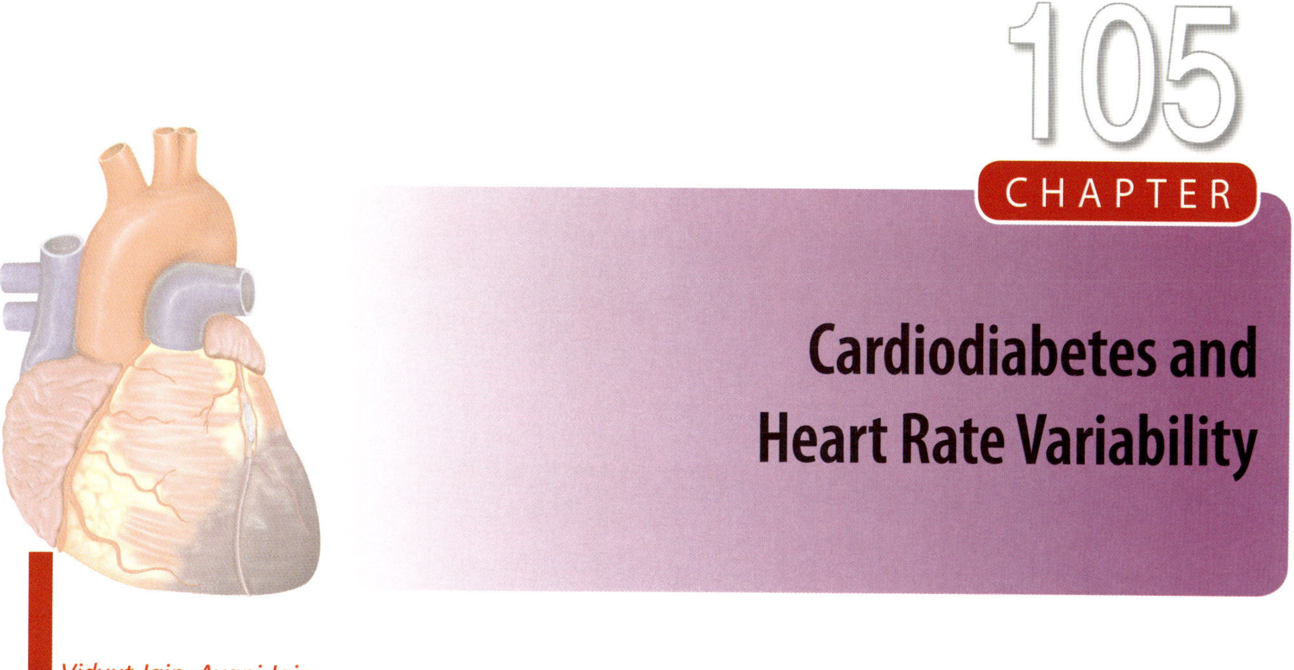

Cardiodiabetes and Heart Rate Variability

Vidyut Jain, Avani Jain

INTRODUCTION

Diabetes mellitus (DM) is a common disease across the globe. DM can cause multisystem involvement including increased cardiovascular morbidity and mortality. It also affects cardiovascular autonomic system involving heart rate variability (HRV). Apart from macro- and microvascular complication of diabetes, the severity of autonomic perturbations in patients with heart failure is affected by the presence of uncontrolled diabetes. Decreased HRV is frequent in diabetic patients free of clinically apparent heart disease and has been invoked as a risk factor for sudden cardiac death. However, reduced HRV is also commonly present in patients with left ventricular dysfunction. The effect of diabetes on autonomic dysfunction in this setting is not known.[1] HRV is considered to be noninvasive index of the neural activity of the heart, and is also influenced by the sympathetic activity of the heart, HRV is usually determined by the vagal stimulation of the heart. Among diabetic patients, who have poor metabolic control (elevated HbA1c) have a low HRV compared to those with good control. Available literature support HRV as diagnostic method as early predictor for future cardiac event; however, there is a need to be further workup for its the utilization of HRV in the clinical practice in understanding cardiac vascular risk among diabetic patients.[2]

Autonomic neuropathy is significant complication of DM. Diabetic autonomic neuropathy (DAN) can increase the cardiovascular morbidity and mortality and at times sudden death. Assessment for autonomic dysfunction of hear can be done by various ways including response of heart rate and blood pressure to maneuvers stimulating the autonomic nervous system, deep breathing, valsalva maneuver, and standing. However, the sensitivity of such tests is relatively less to pick up an early impairment of the autonomic nervous system.[3] HRV is the physiological phenomenon of variation in the time interval between heartbeats. It is measured by the variation in the beat-to-beat interval. HRV is an important noninvasive parameter of the neural activity of the heart but often could not get enough attention. In earlier study, it has been reported that HRV to be useful in assessing the dysfunction of the autonomic nervous system in children and adolescents. HRV is reflection of the sympathetic activity of the heart, but vagal stimulation of the heart also play key role. Reduced HRV has been observed to have correlation with increased mortality after myocardial infarction.[4]

HEART RATE VARIABILITY PHENOMENA

Though HRV is mediated by autonomic nervous system but vagal outflow also has significant impact.[5] HRV based on different frequency characteristics with an insight on respiratory sinus arrhythmia and its transmission by a neural pathway that is different from other components of HRV.[6] In diabetics, neuropathy is characterized by alteration in small nerve fibers, and reduction in time domain parameters of HRV seems not only to carry negative prognostic value may often precede the clinical manifestation of autonomic neuropathy. Among diabetic patients who do not suffer from autonomic neuropathy, decreased absolute power of low frequency and high frequency during controlled conditions was also reported. Thus, diabetic patients can be differentiated from normal controls on the basis of reduction in HRV.[7] Reduced HRV is co-relatable predictor of mortality after myocardial infarction; however, others have shown that mean-heart rate is more relevant to mortality in postacute myocardial infarction survival.[8] Variation in the beat-to-beat interval is a normal physiological phenomenon. The sinoatrial (SA) node receives several signals and the instantaneous heart rate or respiratory rate (RR) interval, and its variation is the effect of these variables. These variables are generated from the sympathetic and the parasympathetic nervous system (PSNS) and humeral factors. Mainly, the factors, which affect the input, are the baroreflex, sleep-wake cycle, meals, physical activity thermoregulation, hormones, and stress. Reduced PSNS activity or heightened sympathetic nervous system activity will result in reduced HR. High-frequency activity (0.15–0.40 Hz), especially, has been linked to parasympathetic nervous system activity. Variation of activity in this range is seen as the respiratory sinus arrhythmia, a vagally mediated modulation of heart rate such that it is augmented during inspiration and falls during expiration. However, the physiological inputs of the low-frequency activity (0.04–0.15 Hz) may not have similar influence. Though previously thought to reflect alone sympathetic activity, it is now believed that it reflects a mixture of both the sympathetic and parasympathetic activity.[9,10]

AUTONOMIC INFLUENCES OF HEART RATE

Although cardiac automaticity is mostly intrinsic to pacemaker tissues, but autonomic nervous system controls heart rate and rhythm are. Acetylcholine is mediator for the parasympathetic influence on heart rate is by its action on the vagus nerve. There is increased in cell membrane K^+ conductance through muscarinic acetylcholine receptors. Muscarinic acetylcholine also inhibits the hyperpolarization activated "pacemaker" current. On the other side, the "if activation" hypothesis suggests that after action potential termination, if provides a slowly activating inward current predominating over decaying outward current (IK), thus initiating slow diastolic depolarization. The sympathetic effects on heart rate are mediated by action of epinephrine and norepinephrine. Activation of β-adrenergic receptors leads to camp-mediated phosphorylation of membrane proteins, and increase in ICaL and in the end result is an acceleration of the slow diastolic depolarization. At rest, it is the vagal tone that prevails and variations in heart rate are largely dependent on vagal modulation. Both vagal and sympathetic activities constantly interact. As sinus node is rich in acetylcholinesterase, the effect of any vagal impulse is for short duration, as the acetylcholine is immediately hydrolyzed. Parasympathetic influences exceed sympathetic effects probably through two independent mechanisms—(1) a cholinergically induced reduction of norepinephrine released in response to sympathetic activity and (2) a cholinergic attenuation of the response to an adrenergic stimulus.[11]

COMPONENTS OF HEART RATE VARIABILITY

The RR interval variations observed in resting conditions denotes variable cardiac autonomic influence. Vagal efferent (parasympathetic) activity plays important role in the high frequency component, as seen in clinical and laboratory observations autonomic maneuvers such as electrical vagal stimulation, vagotomy, and muscarinic receptor blockade. Interpretation of the low-frequency component, considered as a marker of sympathetic modulation (expressed in normalized units) is complex and includes both sympathetic and vagal influences. It has been observed that during sympathetic activation, the resulting tachycardia is accompanied by a marked reduction in total power, and reverse occurs during vagal activation. It is assumed that HRV measures fluctuations in autonomic inputs to the heart rather than the mean level of autonomic inputs. Thus, HRV is reduced by both withdrawal and saturating high-levels of autonomic input to the heart.[12] Many patients suffering from long-term DM have enhanced atherosclerotic disease involving cardiovascular, cerebrovascular accident (CVA), peripheral arterial system in addition to nephropathy and retinopathy. Other significant problems seen are neuropathy and autonomic neuropathy. DAN is not uncommon complication.

Review

Diabetic autonomic neuropathy is seen more in individuals with uncontrolled long-standing type 1 or 2 DM and is due to cholinergic, noradrenergic, and peptidergic fiber involvement (peptides such as pancreatic polypeptide, substance P, etc.). It may manifest by involving multiple system including the cardiovascular, gastrointestinal, genitourinary, sudomotor, and metabolic systems. Common cardiac symptoms of DAN are unexplained resting tachycardia and postural hypotension. Occasionally, sudden cardiac death has also been attributed to autonomic neuropathy. DAN often coexists with the condition of left ventricular compliance abnormality.[13] These hemodynamic changes are partly attributed to cardiac autonomic neuropathy and microangiopathic changes resulting in angina and nonanginal complications from DM. Apart from these, clinical recognition of cardiac hyperfunctions, cardiac autonomic neuropathy, may be used as a prognostic markers of complications.[14] Perioperative cardiac complications are common among patients with long-standing DM, mainly unexplained tachycardia, arrhythmias risk of postoperative myocardial infarction is also more common.[15] Measurement of HRV may serve as an early assessment method to identify and prevent cardiac complications in patients with DM. Analysis of alteration of patterns of HRV provides a sensitive and early indicator of impaired health.

Heart rate variability on higher side is considered to be good sign of adaptation, characterizing a healthy individual with efficient autonomic mechanisms, and low HRV is generally an indicator of abnormal and insufficient adaptation of the autonomic nervous system, which may indicate the presence of physiological malfunction in the individual.[16] Importance of HRV in diagnosis of DAN detecting cardiovascular autonomic neuropathy by HRV is strongly associated with an increased risk of silent myocardial ischemia and mortality. Type I DM also promotes several consequences of micro- and macrovascular changes that lead to dysfunctions and failure in different organs autonomic neuropathy.[17]

HEART RATE VARIABILITY IN DIABETIC AUTONOMIC NEUROPATHY

Diabetic autonomic neuropathy is more common among type I DM patients. In a prospective clinical study with 58 type 1 and 51 type 2 diabetic patients, the results indicated that symptoms accompanied the signs of autonomic neuropathy in type 1 DM, but not in type 2 DM.[18] Autonomic neuropathy causes alteration of parasympathetic and sympathetic functions, which lead heart rate variations. Assessment of diabetic neuropathy can be achieved by assessing heart rate variations. In a study reported by Oikawa et al. comparing 95 patients and 38 controls analyses shows that diabetic patients had lower heart rate during deep breathing. The study affirms that there were significant sympathetic and parasympathetic impairments among patients with diabetic neuropathy.[19]

Routine assessment of HRV in diabetic clinic is useful method to diagnose diabetic neuropathy at the early stage. HRV measurement measured in healthy volunteers as compared to diabetics with autonomic neuropathy was significantly different.[20] DAN often precedes somatic neuropathy and HRV analysis can be helpful in the early stages of DM before the development of somatic neuropathy. Power spectrum analysis of measurement of HRV is considered to be a sensitive indicator in the assessment of autonomic neuropathy related to DM.[21] In another study reported of 27 patient with DAN assessment of HRV using power spectrum analysis, there was reduction of the low-frequency component in the standing position and a significant reduction of the percentage increase compared with the lying position, which was found to discriminate diabetics from controls.[22]

Particularly in diabetic patients without clinical evidence of autonomic neuropathy, lowered absolute power of low frequency and high frequency during controlled conditions was reported. However, when the ratio of low-to-high frequency was considered or when low frequency and high frequency were analyzed in normalized units, no significant difference in comparison to normal was found. Thus, the initial manifestation of this neuropathy is likely to involve both efferent limbs of the autonomic nervous system.[23] It was observed that variation in heart rate during deep breathing proves too simple and sensitive diagnostic index of autonomic neuropathy and was abnormal or borderline in 62 of 64 patients with autonomic symptoms. Abnormal HRV may represent permanent autonomic damage of long duration without the development of autonomic symptoms. It has been noted that HRV on deep breathing over 3–5 years showed little change, although overall there was a small deterioration of autonomic function, with a decrease of HRV score of 1.0 per year.[24]

It has been observed that asymptomatic autonomic neuropathy was more common among patients with type 2 DM as compared to type 1 who becomes more symptomatic with autonomic neuropathy.[25] Majority of patient with DAN will have sudden increase in heart rate in response to standing while other some had a prolonged gradual increase in heart rate on standing.[26] In clinical studies, which assessed the DAN by heart rate variations, suggested that the differences in mean heart rate, standard deviation, and coefficient of HRV was more significant in patients with neuropathy; however, the pulse wave velocity indices did not show noticeable difference.[27] In another study for early diagnosis of DAN shows that simple HRV can detect early subclinical alterations of autonomic nervous system.[28] Considering heart rate reserve and rating of perceived exertion to prescribe exercise intensity in DAN, the results were more in favor of heart rate reserve.[29] In a clinical study of 186 type 2 DM, wherein QTc interval, HRV, and postural hypotension were analyzed as indicators of cardiac autonomic neuropathy yielded and reported that prolonged QTc interval, HRV, and postural hypotension in type 2 DM patients are consistent with cardiac autonomic neuropathy.

Furthermore, once a good glycemic control is obtained, there is chance of a clinical study on the effect of glycemic control on HRV in type 1 diabetic patients with cardiac autonomic neuropathy reported that early diagnosis of DAN has benefit of early treatment and reversible effect on DAN. The results indicated that in patients with early DAN with strict glycemic control there is a potential for reversibility.[30]

CONCLUSION

Importance of HRV in clinical practice was first appreciated in 1965 when Hon and Lee'6' noted that fetal distress was preceded by alterations in interbeat intervals before any appreciable change occurred in the heart rate itself.[31] The clinical importance of HRV became apparent in the late 1980s when it was confirmed that HRV was a strong and independent predictor of mortality following an acute myocardial infarction.[32] Identifying DAN at early stage may be rewarding as good glycemic control can promote reversible effect on the progression of the related cardiac morbidities. HRV may offer a chance to analyze the disease status. This is a simple noninvasive cardiac indicator may prevent morbidity and mortality among patients with DAN. HRV may be considered to be important marker. Devices of new generation now provide automated measurement of HRV, analysis done using frequency-domain contributed to the understanding of the autonomic background of RR interval fluctuations in the heart rate record.[33] Fluctuations in autonomic nervous system are known in normal healthy individuals and in patients with various cardiovascular and noncardiovascular disorders studies done in past have reported that cardiac indicator HRV can be utilized as a significant predictor of cardiac morbidities and DAN among patients with DM. Clinical utility of this test has been proven, as it is a noninvasive assessment method and it is a feasible method, which could be easily used by healthcare professionals. HRV in diabetic to asses for DAN and related cardiovascular morbidity has a diagnostic implication in preventive care, as it is a sensitive indicator of prediction of DAN. Early recognition of abnormal HRV testing provides timely diagnostic and therapeutic action. This test is almost can be practiced in clinical setting, as it is noninvasive technique. Cardiac morbidity and problem related to autonomic neuropathy among diabetic can be properly addressed.

REFERENCES

1. Burger AJ, Aronson D. Effect of diabetes mellitus on heart rate variability in patients with congestive heart failure. Pacing Clin Electrophysiol. 2001;24:53-9.
2. Akinci A, Celiker A, Baykal E, et al. Heart rate variability in diabetic children: sensitivity of the time-and frequency-domain methods. Pediatr Cardiol. 1993;14:140-6.
3. Chessa M, Butera G, Lanza GA, et al. Role of heart rate variability in the early diagnosis of diabetic autonomic neuropathy in children. Herz. 2002;27:785-90.
4. Bigger JT Jr, Kleiger RE, Rottman JN, et al. Frequency domain measures of heart period variability and mortality after myocardial infarction. Circulation. 1992;85:164-1.
5. Porges SW. The Polyvagal Theory: phylogenetic contributions to social behavior. Physiol Behav. 2003;79:503-13.
6. Stephen WP. The polyvagal perspective. Biol Psychol. 2007;74: 116-43.
7. Souza NM, Vanderlei LC, Garner DM, et al. Risk evaluation of diabetes mellitus by relation of chaotic globals to HRV. Complexity. 2015;20:84-92.
8. Bigger JT Jr, Fleiss JL, Steinman RC. Frequency domain measures of heart period variability and mortality after myocardial infarction. Circulation. 1992;85:164-71.
9. George BE. The LF/HF ratio does not accurately measure cardiac sympatho-vagal balance. Front Physiol. 2013;4:26.
10. Vaseghi M, Shivkumar K. Progress in cardiovascular diseases. Prog Cardiovasc Dis. 2008;50:404-19.
11. Bunde A, Havlin S, Kantelhardt JW, et al. Correlated and Uncorrelated Regions in Heart-Rate Fluctuations during Sleep. Phys Rev Lett. 2000;85:3736-9.
12. Beljic T. Frequency of vascular complications in diabetic patients with subclinical cardiac dysfunction. Srp Arh Celok Lek. 1994;122: 40-2.
13. Thuesen L, Christiansen JS, Mogensen CE, et al. Cardiac hyperfunction in insulin-dependent diabetic patients developing microvascular complications. Diabetes. 1988;37:851-6.
14. Valensi P, Paries J, Attali JR. Cardiac autonomic neuropathy in diabetic patients: influence of diabetes duration, obesity, and microangiopathic complications—the French multicenter study. Metabolism. 2003;52:815-20.
15. Zarich SW, Pierce ET, Nesto RW, et al. Age and history of cardiac disease as risk factors for cardiac complications after peripheral vascular surgery in diabetic patients. Mayo Clin Proc. 2001;76:34-8.
16. Pumprla J, Howorka K, Nolan J. Functional assessment of heart rate variability: physiological basis and practical applications. Int J Cardiol. 2002;84:1-14.
17. Rhee SY, Ahn KJ, Kim IJ, et al. Prevalence of chronic complications in Korean patients with Type 2 diabetes mellitus based on the Korean National Diabetes Program. Diabetes Metab J. 2011;35:504-12.
18. Nilsson H, Bergstrom B, Lilja B, et al. Prospective study of autonomic nerve function in type 1 and type 2 diabetic patients: 24 hour heart rate variation and plasma motilin levels disturbed in parasympathetic neuropathy. Diabet Med. 1995;12:1015-21.
19. Oikawa N, Umetsu M, Toyota T, et al. Quantitative evaluation of diabetic autonomic neuropathy by using heart rate variations: relationship between cardiac parasympathetic or sympathetic damage and clinical conditions. Tohoku J Exp Med. 1986;148:125-33.
20. Braune HJ, Geisendorfer U. Measurement of heart rate variations: influencing factors, normal values and diagnostic impact on diabetic autonomic neuropathy. Diabetes Res Clin Pract. 1995;29:179-87.
21. Yoshioka K, Tanaka K. Effect of methylcobalamin on diabetic autonomic neuropathy as assessed by power spectral analysis of heart rate variations. Horm Metab Res. 1995;27:43-4.
22. Lagi A, Cipriani M, Paggetti C, et al. Power spectrum analysis of heart rate variations in the early detection of diabetic autonomic neuropathy. Clin Auton Res. 1994;4:245-8.
23. Pagani M, Malfatto G, Pierini S, et al. Spectral analysis of heart rate variability in the assessment of autonomic diabetic neuropathy. J Auton Nerv Syst. 1988;23:143-53.
24. Mackay JD, Page MM, Cambridge J, et al. Diabetic autonomic neuropathy. The diagnostic value of heart rate monitoring. Diabetologia. 1980;18:471-8.

25. Neil HA, Thompson AV, John S, et al. Diabetic autonomic neuropathy: the prevalence of impaired heart rate variability in a geographically defined population. Diabet Med. 1989;6:20-4.
26. Mitchell EA, Wealthall SR, Elliott RB. Diabetic autonomic neuropathy in children: immediate heart-rate response to standing. Australian Paediatr J. 1983;19:175-7.
27. Matsuto T, Inano K, Miida T, et al. Assessment of diabetic cardiovascular autonomic neuropathy by heart rate variability and pulse wave velocity. Rinsho Byori. 1998;46:1037-42.
28. Chessa M, Butera G, Lanza GA, et al. Role of heart rate variability in the early diagnosis of diabetic autonomic neuropathy in children. Herz. 2002;27:785-90.
29. Colberg SR, Swain DP, Vinik AI. Use of heart rate reserve and rating of perceived exertion to prescribe exercise intensity in diabetic autonomic neuropathy. Diabetes Care. 2003;26:986-90.
30. Khoharo HK, Halepoto AW. QTc-interval, heart rate variability and postural hypotension as an indicator of cardiac autonomic neuropathy in type 2 diabetic patients. J Pak Med Assoc. 2012;62(4):328-31.
31. Hon EH, Lee ST. Electronic evaluations of the fetal heart rate patterns preceding fetal death, further observations. Am J Obstet Gynec. 1965;87:814-26.
32. Kleiger RE, Miller JP, Bigger JT, et al. The Multicenter Post-Infarction Research Group. Decreased heart rate variability and its association with increased mortality after acute myocardial infarction. Am J Cardiol. 1987;59:256-62.
33. Pomeranz M, Macaulay RJB, Caudill MA, et al. Assessment of autonomic function in humans by heart rate spectral analysis. Am J Physiol. 1985;248:H151-3.

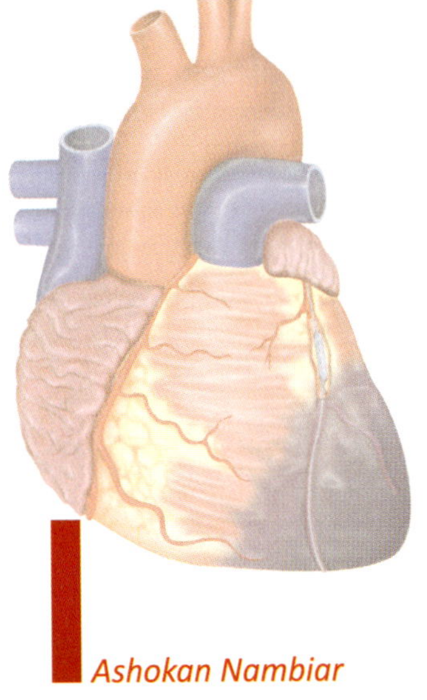

Natural History of Atrial Fibrillation in Cardiodiabetes: Is it Different?

Ashokan Nambiar

INTRODUCTION

Atrial fibrillation (AF) has emerged as a leading cause of morbidity and mortality particularly in the elderly. There is a strong interplay between advancing age and several risk factors such as hypertension, heart failure, history of previous cerebrovascular events, and diabetes. The importance of diabetes as a risk factor for AF has been recognized only more recently. Because of its association with several other risk factors occurring concurrently, the contribution of diabetes by itself to the onset and progression of AF and its complications is difficult to establish. However, the onset of diabetes in a patient with AF definitely points to worse prognosis and newer insights into the molecular basis will shed more light to our understanding about the seriousness of the problem and its management.

The relationship of AF and diabetes mellitus (DM) is mutual and reciprocal. AF is a marker of poor prognosis in diabetics. Conversely, DM is a well-documented risk factor for development of AF and is included prominently in both the $CHADS_2$[1] and $CHADS_2VA_2SC$[2] risk scores. The significance is perhaps more for patients with AF when they are found to be diabetic late in their natural course. This scenario is often associated with many complications of diabetes which were proceeding silently, undetected as its diagnosis is delayed. Such AF patients end up with serious complications like multiple strokes.

The growing epidemic of AF must naturally intersect with many risk factors which also tend to be seen as age advances. Thus advancing age, hypertension, past history of stroke, heart failure, diabetes, and other vascular diseases tend to interact and worsen the overall risk in patients with AF. In an elderly patient with AF, the likelihood of hypertension is there and if both are present, diabetes developing or already diagnosed is a common phenomenon. So it is very difficult to study the impact of one risk factor alone in relation to AF.

EPIDEMIOLOGY

Epidemiological studies point to the importance of each component in the $CHADS_2VA_2SC$ score. The role of inflammatory response in DM predisposing to AF is discussed by Sun.[3] The incidence of AF in patients with DM in survey of hospitalized patients was 14.9% versus 10.3% in controls. In the Framingham study the OR for AF in diabetes was 1.6 for women and 1.4 in men.[4] In 289 patients with persistent AF, logistic regression analysis showed that the duration of AF and the presence of DM were independent predictors of AF recurrence.[5] The incidence of AF is high in many other situations related to lifestyle changes such as obesity, metabolic syndrome, and hypertension. There is a strong interplay between these risk factors and genetic susceptibility.

There have been studies to look into how altered molecular mechanisms in DM may effect initiation and progression of AF.[6] Focal triggers in the pulmonary veins, changes in the refractory period in atria as a result of atrial remodeling, increase in conduction heterogeneity mediated by the angiotensin cascade all may be related to transcription factor kappa signaling pathway. Strategies to develop newer drugs to treat AF have unveiled molecular mechanisms in the genesis of AF.

Oxidative stress, vascular and myocardial dysfunction caused by DM as well as the genetics of AF make transcription factor NF-κB a suitable modifiable target in patients with DM for new drug development. Lower level of PPARγhas shown to increase atrial arrhythmia and its activator thiazolidinedione is found to have protective effect against AF. Ranolazine which acts on the late sodium current is shown to decrease AF in acute cardiac syndrome (ACS) and interestingly it also lowers HbA1C level in these patients. Thus, both genesis and perpetuation of AF as well as its termination could be related to the onset and control of diabetes.[7]

Nicholls et al. described the increased prevalence of AF in DM and also showed a stronger correlation in women. The prolonged intrinsic QT interval in women could be one of the reasons for it. Diabetes appears to remove the protective effect against AF in women as nondiabetic men have AF more frequently.[8] Diabetes is an important predictor of AF progression from paroxysmal to persistent and permanent forms, stroke and cerebrovascular death and progression may occur silently in diabetes.[9] Thromboembolic events are the leading causes of mortality and long-term disability worldwide, and diabetic patients are documented to have an increased stroke risk and poor prognosis.[10] Clinical evidence as well as experimental studies suggest that DM and AF are strongly interconnected.

CONCLUSION

The occurrence of AF portents poses grave additional risk in patients with diabetes. The stroke risk is significantly increased and aggravates incidence of morbidity and mortality in them. However, the relationship of AF to other risk factors which generally coexists with diabetes does not allow us to categorically quantify the excess risk. Newer insights into the molecular basis for the generation and perpetuation of AF in diabetes could enable us to tackle the twin menace successfully.

REFERENCES

1. Gage BF, Waterman AD, Shannon W, et al. Validation of clinical classification schemes for predicting stroke: results from the National Registry of Atrial Fibrillation. JAMA. 2001;285(22):2864-70.
2. Lip GY, Nieuwlaat N, Pisters R, et al. Refining clinical risk stratification for predicting stroke and thromboembolism in atrial fibrillation using a novel risk factor-based approach: the euro heart survey on atrial fibrillation. Chest. 2010;137(2):263-72.
3. Sun Y, Hu D. The Link between diabetes and atrial fibrillation: cause or correlation? J Cardiovasc Dis Res. 2010;1(1):10-11.
4. Benjamin EJ, Levy D, Vaziri SM, et al.Independent risk factors for atrial fibrillation in a population-based cohort. The Framingham Heart Study. JAMA. 1994;271(11):840-4.
5. Soran H, Younis N, Currie P, et al. Influence of diabetes on the maintenance of sinus rhythm after a successful direct current cardioversion in patients with atrial fibrillation. QJM. 2008;101(3):181-7.
6. De Sensi F, De Potter T, Cresti A, et al. Atrial fibrillation in patients with diabetes: molecular mechanisms and therapeutic perspectives. Cardiovasc Diagn Ther. 2015;5(5):364-73.
7. Movahed MR, Hashemzadeh M, Jamal MM. Diabetes mellitus is a strong, independent risk for atrial fibrillation and flutter in addition to other cardiovascular disease. Int J Cardiol. 2005;105(3):315-8.
8. Nicholls GA, Reinin K, ChughSS. Independent contribution of diabetes to increased prevalence and incidence of atrial fibrillation. Diabetes Care. 2009;32(10):1851-6.
9. Papponi C, Zuffada F, Sansinelli V. AF and diabetes—prognosis and prediction. Rijeka: Intech; 2011.
10. Arboix A. Stroke prognosis in diabetes mellitus: new insights but questions remain. Expert Rev Cardiovasc Ther. 2009;7(10):1181-5.

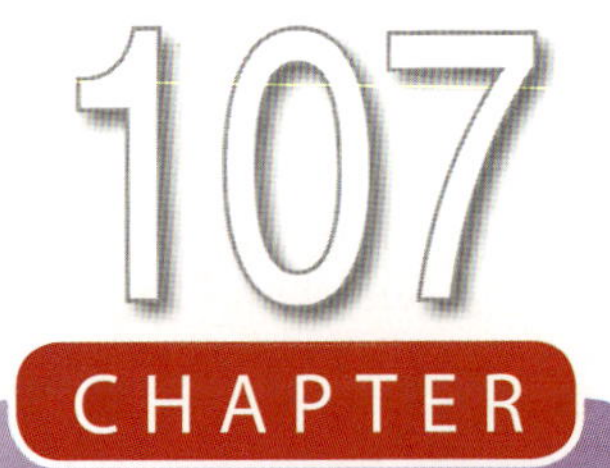

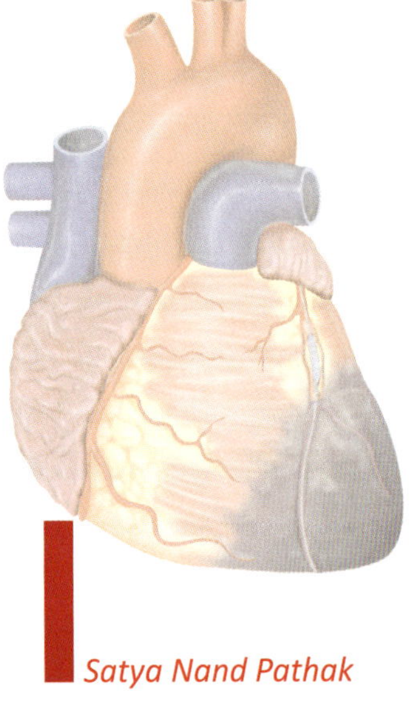

Atrial Fibrillation: Management Strategies in Cardiodiabetics

Satya Nand Pathak

INTRODUCTION

Despite good progress in the management of patients with atrial fibrillation (AF), this arrhythmia remains one of the major causes of stroke, heart failure, sudden death, and cardiovascular morbidity in the world. Its prevalence is more in patients with conditions such as hypertension, heart failure, coronary artery disease (CAD), valvular heart disease, obesity, diabetes mellitus, and chronic kidney disease (CKD).[1-7] The increase in AF prevalence can be attributed both to better detection of silent AF, [8-10] along with increasing age and conditions predisposing to AF.[11]

OVERT AND SILENT ATRIAL FIBRILLATION (TABLES 1 AND 2)

Silent, undetected AF is common,[12,13] with severe consequences such as stroke and death.[14-16] Prompt recording of an electrocardiography (ECG) is a cost-effective method to document chronic forms of AF.[17] Absolutely irregular RR intervals and no discernible, distinct P waves is characteristic finding in ECG. By accepted convention, an episode lasting atleast 30 s is diagnostic. There is good evidence that prolonged ECG monitoring enhances the detection of undiagnosed AF, e.g. monitoring for 72 hours after a stroke.[18]

TABLE 1: Recommendations for screening for atrial fibrillation

Recommendations	*Class*	*Level*
Opportunistic screening for AF is recommended by pulse taking or ECG rhythm strip in patients >65 years of age	I	B
In patients with TIA or ischemic stroke, screening for AF is recommended by short-term ECG recording followed by continuous ECG monitoring for atleast 72 hours	I	B
It is recommended to interrogate pacemakers and ICDs on a regular basis for atrial high rate episodes (AHRE). Patients with AHRE should undergo further ECG monitoring to document AF before initiating AF therapy	I	B

Abbreviations: AF, atrial fibrillation; ECG, electrocardiography; TIA, transient ischemic attack; ICD, implantable cardioverter defibrillator

Source: 2016 ESC guidelines for the mangement of atrial fibrillation develop in collaberation with EACTS

PATIENTS WITH ATRIAL FIBRILLATION AND HEART FAILURE WITH REDUCED EJECTION FRACTION

The general approach to AF management does not differ between heart failure patients and others, but a few considerations are worthwhile. Of note, the only

TABLE 2: Patterens of atrial fibrillation

AF pattern	Definition
First diagnosed AF	AF that has not been diagnosed before, irrespective of the duration of the arrhythmia or the presence and severity of AF-related symptoms
Paroxysmal AF	Self-terminating, in most cases is within 48 hours. Some AF paroxysms may continue for upto 7 days.[a] AF episodes that are cardioverted within 7 days should be considered paroxysmal[a]
Persistent AF	AF that lasts longer than 7 days, including episodes that are terminated by cardioversion, either with drugs or by direct current cardioversion after 7 days or more
Long-standing persistent AF	Continuous AF lasting for ≥1 year when it is decided to adopt a rhythm control strategy
Permanent AF	AF that is accepted by the patient (and physician). Hence, rhythm control interventions are by AF. Should a rhythm control strategy be adopted, the arrhythmia would be re-classified as 'long-standing definition, not pursued in patients with permanent persistent AF'

Source: 2016 ESC guidelines for the mangement of atrial fibrillation develop in collaberation with EACTS.

therapy with proven prognostic value in these patients is anticoagulation. In addition to oral anticoagulation (OAC), standard heart failure therapy should be used in patients with heart failure with reduced ejection fraction (HFrEF). In brief, only beta-blockers and digoxin are suitable in HFrEF because of the negative inotropic potential of verapamil and diltiazem. Beta-blockers are usually the first-line option in patients with clinically stable HFrEF. Digoxin had a neutral effect on mortality in patients with AF and concomitant heart failure.[19] For patients who develop HFrEF as a result of rapid AF (tachycardiomyopathy), a rhythm control strategy is preferred, based on several relatively small patient cohorts and trials reporting improved left ventricular (LV) function after restoration of sinus rhythm.[20-23]

Prevention of Atrial Fibrillation in Heart Failure

Retrospective analyses from large randomized trials have reported a lower incidence of new-onset AF in patients treated with angiotensin-converting enzyme (ACE) inhibitors or angiotensin receptor blockers (ARBs) compared with placebo.[24-26] The reduced incidence of AF with ACE inhibitors or ARBs is less evident in patients with HFpEF[27] and is lost in patients without heart failure.[28-30] Neprilysin inhibition does not seem to add to this effect.[31] Beta-blocker therapy was associated with a 33% reduction in the adjusted odds of incident AF in HFrEF patients pretreated with ACE inhibitors or ARBs, reinforcing the importance of beta-blocker therapy in HFrEF patients in sinus rhythm.[32] Eplerenone, a mineralocorticoid receptor antagonist, also reduced the risk of new-onset AF in patients with LV ejection fraction (LVEF) less than equal to 35%, New York Heart Association (NYHA) Class II, when added to ACE inhibitors or ARBs and beta-blockers (Box 1, Flow charts 1 and 2).[33]

Hypertension

Hypertension is a stroke risk factor in AF; uncontrolled high blood pressure enhances the risk of stroke and bleeding events and may lead to recurrent AF. Therefore, good blood pressure control should form an integral part of the management of AF patients.[34] Inhibition of the renin–angiotensin–aldosterone system can prevent structural remodeling and recurrent AF.[24,35] In patients with established AF, but without LV dysfunction or heart failure, ARBs do not prevent recurrent AF better than placebo.[28,29]

BOX 1: Management of patients presenting acutely with atrial fibrillation and heart failure

Management of patients presenting acutely with AF and heart failure

Acute management | Chronic management

- Cardiovert if unstable
- Anticoagulate according to stroke risk
- Normalize fluid balance with diuretics to improve symptoms
- Control rate: Initial rate target <110 bpm; stricter if persistent HF/AF symptoms
- Inhibit the renin-angiotensin-aldosterone system
- Early consideration of rhythm control
- Advanced HF therapies, including devices
- Treatment of other cardiovascular disease, especially ischemia and hypertension

Flow chart 1: Antithrombotic therapy after an acute coronary syndrome in atrial fibrillation patients requiring anticoagulation

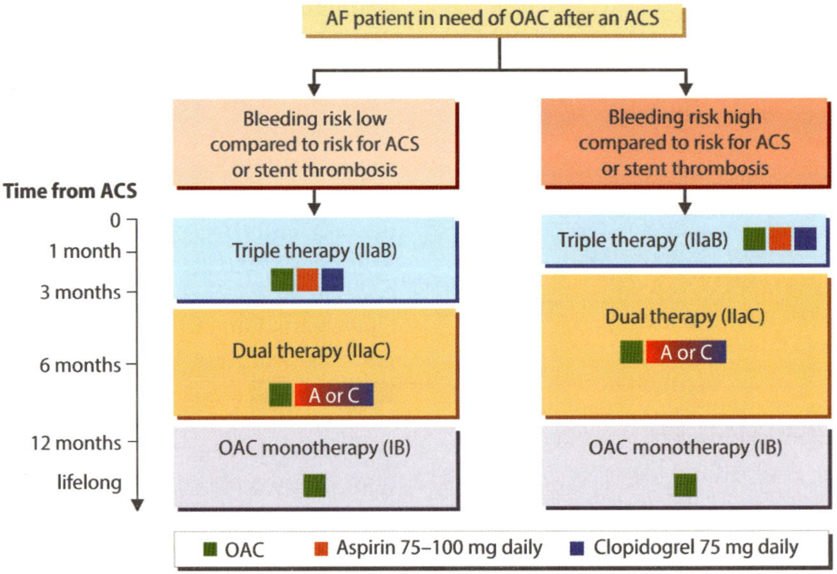

Abbreviations: AF, atrial fibrillation; OAC, oral anticoagulation; ACS, acute coronary syndrome.

Flow chart 2: Antithrombotic therapy after elective percutaneous intervention in atrial fibrillation patients requiring anticoagulation

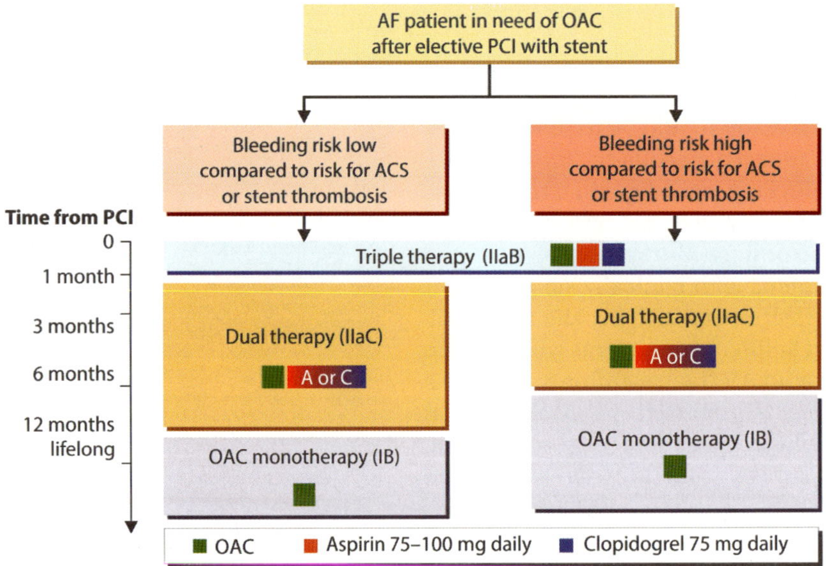

Abbreviations: AF, atrial fibrillation; OAC, oral anticoagulation; ACS, acute coronary syndrome; PCI, percutaneous coronary intervention.

Valvular Heart Disease

Valvular heart disease is independently associated with incident of AF.[36] Approximately 30% of patients with AF have some form of valvular heart disease, often detected only by echocardiogram.[37-39] Valvular AF mainly refers to AF patients that have either rheumatic valvular disease (predominantly mitral stenosis) or mechanical heart valves.

Diabetes

In patients with AF, a longer duration of diabetes appears to confer a higher risk of thromboembolism, albeit without greater risk of OAC-related bleeding.[40] Unfortunately, intensive glycemic control does not affect the rate of new-onset AF,[41] while treatment with metformin seems to be associated with a decreased long-term risk of AF in diabetic patients[42] and may even be associated with a lower long-term stroke risk. Diabetic retinopathy, a measure of disease severity does not increase the risk of ocular bleeding.[43]

INTEGRATED MANAGEMENT OF PATIENTS WITH ATRIAL FIBRILLATION IN ANTICOAGULATED PATIENTS (FIG. 1, TABLE 3, FLOW CHART 3 AND TABLE 4)

Rate Control Therapy in Atrial Fibrillation

For acute rate control, beta-blockers and diltiazem or verapamil are preferred over digoxin because of their rapid onset of action and effectiveness at high sympathetic tone (Flow chart 4).[44-48]

Long-term Pharmacological Rate Control

Beta-adrenoreceptor blocker monotherapy is often the first-line rate-controlling agent,[49] largely based on observations of better acute heart rate control than digoxin. Interestingly, the prognostic benefit of beta-blockers seen in HFrEF patients with sinus rhythm is lost in those with AF. Verapamil or diltiazem provide reasonable rate control in AF patients.[50] They should be avoided in patients with HFrEF because of their negative inotropic effects.[51-53] In the randomized Digitalis Investigation Group (DIG) trial, digoxin had no effect on mortality compared to placebo in HFrEF patients in sinus rhythm (RR 0.99; 95% CI 0.91–1.07), but reduced hospital admissions (RR 0.72; 95% CI 0.66–0.79).[54,55]

Amiodarone can be useful for rate control as a last resort (Flow chart 5 and Table 5).

Rhythm Control Therapy in Atrial Fibrillation

Restoring and maintaining sinus rhythm are an integral part of AF management. Rhythm control therapy is indicated to improve symptoms in AF patients who remain symptomatic on adequate rate control therapy.

Acute Restoration of Sinus Rhythm

In the short-term, electrical cardioversion restores sinus rhythm quicker and more effectively than pharmacological cardioversion and is associated with shorter hospitalization.[56-60] Pharmacological cardioversion, conversely does not require sedation or fasting. Flecainide and propafenone are effective for pharmacological cardioversion,[61,62] but their use is restricted to patients without structural heart disease. Ibutilide is an alternative where available, but carries a risk of torsades de pointes. Vernakalant can be given to patients with mild heart failure (NYHA Class I or II), including those with ischemic heart

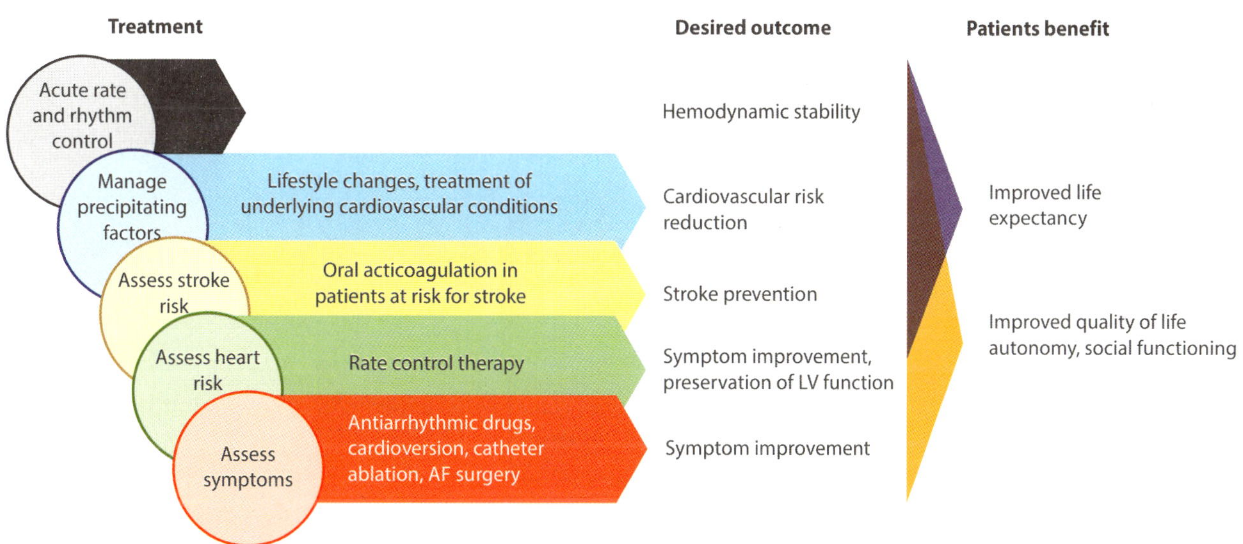

Fig. 1: Management of atrial fibrillation with desired outcomes and patient benefits

Abbreviation: LV, left ventricular.

disease, provided they do not present with hypotension or severe aortic stenosis.[63-65] Amiodarone can be used in patients with heart failure and in patients with ischemic heart disease (although patients with severe heart failure were excluded from most of the AF cardioversion trials). Both amiodarone and flecainide appear more effective than sotalol in restoring sinus rhythm.[66] Outside of Europe, dofetilide is available and can convert recent-onset AF.

TABLE 3: Recommendations for patients with valvular heart disease and atrial fibrillation

CHA_2DS_2-VASc risk factor	*Points*
Congestive heart failure Signs/symptoms of heart failure or objective evidence of reduced left ventricular ejection fraction	+1
Hypertension Resting blood pressure >140/90 mm Hg on atleast two occasions or current antihypertensive treatment	+1
Age 75 years or older	+2
Diabetes mellitus Fasting glucose >125 mg/dL (7 mmol/L) or treatment with oral hypoglycaemic agent and/or insulin	+1
Previous stroke, transient ischemic attack, or thromboembolism	+2
Vascular disease Previous myocardial infarction, peripheral artery disease, or aortic plaque	+1
Age 65–74 years	+1
Sex category (female)	+1

Source: 2016 ESC guidelines for the mangement of atrial fibrillation develop in collaberation with EACTS.

'PILL IN THE POCKET' CARDIOVERSION PERFORMED BY PATIENTS

A single bolus of oral flecainide (200–300 mg) or propafenone (450–600 mg) can be self-administered by the patient at home ('pill in the pocket' therapy) to restore sinus rhythm.

Electrical Cardioversion

Synchronized direct current electrical cardioversion quickly and effectively converts AF to sinus rhythm, and is the method of choice in severely hemodynamically compromised patients with new-onset AF.[67-69] Electrical cardioversion can be performed safely in sedated patients treated with intravenous midazolam and/or propofol. Continuous monitoring of blood pressure and oximetry during the procedure is important. Skin burns may occasionally be observed. Intravenous atropine or isoproterenol, or temporary transcutaneous pacing should be available to mitigate postcardioversion bradycardia. Biphasic defibrillators are more effective than monophasic waveforms, and have become the industry standard.

Anticoagulation in Patients Undergoing Cardioversion

Cardioversion carries an inherent risk of stroke in nonanticoagulated patients,[70] which is reduced substantially

Flow chart 3: Recommendations for patients with valvular heart disease and atrial fibrillation.

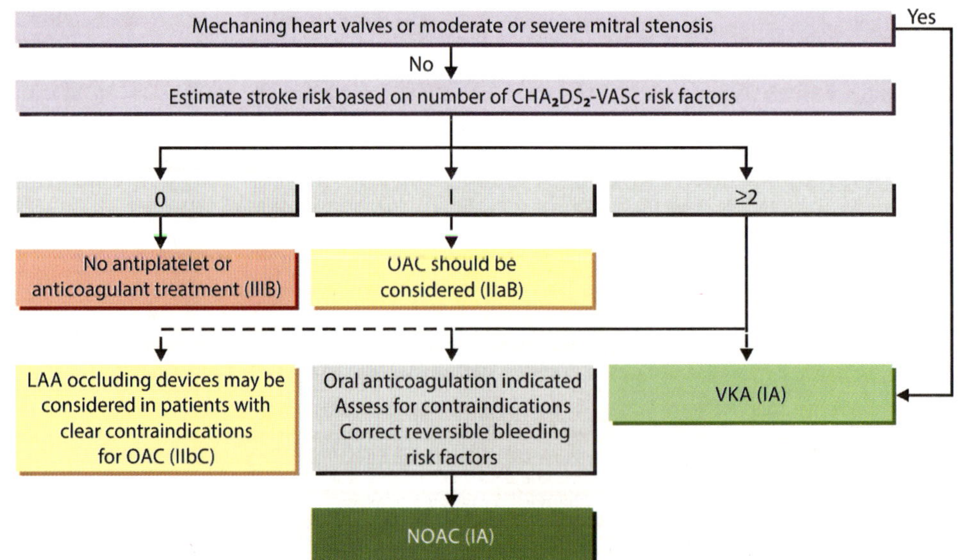

Abbreviations: LLA, lower lingual arch; OAC, oral anticoagulation; VKA, vitamin K antagonists; IA, intraarterial; NOAC, novel oral anticoagulant.

TABLE 4: Recommendations for stroke prevention in patients with atrial fibrillation

Recommendations	*Class*[a]	*Level*[b]	
Oral anticoagulation therapy to prevent thromboembolism is recommended for all male AF patients with a CHA_2DS_2-VASc score of 2 or more	I	A	
Oral anticoagulation therapy to prevent thromboembolism is recommended in all female AF patients with a CHA_2DS_2-VASc score of 3 or more	I	A	
Oral anticoagulation therapy to prevent thromboembolism should be considered in male AF patients with a CHA_2DS_2-VASc score of 1, considering individual characteristics and patient preferences	IIa	B	
Oral anticoagulation therapy to prevent thromboembolism should be considered in female AF patients with a CHA_2DS_2-VASc score of 2, considering individual characteristics and patient preferences	IIa	B	
Vitamin K antagonist therapy (INR 2.0–3.0 or higher) is recommended for stroke prevention in AF patients with moderate-to-severe mitral stenosis or mechanical heart valves	I	B	
When oral anticoagulation is initiated in a patient with AF who is eligible for a NOAC (apixaban, dabigatran, edoxaban, or rivaroxaban), a NOAC is recommended in preference to a Vitamin K antagonist	I	A	
When patients are treated with a vitamin K antagonist, time in therapeutic range (TTR) should be kept as high as possible and closely monitored	I	A	
AF patients already on treatment with a vitamin K antagonist may be considered for NOAC treatment if TTR is not well controlled despite good adherence, or if patient preference without contraindications to NOAC (e.g. prosthetic valve)	IIb	A	
Combinations of oral anticoagulants and platelet inhibitors increase bleeding risk and should be avoided in AF patients without another indication for platelet inhibition	III (harm)	B	
In male or female AF patients without additional stroke risk factors, anticoagulant or antiplatelet therapy is not recommended for stroke prevention	III (harm)	B	
Antiplatelet monotherapy is not recommended for stroke prevention in AF patients, regardless of stroke risk	III (harm)	A	
NOACs (apixaban, dabigatran, edoxaban, and rivaroxaban) are not recommended in patients with mechanical heart valves (Level of evidence B) or moderate-to-severe mitral stenosis (Level of evidence C)	III (harm)	B	C

Source: 2016 ESC guidelines for the mangement of atrial fibrillation develop in collaberation with EACTS

Abbreviations: AF, artrial fibrillation, NOAC, novel oral anticoagulant

Flow chart 4: Acute heart rate control of atrial fibrillation.

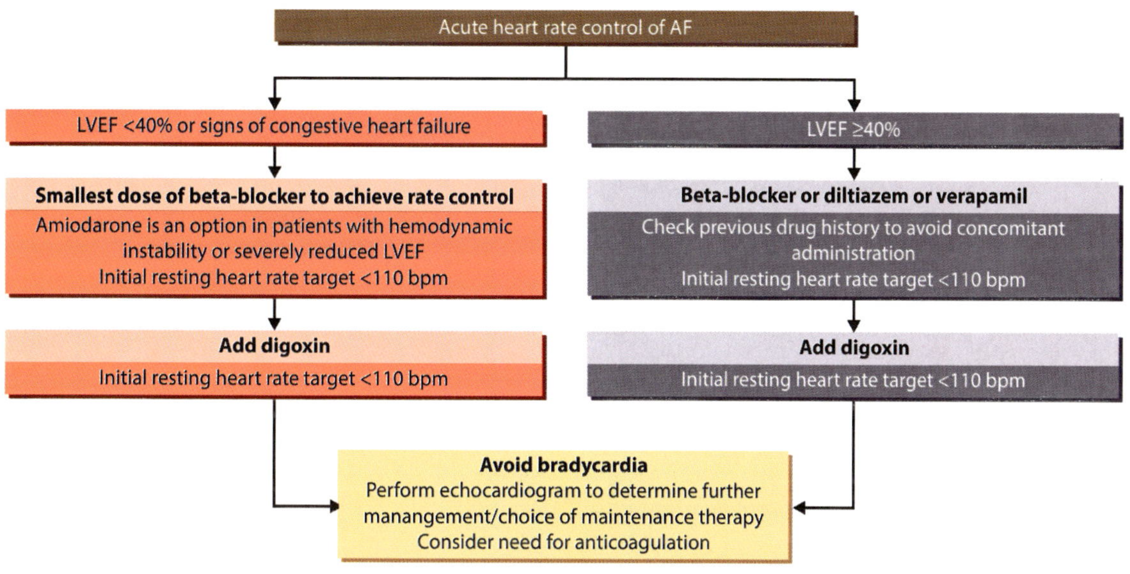

Abbreviations: AF, atrial fibrillation; LVEF, left ventricular ejection fraction.

Flow chart 5: Long-term heart rate control of atrial fibrillation

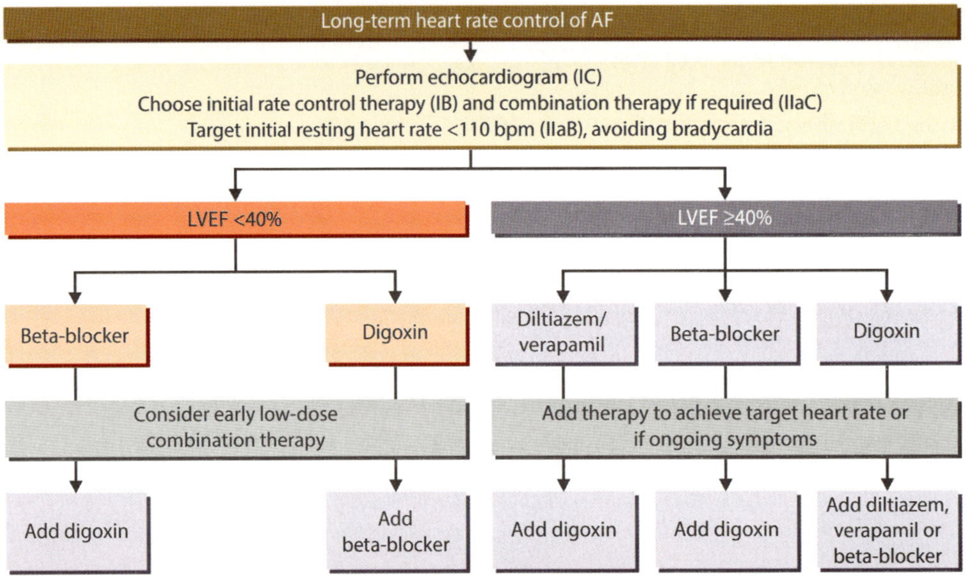

Long-term heart rate control of AF

Perform echocardiogram (IC)
Choose initial rate control therapy (IB) and combination therapy if required (IIaC)
Target initial resting heart rate <110 bpm (IIaB), avoiding bradycardia

LVEF <40%

Beta-blocker

Digoxin

Consider early low-dose combination therapy

Add digoxin

Add beta-blocker

LVEF ≥40%

Diltiazem/ verapamil

Beta-blocker

Digoxin

Add therapy to achieve target heart rate or if ongoing symptoms

Add digoxin

Add digoxin

Add diltiazem, verapamil or beta-blocker

Abbreviations: AF, atrial fibrillation; LVEF, left ventricular ejection fraction

TABLE 5: Recommendation for rate control

Recommendations	*Class[a]*	*Level[b]*
Beta-blockers, digoxin, diltiazem, or verapamil are recommended to control heart rate in AF patients with LVEF ≥40%	I	B
Beta-blockers and/or digoxin are recommended to control heart rate in AF patients with LVEF <40%	I	B
Combination therapy comprising different rate of controlling agents should be considered if a single agent does not achieve the necessary heart rate target	IIa	C
In patients with hemodynamic instability or severely depressed LVEF, amiodarone may be considered for acute control of heart rate	IIb	B

Abbreviations: AF, atrial fibrillation; LVEF, left ventricular ejection fraction

Source: 2016 ESC guidelines for the mangement of atrial fibrillation develop in collaberation with EACTS

by the administration of anticoagulation.[71] Immediate initiation of anticoagulation is important in all patients scheduled for cardioversion.[72-74] Patients who have been in AF for longer than 48 hours should start OAC atleast 3 weeks before cardioversion and continue it for 4 weeks afterwards (in patients without a need for long-term anticoagulation). OAC should be continued indefinitely inpatients at risk of stroke.

Antiarrhythmic effects of nonantiarrhythmic drugs ACE inhibitors or ARBs appear to prevent new-onset AF in patients with LV dysfunction and in hypertensive patients with LV hypertrophy.[75] Compared with placebo, beta-blockers are associated with a reduced risk of new-onset AF in patients with HFrEF and sinus rhythm. Perioperative statin therapy appeared to reduce the risk of postoperative AF in a number of small randomized, controlled trials (RCTs)[76,77] however, an adequately powered placebo-controlled trial has shown no effect of perioperative rosuvastatin therapy on postoperative AF.[78] Statin treatment does not prevent AF in other settings.[79,80] Polyunsaturated fatty acids failed to show convincing benefit.[81] At present there is no robust evidence to make any recommendation for the use of aldosterone antagonists for secondary prevention of AF (Flow charts 6 and 7).[82-33]

CONCLUSION

These strategies of nonpharmacological, pharmacological, mechanical cardioversion such radio frequency ablation has improved outcomes in cardiodiabetes with minimum comorbidities. However, judicial and timely intervention in atrial fibrillation with cardiodiabetes may reduce cardiac inflicted morbidity and mortality. It has been documented that appropriate glycemic control definitely improves the outcome.

Flow chart 6: Rhythm control management of recent onset atrial fibrillation

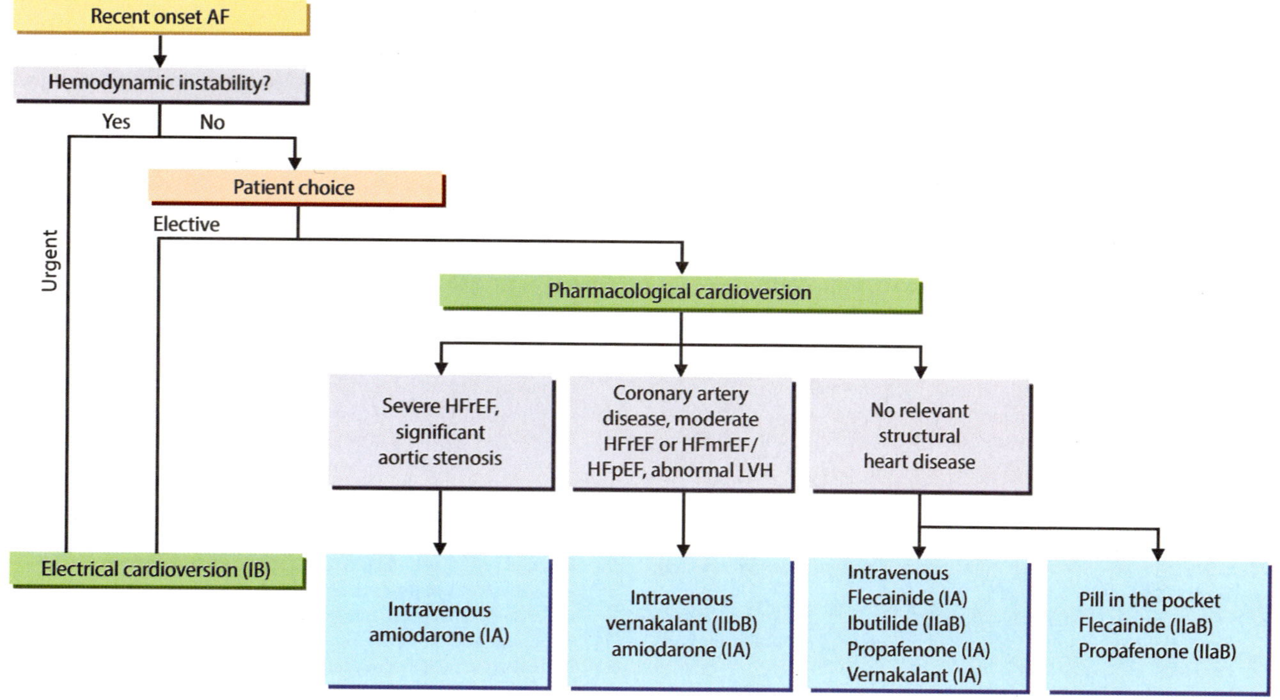

Abbreviations: AF, atrial fibrillation; HFrEF, heart failure with reduced ejection fraction; HFmrEF, heart failure with mildly reduced ejection fraction; HFpEF, heart failure with preserved ejection fraction

Flow chart 7: Initiation of long-term rhythm control therapy to improve symptom in atrial fibrillation

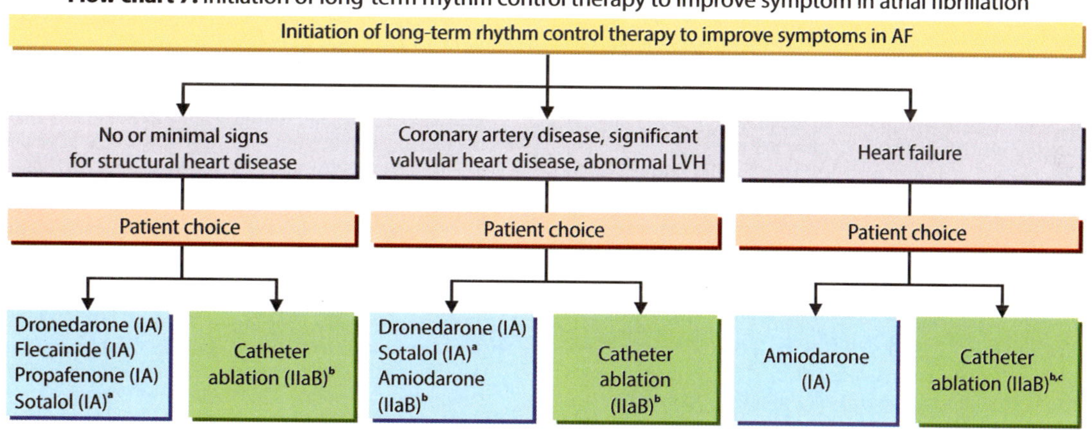

Abbreviations: AF, atrial fibrillation; LVH, left ventricular hypertrophy

REFERENCES

1. Zoni-Berisso M, Lercari F, Carazza T, et al. Epidemiology of atrial fibrillation: European perspective. Clin Epidemiol. 2014;6:213-20.
2. McManus DD, Rienstra M, Benjamin EJ. An update on the prognosis of patients with atrial fibrillation. Circulation. 2012;126(10):e143-146.
3. Ball J, Carrington MJ, McMurray JJ, et al. Atrial fibrillation: profile and burden of an evolving epidemic in the 21st century. Int J Cardiol. 2013;167(5):1807-24.
4. Kannel WB, Wolf PA, Benjamin EJ, et al. Prevalence, incidence, prognosis, and predisposing conditions for atrial fibrillation: population-based estimates. Am J Cardiol. 1998;82(8A):2-9N.
5. Nguyen TN, Hilmer SN, Cumming RG. Review of epidemiology and management of atrial fibrillation in developing countries. Int J Cardiol. 2013;167(6):2412-20.
6. Oldgren J, Healey JS, Ezekowitz M, et al. Variations in cause and management of atrial fibrillation in a prospective registry of 15,400 emergency department patients in 46 countries: the RE-LY Atrial Fibrillation Registry. Circulation. 2014;129(15):1568-76.

7. Chiang CE, Naditch-Brule L, Murin J, et al. Distribution and risk profile of paroxysmal, persistent, and permanent atrial fibrillation in routine clinical practice: insight from the reallife global survey evaluating patients with atrial fibrillation international registry. Circ Arrhythm Electrophysiol. 2012;5(4):632-9.
8. Wang TJ, Larson MG, Levy D, et al. Temporal relations of atrial fibrillation and congestive heart failure and their joint influence on mortality: the Framingham Heart Study. Circulation. 2003;107(23):2920-5.
9. Kishore A, Vail A, Majid A, et al. Detection of atrial fibrillation after ischemic stroke or transient ischemic attack: a systematic review and meta-analysis. Stroke. 2014;45(2):520-6.
10. Sanna T, Diener HC, Passman RS, Et al. Cryptogenic stroke and underlying atrial fibrillation. N Engl J Med. 2014;370(26):2478-86.
11. Schnabel RB, Yin X, Gona P, et al. 50 year trends in atrial fibrillation prevalence, incidence, risk factors, and mortality in the Framingham Heart Study: a cohort study. Lancet. 2015;386(9989):154-62.
12. Kirchhof P, Bax J, Blomstrom-Lundquist C, et al. Early and comprehensive management of atrial fibrillation: executive summary of the proceedings from the 2nd AFNET-EHRA consensus conference 'research perspectives in AF.' Eur Heart J. 2009;30(24):2969-77c.
13. Savelieva I, Camm AJ. Clinical relevance of silent atrial fibrillation: prevalence, prognosis, quality of life, and management. J Interv Card Electrophysiol. 2000;4(2):369-82.
14. Friberg L, Hammar N, Rosenqvist M. Stroke in paroxysmal atrial fibrillation: report from the Stockholm Cohort of Atrial Fibrillation. Eur Heart J. 2010;31(8):967-75.
15. Vanassche T, Lauw MN, Eikelboom JW, et al. Risk of ischaemic stroke according to pattern of atrial fibrillation: analysis of 6563 aspirin treated patients in ACTIVE-A and AVERROES. Eur Heart J. 2015;36(5):281-7a.
16. Steinberg BA, Hellkamp AS, Lokhnygina Y, et al. Higher risk of death and stroke in patients with persistent vs. paroxysmal atrial fibrillation: results from the ROCKET-AF Trial. Eur Heart J. 2015;36(5):288-96.
17. Fitzmaurice DA, Hobbs FD, Jowett S, et al. Screening versus routine practice in detection of atrial fibrillation in patients aged 65 or over: cluster randomised controlled trial. BMJ. 2007;335:383.
18. Grond M, Jauss M, Hamann G. Improved detection of silent atrial fibrillation using 72-hour Holter ECG in patients with ischemic stroke: a prospective multicenter cohort study. Stroke. 2013;44(12):3357-64.
19. Ziff OJ, Lane DA, Samra M, et al. Safety and efficacy of digoxin: systematic review and meta-analysis of observational and controlled trial data. BMJ. 2015;351:h4451.
20. Jones DG, Haldar SK, Hussain W, et al. A randomized trial to assess catheter ablation versus rate control in the management of persistent atrial fibrillation in heart failure. J Am Coll Cardiol. 2013;61(18):1894-1903.
21. Anselmino M, Matta M, D'Ascenzo F, et al. Catheter ablation of atrial fibrillation in patients with left ventricular systolic dysfunction: a systematic review and meta-analysis. Circ Arrhythm Electrophysiol. 2014;7(6):1011-8.
22. Ganesan AN, Nandal S, Luker J, et al. Catheter ablation of atrial fibrillation in patients with concomitant left ventricular impairment: a systematic review of efficacy and effect on ejection fraction. Heart Lung Circ. 2015;24(3):270-80.
23. Khan MN, Jais P, Cummings J, et al. Pulmonary-vein isolation for atrial fibrillation in patients with heart failure. N Engl J Med. 2008;359(174):1778-85.
24. Schneider MP, Hua TA, Böhm M, et al. Prevention of atrial fibrillation by Renin-Angiotensin system inhibition a meta-analysis. J Am Coll Cardiol. 2010;55(21):2299-2307.
25. Healey JS, Baranchuk A, Crystal E, et al. Prevention of atrial fibrillation with angiotensin-converting enzyme inhibitors and angiotensin receptor blockers: a meta-analysis. J Am Coll Cardiol. 2005;45(11):1832-9.
26. Jibrini MB, Molnar J, Arora RR. Prevention of atrial fibrillation by way of abrogation of the renin-angiotensin system: a systematic review and meta-analysis. Am J Ther. 2008;15(1):36-43.
27. Ducharme A, Swedberg K, Pfeffer MA, et al. Prevention of atrial fibrillation in patients with symptomatic chronic heart failure by candesartan in the Candesartan in Heart failure: Assessment of Reduction in Mortality and morbidity (CHARM) program. Am Heart J. 2006;152(1):86-92.
28. GISSI-AF Investigators, Disertori M, Latini R, et al. Valsartan for prevention of recurrent atrial fibrillation. N Engl J Med. 2009;360(16):1606-7.
29. Goette A, Schon N, Kirchhof P, et al. Angiotensin II-antagonist in paroxysmal atrial fibrillation (ANTIPAF) trial. Circ Arrhythm Electrophysiol. 2012;5(1):43-51.
30. Active I Investigators, Yusuf S, Healey JS, et al. Irbesartan in patients with atrial fibrillation. N Engl J Med. 2011;364(10):928-38.
31. McMurray JJ, Packer M, Desai AS, et al. Angiotensin-neprilysin inhibition versus enalapril in heart failure. N Engl J Med. 2014;371(11):993-1004.
32. Kotecha D, Holmes J, Krum H, et al. Efficacy of β-blockers in patients with heart failure plus atrial fibrillation: an individual-patient data meta-analysis. Lancet. 2014;384(9961):2235-43.
33. Swedberg K, Zannad F, McMurray JJ, et al. Eplerenone and atrial fibrillation in mild systolic heart failure: results from the EMPHASIS-HF (Eplerenone in Mild Patients Hospitalization And SurvIval Study in Heart Failure) study. J Am Coll Cardiol. 2012;59(18):1598-1603.
34. Manolis AJ, Rosei EA, Coca A, et al. Hypertension and atrial fibrillation: diagnostic approach, prevention and treatment. Position paper of the Working Group 'Hypertension Arrhythmias and Thrombosis' of the European Society of Hypertension. J Hypertens. 2012;30(2):239-52.
35. Goette A, Staack T, Rocken C, et al. Increased expression of extracellular signal-regulated kinase and angiotensin-converting enzyme in human atria during atrial fibrillation. J Am Coll Cardiol. 2000;35(6):1669-77.
36. Furberg CD, Psaty BM, Manolio TA, et al. Prevalence of atrial fibrillation in elderly subjects (the Cardiovascular Health Study). Am J Cardiol. 1994;74(3):236-41.
37. Vahanian A, Alfieri O, Andreotti F, et al. Guidelines on the management of valvular heart disease (version 2012). Eur Heart J. 2012;33(19):2451-96.
38. Nishimura RA, Otto CM, Bonow RO, et al. 2014 AHA/ACC guideline for the management of patients with valvular heart disease: executive summary: a report of the American College of Cardiology/American Heart Association Task Force on Practice Guidelines. J Am Coll Cardiol 2014;63(22):2438-88.
39. Nieuwlaat R, Capucci A, Camm AJ, et al. Atrial fibrillation management: a prospective survey in ESC member countries: the Euro Heart Survey on Atrial Fibrillation. Eur Heart J. 2005;26(22):2422-34.
40. Overvad TF, Skjøth F, Lip GY, et al. Duration of Diabetes Mellitus and Risk of Thromboembolism and Bleeding in Atrial Fibrillation: Nationwide Cohort Study. Stroke. 2015;46(8):2168-74.
41. Fatemi O, Yuriditsky E, Tsioufis C, et al. Impact of intensive glycemic control on the incidence of atrial fibrillation and associated cardiovascular outcomes in patients with type 2 diabetes mellitus (from the Action to Control Cardiovascular Risk in Diabetes Study). Am J Cardiol. 2014;114(8):1217-22.
42. Chang SH, Wu LS, Chiou MJ, et al. Association of metformin with lower atrial fibrillation risk among patients with type2 diabetes

mellitus: a population-based dynamic cohort and in vitro studies. Cardiovasc Diabetol. 2014;13:123.
43. Lip GY, Clementy N, Pierre B, et al. The impact of associated diabetic retinopathy on stroke and severe bleeding risk in diabetic patients with atrial fibrillation: the Loire valley atrial fibrillation project. Chest. 2015;147(4):1103-10.
44. Segal JB, McNamara RL, Miller MR, et al. The evidence regarding the drugs used for ventricular rate control. In. J Fam Practice. 2000;49(1):47-59.
45. Schreck DM, Rivera AR, Tricarico VJ. Emergency management of atrial fibrillation and flutter: intravenous diltiazem versus intravenous digoxin. Ann Emerg Med. 1997;29(1):135-40.
46. Siu CW, Lau CP, Lee WL, et al. Intravenous diltiazem is superior to intravenous amiodarone or digoxin for achieving ventricular rate control in patients with acute uncomplicated atrial fibrillation. Crit Care Med. 2009;37(7):2174-79.
47. Tisdale JE, Padhi ID, Goldberg AD, et al. A randomized, double-blind comparison of intravenous diltiazem and digoxin for atrial fibrillation after coronary artery bypass surgery. Am Heart J. 1998;135(5 Pt 1):739-47.
48. Scheuermeyer FX, Grafstein E, Stenstrom R, et al. Safety and efficiency of calcium channel blockers versus beta blockers for rate control in patients with atrial fibrillation and no acute underlying medical illness. Acad Emerg Med. 2013;20(3):222-30.
49. National Institute for Health and Care Excellence (NICE). (2014) Atrial fibrillation: management. [online] Available from: http://www.nice.org.uk/guidance/cg180/. [Accessed October, 2017].
50. Ulimoen SR, Enger S, Carlson J, et al. Comparison of four single-drug regimens on ventricular rate and arrhythmia-related symptoms in patients with permanent atrial fibrillation. Am J Cardiol. 2013;111(2):225-30.
51. Ponikowski P, Voors AA, Anker SD, et al. 2016 ESC Guidelines for the diagnosis and treatment of acute and chronic heart failure: The Task Force for the diagnosis and treatment of acute and chronic heart failure of the European Society of Cardiology (ESC) Eur Heart J. 2016;37(27):2129-200
52. Elkayam U. Calcium channel blockers in heart failure. Cardiology. 1998;89(Suppl 1):38-46.
53. Goldstein RE, Boccuzzi SJ, Cruess D, et al. Diltiazem increases late-onset congestive heart failure in postinfarction patients with early reduction in ejection fraction. The Adverse Experience Committee; and the Multicenter Diltiazem Postinfarction Research Group. Circulation. 1991;83(1):52-60.
54. The Digitalis Investigation Group. The effect of digoxin on mortality and morbidity in patients with heart failure. N Engl J Med. 1997;336(8):525-33.
55. Ahmed A, Rich MW, Fleg JL, et al. Effects of digoxin on morbidity and mortality in diastolic heart failure: the ancillary digitalis investigation group trial. Circulation. 2006;114(5):397-403.
56. Gitt AK, Smolka W, Michailov G, et al. Types and outcomes of cardioversion in patients admitted to hospital for atrial fibrillation: results of the German RHYTHM-AF Study. Clin Res Cardiol. 2013;102(10):713-23.
57. Cristoni L, Tampieri A, Mucci F, et al. Cardioversion of acute atrial fibrillation in the short observation unit: comparison of a protocol focused on electrical cardioversion with simple antiarrhythmic treatment. Emerg Med J. 2011;28(11):932-7.
58. Bellone A, Etteri M, Vettorello M, et al. Cardioversion of acute atrial fibrillation in the emergency department: a prospective randomised trial. Emerg Med J. 2012;29(3):188-91.
59. Crijns HJ, Weijs B, Fairley AM, et al. Contemporary real life cardioversion of atrial fibrillation: Results from the multinational RHYTHM-AF study. Int J Cardiol 2014;172(3):588-94.
60. Lip GY, Gitt AK, Le Heuzey JY, et al. Overtreatment and undertreatment with anticoagulation in relation to cardioversion of atrial fibrillation (the RHYTHM-AF study). Am J Cardiol. 2014;113(3):480-4.
61. Reisinger J, Gatterer E, Lang W, et al. Flecainide versus ibutilide for immediate cardioversion of atrial fibrillation of recent onset. Eur Heart J. 2004;25(15):1318-24.
62. Stambler BS, Wood MA, Ellenbogen KA, et al. Efficacy and safety of repeated intravenous doses of ibutilide for rapid conversion of atrial flutter or fibrillation. Ibutilide Repeat Dose Study Investigators. Circulation. 1996;94(7):1613-21.
63. Torp-Pedersen C, Camm AJ, Butterfield NN, et al. Vernakalant: conversion of atrial fibrillation in patients with ischemic heart disease. Int J Cardiol. 2013;166(1):147-51.
64. Savelieva I, Graydon R, Camm AJ. Pharmacological cardioversion of atrial fibrillation with vernakalant: evidence in support of the ESC Guidelines. Europace. 2014;16(2):162-73.
65. Simon A, Niederdoeckl J, Skyllouriotis E, et al. Vernakalant is superior to ibutilide for achieving sinus rhythm in patients with recent-onset atrial fibrillation: a randomized controlled trial at the emergency department. Europace. 2017;19(2):233-40.
66. Reisinger J, Gatterer E, Heinze G, et al. Prospective comparison of flecainide versus sotalol for immediate cardioversion of atrial fibrillation. Am J Cardiol. 1998;81(12):1450-4.
67. Mittal S, Ayati S, Stein KM, et al. Transthoracic cardioversion of atrial fibrillation: comparison of rectilinear biphasic versus damped sine wave monophasic shocks. Circulation. 2000;101(11):1282-7.
68. Kirchhof P, Eckardt L, Loh P, et al. Anterior-posterior versus anterior lateral electrode positions for external cardioversion of atrial fibrillation: a randomised trial. Lancet. 2002;360(9342):1275-9.
69. Kirchhof P, Monnig G, Wasmer K, et al. A trial of self-adhesive patch electrodes and hand-held paddle electrodes for external cardioversion of atrial fibrillation (MOBIPAPA). Eur Heart J. 2005;26(13):1292-7.
70. Airaksinen KE, Gronberg T, Nuotio I, et al. Thromboembolic complications after cardioversion of acute atrial fibrillation: the FinCV (Finnish CardioVersion) study. J Am Coll Cardiol. 2013;62(13):1187-92.
71. Hansen ML, Jepsen RM, Olesen JB, et al. Thromboembolic risk in 16 274 atrial fibrillation patients undergoing direct current cardioversion with and without oral anticoagulant therapy. Europace. 2015;17(1):18-23.
72. Schadlich PK, Schmidt-Lucke C, Huppertz E, et al. Economic evaluation of enoxaparin for anticoagulation in early cardioversion of persisting nonvalvular atrial fibrillation: a statutory health insurance perspective from Germany. Am J Cardiovasc Drugs. 2007;7(3):199-217.
73. Schmidt-Lucke C, Paar WD, Stellbrink C, et al. Quality of anticoagulation with unfractionated heparin plus phenprocoumon for the prevention of thromboembolic complications in cardioversion for non-valvular atrial fibrillation. Subanalysis from the Anticoagulation in Cardioversion using Enoxaparin (ACE) trial. Thromb Res. 2007;119(1):27-34.
74. Stellbrink C, Nixdorff U, Hofmann T, et al. Safety and efficacy of enoxaparin compared with unfractionated heparin and oral anticoagulants for prevention of thromboembolic complications in cardioversion of nonvalvular atrial fibrillation: the Anticoagulation in Cardioversion using Enoxaparin (ACE) trial. Circulation. 2004;109(8):997-1003.
75. Anand K, Mooss AN, Hee TT, et al. Meta-analysis: inhibition of renin-angiotensin system prevents new-onset atrial fibrillation. Am Heart J. 2006;152:217-22.

76. Liakopoulos OJ, Kuhn EW, Slottosch I, et al. Preoperative statin therapy for patients undergoing cardiac surgery. Cochrane Database Syst Rev. 2012;4:Cd008493.
77. Kuhn EW, Liakopoulos OJ, Stange S, et al. Preoperative statin therapy in cardiac surgery: a meta-analysis of 90,000 patients. Eur J Cardiothorac Surg. 2014;45(1):17-26.
78. Zheng Z, Jayaram R, Jiang L, et al. Perioperative Rosuvastatin in Cardiac Surgery. N Engl J Med. 2016;374(18):1744-53.
79. Rahimi K, Emberson J, McGale P, et al. Effect of statins on atrial fibrillation: collaborative meta-analysis of published and unpublished evidence from randomised controlled trials. BMJ. 2011;342:d1250.
80. Pinho-Gomes AC, Reilly S, Brandes RP, et al. Targeting inflammation and oxidative stress in atrial fibrillation: role of 3-hydroxy-3-methylglutaryl-coenzyme a reductase inhibition with statins. Antioxid Redox Signal. 2014;20(8):1268-85.
81. Macchia A, Grancelli H, Varini S, et al. Omega-3 fatty acids for the prevention of recurrent symptomatic atrial fibrillation: results of the FORWARD (Randomized Trial to Assess Efficacy of PUFA for the Maintenance of Sinus Rhythm in Persistent Atrial Fibrillation) trial. J Am Coll Cardiol. 2013;61(4): 463-8.
82. Dabrowski R, Borowiec A, Smolis-Bak E, et al. Effect of combined spironolactone-β-blocker ± enalapril treatment on occurrence of symptomatic atrial fibrillation episodes in patients with a history of paroxysmal atrial fibrillation (SPIR-AF study). Am J Cardiol. 2010;106(11):1609-14.
83. Ito Y, Yamasaki H, Naruse Y, et al. Effect of eplerenone on maintenance of sinus rhythm after catheter ablation in patients with long-standing persistent atrial fibrillation. Am J Cardiol. 2013;111(7):1012-18.

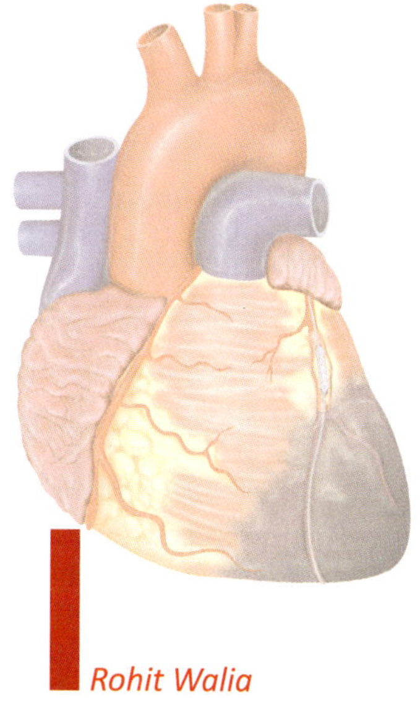

Ventricular Tachycardia in Heart Failure with Cardiodiabetes

Rohit Walia

INTRODUCTION

Diabetes mellitus (DM) is one of the strongest and independent risk factor for cardiovascular morbidity and mortality. DM is almost a synonym for atherosclerosis and coronary artery disease (CAD).[1,2] Not only coronary arteries but also cardiac electrical system is also an important target for diabetic damage. High incidence and extent of atherosclerotic heart disease in diabetics is associated with high incidence of ventricular arrhythmias (VA) and sudden cardiac death (SCD).[1,3]

SCOPE OF PROBLEM

Diabetes and associated ischemic cardiomyopathy are the leading cause of heart failure (HF).[4] Despite remarkable improvements in medical therapy, the prognosis of patients with myocardial failure remains poor, with almost 20% of patients dying within 1 year of initial diagnosis and greater than 80% 8-year mortality. Of the deaths in patients with HF, up to 50% are sudden and unexpected; indeed, patients with HF have 6–9 times the rate of SCD of the general population. Ventricular tachycardia (VT) is common in patients with HF. It is a significant cause of mortality as sustained VT can degenerate into ventricular fibrillation (VF) and cause SCD.[5-8]

PATHOPHYSIOLOGY OF VENTRICULAR ARRHYTHMIA IN DIABETES

Coronary Artery Disease

Acute coronary syndrome remains the most common cause of sudden death in diabetes. Autopsy studies reported findings consistent with acute coronary events including fresh thrombus, recent myocardial infarction or plaque rupture in 57–73% of patients who died suddenly.[9] Apart from CAD, several studies have suggested an electrical instability of diabetic myocardium, which creates a potential substrate for VA independent from the scarred myocardium areas from previous ischemic cardiac damages.[8-12]

Electrical Instability

Ventricular arrhythmia is a multifactorial event, preconditioned by structural abnormalities and modulated by several triggering mechanisms including ischemia, metabolic and hemodynamic alterations, neurohormonal and autonomic factors.[8-20] Noncoronary atherosclerotic processes like autonomic neuropathy, microvascular disease, ventricular structural, and electrical changes may partly play a role in this phenomenon. Diabetes has been associated with ventricular repolarization anomaly which is reflected by marked QTc prolongation.[19-26]

Atypical T wave alternans (TWA) measurements signifying electric instability correlates with significantly elevated hemoglobin A1c (HbA1c) levels. Every 1% rise in HbA1c levels is linked with 13-fold higher risk of having atypical TWA and suboptimal glycemic control is linked with higher risk of spontaneous VA independent of QTc interval duration.[27-29]

Autonomic neuropathy of diabetes results in an unbalanced sympathetic stimulation on myocardium, which may further contribute to this electrical instability and predispose to lethal arrhythmias.[30-36] Cardiac sensory neuropathy of diabetics is an important issue that causes VA and sudden death indirectly via silent ischemia.[37] A study from Chen-Scarabelli et al. investigated if there is a relationship between HbA1c levels and risk of VA in patients with implantable cardioverter defibrillators (ICD) retrospectively. A significant association between HbA1c levels of 8–10% and spontaneous VA incidence in diabetic patients was observed, rather than the diabetic condition and independent from QT prolongation, stating that suboptimal glycemic control and persistent hyperglycemia is related with higher risk of spontaneous VA.[24] The observation that diabetic autonomic neuropathy is associated with a substantial diminution of parasympathetic tone led to the hypothesis that relative predominance of sympathetic activity might predispose patients with diabetes to arrhythmias.[37-39] However, diabetic autonomic neuropathy is associated with both parasympathetic and sympathetic denervation.[40-42] Indeed, evaluation of muscle sympathetic nerve activity,[41] and myocardial m-(123I) iodobenzylguanidine (MIBG) scintigraphy indicate that severe derangements of sympathetic activity and adrenergic cardiac innervation occur concomitantly with parasympathetic dysfunction in diabetic autonomic neuropathy.[29] Therefore, although the protective vagal activity is reduced in patients with diabetes, the absolute sympathetic tone is also substantially diminished. Consequently, the existence and clinical significance of a 'relative' predominance of sympathetic activity in patients with diabetic autonomic neuropathy remains unclear. In fact, the attenuation of sympathetic responses in the setting of HF could be protective with regard to arrhythmias.[32]

Hypoglycemia can trigger ventricular arrhythmia. It is also postulated that hypoglycemia may be triggering VA either with sympathetic overstimulation or QT prolongation.[43,44]

MANAGEMENT

Available options include:

- Antiarrhythmic drugs
- Intracardiac defibrillator
- Radiofrequency ablation.

Antiarrhythmic Drugs

Antiarrhythmic drug (AAD) therapy has been widely used for suppression of VA in patients with HF.[45] These drugs, however, are very poorly tolerated by patients due to their toxic side effects.[46]

Evidence with Amiodarone

Amiodarone is most widely and frequently used. In patients with shock refractory out-of-hospital cardiac arrest and hemodynamically destabilizing ventricular arrhythmia, amiodarone is the most effective drug available to assist in resuscitation. Although the superiority of the transvenous ICD over amiodarone has been well-established in the preventive treatment of patients at high risk of life-threatening VA. Amiodarone combined with beta-blockers is the most effective antiarrhythmic drug to prevent ICD shocks and treat electrical storm.[47-50]

The efficacy of amiodarone in the prevention of SCD had already been well-established in the pre-ICD era. A meta-analysis of all randomized trials showed that amiodarone reduced total mortality by 10–19%.[49] In a pooled database from two similar randomized clinical trials [the European Amiodarone Myocardial Infarction Trial (EMIAT) and the Canadian Amiodarone Myocardial Infarction Trial (CAMIAT)], that evaluated use of amiodarone in primary prevention in patients recovering from myocardial infarction, cardiac death and arrhythmic death or resuscitated cardiac arrest, were significantly lower in patients receiving amiodarone, compared to placebo, if they were also receiving beta-blockers.[47] There appeared to be no benefit of amiodarone over placebo in patients not receiving beta-blockers.[48]

In contrast, the Sudden Cardiac Death in Heart Failure Trial (SCD-HeFT) showed no survival benefit of treatment with amiodarone over placebo in primary prevention in patients with New York Heart Association (NYHA) class II or III congestive heart failure (CHF) and left ventricular ejection fraction (LVEF) less than or equal to 35%, despite a high use of beta-blocker (>70%) in both the placebo and the amiodarone group. The findings were similar for all causes of CHF.[51]

In the Optimal Pharmacological Therapy in Cardioverter Defibrillator Patients (OPTIC) trial, the rate of drug discontinuation at 1 year was 23.5% for patients taking sotalol and 18.2% for those taking amiodarone. Drug toxicity is another concern in patients taking AADs. For example, long-term use of amiodarone is associated with significant pulmonary and thyroid toxicity.[46]

Evidence with Class I Antiarrhythmics

Antiarrhythmic drugs also can increase mortality through a net proarrhythmic effect. Furthermore, they also may interfere with ICD function by altering the defibrillation and pacing thresholds.[52,53] Based on these drawbacks, AADs do not seem to be an effective long-term option and therefore should be used with extreme caution, especially in patients with significant structural heart disease.

Evidence with Beta Blockers

CAPRICORN, MERIT 2, CIBIS-II proved that beta blockers reduced mortality and SCD in HF patients.[54-57]

Intracardiac Defibrillator

Diabetes mellitus patients implanted with a defibrillator have a significantly higher risk for cardiovascular hospitalization or death compared with non-DM patients. Despite the poorer prognosis among DM patients, there was no significant difference in the risk for appropriate or inappropriate ICD therapies compared with non-DM patient.[58-61]

Randomized clinical trials have established the superiority of the transvenous ICD over antiarrhythmic drugs in the preventive treatment of patients at high-risk of life-threatening VA, both in primary and secondary prevention.[59] The ICD has therefore become the treatment of choice for patients at risk of these arrhythmias.

In patients surviving sustained VT or fibrillation the trials of ICD therapy vs amiodarone are consistent with one another and they demonstrate 28% relative reduction in death with the ICD. The ICD prolonged life an average of 4 months during 6 years of follow-up. Assessment of left ventricular ejection fraction appears to stratify those who respond best to the ICD. The ICD is therefore the preferred treatment, especially in those with moderate to severe left ventricular dysfunction.[49]

In the meta-analysis of the ICD secondary prevention trials, patients with LVEF greater than 35% appeared to obtain little or no survival benefit from the ICD compared with amiodarone, whereas those with moderate to severe left ventricular dysfunction obtained a significant benefit from the ICD.[58,59]

Diabetic patients have been found to have increased mortality and morbidity after ICD shock.[60,61] There appears to be no role for amiodarone therapy without concomitant ICD in patients with a stable chronic low LVEF, both in primary and secondary prevention. In secondary prevention, therapy with amiodarone (if used with a beta-blocker) may be a reasonable alternative to ICD in selected patients with LVEF >35%, at least in the short-term. In ICD recipients, amiodarone and ablation therapy may play an important role in the reduction of device therapy.[58-61]

Implantable Cardioverter Defibrillators + Antiarrhythmic Drugs

The Optimal Pharmacological Therapy in Cardioverter Defibrillator Patients (OPTIC) study was a randomized trial that compared amiodarone plus beta-blocker with sotalol alone or beta-blocker alone in 412 patients who had received a dual-chamber ICD for inducible or spontaneous VT or VF and LVEF less than or equal to 40% or syncope. All ICDs were optimally programmed to avoid shocks. During 1 year of follow-up, shocks (appropriate and inappropriate) occurred in 41 patients (38.5%) assigned to beta-blocker alone, in 26 (24.3%) assigned to sotalol alone, and in 12 (10.3%) assigned to amiodarone plus beta-blocker. Amiodarone plus beta-blocker significantly reduced the risk of any shock compared with beta-blocker alone and sotalol. There was a trend for sotalol to reduce shocks compared with beta-blocker alone. The rates of study drug discontinuation at 1 year were 18.2% for amiodarone, 23.5% for sotalol, and 5.3% for beta-blocker alone. The study concluded that despite use of advanced ICD technology and treatment with a beta-blocker, shocks occur commonly in the first year after ICD implant. Amiodarone plus beta-blocker is effective for preventing these shocks and is more effective than sotalol but has an increased risk of drug-related adverse effects.[62]

Killing the Culprit Arrhythmia: Radiofrequency Ablation

It is important to understand that monomorphic VT arises from a focal source or well-defined reentrant circuit which can be eliminated. Also, trigger-induced VA can be eliminated by eliminating the triggers.[58-61,63]

Repeated ICD shocks pose a significant clinical challenge due to pain and hemodynamic deterioration, and they are associated with increased mortality. Furthermore, ICDs do not provide absolute protection against SCD. In one study, the rate of SCD in patients with ICD devices was 5%.[58-61]

It is well-known that a HF patient who receives an appropriate defibrillator shock has a 2- to 5-fold increased mortality rate due to progressive HF.[59-61] Findings from the SCD-HeFT suggest that shock-induced myocardial injury is less likely to be the mechanism of HF, but rather worsening arrhythmia simply reflects progressive HF. Multidisciplinary HF care should be considered an adjunct to catheter ablation procedures for these complex patients to ensure HF medications are optimized, implantable cardiac devices are programmed to avoid right ventricular pacing (noted in 14% of patients in the current study), atrial arrhythmias managed, and assessment for advance HF therapies undertaken at an appropriate time. Such an approach may be necessary to obtain optimal long-term results with VT ablation procedures.[51]

Evidence from Randomized Controlled Trails

- *SMASH-VT* trial enrolled patients with a history of VT or VF, not treated with antiarrhythmic drugs. In that trial, prophylactic substrate-based catheter ablation reduced ICD shocks from 31 to 9% over a mean follow-up of 22.5 ± 5 months ($P = 0.003$), and reduced VT from 33 to 12% ($P = 0.007$). The 30-day mortality rate was zero after ablation. Nearly 50% of the patients were diabetic. The trial delivered an important message that prophylactic VT ablation before defibrillator implantation seemed to prolong time to recurrence of VT in patients with stable VT, previous myocardial infarction, and reduced LVEF. Prophylactic catheter ablation should therefore be considered before implantation of a ICD in such patients.[63]
- *VTACH* trial enrolled patients with a history of stable VT. In both the ablation and control groups, 35% of patients were treated with amiodarone. In this trial, the number of appropriate ICD therapy events per patient and per year was also lower in the ablation group than in the control group ($P = 0.013$). Importantly, no deaths occurred within 30 days after ablation.[64]
- *VANISH* trial also demonstrated the usefulness of catheter ablation. It concluded that in patients with ischemic cardiomyopathy and an ICD who had VT despite antiarrhythmic drug therapy, there was a significantly lower rate of the composite primary outcome of death, VT storm or appropriate ICD shock among patients undergoing catheter ablation than among those receiving an escalation in antiarrhythmic drug therapy.[65]
- *Cooled Radiofrequency (RF) Ablation System* clinical trial enrolled 146 patients who had hemodynamically stable VTs but had failed at least two AAD therapies. The patients were randomized to either radiofrequency catheter ablation (RFCA) or continuation of AADs. Of these patients, 79% either had an ICD at the time of enrolment or had one implanted prior to discharge. The mean number of VT episodes within the preceding 2 months was 25 ± 31. Acute termination of all mappable VTs was achieved in 75% of patients, while 41% of patients had acute termination of all VT types. Clinical success, defined as greater than or equal to 75% reduction of VT frequency at the 2-month follow-up, was observed in 81% of the patients. One or more episodes of VT occurred in 46% of patients, with a median time to first VT episode of 24 days. The Kaplan-Meier recurrence rate of VT was 56% at 1 year. The rate of major complications related to RFCA was 8%, and the mortality rate at 1-year follow-up was 25%. The results of this study demonstrate that catheter ablation of all mappable forms of sustained VT can be performed with high initial success rate.[66]
- *Multicenter Thermocool VT Ablation Trial* was a larger multicenter study with 231 patients. In contrast to the Cooled RF trial, this trial included patients with both mappable and unmappable VTs. Of these patients, 37% had a previous RFA procedure, 70% had failed AAD therapy with amiodarone, and 94% had an ICD at the time of enrolment. A median of 11 VT episodes was recorded in each patient in the preceding 6 months, and 16% of patients had incessant VTs. The primary endpoint of freedom from recurrent incessant VTs at the 6-month follow-up was achieved in 53% of the patients. The median of VT episodes was reduced from 11.5 to 0 at the 6-month follow-up compared to the 6-month period preceding RFCA. While 20% of patients had an increase in their VT episodes, 67% had a greater than or equal to 75% reduction of VT episodes. The procedure mortality rate was 3% and the 1-year rate was 18%. Catheter ablation is a reasonable option to reduce episodes of recurrent VT in patients with prior myocardial infarction, even when multiple and/or unmappable VTs are present.[67]

These trails demonstrated beneficial effect of directly killing the responsible arrhythmia and its triggers and modifying the arrhythmic substrate and the future for ablation therapy looks a lot more promising.

CONCLUSION

Ventricular tachycardia accompanying HF is common with diabetes and requires a multidisciplinary approach. Recent advances and understanding in VT ablation with improved technique and success has potential to be used as first line therapy and also in cases refractory to ICD and antiarrhythmic drugs. Presently, there is lack of dedicated trails of ventricular arrhythmia with HF in cardiodiabetes but the insight from already done trails should also hold true for cardiodiabetes patients with ventricular arrhythmia and HF.

REFERENCES

1. Fox CS, Coady S, Sorlie PD, et al. Trends in cardiovascular complications of diabetes. JAMA. 2004;292(20):2495-9.

2. Cho E, Rimm EB, Stampfer MJ, et al. The impact of diabetes mellitus and prior myocardial infarction on mortality from all causes and from coronary heart disease in men. J Am Coll Cardiol. 2002;40(5):954-60.
3. Balkau B, Jouven X, Ducimetière P, et al. Diabetes as a risk factor for sudden death. Lancet. 1999;354(9194):1968-9.
4. Garcia MJ, McNamara PM, Gordon T, et al. Morbidity and mortality in diabetics in the Framingham population. Sixteen year follow-up study. Diabetes. 1974;23(2):105-11.
5. Curb JD, Rodriguez BL, Burchfiel CM, et al. Sudden death, impaired glucose tolerance, and diabetes in Japanese American men. Circulation. 1995;91(10):2591-5.
6. American Heart Association. Heart Disease and Stroke Statistics—2003 Update. Dallas, Tex: American Heart Association; 2002.
7. Fox CS, Coady S, Sorlie PD, et al. Trends in cardiovascular complications of diabetes. JAMA. 2004;292(20):2495-9.
8. Siscovick DS, Sotoodehnia N, Rea TD, et al. Type 2 diabetes mellitus and the risk of sudden cardiac arrest in the community. Rev Endocr Metab Disord. 2010;11(1):53-9.
9. Lee CD, Folsom AR, Pankow JS, et al. Cardiovascular events in diabetic and nondiabetic adults with or without history of myocardial infarction. Circulation. 2004;109:855-60.
10. Suarez GA, Clark VM, Norell JE, et al. Sudden cardiac death in diabetes mellitus: risk factors in the Rochester diabetic neuropathy study. J Neurol Neurosurg Psychiatry. 2005;76(2):240-5.
11. Junttila MJ, Barthel P, Myerburg RJ, et al. Sudden cardiac death after myocardial infarction in patients with type 2 diabetes. Heart Rhythm. 2010;7(10):1396-403.
12. Jouven X, Lemaître RN, Rea TD, et al. Diabetes, glucose level, and risk of sudden cardiac death. Eur Heart J. 2005;26(20):2142-7.
13. Weston PJ, Gill GV. Is undetected autonomic dysfunction responsible for sudden death in type 1 diabetes mellitus? The 'dead in bed' syndrome revisited. Dibet Med. 1999;16(8):626-31.
14. Page MM, Watkins PJ. Cardiorespiratory arrest and diabetic autonomic neuropathy. Lancet. 1978;1(8054):14-6.
15. O'Brien IA, McFadden JP, Corrall RJ. The influence of autonomic neuropathy on mortality in insulin-dependent diabetes. Q J Med. 1991;79(290):495-502.
16. Ewing DJ, Campbell IW, Clarke BF. Assessment of cardiovascular effects in diabetic autonomic neuropathy and prognostic implications. Ann Intern Med. 1980;92(2 Pt. 2):308-11.
17. McNally PG, Lawrence IG, Panerai RB, et al. Sudden death in type 1 diabetes. Diabetes Obes Metab. 1999;1:151-8.
18. Harris ND, Heller SR. Sudden death in young patients with type 1 diabetes: a consequence of disease, treatment or both? Diabet Med. 1999;16(8):623-5.
19. Montanez A, Ruskin JN, Hebert PR, et al. Prolonged QTc interval and risks of total and cardiovascular mortality and sudden death in the general population: a review and qualitative overview of the prospective cohort studies. Arch Intern Med. 2004;164(9):943-8.
20. Sivieri R, Veglio M, Chinaglia A, et al. Prevalence of QT prolongation in a type 1 diabetic population and its association with autonomic neuropathy. The Neuropathy Study Group of the Italian Society for the Study of Diabetes. Debet Med. 1993;10(10):920-4.
21. Ewing DJ, Boland O, Neilson JM, et al. Autonomic neuropathy, QT interval lengthening, and unexpected deaths in male diabetic patients. Diabetologia. 1991;34(3):182-5.
22. Bellavere F, Ferri M, Guarini L, et al. Prolonged QT period in diabetic autonomic neuropathy: a possible role in sudden cardiac death? Br Heart J. 1988;59(3):379-83.
23. Crow RS, Hannan PJ, Folsom AR. Prognostic significance of corrected QT and corrected JT interval for incident coronary heart disease in a general population sample stratified by presence or absence of wide QRS complex: the ARIC Study with 13 years of follow-up. Circulation. 2003;108(16):1985-9.
24. Chen-Scarabelli C, Scarabelli TM. Suboptimal glycemic control, independently of QT interval duration, is associated with increased risk of ventricular arrhythmias in a high-risk population. Pacing Clin Electrophysiol. 2006;29(1):9-14.
25. Pappachan JM, Sebastian J, Bino BC, et al. Cardiac autonomic neuropathy in diabetes mellitus: prevalence, risk factors and utility of corrected QT interval in the ECG for its diagnosis. Postgrad Med J. 2008;84(990):205-10.
26. Bissinger A, Markuszewski L, Rosiak M. Value and circadian variations of QT dispersion in patients with diabetes mellitus and coronary artery disease. Pol Merkur Lekarski. 2008;24(140):90-4.
27. Molon G, Costa A, Bertolini L, et al. Relationship between abnormal microvolt T-wave alternans and poor glycemic control in type 2 diabetic patients. Pacing Clin Electrophysiol. 2007;30(10):1267-72.
28. Molon G, Costa A, Bertolini L, et al. Relationship between abnormal microvolt T-wave alternans and poor glycemic control in type 2 diabetic patients. Pacing Clin Electrophysiol. 2007;30(10):1267-72.
29. Jouven X, Desnos M, Guerot C, et al. Predicting sudden death in the population. The Paris Prospective Study I. Circulation. 1999;99(15):1978-83.
30. Fox CS, Coady S, Sorlie PD, et al. Trends in cardiovascular complications of diabetes. JAMA. 2004;292(20):2495-9.
31. Wheeler SG, Ahroni JH, Boyko EJ. Prospective study of autonomic neuropathy as a predictor of mortality in patients with diabetes. Diabetes Res Clin Pract. 2002;58(2):131-8.
32. Vinik AI, Ziegler D. Diabetic cardiovascular autonomic neuropathy. Circulation. 2007;115:387-97.
33. Ziegler D, Weise F, Langen KJ, et al. Effect of glycaemic control on myocardial sympathetic innervation assessed by [123I] metaiodobenzylguanidine scintigraphy: a 4-year prospective study in IDDM patients. Diabetologia. 1998;41:443-51.
34. Stevens MJ, Raffel DM, Allman KC, et al. Regression and progression of cardiac sympathetic dysinnervation complicating diabetes: an assessment by C-11 hydroxyephedrine and positron emission tomography. Metabolism. 1999;48(1):92-101.
35. Stevens MJ, Dayanikli F, Raffel DM, et al. Scintigraphic assessment of regionalized defects in myocardial sympathetic innervation and blood flow regulation in diabetic patients with autonomic neuropathy. J Am Coll Cardiol. 1998;31(7):1575-84.
36. Stevens MJ, Raffel DM, Allman KC, et al. Cardiac sympathetic dysinnervation in diabetes: implications for enhanced cardiovascular risk. Circulation 1998;98(10):961-8.
37. Faerman I, Faccio E, Milei J, et al. Autonomic neuropathy and painless myocardial infarction in diabetic patients. Histologic evidence of their relationship. Diabetes. 1977;26(12):1147-58.
38. Bernardi L, Ricordi L, Lazzari P, et al. Impaired circadian modulation of sympathovagal activity in diabetes. A possible explanation for altered temporal onset of cardiovascular disease. Circulation. 1992;86(5):1443-52.
39. Laitinen T, Lyyra-Laitinen T, Huopio H, et al. Electrocardiographic alterations during hyperinsulinemic hypoglycemia in healthy subjects. Ann Noninvasive Electrocardiol. 2008;13(2):97-105.
40. Aronson D, Burger AJ. Diabetes and the occurrence of ventricular arrhythmic events in patients with severe left ventricular dysfunction. Diabetologia. 2002;45(10):1440-5.
41. Israel CW, Lee-Barkey YH. Sudden cardiac death in diabetes mellitus. Herz. 2016;41(3):193-200.
42. Veglio M, Borra M, Stevens LK, et al. The relation between QTc interval prolongation and diabetic complications. The EURODIAB IDDM Complication Study Group. Diabetologia. 1999;42(1):68-75.
43. Stahn A, Pistrosch F, Ganz X, et al. Relationship between hypoglycemic episodes and ventricular arrhythmias in patients with type 2 diabetes and cardiovascular diseases: silent hypoglycemias and silent arrhythmias. Diabetes Care. 2014;37(2):516-20.
44. Pistrosch F, Ganz X, Bornstein SR, et al. Risk of and risk factors for hypoglycemia and associated arrhythmias in patients with type 2 diabetes and cardiovascular disease: a cohort study under real-world conditions. Acta Diabetol. 2015;52(5):889-95.

45. Sim I, McDonald KM, Lavori PW, et al. Quantitative overview of randomized trials of amiodarone to prevent sudden cardiac death. Circulation. 1997;96(9):2823-29.
46. Rakita U, Sobel SM, Mostow N, et al. Amiodarone pulmonary toxicity. Am Heart J. 1983;106(4):906-14.
47. Boutitie F, Boissel JP, Connolly SJ, et al. Amiodarone interaction with beta-blockers: analysis of the merged EMIAT (European Myocardial Infarct Amiodarone Trial) and CAMIAT (Canadian Amiodarone Myocardial Infarction Trial) databases. The EMIAT and CAMIAT Investigators. Circulation. 1999;99(17):2268-75.
48. Connolly SJ, Dorian P, Roberts RS, et al. Comparison of beta-blockers, amiodarone plus beta-blockers, or sotalol for prevention of shocks from implantable cardioverter defibrillators. JAMA. 2006;295(2):165–171.
49. Bokhari F, Newman D, Greene M, et al. Long-term comparison of the implantable cardioverter defibrillator versus amiodarone: eleven-year follow-up of a subset of patients in the Canadian Implantable Defibrillator Study (CIDS). Circulation. 2004;110(2):112-6.
50. Haffajee CI, Love IC, Canada AT, et al. Clinical pharmacokinetics and efficacy of amiodarone for refractory tachyarrhythmias. Circulation. 1983;67(6):1347-55.
51. Bardy GH, Lee KL, Mark DB, Jeanne E, et al. Amiodarone or an implantable cardioverter–defibrillator for congestive heart failure. N Engl J Med. 2005;352(3):225-37.
52. The Cardiac Arrhythmia Suppression Trial II Investigators . Effect of the antiarrhythmic agent moricizine on survival after myocardial infarction. N Engl J Med. 1992;327(4):227-33.
53. Echt DS, Leibson PR, Mitchell LB, et al. Mortality and morbidity in patients receiving encainide, flecainide, or placebo. The Cardiac Arrhythmia Suppression Trial. N Engl J Med. 1991;324(12):781-8.
54. Dargie HJ. Effect of carvedilol on outcome after myocardial infarction in patients with left-ventricular dysfunction: the CAPRICORN randomised trial. The Lancet. 357(9266):1385-90.
55. CIBIS-II Investigators and Committees. The Cardiac Insufficiency Bisoprolol Study II (CIBIS-II): a randomised trial. Lancet. 1999;353(9146):9-13.
56. Tepper D. Frontiers in congestive heart failure: Effect of Metoprolol CR/XL in chronic heart failure: Metoprolol CR/XL Randomised Intervention Trial in Congestive Heart Failure (MERIT-HF). Congest Heart Fail. 1999;5(4):184-5.
57. Connolly SJ, Hallstrom AP, Cappato R, et al. Meta-analysis of the implantable cardioverter defibrillator secondary prevention trial. AVID, CASH and CIDS studies. Antiarrhythmics vs. Implantable Defibrillator study. Cardiac Arrest Study Hamburg. Canadian Implantable Defibrillator Study. Eur Heart J. 2000;21(24):2071-8.
58. Steiner H, Geist M, Goldenberg I, et al. Characteristics and outcomes of diabetic patients with an implantable cardioverter defibrillator in a real world setting: results from the Israeli ICD registry. Cardiovasc Diabetol. 2016;15(1):160.
59. Lee KL, Hafley G, Fisher JD, et al. Effect of implantable defibrillators on arrhythmic events and mortality in the multicenter unsustained tachycardia trial. Circulation. 2002;106(2):233-8.
60. Goldenberg I, Moss AJ, Hall WJ, et al. Causes and consequences of heart failure after prophylactic implantation of a defibrillator in the multicenter automatic defibrillator implantation trial II. Circulation. 2006;113(24):2810-17.
61. Daubert J. Inappropriate implantable cardioverter-defibrillator shocks in MADIT II: frequency, mechanisms, predictors, and survival impact. J Am Coll Cardiol. 2008;51(14):1357-65.
62. Hohnloser SH, Dorian P, Roberts R, et al. Effect of amiodarone and sotalol on ventricular defibrillation threshold: the optimal pharmacological therapy in cardioverter defibrillator patients (OPTIC) trial. Circulation. 2006;114(2):104-9.
63. Reddy VY, Reynolds MR, Neuzil P, et al. Prophylactic catheter ablation for the prevention of defibrillator therapy. N Engl J Med. 2007;357(26):2657-65.
64. Kuck KH, Schaumann A, Eckardt L, et al. Catheter ablation of stable ventricular tachycardia before defibrillator implantation in patients with coronary heart disease (VTACH): a multicentre randomised controlled trial. Lancet. 2010;375(9708):31-40.
65. Sapp JL, Wells GA, Parkash R, et al. Ventricular tachycardia ablation versus escalation of antiarrhythmic drugs. N Engl J Med. 2016;375:111-21.
66. Calkins H, Epstein A, Packer D, et al. Catheter ablation of ventricular tachycardia in patients with structural heart disease using cooled radiofrequency energy: results of a prospective multicenter study. Cooled RF Multi Center Investigators Group. J Am Coll Cardiol. 2000;35(7):1905-14.
67. Stevenson WG, Wilber DJ, Natale A, et al. Irrigated radiofrequency catheter ablation guided by electroanatomic mapping for recurrent ventricular tachycardia after myocardial infarction: the multicenter thermocool ventricular tachycardia ablation trial. Circulation. 2008;118(25):2773-82.

CHAPTER

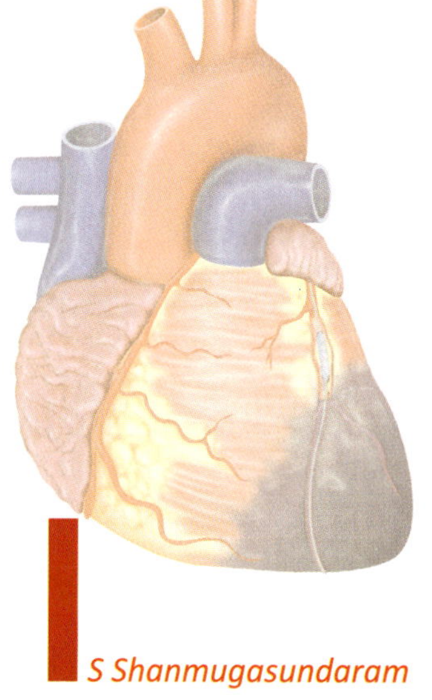

Sudden Cardiac Death in Patients with Diabetes Mellitus: Prevalence, Predictors and Preventive Strategies

S Shanmugasundaram

INTRODUCTION

Truly speaking a satisfactory definition of sudden cardiac death (SCD) does not seem to exist. According to World Health Organization (WHO) criteria, SCD refers to sudden, unexpected, nontraumatic death of cardiac cause, occurring within 1 hour of symptom onset (event witnessed) or within 24 hours of having been seen alive and healthy (unwitnessed).[1] Sudden spontaneous deaths occurring outside the hospital or on arrival to the emergency room (ER) or those who are found dead on arrival to ER are also included in this category. Sudden cardiac arrest (SCA) refers to sudden onset of cardiovascular collapse (witnesses or witnessed) generally due to a very rapid disorganized ventricular rhythm [ventricular tachycardia (VT), ventricular flutter, or ventricular fibrillation (VF)] or electromechanical dissociation (pulseless ventricular rhythm) or rarely due to sudden extreme bradycardia [atrioventricular (AV) block, sinus arrest]. Nearly, 95% of such SCA victims die, if bystander resuscitation and emergency medical services are not promptly available. In communities where bystander initiated resuscitation including automated external defibrillation is well organized, nearly a third survive to reach the hospital. The data derived from emergency medical services suggest that the burden is huge—the rate of out of hospital cardiac arrests per 100,000 patient years ranges from 52.5 in Asia to a maximum of 111.9 Australia, with 86.4 in Europe, and 98.1 in North America. Verbal autopsy conducted in a rural setting in Andhra Pradesh, India revealed that cardiovascular disease (CVD) deaths contributed to 31% of all deaths and 17% experienced sudden nontraumatic deaths—thus half of all CVD deaths are sudden.[2]

CAUSES OF SUDDEN CARDIAC DEATH

Sudden cardiac death is the mode of death in 15–20% of all deaths and 50% of deaths in patients with CVDs [myocardial infarction (MI) both acute and old, heart failure (HF), or left ventricular (LV) dysfunction].[1,3] Roughly in 50%, SCD is the first presentation of heart disease. SCD is mostly due to a serious arrhythmia accounting for 75% of cases. Among the arrhythmic SCDs, 75–80% is due to a shockable rhythm—VT (monomorphic or polymorphic) or VF. In 10–15% of arrhythmic SCDs, bradyarrhythmias namely AV block, sinus bradycardia or asystole seem to be the cause. Pulseless electrical activity (electromechanical dissociation) contributes to roughly 10% and in 5% of cases, the exact arrhythmia is not identifiable.[4] Nonarrhythmic causes of sudden death (25% of all sudden deaths) could be mechanical cardiac causes namely cardiac rupture, cardiac tamponade, acute massive pulmonary embolism, ball valve thrombus, dehiscence or thrombosis of prosthetic valve, etc. or noncardiac causes like massive intracerebral/subarachnoid bleed, midbrain herniation due to increased intracranial pressure, aortic dissection, rupture of aorta or aneurysm, tension pneumothorax, massive visceral bleed, acute respiratory failure, poisoning or severe electrolyte imbalance.

In those with cardiac causes of SCD, the underlying diseases differ according to the age of presentation. In those above 40 years, CAD contributes to 80% (acute MI or scar of previous MI/LV dysfunction or acute ischemia) and the rest caused by dilated cardiomyopathy, myocarditis, aortic stenosis, hypertensive heart diseases, acute psychosocial or economic stress, etc. In those below 40 years, nonatherosclerotic CVD causes like hypertrophic cardiomyopathy (HCM), arrhythmogenic right ventricular cardiomyopathy (ARVC), coronary anomalies, myocarditis, dilated cardiomyopathies, postoperative coronary heart disease (CHD) (TOF), valvular heart diseases like mitral valve prolapse (MVP), AS and channelopathies play a role. Sports related SCD in the general population is most often due to acute coronary event. In professional athletes, HCM is a common cause and other prevalent conditions include ARVC, coronary anomalies, myocarditis, channelopathies, Wolff-Parkinson-White (WPW) syndrome, Marfan syndrome, commotio cordis, heat stroke, etc.

DIABETES AND SUDDEN CARDIAC DEATH

Type 2 diabetes mellitus (T2DM) is an important risk factor for atherosclerotic CVD with a 2- to 3-fold increased risk. Silent myocardial ischemia and MI are also common among patients with T2DM. Seventy-five percent of deaths in patients with T2DM are due to CVDs which include coronary artery disease (CAD) MI and chronic CAD, diabetic cardiomyopathy and hypertensive heart diseases, all of which may lead to left ventricular hypertrophy (LVH), fibrosis, LV remodeling and various degrees of LV dysfunction, and HF (Fig. 1). Diabetes mellitus is associated with two-fold to five-fold increase in risk of HF. For every 1% increase in hemoglobin A1c (HbA1c) there is 8–16% increase in the risk of hospitalization for HF and similarly for every 1 mmol increase in fasting blood glucose levels, there is a 5% increase in the risk of HF admissions. Apart from being a major risk factor for atherosclerotic CAD including MI, diabetes may cause cardiomyopathy as a result of microvessel disease, matrix alterations and metabolic insult to myocardium. Diabetes also predisposes an individual to have higher occurrence of heart failure with preserved ejection fraction (HFpEF), as LVH and diastolic dysfunction are quite prevalent in those with diabetes. Though intensive blood glucose control has not been shown to reduce incident HF, it may help in reducing overall occurrence of cardiovascular events including MI.

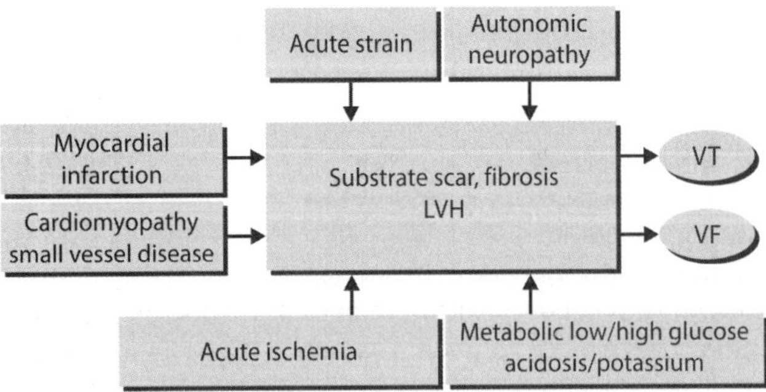

Fig. 1: Proposed mechanisms for sudden cardiac death in diabetics

Abbreviations: VT, ventricular tachycardia; VF, ventricular fibrillation; LVH, left ventricular hypertrophy

Being an important predisposing condition for CAD, acute coronary syndrome (ACS), and HF, it is not surprising to know that DM is an important risk factor for SCD. What remains to be elucidated is whether DM per se contributes to SCD over and above what CAD or HF contributes. The other factors to be considered as causes or triggers are metabolic derangements (hypo or hyperglycemia), cardiac autonomic neuropathy (CAN), acid-base/electrolyte imbalance caused by chronic kidney disease (CKD), obstructive sleep apnea which is common in those with DM/MS, etc.

Chronologically, CAD may develop early in the natural history of DM, even during the prediabetic stage and HF and CAN usually occur in long-standing diabetics. Presumably, the mechanism of SCD may also follow the same pattern—SCD which occurs in the early phase could be caused by CAD and in the later phase by HF and CAN. In a cohort study done in Finland[5] with 10,957 men and women aged 30–59 years enrolled between 1966 and 1972 and followed up till 2007, 52.2% of subjects with normal glucose tolerance, 62.1% of those with impaired glucose tolerance (IGT) and 97.6% of diabetics died. During this follow up, 31.6% of those with normal glucose tolerance, 34.7% of those IGT and 52.4% of diabetics were admitted for CAD. HF admissions for the groups were 14.9%, 16.8%, and 41.5%, respectively. Unadjusted hazard ratio (HR) for SCD was 1.51 for those with IGT and 5.52 for diabetics. HR for nonsudden cardiac death and nonfatal cardiac events was 1.36 and 1.27 for IGT and 8.43 and 6.47 for diabetes. When adjusted for variables like age, sex, body mass index (BMI), systolic blood pressure (SBP), cholesterol, smoking, baseline cardiac disease, HR, QTc, and ECG evidence of CAD, HR for SCD was insignificant for IGT but remained significant (2.40) for DM. QTc and heart rate were insignificantly higher in IGT and diabetics. Thus CAN apparently has not contributed significantly to SCD in this study. In the Paris prospective study,[6] DM carried a hazard ratio of 2.91 for SCD, which got reduced to 1.8 when corrected for other risk factors, but still remaining significant.

In the meta-analysis of 14 studies[7] (10 prospective, 4 case–control) with 346,356 participants and 5,647 SCDs, a relative risk of 2.18 was observed in diabetics when compared to nondiabetics. This risk remained mostly unaltered when confounders like presence of absence of CVD, gender, follow-up duration, number of enrolled patients, and study design were considered. In the Rochester diabetic neuropathy[8] study SCD was encountered in 21 out of 462 patients followed up for 15 years. The identified risk factors were ECG evidence of MI (HR 4.4), bundle branch block (HR 8.6) nephropathy (HR 2.1) and autonomic neuropathy (HR 1.47).

The presence of LV dysfunction and or HF poses a special risk of SCD in diabetics. In a prospective cohort study of ambulant HF patients revealed a higher occurrence of SCD among diabetics—22 SCD occurred among 280 diabetics and 23 SCDs in 811 without diabetes over a follow up period of 960 days. Twenty-four percent of deaths in diabetics were sudden in contrast to 15% of deaths in nondiabetics.[9] In the study performed on 3,276 patients with acute MI, diabetes was present in 19.2%. Incidence of SCD was higher in diabetics (5.9%) than in nondiabetics (1.7%) with a HR of 3.8.[10] In this study, an extraordinarily high-risk has been found to occur in diabetics with LV ejection fraction (LVEF) is less than 35%. Sixteen percent were died suddenly among diabetics with LVEF is less than 35% while only 4.9% of nondiabetics with EF of less than 35%. The incidence of SCD in diabetics with EF is greater than 35% is equal to that of nondiabetics with EF is less than 35% (4.1 vs. 4.9%). Patients with DM and heart failure with reduced ejection fraction (HFrEF) are also not spared from the very high risk. In CHARM study, diabetics with HF, irrespective of EF had higher SCD—40 vs. 25.9 events per 1,000 patient years of follow up.

Intensive blood glucose control has been found to decrease CV risk in some previous studies. In UKPDS, there was significant (25%) reduction of microvascular disease but relative risk (RR) reduction of MI of 16% was insignificant. In ACCORD and VADT trials, intensive glucose control resulted in increased CV death (HR 1.35 and 1.32). This has been attributed to hypoglycemia. Hypoglycemia is believed to cause prolonged QTc, precipitate acute ischemia and worsen electrical instability. Autonomic neuropathy may lead to hypoglycemic unawareness which may worsen the situation.

Autonomic neuropathy is also believed to be an important cause of SCD in diabetics, though the exact role remains to be determined. It may reduce heart rate variability, alter intraventricular conduction and prolong QTc all of which are proarrhythmic. The other possible causes of SCD in diabetics include elevated free fatty acid levels, increased platelet reactivity contributing to coronary thrombosis and distal embolization of microvasculature, insulin resistance, proinflammatory milieu, increased blood levels of oxidants, myocardial steatosis, and so on.[11]

The risk of SCD is increased 20- to 30-fold in hemodialysis patients. CV deaths account for 40% of all deaths in patients with CKD and SCD contributes to 60% of deaths in dialysis patients. LVH, fibrosis associated CAD, acid–base imbalance and electrolyte disturbances may contribute to SCD.

DEAD IN BED SYNDROME

Sudden deaths are known to occur in type 1 DM (T1DM) as well, though rare. The 22–45% of sudden deaths in T1DM, occur in sleep. This type of unexplained death has been termed as dead in bed syndrome. Typically, the patients are in good health when they retire to bed, only to be found dead the next morning. In some instances history of vigorous physical activity has been undertaken by the victims. The bed is often undisturbed indicating that there is no seizure activity. Postmortem studies have been unrevealing in such circumstances.[12] Current evidence suggests a potential role for both hypoglycemia and cardiac autonomic neuropathy. These youngsters are often on multiple doses of insulin with different combinations of short and long acting insulin. Errors in dose or type of insulin could have contributed to hypoglycemic episodes causing unconsciousness progressing to death at nights. It is probable that prolonged QT interval sets the stage for malignant ventricular arrhythmias and QT prolongation in turn may be caused by genetic predisposition, hypoglycemia, and dysautonomia.[13]

PREVENTION OF SUDDEN CARDIAC DEATH IN DIABETICS

Intensive blood glucose control has failed to reduce CV death and actually increased the end point, particularly in elderly individuals with long-standing disease and very high HbA1c on entry. In such individuals the priority is to avoid hypoglycemia and modest glucose control may be accepted. This may help in reducing SCD caused by hypoglycemic episodes. In contrast, in young individuals with recent onset DM and mildly elevated HbA1c, intensive blood glucose control is worthwhile. The drugs of proven CV safety like metformin and newer drugs like liraglutide and gliflozins may be used in preference to others. Though, we have no direct data to document reduction of SCD, total CVD reduction benefit is likely to be reflected in reduction of SCD as well.

Angiotensin converting enzyme inhibitor (ACEI) particularly ramipril should be used in high-risk DM (DM with CVD or DM+1 or more of the following: dyslipidemia, hypertension, smoking) as it has been found to reduce SCD (RR 0.81) in Hope Trial[14] in addition to its beneficial effect in reducing overall death, CV death and HF. Similarly, in PERSPECTIVE trial, a substudy of Europa trial, patients with DM and CAD seem to derive benefit from perindopril in reducing the combined endpoint of CV death, MI and cardiac arrest (RRR 19%). The benefit ACEI in achieving CV protection including reduction of cardiac arrest seems to occur despite minimal effect in BP lowering. Hence, all diabetics with at least one other risk factor should receive ACEI even when there is no LV dysfunction of HF.

Beta-blockers should be used in diabetics with CAD, particularly in those with acute MI and in post MI LV dysfunction/HF. For this indication, metoprolol succinate, bisoprolol, and carvedilol have been proven to reduce overall death (OR 0.65) and SCD.[15] If at all beta-blockers are chosen as additional agents for BP reduction in those with DM and hypertension without CAD or LV dysfunction, carvedilol or nebivolol may be considered.

Statins have potential to reduce SCD in diabetics. In the meta-analysis of 10 randomized controlled trials (RCTs) with 22,275 patients,[16] statin use was found to achieve 19% risk reduction of sudden death (3 vs. 3.8%). In the diabetic subset, the OR of SCD reduction was 0.81. Higher intake and higher levels of omega-3 fatty acid in plasma and red cell membrane are associated with lower risk of SCD. Possibly omega-3 FA supplements may have a role in prevention of SCD.

Aspirin has an established role in secondary prevention, the combined endpoint of nonfatal MI, nonfatal stroke, and CV deaths were reduced by 22%. Despite heightened CV risk in diabetics with CVD, aspirin use resulted in nonsignificant 7% decrease in serious CV events. The role of aspirin in primary prevention is limited or uncertain. In the most recent meta-analysis, combined major CV events were lowered with aspirin therapy with a RR of 0.90.[17] For the other endpoints like overall mortality, CV mortality and sudden death, aspirin was found to have no beneficial outcome. Hence, if at all aspirin is given for primary prevention in diabetics, it has to be done with shared decision making with the well-informed patient. At the most, diabetics with high CV risk as measured by risk prediction models, with no bleeding risk may be prescribed aspirin.

Though dedicated studies assessing the role of optimal medical therapy in diabetics with HF have not been done, all the HFrEF outcome studies have enrolled large numbers of diabetics. Probably the aggressiveness of instituting proven medical therapies—beta-blockers, ACEI, and aldosterone antagonists should be more in those diabetics with HF. ICDs should be offered to those with resuscitated cardiac arrest and documented VT with benefit in mortality reduction being documented in both diabetics and nondiabetics. Those with previous MI of greater than 6 weeks old with LVEF of less than 35% should also receive ICDs (primary prophylaxis) irrespective of the presence of diabetes. Actually analysis of data from MADIT II trial revealed that the HR for risk of death in patients treated with ICD compared with conventional therapy was similar in diabetics (HR 0.61) and nondiabetics (HR 0.71).[18] This benefit was achieved despite the diabetic subset of patients being sicker with advanced functional class, higher percentage with sustained hypertension (SHT), CKD, and higher BMI. Actually diabetic patients are likely to receive less number of inappropriate therapy. In MADIT RIT trial,[19] reprogramming with high rate cut off and delayed therapy, resulted in lesser number of inappropriate shocks both in diabetic and nondiabetic patients. Diabetes mellitus was associated with decreased risk of inappropriate shocks (HR 0.54) and increased risk of appropriate shocks (HR 1.17). The latter is because of vulnerable myocardium resulting from ischemia and scar, altered autonomic function and impaired coronary circulation—both epicardial and microvessels. Lower risk of inappropriate therapy could be due to liberal statin usage, higher prevalence of physical inactivity and autonomic dysfunction resulting in lesser degree of HR variability. Autonomic dysfunction is present in as many as 40% of those with diabetes and may be responsible for a lower maximum heart rate, lower heart rate variability, and reduction of cardiovascular reflexes.

CONCLUSION

Diabetes mellitus increases the vulnerability of an individual to develop SCD. More than the metabolic milieu and autonomic neuropathy, it is the presence of CAD and LV dysfunction that determine the occurrence of CAD. Proven medical therapies which improve the outlook of nondiabetic individuals with CAD and/or LV dysfunction seem to be equally if not more effective in diabetics as well. The threshold for offering ICD has to be low for diabetics with the approved indications. More research is needed to outline the role of dysautonomia and metabolic derangements in causation of SCD in diabetics.

REFERENCES

1. Adabag AS, Luepker RV, Roger VL, et al. Sudden cardiac death: epidemiology and risk factors. Nat Rev Cardiol. 2010;7(4):216-25.
2. Madhavan SR, Reddy S, Panuganti PK, et al. Epidemiology of sudden cardiac death in rural South India - Insights from the Andhra Pradesh rural health initiative. Indian Pacing Electrophysiol J. 2011;11(4):93-102.

3. Hayashi M, Shimizu W, Albert CM. The spectrum of epidemiology underlying sudden cardiac death. Circ Res. 2015;116(12):1887-906.
4. Israel CW. Mechanisms of sudden cardiac death. Indian Heart J. 2014;66(Suppl 1):S10-17.
5. Eranti A, Kerola T, Aro AL, et al. Diabetes, glucose tolerance, and the risk of sudden cardiac death. BMC Cardiovasc Disord. 2016;16:51.
6. Balkau B, Jouven X, Ducimetière P, et al. Diabetes as a risk factor for sudden death. Lancet. 1999:354(9194):1968-9.
7. Zaccardi F, Khan H, Laukkanen JA. Diabetes mellitus and risk of sudden cardiac death: a systematic review and meta-analysis. Int J Cardiol. 2014;177(2):535-7.
8. Suarez GA, Clark VM, Norell JE, et al. Sudden cardiac death in diabetes mellitus: risk factors in the Rochester diabetic neuropathy study. J Neurol Neurosurg Psychiatry. 2005;76(2):240-5.
9. Cubbon RM, Adams B, Rajwani A, et al. Diabetes mellitus is associated with adverse prognosis in chronic heart failure of ischaemic and non-ischaemicaetiology. Diab Vasc Dis Res. 2013;10(4):330-6.
10. Junttila MJ, Barthel P, Myerburg RJ, et al. Sudden cardiac death after myocardial infarction in patients with type 2 diabetes.Heart Rhythm. 2010;7(10):1396-403.
11. Vasiliadis I, Kolovou G, Mavrogeni S. Sudden cardiac death and diabetes mellitus. J Diabet Complic. 2014;28(4):573-79.
12. Tu E, Bagnall RD, Duflou J, et al. Post-mortem pathologic and genetic studies in "dead in bed syndrome" cases in type 1 diabetes mellitus. Human Pathol. 2010;41(3):392-400.
13. Tu E, Twigg SM, Semsarian C. Sudden death in type 1 diabetes: The mystery of the 'dead in bed' syndrome. Int J Cardiol. 2010;138(1):91-3.
14. Teo KK, Mitchell LB, Pogue J, et al. Effect of ramipril in reducing sudden deaths and nonfatal cardiac arrests in high-risk individuals without heart failure or left ventricular dysfunction. Circulation. 2004;110(11):1413-7.
15. Brophy JM, Joseph L, Rouleau J. Beta-blockers in congestive heart failure. A Bayesian meta-analysis. Ann Int Med. 2001;134(7):550-60.
16. Levantesi G, Scarano M, Marfisi R, et al. Meta-analysis of effect of statin treatment on risk of sudden death. Am J Cardiol. 2007;100(11):1644-50.
17. Kunutsor SK, Seidu S, Khunti K. Aspirin for primary prevention of cardiovascular and all-cause mortality events in diabetes: updated meta-analysis of randomized controlled trials. Diabet Med. 2017;34(3):316-27.
18. Wittenberg SM, Cook JR, Hall WJ, et al. Comparison of efficacy of implanted cardioverter-defibrillator in patients with versus without diabetes mellitus. Am J Cardiol. 2005;96(3):417-19.
19. Ruwald MH, Zareba W, Jons C, et al. Influence of diabetes mellitus on inappropriate and appropriate implantable cardioverter-defibrillator therapy and mortality in the Multicenter Automatic Defibrillator Implantation Trial-Reduce Inappropriate Therapy (MADIT-RIT) Trial. Circulation. 2013;128(7):694-701.

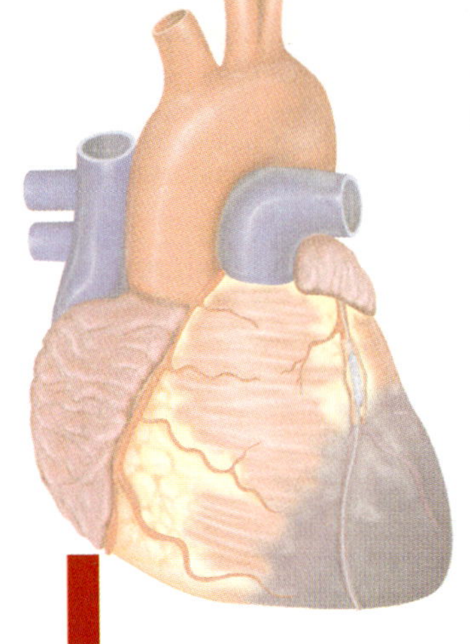

Prevention of Sudden Cardiac Death in Cardiodiabetes

Rabin Chakraborty, Arindam Pande

INTRODUCTION

Sudden cardiac death (SCD) is defined as natural death, in which the time and mode of death is unexpected, in an individual with or without preexisting cardiac diseases, and which occurs within 1 hour of the onset of the heralding symptoms.[1] SCD typically manifests as a structural abnormality coupled with a disturbance in cardiac electrical activity that leads to fatal arrhythmias.[1,2] However, in 5–10% of SCD cases, no definable structural cardiac abnormality exists.[3] Patients may either be asymptomatic or experience symptoms including palpitations, chest pain or discomfort, dyspnea, fatigue, or syncope.[3-5] Sudden cardiac arrest (SCA), in which an electrical malfunction causes the heart to stop abruptly, may occur in these patients; if the heart is not quickly shocked back into rhythm, SCD ensues. At least 90–95% of SCA cases in the community setting end in death before the patient receives any medical assistance.[3,6]

In the United States, the annual number of SCDs is estimated to be between 250,000 and 300,000, with a predominance in males and an increased incidence with age for both genders.[1,3,6,7] SCD is the first cardiac event in approximately 55% of men and 68% of women, while in other cases, SCD follows multiple cardiac events.[2,6] Unfortunately, the prevalence of SCD is difficult to determine since there previously was no unified definition of the condition. In general, SCD is defined as unexpected death occurring within a specific timeframe after initial onset of cardiac symptoms.[8] Depending upon the study being reviewed for SCD, the timeframe between symptom onset and death varies greatly, from less than 1 hour up to 24 hours.

INDIAN CONTEXT

India has faced substantial challenges in employing conventional epidemiological tools to collect mortality data and possibly due to these factors, until recently, there was no contribution to global SCD data from India.[9] In 2004, a study by Gajalakshmi and Peto provided valuable preliminary estimates on SCD using a verbal autopsy methodology, although the primary objective of the study was to assess the classification of deaths using verbal autopsy.[10] The first data of SCD in India was obtained in 2012 by applying the verbal autopsy methodology across Andhra Pradesh.[11] In this study, questionnaires administered by trained health workers were used to collect mortality data in 45 villages. The data was analyzed retrospectively to estimate the prevalence of sudden deaths in this rural population. Analysis of this data revealed that cardiovascular diseases (CVDs) were the leading causes of mortality in rural population. The distribution of causes for SCD in this study was comparable to studies across the globe. However, the proportion of SCD cases in the younger age groups was relatively higher, which was attributed to the higher prevalence of coronary artery disease (CAD) in the young in India.[9]

In India, the levels of coverage of vital registration and the reliability of the cause of death as stated on the death certificate is often low, especially in the rural areas; this has significantly impacted the estimation of SCD incidence. Consequently, surrogate endpoints such as CVD profiles have been extrapolated to estimate the incidence of SCD. In recent years, India has shown an increase in the rates of CAD and a corresponding increase in SCD incidence.

This trend was similar to the increase in prevalence of the major CVDs in the other South Asian countries like China, Thailand, Pakistan, etc.[10] The incidence of SCD is on the rise, especially in the urban regions, which may be largely attributed to the alarming increase in prevalence of CAD, diabetes and hypertension in India.[12]

SUDDEN CARDIAC DEATH AND DIABETES

The most common preventable comorbidities associated with SCD include CAD, myocardial infarction (MI), and heart failure (HF).[1] Since diabetes is a risk factor for these comorbidities, it has been deemed to have an association with SCD. The association between diabetes and SCD may involve a combination of macrovascular and microvascular complications that can affect the electrical system controlling cardiac rhythm, thus increasing the propensity for SCD.[13,14] With the number of diabetes patients growing in epidemic proportions (approximately 29.9 million in the United States), there is an urgent need to determine whether having diabetes increases one's risk for SCD.[15]

Macrovascular Disease

Approximately, 80% of SCD cases have underlying CAD; 90% of cases have arrhythmias which may be caused by CAD.[5,8,16-18] CAD exhibits a direct role in SCD, although the exact mechanism provoking the condition is unclear and may be multifactorial. The study with perhaps the most insight into the relationship between SCD and macrovascular disease is the Framingham Heart Study, in which long-term trends in CAD and SCD were evaluated. A Framingham multivariate risk index combined several CV risk factors (e.g. systolic blood pressure, total cholesterol, and relative weight) with other CAD risk factors [e.g. age, smoking, heart rate (HR), vital capacity, ECG abnormalities] to predict SCD risk.[13] The predicted risk of SCD increased with the addition of each risk factor. However, at 15-year follow-up, the number of SCDs was significantly lower than was predicted through the risk index. Thus, the Framingham risk index may be an acceptable tool overall for risk prediction in the general population, but perhaps less useful for individual risk prediction until more specific predictors of SCD are identified.[3]

Cardiac Autonomic Neuropathy

Chronic hyperglycemia contributes to progressive autonomic neural dysfunction.[19] Patients with cardiac autonomic neuropathy (CAN) typically experience resting tachycardia and less HR variability during exercise.[14] CAN is characterized initially by an early increase of cardiac sympathetic activity which leads to apoptosis and myocardial injury.[15] Patients with diabetes-related CAN have increased mortality compared with patients with nondiabetes-related CAN, and they are more likely to develop arrhythmias, cardiomyopathy, silent ischemia, and subsequent SCD.[13,14,19] Patients would benefit from learning how to recognize less distinct signs of ischemia, such as dyspnea with or without cough, extreme fatigue, and sudden onset of nausea and vomiting. In the Diabetes Control and Complications Trial, intensive glycemic control slowed CAN's development and progression and reduced the progression of atherosclerosis and microvascular disease in patients with type 1 diabetes mellitus (T1DM).[1,13,20] This has not been demonstrated in type 2 diabetes mellitus (T2DM) patients, however. Additionally, SCD was not directly assessed in this trial. Furthermore, it has since been found that glycemic control that is too intensive may increase mortality.[21] Data are inconclusive regarding intensive glycemic control and reduced risk of CAN in patients with T2DM. However, if possible, intensive glycemic control should be recommended in T1DM patients to reduce the risk of CAN.

Silent Ischemia

Silent ischemia is a painless condition in which narrowed or blocked arteries prevent oxygen-rich blood from reaching the heart. Diabetes patients, particularly those with CAN, are at increased risk for developing silent ischemia, which eventually may lead to SCD secondary to arrhythmias.[8,14] However, no studies clearly demonstrate the risk of SCD due to silent ischemia in patients with diabetes.

QT-Interval Prolongation

The Rotterdam Heart Study and the Oregon Sudden Unexpected Death Study provided evidence that prolonged QT intervals heighten the risk of SCD in the general population.[1,4,5,22,23] QT-interval prolongation is common in diabetes, particularly in CAN patients, although the mechanism behind this association is unclear.[8,23] QT-interval prolongation has been indicated as an independent predictor of mortality and has been associated with a suspected increase in risk of SCD in diabetes patients; however, further research is necessary to determine the association between QT prolongation and SCD in patients with diabetes.[8,17]

Heart Failure

Systolic dysfunction—particularly left ventricular ejection fraction (LVEF) below 30% to 35%—increases the risk of

SCD in the general population, but little is known about the effect of diastolic dysfunction on SCD risk.[1,4,8] Patients with less severe HF are more likely to die from SCD, whereas those with more severe HF [i.e. New York Heart Association (NYHA) Class IV] are more likely to die from pump failure.[4,24] However, since the NYHA classification can rapidly fluctuate between Class I and Class IV, this approach only estimates functional consequences, so the usefulness of HF classification as a marker for risk of SCD is minimal. In a posthoc analysis of the Valsartan in Acute Myocardial Infarction Trial, LVEF was a strong predictor of SCD, which increased by 21% with every 5% reduction in ejection fraction.[24,25] Left ventricular systolic dysfunction is established as a strong predictor of SCD.[6,25]

Microvascular Disease

Microvascular disease caused by diabetes may result in autonomic neuropathy, which may lead to QT-interval prolongation. Optimal glycemic control reduces the incidence of microvascular disease, but at the risk of increased hypoglycemic events.[8,20,21,26] Frequent hypoglycemia has been indicated as a potential contributor to SCD.[19]

Hypoglycemia

Intensive glycemic control may reduce the risk of diabetes complications, but it also increases the incidence of hypoglycemia.[8,20,21,26] Even a single hypoglycemic event can impair hormonal and autonomic responses to subsequent events.[8,21] Once hormonal and autonomic responses to hypoglycemia are impaired, hypoglycemia unawareness or asymptomatic hypoglycemia may ensue. This impaired response may induce transient QT prolongation and promote a reduced threshold for arrhythmias, and subsequently, SCD.[8,19]

Prothrombotic State

Based on autopsy reports, thrombus, plaque disruption, or both occur in more than 50% of SCD cases.[18] When stable, atherosclerotic plaques fissure, platelet activation and aggregation occur, resulting in thrombosis.[18] Plaque rupture occurs more often in women, particularly those of advanced age.[18] Distribution of coronary artery lesions does not appear to play a substantial role in SCD development. However, acute thrombosis was observed two to three times more often in smokers than in nonsmokers, likely because of an increase in platelet adhesiveness.[18] SCD was much more likely to occur in current cigarette smokers, underscoring the importance of tobacco cessation. The increased risk of SCD development in diabetes patients through early coronary atherosclerosis and thrombosis appears to be theoretical.[13,14]

GENETIC FACTORS

Family history may be a significant risk factor for SCD, according to the Paris Prospective Study I (PPSI), a 23-year analysis of CV outcomes in 7,746 asymptomatic middle-aged men.[27] In this study, diabetes and parental history of SCD were identified as independent risk factors for SCD.[1,27,28] Multifactorial statistical analyses of PPSI indicated that the relative risk (RR) for development of SCD in offspring was 1.8, if only one parent experienced SCD; however, the RR rose to 9.4 if both parents had a positive family history.[4,17,27,28] Thus, it appears that the risk of SCD is heightened in diabetes patients and in patients with a family history of SCD. Currently, researchers are examining ways to measure genetic susceptibility to SCD, but because of the multifactorial development of SCD, it is likely that no single test will be able to identify at-risk individuals.

RISK PREDICTION

It is understood that most patients with underlying CAD are at greater risk for SCD, and most efforts to stratify SCD risks have focused on patients with known CAD. However, there are no standardized recommendations for predicting risk in patients who have no underlying structural heart disease. Since SCD is multifactorial, prediction of individual risk is more difficult.[3] Researchers have reviewed numerous markers for potential predictors of fatal arrhythmias, including QT dispersion, HR variability, and inflammatory markers, such as C-reactive protein; however, they have not performed well as predictors of SCD.[3] Diabetes, while currently recognized as a clinical risk marker, is not used for risk stratification to predict SCD.[6] Only left ventricular systolic dysfunction is an established clinical risk predictor of SCD, but it is an effective predictor only in patients with a substantial reduction in LVEF.[6]

PREVENTION STRATEGIES

Because of the sudden and unpredictable nature of SCD, risk stratification continues to be an area of interest. The Framingham study revealed a 49% decline in SCD between 1990 and 1999 versus between 1950 and 1969, possibly because of the increased use of preventive agents and/or devices for CV morbidity and mortality.[29] Automated external defibrillators, which became available in the 1970s, may have contributed to the decline in SCD prevalence.[29] Implantable cardioverter defibrillators (ICDs), which were not routinely used until the 1990s, are recommended to prevent SCD in high-risk patients (e.g. prior MI, left ventricular dysfunction).[1,4,13,30] Although the cost-effectiveness of ICDs as a population-based prevention strategy has been questioned, these devices remain a mainstay of SCD prevention.[6] Theoretically, since the vast majority of deaths attributed to SCD involve underlying CAD, controlling the risk factors should indirectly reduce SCD incidence. In fact, many methods of SCD prevention have focused on slowing the progression or development of CV diseases that frequently cause SCD.[6,30] Since patients with diabetes and those who experience SCD share risk factors such as CAD, hypercholesterolemia, and hypertension, controlling the comorbid conditions associated with diabetes should, by default, lessen the risk of SCD in diabetes patients. Pharmacologic agents believed to improve CV longevity include angiotensin-converting enzyme (ACE) inhibitors, beta-blockers, and antiplatelet agents (aspirin).[13,30] Drugs that modulate the renin–angiotensin–aldosterone system, such as ACE inhibitors and angiotensin receptor blockers, are thought to have indirect antiarrhythmic effects and, therefore, may be useful for preventing SCD.[30] Beta blockers—in particular, carvedilol—prevent SCD in CAD and HF.[30] Statins may help reduce SCD incidence by slowing the progression of CV disease; however, few data demonstrate an overall beneficial effect on SCD prevention.[1] Interestingly, Class 1 antiarrhythmics are not recommended for SCD prevention, based on unexpected outcomes of the Cardiac Arrhythmia Suppression Trial (CAST) and CAST II, in which CAD patients using these agents had an increased risk of death.[18,31] Class IV antiarrhythmics have limited use in preventing SCD, but Class III may be considered for this purpose.[31] Nonpharmacologic prevention strategies include weight reduction, dietary education, smoking cessation, stress management, physical activity, and ICDs (in high-risk patients).[1,4,6,13,18,30]

CONCLUSION

It is difficult to ascertain whether diabetes is a direct risk factor for SCD. The notion that diabetes results in enhanced susceptibility to SCD is generally accepted, but is not evidence based. Therefore, although diabetes is recognized as a clinical risk marker for SCD, it is not currently used for risk stratification. If the incidence of SCD is greater in patients with diabetes, the root cause remains unclear. Overall, mortality remains high, most likely owing to the unexpectedness of the event and failure to recognize warning symptoms in a timely manner. Thus, it is critically important to develop prediction and prevention strategies for SCD. The management of SCD in India is conspicuously varied. There is a need for establishing collective measures in estimating the incidence and risk factors of SCD across various regions, using robust methodologies.

REFERENCES

1. Spooner PM. Sudden cardiac death: influence of diabetes. Diabetes Obes Metab. 2008;10(7):523-32.
2. Myerburg RJ, Kessler KM, Castellanos A. Sudden cardiac death: structure, function, and time-dependence of risk. Circulation. 1992;85(Suppl 1):I2-10.
3. Podrid PJ, Myerburg RJ. Epidemiology and stratification of risk for sudden cardiac death. Clin Cardiol. 2005;28(11 Suppl 1):I3-11.
4. Govil AK, Gupta MD, Girish MP, et al. Prediction and prevention in sudden cardiac death. Apollo Med. 2011;8(3):228-37.
5. Chugh SS. Early identification of risk factors for sudden cardiac death. Nat Rev Cardiol. 2010;7(6):318-26.
6. Fishman GI, Chugh SS, DiMarco JP, et al. Sudden cardiac death prediction and prevention: report from a National Heart, Lung, and Blood Institute and Heart Rhythm Society Workshop. Circulation. 2010;122(22):2335-48.
7. Centers for Disease Control and Prevention (CDC). State-specific mortality from sudden cardiac death–United States, 1999. MMWR Morb Mortal Wkly Rep. 2002;51(6):123-26.
8. Bergner DW, Goldberger JJ. Diabetes mellitus and sudden cardiac death: what are the data? Cardiol J. 2010;17(2):117-29.
9. George E, Savitha D, Pais P. Pre-hospital issues in acute myocardial infarction. J Assoc Physicians India. 2001;49:320-3.
10. Lokhandwala Y, Panicker GK, Deshpande S. Sudden cardiac death—an Indian perspective. CVD Prevention and Control. 2009;4(2):103-8.
11. Rao BH, Sastry BK, Chugh SS, et al. Contribution of sudden cardiac death to total mortality in India—a population based study. Int J Cardiol. 2012;154(2):163-7.
12. Honnekeri BS, Lokhandwala D, Panicker GK, et al. Sudden Cardiac Death in India: A Growing Concern. J Assoc Physicians India. 2014;62(12):36-40.
13. El-Atat FA, McFarlane SI, Sowers JR, et al. Sudden cardiac death in patients with diabetes. Curr Diab Rep. 2004;4(3):187-93.
14. El-Menyar AA. Dysrhythmia and electrocardiographic changes in diabetes mellitus: pathophysiology and impact on the incidence of sudden cardiac death. J Cardiovasc Med (Hagerstown). 2006;7(8):580-5.
15. CDC. Number (in millions) of civilian, noninstitutionalized persons with diagnosed diabetes, United States, 1980–2010. [online] Available from www.cdc.gov/diabetes/statistics/prev/national/figpersons.htm. [Accessed October, 2012].
16. Thomas KE, Josephson ME. The role of electrophysiology study in risk stratification of sudden cardiac death. Prog Cardiovasc Dis. 2008;51(2):97-105.
17. Arking DE, Chugh SS, Chakravarti A, et al. Genomics in sudden cardiac death. Circ Res. 2004;94(6):712-23.
18. Zipes DP, Wellens HJ. Sudden cardiac death. Circulation. 1998;98(21):2334-51.
19. Pop-Busui R. Cardiac autonomic neuropathy in diabetes: a clinical perspective. Diabetes Care. 2010;33(2):434-41.
20. The Diabetes Control and Complications Trial Research Group. The effect of intensive treatment of diabetes on the development and progression of long-term complications in insulin-dependent diabetes mellitus. N Engl J Med. 1993;329:977-86.
21. Adler GK, Bonyhay I, Failing H, et al. Antecedent hypoglycemia impairs autonomic cardiovascular function: implications for rigorous glycemic control. Diabetes. 2009;58(2):360-6.

22. Hofman A, Breteler MM, van Duijn CM, et al. The Rotterdam Study: 2010 objectives and design update. Eur J Epidemiol. 2009;24(9):553-72.
23. Chugh SS, Reinier K, Singh T, et al. Determinants of prolonged QT interval and their contribution to sudden death risk in coronary artery disease: the Oregon Sudden Unexpected Death Study. Circulation. 2009;119(5):663-70.
24. Al-Khatib SM, Sanders GD, Bigger JT, et al. Preventing tomorrow's sudden cardiac death today: part I: current data on risk stratification for sudden cardiac death. Am Heart J. 2007;153(6):941-50.
25. Solomon SD, Zelenkofske S, McMurray JJ, et al. Sudden death in patients with myocardial infarction and left ventricular dysfunction, heart failure, or both. N Engl J Med. 2005;352(25):2581-8.
26. UK Prospective Diabetes Study (UKPDS) Group. Intensive blood-glucose control with sulphonylureas or insulin compared with conventional treatment and risk of complications in patients with type 2 diabetes (UKPDS 33). Lancet. 1998;352(913):837-53.
27. Jouven X, Desnos M, Guerot C, et al. Predicting sudden death in the population: the Paris Prospective Study I. Circulation. 1999;99(15):1978-83.
28. Balkau B, Jouven X, Ducimetière P, et al. Diabetes as a risk factor for sudden death. Lancet. 1999;354(9194):1968-9.
29. Fox CS, Evans JC, Larson MG, et al. Temporal trends in coronary heart disease mortality and sudden cardiac death from 1950 to 1999: the Framingham Heart Study. Circulation. 2004;110(5):522-7.
30. Ganz LI. Primary prevention of sudden cardiac death. Curr Cardiol Rep. 2004;6(5):339-47.
31. Das MK, Zipes DP. Antiarrhythmic and nonantiarrhythmic drugs for sudden cardiac death prevention. J Cardiovasc Pharmacol. 2010;55(5):438-49.

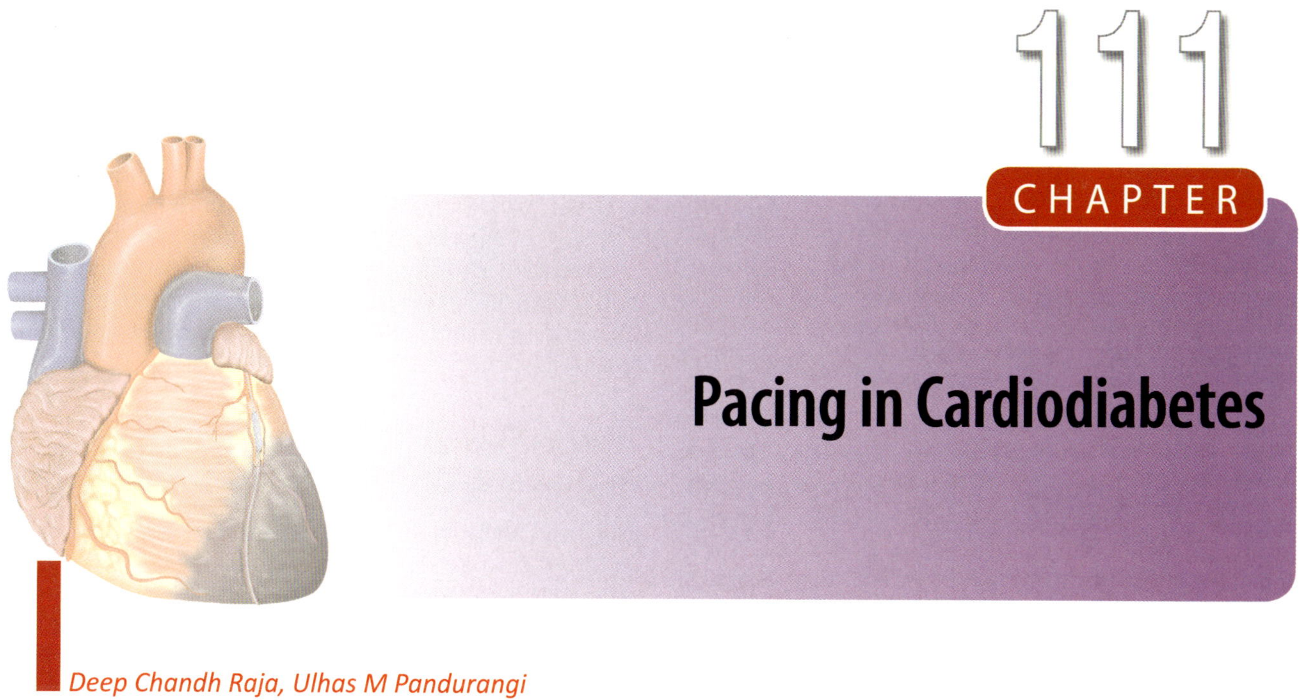

Pacing in Cardiodiabetes

Deep Chandh Raja, Ulhas M Pandurangi

INTRODUCTION

Diabetes mellitus (DM) is one of the most chronic conditions worldwide, with an increasing prevalence of approximately 140 million persons having DM. This number is projected to reach 300 million by the year 2025.[1] Abundant evidence shows that patients with DM are at high-risk for several cardiovascular disorders (CVD) such as coronary heart disease, stroke, peripheral arterial disease, cardiomyopathy, and congestive heart failure (HF). However, the risk of cardiac arrhythmias in DM has been underestimated. These cardiac arrhythmias include bradyarrhythmias ranging from asymptomatic bundle branch blocks (BBB) to symptomatic high degree atrioventricular (HAVB) and complete heart blocks (CHB). Tachyarrhythmias in DM include atrial arrhythmias like atrial fibrillation (AF) and ventricular arrhythmias like ventricular tachycardias (VT). This chapter will elucidate the various mechanisms of arrhythmias in DM followed by discussion of literature showing evidence of CHB and ventricular arrhythmias in DM. The final section will include the treatment aspects for these arrhythmias in DM.

MECHANISMS OF CARDIAC ARRHYTHMIAS IN DIABETES MELLITUS

Cardiovascular Autonomic Neuropathy

Cardiovascular autonomic neuropathy is common among patients with DM and is correlated with an increased five-year mortality rate from CVD.[2] The clinical manifestations of CAN are resting tachycardia, postural hypotension, exercise intolerance, abnormal coronary vasomotor regulation, increased QT interval, and perioperative instability. Collectively, the clinical manifestations of CAN are related to an increased risk of renal disease, stroke, CVD, and sudden death.[3] The development and progression of CAN is likely related to dysregulation of the autonomic nervous system (ANS) with increased sympathetic activity and elevated inflammatory markers. As the ANS is responsible for maintaining the activity of the sinus node, end diastolic volume, end systolic volume and systemic vascular resistance, ANS dysfunction can lead to arterial stiffness, left ventricular (LV) hypertrophy and ventricular diastolic dysfunction. Incidence of CAN increases with age and inadequate glycemic control, which places patients with DM at higher risk of developing both CAN and CVD.[4] Reduced heart rate variability (HRV) has long been associated with increased mortality. In diabetes, a reduction in HRV was associated with increased incidence of inducible ventricular tachyarrhythmias (VT) by programed electrical stimulation.[5] Electrophysiological modeling is likely to be an early event, appearing before structural abnormalities.[6] Comparing abnormal nerve conduction studies with abnormal heart rate beat-to-beat variations and speed of papillary dilatation as a surrogate for autonomic neuropathy. Ziegler et al.[7] found that the incidence of sympathetic peripheral neuropathy was 58% and the incidence of abnormal parasympathetic tests was 35% in patients with DM. Using cardiovascular reflexes, Jermendy et al. found a 44% incidence of definite cardiac autonomic neuropathy and 30% incidence of early signs of autonomic neuropathy in DM patients.[8]

Diabetic Cardiomyopathy

Diabetes mellitus appears to contribute directly to the development of diabetic cardiomyopathy (CMP), rather than solely via coronary atherosclerosis and hypertension. Specifically, diabetics tend to have a greater cardiac mass, particularly LV mass than those without DM. This may be related to an increased adipocyte release of cytokines such as leptin and resistin which have hypertrophic effects on cardiomyocytes.[9] Patients with DM also tend to have a slightly diminished diastolic function.[10] The prevalence of HF, particularly HF and preserved ejection fraction, is higher in diabetic patients (16–31%) than the general population (4–6%).[4] In addition, myocardial fibrosis is increasingly recognized to be a pathogenic factor in diabetic cardiomyopathy.[11] Fibrosis resulting from fibroblast activation is mediated by growth factors such as transforming growth factor-β. This produces conduction abnormalities via two mechanisms: (1) reduced coupling between cardiomyocytes leading to increased axial resistance; (2) increased coupling between fibroblast and cardiomyocyte, increasing membrane capacitance.[11] Both mechanisms lead to a decrease in conduction velocity (CV).

Abnormalities in Conduction

Conduction velocity depends upon sodium channel activation followed by electrotonic spread of the ionic currents via gap junctions, which are electrical coupling pathways located between adjacent cardiomyocytes.[12] Altered gap junction expression or function can produce conduction abnormalities and in turn predisposing to reentrant excitation.[11] There is consistent evidence demonstrating that altered gap junction function or expression in different experimental models of diabetes. Autopsy results of few DM patients with chronic heart block are consistent with direct involvement of DM in the pathogenesis of atrioventricular (AV) block showing conduction system abnormalities typical for DM such as diabetes microangiopathy.[11] Increased incidence and progression of BBB to the high-degree AV block could be one of the explanations for this association. However, the evidence for such a progression is lacking. Ischemia may be a triggering factor of high-degree AV block in DM patients. Autonomic neuropathy and metabolic derangement such as hyperkalemia or acidosis also may explain this association.[6]

QT Prolongation and Dispersion

It has been proposed that autonomic neuropathy in DM could lead to QT interval prolongation and increased mortality rates. Many studies have confirmed the value of QT interval as a predictor of total mortality in both diabetic and non-diabetic patients. Furthermore, several studies have shown a significant correlation between QT interval prolongation and cardiovascular risk factors. Hypoglycemia was not found to increase the risk of QT prolongation. However, the main independent determinant of a prolonged QT dispersion has been ischemia as seen on both ambulatory ST-segment monitoring and Duke treadmill score.[4]

Acute Metabolic Derangements in Diabetes Mellitus

Third and high-degree AV block in DM patients have been reported in case reports during postprandial stress or metabolic derangement such as hyperkalemia or acidosis.[6] High serum potassium levels are thought to impair pulse conduction in Purkinje fibers and ventricles more than that in the AV node. Therefore, although complete AV block can occur, it is a rare initial presentation in patients with DM and underlying chronic kidney disease. However, acute metabolic derangement as a cause of AV block in DM patients should be reversible and does not explain the increased occurrence of chronic AV block in pacemaker patients suggesting another mechanism responsible for this association.

DIABETES AND COMPLETE HEART BLOCKS

Bundle branch blocks are common conduction abnormalities in the population. By analyzing 14,500 electrocardiography (ECGs), Garcia et al.[13] found a high prevalence of bifascicular block (37.5%) in DM patients. Although the prevalence of left bundle branch block (LBBB) was not increased in DM patients, the presence of LBBB in DM signifies advance cardiovascular disease in this population.[6] A higher mortality rate in patients with BBB has been found in the Framingham study.[14] Whether or not the presence of BBB in DM contributes to the increased risk of sudden death in this population requires further investigation.

The prevalence of high-degree AV block in DM patients appears to be significantly higher than that of the normal population. Podlaha et al.[15] studied 258 patients with pacemakers retrospectively. Second- or third-degree AV block was present in 126 (48.8%) of the 258 patients. DM was found in 127 (49.2%) patients. AV block was significantly more prevalent in DM patients (53.9%) and was independent of DM-related risk factors for atherosclerosis. The largest cross-sectional study involving over 800,000 patients was conducted by Movahed et al.[16] DM was found to be independently associated with third-degree AV block in uni- and multivariant analysis with an odds ratio of 3.1 after adjusting for coronary artery disease (CAD), chronic heart failure (CHF), smoking, and hyperlipidemia. However, studies have limitations because of the lack of randomization and the association of bradyarrhythmias with DM needs to be confirmed by a randomized trial. Also, there are no plausible explanations for the increased prevalence of high-degree AV block in DM patients.

In an analysis of 3,115 patients presenting with ST elevation myocardial infarction (STEMI) who underwent primary percutaneous coronary intervention (PCI), high-grade atrioventricular block (HAVB) (second-degree Mobitz II or third-degree atrioventricular block) was present at baseline in 46 patients (1.5%). Diabetes mellitus was one of the independent predictors of HAVB. Mortality rate was significantly higher in patients with versus without HAVB at 1- and 3-year follow-up.[17] The greater risk of AV blocks in diabetics in setting of STEMI could be due to dysautonomic disturbances of the disease or the deleterious effects of hyperglycemia on the conduction system. Most of the elderly patients have many underlying systemic diseases and multiple coronary risk factors. In a paper studying the prevalence of diabetes in elderly patients requiring permanent cardiac pacemaker insertion,[18] there were more number of diabetic population (11.1%). DM conferred an excessive risk of 1.34 ($p < 0.01$) for permanent pacemaker implantation in the elderly. Of the adult individuals with T2DM (2006 patients), age-adjusted chronic kidney disease (CKD) prevalence was 38.3% during 2007–2012. In patients with chronic kidney disease with a pacemaker, higher mortality rates were observed compared with end stage renal disease patients without pacemaker.[19] In 2,778 patients who were on renal replacement therapy (RRT),[20] 110 had a pacemaker implanted. Mortality was higher in the pacemaker group averaging 24.3 deaths per 100 patient-years versus 14.9 deaths per 100 patient-years in the RRT population without pacemaker. This finding is probably related to older age and associated comorbidities.

PACEMAKER THERAPY IN DIABETES MELLITUS

There are no published reports or recommendations for the evaluation of conduction abnormalities in DM patients. The occurrence of high-degree AV block or severe bradycardia in the asymptomatic population is unpredictable, and data for progression of BBB to high-degree AV block in DM patients are lacking. There are no indications for routine 24-hour Holter monitoring of asymptomatic DM patient at this time. The presence of autonomic neuropathy appears to be atleast partially reversible with better glycemic control, which in theory could decrease the risk of arrhythmias in this population.

Treatment with permanent pacemaker insertion for high-grade conduction abnormalities in DM patients should follow the same guidelines as in a non-diabetic population. Reversible cause of BBB and high-degree AV block has been described in case reports of DM patients secondary to electrolytes or metabolic abnormalities or ischemia which needs to be ruled out and treated before considering permanent pacemaker insertion. The most certain indications for permanent pacing include the following—symptomatic bradycardia due to sinus node dysfunction (sick sinus syndrome), symptomatic chronotropic incompetence, second- or third-degree AV block in asymptomatic awake patients in sinus rhythm resulting in periods of asystole longer than 3.0 seconds or ventricular rates less than 40 beats per minute, second- or third-degree AV block in asymptomatic awake patients in AF resulting in pauses of atleast 5 seconds, neurocardiogenic syncope, in the setting of chronic bifascicular block for advanced second-degree AV block or intermittent third-degree AV block or type II second-degree AV block or alternating bundle branch block.[21]

The implant of defibrillators and cardiac resynchronization devices should also follow the same indications as for the normal population. Indications for implantable cardioverter defibrillator (ICD) implant can be divided into two broad categories—secondary prophylaxis against sudden cardiac death (SCD) and primary prophylaxis. An ICD is recommended as therapy in survivors of cardiac arrest due to VF or hemodynamically unstable VT. ICD implantation is appropriate for primary prophylaxis for left ventricular ejection fraction (LVEF) less than 35% and New York Heart Association (NYHA) class I to III symptoms.[22] The SCD Heft trial[23] showed that in patients with NYHA class II or III CHF and LVEF of less than or equal to 35% amiodarone has no favorable effect on survival, whereas single-lead, shock-only ICD therapy reduces overall mortality by 23%. As compared with placebo, amiodarone therapy was associated with a similar risk of death and ICD therapy was associated with a decreased risk of death (hazard ratio, 0.77; 97.5% confidence interval, 0.62–0.96; $P = 0.007$). DM was seen in 32% of the placebo and 31% of the ICD group. The observed benefit of ICD therapy was similar in both DM and non-DM patients.[23] Recent meta-analysis of cardiac resynchronization therapy (CRT) trials have suggested that the benefit of CRT is dependent on QRS duration, with a significant benefit associated with CRT in patients with QRS greater than or equal to 150 ms, but not in patients with QRS less than 150 ms.[23] Clinical response to CRT is also dependent on QRS morphology, with the greatest response for patients with LBBB and QRS greater than or equal to 150 ms.

COMPLICATIONS OF PACEMAKERS IN DIABETES MELLITUS

The most common complication of device implants in the diabetic patients include pocket hematoma (due to concomitant antiplatelet use), lead endocarditis and infection of the pocket (secondary to impaired wound healing and immunity), HF (due to underlying cardiomyopathy). Despite improvements in the design and implantation techniques, infection of the cardiac devices remains a serious problem. A cardiac device infection (CDI) is an important and serious complication of device use. In a study in US with patients with CDI,[24] a total of 189 patients were studied. A 24% of these patients had DM. Generator pocket infection (69%) and device-related endocarditis (23%) were the most common clinical presentations. Coagulase-negative staphylococci and *Staphylococcus aureus*, in 42% and 29% of cases respectively were the leading pathogens for CDI. Most patients (98%) underwent complete device removal. Duration of antibiotic therapy after device removal was based on clinical presentation, causative organism, and comorbidities like renal failure and DM.

CONCLUSION

Cardiac arrhythmias in DM seem to occur at an increased prevalence than in non-DM population, though this finding has not been confirmed with large scale studies. The mechanisms of arrhythmogenesis in DM appear to be secondary to ischemia due to microangiopathy or atherosclerosis in the epicardial vasculature. The underlying substrate of diabetic cardiomyopathy leading to fibrosis and HF also contributes to increased susceptibility to arrhythmias in DM. Cardiac autonomic neuropathy has been investigated in detail to play a significant role in leading to arrhythmias in DM. Treatment guidelines for these arrhythmias remain the same as in non-DM population. However, one has to be aware of the specific complications that one can face while treating these patients with special reference to device infections.

REFERENCES

1. Hart AC, Hopkins CA. Expert for hospitals: international classification of diseases. ninth revision, clinical modification, 6th edition. West Valley City, UT: St. Anthony Publishing; 2001. pp. 29-30.
2. Rolim LC, Sá JRd, Chacra AR, et al. Neuropatia autonômica cardiovascular diabética: fatores de risco, impacto clínico e diagnóstico precoce. Arq Bras Cardiol. 2008;90(4):e24-32.
3. Rolim LC, Sá JR, Chacra AR, et al. Diabetic cardiovascular autonomic neuropathy: risk factors, clinical impact and early diagnosis. Arq Bras Cardiol. 2008;90(4):e24-e31.
4. Leon BM, Maddox TM. Diabetes and cardiovascular disease: Epidemiology, biological mechanisms, treatment recommendations and future research. World J Diabetes. 2015;6(13):1246-58.
5. Koistinen MJ. Prevalence of asymptomatic myocardial ischaemia in diabetic subjects. BMJ. 1990;301(6743):92-5.
6. Movahed MR. Diabetes as a risk factor for cardiac conduction defects: a review. Diabetes Obes Metab. 2007;9(3):276-81.
7. Ziegler D, Cicmir I, Wiefels K, et al. Peripheral and autonomic nerve function in long-term insulin-dependent diabetes. Diabetes Res. 1987;4(1):9-14.
8. Jermendy G, Toth L, Voros P, et al. Correlations between cardiorespiratory reflex impairment and distal neuropathy in diabetics free of clinical symptoms of autonomic neuropathy. Orv Hetil. 1990;131(40):2191-4.
9. Barouch LA, Berkowitz DE, Harrison RW, et al. Disruption of leptin signaling contributes to cardiac hypertrophy independently of body weight in mice. Circulation. 2003;108(6):754-9.
10. Shivalkar B, Dhondt D, Goovaerts I, et al. Flow mediated dilatation and cardiac function in type 1 diabetes mellitus. Am J Cardiol. 2006;97(1):77-82.
11. Tse G, Lai ET, Tse V, et al. Molecular and electrophysiological mechanisms underlying cardiac arrhythmogenesis in diabetes mellitus. J Diabetes Res. 2016;2016:2848759.
12. Tse G, Yeo JM. Conduction abnormalities and ventricular arrhythmogenesis: the roles of sodium channels and gap junctions. Int J Cardiol Heart Vasc. 2015;9:75-82.
13. Garcia Rubi DE, Badui Dergal E. Bifascicular block: long-term follow-up. Report of 40 cases (in Spanish). Arch Inst Cardiol Mex. 1982;52(1):31-8.
14. Schneider JF, Thomas HE Jr, Sorlie P, et al. Comparative features of newly acquired left and right bundle branch block in the general population: the Framingham study. Am J Cardiol. 1981;47(4):931-40.
15. Podlaha R, Falk A. The prevalence of diabetes mellitus and other risk factors of atherosclerosis in bradycardia requiring pacemaker treatment. Horm Metab Res Suppl. 1992;26:84-7.
16. Movahed MR, Hashemzadeh M, Jamal MM. Increased prevalence of third-degree atrioventricular block in patients with type II diabetes mellitus. Chest. 2005;128(4):2611-4.
17. Kosmidou I, Redfors B, Dordi R, et al. Incidence, predictors, and outcomes of high-grade atrioventricular block in patients with ST-segment elevation myocardial infarction undergoing primary percutaneous coronary intervention (from the HORIZONS-AMI trial). Am J Cardiol. 2017;119(9):1295-301.
18. Lear JT, Lawrence IG, Burden AC. Prevalence of diabetes in elderly patients requiring permanent cardiac pacemaker insertion. Acta Diabetol. 1996;33(2):169-70.
19. Bailey RA, Wang Y, Zhu V, et al. Chronic kidney disease in US adults with type 2 diabetes: an updated national estimate of prevalence based on Kidney Disease: improving Global Outcomes (KDIGO) staging. BMC Res Notes. 2014;7:415.
20. Vanerio G, García C, González C, et al. Mortality in patients on renal replacement therapy and permanent cardiac pacemakers. Int J Nephrol. 2014;2014:284172.
21. Brignole M, Auricchio A, Baron-Esquivias G, et al. 2013 ESC guidelines on cardiac pacing and cardiac resynchronization therapy: the task force on cardiac pacing and resynchronization therapy of the European Society of Cardiology (ESC). Developed in collaboration with the European Heart Rhythm Association (EHRA). Europace. 2013;15(8):1070-118.
22. Yancy CW, Jessup M, Bozkurt B, et al. 2013 ACCF/AHA guideline for the management of heart failure: executive summary: a report of the American College of Cardiology Foundation/American Heart Association Task Force on practice guidelines. Circulation. 2013;128(16):e240-327.
23. Steinberg BA, Al-Khatib SM, Edwards R, et al. Outcomes of implantable cardioverter-defibrillator use in patients with comorbidities: results from a combined analysis of 4 randomized clinical trials. JACC Heart Fail. 2014;2(6):623-9.
24. Sohail MR, Uslan DZ, Khan AH, et al. Management and outcome of permanent pacemaker and implantable cardioverter-defibrillator infections. J Am Coll Cardiol. 2007;49(18):1851-9.

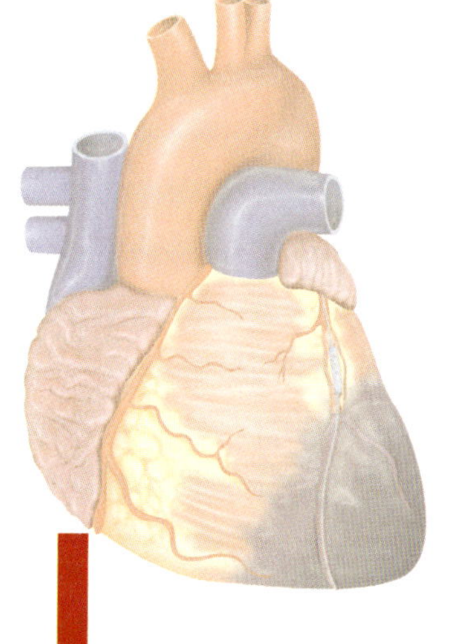

Radiofrequency Ablation in Atrial Fibrillation in Cardiodiabetes

Viveka Kumar, Rajendra Kumar Agarwal

INTRODUCTION

The atrial fibrillation (AF) is a common cardiac rhythm disturbance and increases in prevalence with advancing age. AF is often associated with structural heart disease and other co-occurring chronic conditions. The mechanisms causing and sustaining AF are multifactorial. It can be complex and difficult for clinicians to manage. The role of AF catheter ablation continues to evolve rapidly with improvements in the efficacy and safety of the procedure. Its efficacy for maintaining sinus rhythm is superior to current antiarrhythmic drug therapy (AAD) in selected patient populations. A beneficial effect of radiofrequency catheter ablation (RFA) on quality of life (QoL) has been suggested by several studies,[1,2] but it is unclear whether the effect of RFA on QoL is sustained, because long-term follow-up data have been limited.[3] The evidence supporting the efficacy of catheter ablation is strongest for paroxysmal AF in younger patients with little to no structural heart disease[4] and done at highly experienced centers.

Two randomized controlled trials (RCTs) compared RFA with antiarrhythmic drug therapy as a first-line rhythm control treatment. The *RAAFT* (Radiofrequency Ablation Versus Antiarrhythmic Drug for Atrial Fibrillation Treatment) *II trial* compared the efficacy of AF catheter ablation with that of antiarrhythmic drug therapy as first-line therapy for rhythm control in 127 patients (88% paroxysmal AF) with a higher 1 year freedom from AF (45% versus 28%; $p = 0.02$).[5]

The *MANTRA-PAF* (Medical Antiarrhythmic Treatment or Radiofrequency Ablation in Paroxysmal Atrial Fibrillation) *trial* compared AF catheter ablation with antiarrhythmic drug therapy as first-line therapy in 294 patients.[6] At the 24 month follow-up, more patients in the ablation group were free from any AF or symptomatic AF and quality of life was significantly better.[7] However, total AF burden was not significantly different between the 2 groups and major complications requiring intervention were more common in the ablation group.[8] Meta-analyses have demonstrated the superiority of RFA in maintaining sinus rhythm compared with AAD. A recent meta-analysis[9] indicates that ablation decreases symptoms and improves QoL, but this benefit appears to fade with time. Results on hospitalization rates are heterogeneous with increased risk with RFA when it is used as a first-line AF therapy and decreased risk when it is not used as a first-line therapy. Despite the decrease of AF recurrences and time spent in AF, *RFA perhaps unsurprisingly did not reduce the risk for stroke.* If anything, document edit is that there is an increased stroke risk with RFA which was nevertheless driven by strokes in a single trial. Bleeding and mortality seem unaffected by the procedure compared with AAD (Fig. 1).

On the basis of these data, RFA may be considered as first-line therapy in select patients prior to a trial of antiarrhythmic drug therapy when a rhythm control strategy is desired.Although the outcomes of the invasive management of AF may continue to improve with the use of emerging technologies such as contact-force sensing among others, more definitive evidence on long-term outcomes will be provided by several on-going multicenter RCTs; Catheter Ablation versus Antiarrhythmic Drug

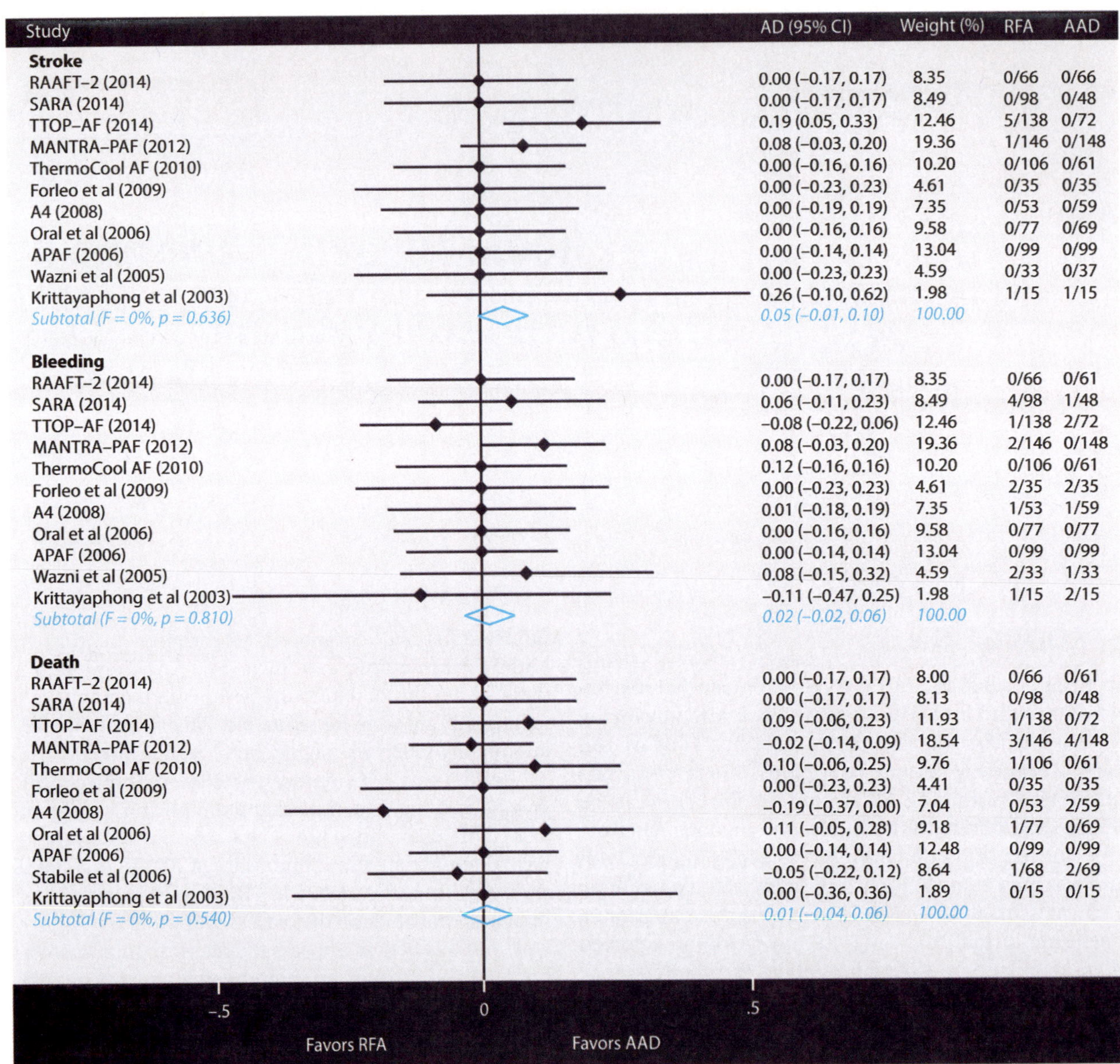

Fig. 1: Summary of arcsine differences (95% confidence intervals) of the effects of radiofrequency ablation and antiarrhythmic drug therapy on stroke, bleeding, and all-cause mortality.

Abbreviations: AAD, antiarrhythmic drug therapy; AD, arcsine difference; CI, confidence interval; RFA, radiofrequency ablation; SMD, standardized mean difference.

Therapy for Atrial Fibrillation (CABANA) trial[10] and Early Treatment of Atrial Fibrillation for Stroke Prevention Trial (EAST)[11] designed to assess the effect of ablation on AF on the clinical end points of stroke, heart failure, hospitalization, and cardiovascular mortality. The new updated guidelines on the role of RFA in the management of AF states, "In patients with recurrent symptomatic paroxysmal AF, RFA is a reasonable initial rhythm-control strategy before therapeutic trials of antiarrhythmic drug therapy, after weighing risks and outcomes of drug and ablation therapy."[12]

CHALLENGES OF ABLATING ATRIAL FIBRILLATION

Catheter ablation reliably and permanently eliminates several types of arrhythmias such as AV nodal reentrant tachycardia (AVNRT) and accessory pathway mediated tachycardias (AVRT). Success rates of more than 95% are attainable when the arrhythmia substrate is well-defined, localized, and temporally stable.[13]

In contrast, the arrhythmia substrate of AF as yet is not well understood, usually is widespread, is variable

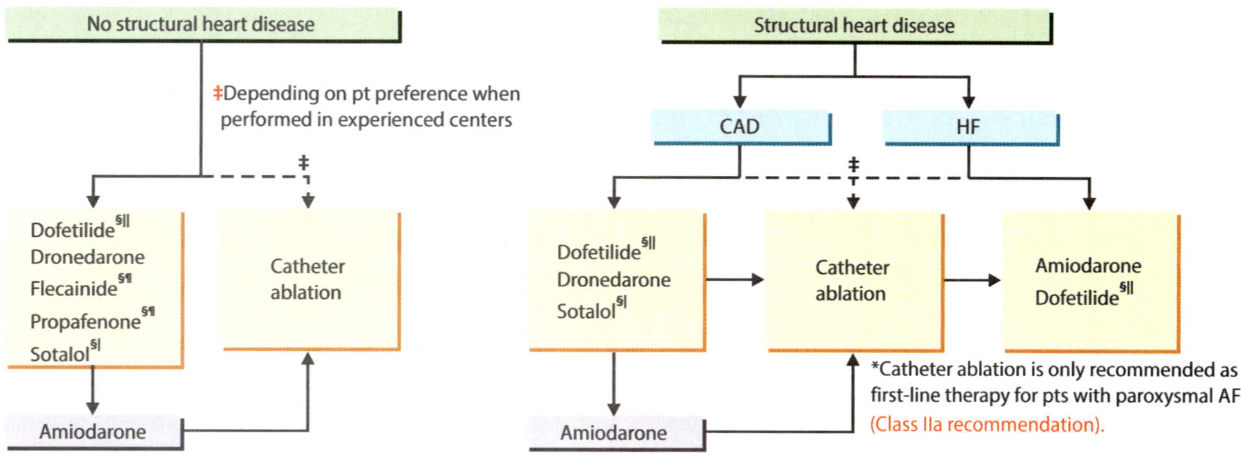

Fig. 2: Strategies for rhythm control in patients with paroxysmal* and persistent AF†.

Abbreviations: AF, atrial fibrillation; CAD, coronary artery disease; HF, heart failure; LVH, left ventricular hypertrophy; pt, patient

between patients and may be progressive.Furthermore, there are several factors that promote AF that cannot be addressed simply by catheter ablation such as hypertension and obstructive sleep apnea, structural remodeling of the atria, inflammatory factors, genetic factors. Therefore, whereas late recurrences of AVNRT or accessory pathway conduction are very rare, AF may recur more than 2 or 3 years after an initially successful ablation procedure.

Patient Selection for Catheter Ablation

Decision whether to pursue catheter ablation depends on a large number of variables including type of AF paroxysmal versus persistent versus longstanding persistent, degree of symptoms, presence of structural heart disease, candidacy for alternative options such as rate control or AAD therapy,likelihood of complications, patient preference. It is important to recognize that most patients enrolled in trials of AF catheter ablation have generally been younger, healthy individuals with symptomatic paroxysmal AF refractory to one or more than one AAD.Safety and efficacy of catheter ablation are less well-established for patients with long-standing persistent AF, very elderly patients,significant heart failure including tachycardia-induced cardiomyopathy. Given the limitations of catheter ablation of AF, it usually is appropriate to treat the patientwith atleast one rhythm-control drug before catheter ablation is considered. This is particularly so if the AF is persistent because the efficacy of catheter ablation is lower for persistent AF than for paroxysmal AF. The most appropriate candidates for catheter ablation have symptomatic AF that is affecting quality of life has not adequately responded to drug therapy. The ideal candidate has lone AF or only minimal structural heart disease. The recommendation for catheter ablation should be influenced by the estimated probability of success, the procedure is least likely to be successful if the left atrium (LA) is markedly dilated and AF has been persistent for more than 4 years.

The strategies for rhythm control in paroxysmal and persistent AF in the new updated guidelines on the role of RFA in the management of AF is summarized in Figure 2.

CONCLUSION

Radiofrequency catheter ablation may be considered as first-line therapy in selected patients prior to a trial of antiarrhythmic drug therapy when a rhythm control strategy is desired. RFA demonstrates an early but nonsustained superiority over antiarrhythmic drug for the improvement of QoL. There are no obvious differences in other clinical outcomes, and the periprocedural stroke risk is non-negligible. However, more data are needed to provide additional insights on the value of catheter ablation for the therapy of AF.

REFERENCES

1. Jais P, Cauchemez B, Daoud E, et al. Catheter ablation versus antiarrhythmic drugs for atrial fibrillation: the A4 study. Circulation. 2008;118(24):2498-505.
2. Wokhlu A, Monahan KH, Hodge DO, et al. Long-term quality of life after ablation of atrial fibrillation the impact of recurrence, symptom relief, and placebo effect. J Am Coll Cardiol. 2010;55(21):2308-16.

3. Pappone C, Vicedomini G, A, et al. Radiofrequency catheter ablation and antiarrhythmic drug therapy: a prospective, randomized 4-year follow-up trial: the APAF study. Circ Arrhythm Electrophysiol. 2011;4:808-14.
4. Leong-Sit P, Zado E, Callans DJ, et al. Efficacy and risk of atrial fibrillation ablation before 45 years of age. Circ Arrhythm Electrophysiol. 2010;3:452-7.
5. Morillo C, Verma A, Connolly SJ, et al. Radiofrequency ablation vs antiarrhythmic drugs as first-line treatment of paroxysmal atrial fibrillation: (RAAFT 2): a randomized trial. JAMA. 2014;311(7):692-700.
6. Jons C, Hansen PS, Johannessen A, et al. The medical antiarrhythmic treatment or radiofrequency ablation in paroxysmal atrial fibrillation (MANTRA-PAF) trial: clinical rationale, study design, and implementation. Europace. 2009;11(7):917-23.
7. Cosedis NJ, Johannessen A, Raatikainen P, et al. Radiofrequency ablation as initial therapy in paroxysmal atrial fibrillation. N Engl J Med. 2012;367(17):1587-95.
8. Khan AR, Khan S, Sheikh MA, et al.Catheter ablation and antiarrhythmic drug therapy as first- or secondline therapy in the management of atrial fibrillation: systematic review and meta-analysis. Circ Arrhythm Electrophysiol. 2014;7:853-60.
9. Siontis KC, Loannidis JPA, Katritsis GD, et al. Radiofrequency ablation versus antiarrhythmic drug therapy for atrial fibrillation: Meta-analysis of quality of life, morbidity, and mortality. JACCCEP. 2016;2(2):170-80.
10. Clinical Trials. Catheter ablation vs anti-arrhythmic drug therapy for atrial fibrillation trial (CABANA). [online] Available from http://clinicaltrials.Gov/ct2/show/ nct00911508. [Accessed October, 2017].
11. Clinical Trials. Early treatment of atrial fibrillation for stroke prevention trial (EAST). [online] Available from http://clinicaltrials.gov/show/NCT01288352. [Accessed October, 2017].
12. January CT, Wann LS, Alpert JS, et al. 2014 AHA/ACC/HRS Guideline for the management of patients with atrial fibrillation: executive summary: a report of the American College of Cardiology/American Heart Association Task Force on Practice Guidelines and the Heart Rhythm Society. JACC. 2014:(14)01739-2.
13. Tracy CM, Epstein AE, Darbar D, et al. 2012 ACCF/AHA/HRS Focused Update Incorporated Into the ACCF/AHA/HRS 2008 Guidelines for device-based therapy of cardiac rhythm abnormalities: a report of the American College of Cardiology Foundation/American Heart Association Task Force on Practice Guidelines and the Heart Rhythm Society. J Am Coll Cardiol. 2013;61:e6-e75.

113

CHAPTER

LA Appendage Closure for AF in Cardiodiabetes: Is the Outcome Different?

Balbir Singh

INTRODUCTION

Atrial fibrillation (AF) is the most common cardiac rhythm disorder seen in clinical practice, affecting 3–5% of the population aged 65–75 years, and increasing to greater than 8% of those older than 80 years in the Western literature. It is associated with substantial mortality and morbidity, particularly due to fatal or disabling stroke. AF is associated with five times higher stroke rates as compared to those without AF.[1] For prevention of this complication, traditional treatment strategies have relied on chronic anticoagulation, either with warfarin or with the newer anticoagulant agents. This anticoagulant therapy has been proven to effectively prevent thromboembolic strokes, but the increased risk of serious bleeding prevents many patients from taking this therapy. Therefore, there is always a need for alternative therapies with lower bleeding risk.[2] Percutaneous left atrial appendage (LAA) occlusion is an evolving therapy, which should be taken into consideration in those patients with AF with a high stroke risk and contraindications for oral anticoagulant (OAC). This chapter aims at discussing the scope for LAA closure, the available LAA occlusion devices and their clinical evidence until now.

EXISTING OPTIONS OF STROKE PREVENTION IN ATRIAL FIBRILLATION

Several randomized controlled trials (RCTs) have demonstrated beyond doubt the efficacy of OACs in preventing strokes and reducing mortality, these trials have also shown that antiplatelets are not useful for this purpose. However, OACs are associated with increased bleeding to the tune of 2–4% per year which is substantial and also with some life-threatening bleeds like intracranial hemorrhage (ICH). There has been a hope that the advent of new oral anticoagulants (NOACs) such as dabigatran, apixaban or rivaroxaban would overcome these disadvantages; however, these drugs still face issues of major bleeding and noncompliance.[3] Table 1 depicts the incidence of bleeds and compliance with these drugs.

RATIONALE FOR LEFT ATRIAL APPENDAGE OCCLUSION

The rationale behind LAA occlusion is that the LAA is the primary site of thrombus formation in patients with nonvalvular AF (NVAF) as has been demonstrated on postmortem studies and transesophageal data. Sixty percent of atrial thrombi in valvular AF were found in the LAA, whereas in NVAF greater than 90% of thrombi were located in the LAA.[4] In view of these data it appears LAA closure will provide protection against thromboembolic episodes in patients with NVAF. Consequently, the European Society of Cardiology (ESC) guidelines for the management of AF (2012) recommend that LAA closure may be considered in patients with a high stroke risk and contraindications for long-term OAC administration (Class: IIb, level of evidence B).

However, one must remember that many patients with NVAF have several comorbidities and could have atheromatous changes in aorta or carotids which could lead to stroke mitigating the benefit of LAA closure.

TABLE 1: The bleeds incidence and drugs compliance

	Warfarin (Protect AF)	*Dabigatran (Rely)*	*Apixaban (Aristotle)*	*Rivaroxaban (Rocket AF)*
Age	71.7	71.5	70	70
Major/minor bleed		16.4	18.1	14.9
Major bleed (%)	4.1	3.1	2.1	3.6
Stroke (%)	2.7	1.1	1.3	1.7
Drug discontinuation	16–34	21		24

Abbreviation: AF, atrial fibrillation

Identifying the Right Patient for Device Closure

Left atrial appendage closure offers an alternative to patients of NVAF who are at risk of thromboembolism and are also at high-risk for bleeds or contraindications to OACs. The patient who could be considered as high-risk for bleeding are: (1) coagulopathies—low platelet counts, or other disorders; (2) severe hepatic or renal dysfunction; (3) known vascular malformations in intestine, brain or retina which could potentially bleed. Other group of patients apart from those with high bleeding risk are:

- Those who develop ischemic stroke despite well-controlled OAC or NOAC therapy
- High probability of therapeutic noncompliance to OAC or NOACs
- Intolerance or contraindications to OAC or NOACs.

Suitability for Left Atrial Appendage Device Closure

Transesophageal echocardiography (TEE) helps to identify the anatomy of LAA and is essential preprocedure and also during the procedure; preprocedural TEE is used to screen suitable candidates and to define LAA morphology and dimensions and exclude LAA thrombus,[2] periprocedural TEE has a major role in guiding delivery and deployment of the device and for assessing procedural complications. Important aspects to assess are the shape and size of the ostium, the width of the 'landing zone' [i.e. area within the LAA where the device will be positioned (Figs 1A to C)].

Device Implantation

Percutaneous LAA occlusion is usually performed under general anesthesia and with TEE and fluoroscopic guidance. Vascular access through a femoral vein is obtained and the delivery system is introduced by transseptal puncture using

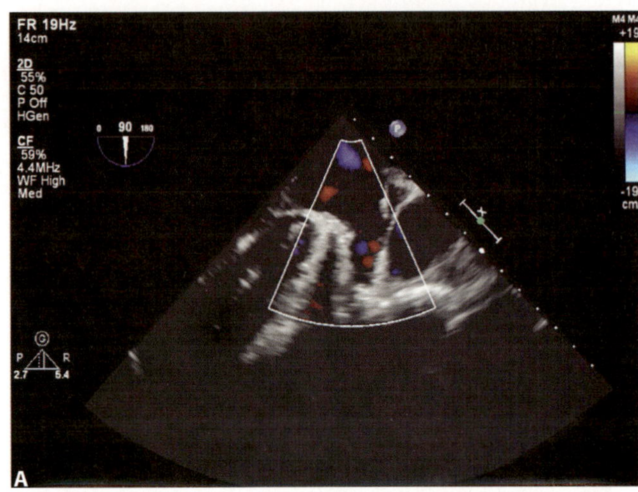

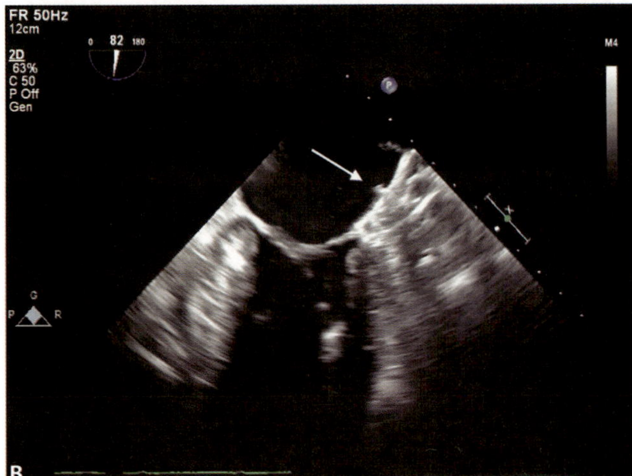

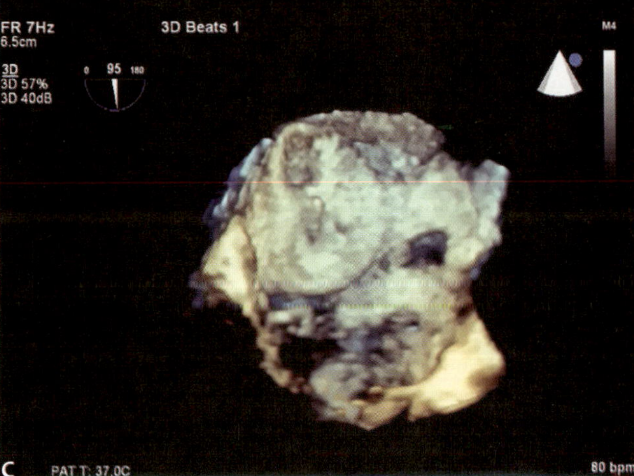

Figs 1A to C: Transesophageal images during the procedure in a patient showing the left atrial appendage (LAA) clearly and dimensions are made from the neck and also help to calculate the length of LAA. 3D image is also seen

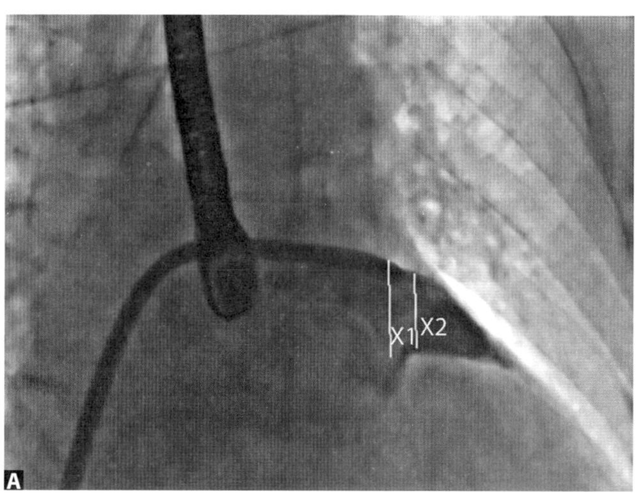

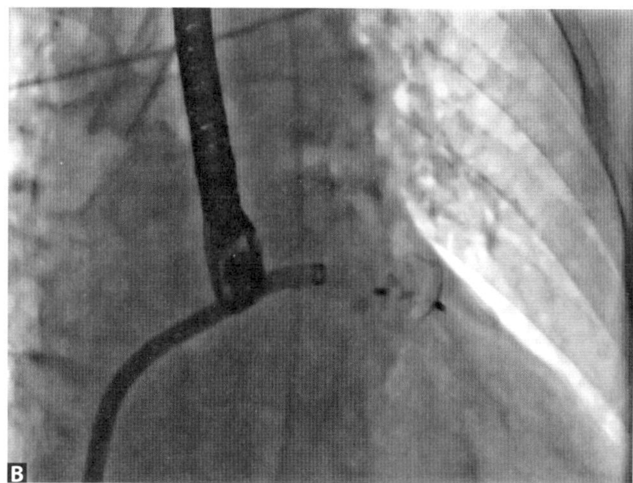

Figs 2A and B: The fluoroscopy images showing the deployment of the device

a standard transseptal puncture techniques. The device is deployed by withdrawing the sheath over the device. Once in position, the device stability is confirmed by a fluoroscopy and TEE imaging. Finally, the device is released from the delivery cable [these are steps for AMPLATZER™ cardiac plug (ACP), St Jude Medical (Figs 2A and B). Until now, the WATCHMAN and ACP device have been most widely used in clinical practice and WATCHMAN device is now US Food and Drug Administration (FDA) approved, in our country only ACP device is available.

POSTPROCEDURAL TREATMENT

Dual antiplatelet therapy (DAPT) (aspirin and clopidogrel) is prescribed for the first 45 days after LAA closure and clopidogrel can then be stopped. After 6 months, ASA treatment may or may not be stopped completely if no other indication for antiplatelet therapy exists. In patients with a very high bleeding risk, it may be considered to give only one antiplatelet drug from right after the procedure. Low dose (NOAC) may be needed if the device indication was recurrent strokes despite (NOACs).

CLINICAL TRIAL RESULTS[4-8]

The only prospective, randomized trial so far published is the PROTECT AF trial in which 707 patients with NVAF were randomly assigned in a 2:1 ratio to either percutaneous LAA occlusion with the WATCHMAN device or to warfarin therapy. The study was designed to assess the noninferiority of the device against chronic OAC therapy. Patients with paroxysmal, persistent or permanent NVAF enrolled if they had a $CHADS_2$ risk score greater than or equal to 1. The trial demonstrated the noninferiority of WATCHMAN LAA occlusion compared with OAC therapy regarding the primary efficacy endpoint—a composite of stroke, systemic embolism, and cardiovascular death (RR = 0.62, 95% CI 0.35–1.25). The probability of noninferiority of the intervention was greater than 99.9%. 4-year follow-up results from the PROTECT AF trial have also been published. The primary efficacy endpoint occurred in 2.3% of the device group versus 3.8% of the warfarin group (RR = 0.60, 95% CI 0.41–1.05), demonstrating a 40% relative risk reduction in primary efficacy in the WATCHMAN group. Cardiovascular death occurred in 1.0% of the device group versus 2.4% of the warfarin group (RR = 0.40, 95% CI 0.21–0.72, $p < 0.05$). The rate of hemorrhagic stroke was 0.2% in the device group versus 1% in the warfarin group (RR = 0.18, 95% CI 0.04–0.60, $p < 0.05$) demonstrating the continued efficacy of the device in long-term follow-up.

More recent data, from the CAP registry (n = 566, WATCHMAN), the PREVAIL study (n = 269, WATCHMAN), and a large multicenter study involving the ACP device (n = 969) show improved procedural safety—complication rates within 7 days were 4.1%, 4.4% and 4.1%, respectively, as compared with greater than 7% in the initial PROTECT AF trial (2009) which had led to initial refusal of FDA to approve the device. These lower rates of complications are due to better operator experience and understanding of device implantation. The PREVAIL study added information to the initial pivotal PROTECT AF trial by using a Bayesian noninferiority design approach. The major findings of this trial were: (1) LAA occlusion with the WATCHMAN device was not noninferior to warfarin for the primary efficacy composite endpoint of all-cause stroke, cardiovascular or unexplained death, and SE, although the event rates with warfarin were significantly lower than expected, affecting the ability of the study to establish non-inferiority; (2) the WATCHMAN device was noninferior to warfarin for the occurrence of late ischemic events such as ischemic stroke or SE occurring after the first 7 days following randomization to isolate the effect of early periprocedural events from a longer term mechanism of action; and (3) the WATCHMAN procedure met the prespecified success criterion for safety events, even with a large proportion of operators without previous experience of implanting the device within a higher risk patient population.

DISCUSSION

Since the first percutaneous LAA closure in 2002, a rapidly growing number of studies have shown that this strategy can be a safe and efficacious therapy in the management of patients with NVAF for whom OAC is indicated but who are at a high-risk of bleeding (Box 1). This has led to FDA approval of WATCHMAN device. Although the only RCTs available until now (PROTECT AF, PREVAIL) included only patients who were eligible for OAC therapy, the current guidelines only justify the use of this in patients with contraindications to OAC therapy. In future studies, it will be important to identify patients who may benefit the most from percutaneous LAA closure apart from those with contraindications to (NOACs).

BOX 1: Potential indications of left atrial appendage (LAA) closure

- Those intolerant to oral anticoagulants (OACs)
- Those who develop a serious bleed with OACs
- Those with contraindications to OACs such underlying coagulopathies
- Those who develop stroke or systemic embolism despite controlled anticoagulation
- Those who are not compliant on drugs

CONCLUSION

Percutaneous LAA occlusion has been shown to be a safe, efficacious, and cost-effective strategy for stroke prevention in patients with NVAF with increased stroke and bleeding risk. It is now a commonly performed procedure in many centers in Europe and US, in our experience success was obtained in all eight patients where it was attempted, however, operator experience and technique is of paramount importance.

REFERENCES

1. Wolf PA, Abbott RD, Kannel WB. Atrial fibrillation as an independent risk factor for stroke: the Framingham Study. Stroke. 1991;22(8):983-8.
2. Camm AJ, Lip GY, De Caterina R, et al. 2012 focused update of the ESC Guidelines for the management of atrial fibrillation: an update of the 2010 ESC Guidelines for the management of atrial fibrillation--developed with the special contribution of the European Heart Rhythm Association. Europace. 2012;14(10):1385-413.
3. Holmes DR, Reddy VY, Turi ZG, et al. Percutaneous closure of the left atrial appendage versus warfarin therapy for prevention of stroke in patients with atrial fibrillation: a randomised non-inferiority trial. Lancet. 2009;374(9689):534-42.
4. Reddy VY, Möbius-Winkler S, Miller MA, et al. Left atrial appendage closure with the Watchman device in patients with a contraindication for oral anticoagulation: the ASAP study (ASA Plavix Feasibility Study with Watchman Left Atrial Appendage Closure Technology). J Am Coll Cardiol. 2013;61(25):2551-6.
5. Plicht B, Konorza TF, Kahlert P, et al. Risk factors for thrombus formation on the Amplatzer Cardiac Plug after left atrial appendage occlusion. JACC Cardiovasc Interv. 2013;6(6):606-13.
6. Reddy VY, Holmes D, Doshi SK, et al. Safety of percutaneous left atrial appendage closure: results from the Watchman Left Atrial Appendage System for Embolic Protection in Patients with AF (PROTECT AF) clinical trial and the Continued Access Registry. Circulation. 2011;123(4):417-24.
7. Holmes D. Preliminary results of the randomized trial of LAA closure vs. warfarin for stroke/thromboembolic prevention in patients with non-valvular atrial fibrillation (PREVAIL)—late breaking clinical trial. San Francisco: American College of Cardiology (ACC) 2013 Scientific Sessions; 2013.
8. Reddy V. Long term results of PROTECT AF: the mortality effects of left atrial appendage closure versus warfarin for stroke prophylaxis in AF—late breaking clinical trial. Denver: Heart Rhythm Society (HRS) 2013 Scientific Sessions; 2013.

114

CHAPTER

AICD after Cardiac Arrest in Cardiodiabetes

Rajeeve Kumar Rajput

INTRODUCTION

Sudden cardiac death (SCD) is a major health problem because it is very common, occurs suddenly and unexpectedly, and is often fatal. Epidemiology of SCD is also very uncertain because it is often unwitnessed, cause is difficult to assess, initial rhythm is often unknown, time since onset can not be certain, and usually the account is based on statement of bystander or rarely on records of emergency medical staff.[1] SCD accounts for nearly half of cardiovascular deaths, occurs in most productive years of life and surprisingly the proportion of SCD in total cardiovascular mortality has not changed over few decades. SCD is defined as irreversible cessation of all biologic function within *1 hour* of onset of acute changes in cardiovascular status. Pre-existing cardiac disease may be known to patient, but the key features of SCD are natural, rapid, and unexpected death. Cardiac arrest is defined as abrupt cessation of cardiac mechanical function which may be reversible with prompt intervention, but will lead to death in its absence.

The incidence of SCD is very difficult to assess due to many reasons, but based on analysis of medical records and epidemiological studies, nearly 350,000 SCDs occur annually in United States alone which corresponds to 1–2 deaths per 1,000 in general population.[2] There is no reliable population based data reincidence of SCD in India. Temporal definition used for SCD strongly influences the epidemiologic data with 2 hours cutoff between onset of symptoms and death nearly 12–14% of all natural deaths are sudden and 90% of these sudden have cardiac cause.[3]

Although, incidence is low at 1–2 per 1,000, most of SCD occurs in general population and fewer SCDs occur in high-risk populations identified by history of prior coronary event, low ejection fraction (EF) less than 30%, cardiac arrest survivors, post-myocardial infarction (MI), or with markers of specific arrhythmias. If we take all SCDs in coronary artery disease (CAD), in 50% cases it is the first manifestation of underlying cardiac disease, 33% have known disease without high feature of SCD or have nonspecific markers, less than 25% have acute coronary syndrome, only 10% have hemodynamic risk markers and only 5–10% have arrhythmia risk markers. This highlights the need of population based measures to have greater impact in reducing SCDs.[4]

Sudden cardiac deaths occur more frequently before 1 year of age [sudden infant death syndrome (SIDS)] or between age group of 50 and 70 years; however, the proportion of SCDs in total mortality due to CAD decreases with age. SCD is more common in blacks, non-Hispanics, and in males apparently because of less CAD in women before menopause.[5]

Conventional risk factors like advanced age, smoking, diabetes, hyperlipidemia, hypertension obesity, and sedentary lifestyle increase risk of SCD and nearly 50% of all SCDs occur in 10% of population who are in the high-risk category. These are also the risk factors for CAD, which is the underlying structural basis in 80% of SCDs in USA. Diabetes mellitus (DM) and prolonged QTc on routine electrocardiography (ECG) are potential markers to predicts SCD.[6] Reduction in EF is the powerful predictor of SCD in chronic ischemic heart disease and EF of less than 30% is the most powerful predictor of SCD. More cardiac deaths are sudden in less severe left ventricular dysfunction (LVD) and in patients with better New York Heart Association (NYHA) class, and more deaths are due to pump failure in more severe heart failure. More SCDs however, would occur in persons with no or mild reductions in EF.[7]

Sudden cardiac death may occur in many cardiac conditions with either functional or structural abnormalities which may cause or contribute to terminal event leading to SCD. Some new markers, like microvolt T wave alternans, contrast enhanced imaging of infarct borders, QT variability, metaiodobenzylguanidine (MIBG) imaging, and genetic study of familial clustering of SCD as a marker of CAD have been evaluated with variable results.

Cardiac arrest typically occurs either due to tachyarrhythmia [ventricular fibrillation (VF or sustained ventricular tachycardia (VT)] or due to bradyarrhythmia, low heart rate less than 20 beats/minute or asystole or persistent electrical activity but no mechanical activity pulseless electrical activity (PEA). The mechanism may change with time beginning as VT/VF and then leading to asystole or vice versa.

The most common rhythm at time of admission following cardiac arrest is asystole or PEA and only 25% have VT/VF. Asystole arrest is common in severely diseased hearts with end stage cardiac and noncardiac diseases and may be due to involvement of subendocardial Purkinje fibers. PEA means presence of electrical activity without mechanical activity. It can be primary due to inability of myocardium to contract due to severe injury because of ischemia or other factors or secondary due to specific mechanical causes like pulmonary embolism, acute malfunctioning of prosthetic valves, exsanguination, and cardiac tamponade.[8]

The potential for successful resuscitation depends upon clinical setting of arrest, the mechanism of arrest, and the underlying clinical status. VT/VF mechanism of cardiac arrest had better survival than asystole or PEA (27% vs 8%). Older age more than 70 years, previous stroke, renal failure, and heart failure are bad prognostic factors for survival. Strategic factors like type and location of hospital, time of arrest (day, night, and weekend) and time to defibrillation were also important.[9] Even amongst survivors recovery of neurological function to allow a meaningful life occurs in only 20–25% cases. 1–2 years survival rates after VT/VF arrest have improved significantly from 1970 to 2010, not only due to automated implantable cardioverter defibrillator (AICD) but also due to better treatment like better heart failure therapies, early and effective reperfusion and beta blockers.

About 80% of out-of-hospital cardiac arrests are due to CAD, 15% due to cardiomyopathies and a small number due to various miscellaneous causes. Patients who survive out of hospital arrest and reach hospital have lesser in hospital and postdischarge mortality than those who have in hospital arrest. Survivors of out-of-hospital cardiac arrest have recurrence of arrhythmias in first 24–48 hours but only 5–10% of deaths are due to arrhythmias and most deaths are due to noncardiac causes like anoxic encephalopathy and sepsis.

The basic response to cardiac arrest is to maintain cardiopulmonary support till the return of spontaneous circulation and quick restoration of spontaneous circulation. The essential steps are initial assessment and summoning emergency response, basic life support, early defibrillation by first responder, advanced life support, post cardiac arrest care, and if successful followed by long-term management.

The survivors of cardiac arrest should have detailed functional assessment for neurological status and those with good recovery should undergo evaluation for cause and conditions leading to cardiac arrest for future management. About 80% of such arrests are due to CAD and require proper workup, anti-ischemic drug therapy, and revascularization in patients with documented ischemia. The beneficial effect of revascularization had not been proven in any large randomized trial, but should be intuitively offered to patients with significant demonstrable ischemia. Optimal guidelines based medical therapy including beta blockers, angiotensin-converting enzyme (ACE) inhibitors, angiotensin-receptor-neprilysin inhibitor (ARNI), and mineralocorticoid receptor antagonist (MRA) should be offered to all suitable candidates.

The risk factors for predicting recurrence like EF, NYHA class, and conventional risk factors for CAD should be found out and addressed to. The neurological and multisystem assessment to assess the useful life expectancy should be done.

Programmed electrical stimulation (PES) has very limited role in secondary prevention and is longer necessary except in cases where ischemia was a trigger and has been corrected and EF is more than 40%.

Various antiarrhythmic agents were used in survivors of cardiac arrest with low to variable success. Class I agents, amiodarone, and beta blockers have been evaluated and the results in secondary prevention have not been good.

The idea of putting a device to diagnose and treat cardiac arrest (AICD) met with lots of resistance initially and many thought it was not an ideal solution.[10] Major technical developments in AICD devices, the refinements in the implant procedures and data from the randomized trials pointed to the usefulness of these devises in secondary prevention of SCD.

The largest of the secondary prevention randomized controlled trials (RCTs) was the antiarrhythmics versus implantable defibrillators (AVID) trial, which enrolled 1,016 patients in North America. Patients had (1) resuscitation from near-fatal VF, (2) syncope with documented sustained VT, or (3) sustained VT with a left ventricular ejection fraction (LVEF) of 40% or less and significant symptoms attributed to the arrhythmia. Patients were randomized to receive an implantable cardioverter defibrillator (ICD) or antiarrhythmic medical therapy with amiodarone. The study population had predominantly white (87%), men (80%) with CAD (81%), with a mean age of 65 and mean LVEF of 31%. The index arrhythmia in nearly half (45%) was VF. After a mean follow-up of 18 months, fewer deaths occurred in the ICD group than in the antiarrhythmic drug group (25% vs 18%) with 27% relative risk reduction and 7% absolute reduction.[11]

Cardiac Arrest Survival in Hamburg (CASH) trial randomized 288 who were resuscitated from cardiac arrest due to documented sustained ventricular arrhythmias. Patients with secondary causes including cardiac arrest within 72 hours of acute MI, severe electrolyte abnormalities or use of proarrhythmic medications were excluded. Patients were randomized to an ICD or antiarrhythmic treatment (amiodarone, metoprolol, and propafenone) in a 1:3 ratio. Most patients were men (80%) with CAD (75%) with a mean age of 57 years and mean LVEF of 45%. After 57 months of follow-up (longer than 18-month follow-up in AVID), the death rates were 44.4% in medical group and 36.4% in the ICD group. Survival free of sudden cardiac arrest (SCA) was significantly higher in patients randomized to ICD although overall survival was not better.[12]

The Canadian Implantable Defibrillator Study (CIDS), enrolled 659 patients if they had documented VF out-of-hospital cardiac arrest requiring defibrillation or cardioversion or syncope resulting from documented sustained VT or documented sustained VT at a rate of more than and equal to 150 beats/min causing presyncope or angina with an LVEF less than and equal to 35% or syncope of undocumented etiology with subsequent documented spontaneous VT more than and equal to 10 seconds or sustained (≥30 seconds) monomorphic VT induced by programmed ventricular stimulation. Patients were randomized to an ICD or amiodarone. Although risks of adverse outcomes were lower in ICD group but the differences were not significant for either arrhythmic death or all cause mortality between ICD and the amiodarone.[13] The main features of major trials of secondary prevention comparing AICD with medical therapy are summarized in Table 1.

The data from these trials were later analyzed in many ways. The first meta-analysis found significant reductions in all death causes and deaths due to arrhythmias in the ICD group versus amiodarone[14] but nonarrhythmic death were similar. In subgroup analysis, patients with LVEF more than 35% and those implanted with an ICD during the 'epicardial era' compared with those randomized after this time had significantly less benefit from the ICD. The second meta-analysis showed a very impressive 7% absolute reduction in arrhythmic death with the ICD with a number needed to treat of 15 to prevent one death at a mean follow-up of 2 years.[15]

Initial trials of ACID in secondary prevention trials showed advantage over amiodarone but even the ACID arm had high mortality as compared to recent trials because of low use of ACE, beta blockers and MRA in these trials. At 3 years follow-up in AVID trial, mortality in ICD group was 16% compared to 24% in patients treated with antiarrhythmic medications and the vast majority of deaths (78%) were related to cardiac causes.[16] In a more contemporary trial, patients undergoing ICD placement for secondary prevention indications had much higher survival of 89.6% and 83.6% at 1 and 2 years, respectively.[17] AICD obviously had no effect on nonarryhmic deaths and noncardiac deaths which are more common in patients

TABLE 1: Brief overview of major secondary prevention trials comparing automated implantable cardioverter defibrillator and medical therapy

Trial	*Patients*	*Follow-up*	*Main inclusion criteria*	*Main findings*
AVID	1016	1.5 years (early termination)	(i) Resuscitation from VF, (ii) VT with syncope and (iii) VT with hemodynamic instability and LVEF ≤ 40%	ICD therapy reduced all-cause death in comparison to amiodarone therapy (relative risk reduction 33%)
CIDS	659	3 years	(i) Resuscitation from VT/VF, (ii) VT with syncope, (iii) VT with hemodynamic instability and LVEF ≤ 35% and (iv) unexplained syncope and VT inducible by PVS	ICD therapy was associated with a non-significant reduction of both all-cause death and arrhythmic death in comparison to amiodarone therapy (relative risk reduction 20 and 33%, respectively)
CASH	288	3 years	Resuscitation from VT/VF	ICD therapy was associated with a non-significant reduction of all-cause death in comparison to therapy with either amiodarone or metoprolol (relative risk reduction 23%)

Abbreviations: AICD, automated implantable cardioverter defibrillator; CIDS, Canadian Implantable Defibrillator Study; CASH, Cardiac Arrest Survival in Hamburg; VF, ventricular fibrillation; VT, ventricular tachycardia; LVEF, left ventricular ejection fraction; PVS, premature ventricular contraction; ICD, implantable cardioverter defibrillator.

BOX 1: Indications of automated implantable cardioverter defibrillator for secondary prevention of sudden cardiac death

Class 1

1. Implantable cardioverter defibrillator (ICD) therapy is indicated in patients who are survivors of cardiac arrest due to VF or hemodynamically unstable sustained VT after evaluation to define the cause of the event and to exclude any completely reversible causes.
2. Implantable cardioverter defibrillator therapy is indicated in patients with structural heart disease and spontaneous sustained VT, whether hemodynamically stable or unstable. (Level of evidence: B).
3. Implantable cardioverter defibrillator therapy is indicated in patients with syncope of undetermined origin with clinically relevant, hemodynamically significant sustained VT or VF induced at electrophysiological study. (Level of evidence: B).

Class 2A

1. Implantable cardioverter defibrillator implantation is reasonable for patients with unexplained syncope, significant LV dysfunction and nonischemic DCM. (Level of evidence: C).
2. Implantable cardioverter defibrillator implantation is reasonable for patients with sustained VT and normal or near-normal ventricular function. (Level of evidence: C).

Class 2B

1. Implantable cardioverter defibrillator therapy may be considered for patients with long-QT syndrome and risk factors for SCD. (Level of evidence: B) (16, 349–354).
2. Implantable cardioverter defibrillator therapy may be considered in patients with syncope and advanced structural heart disease in whom thorough invasive and noninvasive investigations have failed to define a cause. (Level of evidence: C).
3. Implantable cardioverter defibrillator therapy may be considered in patients with a familial cardiomyopathy associated with sudden death. (Level of evidence: C).

Class 3 Indications

1. Implantable cardioverter defibrillator therapy is not indicated for patients who do not have a reasonable expectation of survival with an acceptable functional status for at least 1 year, even if they meet ICD implantation criteria specified in the class I, IIa, and IIb recommendations above. (Level of evidence: C)
2. Implantable cardioverter defibrillator therapy is not indicated for patients with incessant VT or VF. (Level of evidence: C)
3. Implantable cardioverter defibrillator therapy is not indicated in patients with significant psychiatric illnesses that may be aggravated by device implantation or that may preclude systematic follow-up. (Level of evidence: C)
4. Implantable cardioverter defibrillator therapy is not indicated for NYHA class IV patients with drug-refractory congestive heart failure who are not candidates for cardiac transplantation or CRT-D. (Level of evidence: C)
5. Implantable cardioverter defibrillator therapy is not indicated for syncope of undetermined cause in a patient without inducible ventricular tachyarrhythmia and without structural heart disease. (Level of evidence: C)
6. Implantable cardioverter defibrillator therapy is not indicated when VF or VT is amenable to surgical or catheter ablation (e.g. atrial arrhythmias associated with the Wolff-Parkinson-White syndrome, RV or LV outflow tract VT, idiopathic VT, or fascicular VT in the absence of structural heart disease). (Level of evidence: C)
7. Implantable cardioverter defibrillator therapy is not indicated for patients with ventricular tachyarrhythmia due to a completely reversible disorder in the absence of structural heart disease (e.g. electrolyte imbalance, drugs, or trauma). (Level of evidence: B)

Abbreviations: VF, ventricular fibrillation; VT, ventricular tachycardia; LV, Left ventricular; DCM, dilated cardiomyopathy; SCD, sudden cardiac death; NYHA, New York Heart Association; CRT-D, cardiac resynchronization therapy defibrillator; RV, right ventricular

with advanced heart failure. Not all arrhythmic deaths can be prevented by AICD because of failure of detection, VTs occurring below the detection rates, lead fractures, and other device related issues, bradyarrhythmias or due to electromechanical failure in patients with advanced LVD.[18]

No randomized trials of AICD in secondary prevention have been conducted in recent times. This is very important since major improvements have occurred in medical treatment of heart failure since then. Use of ACE/angiotensin receptor blocker (ARB), beta blockers, ARNI, and MRA have been shown to reduce total mortality, CV mortality, and sudden deaths and may reduce the need/usefulness of AICD. Only 44% patients in AVID trial were on beta blockers and MRA use was only 3% and we know that both these groups of drugs have significant effect on SCDs.[11,19] Chan and colleagues in a more recent review identified 1,442 patients who had AICD implantation for a secondary prevention indication, new-onset VT/VF/cardiac arrest. After 3 years of follow-up, patients who received an ICD had significantly lower all-cause and cardiovascular mortality and the reduction was similar to that seen in the AVID trial (31%).[20] The risk reduction was similar in patients on optimal medical therapy and those not receiving optimal therapy, suggesting benefits to the ICD beyond contemporary medical treatment. Current guidelines for AICD use for secondary prevention of SCD are summarized in Box 1.

SPECIAL POPULATION

The benefits of AICD in some special patient subgroups are not so well-established. Patients with advanced LVD and higher NYHA class symptoms are associated with higher risk of death due to progressive heart failure which can potentially reduces the impact of ICD therapy. Similarly, in a meta-analysis of the secondary prevention RCTs, patients with LVEF more than and equal to 35% had significantly less benefit compared with those whose LVEF was severely reduced and in AVID trial maximum benefit was seen in patients with EF between 20 and 35%.[14]

Another group where the benefit is not so sure is elderly patients. Most of the secondary prevention RCTs had small number of elderly patients and the mean age was 63 years. Because the competing risk of noncardiac death is higher with the elderly, the ICD may provide less benefit in these patients. The ratio of sudden death to all-cause death falls from 0.51 before the age of 50 years to 0.26 after age of 80 years among patients with prior MI or heart failure.[21] There is some evidence from pooled data that elderly patients have high mortality due to nonarrhythmic and noncardiac causes, and AICD may be less effective but at present AICD therapy should not be withheld because of age.[22]

Renal disease with or without dialysis is a strong risk factor for mortality due to cardiovascular causes especially SCDs. Most of the RCTs of AICDs have however excluded patients with advanced renal diseases. Procedure related complications like infection, bleeding and access related complications, and venous thrombosis may be higher in these patients, and the benefit of AICD may be less as compared to patients with normal renal function. AICD has been implanted less frequently in patients with renal disease as shown in retrospective cohort study which evaluated 6,042 patients on dialysis who suffered a cardiac arrest or VF episode and survived at least 30 days from the event; only 7.6% underwent ICD implantation.[23] AICD implantation significantly improved the survival as compared to medical treatment; however, unadjusted mortality in this endstage renal disease cohort was higher than that observed among patients enrolled in the RCTs. Current guidelines still recommend an ICD for those that have a reasonable expectation of survival for more than 1 year, but the benefits may be of lesser magnitude.

Women are offered AICD implantation less frequently than males and 75% of patients enrolled in all trials of primary and secondary prevention were males. Women are less likely than men to experience potentially life-saving device therapy suggesting that the current methods of selecting patients for an ICD may be better at identifying men who will benefit from the device than women. Women are more likely than men to experience both major and minor complications from ICD implantation, suggesting that greater care is needed perioperatively. Given the current patient selection protocols and device implantation methods, the net benefit of the ICD is reduced in women because of the lower rates of need of therapies delivered and the increased risk of complications.

The usefulness and safety of testing of defibrillation threshold has been another unsettled issue. All patients enrolled in the RCTs that investigated the efficacy of the ICD underwent defibrillation threshold testing. However, it has been shown that such testing does not improve ICD shock efficacy or reduce mortality.[24] Furthermore, first ICD shocks rarely fail to terminate clinical ventricular arrhythmias (<10%) and defibrillation threshold testing adds complexity, time, and cost of the procedure and creates inconvenience for the patient. The Shockless Implant Evaluation (SIMPLE) trial compared the efficacy and safety of ICD implantation without and with defibrillation testing. Although the majority of patients (73%) had a primary prevention indication, the trial also enrolled patients treated with an ICD for secondary prevention. At a mean follow-up of 3 years, the primary outcome of arrhythmic death or failed appropriate shock occurred in fewer patients in the no-testing group than in those who underwent testing, 7 versus 8%, respectively.[25] Although the primary outcome was similar for all subgroups, there was no separate analysis of the 27% of patients with a secondary prevention indication. The best approach to defibrillation testing among patients undergoing secondary prevention ICD remains unclear and guidelines do not provide specific recommendations.[26]

Given the high-risk substrate of patients receiving an ICD for secondary prevention, it is not surprising that ICD therapies are common in this population; in the AVID trial 51% were treated with either an ICD shock or antitachycardia pacing (ATP) within the first year. By the second year, 62% of patients had received an ICD shock and 77% had received ATP. VT was the first arrhythmia treated in 63% of cases, and VF in 13% of cases.[27] In contrast, among patients in the primary prevention Sudden Cardiac Death in Heart Failure Trial (SCD-HeFT), only a third of patients had received a therapy at median follow-up of 3.75 years.[28] Because of the high frequent use of therapies among patients receiving an ICD for secondary prevention, and because of concerns about the association between ICD shocks and adverse outcomes, contemporary programming strategies to reduce shocks are particularly important in this population.[29] However, patients with secondary prevention ICDs are poorly represented in trials evaluating programming strategies, perhaps due to concerns that interventions to lower the risk of shocks might increase the rate of arrhythmic death among patients who have already experienced episodes of life-threatening ventricular arrhythmias.[30] One quarter (477/1,902) of the population of the ADVANCE III trial had a secondary prevention indication. On follow-up, patients randomized to longer detection intervals had significantly fewer delivered therapies (346 vs 557) without a significant change in total mortality (5.5 vs 6.3) or syncope (1.2 and 1.15 events/patient).[31] A post-hoc analysis of the 477 patients with a secondary prevention indication demonstrated a similar decrease in overall therapies in those randomized to longer detection intervals without a difference in syncope or death.[32] Although, ICD programming should be tailored to previous knowledge of VT/VF (hemodynamic stability and cycle length), these data suggest that programming with longer detection intervals might reduce rates of ICD therapies without increasing risk of adverse outcomes in a secondary prevention population.

Dual-chamber ICDs as compared to standard single chamber AICD have an additional right atrial (RA) lead, thus enabling atrioventricular (AV) sequential (physiological) pacing and holding the potential to improve the differentiation between supraventricular and ventricular tachyarrhythmia based on dual-chamber detection algorithms. Dual chamber ICD systems may provide specific advantage in patients with symptomatic sick-sinus-syndrome and in patients with known slow VT or supraventricular tachycardia not amenable to catheter ablation. In dual-chamber ICDs, however, unnecessary right ventricular (RV) pacing at high rates needs to be avoided as high rate RV pacing is associated with worse outcome.[33] The issue of dual-chamber versus single chamber tachycardia discrimination has been addressed by a number of studies, but with conflicting results. Although, theoretically dual-chamber discrimination should be superior in specificity for VT detection, clinical data do not unanimously demonstrate significant reductions in inappropriate ICD therapies.[34] The performance of tachycardia discrimination algorithms does not only depend on the quality of algorithms per se, but also on the way how VT/VF detection is programmed in individual patient.

Electrical storm defined as more than 3 appropriate VT/VF detection within 24 hours requiring shocks or ATP may occur in up to 25% of ICD patients within 3 years.[35] Common reasons are progression of heart failure/underlying cardiac disease, acute coronary syndrome, electrolyte imbalance, psychological stress, changes in antiarrhythmic medication/proarrhythmia, and infective diseases besides device related issues. Repeated therapies are associated with increased mortality and every effort needs be made to minimize the delivery of therapy. Correction of underlying cause and modifications of ICD programming (e.g. optimization of ATP, overdrive pacing, etc.) are often helpful. Changes in drug therapy, long-term amiodarone combined with beta blocker therapy or ablation of VT may be required in some cases.[36]

Inappropriate shock is an important issue, occurs in nearly 10–15% cases and is associated with adverse outcome. Atrial fibrillation and oversensing due to lead related issues are important causes. Optimal medical therapy for cardiac condition and reprogramming of VT detection zones are usually enough.[37]

TABLE 2: Common primary rhythm disorders causing cardiac arrest and indications of automated implantable cardioverter defibrillator

	Major risk factors for SCD	*Principle recommendations*
Hypertrophic cardiomyopathy	Prior cardiac arrest, spontaneous sustained VT Family history of SCD, unexplained syncope, NSVT, abnormal blood pressure response to exercise, massive LV hypertrophy	ICD implantation is recommended in patients with prior VF or sustained VT. Prophylactic ICD implantation should be considered in high-risk patients. Patients with end-stage hypertrophic cardiomyopathy may have an ICD indication due to heart failure (LVEF≤35%, NYHA II/III)
Arrhythmogenic right ventricular cardiomyopathy	Prior cardiac arrest, spontaneous sustained VT Extensive disease, one or more affected family members with SCD, unexplained syncope	ICD implantation is recommended in patients with prior VF or sustained VT Prophylactic ICD implantation should be considered in high-risk patients
Long QT syndrome	Prior cardiac arrest, spontaneous sustained VT Unexplained syncope, QT duration, genotype, sex	ICD implantation is recommended in patients with prior VF or sustained VT despite adequate medical therapy. Prophylactic ICD implantation should be considered in high-risk patients
Brugada syndrome	Prior cardiac arrest, spontaneous sustained VT Unexplained syncope Role of EP testing controversial	ICD implantation is recommended in patients with prior VF or sustained VT or unexplained syncope. Prophylactic ICD implantation should be considered in high-risk patients
Catecholaminergic polymorphic VT	Prior cardiac arrest, spontaneous sustained VT Unexplained syncope	ICD implantation is recommended in patients with prior VF or sustained VT or unexplained syncope despite beta-blocker therapy
Short QT syndrome	Prior cardiac arrest	ICD implantation is recommended in patients with prior cardiac arrest. Due to the small number of patients, no evidence-based recommendation with respect to the treatment of asymptomatic patients can be made
Idiopathic ventricular fibrillation	Prior cardiac arrest	ICD implantation is recommended in patients with prior cardiac arrest

Abbreviations: SCD, sudden cardiac death; VT, ventricular tachycardia; LV, left ventricular; NSVT, nonsustained ventricular tachycardia; EP, electrophysiological; ICD, implantable cardioverter defibrillator; VF, ventricular fibrillation; LVEF, left ventricular ejection fraction; NYHA, New York Heart Association

Source: Zitron E, Thomas D, Katus HA, et al. Cardioverter defibrillator therapy in the primary and secondary prevention of sudden cardiac death. Appl Cardiopulm Pathophysiol. 2012;16:174-91.

BOX 2: Future investigations of automated implantable cardioverter defibrillator in secondary prevention

Outcomes in populations not represented in trials
- Elderly (>70 years old)
- Women
- Severely symptomatic heart failure (e.g. NYHA class IV symptoms)
- Chronic kidney disease
- Severely depressed LVEF
- Nonwhite race

Impact of care strategies
- ICD programming
- Goal-directed medical therapy (BB, ACEI, MRA) and shock risk models
- Device-related complications
- Competing outcomes of arrhythmic versus nonarrhythmic death
- Outcomes beyond death ICD therapies (shocks and antitachycardia pacing)
- Quality of life

Abbreviations: NYHA, New York Heart Association; LVEF, left ventricular ejection fraction; ICD, implantable cardioverter defibrillator; BB, beta blocker; ACEI, angiotensin-converting enzyme inhibitor; MRA, mineralocorticoid receptor antagonist

Source: Borne RT, Katz D, Betz J, et al. Implantable cardioverter-defibrillators for secondary prevention of sudden cardiac death: a review. J Am Heart Assoc. 2017; 6(3):e005515.

Remote monitoring is also valuable new tool in monitoring patients after AICD implantation. This is more convenient to patients, can detect arrhythmias, atrial fibrillation, and fluid status earlier than conventional in house visits and can reduce inappropriate shocks.[38] Subcutaneous ICDs are also an option in patients who have problems in venous access but these devices do not provide back up pacing (>30 seconds) and do not have option of ATP. Subcutaneous ICDs are more apt for younger patients with increased chance of infection with transvenous procedure.[39] Magnetic resonance imaging (MRI) conditional AICDs are also being increasingly used as many patients, especially elderly, may need MRI for life saving investigations and procedures.

Most of the information regarding AICD in secondary prevention is based on three trials involving 957 patients (AVID, CIDS, and CASH), where most of the patients had underlying CAD. However, observational and registry data support the use of ICDs also in secondary prevention patients with other types of structural heart disease, such as dilated nonischemic cardiomyopathy and hypertrophic cardiomyopathy, and primary electrical disorders such as arrhythmogenic right ventricular dysplasia ARVD, Brugads syndrome, long QT syndrome, short QT syndrome and catecholaminergic polymorphic VT (Table 2). Current guidelines recommend ICD implantation in patients who have survived a cardiac arrest or sustained VT regardless of the type of underlying structural heart disease except with potential reversible causes for cardiac arrest such as acute myocardial infarction and acute myocarditis.[40]

Major advancements have occurred in both AICD technology and implant procedures as well medical treatments of heart failure and more trials are strongly needed to redefine magnitude of benefit of AICD in general and in special subgroups and to address the usefulness of various technical advantages in AICD systems (Box 2).

CONCLUSION

Based on RCTs performed on relatively few patients over two decades ago, in secondary prevention ICDs reduce the risk of death (as compared with antiarrhythmic medications) and are indicated for patients who have survived SCA who have a reasonable expectation of survival for at least a year with good functional status. However, in contemporary practice, patients who receive secondary prevention ICDs do not resemble those enrolled in the trials. Further, advances in medical therapy for left ventricular systolic dysfunction and CAD are likely to attenuate the risk of subsequent SCA in this population, potentially attenuating the benefits of ICD therapy. Observational studies of this population are relatively few compared with those focusing on primary prevention, despite the fact that a substantial proportion (nearly 25%) of ICDs implanted are for secondary prevention. Future investigations are needed to improve the quality of care provided to this large population of patients.

REFERENCES

1. Roger VL, Go AS, Lloyd-Jones DM, et al. Heart disease and stroke statistics—2011 update: a report from the American Heart Association. Circulation. 2011;123(4):e18-e209.
2. Myenberg RJ, Junttila MJ. Sudden Cardiac Death caused by Coronary Aretry Disease. Circulation. 2012;125(8):1043-52.
3. Myerburg RJ, Wellens HJJ. Epidemiology of Cardiac Arrest. In: Priori SG, Zipes DP (Eds). Sudden Cardiac Death: a Handbook of Clinical Practise. Oxford, UK: Blackwell Publishing Ltd; 2006. pp. 3-19.
4. Myerburg RJ. Sudden cardiac death: exploring the limits of our knowledge. J Cardiovasc Electrophysiol. 2001;12(3):369-81.
5. Gillum RF. Sudden cardiac death in Hispanic Americans and African Americans. Am J Public Health. 1997;87(9):1461-6.
6. Chugh SS, Reinier K, Singh T, et al. Determinants of prolonged QT interval and their contribution to sudden death in coronary artery disease: the Oregon Sudden Unexpected Death Study. Circulation. 2009;119(5):663-70.
7. Stecker EC, Vickers C, Waltz J, et al. Population-based analysis of sudden cardiac death with or without left ventricular systolic dysfunction: two-year findings from the Oregon Sudden Unexpected Death Study. J Am Coll Cardiol. 2006;47(6):1161-6.
8. McNally B, Robb R, Mehta M, et al. Out-of-hospital cardiac arrest surveillance—Cardiac Arrest Registry to Enhance Survival (CARES), United States, October 1, 2005–December 31, 2010. MMWR Surveill Summ. 2011;60(8):1-19.
9. Field JM, Hazinski MF, Sayre MR, et al. Part 1: executive summary: 2010 American Heart Association Guidelines for Cardiopulmonary Resuscitation and Emergency Cardiovascular Care. Circulation. 2010;122(18 Suppl 3):S640-56.

10. Lown B, Axelrod P. Implanted standby defibrillators. Circulation. 1972;46(4):637-9.
11. Antiarrhythmics versus Implantable Defibrillators (AVID) Investigators. A comparison of antiarrhythmic drug therapy with implantable defibrillators in patients resuscitated from near-fatal ventricular arrhythmias. N Engl J Med. 1997;337(22):1576-83.
12. Kuck KH, Cappato R, Siebels J, et al. Randomized comparison of antiarrhythmic drug therapy with implantable defibrillators in patients resuscitated from cardiac arrest: the Cardiac Arrest Study Hamburg (CASH). Circulation. 2000;102(7):748-54.
13. Connolly SJ, Gent M, Roberts RS, et al. Canadian Implantable Defibrillator Study (CIDS): a randomized trial of the implantable cardioverter defibrillator against amiodarone. Circulation. 2000;101(11):1297-302.
14. Connolly SJ, Hallstrom AP, Cappato R, et al. Meta-analysis of the implantable cardioverter defibrillator secondary prevention trials. AVID, CASH, and CIDS studies. Antiarrhythmics vs Implantable Defibrillator study. Cardiac Arrest Study Hamburg. Canadian Implantable Defibrillator Study. Eur Heart J. 2000;21(24):2071-8.
15. Lee DS, Green LD, Lui PP, et al. Effectiveness of implantable defibrillators for prevention arrhythmic events and death: a meta-analysis. J Am Coll Cardiol. 2003;41(9):1573-82.
16. AVID Investigators. Causes of death in the antiarrhythmics versus implantable defibrillators (AVID) trial. J Am Coll Cardiol. 1999;34(5):1552-9.
17. Katz DF, Peterson P, Borne RT, et al. Survival after secondary prevention ICD placement: an analysis from the NCDR ICD Registry. JACC Clin Electrophysiol. 2017;3:20-8.
18. Mitchell LB, Pineda EA, Titus JL, et al. Sudden death in patients with implantable cardioverter defibrillators. The importance of postshock electromechanical dissociation. J Am Coll Cardiol. 2002;39:1323-8.
19. Masoudi FA, Gross CP, Wang Y, et al. Adoption of spironolactone therapy for older patients with heart failure and left ventricular systolic dysfunction in the United States, 1998-2001. Circulation. 2005;112:39-47.
20. Chan PS, Hayward RA. Mortality reduction by implantable cardioverter defibrillators in high-risk patients with heart failure, ischemic heart disease, and new-onset ventricular arrhythmia. J Am Coll Cardiol. 2005;45:1474-81.
21. Krahn AD, Connolly SJ, Roberts RS, et al. Diminishing proportional risk of sudden death with advancing age: implications for prevention of sudden death. Am Heart J. 2004;147:837-40.
22. Betz JK, Katz DF, Peterson PN, et al. Outcomes of older patients receiving secondary prevention implantable cardioverter defibrillators: an analysis from the NCDR ICD Registry. J Am Coll Cardiol. 2017;69:265-74.
23. Herzog CA, Li S, Weinhandi ED, et al. Survival of dialysis patients after cardiac arrest and the impact of implantable cardioverter defibrillators. Kidney Int. 2005;68:818-25.
24. Matassini MV, Healey JS. How to manage a high defibrillation threshold in ICD patients: and does it really matter. Curr Treat Options Cardiovasc Med. 2013;15:497-505.
25. Healey JS, Hohnloser SH, Glikson M, et al. Cardioverter defibrillator implantation without induction of ventricular fibrillation: a single-blind, non-inferiority, randomized controlled trial (SIMPLE). Lancet. 2015;385(9970):785-91.
26. Wilkoff BL, Fauchier L, Stiles MK, et al. 2015 HRS/EHRA/APHRS/SOLACECE expert consensus statement on optimal implantable cardioverter-defibrillator programming and testing. Heart Rhythm. 2016;13(2):e50-86.
27. Klein RC, Raitt MH, Wilkoff BL, et al. Analysis of implantable cardioverter defibrillator therapy in the Antiarrhythmics Versus Implantable Defibrillators (AVID) Trial. J Cardiovasc Electrophysiol. 2003;14:940-8.
28. Poole JE, Johnson GW, Hellkamp AS, et al. Prognostic importance of defibrillator shocks in patients with heart failure. N Engl J Med. 2008;359:1009-17.
29. Borne RT, Varosy PD, Masoudi FA. Implantable cardioverter-defibrillator shocks: epidemiology, outcomes, and therapeutic approaches. JAMA Intern Med. 2013;173:859-65.
30. Saeed M, Hanna I, Robotis D, et al. Programming implantable cardioverter-defibrillators in patients with primary prevention indication to prolong time to first shock: results from the PROVIDE study. J Cardiovasc Electrophysiol. 2014;25:52-9.
31. Gasparini M, Proclemer A, Klersy C, et al. Effect of long-detection interval vs standard-detection interval for implantable cardioverter-defibrillators on antitachycardia pacing and shock delivery: the ADVANCE III randomized clinical trial. JAMA. 2013;309(18):1903-11.
32. Kloppe A, Proclemer A, Arenal A, et al. Efficacy of long detection interval implantable cardioverter-defibrillator settings in secondary prevention population. Circulation. 2014;130:308-14.
33. Wilkoff BL, Kudenchuk PJ, Buxton AE, et al. The DAVID (Dual Chamber and VVI Implantable Defibrillator) II trial. J Am Coll Cardiol. 2009;53(10):872-80.
34. Friedman PA, McClelland RL, Bamlet WR, et al. Dual-chamber versus single-chamber detection enhancements for implantable defibrillator rhythm diagnosis: the detect supraventricular tachycardia study. Circulation. 2006;113(25):2871-9.
35. Israel CW, Barold SS. Electrical storm in patients with an implanted defibrillator: a matter of definition. Ann Noninvasive Electrocardiol. 2007;12(4):375-82.
36. Connolly SJ, Dorian P, Roberts RS, et al. Comparison of beta blockers, amiodarone plus beta-blockers, or sotalol for prevention of shocks from implantable cardioverter defibrillators: the OPTIC Study: a randomized trial. JAMA. 2006;295(2):165-71.
37. Germano JJ, Reynolds M, Essebag V, et al. Frequency and causes of implantable cardioverter-defibrillator therapies: is device therapy proarrhythmic? Am J cardiol. 2006;97(8):1255-61.
38. Dubner S, Auricchio A, Steinberg JS, et al. ISHNE/EHRA expert consensus on remote monitoring of cardiovascular implantable electronic devices (CIEDs). Europace. 2012;14(2):278-93.
39. Bardy GH, Smith WM, Hood MA, et al. An entirely subcutaneous implantable cardioverter-defibrillator. N Engl J Med. 2010;363(1):36-44.
40. Zipes DP, Camm AJ, Borggrefe M, et al. ACC/AHA/ESC 2006 guidelines for management of patients with ventricular arrhythmias and the prevention of sudden cardiac death—executive summary: A report of the American College of Cardiology/American Heart Association Task Force and the European Society of Cardiology Committee for Practice Guidelines (Writing Committee to Develop Guidelines for Management of Patients with Ventricular Arrhythmias and the Prevention of Sudden Cardiac Death) Developed in collaboration with the European Heart Rhythm Association and the Heart Rhythm Society. Eur Heart J. 2006;27(17):2099-140.

SECTION 6

Intervention

Coronary Interventions in Cardiodiabetes Prognostication

Harinder K Bali, Hiteshi KC Chauhan

INTRODUCTION

Diabetes mellitus—a chronic and complex multiorgan disease of metabolism characterized by hyperglycemia, insulin resistance, a persistent prothrombotic milieu.[1] and profoundly virulent atherosclerotic potential[2]—has long been recognized as a cardiovascular equivalent.[3] More recently, this lethal amalgamation is referred to as "cardiodiabetes", prompting various guidelines on aggressive risk factor control.[4-6] In the last 40 years since the advent of percutaneous coronary intervention (PCI), the global prevalence (age-standardized) of diabetes has doubled from 4.7% to 8.5% in the adult population.[7] In patients with acute coronary syndrome (ACS) or undergoing PCI, diabetes increases the risk of subsequent myocardial infraction (MI), ACS, congestive heart failure (CHF) and mortality.[8-10]

PCI IN CARDIODIABETES AND FACTORS INFLUENCING PCI OUTCOMES

Over the last 2 decades, as the number of diabetics undergoing percutaneous coronary intervention (PCI) has doubled with a higher proportion of older, sicker patients with more complex coronary lesions;[11] the suboptimal outcomes of PCI in this population have become evident[3,12] with higher rates of in-hospital mortality, MI and need for emergency surgery.[12,13] By 1995, however, the mortality rate in the elective PCI had become equivalent to that of nondiabetics, likely secondary to technological advances.[13] Use of stents and increase in adjunctive medical therapy led to a further decrease in all hard end points in the 1999–2002 NHLBI dynamic registry.[14] However, diabetics tolerate multivessel intervention and acute ischemic complications of angioplasty poorly.[15] The in-hospital mortality amongst diabetics remains higher amongst all undergoing PCI.[16] This is attributable mainly to diabetic traits potentially compromising the short- and long-term outcomes of PCI, namely—diabetic arteriopathy, myocardial dysfunction, diabetic nephropathy, exogenous insulin and altered platelet pharmacokinetics.[17]

Diabetic Arteriopathy and Restenosis

Diabetic arteriopathy compromises long-term success after PCI by higher rates of aggressive restenosis and development of vulnerable plaques outside stented segments.[17] This proliferative restenotic response is multifactorial: aggressive smooth muscle hyperplasia, accelerated fibrosis, enhanced endogenous thrombogenicity and increased recoil have all been implicated.[18] The restenotic process more often results in total vessel occlusion after PCI;[19-21] resulting in MI, ventricular dysfunction and heart failure[22] in diabetics than nondiabetics.[23] Restenosis, especially in its occlusive form, is a major determinant of long-term mortality in diabetic patients after coronary balloon angioplasty:[12,20,24,25] 10-year mortality in patients with no restenosis, nonocclusive restenosis and occlusive restenosis was 24%, 35% and 59%, respectively.[24]

As per the report from the NHLBI Angioplasty Registry, although balloon angioplasty had similar procedural success and relief of angina for patients with diabetes, as in nondiabetics,[12,25] there was a gross variation in the angiographic restenosis rate—47% in diabetic patients compared to 32% in nondiabetics.[26]

A pooled analysis of major stent trials by Cutlip et al. demonstrated that diabetes is the strongest clinical predictor for restenosis, with an almost 50% increased risk for target vessel revascularization (TVR) at 1-year follow-up.[27] HbA1C more than 7% is an independent predictor of TVR.[28] Patients with optimal glycemic control had a TVR of 15%, compared with 34% in individuals with an HbA1C of more than 7%.[28] Although diabetics are at higher risk for restenosis throughout the vessel size range,[29] smaller vessel reference diameter and greater stented length of the vessel are independent predictors of restenosis in diabetics.[30] The Prevention of REStenosis with Tranilast and its Outcomes (PRESTO) trial[31] reiterated that diabetics still had higher 9-month rate of death [relative risk (RR) 1.87, 95% CI 1.31 to 2.68], TVR (RR 1.27, 95% CI 1.14 to 1.42), and the composite of death/MI and TVR (RR 1.26, 95% CI 1.13 to 1.40), even after adjustment for differences in baseline characteristics (older, with more comorbidities and complex coronary lesions). Diabetes is an independent prognosticator of major adverse cardiac and cerebrovascular events (MACCE) and long-term mortality.[32,33]

Chronicles of Percutaneous Coronary Interventions in the Diabetic

Balloon Angioplasty versus Intracoronary Stents

Intracoronary stents are efficacious in decreasing restenosis in diabetics by facilitating greater acute luminal gain, preventing acute vessel recoil and attenuating exaggerated intimal hyperplasia. However, the reported restenosis rates remained in the 24–55% range,[29,34,35] with higher restenosis rates for stents placed in saphenous venous grafts, smaller vessels, and longer lesions. Van Belle et al.[36] reported that for uncomplicated native coronary artery stenting of average vessel size of 3.06 mm and lesion length of 9 mm, there was lesser in-stent restenosis (27% vs 62%; $p < 0.0001$) as compared with balloon angioplasty; with an associated decrease in 4-year cardiac mortality and nonfatal MI (14.8% vs 26%; $p = 0.02$), target lesion revascularization (TLR) (35.4% vs 52.1%; $p = 0.001$) and lower rates of vessel occlusion (4% vs 13%; $p < 0.005$).

Bare-metal versus First-generation Drug-eluting Stents

Multiple randomized trials such as DIABETES,[37] RAVEL,[38] SIRIUS[39] and TAXUS IV[40] have demonstrated that drug-eluting stents use agents like sirolimus and paclitaxel to reduce the antiproliferative response and promote vascular healing. This leads to prevention of neointimal proliferation, a reduction in target segment restenosis[37-42] and major adverse cardiac events (MACE),[37-42] as compared to bare-metal stents (BMS).

Sirolimus-eluting stents (SES) reduced TVR from 59.5% to 17.6% in diabetics (65% reduction).[41] However, the absolute late loss and restenosis remained higher in diabetics receiving SES.[41] Interestingly, in insulin-requiring diabetics, TVR was higher in both SES (35%) and BMS (50%) arms.[41] Among diabetics, PES, as compared to BMS, reduced the rate of 9-month binary angiographic restenosis by 81% (6.4% vs 34.5%, $p < 0.0001$), reduced the 12-month rates of TLR by 65% (7.4% vs 20.9%, $p = 0.0008$), TVR by 53% (11.3% vs 24%, $p < 0.004$), and composite MACE by 44% (15.6% vs 27.7%, $p = 0.01$).[42]

Clinical Outcome with Drug-eluting Stents

Collaborative network meta-analyses by Stettler et al. concluded that compared with BMS, TLR rates were strongly decreased by use of SES and PES in patients with DM.[43,44] Although RCTs are an elegant and scientific approach toward data acquisition, implicit biases exist due to the selection/screening process in patient accrual.[10] Therefore, this data needs to be substantiated by registries, which compile data on patients with various comorbidities, lesion types and personalized preferences for revascularization strategy.[10] The real-world Swedish Coronary Angiography and Angioplasty Registry (SCAAR) registry cast doubts on the unmitigated benefit of DES in diabetics (Table 1).[45] Although DES significantly reduced restenosis to half of that seen with BMS, the numbers needed to treat (NNT) patients with diabetes with DES to avoid one additional restenosis per year with BMS ranged from 21 to 47 lesions in patients treated with one stent and 11 to 27 in patients with multiple stents.[45] Moreover, there was no difference in the combined outcome of death or MI in patients with diabetes treated with DES ($n = 4,754$) or BMS ($n = 4,956$) with upto 4 years of follow-up.[45] Therefore, although the magnitude of restenosis reduction achieved with DES is impressive,[41-44] several randomized trials and meta-analysis[45-47] have shown no significant reduction in the rates of death and MI with DES, as compared with BMS.

TABLE 1: Landmark studies comparing drug-eluting stents in patients with diabetes

S. No	Study	Study, Type	DES, Type	Patients with DM/Total patients	DES, n	Primary endpoint	% DM patients meeting endpoint	Follow-up years	Conculsion in DM
1	SCAAR 2004–2008	Registry	PES-E PES-L ZES SES	8231/19004 43%	Stents per patient PES-E:1.71 PES-L:1.74 ZES:1.74 SES:1.69	Restenosis	PES-E:5.1 PES-L:4.1 ZES:6.5 SES:4.9	2	Risk of restenosis higher with ZES than PES or SES
2	SCAAR 2007–2011	Registry	EES SES PES	4751	Total stents [n] EES:3928 SES:1370 PES:2836	ACM, ST restenosis	EES:3.5 SES:5.4 PES:4.5	1	EES had less ST and mortality, no difference in restenosis
3	ENDEAVOR IV 2005–2006	RCT	ZES PES	477/1548 31%	DM Patients ZES:241 PES:236	ACM, MI, TLR, TVR	ZES:8.6 PES:10.8	1	No difference between ZES and PES
4	SPIRIT II–IV, COMPARE 2005-2008	Pooled RCTs	EES PES	1869/6780 28%	DM Patients EES:241 PES:681	Cardiac death, MI, TLR	EES:10.1 PES:10.3	2	No difference between EES and PES
5	TUXEDO-India 2011–2014	RCT	EES PES	1830/1830 PES:914	DM Patients EES:916	Cardiac death, TVMI, TVR	EES:2.9 PES:5.6	1	EES superior to PES

Abbreviations: SCAAR, Swedish Coronary Angiography and Angioplasty Registry; ENDEAVOR IV, Randomized Comparison of Zotarolimus and Paclitaxel-Eluting Stents in patients with CAD; SPIRIT, Clinical Evaluation of the XIENCE V Everolimus Eluting Coronary Stent System in the Treatment of Patients With de novo Native Coronary Artery Lesions; COMPARE, A Trial of Everolimus-Eluting Stents and Paclitaxel-Eluting Stents for Coronary Revascularization in Daily Practice; TUXEDO, Taxus Element versus XIENCE Prime in a Diabetic Population; RCT, randomized controlled trial; DM, diabetes mellitus; DES, drug-eluting stent; ZES, zotarolimus-eluting stent; EES, everolimus-eluting stent; PES, paclitaxel-eluting stent; PES-E: PES-Express; PES-L: PES- Liberté; SES: sirolimus-eluting stent; ACM, all-cause mortality; MI, myocardial infarction; TLR, target-lesion revascularization; TVR, target-vessel revascularization; ST, stent thrombosis; TVMI, target-vessel myocardial infarction

Sirolimus versus Paclitaxel-eluting Stents

In the three major trials comparing sirolimus-eluting stents (SES) to paclitaxel-eluting stents (PES); sirolimus-eluting stents fared better as they reduced restenosis and major adverse cardiac and cerebrovascular event (MACCE) to a greater extent than PES.[48-50] The Paclitaxel-Eluting Stent versus Sirolimus-Eluting Stent for the Prevention of Restenosis in Diabetic Patients with Coronary Artery Disease (ISAR-DIABETES) trial stated that in-segment late luminal loss was 0.24 mm greater than in PES as compared to SES.[48] SIRTAX (Sirolimus-Eluting and Paclitaxel-Eluting Stents for Coronary Revascularization)[49] revealed that the HR for MACCE was less in SES as compared with PES, especially in the diabetic cohort. Angiographic follow-up in the REALITY trial revealed no difference in rate of binary angiographic in lesion restenosis. However, there was a more robust inhibition of neointimal hyperplasia by SES, while PES, unfortunately, had a higher incidence of in-stent thrombosis.[50] The randomized multicenter intravascular ultrasound (IVUS) study by Jensen et al. reiterated that PES generated more diffuse neointimal hyperplasia than SES.[51]

First (G1-DES) versus Second-generation (G2–DES) Drug-eluting Stents

In the SPIRIT IV trial, Everolimus-eluting Coronary Stent System (EES) compared with PES-reduced target lesion failure (TLF) in non-DM patients (3.1% vs 6.7%, $p < 0.0001$), with significant reductions in MI, stent thrombosis (ST), and TLR.[52] However, there was no difference in TLF (6.4% vs 6.9%, respectively, $p = 0.80$) among DM patients, regardless of insulin use. A SORT OUT III trial sub-study[53] also was not able to show any benefit of G2-DES, endeavor zotarolimus-eluting stent (ZES) on major adverse cardiac events.[53] To the contrary, in diabetics, use of ZES compared to SES was associated with an increased risk of MACE (HR 4.05, 95% CI 1.86–8.82), MI (HR 8.09, 95% CI 1.01–64.7), TVR (HR 4.99, 95% CI 1.90–13.1), and TLR (HR 11.0, 95% CI 2.59–47.1).[53] A pooled analysis of the ENDEAVOR III-IV trials showed that TVF rate estimate was lower for ZES, however, this difference was not statistically significant (20.2% vs 26.9%, $p = 0.065$).[54] The 5-year rate of MACE (17.7% vs 26.6%, $p = 0.012$), death (7.6% vs 15.0%, $p = 0.004$), and MI (1.3% vs 5.1%, $p = 0.011$)

were significantly lower for ZES versus other DES, suggesting that ZES may have favorable long-term outcomes compared to first-generation DES.[54] Kedhi et al.[55] compared Second-Generation Everolimus-Eluting Stents with First-Generation Drug-Eluting Stents in Diabetics. EES was associated with significantly lower event rates compared with SES [SES vs EES hazard ratio (HR): 1.99; 95% confidence interval (CI): 1.19 to 3.08] and PES (PES vs EES HR: 1.33; 95% CI: 0.93 to 1.91). These results were mainly driven by lower incidence of stent thrombosis (ST) (SES vs EES HR: 2.87; 95% CI: 1.08 to 7.61; PES vs EES HR: 1.74, 95% CI: 0.82 to 3.71) and mortality (SES vs EES HR: 2.02; 95% CI: 1.03 to 3.98; PES vs EES HR: 1.69; 95% CI: 1.06 to 2.72). No significant differences in restenosis rates were observed between EES and SES or PES (SES vs EES HR: 1.26; 95% CI: 0.77 to 2.08; PES vs EES HR: 1.05; 95% CI: 0.71 to 1.55).

TUXEDO-India (Taxus Element vs Xience Prime in a Diabetic Population) trial tested the controversy of PES vs EES in diabetic patients presenting with symptomatic (11.6% with STEMI, 53.2% with ACS/NSTEMI, 28.5% with stable angina) or silent (6.7%) ischemia. PES did not meet criterion for noninferiority, while EES met criteria for superiority with a decreased target-vessel failure at 1 year compared to PES by a relative risk of 0.53 (95% CI, 0.33–0.83).[56] A pooled analysis compared 3-year clinical outcomes between G1- and G2-DES according to the presence or absence of DM, using individual patient-level data from the RESET and NEXT trial[57] reiterated that the cumulative incidence of and adjusted hazard ratio (HR) for TLR were not significantly different between G2- and G1-DES in both strata [DM, 8.7% vs 10.1%, adjusted HR: 0.80, 95% confidence interval (CI) 0.59-1.10, p = 0.17; non-DM, 5.7% vs 6.2%, adjusted HR: 0.86, 95% CI 0.62-1.22, p = 0.38]. In the insulin-treated DM (ITDM), G2-DES had a significantly lower adjusted HR for TLR compared with G1-DES, although there was no significant difference in the non-ITDM (ITDM, adjusted HR: 0.54, 95% CI 0.32-0.96, p = 0.04; non-ITDM, adjusted HR: 0.95, 95% CI 0.66-1.42, p = 0.81). G2-DES provided similar risk for TLR in non-ITDM and non-DM patients compared with G1-DES. However, G2-DES compared with G1-DES had a lower risk for TLR among ITDM patients.[57] A meta-analysis comprising 42 trials and 22,884 patient-years of follow-up concluded that among all DES, the EES was the most efficacious and safe in patients with diabetes.[58]

Stent Thrombosis (ST) after DES Implantation in Cardiodiabetes

Although ST is multifactorial,[59] diabetics vs especially insulin-dependent patients—have higher rates of ST.[60-62] Smaller vessel size and longer lesion length are predictors of stent thrombosis.[63] Endothelial dysfunction[64] and platelet dysfunction[65] play a role in the development of ST in diabetics. Insulin-requiring DM is a significant independent predictor of definite or probable ST occurring within 30 days (odds ratio, 2.35; 95% CI, 1.36–4.07).[66] Patients with DM and ACS had a two-fold higher rate of ST than those without DM (2.8% vs 1.4%), with highest rates amongst insulin-dependent diabetics (3.7%).[67]

In a large 2-Institutional Cohort Study, DM was an independent predictor of overall, early, and late definite ST,[68] and the only predictor of early ST. Insulin-treated DM was also an independent predictor of ST in the SCAAR (1.8-fold increase)[69] and the e-Cypher registry (2.8-fold risk increase at 1-year).[60] As diabetics appear to be at a higher risk for ST, dual antiplatelet therapy beyond 1 year may be reasonable in high-risk patients,[70] and any cessation of antiplatelet therapy should be avoided.

G2-DES in Diabetics—Relevant Molecular Biology in Diabetic and Insulin-resistant Patients

Insulin is a potent mitogenic factor leading to cellular proliferation and growth[71] with the help of mTOR, which is a key nutrient and insulin-responsive protein-regulating growth and metabolism. Rapamycin (sirolimus) is an mTOR inhibitor and is known to exhibit immunosuppressive and anti-proliferative properties.[72,73] G2-DES use sirolimus derivatives, primarily everolimus and zotarolimus[74] and one may hypothesize that improved outcomes in diabetic patients with G2-DES are a direct molecular biology consequence of mTOR significance in the endothelium of insulin-resistant coronary arteries.[75]

As biomedical advances translate from the basic sciences laboratory to the catheterization laboratory, we expect more advance stent platforms, which would enhance survival benefit of PCI in the diabetic by decreasing TVR, TLR and ST and reducing MACCE.

CHRONICLES OF THE OPTIMAL REVASCULARIZATION STRATEGY IN THE DIABETIC PATIENT: PCI Vs CABG Vs HYBRID REVASCULARIZATION

Coronary artery bypass grafting (CABG) was the preferred form of revascularization till the dawning of the multivessel PCI era in early 1990s. However, major trials (EAST, RITA, ERACI and GABI) conducted before the historic 1996 Bypass Angioplasty Revascularization Investigation (BARI)[76] had an under-represented diabetic patient subset and, therefore, could derive no conclusions on the mortality benefit of multivessel PCI in diabetic patients.

Coronary Artery Bypass Grafting vs Multivessel PCI with Balloon Angioplasty

The BARI trial[76] was pivotal in establishing the vulnerability of diabetic patients to adverse outcomes after PCI. It demonstrated no significant difference in 5-year mortality (10.7% CABG vs 13.7% PCI, p = 0.19). However, increased frequency of revascularization was observed in the PCI arm (8% vs 54%, p < 0.001). Conversely, the diabetic subset of the BARI trial showed a significantly lower 5-year CABG mortality (19.4% vs 34.5%, p < 0.003) and 7-year mortality (23.6% vs 44%; p = 0.001].[77] The 10-year survival[78] was 71% for PTCA versus 73.5% for CABG.[78] However, in the diabetic subgroup, patients randomized to CABG had higher survival than those who underwent PCI (57.8% vs 45.5%, p = 0.025).[78]

This prompted the NAHBI to issue a clinical alert stating that CABG should be the preferred initial revascularization strategy in diabetics with multivessel CAD.[79] Analyses from multiple trials[80-82] conclude that the survival benefit of CABG is limited to diabetics receiving internal mammary artery (IMA) grafts—cardiac mortality was 2.9% with IMA, as compared with 18.2% with SVG conduits. The latter rate is similar to that in patients undergoing PCI.[79] The PCI subset of the BARI population underwent treatment of two lesions[83] versus the 3.1 graft deployed in the CABG subset.[84] A relook angiogram at 1 year in the diabetic BARI population,[85] as a result, revealed almost double the amount of jeopardized myocardium in the PCI subset than the CABG patient population (42% vs 24%, p = 0.05). The 90% mortality reduction of IMA bypass is mainly related to distal vessel protection from proximal disease progression and more complete revascularization (CR) offered by CABG over PCI.

However, all the BARI patients did not receive the current PCI standard of care, including stents and drugs and, therefore, although significant, the results must not be applied blindly to our current-day practice.

Coronary Artery Bypass Grafting versus Multivessel PCI with Intracoronary Stents (Bare-metal Stents)

The ARTS trial demonstrated that diabetics in PCI group had the lowest 1-year event-free survival (63.4% vs 84% in CABG; p < 0.001), almost entirely due to TVR.[86] At 5-years,[87] MACCE in diabetics treated with stents was 55%, versus 39% in nondiabetes; mainly due to higher rate of repeat revascularization (43% vs 28%). Conversely, no significant difference was found in 5-year MACCE rate between patients with and without diabetes treated with CABG (25% vs 21%).[87] In the stents or surgery trial,[88] incidence of death or Q-wave MI was similar in both groups (PCI 9%, CABG 10%; p = 0.80) at 2 years. However, the need for TVR was higher at 21% in PCI group, as compared with 6% in CABG group (p < 0.0001). The AWESOME study[89] randomized a sicker patient population with one of five high-risk features (prior CABG, MI within last 7 days, ejection fraction less than 35%, age more than 70 years or IABP for hemodynamic stabilization). 30-day survivals for CABG and PCI were 95% and 97%, respectively. Survival rates for CABG and PCI were 90% versus 94% at 6 months and 79% versus 80% at 36 months (log-rank test, p = 0.46). The authors concluded that PCI is an alternative to CABG for patients with medically refractory myocardial ischemia and a high risk of adverse outcomes with CABG.[89] A recent meta-analysis,[90] which included 10 major studies of revascularization (balloon angioplasty/BMS versus CABG), reported that in diabetics (CABG, n = 615; PCI, n = 618), mortality was substantially lower in the CABG group than in the PCI group (HR 0.70, 0.56–0.87 95% CI); unlike nondiabetics where it was similar (HR 0.98, 0.86–1.12; p = 0.014).

Coronary Artery Bypass Grafting vs PCI with Drug-eluting Stents

The landmark SYNergy between percutaneous coronary intervention with TAXus and cardiac surgery (SYNTAX)[91] trial tested G1-DES against CABG in left-main or three-vessel disease based on an anatomic, angiographically derived score. It concluded that in diabetics, the 1-year composite MACCE rate was significantly higher after PES compared with CABG (RR 1.83). The RR of repeat revascularization of PES over CABG was 3.18 in diabetics as compared with 1.94 in nondiabetics. Diabetics had higher mortality after PES use in highly complex lesions, that is, with SYNTAX score > 33, (13.5% vs 4.1%). The authors reported no significant difference in mortality after PCI as compared to CABG in the diabetic subgroup at 5 years (19.5% vs 12.9%; p = 0.065).[92] Arterial Revascularization Therapies Study–Part II[93] concluded that PCI using SES was safer and more efficacious than using BMS in both diabetics and nondiabetics and was a valuable alternative to CABG in patients with diabetes as well. The FREEDOM[94] trial reported a higher rate of the composite of all-cause death, MI, or stroke after PCI than after CABG (26.6% vs 18.7%; p = 0.005), driven by higher rates of MI (13.9% vs 6.0%, p < 0.001) and death from any cause at 5 years (16.3% vs 11.0%; p = 0.049).

Both the old BARI[95] and the new EVENT (Evaluation of Drug-eluting stents and ischemic events)[96] registries have demonstrated that multivessel PCI for diabetics is feasible and safe outside the confines of a randomized clinical trial.[97] Bangalore et al.[98] concluded that survival after implantation of platinum-chromium everolimus-eluting stents might be no different from that after CABG in diabetic patients with multivessel disease. In unprotected left main disease (UPLMS), the EXCEL trial[99] and the NOBLE trial[100] had opposing results, posing a quandary for the physician. Stone et al. concluded[99] that patients with low- or intermediate-SYNTAX scores treated with an everolimus-eluting metallic stent had comparable rates of death, stroke, or MI at 3 years when compared with patients treated with CABG surgery. To the contrary, in the NOBLE trial,[100] treatment with PCI using predominantly a biolimus-eluting stent was associated with a significantly higher rate of MACE at 5 years when compared with CABG surgery (Table 2).

Best of Both Worlds—Hybrid Revascularization in the Diabetic

An alternative strategy to either CABG—or PCI-only approach in multivessel revascularization with the intent of obtaining CR and the survival benefit of an LIMA graft is a "hybrid approach"[101]—a minimally invasive surgical strategy of an LIMA anastomosed to the LAD artery, and PCI of other significant lesions. Advantages are a quicker patient recovery and avoidance of both the risks of an increased systemic inflammatory response to cardiopulmonary bypass and delayed wound healing from a full sternotomy. Although no RCT of hybrid revascularization versus CABG alone or PCI alone has been performed; a retrospective study of 103 diabetic patients,[102] who received hybrid revascularization, propensity matched with 515 patients who underwent CABG,[12] reported similar outcomes of death/MI/stroke at 30 days (4.9% and 3.9%, respectively, p = 0.66), and similar mortality after a 3-year follow-up

TABLE 2: Pivotal studies comparing percutaneous coronary intervention (PCI) with coronary artery bypass grafting (CABG) in diabetic patients

S. No	Study, Year [Reference]	Patient Population	Study Type	Patient with DM/Total Patient	DM patient distribution		PCI, Type	Primary endpoint	% of DM patients meeting primary endpoint		Long-term outcome DM subset [%]		Conclusion
					PCI	CABG			PCI	CABG	PCI	CABG	
1	BARI, 1988–1991 [76]	MVCAD	RCT	353/ 1729 [19%]	173	180	POBA	Survival	65.5	80.6	10-year survival : 57.8	10-year survival : 45.5	CABG associated with better survival in MVD
2	SYNTAX, 2005–2007 [91]	LMD/3VD	RCT	296/1095 [30.7%]	143	153	PES	ACM, stroke, MI, repeat revascular-ization	45.5	23.6	5-year mortality : 19.5	5-year mortality : 12.9	CABG better in patients with 3VD
3	FREEDOM, 2005–2010 [94]	Diabetics with MVCAD	RCT	1900/1900 [100%]	953	947	PES	ACM, MI, stroke	26.6	18.7	5-year mortality: 27	5-year mortality: 19	CABG superior to PCI, however with more stroke
4	EXCEL, 2010–2014 [99]	LMD	RCT	505/1905 [29%]	256	249	EES	ACM, MI, stroke	21.2	19.4	3-year mortality : 20.3	3-year mortality: 19.6	Low - / intermedi-ate—SYNTAX scores with EES had com-parable rates of death/ stroke/MI at 3 years

Abbreviations: BARI, bypass angioplasty revascularization investigation; SYNTAX, synergy between PCI with taxus and cardiac surgery; FREEDOM, Future Revascularization Evaluation in Patients with Diabetes Mellitus: Optimal Management of Multivessel Disease; EXCEL, Evaluation of Xience Prime or Xience V Stents Versus Coronary Artery Bypass Grafting for Effectiveness of Left Main Revascularization; 3VD, three-vessel disease; LMD, left-main disease; MVCAD, multivessel coronary artery disease; POBA, plain old balloon angioplasty; PTCA, percutaneous transluminal coronary angioplasty; PCI, percutaneous coronary intervention; CABG, coronary artery bypass grafting; RCT, randomized-controlled trial; PES, paclitaxel-eluting stent; SES, sirolimus-eluting stent; EES, everolimus-eluting stent; non-MI, nonfatal myocardial infarction; ACM, all-cause mortality

(12.3% and 14.9%, p = 0.86). Hybrid procedures remain rare as of now, however, due to multiple factors: patients are unwilling to undergo randomization for up to two invasive procedures, and most hospitals lack hybrid operating suites with fully capable surgical and interventional modalities.

Which Diabetic Patient is the Ideal Candidate for Percutaneous Coronary Intervention?

In unstable CAD, diabetic patients derive a larger benefit with an early—invasive versus a delayed strategy,[103] as concluded by Norhammar et al.[104] The number needed to treat (NNT) for diabetic patients was 11 to prevent one death or MI, as compared to an NNT of 32 for nondiabetic patients.[104]

REVASCULARIZATION STRATEGY

Revascularization Strategy According to Clinical Presentation

- *Stable ischemic heart disease (SIHD)*:
  - *Low-risk subset*: Diabetic patients with SIHD, who remain symptomatic despite optimal medical therapy (OMT); patients with focal disease, and a low SYNTAX score of more than or equal to 22 can be offered PCI,[105] as long-term outcomes for this subgroup treated with PCI are favorable[92] and there is a lower risk of stroke after PCI than after CABG (2.4% vs 5.2%, p = 0.03].[94]
  - *High-risk subset*: In case of extensive multivessel CAD, especially if left main or proximal LAD is involved, CABG should be the preferred revascularization strategy.[105,106]
- *Acute coronary syndromes (ACS)*:
  - *Acute ST-segment-elevation myocardial infarction (STEMI)*: Diabetic patients presenting with STEMI should have emergent PCI of the culprit lesion, provided coronary anatomy is PCI-amenable. In case of multivessel CAD, the Heart Team comprising cardiologists, cardiac surgeons and imaging specialists should decide the optimal revascularization strategy (OMT/PCI/CABG/hybrid) to tackle the remaining significant obstructive CAD.[105]
  - *ST-segment-elevation myocardial infarction with cardiogenic shock*: Multivessel PCI with/without hemodynamic support may be considered as an option to emergency CABG.[107]
  - *Non-ST-segment-elevation ACS (NSTE-ACS)*:
    - ♦ Diabetics with NSTE-ACS and amenable coronary artery anatomy may benefit from early revascularization with PCI.[105]
    - ♦ Diabetics with NSTE-ACS and multivessel CAD should follow the STEMI protocol underlined above: emergent PCI of the culprit vessel followed by a heart team decision.[107]

From the patient's subjective perspective, relief from ischemic symptoms and subsequent improvement in quality of life (QoL) are perhaps as important as quantification of the survival benefit of one revascularization strategy over another.

Complete versus Incomplete Revascularization in the Patient with Cardiodiabetes

Incomplete revascularization (IR) after PCI occurs in 47% of patients with diabetes and 43% in patients without diabetes.[108] Complete revascularization (CR), as compared to IR, resulted in a greater absolute risk reduction in diabetic patients (14.6%) than nondiabetic patients (8.1%) over 5 years of follow-up.[108] A large meta-analysis of 83,695 patients[109] concluded that in multivessel CAD, as compared with IR, CR confers a clinical benefit that seems larger in cohorts of patients enrolled in more recent studies and with a higher prevalence of diabetes [reduced mortality in either CABG or PCI (overall HR 0.73, 95% CI 0.66–0.81)].

Collectively, the data from CABG versus PCI and complete versus incomplete revascularization strategies suggest that the best possible outcomes for diabetic patients with symptomatic, multivessel CAD is a strategy of durable and complete revascularization.

ANTIPLATELET/ANTITHROMBOTIC STRATEGIES IN THE DIABETIC PATIENTS

Aspirin

Low-dose aspirin is the bedrock of antiplatelet therapy for the management of ACS and for secondary prevention of recurrent ischemic events[110] in patients with cardiovascular disease, including those with DM.[106,111] The CURRENT-OASIS 7 trial, which included ACS patients scheduled to undergo early CAG, did not find any difference in 30-day ischemic events between high-dose versus low-dose aspirin. However, higher rates of GI bleed were observed in high-dose versus low-dose group (0.38% vs 0.24%, p = 0.051).[112,113]

P2Y12 Inhibitors

- *Clopidogrel*: It remains the most commonly prescribed antiplatelet drug. However, low response to clopidogrel or "clopidogrel resistance" and atherothrombotic events in high-risk patients with ACS or those treated with PCI,[114] has led to the conclusion that high-dose clopidogrel (600 mg loading or 150 mg daily maintenance) strategy is associated with enhanced platelet inhibition and reduced risk for high platelet reactivity.[115] The impaired metabolism of clopidogrel in some diabetic patients has led to subgroup analyses of RCTs to evaluate alternative P2Y2 inhibitors and a class IIb recommendation for treatment with these drugs in patients identified with HPR on clopidogrel.[116]

- *Prasugrel*: The TRITON TIMI 38[117,118] trial revealed lower rates of cardiovascular death, nonfatal MI, or nonfatal stroke with prasugrel than clopidogrel in diabetics (12.2% vs 17.0%), without DM (9.2% vs 10.6%), and without increased major bleeding (2.6% vs 2.5%).
- *Ticagrelor*: The groundbreaking PLATelet inhibition and patient Outcomes (PLATO) trial compared ticagrelor versus clopidogrel for 18,624 patients admitted with ACS and reported a decrease in the primary combined endpoint of death, MI, or stroke at 1 year for ticagrelor compared to clopidogrel (hazard ratio 0.84, 95% CI 0.77–0.92, $p < 0.001$).[119] Patients with high HbA1 C levels benefited the most from ticagrelor with reductions in primary endpoint, death, and ST (HR 0.80, 95% CI 0.7–0.91; HR 0.78, 95% CI 065–0.93; and HR 0.62, 95% CI 0.39–1, respectively) and similar bleeding rates.[120]

The current guidelines do not recommend any one P2Y12 drug over the others in the diabetic subset.[106,111,116]

Duration of Dual Antiplatelet Therapy

In patients with stable ischemic heart disease (SIHD) treated with DAPT after DES implantation, $P2Y_{12}$ inhibitor therapy with clopidogrel should be given for atleast 6 months (Class I).[121] In patients with ACS (NSTE-ACS or STEMI) treated with PCI, who have tolerated DAPT without a bleeding complication and who are not at high bleeding risk (e.g. prior bleeding on DAPT, coagulopathy, oral anticoagulant use), continuation of DAPT (clopidogrel, prasugrel, or ticagrelor) for longer than 12 months may be reasonable (Class IIb).[121] A new risk score (the "DAPT score"), derived from the Dual Antiplatelet Therapy study, may be useful for decisions about whether to continue (prolong or extend) DAPT in patients treated with coronary stent implantation.[121]

Gp IIb-IIIa Inhibitors

A meta-analysis of 16 randomized trials including 10,085 patients showed that Gp IIb-IIIa inhibitors did not reduce 30-day mortality (2.8% vs 2.9%, $p = 0.75$) or re-infarction (1.5% vs 1.9%, $p = 0.22$). However, they were associated with higher risk of major bleeding complications (4.1% vs 2.7%, $p = 0.0004$).[122] However, high-risk ACS patients associated with benefits in terms of death ($p = 0.008$) but not re-infarction ($p = 0.25$). In contrast, the CADILLAC trial conducted in low-risk ACS patients with DM ($n = 346$) did not find a benefit in terms of death, reinfarction, or stroke with the use of abciximab after balloon angioplasty or stenting.[123] In the current era of routine thienopyridine and direct thrombin inhibitor use; GPI usage should be limited to patients undergoing PCI for NSTEMI, primary PCI, and undergoing PCI without appropriate preloading with a thienopyridine. Moreover, strategies to minimize bleeding should be applied in these patients, such as shorter GPI infusions and dose adjustments of heparin and GPI.[124]

Potent anticoagulation in diabetic patients undergoing PCI with potent P2Y12 inhibitors with/without GPIIb-IIIA inhibitors should be used on an individualized basis after a careful risk–benefit assessment. Diabetics remain at a higher risk of ischemic events, regardless of the antiplatelet strategy used.

CONCLUSION

Diabetes is a complex and systemic disorder of metabolism, proliferation and inflammation, which has attained pandemic proportion. Diabetics have more aggressive CAD and increased CV events than their nondiabetic counterparts and would benefit the most from early and complete revascularization. However, unfortunately, incident diabetes is underdiagnosed and undertreated in patients hospitalized with ACS. As physicians, we must understand that a revascularization procedure is a vital component of a comprehensive treatment strategy, which includes compliance with the drug therapy, cardiac rehabilitation, aggressive risk factor control and stress management.

Coronary artery bypass grafting, preferentially with an LIMA to LAD anastomosis, is the Class I recommendation for revascularization in diabetics with multivessel CAD. However, substantial equipoise and controversy exist amidst the choice between CABG versus PCI as progressively newer DESs enter the terrain. From a futuristic perspective; basic science would further target elucidation of molecular mechanisms, which prompt aggressive atherosclerosis in the diabetic patients. Biomedical leaders would translate this data into designing novel stent designs and novel platforms, including the third generation of DES consisting of drug-eluting bioresorbable vascular scaffolds or polymer-free drug-eluting coatings on metal alloys. Data would emerge on the outcomes of these new players on the block and science would continue to evolve. However, amidst all the novelty and change, one thing remains consistent for the practicing physician. The approach to each diabetic patient requiring coronary revascularization must be personalized taking into account his clinical presentation, coronary tree anatomy and a constructive discussion between the multidisciplinary Heart Team and each individual's priorities and preferences. We must bear in mind that from the patient's subjective perspective, relief from ischemic symptoms and subsequent improvement in quality of life (QoL) are perhaps as important as quantification of the survival benefit of one revascularization strategy over another.

REFERENCES

1. Mathewkutty S, McGuire DK. Platelet perturbations in diabetes: implications for cardiovascular disease risk and treatment. Expert Rev Cardiovasc Ther. 2009;7(5):541-9.
2. Kannel WB, McGee DL. Diabetes and cardiovascular disease. The Framingham study. JAMA. 1979;241(19):2035-8.
3. Haffner SM, Lehto S, Ronnemaa T, et al. Mortality from coronary heart disease in subjects with type 2 diabetes and in nondiabetic subjects with and without prior myocardial infarction. N Engl J Med. 1998;339:229-34.
4. National Institute for Health and Clinical Excellence. Clinical Guideline 67. Lipid Modification. Cardiovascular risk assessment and the modification of blood lipids for the primary and secondary prevention of cardiovascular disease. May 2008.
5. National Institute for Health and Clinical Excellence. Clinical Guideline 66. Type 2 diabetes. May 2008.
6. Ryden L, Standl E, Bartnik M, et al. Guidelines on diabetes, pre-diabetes, and cardiovascular diseases: executive summary. The Task Force on Diabetes and Cardiovascular Diseases of the European Society of Cardiology (ESC) and of the European Association for the Study of Diabetes (EASD). Eur Heart J. 2007;28:88-136.
7. Ogurtsova K, da Rocha Fernandes JD, Huang Y, et al. IDF Diabetes Atlas: Global estimates for the prevalence of diabetes for 2015 and 2040. Diabetes Res Clin Pract. 2017;128:40-50.
8. Beckman JA, Creager MA, Libby P. Diabetes and atherosclerosis: epidemiology, pathophysiology, and management. JAMA. 2002;287(19):2570-81.
9. Norhammar A, Malmberg K, Diderholm E, et al. Diabetes mellitus: the major risk factor in unstable coronary artery disease even after consideration of the extent of coronary artery disease and benefits of revascularization. J Am Coll Cardiol. 2004;43(4):585-91.
10. Martinez SC, Holmes DR. Controversies surrounding percutaneous coronary intervention in the diabetic patient. Expert Rev Cardiovasc Ther. 2016;14(5):633-48.
11. Williams DO, Holubkov R, Yeh W, et al. Percutaneous coronary intervention in the current era compared with 1985–1986: the National Heart, Lung, and Blood Institute Registries. Circulation. 2000;102(24):2945-51.
12. Kip KE, Faxon DP, Detre KM, et al. Coronary angioplasty in diabetic patients. The National Heart, Lung, and Blood Institute Percutaneous Transluminal Coronary Angioplasty Registry. Circulation. 1996;94(8):1818-25.
13. Marso SP, Giorgi LV, Johnson WL, et al. Diabetes mellitus is associated with a shift in the temporal risk profile of in-hospital death after percutaneous coronary intervention: an analysis of 25,223 patients over 20 years. Am Heart J. 2003;145(2):270-7.
14. Freeman AM, Abbott JD, Jacobs AK, et al. Marked improvements in outcomes of contemporary percutaneous coronary intervention in patients with diabetes mellitus. J Interv Cardiol. 2006;19(6):475-82.
15. Goldberg S, Savage MP, Fischman DL. The interventional cardiologist and the diabetic patient. Have we pushed the envelope too far or not far enough? Circulation. 1996;94(8):1804-6.
16. Abizaid A, Kornowski R, Mintz GS, et al. The influence of diabetes mellitus on acute and late clinical outcomes following coronary stent implantation. J Am Coll Cardiol. 1998;32(3):584-9.
17. Bittl JA. Percutaneous coronary interventions in the diabetic patient: where do we stand? Circ Cardiovasc Interv. 2015;8(4):e001944.
18. Lorenz DP, Carrozza JP, Garcia L. Diabetes and Percutaneous Interventional Therapy. Diabetes and percutaneous interventional therapy. In: Johnstone MT, Veves A (Eds). Diabetes and cardiovascular disease. Boston: Humana Press; 2005. pp. 519-41.
19. Van Belle E, Bauters C, Hubert E, et al. Restenosis rates in diabetic patients: a comparison of coronary stenting and balloon angioplasty in native coronary vessels. Circulation. 1997;96:1454-60.
20. Elezi S, Kastrati A, Pache J, et al. Diabetes mellitus and the clinical and angiographic outcome after coronary stent placement. J Am Coll Cardiol. 1998;32:1866-73.
21. Schofer J, Schluter M, Rau T, et al. Influence of treatment modality on angiographic outcome after coronary stenting in diabetic patients: a controlled study. J Am Coll Cardiol. 2000;35:1554-9.
22. Van Belle E, Abolmaali K, Bauters C, et al. Restenosis, late vessel occlusion and left ventricular function six months after balloon angioplasty in diabetic patients. J Am Coll Cardiol. 1999;34:476-85.
23. Mak KH, Faxon DP. Clinical studies on coronary revascularization in patients with type 2 diabetes. Eur Heart J. 2003;24:1087-103.
24. Van Belle E, Ketelers R, Bauters C, et al. Patency of percutaneous transluminal coronary angioplasty sites at 6- month angiographic follow-up: A key determinant of survival in diabetics after coronary balloon angioplasty. Circulation. 2001;103(9):1218-24.
25. Stein B, Weintraub WS, Gebhart SP, et al. Influence of diabetes mellitus on early and late outcome after percutaneous transluminal coronary angioplasty. Circulation. 1995;91(4):979-89.
26. Holmes DR Jr, Vlietstra RE, Smith HC, et al. Restenosis after percutaneous transluminal coronary angioplasty (PTCA): a report from the PTCA Registry of the National Heart, Lung, and Blood Institute. Am J Cardiol. 1984;53(12):77C-81C.
27. Cutlip DE, Chauhan MS, Baim DS, et al. Clinical restenosis after coronary stenting: perspectives from multicenter clinical trials. J Am Coll Cardiol. 2002;40:2082-9.
28. Corpus RA, George PB, House JA, et al. Optimal glycemic control is associated with a lower rate of target vessel revascularization in treated type II diabetic patients undergoing elective percutaneous coronary intervention. J Am Coll Cardiol. 2004;43:8-14.
29. Elezi S, Kastrati A, Pache J, et al. Diabetes mellitus and the clinical and angiographic outcome after coronary stent placement. J Am Coll Cardiol 1998;32(7):1866-73.
30. West NE, Ruygrok PN, Disco CM, et al. Clinical and angiographic predictors of restenosis after stent deployment in diabetic patients. Circulation. 2004;109:867-73.
31. Mathew V, Gersh BJ, Williams BA, et al. Outcomes in patients with diabetes mellitus undergoing percutaneous coronary intervention in the current era: a report from the Prevention of REStenosis with Tranilast and its Outcomes (PRESTO) Trial. Circulation. 2004;109:476-80.
32. Laskey WK, Selzer F, Vlachos HA, et al. Comparison of in-hospital and one-year outcomes in patients with and without diabetes mellitus undergoing percutaneous catheter intervention (from the National Heart, Lung, and Blood Institute Dynamic Registry). Am J Cardiol. 2002;90:1062-7.

33. Srinivas VS, Brooks MM, Detre KM, et al. Contemporary percutaneous coronary intervention versus balloon angioplasty for multivessel coronary artery disease: a comparison of the National Heart, Lung and Blood Institute Dynamic Registry and the Bypass Angioplasty Revascularization Investigation (BARI) study. Circulation. 2002;106:1627-33.
34. Carrozza JP Jr, Kuntz RE, Fishman RF, et al. Restenosis after arterial injury caused by coronary stenting in patients with diabetes mellitus. Ann Intern Med. 1993;118(5):344-9.
35. Savage MP, Fischman DL, Schatz RA, et al. Coronary intervention in the diabetic patient: improved outcome following stent implantation compared with balloon angioplasty. Clin Cardiol. 2002;25(5):213-7.
36. Van Belle E, Périé M, Braune D, et al. Effects of coronary stenting on vessel patency and long-term clinical outcome after percutaneous coronary revascularization in diabetic patients. J Am Coll Cardiol. 2002;40(3):410-7.
37. Sabate M, Jimenez-Quevedo P, Angiolillo DJ, et al. Randomized comparison of sirolimus-eluting stent versus standard stent for percutaneous coronary revascularization in diabetic patients: the diabetes and sirolimus-eluting stent (DIABETES) trial. Circulation. 2005;112:2175-83.
38. Morice MC, Serruys PW, Sousa JE, et al. A randomized comparison of a sirolimus-eluting stent with a standard stent for coronary revascularization. N Engl J Med. 2002;346(23):1773-80.
39. Leon M. The SIRIUS trial. Presented at the Transcatheter Therapeutics meeting, September 24, 2002, Washington, DC.
40. Stone G. TAXUS-IV. The pivotal, prospective, randomized trial of the slow-rate release polymer- based paclitaxel-eluting TAXUS stent. Clinical overview and subset analysis. Presented at the Transcatheter Therapeutics Meeting, September 16, 2003, Washington, DC.
41. Moussa I, Leon MB, Baim DS, et al. Impact of sirolimus-eluting stents on outcome in diabetic patients: a SIRIUS (SIRolImUS-coated Bx Velocity balloon-expandable stent in the treatment of patients with de novo coronary artery lesions) substudy. Circulation. 2004;109:2273-8.
42. Hermiller JB, Raizner A, Cannon L, et al. Outcomes with the polymer-based paclitaxel-eluting TAXUS stent in patients with diabetes mellitus: the TAXUS-IV trial. J Am Coll Cardiol. 2005;45:1172-9.
43. Stettler C, Allemann S, Wandel S, et al. Drug-eluting and bare-metal stents in people with and without diabetes: collaborative network meta-analysis. BMJ. 2008;337:a1331.
44. Stettler C, Wandel S, Allemann S, et al. Outcomes associated with drug-eluting and bare-metal stents: a collaborative network meta-analysis. Lancet. 2007;370:937-48.
45. Stenestrand U, James SK, Lindback J, et al. Safety and efficacy of drug-eluting vs. bare-metal stents in patients with diabetes mellitus: long-term of follow-up in the Swedish Coronary Angiography and Angioplasty Registry (SCAAR). Eur Heart J. 2010;31(2):177-86.
46. Babapulle MN, Joseph L, Belisle P, et al. A hierarchical Bayesian meta-analysis of randomised clinical trials of drug-eluting stents. Lancet. 2004;364:583-91.
47. Trikalinos TA, Alsheikh-Ali AA, Tatsioni A, et al. Percutaneous coronary interventions for non-acute coronary artery disease: a quantitative 20-year synopsis and a network meta-analysis. Lancet. 2009;373:911-8.
48. Dibra A, Kastrati A, Mehilli J, et al. Paclitaxel-eluting or sirolimus-eluting stents to prevent restenosis in diabetic patients. N Engl J Med. 2005;353:663-70.
49. Windecker S, Remondino A, Eberli FR, et al. Sirolimus-eluting and paclitaxel-eluting stents for coronary revascularization. N Engl J Med. 2005;353:653-62.
50. Morice MC, Colombo A, Meier B, et al. Sirolimus- vs paclitaxel-eluting stents in de novo coronary artery lesions: the REALITY trial: a randomized controlled trial. JAMA. 2006;295(8):895-904.
51. Jensen LO, Maeng M, Thayssen P, et al. Neointimal hyperplasia after sirolimus-eluting and paclitaxel-eluting stent implantation in diabetic patients: the Randomized Diabetes and Drug-Eluting Stent (DiabeDES) Intravascular Ultrasound Trial. Eur Heart J. 2008;29:2733-41.
52. Kereiakes DJ, Cutlip DE, Applegate RJ, et al. Outcomes in diabetic and nondiabetic patients treated with everolimus- or paclitaxel-eluting stents: results from the SPIRIT IV clinical trial (Clinical Evaluation of the XIENCE V Everolimus-Eluting Coronary Stent System). J Am Coll Cardiol. 2010;56:2084-9.
53. Maeng M, Jensen LO, Tilsted HH, et al. Outcome of sirolimus-eluting versus zotarolimus-eluting coronary stent implantation in patients with and without diabetes mellitus (a SORT OUT III Substudy). Am J Cardiol. 2011;108:1232-7.
54. Vardi M, Burke DA, Bangalore S, et al. Long-term efficacy and safety of Zotarolimus-eluting stent in patients with diabetes mellitus: pooled 5-year results from the ENDEAVOR III and IV trials. Catheter Cardiovasc Interv. 2013;82:1031-8.
55. Kedhi E, Gomes ME, Lagerqvist B, et al. Clinical Impact of Second-Generation Everolimus-Eluting Stent Compared With First-Generation Drug-Eluting Stents in Diabetes Mellitus Patients. JACC: Cardiovascular Interventions. 2012;5(11):1141-9.
56. Kaul U, Bangalore S, Seth A, et al. Paclitaxel-eluting versus everolimus-eluting coronary stents in diabetes. N Engl J Med. 2015;373(18):1709-19.
57. Nakatsuma K, Shiomi H, Natsuaki M, et al. Second-generation versus first-generation drug-eluting stents in patients with and without diabetes mellitus: pooled analysis from the RESET and NEXT trials. Cardiovasc Interv Ther. 2017 Feb 1.
58. Bangalore S, Kumar S, Fusaro M, et al. Outcomes with various drug-eluting or bare-metal stents in patients with diabetes mellitus: mixed treatment comparison analysis of 22,844 patient years of follow-up from randomised trials. BMJ. 2012;345:e5170.
59. Windecker S, Meier B. Late coronary stent thrombosis. Circulation. 2007;116:1952-65.
60. Urban P, Gershlick AH, Guagliumi G, et al. Safety of coronary sirolimus-eluting stents in daily clinical practice: one-year follow-up of the e-Cypher registry. Circulation. 2006;113:1434-41.
61. Iakovou I, Schmidt T, Bonizzoni E, et al. Incidence, predictors, and outcome of thrombosis after successful implantation of drug-eluting stents. JAMA. 2005;293:2126-30.
62. Machecourt J, Danchin N, Lablanche JM, et al. Risk factors for stent thrombosis after implantation of sirolimus-eluting stents in diabetic and nondiabetic patients: the EVASTENT Matched-Cohort Registry. J Am Coll Cardiol. 2007;50:501-8.
63. Daemen J, Wenaweser P, Tsuchida K, et al. Early and late coronary stent thrombosis of sirolimus-eluting and paclitaxel-eluting stents in routine clinical practice: data from a large two-institutional cohort study. Lancet. 2007;369:667-78.
64. Rask-Madsen C, King GL. Mechanisms of Disease: endothelial dysfunction in insulin resistance and diabetes. Nat Clin Pract Endocrinol Metab. 2007;3:46-56.
65. Colwell JA, Nesto RW. The platelet in diabetes: focus on prevention of ischemic events. Diabetes Care. 2003;26:2181-8.
66. Aoki J, Lansky AJ, Mehran R, et al. Early stent thrombosis in patients with acute coronary syndromes treated with drug-eluting and bare metal stents: the Acute Catheterization and Urgent Intervention Triage Strategy trial. Circulation. 2009;119:687-98.
67. Wiviott SD, Braunwald E, Angiolillo DJ, et al. Greater clinical benefit of more intensive oral antiplatelet therapy with prasugrel in patients with diabetes mellitus in the trial to assess improvement in therapeutic outcomes by optimizing platelet inhibition with prasugrel-Thrombolysis in Myocardial Infarction 38. Circulation. 2008;118:1626-36.

68. Wenaweser P, Daemen J, Zwahlen M, et al. Incidence and correlates of drug-eluting stent thrombosis in routine clinical practice. 4-year results from a large 2-institutional cohort study. J Am Coll Cardiol. 2008;52:1134-40.
69. Lagerqvist B, Carlsson J, Frobert O, et al. Stent thrombosis in Sweden: a report from the Swedish coronary angiography and angioplasty registry. Circ Cardiovasc Interv. 2009;2:401-8.
70. King SB 3rd, Smith SC Jr, Hirshfeld JW Jr, et al. 2007 Focused Update of the ACC/AHA/SCAI 2005 Guideline Update for Percutaneous Coronary Intervention: a report of the American College of Cardiology/American Heart Association Task Force on Practice Guidelines: 2007 Writing Group to Review New Evidence and Update the ACC/AHA/SCAI 2005 Guideline Update for Percutaneous Coronary Intervention, Writing on Behalf of the 2005 Writing Committee. Circulation. 2008;117:261-95.
71. Bedinger DH, Adams SH. Metabolic, anabolic, and mitogenic insulin responses: a tissue-specific perspective for insulin receptor activators. Mol Cell Endocrinol. 2015;415:143-56.
72. Strimpakos AS, Karapanagiotou EM, Saif MW, et al. The role of mTOR in the management of solid tumors: an overview. Cancer Treat Rev. 2009;35(2):148-59.
73. Sabatini DM, Erdjument-Bromage H, Lui M, et al. RAFT1: a mammalian protein that binds to FKBP12 in a rapamycin-dependent fashion and is homologous to yeast TORs. Cell. 1994;78(1):35-43.
74. Gogas BD, McDaniel M, Samady H, et al. Novel drug-eluting stents for coronary revascularization. Trends Cardiovasc Med. 2014;24 (7):305-13.
75. Kedhi E, Gomes ME, Lagerqvist B, et al. Clinical impact of second-generation everolimus-eluting stent compared with first-generation drug-eluting stents in diabetes mellitus patients: insights from a nationwide coronary intervention register. JACC Cardiovasc Interv. 2012;5(11):1141-9.
76. Comparison of coronary bypass surgery with angioplasty in patients with multivessel disease. The Bypass Angioplasty Revascularization Investigation (BARI) Investigators. N Engl J Med. 1996;335(4):217-25.
77. BARI Investigators. Seven-year outcome in the Bypass Angioplasty Revascularization Investigation (BARI) by treatment and diabetic status. J Am Coll Cardiol. 2000;35(5):1122-9.
78. The final 10-year follow-up results from the BARI randomized trial. J Am Coll Cardiol. 2007;49:1600-6.
79. Ferguson JJ. NHBLI BARI clinical alert on diabetics treated with angioplasty. Circulation. 1995;92(12):3371.
80. Hirotani T, Kameda T, Kumamoto T, et al. Effects of coronary artery bypass grafting using internal mammary arteries for diabetic patients. J Am Coll Cardiol. 1999;34(2):532-8.
81. Morris JJ, Smith LR, Jones RH, et al. Influence of diabetes and mammary artery grafting on survival after coronary bypass. Circulation. 1991;84(5 Suppl):III275-III284.
82. Farinas JM, Carrier M, Hébert Y, et al. Comparison of long-term clinical results of double versus single internal mammary artery bypass grafting. Ann Thorac Surg. 1999;67(2):466-70.
83. Influence of diabetes on 5-year mortality and morbidity in a randomized trial comparing CABG and PTCA in patients with multivessel disease: the Bypass Angioplasty Revascularization Investigation (BARI). Circulation. 1997;96(6):1761-9.
84. Schaff HV, Rosen AD, Shemin RJ, et al. Clinical and operative characteristics of patients randomized to coronary artery bypass surgery in the Bypass Angioplasty Revascularization Investigation (BARI). Am J Cardiol. 1995;75(9):18C-26C.
85. Kip KE, Alderman EL, Bourassa MG, et al. Differential influence of diabetes mellitus on increased jeopardized myocardium after initial angioplasty or bypass surgery: bypass angioplasty revascularization investigation. Circulation. 2002;105(16):1914-20.
86. Serruys PW, Unger F, Sousa JE, et al. Comparison of coronary-artery bypass surgery and stenting for the treatment of multivessel disease. N Engl J Med. 2001;344(15):1117-24.
87. Serruys PW, Ong AT, van Herwerden LA, et al. Five-year outcomes after coronary stenting versus bypass surgery for the treatment of multivessel disease: the final analysis of the Arterial Revascularization Therapies Study (ARTS) randomized trial. J Am Coll Cardiol. 2005;46:575-81.
88. Coronary artery bypass surgery versus percutaneous coronary intervention with stent implantation in patients with multivessel coronary artery disease (the Stent or Surgery trial): a randomized controlled trial. Lancet. 2002;360(9338):965-70.
89. Sedlis SP, Morrison DA, Lorin JD, et al. Percutaneous coronary intervention versus coronary bypass graft surgery for diabetic patients with unstable angina and risk factors for adverse outcomes with bypass: outcome of diabetic patients in the AWESOME randomized trial and registry. J Am Coll Cardiol. 2002;40(9):1555-66.
90. Hlatky MA, Boothroyd DB, Bravata DM, et al. Coronary artery bypass surgery compared with percutaneous coronary interventions for multivessel disease: a collaborative analysis of individual patient data from ten randomized trials. Lancet. 2009;373:1190-7.
91. Banning AP, Westaby S, Morice MC, et al. Diabetic and Nondiabetic Patients With Left Main and/or 3-Vessel Coronary Artery Disease Comparison of Outcomes With Cardiac Surgery and Paclitaxel-Eluting Stents. J Am Coll Cardiol. 2010;55(11):1067-75.
92. Kappetein AP, Head SJ, Morice MC, et al. Treatment of complex coronary artery disease in patients with diabetes: 5-year results comparing outcomes of bypass surgery and percutaneous coronary intervention in the SYNTAX trial. Eur J Cardiothorac Surg. 2013;43:1006-13.
93. Daemen J, Kuck KH, Macaya C, et al. Multivessel coronary revascularization in patients with and without diabetes mellitus 3-year follow-up of the ARTS-II (Arterial Revascularization Therapies Study–Part II) trial. J Am Coll Cardiol. 2008;52;1957-67.
94. Farkouh ME, Domanski M, Sleeper LA, et al. FREEDOM Trial Investigators. Strategies for multivessel revascularization in patients with diabetes. N Engl J Med. 2012;367:2375-84.
95. Feit F, Brooks MM, Sopko G, et al. Long-term clinical outcome in the Bypass Angioplasty Revascularization Investigation Registry: comparison with the randomized trial. BARI Investigators. Circulation. 2000;101:2795-802.
96. Novack V, Tsyvine D, Cohen DJ, et al. Multivessel drug-eluting stenting and impact of diabetes mellitus—a report from the EVENT registry. Catheter Cardiovasc Interv. 2009;73:874-80.
97. Dauerman HL. Percutaneous Coronary Intervention, Diabetes Mellitus, and Death. J Am Coll Cardiol. 2010;55(11):1076-9.
98. Bangalore S, Toklu B, Feit F. Outcomes with coronary artery bypass graft surgery versus percutaneous coronary intervention for patients with diabetes mellitus: Can newer generation drug-eluting stents bridge the gap? Circ Cardiovasc Interv. 2014;7:18-25.
99. Stone GW, Sabik JF, Serruys PW, et al. EXCEL Trial Investigators. Everolimus-Eluting Stents or Bypass Surgery for Left Main Coronary Artery Disease. N Engl J Med. 2016;375(23):2223-5.
100. Mäkikallio T, Holm NR, Lindsay M, et al. NOBLE study investigators. Percutaneous coronary angioplasty versus coronary artery bypass grafting in treatment of unprotected left main stenosis (NOBLE): a prospective, randomised, open-label, non-inferiority trial. Lancet. 2016;388(10061):2743-52.
101. Reicher B, Poston RS, Mehra MR, et al. Simultaneous "hybrid" percutaneous coronary intervention and minimally invasive surgical bypass grafting: feasibility, safety, and clinical outcomes. Am Heart J. 2008;155(4):661-7.
102. Harskamp RE, Walker PF, Alexander JH, et al. Clinical outcomes of hybrid coronary revascularization versus coronary artery

bypass surgery in patients with diabetes mellitus. Am Heart J. 2014;168(4):471-8.

103. Bittl JA. Percutaneous coronary interventions in the diabetic patient: where do we stand? Circ Cardiovasc Interv. 2015;8(4):e001944.
104. Norhammar A, Malmberg K, Diderholm E, et al. Diabetes mellitus: the major risk factor in unstable coronary artery disease even after consideration of the extent of coronary artery disease and benefits of revascularization. J Am Coll Cardiol. 2004;43(4):585-91.
105. Windecker S, Kolh P, Alfonso F, et al. 2014 ESC/EACTS guidelines on myocardial revascularization: The Task Force on Myocardial Revascularization of the European Society of Cardiology (ESC) and the European Association for Cardio-Thoracic Surgery (EACTS) developed with the special contribution of the European Association of Percutaneous Cardiovascular Interventions (EAPCI). Eur Heart J. 2014;35:2541-619.
106. Fihn SD, Blankenship JC, Alexander KP, et al. 2014 ACC/AHA/AATS/PCNA/SCAI/STS focused update of the guideline for the diagnosis and management of patients with stable ischemic heart disease: a report of the American College of Cardiology/American Heart Association Task Force on Practice Guidelines, and the American Association for Thoracic Surgery, Preventive Cardiovascular Nurses Association, Society for Cardiovascular Angiography and Interventions, and Society of Thoracic Surgeons. Circulation. 2014;130:1749-67.
107. O' PT, Kushner FG, Ascheim DD, et al. 2013 ACCF/AHA guideline for the management of ST-segment myocardial infarction: a report of the American College of Cardiology Foundation/American Heart Association Task Force on Practice Guidelines. Circulation. 2013;127:529-55.
108. Jiménez-Navarro MF, López-Jiménez F, Barsness G, et al. Long-term prognosis of complete percutaneous coronary revascularisation in patients with diabetes with multivessel disease. Heart. 2015;101(15):1233-9.
109. Zimarino M, Ricci F, Romanello M, et al. Complete myocardial revascularization confers a larger clinical benefit when performed with state-of-the-art techniques in high-risk patients with multivessel coronary artery disease: A meta-analysis of randomized and observational studies. Catheter Cardiovasc Interv. 2015 Apr 2.
110. Simpson SH, Gamble JM, Mereu L, et al. Effect of aspirin dose on mortality and cardiovascular events in people with diabetes: a meta-analysis. J Gen Intern Med. 2011;26(11):1336-44.
111. Amsterdam EA, Wenger NK, Brindis RG, et al. AHA/ACC guideline for the management of patients with Non-ST-elevation acute coronary syndromes. J Am Coll Cardiol. 2014;64(24):e139-228.
112. CURRENT-OASIS 7 Investigators, Mehta SR, Bassand JP, et al. Dose comparisons of clopidogrel and aspirin in acute coronary syndromes. N Engl J Med. 2010;363:930-42.
113. Mehta SR, Tanguay JF, Eikelboom JW, et al. Double-dose versus standard-dose clopidogrel and high-dose versus low-dose aspirin in individuals undergoing percutaneous coronary intervention for acute coronary syndromes (RENT-OASIS 7): a randomised factorial trial. Lancet. 2010;376:1233-43.
114. Tantry US, Bonello L, Aradi D, et al. Consensus and update on the definition of on-treatment platelet reactivity to adenosine diphosphate associated with ischemia and bleeding. J Am Coll Cardiol. 2013;62:2261-73.
115. Jeong YH, Kim IS, Park Y, et al. Carriage of cytochrome 2C19 polymorphism is associated with risk of high post-treatment platelet reactivity on high maintenance-dose clopidogrel of 150 mg/day: results of the ACCEL-DOUBLE (Accelerated Platelet Inhibition by a Double Dose of Clopidogrel According to Gene Polymorphism) study. JACC Cardiovasc Interv. 2010;3:731-41.
116. Levine GN, Bates ER, Blankenship JC, et al. ACCF/AHA/SCAI guideline for percutaneous coronary intervention. A report of the American College of Cardiology Foundation/American Heart Association Task Force on Practice Guidelines and the Society for Cardiovascular Angiography and Interventions. J Am Coll Cardiol. 2011;58(24):e44-122.
117. Wiviott SD, Braunwald E, Angiolillo DJ, et al. Greater clinical benefit of more intensive oral antiplatelet therapy with prasugrel in patients with diabetes mellitus in the trial to assess improvement in therapeutic outcomes by optimizing platelet inhibition with prasugrel-Thrombolysis in Myocardial I. Circulation. 2008;118(16):1626-36.
118. Wiviott SD, Braunwald E, McCabe CH, et al. Prasugrel versus clopidogrel in patients with acute coronary syndromes. N Engl J Med. 2007;357(20):2001-15.
119. Wallentin L, Becker RC, Budaj A, et al. Ticagrelor versus clopidogrel in patients with acute coronary syndromes. N Engl J Med. 2009;361(11):1045-57.
120. James S, Angiolillo DJ, Cornel JH, et al. Ticagrelor vs. clopidogrel in patients with acute coronary syndromes and diabetes: a substudy from the PLATelet inhibition and patient Outcomes (PLATO) trial. Eur Heart J. 2010;31(24):3006-16.
121. Levine GN, Bates ER, Bittl JA, et al. 2016 ACC/AHA Guideline Focused Update on Duration of Dual Antiplatelet Therapy in Patients With Coronary Artery Disease: A Report of the American College of Cardiology/American Heart Association Task Force on Clinical Practice Guidelines. An Update of the 2011 ACC/AHA/SCAI PCI Guideline, 2011 ACC/AHA CABG Guideline, 2012 ACCF/AHA/ACP/AATS/PCNA/SCAI/STS SIHD Guideline, 2013 ACC/AHA STEMI Guideline, 2014 ACC/AHA NSTE-ACS Guideline, and 2014 ACC/AHA Perioperative Guideline. J Am Coll Cardiol. 2016;134(10):e123-55.
122. Boersma E, Harrington RA, Moliterno DJ, et al. Platelet glycoprotein IIb/IIIa inhibitors in acute coronary syndromes: a meta-analysis of all major randomised clinical trials. Lancet. 2002;359:189-98.
123. Stone GW, Grines CL, Cox DA, et al. Comparison of angioplasty with stenting, with or without abciximab, in acute myocardial infarction. N Engl J Med. 2002;346:957-66.
124. Hanna EB, Rao SV, Manoukian SV, et al. The Evolving Role of Glycoprotein IIb/IIIa Inhibitors in the Setting of Percutaneous Coronary Intervention. JACC: Cardiovascular Interventions. 2010;3(12):1209-19.

CHAPTER

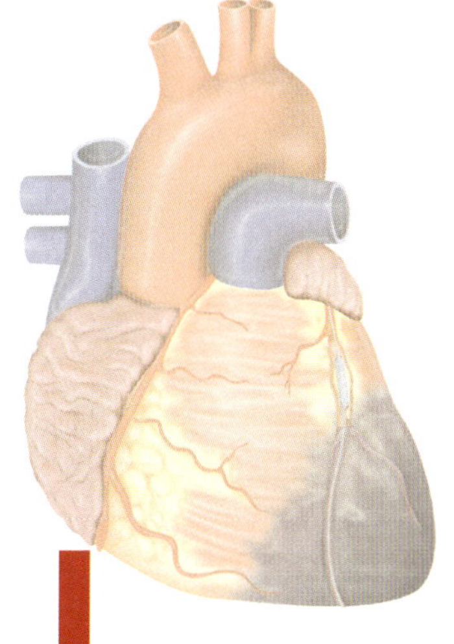

Primary PCI for STEMI in Cardiodiabetes: What is the Outcome?

Shirish (MS) Hiremath, Gaurav M Ganeshwala

INTRODUCTION

An estimated 422 million people worldwide suffer from diabetes according to the 2016 data from the World Health Organization and the prevalence is growing rapidly particularly in the developing countries. In 2015, around 69.2 million people in India had diabetes (8.7%). Acute coronary syndrome (ACS) is the leading cause of mortality and morbidity in diabetics. The mortality during acute myocardial infarction (MI) and in the postinfarction period is significantly higher compared to nondiabetics.[1,2]

How Does Diabetics with Acute Myocardial Infarction Differ from Nondiabetics?

Several studies have proven that patients with diabetes without prior cardiovascular disease (CVD) are at a similar risk of MI as nondiabetic subjects with an acute coronary event in their medical history (Fig. 1) and these correlates with the burden of *vulnerable plaques* in diabetes subjects.[3] Marso et al. noted that plaque volume was not statistically different between diabetes and nondiabetes subjects, however, there was a significant two fold increase in thin cap fibroatheroma in the diabetics (Fig. 2).[4]

The vulnerable myocardium: Various alterations of the myocardium such as cardiac metabolism (e.g. insulin resistance, increased oxygen demand), microangiopathy with endothelial dysfunction, and autonomic neuropathy—lead to the development of ACS and heart failure.[5]

The vulnerable blood: Patients with diabetes exhibit a prothrombotic milieu consisting of hyperreactive platelets, a tight and rigid clot structure which is due to upregulation of coagulation factors and prolongation of clot lysis, along with marked rise in inflammatory mediators contribute to cardiovascular events (Table 1).[6]

These pathological changes in diabetes subjects lead to all phases of vascular damage from early endothelial dysfunction through to plaque formation, rupture and occlusive thrombus formation. The specific changes in thrombus constitution generates a platelet-rich clot which is more dense, resistant to lysis and associated with higher chances of ACS, i.e. *vulnerable patient.*[7]

Apart from the pathological alterations, the potentially worse clinical outcome of ST elevation myocardial infarction (STEMI) in diabetics might result from their later hospitalization and differences in pain quality due to impaired pain perception. In a study from Croatia, while the majority of nondiabetic STEMI patients experienced 'moderate' and 'severe' chest pain, even 51.7% of diabetics experienced 'slight' or 'no pain'—predominantly symptom of dyspnea—which seemed equally indicative of serious disease as severe pain in nondiabetics.[8] Peak cardiac troponin levels were significantly higher in diabetics than nondiabetic patients which corresponds to larger areas of myocardial necrosis and multivessel disease.[8]

Typical features of coronary arteries in diabetics include:

- Multivessel coronary artery disease (Figs 3A and B)
- Multiple vulnerable plaques with diffuse involvement even in single vessel disease

TABLE 1: Factors affecting platelet function and thrombosis in diabetes subjects[7]

Endothelial dysfunction	*Metabolic changes*	*Oxidative stress*
Reduced nitric oxide production	Increased thromboxane synthesis	Increased platelet nitric oxide production
Increased reactive oxygen species (ROS)	Enhanced sensitivity to agonists	Elevated intracellular Ca^{2+} concentration
Upregulation of proinflammatory cytokines	Activation of protein kinase C	Platelet membrane sodium-potassium-ATP activity decreased
Increased platelet adhesion molecules	• Reduced nitric oxide production • Increased superoxide formation • Nonenzymatic glycation of platelet membrane proteins • Enhanced expression of p-selectin and glycoprotein receptors • Diminished insulin sensitivity • Upregulation of ROS	Activation of protein kinase C and nuclear factor-κB Formation of 8-iso-prostaglandin F2

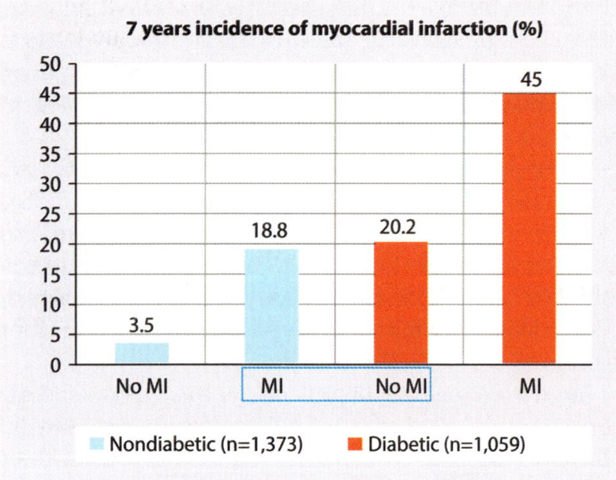

Fig. 1: Risk of acute coronary syndrome in diabetes mellitus[3]

- More small vessels and microvascular involvement
- High thrombogenicity
- Higher incidence of slow flow/no reflow and stent thrombosis after percutaneous coronary intervention (PCI)
- High rate of restenosis after PCI
- More total occlusions and calcific plaques compared to nondiabetics (Figs 3A and B).

PRIMARY PCI IN CARDIODIABETICS WITH STEMI

Prompt and complete restoration of coronary flow is the principal mechanism by which reperfusion therapy improves survival and other clinical outcomes in patients with acute STEMI. The efficacy of thrombolysis is likely to be lesser in diabetics due to enhanced platelet activity, elevated procoagulant activity and impaired intrinsic fibrinolysis. Results of *the Primary Coronary Angioplasty versus Thrombolysis-2 Trial* showed that the 30 days and long-term mortality was lower after primary PCI compared with fibrinolysis in both patients with diabetes (odds ratio, 0.49; 95% confidence interval, 0.31–0.79; $p = 0.004$) and without diabetes (odds ratio, 0.69; 95% confidence interval, 0.54–0.86, $p = 0.001$), with significant lower rates of recurrent infarction and stroke. Despite achieving similar patency rates (70%) as nondiabetics, the mortality is higher in diabetics (17.3% vs 10.2%), probably because of impaired endothelial function and diminished myocardial flow reserve.[9] Reocclusion with recurrent ischemia was also higher in diabetics (9.2% vs 5.3%) in *the Global Utilization of Streptokinase and Tissue Plasminogen Activator for Occluded Coronary Arteries (GUSTO) study.*[10]

Primary PCI has been shown to improve survival and the risk of recurrent MI, stroke, and intracranial hemorrhage compared with systemic thrombolysis in patients with STEMI—especially in diabetics.[11,12] A subset analysis of clinical trials[12-14] comparing primary PCI with thrombolysis in diabetic patients showed a significant reduction in death

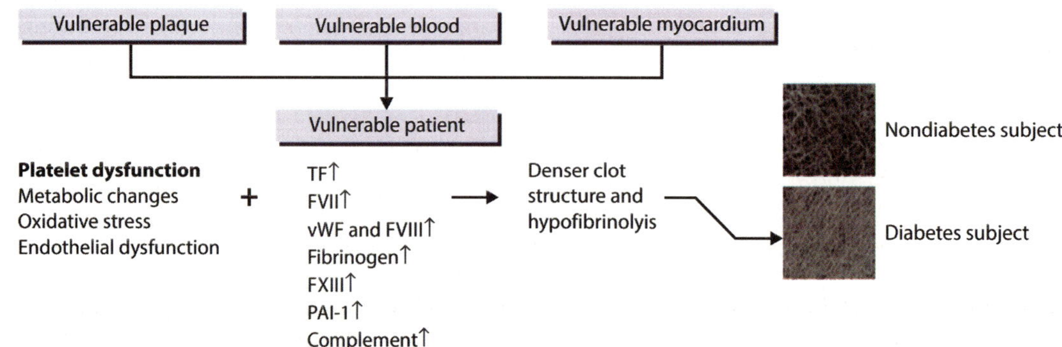

Fig. 2: Pathophysiological alterations in cardiodiabetics

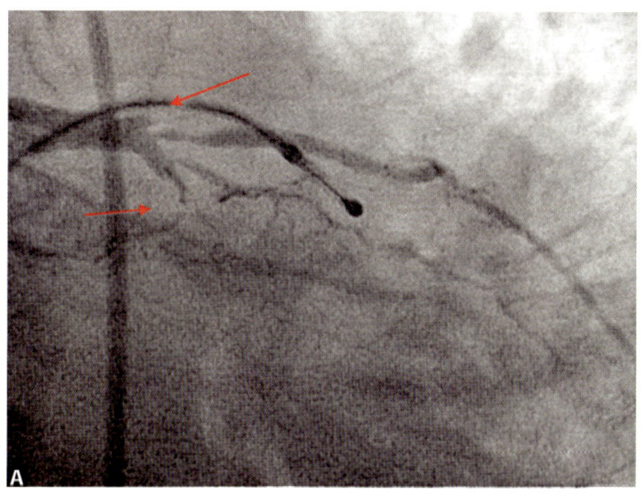

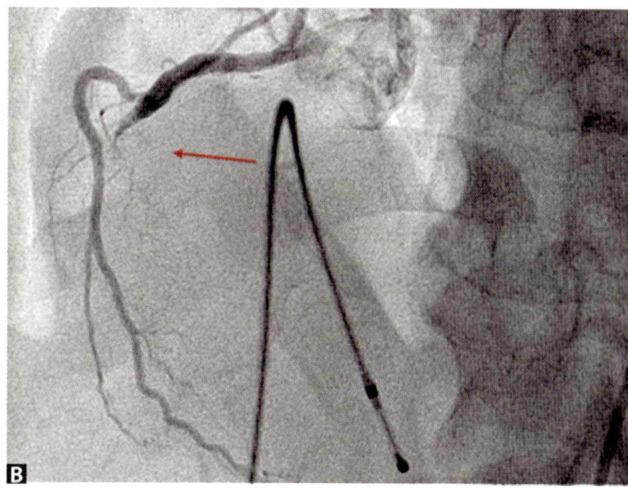

Figs 3A and B: Diabetic patient with acute anterior wall STEMI with cardiogenic shock. (A) Totally occluded LAD and LCX with critical stenosis of ramus intermedius; (B) Totally occluded mid RCA. Angiographic picture unfavorable for PCI. Patient underwent emergency CABG surgery with IABP

Abbreviations: IABP, intra-aortic balloon pump; STEMI, segment elevation myocardial infarction; LAD, left anterior descending artery; RCA, right coronary artery; LCX, left circumflex; PCI, percutaneous coronary intervention; CABG, coronary artery bypass grafting

or MI at 30 days (9.2% vs. 19.3%; $p < 0.05$),[12] a higher infarct-related artery patency rate (88% vs 31%; $p < 0.001$), and improved left ventricular function (left ventricular ejection fraction 49% vs 36%; $p < 0.05$) and long-term survival.[13] Diabetes along with other factors such as left ventricular function, left anterior descending artery involvement, and low thrombolysis in myocardial infarction (TIMI) flow are risk factors of major adverse cardiac event (MACE) in patients undergoing primary PCI.

In the angiographic substudy of the *GUSTO-IIb trial*,[15] despite the worse baseline clinical and angiographic profiles, more severe stenosis and poorer flow in the culprit artery in diabetics, procedural success with angioplasty was similar for both diabetics (n = 81; 70.4%) and nondiabetics (n = 391; 72.4%).The study was convincing in showing a reduction in death, reinfarction or disabling stroke in the nondiabetic group. The composite endpoint was somewhat lower at 30 days in the angioplasty group (11 of 99) as compared with the thrombolysis group (13 of 78) in the diabetics, however, this did not reach statistical significance. The predominant balloon angioplasty, lower rates of stenting and GPIIb/IIIa inhibitors use in this study was the possible reason for the same.

In *the STENT PAMI trial*,[16] the noninsulin dependent diabetic who underwent primary PCI with stenting demonstrated benefits from this strategy with a significant reduction in the combined incidence of occurrence of MACE at 1-year clinical follow-up and a lower rate of target vessel revascularization (TVR) (10 vs 21%, $p = 0.001$) compared to balloon angioplasty alone. The angiographic follow-up demonstrated that primary stenting in diabetic patients did not prevent them from having a higher restenosis rate (38%), twice as high compared with that in nondiabetic patients (18%, $p < 0.001$).[16] Diabetic patients developed greater intimal hyperplasia with significantly greater late lumen loss especially when stents were implanted, compared with nondiabetic patients.The analysis of long-term outcome of primary PCI in diabetics from *DESERT cooperation*[17] revealed that diabetes was associated with higher rates of death (19.1% vs 7.4%; $p = 0.0001$), reinfarction (10.4% vs 7.5%; $p = 0.001$), stent thrombosis (7.6% vs 4.8%; $p = 0.002$), and TVR (18.6% vs 15.1%; $p = 0.006$) in over 3 years follow-up. In another study, after primary PCI for STEMI, the 1-year mortality rate is 7.2% for patients without and 17.8% for patients with diabetes. For diabetic patients taking oral hypoglycemic agents at the time of admission for STEMI, the 1-year mortality is 14.3% and for those taking insulin mortality is 27.1%.[18]

Overall, primary PCI is proven to be superior to thrombolysis in diabetics with STEMI with better acute and long-term clinical outcomes even though the long-term restenosis and TVR rates are high. When consider a primary PCI in a diabetic, it must end up with a stent implantation compared to balloon angioplasty alone.

Difficulties in Primary PCI in Cardiodiabetics

Diabetic patients presenting with STEMI are overall at high-risk of mortality and mortality owing to their risk factors and more severe and late presentation. DESERT cooperation[17] database observed that diabetics with acute STEMI were older ($p < 0.001$), more likely to be female ($p < 0.001$), with higher prevalence of hypertension

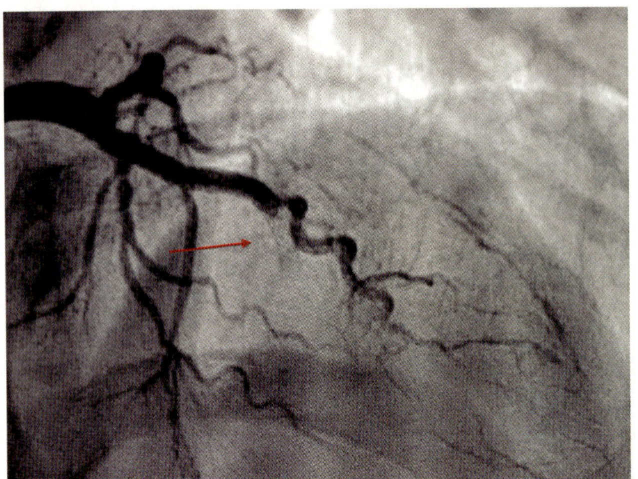

Fig. 4: Acute stent thrombosis of LAD—3 days after primary PCI in a cardiodiabetic patient

Abbreviations: LAD, left anterior descending artery; PCI, percutaneous coronary intervention

($p < 0.001$), hypercholesterolemia ($P < 0.001$), and longer ischemia time ($p < 0.001$). Diabetics with STEMI are also found to have higher Killip class, poor left ventricle(LV) ejection fraction, cardiogenic shock, multivessel involvement, ventricular arrhythmia, and higher atrioventricular (AV) block on presentation compared to nondiabetics.[19] Left ventricular failure out of proportion to myocardial infarct size could be due in part to concomitant subclinical diabetic cardiomyopathy (Fig. 4).[20]

Angiographic picture of diabetics with STEMI undergoing primary PCI is often unfavorable for angioplasty due to multivessel involvement, chronic total occlusions, higher calcium burden, more diffuse, and long stenotic lesions and at times difficult anatomies including left main or bifurcation disease. These lead to either inability to continue with the angioplasty or make the angioplasty procedure extremely difficult and increases the PCI related mortality. The longer procedure time and higher contrast volume also adds to the mortality and morbidity. Many of these patients may require early coronary artery bypass grafting(CABG) surgery.

Diabetics with STEMI more often have lower TIMI flow grades and even after attaining TIMI III flows, the myocardial blush is absent or suboptimal leading to incomplete resolution of ST segments in ECG and higher probability of stunned myocardium compared to nondiabetics. Prasad et al. noted that diabetics had more frequent absent myocardial perfusion (myocardial blush grade, MBG 0/1, 56.0% vs 47.1%, $p = 0.01$) and absent ST segment resolution (STR) (20.3% vs 8.1%, $p = 0.002$) compared to nondiabetics, after primary PCI despite similar postprocedural TIMI flow grade.[21]

Higher thrombus burden is likely to be encountered during primary PCI in diabetics due to platelet dysfunction, hypercoagulability, and altered fibrinolysis. These patients may require more frequent use of mechanical thrombus aspiration and GPIIb/IIIa inhibitors to minimize the complications of distal microembolization and potential risk of no-reflow phenomenon. Shehata et al. concluded that patients undergoing primary PCI with thrombus aspiration had higher probability of final TIMI III flow, lesser incidence of no-reflow phenomenon and reduced incidence of in-stent restenosis.[22] Use of intracoronary vasodilators including adenosine, sodium nitroprusside, verapamil, nicorandil, or adrenaline may help in improving the microvascular flow and function.Frequent need of left ventricular assist devices (LVADs) including intra-aortic balloon pump (IABP) is warranted during primary PCI in diabetics due to late presentation with higher Killip class and cardiogenic shock.

Choice of Antiplatelet Agents

There is no clear recommendation on the choice of antiplatelet regimen in diabetics undergoing primary PCI. Dual antiplatelet therapy (DAPT) with prasugrel or ticagrelor in combination with aspirin is preferred over clopidogrel and aspirin combination in diabetics based on the data available.[23,24]

Prasugrel was found to be superior to clopidogrel in reducing the composite endpoint o fcardiovascular death or MI or stroke (12.2% vs 17.0%; HR = 0.70; $p < 0.001$) without excess major bleeding in the TRITON-TIMI 38 trial.[25] This benefit was consistent in patients with (14.3% vs 22.2%; HR = 0.63; $p = 0.009$) and without (11.5% vs 15.3%; HR = 0.74; $p = 0.009$) insulin treatment. Prasugrel was also shown to reduce the risk of stent thrombosis in the diabetes mellitus (DM) subgroup (overall DM cohort: 2.0% vs 3.6%; HR = 0.52; $p = 0.007$; insulin-dependent patients: 1.8% vs 5.7%; HR = 0.31; $p = 0.008$).[25]

Ticagrelor compared with clopidogrel in the platelet inhibition and patient outcomes (PLATO) trial reduced the composite endpoint of cardiovascular death or MI or stroke in diabetic patients by 2.1% (23% relative) which did not reach statistical significance.[26] However, patients with high HbA1c (>6%) at randomization experienced a significant 2.8% absolute (30% relative) reduction in the primary composite endpoint and 1.8% absolute (21% relative) reduction in rate of MI with ticagrelor versus clopidogrel.[26]

Role of GPIIb/IIIa Inhibitors in Cardiodiabetics

The ADMIRAL trial[27] revealed a significant reduction in death (0% vs 16.7%; $p = 0.02$) as well as the combined endpoint of death, reinfarction, or revascularization (20.7% vs 50.0%, $p = 0.02$) at 6 months in diabetic patients when abciximab was added to the antiplatelet regimen. Montalescot et al.[28] in a meta-analysis of diabetic patients with STEMI, reported improved survival at 3 years in patients treated with abciximab (22% vs 40%, $p = 0.02$). The CADILLAC trial,[29] assessing the benefit of adjunctive therapy with abciximab in diabetic patients, did not show any benefit in terms of survival or recurrent MI, although the risk of repeat revascularization procedures was significantly improved. A substudy of the EPISTENT trial reported the nondiabetic AMI patients demonstrating a more than 50% reduction in the need for new revascularization procedures for the target vessel at the end of the 6-month follow-up period.

In the context of PCI, *eptifibatide* has demonstrated its effectiveness in reducing events in the short, intermediate, and long-term in ACS. In diabetics, they reduce the incidence of events at 1 year of angioplasty almost twice as much (78% more) as in nondiabetics, so the spread of the use of these drugs has undoubtedly been one of the most important advances to improve the outcomes of primary PCI in diabetics.[30]

Choice of Stents in Diabetics Undergoing PCI

There is no randomized controlled trials (RCTs) comparing different drug-eluting stent (DES) in primary PCI assessing the acute and long-term results. In a meta-analysis, comparing DES versus BMS (bare-metal stents) in diabetics, a DES (paclitaxel and sirolimus) proved to be at least as safe as a BMS for incidence of stent thrombosis and MI, provided that DAPT is continued for greater than 6 months. Repeat TVR was considerably less frequent with a DES than a BMS (OR 0.29 for sirolimus eluting; 0.38 for paclitaxel-eluting).[31]In diabetics enrolled in the TUXEDO trial,[32] compared with paclitaxel-eluting stents, everolimus-eluting stents reduced the rates of target vessel failure, MACE, MI, any stent thrombosis, definite stent thrombosis, target lesion revascularization, and TVR.

Glycemic Control in Patients Undergoing Primary PCI

Glucose level should be a part of the initial laboratory evaluation in all patients with MI. The precise goal of treatment has not yet been defined. However, until further data are available, achieving glucose levels close to normoglycemia appears to be a reasonable goal (suggested range for plasma glucose 90–140 mg/dL), as long as hypoglycemia is avoided.[24] Until more data become available the treatment target should be to avoid severe hyperglycemia (>180–200 mg/dL) as well as hypoglycemia (<90 mg/dL).[33] There is no evidence that glucose-insulin-potassium improves outcome, but may be even deleterious.[34]

OTHER PHARMACOLOGICAL THERAPIES IN CARDIODIABETES WITH MYOCARDIAL INFARCTION

The available evidence from multiple studies evaluating the effect of beta-blockers in MI have demonstrated a two-fold reduction in the relative risk in terms of mortality benefit after MI in diabetics as compared to nondiabetics. With early initiation of beta-blockers, the percentage reduction in mortality was higher in diabetics (37%) compared to nondiabetics (13%). There were similar trends for reinfarction rates with a 55% reduction in patients with DM versus 21% reduction in nondiabetics. Theoretical concerns about diminished awareness of hypoglycemia and adverse effects on lipid profiles are of little clinical significance and should not deter the use of beta-blockers.[35]

The GISSI-3 investigators[36] compared the effect of early administration (within 24 hours of admission) of *ACE inhibitor* (lisinopril) in patients with and without diabetes in MI. Lisinopril significantly reduced both 6-week and 6-month mortality in diabetics versus nondiabetics (6 weeks, 30% vs 5% and 6 months, 20% and 0%, respectively). The incidence of drug-related adverse effects was similar between the two groups. In addition to beneficial effects on ventricular remodeling, ACE inhibitors can further improve outcomes by reducing recurrent ischemic events (reduction in recurrent MI by 25% in the SAVE trial[37] and by 37% in CATS trial).[38] In CONSENSUS II, hypotension in the enalapril-treated group negated any potential benefit of early ACE inhibition. Still the available cumulative evidence strongly supports the early administration of ACE inhibitors post-MI.

CONCLUSION

Overall, the available literature strongly supports the role of primary PCI in diabetics with MI despite of technical difficulties and unfavorable long-term results in diabetics compared to those without diabetes. The use of potent antiplatelet agents, high dose statin, special angioplasty techniques, long-term ACE inhibitor, and beta-blockers certainly improve the acute and long-term clinical outcome.

REFERENCES

1. Jacoby RM, Nesto RW. Acute myocardial infarction in the diabetic patient:pathophysiology, clinical course and prognosis. J Am Coll Cardiol. 1992;20(3):736-44.

2. Aronson D, Rayfield EL, Cheseboro JH. Mechanisms determining course and outcome of diabetic patients who have had acute myocardial infarction. Ann Intern Med. 1997;126(4):296-306.
3. Haffner SM, Lehto S, Rönnemaa T, et al. Mortality from coronary heart disease in subjects with type 2 diabetes and in nondiabetic subjects with and without prior myocardial infarction. N Engl J Med. 1998;339(4):229-34.
4. Marso SP, House JA, Klauss V, et al. Diabetes mellitus is associated with plaque classified as thin cap fibroatheroma: an intravascular ultrasound study. Diab and Vasc Dis Res. 2010;7(1):14-9.
5. Hess K, Marx N, Lehrke M. Cardiovascular disease and diabetes: the vulnerable patient. Eur Heart J. 2012;14(Suppl B):B4-B13.
6. Hess K. The vulnerable blood. Coagulation and clot structure in diabetes mellitus. Hämostaseologie.2015;35(1):25-33.
7. Hess K, Grant PJ. Inflammation and thrombosis in diabetes. Thromb Haemost. 2011;105(Suppl 1):S43-S54.
8. Gradišer M, Dilber D, Cmrečnjak J, et al. Comparison of the hospital arrival time and differences in pain quality between diabetic and non-diabetic STEMI patients. Int J Environ Res Public Health. 2015;12(2):1387-96.
9. Fibrinolytic Therapy Trialists (FTT) Collaborative Group. Indications for fibrinolytic therapy in suspected acute myocardial infarction: collaborative overview of early mortality and major morbidity results from all randomised trials of more than 1000 patients. Lancet. 1994;343(8893):311-22.
10. Woodfield SL, Lundergan CF, Reiner JS, et al. Angiographic findings and outcome in diabetic patients treated with thrombolytic therapy for acute myocardial infarction: the GUSTO-I experience. J Am Coll Cardiol.1996;28(7):1661-9.
11. Keeley EC, Boura JA, Grines CL. Primary angioplasty versus intravenous thrombolytic therapy for acute myocardial infarction: A quantitative review of 23 randomised trials. Lancet. 2003;361(9351):13-20.
12. Grines C, Patel A, Zijlstra F, et al. Primary coronary angioplasty compared with intravenous thrombolytic therapy for acute myocardial infarction: Six-month follow up and analysis of individual patient data from randomized trials. Am Heart J. 2003;145(1):47-57.
13. Timmer JR, Ottervanger JP, Thomas K, et al. Long-term, cause-specific mortality after myocardial infarction in diabetes. Eur Heart J. 2004;25(11):926-31.
14. Hsu LF, Mak KH, Lau KW, et al. Clinical outcomes of patients with diabetes mellitus and acute myocardial infarction treated with primary angioplasty or fibrinolysis. Heart. 2002;88(3):260-5.
15. Hasdai D, Granger CB, Srivatsa SS, et al. Diabetes mellitus and outcome after primary coronary angioplasty for acute myocardial infarction: Lessons from the GUSTO-IIb angioplasty substudy. J Am Coll Cardiol. 2000;35(6):1502-12.
16. Mattos LA, Grines CL, de Sousa JE, et al. One-year follow-up after primary coronary intervention for acute myocardial infarction in diabetic patients. A substudy of the STENT PAMI Trial. Arq Bras Cardiol. 2001;77(6):556-61.
17. Luca GD, Dirksen MT, Spaulding C, et al. Impact of diabetes on long-term outcome after primary angioplasty: Insights from the DESERT cooperation. Diabetes Care. 2013;36(4):1020-25.
18. van der Schaaf RJ, Henriques JPS, WiersmaJJ, et al. Primary percutaneous coronary intervention for patients with acute ST elevation myocardial infarction with and without diabetes mellitus. Heart. 2006;92(1):117-8.
19. Vasilupă L, Petrescu L. The impact of primary angioplasty in diabetics versus non-diabetics patients with myocardial infarction with ST elevation at 12 hours after the acute event. J Exp Med Surg Res. 2013;112-5.
20. Zarich SW, Nesto RW. Diabetic cardiomyopathy. Am Heart J. 1989;118(5 Pt 1):1000-12.
21. Prasad A, Stone GW, Stuckey TD, et al. Impact of diabetes mellitus on myocardial perfusion after primary angioplasty in patients with acute myocardial infarction. J Am Coll Cardiol. 2005;45(4):508-14.
22. Shehata M. Angiographic and clinical impact of successful manual thrombus aspiration in diabetic patients undergoing primary PCI. Int J Vasc Med. 2014;2014(263926):1-8.
23. Saeid S, Masoud P, Mahmoud H, et al. Factors affecting outcome of primary percutaneous coronary intervention for acute myocardial infarction. ARYA Atheroscler. 2013;9:241-6.
24. Mehta SR, Tanguay JF, Eikelboom JW, et al. CURRENT-OASIS 7 trial investigators. Double-dose versus standard-dose clopidogrel and high-dose versus low-dose aspirin in individuals undergoing percutaneous coronary intervention for acute coronary syndromes (CURRENT-OASIS 7): a randomised factorial trial. Lancet. 2010;376(9748):1233-43.
25. Wiviott SD, Braunwald E, Angiolillo DJ, et al. Greater clinical benefit of more intensive oral antiplatelet therapy with prasugrelin patients with inhibition with prasugrel-Thrombolysis in Myocardial Infarction 38. Circulation. 2008;118(16):1626-36.
26. James S, Angiolillo DJ, Cornel JH, et al. Ticagrelor vs. clopidogrel in patients with acute coronary syndromes and diabetes: a substudy from the PLATelet inhibition and patient Outcomes (PLATO) trial. Eur Heart J. 2010;31(24):3006-16.
27. Montalescot G, Barragan P, Wittenberg O, et al. Platelet glycoprotein IIb/IIIa inhibition with coronary stenting for acute myocardial infarction. New Engl J Med. 2001;344(25): 1895-903.
28. Montalescot G, Antoniucci D, Kastrati A, et al. Abciximab in primary coronary stenting of ST-elevation myocardial infarction: A European meta-analysis on individual patients' data with long-term follow-up. Eur Heart J. 2007;28(4):443-9.
29. Stuckey TD, Stone GW, Cox DA, et al. Impact of stenting and abciximab in patients with diabetes mellitus undergoing primary angioplasty in acute myocardial infarction (the CADILLAC trial). Am J Cardiol. 2005;95(1):1-7.
30. Alonso JJ, Durán JM, Gimeno F, et al. Coronary angioplasty in diabetic patients. Current and futureperspectives. Rev Esp Cardiol. 2002;55(11):1185-200.
31. Stettler C, Allemann S, Wandel S, et al. Drug eluting and bare metal stents in people with and without diabetes: collaborative network meta-analysis. BMJ. 2008;337:a1331.
32. Bangalore S, Bhagwat A, Pinto B, et al. Percutaneous coronary intervention in patients with insulin-treated and non-insulin-treated diabetes mellitus secondary analysis of the TUXEDO trial. JAMA Cardiol. 2016;1(3):266-73.
33. Finfer S, Chittock DR, Su SY, et al. Intensive versus conventional glucose control in critically ill patients. N Engl J Med. 2009;360(13):1283-97.
34. Diaz R, Goyal A, Mehta SR, et al. Glucose-insulin-potassium therapy in patients with ST-segment elevation myocardial infarction. JAMA. 2007;298(20):2399-405.
35. Kendall MJ, Lynch KP, Hjalmarson A, et al. Beta-blockers and sudden cardiac death. Ann Intern Med. 1995;123(5):358-67.
36. Zuanetti G, Latini R, Maggioni A, et al. Effect of the ACE-inhibitor lisinopril on mortality in diabetic patients with acute myocardial infarction: the data from the GISSI-3 study. Circulation. 1997;96(12):4239-45.
37. Moye LA, Pfeffer MA, Wun CC, et al. Uniformity of captopril benefit in the SAVE study: subgroup analysis. Eur Heart J. 1994;15(Suppl B):2-8.
38. Torp-Pedersen C, Kober L, Carlsen J, et al. Angiotensin-converting enzyme inhibition after myocardial infarction: the Trandolapril Cardiac Evaluation study. Am Heart J. 1996;132(Suppl):235-43.

117

CHAPTER

Optimizing Results of Percutaneous Coronary Intervention in Multivessel Disease with Diabetes

Dev Pahlajani

INTRODUCTION

Diabetes and coronary artery disease (CAD) are lifestyle diseases and both account for large number of patients who visit the cardiology or diabetes clinics of the physicians or a busy hospital. It is estimated that more than 170 million patients all over the world suffer from diabetes. There is an increasing burden of diabetes particularly in India. It is projected to be the world capital of diabetes and will account for approximately 100 million diabetic patients by the year 2020. The incidence of CAD is also exponentially rising and it is estimated that over 60 million individuals, suffer from one or the other clinical form of CAD. More than 25% patients with CAD have diabetes and about 75% diabetics succumb to death due to cardiovascular event. Choice and optimum treatment of CAD particularly multivessel disease (MVD) has been a subject of various randomized controlled trials and registries and attracted several debates during various national and international scientific conferences. Large scale data regarding the benefit and outcomes of medical versus percutaneous coronary intervention (PCI) versus coronary artery bypass graft (CABG) surgery is available that has formed a ground work for the current guidelines.

PATHOPHYSIOLOGY OF DIABETES AND ATHEROSCLEROTIC CORONARY ARTERY DISEASE

Diabetic patients usually have MVD which is diffuse in nature. Coronary arteries more often than not are of smaller diameter as compared to those of nondiabetics. The disease also involves smaller arteries and several of diabetics have microvessel disease and associated cardiomyopathy. Thus the results of PCI and CABG surgery in diabetics are associated with unfavorable outcomes as compared to those in nondiabetics. CAD and diabetes are linked to altered inflammatory pathways with insulin resistance and defective free fatty acid metabolism. Both of them have endothelial dysfunction. There is an increased thrombogenicity and altered smooth muscle cell migration. Plaque burden in patients with diabetes and MVD is larger than in nondiabetics. There is an increased platelet activity and decreased nitric oxide production. In diabetes there is an increased production of proinflammatory cytokines and there is altered monocyte and leucocyte binding on the platelets and increased platelet reactivity that predisposes diabetics to thrombosis.[1,2] All these factors combined together predispose diabetic with CAD to new adverse cardiac events following revascularization procedure—be it CABG surgery or PCI. Diabetics are also prone to develop restenosis, stent thrombosis, and increased risk of death following PCI.

With such unfavorable pathology it can be anticipated that patients of CAD with diabetes would achieve suboptimal results of revascularization.

REVASCULARIZATION IN DIABETICS AND MULTIVESSEL DISEASE

Several large scale randomized control trials have been undertaken in last 30 years to assess the efficacy and safety of CABG Surgery versus PCI. One of the earliest trials, bypass angioplasty revascularization investigation (BARI) compared the results of percutaneous transluminal coronary angioplasty (PTCA) versus CABG surgery in patients with CAD. The trial enrolled 1,829 patients and randomized them to PTCA versus CABG surgery. The initial results of trial reported that patients with diabetes who underwent PTCA had increased risk of death, myocardial infarction (MI), and target vessel revascularization (TVR) than those treated with CABG surgery.[3] Ten years follow-up data has further strengthened the initial results of the trial.[4] However, the trial has attracted criticism since majority of PCI procedures were performed with balloon angioplasty.

Arterial Revascularization Therapy Study-I (ARTS I) trial compared the outcomes of PCI with bare metal stent (BMS) versus CABG surgery in patients with CAD and diabetes. However, the results of trial also demonstrated superiority of CABG surgery over PCI in diabetics even after stent deployment. Subsequently, ARTS I and II reported the safety and efficacy of PCI with sirolimus-eluting stent (SES) versus CABG surgery in patients with and without diabetes mellitus (DM). This was a historical comparison and showed the superiority of SES over BMS. In ARTS I and II studies, 367 diabetic patients were included. Out of these 159 received SES and 112 received BMS while 96 patients underwent CABG surgery. Five year follow-up showed that the major adverse cardiac and cerebrovascular events (MACCE) were higher in the BMS treated patients versus SES treated patients. However, the rate of TVR was significantly higher in the SES treated patients as compared to those subjected to CABG Surgery (SES 32.2% versus CABG 10.7%) ($p = <0.001$). The revascularization rate of SES treated patients at 5 years was more or less similar but numerically lower than the BMS treated patients. The 5-year follow-up showed that SES treated patients had better outcomes than the patients randomized to BMS. However, in both these trials CABG Surgery was associated with decreased rate of TVR as compared to PCI treated patients.[5]

Coronary Artery Revascularization in Diabetes (CARDia) trial enrolled 510 patients with complex CAD or MVD with diabetes. Out of these 71% patients in PCI treated group received SES and 29% received BMS. The trial was noninferior trial. The primary end point of death was 14% for PCI and 12.6% for CABG. However, nonfatal MI and repeat revascularization were significantly higher for PCI group as compared to CABG surgery at 5 years.[6]

Subsequently, a large scale FREEDOM trial was conducted.[7] The trial was a prospective randomized multicenter trial. It was a superiority trial that compared PCI to CABG Surgery patients on optimum medical therapy. Investigators of FREEDOM trial enrolled 1,900 patients at 140 international centers to ascertain whether aggressive medical therapy and the use of drug-eluting stents (DES) could alter the revascularization approach for patients with diabetes and CAD.

The primary outcome was composite of death, nonfatal MI from any cause, and nonfatal stroke. The primary outcome occurred in 26.6% in PCI group and 18.7% in CABG surgery group. The CABG surgery benefit was mainly driven by difference in death and MI and death from any cause. However, incidence of stroke was higher in CABG surgery group at 5 years. Again CABG surgery proved to be superior to PCI by reduction of all-cause mortality, nonfatal MI.

SYNTAX trial has been one of the landmark trial that enrolled 1800 patients to see if PCI performed with paclitaxel coated stent was not inferior to CABG surgery.[8] Amongst the patients enrolled in the study, 30% had diabetes. At the end of 5 years, the overall rates of adverse events were lower with the CABG surgery patients (27%) than PCI treated patients (37%) ($p = <0.01$). While the all-cause mortality did not differ significantly between the two groups the rates of MI and repeat revascularization were higher with PCI than CABG Surgery (9.7% vs 3.8% and 26% vs 14%, respectively). The advantage of CABG surgery was mainly driven by patients with higher SYNTAX score of greater than 33 and anatomical complexity. Patients with low and intermediate SYNTAX score of less than 33 fared equally well when compared with CABG surgery. In the patients with high SYNTAX score CABG surgery had distinct advantage over PCI with overall event rate of 27% in as against 44% in the PCI arm. In the subgroup analysis of 452 medically treated diabetics patients treated with paclitaxel coated stent had higher 1 year MACCE as compared those who underwent CABG Surgery. The higher event rate was mainly driven by increased repeat revascularization rate (6.4% vs 20.3%). Diabetics with higher SYNTAX score and highly complex lesions had higher mortality with PCI as compared to CABG surgery (4.1% vs 13.5%).

Can we Improve upon the results of PCI to match CABG surgery outcomes?

The wealth of data has repeatedly shown the superiority of CABG Surgery over PCI in CAD patients with diabetes. This is particularly true of the trials and registries during the balloon, BMS, and first generation stents era.

However, one could look forward to optimizing the results of PCI with second generation DES with newer antiplatelet regimens.

STENT TYPE AND OUTCOMES: ROLE OF NEWER GENERATION STENTS

Earlier trials have been criticized for having compared the data of BMS or first generation stents to CABG surgery. First generation DES and paclitaxel coated stents have been shown to be inferior to newer generation stents made up of cobalt chromium and coated with new biocompatible or bioabsorbable polymer or no polymer. These stents have low strut thickness stents shown to have low restenosis rates.[9,10] BEST trial compared the outcomes of everolimus-eluting second generation stent (EES) with CABG surgery.[11] It was an open label randomized trial and enrolled 880 patients and randomized them to PCI with EES or CABG surgery. Amongst these more than 40% had diabetes. Overall the study showed that during long-term follow-up primary end point of composite of death, MI or TVR occurred more frequently in PCI arm than in CABG surgery arm (15.3 vs 10.6%). Patients with diabetes had worse outcome with PCI with the primary end point occurring in 19.2% in PCI treated patients as opposed to 9.1% in CABG surgery treated patients.

Kaul et al. from India reported their data from TUXEDO trial that compared paclitaxel coated stent with EES stents in diabetics.[12] At one year, paclitaxel stent did not meet then on inferiority criteria to EES. The adverse events were two times higher in paclitaxel stent arm as compared to EES arm.

While comparing the adverse outcomes in insulin versus noninsulin treated diabetics who were randomized to PCI with EES stent versus paclitaxel stent in the TUXEDO trial, Bangalore et al. found no difference in the combined events of cardiac death, target vessel MI, TVR after risk adjustment. In propensity adjusted analysis the differences in outcomes were no longer significant. However, the event rate was far lower in the EES treated arm when compared with the PES. There was a significant increase in the risk of cardiovascular events when the insulin treated diabetics were compared with noninsulin diabetics in unadjusted model.[13]

Zotarolimus stent was the first stent amongst the second generation DES to have received FDA approval for diabetics. However Park et al. reported their analysis of 1855 diabetic patients from EXCELLENT and RESOLUTE Korea trial that used second generation DES in all comers. EES and zotarolimus-eluting stents (ZES) showed comparable efficacy and safety up to 1 year follow-up. Overall incidence of TLF was low even in patients with diabetes establishing safety and efficacy of second generation DES in DM.[14-16]

WILL NEWER DUAL ANTIPLATELET THERAPY REDUCE ADVERSE EVENTS?

Dual antiplatelet therapy (DAPT) is the cornerstone of management of patients who have undergone stent deployment. Recommended duration of P2Y12 inhibitor is 6–12 months while aspirin is recommended to be continued indefinitely.

While clopidogrel has been the longest surviving P2Y12 agent with millions of patients having been treated over last two decades, newer antiplatelet drugs like prasugrel and ticagrelor have found favors among patients with ST-elevation myocardial infarction (STEMI), high-risk acute coronary syndrome (ACS) and diabetics.

Earlier trials like CURE trial documented a 20% relative risk reduction (RRR) in composite of vascular death, MI or stroke at a median of 1.9 years follow-up in the clopidogrel plus aspirin arm versus aspirin alone. TRITON-TIMI 38 demonstrated 19% RRR in primary composite end point of death, nonfatal MI or nonfatal stroke in prasugrel treated patients as compared to clopidogrel arm in ACS patients treated invasively over more than 1 year. However, prasugrel was associated with a slightly increased risk of bleeding.[17,18]

Lately ticagrelor has been widely recommended for patients with STEMI and diabetics. In PLATO trial ticagrelor was found to be superior to clopidogrel in platelet inhibition and reduction of major adverse cardiac events. PLATO substudy involved 4,662 patients with preexisting diabetes of whom 1,036 patients were on insulin.[19] The primary composite end point of cardiovascular death, MI or stroke was lower in ticagrelor treated patients as compared to those treated with clopidogrel. Results were consistent with those of the main PLATO trial. Beneficial effect of ticagrelor was maintained in the diabetic patients with no increase in the major bleeding. It also provided benefit in patients with insulin treated patients. The ischemic complications in STEMI patients were reduced as compared to clopidogrel irrespective of diabetic status without any increase in major bleeding events.

OPTIMUS-3 compared the pharmacodynamics of standard dose prasugrel versus high dose clopidogrel in diabetics.[20] Prasugrel had greater platelet inhibition and better response profile as compared to double dose clopidogrel.

OPTIMUS-4 trial compared the pharmacodynamics of prasugrel versus ticagrelor in patients with type II DM and CAD. Fifty aspirin treated diabetic patients with CAD were randomly assigned to prasugrel or ticagrelor. The primary end point was effect on P2Y12 reaction units determined by verify now at 1 week.[21]

At 1 week, ticagrelor exerted similar or greater inhibition of ADP induced platelet reactivity as compared to prasugrel (52 vs 83). Thus the study indicated that both these agents do inhibit ADP but ticagrelor exerts a higher platelet inhibition as compared to prasugrel.

In PEGASUS-TIMI 54 trial, 21,162 patients were randomly assigned in 1:1:1 fashion to receive ticagrelor—(a) 90 mg twice a day, (b) 60 mg twice a day and (c) placebo.[22] The eligible patients had MI and had additional features which included diabetes requiring medication. More than

30% patients had diabetes out of these 87% were treated with hypoglycemic pharmacologic therapy.

The primary efficacy end point was composite of vascular death, MI or stroke. The primary safety end point was bleeding. Both doses of ticagrelor reduced the rate of primary efficacy end point as compared to placebo at 3 years. There was slight increase in the TIMI major bleeding as compared to placebo with both the doses.

Whether the diabetics should receive longer duration of DAPT as compared to nondiabetics has been a matter of several discussions and debates. Case for longer duration is based on the clinical observations that diabetics have higher platelet reactivity, increased inflammation, and therefore more prone to develop stent thrombosis and death. A recent meta-analysis of short-term (less than 6 months) versus long-term DAPT (6–12 months) after implantation of DES analyzed the results of 11,473 patients from six trials. Amongst these 3681, 32.1% had diabetes. Diabetes was found to be an independent predictor of major cardiovascular events (MACE). Long-term DAPT was not associated with decreased risk of MACE as compared to short-term DAPT in patients with or without diabetes. There was no difference in the risk of MI. However, there was a lower risk of stent thrombosis with long-term DAPT amongst patients with diabetes. There was an increased risk of bleeding irrespective of diabetes with long-term administration.

CONCLUSION

In the light of current data available how do we optimize PCI outcomes in patients with diabetes and MVD? Patient with MVD and diabetes should preferably be treated with CABG surgery if the surgical risk is acceptable. A heart team approach to decide on the revascularization strategy would be an appropriate initial strategy.

- However, when EURO score or Society of Thoracic Surgeons (STS) score is forbidding for surgery, and revascularization is indicated, PCI should not be denied so as to offer symptom relief and improve quality of life. It should be performed with a second generation EES or ZES. Though not enough data is available it will make sense to use a stent with absorbable polymer. First generation SES though better than BMS should be avoided in favor of second generation DES. Paclitaxel stent has been found to be inferior to EES in TUXEDO trial. In the light of current data of increased risk of stent thrombosis bioresorbable vascular scaffold (BVS) should be avoided.
- The data from TUXEDO trial indicates that insulin treated diabetics after adjustment were made for clinical comorbidities would have similar outcomes when treated with EES stent as compared to paclitaxel stent. Therefore, if the clinical situation warrants PCI with second generation should not be denied to insulin treated diabetics.
- First generation stents like cypher and taxus are better avoided. BMS would have higher rates of restenosis.
- Longer duration of DAPT has not been shown to provide any additional benefit and may be associated with greater risk of bleeding. One may stick to guideline recommended duration of 6–12 months.
- Drugs like ticagrelor and prasugrel could have advantage over clopidogrel in preventing MACE rates. OPTIMUS trial results favor ticagrelor as compared to prasugrel.

REFERENCES

1. Hartge MM, Unger T, Kintscher U. The endothelium and vascular inflammation in diabetes. Diab Vasc Dis Res. 2007;4(2):84-8.
2. Vinik AI, Erbas T, Park TS, et al. Platelet dysfunction in type 2 diabetes. Diabetes Care. 2001;24(8):1476-85.
3. Rogers WJ, Baxley WA, Dean LS, et al. Influence of diabetes on 5-year mortality and morbidity in a randomized trial comparing CABG and PTCA in patients with multivessel disease: the Bypass Angioplasty Revascularization Investigation (BARI). Circulation. 1997;96(6):1761-9.
4. BARI Investigators. The final 10-year follow-up results from the BARI randomized trial. J Am Coll Cardiol. 2007;49(15):1600-6.
5. Onuma Y, Wykrzykowska JJ, Garg S, et al. 5-year follow-up of coronary revascularization in diabetic patients with multivessel coronary artery disease: Insights from ARTS (arterial revascularization therapy study)-II and ARTS-I trials. JACC Cardiovasc Interv. 2011;4(3):317-23.
6. Kapur A, Hall RJ, Malik IS, et al. Randomized comparison of percutaneous coronary intervention with coronary artery bypass grafting in diabetic patients. 1-year results of the CARDia (Coronary Artery Revascularization in Diabetes) trial. J Am Coll Cardiol. 2010;55(5):432-40.
7. Farkouh ME, Domanski M, Sleeper LA, et al. Strategies for multivessel revascularization in patients with diabetes. N Engl J Med. 2012;367(25):2375-84.
8. Kappetein AP, Head SJ, Morice MC, et al. Treatment of complex coronary artery disease in patients with diabetes: 5-year results comparing outcomes of bypass surgery and percutaneous coronary intervention in the SYNTAX trial. Eur J Cardiothorac Surg. 2013;43(5):1006-13.
9. Stone GW, Kedhi E, Kereiakes DJ, et al. Differential clinical responses to everolimus-eluting and paclitaxel-eluting coronary stents in patients with and without diabetes mellitus. Circulation. 2011;124(8):893-900.
10. Kim WJ, Lee SW, Park SW, et al. Randomized comparison of everolimus-eluting stent versus sirolimus-eluting stent implantation for de novo coronary artery disease in patients with diabetes mellitus (ESSENCE-DIABETES): Results from the ESSENCE-DIABETES trial. Circulation. 2011;124(8):886-92.
11. Park SJ, Ahn JM, Kim YH, et al. Trial of everolimus-eluting stents or bypass surgery for coronary disease. N Eng J Med. 2015;372(13):1204-12.
12. Kaul U, Bangalore S, Seth A, et al. Paclitaxel-eluting versus everolimus-eluting coronary stents in diabetes. N Engl J Med. 2015;373(18):1709-19.
13. Bangalore S, Bhagwat A, Pinto B, et al. Percutaneous Coronary Intervention – patients with insulin treated and non-insulin treated

diabetes mellitus secondary analysis of the TUXEDO trial. JAMA Cardiol. 2016;1(3):266-73.
14. Park KW, Lee JM, Kang SH, et al. Everolimus-eluting Xience V/ Promus versus zotarolimus-eluting resolute stents in patients with diabetes mellitus. JACC Cardiovasc Interv. 2014;7(5): 471-81.
15. Jain AK, Lotan C, Meredith IT, et al. Twelve-month outcomes in patients with diabetes implanted with a zotarolimus-eluting stent: results from the E-Five Registry. Heart. 2010;96(11):848-53.
16. von Birgelen C, Basalus MW, Tandjung K, et al. A randomized controlled trial in second-generation zotarolimus-eluting Resolute stents versus everolimus-eluting Xience V stents in real-world patients: The TWENTE trial. J Am Coll Cardiol. 2012;59(15):1350-61.
17. Wiviott SD, Braunwald E, McCabe CH, et al. Intensive oral antiplatelet therapy for reduction of ischaemic events including stent thrombosis in patients with acute coronary syndromes treated with percutaneous coronary intervention and stenting in the TRITON-TIMI 38 trial: a subanalysis of a randomised trial. Lancet. 2008;371(9621):1353-63.
18. Wiviott SD, Braunwald E, Angiolillo DJ, et al. Greater clinical benefit of more intensive oral antiplatelet therapy with prasugrel in patients with diabetes mellitus in the trial to assess improvement in therapeutic outcomes by optimizing platelet inhibition with prasugrel-thrombolysis in myocardial infarction 38. Circulation. 2008;118(16):1626-36.
19. James S, Angiolillo DJ, Cornel JH, et al. Ticagrelor vs. Clopidogrel in patients with acute coronary syndromes and diabetes: a substudy from the platelet inhibition and patient outcomes (PLATO) trial. Eur Heart J. 2010;31(24):3006-16.
20. Angiolillo DJ, Badimon JJ, Saucedo JF, et al. A pharmacodynamics comparison of prasugrel vs. high-dose clopidogrel in patients with type 2 diabetes mellitus and coronary artery disease: results of optimizing antiplatelet therapy in diabetes mellitus (OPTIMUS)-3 trial. Eur Heart J. 2011;32(7):838-46.
21. Franchi F, Rollini F, Aggarwal N, et al. Pharmacodynamic comparison of prasugrel versus ticagrelor in patients with type 2 diabetes mellitus and coronary artery disease: the OPTIMUS (Optimizing Antiplatelet Therapy in Diabetes Mellitus)-4 study. Circulation. 2016;134(11):780-92.
22. Bonaca MP, Bhatt DL, Cohen M, et al. Long-term use of ticagrelor in patients with prior myocardial infarction. N Eng J Med. 2015;372(19):1791-800.

STEMI Management in Diabetes Mellitus: Is it Different?

Santanu Guha, Sumanta Chatterjee

INTRODUCTION

The main cause of death in the industrialized countries is the coronary artery disease (CAD). The risk of myocardial infarction is high in patients with diabetes mellitus (DM). In the United States, diabetes is the most prevalent risk factor for cardiovascular events.[1] The patients with DM have increased risk for cardiovascular disease (CVD), a risk that contributes to a significant decrease in life expectancy. The patients with diabetes have a risk for myocardial infarction (MI) comparable to that of the risk of recurrent MI in a patient without diabetes. The association between diabetes and CVD has been well identified, and the increased of risk for acute coronary syndromes and the poor outcome linked to raise blood glucose levels has been studied in many trials. CVD is the leading cause of morbidity and mortality in individuals with diabetes, for which 65% of deaths are attributable to heart disease or stroke. Hyperglycemia is encountered in up to 50% of all ST-segment elevation myocardial infarction (STEMI) patients, whereas previously diagnosed DM is present in only 20–25% of STEMI patients.[2] When admission glucose level exceeds 200 mg/dL, mortality is similar in non-DM and DM subjects with MI. Admission glucose has been identified as a major independent predictor of both in-hospital congestive heart failure and mortality in STEMI.[3] A Finnish population-based study has shown that patients with diabetes without a previous MI have as great risk for infarction as individuals without diabetes with a previous MI (Fig. 1). The 7-year incidence rates of MI (fatal and nonfatal) in subjects without diabetes were 18.8% in those with a previous MI and 3.5% in those without a history of infarction; the corresponding rates in individuals with diabetes were 45.0% and 20.2%, respectively[4] (Fig. 1).

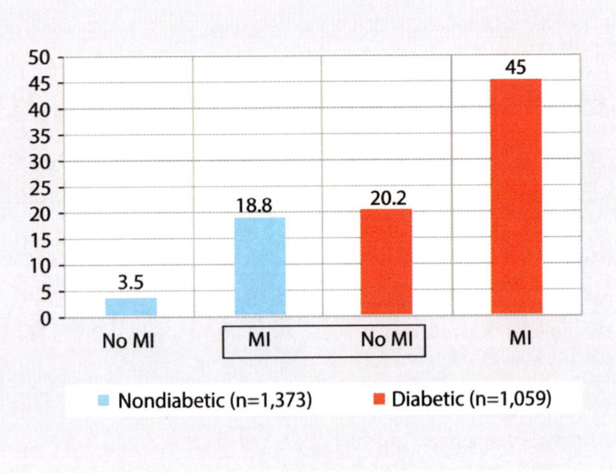

Fig. 1: A 7-year incidence rates of myocardial infarction

PATHOLOGICAL CORRELATION BETWEEN DIABETES MELLITUS AND STEMI

The possible mechanisms that influence the increased risk in diabetes for cardiovascular events include insulin resistance, changes in endothelial function, dyslipidemia, chronic inflammation and release of mediators of inflammation, procoagulability and impaired fibrinolysis.

Insulin Resistance

Insulin resistance is a hallmark in type 2 DM and obesity, the resistance to action of insulin in skeletal muscle leads to a decrease in the glucose disposal and the use of fatty acids and compensatory hyperinsulinemia. The SMART study group published a prospective cohort study in 2,611 patients with manifest arterial disease without known diabetes. Homeostasis model of insulin resistance (HOMA-IR) was used to quantify insulin resistance. The relation of HOMA-IR with cardiovascular events (vascular death, MI or stroke) and all causes of mortality were assessed. In patients with manifest arterial disease without known diabetes, the results of this trial concludes that insulin resistance increases with the number of metabolic syndrome components, and elevated insulin resistance increases the risk of new cardiovascular events.[5]

Endothelial Dysfunction

Acute coronary syndromes are associated to unstable atheromatous plaques in which inflammation and endothelial dysfunction play key roles, as well as in subsequent occlusive coronary thrombosis a global flow abnormality affecting the entire coronary tree is associated with adverse clinical outcomes in patients with ACS and might be caused by a combination of global inflammation and vasoconstriction.

Dyslipidemia

Overproduction of triglyceride-rich lipoproteins and impaired clearance by lipoprotein lipase lead to the hypertriglyceridemia common in diabetes. Low levels of high-density lipoprotein (HDL) represent the second common abnormality in type 2 diabetes. Elevated levels of triglyceride-rich lipoproteins lower HDL levels by promoting exchanges of cholesterol from HDL to very low-density lipoprotein (VLDL) via cholesteryl ester transfer protein. Diabetic patients with CAD more commonly have the combination of elevated triglycerides and low HDL than elevated total and low-density lipoprotein (LDL) cholesterol levels.

Procoagulability and Impaired Fibrinolysis

Hyperglycemia also stimulates coagulation and platelet aggregation. It has been reported that hyperglycemia elevates coagulant activation markers, including thrombin-antithrombin complexes and soluble tissue factor, whereas hyperinsulinemia inhibits fibrinolysis. Patients with type 2 diabetes have impaired fibrinolytic capacity because of elevated levels of plasminogen activator inhibitor type 1 in atherosclerotic lesions and in non-atheromatous arteries.[6] Diabetes increases the expression of tissue factor, a potent procoagulant, and plasma coagulation factors such as factor VII and decreases levels of endogenous anticoagulants such as antithrombin III and protein C.[7]

OUTCOME OF ACUTE MYOCARDIAL INFARCTION IN DIABETES MELLITUS PATIENTS

Acute hyperglycemia is associated with multiple biological effects that contribute to a poor outcome of the acute coronary syndromes. In the OASIS registry, a 6-nation study of unstable angina and non-Q-wave MI, diabetes independently increased the risk of death by 57%. Elevated plasma glucose and glycated hemoglobin levels on admission are independent prognosticators of both in-hospital and long-term outcome regardless of diabetic status. For every 18 mg/dL increase in glucose level, there is a 4% increase in mortality in nondiabetic subjects.[8] Diabetes has been a consistently powerful risk factor for development of post-infarction heart failure, accounting for 66% of mortality during the first year. The combination of diabetes and HF after MI requires preventive action because it is usually not associated with the characteristic left ventricular remodeling. If left ventricular remodeling does develop, it requires appropriate treatment that includes revascularization and metabolically and hemodynamically effective treatment strategies that limit infarct size, cardiac dysfunction, and left ventricle remodeling. In patients without a history of diabetes, there was a linear relation between admission blood glucose level and in-hospital mortality (Figs 2 and 3).

MANAGEMENT OF STEMI IN DIABETES MELLITUS

It is clearly established that DM is a well-established risk factor for death and cardiac complications such as cardiogenic shock in patients with acute STEMI. Although the use of reperfusion therapy in the treatment of STEMI has resulted in a considerable improvement in survival, diabetes remains an important predictor of mortality. Patients with abnormal fasting glycemia represent a large proportion of the MI population (53%) and the effects of such abnormal glucose metabolism during acute MI are

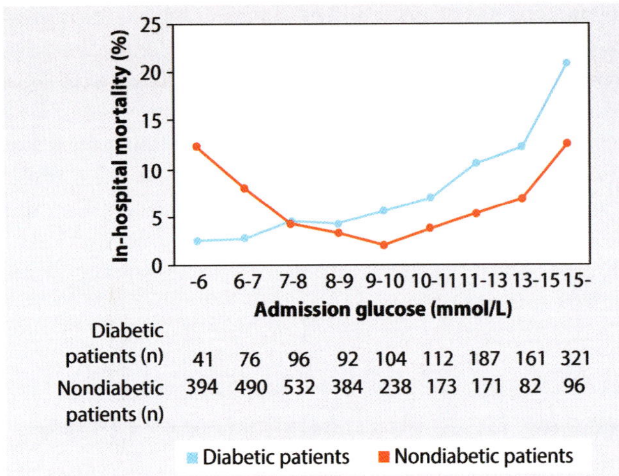

Fig. 2: A linear relation between admission blood glucose level and in-hospital mortality

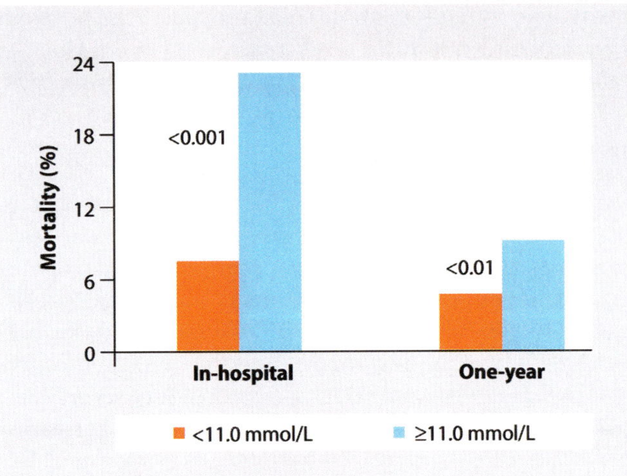

Fig. 3: Blood glucose at admission as an independent predictor of short-term and long-term mortality in acute myocardial infarction in the thrombolytic era (n=1,664)

deleterious with regard to short-term clinical outcomes. Improving microvascular perfusion within the ischemic myocardium remains the ultimate goal of managing STEMI patients with impaired glucose metabolism. Identification of defective myocardial perfusion together with an aggressive antithrombotic regimen, reduction of the inflammatory response of the ischemic myocardium and improvement of glycemia control represent promising therapeutic approaches.[9]

In patients with the clinical presentation of MI and with persistent ST-segment elevation or new or presumed new left bundle branch block, early mechanical or pharmacological reperfusion should be performed to limit the extent of myocardial damage unless clear contraindications are present.

ROLE OF FIBRINOLYSIS IN STEMI PATIENTS WITH DIABETES MELLITUS

Fibrinolytic therapy has undoubtedly improved the outcome of patients after acute myocardial infarction (AMI), saving 35 lives per 1,000 diabetic patients at 35 days compared with 15 per 1,000 nondiabetic patients.[10] Thus, the absolute benefit is more than doubled for fibrinolytic therapy among diabetics. Unfortunately, there are major drawbacks, which may account for the poor outcomes of STEMI patients with abnormal glucose metabolism as compared to those with normal fasting glycemia.[11]

In 1998, the National Registry of Myocardial Infarction reported that among the 84,663 patients eligible for reperfusion therapy, out of a total of 272,651, the odds of patients with DM receiving reperfusion therapy were only half of those of nondiabetics. The presence of DM remained an independent factor associated with failure to use reperfusion therapy in multivariate analysis [odds ratio (OR) 0.67; 95% confidence interval (CI) 0.52–0.87]. Similar findings were recently reported in a contemporary French survey (39% vs 51%; p = 0.0001).[12]

Diabetic patients, when they receive fibrinolytic therapy, receive it later than nondiabetics. The impaired sensation of pain may account for atypical and late presentation of diabetic patients. Diabetes, in common with age, female gender, history of heart failure and history of previous MI, was a predictive factor of non-revascularization of STEMI in the large Global Registry of Acute Coronary Events (GRACE). Fibrinolytic agents may have reduced efficacy in patients with impaired glucose tolerance. Indeed, the propensity for platelet activation and aggregation, coupled with a tendency for coagulation and impaired intrinsic fibrinolysis, are common features in diabetic patients.[13] Reassessment of epicardial flow in the Thrombolysis in Myocardial Infarction (TIMI)-4, 10, 10A, 10B and 14 studies (n=2,588) demonstrated no relationship between diabetes and TIMI-3 flow at 90 minutes (55.4%, vs 59.0% in those without diabetes). These findings are concordant with the GUSTO-1 trial. However, complete ST-segment resolution occurred less frequently in diabetic patients after fibrinolysis (38.6% vs 49.2%, adjusted p=0.04), suggesting impaired microvascular flow (Fig. 4).

ROLE OF PRIMARY PERCUTANEOUS CORONARY INTERVENTION IN STEMI PATIENTS WITH DIABETES MELLITUS

Thrombolytic therapy was the first effective treatment to reduce mortality in STEMI. Although accessible to virtually

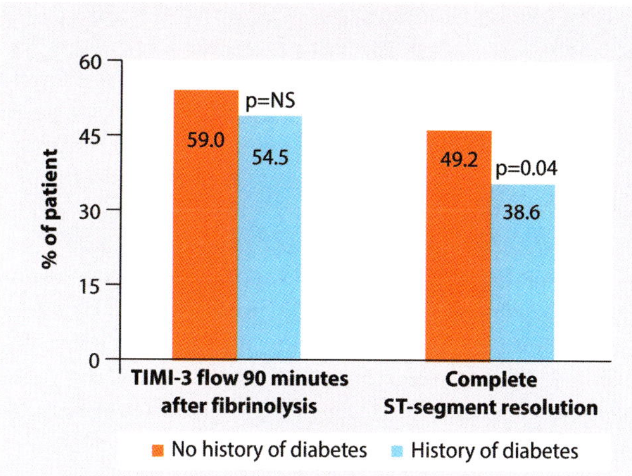

Fig. 4: Epicardial and microvascular flow after fibrinolytic therapy for STEMI. TIMI (Thrombolysis in Myocardial Infarction)-3 flow indicates normal flow in the coronary artery. A complete ST-segment resolution indicates a normal microvascular flow

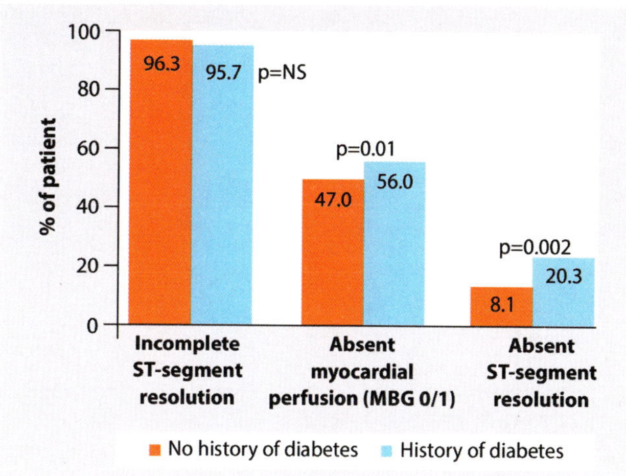

Fig. 6

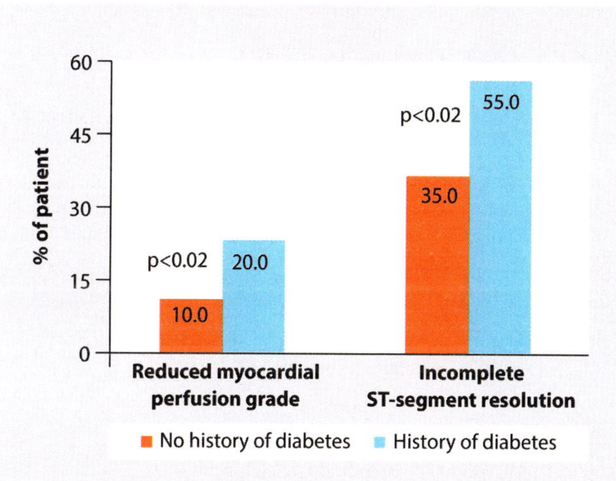

Fig. 5: PCI for STEMI with and without diabetes

all patients, fibrinolysis fails to reopen occluded arteries in 50% of cases. Primary stent percutaneous coronary intervention (PCI) has now become the reperfusion strategy of choice since it is superior to fibrinolysis in preventing death, regardless of time from symptom onset.[14] Impaired microvascular flow in diabetics was recently confirmed by the Zwolle Myocardial Infarction Study Group.

This group reported on 386 patients who underwent successful primary PCI for STEMI of whom, 64 had DM (Fig. 5). These patients had reduced myocardial perfusion grade (MPG) and incomplete ST-segment resolution more often compared with patients without DM. DM was still associated with impaired ST resolution (OR 2.1, p <0.03) and reduced MPG (OR 2.2, p <0.03) after the inclusion of all variables, with trends toward a significant difference between patients with and without DM. This was further confirmed in a substudy of the CADILLAC randomized trial (Controlled Abciximab and Device Investigation to Lower Late Angioplasty Complications). Despite similar high rates of TIMI flow grade 3 after primary PCI in patients with and without diabetes, DM was an independent predictor of absent myocardial perfusion (MPG 0/1) [Hazard ratio (HR) 1.63, 95% confidence interval (CI) 1.17-2.28], (p=0.004) and absent ST-segment resolution (HR 2.94, 95% CI 1.64-5.37), (p=0.005) by multivariate modeling (Fig. 6). Diminished microvascular perfusion in diabetics after primary PCI may contribute to adverse outcomes.

WHAT COULD BE BETTER ANTI-THROMBOTIC OPTIONS FOR STEMI PATIENTS HAVING DIABETES MELLITUS?

Improvement of myocardial perfusion is obviously a key issue to improve outcomes of AMI patients with abnormal glucose metabolism. Methods of improving coronary flow before primary PCI or fibrinolysis in these patients are warranted. Glycoprotein (GP) IIb/IIIa receptor inhibitors may answer this challenge. These agents block the final pathway of platelet aggregation and have been tested successfully in the prevention of coronary complications

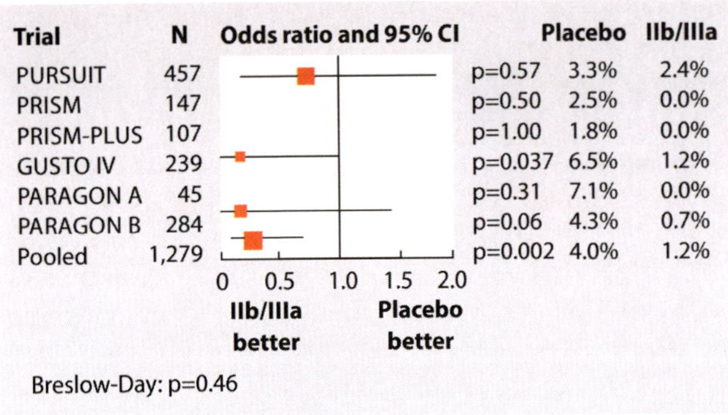

Fig. 7: Odds ratios with 95% confidence intervals and corresponding p values for GpIIb/IIIa treatment effect on 30-day mortality among diabetic patients with acute coronary syndrome undergoing percutaneous coronary intervention

of elective percutaneous coronary revascularization. These agents have been shown to reduce mortality in DM patients undergoing elective PCI[15] (Fig. 7).

Fewer and smaller randomized studies have been conducted in primary PCI of STEMI. A meta-analysis of this heterogeneous population, including balloon and stent studies, primary and rescue PCI, showed a significant effect of GP IIb/IIIa inhibition on mortality (4.4% vs 6.2%; OR 0.69; 95% CI 0.52–0.92; p=0.01). Early administration of these agents, especially during the prehospital management phase, has been shown to improve coronary patency, with favorable trends for clinical outcome. Importantly, a recent analysis obtained in a more homogeneous study population representative of modern primary PCI practice (n=1,101) providing for the first time long-term follow-up to 3 years, confirmed a reduction in hard clinical outcomes with the use of GP IIb/IIIa receptor antagonists. This risk reduction translates into 50 major events (death or re-infarction) prevented for every 1,000 patients treated—this benefit increases five-fold in diabetics, with 250 deaths or MIs prevented for every 1,000 diabetic patients treated.[16]

Clopidogrel has shown significant mortality reduction with lesser bleeding in trials like CLARITY-COMMIT. In CLARITY trial, out of 3,491 patients, 13% patients were having DM. In this group of patients, 300 mg clopidogrel followed by 75 mg OD had shown significant mortality reduction against placebo. The large TRITON TIMI 38 randomized trial compared clopidogrel to prasugrel in the setting of percutaneous coronary intervention for acute coronary syndromes. The diabetic subgroup (n = 3,146) experienced considerable incremental benefit with a 4.8% reduction in cardiovascular death, nonfatal MI, and nonfatal stroke at 15-month follow-up with prasugrel treatment. Early 32% (6,806/21,162) of the patients in the PEGASUS TIMI 54 trial had diabetes, out of whom 87% (5,960/6,806) were treated with hypoglycemic pharmacological therapy. In diabetic patients, the absolute difference in primary outcome was 4% higher in the placebo arm as compared to nondiabetics at 3-year follow up. Antiplatelet therapy has shown significant advantage in diabetic subgroup patients of ACS. Other major issues may be critical for DM patients.[15] Post-fibrinolysis strategies are important given the fact that fibrinolysis fails to reopen the occluded artery in 50% of patients. Whether all DM patients should undergo rapid catheterization is a real question given the fact that complete ST-segment resolution occurs less frequently among diabetic patients after fibrinolysis. Acute and late stent thrombosis is another question. Indeed, DM is an independent predictor of stent thrombosis and the question arises whether the dual oral antiplatelet aggregation regime of aspirin + clopidogrel should ever be withheld from these patients.[16]

ROLE OF CORONARY ARTERY BYPASS GRAFTING IN STEMI PATIENTS WITH DIABETES MELLITUS

Percutaneous coronary intervention promised a less invasive approach to revascularization, but early clinical trials showed surgical revascularization [coronary artery bypass graft (CABG) yielded better outcomes for patients with DM]. Restenosis is a classic response to mechanical injury of the vessel wall. Endothelial damage causes local thrombosis; superficial and then deep inflammation, which trigger smooth muscle cell proliferation; and eventually matrix remodeling and extracellular matrix deposition. Each of these events can be exacerbated by hyperglycemia, hyperinsulinemia, insulin or DM.[17] The Bypass Angioplasty Revascularization Investigation (BARI) trial compared patients who were randomly assigned to treatment of multivessel CAD with percutaneous transluminal coronary angioplasty (PTCA) (without stent) or CABG. Results showed superiority for CABG over balloon angioplasty (PTCA) and a very high rate of reintervention [target vessel revascularization (TVR)] after PTCA (76.8% vs 20.3%, p<0.001). Specifically for patients with DM, survival was significantly better after CABG (57.8% vs PTCA 45.5%, p=0.025).[18] The SYNTAX study (Synergy between PCI with Taxus and Cardiac Surgery) was a seminal multicenter randomized trial of three-vessel or left main coronary disease treated by DES or CABG. SYNTAX established a new standardized score to compare the distribution and severity of CAD. At 4 years, all cause and cardiac mortality were each lower after CABG, mainly in patients in the moderate or high SYNTAX score tertiles. SYNTAX prespecified a DM subgroup. Among this cohort (n=452), PCI patients had significantly more cardiac deaths at 5 years than CABG (12.7% versus 6.5%, respectively, p=0.034).[19] The Future Revascularization Evaluation in Patients with Diabetes Mellitus: Optimal Management of Multivessel Disease (FREEDOM) trial was specifically designed to identify the optimal revascularization strategy for patients with DM and multivessel CAD. Enrolled were patients with DM who had double (17%) or triple vessel disease (83%) but without left main stenosis. Between 2005–2010, 33,000 patients were screened; 3,300 were eligible and 1,900 consented and were randomized to revascularization with CABG or PCI (DES 94%). The primary outcome was a composite of all cause death, nonfatal MI, and nonfatal stroke. Mean age was 63.1 ± 9.1 years and mean hemoglobin A1c as an index of blood sugar control was 7.8%. Most patients had normal left ventricular function (mean ejection fraction 66%) and median follow-up was 3.8 years. The mean SYNTAX score was 26.2 ± 8.6 (middle tertile) and the SYNTAX score did not predict outcomes after CABG, but did predict worse outcomes after PCI.

At 30 days, the primary outcome favored PCI patients, but at all points after 30 days, the primary outcome favored CABG (PCI 26.6% vs CABG 18.7%; p=0.005), and the relative risk (RR) reduction was 30% for CABG. Results were mainly driven by differences between PCI and CABG in MI (13.9% vs 6.0%, respectively; p<0.001) and death from any cause (16.3% vs 10.9%, respectively; p<0.049).[20]

GUIDELINE RECOMMENDATIONS

Guidelines for the management of patients with ACS have been developed by the American College of Cardiology (ACC) or American Heart Association (AHA) and the European Society of Cardiology. In most situations, there are no clinical trials that specifically address management of the patient with diabetes and ACS. However, subgroup analyses in patients with diabetes and ACS show either a similar or an enhanced benefit from treatment compared to the overall group. The availability of more potent and reliable antiplatelet agents for the management of patients with ACS provides an opportunity to further reduce recurrent ACS and mortality. High-risk patients with diabetes with either STEMI or non-ST elevation acute coronary syndromes (NSTE-ACS) should be considered for treatment with either prasugrel (after the coronary disease anatomy has been defined) or ticagrelor. Platelet aggregation is largely mediated by the GPIIb/IIIa receptor through its binding to fibrinogen. The GPIIb/IIIa receptor inhibitors abciximab, eptifibatide and tirofiban were shown to be effective for the management of ACS in patients with diabetes in a meta-analysis of six clinical trials. GPIIb/IIIa inhibitors were shown to reduce 30-day mortality by 26% (4.6% vs 2.6%; p=0.007). In contrast, patients without diabetes had no mortality benefit. Patients with diabetes and ACS undergoing PCI should receive antiplatelet therapy with prasugrel (if clopidogrel naïve, <75 years of age, weight >65 kg, and no history of stroke) (Grade A, level 1) or ticagrelor (Grade B, level 1), rather than clopidogrel, to further reduce recurrent ischemic events. Patients with diabetes and non-STE ACS and higher-risk features destined for a selective invasive strategy should receive ticagrelor rather than clopidogrel (Grade B, level 2). Patients with diabetes and non-STE ACS and high-risk features should receive an early invasive strategy rather than a selective invasive approach to revascularization to reduce recurrent coronary events, unless contraindicated (Grade B, level 2). An appropriate protocol should be developed and staff trained to ensure the safe and effective implementation of this therapy and to minimize the complications of ACS in DM patients.[21] American Diabetes Association recommends to use aspirin therapy (75–162 mg/day) as secondary prevention in those with diabetes and history of atherosclerotic cardiovascular disease (ASCVD) (A). For patients with ASCVD and aspirin allergy, clopidogrel (75 mg/day) should be used (B). Dual antiplatelet therapy is reasonable for up to a year after an acute coronary syndrome (B).[22]

CONCLUSION

Patients with DM develop worse forms of atherosclerotic CAD and medical management of such coronary disease has consistently yielded results inferior to revascularization. Notwithstanding developments in PCI, diabetics still do less well with PCI than patients who do not have DM. PCI is established as the appropriate treatment for patients with DM presenting with acute coronary syndromes (non-ST segment elevation MI and ST-elevation MI). Diabetic patients benefit from the same medical management and secondary risk modification as patients without DM. Level 1 evidence from the SYNTAX trial establishes CABG as the revascularization option of choice in patients with more complex CAD. Level 1 evidence from the FREEDOM trial has confirmed that diabetic patients with multivessel CAD benefit from revascularization by CABG. Improvements in surgical revascularization benefiting patients with DM include wider use of the radial artery as a bypass conduit in place of the saphenous vein, and improved perioperative glucose management.

REFERENCES

1. Thom T, Haase N, Rosamond W, et al. For the American Heart Association Statistics Committee and Stroke Statistics Subcommittee. Heart disease and stroke statistics— 2006 update: a report from the AHA Statistics Committee and Stroke Statistics Subcommittee. Circulation. 2006;113:e85-e151.
2. Wahab NN, Cowden EA, Pearce NJ, et al. Is blood glucose an independent predictor of mortality in acute myocardial infarction in the thrombolytic era? J Am Coll Cardiol. 2002;40:1748-54.
3. Zeller M, Steg P, Ravisy J, et al. Prevalence and impact of metabolic syndrome on hospital outcomes in acute myocardial infarction. Arch Intern Med. 2005;165:1192-8.
4. Haffner SM, Lehto S, Ronnemaa T, et al. Mortality from coronary heart disease in subjects with type 2 diabetes and in nondiabetic subjects with and without prior myocardial infarction. N Engl J Med. 1998;339:229-34.
5. Verhagen SN, Wassink AM, van der Graaf Y, et al. Insulin resistance increases the occurrence of new cardiovascular events in patients with manifest arterial disease without known diabetes. the SMART study. Cardiovasc Diabetol. 2011;10:100.
6. Carr ME. Diabetes mellitus: a hypercoagulable state. J Diabetes Complications. 2001;15:44-54.
7. Ceriello A, Giugliano D, Quatraro A, et al. Evidence for a hyperglycemia-dependent decrease of antithrombin III-thrombin complex formation in humans. Diabetologia. 1990;33:163-7.
8. Malmberg K, Yusuf S, Gerstein HC, et al. Impact of diabetes on long-term prognosis in patients with unstable angina and non-Q-wave myocardial infarction: results of the OASIS (Organization to Assess Strategies for Ischemic Syndromes) Registry. Circulation. 2000;102:1014-9.
9. Collete JP, Montalescot G. The acute reperfusion management of STEMI in patients with impaired glucose tolerance and type 2 diabetes. Diabetes Vasc Dis Res. 2005;2:136-43.
10. Fibrinolytic Therapy Trialists (FTT) Collaborative Group. Indications for fibrinolytic therapy in suspected acute myocardial infarction: collaborative overview of early mortality and major morbidity results from all randomized trials of more than 1,000 patients. Lancet. 1994;343:311-22.
11. Wahab NN, Cowden EA, Pearce NJ, et al. Is blood glucose an independent predictor of mortality in acute myocardial infarction in the thrombolytic era? J Am Coll Cardiol. 2002;40:1748-54.
12. Vaur L, Danchin N, Hanania G, et al. Management and short-term outcome of diabetic patients hospitalized for acute myocardial infarction: results of a nationwide French survey. Diabetes Metab. 2003;29:241-9.
13. Eagle KA, Goodman SG, Avezum A, et al. Practice variation and missed opportunities for reperfusion in ST-segment-elevation myocardial infarction: findings from the Global Registry of Acute Coronary Events (GRACE). Lancet. 2002;359:373-7.
14. Silber S, Albertsson P, Aviles FF, et al. Guidelines for percutaneous coronary interventions. The task force for percutaneous coronary interventions of the European Society of Cardiology. Eur Heart J. 2005;26:804-47.
15. Ferreiro JL, Angiolillo DJ. Diabetes and antiplatelet therapy in acute coronary syndrome. Circulation. 2011;123:798-813.
16. Iakovou I, Schmidt T, Bonizzoni E, et al. Incidence, predictors, and outcome of thrombosis after successful implantation of drug-eluting stents. JAMA. 2005;293:2126-30.
17. Hoffman D, Tranbaugh RF. Coronary artery bypass graft (CABG) and the diabetic patient: current perspectives. Dove Press. 2014;(2014):57-67.
18. BARI Investigators. The final 10-year follow-up results from the BARI randomized trial. J Am Coll Cardiol. 2007;49(15):1600-06.
19. Kappetein P, Head SJ, Morice MC, et al. SYNTAX Investigators. Treatment of complex coronary artery disease in patients with diabetes: 5-year results comparing outcomes of bypass surgery and percutaneous coronary intervention in the SYNTAX trial. Eur J Cardiothorac Surg. 2013;43(5):1006-13.
20. Farkouh ME, Domanski M, Sleeper LA, et al. Strategies for multivessel revascularization in patients with diabetes. N Engl J Med. 2012;367(25):2375-84.
21. Harper W, Clement M, Goldenberg R, et al. Canadian Diabetes Association 2013 Clinical Practice Guidelines for the Prevention and Management of Diabetes in Canada: pharmacologic management of type 2 diabetes. Can J Diabetes. 2013;37(Suppl 1):S61-8.
22. American Diabetes Association Standards of Medical Care in Diabetes. Cardiovascular disease and risk management. Diabetes Care. 2017;40 (Suppl 1):S75-87.

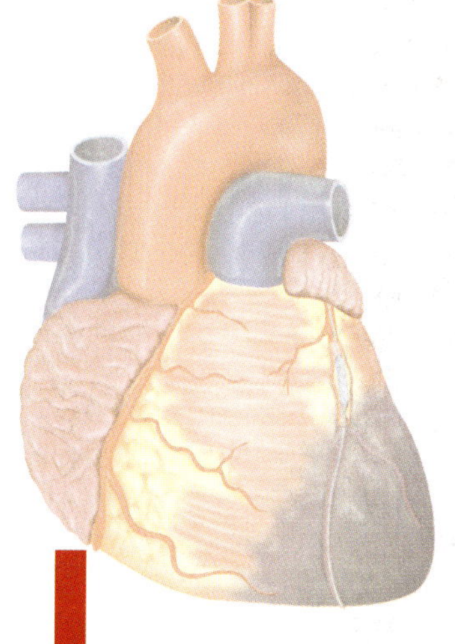

CTO with STEMI in Cardiodiabetes: Is the Outcome Different?

Satyendra Tewari, Ankit Kumar Sahu

INTRODUCTION

A coronary chronic total occlusion (CTO) is defined as a 100% occlusion with thrombolysis in myocardial infarction (TIMI) grade 0 flow for atleast 3 months. This 3 month period is an arbitrary cutoff as the chronology of intracoronary lesion organization is different from myocardial infarct healing. It is worthwhile to note the chronicity of a coronary lesion and its morphology has nothing to do with the quantum of myocardial damage. Its inflict proven by the observation that in many patients with ST-elevation myocardial infarction (STEMI), who present late, the acute total occlusion progresses to CTO silently without any clinical demarcation or progressive myocardial damage. CTO are commonly encountered complex lesions that are most frequently treated with medical therapy or surgical revascularization rather than with percutaneous coronary intervention (PCI). CTOs are regarded as very complex lesions with relatively low procedural success rates, and even after successful PCI, restenosis rates are 1.5- to 4-times higher compared with nonoccluded coronary artery lesions. In the past 5 years, important advancements have been made in techniques that safely and more predictably overcome this essential challenge.[1] These complex lesions are found in 18% of patients with significant coronary artery disease (CAD) at angiography; evidence of myocardial infarction (MI) in the territory subtended by the CTO is present in only 25% of cases.[2] Despite this frequent finding, only 13.7% of eligible CTOs are treated with PCI,[3] and CTOs account for only 5% of all vascular interventions.[4]

EPIDEMIOLOGY, CLINICAL PROFILE, AND PRESENTATION

Approximately 10–15% of STEMI patients undergoing primary percutaneous coronary intervention (pPCI) are found to have a CTO in a noninfarct related artery (IRA).[5,6] When compared with a cohort of patients of CAD patients without CTO, cohorts of CAD patients with CTO have more advanced stages of atherosclerosis, more likely to be male, elderly, diabetic, hypertensive, have associated multivessel disease (MVD), peripheral arterial disease, and cerebrovascular disease. A two-fold excess in history of prior MI was observed among CTO patients in both Canadian[2] and Swedish[7] registries (40% vs 23% and 37% vs 17% respectively; $p < 0.01$). Acute coronary syndrome (ACS) immediately preceded CTO detection in 46% of Canadian[2] and 40% of Swedish[7] cohort. However, the relationship between a CTO, the presence and extent of infarction in the subtended territory and the degree of left ventricular (LV) dysfunction attributable to CTO is not well-established. Conversely, in a prospective single center registry of nearly 3,000 consecutive pPCI procedures for STEMI, the prevalence of a preexisting CTO was 12.8%. Moreover, patients with CTO detected at pPCI had significantly worse prognosis than patients with single-vessel CAD (infarct vessel only) or those with MVD without a CTO.[8] A study in 170 consecutive patients with an angiographically documented CTO undergoing late gadolinium enhancement cardiac magnetic resonance imaging (cMRI) also reported that while only 42% of patients had previous ischemic symptoms consistent with MI, yet cMRI showed that 86% of patients had evidence of a prior MI.[9]

DIABETES AND CTO IN THE SETTING OF STEMI

Patients with diabetes mellitus (DM) constitute a patient group with a high prevalence of MVD and high mortality after STEMI. Approximately 35–45% of nondiabetic STEMI patients have MVD compared with 60–70% of patients with DM. Diabetic patients with MVD (both with and without a CTO) were older, more often had a previous MI and cardiogenic shock at presentation were more often treated with intra-aortic balloon pump counter pulsation and were less frequently treated with coronary stents and thrombosuction than patients with single vessel disease (SVD). Furthermore, patients with a CTO in a non-IRA more often had a previous MI and cardiogenic shock at presentation than those with MVD without a CTO. According to a study by Claessen et al.[10] the prevalence of a CTO in a non-IRA was 21% in diabetic patients with STEMI as compared to 12% in nondiabetic patients with STEMI (p<0.01) (Figs 1A and B).

PROGNOSIS AND OUTCOMES

Patients with MVD have two-fold higher morbidity and mortality rates compared with patients with SVD in STEMI setting,[11,12] mainly attributable to the increased mortality caused by heart failure.[5,12] Although, several observational studies[13-15] suggest that CTO-PCI leads to higher LV ejection fraction (mean 4.4%), significant reduction in residual or recurrent angina, reduced need for coronary artery bypass graft (CABG) surgery, and improved survival, yet CTO-PCI is attempted only in 10% of all CTO lesions, that too in elective setting despite the success rate of 80–90% in high-volume center and experienced operator in current modern times.[3] Patients with CTO have a higher prevalence of comorbidities including diabetes and previous MI, nevertheless, the presence of a CTO is an independent predictor of mortality.

A Netherlands registry[16] of 4,506 STEMI patients from 1997 to 2007 evaluated the prevalence of CTO in a non-IRA and its impact on long-term mortality in diabetics. MVD with or without CTO was present in 33% of nondiabetic patients and in 51% of diabetic patients. Kaplan-Meier estimates for 5-year mortality in STEMI patients with diabetes were 25%, 21%, and 47% in patients with SVD, MVD without CTO and MVD with non-IRA CTO, respectively. CTO in a non-IRA was an independent predictor of 5-year mortality [HR 2.2, 95% confidence interval (CI), 1.3–3.5, p<0.01]. Diabetic patients with MVD without a CTO had a 5-year mortality rate which was comparable to diabetic patients with SVD and also comparable to nondiabetic patients with MVD without a CTO (Fig. 2).

Zhang et al.[17] evaluated the effect of non-IRA CTO on the cardiovascular outcomes in patients undergoing

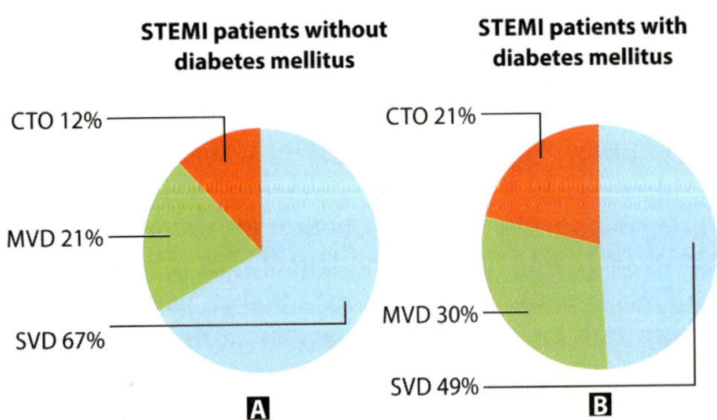

Figs 1A and B: Prevalence of single vessel disease, multivessel disease without a CTO and CTO in (A) patients with STEMI without diabetes mellitus and (B) patients with STEMI with diabetes mellitus

Abbreviations: CTO, chronic total occlusion; MVD, multivessel disease; STEMI, ST-elevation myocardial infarction; SVD, single vessel disease

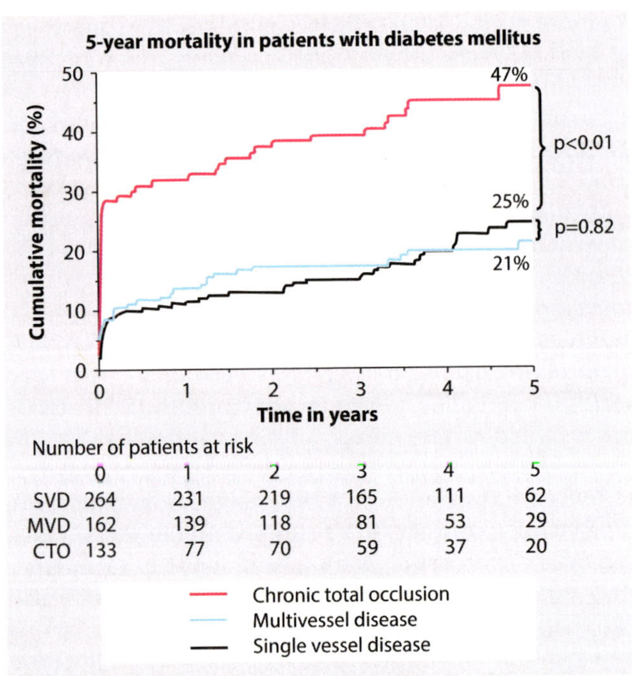

Fig. 2: Kaplan-Meier estimates of 5-year mortality in patients with ST-elevation myocardial infarction with diabetes mellitus treated with primary percutaneous coronary intervention

Abbreviations: CTO, chronic total occlusion; MVD, multivessel disease; SVD, single vessel disease

pPCI and found out that patients with CTO in a non-IRA who underwent pPCI for acute STEMI had a higher cardiac mortality. After adjusted for differences in clinical, angiographic, and procedure variables, the presence of CTO in a non-IRA, cardiogenic shock on admission, and 3-vessel disease remained an independent predictor of greater 1-year cardiac mortality (Fig. 3).

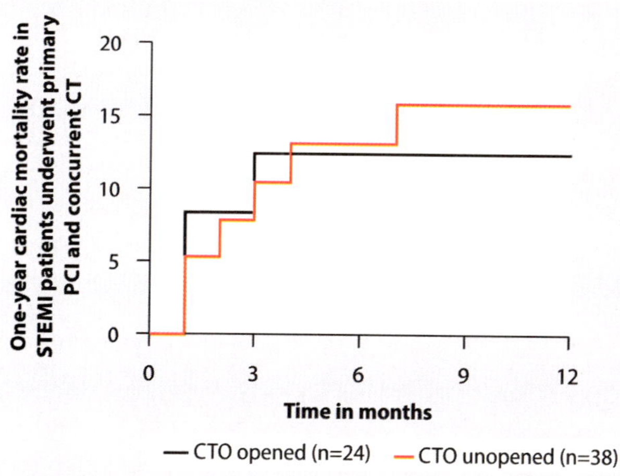

Fig. 3: One-year cardiac mortality rate in STEMI patients underwent primary PCI and concurrent CTO. Patients with CTO being opened versus patients with CTO being unopened, Log-rank P = 0.744.

Abbreviations: CTO, chronic total occlusion; PCI, percutaneous coronary intervention; STEMI, ST-elevation myocardial infarction; CT, computer tomography

A number of mechanisms may be responsible for this worsened prognosis includes:

1. Impaired healing at the infarct border zone
2. Decreased protection against future cardiovascular events
3. Increased risk of arrhythmias
4. Larger completed infarct size in patients with a CTO in a non-IRA, particularly if the distal coronary bed of the CTO depends upon collateral flow from IRA. In this situation, the area at risk of the IRA territory would extend beyond its own supply territory and extend to the collateralized non-IRA CTO area[18]
5. Higher rate of incomplete ST segment resolution
6. Reduced myocardial blush grade after pPCI for STEMI suggesting impaired reperfusion at the myocardial tissue level
7. Adverse metabolic changes in endothelium due to longstanding hyperglycemia, hyperinsulinemia, and increased free fatty acids
8. Intrinsic myocardial dysfunction in diabetic patients, probably as a result of autonomic neuropathy and microvascular dysfunction.

In the multicenter, randomized, prospective, two-arm EXPLORE[19] trial, participants were randomly assigned at a 1:1 ratio to treatment with PCI for CTO (n = 148) within 7 days of STEMI or no CTO intervention after STEMI (n = 154). In the CTO-PCI group, there were 13 patients (9%) with multiple CTOs, and 22 patients (14%) in the no CTO-PCI group (Table 1). The (mean, SD) pre-pPCI MI SYNTAX

TABLE 1: Imaging related outcomes included in EXPLORE trial

	CTO PCI	*No CTO PCI*	*Difference (95% CI)*	*p value*
Primary endpoint	136	144		
Left ventricular ejection fraction, %	44.1 (12.2)	44.8 (11.9)	−0.8 (−3.6 to 2.1)	0.60
Left ventricular end-diastolic volume, mL	215.6 (62.5)	212.8 (60.3)	2.8 (−11.6 to 17.2)	0.70
MRI or other imaging	132	143		
Left ventricular ejection fraction, %	45.1 (10.9)	45.1 (11.6)	0.1 (−2.7 to 2.7)	1.00
Left ventricular end-diastolic volume, mL	209.9 (53.8)	211.5 (58.3)	−1.6 (−14.9 to 11.8)	0.82
Left ventricular end-diastolic volume index, mL/m^2	102.9 (23.9)	104.3 (25.4)	−1.4 (−7.3 to 4.4)	0.63
Left ventricular end-systolic volume index, mL/m^2	57.9 (22.6)	58.9 (24.8)	−1.1 (−6.7 to 4.6)	0.71
MRI only	124	135		
Left ventricular ejection fraction, %	45.0 (10.6)	45.2 (11.5)	−0.2 (−2.9 to 2.5)	0.88
Left ventricular end-diastolic volume, mL	213.8 (51.8)	214.8 (56.4)	−1.0 (−14.2 to 12.3)	0.89
Left ventricular end-diastolic volume index, mL/m^2	104.9 (22.6)	105.9 (24.2)	−1.0 (−6.7 to 4.7)	0.73
Left ventricular end-systolic volume index, mL/m^2	59.0 (22.4)	59.7 (24.5)	−0.7 (−6.5 to 5.0)	0.81
Left ventricular end-diastolic mass index, g/m^2	51.6 (9.2)	52.4 (12.0)	−0.8 (−3.5 to 2.0)	0.58
Dysfunctional segment, %*	58.0 (26.6)	61.5 (27.0)	−3.6 (−10.4 to 3.2)	0.30
Total infarct size, g†	7.6 (6.0)	7.2 (5.6)	0.4 (−11 to 2.0)	0.59

Value are n or n (%), unless otherwise indicated * Data available in n = 113/n = 130. †Data available in n = 95/n = 114.

Abbreviations: CTO, chronic total occlusion; PCI, percutaneous coronary intervention; MRI, magnetic resonance imaging; CI, confidence interval

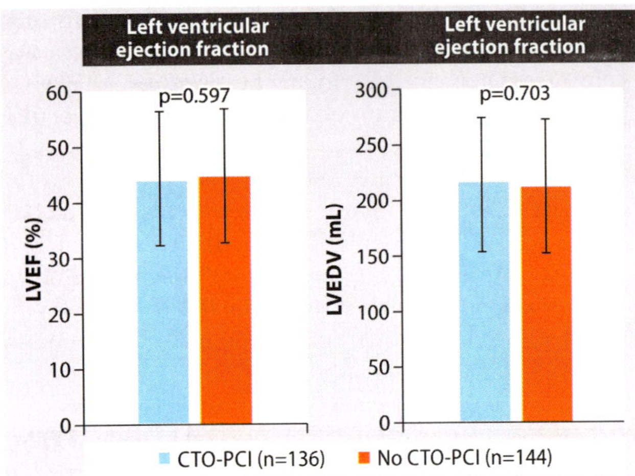

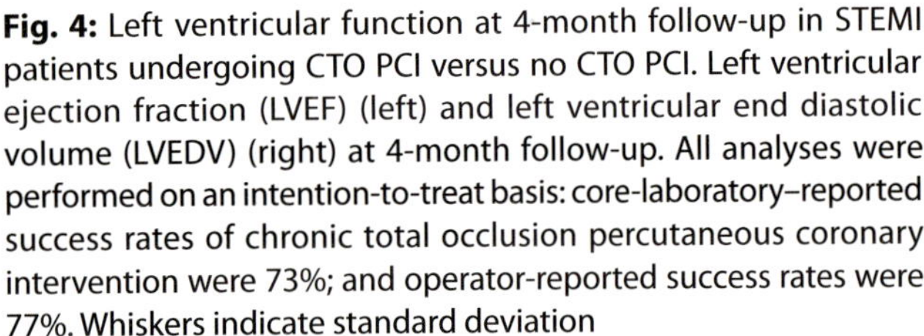

Fig. 4: Left ventricular function at 4-month follow-up in STEMI patients undergoing CTO PCI versus no CTO PCI. Left ventricular ejection fraction (LVEF) (left) and left ventricular end diastolic volume (LVEDV) (right) at 4-month follow-up. All analyses were performed on an intention-to-treat basis: core-laboratory–reported success rates of chronic total occlusion percutaneous coronary intervention were 73%; and operator-reported success rates were 77%. Whiskers indicate standard deviation

Abbreviations: CTO, chronic total occlusion; PCI, percutaneous coronary intervention; STEMI, ST-elevation myocardial infarction

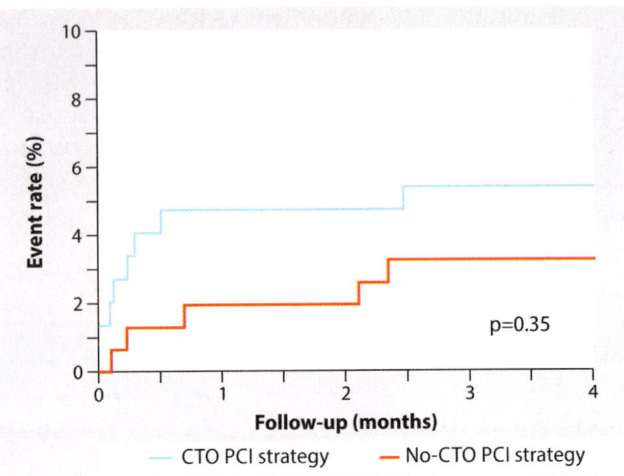

Fig. 5: Major adverse cardiac events event rates at 4 months follow-up. Major adverse cardiac events consisted of cardiac death, myocardial infarction, and coronary artery bypass graft operation

Abbreviations: CTO, chronic total occlusion; PCI, percutaneous coronary intervention

score was 29 ± 8 in the CTO-PCI group, and 29 ± 10 in the no CTO-PCI group found no significant difference in 4 month percent LV ejection fraction [CTO-PCI 44.1 (12.2) vs. no CTO-PCI, 44.8 (11.9); difference, -0.8; 95% CI, -3.6–2.1] or LVEDV in mL [CTO-PCI, 215.6 (62.5) vs. no CTO-PCI, 212.8 (60.3); difference, 2.8; 95% CI, -11.6–17.2] (Fig. 4). In terms of major adverse CV events at 4 months, the rate was 5.4% in the CTO-PCI group and 2.6% in the no CTO-PCI group (P = 0.212). However, on subgroup analysis, there was a significant improvement in LVEF (p = 0.002) and LV end diastolic volume (LVEDV) (p = 0.039) in the left anterior descending (LAD) CTO subset. One major drawback of this trial was that it was not powered enough to predict clinical outcomes (Fig. 5).

Another trial DECISION-CTO[20] was conducted to assess the safety and efficacy of CTO-PCI compared with optimal medical therapy (OMT) among patients with atleast one CTO. The primary endpoint for CTO-PCI with OMT versus OMT alone, major adverse cardiac events (MACE) at 3 years (all-cause mortality, MI, stroke, and repeat revascularization) was 20.6% versus 19.6% ($P_{noninferiority}$ = 0.008), thereby concluding that routine CTO-PCI with OMT is not superior to OMT alone in reducing cardiovascular outcomes among patients with atleast one CTO.

The EURO-CTO trial[21] randomized 396 patients from 26 centers on a 2:1 basis to PCI or OMT. Half (50%) of the patients had single vessel CTOs and 30% had a non-CTO lesion treated before randomization. Results showed a high procedural success rate with PCI and low procedural risk. The CTO was successfully opened in 86.3% of patients treated with PCI. There were no procedural deaths and the overall 12-month major adverse cardiac and cerebrovascular events (MACCE) rate was 0.4%. Improvement in clinical symptoms was more pronounced in patients treated with PCI than with OMT, based on the Seattle Angina Questionnaire (SAQ) subscales of physical limitation and angina frequency. The PCI group also showed a trend to improved quality of life and significantly greater absolute freedom from angina.

SHINE-CTO (NCT02784418) an ongoing single center, double-blind, sham-controlled trial will address the clinical benefit in terms of functional capacity as assessed by the 7-item SAQ. In this trial, randomization of symptomatic patients with a coronary CTO to CTO-PCI or a sham-procedure is done in 1:1 ratio. Patients randomized to sham-procedure will undergo only bilateral arterial access, without angiography or PCI being performed.

CONCLUSION

Angiographically coronary CTO are one of the pinnacles of interventional cardiology. CTO in non-IRA are seen in about one-eighth of the patients undergoing primary PCI for STEMI although, the success rate was 60–70%. Diabetic patients enhance the complexity of the lesion (heavy calcification, high thrombus burden, distal vessel (microvascular) disease, and diffuse nature of CAD), besides technically challenging interventional procedure, delayed presentation and LV dysfunction (diabetic cardiomyopathy), and therefore, have poor survival as compared to nondiabetics. Also based on the findings of EXPLORE trial, CTO-PCI of non-IRA within 1 week of pPCI is safe, but does not result in improved LV function or clinical outcomes over a follow-up of 4 months. Although, PCI of a CTO located in the LAD may improve LV ejection fraction and potentially improve clinical outcome during follow-up, despite of relatively low procedural success (~70%) in this trial for CTO-PCI. There should be ample evidence of inducible ischemia and viability before attempting non-IRA CTO-PCI. Therefore, the outcomes of intervention and prognosis for CTO-PCI are poorer in diabetic patients. Further large randomized trials are needed to evaluate long-term clinical efficacy and outcomes of non-IRA CTO-PCI in diabetic patients in the setting of STEMI as a staged procedure.

REFERENCES

1. Christofferson RD, Lehmann KG, Martin GV, et al. Effect of chronic total coronary occlusion on treatment strategy. Am J Cardiol. 2005;95(9):1088-91.
2. Fefer P, Knudtson ML, Cheema AN, et al. Current perspectives on coronary chronic total occlusions: the Canadian multicenter chronic total occlusions registry. J Am Coll Cardiol. 2012;59(12):991-7.
3. Grantham JA, Marso SP, Spertus JA, et al. Chronic total occlusion angioplasty in the United States. JACC Cardiovasc Interv. 2009;2(6):479-86.
4. Abbott JD, Kip KE, Vlachos HA, et al. Recent trends in the percutaneous treatment of chronic total coronary occlusions. Am J Cardiol. 2006;97(12):1691-6.
5. Tajstra M, Gasior M, Gierlotka M, et al. Comparison of five-year outcomes of patients with and without chronic total occlusion of noninfarct coronary artery after primary coronary intervention for ST-segment elevation acute myocardial infarction. Am J Cardiol. 2012;109(2):208-13.
6. Van der Schaaf RJ, Vis MM, Sjauw KD, et al. Impact of multivessel coronary disease on long-term mortality in patients with ST-elevation myocardial infarction is due to the presence of a chronic total occlusion. Am J Cardiol. 2006;98(9):1165-9.
7. Ramunddal T, Hoebers L, Henriques JP, et al. Chronic total occlusions in Sweden: a report from the Swedish Coronary Angiography and Angioplasty Registry (SCAAR). PLoS One. 2014;9(8):e103850.
8. Claessen BE, van der Schaaf RJ, Verouden NJ, et al. Evaluation of the effect of a concurrent chronic total occlusion on long-term mortality and left ventricular function in patients after primary percutaneous coronary intervention. JACC Cardiovasc Interv. 2009;2(11):1128-34.
9. Choi JH, Chang SA, Choi JO, et al. Frequency of myocardial infarction and its relationship to angiographic collateral flow in territories supplied by chronically occluded coronary arteries. Circulation. 2013;127(6):703-9.
10. Claessen BE, Hoebers LP, van der Schaaf RJ, et al. Prevalence and impact of a chronic total occlusion in a non-infarct-related artery on long-term mortality in diabetic patients with ST elevation myocardial infarction. Heart. 2010;96(24):1968-72.
11. Park DW, Clare RM, Schulte PJ, et al. Extent, location, and clinical significance of non-infarct related coronary artery disease among patients with ST-elevation myocardial infarction. JAMA. 2014;312(19):2019-27.
12. Van der Schaaf RJ, Timmer JR, Ottervanger JP, et al. Long-term impact of multivessel disease on cause-specific mortality after ST elevation myocardial infarction treated with reperfusion therapy. Heart. 2006;92(12):1760-3.
13. Joyal D, Afilalo J, Rinfret S. Effectiveness of recanalization of chronic total occlusions: a systematic review and meta-analysis. Am Heart J. 2010;160(1):179-87.
14. Christakopoulos GE, Christopoulos G, Carlino M, et al. Meta-analysis of clinical outcomes of patients who underwent percutaneous coronary interventions for chronic total occlusions. Am J Cardiol. 2015;115(10):1367-75.
15. Hoebers LP, Claessen BE, Elias J, et al. Meta-analysis on the impact of percutaneous coronary intervention of chronic total occlusions on left ventricular function and clinical outcome. Int J Cardiol. 2015;187:90-6.
16. Claessen B, Hoebers L, Henriques J. Coronary chronic total occlusions in the setting of acute myocardial infarction. EMJ Int Cardiol. 2014;1:38-43.
17. Zhang HP, Zhao Y, Li H, et al. Impact of chronic total occlusion in a noninfarct-related artery on clinical outcomes in patients with acute ST-elevation myocardial infarction undergoing primary percutaneous coronary intervention. Medicine (Baltimore). 2016;95(2):e2441.
18. Mozid AM, Mohdnazri S, Mannakkara NN, et al. Impact of a chronic total occlusion in a non-infarct related artery on clinical outcomes following primary percutaneous intervention in acute ST-elevation myocardial infarction. J Invasive Cardiol. 2014;26(1):13-6.
19. Henriques JP, Hoebers LP, Råmunddal T, et al. Percutaneous intervention for concurrent chronic total occlusions in patients with STEMI: the EXPLORE trial. J Am Coll Cardiol. 2016;68(15):1622-32.
20. Park SJ. Optimal medical therapy with or without stenting for coronary chronic total occlusion: DECISION-CTO. J Am Coll Cardiol, 2017.
21. Werner G. EuroCTO trial: better quality of life for patients with CTO PCI compared with OMT. EuroPCR, 2017.

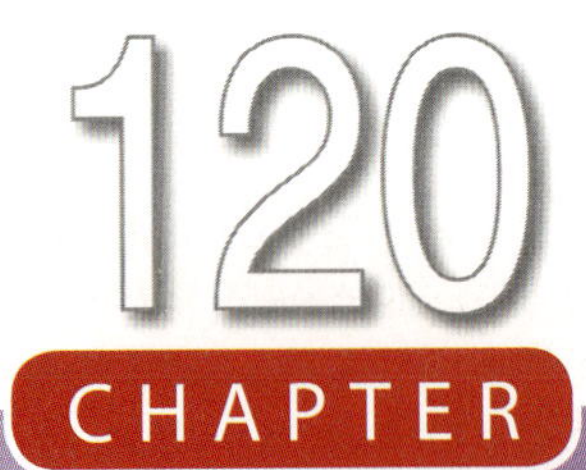

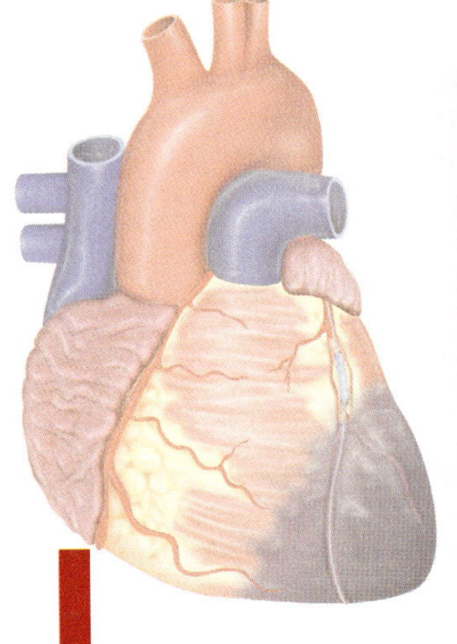

Coronary Intervention in Venous Grafts in Diabetes

Aniruddha Pawar, Prafulla Kerkar

INTRODUCTION

Diabetes is a major determinant of atherosclerosis and adverse cardiac events, and portends an adverse prognosis in patients with coronary artery disease regardless of treatment strategy. There is significant association between the HbA1C levels and severity of coronary artery disease (CAD).[1] It is shown in multiple trials that coronary artery bypass grafting (CABG) has significant mortality benefit over percutaneous coronary intervention (PCI) in diabetic population with multivessel disease.[2] The percutaneous treatment of patients with obstructive atherosclerotic disease in coronary saphenous vein bypass grafts (SVGs) remains a challenge in interventional cardiology. Patients undergoing SVG intervention are often older with significant comorbidities. Saphenous vein graft interventions carry a higher risk of acute complications, mainly distal embolization, and poorer long-term outcomes, mainly restenosis, than do native coronary vessel interventions.[3,4] Recurrent ischemic events and SVG stenosis have been shown to be higher among diabetic patients compared with nondiabetic patients at long-term follow-up with many such patients requiring vein graft interventions at follow-up. Important reason for poorer outcomes of PCI in SVGs is the embolization of atherothrombotic debris into the native coronary circulation, often resulting in periprocedural myocardial infarction (MI) or reduced antegrade flow (no-reflow). The occurrence of such events can be decreased by use of proximal and distal protection devices, adjunctive pharmacology and stenting with newer generation drug-eluting stents.

NATURAL HISTORY AND PATHOPHYSIOLOGY OF SAPHENOUS VEIN GRAFT DISEASE

The rate of SVG graft attrition is up to 40% during the first year; 1–2% of grafts occlude annually 1–5 years after surgery, and 4–5% occlude each year over the next 5 years. At 10 years, one-half of all SVGs are occluded, and half of the patent SVGs are diseased.[5] The SVG disease process involves three interlinked pathophysiological phenomena which lead to progressive degeneration: thrombosis, intimal hyperplasia, and atherosclerosis. Pathological studies have shown that because the medial layer of the SVG is thinner than that of the native coronary arteries, it is likely to be more susceptible to the mechanical damage caused by stents leading to more aggressive neointimal proliferation.

Thrombosis

About 10% of SVGs occlude, with or without symptoms, within the first month after CABG surgery. This early phenomenon is related to severe endothelial cell loss and medial damage during harvesting. In addition, this prothrombotic stage of SVG may be amplified by anastomosis stricture, and graft anastomosis proximal to diseased segments.

Intimal Hyperplasia

Intimal hyperplasia is the main disease process that occurs during the first months after venous bypass grafting. The pronounced increase in wall stress by exposure to arterial pressures seems to be an important factor inducing this phenomenon. This process represents the foundation for later development of SVG atherosclerosis.

Atherosclerosis

In the first years after CABG, atherosclerosis is the dominant process involved in SVG disease, but recurrent symptoms due to SVG disease rarely occur before three years after grafting. Morphologically, vein graft atherosclerosis tends to be diffuse, concentric, and friable with a poorly developed or absent fibrous cap and little evidence of calcification.

PATHOPHYSIOLOGY IN DIABETIC POPULATION

The graft atherosclerosis in patients with diabetes mellitus has more of a necrotic core with unstable plaques.[6] Pathophysiology in patients with diabetes mellitus has been attributed to exaggerated neointimal response, negative vessel remodeling and increased platelet aggregation.[7] DM is associated with both, systemic inflammation and atherosclerosis . Various cytokines and inflammatory mediators such as IFN-γ, IL-1, IL-6, and TNFα contribute to the pathogenesis of inflammation observed in atherosclerosis in patients with DM. The greater plaque instability with more particulate debris release appears to account for the greater microvascular obstruction immediately after stent implantation. The higher concentration of TNFα in particulate debris and coronary aspirate plasma of patients with DM possibly reflects the activity of the atherosclerotic process and could potentially serve as a biomarker for the incidence and extent of restenosis.[8,9]

INDICATIONS OF PCI IN VENOUS GRAFTS

Due to the increased risk of periprocedural MI related to SVG interventions, PCI of the native grafted vessel if technically feasible is usually preferred over PCI of the degenerated SVG. However, when PCI of the native vessel is not possible, the benefit of a high-risk SVG intervention should be balanced against the risk of morbidity and mortality of repeat CABG. The latest updated guidelines on this topic recommend PCI in the following circumstances:[7] Early ischemia (usually within 30 days) after CABG, when technically feasible. Ischemia occurs one to three years after CABG in patients with discrete lesions and preserved LV function. It is also reasonable in patients with diseased SVGs older than three years and, if feasible, in patients with patent left internal mammary artery (IMA) and significant obstruction in other vessels. PCI is not recommended in patients with total SVG occlusions, or multiple target lesions (native/SVG disease) and impaired LV function, unless repeat CABG poses excessive risk. CABG is usually reserved for patients who cannot have adequate percutaneous revascularization or for those who may gain an additional benefit from CABG, such as those with previously unused left IMA to left anterior descending artery.

PERCUTANEOUS INTERVENTIONS IN VENOUS GRAFTS

Redo-CABG is associated with a marked increase in morbidity and mortality compared with initial surgery[10] and is, therefore, used as a last resort. Percutaneous transluminal coronary angioplasty (PTCA) alone also proved to be inadequate therapy with unacceptably high rates of restenosis and major adverse coronary events (MACE).[11] The Saphenous Vein De Novo (SAVED) trial was the seminal study that compared balloon angioplasty with bare-metal stents (BMS) in SVG lesions.[12] This demonstrated that the use of BMS had a better composite outcome of freedom from death, MI, repeat CABG, and target lesion revascularization (TLR). Some observational studies comparing drug-eluting stents (DES) to BMS in SVG PCI suggest that DES was associated with reduction in TLR and death.[13,14] Other studies, however, showed no difference between DES and BMS in terms of death, MI, and target vessel revascularization (TVR).[15,16] The moderate VEin graft LEsion stenting with the Taxus stent and Intravascular ultrasound (VELETI) trial showed that stenting moderate SVG lesions with DES showed better luminal area, no progression to occlusion, and a trend toward lower incidence of MACE compared to medical treatment alone.[17]

PHARMACOLOGIC AND MECHANICAL STRATEGIES TO MINIMIZE COMPLICATIONS DURING SVG PCI

Intra/periprocedural complications associated with SVG PCI:

1. Slow flow/no flow phenomenon.
2. Periprocedural. As described earlier, since the graft atherosclerosis in patients with diabetes mellitus has more necrotic core with unstable plaques, this subgroup of patients has higher risk of such events. Various pharmacological and mechanical strategies have been developed in an attempt to decrease complications in SVG PCI.

Pharmacological Strategies

GP IIb/IIIa Inhibitors

There are no prospective randomized trials clearly demonstrating the benefits of GP IIb/IIIa inhibitors in SVG PCI. There may be a role in their usage as adjuncts with certain embolic protection devices, such as the distal filtration devices.

Vasodilators

Vasodilators that have been studied in the no-reflow phenomenon include adenosine, verapamil, and nicardipine. Fischell et al. showed promising results with adenosine in reversing slow-flow and no-reflow phenomenon among patients undergoing SVG PCI.[18] The Vasodilator Prevention of No-Reflow (VAPOR) trial, showed that there was a significant reduction in no-reflow with prophylactic intragraft administration of verapamil during SVG PCI.[19] Fischell et al. showed promising results with nicardipine to prevent no-reflow in SVG PCI.[20] Although the available data are limited and not enough to support the routine use of adjunctive pharmacotherapy in SVG PCI, the above studies are promising. Currently, aspirin, thienopyridine, and anticoagulation with heparin are the only recommended adjuvant pharmacotherapy in SVG interventions.

Covered Stents

The Stents IN Grafts (STING) trial showed that death, MI, and TLR were comparable in the polytetrafluoroethylene (PTFE)-membrane covered stents versus conventional stents.[21] The Symbiot III trial further confirmed that there was no advantage of the Symbiot PTFE-covered stent over BMS in terms of restenosis rates and clinical outcomes.[22] The more recent Barrier Approach to Restenosis: Restrict Intima to Curtail ADverse Events (BARRICADE) trial in fact demonstrated more target vessel failure in patients treated with covered stents compared to BMS.[23]

Embolic Protection Devices

Mechanical embolic protection devices (EPDs) were developed and proved to be the first treatment modality to reduce MACE during SVG PCI. Currently, there are three types of EPDs: the distal balloon occlusion/aspiration system; distal filter system; and the proximal occlusion/aspiration system.

Distal Occlusion/Aspiration System

The PercuSurge GuardWire® system (Medtronic Inc.) occludes the target vessel several centimeters distal to the target lesion during SVG PCI in order to provide myocardial protection. After the intervention, aspiration removes debris-laden blood prior to balloon deflation and restoration of antegrade blood flow (Fig. 1).This was the first EPD to gain US Food and Drug Administration (FDA) approval following the results of the Saphenous Vein Graft Angioplasty Free of Emboli Randomized (SAFER) trial.[24]

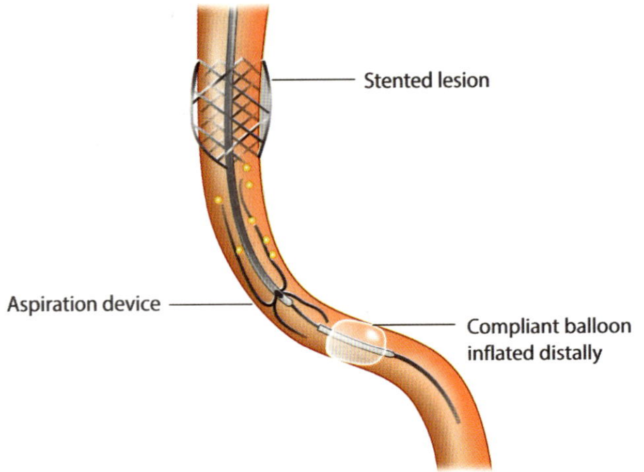

Fig. 1: Distal occlusion system[25]

Distal Filtration System

The FilterWire EX (Boston Scientific) Randomized Evaluation (FIRE) study showed noninferiority of the FilterWire EX System to the GuardWire balloon occlusion and aspiration system and led to FDA approval of the first distal filtration device (Figs 2A to C).[26]

Proximal Occlusion/Aspiration System

Proximal occlusion devices occlude the vessel proximal to a target lesion and suspend antegrade flow. The only FDA-approved proximal occlusion/flow reversal device is the Proxis system (St Jude Medical) (Figs 3A to C). This was based on the Proximal Protection during Saphenous Vein Graft Intervention Using the Proxis Embolic Protection System (PROXIMAL) trial that showed the Proxis system to be non-inferior to distal EPD.[27]

EARLY AND LATE CLINICAL OUTCOMES IN SAPHENOUS VEIN GRAFT STENTING IN DIABETIC PATIENTS

Diabetes remains an independent risk factor for worse clinical and angiographic outcomes after both balloon angioplasty and stenting in native coronary arteries.[28] Recurrent ischemic events and SVG stenosis have been shown to be higher among diabetic patients compared

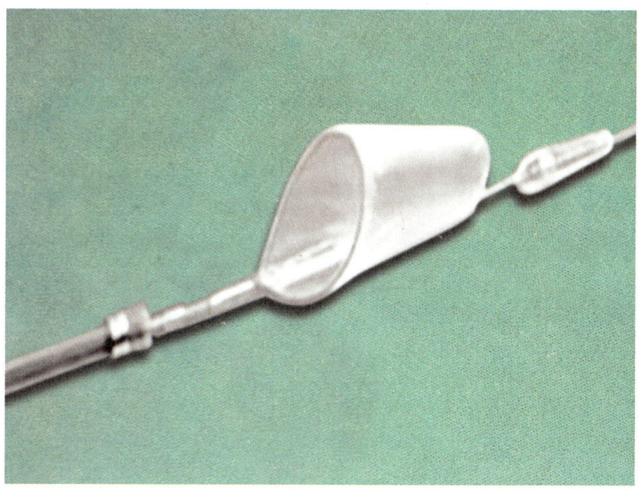

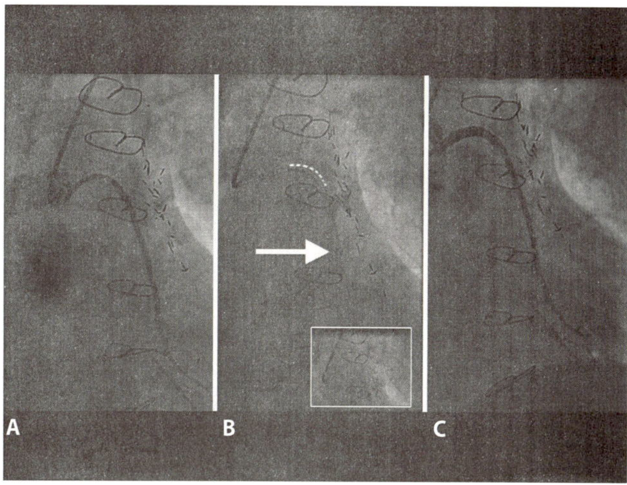

Figs 2A to C: Distal filter mechanism of action. (A) Long severe proximal stenosis of a saphenous vein graft to the left circumflex coronary artery; (B) Distal filter (arrow) and stent in place (dotted line). In the small bottom left quadrant, a second stent is deployed in proximal overlap with the first one, still with the filter in place; (C) Final result[25]

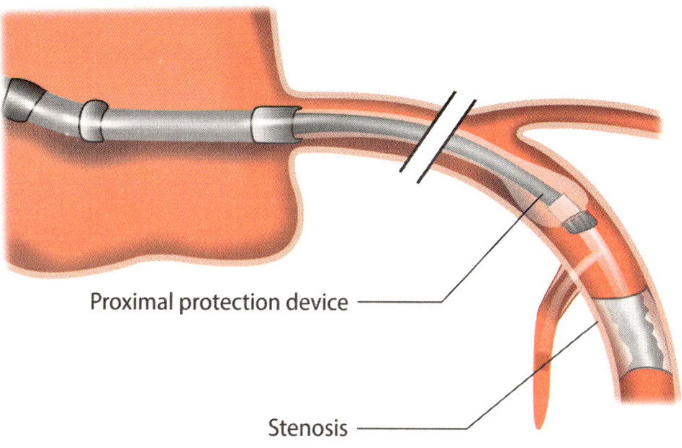

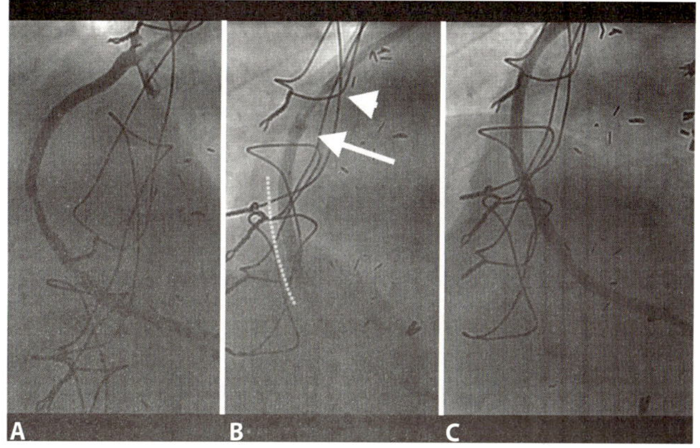

Figs 3A to C: Proximal occlusion device mechanism of action. (A) Severe stenosis in the mid-portion of a saphenous vein graft to the right coronary artery; (B) Proximal protection device in place with balloon inflated (arrow: distal tip of the device, where the non-compliant balloon is; arrowhead: distal tip of the guiding catheter) and stent in place and inflated (white dotted line); (C) Final result[25]

with nondiabetic patients at long-term follow-up with many such patients requiring vein graft interventions at follow-up.[29,30] Study done by Ahmed et al.,[31] showed that patients with diabetes undergoing stent implantation in SVG have: Higher in-hospital and late mortality, Higher 1-year TLR rates, significantly lower 1-year cardiac event-free survival (Figs 4 and 5).

Thus, diabetic patients have less favorable acute and late clinical outcomes after stent implantation in SVG lesions. High prevalence of in-hospital mortality could be related to the presence of complex SVG lesion morphology, generalized atherosclerotic disease, reduced left ventricular function and frequently associated comorbid conditions in diabetic patients. During follow-up, the overall clinical outcome was worse for diabetic patients due to higher rates of TLR and increased 1-year mortality. Consequently, diabetic patients had lower event-free survival. On subgroup analysis there was no difference in mortality between the two diabetic populations. By multivariate regression analysis, presence of diabetes was found to be the only predictor of in-hospital mortality.

Another study done by Mehta et al., showed that compared with patients without diabetes, diabetic patients undergoing SVG intervention have significantly worse long-term outcomes with one-third dying at median follow-up of 4 years.[32] The study demonstrated that 88% of patients without heart rate 80 beat/min, congestive heart failure, renal insufficiency, or hypertension survived after SVG intervention at median follow-up of 4 years. In contrast, none of the few patients with all these 4 factors survived at follow-up.

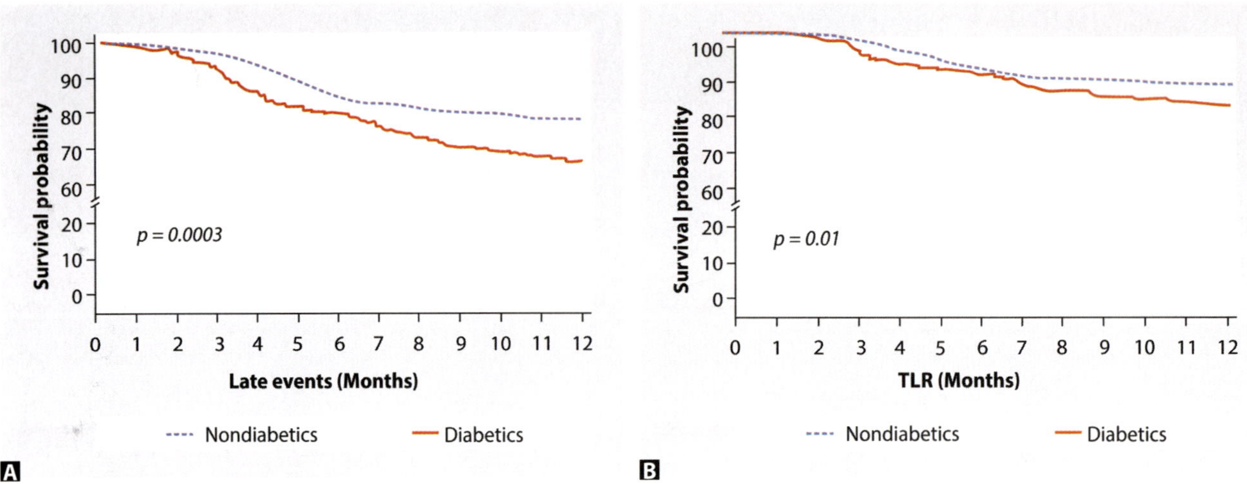

Figs 4A and B: (A) Actuarial event-free survival curves for any adverse cardiac events (death, Q-wave infarction, angioplasty and coronary artery bypass surgery (A), and (B) TLR for 12 months after stenting in diabetic versus nondiabetic patients

Abbreviation: TLR, target lesion revascularization

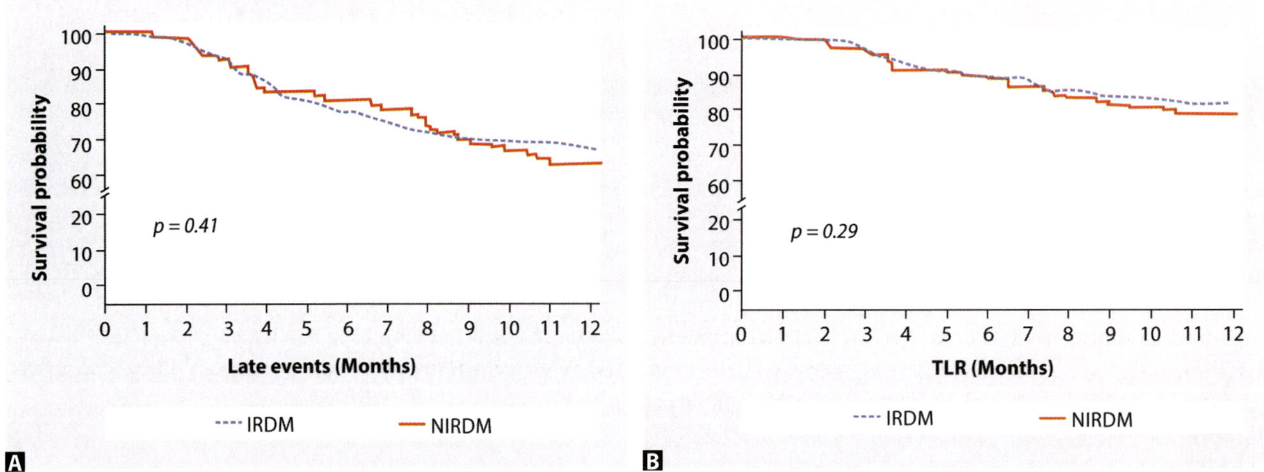

Figs 5A and B: (A) Actuarial event-free survival curves for any adverse cardiac events (death, Q-wave infarction, angioplasty and coronary artery bypass surgery, (A), and (B) TLR for 12 months after stenting

Abbreviations: IRDM, insulin-requiring diabetics; NIRD, noninsulin-requiring diabetics; TLR, target lesion revascularization

Pendyala et al. studied early and late clinical outcomes in diabetic and non-diabetic patients who underwent SVG PCI with the use of DES.[33] Patients with diabetes mellitus are shown to have less favorable outcomes after SVG intervention with the use of bare-metal stents. However, In the present era, a better understanding of the pathology of SVG disease, aggressive risk factor modification, improved PCI pharmacotherapy, advances in stent technology, development of aspiration and protective devices to avoid distal embolization, and optimal stent deployment techniques, have made a significant impact on outcomes of this high-risk patient subset. A large, prospective, multicenter, randomized study, Is Drug-Eluting-Stenting Associated with improved Results in Coronary Artery Bypass Grafts (ISAR-CABG)? is the first study to convincingly show the benefit use of DES compared to bare-metal stents for SVG intervention. Major adverse coronary events at 1-year was significantly lower in the DES group and was mainly driven by a nearly 50% relative reduction in the risk of TLR. Drug-eluting stents, when used for the treatment of vein graft lesions, equate the short- and long-term outcomes between diabetic and nondiabetic patients, suggesting that DES should be considered the default stent in diabetic populations undergoing PCI for the treatment of SVG lesions (Figs 6A and B).

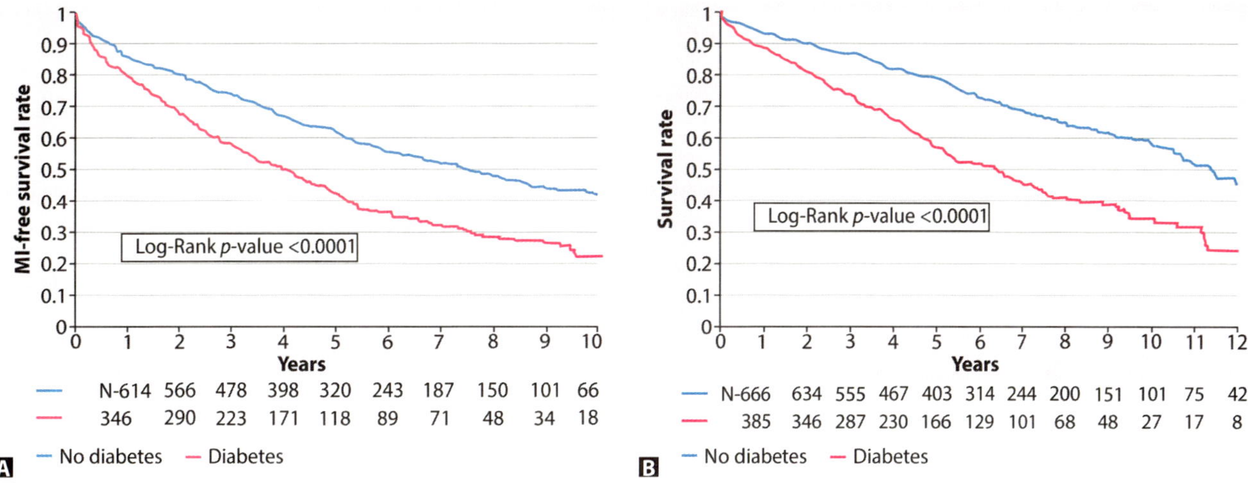

Figs 6A and B: Kaplan-Meier estimates of myocardial infarction, survival in patients with and without diabetes mellitus undergoing percutaneous interventions of saphenous vein grafts

GLYCEMIC CONTROL AND REVASCULARIZATION

Impact of good glycemic control on macrovascular events remains controversial, i.e. no significant reduction in cardiovascular disease (CVD) outcomes with intensive glycemic control except in few subsets.[34] Although few studies show that diabetic patients with HbA1c – 7% at the time of PCI had a significantly lower rate of TVR than did those with HbA1c – 7%, despite similar baseline clinical and angiographic characteristics. Furthermore, optimally controlled diabetic patients had rates of TVR similar to those of nondiabetic patients.[35] Thus aggressive treatment of diabetes to achieve HbA1c levels 7% may be beneficial in reducing the risk of restenosis and may improve the clinical outcome after PCI.

CONCLUSION

Diabetic patients undergoing SVG intervention have significantly worse long-term outcomes than nondiabetics interventions are particularly challenging due to plaque embolization and the no-reflow phenomenon. Drug-eluting stents, when used for the treatment of vein graft lesions, equate the short- and long-term outcomes between diabetic and non-diabetic patients, suggesting that DES should be considered the default stent in diabetic populations undergoing PCI for the treatment of SVG lesions.

REFERENCES

1. Ma J, Wang X, Wang Y, et al. The relationship between glycated hemoglobin and complexity of coronary artery lesions among older patients with diabetes mellitus. Plos One. 2014;9:e91972.
2. Hannan EL, Wu C, Walford G, et al. Long-term outcomes of coronary artery bypass grafting versus stent implantation. New Engl J Med. 2005;352:2174-83 .
3. Frimerman A, Rechavia E, Eigler N, et al. Long-term follow-up of a high-risk cohort after stent implantation in saphenous vein grafts. J Am Coll Cardiol. 1997;30(5):1277-83.
4. Pucelikova T, Mehran R, Kirtane AJ, et al. Short- and long-term outcomes after stent-assisted percutaneous treatment of saphenous vein grafts in the drug-eluting stent era. Am J Cardiol. 2008;101(1):63-8.
5. Goldman S, Zadina K, Moritz T, et al. Long-term patency of saphenous vein and left internal mammary artery grafts after coronary artery bypass surgery: results from a Department of Veterans Affairs Cooperative Study. J Am Coll Cardiol. 2004;44(11):2149-56.
6. Baars T, Konorza T, Kahlert P, et al. Coronary aspirate TNF-α reflects saphenous vein bypass graft restenosis risk in diabetic patients. Cardiovasc Diabetol. 2013;12:12.
7. Mathew V, Holmes DR. Outcomes in diabetics undergoing revascularization: the long and the short of it. J Am Coll Cardiol. 2002;40(3):424-7.
8. Boese D, Leineweber K, Konorza T, et al. Release of TNF-α during stent implantation into saphenous vein aortocoronary bypass grafts and its relation to plaque extrusion and restenosis. Am J Physiol Heart Circ Physiol. 2007;292(5):H2295-9.
9. Kleinbongard P, Heusch G, Schulz R. TNF-alpha in atherosclerosis, myocardial ischemia/reperfusion and heart failure. Pharmacol Ther. 2010;127(3):295-314.
10. Cameron A, Kemp Jr HG, Green GE. Reoperation for coronary artery disease: 10 years of clinical follow-up. Circulation. 1988;78(3 Pt 2):1158-62.
11. de Feyter PJ, van Suylen RJ, de Jaegere PP, et al. Balloon angioplasty for the treatment of lesions in saphenous vein bypass grafts. J Am Coll Cardiol. 1993;21(7):1539-49.
12. Savage MP, Douglas JS Jr, Fischman DL, et al. Stent placement compared with balloon angioplasty for obstructed coronary bypass grafts. Saphenous Vein De Novo Trial Investigators. N Engl J Med. 1997;337(11):740-7.
13. Hiscock M, Oqueli E, Dick R. Percutaneous saphenous vein graft intervention—a review. Heart Lung Circ. 2007;(16 Suppl 3):S51-S55.
14. Ge L, Lakovou L, Sangiorgi GM, et al. Treatment of saphenous vein graft lesions with drug-eluting stents: immediate and midterm outcome. J Am Coll Cardiol. 2005;45(7):989-94.

15. Ramana RK, Ronan A, Cohoon K, et al. Long-term clinical outcomes of real-world experience using sirolimus-eluting stents in saphenous vein graft disease. Catheter Cardiovasc Interv. 2008;6(7):886-93.
16. Assali A, Raz Y, Vaknin Assa H, et al. Beneficial 2 years results of drug eluting stents in saphenous vein graft lesions. Eurointervention. 2008;4(1):108-14.
17. Rodes Cabau J, Bertrand OF, Larose E, et al. Comparison of plaque sealing with paclitaxel-eluting stents versus medical therapy for the treatment of moderate nonsignificant saphenous vein graft lesions: the moderate vein graft lesion stenting with the taxus stent and intravascular ultrasound (VELETI) pilot trial. Circulation. 2009;120(20):1978-86.
18. Fischell TA, Carter AJ, Foster MT, et al. Reversal of "no reflow" during vein graft stenting using high velocity boluses of intracoronary adenosine. Cathet Cardiovasc Diagn. 1998;45(4):360-5.
19. Michaels AD, Appleby M, Otten MH, et al. Pretreatment with intragraft verapamil prior to percutaneous coronary intervention of saphenous vein graft lesions: results of the randomized, controlled vasodilator prevention on no-reflow (VAPOR) trial. J Invasive Cardiol. 2002;14(6):299-302.
20. Fischell TA, Subraya RGf, Ashraf K, et al. "Pharmacologic" distal protection using prophylactic, intragraft nicardipine to prevent no-reflow and non-Q-wave myocardial infarction during elective saphenous vein graft intervention. J Invasive Cardiol. 2007;19(2): 58-62.
21. Schachinger V, Hamm CW, Munzel T, et al. STING (STents IN Grafts) Investigators. A randomized trial of polytetrafluoroethylene membrane covered stents compared with conventional stents in aortocoronary saphenous vein grafts. J Am Coll Cardiol. 2003;42(8):1360-9.
22. Turco MA, Buchbinder M, Popma JJ, et al. Pivotal, randomized U.S. study of the Symbiot-TM-covered stent system in patients with saphenous vein graft disease: eight-month angiographic and clinical results from the Symbiot III trial. Catheter Cardiovasc Interv. 2006;68(3):379-88.
23. Stone GW, Goldberg S, O'Shaughnessy C, et al. 5-year-follow-up of polytetrafluoroethylene covered stents compared with bare-metal stents in aortocoronary saphenous vein grafts the randomized BARRICADE (barrier approach to restenosis: restrict intima to curtail adverse events) trial. JACC Cardiovasc Interv. 2011;4(3):300-9.
24. Carrozza Jr JP, Mumma M, Breall JA, et al. The PRIDE Study Investigators. Randomized evaluation of the TriActiv balloon-protection flush and extraction system for the treatment of saphenous vein graft disease. J Am Coll Cardiol. 2005;46(9):1677-83.
25. Agostoni P, Voskuil M, Onsea K, et al. Tools and techniques: percutaneous intervention of saphenous vein graft lesions. Utrecht/Belgium: The Netherlands: Department of Cardiology, University Medical Center/Antwerp Cardiovascular Institute; 2011.
26. Stone G, Rogers C, Hermiller J, et al. Randomized comparison of distal protection with a filter-based catheter and a balloon occlusion and aspiration system during percutaneous intervention of diseased saphenous vein aortocoronary bypass grafts. Circulation. 2003;108(5):548-53.
27. Mauri L, Cox DA, Hermiller J, et al. The PROXIMAL trial: proximal protection during saphenous vein graft intervention using the proxis embolic protection system: a randomized, prospective, multicenter trial. J Am Coll Cardiol. 2007;50(15):1142-449.
28. Waller B, Palumbo B, Roberts W. Status of the coronary arteries at necropsy in diabetes mellitus with onset after age 30 years: analysis of 229 diabetic patients with and without clinical evidence of coronary heart disease and comparison to 183 control subjects. Am J Med. 1980;69:498-506.
29. Detre KM, Lombardero MS, Brooks MM, et al. The effect of previous coronary bypass surgery on the prognosis of patients with diabetes mellitus who have acute myocardial infarction. N Engl J Med. 2000;342:989-97.
30. The Bypass Angioplasty Revascularization Investigation (BARI). Influence of diabetes on 5-year mortality and morbidity in a randomized comparing CABG with PTCA in patients with multivessel disease. Circulation. 1997;96:1761-9.
31. Ahmed JM, Hong MK, Mehran R, et al. Influence of diabetes mellitus on early and late clinical outcomes in saphenous vein graft stenting. J Am Coll Cardiol. 2000;36(4).
32. Mehta RH, Honeycutt E, Shaw LK, et al. Clinical characteristics associated with poor long-term survival among patients with diabetes mellitus undergoing saphenous vein graft interventions. Am Heart J. 2008;156:728-35.
33. Pendalya LK, Loh JP. The impact of diabetes mellitus on long-term clinical outcomes after percutaneous coronary saphenous vein graft interventions in the drug-eluting stent era. New Jersey: Wiley Periodicals, Inc; 2014.
34. Gerstein HC, Miller ME, Byington RP, et al. Effects of intensive glucose lowering in type 2 diabetes. New Engl J Med. 2008;358: 2545-59.
35. Corpus RA, George PB, House LA, et al. Optimal glycemic control is associated with a lower rate of target vessel revascularization in treated type II diabetic patients undergoing elective percutaneous coronary intervention. JACC. 2004;43(1):8-14.

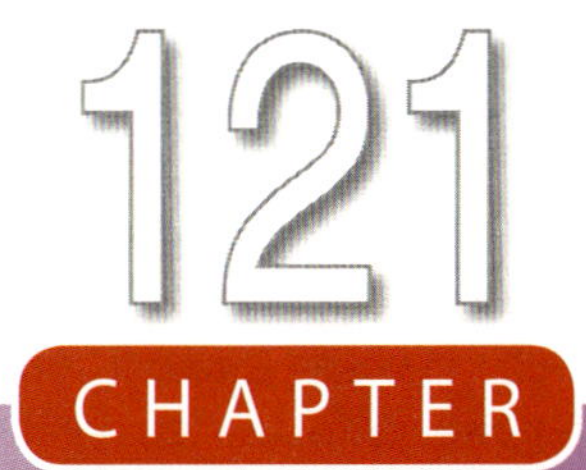

CHAPTER

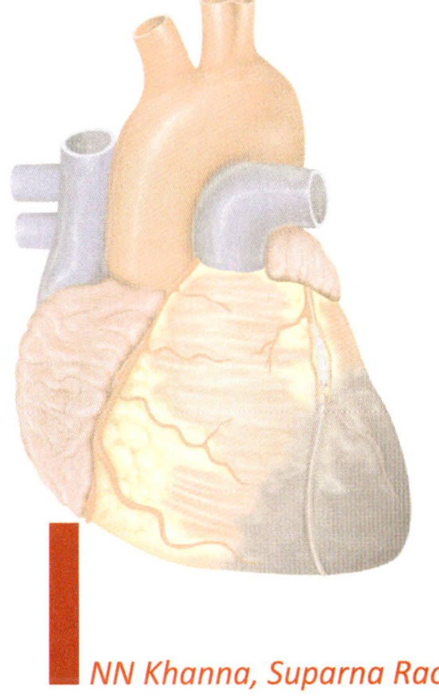

Cardiodiabetes and Peripheral Vascular Interventions

NN Khanna, Suparna Rao

INTRODUCTION

Diabetes mellitus is a condition with a wide-ranging secondary effect on multiple organ systems, including the cardiac, vascular, renal, and nervous systems. Diabetic patients have an increased risk of atherosclerotic disease, in addition to other cardiovascular risk factors. Atherosclerosis is one of the main causes of the morbidity and mortality in patients with diabetes, especially in the type 2 diabetic patient population.[1] Peripheral arterial disease (PAD) in diabetics is the main cause of lower limb amputation. Cardiovascular disease accounts for 44% of all-cause fatalities in the diabetic patients, according to the Verona Diabetes Study.[2] Factors such as increased age and longer duration of diabetes increases the incidence of PAD and risk of death from cardiovascular disease, independent of coexisting risk factors.[3] Insulin resistance plays a major role in the pathogenesis of diabetes. It is estimated that worldwide, diabetes mellitus is associated with 25–90% of all amputations.[4] Conservative treatment and vascular bypass surgery have failed to yield good results in managing patients with diabetic PAD. Novel treatments such as percutaneous transluminal angioplasty (PTA) and luminal stenting have emerged in recent years. Both of these are endovascular treatments.

EPIDEMIOLOGY

Epidemiological studies have confirmed an association between diabetes and an increased prevalence of PAD.[5,6] In a study by Dormandy et al.[7], prevalence of PAD varies from 0% to 2% below 40 years of age, 0.5% to 2.5% at 50 years, 1% to 4.5% at 60 years, and 2% to 9% at age of 70 years. Schroll M noted that asymptomatic diseases were present in 0.9–22% cases of diabetes.[8] V Mohan et al. observed that in India, the incidence of PAD is less (3.9%), though prevalence increases with age.[9] In India, the lower incidence of PAD may be attributed to lower lifespan of diabetic patients. Advances in the management of diabetes leading to better diabetic control and increased longevity in future may lead to increased prevalence of PAD.

PATHOPHYSIOLOGY OF DIABETIC VASCULAR DISEASE AND DIABETIC FOOT

Diabetic PAD and diabetic foot are caused due to the effect of hyperglycemia on the vascular, immune, and nervous systems, which ultimately affect the musculoskeletal architecture of the foot. The altered metabolic state that occurs in diabetes directly contributes to the development of atherosclerosis, by increase in vascular inflammation and alterations in multiple cell types.[10] A triad of insulin resistance, hyperglycemia, and dyslipidemia alters function of the endothelium and smooth muscles. Insulin resistance leads to excess liberation of free fatty acids (FFA) from the adipocytes, which increase reactive oxygen species (through protein kinase pathway), thus impairing nitric oxide (NO) production. In healthy vessels of nondiabetic patients, endothelial cells synthesize NO, a potent vasodilator that inhibits platelet activation and impairs vascular smooth muscle cell migration. Diabetes impairs endothelium dependent (NO mediated) vasodilatation.

In addition, the production of vasoconstrictors like endothelin 1 is increased, which in turn induces vascular smooth muscle hypertrophy, increases renal salt and water retention and stimulates renin angiotensin system. Endothelium-derived vasoactive substances such as vasoconstrictor prostanoids and angiotensin II are also increased.[11] Hyperglycemia inhibits production of NO by blocking endothelial NO synthetase activation and increasing production of reactive oxygen species (by activating protein kinase C and nuclear factor kappa B), which in turn promotes the formation of atherosclerotic lesions.[12] In diabetes, platelets have an increased expression of glycoprotein Ib and IIb/IIIa receptors, increasing their thrombotic potential.[13] Blood coagulability is increased by increased expression of tissue factor and decreased levels of anticoagulants (such as antithrombin III). Overall, the effects of endothelial cell dysfunction increase arterial susceptibility to atherosclerosis. Motor and sensory neuropathy plays a major role in the pathogenesis of diabetic foot. Motor neuropathy contributes to altered weight distribution and repeated painless fractures that result in Charcot foot deformity. The altered weightload on the foot, peripheral vascular disease, and microcirculation disorders cause further pressure ulceration and delayed healing. Sensory neuropathy in diabetics results in neglect of minor traumatic events, triggering ulcer formation. Increased susceptibility to infection results from the poor circulation in combination with the inhibitory effects of hyperglycemia on the immune system.[14,15]

CLINICAL FEATURES OF PERIPHERAL ARTERIAL DISEASE

Patients with PAD present with intermittent claudication, cramping or aching pain in the lower limbs aggravated by walking and relived with rest, which occurs due to metabolic mismatch between demand and supply because of vascular compromise. This symptom may be absent if the patient suffers from sensory neuropathy. Claudication typically occurs in the muscles distal to occlusion. Femoropopliteal disease causes calf claudication, and aortoiliac disease causes bilateral thigh and buttock claudication. Other features of PAD include skin atrophy, hair loss, nail dystrophy, and coldness of toes (Figs 1A and B). All the peripheral pulses should be palpated individually. Ultimately, patient complains of rest pain due to severe multilevel multivessel disease. Peripheral nerve ischemia is the cause of rest pain. Pain is worse at night, often precipitated by elevation of limb and exertion, and relieved by dependent position.

DIAGNOSIS AND ASSESSMENT OF PERIPHERAL ARTERIAL DISEASE IN DIABETICS

Diagnosing PAD in diabetic individuals is important to initiate therapies that improve quality of life and decrease disability. The presence of PAD indicates the presence of systemic atherosclerosis, which is an additional cardiovascular risk to the patient with diabetes. It mandates aggressive management of vascular risk factors in this high-risk group. It is imperative to know the thorough medical history and perform proper physical examination to evaluate a diabetic patient for the presence of PAD. The onset and duration of symptoms, pain characteristics, and any alleviating factors should be asked. The clinical stage of symptomatic PAD can be classified using the Fontaine and Rutherford staging system (Tables 1 and 2).[16]

Typical symptom of claudication has a low sensitivity, but a high specificity for PAD.[17] Complete physical examination

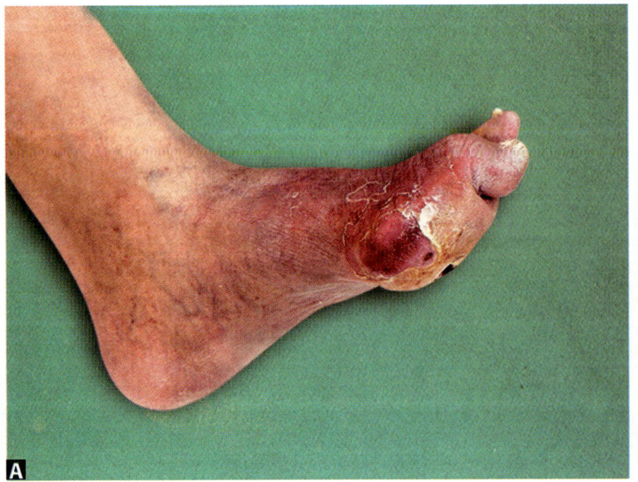

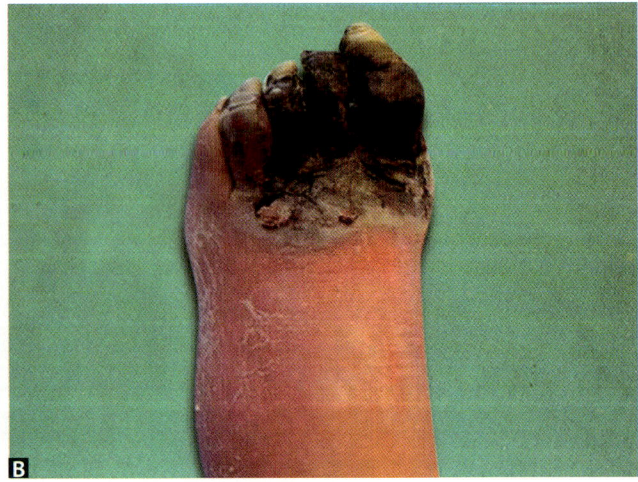

Figs 1A and B: Diabetic foot with (A) ulcer and (B) gangrene

TABLE 1: Fontaine classification

Stages	Clinical features
Stage I	Have peripheral arterial disease (PAD), but asymptomatic
Stage IIa, IIb	Mild and moderate-severe intermittent claudication
Stage III	Ischemic rest pain
Stage IV	Distal ulceration and gangrene

TABLE 2: Rutherford classification

Grade	Category	Clinical
0	0	Asymptomatic
I	1	Mild claudication
I	2	Moderate claudication
I	3	Severe claudication
II	4	Ischemic rest pain
III	5	Minor tissue loss
III	6	Major tissue loss

TABLE 3: Correlation of PAD with ankle brachial pressure index (ABI)

ABI	Severity of PAD
0.90–1.30	Normal
0.70–0.89	Mild PAD
0.40–0.69	Moderate PAD
<0.40	Severe PAD

TABLE 4: Features of critical limb ischemia (CLI)

Noninvasive vascular laboratory test for CLI	
Ankle-brachial index	≤0.4
Ankle systolic pressure	≤50 mm Hg
Toe systolic pressure	≤30 mm Hg
Measures of skin microcirculation	
Capillary density	≤20/mm^2
Absent reactive hyperemia on capillary microscopy	
$TcpO_2$	<10 mm Hg

should include blood pressure measurement, palpation of peripheral pulses, and auscultation of pulses and bruits. All peripheral pulses including femoral, popliteal, and pedal vessels should be assessed.[18] PAD is strongly suggested by absence of both dorsalis pedis pulse and the posterior tibial pulse, but further diagnostic testing is required to confirm the diagnosis.

Ankle-brachial Pressure Index

It is a simple, noninvasive method to assess lower extremity circulation. Using a blood pressure cuff and a Doppler ultrasound probe, the systolic pressure in the brachial arteries of both arms is measured; and the systolic pressure in the dorsalis pedis and posterior tibial arteries of both lower extremities is measured. The higher of two readings between the dorsalis pedis and posterior tibial artery determines the ankle pressure. Ankle-brachial pressure index (ABI) is calculated by dividing the ankle pressure by higher of two brachial artery pressures. The American Diabetes Association consensus statement recommends that a screening ABI be performed in all diabetic individuals greater than 50 years of age. If normal (0.91–1.40), the test should be repeated every five years. A screening ABI should be performed in any patient with symptoms of PAD.[18] Table 3 shows the correlation of PAD with ABI. Other features of critical limb ischemia (CLI) are shown in Table 4. There are some drawbacks to the measurement of ankle-brachial index. It may be of limited value in some patients with diabetes, since the arteries become non-compressible due to calcification, resulting in unusually high ABI values (>1.40).[19]

After confirming the diagnosis of PAD, further investigation is required, usually for planning a revascularization procedure. A vascular laboratory evaluation for segmental pressure and pulse volume recordings can be performed, which aid in the localization of arterial occlusive lesions.[18]

Duplex Ultrasound

Cross-sectional imaging of arteries and veins with simultaneous color flow and spectral Doppler information is available by duplex ultrasound. Duplex scanning directly visualizes vessels and provides information on thickness of artery wall, degree of flow turbulence, and records the blood flow velocity changes at specific sites within the vessels.[20] It detects hemodynamically significant stenosis with high degree of sensitivity and specificity.

Magnetic Resonance Angiography

Magnetic resonance angiography (MRA) is a noninvasive imaging tests which can be used when details of the morphological features of occlusions are required. MRA looks at the blood flowing in the vessels and not at the vessel itself. If a stenotic lesion is present, then it may appear as a narrowed area, and a very tight lesion is shown as a signal void (Fig. 2). It is often possible to image distal arteries with this technique, since the blood flow is imaged.

Invasive Conventional Angiography

Invasive conventional angiography is the only tool which is used for comprehensive imaging of the peripheral

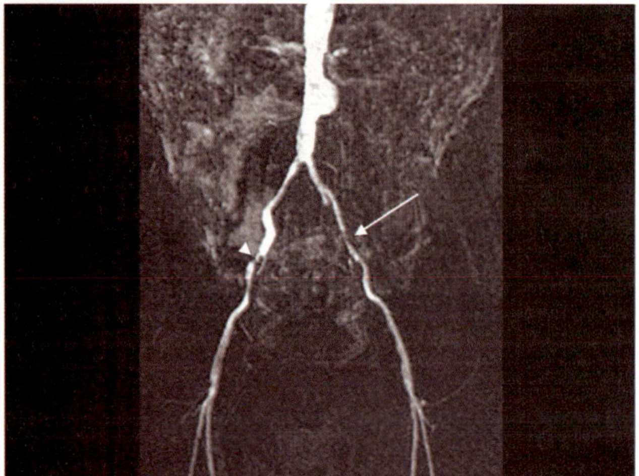

Fig. 2: Magnetic resonance angiography (MRA) showing bilateral iliac disease within the right external (arrowhead) and left external (white arrow) iliac arteries

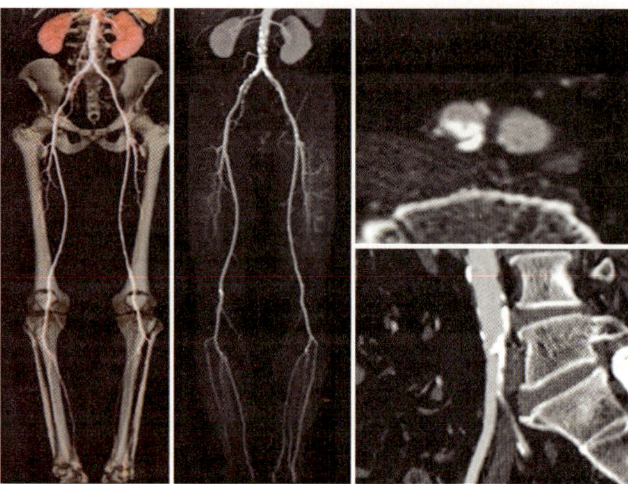

Fig. 3: Diffuse aortoiliac calcified plaques hindering lumen visualization. Axial-base images and multiplanar reconstruction images are better suited for lumen assessment

vasculature. This is usually done by transfemoral or transbrachial approach.

Recently, with the introduction of magnetic resonance angiography (MRA) and computed tomographic angiography (CTA), noninvasive imaging can now be done, with images that are comparable with conventional angiography.[21] Consequently, The CTA is replacing conventional angiography in many PAD imaging studies.[22]

Computed Tomographic Angiography

Computed tomography angiography has revolutionized vascular imaging in recent years. With the evolution of multidetector computed tomography (MDCT) technology, high-resolution imaging of the peripheral vasculature has become possible. With the evolution of this technology, imaging the entire inflow and runoff vessels with a single acquisition and a single intravenous contrast medium injection is now possible (Figs 3 and 4). CT angiography is preferable due to its shorter acquisition times and thinner slices with higher spatial and temporal resolutions.

MANAGEMENT OF PERIPHERAL ARTERIAL DISEASE IN DIABETES

The aim of medical management in diabetic patients is to aggressively modify cardiovascular risk factors and to prescribe antiplatelet therapy. In order to improve functional status and quality of life, the symptoms of intermittent claudication should be relieved. Multidisciplinary care involves:

- Control of risk factors
- Medical management
- Optimization of wound care
- Revascularization
- Rehabilitation.

Risk Factor Modification

This is one of the most important measures in the management of PAD in diabetes. Atherosclerotic risk factors for PAD in diabetics include cigarette smoking, dyslipidemia, and hypertension. Cigarette smoking is the main risk factor for the development and progression of PAD. The progression of PAD directly correlates with the amount and duration of tobacco use.[23] Smoking cessation increases long-term survival in patients with PAD.

As per the National Cholesterol Education Program/ Adult Treatment Panel III guidelines, diabetes is classified as a coronary heart disease equivalent and recommend a targeted low-density lipoprotein (LDL) cholesterol level of less than 70 mg/dL for very high risk patients.[24]

Aggressive hypertension management leading to a marked reduction in vascular events has been demonstrated in diabetic individuals.[25] The American Diabetes Association (ADA) guidelines supports intensive blood pressure control (<130/80 mm Hg) in patients with diabetes and PAD to reduce cardiovascular risk.[18]

Management of Diabetes

In the UK Prospective Diabetes Study (UKPDS), it was seen that intensive glycemic control with a sulfonylurea or insulin produced a nonsignificant 16% risk reduction for

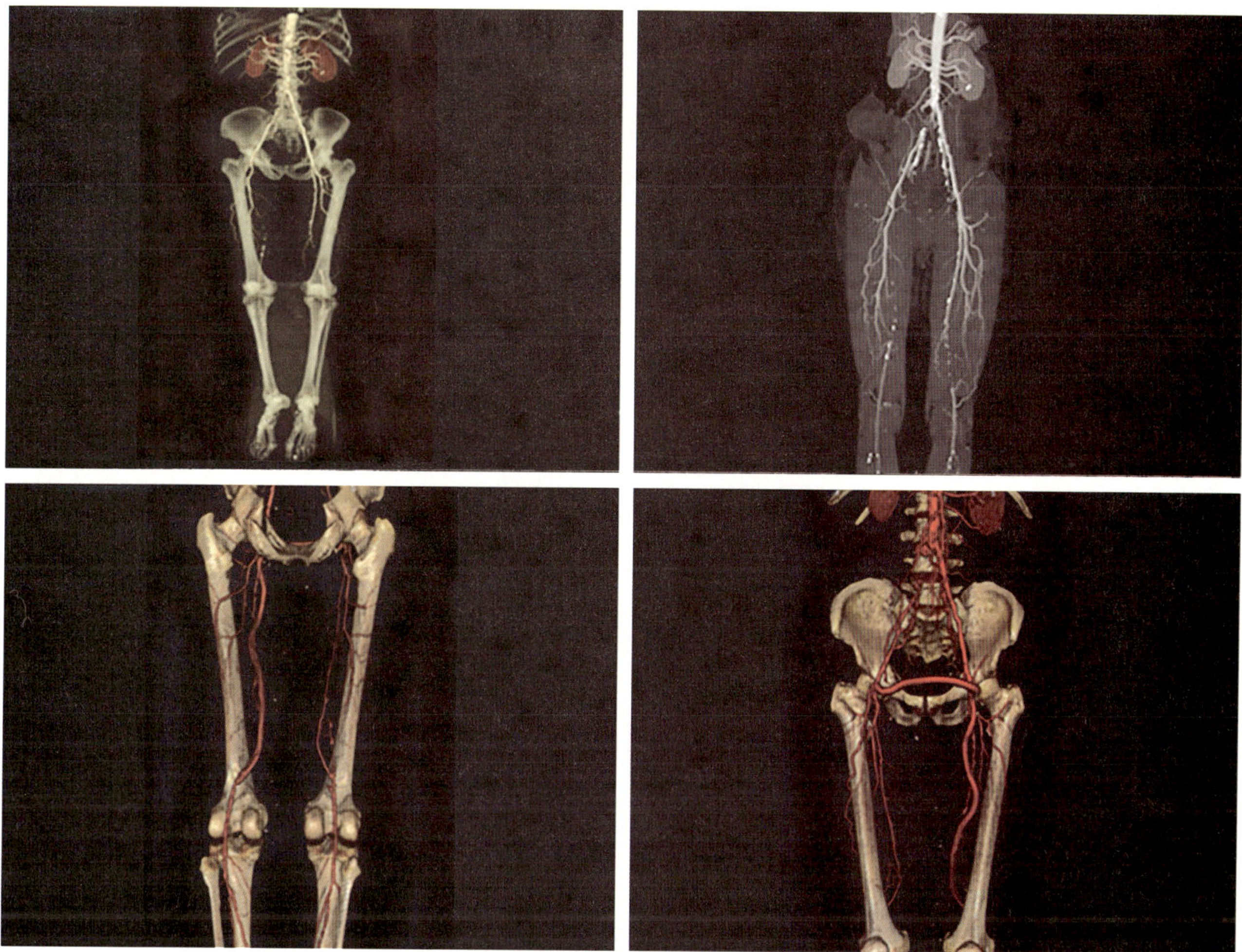

Fig. 4: Patient with severe atherosclerotic vaso-occlusive disease (Pre- and postoperative status). Computed tomographic angiography (CTA) nicely depicts multiple patent grafts

myocardial infarction (MI) and sudden death as compared to diet-controlled diabetes,[26] although no significant differences were noted in diabetes related mortality or all-cause mortality between the intensive and conventional groups. Current guidelines from the ADA recommend a target glycosylated hemoglobin level of less than 7.0% in diabetic individuals in order to prevent microvascular complications.[27]

Antiplatelet Therapy

According to the US Food and Drug Administration (FDA), there is insufficient evidence to approve the use of aspirin for the secondary prevention of atherosclerotic events in patients with PAD.[28] However, its use in these patients has received a guideline recommendation.[29] There has been a significant improvement in vascular graft patency in greater than 3,000 patients with PAD treated with bypass surgery or peripheral angioplasty due to aspirin use.[30] The recommendation of aspirin at dosages of 80–325 mg/day for all diabetic individuals greater than 21 years of age,[31] is not fully supported by clinical trial evidence. Aspirin has an established role in secondary prevention in patients at high risk, with clinical evidence of either coronary artery disease (CAD) or stroke.

The Clopidogrel versus Aspirin in Patients at Risk of Ischemic Events (CAPRIE) study[32] evaluated aspirin (at 325 mg/day) versus clopidogrel (at 75 mg/day) in patients with recent stroke, recent MI, or established PAD. The study was performed with greater than 19,000 patients (approximately 20% with diabetes). In a subset analysis of 6,452 patients with PAD, those treated with clopidogrel showed a 23.8% relative-risk reduction compared with aspirin recipients ($p = 0.0028$). In the PAD subgroup (with approximately one-third of the patients having diabetes), clopidogrel was found to be superior to aspirin.[33] These results proved that clopidogrel use reduced the incidence of ischemic events in patients with PAD and its use was approved by FDA.

Management of Symptomatic Peripheral Arterial Disease

Supervised exercise therapy plays an important role in the management of PAD. Symptoms of intermittent claudication are relieved by regular exercise.

Currently, there are two medications which are used for the symptomatic treatment of intermittent claudication: pentoxifylline and cilostazol.

Pentoxifylline was the first drug approved by the FDA for intermittent claudication in 1984. It improves blood flow and increases tissue oxygenation by reducing blood viscosity and retarding platelet aggregation.[34] *Cilostazol* is a phosphodiesterase inhibitor which acts by suppressing platelet aggregation and is a direct vasodilator. Patients have seen an improvement in maximal walking distance by 40–50%, in as short as 4 weeks, compared with placebo.[35]

Management of Critical Limb Ischemia in Diabetes (Diabetic Foot)

Critical limb ischemia requires urgent treatment. It is the precursor of limb loss. Conservative management includes debridement of ulcers, wearing appropriate footwear, use of non-adherent dressings, and treatment of infection with antibiotics. Revascularization is mostly indicated in CLI (Figs 5A and B), while surgical drainage and debridement are performed to resolve the infection.[18] Without revascularization, surgical debridement leads to larger nonhealing wounds.

Podiatric Wound Care in Diabetes

Adequate perfusion to ischemic limb and adequate nutrition are essential for proper wound care of diabetic foot. Surgical debridement of infected wound is often required before healing can be expected. Debridement can be done by different means, such as hydrotherapy, negative pressure therapy, and repeated wound dressing. Adjunctive therapies which may be beneficial include low intensity-low frequency, ultrasound therapy, hyperbaric oxygen, topical therapy of platelet-derived growth factors, and low-dose diode laser therapy at the wound margins. Biosurgery (myiasis) with sterile maggots have been shown to be beneficial by debriding and increasing vascularity.

EMERGING VASCULAR INTERVENTIONS

Revascularization is an important strategy for management of patients of PAD with diabetes. With advancements in modern vascular surgical reconstruction strategies and improvements in endovascular techniques, limb salvage in patients with PAD has been greatly aided. The techniques of revascularization include endovascular intervention or open surgical repair.

The aim of treatment for patients with limb-threatening ischemia is to re-establish continuous straight line inflow to the distal limb vessels and plantar arch. Adequate inflow and outflow are required to keep the revascularized segment functioning. The appropriate revascularization strategy, whether endovascular, surgical or hybrid procedure, has to be selected on an individual basis based upon the balance between risk of a specific intervention and the degree and

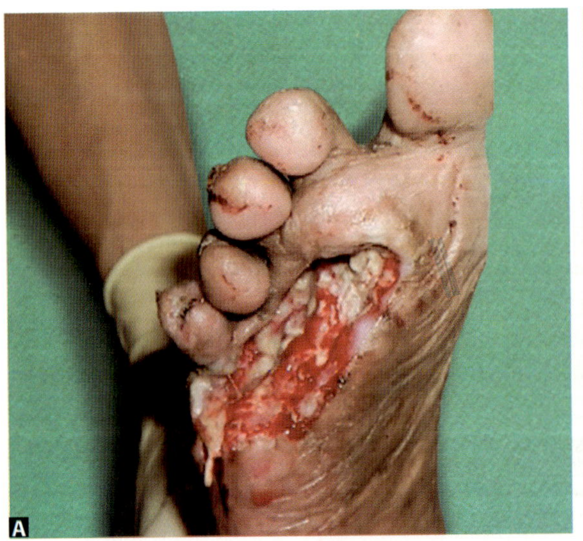

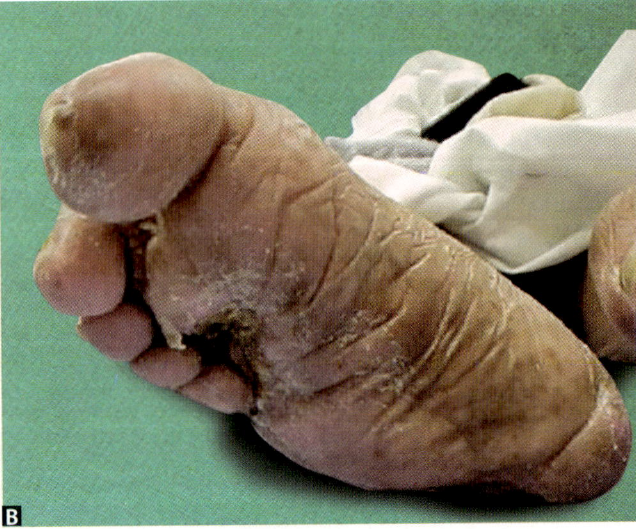

Figs 5A and B: Pre- and postrevascularization images of the foot

durability of the improvement that can be expected from this intervention. Other factors that determine the approach to revascularization include urgency of treatment, anatomic suitability, comorbidities, and available level of expertise.

Revascularization is the definitive therapy for the management of patients with CLI, as it helps in healing ischemic ulcers and preventing limb loss. Due to lack of trials comparing endovascular treatment to surgery, the benefit of one procedure over other is not conclusively established. However, surgical grafts are generally considered to have better long-term patency rates. According to TASC-II (Table 5) for type A aortoiliac and femoropopliteal lesions, endovascular revascularization is considered as treatment of choice, while for type D lesions surgery is treatment of choice. In cases with type B or C lesions, the choice should be individualized based on comorbidities, patient preference, and success rate of operator, with endovascular therapy having preference in type B lesions and surgery in type C lesions.[36]

Endovascular treatment for diabetic PAD has the following advantages:

- There are lesser chances of trauma and a faster recovery speed.
- Local anesthesia is used in endovascular interventions, which has fewer side effects and is more suitable for elderly and frail patients.[37]
- The treatment can be repeated similarly for other diseased or occluded vessels. With repeated balloon dilatation, the lesion can be re-expanded with the same safety and effectiveness.
- It has a higher rate of limb salvage. The diabetic foot ulcers after interventional treatment gradually heal with the recanalization of blood vessels.
- The technical success rate is high with a low mortality rate. The result can be immediately seen after treatment.

SURGICAL REVASCULARIZATION

Surgical revascularization has the highest patency rates in patients with PAD and CLI. Bypass grafts are significant in complex and calcified lesions that are not amenable to catheter-based intervention, and for younger patients with life expectancy of more than 2 years who require a more durable revascularization. Extra-anatomical bypass is generally reserved for older patients with advanced ischemia, previous aortofemoral bypasses, renal insufficiencies, and chronic obstructive airway disease. Aortobifemoral bypasses can be performed laparoscopically but this approach does not appear to alter the overall morbidity and mortality. Despite superiority and durability of surgical anatomical bypasses compared with angioplasty and stenting, there has been 850% increase in endovascular approach to treat CLI.

ENDOVASCULAR INTERVENTIONS

Procedure of PTA involves disruption of the atheromatous plaque. There has been an increase in the use of PTA for tibial vessels in diabetes in the past 5 years.

Endovascular interventions are undergoing constant evolution and refinement. The following techniques are now available to the vascular interventionalist:

- *Percutaneous transluminal balloon angioplasty (PTA)*
  - Plain balloon angioplasty (POBA)
  - Cutting balloon angioplasty
  - Drug-coated balloons (DCB)
  - Scoring balloons
- *Stents:*
  - Bare metal balloon expandable stent (BMS)
  - Self-expanding stents {Stainless steel, Nitinol} (SES)
  - Drug-eluting stents (DES)
  - Covered stents
  - Bioabsorbable vascular scaffolds (BVS)
- *Debulking devices:*
  - Rotablation
  - *Atherectomy devices:*
    - Directional atherectomy
    - Silver hawk
    - Orbital atherectomy device
- LASER
- *Re-entry devices:*
  - Pioneer
  - Outback catheter
  - Front runner
- *Other modalities:*
  - Cryoplasty
  - Photodynamic therapy
  - Gene therapy
  - Autologous stem cell implantation.

PTA versus Stents

Percutaneous transluminal balloon angioplasty (PTA) is found to be better than optimal medical therapy for CLI. Stents are superior to PTA alone as is seen in ABSOLUTE trial (Fig. 6). In an article published in New England Journal of Medicine in 2006, Schillinger et al. reported significant restenosis rates in patients treated with stents. RESILIENT trial confirmed the superiority of stents over PTA.

Drug-coated Balloons

PACIFIER, LEVANT-I, FEM-PAC, and THUNDER trials were one of the first randomized controlled trials for treating superficial femoral artery (SFA) disease by drug (paclitaxel)-coated balloons (Table 6). Drug-coated balloons (DCBs) were found to have higher patency rates

TABLE 5: Lesion Classification according to the Trans-Atlantic Inter-Society Consensus (TASC II) for the Management of Peripheral Arterial Disease

Aortoiliac lesions	
Type A	• Unilateral or bilateral stenosis of CIA • Unilateral or bilateral single short (≤3 cm) stenosis of EIA
Type B	• Short (≤3 cm) stenosis of infrarenal aorta • Unilateral CIA occlusion • Single or multiple stenosis totaling 3–10 cm involving the EIA not extending into the CFA • Unilateral EIA occlusion not involving the origins of internal iliac or CFA
Type C	• Bilateral CIA occlusions • Bilateral EIA stenosis 3–10 cm long not extending into the CFA • Unilateral EIA stenosis extending into the CFA • Unilateral EIA occlusion that involves the origins of internal iliac and/or CFA • Heavily calcified unilateral EIA occlusion with or without involvement of origins of internal iliac and/or CFA
Type D	• Infra-renal aortoiliac occlusion • Diffuse disease involving the aorta and both iliac arteries requiring treatment • Diffuse multiple stenosis involving the unilateral CIA, EIA, and CFA • Unilateral occlusions of both CIA and EIA • Bilateral occlusions of EIA • Iliac stenosis in patients with abdominal aortic aneurysm (AAA) requiring treatment and not amenable to endograft placement or other lesions requiring open aortic or iliac surgery
Femoropopliteal lesions	
Type A	• Single stenosis ≥10 cm in length • Single occlusion ≤5 cm in length
Type B	• Multiple lesions (stenoses or occlusions), each ≤5 cm • Single stenosis or occlusion ≤15 cm not involving the infrageniculate popliteal artery • Single or multiple lesions in the absence of continuous tibial vessels to improve inflow for a distal bypass • Heavily calcified occlusion ≤5 cm in length • Single popliteal stenosis
Type C	• Multiple stenoses or occlusions totaling >15 cm with or without heavy calcifications • Recurrent stenoses or occlusions that need treatment after two endovascular interventions
Type D	• Chronic total occlusion of CFA or SFA (>20 cm, involving the popliteal artery) • Chronic total occlusion of popliteal artery and proximal trifurcation vessels

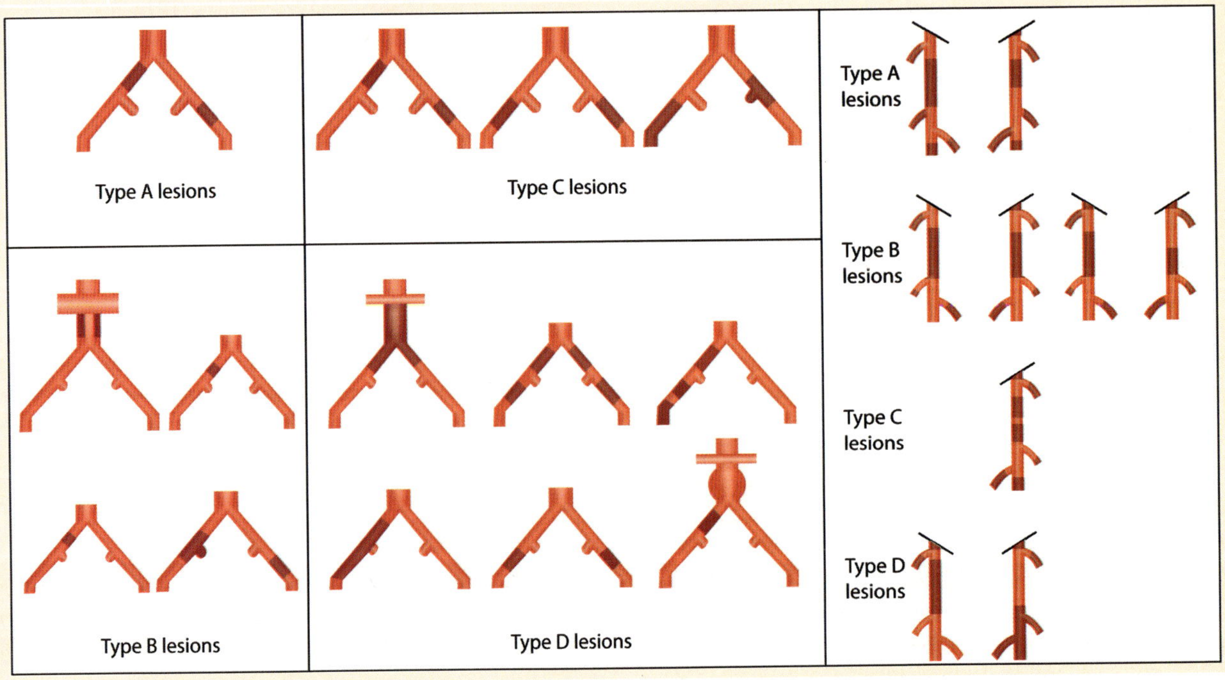

Abbreviations: EIA, external iliac artery; CIA, common iliac artery; CFA, common femoral artery; SFA, superficial femoral artery.

TABLE 6: Comparison of various trials of drug coated balloons (DCBs) and drug-eluting stents (DES)

	Absolute	*Resilient*	*Sirocco*	*Strides*	*Zilver PTX*	*Thunder*	*FEM-PAC*	*Levant*
Lesion length (cm)	~10	~6.7	~8.4	9.0	5.4	7.5	4.5	8.1
Diabetes mellitus	~38%	38%	~47%	39%	46%	50%	47%	47%
Ca^{2+} (mod/sev)	~82%	~35%	~77%	78%	72%	46%	52%	N/A
Occlusion	~18%	~18%	~57%	47%	25%	50%	13%	41%
Restenosis	N/A	~3%	~7%	10%	6%	22% 14% ISR	27% 7% ISR	11%
12 month patency	63%	81%	82% (18 month)	63%	76%	75%	81% (6 month)	72% (6 month)

Abbreviation: ISR: in-stent restenosis.

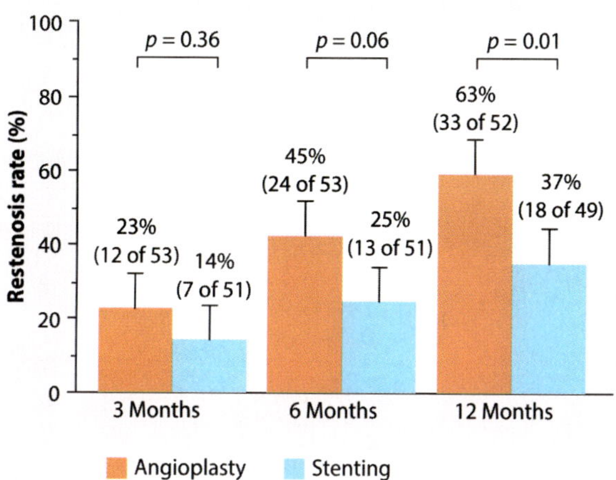

Fig. 6: Results of ABSOLUTE trial at 3, 6, and 12 months follow-up

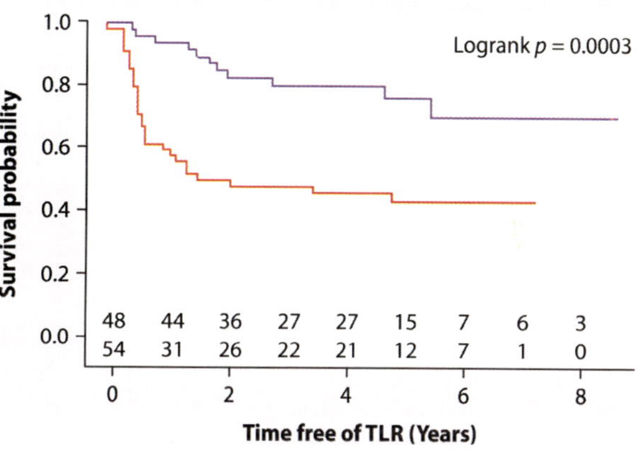

Fig. 7: Freedom from target lesion revascularization (TLR) in THUNDER trial, Kaplan–Meir curve

and lower incidence of target lesion revascularization (TLR) in all these trials (Fig. 7). The DCBs were used to treat in-stent restenosis (ISR) in SFA lesions in the IN.PACT trial. 12-month TLR and restenosis rates were 7.8%. Two types of coatings—crystalline or amorphous are done on DCBs. Amorphous coatings have higher uptake and lower retention. Sirolimus-based nanocrystal balloon coating technology are also in the pipeline.

Drug-eluting Stents

Drug-eluting stents have been increasingly used in CLI to reduce neointimal hyperplasia and ISR in both SFA and below knee lesions. Zilver PTX (paclitaxel-eluting stent from Cook Medical Inc.) and sirolimus-eluting SMART stent (from Cordis, Johnson and Johnson Ltd.) were used in Zilver PTX and sirolimus coated cordis self-expandable stent (SIROCCO) trials, respectively, for treating SFA lesions. Zilver PTX and SIROCCO trials are the only two large randomized trials which have unequivocally demonstrated superiority of DES over PTA/BMS in terms of higher primary patency and lower restenosis at 12 months. Scheinert et al. in the ACHILLES trial (prospective randomized multicentric trial comparing PTA versus sirolimus-eluting stent for infrapopliteal artery) reported a higher vessel patency (75% vs 57.1%) and lower angiographic restenosis (22.4% vs 41.9%).

Subintimal Angioplasty

Subintimal angioplasty is a technique used to treat occlusions, in which a deliberate attempt is made to cause a dissection in the arterial wall, commenced above the occlusion. The guidewire is passed in the subintimal layer beyond the occlusion where re-entry into the vessel lumen is then achieved. The potential space in the subintimal layer is then dilated by balloon angioplasty to form a new lumen (Figs 8A to D).

Aortoiliac Disease

With improvements in technology and endovascular techniques, endovascular therapy has replaced open surgical bypass as a primary treatment for both focal and advanced aortoiliac occlusive disease in many cases.

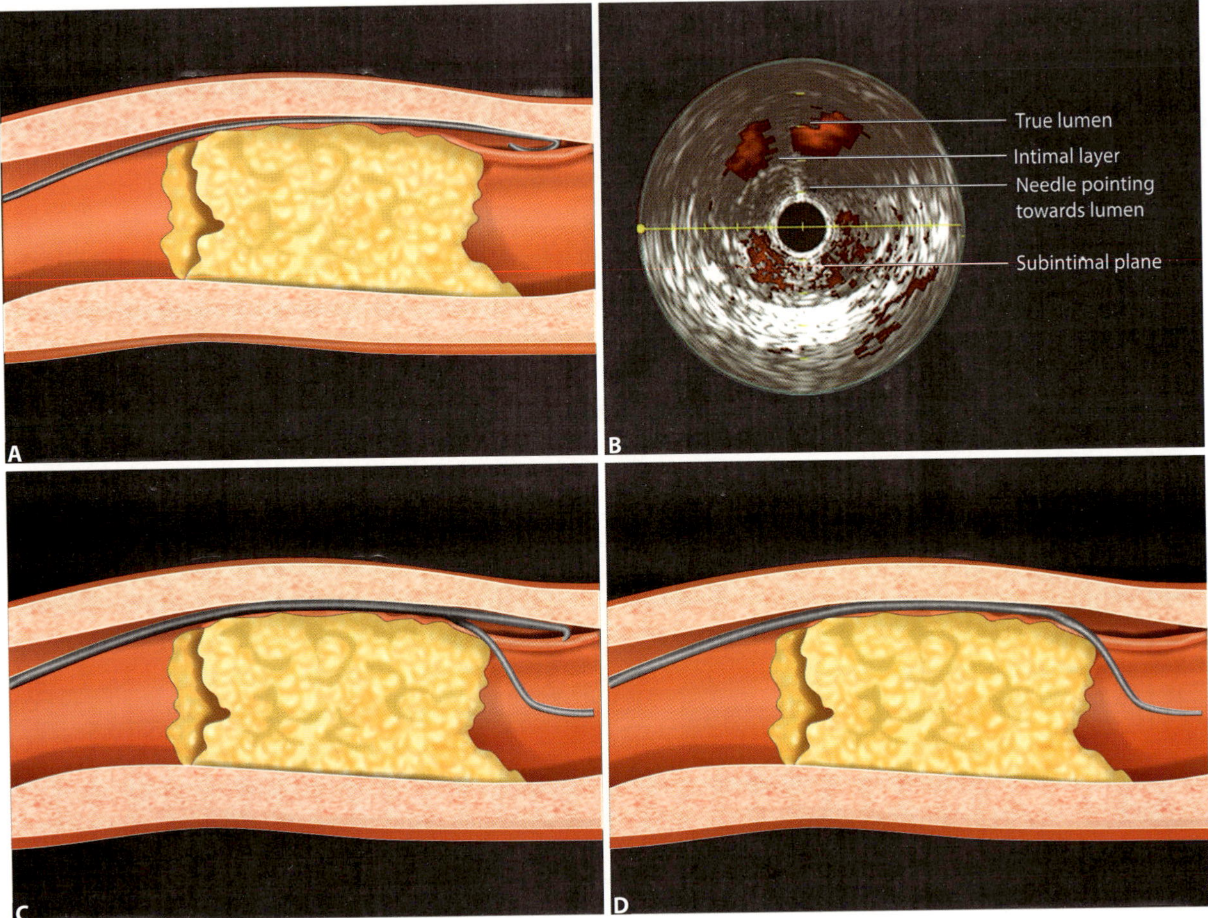

Figs 8A to D: (A) Subintimal entry of device; (B) Pioneer catheter pointing towards true lumen; (C) Outback catheter-guided reentry; (D) Wire reentry into the true lumen.

For iliac angioplasty using stents, long-term results are comparable with open surgery.[38,39] Other techniques include devices for crossing long-segment total occlusions, stent grafts, and hybrid procedures (combining iliac stenting with femoral endarterectomy) as alternatives to aortofemoral surgical reconstructions in appropriate with suitable anatomy.

Technical success rates for intervention vary from 90% to 100%, with 1-year primary patency rates ranging from 75% to 100% and 4-year primary patency rates from 60% to 80%. Secondary patency can be maintained with repeat percutaneous intervention, with 1-year and 5-year secondary patency noted to be 90–100% and 60–100%, respectively.[40,41] Percutaneous approach can be achieved through a femoral or brachial approach or a combination of the two. The types of stents used include balloon-expandable and SES. The choice of stent used depends on the type of disease and size of stent available. Calcific disease usually requires balloon-expandable stents. The aortic bifurcation is treated with *"kissing stents"* at the origin of the iliac arteries. Alternatively, an aortic stent is placed down to the bifurcation followed by kissing stents placed at the iliac vessel origins.

Mortality rate due to endovascular interventions in the aorta can range from 1% to 3%, and morbidity ranges from 5% to 20%, with aortic rupture a possibility.[40,41] Aortic rupture is a potential complication encountered when embarking on treatment for an aortic lesion.

Iliac Disease

Primary stenting is now the mainstay of therapy for treatment of iliac artery disease. More extensive and complex occlusive diseases are better treated by a primary stent approach with improved patency. The percutaneous access can vary from ipsilateral or contralateral groin or brachial. One should be certain that devices with an appropriate length should be available before initiating a procedure. If the brachial approach is used, longer delivery systems should be available. Uncovered stents across the

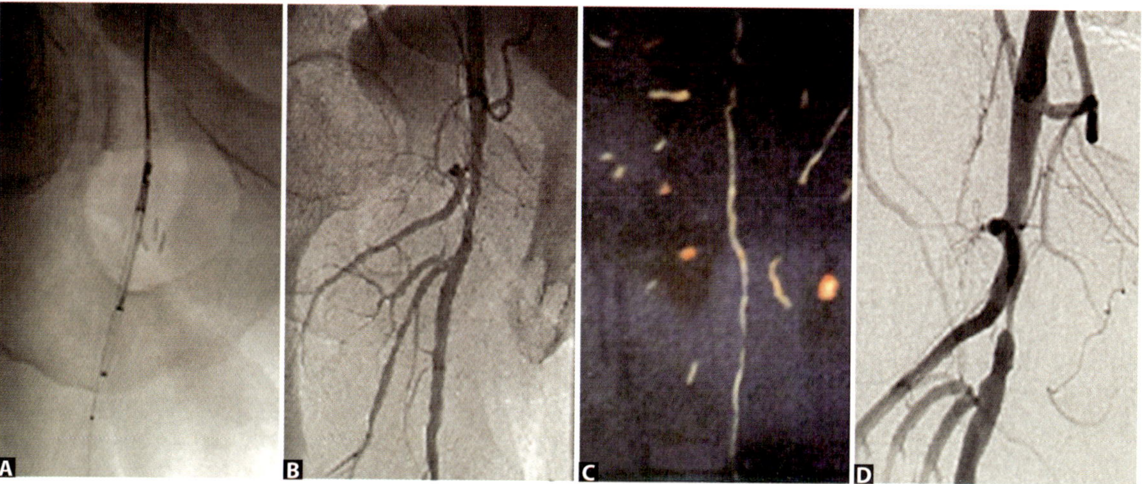

Figs 9A to D: (A) Lesion in ostial superficial femoral artery (SFA) been treated with atherectomy device, (B) final result, (C and D) picture of actual atheroma removed.

orifice of the internal iliac artery maintains adequate hypogastric artery perfusion. Covered balloon-expandable stents was found to have better primary patency rates when used in more complex lesions in the iliac artery.[42]

An important factor in the treatment of iliac occlusive disease is the extension of the disease into the femoral artery. Stents are not preferably used in the common femoral artery (CFA) since they are more likely to fracture or fail due to flexion of the artery that occurs with hip flexion. As such, when the disease extends into the CFA, the use of a hybrid approach combining femoral endarterectomy with iliac stenting is a better alternative. Covered stents have been used in the treatment of iliac occlusive disease.

Femoropopliteal Occlusive Disease

Endovascular treatment options for femoropopliteal occlusive disease include PTA alone, especially for short focal lesions less than 4 cm, angioplasty with SES, balloon-expandable stents, covered stent grafts, use of atherectomy devices (Figs 9A to D) drug-coated balloons,[43] and DESs.[44] While atherectomy is not a novel technique, the introduction of new technology has generated interest in interventional circles, with the FDA approving four new atherectomy devices over the last decade.

The SFA is the most common site of atherosclerotic occlusive disease resulting in lower limb claudication. The severity of symptoms from occlusive disease in the SFA is based on the extent of collateralization from the profunda femoral artery to the geniculate collateral arteries at the popliteal artery. After failure of a supervised exercise training program and optimal medical therapy, endovascular intervention can be considered.

Catheter-directed Thrombolytic Therapy

Catheter-directed intra-arterial thrombolytic therapy (CDTT) is a technique that has been developed to treat thrombotic occlusion of the peripheral arteries. It has an important role in the management of CLI, when a stenosed lesion is occluded with thrombus. The technique consists of intra-arterial infusion of a concentrated dose of fibrinolytic agents (recombinant tissue plasminogen activator) into the thrombus to restore blood flow to the ischemic limb. This uncovers underlying stenotic lesions which are then treated by an endovascular or surgical approach. Since the lytic agent is infused locally, the risk of bleeding is drastically reduced and the systemic effects of the drug are also reduced.

Modalities on the Horizon: Vascular Grafts, Stem Cell Therapy

Newer innovations are being brought to the forefront. Newer experimentation includes the creation of artificial biological blood vessels; signaling manipulations in ischemic limbs to increase collateralization and possibly help in new blood vessel formation. Advances in vascular grafting technology are leading towards the creation of synthetic bypass conduits utilizing autologous cells and tissues from the affected patient. Increasing limb salvage in patients who are otherwise unfit for intervention has led to the concept of increasing the body's native adaptation to ischemia by collateralization. Experimental ischemia models in animals have demonstrated that direct injection of growth factors, bone marrow derived stem cells, or progenitor cells into affected limbs have promoted angiogenesis.[45, 46]

CONCLUSION

A multidisciplinary team consisting of a diabetologist, interventional cardiologist, vascular surgeon, and podiatrist are required to maximize the chances of successful outcomes for diabetic patients with PAD. Diabetic PAD is one of the main causes of lower limb amputation in patients with diabetes. PTA is a feasible technique for diabetic peripheral artery disease. Endovascular treatment has good results in treating diabetic PAD, with higher safety, less chances of trauma and fewer complications. Traditional surgical techniques such as arterial bypass was the mainstay and gold standard for therapy in patients with peripheral vascular compromise. However, the emergence of endovascular therapies has resulted in increasing rates of limb salvage in patients who cannot undergo surgery. Through advances in endovascular technologies advance with techniques such as subintimal angioplasty and excisional atherectomy, those patients who would have otherwise been referred for amputation, are now being successfully treated with the limb being preserved. The future may show a revolution in graft technology engineered from patient-derived tissues, probably allowing for superior graft patency and limb salvage rates. New modalities for treating limb ischemia by increasing blood flow without the need for surgical or endovascular intervention may also emerge. Ultimately, the role of risk factor prevention, proper glycemic control, and careful surveillance plays the most significant role in the maintenance of overall well-being.

REFERENCES

1. Beckman JA, Creager MA, Libby P. Diabetes and atherosclerosis. Epidemiology, pathophysiology, and management. JAMA. 2002;287(19):2570-81.
2. Brun E, Nelson RG, Bennett PH, et al. Diabetes duration and cause-specific mortality in the Verona Diabetes Study. Diabetes Care. 2000;23(8):1119-23.
3. Fox CS, Sullivan L, D'Agostino RB, et al. The significant effect of diabetes duration on coronary heart disease mortality: the Framingham Heart Study. Diabetes Care. 2004;27(3):704-8.
4. Global Lower Extremity Amputation Study Group. Epidemiology of lower extremity amputation in centres in Europe, North America and East Asia. Br J Surg. 2000;87(3):328-37.
5. Pyorala K, Laakso M, Uusitupa M. Diabetes and atherosclerosis: an epidemiologic view. Diabetes Metab Rev. 1987;3(2):463-524.
6. Donahue RP, Orchard TJ. Diabetes mellitus and macrovascular complications: an epidemiological perspective. Diabetes Care. 1992;15(9):1141-55.
7. Dormandy IA, Rutherford RB, Bakal C, et al. Management of peripheral arterial disease. Int Angiol. 2000;19(Suppl 1):1-310.
8. Schroll M, Munck O. Estimation of peripheral arteriosclerotic disease by ankle blood pressure measurements in a population study of 60-year-old men and women. J Chron Dis. 1981;334(6):261-9.
9. Ramachandran A. Burden of Diabetes and its complications in India. In: Proceeding Novo Nordisk Update (NNDU), February 18-20. Mumbai: NNDU; 2000. pp. 51-7.
10. Beckman JA, Creager MA, Libby P. Diabetes and atherosclerosis. Epidemiology, pathophysiology, and management. JAMA. 2002;287(19):2570-81.
11. Zou M, Yesilkaya A, Ultrich V. Peroxynitrite inactivates prostacyclin synthase by heme-thiolate-catalyzed tyrosine nitration. Drug Metab Rev. 1999;31(2):343-9.
12. Milstein S, Katisic Z. Oxidation of tetrahydrobiopterin by peroxynitrite: implications for vascular endothelial function. Biochem Biophys Res Common. 1999;263(3):681-4.
13. Vinik AI, Erbas T, Park TS, et al. Platelet dysfunction in type 2 diabetes. Diabetes Care. 2001;24(8):1476-85.
14. Sumpio BE, Paszkowiak J, Aruny JA, et al. Vascular Medicine, 3rd edn. Philadelphia: Elsevier; 2005, pp. 880-93.
15. Sumpio BE. Foot ulcers. N Engl J Med. 2000;343(11):787-93.
16. Dormandy JA, Rutherford RB. Management of peripheral arterial disease. TASC Working Group. TransAtlantic Inter-Society Consensus. J Vasc Surg. 2000;31:S1-296.
17. Criqui MH, Fronek A, Klauber MR, et al. The sensitivity, specificity, and predictive value of traditional clinical evaluation of peripheral arterial disease: results from noninvasive testing in a defined population. Circulation. 1985;71:516-22.
18. American Diabetes Association. Peripheral arterial disease in people with diabetes. Diabetes Care. 2003;26(12):3333-41.
19. Hiatt WR, Hoag S, Hamman RF. Effect of diagnostic criteria on the prevalence of peripheral arterial disease. The San Luis Valley Diabetes Study. Circulation. 1995;91(5):1472-9.
20. Hiatt WR, Jones DN. The role of hemodynamics and duplex ultrasound in the diagnosis of peripheral arterial disease. Curr Opin Cardiol. 1992;7(5):805-10.
21. Ouriel K. Peripheral arterial disease. Lancet. 2001;358(9289):1257-64.
22. CTisus. (2004). CT Angiography: The State of the Art in 2004 (Fishman EK). [online] Available from http://www.ctisus.org/cta_web/7_04/pdfs/AR_07_04_CTA_FishmanOver.pdf. [Accessed October, 2014].
23. Freund KM, Belanger AJ, D'Agostino RB, et al. The health risks of smoking. The Framingham Study: 34 years of follow-up. Ann Epidemiol. 1993;3(4):417-24.
24. Grundy SM, Cleeman JI, Bairey Merz CN, et al. Implications of recent clinical trials for the National Cholesterol Education Program Adult Treatment Panel III Guidelines. J Am Coll Cardiol. 2004;44(3):720-32.
25. Hansson L, Zanchetti A, Carruthers SG, et al. Effects of intensive blood-pressure lowering and low-dose aspirin in patients with hypertension: principal results of the Hypertension Optimal Treatment (HOT) randomised trial. HOT Study Group. Lancet. 1998;351(9118):1755-62.
26. UK Prospective Diabetes Study (UKPDS) Group. Intensive blood-glucose control with sulfonylureas or insulin compared with conventional treatment and risk of complications in patients with type 2 diabetes (UKPDS 33). Lancet. 1998;352(9131):837-53.
27. American Diabetes Association. Standards of medical care for patients with diabetes mellitus. Diabetes Care. 2001,24(Suppl 1):S33-43.
28. Food and Drug Administration. Internal analgesic, antipyretic, and antirheumatic drug products for over-the-counter human use: final rule for professional labeling of aspirin, buffered aspirin, and aspirin in combination with antacid drug products. Fed Regist. 1998;63:56802-19.
29. Clagett GP, Sobel M, Jackson MR, et al. Antithrombotic therapy in peripheral arterial occlusive disease: the Seventh ACCP Conference on Antithrombotic and Thrombolytic Therapy. Chest. 2004;126(3 Suppl):609S-26S.
30. Antiplatelet Trialists Collaboration. Collaborative overview of randomised trials of antiplatelet therapy, II: maintenance of vascular graft or arterial patency by antiplatelet therapy. BMJ. 1994;308(6922):159-68.

31. American Diabetes Association. Aspirin therapy in diabetes. Diabetes Care. 2003;26:S87-8.
32. CAPRIE Steering Committee. A randomised, blinded trial of clopidogrel versus aspirin in patients at risk of ischemic events (CAPRIE). Lancet. 1996;348(9038):1329-39.
33. Bhatt DL, Marso SP, Hirsch AT, et al. Amplified benefits of clopidogrel versus aspirin in patients with diabetes mellitus. Am J Cardiol. 2002;90(6):625-8.
34. Angelkort B, Spurk P, Habbaba A, et al. Blood flow properties and walking performance in chronic arterial occlusive disease. Angiology. 1985;36(5):285-92.
35. Money SR, Herd JA, Isaacsohn JL, et al. Effect of cilostazol on walking distances in patients with intermittent claudication caused by peripheral vascular disease. J Vasc Surg. 1998;27(2):267-74.
36. Norgren L, Hiatt WR, Dormandy JA, et al. Inter-society consensus for the management of peripheral arterial disease (TASC II). J Vasc Surg. 2007;45 (Suppl. 1):S5-67.
37. Yongquan G, Jian Z, Xiheng Y. Infrapopliteal artery endoluminal angioplasty for the treatment of severe limb ischemia. Chin J Gen Sur. 2007, 22(1):123-25.
38. Galaria II, Davies MG. Percutaneous transluminal revascularization for iliac occlusive disease: long-term outcomes in Trans-Atlantic Inter-Society Consensus A and B lesions. Ann Vasc Surg. 2005;19(3):352-60.
39. Schurmann K, Mahnken A, Meyer J, et al. Long-term results 10 years after iliac arterial stent placement. Radiology. 2002;224(3):731-8.
40. Feugier P, Toursarkissian B, Chevalier JM, et al. Endovascular treatment of isolated atherosclerotic stenosis of the infrarenal abdominal aorta: long-term outcome. Ann Vasc Surg. 2003;17(4):375-85.
41. Kim TH, Ko YG, Kim U, et al. Outcomes of endovascular treatment of chronic total occlusion of the infrarenal aorta. J Vasc Surg. 2011;53(6):1542-9.
42. Mwipatayi BP, Thomas S, Wong J, et al. A comparison of covered vs bare expandable stents for the treatment of aortoiliac occlusive disease. J Vasc Surg. 2011;54(6):1561-70.
43. Werk M, Langner S, Reinkensmeier B, et al. Inhibition of restenosis in femoropopliteal arteries: paclitaxel-coated versus uncoated balloon: femoral paclitaxel randomized pilot trial. Circulation. 2008;118(13):1358-65.
44. Dake MD, Ansel GM, Jaff MR, et al. Paclitaxel-eluting stents show superiority to balloon angioplasty and bare metal stents in femoropopliteal disease: twelve-month Zilver PTX randomized study results. Circ Cardiovasc Interv. 2011;4(5):495-504.
45. Lawall H, Bramlage P, Amann B. Treatment of peripheral arterial disease using stem and progenitor cell therapy. J Vasc Surg. 2011;53(2):445-53.
46. Horio T, Fujita M, Tanaka Y, et al. Efficacy of fragmin/protamine microparticles containing fibroblast growth factor-2) F/PMPs/FGF-2) to induce collateral vessels in a rabbit model of hindlimb ischemia. J Vasc Surg. 2011;54(3):791-98.

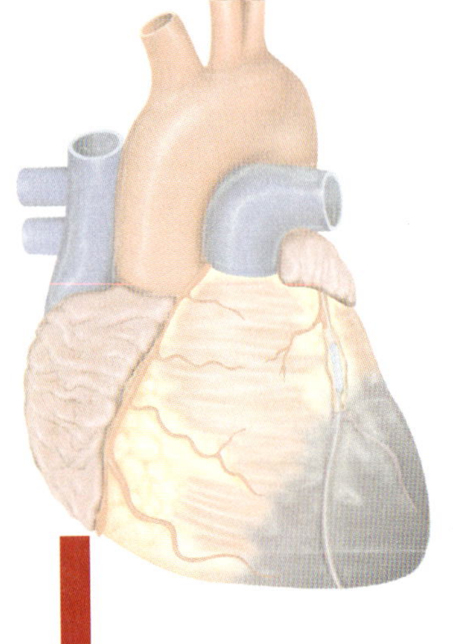

Cardiodiabetes and Vasculopathy

Sameer Shrivastava, Biswajit Paul

INTRODUCTION

According to the World Health Organization (WHO), an estimated 422 million adults were living with diabetes in 2014 compared to 108 million in 1980. The global prevalence of diabetes in adult population has moved up from 4.7% in 1980 to 8.5% in 2014. In 2012, diabetes caused 1.5 million deaths. An additional 2.2 million deaths were caused by higher than optimal blood glucose by increasing the risk of cardiovascular disease. About 4.3% of these 3.7 million deaths occurred before the age of 70 years. Additionally, a higher percentage of deaths were seen in low and middle-income countries than in high-income countries.[1] It is, therefore obvious that the financial burden of the disease would be borne by the less affluent population of the world. While in Asia and Africa, the rising prevalence is unchallenged; the epidemic seems to have leveled off in the US and European countries.[2] A pertinent question that comes to one's mind is why this epidemic? The roots of the cause have been traced to our lifestyle changes. The problem has been compounded with the additional burden of cardiovascular disease, a manifestation of macrovascular complication. The microvascular complications of diabetes—neuropathy, nephropathy, and retinopathy have a severe impact on morbidity and mortality. Cardiovascular disease in diabetes increases the rate of all-cause morbidity by three-fold and the rate of all-cause cardiovascular death by five-fold.[3] This chapter aims to discuss the pathophysiology of diabetic vasculopathy and its management.

PATHOPHYSIOLOGY OF VASCULAR DISEASE IN DIABETICS

Role of Insulin Resistance and Hyperglycemia

The vasculopathy in diabetes is induced by a proinflammatory thrombotic state which leads to atherosclerosis. The inciting event is insulin-resistance mediated hyperglycemia with clustering of other factors such as hypertension, dyslipidemia, sedentary lifestyle, genetic susceptibility, etc. The detrimental effects of glucose occur even before the threshold of diagnosis of diabetes is attained. This is explained by the phenomenon of "'glycemic continuum," i.e. a spectrum of prediabetes to diabetes and cardiovascular disease.[4] Hyperglycemia creates imbalance between nitric oxide (NO) bioavailability and accumulation of reactive oxygen species (ROS) leading to endothelial dysfunction. The generation of superoxide anion (O^{2-}) inactivates NO to form peroxynitrite ($ONOO^-$) which is a powerful oxidant. It penetrates across phospholipid membranes and induces substrate nitration thereby blunting the activity of endothelial NO synthase (eNOS). Reduced bioavailability of NO is a harbinger of cardiovascular disease.[5] Excess ROS production activates the polyol pathway, production of advanced glycation end products (AGE), activation of protein kinase C, and NF-kβ-mediated vascular inflammation.[6] All these are responsible for alteration in cell permeability, inflammatory angiogenesis, and apoptosis. In other words, hyperglycemia mediates vascular inflammation, vasoconstriction, and platelet aggregation. The atherogenic effect of insulin resistance has also been ascribed to the dyslipidemia associated with it—high triglyceride, low level of high-density lipoprotein (HDL), elevated ApoB, and small dense low-density lipoprotein (LDL).[7] Micro-RNA (miRs), have been defined as key players in the pathogenesis of hyperglycemia induced vascular damage. Diabetics display a deregulation of miRs involved in angiogenesis, vascular repair, and endothelial hemostasis.[8]

Thrombotic Milieu in Diabetes

Insulin resistance increases plasminogen activator inhibitor-1 (PAI-1) and fibrinogen levels and reduces tissue plasminogen activator (tPA) activity.[9] Hyperglycemia alters platelet-Ca^{2+} homeostasis leading to cytoskeletal abnormalities and increased secretion of proaggregant factors. Upregulation of Gp 2b/3a and Gp 1b receptor trigger thrombus formation in diabetic patients.[10]

Hyperglycemic Memory

Despite achieving normoglycemia in diabetic patients cardiovascular risk may be unaltered. This has been attributed to "hyperglycemia memory" wherein the vasculature remembers the insult borne by it. Vascular inflammation, once initiated, is not restored by normoglycemia.[11]

Coronary Artery Disease

There is ample data to suggest that diabetes increases the risk of coronary events. The *Finnish* study documented that in diabetics the risk of myocardial infarction (MI) and death were higher as compared to nondiabetics. The concept of diabetes as a coronary artery disease (CAD) risk equivalent evolved and recommended by Adult Treatment Panel III (ATP 3) of the National Cholesterol Education Program (NCEP).[12] There has been data to the contrary questioning the risk equivalence.[13] In non-ST segment elevation acute coronary syndromes (ACS) subjects with diabetes had higher rates of the composite end points of cardiovascular deaths, MI or recurrent ischemia. Trial to Assess Improvement in Therapeutic Outcomes-Thrombolysis in Myocardial Infarction (TRITON-TIMI) 38 showed that prasugrel lowered adverse event rate in patients with ACS. But patients with diabetes still had higher levels of MI, stent thrombosis, and cardiovascular deaths. In patients with ST-segment elevation MI treated with percutaneous coronary intervention (PCI), diabetes was associated with a higher rate of MI and all-cause mortality.[14] Using the United Kingdom Prospective Diabetes Study (UKPDS) risk calculator, the estimated 10-year risk for CAD decreased from 21.1% in 1999–2000 to 16.4% in 2007–2008.[15] A decline in cardiovascular death rates in recent years in diabetics have been attributed to better medical therapy which includes statins.[16]

Stroke

The *interstroke* case-controlled study was performed in 22 nations. Diabetes increases the risk of stroke by 35%.[17] The Emerging Risk Factor Collaboration analyzed almost 700,000 people from 102 prospective studies and found that diabetes was associated with 2.27-fold increase in the risk of ischemic stroke and 56% excess rate of hemorrhagic stroke.[18] In the Life and Longevity After Cancer (LILAC) cohort study, diabetes increased the risk of fatal and nonfatal stroke more than two-fold.[19] Improvements in the control of hypertension, dyslipidemia, and treatment of diabetes have been demonstrated to contribute to more favorable outcomes of stroke and a lower rate of recurrence.

Peripheral Artery Disease

Patients with diabetes have a higher prevalence of peripheral artery disease (PAD) and intermittent claudication. Diabetes increases the risk of critical limb ischemia in patients with PAD.[20] In those with critical limb ischemia, 50% patients will develop critical limb ischemia in the contralateral limb within 5 years.[21] The results of revascularization are worse in diabetics and there is a higher rate of cardiovascular morbidity associated with the procedure. It is not established whether aggressive risk facto modification decreases the risk of PAD in patients with diabetes.

TREATMENT OF ATHEROSCLEROSIS IN DIABETES

Hyperglycemia

Tight glucose control produced statistical significant reduction in MI in the UKPDS trial.[22] However, in ACCORD study, there was a significant increase in all-cause mortality.[23] Similarly in ADVANCE, intensive glucose control did not reduce major macrovascular events, deaths from cardiovascular causes, and deaths from any cause.[24] Based on these studies, the American Diabetes Association (ADA) recommended a HbA1C goal of 7%.[25] Improving insulin sensitivity with metformin—a biguanide has been shown to have a significant reduction in mortality and reduction of MI in UKPDS and Reduction of Atherothrombosis for Continued Health (REACH) registry.[26,27] Pioglitazone—a thiazolidinedione has shown benefit in secondary composite endpoint (all-cause mortality, nonfatal MI, and stroke).[28] Rosiglitazone has been associated with an increase in MI but not all-cause mortality. Several other hypoglycemic drugs are used in diabetes.[29] There is lack of enough data to recommend their use as treatments to reduce cardiovascular events.

Hypertension

In UKPDS, tight control of blood pressure (BP) produced a significant reduction in stroke (44%) and diabetes-related death (32%).The choice of beta blocker or ACE inhibitor made no difference and the majority required more than one antihypertensive drug.[30] Based on the Appropriate Blood Pressure Control in Diabetes (ABCD) trial where aggressive control of diastolic blood pressure lowered all-cause mortality, Seventh Joint National Committee (JNC7) recommended that diabetics should have their BP controlled to 130/80 mm Hg or lower. The ACCORD trial did not show a significant reduction in primary outcome (nonfatal MI, nonfatal stroke, death from cardiovascular cause) by intensive BP control. A significant (40%) reduction in stroke was notice-worthy.[31] The ALLHAT demonstrated no differences in the primary outcome of fatal CAD or nonfatal MI among chlorthalidone, amlodipine, and lisinopril arms in patients with diabetes.[32] When the consideration for antihypertensive agents are to be made, the following points need to be considered. First, if the primary goal of treatment is reduction of BP, thiazide diuretic, dihydropyridine calcium channel blockers or ACE inhibitors are acceptable first choice. Second, in the setting of post-MI, angina, left ventricular dysfunction, beta-blockers are preferred agents. For secondary prevention of atherosclerotic events, ACE inhibitors or angiotensin receptor blockers (ARBs) take precedence and have been highlighted in several trials.

Dyslipidemia

The cornerstone of dyslipidemia management in diabetes has been statins since the results of heart protection study were published.[33] However, in patients with renal failure, they have failed to show any consistent efficacy in diabetic patients undergoing hemodialysis.[34] More potent statins in high doses have been found to be more favorable.

Antiplatelet Therapy

The recommendation of low-dose aspirin for primary prevention by the US Preventive Services Task Force and American College of Chest Physicians (ACCP) has been questioned by JAPAD[35] and POPADAD[36] trials. However, when the cardiovascular risk exceeds 1% per year, low-dose aspirin may gain the small benefit in primary prevention.[37] In patients with ACS, the addition of clopidogrel to aspirin provides incremental benefit and has been highlighted in CAPRIE,[38] CHARISHMA,[39] and CORE[40] trials. Patients of ACS undergoing PCI, the addition of prasugrel to aspirin provides incremental benefit in TRITON-TIMI 38 trial[14] but not in TRILOGY-ACS[41] trial. Another P2Y12 inhibitor ticagrelor was superior to clopidogrel in PLATO[42] trial, but provided no significant benefit for diabetes subjects.

Risk Factor Modification

Modification of risk factors is the foremost approach to reduce cardiovascular complications. Intensive modification of risk factors and treatment with low-dose aspirin and renin-angiotensin-aldosterone system (RAAS) antagonist have been shown to lower cardiovascular and total mortality.[43] In fact, detection of ischemia by radionuclide imaging did not prove to be of much significance.[44] However, it needs mentioning that intensive control of hyperglycemia and hypertension may be associated with increased cardiovascular events in the diabetic population.

Coronary Revascularization

In the COURAGE trial, the addition of PCI to medical therapy did not reduce death and MI as compared to medical therapy alone. The results were the same in diabetic subgroup.[45] The Bypass Angioplasty Revascularization Investigation 2 Diabetes (BARI 2D) trial failed to show any incremental benefit of revascularization over medical therapy alone.[46] The FREEDOM trial compared the outcome of PCI and coronary artery bypass grafting (CABG) in 1,900 diabetic patients with multivessel CAD. The CABG arm produced a significant reduction in mortality. Thus, in patients with diabetes and multivessel CAD who require revascularization, CABG is preferred over PCI.[47]

CONCLUSION

The process of vasculopathy is complex and is initiated at a stage much before the onset of frank diabetes. It can be improved by lifestyle modification, lowering BP by drugs, using statins and antiplatelet therapy in appropriately chosen subjects to minimize atherosclerosis and vascular thrombosis.

REFERENCES

1. NCD risk factor collaboration (NCD-RisC). Worldwide trends in diabetes since 1980: a pooled analysis of 751 population- based studies with 4.4 million participants. Lancet. 2016;387(10027): 1513-30.
2. Doak CM, Winhoven TM, Schokker DF, et al. Age standardization in mapping adult overweight and obesity trends in the WHO European Region. Obes Rev. 2012;13(2):174-91.
3. Preiss D, Sattar N, McMurray JJ, et al. A systematic review of event rates in clinical trials in diabetes mellitus: the importance of quantifying baseline cardiovascular disease history and proteinuria and implications for clinical trial design. Am heart J. 2011;161(1):210-219.e1.
4. Wei M, Gaskill SP, Haffner SM, et al. Effects of diabetes and level of glycemia on all-cause and cardiovascular mortality. The San Antonio Heart Study. Diabetes Care. 1998;21:1167-72.
5. LermanA, Zeller AM. Endothelial function: cardiac events. Circulation. 2005;111(3):363-8.
6. Nishikawa T, Edelstein D, Du XL, et al. Normalizing mitochondrial superoxide production blocks three pathways of hyperglycemic damage. Nature. 2000;404(6779):787-90.
7. Zhang H, Dellsperger KC, Zhang C. The link between metabolic abnormalities and endothelial dysfunction in type 2 diabetes: an update. Basic Res Cardiol. 2012:107(1):237.
8. Zampetaki A, Kiechl S, Drozdov I, et al. Plasma microRNA profiling reveals loss of endothelial mir-126 and other microRNAs in type 2 diabetes. Circ Res. 2010;107(6):810-7.
9. Lemkes BA, Hermanides J, Devries JH, et al. Hyperglycemia: a prothrombotic factor? J Thromb Haemost. 2010;8(8):1663-9.
10. Vinik AL, Erbas T, Park TS, et al. Platelet dysfunction in type 2 diabetes. Diabetes Care. 2001;24:1476-85.
11. Ceriello A. Hypothesis: the "metabolic memory", the new challenge of diabetes. Diabetes Res Clin Pract. 2009;86 (Suppl 1):S2-S6.
12. Haffner SM, Lehto S, Ronnemaa T, et al. Mortality from coronary heart disease in subjects with type 2 diabetes and in nondiabetic subjects with and without prior myocardial infarction. N Engl J Med. 1998;339(4):229-34.
13. SchrammTK, Gislason GH, Kober L, et al. Diabetes patients requiring glucose-lowering therapy and nondiabetics with a prior myocardial infarction carry the same cardiovascular risk: a population study of 3.3 million people. Circulation. 2008;117(15):1945-54.
14. Wiviott SD, Braunwald E, Angiollilo DJ, et al. Greater clinical benefit of more intensive oral antiplatelet therapy with prasugrel in patients with diabetes mellitus in the trial to assess improvement in therapeutic outcomes by optimizing platelet inhibition with prasugrel. Thrombolysis in Myocardial Infarction 38. Circulation. 2008;118(16):1626-36.
15. Ford ES. Trends in the risk for coronary heart disease among adults with diagnosed diabetes in the US: findings from the National Heart and Nutrition Examination Survey,1998-2008. Diabetes Care. 2011;34(6):1337-43.
16. Collins R, Armitage J, Parish S, et al. MRC/BHF Heart Protection Study of cholesterol lowering with simvastatin in 20,536 high-risk individuals: a randomised placebo-controlled trial. Lancet. 2002; 360(9326):7-22.
17. O'Donnell MJ, Xavier D, Liu L, et al. Risk factors for ischaemic and intracerebral haemorrhagic stroke in 22 countries (the INTERSTROKE study): a case-control study. Lancet. 2010;376(9735):112-23.
18. Sarwar N, Gao P, Seshasai SR, et al. Diabetes mellitus, fasting blood glucose concentrations, and risk of vascular disease: a collaborative meta-analysis of 102 prospective studies. Lancet. 2010;375(9733):2215-22.
19. van Wijk I, Kappelle LJ, van Gijn J, et al. Long-term survival and vascular event risk after transient ischemic attack or minor ischemic stroke: a cohort study. Lancet. 2005;365(9477):2098-104.
20. Lange S, Diehn C, Darius H, et al. High prevalence of peripheral arterial disease but low antiplatelet treatment rates in elderly primary care patients with diabetes. Diabetes Care. 2003;26(12): 3357-8.
21. Diehn C, Schuster A, Allenberg JR, et al. High prevalence of peripheral arterial disease and comorbidity in 6,880 primary care patients: cross-sectional study. Atherosclerosis. 2004;172(1):95-105.
22. Effect of intensive blood-glucose control with metformin on complications in overweight patients with type 2 diabetes (UKPDS 34). UK prospective diabetes study group. Lancet. 1998;352(9131):854-65.
23. Gerstein HC, Miller ME, Byington RP, et al. Effects of intensive glucose lowering in type 2 diabetes. N Engl J Med. 2008;358(24):2545-59.
24. Patel A, MacMohan S, Chalmers J, et al. Intensive blood glucose control and vascular outcomes in patients with type 2 diabetes. N Engl J Med. 2008;358(24):2560-72.
25. Skyler JS, Bergenstel R, Bonow RO, et al. Intensive glycemic control and the prevention of cardiovascular events: implications of the ACCORD, ADVANCE, and VA Diabetes Trials: a position statement of the American Diabetes Association and a Scientific Statement of the American College Cardiology Foundation and the American Heart Association. J Am Coll Cardiol. 2009;53(3):298-304.
26. Holman RR, Paul SK, Bethel MA, et al. 10-year follow-up of intensive glucose control in type 2 diabetes. N Engl J Med. 2008;359 (15):1577-89.
27. Roussel R, Travert F, Pasquet B, et al. Metformin use and mortality in patients with diabetes and atherothrombosis. Arch Intern Med. 2010;170(21):1892-99.
28. Dormandy JA, Charbonnel B, Eckland DJ, et al. Secondary prevention of macrovascular events in patients with type 2 diabetes in the PROactive study (PROspective pioglitaZone Clinical Trial in macroVascular Events): a randomised controlled trial. Lancet. 2005;366(9493):1279-89.
29. Nissen SE, Wolski K. Rosiglitazone revisited: an updated meta-analysis of risk for myocardial infarction and cardiovascular mortality. Arch Intern Med. 2010;170(14):1191-201.
30. Robert T, Holman R, Stratton I, et al. Tight blood pressure control and risk of macrovascular and microvascular complications in type 2 diabetes: UKPDS 38. UK Prospective Diabetes Study Group. BMJ. 1998;317(7160):703-13.
31. Estacio RO, Schrier RW. Antihypertensive therapy in type 2 diabetes: implications of the appropriate blood pressure control in diabetes (ABCD) trial. Am J Cardiol. 1998;82(9):9R-14R.
32. Furberg CD, Wright JT, Davis BR, et al. Major outcomes in high-risk hypertensive patients randomized to ACE inhibitor or calcium channel blocker vs. diuretic. The Antihypertensive and Lipid Lowering Treatment to Prevent Heart Attack Trial (ALLHAT). JAMA. 2002;288(23):2981-97.
33. Collins R, Armitage J, Parish S, et al. MRC/BHF Heart Protection Study of cholesterol-lowering with simvastatin in 5,963 people with diabetes: a randomised placebo-controlled trial. Lancet. 2003;361(9374):2005-16.

34. Fellstrom BC, Jardine AG, Schmieder RE, et al. Rosuvastatin and cardiovascular events in patients undergoing hemodialysis. N Engl J Med. 2009;360(14):1395-407.
35. Ogawa H, Nakayama M, Morimoto T, et al. Low-dose aspirin for primary prevention of atherosclerotic events in patients with type 2 diabetes: a randomized controlled trial. JAMA 2008;300(18):2134-41.
36. Beich J, MacCuish A, Campbell I, et al. The prevention of progression of arterial disease and diabetes (POPADAD) trial: factorial randomised placebo-controlled trial of aspirin and antioxidants in patients with diabetes and asymptomatic peripheral arterial disease. BMJ. 2008;337:a1840.
37. Pignone M, Alberts MJ, Colwell JA, et al. Aspirin for primary prevention of cardiovascular events in people with diabetes. Diabetes Care. 2010;33(6):1395-402.
38. Gent M, Beaumont D, Bianchard J, et al. A randomised blinded trial of clopidogrel versus aspirin in patients at risk of ischemic events (CAPRIE). CAPRIE Steering Committee. Lancet. 1996;348(9038):1329-39.
39. Bhatt DL, Fox KA, Hacke W, et al. Clopidogrel and aspirin versus aspirin alone for the prevention of atherothrombotic events. N Engl J Med. 2006;354(16):1706-17.
40. Yusuf S, Zhao F, Mehta SR, et al. Effects of clopidogrel in addition to aspirin in patients with acute coronary syndromes without ST-segment elevation. N Engl J Med. 2001;345(7):494-502.
41. Roe MT, Armstrong PW, Fox KA, et al. Prasugrel versus clopidogrel for acute coronary syndromes without revascularization. N Engl J Med. 2012;367(14):1297-309.
42. James S, Angiolilio DJ, Cornell JH, et al. Ticagrelor vs. Clopidogrel in patients with acute coronary syndromes and diabetes: a substudy from the PLATelet inhibition and patient Outcome (PLATO) trial. Eur Heart J. 2010;31(24):3006-16.
43. Gaede P, Lund-Anderson H, Parving HH, et al. Effect of a multifactorial intervention on mortality in type 2 diabetes. N Engl J Med. 2008;358(6):580-91.
44. Young LH, Wacker FJ, Chyun DA, et al. Cardiac outcomes after screening for asymptomatic coronary artery disease in patients with type 2 diabetes: the DIAD study: a randomized control trial. JAMA. 2009;301(15):1547-55.
45. Boden WE, O'Rourke RA, Teo KK, et al. Optimal medical therapy for patients with or without PCI for stable coronary artery disease. N Engl J Med. 2007;356:1503-16.
46. Frye RL, August P, Brooks MM, et al. A randomized trial of therapies for type 2 diabetes and coronary artery disease. N Engl J Med. 2009;360(24):2503-15.
47. Farkouh ME, Domanski M, Sleeper LA, et al. Strategies for multivessel revascularization in patients with diabetes. N Engl J Med. 2012;367(25):2375-84.

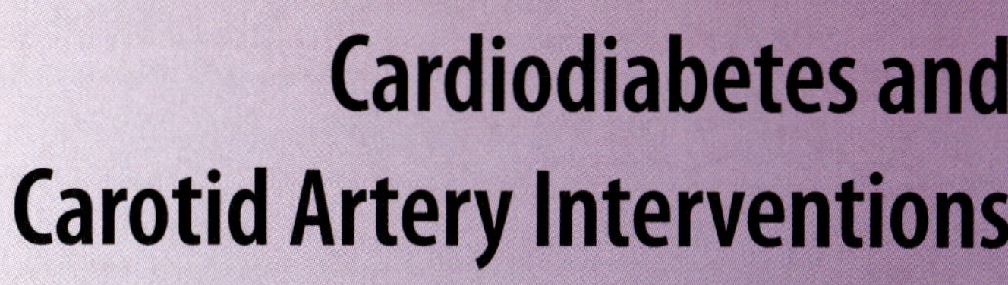

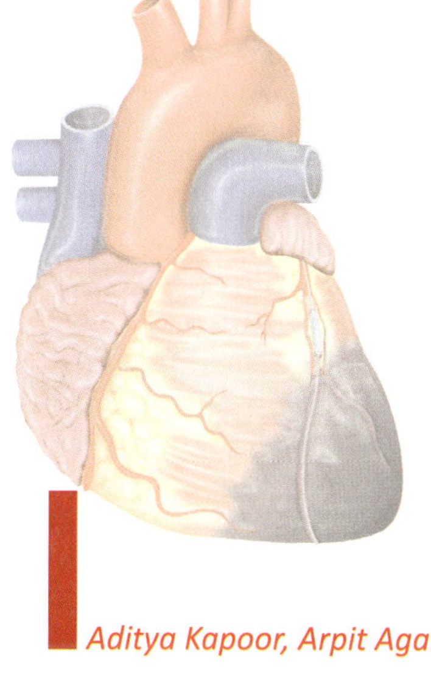

Cardiodiabetes and Carotid Artery Interventions

Aditya Kapoor, Arpit Agarwal

INTRODUCTION

Diabetes mellitus (DM) is a chronic metabolic disorder that requires intensive multifactorial risk management beyond strict glycemic control. The adverse effects of hyperglycemia are usually categorized as microvascular (retinopathy, nephropathy, and neuropathy) and macrovascular [coronary artery disease (CAD), peripheral arterial disease, and cerebrovascular disease]. Atherosclerosis is generally more extensive and occurs prematurely in diabetic subjects than in the general population leading to a 1.5- to 2-fold increased risk of cardiovascular (CV) events, including CAD, stroke, and heart failure.[1] Patients with diabetes are not only more likely to have a stroke as compared to nondiabetics (relative risk 1.8- to 6-fold), but also tend to have worse functional outcome and higher mortality rates following a stroke.[2-5] Increased carotid intima-media thickness (cIMT), occurrence of carotid plaques, total plaque area and volume are reliable suurogate markers to detect early atherosclerosis and are associated with prevalent and incident coronary heart disease and stroke, with the presence of plaque generally having a stronger association with cardiovascular disease (CVD) compared to cIMT alone. Since DM is an independent determinant of presence as well as progression of asymptomatic and symptomatic carotid artery disease (CARD), the following section addresses issues related to CARD in the diabetic subgroup with special focus on results of carotid interventions.

PREVALENCE OF CAROTID ARTERY DISEASE IN DIABETES AND ITS SIGNIFICANCE

The prevalence of CARD (symptomatic or asymptomatic) in studies of population with DM (especially type 2 DM) is reported to range from 50% to 70%.[6-9] The odds risk of developing carotid disease in patients with diabetes varies from 1.4 to 5.3.[10-12] Carotid IMT is reported to be increased not only in adults but even in children and adolescents with type 1 and type 2 diabetes compared with those without diabetes. Haffner et al. compared the IMT in the common carotid artery (CCA) and internal carotid artery (ICA) in 43 diabetics with CAD, 446 diabetics without CAD, 47 nondiabetics with CAD, and 975 nondiabetics without CAD (subjects aged 40–70 years) in the Insulin Resistance Atherosclerosis Study.[13] Both DM and CAD were associated with increased atherosclerosis in the CCA. While DM was significantly associated with increased ICA-IMT; CAD was not associated with ICA intima-media wall thickness. Göksan et al., in a Doppler ultrasonography study of 1,058 patients with DM, reported high-grade carotid artery stenosis (CS, diameter reduction of 70–99%) in 89/1058 (8.4%), while moderate (40–69%) and mild (0–39%) stenosis was observed in 85 (8%) and 884 (83.5%) patients, respectively. Diabetes mellitus (odds ratio [OR] = 2.77), ischemic heart disease (OR = 1.67), age (OR = 1.02), and male gender (OR = 1.75) were found to be significantly associated with high-grade carotid stenosis.[14] Bosevski et al. assessed 340 patients with type 2 diabetes mellitus (T2DM) and CAD; 68.5% had some evidence of CARD on Doppler ultrasound, 41.5% had bilateral plaques, 20% had unilateral CS, and 9.4% had bilateral CS.[15]

In a prospective study of 1500 subjects (> 40 years and asymptomatic for cerebrovascular disease) Kaul et al. found that the prevalence of significant carotid stenosis, as detected by Doppler ultrasound, was 5.2%. Risk factors significantly associated with greater than 50% stenosis included age greater than 70 years (OR = 2.0), hypertension (OR = 1.8), diabetes (OR = 2.3), smoking (OR = 3.6), and dyslipidemia (OR = 4.0). Duration (>15 years) of hypertension (OR = 2.5), diabetes (OR = 6.2), and smoking (OR = 5.2) markedly worsened the risk.[16]

The risk of future major adverse cardiovascular event (MACE) is significantly greater in patients with T2DM and CARD, especially with long duration of DM and significant CS, compared with those who have a shorter duration and/or nonsignificant CS. Patients of T2DM without any underlying CVD or previous CV event who develop future CV events during prospective follow-up, are often reported to have higher carotid artery plaque burden as compared to those who remain free from CV events.[8,9] Noh et al. reported that diabetics (without underlying CVD) with both a longer diabetes duration and significant carotid artery stenting (CAS) had additive and high risks of MACE [hazard ratio (HR), 2.07; $p = 0.012$] and stroke (HR, 3.38; $p = 0.002$).[17]

RISK FACTORS OF CAROTID ARTERY DISEASE IN DIABETES

In the general population, the risk of symptomatic or asymptomatic CARD incerases exponentially with age. The annual risk of population aged between 50 and 59 years is ~1.5–2% and for the population between 80 and 89 years is 20–25%.[18-20] The Chennai urban population study (CUPS) from South India also reported higher IMT values with increasing age, both in diabetic and nondiabetic subjects.[21] Studies from the West on prevalence of CARD in diabetic patients have also concluded that IMT is directly related with age in diabetic subjects.

Postprandial hyperglycemia also directly correlates with increase in CIMT and as the level of postprandial blood sugar increases, there is proportionate increase in the IMT. Experimental studies in obese models of rats have shown that hyperglycemia accelerates the progression of CAS. Although hyperglycemia and duration of diabetes have been determined as factors for development of CARD, studies have also reported a direct correlation between arterial hypertension, hypercholesterolemia and inflamatory biomarkers, and CARD in patients with DM. Associated diabetic neuropathy has also been shown to be an independent factor for the developement of carotid plaques and developement of ischemic stroke in the T2DM population. The underlying pathophysiology could either be due to the dysmetabolic state in diabetes or an expression of diabetic vascular disease. In diabetics, chronic kidney disease (CKD), defined as an estimated glomerular filtration rate (eGFR) less than 60 mL/min, is known to be an independent risk factor for the presence of carotid plaques and CARD, independent of albuminuria.[22,23] Associated fatty liver disease and steatohepatitis in DM is also postulated to be a risk factor for CARD. Casoinic et al. assessed the presence of significant CS (symptomatic or asymptomatic) in type 2 DM patients with steatohepatitis, compared to diabetics without evidence of fatty liver [Non-alcoholic fatty liver disease (NAFLD)].[24] A high prevalence of carotid atherosclerosis was noted in diabetic patients with steatohepatitis (92.5%) as compared to controls (52.73%). Significant CS (≥ 60%), was noted in 30% of diabetics with steatohepatitis vs. 10% in controls ($p < 0.001$). Those with long duration of DM and poor metabolic control were especially likely to have CARD. A high level of high-sensitivity C-reactive protein (hs-CRP) was also observed in DMT2 patients with steatohepatitis. The authors concluded that patients with type 2 diabetes and steatohepatitis had a higher prevalence of CARD as compared to controls, and severe disease was more frequent in the high-risk group of patients, especially those with high levels of hs-CRP. Presence of diabetic retinopathy (DR) in T2DM patients without manifest CVD is also reported to be associated with higher atherosclerotic plaque burden in the carotid arteries. In a study of 312 patients with T2DM, the percentage of carotid plaques (68% vs. 52.2%, $p = 0.004$), and prevalence of greater than or equal to 2 carotid plaques (44.4% vs. 21.4%; $p < 0.0001$) was significantly higher in diabetics with DR as compared to those without DR.[25] Interestingly, no differences in cIMT (measured at various carotid regions), was reported between the two groups. By multivariate logistic regression, DR was independently associated with the presence of carotid plaques ($p = 0.0366$) and carotid plaque burden (≥2 plaques; $p < 0.0001$).

CAROTID INTERVENTION IN DIABETICS

Carotid plaque predominantly occurs at sites of non-laminar turbulent flow, such as the carotid bulb and the proximal ICA, but rarely in the CCA, except in advanced atherosclerotic disease. The bifurcation point of the CCA, or carotid bulb, is predisposed to the development of atherosclerosis owing to low wall shear stress and resulting flow stagnation.

Carotid Endarterectomy

Carotid endarterectomy (CEA) represents the gold standard for the treatment of extracranial carotid disease, especially when performed with low perioperative morbidity and mortality rates at high volume centers with good operator experience. Presence of DM has been suggested as an adverse marker of higher operative risk during carotid artery revascularization whereas other studies have reported conflicting results. The increased risk in diabetics is thought to be primarily due to higher perioperative mortality secondary to cardiac causes (silent myocardial ischemia) or unstable carotid plaque (with associated perioperative neurological complications).

Studies of Carotid Endarterectomy Reporting Inferior Outcomes in Diabetics vs. Nondiabetics

Axelrod et al. studied the impact of DM on perioperative outcomes and length of stay in patients undergoing all types of major vascular surgery [including carotid endarterectomy ($n = 5522$)].[26] *Patients with DM on treatment with insulin were at increased risk* for CV complications (OR = 1.48) although this was not associated with increased risk for death. Data from the Ontario Carotid Endarterectomy Registry ($n = 6038$ CEAs) was analyzed for predictors of 30-day death or stroke rate after surgery.[27] A history of transient ischemic attack or stroke (OR = 1.75), atrial fibrillation (OR = 1.89), contralateral carotid occlusion (OR = 1.72), congestive heart failure (OR = 1.80), and *diabetes (OR = 1.28) were significant independent predictors for 30-day death or stroke.* The prospective National Surgical Quality Improvement Program database used multivariate models to identify risk factors associated with the composite (stroke, death, or cardiac event) endpoint from 13622 CEA procedures.[28] Associated adverse factors included deciles of age (OR = 1.13, $p = 0.018$), *insulin-requiring diabetes (OR = 1.73, p = <0.001), oral agent-controlled diabetes (OR = 1.39, p = 0.003),* decade of pack-years smoking (OR = 1.04, $p < 0.001$), history of transient ischemic attack (OR = 1.41, $p < 0.001$), history of stroke (OR = 1.51, $p < 0.001$), creatinine > 1.5 mg/dL (OR = 1.48, $p < 0.001$), and hypoalbuminemia (OR = 1.49, $p < 0.001$). Halm et al. analyzed predictors of death or stroke in 9308 carotid endarterectomies at 30 days.[29] These included: age greater than or equal to 80 years (OR = 1.30), previous history of stroke/transient ischemic attack (TIA) (OR = 1.40), TIA as an indication for surgery (OR = 1.81), stroke as an indication (OR = 2.40), crescendo TIA/stroke-in-evolution (OR = 3.61), contralateral carotid stenosis greater than or equal to 50% (OR = 1.44), CAD (OR = 1.51), and *diabetes on insulin (OR = 1.55).* Dorigo et al. (2011) analyzed the results of CEA in 3,573 patients (total of 4,305 consecutive CEAs performed, diabetic patients: 883, 20.5% and nondiabetics: 3,422, 79.5%).[30] Diabetic patients were more likely to be females and have CAD, peripheral vascular disease, dyslipidemia, and hypertension. The two groups had similar neurological outcomes, while the *mortality rate was 3.5 times higher in those with DM. The combined 30-day stroke and death rate were also significantly higher in diabetics (2% vs. 0.9%, p = 0.006, OR = 2.2).* Performing CEA under general anesthesia with somatosensory-evoked potentials (SEPs) monitoring increased the perioperative risk of stroke and death in diabetic patients (OR = 5.9; $p = 0.01$). At follow-up (mean 40 months, range 1–166 months), there was no difference between the two groups in estimated 7-year survival (87.3 and 88.8%) and stroke-free survival (86.8 and 88.1%). The restenosis-free survival rate at 7 years was significantly lesser in diabetics (77.4 and 82.2%, $p = 0.05$). The authors concluded that though the perioperative stroke rates were similar with CEA, *diabetics undergoing intervention under general anesthesia represent a subgroup with higher perioperative risk,* suggesting the need for neurologic monitoring in them, whenever possible. Data analyzing medical management of DM has suggested an *increased operative risk for those on insulin.*[26-29] The need for insulin might be associated with more than 7-fold increased risks of perioperative stroke and deaths after CEA: 6.5% vs. 1.7% in patients with and without insulin, respectively (OR = 7.55; 95% CI, 2.50–22.87; $p < 0.0001$, multivariate analysis).[31] This may suggest that a more advanced diabetic disease, or a different metabolic status requiring more aggressive glycemic control in diabetic patients requiring insulin could lead to higher ischemic events and mortality.

Studies of CEA Reporting Similar Outcomes in Diabetics and Nondiabetics

Amongst 781 carotid endarterectomies (734 patients), of whom, 181 were diabetics, Pistolese et al. reported that surgery was characterized by significantly longer carotid arteriotomies ($p = 0.03$) and clamp times ($p < 0.003$).[32] *Operative mortality (1.5% vs. 0.5%) and stroke rates (1.5% vs. 0.5%) were not significantly different.* Long-term survival (5 years) was also similar among the two groups. The study concluded that DM did not increase the surgical risk for CEA. Rockman et al. performed a retrospective review of 2151 CEAs ($n = 507$, 23.6%).[33] *Diabetic patients had similar perioperative outcomes compared with non-diabetics,* including perioperative myocardial infarction (MI) (0.6% vs. 0.4%, p = NS), perioperative death (0.8% vs. 0.5%, p = NS), and perioperative neurologic events such as transient ischemic attack and stroke (3.2% vs. 2.4%, p = NS). History of smoking, use of general anesthesia or shunt, and the lack of clamp tolerance while under regional anesthesia predicted adverse perioperative neurologic outcome, while contralateral occlusion was associated with increased perioperative mortality.

Carotid Artery Stenting

Carotid artery stenting is now endorsed by international guidelines as a valid alternative to CEA for treatment of carotid stenosis in subgroups of patients less suitable or at higher risks for CEA.[34]

Gurm et al. analyzed the short-term outcomes (30-day incidence of stroke, MI, and death) in 833 patients (n = 311 with diabetes) who underwent CAS.[35] There was no difference in the incidence of stroke (1.9% versus 2.7%,), MI (2.6% versus 1.9%), death (3.9% versus 2.5%), or the composite of death stroke or MI (6.8% versus 5.9%) at 30 days between diabetics and nondiabetics. No difference in outcomes was observed whether or not an emboli protection device was used. Despite the fact that diabetics undergoing CAS were more likely to have associated comorbidities, short term outcomes after CAS were similar to that of nondiabetics.

Siewiorek et al., analyzed the clinical variables and 30-day outcomes in 203 CAS procedures and reported that diabetes (OR = 2.8; p = 0.04) and prior CEA (OR = 1.8; p = 0.03) were significantly associated with adverse outcome (increased combined rate of stroke, TIA, and death within 30 days).[36] Probably, the inclusion of minor neurologic complications (like TIA) might have influenced the combined outcomes since the individual rates of stroke alone (p = 0.28) or mortality alone (p = 0.41) were not significantly higher in diabetic patients.

Data from the pooled analysis of outcomes from International Carotid Stenting Study [ICSS], Endarterectomy Versus Angioplasty in Patients with Symptomatic Severe Carotid Stenosis [EVA-3S], Stent-Protected Angioplasty versus Carotid Endarterectomy [SPACE]) comparing CAS vs. CEA in 3,454 symptomatic patients, revealed that CAS was associated with increased perioperative risk only in the nondiabetics (OR = 1.67) and not in diabetics (OR = 1.21).[37] The cumulative stroke and death rate in diabetics vs. non-diabetics within 120 days were 9.8% vs. 8.5% in the CAS group and 8.0% vs. 5.1% in the CEA group, respectively. Parlani et al. investigated early and 6-year outcomes of diabetic patients undergoing carotid revascularization with CAS and CEA (n = 2,196 procedures, 1,116 CEA, and 1080 CAS).[31] Diabetes was prevalent in 630 (28.7%). The perioperative stroke/death rate was 2.7% vs. 2.3%, p = NS in diabetics vs. nondiabetics [3.4% in diabetic CEA group vs. 2.1% in diabetic CAS group, p = NS]. At multivariate analyzes, diabetes was a significant predictor of perioperative stroke/death in the CEA group (OR = 2.83, p = 0.04) but not in the CAS group (p = NS). The 6-year survival (76% vs. 80.8%, p = NS), stroke estimates (3.2% vs. 4.6%, p = NS), and risk of restenosis (4.6% vs. 4.2%, p = NS) were similar in diabetic and nondiabetic patients. Survival, late stroke, and restenosis rates between diabetics and nondiabetics were also similar in CAS and CEA groups. The authors concluded that diabetic patients are not at greater risk of perioperative morbidity and mortality or late stroke after CAS, although the perioperative risk may be slightly higher after CEA. Therefore, it is important to select the appropriate technique for carotid revascularization in patients who are best suited for the type of procedure (whether CEA or CAS). *Restenosis after CAS*: Diabetics have accelerated neointimal hyperplasia and faster development of neo-plaques at the site of arterial injury, therefore, theoretically leading to increased risk of restenosis risk after revascularization. However, clinical data shows that diabetic patients have similar restenosis rates compared with non-diabetics irrespective of the revascularization strategy.[38-40]

META-ANALYSIS

Hussain et al. conducted a systematic analysis of various studies comparing clinical outcomes of diabetic vs. nondiabetic patients undergoing CEA or CAS.[41] Of the 14 observational studies (n = 16,264 patients), while CEA was used in 10 studies, 3 studies reported on the results of CAS, and 1 study used both CEA and CAS. The authors reported that carotid revascularization in diabetic patients was associated with a higher risk of perioperative stroke (OR = 1.38; 95% CI, 1.02–1.88; p = 0.04), death (OR = 1.94; 95% CI, 1.36–2.75; p = 0.0002), composite risk of stroke or death (OR = 1.80; 95% CI, 1.32–2.47; p = 0.0002), and long-term risk of death (OR = 1.57; 95% CI, 1.22–2.03; p = 0.0005). No association was found between diabetes and perioperative risk of MI; composite risk of MI, stroke, or death; and long-term risk of stroke. The study concluded that future studies should focus on evaluating which mode of revascularization (CEA or CAS) is more effective in diabetic patients with carotid artery stenosis.

CONCLUSION

Presence of DM confers an increased risk of occurrence of stroke with worse functional outcomes and higher mortality as compared to nondiabetics. Many studies have suggested an increased perioperative risk of stroke and death during CEA in the diabetic patient population. Hence, it is thought that the benefit of the procedure in stroke prevention might be marginally decreased in this subgroup of patients with carotid stenosis. Perhaps this is related to the more diffuse intracranial small vessel disease and the lower clamping tolerance to ischemia, higher risk of general anesthesia and worse response to surgical stress in diabetics. However, after the immediate perioperative period, the rate of stroke is 4–5% at 5–6 years with both procedures, confirming that the efficacy of carotid revascularization in stroke prevention may persist in the long-term also in diabetic settings. Therefore, long-term stroke prevention may be achieved even in diabetes by optimal carotid revascularization, despite the fact that DM may be considered an important risk factor during the perioperative period for patients undergoing CEA. It also needs to be remembered that even in the presence of DM, the perioperative risk remains well below the limits recommended by published guidelines, confirming the feasibility and safety of CEA in diabetic patients. Due to the proportionally higher surgical risks of CEA in diabetics, more studies are needed to identify subgroups of patients better suited for CAS than for CEA.

REFERENCES

1. Rosenson RS, Fioretto P, Dodson PM. Does microvascular disease predict macrovascular events in type 2 diabetes? Atherosclerosis. 2011;218(1):13-8.
2. Stegmayr B, Asplund K. Diabetes as a risk factor for stroke. A population perspective. Diabetologia. 1995;38(9):1061-8.
3. Tuomilheto J, Rastentye D, Jousilahti P, et al. Diabetes mellitus as a risk factor for death from stroke. Prospective study of the middle-aged Finnish population. Stroke. 1996;27(2):210-5.
4. Bond R, Rerkasem K, Rothwell PM. Systematic review of the risks of carotid endarterectomy in relation to the clinical indication for and timing of surgery. Stroke. 2003;34(9):2290-301.
5. Tuomilehto J, Rastenyte D, Jousilahti P, et al. Diabetes mellitus as a risk factor for death from stroke. Prospective study of the middle-aged Finnish population. Stroke. 1996;27(2):210-5.
6. De Angelis M, Scrucca L, Leandri M, et al. Prevalence of carotid stenosis in type 2 diabetic patients asymptomatic for cerebrovascular disease. Diabetes Nutr Metab. 2003;16(1);48-55.
7. Lacroix P, Aboyyans V, Criqui MH, et al. Type-2 diabetes and carotid stenosis: a proposal for a screening strategy in asymptomatic patients. Vasc Med. 2006;11(2):93-9.
8. Bernard S, Sérusclat A, Targe F, et al. Incremental predictive value of carotid ultrasonography in the assessment of coronary risk in a cohort of asymptomatic type 2 diabetic subjects. Diabetes Care. 2005;28(5):1158-62.
9. Lau KK, Wong YK, Chan YH, et al. Prognostic implications of surrogate markers of atherosclerosis in low to intermediate risk patients with type 2 diabetes. Cardiovasc Diabetol. 2012;11:101.
10. Roh YN, Woo SY, Kim N, et al. Prevalence of asymptomatic carotid stenosis in Korea, based on health screening population. J Korean Med Sci. 2011;26(9):1173-7.
11. De Angelis M, Scrucca L, Leandri M, et al. Prevalence of carotid stenosis in type 2 diabetic patients asymptomatic for cerebrovascular disease. Diabetes Nutr Metab. 2003;16(1):48-55.
12. Fabris F, Zanocchi M, Bo M, et al. Carotid plaque, aging, and risk factors. A study of 457 subjects. Stroke. 1994;25(6):1133-40.
13. Haffner SM, Agostino RD Jr., Saad MF, et al. Carotid artery atherosclerosis in type-2 diabetic and nondiabetic subjects with and without symptomatic coronary artery disease (The Insulin Resistance Atherosclerosis Study). Am J Cardiol. 2000;85(12):1395-400.
14. Göksan B, Erkol G, Bozluolcay M, et al. Diabetes as a determinant of high-grade carotid artery stenosis: Evaluation of 1,058 cases by Doppler sonography. J Stroke Cerebrovasc Dis. 2001;10(6):252-6.
15. Bosevski M, Lazarova-Trajkovska E. Carotid artery disease in patients with type 2 diabetes. Angiol Sosud Khir. 2015;21(3):17-26.
16. Kaul S, Alladi S, Mridula KR, et al. Prevalence and risk factors of asymptomatic carotid artery stenosis in Indian population: An 8-year follow-up study. Neurol India. 2017;65(2):279-85.
17. Noh M, Kwon H, Jung CH, et al. Impact of diabetes duration and degree of carotid artery stenosis on major adverse cardiovascular events: a single-center, retrospective, observational cohort study. Cardiovasc Diabetol. 2017;16(1):74.
18. Go AS, Hylek EM, Phillips KA, et al. Prevalence of diagnosed atrial fibrillation in adults: national implications for rhythm management and stroke prevention: the Anticoagulation and Risk Factors in Atrial Fibrillation (ATRIA) Study. JAMA. 2001;285(18):2370-75.
19. Lernfelt B, Forsberg M, Blomstrand C, et al. Cerebral atherosclerosis as predictor of stroke and mortality in representative elderly population. Stroke. 2002;33:224-9.
20. Hillen T, Nieczaj R, Munzberg H, et al. Carotid atherosclerosis, vascular risk profile and mortality in a population-based sample of functionally healthy elderly subjects: the Berlin ageing study. J Intern Med. 2000;247(6):679-88.
21. Mohan V, Ravikumar R, Shenathi Rani S, et al. Intimal medial thickness of the carotid artery in South Indian diabetic and non-diabetic subjects: the Chennai Urban Population Study (CUPS). Diabetologia. 2000;43(4);494-9.
22. Choi SW, Kim HY, Lee YH, et al. eGFR is associated with subclinical atherosclerosis independent of albuminuria: the Dong-gu Study. Atherosclerosis. 2010;212(2):661-7.
23. Betriu A, Martinez-Alonso M, Arcidiacono MV, et al. Prevalence of subclinical atheromatosis and associated risk factors in chronic kidney disease: the NEFRONA study. Nephrol Dial Transplant. 2014;29(7):1415-22.
24. Casoinic F, Baston D, Sampelean D, et al. Symptomatic and asymptomatic significant carotid artery disease in type 2 diabetes patients with nonalcoholic steatohepatitis. Hum Vet Med. 2015; 7(4):341-5.
25. Alonso N, Traveset A, Rubinat E, et al. Type 2 diabetes-associated carotid plaque burden is increased in patients with retinopathy compared to those without retinopathy. Cardiovasc Diabetol. 2015;14:33.
26. Axelrod DA, Upchurch GR Jr., DeMonner S, et al. Perioperative cardiovascular risk stratification of patients with diabetes who undergo elective major vascular surgery. J Vasc Surg. 2002;35(5):894-901.
27. Tu JV, Wang H, Bowyer B, et al. Risk factors for death or stroke after carotid endarterectomy: observations from the Ontario Carotid Endarterectomy Registry. Stroke. 2003;34(11):2568-73.
28. Stoner MC, Abbott WM, Wong DR, et al. Defining the high-risk patient for carotid endarterectomy: an analysis of the prospective National Surgical Quality Improvement Program database. J Vasc Surg. 2006;43(2):285-96.
29. Halm EA, Tuhrim S, Wang JJ, et al. Risk factors for perioperative death and stroke after carotid endarterectomy: results of the New York carotid artery surgery study. Stroke. 2009;40(1): 221-9.
30. Dorigo W, Pulli R, Pratesi G, et al. Early and long-term results of carotid endarterectomy in diabetic patients. J Vasc Surg. 2011;53(1):44-52.
31. Parlani G, De Rango P, Cieri E, et al. Diabetes is not a predictor of outcome for carotid revascularization with stenting as it may be for carotid endarterectomy. J Vasc Surg. 2012;55(1): 79-89.
32. Pistolese GR, Appolloni A, Ronchey S, et al. Carotid endarterectomy in diabetic patients. J Vasc Surg. 2001;33(1):148-54.
33. Rockman CB, Saltzberg SS, Maldonado TS, et al. The safety of carotid endarterectomy in diabetic patients: clinical predictors of adverse outcome. J Vasc Surg. 2005;42(5):v878-83.
34. Brott TG, Halperin JL, Abbara S, et al. ASA/ACCF/AHA/AANN/ AANS/ACR/ASNR/CNS/ SAIP/SCAI/SIR/SNIS/SVM/SVS Guideline

on the Management of Patients with Extracranial Carotid and Vertebral Artery Disease. J Am Coll Cardiol. 2011;2011:1002-44.

35. Gurm HS, Rajagopal V, Sachar R, et al. Impact of Diabetes Mellitus on Outcome of Patients Undergoing Carotid Artery Stenting: Insights From a Single Center Registry. Catheter Cardiovasc Interv. 2007;69(4):541-5.

36. Siewiorek GM, Krafty RT, Wholey MH, et al. The association of clinical variables and filter design with carotid artery stenting thirty-day outcome. Eur J Vasc Endovasc Surg. 2011;42(3):282-91.

37. Carotid Stenting Trialists' Collaboration. Bonati LH, Dobson J, et al. Short-term outcome after stenting versus endarterectomy for symptomatic carotid stenosis: a preplanned meta-analysis of individual patient data. Lancet. 2010;376(9746):1062-73.

38. Paraskevas KI, Baker DM, Pompella A, et al. Does diabetes mellitus play a role in restenosis and patency rates following lower extremity peripheral arterial revascularization? A critical overview. Ann Vasc Surg. 2008;22(3):481-91.

39. Goodney PP, Nolan BW, Eldrup-Jorgensen J, et al. Restenosis after carotid endarterectomy in a multicenter regional registry. J Vasc Surg. 2010;52(4):897-904, 905.e1-2

40. Cosottini M, Michelassi MC, Bencivelli W, et al. In stent restenosis predictors after carotid artery stenting. Stroke Res Treat. 2010;2010:864724.

41. Hussain MA, Bin-Ayeed SA, Saeed OQ, et al. Impact of diabetes on carotid artery revascularization. J Vasc Surg. 2016;63(4): 1099-107.e4.

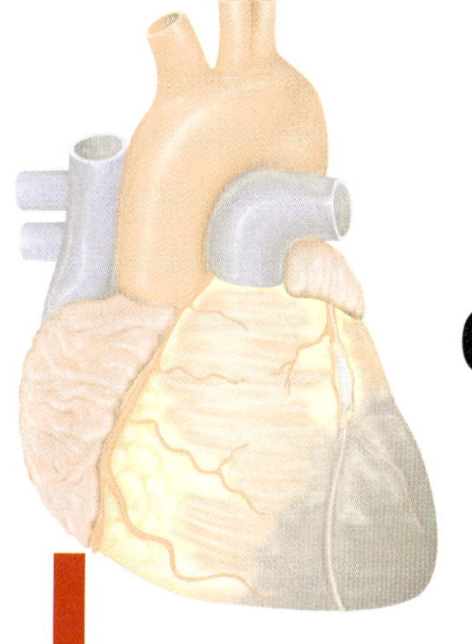

Coronary Revascularization in Diabetics

Brian Pinto, Neeraj Desai, Kunal Sinkar, Dinesh Parikh

INTRODUCTION

Cardiovascular disease is the leading cause of morbidity and mortality in people with diabetes mellitus. Patients with diabetes mellitus have a two- to four-fold increase in risk of developing cardiovascular disease than those without diabetes mellitus, and also a two- to five-fold increase in mortality attributable to cardiovascular disease when compared with age- and sex-matched nondiabetic persons.[1] Diabetic patients currently comprise approximately one-quarter of patients referred for PCI.[2,3] Diabetic patients experience worse outcomes than nondiabetic patients undergoing either coronary artery bypass grafting (CABG) or PCI. There are several pathophysiological features of atherosclerosis (Box 1) in diabetic patients that contribute to their poorer prognosis and unique response to coronary revascularization.

Diabetes mellitus (DM) has been associated with accelerated atherosclerosis due to a number of factors, such as endothelial dysfunction,[4] decreased coronary flow reserve,[5] increased platelet activity[6-8] increased levels of fibrinogen and factor VII[9] decreased fibrinolytic activity and of antithrombin III[9] and increased levels of plasminogen activator inhibitor 1.[10] Morphologic characterization of the coronary arteries of diabetic patients who died suddenly, has found a greater burden of atherosclerotic plaque, increased lipid cores, as well as increased macrophage and T-lymphocyte infiltration when compared to nondiabetics with sudden death.[11]

In asymptomatic diabetics, significant coronary artery obstructions have been found in over 75% of the patients, and multivessel involvement in over 50%.[11,12] Moreover, DM is associated with a higher prevalence of left main coronary artery disease but less collateral circulation.[13,14] Coronary lesions in diabetics are generally more calcified than in nondiabetics,[14] and compensatory arterial remodeling is often inadequate.[15] All of the former contribute to the peculiar angiographic aspects of DM (diffuse and often distal atherosclerotic involvement of coronary arteries), to the increased risk of adverse coronary events and of incomplete coronary revascularization, either surgical or percutaneous.[16-20] The presence of diabetic nephropathy identifies a subgroup of patients with reduced survival after

BOX 1: Pathophysiological features of atherosclerosis in diabetes conferring high risk

- Metabolic abnormalities
  - Hyperinsulinemia and insulin resistance
  - Hyperglycemia
  - Increased prevalence of small, dense, low-density lipoprotein and triglyceride-rich lipoproteins
  - Increased advanced glycation end-product formation
  - Increased oxidative stress and enhanced lipoprotein susceptibility to oxidation
- Endothelial dysfunction
- Hematological abnormalities
  - Abnormal platelet function
  - Abnormal coagulation system
    - Increased plasma fibrinogen
  - Impaired fibrinolytic system
    - Increased plasminogen activator inhibitor-1
- Impaired ability to form collaterals
- Higher prevalence of obesity, hypertension and dyslipidemia

coronary artery bypass.[21] Moreover, after bypass surgery, vascular grafts (especially venous) occlude more frequently in diabetics than in nondiabetics.[22,23]

In coronary artery disease (CAD), atherosclerotic plaques can cause damage either with progressive evolution of the plaque volume leading to the narrowing of the lumen of the coronary arteries with subsequent ischemia, or with an unstable fissured plaque triggering local thrombosis, leading to an acute coronary syndrome.

Primary and secondary prevention of CAD remain unmet therapeutic challenges in diabetic patients. Drug management of CAD has evolved similarly for diabetic and nondiabetic patients, although the risk of complications and the long-term prognosis differ (Box 2).

The presence of symptoms (typical angina or equivalents) in patients with type 2 diabetes mellitus has been associated with worse outcomes than in nondiabetic patients because it may indicate severe CAD. Silent myocardial ischemia discovered through resting ECG abnormalities, wall motion abnormalities in echocardiography, screening ischemic stress test, or *fractional flow reserve* **(FFR)** during coronary angiography, is more frequent in diabetic patients than nondiabetic patients and is associated with a worse prognosis. The management of CAD ranges from optimal medical therapy (OMT) to coronary revascularization with percutaneous coronary intervention (PCI) or coronary artery bypass graft (CABG) surgery (Fig. 1).

BOX 2: Characteristics of diabetic patients with coronary artery disease compared with nondiabetic patients

- More frequent asymptomatic ischemic disease or silent ischemia attributable to diabetic neuropathy which appears early in the development of diabetes
- More severe coronary artery lesions that are often multiple, with extensive and diffuse lesions attributable to accelerated atherogenesis
- Increased platelet reactivity and decreased platelet inhibition in response to antiplatelet agents used for primary or secondary prevention
- More severe acute coronary syndrome with higher risk of mortality after a myocardial infarction, regardless of the treatment
- Higher rate of in-stent restenosis and stent thrombosis
- More frequent comorbidities (renal insufficiency, other localization of atherosclerotic disease), leading to higher surgical risk when considering surgical coronary revascularization.

COMPARING MEDICAL THERAPY TO REVASCULARIZATION IN STABLE CAD

Until recently, little if any, data were available on revascularization vs. medical management in DM patients with stable CAD.[24] The Bypass Angioplasty Revascularization Investigation (BARI) 2D trial randomly assigned 2368 DM

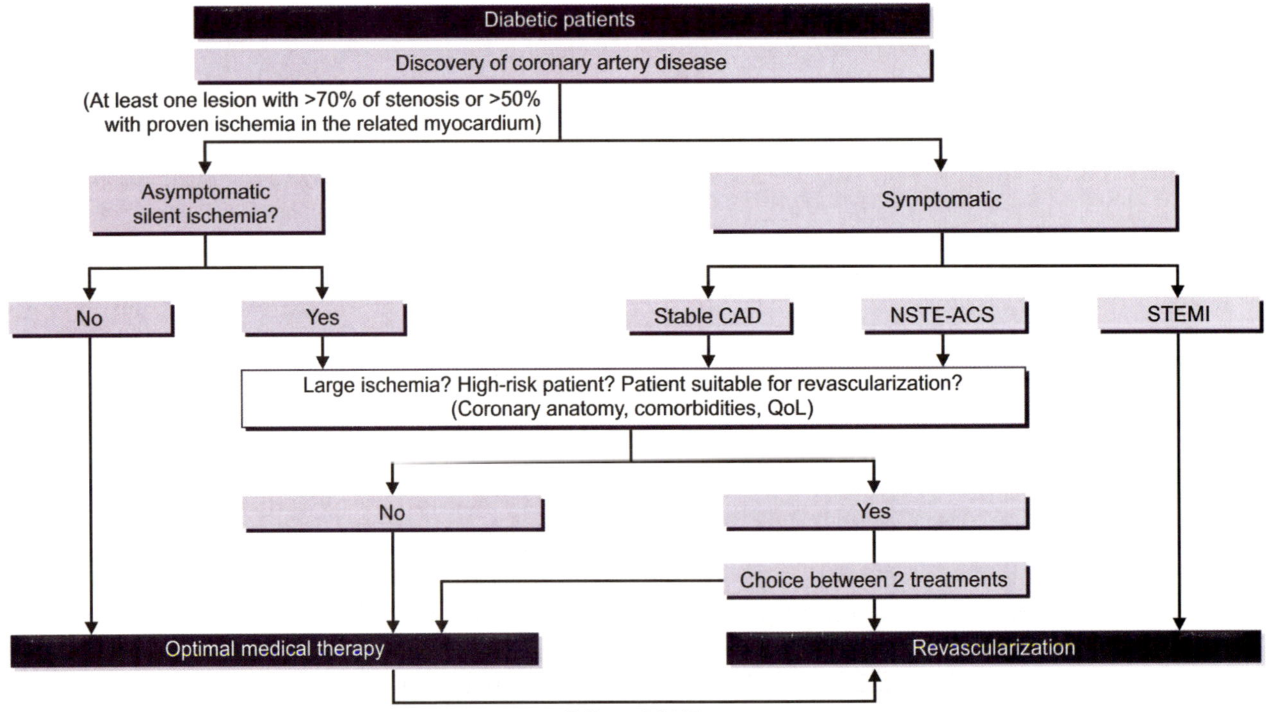

Fig. 1: Management of coronary artery disease under optimal medical therapy (OMT)

Abbreviations: CAD, coronary artery disease; OMT, optimal medical therapy; STEMI, ST-elevation myocardial infarction; NSTE-ACS, non-ST elevation acute coronary syndrome; QoL, quality of life

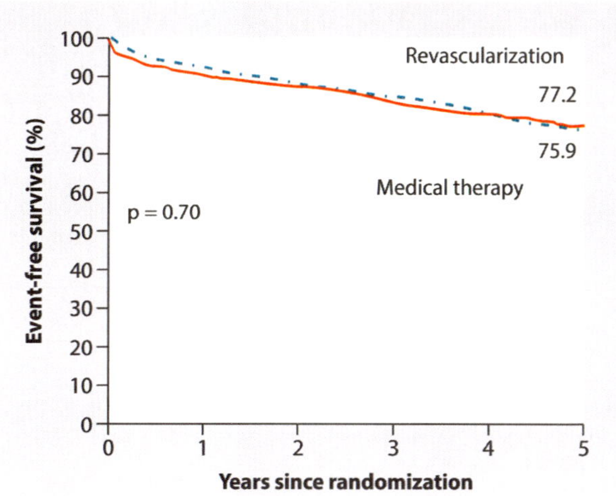

Fig. 2: Medical therapy vs revascularization

patients with stable CAD to either prompt revascularization with intensive medical therapy or intensive medical therapy alone.[25] Primary endpoints were the 5-year rate of death and of MACE defined as a composite of death, MI, or stroke. Randomization was stratified according to the choice of PCI or CABG as the more appropriate intervention. Survival as well as MACE did not differ between the two groups (Fig. 2). At 5 years, 42% of patients randomized in the conservative arm crossed over to revascularization. With respect to subgroups, while in the PCI stratum there was no significant difference in the primary endpoints between the revascularization group and the medical therapy group, in the CABG stratum the MACE rate was significantly lower in the revascularization group (22.4%) than in the medical therapy group (30.5%, p = 0.01; p = 0.002 for interaction between stratum and study group).[25] Importantly, the CABG stratum included patients with a higher risk profile. Therefore, no conclusion should be drawn on the efficacy of PCI versus CABG based on those results. Overall, the BARI 2D trial shows that in DM patients with stable CAD and no high-risk features on coronary angiography medical therapy may be a valuable initial strategy.

PCI VS CABG

In the absence of multivessel disease or a lesion involving the left main, PCI is a simple and efficient technique to revascularize one vessel. As soon as the left main artery or 2 major epicardial vessels are involved, especially the LAD, discussion for the technique of revascularization must occur. The benefit of off-pump CABG in diabetics is still debated.[26]The failure of PCI to show superiority over CABG in multivessel disease was initially attributed to the use of bare-metal stents, inadequate antiplatelet therapy to prevent stent thrombosis, and absence of optimal OMT for secondary prevention. The Synergy between PCI with Taxus and Cardiac Surgery (SYNTAX) trial (n = 1800) comparing PCI with the first generation of drug (paclitaxel), eluting stent (DES) with CABG for treating patients with previously untreated 3-vessel or left main coronary artery disease (or both) concluded that CABG was the best option for patients with 3-vessel with or without associated left main CAD.[27] In the 452 diabetic patients of the SYNTAX trial, the 1-year major adverse cardiac and cerebrovascular event rate was higher with PCI-DES than with CABG, a difference driven by an increase in repeat revascularization that reached 20.3% in diabetic PCI patients versus 6.4% in diabetic CABG patients (p < 0.001). Moreover, mortality in diabetic patients was higher in the PCI arm when compared with CABG (13.5% versus 4.1%, p = 0.04).[28] In the more recently published Future Revascularization Evaluation in Patients with Diabetes Mellitus: Optimal Management of Multivessel Disease (FREEDOM) trial, 1900 diabetic patients with multivessel disease eligible for both revascularization techniques were randomized to PCI with DES (paclitaxel and sirolimus) versus CABG.[29] The primary endpoint of all-cause mortality, nonfatal MI, or stroke over a mean 3.8 years follow-up favored CABG, with 18.7% of events at 5 years with CABG versus 26.6% with PCI (p = 0.005). All-cause mortality was lower with CABG at 5 years (10.3% versus 16.3% p = 0.049). Repeat revascularization (13% versus 5% p < 0.001) and nonfatal MI (13.9% versus 6.0% p < 0.001) were higher with PCI. PCI had a lower rate of stroke (2.4% versus 5.2% p < 0.001). These results from SYNTAX and FREEDOM are compelling in favor of CABG for patients with triple, vessel disease (only 15% had 2-vessel disease in FREEDOM). The only subgroup of patients in whom PCI seems to do equally well with PCI, albeit with a higher rate of repeat revascularization, is the group with left main disease when isolated or with 1-vessel disease (Table 1).[30]

The EXCEL trial (Evaluation of XIENCE versus Coronary Artery Bypass Surgery for Effectiveness of Left Main Revascularization) enrolled 1,905 patients with significant left main disease eligible for both PCI or CABG who had low or intermediate SYNTAX scores (<32) and randomized 948 patients to PCI using second-generation drug-eluting stents and 957 patients to CABG.[31] The primary endpoint of the study was the combined endpoint of death from any cause, stroke, or MI at 3 years. Secondary endpoints were the combined endpoint at 30 days and the combined endpoint plus target vessel revascularization (TVR) at 3 years. The primary endpoint was achieved in 15.4% of PCI patients and 14.7% of CABG patients, achieving statistical noninferiority of PCI. The prespecified secondary endpoint

TABLE 1: Diabetic patients with coronary artery disease need revascularization

Diabetic patient with CAD and needing revascularization	
Single or two-vessel disease, (nonproximal LAD, non-left main)	PCI preferred
High surgical risk (comorbidities)	
Contraindication to surgery	
Elderly patients (> 80 years old) or frailty	
MV disease	CABG preferred
Proximal LAD	
Left main involved	
In-stent restenosis (with DES in major arteries)	

Abbreviations: CAD, coronary artery disease; LAD, left anterior descending; DES, drug-eluting stent; PCI, percutaneous coronary intervention; CABG, Coronary artery bypass grafting

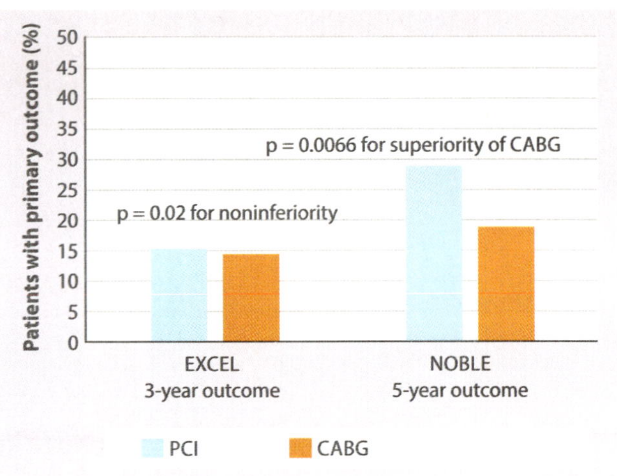

Fig. 3: PCIs CABG for left main artery

Abbreviations: EXCEL, Evaluation of XIENCE versus coronary artery bypass surgery for effectiveness of left main revascularization; NOBLE, Nordic-Baltic-British left main revascularization study; CABG, coronary artery bypass grafting; PCI, percutaneous coronary intervention

of the combined endpoint at 30 days was lower in the PCI group (4.9% for PCI vs 7.9% for CABG). The 3-year combined endpoint (including TVR) again showed noninferiority for PCI (23.1% for PCI vs 19.1% for CABG). Ischemia-driven revascularization was more common during follow-up for PCI patients (12.6% for PCI vs 7.5% for CABG).

The EXCEL trial consisted primarily of patients with preserved ejection fraction. Of those patients, 60% had stable syndromes, and 30% were diabetic. The majority (80.5%) had disease involving the distal bifurcation. The site-designated average SYNTAX score was 20; 60.5% had low scores (<22), and 39.5% had intermediate scores (23–32). However, by core laboratory analysis, the average score was higher (26.5), fewer had low scores (35.8%), and 24.2% had scores greater than 33, which should have been excluded. Little data were provided regarding technical aspects of PCI such as use of support devices, bifurcation strategy, or need for rotational atherectomy. An average of 1.9 lesions were treated per patient. The procedure was guided by intravascular ultrasound in 77% of cases. The study did not report on the rate of complete revascularization achieved.

NOBLE (Nordic-Baltic-British Left Main Revascularization Study) enrolled 1,201 patients with left main disease and no more than 3 additional noncomplex lesions (defined as chronic total occlusions, bifurcations requiring 2-stent strategies, or extensive coronary calcification or tortuosity); the SYNTAX score was not used.[32] Of those patients, 598 were randomized to PCI and 603 to CABG. The primary study endpoint was a combined endpoint of all-cause mortality, nonprocedure related MI, stroke, and repeat revascularization at 5 years. The primary endpoint was achieved in 29% of PCI patients and 19% of CABG patients, indicating statistical superiority of CABG. Regarding the individual endpoints, all-cause death was not different, but the individual rates of MI, revascularization, and stroke were each higher in PCI patients compared with CABG patients. The SYNTAX score was not related to outcomes, and even patients with low SYNTAX scores did better with CABG.

NOBLE patients had preserved ejection fraction; 82% had stable syndromes, and 15% were diabetic. Disease complexity appeared similar to EXCEL with an average SYNTAX score of 22.5 and 81% with distal left main disease. The distal bifurcation was treated using a 2-stent strategy in 35% of patients. The median number of lesions was 2.0, intravascular ultrasound was used in 74%, and complete revascularization was achieved in 92% of patients.

These two randomized trials of PCI versus CABG for left main disease are interesting in that they enrolled similar patients yet came to different conclusions. The primary endpoints for both studies are shown in Figure 3.

These two trials included very similar patients who are representative of this subset. The most important difference is that the primary endpoints differed. The EXCEL trial's primary endpoint consisted of only death, MI, and stroke at 3 years. NOBLE's primary endpoint consisted of death, MI, stroke, and revascularization at 5 years. When you add revascularization to the EXCEL trial's endpoint, that trial starts looking more like NOBLE, and the p-value for superiority of CABG approaches significance at 0.10 (Fig. 4). The rate of repeat revascularization will likely increase in the PCI group from 3 to 5 years, and it is possible that by 5 years the rates of achieving the combined endpoint that includes repeat revascularization will be similar to NOBLE.

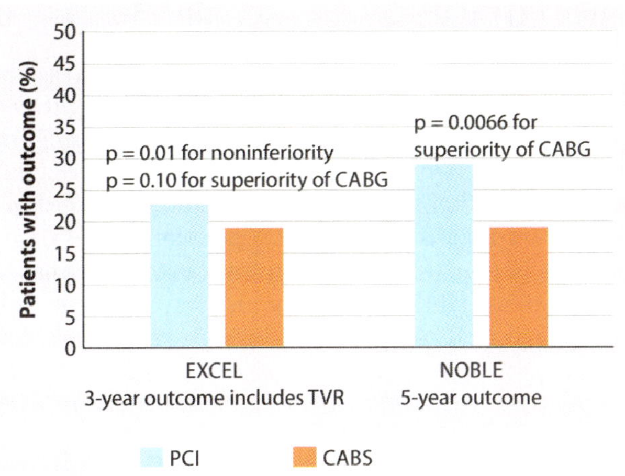

Fig. 4: EXCEL versus NOBLE trials

Abbreviations: EXCEL, evaluation of XIENCE versus coronary artery bypass surgery for effectiveness of left main revascularization; NOBLE, Nordic-Baltic-British left main revascularization study; CABG, coronary artery bypass grafting; PCI, percutaneous coronary intervention

WHICH IS BETTER?

Theoretically, coronary artery bypass grafting surgery is advantageous since grafts bypass the proximal two-thirds of the coronary arteries, where most plaque ruptures occur, generating clinical events, while PCI offers target-lesion treatment, leaving other plaques unprotected.[33] In addition, CABG also provides complete revascularization more often than PCI, what may lead to less repeat revascularization procedures and less angina during follow-up.[34] On the other side, CABG may have complications, and even those considered mild and reversible may prolong hospitalization;[35,36] the short-term risk of cerebrovascular accidents (CVA) is also increased.[37]

The Bypass Angioplasty Revascularization Investigation (BARI) Study has demonstrated that in 10 years of follow-up, diabetics patients had the highest benefit with CABG (57.9% of survival) compared to balloon PCI (45.5%). However, that was true only for patients who received internal mammary grafts in the LAD artery.[38] Other two randomized trials, ARTS[39] and SoS[40] in which bare-metal stents were used, have shown similar results, that is, diabetic patients who underwent CABG had lower 5-year mortality than those who had PCI. In the ARTS study, 5-year mortality in diabetics was 13.4% for those who underwent PCI and 8.3% for those who had CABG, while in SoS, the 6-year mortality was 17.6% for PCI and 5.4% for CABG. Also, in a substudy of 452 patients from the SYNTAX study, CABG determined a lower incidence of composite endpoints (death, AMI, CVA or repeat revascularization) compared to PCI, but there was no difference regarding the incidence of death or AMI.[41]However, even though these 4 studies suggest that CABG is the best revascularization strategy for diabetics, they were not designed to evaluate specific revascularization strategies in this patient group, and, therefore, did not have enough statistical power to draw definitive conclusions about that issue.

Recently, the Coronary Artery Revascularization in Diabetes (CARDia) study tried to address the efficacy and safety of PCI compared to CABG in diabetics with symptomatic, multivessel or complex single-vessel CAD.[42] Patients were followed for a median of 1 year; 65% of those undergoing PCI had 3-vessel CAD, and of these, 88% had complete myocardial revascularization, with pharmacologic stents in 69% of cases and a mean of 3.6 stents per patient. In the CABG group, 60% had 3-vessel CAD, 90% of whom had complete myocardial revascularization, with 94% with internal mammary grafts to the LAD artery and a mean of 2.9 grafts per patient. The primary endpoint of the study was the combination of death, nonfatal AMI or CVA, and the secondary endpoint included repeat revascularization. At 1 year, no statistically significant difference was found between treatment strategies regarding the primary endpoint, but considering the secondary endpoint a significant difference in favor of CABG was found, due to increased repeat revascularization procedures in the PCI group. Nonetheless, the short follow-up and small patients number somewhat limit the study's conclusions.

The major limitations of most of the trials especially FREEDOM, were the inclusion of only approximately 10% of the screening population due to stringent exclusion criteria. The alarming revelation to this point was that most of the excluded cohort would have made CABG a less favorable outcome. These exclusion criteria were as follows:

- Class III or IV heart failure
- Prior CABG/prior PCI
- Stroke with significant neurological involvement
- In stent restenosis
- Chronic total occlusion
- Left main disease
- STEMI/NSTEMI
- Severe comorbidities

This was confirmed on the fact that the mean EURO score for patients undergoing CABG in FREEDOM was 2.8, which was way below the mean in most registries of CABG in the real world population. The direct consequence of these various shortcomings has a significant impact on the treatment modalities for complex multivessel disease in DM as it is not up to date. The longer trials still incorporate older techniques not relevant in present scenario, and the newer shorter trials are dismissed due to the smaller sample size with reduced significance.

This leaves void in the treatment of diabetic patients who fall in the grey zone. For such patients a functional Syntax

TABLE 2: Specific recommendations for revascularization in patients with diabetes

Recommendations	*Class*[a]	*Level*[b]
In patients presenting with STEMI. Primary PCI is recommended over fibrinolysis if it can be performed within recommended time limits	I	A
In patients with NSTE-ACS, an early invasive strategy is recommended over noninvasive management	I	A
In stable patients with multivessel CAD and/or evidence of ischemia, revascularization is indicated in order to reduce cardiac adverse events	I	B
In patients with stable multivessel CAD and an acceptable surgical risk, CABG is recommended over PCI	I	A
In patients with stable multivessel CAD and SYNTAX score ≤22, PCI should be considered as alternative to CABG	IIa	B
New-generation DES are recommended over BMS	I	A

score can be of some help in stratifying risk and classifying patients to treat coronary artery disease. Functional syntax can help downgrade a patient of high syntax score to a relatively lower score depending upon the FFR of certain borderline lesions.[43] Based on various RCTs, the European society of Cardiology has set up certain recommendations for revascularization in Diabetics (Table 2).[44]

Improvements in rates of repeat revascularization and lower rates of stent thrombosis with DES have influenced physician's choice in the type of revascularization for diabetic patients. This is particularly true with the second-generation of DES using everolimus.[45] PCI is also more attractive to patients with its percutaneous approach, its lower rate of stroke, and shorter length of hospital stay. According to the results of registries and randomized studies comparing the 2 techniques and in the absence of contraindication to surgery, PCI can be envisioned in diabetic patients with single or 2-vessel disease without complex lesions, when the proximal LAD is not involved.[46,47] Patients presenting with STEMI should undergo primary PCI of the culprit lesion only and then be reconsidered once stabilized for CABG if there is multivessel disease involving the LAD. For non-ST-elevation acute coronary syndrome, the choice is more difficult. These patients can be considered like stable CAD patients in terms of revascularization. Based on the recent results of the FAME-2 trial supporting the use of FFR measurement in stable CAD,[48] FFR-guided PCI should be used more thoroughly to evaluate lesions in diabetic patients who are identified with multivessel disease.

CONCLUSION

What the future holds? An aggressive cardiovascular prevention strategy and adequate blood glucose control remain cornerstones of the management of DM patients and the decision when and how to proceed to coronary revascularization should be based on multiple parameters including clinical presentation, coronary anatomy, ischemic burden, left ventricular function, and comorbidities. All DM patients with complex multivessel CAD should be discussed within a heart team, consisting of cardiologists, cardiac surgeons, and anesthesiologists. Overall, the threshold for CABG should be lower in DM patients than in non-DM individuals. In DM patients undergoing PCI, the use of DES is recommended while in ACS, an early invasive strategy should be favored Diabetic patients with CAD are at high risk of complications, and irrespective of the chosen revascularization strategy, they continue to have poorer outcomes after revascularization compared to nondiabetics. Consequently, considerable work is still needed to better understand the specific underlying mechanisms of CAD in the setting of diabetes. Further characterization of the signaling mechanisms that link diabetes to restenosis after percutaneous intervention could lead to development of novel antirestenotic agents specific to diabetic patients. While CABG remains superior to PCI among patients with diabetes who are candidates for surgical revascularization (and particularly for those with higher angiographic disease complexity), the gap between CABG and PCI has reduced. As the prevalence of diabetes continues to rise, the development of new treatment strategies will hopefully improve the outcomes for this high-risk cohort of patients.

REFERENCES

1. American Diabetes Association. Statistics About Diabetes. [online] Available from http://www.Diabetes.Org/diabetes-basics/diabetes-statistics/. [Accessed October, 2017].
2. Van Belle E, Périé M, Braune D, et al. Effects of coronary stenting on vessel patency and long-term clinical outcome after percutaneous coronary revascularization in diabetic patients. J Am Coll Cardiol. 2002;40:410-7.
3. Kip KE, Faxon DP, Detre KM, et al. Coronary angioplasty in diabetic patients. The National Heart, Lung, and Blood Institute Percutaneous Transluminal Coronary Angioplasty Registry. Circulation. 1996;94:1818-25.
4. Aronson D, Bloomgarden Z, Rayfield EJ. Potential mechanisms promoting restenosis in diabetic patients. J Am Coll Cardiol. 1996;27:528-35.
5. Nahser PJ, Brown RE, Oskarsson H, et al. Maximal coronary flow reserve and metabolic coronary vasodilation in patients with diabetes mellitus. Circulation. 1995;91:635-40.
6. Winocour PD. Platelet abnormalities in diabetes mellitus. Diabetes. 1992;41(Suppl 2):26-31.

7. Strano A, Davi G, Patrono C. In vivo platelet activation in diabetes mellitus. (review) Semin Thromb Haemost. 1991;17:422-5.
8. Creager MA, Luscher TF, Cosentino F, et al. Diabetes and vascular disease pathophysiology, clinical consequences, and medical therapy: part I. Circulation. 2003;108(12):1527-32.
9. Ceriello A. Coagulation activation in diabetes mellitus: a role of hyperglycemia and therapeutic prospects. Diabetologia. 1993;36(11):1119-25.
10. Sobel BE, Woodcock-Mitchell J, Schneider DJ, et al. Increased plasminogen activator inhibitor type-1 in coronary artery atherectomy specimens from type-2 diabetic compared with nondiabetic patients. Circulation. 1998;97(22):2213-21.
11. Burke AP, Kolodgie FD, Zieske A, et al. Morphologic findings of coronary atherosclerotic plaques in diabetics. A postmortem study. Arterioscler Thromb Vasc Biol. 2004;24:1266-71.
12. Goraya TY, Leibson CL, Palumbo PJ, et al. Coronary atherosclerosis in diabetes mellitus. A population-based autopsy study. J Am Coll Cardiol. 2002;40(5):946-53.
13. Berry C, Tardif JC, Bourassa MG. Coronary heart disease in patients with diabetes. Part I: recents advances in prevention and non-invasive management. J Am Coll Cardiol. 2007;49(6):631-42.
14. Stone KE, Chiquette E, Chilton RJ. Diabetic endovascular disease: role of coronary artery revascularization. Am J Cardiol. 2007;99(Suppl I):105B-112B.
15. Nicholls SJ, Tuzcu M, Kalidindi S, et al. Effect of diabetes on progression of coronary atherosclerosis and arterial remodeling. A pooled analysis of 5 intravascular ultrasound trials. J Am Coll Cardiol. 2008;52:255-62.
16. Ledru F, Ducimetière P, Battaglia S, et al. New diagnostic criteria for diabetes and coronary artery disease: insights from an angiographic study. J Am Coll Cardiol. 2001;37(6):1543-50.
17. Barsness GW, Peterson ED, Ohman EM, et al. Relationship between diabetes mellitus and long-term survival after coronary bypass and angioplasty. Circulation. 1997;96:2551-6.
18. Alderman EL, Corley SD, Fisher LD, et al. Five-year angiographic follow-up of factors associated with progression of coronary artery disease in the coronary artery surgery study (CASS). CASS participating investigators and staff. J Am Coll Cardiol. 1993;22:1141-51.
19. Thourani VH, Weintraub WS, Stein B, et al. Influence of diabetes mellitus on early and late outcome after coronary artery bypass grafting. Ann Thorac Surg. 1999;67:1045-52.
20. Kip KE, Faxon DP, Detre KM, et al. Coronary angioplasty in diabetic patients. The National Heart, Lung, and Blood Institute Percutaneous Transluminal Coronary Angioplasty Registry. Circulation. 1996;94:1818-25.
21. Reeder GS, Holmes DR, Lennon RJ, et al. Proteinuria, serum creatinine, and outcome of percutaneous coronary intervention in patients with diabetes mellitus. Am J Cardiol. 2002;89:760-4.
22. Singh SK, Desai ND, Petroff SD, et al. The impact of diabetic status on coronary artery bypass graft patency. Insights from the radial artery patency study. Circulation. 2008;118:S222-5.
23. Leavitt BJ, Sheppard L, Maloney C, et al. Effect of diabetes and associated conditions on long-term survival after coronary artery bypass graft surgery. Circulation. 2004;110(Suppl I):II41-4.
24. Soares PR, Hueb WA, Lemos PA, et al. Coronary revascularization (surgical or percutaneous) decreases mortality after the first year in diabetic subjects but not in nondiabetic subjects with multivessel disease: an analysis from the Medicine, Angioplasty, or Surgery Study (MASS II). Circulation 2006;114:I420-4.
25. Frye RL, August P, Brooks MM, et al. A randomized trial of therapies for type 2 diabetes and coronary artery disease. N Engl J Med. 2009;360:2503-15.
26. Srinivasan AK, Grayson AD, Fabri BM. On-pump versus off-pump coronary artery bypass grafting in diabetic patients: a propensity score analysis. Ann Thorac Surg. 2004;78:1604-9.
27. Serruys PW, Morice MC, Kappetein AP, et al. SYNTAX investigators. Percutaneous coronary intervention versus coronary-artery bypass grafting for severe coronary artery disease. N Engl J Med. 2009;360:961-72.
28. Kappetein AP, Head SJ, Morice MC, et al. SYNTAX Investigators. Treatment of complex coronary artery disease in patients with diabetes: 5-year results comparing outcomes of bypass surgery and percutaneous coronary intervention in the SYNTAX trial. Eur J Cardiothorac Surg. 2013;43(5):1006-13.
29. Farkouh ME, Domanski M, Sleeper LA, et al. FREEDOM Trial Investigators. Strategies for multivessel revascularization in patients with diabetes. N Engl J Med. 2012;367(25):2375-84.
30. Morice MC, Serruys PW, Kappetein AP, et al. Outcomes in patients with de novo left main disease treated with either percutaneous coronary intervention using paclitaxel-eluting stents or coronary artery bypass graft treatment in the Synergy between Percutaneous Coronary Intervention with TAXUS and Cardiac Surgery (SYNTAX) trial. Circulation. 2010;121:2645-53.
31. Stone GW, Sabik JF, Serruys PW, et al. Everolimus-eluting Stents or Bypass Surgery for Left Main Coronary Artery Disease. N Eng J Med. 2016;375:2223-35.
32. Mäkikallio T, Holm NR, Lindsay M, et al. Percutaneous coronary angioplasty versus coronary artery bypass grafting in treatment of unprotected left main stenosis (NOBLE): a prospective, randomised, open-label, non-inferiority trial. Lancet. 2016;388:2743-52.
33. Gersh BJ, Frue RL. Methods of coronary revascularization-things may not be as they seem. N Engl J Med. 2005;352:2235-7.
34. Ong ATL, Serruys PW. Complete revascularization. Coronary artery bypass graft surgery versus percutaneous coronary intervention. Circulation. 2006;114:249-55.
35. Di Carlo A, Perna AM, Pantoni L, et al. Clinically relevant cognitive impairment after cardiac surgery: a 6-month follow-up study. J Neurol Sci. 2001;188:85-93.
36. Barber PA, Hach S, Tippen LJ, et al. Cerebral ischemic lesions on diffusion-weighted imaging are associated with neurocognitive decline after cardiac surgery. Stroke. 2008;39:1427-33.
37. MaKhann GM, Grega MA, Borowicz Jr LM, et al. Stroke and encephalopathy after cardiac surgery. An update. Stroke. 2006;37(2):562-71.
38. The BARI investigators. The final 10-year follow-up results from the BARI randomized trial. J Am Coll Cardiol. 2007;49:1600-6.
39. Serruys PW, Ong AT, van Herwerden LA, et al. Five-year outcomes after coronary stenting versus bypass surgery for the treatment of multivessel disease: the final analysis of the Arterial Revascularization Therapies Studies (ARTS) randomized trial. J Am Coll Cardiol. 2005;46:575-81.
40. Booth J, Clayton T, Pepper J, et al. Randomized, controlled trial of coronary artery bypass surgery versus percutaneous coronary intervention in patients with multivessel coronary artery disease. Six-year follow-up for the Stent or Surgery Trial (SOS). Circulation. 2008;118:381-8.
41. Banning AP, Wetaby S, Morice MC, et al. Diabetic and nondiabetic patients with left main and/or 3-vessel coronary artery disease: comparison of outcomes with cardiac surgery and paclitxel-eluting stents. J Am Coll Cardiol. 2010;55:1067-75.
42. Kapur A, Hall RJ, Malik IS, et al. Randomized comparison of percutaneous coronary intervention with coronary artery bypass grafting in diabetic patients. 1-year results of the CARDia (Coronary Artery Revascularization in Diabetes) trial. J Am Coll Cardiol. 2010;55:432-40.

43. Nam CW, Mangiacapra F, Entjes R, et al. Functional SYNTAX score for risk assessment in multivessel coronary artery disease. J Am CollCardiol. 2011;58(12):1211-8.
44. 2014 ESC guidelines for myocardial revascularization. Eur Heart J. 2014;35:2541-619.
45. Sabate M, Cequier A, Iñiguez A, et al. Everolimus-eluting stent versus bare-metal stent in ST-segment elevation myocardial infarction (EXAMINATION): 1-year results of a randomised controlled trial. Lancet. 2012;380:1482-90.
46. Reeves BC, Angelini GD, Bryan AJ, et al. A multi-centre randomised controlled trial of minimally invasive direct coronary bypass grafting versus percutaneous transluminal coronary angioplasty with stenting for proximal stenosis of the left anterior descending coronary artery. Health Technol Assess. 2004;8(16):1-43.
47. Jaffery Z, Kowalski M, Weaver WD, et al. A meta-analysis of randomized control trials comparing minimally invasive direct coronary bypass grafting versus percutaneous coronary intervention for stenosis of the proximal left anterior descending artery. Eur J Cardiothorac Surg. 2007;31:691-7.
48. De Bruyne B, Pijls NH, Kalesan B, et al. Fractional flow reserve-guided PCI versus medical therapy in stable coronary disease. N Engl J Med. 2012;367:991-1001.

CHAPTER

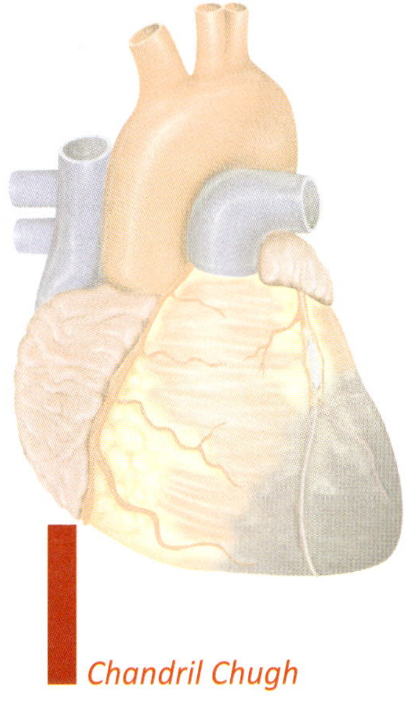

Endovascular Intervention in Stroke in Cardiodiabetes: New Frontiers

Chandril Chugh

INTRODUCTION

Stroke is defined by the World Health Organization as a clinical syndrome consisting of rapidly developing clinical signs of focal (or global in case of coma) disturbance of cerebral function lasting more than 24 hours or leading to death with no apparent cause other than a vascular origin.[1] Stroke is classified broadly into three categories: ischemic stroke, hemorrhagic stroke, and subarachnoid hemorrhage. Ischemic stroke occurs due to blockage of blood vessel which limits the blood supply to the brain whereas hemorrhagic stroke occurs due to rupture of blood vessel leading to spillage of blood in the intracranial cavity.[2] Depending on the site of blood spillage, the hemorrhagic stroke could be classified as intracerebral hemorrhage or subarachnoid hemorrhage. Approximately 60–80% of all strokes are ischemic and are more common in cardiovascular patients as well. Hence, this chapter is dedicated to acute ischemic strokes and their endovascular management.

EPIDEMIOLOGY

Stroke is the second most common cause of mortality and third most common cause of disability worldwide.[3] Globally, 68% of all strokes are ischemic and 32% are hemorrhagic.[3] Numbers from the USA differ a little with 87% of all strokes being ischemic, 10% hemorrhagic and about 3% being subarachnoid hemorrhage.[4,5] Data regarding prevalence of stroke in India is lacking, however, it can be extrapolated from the data available from the West. In a study done by Banerjee et al. in 2001 crude prevalence rate of stroke in India was 147/100,000 and the annual incidence rate was 36/100,000. Women had substantially higher age-adjusted prevalence rate (564/100,000 for women versus 196/100,000 for men) and incidence rate (204/100,000 for women versus 36/100,000 for men).[6,7] Overall prevalence of stroke ranges from 147 to 922/100,000 in various studies.[8,9] India has the highest burden of acute coronary syndrome (ACS) in the world and the three most common risk factors for ACS are smoking (40%), high blood pressure (38%), and diabetes (30%).[10] Taking account of the above mentioned data and considering the fact that stroke shares common risk factors with ACS, we can safely assume that India has a very high incidence of stroke as well.

RISK FACTORS

Majority of the ischemic strokes seen in patients with cardiovascular disease are embolic. Embolic strokes may arise directly from the heart or the aorta. Following is the list of conditions that carry a high risk for embolic strokes:[11,12]

Arrhythmias

- Atrial fibrillation and paroxysmal atrial fibrillation
- Sick sinus syndrome
- Sustained atrial flutter.

Valvular Heart Disease

- Rheumatic mitral or aortic valve disease
- Bioprosthetic and mechanical heart valves
- Fibrous nonbacterial endocarditis (i.e. Libman-Sacks endocarditis), antiphospholipid syndrome, and cancer (marantic endocarditis), systemic lupus erythematosus
- Infective endocarditis.

Thrombus and Structural Lesion

- Papillary fibroelastoma
- Left atrial myxoma
- Atrial or ventricular thrombus.

Structural Heart Disease

- Recent myocardial infarction (within one month)
- Chronic myocardial infarction together with ejection fraction < 28 %
- Congestive heart failure with ejection fraction < 30%
- Dilated cardiomyopathy.

Surgical

Coronary artery bypass graft (CABG) surgery conditions which have been associated with embolic stroke but lack definitive evidence are mitral annular calcification, patent foramen ovale, left atrial smoke on echocardiogram, atrial septal aneurysm, left ventricular aneurysm, and aortic arch atheroma.

Systemic diseases like hypertension, diabetes mellitus, hyperlipidemia and risk factors like smoking and obesity have well-established association with stroke.

CLINICAL PRESENTATION

Clinical presentation of stroke depends on the area of the brain affected by occlusion of the arteries. American Heart Association/American Stroke Association (AHA/ASA) have popularized the FAST algorithm to diagnose stroke. FAST acronym stands for Facial droop, Arm weakness, Slurred speech and Time of onset. Another easy way to remember to signs of stroke is the 6S method.

STROKE: REMEMBER THE 6S METHOD TO DIAGNOSE STROKE

1. **S**udden (symptoms usually start suddenly)
2. **S**lurred speech (speech is not clear, as if drunk)
3. **S**ide weak (face, arm or leg or all three can get weak)
4. **S**pinning (vertigo)
5. **S**evere headache
6. **S**econds (note the time when the symptoms start and rush to the hospital).

All the symptoms need not be present to diagnose stroke. Any of the above mentioned symptoms can be present and is helpful in diagnosing ischemic as well as hemorrhagic stroke.

TREATMENT

The most important factor in the treatment of acute ischemic stroke is time. Patient with ischemic stroke loses 19,00,000 brain cells every minute, about 14,000,000,000 nerve connections are destroyed every minute and 12 km (7.5 miles) of nerve fibers are lost every minute. The brain ages 3.6 years for every hour it is deprived of blood supply.[13] There are two modalities of treatment available for treatment of acute ischemic stroke. Intravenous thrombolysis and mechanical thrombectomy.

Intravenous Thrombolysis

As recommended by AHA/ASA intravenous tPA infusion is treatment modality of choice for patients presenting within first 3 hours of onset of symptoms. The treatment window can be extended to 4.5 hours for eligible patients.[14,15] Use of intravenous alteplase is based on the landmark National Institute of Neurological Disorders and Stroke (NINDS) tPA trial which showed that patients who received tPA were at least 30% more likely to have minimal or no disability at three months on the assessment scales. Outcome measures were in favor of the group that received tPA (global odds ratio for a favorable outcome, 1.7; 95% confidence interval, 1.2 to 2.6).[16]A pooled analysis of ATLANTIS, ECASS, and NINDS was published in 2004 which showed that the tPA window could be extended to 4.5 hours with reasonable benefit to the patient.[17] The European Cooperative Acute Stroke Study III (ECSASS-III) definitively established the efficacy of tPA within 3–4.5 hours window. ECASS-III showed that patients who received tPA within 3 to 4.5 hours window had a better chance to a favorable outcome with an odds ratio of 1.42 (95% CI: 1.02–1.98, $p = 0.04$).[18,19]

Intravenous tPA infusion can only be given to eligible patients and there are strict inclusion and exclusion criteria as per stroke guidelines published in 2013 (Box 1).[14]

BOX 1: Strict inclusion and exclusion criteria of intravenous tPA infusion

Inclusion criteria

- Diagnosis of ischemic stroke causing measurable neurological deficit
- Onset of symptoms < 3 hours before beginning treatment
- Age ≥ 18 years

Exclusion criteria

- Significant head trauma or prior stroke in previous 3 months
- Symptoms suggest subarachnoid hemorrhage
- Arterial puncture at noncompressible site in previous 7 days
- History of previous intracranial hemorrhage
- Intracranial neoplasm, arteriovenous malformation, or aneurysm
- Recent intracranial or intraspinal surgery
- Elevated blood pressure (systolic >185 mm Hg or diastolic >110 mm Hg)
- Active internal bleeding
- Acute bleeding diathesis, including but not limited to
- Platelet count <100,000/mm^3
- Heparin received within 48 hours, resulting in abnormally elevated aPTT greater than the upper limit of normal
- Current use of anticoagulant with INR >1.7 or PT >15 seconds
- Current use of direct thrombin inhibitors or direct factor Xa inhibitors with elevated sensitive laboratory tests (such as aPTT, INR, platelet count, and ECT; TT; or appropriate factor Xa activity assays)
- Blood glucose concentration <50 mg/dL (2.7 mmol/L)
- CT demonstrates multilobar infarction (hypodensity >1/3 cerebral hemisphere)

Relative exclusion criteria

- Recent experience suggests that under some circumstances: with careful consideration and weighing of risk to benefit, patients may receive fibrinolytic therapy despite 1 or more relative contraindications. Consider risk to benefit of IV rtPA administration carefully if any of these relative contraindications are present:
- Only minor or rapidly improving stroke symptoms (clearing spontaneously)
- Pregnancy
- Seizure at onset with postictal residual neurological impairments
- Major surgery or serious trauma within previous 14 days
- Recent gastrointestinal or urinary tract hemorrhage (within previous 21 days)
- Recent acute myocardial infarction (within previous 3 months)

Note:

- The checklist includes some FDA-approved indications and contraindications for administration of IV rtPA for acute ischemic stroke. Recent guideline revisions have modified the original FDA-approved indications. A physician with expertise in acute stroke care may modify this list.
- Onset time is defined as either the witnessed onset of symptoms or the time last known, normal if symptom onset was not witnessed.
- In patients without recent use of oral anticoagulants or heparin, treatment with IV rtPA can be initiated before availability of coagulation test results but should be discontinued if INR > 1.7 or PT is abnormally elevated by local laboratory standards.
- In patients without history of thrombocytopenia, treatment with IV rtPA can be initiated before availability of platelet count but should be discontinued if platelet count is < 100,000/mm^3.

Abbreviations: aPTT, activated partial thromboplastin time; CT, computed tomography; ECT, ecarin clotting time; FDA, Food and Drug Administration; INR, international normalized ratio; IV, intravenous; PT, partial thromboplastin time; rtPA, recombinant tissue plasminogen activator; TT, thrombin time.

BOX 2: Additional relative exclusion criteria of patients for tPA

- Age > 80 years
- Severe stroke (NIHSS > 25)
- Taking an oral anticoagulant regardless of INR
- History of both diabetes and prior ischemic stroke

Note: Dose of tPA: As per the guidelines, infuse 0.9 mg/kg (maximum dose 90 mg) over 60 minutes, with 10% of the dose given as a bolus over 1 minute.

There are additional relative exclusion criteria for patients in 3–4.5 hours window that determine if the patients are eligible for tPA or not (Box 2).

Endovascular Treatment for Stroke

Intravenous tPA has been the backbone of stroke treatment for almost 20 years. Intravenous therapy, although effective, has specific inclusion and exclusion criteria which limit its use in a large number of patients. Moreover, the intravenous tPA cannot be used after the 4.5 hourrs window and has limited efficacy in patients with large vessel occlusion. Riedel et al. showed that it is almost impossible to dissolve large clots with intravenous therapy.[20] In another study by Alexandrov and Grotta up to one-third of patients had reocclusion of blood vessels after initial recanalization.[21]

Over the last two decades, the field of endovascular stroke intervention has grown exponentially. From initial trials of intra-arterial tPA infusion to initial clot retrieval devices and now to stent retriever technology, the field has come a long way indeed. Initial trials, PROACT I and II showed promise with intra-arterial pro-urokinase infusion with improved outcomes and recanalization rates, however, pro-urokinase was never approved by the US Food and Drug Administration (FDA) citing need for further confirmatory trials.[22,23] Intra-arterial therapy theoretically sounds promising but has never been shown to improve outcomes or decrease mortality in randomized trials, thus is not the preferred approach today.

First-generation device, the MERCI device, was approved for mechanical thrombectomy by the FDA and marked the beginning of era of endovascular stroke intervention. The MERCI device was tested in the MERCI and MULTI-MERCI trials both of which had significantly high mortality (44% and 34% respectively), despite that the patients who had successful recanalization had a better chance at achieving good functional outcome.[24,25] These trials laid the foundation for further research in the field of acute stroke intervention.[26]

In 2013, three landmark trials SYNTHESIS, MR RESCUE, and IMS III were published and disappointingly all three trials ruled against endovascular stroke intervention. The SYNTHESIS trial compared treatment with intravenous tPA alone to intra-arterial thrombolysis with rtPA, mechanical clot disruption or retrieval or a combination of these approaches. There was no difference in good clinical outcome (42%) in the endovascular arm versus (46%) in the intravenous tPA arm. Mechanical device was used in only 56/181 patients and stent retrievers were only used in 23 patients.[27] MR RESCUE trial compared patients receiving standard care versus endovascular therapy using the MERCI device and the PENUMBRA system. Patients with intracranial ICA or M1 occlusion, NIHSS greater or equal to 6 and within 8 hours of symptoms onset were enrolled. This trial showed no difference in outcomes of patients in the two groups.Reperfusion, defined as modified thrombolysis in cerebral infarction score (mTICI) 2a/3, was 67% and defined as mTICI 2b/3 was only 27%. Good clinical outcome (mRS 0–2) was only demonstrated in 14%.[28] IMS III trial showed a similar outcome with 41% good clinical outcome (mRS 0–2) in the combined intravenous therapy (IVT)/endovascular therapy arm versus 39% in the IVT-only arm.[29] IMS III did not require demonstration of vascular occlusion until the trial was midway when CT angiogram was included in the study protocol. IMS III also did not standardize the endovascular therapy as a result; the methods were a mix of pharmacological thrombolysis, manipulation of clot with use of a guidewire or microcatheter, mechanical and aspiration thrombectomy, and stent-retriever technology.[29] These trials failed to show any benefit of endovascular intervention over the intravenous therapy for a variety of reasons. These trials did not standardize the noninvasive vascular imaging, thus, in IMS III more than 50% patients did not undergo vascular imaging. The endovascular therapy was performed using older devices and thus the results were often not promising. There were long delays from stroke onset to revascularization, in part due to lack of rapid workflow.[26]

Learning from the shortcomings of the trials done in 2013, multiple trials were started using standardized endovascular and imaging approaches. Six trials published from 2014 to 2016 showed statistically significant benefit of patients with anterior circulation strokes who presented within 6 hours of onset of symptoms.[30-37] These trials have established the efficacy of mechanical thrombectomy over intravenous therapy with patients doing considerably well in the endovascular arm. The meta-analysis of the trials, including the three negative trials IMSIII, SYNTHESIS, and MR Rescue trial have shown benefit of endovascular intervention. The adjusted combined odds ratio for reduced disability at 90 days was 2.49, 95% CI: 1.76–3.53, $p < 0.0001$ and number needed to treat (NNT) to reduce the disability by at least one point was 2.6. The largest meta-analysis to date included the above eight trials and also preliminary data from THERAPY and THRACE trial, and showed similar benefit with risk ratio for good functional outcome (mRS 0–2) at 90 days reported as 1.37; 95% CI: 1.14–1.64. Details of the above mentioned trials have been given in the Tables 1 and 2.[26]

CONCLUSION

Endovascular stroke intervention is a rapidly evolving field. Last couple of years have changed the entire treatment profile for acute stroke patients with mechanical thrombectomy offering a new lease of life of the patients. New devices have made the stroke thrombectomy more feasible and safe. The entire stroke treatment protocol

TABLE 1: Baseline characteristics

	Age (median)	*Male (%)*	*NIHSS (median)*	*Vessel occlusion*	*Tandem lesion (extracranial ICA occlusion)*	*ASPECTS (median)*	*IVT (%)*	*Retrievable stent (%)*
MR RESCUE	66	50	16	71% ICA or M1*	nr	Predicted core 36 mL*	47*	0
IMS III	69	50	17	18% of EVT group had no occlusion	nr	nr	100	4
SYNTHESIS	66	59	13	2% no occlusion	nr	nr	0	41
PISTE	67	39	18	90% carotid T/L or M1	3%	9	100	68
THERAPY	67	62	17	89% I-ICA or M1	excluded	7.5	100	13% (majority used aspiration thrombectomy)
MR CLEAN	66	58	17	92% I-ICA, carotid T or M1	32%	9	87 (44% drip & ship)	82
ESCAPE	71	48 (87% white)	16	96% carotid T/L or M1	13%	9	73	73
EXTEND_IA	69	49	17	88% I-ICA or M1	n/r	n/r (median core 12 mL)	100	100
SWIFT PRIME	65	55 (89% white)	17	86% carotid T/L or M1	excluded	9	100 (44% drip & ship)	100
REVASCAT	65	55	17	90% carotid T/L or M1	19	7	70	70
THRACE	66	57	18	98% ICA or M1	excldued	nr	100 (100% mothership)	77

*MR RESCUE values reported for penumbral group receiving embolectomy

TABLE 2: Outcomes

	Recanalization (%, EVT v control)	*Reperfusion (mTICI 2b/3, %)*	*Primary outcome*	*mRS at day 90*	*mRS 0-2 at day 90*	*Final infarct volume (mL)*	*sICH (PH-2, %)*	*Death at day 90 (%)*	*New AIS in a different territory (%)*
MR RESCUE	69	27	mRS 3.8 v 3.4	3.8 v 3.4	21 v 26	32 v 32	9 v 6	18 v 21	1.4
IMS III	81 ICA; 86 M1; 88 M2	38 ICA; 44 M1; 44 M2	mRS 0-2 41 v 39%	nr	41 v 39	nr	6 v 6	19 v 21	nr
SYNTHESIS	nr	nr	mRS 0-1 30 v 35%	nr	42 v 46	nr	6 v 6	8 v 6	nr
PISTE	69	87	OR 2.12 mRS 0-2 p=0.2	nr	51 v 40 NNT=9	nr	0 v 0	7 v 4	nr
THERAPY	nr	70	mRS 0-2 38 v 30% p=0.44	nr	38 v 30 ns	nr	9.3 v. 9.7	12 v 24	nr
MR CLEAN	75 v 33	59	mRS 3 v 4 day 90	3 v 4	33 v 19 NNT=7	49 v 79	6 v 5	21 v 22	5.6
ESCAPE	nr v 31 (mAOL 2-3)	72	cOR 2.6	2 v 4	53 v 29 NNT=4	nr	4 v 3	10 v 19 (significant)	nr
EXTEND_IA	94 v 43 (TIMI 2-3)	86	24 hrs reperfusion 100 v 37% Early neurological recovery 82 v 37%	1 v 3	71 v 40 NNT=3	23 v 53	0 v 6	9 v 20 (p=0.18)	5.7
SWIFT PRIME	nr	88	Shift analysis p=0.0002	2 v 3	60 v 36 NNT=4	nr	1 v 3	9 v 12 (p=0.5)	nr
REVASCAT	nr	66	cOR 1.7	nr	44 v 28 NNT=6	16 v 39	5 v 2	18 v 16	5
THRACE	78	69	mRS 0-2 at day 90 53 v 42%	nr	53 v 42 NNT =9	nr	2 v 2	12 v 13	6

depends on the time of onset of symptoms and how fast the clot can be removed. To achieve a good functional outcome, there is a huge need for a well-regulated stroke team headed by an endovascular stroke specialist that can deliver good care expeditiously. As stroke care is time-dependent, it is extremely important that centers of excellence are identified which can deliver such high acuity care in a reasonable time. Peripheral centers need to identify and transfer acute stroke patients in time to higher care centers. As with life, with brain too, "Time is everything".

REFERENCES

1. Hatano S. Experience from a multicentre stroke register: a preliminary report. Bull World Health Organ.1976;54(5):541-53.
2. Caplan LR. Basic pathology, anatomy, and pathophysiology of stroke. In: Caplan's stroke: a clinical approach, 4th edition.Philadelphia: Saunders Elsevier; 2009. p.22.
3. Lozano R, Naghavi M, Foreman K, et al. Global and regional mortality from 235 causes of death for 20 age groups in 1990 and 2010: a systematic analysis for the Global Burden of Disease Study 2010. Lancet. 2012;380(9859):2095.
4. Krishnamurthi RV, Feigin VL, Forouzanfar MH, et al. Global and regional burden of first-ever ischaemic and haemorrhagic stroke during 1990-2010: findings from the Global Burden of Disease Study 2010. Lancet Glob Health. 2013;1(5):e259.
5. Benjamin EJ, Blaha MJ, Chiuve SE, et al. Heart disease and stroke statistics-2017 update: a report from the American Heart Association. Circulation. 2017;135(10):e146.
6. Banerjee TK, Mukherjee CS, Sarkhel A. Stroke in the urban population of Calcutta—and epidemiological study. Neuroepidemiology. 2001;20(3):201-7.
7. Pandian JD, Sudhan P. Stroke epidemiology and stroke care services in India. J Stroke. 2013;15(3):128-34. doi:10.5853/jos.2013.15.3.128.
8. Prasad K, Vibha D, Meenakshi cerebrovascular disease in South Asia - Part I: a burning problem. JRSM Cardiovasc Dis. 2012;1(7):20.
9. Bharucha NE, Bharucha EP, Bharucha AE, et al. Prevalence of stroke in the Parsi community of Bombay. Stroke.1988;19:60-2.
10. Xavier D, Pais P, Devereaux PJ, et al. Treatment and outcomes of acute coronary syndromes in India (CREATE): a prospective analysis of registry data.Lancet. (Apr 26) 2008;371(9622):1435-42.
11. Ay H, Furie KL, Singhal A, et al. An evidence-based causative classification system for acute ischemic stroke. Ann Neurol. 2005;58(5):688.
12. Doufekias E, Segal AZ, Kizer JR. Cardiogenic and aortogenic brain embolism. J Am Coll Cardiol. 2008;51:1049.
13. Saver JL. Time is brain-quantified.Stroke. 2006;37(1):263-6.
14. Jauch EC, Saver JL, Adams HP Jr, et al. Guidelines for the early management of patients with acute ischemic stroke: a guideline for healthcare professionals from the American Heart Association/American Stroke Association. Stroke. 2013;44(3):870.
15. Lansberg MG, O'Donnell MJ, Khatri P, et al. Antithrombotic and thrombolytic therapy for ischemic stroke: antithrombotic therapy and prevention of thrombosis, 9th edn: American College of Chest Physicians Evidence-based Clinical Practice Guidelines. Chest. 2012;141(2 Suppl):e601S.
16. Group NS. Tissue plasminogen activator for acute ischemic stroke. The National Institute of Neurological Disorders and Stroke rt-PA stroke study group. N Engl J Med. 1995;333(24):1581-7.
17. Hacke W, Donnan G, Fieschi C, et al. Association of outcome with early stroke treatment: pooled analysis of ATLANTIS, ECASS, and NINDS rt-PA stroke trials.Lancet. 2004;363(9411):768-74.

18. Hacke W, Kaste M, Bluhmki E, et al. Thrombolysis with alteplase 3 to 4.5 hours after acute ischemic stroke. N Engl J Med. 2008;359(13):1317-29.
19. Saver JL, Gornbein J, Grotta J, et al. Number needed to treat to benefit and to harm for intravenous tissue plasminogen activator therapy in the 3- to 4.5-hour window: joint outcome table analysis of the ECASS 3 trial. Stroke. 2009;40(7):2433-7.
20. Riedel CH, Zimmermann P, Jensen-Kondering U, et al. The importance of size: successful recanalization by intravenous thrombolysis in acute anterior stroke depends on thrombus length. Stroke.2011;42(6):1775-7.
21. Alexandrov AV, Grotta JC. Arterial reocclusion in stroke patients treated with intravenous tissue plasminogen activator. Neurology. 2002;59(6):862-7.
22. Del Zoppo G, Higashida R, Furlan A, et al. PROACT: a phase II randomized trial of recombinant pro-urokinase by direct arterial delivery in acute middle cerebral artery stroke. Stroke. 1998;29(1):4-11.
23. Furlan A, Higashida R, Wechsler L, et al. Intra-arterial prourokinase for acute ischemic stroke–the PROACT II study: a randomized controlled trial. JAMA. 1999;282(21):2003-11.
24. Smith W, Sung G, Starkman S, et al. Safety and efficacy of mechanical embolectomy in acute ischemic stroke: results of the MERCI trial. Stroke. 2005;36(7):1432-8.
25. Smith W, Sunf G, Saver J, et al. Mechanical thrombectomy for acute ischemic stroke: final results of the multi-MERCI trial. Stroke. 2008;39(4):1205-12.
26. Boyle K, Joundi RA, Aviv RI. An historical and contemporary review of endovascular therapy for acute ischemic stroke.Neurovascular Imaging. 2017;3(1):1.
27. Ciccone A, Valvassori L, Nichelatti M, et al. SYNTHESIS expansion investigators. Endovascular treatment for acute ischemic stroke. N Engl J Med. 2013;368:904-13.
28. Kidwell CS, Jahan R, Gornbein J, et al. MR RESCUE Investigators. A trial of imaging selection and endovascular treatment for ischemic stroke. N Engl J Med. 2013;368:914-23.
29. Broderick JP, Palesch YY, Demchuk AM, et al. Interventional Management of Stroke (IMS) III Investigators. Endovascular therapy after intravenous t-PA versus t-PA alone for stroke. N Engl J Med. 2013;368:893-903.
30. Berkhemer O, Beumer F, van den Berg L, et al. A randomized trial of intra-arterial treatment for acute ischemic stroke (MR CLEAN). NEJM. 2015;372:11-20.
31. Goyal M, Demchuk A, Menon B. Randomized assessment of rapid endovascular treatment of ischemic stroke (ESCAPE). NEJM. 2015;372:1019-30.
32. Campbell B, Mitchell P, Kleinig T, et al. Endovascular therapy for ischemic stroke with perfusion-imaging selection (EXTEND-IA). NEJM. 2015;372:1009-18.
33. Saver J, Goyal M, Bonafe A, et al. Stent-retriever thrombectomy after intravenous t-PA vs. t-PA alone in stroke (SWIFT-PRIME). NEJM. 2015;372:2285-95.
34. Jovin T, Chamorro A, Cobo E, et al. Thrombectomy within 8 hours after symptom onset in ischemic stroke (REVASCAT). NEJM. 2015;372(24):2296-306.
35. Baccard S, Ducrocq X, Mas J, et al. Mechanical thrombectomy after intravenous alteplase versus alteplase alone after stroke (THRACE): a randomized controlled trial. Lancet Neurol. 2016;15:1138-47.
36. Goyal M, Menon B, van Zwam W, et al. Endovascular thrombectomy after large-vessel ischaemic stroke: a meta-analysis of individual patient data from five randomized controlled trials (HERMES collaboration). Lancet. 2016;387(10029):1723-31.
37. Rodrigues F, Neves J, Caldeira D, et al. Endovascular treatment versus medical care alone for ischaemic stroke: systematic review and meta-analysis. BMJ. 2016;353:i1754.

SECTION 7

Cardiac Surgery

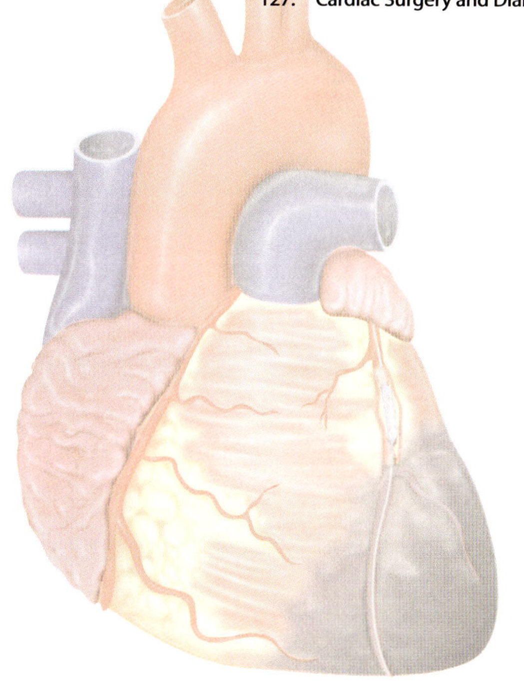

Coronary Artery Bypass Grafting in Cardiodiabetes

OP Yadava

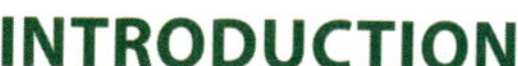

INTRODUCTION

Diabetes mellitus (DM) has ubiquitous presence in Indian subcontinent with overall prevalence of cardiovascular diseases as high as 77% among adult diabetic patients compared with 2–4% in the general population.[1] Conversely DM is preset in 25–30% of patients with acute coronary syndrome (ACS) and in those undergoing coronary revascularization in the developed world.[2] This sinister coexistence has a far higher incidence in Asian countries.[3] Over the past few decades, age adjusted mortality, especially cardiovascular mortality, has declined, which has been attributed to the reduction in cardiovascular risk factors and improvement in treatment of heart diseases. Paradoxically, mortality attributable to diabetes has increased sharply[4] and this may be related to the fact that diabetics are altogether a different subset—clinically, anatomically, biologically, rheologically, and etiopathologically.

CLINICAL CHARACTERISTICS

Diabetics with cardiovascular manifestations may be asymptomatic, present with atypical symptoms or with ACS. Evaluating the preoperative variables in diabetic patients in various studies,[5-8] patients were more often women and elderly. A higher proportion of those with treated DM, as against nondiabetics had a history of congestive heart failure (19% vs 6%), hypertension (65% vs 45%), chronic renal failure (6% vs 2%), carotid disease (17% vs 11%), and peripheral vascular disease (23% vs 15%). In addition, they have higher triglyceride levels, body mass index, and more LV dysfunction. They are more likely to have left main (LM) or multivessel disease (MVD), especially involving distal segments and small vessels.[9] They have higher atherosclerotic burden in form of diffused disease, more vulnerable plaques[10,11] and intracoronary thrombi.[12] Diabetics have higher vascular inflammation[13] and less collateralization.[14] Impaired platelet reactivity and responsiveness to antiplatelet drugs[15] along with endothelial vasomotion abnormalities and microvascular dysfunction[16,17] make matters worse and contribute to an unfavorable prognosis. The relative risk of myocardial infarction (MI) and sudden death is 50% greater in diabetic men and 150% greater in diabetic women, than their age-matched nondiabetic counter parts.[18]

PREOPERATIVE

No wonder then, results of any form of myocardial revascularization in diabetics, be it percutaneous coronary intervention (PCI) or coronary artery bypass graft (CABG) surgery, and have been historically inferior to nondiabetics (Table 1). These patients therefore need to be prepared well for surgery. Glycemic control should be adequate with a target HbA1C of less than 7%.[19] Hypertension and dyslipidemia too should be targeted with a systolic blood pressure goal of less than 140 mm Hg and diastolic of less than 85 mm Hg[20] with special preference for use of renin-angiotensin blockers, especially in patients with chronic kidney disease.[21] Statins should be continued to the point

TABLE 1: Clinical outcomes for diabetes after coronary artery bypass graft/percutaneous transluminal coronary angioplasty.

Trials	Follow-up (years)	n		Mortality (%)		Cerebrovascular Events (%)		Repeat Revascularization (%)		Event free(%)	
		CABG	PTCA	CABG	PTCA	CABG	PTCA	CABG	PTCA	CABG	PTCA
BARI	5	173	170	19.1	34.7	2.3	0.6	8.0	54.5	75	22.1
ARTS	1	96	112	3.1	6.3	6.3	1.8	3.1	22.3	84.4	63.4
EAST	8	30	29	24.5	39.9	NR	NR	26.5	65.3	NR	NR
CABRI	4	63	62	12.5	22.6	NR	NR	NR	NR	NR	NR
Duke	5	626	144	19	20	NR	NR	7.0	57	70	32

Abbreviations: PTCA, percutaneous transluminal coronary angioplasty; BARI, bypass angioplasty revascularization investigation; ARTS, arterial revascularization therapy study; EAST, emory angioplasty vs surgery trial; CABRI, coronary angioplasty and bypass revascularization investigation; NR, not reported.

of surgery[22] with a low-density lipoprotein (LDL) target of less than 100 mg/dL, and even less than 70 mg/dL for those at high CV risk.[19,23] Smoking cessation, weight control, chest physiotherapy, and infection control measures assume special importance.

REVASCULARIZATION STRATEGIES: CABG VERSUS PCI

Starting in 1980s and 1990s, several studies have compared outcomes of PCI, albeit with outdated technology versus CABG in diabetics and reported same or reduced early adverse outcomes with PCI but higher repeat revascularization and lower long-term survival as compared to CABG (Table 1). Closer in time, the SYNTAX trial (Diabetes Substudy)[24] looked at PCI with Paclitaxel eluting stent (again obsolete) against CABG. At 5 years follow-up, major adverse cardiac or cerebrovascular events (MACCE) were higher with PCI as compared with CABG (HR 1.81, 95% CI: 1.31–2.48, $p < 0.001$), driven mainly by repeat revascularization (HR 2.01, 95% CI: 1.04–3.88, $p < 0.001$) and cardiac death (HR 2.01, 95% CI: 1.04–3.88, $p = 0.034$). However, there was no difference in composite safety end-points of all cause death/stroke/myocardial infarction (MI): (HR 1.27, 95% CI: 0.84–1.92, $p = 0.26$).

When analyzed according to SYNTAX scores, the ones in greater than or equal to 33 tertile had a still higher 5 years MACCE (56.7% vs 25.5% respectively, $p < 0.001$) and even adverse safety endpoint outcomes (Death/MI/Stroke: 31% vs 16% respectively, $p = 0.034$). Superiority of CABG over PCI was demonstrated for both the oral drug-dependent and insulin-dependent diabetics.[24] Arterial revascularization therapy study (ARTS) I and II showed that Sirolimus eluting stents reduced MACCE compared to bare metal stents (BMS) but had no impact on mortality and barring reduced repeat revascularization, even CABG could not demonstrate improved hard endpoints over PCI.[25-27] This study however, was criticized as ARTS II was a single arm study and compared to the historical ARTS I Trial. Coronary artery revascularization in diabetes (CARDia) trial[28] too failed to demonstrate non-inferiority of PCI. Though there was no difference in primary endpoints at 5 years, repeat revascularization (21.9% vs 8.3%, HR 2.87, 95% CI: 1.74–4.74, $p < 0.001$) and composite of MACCE (37.5% vs 26%, HR 1.56, 95% CI: 1.14–2.14, $p = 0.0048$) were significantly higher for PCI. There were marginally increased strokes in CABG (4.3% vs 3.1%, $p = 0.48$) but countervailing higher MI in PCI (14% vs 6.3%, $p = 0.007$).

VA CARDS study,[29] a prospective randomized multicenter study, showed a reduced 2-year mortality of 5% with CABG as against 21% with PCI (HR 0.30, 95% CI: 0.11–0.80). However, MI was higher in CABG (15% vs 6.2%) due to a flawed definition of MI used in the study. Further the trial was terminated prematurely due to slow recruitment and was underpowered, and hence not much can be read from this trial. More meaningful is the relatively recent future revascularization evaluation in patients with diabetes mellitus: optimal management of multivessel disease (FREEDOM)[30] trial, a prospective randomized trial of 1900 diabetics comparing PCI with drug eluting stents (DES) (n-953) with CABG (n-947).

The 5 years MACCE rate was 26.6% in PCI versus 18.7% in CABG (95% CI: 3.3 to 12.5; $p = 0.005$): Table 2 showing divergence of curves beginning at 2 years (Fig. 1), and outcomes similar across all three SYNTAX score subgroups.

Even the BEST trial,[31] another multicenter randomized control trial (RCT) from Asia, using the contemporary Everolimus: eluting stent showed that the primary end-points of Death/MI or target vessel revascularization (TVR) were significantly higher in PCI as compared to CABG in diabetics (19.2% vs 9.1%, $p = 0.007$).

Superiority of CABG over PCI seems to be a universal truth as exemplified by numerous other studies[32,33] and meta-analyses.[34,35] Herbison and Wong in a recent meta-analysis of 14 studies showed CABG to have a 30% mortality advantage over PCI despite various eras that the studies spanned across; and irrespective of insulin status of these patients.

TABLE 2: Coronary artery bypass graft versus percutaneous coronary intervention: Diabetes[30]

Outcomes (5 years)	*PCI (%)*	*CABG (%)*	*'p'*
Primary endpoints	26.6	18.7	0.005
All cause mortality	16.3	10.9	0.049
MI	13.9	6.0	<0.001
CVA	2.4	5.2	0.03
Cardiovascular mortality	10.9	6.8	0.12

Abbreviations: CVA, cerebrovascular accidents; MI, myocardial infarction; CABG, coronary artery bypass graft; PCI, percutaneous coronary intervention.

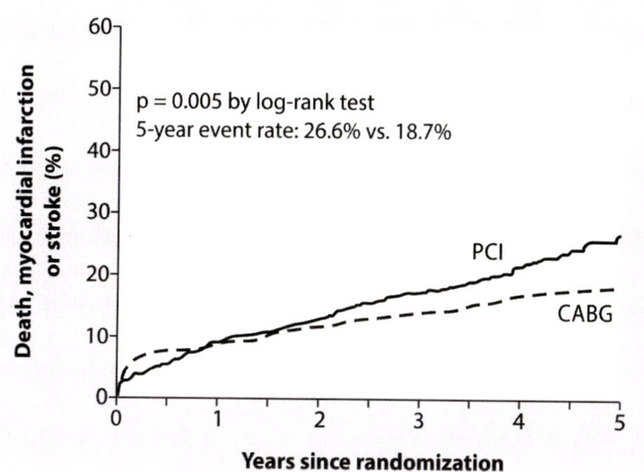

Fig. 1: Coronary artery bypass graft (CABG) versus percutaneous coronary intervention (PCI): Survival/major adverse cardiac or cerebrovascular events[30]

Ikeno et al.[36] revisited the BARI 2D trial and looked at MACE according to retrospectively calculated SYNTAX score in 1,500 patients. In the group with SYNTAX score greater than or equal to 23, MACE was lowest with CABG (15.3%) as compared to medical therapy (30.3%), and PCI (35.6%). Heart team approach is recommended for evaluating a patient for eligibility for CABG or PCI. The ESC/EACTS guidelines[37] recommend CABG as the revascularization modality of choice for improved survival in DM and multivessel or complex (SYNTAX score >22) CAD. PCI can be considered as an alternative in DM with low SYNTAX score (<22). The ACC/AHA guidelines[38] too recommend CABG over PCI for multivessel CAD for improved survival and accord class I recommendation to CABG.

CHOICE OF CONDUITS

Even though results of CABG may be better than PCI, diabetic patients far worse than their nondiabetic counter parts with higher proclivity for recurrent ischemia, graft occlusion and reduced survival.[39] It has been reasoned that these patients may benefit from a conduit most resistant to the augmented diabetic vascular process.[40] Out of various arterial conduits tried,[41,42] the internal mammary artery (IMA) has the best histologic[43] and vasoreactive credentials,[44] clinically translating into improved survival.[45] However, use of multiple arterial conduits, beyond the Left IMA to LAD, has not found widespread acceptance in the cardiac surgery community. This is partially due to technical complexities and increased time spent on harvesting these conduits, but possibly more related to the fear of sternal devascularization and increased wound infection rates, thus prompting the ACC/AHA guidelines[38] to grant Class II (b) recommendation to bilateral IMAs in DM. However, Dorman et al.[46] found bilateral IMA grafting to be as safe as single IMA in diabetics with no increase in either operative mortality (3.1% vs 2.4%, $p = 0.279$), sternal infection (3.1% vs 1.7%, $p = 0.179$) or total complication rates (17.1% in each, $p = 1.0$), respectively. The risk of sternal infection with bilateral IMA can be obviated to some extent with skeletonization.[40,47,48] Will the goodness of a single IMA translate into double benefits with bilateral IMAs is a matter of debate. Late survival was significantly enhanced with bilateral IMA (Median Survival: Single IMA 9.8 years versus Bilateral IMA 13.1 years, $p = 0.001$) in experience of Dorman et al.[46] Lev-Ran et al.[40] demonstrated improved 7 years survival with bilateral IMA to left sided arteries versus single IMA + Saphenous Vein (Kaplan-Meier, 75% vs 59%, $p = 0.006$) (Fig. 2); freedom from cardiac mortality (92% vs 68%, $p < 0.0001$) and freedom from MACE (70% vs 59%, $p = 0.004$) in oral drugs-treated diabetics. Multivariate analysis identified use of bilateral IMAs as a protective correlate of improved long-term cardiac outcomes. However, Calafiore et al.[49] ring a contrarian view point suggesting that extensive use of arterial grafting do not

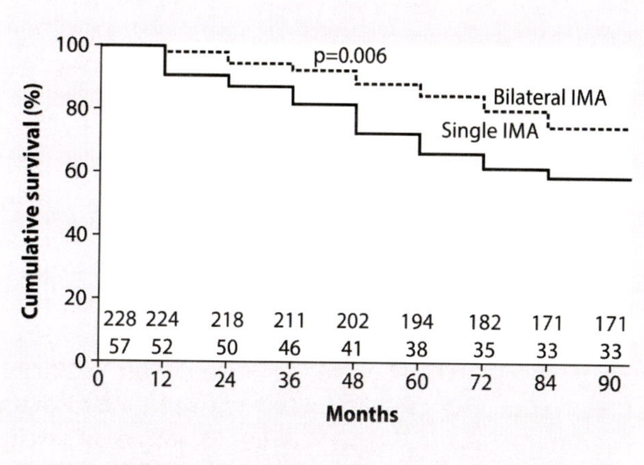

Fig. 2: Cumulative survival: Bilateral internal mammary artery versus single internal mammary artery[40]

influence late cardiac mortality in diabetics. Obesity, Chronic obstructive airway disease and friable sternum especially in Insulin-treated diabetics still remain relative contraindications to use of bilateral IMAs. In such cases, radial artery may be the second conduit of choice,[50] though it is less resistant to arteriosclerosis, intimal hyperplasia and medial calcification as compared to IMA[43] and even long-term impact of non-IMA arterial grafts is not confirmed.[40]

PUMP VERSUS OFF-PUMP CABG

Despite all the brouhaha in the western literature against off-pump CABG, Indian surgical diaspora have been nonchalant and unequivocally committed to its use as a default strategy. Sporadic support poured in from western literature too. Calafiore et al.[49] and Zapolanski et al.[51] have reported that off pump CABG reduces early mortality from 4.0% to 2.0% in diabetics when compared with patients operated on cardiopulmonary bypass (CPB). Thus this strategy would further improve results in management of diabetic patients with coronary disease (CAD). At National Heart Institute, where we use off-pump technique routinely for all patients undergoing surgical myocardial revascularization, the 30 days mortality rate in diabetics was 1.67% vs 1.37% in nondiabetics, a significant reduction from the historical data from 1990 to 2001 (Diabetics: 3.5%; Nondiabetics: 2.8%): $p < 0.01$ for both groups.

OUTCOMES

There is a conflicting evidence on the effect of DM on outcomes following CABG. Calafiore et al. found that though DM was a predictor of early death after CABG, it had no adverse impact on subsequent 5 year survival. Others however, find DM is linked to worse outcomes after CABG.[52-54] Mohammadi et al.[55], in an age-adjusted survival analysis, found insulin-treated diabetics to have two-fold increased long-term risk of death as compared to noninsulin-treated diabetes and nondiabetics. Holzmann et al.[54] found type 1 Diabetes to more than double the long-term risk of death after CABG (HR 2.04, 95% CI: 1.72–2.42) with only a marginal increase with Type 2 DM (HR 1.11, 95% CI: 1.05–1.18). Corroborating the above and going a step further, Alserius et al.[56] found an association with death and MI in both Type 1 and 2 DM.

Though a higher incidence of wound infections has been reported in diabetic patients than in nondiabetics,[58] Hirotani et al.[57] found that the rate of major chest wound infection that required reexploration and refixation of the sternum was not significantly different in the two groups. Further, in a study by Furnary et al.,[58] it was observed that tighter perioperative and postoperative glucose management (target blood glucose: 100–150 mg/dL) by continuous insulin infusion improved outcomes and reduced mortality in diabetic patients undergoing CABG. Observed mortality with continuous insulin infusion was significantly lower than with subcutaneous insulin (2.5% vs 5.3%). Lately a more liberal target of postoperative blood sugar of around 200 mg% or less for 48 hours has been shown to be optimum.[59]

Postoperatively diabetic patients appear to have a higher incidence of cerebrovascular accidents (CVA), than nondiabetics (6.3% vs 1.2%), as shown in the ARTS trial.[25] Infact diabetes has been demonstrated to be an independent risk factor for CVA after CABG. However, controversy surrounds the impact of left ventricular (LV) dysfunction and gender on the outcomes. In the CABG Patch Trial,[60] diabetes was not a predictor of mortality after CABG in patients with LV dysfunction, but was associated with increased postoperative complications and rehospitalization. However, others[52] have identified diabetes as a risk factor for mortality in LV dysfunction. As for gender, against conventional thinking that outcomes are worse in women, recent studies have found no gender difference in outcomes of both Type 1 and 2 DM.[61]

FOLLOW-UP

No form of myocardial revascularization is a panacea to all the ills of DM. CABG is only a minor part of the larger picture. Adequate follow-up with lifestyle modification[62] and optimum pharmacotherapy, especially use of antiplatelet drugs, high-dose statins titrated to the dyslipidemic profile, Beta blockers, Angiotensin-converting enzyme inhibitors, Angiotensin II receptor blockers and antianginals, depending on the clinical profile and needs of the patient cannot be over emphasized. Lifestyle modification in terms of regular and adequate physical activity—both aerobic and resistance, weight control, reduction of visceral obesity, total abstinence from tobacco, diet control[63] relief of stress and depression are of paramount importance. Needless to say, blood sugar needs to be controlled meticulously. Risk factor modification goals are mentioned in Table 3 as per EXCEL Study[63] protocols. Adequate stress should be paid to rehabilitation of these patients and early return to gainful employment. Patients should be monitored for recurrence of angina and there should be a low threshold for investigating the same. They may need follow-up interventions both percutaneous and surgical and recurrent ischemia may manifest in a subtle and varied form and may need high end imaging. Role of primary physicians in getting the best results following a CABG cannot be over emphasized and they should be an integral part of the heart team managing these patients postoperatively.

TABLE 3: Risk factor goals following myocardial revascularization

Risk Factor	*Goal*	
Smoking	Cessation	
Total dietary fat/ saturated fat	<30% calories/<7% calories	
Dietary cholesterol	<200 mg/day	
Sodium	<2,400 mg/day	
Fish	≥2 servings per week	
Physical activity	≥ 30 minutes of moderate intensity, ≥ 5 times/week	
Body weight by body mass index (kg/m²)	Initial BMI	Weight loss goal
	25–27.5 kg/m²	BMI < 25 kg/m²
	>27.5 kg/m²	10% relative weight loss
Blood pressure	<130/80 mm Hg	
LDL cholesterol (primary goal)	<70 mg/dL (<1.8 mmol/L)	
Non-HDL cholesterol (secondary goal)	<100 mg/dL (<2.6 mmol/L) if TG>150	
	(>1.59 mmol/L)	
Triglycerides (secondary goal)	<150 mg/dL (<1.7 mmol/L)	
HDL cholesterol (secondary goal)	>40 mg/dL (>1.0 mmol/L for men)	
	>50 mg/dL (>1.3 mmol/L for women)	
Diabetes	HbA_{1c} < 7.0%	
Influenza vaccination	All subjects annually	

Abbreviations: BMI, body mass index; LDL, low-density lipoprotein; HDL, high-density lipoprotein.

CONCLUSION

Cardiodiabetics are a challenging subset of patients with a distinct identity—clinically, rheologically and etiopathologically. Their early and long-term outcomes are worse as compared to their nondiabetic counter parts. Barring simple coronary lesions, majority of patients would need CABG in preference to PCI. Multiarterial grafting with good preoperative preparation and perioperative care of blood sugar improve overall results of surgical myocarcardial revascularization. CABG is just a part of a continuum of holistic care that these patients need and postoperative close follow-up, with a view to optimizing outcomes and early diagnosis of recurrent ischemia are of supreme importance.

REFERENCES

1. Mooradian AD. Cardiovascular disease in Type 2 diabetes mellitus. Current management guidelines. Arch Intern Med. 2003:163(1);33-40.
2. Luscher TF, Creager MA, Beckman JA, et al. Diabetes and vascular disease: pathophysiology, clinical consequences, and medical therapy: part II. Circulation 2003;108(13):1655-61.
3. Taggart DP. Impact of Type 1 and 2 diabetes mellitus on long- term outcomes after CABG. J Am Coll Cardiol. 2015;65(16):1653-4.
4. Gu K, Cowie CC, Harris MI. Diabetes and decline in heart disease mortality in US adults. JAMA. 1999;281(14):1291-7.
5. The Bypass Angioplasty Revascularisation Investigation (BARI). Influence of diabetes on 5-year mortality and morbidity in a randomized trial comparing CABG and PTCA in patients with multivessel disease. Circulation. 1997;96(6):1761-9.
6. King SBI, Kosinski AS, Guyton RA, et al. Eight year mortality in the Emory angioplasty vs surgery trial (EAST). J Am Coll Cardiol. 2000;35:1116-21.
7. Kurbaan AS, Bowker TJ, Ilsley CD, et al. Differences in the mortality of the CABRI diabetic and nondiabetic population and its relation to CAD and the revascularisation mode. Am J Cardiol. 2001;87:947-50.
8. Barsness GW, Peterson ED, Ohman EM, et al. Relationship between diabetes mellitus and long-term survival after coronary artery bypass and angioplasty. Circulation. 1997;96(8):2551-6.
9. Ledru F, Ducimetiere P, Battaglia S, et al. New diagnostic criteria for diabetes and coronary artery disease: insights from an angiographic study. J Am Coll Cardiol. 2001;37(6):1543-50.
10. Moreno PR, Murcia AM, Palacios IF, et al. Coronary composition and macrophage infiltration in atherectomy specimens from patients with diabetes mellitus. Circulation. 2000;102(18):2180-4.
11. Marso SP, Mercado N, Maehara A, et al. Plaque composition and clinical outcomes in acute coronary syndrome patients with metabolic syndrome or diabetes. JACC Cardiovasc Imaging. 2012;5(3 Suppl):S42-52.
12. Silva JA, Escobar A, Collins TJ, et al. Unstable angina: a comparison of angioscopic findings between diabetic and non-diabetic patients. Circulation. 1995;92(7):1731-6.
13. Kim TN, Kim S, Yang SJ, et al. Vascular inflammation in patients with impaired glucose tolerance and type 2 diabetes: analysis with[18] F-fluorodeoxyglucose positron emission tomography. Circ Cardiovasc Imaging. 2010;3:142-8.
14. Abaci A, Oguzhan A, Kahraman S, et al. Effect of diabetes mellitus on formation of coronary collateral vessels. Circulation. 1999;99(17):2239-42.
15. Angiolillo DJ, Jakubowski JA, Ferreiro JL, et al. Impaired responsiveness to the platelet P2Y12 receptor antagonist clopidogrel in patients with type 2 diabetes and coronary artery disease. J Am Coll Cardiol. 2014;64(10):1005-14.
16. Topol EJ. Textbook of cardiovascular medicine, 2nd edition. Philadelphia: Lippincott Williams and Wilkins; 2002.
17. Kornowski R, Lansky AJ. Current perspectives on interventional treatment strategies in diabetic patients with coronary artery disease. Cather Cardiovasc Interv. 2000;50(2):245-54.
18. Jacoby RM, Nerto RW. Acute MI in diabetic patients, pathophysiology clinical course and progress. J Am Coll Cardiol. 1992;20(3):736-44.
19. Rydén L, Grant PJ, Anker SD, et al. ESC Guidelines on diabetes, pre-diabetes, and cardiovascular diseases developed in collaboration with the EASD: the Task Force on diabetes, pre-diabetes, and cardiovascular diseases of the European Society of Cardiology (ESC) and developed in collaboration with the European Association for the Study of Diabetes (EASD). Eur Heart J. 2013;34 3035-87.
20. Kassimis G, Bourantas CV, Tushar R, et al. Percutaneous coronary intervention Vs Cardiac surgery in diabetic patients. Where are we now and where should we be going. Hellenic J Cardiol. 2017;pii :S1109-9666(16)30243-3.
21. Mancia G, Fagard R, Narkiewicz K, et al. 2013 ESH/ESC Guidelines for the management of arterial hypertension: The Task Force for the management of arterial hypertension of the European Society of Hypertension (ESH) and of the European Society of Cardiology (ESC). Eur Heart J. 2013;34:2159-219.

22. Curtis M, Deng Y, Lee VV, et al. Effect of dose and timing of preoperative statins on mortality after coronary artery bypass surgery. Ann Thorac Surg. 2017;104(3):782-9.
23. Reiner Z, Catapano AL, De Backer G, et al. ESC/EAS guidelines for the management of dyslipidaemias: the Task Force for the management of dyslipidaemias of the European Society of Cardiology (ESC) and the European Atherosclerosis Society (EAS). Eur Heart J. 2011;32(14):1769-818.
24. Kappetein AP, Head SJ, Morice MC, et al. SYNTAX investigators. Treatment of complex coronary artery disease in patients with diabetes: 5-year results comparing outcomes of bypass surgery and percutaneous coronary intervention in the SYNTAX trial. Eur J Cardiothorac Surg. 2013;43:1006-13.
25. Abizaid A, Costa MA, Centemero M, et al. Clinical and economic impact of diabetes mellitus on percutaneous and surgical treatment of multivessel coronary disease. Insights from the arterial revascularisation therapy study (ARTS) trial. Circulation. 2001;104:533-8.
26. Serruys PW, Onuma Y, Garg S, et al. for the ARTS II Investigators. 5-year clinical outcomes of the ARTS II (Arterial Revascularization Therapies Study II) of the sirolimus-eluting stent in the treatment of patients with multivessel de novo coronary artery lesions. J Am Coll Cardiol. 2010;55:1093-101.
27. Onuma Y, Wykrzykowska JJ, Garg S, et al. ARTS I and II investigators. 5-year follow-up of coronary revascularization in diabetic patients with multivessel coronary artery disease: insights from ARTS (arterial revascularization therapy study)-II and ARTS-I trials. JACC Cardiovasc Interv. 2011;4:317-23.
28. Hall RJ. CARDia investigators. 5 years follow up. ESC Congress 2012. 2012.
29. Kamalesh M, Sharp TG, Tang XC et al. VA CARDS investigators. Percutaneous coronary intervention versus coronary bypass surgery in United States veterans with diabetes. J Am Coll Cardiol. 2013;61:808-16.
30. Farkouh ME, Domanski M, Sleeper LA, et al. Strategies for multivessel revascularization in patients with diabetes. N Engl J Med. 2012;367(25):2375-84.
31. Park SJ, Ahn JM, Kim YH, et al. Trial of everolimus-eluting stents or bypass surgery for coronary disease. N Engl J Med. 2015;372:1204-12.
32. Hlatky MA, Boothroyd DB, Baker L, et al. Comparative effectiveness of multivessel coronary bypass surgery and multivessel percutaneous coronary intervention: a cohort study. Ann Intern Med. 2013;158(10):727-34.
33. Weintraub WS, Grau-Sepulveda MV, Weiss JM, et al. Comparative effectiveness of revascularization strategies. N Engl J Med. 2012;366:1467-76.
34. Hakeem A, Garg N, Bhatti S, et al. Effectiveness of percutaneous coronary intervention with drug-eluting stents compared with bypass surgery in diabetics with multivessel coronary disease: comprehensive systematic review and meta-analysis of randomized clinical data. J Am Heart Assoc. 2013;2:e000354.
35. Herbison P, Wong CK. Has the difference in mortality between percutaneous coronary intervention and coronary artery bypass grafting in people with heart disease and diabetes changed over the years? A systematic review and metaregression. BMJ Open. 2015;5:e010055.
36. Ikeno F, Brooks MM, Nakagawa K, et al. SYNTAX Score and long-term outcomes: the BARI-2D Study. J Am Coll Cardiol. 2017;69(4):395-403.
37. Windecker S, Kolh P, Alfonso F, et al. 2014 ESC/EACTS Guidelines on myocardial revascularization: The Task Force on Myocardial Revascularization of the European Society of Cardiology (ESC) and the European Association for Cardio-Thoracic Surgery (EACTS). Developed with special contribution of the European Association of Percutaneous Cardiovascular Interventions (EAPCI). Eur Heart J. 2014;37:2541-619.
38. Hillis LD, Smith PK, Anderson JL, et al. 2011 ACCF/AHA guidelines for Coronary Artery Bypass Graft surgery. A report of the American College of Cardiology Foundation/American Heart Association Task Force on Practice Guidelines. Circulation. 2011;124:e652-e735.
39. Lawrie GM, Morris GC Jr, Glaeser DH. Influence of diabetes mellitus on the results of coronary bypass surgery. Follow-up of 212 diabetic patients ten to 15 years after surgery. JAMA. 1986;256:2967-71.
40. Lev-Ran O; Braunstein R, Nesher N, et al. Bilateral versus single internal thoracic artery grafting in oral treated diabetic subsets: comparative seven - year outcome analysis. Ann Thorac Surg. 2004;77:2039-45.
41. Abizaid A, Costa MA, Centemero M, et al. Clinical and economic impact of diabetes mellitus on percutaneous and surgical treatment of multivessel coronary artery disease. Insights from the Arterial Revascularization Therapy Study (ARTS) trial. Circulation. 2001;104(5):553-8.
42. Szabo Z, Hakanson E, Svedjeholm R. Early postoperative outcome and medium-term survival in 540 diabetic and 2239 non-diabetic patients undergoing coronary artery bypass grafting. Ann Thorac Surg. 2002;74:712-9.
43. Ruengsakulrach P, Sinclair R, Komeda M, et al. Comparative histopathology of radial artery versus internal thoracic artery and risk factors for development of intimal hyperplasia and atherosclerosis. Circulation. 1999;100(Suppl 19):II139-44.
44. Wendler O, Landwehr P, Bandner-Risch D, et al. Vasoreactivity of arterial grafts in the patient with diabetes mellitus: investigations on internal thoracic artery and radial artery conduits. Eur J Cardiothorac Surg. 2001;20(2):305-11.
45. Hirotani T, Kameda T, Kumamoto T, et al. Effects of coronary artery bypass grafting using internal mammary arteries in diabetic patients. J Am Coll Cardiol. 1999;34(2):532-8.
46. Dorman MJ, Kurlansky PA, Traad EA et al. Bilateral Internal Mammary Artery grafting enhances survival in diabetic patients: a 30 year follow up of propensity score matched cohorts. Circulation. 2012;126(5):2935-42.
47. Taggart DP, D'Amico R, Altman DG. Effect of arterial revascularization on survival: a systematic review of studies comparing bilateral and single internal mammary arteries. Lancet. 2001;358(9285):870-5.
48. Cohen AJ, Lockman J, Lorberboym M, et al. Assessment of sternal vascularity with single photon emission computed tomography after harvesting of the internal thoracic artery. J Thorac Cardiovasc Surg. 1999;118:(3)496-502.
49. Calafiore AM, Mauro MDi, Giammarco GDi, et al. Effect of diabetes on early and late survival after isolated first coronary bypass surgery in multivessel disease. J Thorac Cardiovasc Surg. 2003;125(1):144-54.
50. Singh SK, Desai ND, Stephanie D, et al. The impact of diabetic status on Coronary Artery Bypass Graft patency. Insights from the radial artery patency study. Circulation. 2008;118(suppl1):S222-5.
51. Zapolanski A, Mengarelli L, Pilam MB, et al. Diabetes undergoing beating heart surgery have better outcomes compared with conventional CABG. Heart Surg Forum. 2003;6(Suppl 1):S41.
52. Morris JJ, Smith R, Jones RH, et al. Influence of diabetes and mammary artery grafting on survival after coronary bypass. Circulation. 1991;84(Suppl III):275-84.
53. Herlitz J, Wognses GB, Emanuelsson H, et al. Mortality and morbidity in diabetic and nondiabetic patients during a two year period after Coronary Artery Bypass Grafting. Diabetes Care. 1996;19:698-703.
54. Holzmann MJ, Rathsman B, Eliasson N, et al. Long term prognosis in patients with type 1 and 2 diabetes mellitus after Coronary Artery Bypass Grafting. J Am Coll Cardiol. 2015;65(16):1644-52.

55. Mohammadi S, Dagenais F, Mathieu P, et al. Long term impact of diabetes and its co-morbidities in patients undergoing isolated primary Coronary Artery Bypass Graft Surgery. Circulation. 2007;116:1220-25.
56. Alserius T, Hammar N, Nordqvist T, et al. Risk of death or acute myocardial infarction. 10 years after Coronary Artery Bypass Surgery in relation to type of diabetes. Am Heart J. 2006;152:599-605.
57. Fietsam R Jr, Bassett J, Glower JL. Complication of coronary artery surgery in diabetic patients. Ann Surg. 1991;57:551-7.
58. Furnary AP, Gao G, Grunkemier GL, et al. Continuous insulin infusion reduces mortality in patients with diabetes undergoing CABG. J Thorac Cardiovasc Surg. 2003;125(5):1007-21.
59. Furnary AP, Zerr KJ, Grunkemeier GL, et al. Continuous intravenous insulin infusion reduces the incidence of deep sternal wound infection diabetic patients after cardiac surgical procedures. Ann Thorac Surg. 1999;67(2):352-60.
60. Whang W, Bigger JT. Diabetes and outcomes of Coronary Artery Bypass Graft surgery in patients with severe left ventricular dysfunction: results from the CABG Patch Trial Database. J Am Coll Cardiol. 2000;36(4):1166-72.
61. Livingstone SJ, Looker HC, Hothersall EJ, et al. Risk of cardiovascular disease and total mortality in adults with type I diabetes: Scottish Registry Linkage Study. PLoS Med. 2012;9(10):e1001321.
62. Eckel RH, Jakicic JM, Ard JD, et al. 2013 AHA/ACC Guidelines on lifestyle management to reduce cardiovascular risk–a report of the American College of Cardiology/American Heart Association Task Force on Practice Guidelines. Circulation. 2014;129(25 Suppl 2): S76-99.
63. Kappetein AP, Serruys PW, Sabik JF, et al. Design and rationale for a randomized comparison of everolimus-eluting stents and coronary artery bypass surgery in selected patients with Left Main Coronary Artery Disease: the EXCEL Trial. Euro intervention. 2016;104:861-72.

CHAPTER 127

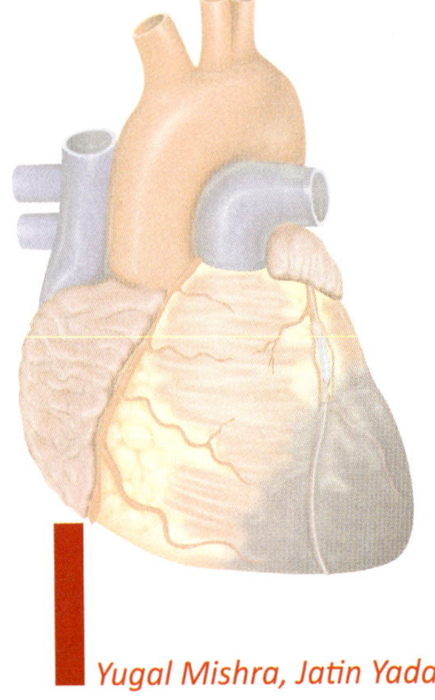

Cardiac Surgery and Diabetes

Yugal Mishra, Jatin Yadav

INTRODUCTION

Diabetes is among the most common chronic diseases in the world, affecting an estimated 285 million adults in 2010 (6.4% of the global adult population). The mounting incidence and prevalence of type 2 diabetes, driven by increasing population age, obesity, and physical inactivity, compound this high global burden, as does the increasing longevity of patients with diabetes. Estimates project that diabetes will affect more than 430 million persons (7.7% of the global adult population) by 2030.[1] Diabetes mellitus is a group of diseases characterized by insufficient production of insulin or by the failure to respond appropriately to insulin, resulting in hyperglycemia. The diagnostic criteria are summarized in Table 1. Diabetes typically is classified as either type 2 diabetes, characterized by insulin resistance and relative insulin deficiency, representing greater than 90% of all diabetes cases, or type 1 diabetes, characterized by absolute insulin deficiency. In view of the excess and increasing prevalence of type 2 diabetes and its incremental cardiovascular risk compared with type 1 diabetes, the focus of this chapter is on type 2 diabetes and its relevance in cardiac surgery.[2]

Diabetes is a well-established risk factor for atherosclerotic coronary heart disease. Coronary artery disease is not only more prevalent in diabetic patients (55%) compared with the rest of the population (2–4%) but tends to be more extensive, involving multiple vessels, and being rapidly progressive.[3] Moreover, diabetes is also a significant risk factor for early and late adverse outcome after myocardial revascularization with coronary artery bypass grafting (CABG).[4] Type 2 diabetes is highly prevalent in India[5] and its management poses challenges especially in hospitalized patients. Patients undergoing CABG surgery suffer from type 2 diabetes in 30–40%[6] cases and another 50% of those without preexisting diabetes develop hyperglycemia in the postoperative period.[7] Presence of diabetes is a risk factor for deep sternal wound infections (DSWI).[8,9] Although, earlier studies showed an association of diabetes with short-term morbidity and mortality in patients undergoing CABG, with improved hyperglycemia management, the immediate outcome in patients with diabetes is similar to those without diabetes.[10,11]

PATHOPHYSIOLOGY OF DETRIMENTAL EFFECTS OF HYPERGLYCEMIA ON CARDIOVASCULAR SYSTEM

In order to understand the beneficial effects of glycemic control during CABG surgery in patients with hyperglycemia, it is important to understand the detrimental effects of hyperglycemia on the cardiovascular system. In the nonischemic myocardium, the primary energy substrate is free fatty acids.[12] However, during ischemia when free fatty acids cannot be metabolized, increased levels of free fatty acids can be detrimental to the myocardium because they increase oxygen consumption, depress contractility, and increase arrhythmias and oxygen free radicals, which ultimately impair endothelial function.[13] Increased levels

TABLE 1: American Diabetes Association diagnostic criteria for diabetes mellitus[2]

1. Fasting plasma glucose ≥7.0 mmol/L (126 mg/dL) or
2. 2-hour plasma glucose ≥11.1 mmol/L (200 mg/dL) during standardized 75-g oral glucose tolerance test or
3. Symptoms of hyperglycemia plus nonfasting plasma glucose ≥11.1 mmol/L (200 mg/dL) or
4. HbA1c ≥6.5%

Abbreviation: HbA1c, glycated hemoglobin

of free fatty acids also impair glucose metabolism which is the preferred myocardial substrate during periods of ischemia.[12] In the nondiabetic ischemic myocardium, the change from the oxidative metabolism of free fatty acids to that of glucose is protective since it allows the ischemic myocardium to more efficiently utilize oxygen to generate the ATP necessary to preserve cellular transport systems and prevent cell death. However, the diabetic myocardium, because of impaired glucose transport into the myocardium, cannot metabolize this energy source and therefore there is decreased energy production and increased serum glucose levels.[14] Hyperglycemia also directly affects pathways responsible for changes in endothelial function, inflammation, and oxidative stress by altering the polyol pathway and increasing the synthesis of diacylglycerol, which activates protein kinase-C.[15,16] These changes in endothelial function contribute to decreased nitric oxide activity and increase production of superoxide radicals in diabetic internal mammary artery and saphenous vein grafts (SVGs).[17,18] Ultimately, this increased inflammatory response results in oxidative vascular stress, which contributes to vascular thrombosis, plaque rupture, and impaired platelet function.[19,20] These all contribute to reduced graft patency, recurrent ischemic events, and increased need for revascularization procedures in CABG patients with diabetes mellitus.

Pathophysiological Features of Atherosclerosis in Diabetes Conferring High Risk

- Metabolic abnormalities
- Hyperinsulinemia and insulin resistance
- Hyperglycemia
- Increased prevalence of small, dense, low-density lipoprotein, and triglyceride-rich lipoproteins
- Increased advanced glycation end product formation
- Increased oxidative stress and enhanced lipoprotein susceptibility to oxidation
- Endothelial dysfunction
- Hematological abnormalities
- Abnormal platelet function
- Abnormal coagulation system
- Increased plasma fibrinogen
- Impaired fibrinolytic system
- Increased plasminogen activator inhibitor-1
- Impaired ability to form collaterals
- Higher prevalence of obesity, hypertension, and dyslipidemia.[21]

STRESS HYPERGLYCEMIA

Stress hyperglycemia is defined as an elevation of plasma glucose levels (above 126 mg/dL in fasting condition or 200 mg/dL at any time) in critically ill or hospitalized patients, with or without history of diabetes.[22] More specifically, elevated values of blood glucose in presence of normal levels of glycosylated hemoglobin (HbA1c), regardless of diabetes status, may be considered a stress response; this kind of hyperglycemia is developed during any physiological reaction to a situation of high metabolic demand or injury, in which diverse mechanisms become active for maintaining homeostasis, for example: major burns, severe trauma, hemorrhage, septicemia, and major surgery, in which it is very common for blood sugar to reach levels up to 370 mg/dL.[23]

Predisposing Factors

Although stress hyperglycemia is mainly caused by six events: severe trauma, bleeding, hypothermia, septicemia, severe burns, and great-magnitude surgeries, there are several factors that may contribute to this alteration, which could and should be explored in the preoperative examinations (Table 2). Some of these factors are:

- *Endogenous factors:* Endogenous factor is an acute pain which inhibits the suppression of endogenous glucose by insulin; in addition, it releases diverse acute-stress hormones that contribute hyperglycemia, such as cortisol, glucagon, growth hormone, etc.[24] Elderly patients represent an important group that undergoes cardiac surgeries; it is well known that insulin secretion is diminished in this group of age.
- *Exogenous factors:*
  - Hypothermia, especially present in coronary bypass surgery due to cardioplegic solutions. Also, desaturation and arterial hypoxemia, increase a sympathetic autonomous response that favors glucagon release by an alpha-receptor action[25]
  - Many drugs commonly used with inpatient care might modify glucose metabolism. Some of them are well known as "diabetogenic" medications such as glucocorticoids and opiates; others are used for treating hypertension such as calcium channel

TABLE 2: Predisposing factors for developing stress hyperglycemia[29]

Action	Factor
Insulin deficiency (relative or absolute)/insulin resistance	Diabetes mellitus
Higher counterregulatory hormone levels	Acute pain Elevated acute physiology and chronic health evaluation (APACHE) score
Insulin peripheral resistance	Catecholamine-infusion Glucocoticoid treatment Overweight Septicemia/sepsis/septic shock Uremia Bed rest Fasting
Insulin impaired secretion	Elderly Hypothermia Hypoxemia

blockers, chlorthalidone, and prazosin. Every synthetic catecholamine or catecholamine-agonist or blocker (such as epinephrine, norepinephrine, salbutamol, metoprolol, and propranolol) and tricyclic antidepressants, might elevate glucose levels. Particularly, catecholamine-infusion during cardiac surgery contributes greatly to this metabolic state during surgery, as well as in the early postoperative period; it might also overlap and/or worsen stress response

- All volatile anesthetic agents, including halothane, enflurane, and isoflurane inhibit the insulin response to glucose in a dose-dependent manner in vitro.[26] The hyperglycemic response during inhaled anesthesia with isoflurane is a consequence of both impaired glucose clearance and increased glucose production (Fig. 1).[27,28]

BENEFICIAL EFFECTS OF INSULIN IN ISCHEMIC MYOCARDIUM

Insulin reverses the harmful effects of hyperglycemia on vascular oxidative stress by increasing myocardial glucose uptake, diminishing the inflammatory response, and decreasing apoptosis. Insulin enhances myocardial glucose metabolism by facilitating glucose transport into the myocyte, inhibiting the release of free fatty acids, and augmenting aerobic metabolism by stimulating pyruvate dehydrogenase.[30] It acts as an anti-inflammatory agent by suppressing the proinflammatory transcription factors and nuclear factor kappa-light-chain-enhancer of activated B cells (NFKB), early growth response protein 1 (EGR-1), and activator protein 1 (AP-1) and reduces inflammatory mediators such as interleukin 6 (IL-6), tumor necrosis factor-alpha (TNF-alpha), intercellular adhesion molecule 1 (ICAM-1), and E-selectin.[31,32] Insulin up, regulates the L-arginine nitric oxide pathway, thus promoting vasodilatation and enhancing endothelial function, improving platelet function by decreasing PA-1, and increasing prostacyclin release, and reducing apoptosis by increasing nitric oxide levels by a P-13 kinase dependent pathway.[33,34] In clinical studies, insulin has been shown to decrease levels of free fatty acids following CABG, improves aerobic metabolism when added to cardioplegic solutions, and decreases levels of reactive oxygen species, adhesion molecules, and C-reactive protein.[35-37]

PERIOPERATIVE MANAGEMENT OF HYPERGLYCEMIA

The following are the current recommendations of the Society of Thoracic Surgery regarding blood glucose management during adult cardiac surgery.[38]

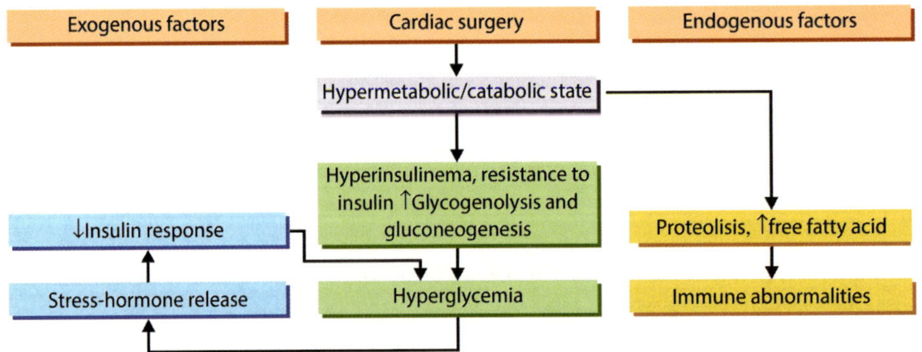

Fig. 1. It is showed how endogenous and exogenous predisposing factors may trigger the developing of stress hyperglycemia, adding cardiac surgery's aggression. Physiological stress triggers a catabolic state that results in stress hyperglycemia; the appearance of stress released hormones and a diminished peripheral response to insulin augment glycemia, and condition the release of proteins and free fatty acids that in addition to hyperglycemia entail an abnormal immune response

- All patients with diabetes undergoing cardiac surgical procedures should receive an insulin infusion in the operating room (OR) and for at least 24 hours postoperatively to maintain serum glucose levels less than 180 mg/dL (Class I; level of evidence B)
- An HbA1c level should be obtained prior to surgery in patients with diabetes, and those patients at risk for postoperative hyperglycemia to characterize the level of postoperative glycemic control (Class I; level of evidence C)
- Glucose levels more than 180 mg/dL that occur in patients without diabetes only during cardiopulmonary bypass may be treated initially with a single intermittent dose of intravenous (IV) insulin as long as the levels remain less than 180 mg/dL. However, in those patients with persistently elevated glucose (>180 mg/dL) after cardiopulmonary bypass, a continuous insulin drip should be instituted (Class I; Level of Evidence B)
- Patients with and without diabetes with persistently elevated serum glucose (>180 mg/dL) should receive IV insulin infusions to maintain serum glucose less than 180 mg/dL for the duration of their intensive care unit (ICU) care (Class I; Level of Evidence A)
- All patients who require more than or equal to 3 days in the ICU because of ventilatory dependency requiring the need for inotropes, intra-aortic balloon pump or left ventricular assist support, antiarrhythmics, dialysis, or continuous veno-venous hemofiltration should have a continuous insulin infusion to keep blood glucose less than or equal to 150 mg/dL, irregardless of their diabetic status (Class I; Level of Evidence B).

Intraoperative Management Recommendations: Class I

- Glucose levels more than 180 mg/dL that occur in patients without diabetes only during cardiopulmonary bypass may be treated initially with a single or intermittent dose of IV insulin as long as levels remain less than equal to 180 mg/dL. However, in those patients with persistently elevated serum glucose (>180 mg/dL) after cardiopulmonary bypass, a continuous insulin drip should be instituted, and an endocrinology consult should be obtained (level of evidence = B)
- If an IV insulin infusion is initiated in the preoperative period, it should be continued throughout the intraoperative and early postoperative period according to institutional protocols to maintain serum glucose less than 180 mg/dL (level of evidence = C).

Patients with IV insulin infusions initiated in the preoperative period should have them continued in the OR to maintain serum glucose less than equal to 180 mg/dL. Patients with no history of diabetes prior to surgery, may exhibit transient elevation of blood glucose more than 180 mg/dL during cardiopulmonary bypass. These patients may have insulin resistance and should be treated with a single or intermittent dose of IV insulin to maintain glucose less than or equal to 180 mg/dL.

Glycemic Control in the Intensive Care Unit Postoperatively Recommendation: Class I

- Patients with and without diabetes with persistently elevated serum glucose (>180 mg/dL) should receive IV insulin infusions to maintain serum glucose less than 180 mg/dL for the duration of their ICU care (level of evidence = A)
- All patients who require more than or equal to 3 days in the ICU because of ventilatory dependency or requiring the need for inotropes, intra-aortic balloon pump, or left ventricular assist device support, antiarrhythmics, dialysis, or continuous veno-venous hemofiltration should have a continuous insulin infusion to keep blood glucose less than or equal to 150 mg/dL, regardless of diabetic status (level of evidence = B)
- Before IV insulin infusions are discontinued, patients should be transitioned to a subcutaneous insulin schedule using institutional protocols (level of evidence = B).

Glycemic Control in the Step-down Units and on the Floor Recommendations: Class I

- A target blood glucose level less than 180 mg/dL should be achieved in the peak postprandial state (level of evidence = B)
- A target blood glucose level less than or equal to 110 mg/dL should be achieved in the fasting and premeal states after transfer to the floor (level of evidence = C)
- Oral hypoglycemic medications should be restarted in patients who have achieved target blood glucose levels if there are no contraindications. Insulin dosages should be reduced accordingly (level of evidence = C)
- According to the American Association of Clinical Endocrinologists, a reasonable goal for a noncritically ill patient on a regular hospital ward is less than 110 mg/dL premeal and less than 180 mg/dL postprandial or randomly.[24] The best method to achieve this control is with scheduled subcutaneous basal and, or bolus insulin therapy, such as glargine or detemir (basal) and lispro, aspart, or glulisine (bolus). Patients with type 2 diabetes who have used oral diabetes medications preoperatively can be restarted on those medications

once they have reached their targeted glucose goals and are eating a regular diet. Metformin should not be restarted until stable renal function has been documented. Thiazolidinediones (e.g. pioglitazone and rosiglitazone) can be restarted in patients without congestive heart failure or liver dysfunction.

PREPARATION FOR HOSPITAL DISCHARGE RECOMMENDATIONS: CLASS I

- Prior to discharge, all patients with diabetes and those who have started a new glycemic control regimen, should receive in-patient education regarding glucose monitoring, medication administration (including subcutaneous insulin injection if necessary), nutrition, and lifestyle modification (level of evidence = C)
- Upon discharge, changes in therapy for glycemic control should be communicated to primary care physicians, and follow-up appointments should be arranged with an endocrinologist when appropriate (level of evidence = C).[38]

REVASCULARIZATION STRATEGIES IN DIABETICS

Recent large, well-conducted randomized trials and exhaustive meta-analyses have clearly shown superior long-term survival for diabetic patients revascularized by CABG surgery by comparison with percutaneous coronary intervention (PCI).[39,40] For diabetic patients having CABG, there is emerging evidence that those having multiple arterial grafts may have even greater long-term prognostic benefits (with similar perioperative mortality and morbidity) over those having conventional CABG with a left internal thoracic artery (LITA) graft and SVG.[41-43]

ARTERIAL REVASCULARIZATION THERAPIES STUDY–PART II TRIAL[44]

Arterial Revascularization Therapies Study–Part II (ARTS II) trial studied the 3-year outcome of CABG surgery and PCI using sirolimus-eluting stents (SES) in patients who had multivessel coronary artery disease with and without diabetes mellitus. At 3 years, among nondiabetic patients, the incidence of the primary composite of death, cerebrovascular accident (CVA), myocardial infarction (MI), and repeat revascularization [major adverse cardiac and cerebrovascular events (MACCE)], was significantly lower in ARTS-II than in ARTS-I PCI [adjusted odds ratio (OR): 0.41; 95% confidence interval (CI): 0.26–0.64] and similar to ARTS-I CABG. The ARTS-II patients were at significantly lower risk for death, CVA, and MI as compared with both the ARTS-I PCI (adjusted OR: 0.55; 95% CI: 0.34–0.91) and ARTS-I CABG patients (adjusted OR: 0.56; 95% CI: 0.35–0.92). Among diabetic patients, the incidence of MACCE in ARTS-II was similar to that of both PCI and CABG in ARTS-I. Conversely, the incidence of death, CVA, and MI was significantly lower in ARTS-II than in ARTS-I PCI (adjusted OR: 0.67; 95% CI: 0.27–1.65) and was similar to that of ARTS-I CABG.

SYNERGY BETWEEN PERCUTANEOUS CORONARY INTERVENTION WITH TAXUS AND CARDIAC SURGERY TRIAL[45]

This study was designed to compare contemporary surgical revascularization (CABG surgery) versus TAXUS Express (Boston Scientific, Natick, Massachusetts) paclitaxel-eluting stents (PES) in diabetic and nondiabetic patients with left main and/or 3-vessel disease. The SYNTAX (SYNergy between PCI with TAXus and cardiac surgery) study randomly assigned 1,800 patients (452 with medically treated diabetes) to receive PES or CABG. The overall 1-year MACCE rate was higher among diabetic patients treated with PES compared with CABG, but the revascularization method did not impact the death or stroke or MI rate for nondiabetic patients (6.8% CABG vs 6.8% PES, $p < 0.97$) or for diabetic patients (10.3% CABG vs. 10.1% PES, $p < 0.96$). The presence of diabetes was associated with significantly increased mortality after either revascularization treatment. The incidence of stroke was higher among nondiabetic patients after CABG (2.2% vs PES 0.5%, $p < 0.006$). Compared with CABG, mortality was higher after PES use for diabetic patients with highly complex lesions (4.1% vs 13.5%, $p < 0.04$). Revascularization with PES resulted in higher repeat revascularization for nondiabetic patients (5.7% vs 11.1%, $p < 0.001$) and diabetic patients (6.4% vs 20.3%, $p < 0.001$).

FUTURE REVASCULARIZATION EVALUATION IN PATIENTS WITH DIABETES MELLITUS: OPTIMAL MANAGEMENT OF MULTIVESSEL DISEASE TRIAL[39]

In this randomized trial, they assigned patients with diabetes and multivessel coronary artery disease to undergo either PCI with drug-eluting stents or CABG. The patients were followed for a minimum of 2 years (median among survivors, 3.8 years). The primary outcome measure was a composite of death from any cause, nonfatal MI, or nonfatal stroke. From 2005 through 2010, they enrolled 1,900 patients at 140 international centers. The patients' mean age was 63.1 ± 9.1 years, 29% were women, and 83% had three vessel diseases. The primary outcome occurred more frequently in the PCI group (P = 0.005), with 5-year rates of 26.6% in the PCI group and 18.7% in the CABG group. The benefit of CABG was driven by differences in rates of both MI (P< 0.001) and death from any cause (P = 0.049). Stroke was more frequent in the CABG group, with 5-year rates of 2.4% in the PCI group and 5.2% in the CABG group (P = 0.03). This trial concluded that for patients with diabetes and advanced coronary artery disease, CABG was superior to PCI in that it significantly reduced rates of death and MI, with a higher rate of stroke.[39]

In a recent study by Tatoulis et al. out of the 11,642 diabetic patients who underwent CABG from 2001 to 2012, total arterial revascularization (TAR) was performed in 3,795 (32.6%) and non-TAR in 7,847 (67.4%). Mean follow-up was 4.9 years. Perioperative mortality, including 30-day mortality, was similar: 1.2% (24 of 2,017) for TAR and 1.4% (28 of 1,967) for non-TAR (p < 0.506). Late mortality was less among diabetic patients who underwent TAR, 10.2% (205 of 2,017), than no TAR, 12.2% (240 of 1,967; p < 0.041). Kaplan-Meier survival for the diabetic TAR group at 1, 5, and 10 years was 96.2%, 88.9%, and 82.2%, respectively, versus 95.4%, 87.5%, and 78.3% for the diabetic non-TAR group (log rank, p < 0.036). In this study of diabetic patients undergoing CABG, there were two major findings: that TAR confers a significant survival benefit for diabetic patients who did not have TAR; and that the long-term benefits from TAR did not compromise perioperative outcomes, especially 30-day mortality and DSWI. Diabetic patients having TAR had low and similar 30-day mortality and low and similar perioperative major morbidity, including stroke, MI, septicemia, and reoperation for bleeding, compared with diabetic patients who did not have TAR but, rather, more conventional CABG. An important finding was that DSWI among diabetic patients was extremely low and similar, 0.8% for TAR and 1.2% for non-TAR, emphasizing that TAR can be achieved, even for diabetic patients, without compromising sternal integrity.[46] The factors for better outcomes of bilateral internal thoracic artery (BITA) harvesting are Skeletonized ITA harvest.[46,42,47] There is less chest wall trauma, the endothoracic fascia, which is partly vascular, covers the ITA bed, and the small branches between the ITAs and the intercostal arteries are divided in a manner that preserves the terminal intercostals and vascular supply to the sternum.[47] In addition, the skeletonized ITAs are longer, more dilated, and more versatile.[46,47]

Diabetic patients have a greater incidence of coronary risk factors—such as obesity, hypercholesterolemia, and hypertension—that further affect the development of atherosclerosis within the SVG and diffuse distal disease in the coronary artery, further compromising SVG patency and leading to poorer outcomes for diabetic patients compared with nondiabetic patients.[43,46,42] Hence, TAR and avoiding the SVG specifically address graft patency and long-term survival of diabetic patients in several ways:

- Arterial grafts, especially the ITA, are resistant to developing atheroma, even in diabetic patients, despite the greater prevalence of comorbid risk factors
- Quality of SVG in diabetic patients may be compromised by chronic or recurrent lower limb infections
- With diabetes, coronary arteries often have diffuse distal disease and poor runoff, which may also negatively impact SVG patency. Arterial graft endothelium produces nitric oxide, prostacyclin, and other favorable vasoactive factors that may be protective and help ameliorate progression of the distal coronary disease so prevalent among diabetic patients.[48]

CONCLUSION

Total arterial revascularization in large numbers of diabetic patients is achievable, by senior trainees and attending surgeons in many institutions, with low perioperative mortality and morbidity, including DSWI, identical to conventional CABG but resulting in superior long-term survival. These findings will gain increasing importance with the progressive longevity of the population and the increasing proportion of diabetic patients who may require CABG.

REFERENCES

1. Shaw JE, Sicree RA, Zimmet PZ. Global estimates of the prevalence of diabetes for 2010 and 2030. Diabetes Res Clin Pract. 2010;87(1): 4-14.
2. American Diabetes Association: Diagnosis and classification of diabetes mellitus. Diabetes Care. 2010;33(Suppl 1):S62-9.
3. Stewart RD, Campos CT, Jennings B, et al. Predictors of 30-day hospital readmission after coronary artery bypass. Ann Thorac Surg. 2000;70(1):169-74.
4. Herlitz J, Caidahl K, Wiklund I, et al. Impact of a history of diabetes on the improvement of symptoms and quality of life during 5 years after coronary artery bypass grafting. J Diabetes Complications. 2000;1(6):314-21.
5. Anjana RM, Pradeepa R, Deepa M, et al. The Indian Council of Medical Research-India Diabetes (ICMR-INDIAB) study: Methodological details. J Diabetes Sci Technol. 2011;5(4):906-14.
6. Lazar HL. Glycemic control during coronary artery bypass graft surgery. ISRN Cardiol. 2012;2012:292490.
7. Azarfarin R, Alizadeh Asl A. Prevalence and intensity of hyperglycemia in non-diabetic patients undergoing coronary artery bypass graft surgery with and without cardiopulmonary bypass. Saudi Med J. 2008;29(9):1294-8.
8. Antunes PE, de Oliveira JF, Antunes MJ. Coronary surgery in patients with diabetes mellitus: A risk-adjusted study on early outcome. Eur J Cardiothorac Surg. 2008;34(2):370-5.
9. Bryan CS, Yarbrough WM. Preventing deep wound infection after coronary artery bypass grafting: A review. Tex Heart Inst. J 2013;40(2):125-39.
10. Mediratta N, Chalmers J, Pullan M, et al. In-hospital mortality and long-term survival after coronary artery bypass surgery in young patients. Eur J Cardiothorac Surg. 2013;43(5):1014-21.

11. Movahed MR, Ramaraj R, Khoynezhad A, et al. Declining in-hospital mortality in patients undergoing coronary bypass surgery in the United States irrespective of presence of type 2 diabetes or congestive heart failure. Clin Cardiol. 2012;35(5):297-300.
12. Opie LH. Effects of regional ischemia on metabolism of glucose and fatty acids. Relative rates of aerobic and anaerobic energy production during myocardial infarction and comparison with effects of anoxia. Circulation Res. 1976;38(5):52-74.
13. Liu Q, Docherty JC, Rendell JC, et al. High levels of fatty acids delay the recovery of intracellular pH and cardiac efficiency in post ischemic hearts by inhibiting glucose oxidation. J Am Coll Cardiol. 2002;39(4):718-25.
14. Sowers JR, Epstein M. Diabetes mellitus and associated hypertension, vascular disease, and nephropathy. Hypertension. 1995;26(6):869-79.
15. Guerci B, Bohme P, Kearney-Schwartz A, et al. Endothelial dysfunction and type 2 diabetes. Part 2: altered endothelial function and the effects of treatments in type 2 diabetes mellitus. Diabetes Metab. 2001;27(4 Pt 1):436-47.
16. Park JY, Takahara N, Gabriele A, et al. Induction of endothelin-1 expression by glucose an effect of protein kinase C activation. Diabetes. 2000;49(7):1239-48.
17. Lazar HL, Joseph L, San Mateo C, et al. Expression of inducible nitric oxide synthase in conduits used in patients with diabetes mellitus undergoing coronary revascularization. Journal of Cardiac Surgery. 2010;25(1):120-6.
18. Guzik TJ, Mussa S, Gastaldi D, et al. Mechanisms of increased vascular superoxide production in human diabetes mellitus: role of NAD(P)H oxidase and endothelial nitric oxide synthase. Circulation. 2002;105(14):1656-62.
19. Davi G, Catalano I, Averna M, et al. Thromboxane biosynthesis and platelet function in type II diabetes mellitus. N Engl J Med. 1990;322(25):1769-74.
20. Marfella R, Esposito K, Gionata R, et al. Circulating adhesion molecules in humans: role of hyperglycemia and hyperinsulinemia. Circulation. 2000;101(19):2247-51.
21. Singh M, Arora R, Kodumuri V, et al. Coronary revascularization in diabetic patients: current state of evidence. Exp Clin Cardiol. 2011;16(1):16-22.
22. Fahy BG, Sheehy AM, Coursin DB. Glucose control in the intensive care unit. Crit Care Med. 2009;37(5):1769-76.
23. Luna-Ortiz P, Carbó R, Rojas E, et al. Strict control of glycemia and cardioprotection. Rev Mex Anest. 2008;31(4):298-310.
24. Greisen J, Juhl CB, Grofte T, et al. Acute pain induces insulin resistance in humans. Anesthesiology. 2001;95:578-84.
25. Baum D, Porte D Jr. Stress hyperglycemia and the adrenergic regulation of pancreatic hormones in hypoxia. Metabolism.1980;29(11 Suppl 1):1176-85.
26. Desborough JP, Jones PM, Persaud SJ, et al. Isoflurane inhibits insulin secretion in isolated rat pancreatic islets of Langerhans. Br J Anaesth. 1993;71(6):873-6.
27. Lattermann R, Schricker T, Wachter U, et al. Understanding the mechanisms by which isoflurane modifies the hyperglycemic response to surgery. Anesth Analg. 2001;93(1):121-7.
28. Tanaka K, Kawano T, Tomino T, et al. Mechanisms of impaired glucose tolerance and insulin secretion during isoflurane anesthesia. Anesthesiology. 2009;111(5):1044-51.
29. McCowen KC, Malhotra A, Bistrian BR. Stress-induced hyperglycemia. Crit Care Clin. 2001;17:107-24.
30. Suzuki K, Kono T. Evidence that insulin causes translocation of glucose transport activity to the plasma membrane from an intracellular storage site. Proc Natl Acad Sci USA. 1980;77(5):2542-5.
31. Jeschke MG, Klein D, Bolder U, et al. Insulin attenuates the systemic inflammatory response in endotoxemic rats. Endocrinology. 2004;145(9):4084-93.
32. Langovche L, Vanhorebeek I, Vlaselaers D, et al. Intensive insulin therapy protects the endothelium of critically ill patients. J Clin Invest. 2005;115(8):1177-86.
33. Jonassen AK, Sack MN, Mjøs OD, et al. Myocardial protection by insulin at reperfusion requires early administration and is mediated via Akt and p70s6 kinase cell-survival signaling. Circulation Research. 2001;89(12):1191-8.
34. Gao F, Gao E, Yue TL, et al. Nitric oxide mediates the antiapoptotic effect of insulin in myocardial ischemia-reperfusion: the roles of PI3-kinase, Akt, and endothelial nitric oxide synthase phosphorylation. Circulation. 2002;105(12):1497-1502.
35. Svensson S, Svedjeholm R, Ekroth R. et al. Trauma metabolism and the heart. Uptake of substrates and effects of insulin early after cardiac operations. J Thorac Cardiovasc Surg. 1990;99(6):1063-73.
36. Rao V, Merante F, Weisel RD, et al. Insulin stimulates pyruvate dehydrogenase and protects human ventricular cardiomyocytes from simulated ischemia. J Thorac Cardiovasc Surg. 1998;116(3):485-94.
37. Dandona P, Aljada A, Mohanty P, et al. Insulin inhibits intranuclear nuclear factor kappaB and stimulates IkappaB in mononuclear cells in obese subjects: evidence for an anti-inflammatory effect? J Clin Endocrinol Metab. 2001;86(7):3257-65.
38. Lazar HL, McDonnell M, Chipkin SR, et al. The Society of Thoracic Surgeons Practice Guideline Series: blood glucose management during adult cardiac surgery. Ann Thorac Surg. 2009;87(2):663-9.
39. Farkouh ME, Domanski M, Sleeper LA, et al. Strategies for multivessel revascularization in patients with diabetes. N Engl J Med. 2012;367(25):2375-84.
40. Verma S, Farkouh ME, Yanagawa B, et al. Comparison of coronary artery bypass surgery and percutaneous coronary intervention in patients with diabetes: a meta-analysis of randomised controlled trials. Lancet Diabetes Endocrinol. 2013;1(4):317-28.
41. Puskas JD, Sadiq A, Vassiliades TA, et al. Bilateral internal thoracic artery grafting is associated with significantly improved long term survival, even among diabetic patients. Ann Thorac Surg. 2012;94(3):710-6.
42. Raza S, Sabik JF, Masabni K, et al. Surgical revascularization techniques that minimize surgical risk and maximize late survival after coronary artery bypass grafting in patients with diabetes mellitus. J Thorac Cardiovasc Surg. 2014;148(4):1257-66.
43. Dorman MJ, Kurlansky PA, Traad EA, et al. Bilateral internal mammary artery grafting enhances survival in diabetic patients. A 30-year follow-up of propensity score-matched cohorts. Circulation. 2012;126(25):2935-42.
44. Abizaid A, Costa MA, Centemero M, et al. Clinical and economic impact of diabetes mellitus on percutaneous and surgical treatment of multivessel coronary disease patients: insights from the Arterial Revascularization Therapy Study (ARTS) trial. Circulation. 2001;104(5):533-8.
45. Mohr FW, Morice MC, Kappetein AP, et al. Coronary artery bypass graft surgery versus percutaneous coronary intervention in patients with three-vessel disease and left main coronary disease: 5-year follow up of the randomised, clinical SYNTAX trial. Lancet. 2013;381(9867):629-38.
46. Tatoulis J, Wynne R, Skillington PD, et al. Total arterial revascularization: achievable and prognostically effective. A multicenter analysis. Ann Thorac Surg. 2015;100(4):1268-75.
47. Sasso S, James D, Vecht JA, et al. Effect of skeletonization of the internal thoracic artery for coronary revascularization on the incidence of sternal wound infection. Ann Thorac Surg. 2010;89(2):661-70.
48. Dimitrova KR, Hoffman DM, Geller CM, et al. Arterial grafts protect the native coronary vessels from atherosclerotic disease progression. Ann Thorac Surg. 2012;94(2):475-81.

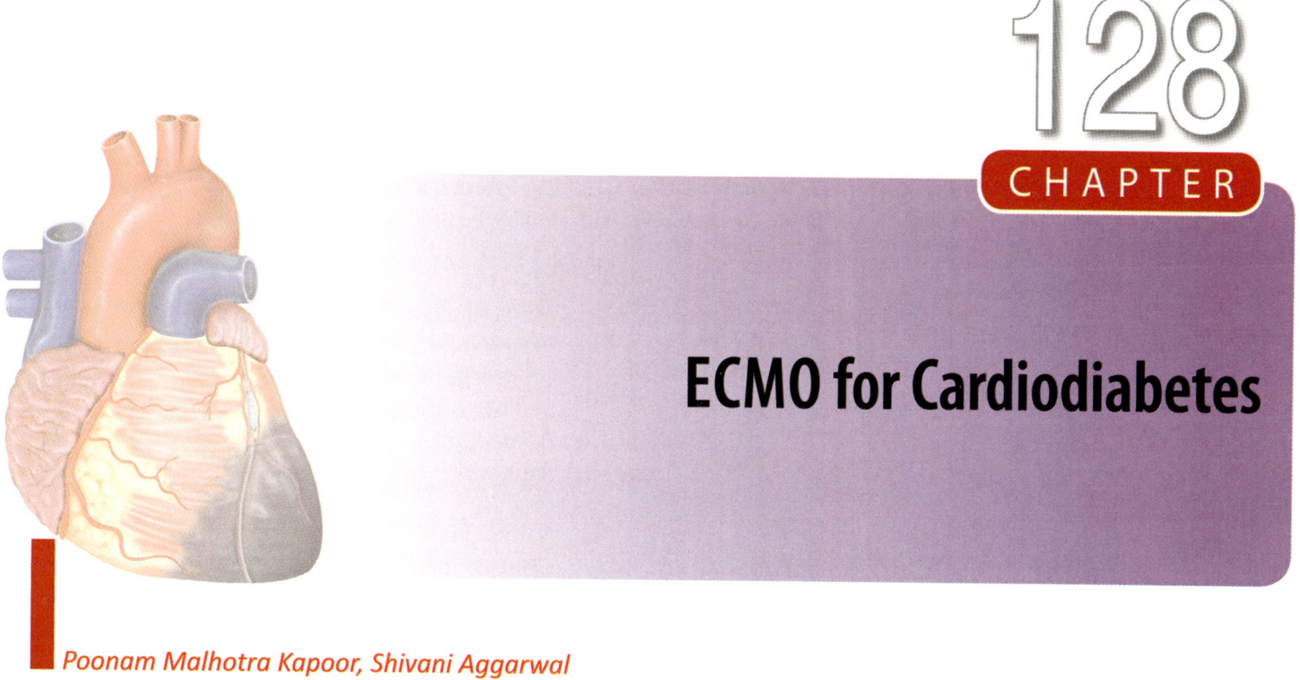

ECMO for Cardiodiabetes

Poonam Malhotra Kapoor, Shivani Aggarwal

INTRODUCTION

Extracorporeal membrane oxygenation (ECMO) traditionally is used in cases of respiratory failure (venovenous or VV-ECMO) and severe cardiac failure (venoarterial or VA-ECMO). In addition, ECMO is also used for providing postoperative support following cardiac surgery, short-term therapy in postcardiotomy syndrome, acute myocarditis and refractory severe decompensated heart failure as a bridge to recovery or as a bridge to decision (heart transplant). The results have been encouraging in neonates and infants[1] but not so in adults.[2]

Options for managing heart failure in patients with refractory cardiogenic shock are limited. Given the circumstances, with dearth of randomized trials and lack of consensus for standard practices, survival has improved only slightly over the years. Cardiogenic shock is still associated with high mortality in adults (50–80%)[3-6] despite revascularization and pharmacologic therapies.

With increasing technological advancements in designs of circuit, pumps, oxygenators, recent years have witnessed an increasing use of ECMO as a bridge to definitive therapy in cases of cardiogenic shock from acute coronary syndromes and as a bridge to transplant with or without the use of other ventricular assist devices (VADs). Use of ECMO following cardiac arrest is rapidly growing in popularity. Our basic focus in this chapter would mainly be use of ECMO in cardiogenic shock and heart failure.

INDICATIONS OF ECMO IN CARDIAC PATIENTS WITH DIABETES

People with cardiovascular disease have a higher incidence of development of diabetes particularly in patients when develop diabetic cardiomyopathy. ECMO can be used in diabetic patients who are more prone to develop the following:

- Bridge to decision for transplant or VAD [left ventricular assist device (LVAD)/biventricular assist device (BiVAD)]
- Support postcardiac surgery in low output
- Cardiogenic shock
- Fulminant myocarditis
- Pulmonary hypertension and right heart failure
- Pulmonary embolus with hemodynamic compromise
- Cardiac arrest
- Drug overdose
- Nonischemic cardiomyopathy including sepsis-induced cardiomyopathy.

Indications for ECMO in cardiodiabetes are:

- Cardiogenic shock
- Heart failure
- ST-elevation myocardial infarction (STEMI)
- Extracorporeal cardiopulmonary resuscitation (E-CPR)
- ECMO in infants and diabetes.

Risk Factors for heart failure and diabetes are:

- Increasing age
- Hypertension
- Hyperlipidemia
- Obesity
- Atherosclerosis
- Coronary artery disease.

Numerous clinical trials report increased correlation between occurrence of heart failure and diabetes but exact pathophysiology is still unknown.

ECMO IN HEART FAILURE: WHY THE NEED FOR ECMO?

Diabetic patients are more prone to develop acute heart failure (AHF). According to the European Society of Cardiology (ESC) guidelines,[7] AHF is rapid onset or worsening of symptoms and/or signs of heart failure requiring urgent evaluation and treatment. AHF may appear de novo or mostly as acute or chronic heart failure. It may be primarily because of cardiac dysfunction or precipitated by extrinsic factors in chronic heart failure. Acute myocardial dysfunction (ischemic, inflammatory or toxic), acute valve insufficiency or pericardial tamponade are among the most frequent acute primary cardiac causes of AHF. Decompensation of chronic heart failure can occur because of infection, uncontrolled hypertension, rhythm disturbances or nonadherence with drugs/diet.

With advancement in cardiovascular sciences, challenges have grown in terms of the disease spectrum available for treatment. Various permutation and combinations can be seen such as chronic systolic dysfunction and acute decompensated heart failure, high-risk multivessel disease requiring percutaneous coronary intervention (PCI) or other procedures, patients having coexisting cardiac dysfunction after myocardial infarction (MI) despite successful reperfusion and so on. The prognosis is grave if associated with diseases like diabetes. Such patients who are not stabilized with medical therapy alone can be supported using mechanical circulatory devices. These serve to unload the failing ventricle and maintain end-organ perfusion. BiVADs, extracorporeal life support (ECLS)[8] and intra-aortic balloon pump (IABP) are usually used. According to 2011 American College of Cardiology/American Heart Association/Society for Cardiovascular Angiography and Interventions (ACC/AHA/SCAI) Guidelines[9] for PCI, percutaneous mechanical circulatory support is recommended in two clinical settings: (1) high-risk PCI (Class IIb) and (2) cardiogenic shock with STEMI (Class Ib).

High-risk PCI is characterized as follows:

1. *Patient-specific variables*
   i. Increased age
   ii. Symptoms of heart failure
   iii. Diabetes mellitus
   iv. Chronic kidney disease
   v. Prior MI
   vi. Multivessel or left main disease
   vii. Peripheral arterial disease
2. *Lesion-specific variables*
   i. Left main stenosis
   ii. Bifurcation disease
   iii. Saphenous vein graft
   iv. Ostial stenosis
   v. Heavy calcified lesions
   vi. Chronic total occlusions
   vii. Dissection or occlusion during PCI
3. *Left ventricular (LV) dysfunction especially acute decompensated heart failure with difficult lesions.*

ECMO in Heart Failure

Diastolic dysfunction is more common in elderly persons, partly because of increased collagen cross-linking, increased smooth muscle content, and loss of elastic fibers. These changes tend to decrease ventricular compliance, making more susceptible to the adverse effects of hypertension, tachycardia, and atrial fibrillation. It worsens in diabetes, leading to acute decompensated heart failure and patient may be required to be put in a mechanical device like ECMO for a short while.

Pathophysiology of Diabetes and Heart Failure

Framingham Heart Study reports higher incidence of heart failure in diabetics compared to controls (men—two times more and women—five times more).[10] Idiopathic cardiomyopathy has also increased the incidence of diabetes (22%) compared to normal population (11%).[11,12] Increasing age, duration of disease,[13] extent of metabolic disturbances and requirement of drug therapy (regardless of drug used) are strongly correlated with development of increased risk of heart failure in diabetic patient.[14] Since diabetes is associated with silent MI and sudden cardiac death, it is important to periodically screen diabetic patients for development of heart failure so that appropriate therapy may be initiated at the earliest (Flow chart 1).

Management is same as for other heart failure patients with special attention to the following:

- Strict glycemic control

- Monitoring of renal dysfunction and need for renal replacement therapy
- Atherosclerosis in peripheral and central arteries may affect the decision in case mechanical support is required in advanced cases
- Autonomic dysfunction may affect hemodynamic management.

Flow chart 1: Pathophysiology of heart failure

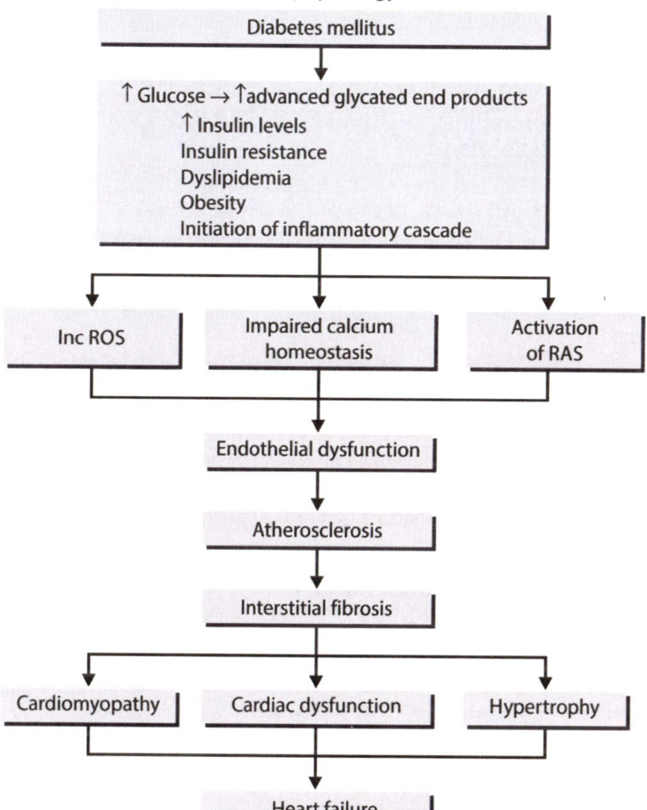

Initiation of ECMO

Since cardiac dysfunction is primary pathology in heart failure and cardiogenic shock, VA-ECMO is invariably used. Usually VA-ECMO initiated peripherally is adequate for majority of cases of cardiogenic shock (Fig. 1 and Box 1).

It however, requires frequent echocardiographic monitoring for progressive ventricular dilatation because ECMO does not allow for venting of left ventricle. If ventricular dilatation occurs then either configuration of ECMO circuit can be changed or a percutaneous atrial septostomy needs to be performed.

Another pitfall associated with the use of peripheral ECMO stems from the fact that native cardiac output generated from the dysfunctional heart theoretically may mechanically oppose the cardiac output generated by the ECMO in the femoral aortic cannula. This may lead to increased LV stress. If an added respiratory insult ensues, there is inadequate oxygenation with deterioration in the medical condition of the patient despite optimal ECMO flows.

BOX 1: Objective parameters to target of cardiogenic shock (CS) on ECMO

- $ScVO_2$ >70%
- MAP >60 mm Hg (in case of full support with non-pulsatile flow)
- MAP >70 mm Hg (in case of partial support with pulsatile flow)
- Avoid full flow and give partial flow about 2/3 through ECMO
- Maintain oxygen saturation of 90% or PaO_2 of >50 mm Hg (in young patient) and >60 (in elderly and with CAD or CVA)
- Maintain coronary saturation of >70%

Abbreviations: $ScVO_2$, central venous saturation; MAP, mean arterial pressure; CAD, coronary artery disease; CVA, central nervous system vascular accidents.

Source: Adapted with permission from Sharma J, Mehta Y. Extracorporeal membrane oxygenation in cardiogenic shock. In: Kapoor PM (Ed). Manual of Extracorporeal Membrane Oxygenation (ECMO) in ICU, 1st edition. New Delhi: Jaypee Brothers Medical Publishers Pvt. Ltd., India; 2014.

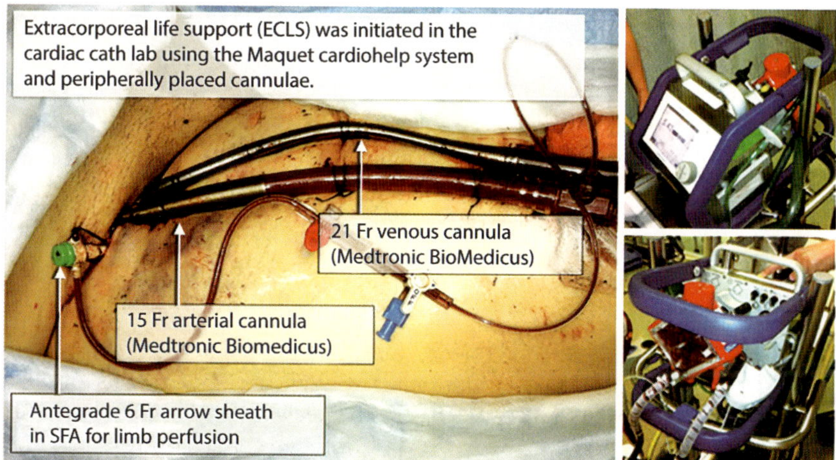

Fig. 1: ECMO cannula placement: femoral approach with antegrade sheath

Source: Adapted with permission from Chopra HK, Kapoor PM. Role of extracorporeal membrane oxygenation for acute decompensated heart failure. In: Kapoor PM (Ed). Manual of Extracorporeal Membrane Oxygenation (ECMO) in ICU, 1st edition. New Delhi: Jaypee Brothers Medical Publishers Pvt. Ltd., India; 2014

TYPES OF ECMO

Extracorporeal membrane oxygenation was first used successfully for life-threatening respiratory failure in an adult in 1971 and in a neonate with meconium aspiration in 1975.

There are two types of ECMO:

1. *Venoarterial ECMO*: It allows gas exchange and hemodynamic support while blood is pumped from the venous to the arterial side (Fig. 2A).
2. *Venovenous ECMO*: It facilitates gas exchange; blood is removed from the venous side and then pumped back into it, but does not provide hemodynamic support (Fig. 2B).

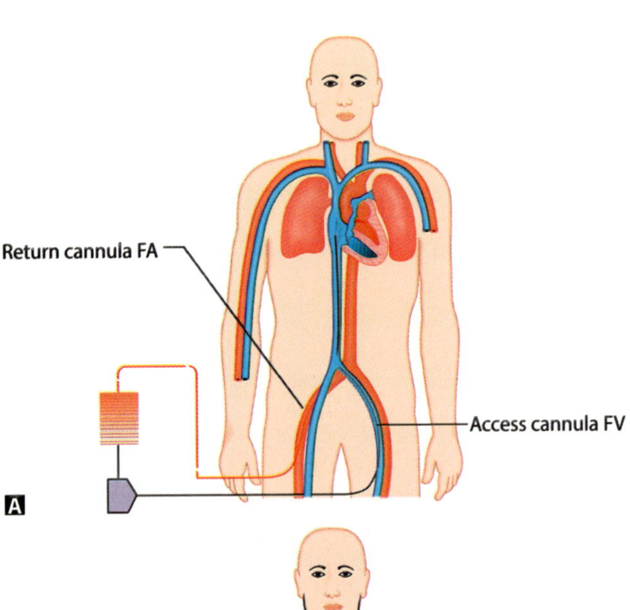

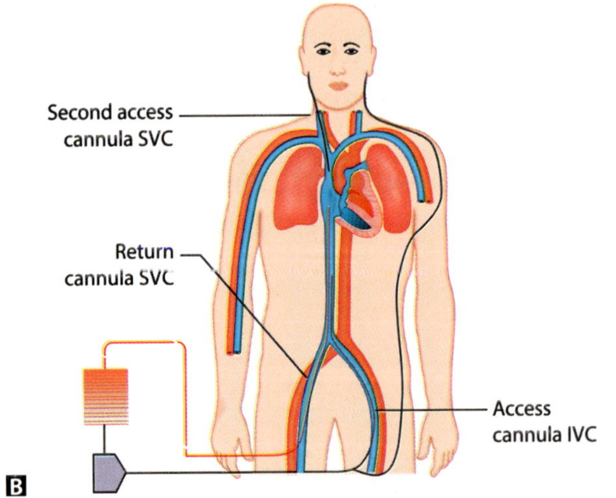

Figs 2A and B: (A) Venoarterial (VA) ECMO; (B) Venovenous (VV) ECMO

The circuit setup for VA or VV is almost identical. Blood movement is facilitated by an external pump that then pushes the blood through a membrane allowing gas exchange (oxygenation and CO_2 removal), before returning the blood to the patient's circulation via a warmer. Due to its configuration, VA-ECMO bypasses the patient's heart and lung and part or all of the blood flow is diverted through the ECMO circuit (Fig. 3). In contrast, VV-ECMO returns the blood before it enters the pulmonary circulation. So, VA-ECMO is ideal for STEMI patients. In fact, in a study done by Chung et al. patients included for ECMO support (>85% of the total) were those with profound cardiogenic shock undergoing CPCR and in whom a prompt ECMO was instituted.

The ECMO timing for initiation and weaning has always been crucial and controversial. For patients with advanced heart failure, the Interagency Registry for Mechanically Assisted Circulatory Support (INTERMACS)[7] has defined seven clinical profiles (Table 1).

Interagency Registry for Mechanically Assisted Circulatory Support

Out of seven levels, one and two patients are considered for mechanical circulatory support. Availability of advanced mechanical support systems has resulted in improvements in survival and quality of life in patients with advanced cardiac failure.[15]

Although human studies demonstrating benefits of ECMO for myocardial protection are limited, increasing

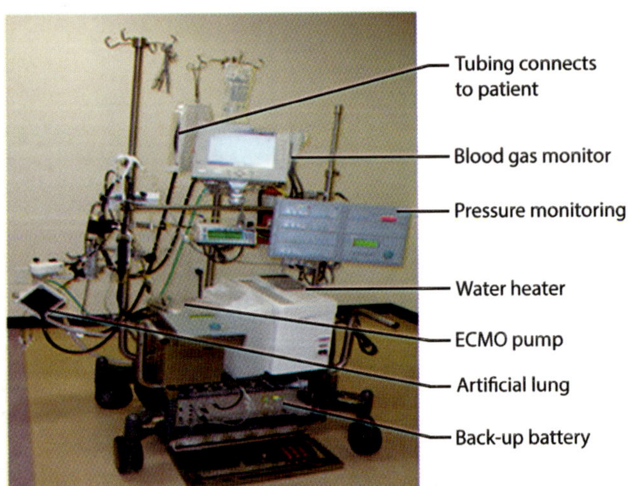

Fig. 3: ECMO circuit machine

TABLE 1: Interagency Registry for Mechanically Assisted Circulatory Support stages for classifying patients with advanced heart failure

INTERMACS	NYHA Class	Description	Device	Life year (LY) survival with LVAD therapy
Cardiogenic Shock 'Crash and run'	IV	Hemodynamic instability in spite of increases doses of catecholamine's and/or mechanical circulatory support with critical hypoperfusion of target organs	ECLS, ECMO, percutaneous support devices	52.6 ± 5.6%
Progressive decline despite inotropic support 'Sliding on inotropes'	IV	Intravenous inotropic support with acceptable blood pressure but rapid deterioration of renal function, nutritional state or signs of congestion	ECLS, ECMO, LVAD	63.1 ± 3.1%
Stable but inotrope-dependent 'Dependent stability'	IV	Hemodynamic stability with low or intermediate doses of inotropic but necessary due to hypotension, worsening of symptoms or progressive renal failure	LVAD	78.4 ± 2.5%
Resting symptoms 'Frequent flyer'	IV ambulatory	Temporary cessation of inotropic treatment is possible but patient presences with frequent symptom recurrences and typically with fluid overload	LVAD	78.7 ± 3.0%
Exertion intolerant 'Housebound'	IV Ambulatory	Complete cessation of physical activity, stable at rest, but frequently with moderate fluid retention and some level of renal dysfunction	LVAD	93.0 ± 3.9%
Exertion limited 'walking wounded'	III	Minor limitation on physical activity and absence of congestion while at rest. Easily fatigued by light activity	LVAD as option	-
'Placeholder'	III	Patient in NYHA Class III with no current or recent unstable fluid balance	Discuss LVAD as option	-

use is based on the hypothesis that ventricular support may provide myocardial preservation during periods of acute ischemic insult. It serves to improve hemodynamic condition with reduction of infarct size.

BENEFICIAL HEMODYNAMIC EFFECTS OF ECMO

Whether it is VV-ECMO or VA-ECMO, the overall benefits accrued from ECMO use are:

- Decreased LV volume, wall stress and oxygen consumption
- Limits the infarct size
- Improves coronary perfusion
- Maintenance of perfusion to other vital organs
- Decreased cardiac filling pressures.

Contraindications for initiation of VA-ECMO in cardiac failure are:

- Irreversible disease (malignancy, cardiac dysfunction)
- Chronic multiorgan dysfunction [chronic obstructive pulmonary disease (COPD), renal dysfunction, hepatic dysfunction]
- Prolonged CPR without adequate tissue perfusion or unwitnessed cardiac arrest
- Compliance limitation (financial, cognitive, psychiatric, social)
- Bleeding diathesis
- Central nervous system (CNS) injury (intracranial bleed, encephalitis, persistent vegetative state, hypoxic ischemic encephalopathy, intractable seizures).

ECMO in cardiogenic shock associated with sepsis is controversial due to concerns about bacteremia, inflammation and bleeding following disseminated intravascular coagulopathy. VA-ECMO might be considered for mixed cardiogenic and septic shock provided benefits outweigh the risks of bleeding and thrombosis.[16]

Cardiodiabetes and Role of ECMO

Diabetes is multifactorial metabolic disease with a myriad of causative factors. Association of diabetes with heart failure is independent of other risk factors.[15]

ECMO IN CARDIOGENIC SHOCK

Systemic tissue hypoperfusion occurring as a result of inadequate cardiac output circulatory volume and LV filling pressures are adequate is known as cardiogenic shock.[17] Diagnostic criteria include: a systolic blood pressure less

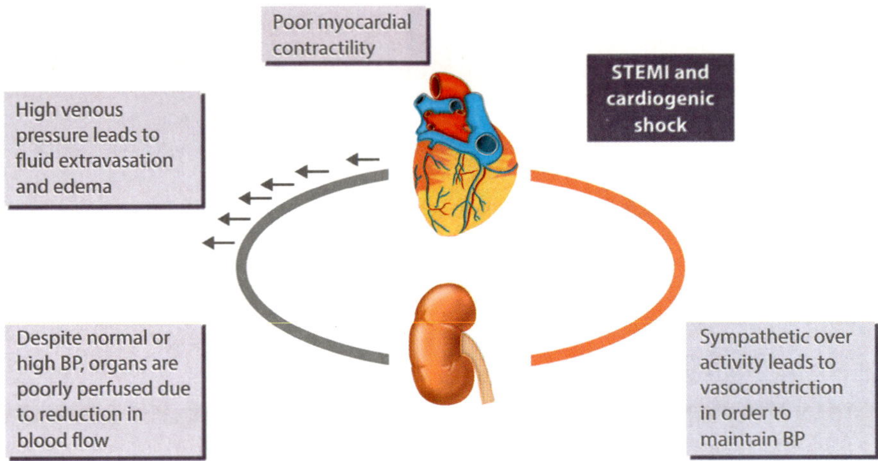

Fig. 4: Sequence of events leading to cardiogenic shock in STEMI

Source: Adapted with permission from Chopra HK, Kapoor PM. Role of extracorporeal membrane oxygenation for acute decompensated heart failure. In: Kapoor PM (Ed). Manual of Extracorporeal Membrane Oxygenation (ECMO) in ICU, 1st edition. New Delhi: Jaypee Brothers Medical Publishers Pvt. Ltd., India; 2014.

than 90 mm Hg for 30 minutes; a drop in mean arterial blood pressure greater than 30 mm Hg below baseline, with a cardiac index (CI) less than 1.8 L/min/m^2 without hemodynamic support or less than or equal to 2.2 L/min/m^2 with support; and a pulmonary capillary wedge pressure greater than 15 mm Hg. It most commonly occurs after acute MI due to myocardial dysfunction or result of mechanical complications like acute ventricular septal defect, cardiac rupture, papillary muscle rupture, cardiac tamponade, etc. Consequently, inability to maintain tissue perfusion and oxygenation is associated with poor prognosis[18] (Fig. 4 and Flow chart 2).

Treatment consists of initial medical stabilization with oxygen, aspirin, morphine, fluids, inotropes, vasopressors, diuretics in pulmonary edema and vasodilators according to patient's hemodynamic status. Supportive measures include mechanical support (IABP, VADs, ECLS), reperfusion therapy [fibrinolytics, PCI and surgery (coronary artery bypass grafting)].

Use of IABP in refractory cases of cardiogenic shock is controversial as it is not effective when CI is less than 1.2 L/min/m^2.[19,20] Other partial support therapies like VADs have also been used.[21] However, VADs have not shown to improve mortality in severe cases.[22]

Significant limitations of IABP and VAD include availability, cost, and time delay during initiation and need for personnel trained in providing specialized support according to the degree of hemodynamic compromise. The situation is further complicated with the development of respiratory compromise following hypoxemia, hypercarbia and consequent pulmonary edema. ECMO emerges as a rescue therapy in such a scenario.

Flow chart 2: The downward spiral in cardiogenic shock

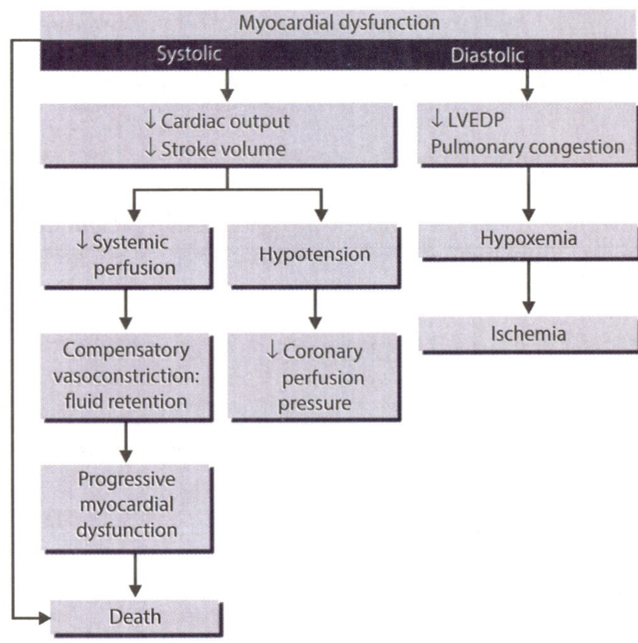

Abbreviation: LVEDP, left ventricular end-diastolic pressure.

Source: Adapted with permission from Chopra HK, Kapoor PM. Role of extracorporeal membrane oxygenation for acute decompensated heart failure. In: Kapoor PM (Ed). Manual of Extracorporeal Membrane Oxygenation (ECMO) in ICU, 1st edition. New Delhi: Jaypee Brothers Medical Publishers Pvt. Ltd., India; 2014.

ECMO has been used in acute cardiogenic shock with left or biventricular failure for initial short-term assistance till the time cardiac and other organ functions have recovered and more definitive therapy can be planned. Time duration is usually restricted from few days to weeks.

Percutaneous cardiopulmonary bypass can also be used to provide support.[23]

ECMO for Cardiogenic Shock

The European Society of Cardiology (ESC) guidelines for the diagnosis and treatment of acute and chronic heart failure recommend short-term mechanical circulatory support (as a 'bridge to recovery') in patients remaining severely hypoperfused despite inotropic therapy and with a potentially reversible cause (e.g. viral myocarditis) or a potentially surgically correctable cause (e.g. acute interventricular septal rupture)[15] (Box 2).

ECMO and STEMI

Patients who present with STEMI complicated by cardiogenic shock that suffer a cardiac arrest have high-mortality rates. Little data exist on using ECMO as a rescue device during CPR in the cardiogenic shock patient.

ECMO and Hypothermia as Rescue Therapy

ECMO can be a lifesaving rescue technique when instituted by an experienced Shock Team in the CV lab for refractory PEA arrest occurring in the CV lab. Lucas CPR was a valuable adjunct. Striking recovery of LV function can also occur in several days. The combination of ECMO and therapeutic hypothermia was associated with excellent neurologic outcomes as well. ECMO may have a role in selected PCI centers with advanced specialized teams. The use of ECMO accompanied by mechanical CPR, in patients with massive MIs can lead to unexpected survival. ECMO is an advanced technology that functions as a replacement for a critically ill patient's heart and lungs.

'For many patients who present with a severe heart attack, or STEMI, complicated by cardiogenic shock that progresses to cardiac standstill, the result is almost uniformly fatal,' says Michael R Mooney, MD, a research cardiologist at the Minneapolis Heart Institute Foundation (MHIF) and a physician at the Minneapolis Heart Institute at Abbott Northwestern Hospital in Minneapolis. 'This aggressive approach despite its complexity extends our ability to salvage the most devastating complication of acute MI.'

Early and Timely ECMO Alone

Early and timely ECMO alone is beneficial. Early ECMO-assisted primary PCI improved 30 days outcome in STEMI patients complicated with profound cardiogenic shock.

BOX 2: The European Society of Cardiology (ESC) guidelines for the diagnosis and treatment of acute and chronic heart failure

Indications
- Cardiogenic shock secondary to acute coronary syndrome
- Viral myocarditis
- Cardiogenic shock with acute severe mitral regurgitation and aortic regurgitation
- Postcardiotomy cardiogenic shock
- Failure to wean off from cardiopulmonary bypass
- Poisoning—beta-blocker, calcium channel blocker, aluminum phosphide
- Patient waiting for left ventricular assist device
- Patient is waiting for cardiac transplant

Criteria for initiation of ECMO

Presence of any two criteria mentioned here observed over a period of 4–6 hour after maximum medical resuscitation:
- Refractory arrhythmias
- Cardiogenic shock with high inotropic requirements
- Lactate level >5 mmol/L or rising titer or $ScVO_2$ <65% with maximum medical management
- Signs of poor tissue perfusion

Contraindications
- Irreversible disease e.g. malignancy
- Dilated cardiomyopathy except for waiting for final destination therapy or transplant
- Age >75 years
- Patient on ventilator from 15 days
- Intracranial bleed
- Active bleeding from noncompressive site
- Patient of gross multiorgan failure
- Severe CNS injury including encephalitis, persistent vegetative state, hypoxic ischemic encephalopathy, intractable seizures
- Unwitnessed arrest or arrest >30 minutes

Echocardiography criteria for contraindications
- Severe aortic regurgitation (AR)
- Severe aortic stenosis (AS)
- Coarctation of aorta
- Aortic dissection

Objective parameters to target of cardiogenic shock on ECMO
- $ScVO_2$ >70%
- MAP >60 mm Hg (in case of full support with nonpulsatile flow)
- MAP >70 mm Hg (in case of partial support with pulsatile flow)
- Avoid full flow and give partial flow about two-third through ECMO
- Maintain oxygen saturation of 90% or PaO_2 of >50 mm Hg (in young patient) and >60 mm Hg (in elderly and with CAD or CVA)
- Maintain coronary saturation of >70%

Abbreviations: $ScVO_2$, central venous saturation; MAP, mean arterial pressure; CAD, coronary artery disease; CVA, central nervous system vascular accidents.

Extracorporeal Cardiopulmonary Resuscitation

ECMO can also be initiated percutaneously with ongoing CPR, i.e. E-CPR. It aims to restore circulation during cardiac arrest in conjunction with ongoing advanced life support strategies. E-CPR has resulted in improved in-hospital survival free from major neurologic impairment.[24,25] Surgical assistance is not always necessary. Financial implications are difficult to determine due to the complexity of the intervention.

Disadvantages of Intra-Aortic Balloon Pump and Ventricular Assist Devices

ECMO bypasses all the disadvantages of IABP and VAD. In ECMO, optimal gas exchange is possible as lungs are bypassed. It can provide upto 7 L/minute of flow if required. With increasing use of peripheral cannulation techniques, availability of integrated portable pump systems and development of management guidelines has drastically reduced the time required for initiation of ECMO and can be performed bedside. In fact, the time for initiating ECMO is comparable to that required for percutaneous/catheter-directed therapies performed in cardiac catheterization laboratory or hybrid operating rooms.[26,27] A nonrandomized study by Tyara et al. depict survival advantage when mechanical support including ECMO is initiated early in acute MI with cardiogenic shock, as an initial therapy for cardiopulmonary stabilization (in-hospital mortality—33%, 5-year survival—81%) compared to early PCI or coronary artery bypass graft alone (in-hospital mortality—81%, 5-year survival—6.2%).[28] Selection bias, nonrandomization, and variable management protocols were major drawbacks in this study. This study clearly demonstrates that ECMO when used early in carefully selected suitable candidates before the onset of a reversible shock and organ failure can improve outcomes. Early identification and resuscitation is the key for improving outcomes.[17,29] Studies have also demonstrated beneficial role of extracorporeal support for high-risk PCI, particularly in cases of acute cardiogenic shock.[30]

Venoarterial ECMO in acute MI with cardiogenic shock has shown improved in-hospital survival and reduced 30-day mortality in conjunction with revascularization.[31,19] Careful selection of candidates for early initiation of VA-ECMO at first sign of cardiogenic shock provides the greatest chance for survival before development of irreversible multiple end-organ failure.[32,33] This allows for hemodynamic stabilization and optimization of reperfusion via PCI or surgery.

Cardiogenic shock may also occur as part of nonischemic process in the form of fulminant myocarditis and sepsis-associated cardiomyopathy. Patients with fulminant myocarditis stabilized with VA-ECMO have similar outcomes as myocarditis patients without shock.[34]

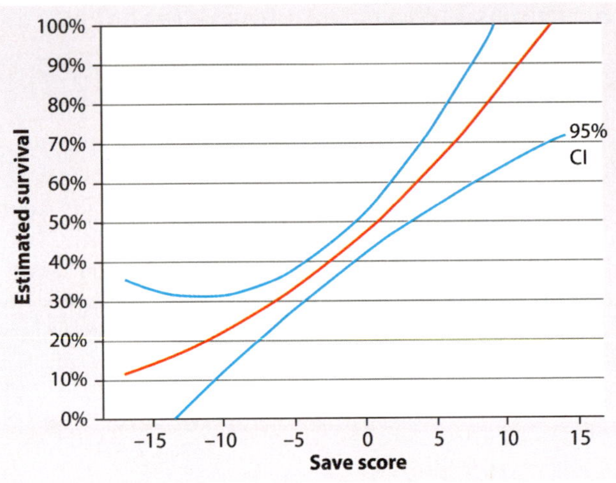

Fig. 5: Survival after venoarterial ECMO (SAVE) score

SURVIVAL AFTER VENOARTERIAL ECMO

The survival after venoarterial ECMO (SAVE) score can help to predict survival for patients receiving ECMO for refractory cardiogenic shock.[17] It should be used in conjunction with clinical assessment and not solely for decision-making for ECMO (Fig. 5).

COMPLICATIONS OF ECMO

- Bleeding (30–60%)—with newer pumps and circuitry, comparatively low levels of anticoagulation may suffice in reducing the incidence of bleeding.
- Neurological complications: These either result from intracranial bleed or emboli in the circuit (clot/air bubble). Overall incidence of stroke is 3–12%.
- Nosocomial infection: 50–60%.
- Mechanical complications due to device failure.
- Multiorgan dysfunction: 33%.
- Others—limb ischemia, hepatic dysfunction, renal dysfunction, hemolysis, and anemia.

NEWER DEVELOPMENTS IN ECMO

Maquet Cardiohelp® system, a portable version has revolutionized the ECMO era. The ease of insertion and increased mobility of patients may permit its use in cardiac catheterization laboratories in future (Figs 6A and B and Box 3).

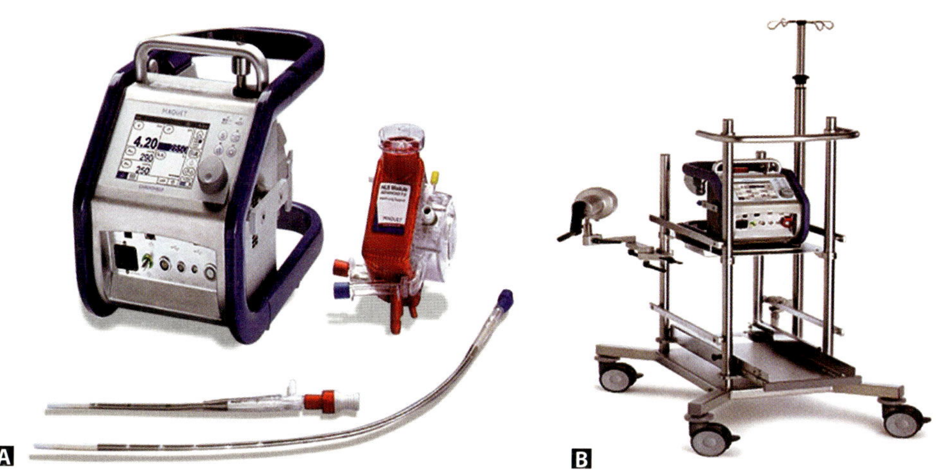

Figs 6A and B: The Cardiohelp from Maquet

Source: Adapted with permission from Kapoor PM. ECMO in STEMI management. In: Chopra HK (Ed). STEMI: A Cardiology Update, 1st edition. New Delhi: Jaypee Brothers Medical Publishers Pvt. Ltd., India; 2014.

BOX 3: Maquet Cardiohelp extracorporeal life support (ECLS)

Smallest commercially available, pump and integrated oxygenator (All in one heart-lung support system)

- Biocompatible surface coatings for optimum protection
- Extracorporeal mechanical circulatory support
- Partial or complete cardiac output
- Support for CO_2 removal and oxygenation
- 10 kg (22 lbs)
- 14 × 10 × 17 inches
- Optional Sprinter Cart for in-hospital mobility

Source: Adapted with permission from Chopra HK, Kapoor PM. Role of extracorporeal membrane oxygenation for acute decompensated heart failure. In: Kapoor PM (Ed). Manual of Extracorporeal Membrane Oxygenation (ECMO) in ICU, 1st edition. New Delhi: Jaypee Brothers Medical Publishers Pvt. Ltd., India; 2014.

CONCLUSION

The availability of ECMO has increased the horizon of therapeutic options available for patients requiring high level of hemodynamic support. Early initiation of ECMO in cases of impaired oxygenation in acute decompensated heart failure or large acute MI requiring revascularization may reduce mortality and morbidity. More randomized controlled trials for testing the efficacy of routine use of ECMO for salvaging the myocardium are needed. Introduction of portable ECMO devices may play an important role in future.

REFERENCES

1. Lowry AW, Morales DL, Graves DE, et al. Characterization of extracorporeal membrane oxygenation for pediatric cardiac arrest in the United States: analysis of the kids' inpatient database. Pediatr Cardiol. 2013;34(6):1422-30.
2. Smedira NG, Moazami N, Golding CM, et al. Clinical experience with 202 adults receiving extracorporeal membrane oxygenation for cardiac failure: survival at five years. J Thorac Cardiovasc Surg. 2001;122(1):92-102.
3. Killip T, Kimball JT. Treatment of myocardial infarction in a coronary care unit. A two-year experience with 250 patients. Am J Cardiol. 1967;20(4):457-64.
4. Goldberg RJ, Gore JM, Alpert JS, et al. Cardiogenic shock after acute myocardial infarction. Incidence and mortality from a community-wide perspective, 1975 to 1988. N Engl J Med. 1991;325(16):1117-22.
5. Tipoo FA, Quraishi AR, Najaf SM, et al. Outcome of cardiogenic shock complicating acute myocardial infarction. J Coll Physicians Surg Pak. 2004;14:6-9.
6. Hochman JS, Boland J, Sleeper LA, et al. Current spectrum of cardiogenic shock and effect of early revascularisation on mortality. Results of an international registry. SHOCK registry investigators. Circulation. 1995;91(3):873-81.
7. Ponikowski P, Voors AA, Anker SD, et al. 2016 ESC Guidelines for the diagnosis and treatment of acute and chronic heart failure: the Task Force for the diagnosis and treatment of acute and chronic heart failure of the European Society of Cardiology (ESC) developed with the special contribution of the Heart Failure Association (HFA) of the ESC. Eur Heart J. 2016;37:2129-200.
8. Bartlett RH, Roloff DM, Custer JR, et al. Extracorporeal life support: the University of Michigan experience. JAMA. 2000;283:904-8.
9. Levine GN, Bates ER, Blankenship JC, et al. 2011 ACCF/AHA/SCAI Guideline for Percutaneous Coronary Intervention: executive summary: a report of the American College of Cardiology Foundation/American Heart Association Task Force on Practice Guidelines and the Society for Cardiovascular Angiography and Interventions. Circulation. 2011;124(23):2574-609.
10. Kannel WB, McGee DL. Diabetes and cardiovascular disease: the Framingham study. JAMA. 1979;241(19):2035-8.
11. Bertoni AG, Tsai A, Kasper EK, et al. Diabetes and idiopathic cardiomyopathy: a nationwide case-control study. Diabetes Care. 2003;26:2791-5.

12. Hamby RI, Zoneraich S, Sherman L. Diabetic cardiomyopathy. JAMA. 1974;229:1749-54.
13. Lind M, Bounias I, Olsson M, et al. Glycaemic control and incidence of heart failure in 20,985 patients with type 1 diabetes: an observational study. Lancet. 2011;378:140-6.
14. Kasznicki J, Drzewoski J. Heart failure in the diabetic population—pathophysiology, diagnosis and treatment. Arch Med Sci. 2014;10:546-56.
15. Rose EA, Gelijins AC, Moskowitz AJ, et al. Long-term use of a left ventricular assist device for end-stage heart failure. N Engl J Med. 2001;345(20):1435-43.
16. Brechot N, Luyt CE, Schmidt M, et al. Venoarterial extracorporeal membrane oxygenation support for refractory cardiovascular dysfunction during severe bacterial septic shock. Crit Care Med. 2013;41(7):1616-26.
17. Rihal CS, Naidu SS, Givertz MM, et al. 2015 SCAI/ACC/HFSA/STS Clinical Expert Consensus Statement on the Use of Percutaneous Mechanical Circulatory Support Devices in Cardiovascular Care. Endorsed by the American Heart Association, the Cardiological Society of India, and Sociedad Latino Americana de Cardiologia Intervencion; Affirmation of Value by the Canadian Association of Interventional Cardiology-Association Canadienne de Cardiologie d'intervention. J Am Coll Cardiol. 2015;65(19):e7-e26.
18. Menees DS, Peterson ED, Wang Y, et al. Door-to-balloon time and mortality among patients undergoing primary PCI. N Engl J Med. 2013;369:901-9.
19. Thiele H, Zeymer U, Neumann F-J, et al. Intraaortic balloon support for myocardial infarction with cardiogenic shock. N Engl J Med. 2012;367:1287-96.
20. Thiele H, Zeymer U, Neumann F-J, et al. Intraaortic balloon counterpulsation in acute myocardial infarction complicated by cardiogenic shock (IABP-SHOCK II): final 12 month results of a randomised, open-label trial. Lancet. 2013;382(9905):1638-45.
21. Norman JC, Cooley DA, Igo SR, et al. Prognostic indices for survival during postcardiotomy intra-aortic balloon pumping. Methods of scoring and classification, with implications for left ventricular assist device utilization. J Thorac Cardiovasc Surg. 1977;74(5):709-20.
22. Myat A, Patel N, Tehrani S, et al. Percutaneous circulatory assist devices for high-risk coronary intervention. JACC Cardiovasc Interv. 2015;8(2):229-44.
23. Vogel RA, Shawl F, Tommaso C, et al. Initial report of the National registry of elective cardiopulmonary bypass supported coronary angioplasty. J Am Coll Cardiol. 1990;15:23-9.
24. Shin TG, Jo IJ, Sim MS, et al. Two-year survival and neurological outcome of in-hospital cardiac arrest patients rescued by extracorporeal cardiopulmonary resuscitation. Int J Cardiol. 2013;168:3424-30.
25. Maekawa K, Tanno K, Hase M, et al. Extracorporeal cardiopulmonary resuscitation for patients with out-of-hospital cardiac arrest of cardiac origin: a propensity-matched study and predictor analysis. Crit Care Med. 2013;41(5):1186-96.
26. Brodie D, Bacchetta M. Extracorporeal membrane oxygenation for ARDS in adults. N Engl J Med. 2011;365(20):1905-14.
27. Arlt M, Philipp A, Voelkel S, et al. Early experiences with miniaturized extracorporeal life-support in the catheterization laboratory. Eur J Cardiothorac Surg. 2012;42:858-63.
28. Tayara W, Starling RC, Yamani MY, et al. Improved survival after acute myocardial infarction complicated by cardiogenic shock with circulatory support and transplantation: comparing aggressive intervention with conservative treatment. J Heart Lung Transplant. 2006;25:504-9.
29. Abrams D, Combes A, Brodie D, et al. Extracorporeal membrane oxygenation in cardiopulmonary disease in adults. J Am Coll Cardiol. 2014;63:2769-78.
30. Spina R, Forrest AP, Adams MR, et al. Veno-arterial extracorporeal membrane oxygenation for high-risk cardiac catheterisation procedures. Heart Lung Circ. 2010;19(2):736-41.
31. Hochman JS, Sleeper LA, Webb JG, et al. Early revascularization in acute myocardial infarction complicated by cardiogenic shock investigators. Should we emergently revascularize occluded coronaries for cardiogenic shock. N Engl J Med. 1999;341: 625-34.
32. Takayama H, Truby L, Koekort M, et al. Clinical outcome of mechanical circulatory support for refractory cardiogenic shock in the current era. J Heart Lung Transplant. 2013;32(1):106-11.
33. Rastan AJ, Dege A, Mohr M, et al. Early and late outcomes of 517 consecutive adult patients treated with extracorporeal membrane oxygenation for refractory postcardiotomy cardiogenic shock. J Thorac Cardiovasc Surg. 2010;139(2):302-11.
34. Asaumi Y, Yasuda S, Morii I, et al. Favourable clinical outcome in patients with cardiogenic shock due to fulminant myocarditis supported by percutaneous extracorporeal membrane oxygenation. Eur Heart J. 2005;26(20):2185-92.

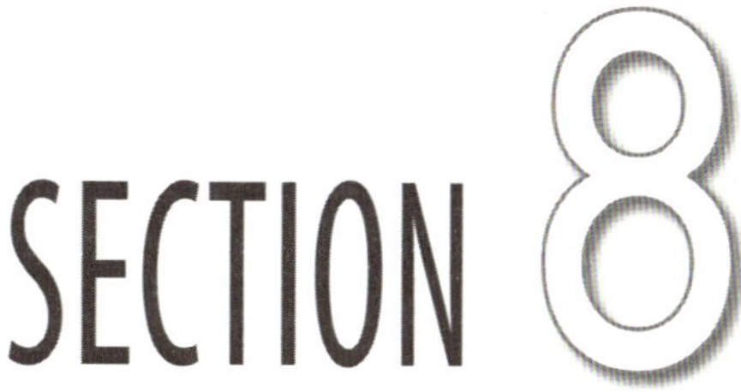

SECTION 8

Rehabilitation

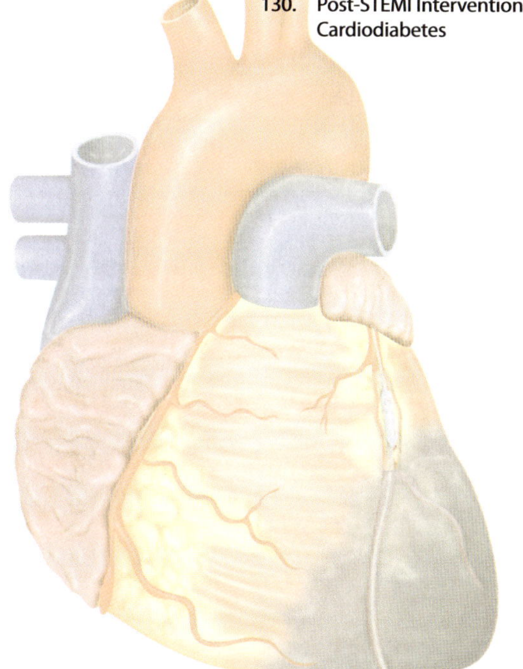

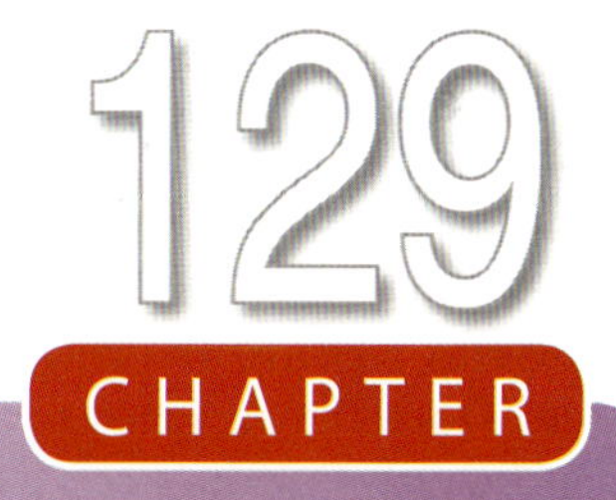

Cardiac Rehabilitation in Cardiodiabetes

Aashish Contractor, Sagri Negi

INTRODUCTION

Coronary heart disease (CHD) is a major cause of mortality and morbidity in India.[1] The reported prevalence of CHD in Indian adults has risen four-fold over the last 40 years (to a present level of around 10%), and even in rural areas the prevalence has doubled over the past 30 years (to a present level of around 4%).[2] Within the spectrum of CHD, Myocardial infarction (MI) is the leading cause of death. A study by Sharma et al. (2014) in Karnataka found that MI was the most common presentation amongst 1,562 patients having acute coronary syndrome and that the mean age of occurrence of acute coronary syndrome was approximately a decade lower than that of Western population.[3] Eight factors that accounted for 89% of all acute MI in Indians in the INTERHEART-South Asia study were: abnormal lipids, smoking, hypertension, diabetes, abdominal obesity, psychosocial factors, low fruit and vegetable consumption, and lack of physical activity.[4]

For those who survive a CHD event, the prevention of subsequent coronary events and the maintenance of physical functioning are the major challenges.[5,6] Cardiac rehabilitation is an essential component of the continuum of care for patients with CHD.[6-9] The American Health Association (AHA) and the American College of Cardiology (ACC) endorse cardiac rehabilitation/secondary prevention programs to treat patients with CHD.[10-12]

WHAT IS CARDIAC REHABILITATION?

The AHA adopted the definition by Taylor et al. (2004) for cardiac rehabilitation in their scientific statement on cardiac rehabilitation and secondary prevention of coronary health disease,[6] i.e. 'cardiac rehabilitation refers to coordinated, multifaceted interventions designed to optimize a cardiac patient's physical, psychological, and social functioning, in addition to stabilizing, slowing, or even reversing the progression of the underlying atherosclerotic processes, thereby reducing morbidity and mortality.'[13] Key components of cardiac rehabilitation programs are evaluation of medical status, nutritional counseling, blood pressure and lipid management, lifestyle modification through counseling (tobacco cessation etc.), and physical activity counseling and plan.[8] These programs have been designed to decrease risk of mortality and/or recurrence of a cardiac event and to have positive effects on a patient's physiological and psychological make-up.[14] Cardiac rehabilitation is prescribed for patients who have had MI, coronary artery bypass graft (CABG) surgery, chronic stable angina pectoris, percutaneous transluminal coronary angioplasty (PTCA), cardiomyopathy, heart failure, heart transplantation, and for all patients diagnosed with CHD. Cardiac rehabilitation services are a continuum of care delivered in three phases, beginning during hospitalization (Phase I), followed by a supervised ambulatory outpatient program lasting 3–6 months (Phase II), and continuing in a lifetime maintenance stage (Phase III).

Inpatient Cardiac Rehabilitation

After a MI or any revascularization, the key focus is to mobilize the patient as soon as he/she is clinically stable.[15] A patient is considered stable if there is no new or recurrent chest pain in the past eight hours; creatine kinase and/or troponin levels are not rising; no new signs of uncompensated heart failure and no new significant, abnormal rhythm or ECG changes in the past eight hours. Once the patient is stable, he should be made to sit at the edge of the bed during the first day, and then gradually mobilized throughout the hospital stay. During mobilization the goal should be to keep the heart rate below 120 beats/min, or if the patient has a high resting heart rate, then the goal should be to keep the heart rate within 20 beats above resting heart rate (within 30 beats for post-CABG surgery patients). The patient should be made to walk within the room at first, and then in the corridors for about 2–5 minutes, three to four times a day. Progression of activity depends on the initial assessment as well as the daily assessment of the patient and may vary from a rapid increase in activity tolerance in the low-risk patient (uncomplicated MI or a patient without left ventricular dysfunction) to a slower progression in higher risk or more debilitated patients, such as those with heart failure.[16]

The goals of inpatient rehabilitation are to assist the patient in becoming ambulatory; to prepare the patient and family to cope with the psychological and emotional stress that accompanies a coronary event; and to educate the patient about coronary risk factor modification. The guidelines for patient mobilization for inpatient cardiac rehabilitation are enlisted in Table 1.

Outpatient Cardiac Rehabilitation

The outpatient program can be begun once the patient has left hospital and has clearance from his/her physician. Depending on the patient's clinical condition postevent, the outpatient program is typically begun 2–4 weeks after the event. Cardiac rehabilitation programs were first developed in the 1960s, once the benefits of ambulation during prolonged hospitalization for coronary events had been recognized. Safety of discharged patients while exercising unsupervised was the leading motivation behind development of physician-supervised structured rehabilitation programs which included electrocardiographic monitoring.[5] The focus of these programs was almost exclusively on exercise.[17] A meta-analysis based on a review of 48 randomized trials ($n = 8,940$) that compared outcomes of exercise-based rehabilitation with usual medical care, showed a reduction of 20% in total mortality and 26% in cardiac mortality rates, with exercise-based rehabilitation compared with usual medical care.[13] Over time, cardiac rehabilitation programs have evolved, to comprehensive cardiovascular risk reduction programs, with exercise being an integral component of the program, but not the only component. Since, hospital stays for MI and revascularization has dramatically decreased over time, it has reduced opportunities for in-hospital risk factor interventions. Outpatient cardiac rehabilitation programs have gradually broadened their scope to become an important avenue for secondary prevention.[5]

TABLE 1: Patient mobilization guidelines for inpatient cardiac rehabilitation

S. No.	Exercise parameters	Guidelines
1.	Frequency	Early mobilization: 2–4 times per day
2.	Intensity	Post-MI: Maintain heart rate (HR) less than 120 beats/min or HR at rest + 20 beats/min Post CABG surgery: HR at rest + 30 beats/min Rate of perceived exertion (RPE) < 13 on a 6–20 Borg scale
3.	Type	Walking
4.	Duration	Intermittent bouts lasting 2–5 minutes

Abbreviation: CABG, coronary artery bypass graft

COMPONENTS OF CARDIAC REHABILITATION

A comprehensive cardiac rehabilitation program should aim to identify each patient's risk factors, establish risk reduction goals and then help the patient to achieve these goals through lifestyle modification, supervised exercise, and medications. Table 2 lists the major risk factors, their evaluation, goals values, and suggested intervention. For maximum efficacy the program staff should coordinate their efforts with the patient's personal physician.

Physical Activity/Exercise

World Health Organization (WHO)[18] and National Institutes of Health (NIH)[19] use the following definitions of physical activity and exercise respectively, 'bodily movement produced by skeletal muscle that requires energy expenditure and promotes health benefits.' and 'planned, structured, and repetitive bodily movement done to improve or maintain one or more components of physical fitness.' Over the years research has shown that an increase in leisure time physical activity, as well as structured exercise training play an important role in reducing CHD mortality.[20]

Exercise Prescription

A comprehensive exercise prescription for the cardiac patient includes activities performed in formal supervised programs as well as everyday physical activities. The exercise program should prescribe the appropriate mode, frequency, intensity, and duration of exercise which should

TABLE 2: Comprehensive risk reduction guidelines for patients with coronary heart disease (CHD)

	Criteria	*Guidelines*
1.	Lipid management	
1.1	Evaluation	• Obtain fasting measures of total cholesterol, HDL, LDL, and triglycerides • Repeat lipid profiles at 4–6 weeks after hospitalization and at 2 months after initiation of, or change in lipid-lowering medications
1.2	Goal	• Primary goal: LDL < 100 mg/dL; further reduction of LDL < 70 mg/dL is reasonable • Secondary goals: HDL > 40 mg/dL, total cholesterol < 200 mg/dL, triglycerides < 150 mg/dL
1.3	Intervention	• In patients with LDL > 100 mg/dL, provide nutritional counseling and weight management; consider adding drug therapy. Statins are the drug of choice unless contraindicated • In patients with HDL < 40 mg/dL, emphasize exercise, smoking cessation, and consider targeted drug therapy
2.	*Hypertension management*	
2.1	Evaluation	• Measurement of resting BP on two or more visits • Assess current treatment and compliance
2.2	Goal	• Optimal BP is < 120/80 mm Hg
2.3	Intervention	• For patients with systolic BP ≥ 130 mm Hg or diastolic BP ≥ 85 mm Hg initiate lifestyle modification (including exercise, weight management, moderate sodium restriction, alcohol moderation, and smoking cessation). Add drug therapy for patients with diabetes, heart failure, or renal failure • For patients with systolic BP ≥ 140 mm Hg or diastolic BP ≥ 90 mm Hg initiate lifestyle modification and drug therapy.
3.	Diabetes management	
3.1	Evaluation	• Obtain fasting plasma glucose measurements in all patients and HbA1C in diabetic patients to monitor therapy.
3.2	Goal	• Near normal fasting plasma glucose(< 100 mg/dL)and near normal HbA1C (<7)
3.3	Intervention	• Appropriate hypoglycemic therapy (including weight control, exercise, and if needed oral hypoglycemic agents and/or insulin) • Monitor glucose levels before and/or after exercise sessions. Instruct patient regarding identification and treatment of post exercise hypoglycemia. Exercise with caution if blood glucose > 300 mg/dL (evaluate for urine ketones as well), after consulting with a physician
4.	Smoking/Tobacco	
4.1	Evaluation	• Document smoking and/or tobacco consumption habits in detail including amount and duration • Assess the readiness to change on the part of the patient
4.2	Goal	• Complete cessation
4.3	Intervention	• Provide individual education and counseling. Encourage patient to quit at each and every visit • Provide nicotine replacement and pharmacological therapy as appropriate
5.	Weight management	
5.1	Evaluation	• Measure weight, height, and waist circumference. Calculate body mass index (BMI)
5.2	Goal	• BMI 21–25 kg/m^2, waist < 35 inches in men and < 31 inches in women
5.3	Intervention	• For patients who do not meet the goal criteria, advice a reduction in total caloric intake, and increase in energy expenditure through a combined program of diet, and exercise • The initial goal of weight loss therapy should be to reduce body weight by approximately 10% from baseline. With success, further weight loss can be attempted, if indicated
6.	Psychosocial management	
6.1	Evaluation	• Identify patients with clinically significant depression, anxiety, anger, and substance abuse
6.2	Goal	• To minimize the patient's psychosocial distress
6.3	Intervention	• Stress management and individual or group education to help the patient adjust to his/her disease • When needed, refer the patient to appropriate mental health specialists for further treatment

Abbreviations: HDL, high-density lipoprotein; LDL, low-density lipoprotein; BP, blood pressure

Source: Adapted from references 8 and 28.

be tailored to the individual's cardiovascular and general medical status. However, there are some patients for whom exercise is contraindicated as listed in Table 3.

A summary of the exercise prescription is given in Table 4. After 2–4 weeks of participation in a traditional aerobic exercise program, low to moderate risk patients should

TABLE 3: Contraindications for exercise in outpatient cardiac rehabilitation[10]

S. No.	Contraindications
1.	Unstable angina
2.	Resting systolic BP (SBP) > 200 mm Hg or resting diastolic BP (DBP) > 110 mm Hg that should be evaluated on a case by case basis
3.	Orthostatic BP drop of > 20 mm Hg with symptoms
4.	Critical aortic stenosis (i.e. peak SBP gradient of > 50 mm Hg with an aortic valve orifice area of < 0.75 cm^2 in an average-size adult
5.	Acute systemic illness or fever
6.	Uncontrolled atrial or ventricular dysrhythmias
7.	Uncontrolled sinus tachycardia (> 120 beats per min)
8.	Uncompensated CHF
9.	Third-degree atrioventricular (AV) block without pacemaker
10.	Active pericarditis or myocarditis
11.	Recent Embolism
12.	Thrombophlebitis
13.	Resting ST-segment depression or elevation (> 2 mm)
14.	Uncontrolled diabetes mellitus
15.	Severe orthopedic conditions that would prohibit exercise
16.	Other metabolic conditions such as acute thyroiditis, hypokalemia, hyperkalemia or hypovolemia

Source: American College of Sports Medicine's Guidelines for Exercise Testing and Prescription.

TABLE 4: Summary of aerobic exercise and resistance training recommendations for patients with coronary heart disease (CHD)

S. No.	Exercise parameters	Guidelines
1.	Frequency	Aerobic: Structured exercise 3–5 days per week (lifestyle physical activity daily) Resistance: 2–3 days per week
2.	Intensity	Aerobic: 60–85% of HRmax (Predicted HRmax = 220 – age of person). Resistance: Moderate (avoid breath holding and excessive straining)
3.	Type	Aerobic: Walking, running, cycling, swimming, etc. Resistance: Hand weights, elastic bands, machine weights
4.	Duration	Aerobic: 20–60 minutes Resistance: 10–15 repetitions; 3 sets of 8–10 different exercises for both upper and lower body
5.	Special considerations	Monitor for abnormal signs and symptoms, i.e., chest pain or pressure, dizziness, and dysrhythmias High-intensity exercise may precipitate cardiovascular complications in post-MI patients. Patients with stable angina should always carry nitroglycerin and be educated in its use Heart rate guidelines may not be applicable to patients taking drugs, which slow down the heart rate, e.g. beta-blockers Lift weights through a full range of motion and avoiding breath-holding

initiate resistance training that is prescribed by a physician and supervised by trained personnel. Resistance training increases muscular strength and endurance, functional capacity and independence as well as reducing disability. Those who have had CABG surgery should consult with their surgeon, before lifting heavy weights, since it takes a few months for complete sternal healing. Light resistance training, using resistance bands and hand weights can be begun, along with initiation of the aerobic exercise program.

Prescribed and supervised resistance training enhances muscular strength and endurance, functional capacity and independence, and quality of life while reducing disability in persons with CHD.[21] Both endurance and strength training can elicit substantial increases in physical fitness. Table 5 summarizes many of these benefits and attempts to weigh them according to the current literature. Endurance training induces greater improvements in aerobic capacity and associated cardiopulmonary and metabolic variables and more effectively modifies CHD risk factors. Resistance training enhances muscular strength, endurance, and muscle mass to a greater extent.[21]

Nutrition Counseling

It is necessary to assess the dietary habits of the patient to obtain an estimate of total caloric intake, as well as daily consumption of saturated fat, cholesterol, sodium, and other nutrients. Patients should be recommended a diet low to moderate in fat (especially saturated fat), and include a good amount of fruits and vegetables.[8] As a general guidelines the diet should consist of 50–60% calories from carbohydrates, up to 30% from fat (with saturated fat forming 10% or less), and 10–15% from protein. Individualized plans should be formulated depending on the presence of risk factors such as diabetes, hypertension, and hypercholesterolemia. Nutrition guidelines are undergoing reevaluation with the role of fats in causation of CHD being debated, but as of present, the majority of evidence supports these recommendations.

Psychosocial Rehabilitation

After a CHD event, some of the common psychological reactions that patients may experience are: low mood, tearfulness, sleep disturbance, irritability, anxiety, acute awareness of minor somatic sensations or pains, poor concentration, and memory. The patients should be made aware of the normality and universality of these symptoms as a part of the process of recovery from a life-threatening event.[14]

Psychological factors are strong risk factors for CHD and adversely affect recovery after major CHD events.[22] Besides depression, anxiety, hostility, and psychosocial stress may also be significant CHD risk factors.[23] Studies

TABLE 5: Comparison of effects of aerobic endurance training with strength training on health and fitness variables[11]

S. No.	Variable	Aerobic exercise	Resistance exercise
1.	Body composition		
1.1	Bone mineral density	↑↑	↑↑
1.2	Percent body fat	↓↓	↓
1.3	Lean body mass	0	↑↑
1.4	Muscle strength	0↑	↑↑↑
2.	Glucose metabolism		
2.1	Insulin response to glucose challenge	↓↓	↓↓
2.2	Basal insulin levels	↓	↓
2.3	Insulin sensitivity	↑↑	↑↑
3.	Plasma lipids and lipoproteins		
3.1	HDL cholesterol	↑0	↑0
3.2	LDL cholesterol	↓0	↓0
3.3	Triglycerides	↓↓	↓0
4.	Cardiovascular dynamics		
4.1	Resting heart rate	↓↓	0
4.2	Stroke volume, resting and maximal	↑↑	0
4.3	Cardiac output, rest	0	0
4.4	Cardiac output, maximal	↑↑	0
4.5	SBP at rest	↓0	0
4.6	DBP at rest	↓0	0
4.7	VO_2max	↑↑↑	↑0
4.8	Submaximal and maximal endurance time	↑↑↑	↑↑
4.9	Submaximal exercise rate-pressure product	↓↓↓	↓↓
4.10	Basal metabolic rate	↑0	↑
5.	Health-related quality of life	↑0	↑0

Note: ↑ Indicates values increase; ↓, values decrease; 0, values remain unchanged; 1 arrow, small effect; 2 arrows, moderate effect; 3 arrows, large effect.

Abbreviations: HDL, high-density lipoprotein cholesterol; LDL, low-density lipoprotein cholesterol

Source: Adapted from Williams MA, Haskell WL, Ades PA, et al. Resistance exercise in individuals with and without cardiovascular disease: 2007 Update. Circulation. 2007;116(5):572-84.

have demonstrated reductions of between 40% and 70% in the prevalence of depression, anxiety, and hostility after cardiac rehabilitation as well as a 70% reduction in the risk of mortality amongst depressed patients.[23,24] It has been found that only small improvements in exercise capacity may produce profound improvements in depression and depression-related mortality.[19,24,25]

SAFETY

Risk stratification helps identify patients who are at increased risk for exercise-related cardiovascular events and who may require more intensive cardiac monitoring in addition to the medical supervision provided for all cardiac rehabilitation program participants.[6] Risk stratification schema are essential for optimizing patient management and minimizing potential risk.[8]

Cardiac rehabilitation programs that are directed by the physician and supervised by trained medical staff are well-established for their relative safety.[6] The occurrence of major cardiovascular events during supervised exercise ranges from 1/50,000 to 1/120,000 patient-hours of exercise, with only two fatalities reported per 1.5 million patient-hours of exercise.[26]

RETURN TO WORK

Although improvement in functional capacity and the associated reduction in cardio-respiratory symptoms may enhance a cardiac patient's ability to return to work, factors unrelated to physical fitness appear to have a greater influence on whether a patient returns to work after a cardiac event. These include socioeconomic and worksite-related issues and previous employment status. The educational and vocational counseling components of cardiac rehabilitation programs should further improve the ability of a patient to return to work.[6] Therefore, the time to return to work, after an MI can vary greatly from about 2 weeks, to upward of 6 weeks.[27-29]

CONCLUSION

Despite available evidence, and the Class I recommendation by the AHA and ACC, participation rates in cardiac rehabilitation are very low worldwide. A systematic review of the literature revealed that participation rates vary between 21% and 75%, but are usually less than 50%.[30,31] This type of analysis has not been performed in India. In India, most programs are performed at the hospital during phase I. However, subsequent phase II programs have not gained widespread acceptance due to various feasibility issues. Nevertheless, there are few reports of institution based and home-based cardiac rehabilitation programs for those with CHD, and their numbers are increasing steadily.[32]

REFERENCES

1. Institute for Health Metrics and Evaluation. (2016). GBD India Country Profile. [online]. Available from http://www.healthdata.org/india. [Accessed October, 2017].
2. Reddy KS. India wakes up to the threat of cardiovascular diseases. J Am Coll Cardiol. 2007;50(14):1370-2.
3. Sharma R, Bhairappa S, Prasad S, et al. Clinical characteristics, angiographic profile and in hospital mortality in acute coronary syndrome patients in south Indian population. Heart India. 2014;2(3):65-9.

4. Yusuf S, Hawken S, Ounpuu S, et al. Effect of potentially modifiable risk factors associated with myocardial infarction in 52 countries (the INTERHEART study): case-control study. Lancet. Lond Engl. 2004;364(9438):937-52.
5. Ades PA. Cardiac rehabilitation and secondary prevention of coronary heart disease. N Engl J Med. 2001;345(12):892-902.
6. Leon AS, Franklin BA, Costa F, et al. Cardiac rehabilitation and secondary prevention of coronary heart disease. Circulation. 2005;111(3):369-76.
7. Wenger NK, Froelicher ES, Smith LK, et al. Cardiac rehabilitation as secondary prevention. Agency for Health Care Policy and Research and National Heart, Lung, and Blood Institute. Clin Pract Guidel Quick Ref Guide Clin. 1995;17:1-23.
8. Balady GJ, Williams MA, Ades PA, et al. Core components of cardiac rehabilitation/secondary prevention programs: 2007 update: a scientific statement from the American Heart Association Exercise, Cardiac Rehabilitation, and Prevention Committee, the Council on Clinical Cardiology; the Councils on Cardiovascular Nursing, Epidemiology and Prevention, and Nutrition, Physical Activity, and Metabolism; and the American Association of Cardiovascular and Pulmonary Rehabilitation. Circulation. 2007;115(20):2675-82.
9. Mishra S, Ramakrishnan S, Babu AS, et al. Management algorithms for acute ST elevation myocardial infarction in less industrialized world. Indian Heart J. 2017;69(Suppl 1):S98-103.
10. Antman EM, Anbe DT, Armstrong PW, et al. ACC/AHA guidelines for the management of patients with ST-elevation myocardial infarction: executive summary: a report of the American College of Cardiology/American Heart Association Task Force on Practice Guidelines (Committee to Revise the 1999 Guidelines for the Management of Patients with Acute Myocardial Infarction). Circulation. 2004;110(9):e82-292.
11. Braunwald E, Antman EM, Beasley JW, et al. ACC/AHA guidelines for the management of patients with unstable angina and non-ST-segment elevation myocardial infarction: executive summary and recommendations. A report of the American College of Cardiology/American Heart Association task force on practice guidelines (committee on the management of patients with unstable angina). Circulation. 2000;102(10):1193-209.
12. Gibbons RJ, Abrams J, Chatterjee K, et al. ACC/AHA 2002 guideline update for the management of patients with chronic stable angina–summary article: a report of the American College of Cardiology/American Heart Association Task Force on Practice Guidelines (Committee on the Management of Patients With Chronic Stable Angina). Circulation. 2003;107(1):149-58.
13. Taylor RS, Brown A, Ebrahim S, et al. Exercise-based rehabilitation for patients with coronary heart disease: systematic review and meta-analysis of randomized controlled trials. Am J Med. 2004;116(10):682-92.
14. Thompson D, Lewin R. Management of the post-myocardial infarction patient: rehabilitation and cardiac neurosis. Heart. 2000;84(1):101-5.
15. Guha S, Sethi R, Ray S, et al. Cardiological Society of India: position statement for the management of ST elevation myocardial infarction in India. Indian Heart J. 2017;69(Suppl 1):S63-97.
16. American Association of Cardiovascular & Pulmonary Rehabilitation. Guidelines for cardiac rehabilitation and secondary prevention programs. Illinois: Human Kinetics; 2004. pp. 294.
17. Pashkow FJ. Issues in contemporary cardiac rehabilitation: a historical perspective. J Am Coll Cardiol. 1993;21(3):822-34.
18. WHO. (2016). Physical Activity-Global Strategy on Diet, Physical Activity and Health. [online] Available from: http://www.who.int/dietphysicalactivity/pa/en/. [Accessed October, 2017].
19. NIH. Physical activity and cardiovascular health: NIH consensus development panel on physical activity and cardiovascular health. JAMA. 1996;276(3):241-6.
20. Wen CP, Wai JP, Tsai MK, et al. Minimum amount of physical activity for reduced mortality and extended life expectancy: a prospective cohort study. Lancet. 2011;378(9798):1244-53.
21. Williams MA, Haskell WL, Ades PA, et al. Resistance exercise in individuals with and without cardiovascular disease: 2007 update. Circulation. 2007;116(5):572-84.
22. Lavie CJ, Milani RV, Artham SM, et al. Psychological factors and cardiac risk and impact of exercise training programs—a review of Ochsner studies. Ochsner J. 2007;7(4):167-72.
23. Lavie CJ, Thomas RJ, Squires RW, et al. Exercise training and cardiac rehabilitation in primary and secondary prevention of coronary heart disease. Mayo Clin Proc. 2009;84(4):373-83.
24. Milani RV, Lavie CJ. Impact of cardiac rehabilitation on depression and its associated mortality. Am J Med. 2007;120(9):799-806.
25. Lichtman JH, Bigger JT, Blumenthal JA, et al. Depression and coronary heart disease: recommendations for screening, referral, and treatment: a science advisory from the American Heart Association Prevention Committee of the Council on Cardiovascular Nursing, Council on Clinical Cardiology, Council on Epidemiology and Prevention, and Interdisciplinary Council on Quality of Care and Outcomes Research: endorsed by the American Psychiatric Association. Circulation. 2008;118(17):1768-75.
26. Franklin BA, Bonzheim K, Gordon S, et al. Safety of medically supervised outpatient cardiac rehabilitation exercise therapy: a 16-year follow-up. Chest. 1998;114(3):902-6.
27. Witt BJ, Jacobsen SJ, Weston SA, et al. Cardiac rehabilitation after myocardial infarction in the community. J Am Coll Cardiol. 2004;44(5):988-96.
28. Smith SC, Allen J, Blair SN, et al. AHA/ACC guidelines for secondary prevention for patients with coronary and other atherosclerotic vascular disease: 2006 update. Circulation. 2006;113(19):2363-72.
29. ACSM. American College of Sports Medicine's Guidelines for Exercise Testing and Prescription. Philadelphia: Lippincott Williams & Wilkins; 2010.
30. Cooper AF, Jackson G, Weinman J, et al. Factors associated with cardiac rehabilitation attendance: a systematic review of the literature. Clin Rehabil. 2002;16:541.
31. Neubeck L, Freedman B, Clark AM, et al. Participating in cardiac rehabilitation: a systematic review and metasynthesis of qualitative data. Eur J Prev Cardiol. 2012;19(3):494-503.
32. Madan K, Babu AS, Contractor A, et al. Cardiac rehabilitation in India. Prog Cardiovasc Dis. 2014;56(5):543-50.

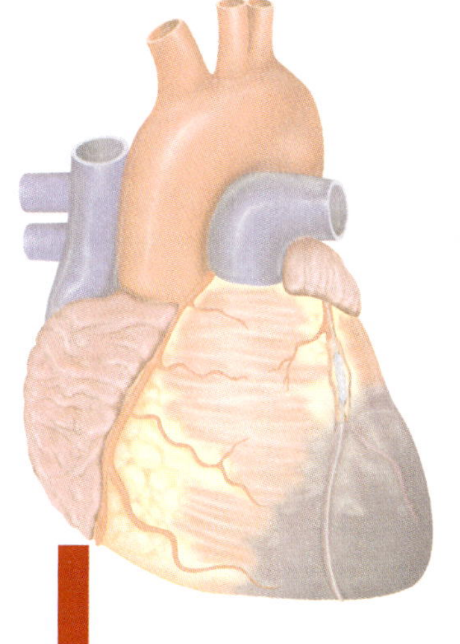

Post-STEMI Intervention: Rehabilitation in Cardiodiabetes

JPS Sawhney, Kushal Madan, Simran Sawhney

INTRODUCTION

Cardiac rehabilitation (CR) is a medically supervised multidisciplinary program of exercise and education designed to assist patients with cardiovascular diseases to achieve optimal physical, psychological and functional status. In 1993, World Health Organization defined cardiac rehabilitation as "The rehabilitation of cardiac patients is the sum of activities required to influence favorably the underlying cause of the disease, as well as to ensure the patients best possible physical, mental and social conditions so that they may, by their own efforts, preserve, or resume when lost, as normal a place as possible in the life of the community. Rehabilitation cannot be regarded as an isolated form of therapy, but must be integrated with the whole treatment, of which it forms only a facet." [1] that means a cardiac rehabilitation program includes: Education of the patient and family in the recognition, prevention, and treatment of cardiovascular disease, helping the patient modify risk factors such as high blood pressure, high blood cholesterol, physical inactivity, diabetes and obesity, beginning an exercise program tailored according to the abilities and needs of the patient, counseling on nutrition and also guidance to enable the patient to return to work. Cardiac rehabilitation is primarily indicated for patients who have received a diagnosis of acute myocardial infarction, have undergone coronary revascularization, or have chronic stable angina.[2,3] Cardiac rehabilitation with exercise training after myocardial infarction (MI) significantly reduces cardiovascular morbidity and mortality,[4] and CR is recommended as class 1 in most cardiovascular clinical practice guidelines.[5] Patients with type 2 diabetes mellitus (T2DM) have a 2–4 times higher risk of cardiovascular disease, particularly coronary artery disease (CAD), than nondiabetic patients.[6] Type 2 diabetes mellitus doubles mortality due to a cardiovascular event, even after adjustment for other cardiovascular risk factors.[7] In addition, prognosis after MI is worse in diabetic patients than in nondiabetic subjects.[8-11] Due to their high cardiovascular risk, patients with type 2 diabetes are highly recommended for cardiac rehabilitation. Cardiovascular rehabilitation through exercise training helps diabetic patients to improve their reduced post-MI exercise capacity.[12-14] The World Health Organization has declared that diabetes mellitus (DM) is a major public health issue, and that it is necessary to implement health education measures, given that there are predicted to be 366 million diabetic individuals worldwide by 2030.[15] Of patients referred for CR, 20–30% has DM[16] but few studies have assessed the efficacy of CR specifically in diabetic patients, even though CR may be especially valuable in this patient population. Although diabetes is associated with a high cardiovascular risk, very little information is available about diabetic patients enrolled in cardiac rehabilitation.

EVIDENCE

Aerobic training, which forms a primary component of CR, is especially beneficial to patients with diabetes. Aerobic exercise improves insulin action, blood glucose control, and fat oxidation and storage in the muscle in people with diabetes.[17] There have been inconsistencies in the studies comparing improvement in exercise capacity after post-MI cardiovascular rehabilitation in DM and non-DM patients. Previous studies demonstrated that the effect of CR was lower among DM than in non-DM patients in relation to exercise capacity after acute ischemic heart disease.[18] Some studies have reported similar benefits and similar degrees of exercise capacity improvement in DM and non-DM patients after cardiovascular rehabilitation.[12] In a study conducted on coronary heart disease patients including 413 patients with DM and 614 patients with non-DM before and after a 6 week multidisciplinary cardiac rehabilitation program, it was shown that DM patients with coronary heart disease had a higher prevalence of cardiovascular disease risk factors (hypertension, hypercholesterolemia, hypertriglyceridemia, obesity, excess abdominal fat, and depression) as well as lower physical capacity than non-DM (NDM) patients at the beginning of rehabilitation. The extent of the improvement was similar in DM and NDM patients.[19] Madssen et al. [20] reported that exercise capacity stayed constant without significant change in patients who continued with community-based self-exercise for a year after the post-MI hospital-based CR compared with the patients who completed only the hospital-based rehabilitation. In a prospective study consisting of 682 patients (253 diabetic and 429 nondiabetic), diagnosed with ischemic heart disease referred for a cardiac rehabilitation program, patients were assessed at the beginning of phase II and 3 months later. It was shown that diabetic patients were significantly older, had a worse cardiovascular risk profile (higher prevalence of overweight, dyslipidemia, hypertension and sedentary lifestyle) and lower functional capacity. At the end of phase II, there was a statistically significant improvement ($p < 0.05$) in all risk factors and functional capacity, which was similar in both groups, except for body mass index, triglycerides and functional capacity.[21]

Kim et al. investigated the long-term outcomes of CR on exercise capacity in DM and non-DM patients with MI. Exercise capacity of 37 patients (12 with DM and 25 without DM) was measured before and after hospital-based CR and 1 year after the onset of MI. Before the CR, the DM group had significantly lower exercise capacity in exercise times, peak oxygen consumption (VO2peak), and metabolic equivalent tasks (METs) than did the non-DM group. After the CR, both groups showed significantly improved exercise capacity, but the DM group had significantly lower exercise capacity in exercise times, submaximal rate pressure products (RPPsubmax), VO2peak, and METs. One year after the onset of the MI, the DM group had significantly lower exercise capacity in exercise times, RPPsubmax, and VO2peak than did the non-DM group, but both groups maintained their improved exercise capacity following hospital-based CR.[22] In another study aimed to investigate patients of metabolic syndrome who were referred to cardiac rehabilitation after myocardial revascularization following a ST elevation of MI concluded patients with and without metabolic syndrome benefited substantially from the participation in cardiac rehabilitation, as their lipid profile, blood pressure, and physical fitness improved.[23] Treatment effects were similar in the two groups.

STRUCTURE OF CARDIAC REHABILITATION

Phase 1: This phase refers to the inpatient cardiac rehabilitation program comprising mainly of early mobilization and patient education. Nowadays because of the shorter duration of hospital stay, these programs are uncommon but remain useful in mobilizing patients after coronary artery bypass graft (CABG), elderly patients after ST-elevation myocardial infarction or sicker patients with complications. This is routinely carried out by trained physiotherapists or dedicated cardiac rehabilitation staff. During hospitalization there is an educational class for all appropriate surgical and medical patients. During this session, patients and their family members are taught about the causes, risk factors and management of CAD. Inpatient rehabilitation programs also assist the patients and family in coping with the psychological stress that accompanies such coronary event. Phase I service is usually included in the package charges for the acute event.

Phase 2: It is a supervised exercise based outpatient program in the post discharge period. Patients exercise for 3–4 times/week for a total of 36 sessions over 3–4 months. Many patients who do not attend supervised exercise training program should be advised about home-based, unsupervised exercises to the onset of mild dyspnea. Nowadays home-based telephonically monitored electrocardiogram (ECG) based exercise programs have been researched with standard supervised programs and found to be favorable in research settings. Medicare in the Unites States routinely covers for a total of 36 exercise sessions for patients who have suffered acute MI or have undergone CABG or PTCA.

Phase 3: It is a non-supervised, non-ECG monitored maintenance program at least 6 months after the cardiovascular event. During this phase exercise prescription becomes closer to that recommended for the healthy adult. It is generally used to maintain the results achieved during the earlier phases of rehabilitation.

PRE-EXERCISE HYPOGLYCEMIA CARE[24]

- Assess patient for individual risks for low blood glucose: medication use, time and content of last meal or snack.
- Assess patient level of understanding and discuss signs and symptoms of low blood glucose and treatment if needed.
- Patients using insulin or oral agents that increase the risk of hypoglycemia should maintain blood glucose levels during exercise at 100 mg/dL or higher.
- Blood glucose should be taken immediately before exercise.
- Increase or maintain appropriate blood glucose levels during exercise by eating a meal or snack of 15 g carbohydrate with some fat and protein before exercising.
- Individual blood glucose targets should be set.
- Every effort should be made to set appropriate blood glucose targets to prevent hypoglycemia from interfering with the exercise session and performance.

POST-EXERCISE HYPOGLYCEMIA CARE[24]

- Glycemic goal post-exercise should be individualized.
- Blood glucose should be taken within 15 minutes after exercise.
- A post-exercise blood glucose goal of 100 mg/dL or higher can be used to discharge an asymptomatic patient until a blood glucose pattern and response have been established.
- Encourage patients to test blood glucose frequently after exercise to be aware of the potential for a hypoglycemic response that can last 24–48 hours after exercise session.
- Carbohydrate snacks to prevent hypoglycemia may contain some protein, fat or both; carbohydrate snacks to treat hypoglycemia are rapidly digested and absorbed if they are pure carbohydrate to prevent hypoglycemia during extended activity, a snack of 15 to 30 g carbohydrate should be eaten for every 30–60 minutes of physical activity.

HYPOGLYCEMIA: POINTS FOR CONSIDERATION[24]

- Treatment of hypoglycemia requires ingestion of glucose-or-carbohydrate containing foods.
- The '15 g of a rapidly digested carbohydrate, wait for 15 minutes' rule, that is giving 15–20 g of a rapidly digested carbohydrate for the conscious individual with hypoglycemia; if blood glucose 15 minutes after treatment shows continued hypoglycemia, the treatment should be repeated; once blood glucose returns to normal, the individual should consume a meal or snack to prevent recurrence of hypoglycemia.
- Examples of 15 g glucose: ½ cup of fruit juice, 1 cup of milk, 5 or 6 pieces of hard candy.

There are a number of precautions and special instructions for exercise in persons with diabetes. Complications involving the feet are common in people with diabetes; therefore foot care is an important consideration.

GENERAL PRECAUTIONS FOR PATIENTS WITH DIABETES[24]

- Avoid vigorous exercise before blood glucose has been adequately controlled.
- Have knowledge and awareness of the signs, symptoms, and management of hypoglycemia and hyperglycemia; exercise late in the evening may increase risk of nocturnal hypoglycemia.
- Some medications may mask or exacerbate exercise-related hypo- or hyperglycemia including beta-blockers, diuretics, calcium channel blockers, and warfarin.
- Take appropriate precautions.
- Always carry a carbohydrate (CHO) source.
- Avoid exercise at time of peak insulin effect alternatively, consume a CHO snack 30 minutes before exercise or decrease insulin or oral hypoglycemic dose before exercise; schedule exercise 1–2 hours after meals.
- Test blood glucose frequently; responses may vary with each individual and day-to-day.
- Hydrate adequately before, during, and after exercise.
- Public or cell phone access is important.
- Inject insulin abdominally before exercise commencing within 30 minutes; do not use active muscles as injection sites for insulin pre-exercise.
- Patients with neuropathy may have abnormal heart rate and blood pressure responses to exercise, are at increased risk of orthostatic hypotension, and should routinely care for their feet and hands.
- Buy comfortable shoes made of materials that provide protection for your feet and keep your feet dry.

GROUP EDUCATION FOR CARDIODIABETES[25]

The type 2 diabetes education in the comprehensive cardiac rehabilitation program comprises of patients who have had type 2 diabetes for many years and ones who have been diagnosed recently. The purpose is to educate patients and family members on the causes and symptoms of type 2 diabetes and late arteriosclerotic complications. The message communicated is that the progression of type 2 diabetes can optimally be prevented by changing lifestyle and by strictly controlling blood sugar, blood pressure, serum cholesterol, and other parameters.

CONCLUSION

The number of cardiodiabetic patients in cardiac rehabilitation set ups is increasing, a trend that is likely to continue in view of the predicted rise in the prevalence of DM. Cardiodiabetes patients are benefited from a cardiac rehabilitation and achieve comparable benefits to nondiabetic patients in terms of improvements in their cardiovascular risk profile. Diabetic patients are at increased risk of cardiovascular events and thus need more aggressive secondary prevention measures. Referral of cardiodiabetes patients to cardiac rehabilitation becomes important given their proven benefits in improving their quality of life. Considering the available evidence on the benefits of CR, it is alarming that CR is markedly underutilized. Given the clinical, effective and cost-saving benefits of cardiac rehabilitation, particularly in those with diabetes, greater emphasis must be placed on improving referral and attendance of cardiodiabetes patients to cardiac rehabilitation after major cardiovascular events.

REFERENCES

1. World Health Organization. Needs and action priorities in cardiac rehabilitation and secondary prevention in patients with coronary heart disease. Geneva: WHO Regional Office for Europe; 1993.
2. Ades PA. Cardiac rehabilitation and secondary prevention of coronary heart disease. N Engl J Med. 2001;345(12):892-902.
3. Karoff M, Held K, Bjarnason-Wehrens B. Cardiac rehabilitation in Germany. Eur J Cardiovasc Prev Rehabil. 2007;14(1):18-27.
4. O'Connor GT, Buring JE, Yusuf S, et al. An overview of randomized trials of rehabilitation with exercise after myocardial infarction. Circulation. 1989;80(2):234-44.
5. Wenger NK. Current status of cardiac rehabilitation. J Am Coll Cardiol. 2008;51(17):1619-31.
6. Juutilainen A, Lehto S, Ronnemaa T, et al. Type 2 diabetes as a "coronary heart disease equivalent": an 18-year prospective population-based study in Finnish subjects. Diabetes Care. 2005;28(12):2901-7.
7. Rytter L, Troelsen S, Beck-Nielsen H. Prevalence and mortality of acute myocardial infarction in patients with diabetes. Diabetes Care. 1985;8(3):230-4.
8. Krempf M, Parhofer KG, Steg PG, et al. Cardiovascular event rates in diabetic and nondiabetic individuals with and without established atherothrombosis (from the reduction of atherothrombosis for continued health [REACH] registry). Am J Cardiol. 2010;105(5):667-71.
9. Abbud ZA, Shindler DM, Wilson AC. Effect of diabetes mellitus on short- and long-term mortality rates of patients with acute myocardial infarction: a statewide study. Myocardial infarction data acquisition system study group. Am Heart J. 1995;130:51-8.
10. Behar S, Boyko V, Reicher-Reiss H, et al. Ten-year survival after acute myocardial infarction: comparison of patients with and without diabetes. Secondary Prevention Reinfarction Israeli Nifedipine Trial. Am Heart J. 1997;133:290-6.
11. Zuanetti G, Latini R, Maggioni AP, et al. Influence of diabetes on mortality in acute myocardial infarction: data from the GISSI-2 study. J Am Coll Cardiol. 1993;22:1788-94.
12. Banzer JA, Maguire TE, Kennedy CM, et al. Results of cardiac rehabilitation in patients with diabetes mellitus. Am J Cardiol. 2004;93(1):81-4.
13. Milani RV, Lavie CJ. Behavioral differences and effects of cardiac rehabilitation in diabetic patients following cardiac events. Am J Med. 1996;100:517-23.
14. Hindman L, Falko JM, LaLonde M, et al. Clinical profile and outcomes of diabetic and non-diabetic patients in cardiac rehabilitation. Am Heart J. 2005;150:1046-51.
15. Wild S, Roglic G, Green A, et al. Global prevalence of diabetes: estimates for the year 2000 and projections for 2030. Diabetes Care. 2004;27(5):1047-53.
16. Soja AM, Zwisler AD, Frederiksen M, et al. Use of intensified comprehensive cardiac rehabilitation to improve risk factor control in patients with type 2 diabetes mellitus or impaired glucose tolerance—the randomized DANishStUdy of impaired glucose metabolism in the settings of cardiac rehabilitation (DANSUK) study. Am Heart J. 2007;153:621-8.
17. Colberg SR, Albright AL, Blissmer BJ, et al. Exercise and type 2 diabetes: American College of Sports Medicine and the American Diabetes Association: joint position statement. Exercise and type 2 diabetes. Med Sci Sports Exerc. 2010;42(12):2282-303.
18. Verges B, Patois-Verges B, Cohen M, et al. Effects of cardiac rehabilitation on exercise capacity in Type 2 diabetic patients with coronary artery disease. Diabet Med. 2004;21(8):889-95.
19. Mourot L, Boussuges A, Maunier S, et al. Cardiovascular rehabilitation in patients with diabetes. J Cardiopulm Rehabil Prev. 2010;30(3):157-64.
20. Madssen E, Arbo I, Granoien I, et al. Peak oxygen uptake after cardiac rehabilitation: a randomized controlled trial of a 12-month maintenance program versus usual care. PLoS One. 2014;9(9):e107924.
21. Toste S, Viamonte S, Barreira A, et al. Cardiac rehabilitation in patients with type 2 diabetes mellitus and coronary disease: a comparative study. Rev Port Cardiol. 2014 (Oct);33(10):599-608.
22. Kim HJ, Joo MC, Noh SE, et al. Long-term outcomes of cardiac rehabilitation in diabetic and non-diabetic patients with myocardial infarction. Ann Rehabil Med. 2015;39(6):853-62.
23. Gitt A, Jannowitz C, Karoff M, et al. Treatment patterns and risk factor control in patients with and without metabolic syndrome in cardiac rehabilitation. Vasc Health Risk Manag. 2012;8:265-74.
24. Lopez-Jimenez F, Kramer VC, Masters B, et al. Recommendations for managing patients with diabetes mellitus in cardiopulmonary rehabilitation: an American Association of Cardiovascular and Pulmonary Rehabilitation statement. J Cardiopulm Rehabil Prev. 2012;32(2):101-12.
25. Soja AMB, Ejlertsen M. Type 2 diabetes mellitus. Cardiac rehabilitation. Rationale, methods and experience from Bispebjerg Hospital. Cardiac Rehabilitation Unit, Department of Cardiology. H:S Bispebjerg Hospital, Copenhagen Hospital Corporation; 2004. pp. 135-46.

131

CHAPTER

Role of Nurses in a Structured Manner for Cardiac Rehabilitation in Cardiodiabetes

Harvinder Kaur

INTRODUCTION

In most developed countries worldwide, the number of patients with chronic heart failure is growing, with 1–3% of the adult population suffering from this syndrome, rising to about 10% in the very elderly. Because the incidence of heart failure increases with age, its prevalence will greatly increase as our population ages. In the near future a large part of the population will suffer from heart failure and society will be faced with the financial consequences. Heart failure is consuming about 1.5–2.5% of the health care budget, with approximately 70% of this being spent on hospitalization. On an average one in five patients is readmitted within 12 months, making heart failure one of the most common causes of hospitalization in people over 65 years of age. These older patients are challenged with a difficult recovery after hospitalization due to the concomitant occurrence of comorbidity, frailty, and restricted activity during the hospital stay. The consequence is that older adults after cardiac events often require additional post-acute rehabilitation at a skilled nursing facility (SNF).

Diabetes mellitus (DM) is increasing in prevalence in the United States[1] and is now more common in patients entering cardiac rehabilitation (CR).[2] The association between DM and cardiovascular disease is well established,[3-6] and diabetic patients who have suffered with myocardial infarction (MI) have worse outcomes than no diabetics.[4,5] Despite improvements in cardiovascular disease treatments, diabetic outcomes after a MI continue to lag.[4]

WHAT IS CARDIAC REHABILITATION?

It is defined as, 'all measures used to help cardiac patients return to an active and satisfying life and to prevent re-occurrence of cardiac events'. Cardiac Rehabilitation includes exercise, education, and social and emotional support. Rehabilitation can be hospital or home-based. Services should include physical activity, health education, counseling, behavior modification strategies and support for self-management. They should be tailored to meet the individual and cultural needs of the patient and their family. Cardiac rehabilitation services are available across a continuum that includes inpatient, outpatient and ongoing prevention approaches.

Barriers to Rehabilitation

Lack of knowledge, poor motivation, insufficient understanding, lower perceived self-efficacy, forgetfulness, decrease support from family and other caregivers, cost, poor patient referral by nurses and doctors, time conflict between work and rehabilitation program.

Rehabilitation Outcome and Quality of Life

Improves exercise tolerance, coronary risk factors, psychological well-being, reduction in mortality, improvement in quality of life, and lowering of hospital re-admission rates, with the prevention of reoccurrence of future cardiac events.[7-10]

Standard Interventions

Cardiac rehab staff nurse will meet patient prior to discharge from hospital and address the rehabilitation program protocol. Rehabilitation consists of forty exercise sessions; 24 sessions (3 per week) endurance training on a cycle ergometer (with 5 minutes warm up); 20 minutes training with constant workload, 5 minutes cool down, and 5 minutes post-exercise monitoring, and in addition, 16 (2 per week) 1-hour sessions of stretching and flexibility exercises. At discharge, patients receive risk factor management counseling, instructions on session procedures, and cardiovascular risk factor management during exercise. Patients also receive exercise prescriptions both home and hospital based, physical therapists are assigned for home visits to patients every other week. Information is also given to those patients who are in need of advice for smoking cessation, weigh loss in the overweight or obese, adequate physical activity, and lower dietary fat intake, in order to obtain optimal health benefits from engaging in positive health behavior.

Outcome Measuring Tools

Establish a baseline evaluation for cardiac rehabilitation, vital signs, pulse oximetry, EKG, BMI; pulse oximetry with activities to monitor the need for oxygen. Re-hospitalization due to reoccurrence of a cardiac event. Establish daily patient journal to monitor patient impression of daily improvement and level of performance of ADL. Pre-, intra-, post-echocardiogram to evaluate ejection fraction.[11-14]

PHASES OF REHABILITATION FOLLOWING ACUTE CORONARY SYNDROME

Phase I: Hospital

It occurs while the patient is still hospitalized. Till patient discharge, activity level depends on severity of angina or MI. Patient may initially sit up in bed or chair, perform range-of-motion exercises and self-care (e.g. washing, shaving), and progress to ambulation in hallway and limited stair climbing.

Phase II: Early Recovery

Being after the patient is discharged. Usually lasts from 2 weeks to 12 weeks, activity level is gradually increased and Information regarding risk factor reduction is provided.

Phase III: Late Recovery

Long-term maintenance program. Individual physical activity programs and lifestyle changes that can be designed and implemented at home, a local gym or the rehabilitation center.

> ***Note:*** Teaching the patient to check the pulse rate is nursing responsibility. The patient should be told the maximum HR that should be present at any point. The ideal training target HR is 80% of maximum HR. If the HR exceeds this level or does not return to the rate of the resting pulse within a few minutes, the patient should stop and rest. The patient should also be instructed to stop exercising if angina or dyspnea occurs.

FACTORS ASSOCIATED WITH CARDIOVASCULAR DISEASE

Major factors associated with cardiovascular disease are diabetes, hypertension, obesity, dyslipidemia smoking.

- Control of glucose is important to prevent recurrent CAD.
- Self-monitoring of glucose is an important tool to achieve good glucose control.

Self-monitoring of Blood Glucose

Importance of Self-monitoring Blood Glucose

It gives diabetics an idea as to how exercise and food affect their blood sugar, and prevent hypoglycemia or hyperglycemia.

When Glucose Needs to be Checked?

Fasting: Test taken after 8 hours of fasting 80–130 mg%.

Postprandial: Test taken after 2 hours of meals less than 180 mg% (prelunch and predinner).

What are the Symptoms of Hypoglycemia?

Shaky, nauseated, nervous, irritable, hungry, sweaty, headache, weak and drowsy.

What You Need to do?

15 m glucose in the form of glucose tablets. 15 cc (1 tablespoon) or 3 packets of table sugar dissolved in water. 175 cc (3/4 cup) of juice or regular soft drinks. Record such episode and inform doctor about same.

Keeping Record

Note down all records in logbook. Show logbook to doctor every time. If greater than 240 mg%, check urine for ketone, if ketones are present. Do not exercise, record and inform your doctor.

What to Record?

Blood sugar recorded, food, exercise, medicine, stress, sickness history, etc.

SICK DAY GUIDELINES

'Sick days' refer to periods of minor intercurrent illness usually of only 1–4 days' duration that require changes to the person's usual diabetes self-management practices. Intercurrent illness in people with diabetes, if not managed appropriately and expediently, can result in hyperglycemia, diabetic ketoacidosis (DKA), hyperosmolar hyperglycemic state (HHS), hypoglycemia or other adverse outcomes.

Steps to Take During an Illness

Continue taking your diabetes medicine even if you are vomiting and having trouble eating or drinking. Your blood sugar may continue to rise because of your illness. If you cannot take your medicines, call your doctor and discuss whether you need to adjust your insulin dose or other medicine. Try to eat your normal types and amounts of food and to drink extra fluids, such as water, broth, carbonated drinks, and fruit juice. If your blood sugar level is higher than the blood sugar level your doctor recommends, for example, 240 mg/dL, drink extra liquids that do not contain sugar, such as water or sugar-free cola. If you cannot eat the foods in your regular diet, try to eat or drink 50 g of carbohydrate every 3–4 hours. Some ideas include broth, juice, soup, crackers, gelatin, and applesauce. Check your blood sugar atleast every 3–4 hours, or more often if it is rising quickly, even through the night. If your doctor has told you to take an extra insulin dose for high blood sugar levels, take the appropriate amount. If you take insulin and your doctor has not told you to take a specific amount of additional insulin, call him or her for advice. If you take insulin, do a test for ketones, especially when you have high blood sugar. Weigh yourself and check your temperature, breathing rate, and pulse frequently. If you are losing weight and your temperature, breathing rate, and pulse are increasing, contact a doctor. You may be getting worse. Do not take any nonprescription medicines without talking with your doctor. Many nonprescription medicines affect your blood sugar level. The presence of comorbidities and/or end-stage organ failure will require the individual to seek prompt medical attention regardless of blood glucose levels. People with renal impairment should be advised to cease metformin promptly if an intercurrent illness is leading to dehydration. Ketoacidosis is considered uncommon in individuals with type 2 diabetes, however, it may occur in with people with type 2 diabetes who are lean, pregnant women or known to have previously shown ketones.

GENERAL PRECAUTIONS FOR PATIENTS WITH DIABETES

Avoid vigorous exercise before blood glucose has been adequately controlled. Have knowledge and awareness of the signs, symptoms, and management of hypoglycemia and hyperglycemia; exercise late in the evening may increase risk of nocturnal hypoglycemia. Some medications may mask or exacerbate exercise-related hypo- or hyperglycemia, including beta-blockers, diuretics, calcium channel blockers, and warfarin. Always carry a carbohydrate (CHO) source. Avoid exercise at time of peak insulin effect; alternatively, consume a CHO snack 30 minutes before exercise or decrease insulin or oral hypoglycemic dose before exercise; schedule exercise 1–2 hour after meals. Test blood glucose frequently; responses may vary with each individual and day to day. Hydrate adequately before, during, and after exercise. Carry a personal ID at all times specifying diabetes along with emergency contacts.

Instructions for Foot Care to Patients with Diabetes Foot Hygiene

Inspect your feet daily for blisters, cuts, and scratches; report any issues to your healthcare provider immediately. If appropriate, a family member may assist with foot inspection. Inspect the interior and the soles of your shoes on a daily basis for roughness or inconsistent wear. It is helpful to have and alternate two pairs of shoes on a daily basis for exercise. Wash and dry the feet carefully every day, giving special attention to areas between the toes. Dry skin may be relieved with application of baby oil after bathing and drying feet or hands. Do not soak your feet. Avoid bathing in extreme temperatures. Cut toenails straight across. Do not cut or trim corns; do not treat corns and calluses with chemical agents. Do not use adhesive tape on feet.

Note: The nurse should examine feet at each visit.

Pre-exercise Hypoglycemia Care

Pre-exercise: Patient using insulin or oral agents that increase the risk of hypoglycemia should maintain blood glucose (BG) levels during exercise at 100 mg/dL or higher.

Intervention: Increase or maintain appropriate BG levels during exercise by eating meal or a snack of 15 g carbohydrate (with some fat and protein, e.g. 1 tablespoon peanut butter and six crackers) before exercising if blood glucose blues are less than 100 mg/dL.

Post-exercise Hypoglycemia Care

Other Precautions

Hypertension:
- ↓ salt intake
- Check blood pressure regularly
- Avoid smoking
- ↓ fat intake
- Keep ↓ BMI by regularly exercising.

Resumption of sexual activity: This is often a neglected area of discussion may be difficult for both patient and health care providers to approach. However, the patient's concern about resumption of sexual activity after hospitalization for ACS often produces more stress than the physiologic act itself. About one-third of men and women do not resume sexual activity or have a decrease in sexual activity after MI. The majority of these patients changed their sexual behavior not because of physical problems, but because they were concerned about sexual inadequacy, Death during coitus, and impotence.[15-19]

Patient and family teaching guide—sexual activity after acute coronary syndrome: Planning of resumption of sexual activity should correspond to sexual activity before hospitalization for acute coronary syndrome. Physical training seems to improve the physiologic response to coitus; therefore, daily physical activity during recovery should be encaged. Consumption of food and alcohol should be reduced before intercourse is anticipated (e.g. waiting 3–4 hours after ingesting a large meal before engaging in sexual activity). Familiar surroundings and a familiar partner reduce anxiety. Masturbation may be a useful sexual outlet and may reassure the patient that sexual activity is still possible. Hot or cold showers should be avoided just before and just after intercourse. Foreplay is desirable because it allows a gradual increase in heart rate before orgasm. Positions during intercourse are a matter of individual choice. Orogenital sex place no undue strain on the heart. A relaxed atmosphere free of fatigue and stress is optimal. Prophylactic use of nitrates is effective in decreasing angina during sexual activity. Use of erectile agents (e.g. sildenafil) is contraindicated if taking nitrates in any form. Anal intercourse may cause undue cardiac stress because of the possibility of inducing a vasovagal response.

CONCLUSION

In considering rehabilitation, the nurse and patient must recognize that CAD is a chronic disease. It will not be cured, nor will it disappear by itself. Therefore, basic changes in lifestyle must be made to promote recovery and health. These changes must frequently be made at a time when a person is middle-aged or older. The patient must also realize that recovery takes time. Resumption of physical activity after acute coronary syndrome (ACS) or coronary artery bypass grafting (CABG) surgery is slow and gradual. However, with appropriate and adequate supportive care, recovery is more likely to occur. Monitoring BG levels is vital for the long-term maintenance of glycemic control and is especially important during exercise given that beta blocker therapy can mask the onset of an impending insulin reaction. Monitoring BG levels during exercise may also provide positive feedback regarding the regulation or progression of the exercise prescription, which may result in subsequent long-term adherence to exercise. This is particularly important since exercise is a cornerstone of treatment for diabetes.

REFERENCES

1. Marchionni N, Fattirolli F, Fumagalli S, et al. Improved exercise tolerance and quality of with cardiac rehabilitation of older patients after myocardial infarction: result of a random control trial. J Am Heart Assoc. 2003;107;2201-6.
2. Thomas RJ, Miller NH, Lamendola C, et al. National survey on gender differences in cardiac rehabilitation programs: patient characteristics and enrollment patterns. J Cardiac Rehabil. 1996;16(2);402-12.
3. Roblin D, Diseker RA, Orenstein D, et al. Delivery of outpatient cardiac rehabilitation in a managed care organization. J Cardiopulm Rehabil. 2004;24(3):157-64.
4. Caulin-Glaser T, Blum M, Schmeizl R, et al. Gender differences in referral to cardiac rehabilitation programs after revascularization. J Cardiopulm Rehabil. 2001;21(1): 24-30.
5. Donker Frank. Cardiac rehabilitation: a review of current developments. Clin Psychol Rev. 2000;20(7):923-43.
6. Goble AJ, Worcester MU. Best practice guidelines for cardiac rehabilitation and secondary prevention: a synopsis. Heart Res Cent. 1999.
7. Daoud G, Dabir R, Archambeau M, et al. Randomized, double-blind trial of simultaneous right and left atrial epicardial pacing for prevention of post-open heart surgery atrial fibrillation. Circulation. 2000;102:761-5.
8. Barber K, Stommel M, Kroll J, et al. Cardiac rehabilitation for community-based patients with myocardial infarction: factors predicting discharge recommendation and participation. J Clin Epidemiol. 2001;54(10):1025-30.
9. Hasnain D, Philip HE, John LC. Recent development in secondary prevention and cardiac rehabilitation after acute myocardial infarction. BMJ Publishing Group. 2004;328:693-7.
10. Kate JR. Home-based versus hospital-based cardiac rehabilitation after myocardial infarction or revascularization: design and rationale of the Birmingham rehabilitation uptake maximization study: a randomized controlled trial. BMC Cardiovasc Disord. 2003;3(10):1471-2261.
11. Evenson KR, Johnson A, Aytur SA. Five-year changes in North Carolina outpatient cardiac rehabilitation. J Cardiopulm Rehabil. 2006;26:366-76.
12. Mittag O, China C, Hoberg E, et al. Outcomes of Cardiac Rehabilitation with versus without Follow-up Intervention Rendered by Telephone

(Luebeck Follow-up Trial): Overall and Gender-specific Effects. Int J Rehabil Res. 2006;29:295-302.

13. Pierson LM. Norton HJ, Herbert WG, et al. Recovery of self-reported functional capacity after coronary artery bypass surgery. Chest. 2003;123(5):1367-74.
14. Goodman JM, Pallandi DV, Reading JR, et al. Central and peripheral adaptations after 12 weeks of exercise training in post-coronary artery bypass surgery patients. J Cardiopulm rehabil. 1999;19(3):144-50.
15. Evenson KR, Johnson A, Aytur SA. Five-year changes in North Carolina outpatient cardiac rehabilitation. [Electronic Version]. J Cardiopulm Rehabil. 2006;26:366-76.
16. Association of Rehabilitation Nurses. (2013). White paper by the Association of Rehabilitation Nurse Executive Summary "The essential role the rehabilitation nurse in facilitating care transitions". [online] Available from http://www.rehabnurse.org/uploads/files/healthpolicy/ARN_Care_Transitions_White_Paper_Journal_Copy_FINAL.pdf. [Accessed October, 2017].
17. King Saud University. Cardiac Rehabilitation. [online] Available from faculty.ksu.edu.sa/26348/Documents/Cardiac%20Rehabilitation%20by%20albarati.ppt. [Accessed October, 2017].
18. Fridlund B. The role of the nurse in cardiac rehabilitation programmes. Eur J Cardiovasc Nurs. 2002 Feb;1(1):15-8.
19. Dolansky MA, Zullo MD, Hassanein S, et al. Cardiac rehabilitation in skilled nursing facilities: a missed opportunity. Heart Lung. 2012;41(2):115-24.

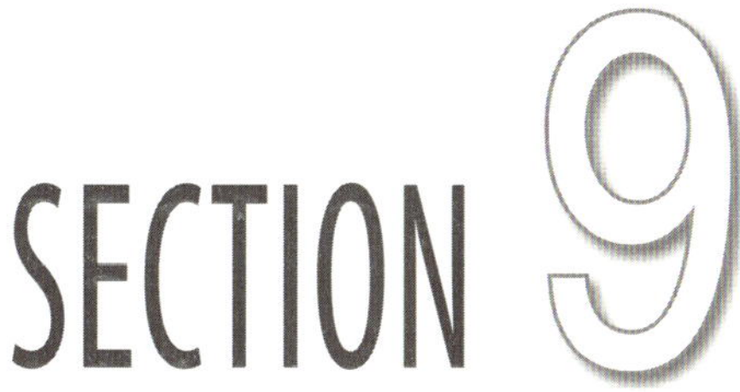

Future Directions

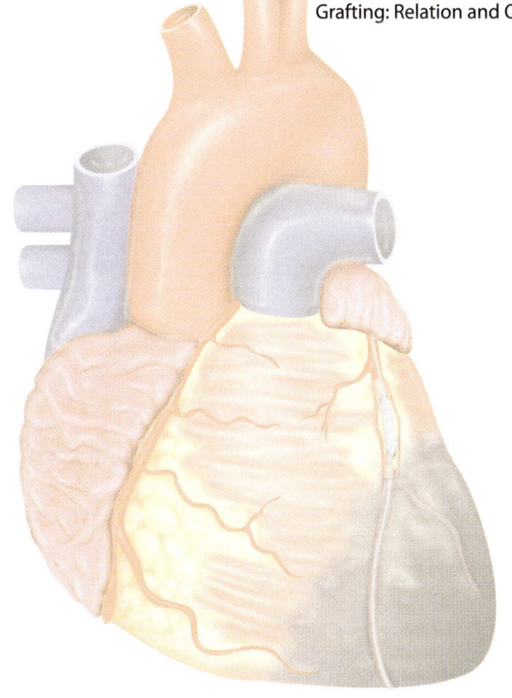

132 CHAPTER

Type 2 Diabetes and Coronary Artery Bypass Grafting: Relation and Outcomes

Naresh Trehan, Jasjeet S Wasir, Tarannum Bano, Paras Aggarwal

INTRODUCTION

At present, there is an ever-increasing incidence of diabetes mellitus (DM) globally. The worldwide burden of DM has increased from 30 million in 1985 to 382 million in 2014, with current estimates indicating that these rates will only continue to rise and reach epidemic proportion not just in the developed, but also in the developing countries.[1] As per the International Diabetes Federation (IDF), 1 in 10 persons throughout the world will have DM by 2035.[2] Occurrences of both type 1 DM (T1DM) and type 2 DM (T2DM) are increasing; however, T2DM has a disproportionately greater contribution to the increased incidence and prevalence of DM.[1] The important consequence of the increasing prevalence of DM is a considerable increment in the economic burden both on the patient and already overburdened the healthcare systems, especially in the developing countries. In the United States, the total cost of DM averages $2108/patient per year, which is nearly twice that of nondiabetic patients.[3] This economic burden associated with DM is both in terms of the direct costs of medical care as well as indirect costs of diminished productivity of patients with diabetes and its complications and the subsequent effect on morbidity and mortality.[4] The greatest expense of DM is attributed to both macrovascular and microvascular complications such as coronary artery disease (CAD), myocardial infarction (MI), hypertension, peripheral vascular disease, retinopathy, end-stage renal disease, and neuropathy.[3,4] DM and cardiovascular disease (CVD) have a very close link by virtue of the following facts. DM is considered to be a cardiovascular risk equivalent as subjects with DM without previous MI carry the same risk of subsequent coronary events and related morbidity and mortality as patients without diabetes but with history of previous MI. It is reported that a very large percentage of patients with diabetes die from CVDs, while CAD is responsible for two-thirds of these deaths.[5] CVD is the most common cause of mortality and morbidity in diabetic populations.[6] CVD death rates are 1.7 times greater among adults (>18 years) with DM than those without diagnosed DM; this increase is primarily driven by greater occurrence of cerebrovascular disease and MI in DM patients.[7] Increased CVD mortality in diabetic patients is found in both men and women. The relative risk for CVD morbidity and mortality in adults with diabetes ranges from 1 to 3 in men and from 2 to 5 in women compared to those without DM.[8] In most studies, clinical outcomes of CVD are worse in patients with diabetes as compared to nondiabetic subjects.[9,10] Important and interesting facts about CVD and DM are that over 25% of all percutaneous coronary interventions (PCI)[11] and greater than 30% of the patients undergoing coronary artery bypass graft (CABG) surgery have DM.[12] These percentages are in reality much higher in certain ethnic and racial populations like Asian Indians, where they may reach as high as 50–60% at specialized centers.

PATHOPHYSIOLOGY OF CARDIOVASCULAR DISEASE IN DIABETES

The increased risk of CVD among diabetes is majorly due to the increased atherosclerotic burden (starting from endothelial dysfunction; birthplace for atherosclerosis), metabolic derangements, and the proinflammatory/thrombotic state associated with diabetes.[13] DM subjects have highly increased aggregation risk factors of atherosclerosis/CVD: hypertension, overweight/obesity, abdominal obesity, dyslipidemia, disorders of increased clotting increased platelet adhesion, increased fibrinogen, increased plasminogen activator inhibitor-1 and von Willebrand factor.[14]

In uncontrolled DM, there is a disturbance of the metabolism of arachidonic acid, which is one of the major reasons of improper platelet function.[15] Smoking in another very important modifiable risk factor for CVD in patients with DM. Smoking majorly increases to the already increased risk for CVD mortality and morbidity by virtue of presence of DM. It causes damage to vascular endothelium; it creates proatherogenic changes in lipoproteins and increases the tendency for clotting.[16-19] Atheromatous changes in diabetes are diffuse and they are also located even in the small arteries.[20]

MANAGEMENT OF CORONARY ARTERY DISEASE IN DIABETES MELLITUS

Very briefly, in this section, we will discuss the basic concepts of prevention/management of CAD in patients with DM. We will discuss the important landmark trials which are the basis of the current-day therapeutics.[21] CAD may be managed medically (recent advances in drug therapy of diabetes for CVD reduction is discussed in the concluding section) or with interventions (percutaneous coronary interventions, PCI; or coronary artery bypass surgery, CABG).

Medical Management

Landmark clinical trials in the recent decades have investigated the effect of intensive treatment of hyperglycemia on cardiovascular risk reduction, in DM[22-26] and have presented conflicting results. These differences in the benefits of CAD prevention (primary or secondary) may be explained by the clinical profile of the study population, presence or absence of CVD, the duration of diabetes as well as the type of intensive intervention performed and the treatment targets for glycemic control to be achieved.

The *United Kingdom Prospective Diabetes Study* (UKPDS)[22] was carried out in newly diagnosed type 2 diabetes patients at a relatively low risk for CAD; the early intensive treatment of hyperglycemia within the first 5 years of disease resulted in a long-term microvascular and macrovascular (CVD reduction, including incident MI) complication prevention benefit, compared with patients in the conventional treatment group. This clinical benefit of prevention of complications was maintained even after the loss of difference in glycemic control between the two groups that was observed (post-trial termination follow-up) during the further follow-up. However, the results of the *UKPDS* could not be duplicated in the three other large, long-term clinical trials conducted in patients with DM. The *Veterans Affairs Diabetes Trial* (VADT)[23] subjects were older in age and had a 10 years mean duration of diabetes; this trial did not show CAD benefits when the glycemic control was intensively controlled. The VADT cohort had ~40% of subjects with a previous history of CVD. Similar to the *VADT*, the *Action in Diabetes and Vascular Disease: Preterax and Diamicron Modified Release Controlled Evaluation* (ADVANCE) trial[24] in which the aim was to achieve an HbA1c of A1c of 6.5% through intensive treatment did not reduce the rate of major macrovascular events or death, despite a reduction in the incidence of diabetic nephropathy. As in previous trial, study subjects were older (mean age of 66 years) and had a longer duration of diabetes (8 years) than the UKPDS patients, when the intensive treatment was started. In contrast, intensive glycemic control aimed to reduce HbA1c below 6% in DM patients, in the *Action to Control Cardiovascular Risk in Diabetes* (ACCORD) trial,[25] in addition to demonstrating no benefit in reducing macrovascular events the trial resulted in increased mortality (trial prematurely terminated), weight gain, and high risk of hypoglycemia. Patients in this study had a high cardiovascular risk profile when first started on intensive glycemic treatment.

Even after losing the strict glycemic control, represented by an HbA1c < 7%, during the observational period, the group previously intensively treated presented a reduction of any cardiovascular (including MI) event by 42% (UKPDS).

In summary, these trial results indicate that early intensive control of blood glucose levels, targeting HbA1c levels below 7%, when initiated promptly in patients with short duration of diabetes and low cardiovascular risk, results in significant cardiovascular benefits. The same is not true when we target lower (stricter) blood glucose targets in a DM population who are older patients exposed to ill effects of hyperglycemia for years before the intervention and have a higher cardiovascular risk profile.

This mechanism of early intervention for CVD/CAD protection is termed as "metabolic memory/legacy effect", which means that the effect of the early glycemic control is remembered later on in the target organs[26] resulting in long-term protection. The mechanism of this protection is related to epigenetic changes and intracellular metabolic/gene expression changes that result in lesser endothelial dysfunction, oxidative stress, and low-grade inflammation.

And finally, a multipronged risk factor (glycemic control, cholesterol control, blood pressure control, weight reduction, therapeutic lifestyle changes, smoking cessation, alcohol limitation, and use of cardiovascular safe/beneficial drugs when indicated) intervention should be adopted as shown by the results of the STENO-2 trial. The results of the intervention and the follow-up indicated that at 21.2 years of follow-up of 7.8 years of intensified, multifactorial, target-driven treatment of DM subjects with microalbuminuria, a median of 7.9 years gain of life was attained, and the increase in lifespan is matched by time free from incident CVD/CAD.[27]

Intervention Management (Percutaneous Coronary Intervention and Coronary Artery Bypass Graft)

In patients with DM, CAD is more likely to be a complex disease characterized by small, diffuse, calcified, and multivessel disease (MVD)[28,29] and often requires coronary revascularization in addition to optimal medical therapy to control the CAD process or its symptoms.[30]

Advances in PCI have enabled its use in more complex lesions that were earlier treated with CABG. However, MVD in DM patients is associated with a high incidence of repeat revascularization after PCI even with use of drug-eluting stents (DESs); therefore, CABG remains superior to PCI in patients with such lesions. A recent meta-analysis has clearly suggested the superiority of CABG to PCI with balloon angioplasty or bare-metal stents with respect to all-cause mortality in patients with DM.[31]

In the recent past, numerous randomized control clinical trials (RCTs) have compared CABG with PCI using DES. In this section, we will briefly discuss the recent and important trials of PCI versus CABG in DM:

- In the SYNergy trial, comparison was made between percutaneous coronary intervention with TAXus and cardiac surgery (SYNTAX) study, CABG and PCI with paclitaxel-eluting stents (PES) were compared in patients with *de novo* left main coronary disease, three-vessel disease, or both, which were considered equally suitable for CABG or PCI by both a cardiac surgeon and an interventional cardiologist.[32] Of the total enrolments ~25% subjects had DM and were included in a prespecified subgroup analysis. The results indicated the following:
  - A lesser 3-year major adverse cardiac and cerebrovascular events in the DM subgroup (37.0% and 22.9%) in the PCI group and CABG group (p = 0.002), respectively.
  - The rate of revascularization was also higher in the PCI group (PCI, 28.0% vs CABG, 12.9%; p < 0.001).[33]
- In the second large trial, the Future Revascularization Evaluation in Patients with Diabetes Mellitus (FREEDOM) trial which enrolled ~2,000 DM patients with MVD who were randomly allotted to undergo either CABG or PCI with DES.[34] Results of the FREEDOM trial include:
  - Significantly increased all-cause mortality and MI were observed in the PCI group during the mean follow-up of 5 years compared with the CABG group (PCI, 26.6% vs CABG, 18.7%).
  - Based on these results, the updated guidelines from the ECS for the management of DM patients stated that PCI for MVD was a Class IIb indication for disease control/relieving symptoms as an alternative to CABG in patients with low complexity lesions that were defined by SYNTAX scores.[35]
- The latest generation DESs have partially overcome the critical issue of in-stent thrombosis as compared to the earlier DES, in particular, the everolimus-eluting stent (EES).[36] In a recent meta-analysis of 68 RCTs comparing clinical outcomes in CAD patients with DM between those who received CABG and DESs, including SES, PES, and EES[37] it was shown that:
  - All-cause mortality was higher in the patients who received SES and PES compared with CABG, whereas the mortality rates in the EES group were similar to those of the CABG group (reference rate ratio to CABG, 1.31, 95% confidence interval; 0.74–2.29).
- Results of two recent clinical trials comparing EES and CABG in patients with a left main lesion [the Evaluation of XIENCE versus CABG for Effectiveness of Left Main Revascularization (EXCEL) trial][38] or MVD [the randomized comparison of CABG and EES implantation in the treatment of patients with multivessel coronary artery disease (BEST)][23,39] provided contradictory results.
  - The randomized EXCEL trial[38] compared the efficacy between EES and CABG in patients with low to intermediate SYNTAX scores; it enrolled ~1,900 subjects. The composite of all-cause mortality, stroke, or MI at 3 years (primary endpoint) occurred in 15.4% and 14.5% in EES group and CABG group (p = 0.02 for noninferiority), respectively. Importantly, the short-term events (30-day mortality, stroke, or MI) were shown to be lower in the EES group (4.9% vs 7.9%; HR 0.61; 95% CI: 0.42–0.88). These differences were mainly driven by the lesser occurrence of MI in the EES group in the short term. The treatment effect for the primary endpoint was consistently similar in subjects with DM.

- Finally, the BEST trial[39] enrolled ~900 subjects including a subgroup of DM subjects and compared EES and CABG in MVD.
  - In the total study cohort, the composite of 2-year mortality, target vessel revascularization, and MI (primary endpoint) ensued in 11.0% and 7.9% in the EES and CABG groups (p = 0.32 for noninferiority), respectively.
  - In the DM subgroup, the rate of the primary endpoint was significantly greater in the EES group as compared to the CABG group. Hence, indicating significantly better outcomes of coronary revascularization with CABG in subjects with MVD and DM.
- The incongruity of the two above mentioned RCTs might be explained by:
  - Differences in the populations (left main lesion or MVDs)
  - Complexity of the lesions
  - Dissimilar primary endpoints.

In conclusion, CABG should be the preferred procedure for coronary revascularization in multivessel and complex coronary diseases lesions, considering the higher frequency of complete revascularization in CABG-treated patients and lesser morbidity and mortality in the CABG group.

CORONARY ARTERY BYPASS GRAFT OUTCOMES IN DIABETES MELLITUS

In spite of the recent scientific advances, greater expertise at advanced cardiac centers, and improved skills, CABG surgery is still associated with inherent risks and possible complications. In this section, we will review and discuss the heterogeneity in outcomes of CABG in subjects with DM. Treatment of DM entails three major modalities—lifestyle changes, oral antidiabetic drugs [noninsulin requiring DM (NIDM)], and insulin therapy [insulin requiring DM (IDM)]; these may be used alone or in various permutations or combinations based on individual patient profiles. We will discuss the outcomes in the total DM population as well as in the subgroups of DM patients who are on NIDM or IDM and look at the possible differences. The possible risk factors which may lead to greater occurrence of complication following CABG in DM subjects include preexisting cerebrovascular disease, chronic obstructive pulmonary disease, diabetes, smoking, hypertension, dyslipidemia, generalized or abdominal obesity, prior occurrence of pulmonary hypertension, peripheral vascular disease, or MI.[40]

Various studies have reported graft occlusion and MI post-CABG to be in tune of 5–10% (these percentages are lower in specialized centers dealing with larger numbers of annual CABGs). This graft occlusion or postoperative ACS is associated with a high in-hospital mortality rate (up to 68%).[41]

Graft occlusion early on following CABG is usually caused by technical failure and is almost always thrombotic in nature.[42] Whereas late graft occlusion is due to the similar process of coronary occlusion as is present in the diseased native coronaries.[43]

Low cardiac output syndrome is a serious complication of CABG surgery. Mortality rates from this condition can be as high as 38% and is considered the largest cause of mortality in patients following CABG surgery.[44]

Superficial sternal wound infections affect 3–10% of median sternotomies. However, deep sternal wound infections (DSWI) are less common and it affects 1–2% of patients after CABG surgery.[45]

Arrhythmias are common phenomenon after CABG surgery. Atrial fibrillation is usually of benign nature and occurs in about 25% of patients postoperatively after CABG.[46] Postoperative causes of arrhythmias include ongoing myocardial ischemia, hypoxia, infections (e.g. pneumonia, wound infection), pericardial collections, electrolyte disturbances, coronary spasm, hypervolemia, pulmonary artery catheter irritation, and drug withdrawal/toxicity (e.g. beta-blockers, digoxin, and alcohol).

Perioperative stroke is rare and affects 1–2% of patients undergoing CABG surgery. Perioperative stroke can be embolic (two-thirds of all strokes), or it can be due to cerebral hemorrhage or generalized cerebral hypoperfusion (e.g. during cardiopulmonary bypass).[47]

The incidence of gastrointestinal complications following CABG surgery has been reported to be between 1.6% and 2.3%. Various complications associated are gastric perforations, intra-abdominal bleeding, pancreatitis, acute cholecystitis, and intestinal ischemia.[48,49]

Renal dysfunction following CABG surgery has many potential causes and is associated with increased mortality, hospital stay, and costs. Off-pump CABG surgery was not independently associated with a reduction in the occurrence of renal dysfunction.[50] The possible risk factors for postoperative renal insufficiency are preoperative renal insufficiency, increasing age, poor glycemic control, and longer duration of DM.[51]

The next important section is centered on differences in outcomes of CABG based on the type of ongoing treatment for DM prior to surgery (NIDM vs IDM).[52] Patients with IDM are expected to be associated with higher comorbidities and a longer duration of DM when compared with patients with NIDM. Generally, due to the clinical inertia, insulin treatment is often delayed and hence is started late in the course of diabetes at a time when complications of diabetes have already set in or there is a failure of oral agents, hence by virtue of this delay in glycemic control and increased duration of diabetes the patients shift to a high-risk category development of complications following CABG.

In DM patients undergoing PCI, it has been clearly documented that adverse clinical outcomes postprocedure are significantly higher in patients with IDM compared with DM patients without insulin therapy.[53] However, in post-CABG patients, these differences in outcomes are not so clearly defined.

The Emory Angioplasty versus Surgery Trial (EAST) reported no significant differences morbidity or mortality of CABG in patients with DM at 3 years,[54] whereas the Coronary Artery Bypass Revascularization Investigation (CABRI) demonstrated positive outcomes of CABG in a similar cohort of DM patients.[55] Previously discussed FREEDOM trial which compared CABG and PCI with DES in patients with IDM and NIDM found CABG to be beneficial compared with PCI in patients with NIDM, importantly, its results could not provide enough proof to show any statistically significant positive befits of CABG in the IDM group.[34]

A recent meta-analysis (2017)[56] of studies compared CABG outcomes in the two groups, including NDM versus IDM. The results indicated that during the short-term follow-up period post-CABG, mortality was statistically higher in the IDM group (OR: 1.47, 95% CI: 1.33–1.61, p < 0.00001). Also, major adverse events post-CABG were significantly lower in the NIDM cohort (OR: 1.66, 95% CI: 1.48–1.87, p < 0.00001). Also, the short-term incidence of cerebrovascular events was not different between the two groups (OR: 1.12, 95% CI: 0.99–1.27, p < 1⁄4 0.08).

In long-term outcomes (>1 year) post-CABG, IDM was associated with a greater mortality (OR: 1.23, 95% CI: 1.09–1.42, p = 0.03), and a higher rate of major adverse events including CAD and CVA (OR: 1.50, 95% CI: 1.07–2.12, p = 0.02). The long-term chances of occurrence of stroke post-CABG are lower in the NIDM subject groups (OR: 1.39, 95% CI: 1.22–1.59, p < 0.00001). However, MI and repeated revascularization rates between the IDM and NIDM groups (OR: 1.18, 95% CI: 0.85–1.65, p = 0.31 and OR: 1.31, 95% CI 0.81–2.12, p = 0.27, respectively) were similar in the long term.[56]

Further, in the SYNTAX trial, results indicate that during a long-term (5-year) follow-up period, CABG is associated with a far lesser rate of combined adverse outcomes and revascularization in both categories (IDM and NIDM) of patients when compared with PCI.[57]

In another meta-analysis which included 10 RCTs comparing CABG and PCI in patients with DM reinforced the earlier association of CABG to better outcomes in the long-term follow-up.[58] The American College of Cardiology Foundation and the Society of Thoracic Surgeons Collaboration on the Comparative Effectiveness of Revascularization Strategies (ASCERT) study showed that CABG is associated with a significantly lower rate of mortality compared with PCI, irrespective of the treatment for DM (NIDM and IDM considered together) in patients with MVDs. Importantly, the above discussed meta-analysis,[59] the adverse clinical outcomes have been compared by subgroups of NIDM versus IDM, after CABG. IDM patients both in the short term and long term have a significantly greater rate of mortality, and major adverse cardiovascular and cerebrovascular events after CABG. The long-term rate of stroke was also significantly higher in the IDM group, whereas MI and repeated revascularization are not different between these two groups after CABG. The FREEDOM trial also showed a significantly higher 5-year mortality, stroke, and MI in the IDM group after CABG compared with the NIDM group. Also, occurrence of short-term (30-day) major adverse events was observed to be lesser in the NIDM group after CABG in the FREEDOM trial.[34] Another clinical trial[60] indicated similar results of worse clinical outcomes in IDM patients undergoing CABG because of a poor prior glycemic control and overall worse health status in them. Finally, the PRoject of Ex-vivo Vein graft ENgineering via Transfection IV Trial, which included a total of 3,014 patients (with and without DM) also concluded that IDM patients had poor clinical outcomes compared to patients with NIDM after CABG.[61]

NEWER DRUG THERAPY FOR CARDIOVASCULAR RISK REDUCTION

The landmark studies (cited in the earlier section; ACCORD, ADVANCE, and VADT) which were done in the early 2000s showed no cardiovascular benefits of intensive glycemic control in subjects with DM. Also, in the early 2000s an important meta-analysis by Nissen et al.[62] showed that the antidiabetic drug rosiglitazone was associated with increased cardiovascular death and MI in subjects with DM. It was following this article that FDA mandated that for any new drug therapy to be approved for treatment of DM, it first has to undergo rigorous RCTs to prove its cardiovascular safety. In this final section, we share evidence of CVD reduction in patients with DM (in patients with high CAD risk factors or with established CAD) with newer antidiabetic drugs, i.e. glucagon-like peptide-1 receptor antagonists (GLP-1RA) and sodium glucose transporter-2 inhibitors (SGLT-2i).

- *Glucagon-like peptide-1 receptor antagonists (GLP-1RA)*: The two recently published large clinical trial programs LEADER (Liraglutide Effect and Action in Diabetes: Evaluation of Cardiovascular Outcome Results) trial[63] and SUSTAIN-6 (Evaluate Cardiovascular and Other Long-term Outcomes with Semaglutide in Subjects with Type 2 Diabetes)[64] have evaluated the primary/secondary prevention of CVD effect of

GLP-1RAs. These two trials strongly prove a primary and secondary prevention potential of this group of drugs by significant reduction in a combined outcome, including cardiovascular death, nonfatal MI, and nonfatal stroke. In the LEADER trial, a total of 9,340 patients with type 2 diabetes were randomly assigned to liraglutide with standard care or placebo. The primary endpoint (a combined outcome of cardiovascular death, nonfatal MI, or nonfatal stroke) occurred in 13.0% and 14.9% in the liraglutide group and the placebo group during the median follow-up of 3.8 years (hazard ratio 0.87; 95% confidence interval 0.78–0.97).[63] In the SUSTAIN-6 trial, a total of 3,297 patients with type 2 diabetes, 83.0% of the study population had established CVD, the study population was randomly allocated to semaglutide added to standard care or placebo. The rate of a combined outcome (cardiovascular death, nonfatal MI, or nonfatal stroke) was demonstrated to be lower in the semaglutide group (hazard ratio 0.74, 95% CI 0.58–0.95).[64]

- *Sodium glucose transporter-2 inhibitors (SGLT-2i):* The novel drug Empagliflozin was evaluated in the recently published EMPA-REG OUTCOME trial.[65] This trial included over 7,000 subjects (97% study completion rates) from 42 countries including ~200 DM patients form our country; all the patients in the study were at high risk of future cardiovascular events. The results strongly prove the drugs efficacy in primary/secondary prevention of CVD in high CV risk DM subjects. The important results were as follows:
  - Three-point MACE reduction by 14% in the study group as compared to placebo when added to the standard of care treatment.
  - Reduction in the risk of CV death by 38%.
  - Improved survival by reducing the rate of all-cause mortality by 32%.
  - Empagliflozin prevented hospitalization for heart failure by reducing the heart failure hospitalization events by 35% when compared to placebo.

CONCLUSION

Rapid sociodemographic, nutrition, and environmental changes are fueling an ever-increasing epidemic of noncommunicable disease, including DM and CVD, especially in developing countries like ours. The relation of DM and CVD is so strong that DM has been termed as a CAD risk equivalent. The most common reason for death in subjects with DM is CVD. These two facts of increasing burden of noncommunicable diseases and CVD being the most important reason for morbidity and mortality in subjects with DM are overstressing the already overburdened healthcare systems globally. CAD in diabetics is more likely to involve multiple vessels and may be more complex in its anatomy as compared to nondiabetics. Data suggest that CABG may be a better option of revascularization as compared to PCI (±DES) in subjects with DM as compared to nondiabetics, as greater revascularization may be attained with CABG. However, the final decision for the preferred revascularization must be taken by the cardiac surgeon and cardiologist together keeping in mind not only the complexity of the CAD but also of the patients overall profile. The overall mortality and morbidity outcomes after CABG in DM are poorer than in nondiabetic subjects. In the cohort of DM subjects, patients treated with only oral agents for glucose control have better outcomes when compared to insulin-treated DM subjects. For better outcomes of CABG in diabetics, a multipronged approach, including lifestyle changes, early and aggressive glycemic control, weight reduction, control of blood pressure and lipids, alcohol and cigarette cessation, and greater use of cardioprotective drugs, including aspirin, statins, and angiotensin-converting enzyme inhibitors/angiotensin receptor blockers (ACEi/ARBs) is advocated. Despite use of all of the above mentioned interventions a residual risk of poor outcomes in CABG patients with DM may still remain; this may be further addressed by using the newer antidiabetic agents like GLP-1RAs and SGLT-2i, aiming at further mitigation of the risk of adverse outcomes beyond the conventional approaches.

REFERENCES

1. Wild S, Roglic G, Green A, et al. Global prevalence of diabetes: estimates for the year 2000 and projections for 2030. Diabetes Care. 2004;27:1047-53.
2. Aguiree F, Brown A, Cho NH, et al. IDF Diabetes Atlas, 6th edition. Basel, Switzerland: International Diabetes Federation; 2013. pp. 155.
3. Bahia LR, Araujo DV, Schaan BD, et al. The costs of type 2 diabetes mellitus outpatient care in the Brazilian public health system. Value Health. 2011;14:S137-40.
4. American Diabetes Association. Economic costs of diabetes in the U.S. In 2007. Diabetes Care. 2008;31:596-615.
5. Pitsavos CH, Xenakis KE, Vavouranakis EM, et al. Diabetes and coronary artery disease. Hellenic J Cardiol. 2001;42:302-26.
6. Matheus AS, Tannus LR, Cobas RA, et al. Impact of diabetes on cardiovascular disease: an update. Int J Hypertens. 2013;2013:653789.
7. Centers for Disease Control and Prevention. National diabetes statistics report: Estimates of diabetes and its burden in the United States, 2014. Atlanta, GA: US Department of Health and Human Services; 2014.
8. Rivellese AA, Riccardi G, Vaccaro O. Cardiovascular risk in women with diabetes. Nutr Metab Cardiovasc Dis. 2010;20:474-80.
9. Tierney EF, Geiss LS, Engelgau MM, et al. Population-based estimates of mortality associated with diabetes: use of a death certificate check box in North Dakota. Am J Public Health. 2001;91(1):84-92.
10. Pasterkamp G. Methods of accelerated atherosclerosis in diabetic patients. Heart. 2013;99:743-9.
11. Aronson D, Edelman ER. Revascularization for coronary artery disease in diabetes mellitus: Angioplasty, stents and coronary artery bypass grafting. Rev Endocr Metab Disord. 2010;11:75-86.

12. Thourani VH, Weintraub WS, Stein B, et al. Influence of diabetes mellitus on early and late outcome after coronary artery bypass grafting. Ann Thorac Surg. 1999;67(4):1045-52.
13. Beckman JA, Creager MA, Libby P. Diabetes and atherosclerosis. Epidemiology, pathophysiology and management. JAMA. 2002;287:2570-81.
14. Donahue RP, Orchard TJ. Diabetes millitus and macrovascular complications. An epidemiological perspective. Diab Care. 1992;15:1141-55.
15. Jones DB, Carter RD, Mann JI. Indirect evidence of impairment of platelet desaturase enzymes in diabetes mellitus. Hormone Metab Res. 1986;18:341-4.
16. Wald N, Howard S, Smith PG, et al. Association between atherosclerotic diseases and carboxyhaemoglobin levels in tobacco smokers. Br Med J. 1973;1(856):761-5.
17. Brischetto CS, Connor WE, Connor SL, et al. Plasma lipid and lipoprotein profiles of cigarette smokers from randomly selected families: enhancement of hyperlipidemia and depression of high-density lipoprotein. Am J Cardiol. 1983;52(7):675-80.
18. Belch JJ, McArdle BM, Burns P, et al. The effects of acute smoking on platelet behaviour, fibrinolysis and haemorheology in habitual smokers. Thromb Haemost. 1984;51(1):6-8.
19. Levine PH. An acute effect of cigarette smoking on platelet function: a possible link between smoking and arterial thrombosis. Circulation. 1973;48:619-23.
20. Alderman EL, Corley SD, Fisher LD, et al. Five-year angiographic follow-up of factors associated with progression of coronary artery disease in the Coronary Artery Surgery Study (CASS). J Am Coll Cardiol. 1993;22:1141-54.
21. Matheus AS de M, Tannus LRM, Cobas RA, et al. Impact of diabetes on cardiovascular disease: an update. Int J Hypertens. 2013;2013:15.
22. Holman RR, Paul SK, Bethel MA, et al. 10-Year follow-up of intensive glucose control in type 2 diabetes. N Engl J Med. 2008;359(15):1577-89.
23. Duckworth W, Abraira C, Moritz T, et al. Glucose control and vascular complications in veterans with type 2 diabetes. N Engl J Med. 2009;360(2):129-39.
24. Patel A, MacMahon S, Chalmers J, et al. Intensive blood glucose control and vascular outcomes in patients with type 2 diabetes. N Engl J Med. 2008;358(24):2560-72.
25. The Action to Control Cardiovascular Risk in Diabetes Study Group. Effects of intensive glucose lowering in type 2 diabetes. N Engl J Med. 2008;358:2545-59.
26. Ceriello A, Ihnat MA, Thorpe JE. The 'Metabolic memory': is more than just tight glucose control necessary to prevent diabetic complications?" J Clin Endocrinol Metabol. 2009;94(2):410-5.
27. Gæde P, Oellgaard J, Carstensen B, et al. Years of life gained by multifactorial intervention in patients with type 2 diabetes mellitus and microalbuminuria: 21 years follow-up on the Steno-2 randomised trial. Diabetologia. 2016;59(11):2298-307.
28. Norhammar A, Malmberg K, Diderholm E, et al. Diabetes mellitus: the major risk factor in unstable coronary artery disease even after consideration of the extent of coronary artery disease and benefits of revascularization. J Am Coll Cardiol. 2004;43:585-91.
29. Creager MA, Lüscher TF, Cosentino F, et al. Diabetes and vascular disease: pathophysiology, clinical consequences, and medical therapy: Part I. Circulation. 2003;108:1527-32.
30. Dagenais GR, Lu J, Faxon DP, et al. Bypass Angioplasty Revascularization Investigation 2 Diabetes (BARI 2D) Study Group. Effects of optimal medical treatment with or without coronary revascularization on angina and subsequent revascularizations in patients with type 2 diabetes mellitus and stable ischemic heart disease. Circulation. 2011;123:1492-500.
31. Hlatky MA, Boothroyd DB, Bravata DM, et al. Coronary artery bypass surgery compared with percutaneous coronary interventions for multivessel disease: a collaborative analysis of individual patient data from ten randomised trials. Lancet. 2009;373:1190-7.
32. Serruys PW, Morice MC, Kappetein AP, et al. SYNTAX investigators. Percutaneous coronary intervention versus coronary-artery bypass grafting for severe coronary artery disease. N Engl J Med. 2009;360:961-72.
33. Mack MJ, Banning AP, Serruys PW, et al. Bypass versus drug- eluting stents at three years in SYNTAX patients with diabetes mellitus or metabolic syndrome. Ann Thorac Surg. 2011;92:2140-6.
34. Farkouh ME, Domanski M, Sleeper LA, et al. Strategies for multivessel revascularization in patients with diabetes. N Engl J Med. 2012;367:2375-84.
35. Rydén L, Grant PJ, Anker SD, et al. ESC Guidelines on diabetes, pre-diabetes, and cardiovascular diseases developed in collaboration with the EASD: the Task Force on diabetes, prediabetes, and cardiovascular diseases of the European Society of Cardiology (ESC) and developed in collaboration with the European Association for the Study of Diabetes (EASD). Eur Heart J. 2013;34:3035-87.
36. Baber U, Mehran R, Sharma SK, et al. Impact of the everolimus-eluting stent on stent thrombosis: a meta-analysis of 13 randomized trials. J Am Coll Cardiol. 2011;58:1569-77.
37. Bangalore S, Toklu B, Feit F. Outcomes with coronary artery bypass graft surgery versus percutaneous coronary intervention for patients with diabetes mellitus: can newer generation drug-eluting stents bridge the gap? Circ Cardiovasc Interv. 2014;7:518-25.
38. Stone GW, Sabik JF, Serruys PW, et al. Everolimus-eluting stents or bypass surgery for left main coronary artery disease. N Engl J Med. 2016;375:2223-35.
39. Park SJ, Ahn JM, Kim YH, et al. Trial of everolimus-eluting stents or bypass surgery for coronary disease. N Engl J Med. 2015;372:1204-12.
40. Kshettry VR, Flavin TF, Emery RW, et al. Does multivessel, off-pump coronary artery bypass reduce postoperative morbidity? Ann Thorac Surg. 2000;69:1725-31.
41. Rasmussen C, Thiis JJ, Clemmensen P, et al. Significance and management of early graft failure after coronary artery bypass grafting: feasibility and results of acute angiography and re-re-vascularization. Eur J Cardiothorac Surg. 1997;12(6):847-52.
42. Blessing F, Jaeger BR, Oberhoffer M, et al. Prevention of early graft occlusion after coronary bypass grafting by postoperative reduction of plasma fibrinogen by H.E.L.P apheresis. Z Kardiol. 2003;92(Suppl 3): 42-7.
43. Walts AE, Fishbein MC, Sustaita H, et al. Ruptured atheromatous plaques in saphenous vein coronary artery bypass grafts: a mechanism of acute, thrombotic, late graft occlusion. Circulation. 1982;65(1):197-201.
44. de Oliveira Sa MPB, Nogueira JRC, Ferraz PE, et al. Risk factors for low cardiac output syndrome after coronary artery bypass grafting surgery. Rev Bras Cir Cardiovasc. 2012;27(2):217-23.
45. Mauerman WJ, Sampathkumar P. Sternal wound infections. Best Pract Res Clin Anaesthesiol. 2008;22(3):423-36.
46. Pires LA, Wagshal AB, Lancey R, et al. Arrhythmias and conduction disturbances after coronary artery bypass graft surgery: epidemiology, management, and prognosis. Am Heart J. 1995;129(4):799-808.
47. Tarakji KG, Sabik JF, Bhudia SK, et al. Temporal onset, risk factors, and outcomes associated with stroke after coronary artery bypass grafting. JAMA. 2011;305(4):381-90.
48. Wallwork J, Davidson KG. The acute abdomen following cardiopulmonary bypass surgery. Br J Surg. 1980;67:410-2.
49. Christenson JT, Schmuziger M, Maurice J, et al. Gastrointestinal complications after coronary artery bypass grafting. J Thorac Cardiovasc Surg. 1994;108:899-906.
50. Gamoso MG, Phillips-Bute B, Landolfo KP, et al. Off-pump versus on-pump coronary artery bypass surgery and postoperative renal dysfunction. Anesth Analg. 2000;91:1080-4.
51. Conlon PJ, Stafford-Smith M, White WD, et al. Acute renal failure following cardiac surgery. Nephrol Dial Transplant. 1999;14(5): 1158-62.

52. Munnee K, Bundhun PK, Quan H, et al. Comparing the clinical outcomes between insulin-treated and non-insulin-treated patients with type 2 diabetes mellitus after coronary artery bypass surgery: a systematic review and meta-analysis. Medicine (Baltimore). 2016;95(10):e3006.
53. Bundhun PK, Li N, Chen MH. Adverse cardiovascular outcomes between insulin-treated and non-insulin treated diabetic patients after percutaneous coronary intervention: a systematic review and meta-analysis. Cardiovasc Diabetol. 2015;14:135.
54. King SB 3rd, Lembo NJ, Weintraub WS, et al. A randomized trial comparing coronary angioplasty with coronary bypass surgery. Emory Angioplasty versus Surgery Trial (EAST). N Engl J Med. 1994;331:1044-50.
55. CABRI Investigators. Long-term follow-up of European revascularization trial. Presented at the 68th Scientific Sessions of the American Heart Association, Plenary Session XII; November 16, 1995; Anaheim, CA.
56. Naito R, Kasai T. Coronary artery disease in type 2 diabetes mellitus: Recent treatment strategies and future perspectives. World J Cardiol. 2015;7(3):119-24.
57. Serruys PW, Morice MC, Kappetein AP, et al. Percutaneous coronary intervention versus coronary-artery bypass grafting for severe coronary artery disease. N Engl J Med. 2009;360:961-72.
58. Hlatky MA, Boothroyd DB, Bravata DM, et al. Coronary artery bypass surgery compared with percutaneous coronary interventions for multivessel disease: a collaborative analysis of individual patient data from ten randomised trials. Lancet. 2009;373:1190-7.
59. Weintraub WS, Grau-Sepulveda MV, Weiss JM, et al. Comparative effectiveness of revascularization strategies. N Engl J Med. 2012;366:1467-76.
60. Deaton C, Thourani V. Patients with type 2 diabetes undergoing coronary artery bypass graft surgery: predictors of outcomes. Eur J Cardiovasc Nurs. 2009;8:48-56.
61. Koshizaka M, Lopes RD, Reyes EM, et al. Long-term clinical and angiographic outcomes in patients with diabetes undergoing coronary artery bypass graft surgery: results from the Project of Ex-vivo Vein Graft Engineering via Transfection IV trial. Am Heart J. 2015;169:175-84.
62. Nissen SE, Wolski K. Effect of rosiglitazone on the risk of myocardial infarction and death from cardiovascular causes. N Engl J Med. 2007;356(24):2457-71.
63. Marso SP, Daniels GH, Brown-Frandsen K, et al. Liraglutide and cardiovascular outcomes in type 2 diabetes. N Engl J Med. 2016;375:311-22.
64. Marso SP, Bain SC, Consoli A, et al. Semaglutide and cardiovascular outcomes in patients with type 2 diabetes. N Engl J Med. 2016;375:1834-44.
65. Zinman B, Wanner C, Lachin JM, et al. Empagliflozin, cardiovascular outcomes, and mortality in type 2 diabetes. N Engl J Med. 2015;373:2117-28.

Index

Page numbers followed by *b* refer to box, *f* refer to figure, *fc* refer to flow chart, and *t* refer to table.

A

B

C

D

E

F

G

H

I

J

K

L

M

N

O

P

Q

R

S

T

U

V

W

X

Y

Z